1989

CONN'S CURRENT THERAPY

Edited by ROBERT E. RAKEL, M.D.

Chairman, Department of Family Medicine
Associate Dean for Academic and Clinical Affairs
Baylor College of Medicine, Houston, Texas

LATEST APPROVED METHODS OF TREATMENT FOR THE PRACTICING PHYSICIAN

W.B. SAUNDERS COMPANY
Harcourt Brace Jovanovich, Inc.
Philadelphia   London   Toronto   Montreal   Sydney   Tokyo

W. B. SAUNDERS COMPANY
Harcourt Brace Jovanovich, Inc.

The Curtis Center
Independence Square West
Philadelphia, PA 19106

Library of Congress Cataloging-in-Publication Data

Current therapy; latest approved methods of treatment for the practicing physician. 1949–

v. 28 cm. annual.

Editors: 1949–   H. F. Conn and others.

1. Therapeutics.   2. Therapeutics, Surgical.
  3. Medicine—Practice.   I. Conn, Howard Franklin, 1908–1982 ed.

RM101.C87   616.058   49–8328 rev*

ISBN 0–7216–2581–9

Editor: John Dyson
Developmental Editor: Kathleen McCullough
Designer: W. B. Saunders Staff
Production Manager: Bob Butler
Manuscript Editor: Mark Coyle
Illustration Coordinator: Lisa Lambert
Indexer: Dennis Dolan

Conn's Current Therapy 1989   ISBN 0–7216–2581–9

Last digit is the print number: 9   8   7   6   5   4   3   2   1

Contributors

CHARLES FOUAD ABBOUD, M.B., B.CH.
Mayo Medical School, Rochester, Minnesota
Hyperprolactinemia

JONATHAN ABRAMS, M.D.
Professor of Medicine and Chief, Division of Cardiology, University of New Mexico School of Medicine, Albuquerque, New Mexico
Congestive Heart Failure

SUHAIL AHMAD, M.D.
Associate Professor of Nephrology/Medicine, University of Washington; Attending Physician, University Hospital; Medical Director, Scribner Kidney Center, Seattle, Washington
Chronic Renal Failure

DANIEL A. ALBERT, M.D.
Assistant Professor of Medicine and Program Director, Internal Medicine, University of Chicago; Attending Staff, University of Chicago Hospitals and Clinics, Chicago, Illinois
Polymyalgia Rheumatica and Giant Cell Arteritis

MICHAEL J. ALBOM, M.D.
Associate Clinical Professor, Department of Dermatology, New York University Medical Center; Attending Physician, University Hospital (New York University Medical Center) and Belleview Hospital Medical Center; Director of Mohs Micrographic Surgery and Associate Attending Surgeon, Department of Plastic Surgery, Manhattan Eye, Ear and Throat Hospital, New York, New York
Cancer of the Skin

ROBERT H. ALFORD, M.D.
Clinical Professor of Medicine, Vanderbilt University Medical School; Medical Director, Parkview Medical Center, Nashville, Tennessee
Histoplasmosis

KARL M. ALTENBURGER, M.D.
Staff Physician, Munroe Regional Medical Center and Marion Community Hospital, Ocala, Florida
Asthma in Children

ROY D. ALTMAN, M.D.
Professor of Medicine, University of Miami Medical School; Chief, Arthritis Section, Miami Veterans Administration Medical Center, Miami, Florida
Paget's Disease of Bone

CRAIG L. ANDERSON, M.D.
Associate Professor of Pediatrics and Director of Newborn Medicine, Loyola University Medical Center; Attending Staff, Foster G. McGaw Hospital–Loyola University Medical Center, Maywood, Illinois
Neonatal Resuscitation

MARION C. ANDERSON, M.D.
Professor and Chairman, Department of Surgery, Medical University of South Carolina; Chief of Surgery, Medical University of South Carolina Medical Center; Consulting Surgeon, Charleston Veterans Administration Medical Center and Charleston Memorial Hospital, Charleston, South Carolina
Acute Pancreatitis

PHILIP C. ANDERSON, M.D.
Professor, Division of Dermatology, Department of Medicine, University of Missouri–Columbia; Attending Staff, University of Missouri Hospital and Clinics, Columbia, Missouri
Spider Bites and Scorpion Stings

THOMAS F. ANDERSON, M.D.
Associate Professor, University of Michigan Medical School; Attending Staff, University Hospital, Ann Arbor, Michigan
Bacterial Diseases

AUGUSTO AQUIRRE, M.D.
Clinical Assistant Professor of Pathology, Ohio State University; Senior Attending Pathologist, Riverside Methodist Hospitals, Columbus, Ohio
Tetanus

EDUARDO G. ARATHOON, M.D.
Assistant Professor of Infectious Diseases, Hospital General San Juan de Dios, Guatemala City, Guatemala
Coccidioidomycosis

MURAT ARCASOY, M.D.
Postdoctoral Research Fellow, Sleep Disorders and Research Center, Baylor College of Medicine, Houston, Texas; Resident in Internal Medicine, New York Medical College, New York, New York
Insomnia

JAMES O. ARMITAGE, M.D.
Professor and Vice Chairman, Department of Internal Medicine, and Chief, Section of Oncology/Hematology, University of Nebraska Medical Center, Omaha, Nebraska
Non-Hodgkin's Lymphomas

DONALD ARMSTRONG, M.D.
Professor of Medicine, Cornell University Medical College; Chief, Infectious Disease Service, and Director, Microbiology Laboratory, Memorial Sloan-Kettering Cancer Center, New York, New York
Acquired Immunodeficiency Syndrome (AIDS)

SANJEEV ARORA, M.D.
Assistant Professor of Medicine, Tufts University School of Medicine; Staff Physician, New England Medical Center, Boston, Massachusetts
Cirrhosis

ANN M. ARVIN, M.D.

Associate Professor of Pediatrics, Stanford University School of Medicine; Attending Staff, Stanford University Medical Center and Children's Hospital at Stanford, Stanford, California
Chickenpox (Varicella)

MICHAEL E. ASSEY, M.D.

Associate Professor of Medicine (Cardiology) and Director, Adult Cardiac Catheterization Laboratories, Medical University of South Carolina, Charleston, South Carolina
Atrial Fibrillation

ROBERTO BADARÓ, M.D.

Associate Professor, Faculty of Medicine, University of Bahia; Attending Physician in Infectious Diseases, Hospital Professor Edgard Santos, Federal University of Bahia, Canela/Salvador, Bahia, Brazil
Leishmaniasis

HOWARD P. BADEN, M.D.

Professor of Dermatology, Harvard Medical School; Dermatologist, Massachusetts General Hospital, Boston, Massachusetts
Diseases of the Nails

WILLIAM C. BAILEY, M.D.

Professor of Medicine, Division of Pulmonary and Critical Care Medicine, University of Alabama at Birmingham School of Medicine; Associate Chief of Staff for Education, Veterans Administration Medical Center, Birmingham, Alabama
Tuberculosis and Nontuberculous Mycobacterial Diseases

JI BAOHONG, M.D.

Secretary, Chemotherapy of Leprosy (THELEP) Steering Committee, Special Programme of Research and Training in Tropical Diseases, World Health Organization, Geneva, Switzerland
Leprosy (Hansen's Disease)

JOHN B. BARLOW, M.D.

Professor of Cardiology, University of Witwatersrand; Chief Physician, Department of Cardiology, Johannesburg Hospital, Johannesburg, South Africa
Mitral Value Billowing and Prolapse

JOHN G. BARTLETT, M.D.

Professor of Medicine, Johns Hopkins University School of Medicine; Chief of Infectious Disease Division, Johns Hopkins Hopsital, Baltimore, Maryland
Primary Lung Abscess

JAMES W. BASS, M.D., M.P.H.

Professor of Pediatrics, Uniformed Services University of the Health Sciences, Bethesda, Maryland; Clinical Professor of Pediatrics, University of Hawaii School of Medicine, and Chairman, Department of Pediatrics, Tripler Army Medical Center, Honolulu, Hawaii
Streptococcal Pharyngitis

ROBERT P. BAUGHMAN, M.D.

Assistant Professor of Medicine, University of Cincinnati Medical Center, Cincinnati, Ohio
Sarcoidosis

WILLIAM B. BEAN, M.D.

Sir William Osler Professor, Emeritus Professor of Medicine, Department of Internal Medicine, University of Iowa, Iowa City, Iowa
Scurvy and Vitamin C Deficiency

WELDEN E. BELL, D.D.S.

Clinical Professor of Oral Surgery, University of Texas Southwestern Medical School; Consultant, Parkland Memorial Hospital, Dallas, Texas
Disorders of the Temporomandibular Joint

ROBIN BENNETT, M.D.

Nephrologist, Freedman Clinic of Internal Medicine; Staff Physician, St. Francis Cabrini Hospital and Rapides General Hospital, Alexandria, Louisiana
Pyelonephritis

JOHN J. BERGAN, M.D.

Magerstadt Professor of Surgery, Northwestern University Medical School; Attending Surgeon, Northwestern Memorial Hospital, Chicago, Illinois
Acquired Aortic Disease

CHERYL BERGER, M.D.

Resident in Dermatology, Oregon Health Sciences University, Portland, Oregon
Herpes Simplex and Herpes Zoster

WILMA F. BERGFELD, M.D.

Head of Dermatopathology and Clinical Dermatology Research, and Senior Staff Dermatologist, Cleveland Clinic Foundation, Cleveland, Ohio
Hair Disorders

DANIEL E. BERGSAGEL, M.D., D.PHIL.

Professor of Medicine, University of Toronto; Chief of Medicine, Princess Margaret Hospital, Toronto, Ontario, Canada
Multiple Myeloma

DAVID E. BERMAN, M.D.

Instructor, Department of Plastic Surgery, University of Virginia School of Medicine, Charlottesville, Virginia
Gas-Forming Infections

ROBERT F. BETTS, M.D.

Professor of Medicine, University of Rochester; Associate Physician, Strong Memorial Hospital; Consultant, Highland Hospital, Rochester, New York
Influenza

PHILIP BIERMAN, M.D.

Assistant Professor, University of Nebraska Medical Center, Omaha, Nebraska
Non-Hodgkin's Lymphomas

E. G. BIGLIERI, M.D.

Professor of Medicine, University of California, San Francisco; Director, Clinical Study Center, San Francisco General Hospital, San Francisco, California
Adrenocortical Insufficiency

JACOB D. BITRAN, M.D.

Professor of Medicine, University of Chicago Pritzker School of Medicine; Attending Staff, Michael Reese Medical Center,

University of Chicago, Bernard Mitchell Hospital, Chicago, Illinois
Carcinoma of the Lung

JOHN H. BLAND, M.D.

Professor of Medicine (Rheumatology), University of Vermont College of Medicine; Attending Physician in Medicine and Rheumatology, Medical Center Hospital of Vermont, Burlington, Vermont
Ankylosing Spondylitis

MARIAN BLOCK, M.D.

Associate Professor and Chief, Division of Family Medicine, University of Pittsburgh School of Medicine; Attending Staff, Shadyside Hospital, Pittsburgh, Pennsylvania
Contraception

W. KLINE BOLTON, M.D.

Professor of Medicine, University of Virginia School of Medicine, Charlottesville, Viriginia
Glomerular Disorders

GEORGE A. BRAY, M.D.

Professor of Medicine, University of Southern California School of Medicine; Chief, Division of Diabetes and Clinical Nutrition, Los Angeles County–University of Southern California Medical Center, Los Angeles, California
Obesity

JOSEPH L. BREAULT, M.S., M.D., M.P.H.T.M.

Department of Family Practice, Montefiore Medical Center, New York, New York
Acute Diarrhea

STEVEN F. BRENA, M.D.

Clinical Professor of Rehabilitation Medicine, Emory University; Board Chairman, Pain Control and Rehabilitation Institute of Georgia, Atlanta, Georgia
Pain

KENNETH R. BRIDGES, M.D.

Assistant Professor of Medicine, Harvard Medical School; Associate Physician, Brigham and Women's Hospital, Boston, Massachusetts
Hemochromatosis

BRUCE BROECKER, M.D.

Associate Professor of Surgery and Director of Pediatric Urology, Emory University School of Medicine; Attending Staff, Henrietta Egleston Hospital for Children and Emory University Hospital, Atlanta, Georgia
Urinary Tract Infections in Female Children

SHELDON BROWN, M.D.

Instructor in Medicine, Cornell University School of Medicine; Fellow, Infectious Disease Service, Memorial Sloan-Kettering Cancer Center, New York, New York
Acquired Immunodeficiency Syndrome (AIDS)

THOMAS R. BROWNE, M.D.

Professor and Vice Chairman, Department of Neurology, Boston University School of Medicine; Associate Chief, Neurology Service, Boston Veterans Administration Medical Center, Boston, Massachusetts
Epilepsy in Adolescents and Adults

RICHARD E. BRYANT, M.D.

Professor of Medicine and Director of Infectious Diseases Division, Oregon Health Sciences University; Attending Staff, Oregon Health Sciences University Hospital, Portland, Oregon
Bacteremia

DENISE M. BUNTIN, M.D.

Associate Professor, Division of Dermatology, Department of Medicine, University of Tennessee; Chief, Dermatology Section, Memphis Veterans Administration Medical Center, Memphis, Tennessee
Urticaria

WALTER H. C. BURGDORF, M.D.

Professor and Chairman, Department of Dermatology, University of New Mexico School of Medicine, Albuquerque, New Mexico
Papulosquamous Eruptions

WILLIAM R. BYRNE, M.D.

Staff Physician, St. Mary's Hospital, Henrico Doctors' Hospital, and Retreat Hospital, Richmond, Virginia; formerly Chief, Infectious Disease Service, Letterman Army Medical Center, San Francisco, California
Bacterial Meningitis

DONALD B. CALNE, D.M.

Professor of Medicine, University of British Columbia; Head, Division of Neurology, University Hospital, Vancouver, British Columbia, Canada
Parkinsonism

ROBERT CANCRO, M.D.

Professor and Chairman, Department of Psychiatry, New York University Medical Center; Director, Department of Psychiatry, New York University Hospital; Director, Nathan S. Kline Institute for Psychiatric Research, New York, New York
Schizophrenic Disorders

THOMAS R. CARACCIO, Pharm.D., R.P.H.

Adjunct Assistant Professor of Clinical Pharmacy, St. John's University College of Pharmacy, Jamaica, New York; Visiting Assistant Clinical Professor of Pharmacology and Toxicology, New York College of Osteopathic Medicine, Old Westbury, New York; Clinical Coordinator, Long Island Regional Poison Control Center, and Clinical Pharmacist, Department of Pediatric Pharmacology, Nassau County Medical Center, East Meadow, New York
Acute Poisonings

SANDRA ANN CARSON, M.D.

Assistant Professor of Obstetrics and Gynecology, University of Tennessee, Memphis; Attending Staff, William F. Bowld Hospital, Baptist Memorial Hospital, St. Jude's Children's Hospital, and Le Bonheur Children's Hospital, Memphis, Tennessee
Amenorrhea

EDGAR M. CARVALHO, M.D.

Associate Professor, Faculty of Medicine, Federal University of Bahia; Head of Immunology Division, Hospital Professor Edgard Santos, Canela/Salvador, Bahia, Brazil
Leishmaniasis

THOMAS B. CASALE, M.D.

Assistant Professor, University of Iowa College of Medicine; Staff Physician, University of Iowa Hospitals and Clinics and Veterans Administration Medical Center, Iowa City, Iowa
Asthma in the Adolescent and the Adult

DAN K. CHALKER, M.D.

Professor of Dermatology, Medical College of Georgia; Chief, Division of Dermatology, Veterans Administration Hospital; Consultant, Augusta Correctional and Medical Institute, Augusta, Georgia
Acne Vulgaris and Rosacea

DONALD C. CHAMBERS, M.D.

Assistant Professor of Obstetrics and Gynecology, Howard University College of Medicine, Washington, D.C.; Attending Staff, Sinai Hospital of Baltimore and Liberty Medical Center, Baltimore, Maryland
Leiomyomas of the Uterus

THOMAS A. CHAPEL, M.D.

Clinical Professor of Dermatology and Syphilology, Wayne State University, Detroit, Michigan; Chief, Subsection of Dermatology, Oakwood Hospital, Dearborn, Michigan
Granuloma Inguinale (Donovanosis); Lymphogranuloma Venereum

CHARLES W. CHAPPUIS, M.D.

Assistant Professor of Surgery, Louisiana State University School of Medicine; Visiting Surgeon, Charity Hospital at New Orleans and Veterans Administration Medical Center, New Orleans, Louisiana
Tumors of the Stomach

CLARE L. CHERNEY, M.D.

Instructor in Medicine, St. Francis Medical Center, Trenton, New Jersey; formerly Instructor in Medicine, Medical College of Pennsylvania, Philadelphia, Pennsylvania
Salmonellosis

INDER J. CHOPRA, M.D.

Professor of Medicine, University of California, Los Angeles, School of Medicine; Attending Physician, Department of Medicine, UCLA Center for Health Sciences, Los Angeles, California
Hypothyroidism

ANTHONY W. CHOW, M.D.

Professor of Medicine and Head, Division of Infectious Diseases, University of British Columbia and Vancouver General Hospital, Vancouver, British Columbia, Canada
Toxic Shock Syndrome

ARNOLD C. CINMAN, M.D.

Clinical Assistant Professor of Urology, University of California, Los Angeles, School of Medicine; Attending Urologist, Cedars-Sinai Medical Center, Los Angeles, California
Genitourinary Tuberculosis

DAVID P. CLARK, M.D.

Assistant Professor of Dermatology, University of Missouri–Columbia School of Medicine; Attending Staff, University of Missouri Hospital and Clinics, Columbia, Missouri
Verruca Vulgaris (Warts)

KEITH F. CLARK, M.D.

Assistant Professor, University of Oklahoma Health Sciences Center; Attending Staff, Oklahoma Memorial Hospital, Oklahoma Children's Hospital, Veterans Administration Hospital, O'Donoghue Rehabilitation Institute, and Central State Hospital; Courtesy Staff, Presbyterian Hospital, Oklahaoma City, Oklahoma
Hoarseness and Laryngitis

REBECCA A. CLARK, R.N.

Clinical Research Nurse, Memorial Sloan-Kettering Cancer Center, New York, New York
Nausea and Vomiting

MARC D. COHEN, M.D.

Associate Professor of Internal Medicine, Mayo Medical School; Consultant, Division of Rheumatology and Internal Medicine, Mayo Clinic and Mayo Foundation, Rochester, Minnesota; Consultant in Internal Medicine and Rheumatology, St. Luke's Hospital, Jacksonville, Florida
Rheumatoid Arthritis

MARC S. COHEN, M.D.

Associate Professor of Surgery (Urology) and Microbiology, University of Texas Medical Branch at Galveston; Attending Staff, University of Texas Medical Branch Affiliated Hospitals; Courtesy Staff, St. Mary's Hospital, Galveston, Texas
Nongonococcal Urethritis

ISIDORE COHN, JR., M.D., D.S.C. (MED.)

Professor and Chairman, Department of Surgery, Louisiana State University School of Medicine; Surgeon-in-Chief, LSU Surgical Service, Charity Hospital, New Orleans, Louisiana
Tumors of the Stomach

PAUL G. COLAVITA, M.D.

Faculty, The Carolinas Heart Institute; Cardiologist, Charlotte Memorial Hospital, Charlotte, North Carolina
Heart Block

NEVILLE COLMAN, M.D., PH.D.

Associate Professor of Pathology and Associate Director, Center for Clinical Laboratories, Mount Sinai School of Medicine; Medical Director, Blood Bank and Hematology Laboratory, Bronx Veterans Administration Medical Center; Attending in Pathology, Mount Sinai Medical Center, New York, New York
Pernicious Anemia and Other Megaloblastic Anemias

ANTHONY J. COMEROTA, M.D.

Associate Professor, Temple University School of Medicine; Chief, Section of Vascular Surgery, Temple University Hospital, Philadelphia, Pennsylvania
Deep Venous Thrombosis of the Lower Extremities

REX B. CONN, M.D.

Professor of Pathology, Jefferson Medical College of Thomas Jefferson University; Director, Clinical Laboratories, Thomas Jefferson University Hospital, Philadelphia, Pennsylvania
Laboratory Values of Clinical Importance

DAVID S. COOPER, M.D.

Associate Professor of Medicine, Johns Hopkins University School of Medicine; Chief, Division of Endocrinology, Sinai Hospital of Baltimore; Physician, Johns Hopkins Hospital, Baltimore, Maryland
Simple Goiter

JOSHUA A. COPEL, M.D.

Assistant Professor and Director of Resident Education, Department of Obstetrics and Gynecology, Yale University School of Medicine; Attending Physician, Yale–New Haven Hospital, New Haven, Connecticut
Antepartum Care

LARRY J. COPELAND, M.D.

Professor of Obstetrics and Gynecology, and Director of Gynecologic Oncology, Ohio State University College of Medicine and Ohio State University Hospital, Columbus, Ohio
Neoplasms of the Vulva

RALPH COREY, M.D.

Associate Professor and Program Director, Department of Medicine, and Infectious Disease Consultant, Duke University Medical Center, Durham, North Carolina
Osteomyelitis

RANDLE S. CORFMAN, PH.D., M.D.

Associate Professor, Department of Obstetrics and Gynecology, Yale University School of Medicine; Attending Staff, Department of Obstetrics and Gynecology, Yale–New Haven Hospital, New Haven, Connecticut
Dysfunctional Uterine Bleeding

JAMES J. CORRIGAN, JR., M.D.

Professor of Pediatrics and Internal Medicine, University of Arizona Health Sciences Center; Chief, Pediatric Hematology-Oncology, and Director, Hemophilia Center, University Medical Center, Tucson, Arizona
Vitamin K Deficiency

JAMES P. CROWLEY, M.D.

Associate Professor of Medicine, Brown University; Associate Director, Division of Clinical Hematology, Rhode Island Hospital, Providence, Rhode Island
Nonimmune Hemolytic Anemia

JAMES J. CURRAN, M.D.

Associate Professor of Medicine, University of Chicago Pritzker School of Medicine, Chicago, Illinois
Polymyalgia Rheumatica and Giant Cell Arteritis

SADY S. DA COSTA, M.D.

Research Fellow, International Hearing Foundation, Minneapolis, Minnesota
Meniere's Disease

KIRON M. DAS, M.D., PH.D.

Professor of Medicine, Microbiology, and Molecular Genetics, University of Medicine and Dentistry of New Jersey–Robert Wood Johnson Medical School, Piscataway, New Jersey; Chief, Division of Gastroenterology and Hepatology, Robert Wood Johnson University Hospital, New Brunswick, New Jersey
Ulcerative Colitis

RICHARD J. DAVEY, M.D.

Department of Transfusion Medicine, National Institutes of Health, Bethesda, Maryland
Autoimmune Hemolytic Anemia

RICHARD A. DAVIDSON, M.D., M.P.H.

Associate Professor, Department of Medicine, University of Florida; Attending Staff, Shands Hospital of the University

of Florida and Gainesville Veterans Administration Medical Center, Gainesville, Florida
Amebiasis

STARKEY D. DAVIS, M.D.

Professor and Chairman, Department of Pediatrics, and Professor of Microbiology, Medical College of Wisconsin; Pediatrician-in-Chief, Children's Hospital of Wisconsin, Milwaukee, Wisconsin
Viral and Mycoplasmal Pneumonia

ALAN H. DeCHERNEY, M.D.

John Slade Ely Professor of Obstetrics and Gynecology, Yale University School of Medicine; Director of Reproductive Endocrinolgy, Yale–New Haven Hospital, New Haven, Connecticut
Dysfunctional Uterine Bleeding

LEONARD J. DEFTOS, M.D.

Professor of Medicine, University of California, San Diego, School of Medicine; Chief, Section on Bone and Mineral Research, San Diego Veterans Administration Medical Center, San Diego, California
Hyperparathyroidism and Hypoparathyroidism

DAVID T. DENNIS, M.D., M.P.H.

Adjunct Assistant Professor of Medicine, Dartmouth Medical College, Hanover, New Hampshire; Centers for Disease Control, Atlanta, Georgia
Typhus Fevers

JESS DIAMOND, M.D.

Adjunct Associate Professor, Department of Pediatrics, University of California, Los Angeles, School of Medicine, Los Angeles, California; Clinical Associate Professor, Department of Pediatrics, University of California, Irvine, School of Medicine, Irvine, California; Clinical Professor, Department of Nursing, California State University, and Chairman, Department of Pediatrics, Kern Medical Center, Bakersfield, California
Measles (Rubeola)

LUIS A. DIAZ, M.D.

Professor and Chairman, Department of Dermatology, Medical College of Wisconsin, Milwaukee, Wisconsin; Consulting Physician, Johns Hopkins Hospital, Baltimore, Maryland
Bullous Diseases

JOSÉ ERNESTO DOS SANTOS, M.D.

Associate Professor, Universidade de São Paulo School of Medicine, Ribeirão Preto, São Paulo, Brazil
Pellagra

EUGENIE F. DOYLE, M.D.

Professor of Pediatrics, New York University School of Medicine; Director, Division of Pediatric Cardiology, New York University Medical Center, New York, New York
Rheumatic Fever

DONALD J. DUDLEY, M.D.

Fellow, Department of Obstetrics and Gynecology, University of Utah, Salt Lake City, Utah
Vaginal Bleeding in Late Pregnancy

DAVID L. DUNNER, M.D.

Professor of Psychiatry and Behavioral Sciences, University of Washington; Chief of Psychiatry, Harborview Medical Center, Seattle, Washington
Affective Disorders

RICHARD F. EDLICH, M.D., PH.D.

Distinguished Professor of Plastic Surgery and Biomedical Engineering, University of Virginia School of Medicine, Charlottesville, Virginia
Gas-Forming Infections

STAFFAN EDSTRÖM, M.D., PH.D.

Assistant Professor, Department of Otolaryngology, Sahlgrenska Sjukhuset, University of Göteborg, Göteborg, Sweden
Acute Facial Paralysis

JAMES M. EDWARDS, M.D.

Assistant Professor of Surgery, Division of Vascular Surgery, Oregon Health Sciences University, Portland, Oregon
Peripheral Arterial Disease

MORVEN S. EDWARDS, M.D.

Associate Professor of Pediatrics, Baylor College of Medicine; Active Staff, Texas Children's Hospital, Ben Taub General Hospital, and Jefferson Davis Hospital, Houston, Texas
Rubella and Congenital Rubella

MERVYN L. ELGART, M.D.

Professor and Chairman, Department of Dermatology, and Professor, Department of Medicine and Department of Child Health, George Washington University School of Medicine; Chief, Dermatology Service, George Washington University Hospital; Attending Physician and Chief of Dermatology Service, Children's Hospital National Medical Center; Consultant, Washington Hospital Center, Washington, D.C., and Andrews Air Force Base Hospital, Andrews A.F.B., Maryland
Fungal Diseases

M. A. EMANUELE, M.D.

Associate Professor of Medicine, Loyola University of Chicago Stritch School of Medicine; Staff Endocrinologist, Loyola University Medical Center, Maywood, Illinois; Consulting Endocrinologist, Hines Veterans Administration Medical Center, Hines, Illinois
Diabetes Mellitus in Adults

N. V. EMANUELE, M.D.

Associate Professor of Medicine, Loyola University of Chicago Stritch School of Medicine, Maywood, Illinois; Associate Chief of Medicine, Hines Veterans Administration Hospital, Hines, Illinois
Diabetes Mellitus in Adults

THOMAS R. ENG, V.M.D., M.P.H.

Viral and Rickettsial Zoonoses Branch, Division of Viral Diseases, Centers for Disease Control, Atlanta, Georgia
Rabies

GORDON A. EWY, M.D.

Professor and Associate Head, Department of Internal Medicine, and Chief, Section of Cardiology, University of Arizona College of Medicine; Medical Director, Diagnostic Cardiology, University Medical Center, Tucson, Arizona
Cardiac Arrest

VINCENT FALANGA, M.D.

Assistant Professor of Medicine and Dermatology, University of Miami School of Medicine; Attending Physician, Jackson Memorial Hospital and University of Miami School of Medicine, Miami, Florida
Venous Ulcers and Other Cutaneous Ulcerations

GARY W. FALK, M.D.

Staff Physician, Department of Gastroenterology, Cleveland Clinic Foundation and Hospital, Cleveland, Ohio
Diverticula of the Alimentary Tract

MICHAEL D. FALLON, M.D.

Surgical Pathologist, Department of Pathology and Laboratory Medicine, Hospital of the University of Pennsylvania, Philadelphia, Pennsylvania
Rickets and Osteomalacia

WILLIAM E. FANN, M.D.

Professor of Psychiatry and Associate Professor of Pharmacology, Baylor College of Medicine; Chief, Psychiatry Service, Houston Veterans Administration Medical Center; Consultant in Psychiatry, Methodist Hospital, Houston, Texas
Anxiety Disorders

NADIR R. FARID, M.B., B.S.

Professor of Medicine, Memorial University of Newfoundland; Chief, Division of Endocrinology and Metabolism, Memorial University Health Sciences Centre, St. John's, Newfoundland, Canada
Thyroiditis

SEBASTIAN FARO, M.D., PH.D.

Professor, Baylor College of Medicine; Attending Staff, St. Luke's Episcopal Hospital, Methodist Hospital, Jefferson Davis Hospital, and Ben Taub General Hospital, Houston, Texas
Vulvovaginitis

MARK S. FEDDER, M.D.

Associate in Medicine, University of Illinois at Chicago; Fellow in Gastroenterology, University of Illinois Hospital, Chicago, Illinois
Constipation

PETER F. FEDULLO, M.D.

Assistant Professor of Medicine, Pulmonary/Critical Care Division, University of California, San Diego, School of Medicine; Attending Staff, University of California, San Diego, Medical Center, and Veterans Administration Medical Center, San Diego, California
Pulmonary Embolism

LAWRENCE J. FENTON, M.D.

Professor and Chairman, Department of Pediatrics, University of South Dakota School of Medicine; Attending Staff and Director, Newborn Intensive Care Unit, Sioux Valley Hospital, Sioux Falls, South Dakota
Care of the High-Risk Neonate

ROBERT FERRARO, M.D.

Senior Clinical Fellow in Endocrinology, Metabolism, and Nutrition, St. Luke's/Roosevelt Hospital, New York, New York
Parenteral Nutrition in Adults

JO-DAVID FINE, M.D.

Associate Professor of Dermatology and Director of Dermatologic Research, University of Alabama at Birmingham; Attending Staff, University of Alabama Hospital; Chief, Dermatology Section, Medical Service, Birmingham Veterans Administration Medical Center, Birmingham, Alabama
Skin Diseases of Pregnancy

SYDNEY M. FINEGOLD, M.D.

Professor of Medicine and Professor of Microbiology and Immunology, University of California, Los Angeles, School of Medicine; Attending Staff, Wadsworth Veterans Administration Medical Center–West Los Angeles and UCLA Medical Center, Los Angeles, California
Brain Abscess

JOHN FLAHERTY, M.D.

Instructor, Department of Medicine, University of Chicago Pritzker School of Medicine; Attending Staff, Michael Reese Hospital and Medical Center, and University of Chicago Hospitals and Clinics, Chicago, Illinois
Q Fever

T. RAYMOND FOLEY, M.D.

Fellow in Gastroenterology, Milton S. Hershey Medical Center of Pennsylvania State University, Hershey, Pennsylvania
The Malabsorption Syndromes

JERRY E. FOOTE, M.D.

Attending Staff, Boone Hospital Center and Columbia Regional Hospital, Columbia, Missouri
Parasitic Diseases

NOBLE O. FOWLER, M.D.

Emeritus Professor of Medicine, Pharmacology, and Cell Biophysics, University of Cincinnati College of Medicine; Attending Staff, University of Cincinnati Hospitals and Christ Hospital; Consultant Staff, Jewish Hospital, Cincinnati, Ohio
Pericarditis

ANDREW G. FRANTZ, M.D.

Professor of Medicine, Columbia University College of Physicians and Surgeons; Attending Physician, Presbyterian Hospital, New York, New York
Hypopituitarism

EDWARD D. FROHLICH, M.D.

Alton Ochsner Distinguished Scientist, Vice President for Academic Affairs, and Professor, Department of Medicine and Department of Physiology, Louisiana State University School of Medicine; Clinical Professor of Medicine and Adjunct Professor of Pharmacology, Tulane University School of Medicine; Staff Member, Section of Hypertensive Diseases, Ochsner Clinic, New Orleans, Louisiana
Hypertension

WESLEY FURSTE, M.D.

Clinical Professor Emeritus of Surgery, Ohio State University; Senior Attending Surgeon, Mt. Carmel Medical Center and Riverside Methodist Hospitals, Columbus, Ohio
Tetanus

JOHN I. GALLIN, M.D.

Director, Intramural Research Program, National Institute of Allergy and Infectious Diseases; Attending Medical Officer, Warren Grant Magnuson Clinical Center of the National Institutes of Health, Bethesda, Maryland
Neutropenia

MAREK J. GAWEL, M.D.

Assistant Professor of Medicine (Neurology), University of Toronto; Staff Neurologist, Sunnybrook Medical Center, Toronto, Ontario; Staff Neurologist, Centenary Hospital, Scarborough, Ontario, Canada
Ischemic Cerebrovascular Disease

HARRIET S. GILBERT, M.D.

Professor of Medicine, Albert Einstein College of Medicine of Yeshiva University; Lecturer, Mount Sinai Medical School of City University of New York; Attending Staff, Weiler Hospital of the Albert Einstein College of Medicine, Bronx Municipal Hospital Center, and Mount Sinai Hospital, New York, New York
Polycythemia Vera and Other Polycythemic Conditions

MICHAEL T. GOLDFARB, M.D.

Lecturer, University of Michigan Medical School; Attending Staff, University of Michigan Hospital, Ann Arbor, Michigan
Bacterial Diseases

LOU GOLDMAN, M.B., B.S.

State Director, New South Wales Family Medicine Programme, Royal Australian Conference of General Practitioners; Director, Drug and Alcoholic Unit, Northside Clinic, Greenwich, New South Wales, Australia
Alcohol-Related Problems

DAVID E. GOLDSTEIN, M.D.

Associate Professor of Child Health, Medicine, and Pathology, University of Missouri–Columbia School of Medicine; Associate Physician, University of Missouri–Columbia Hospital and Clinics, Columbia, Missouri
Diabetes Mellitus in Children and Adolescents

JAY L. GOLDSTEIN, M.D.

Assistant Professor of Medicine, University of Illinois at Chicago; Attending Physician, University of Illinois Hospital and West Side Veterans Administration Medical Center, Chicago, Illinois
Constipation

W. ROBERT GRAHAM, M.D.

Assistant Clinical Professor, University of California, San Diego, School of Medicine; Director, Admissions/Triage, Veterans Administration Medical Center, San Diego, California
Hyperparathyroidism and Hypoparathyroidism

PETER A. T. GRANNUM, M.D.

Associate Professor, Director of Medical Studies, Yale University School of Medicine; Director of Clinical High Risk Obstetrics, Yale–New Haven Hospital, New Haven, Connecticut
Antepartum Care

J. THOMAS GRAYSTON, M.D.

Professor of Epidemiology, School of Public Health and Community Medicine, University of Washington, Seattle, Washington
Psittacosis (Ornithosis)

GEORGE R. GREEN, M.D.

Clinical Professor of Medicine, University of Pennsylvania School of Medicine and Hospital of the University of Pennsylvania, Philadelphia, Pennsylvania; Chief, Allergy and Immunology, Abington Memorial Hospital, Abington, Pennsylvania
Adverse Reactions to Drugs

ARTHUR GREENBERG, M.D.

Associate Professor of Medicine, Renal-Electrolyte Division, Department of Medicine, University of Pittsburgh School of Medicine; Active Staff, Presbyterian–University of Pittsburgh Hospital; Attending Physician, Oakland Veterans Administration Hospital, Pittsburgh, Pennsylvania
Diabetes Insipidus

JOSEPH GREENSHER, M.D.

Professor of Clinical Pediatrics, State University of New York at Stony Brook, Stony Brook, New York; Associate Chairman, Department of Pediatrics, Winthrop-University Hospital, Mineola, New York; Associate Director, Long Island Regional Poison Control Center, Nassau County Medical Center, East Meadow, New York
Acute Poisonings

DARYL R. GRESS, M.D.

Instructor in Neurology, Harvard Medical School; Assistant in Neurology, Massachusetts General Hospital, Boston, Massachusetts
Intracerebral Hemorrhage

JOHN H. GROSSMAN, III, M.D., PH.D.

Professor of Obstetrics, Gynecology, and Microbiology, and Director, Division of Maternal-Fetal Medicine, Department of Obstetrics and Gynecology, George Washington University School of Medicine and Health Sciences, Washington, D.C.
Chlamydia Trachomatis

SHARON GRUNDFEST-BRONIATOWSKI, M.D.

Staff, Department of General Surgery, Cleveland Clinic, Cleveland, Ohio
Diseases of the Breast

A. JULIANNA GULYA, M.D.

Associate Professor of Surgery (Otolaryngology), George Washington University School of Medicine and Health Sciences; Associate Surgeon, George Washington University Hospital Medical Center; Courtesy Staff, Children's Hospital National Medical Center, Washington, D.C., Consultant in Otology/Neurotology, Bethesda Naval Hospital, Bethesda, Maryland
Otitis Media

GARY R. GUTCHER, M.D.

Professor of Pediatrics, Medical College of Virginia; Attending Staff, Medical College of Virginia Hospital, Richmond, Virginia
Hemolytic Disease of the Newborn

PHILIP H. GUTIN, M.D.

Associate Professor, Department of Neurological Surgery, University of California, San Francisco, School of Medicine, San Francisco, California
Brain Tumors

LEWIS H. HAMNER, III, M.D.

Assistant Professor of Gynecology and Obstetrics, Emory University School of Medicine, Grady Memorial Hospital, and Crawford Long Hospital of Emory University, Atlanta, Georgia
Chlamydia Trachomatis

PHILIP M. HANNO, M.D.

Associate Professor of Urology, University of Pennsylvania School of Medicine; Chief of Division of Urology, Philadelphia Veterans Administration Medical Center, Philadelphia, Pennsylvania
Bacterial Infections of the Urinary Tract in Males; Trauma to the Genitourinary Tract

T. MICHAEL HARRINGTON, M.D.

Associate Professor, University of Alabama at Birmingham School of Medicine; Attending Staff, University of Alabama Hospital and Children's Hospital, Birmingham, Alabama
Disturbances due to Heat

WILLIAM O. HARRISON, M.D.

Associate Clinical Professor, Department of Medicine, University of California, San Diego, School of Medicine; Staff Consultant, U.S. Naval Hospital, San Diego, California
Gonorrhea

GRIFFITH R. HARSH, IV, M.D.

Assistant Adjunct Professor, Department of Neurological Surgery, University of California, San Francisco, School of Medicine, San Francisco, California
Brain Tumors

WILLIAM S. HAUBRICH, M.D.

Clinical Professor of Medicine, University of California, San Diego, School of Medicine, San Diego, California; Senior Consultant in Gastroenterology, Scripps Clinic and Research Foundation, La Jolla, California
Gastritis

DAVID M. HEIMBACH, M.D.

Professor of Surgery, University of Washington; Director, University of Washington Burn Center at Harborview Medical Center, Seattle, Washington
Burns

STANLEY HELLERSTEIN, M.D.

Professor of Pediatrics, University of Missouri–Kansas City School of Medicine; Chief, Section of Pediatric Nephrology, Children's Mercy Hospital, Kansas City, Missouri
Parenteral Fluid Therapy for Infants and Children

ROBERT E. HERMANN, M.D.

Clinical Professor of Surgery, Case Western Reserve University School of Medicine; Chairman, Department of General Surgery, Cleveland Clinic, Cleveland, Ohio
Diseases of the Breast

CHRISTIAN HERRMANN, JR., M.D.

Professor Emeritus of Neurology, University of California, Los Angeles, School of Medicine; Honorary Consultant, Neuropsychiatric Institute and Hospitals, University of California, Los Angeles, Los Angeles, California
Myasthenia Gravis

HENRY G. HERROD, M.D.

Professor, Department of Pediatrics, University of Tennessee, Memphis; Vice President, Medical Affairs, Le Bonheur Children's Medical Center, Memphis, Tennessee
Anaphylaxis, Anaphylactoid Reactions, and Serum Sickness

STEVEN B. HEYMSFIELD, M.D.

Associate Professor of Medicine, Columbia University College of Physicians and Surgeons; Director of Outpatient Research and Body Composition Units, Obesity Research Center, St. Luke's–Roosevelt Hospital Center, New York, New York
Parenteral Nutrition in Adults

JAMES R. HIGGINS, M.D.

Associate Clinical Professor of Medicine, University of Oklahoma School of Medicine and Tulsa Medical School; Staff Cardiologist and Director of Electrophysiology and Pacemaker Laboratory, St. Francis Hospital, Tulsa, Oklahoma
Angina Pectoris

JOHN L. HO, M.D.

Assistant Professor of Medicine, Cornell University Medical College; Attending Staff, New York Hospital, New York, New York
Food-Borne Illness

MELBA R. HOEPER, R.N., M.S.

Clinical Instructor, University of Missouri–Columbia School of Nursing; Clinical Nurse Specialist, University of Missouri Health Sciences Center, University of Missouri–Columbia Hospital and Clinics, Columbia, Missouri
Diabetes Mellitus in Children and Adolescents

JAMES S. HOFFMAN, M.D.

Assistant Professor of Obstetrics and Gynecology, University of Connecticut Health Center; Attending Staff, New Britain General Hospital and Mount Sinai Hospital, New Britain, Connecticut
Cancer of the Endometrium

EDWARD W. HOOK III, M.D.

Associate Professor of Medicine, Johns Hopkins University School of Medicine; Chief, STD Clinical Services, Baltimore City Health Department, Baltimore, Maryland
Syphilis

W. KEITH HOOTS, M.D.

Associate Pediatrician and Associate Professor of Pediatrics, M.D. Anderson Hospital and Tumor Institute; Associate Professor of Pediatrics and Internal Medicine, University of Texas Medical School at Houston; Attending Staff, Gulf States Hemophilia Center, Hermann Hospital, Houston, Texas
Hemophilia and Related Conditions

RICHARD T. HOPPE, M.D.

Associate Professor of Radiation Oncology, Stanford University, Stanford, California
Mycosis Fungoides

JAMES I. HUDSON, M.D.

Assistant Professor of Psychiatry, Harvard Medical School, Boston, Massachusetts; Staff Psychiatrist, McLean Hospital, Belmont, Massachusetts
Bulimia Nervosa

DUANE G. HUTSON, M.D.

Professor of Surgery, University of Miami School of Medicine; Staff Surgeon, Veterans Administration Medical Center, Miami, Florida
Bleeding Esophageal Varices

AKIHIRO IGATA, M.D.

President, University of Kagoshima, Kagoshima, Japan
Beriberi (Thiamine [Vitamin B₁] Deficiency)

ANDREW F. IPPOLITI, M.D.

Associate Professor in Medicine/Gastroenterology, University of California, Los Angeles, Center for Health Sciences, Los Angeles, California
Flatulence and Indigestion

I. IRONY, M.D.

Research Associate Physician, University of California, San Francisco, Medical Service and San Francisco General Hospital, San Francisco, California
Adrenocortical Insufficiency

JAN JANSEN, M.D., PH.D.

Associate Professor of Medicine and Pediatrics, Indiana University School of Medicine; Director, Bone Marrow Transplantation Program, Division of Hematology/Oncology, Indiana University Hospitals, Indianapolis, Indiana
Aplastic Anemia

STEVEN R. JARRETT, M.D.

Clinical Associate Professor of Physical Medicine and Rehabilitation, Albany Medical College, Albany, New York; Chief of Physical Medicine and Rehabilitation, Sunnyview Rehabilitation Hospital; Consultant in Physical Medicine and Rehabilitation, Ellis Hospital and St. Clare's Hospital, Schenectady, New York
Rehabilitation of the Patient with Hemiplegia

GEORGE L. JORDAN, JR., M.D., M.S.

Distinguished Service Professor of Surgery, Baylor College of Medicine; Chief of Staff, Harris County Hospital District; Attending in Surgery, Ben Taub General Hospital and Methodist Hospital; Consultant in Surgery, Veterans Administration Medical Center, St. Luke's Episcopal Hospital, and Texas Children's Hospital, Houston, Texas
Chronic Pancreatitis

J. MICHAEL JORDAN, M.D.

Attending Staff, Baylor Hospital, Dallas, Texas
Acute Respiratory Failure

JOSEPH L. JORIZZO, M.D.

Professor and Chairman, Department of Dermatology, Bowman Gray School of Medicine, Wake Forest University; Attending Staff, North Carolina Baptist Hospital, Winston-Salem, North Carolina
Connective Tissue Disorders: Lupus Erythematosus, Dermatomyositis, and Scleroderma

JONATHAN JUI, M.D.

Assistant Professor of Medicine and Emergency Medicine, Oregon Health Sciences University, Portland, Oregon
Bacteremia

ROBERT I. KAHN, M.D.

Active Staff, Pacific Presbyterian Medical Center and Children's Hospital; Courtesy Staff, Mount Zion Hospital and Chinese Hospital, San Francisco, California, and Peralta Hospital, Oakland, California
Renal Calculi

BALU KALAYAM, M.D.

Assistant Professor of Psychiatry, Cornell University Medical College, New York, New York; Assistant Attending Psychiatrist, New York Hospital–Cornell Medical Center, Westchester Division, White Plains, New York
Alzheimer's Disease

MARSHALL M. KAPLAN, M.D.

Professor of Medicine, Tufts University School of Medicine; Chief, Division of Gastroenterology, New England Medical Center Hospital, Boston, Massachusetts
Cirrhosis

ISMET KARACAN, M.D., D.Sc. (MED.)

Professor of Psychiatry and Director, Sleep Disorders and Research Center, Baylor College of Medicine; Associate Chief of Staff for Research and Development, Veterans Administration Hospital; Senior Attending Physician, Methodist Hospital; Consultant, St. Luke's Hospital, Texas Children's Hospital, Spring Shadows Glen, and Bellaire General Hospital, Houston, Texas
Insomnia

ADRIAN I. KATZ, M.D.

Professor of Medicine, University of Chicago Pritzker School of Medicine; Attending Physician, University of Chicago Medical Center, Chicago, Illinois
Hypertensive Disorders of Pregnancy

BARRETT KATZ, M.D.

Associate Professor of Ophthalmology and Neurosciences, University of California, San Diego, School of Medicine; Director, Neuro-Ophthalmology Unit, University of California, San Diego, Medical Center, San Diego, California
Optic Neuritis

JOHN J. KELLY, JR., M.D.

Associate Professor and Director of Electromyography Laboratory, New England Medical Center, Boston, Massachusetts
Polyneuropathies

ELIZABETH T. KHURI, M.D.

Associate Professor of Clinical Public Health and Pediatrics, Cornell University Medical College; Clinical Affiliate, New York Hospital; Visiting Physician, Rockefeller University Hospital, New York, New York
Narcotic Poisoning

J. PHILIP KISTLER, M.D.

Associate Professor of Neurology, Harvard Medical School; Associate Neurologist, Massachusetts General Hospital, Boston, Massachusetts
Intracerebral Hemorrhage

K. WILLIAM KITZMILLER, M.D.

University of Cincinnati School of Medicine, Cincinnati, Ohio
Pruritus Ani and Vulvae

FELIX O. KOLB, M.D.

Clinical Professor of Medicine, University of California, San Francisco, School of Medicine; Active Staff, Pacific Presbyterian Medical Center; Consultant Staff, Children's Hospital, Mt. Zion Hospital, and Marshall Hall Hospital; Courtesy Staff, University of California, San Francisco, Hospital, San Francisco, California
Renal Calculi

MARY KORYTKOWSKI, M.D.

Instructor, Johns Hopkins University School of Medicine; Fellow in Endocrinology, Johns Hopkins Hospital, Baltimore, Maryland
Simple Goiter

FRANKLIN KOZIN, M.D.

Staff Physician, Scripps Clinic and Research Foundation and Green Hospital of Scripps Clinic, La Jolla, California
Fibrositis, Bursitis, and Tendinitis

BERNICE R. KRAFCHIK, M.B., Ch.B.

Associate Professor, University of Toronto; Active Staff, Hospital for Sick Children, Toronto, Ontario, Canada
Atopic Dermatitis

MARK G. KRIS, M.D.

Assistant Professor of Medicine, Cornell University Medical College; Assistant Attending Physician, Memorial Sloan-Kettering Cancer Center, New York, New York
Nausea and Vomiting

A. M. LAWRENCE, M.D., Ph.D.

Professor of Medicine, Loyola University of Chicago Stritch School of Medicine, Maywood, Illinois; Associate Chief of Staff for Education and Program Director in Endocrinology, Hines Veterans Administration Hospital, Hines, Illinois
Diabetes Mellitus

LaSALLE D. LEFFALL, Jr., M.D.

Professor and Chairman, Department of Surgery, Howard University College of Medicine; Surgeon-in-Chief, Howard University Hospital, Washington, D.C.
Tumors of the Colon and Rectum

BERNARD I. LEMAN, M.D.

Fellow in Gastroenterology, University of California, Los Angeles, Center for the Health Sciences, Los Angeles, California
Flatulence and Indigestion

MYRON J. LEVIN, M.D.

Professor of Pediatrics and Medicine, and Chief, Section of Pediatric Infectious Diseases, University of Colorado School of Medicine, Denver, Colorado
Viral Meningoencephalitis

MACY I. LEVINE, M.D.

Clinical Professor of Medicine, University of Pittsburgh School of Medicine; Chief, Allergy Clinic, Veterans Administration Hospital; Active Staff, Montefiore Hospital, Presbyterian-University Hospital, and St. Margaret's Hospital, Pittsburgh, Pennsylvania
Allergic Reactions to Insect Stings

MATTHEW E. LEVISON, M.D.

Professor of Medicine and Chief, Division of Infectious Diseases, Medical College of Pennsylvania, Philadelphia, Pennsylvania
Salmonellosis

D. BETTY LEW, M.D.

Assistant Professor, University of Tennessee, Memphis, College of Medicine, Memphis, Tennessee
Anaphylaxis, Anaphylactoid Reactions, and Serum Sickness

JAMES H. LEWIS, M.D.

Associate Professor of Medicine, Division of Gastroenterology, Georgetown University School of Medicine; Attending Physician, Georgetown University Hospital, Washington, D.C.
Peptic Ulcer

TIMOTHY J. LEY, M.D.

Assistant Professor of Medicine and Genetics, Washington University Medical School; Assistant Physician, Jewish Hospital of St. Louis, St. Louis, Missouri
Thalassemia

JENNIFER LI, M.D.

Pediatric Resident, Children's Hospital of Philadelphia, Philadelphia, Pennsylvania
Osteomyelitis

CLAUDIA R. LIBERTIN, M.D.

Assistant Professor of Medicine and Pathology, Loyola University Stritch School of Medicine, Chicago, Illinois; Director, Infectious Diseases Laboratory, and Assistant Director, Clinical Microbiology Laboratory, Foster G. McGaw Hospital, Maywood, Illinois
Infective Endocarditis

MICHAEL R. LIEBOWITZ, M.D.

Associate Professor of Clinical Psychiatry, College of Physicians and Surgeons of Columbia University; Director, Anxiety Disorders Clinic, New York State Psychiatric Institute, New York, New York
Panic Disorders and Agoraphobia

HENRY W. LIM, M.D.

Associate Professor of Dermatology, New York University School of Medicine; Chief, Dermatology Service, New York Veterans Administration Medical Center, New York, New York
Dermatoses Induced by Sunlight

MARSHALL D. LINDHEIMER, M.D.

Professor of Medicine and of Obstetrics and Gynecology, University of Chicago Pritzker School of Medicine; Attending Physician, University of Chicago Hospitals and Clinics; Director, Medical High Risk Clinic, Chicago Lying-in Hospital, Chicago, Illinois
Hypertensive Disorders of Pregnancy

ROBERT LINDSAY, M.B., CH.B., PH.D.

Professor of Clinical Medicine, College of Physicians and Surgeons of Columbia University, New York, New York; Chairman, Department of Medicine, and Director of Research, Helen Hayes Hospital, West Haverstraw, New York
Osteoporosis

JOHN A. LINFOOT, M.D.

Director, Diabetes and Endocrine Institute, Providence Hospital, Oakland, California
Acromegaly

MARTA M. LITTLE, M.D.

Fellow Associate Physician, University of Iowa Hospitals and Clinics, Iowa City, Iowa
Asthma in the Adolescent and the Adult

RICHARD K. LO, M.D.

Assistant Professor of Surgery, Stanford University School of Medicine; Attending Staff, Stanford University Hospital, Stanford, California, and Palo Alto Veterans Administration Hospital, Palo Alto, California
Prostatitis

ROBERT G. LOUDON, M.B., CH.B.

Professor of Medicine and Director of Pulmonary Disease Division, University of Cincinnati College of Medicine; Attending Physician, University Hospital, Cincinnati, Ohio
Cough

FRANKLIN D. LOWY, M.D.

Associate Professor of Medicine, Albert Einstein College of Medicine of Yeshiva University; Attending Staff, Montefiore Hospital, New York, New York
Rat-Bite Fever

JOHN N. LUKENS, M.D.

Professor of Pediatrics, Vanderbilt University School of Medicine; Director, Pediatric Hematology-Oncology, Vanderbilt Children's Hospital, Nashville, Tennessee
Acute Leukemia in Childhood

SEAN R. LYNCH, M.D.

Professor of Medicine, University of Kansas Medical Center School of Medicine; Attending Physician, University of Kansas Medical Center, Kansas City, Kansas
Iron Deficiency

PIRZADA A. MAJID, M.B., B.S., PH.D.

Associate Professor of Medicine, Baylor College of Medicine; Chief, Section of Cardiology, Ben Taub General Hospital, Houston, Texas
Acute Myocardial Infarction

HARRY L. MALECH, M.D.

Head, Bacterial Diseases Section, Laboratory of Clinical Investigation, National Institute of Allergy and Infectious Diseases; Attending Medical Officer, Warren Grant Magnuson Clinical Center of the National Institutes of Health, Bethesda, Maryland
Neutropenia

SANFORD M. MARKHAM, M.D.

Chairman, Department of Obstetrics and Gynecology, David Grant USAF Medical Center, Travis Air Force Base, California
Endometriosis

JAMES G. MARKS, JR., M.D.

Associate Professor of Medicine, Pennsylvania State University School of Medicine; Staff Dermatologist, Milton S. Hershey Medical Center, Hershey, Pennsylvania
Contact Dermatitis

JOHN A. MATA, M.D.

Assistant Professor of Urology, Louisiana State University Medical School, Shreveport; Pediatric Urologic Consultant, Shriner's Hospital for Crippled Children; Attending Staff, University Hospital, LSU Medical Center, and Veterans Administration Medical Center, Shreveport, Louisiana
Bacterial Infections of the Urinary Tract in Females

MICHAEL E. MAYO, M.B., B.S.

Professor of Urology, University of Washington School of Medicine; Attending Staff, University Hospital, Children's Hospital and Medical Center, and Harborview Medical Center, Seattle, Washington
Benign Prostatic Hyperplasia

PAUL L. McCARTHY, M.D.

Professor of Pediatrics, Yale University School of Medicine; Head, Section of General Pediatrics, Yale–New Haven Hospital, New Haven, Connecticut
Fever

PHILIP L. McCARTHY, JR., M.D.

Research Fellow in Medicine, Harvard Medical School and Division of Hematology, Department of Medicine, Brigham and Women's Hospital, Boston, Massachusetts
Acute Leukemia in Adults

WALTER J. McCARTHY, M.D.

Assistant Professor of Surgery, Northwestern University Medical School; Attending Staff, Northwestern Memorial Hospital, Chicago, Illinois
Acquired Aortic Disease

EDWARD J. McGUIRE, M.D.

Head, Section of Urology, University of Michigan Medical School and University Hospital, Ann Arbor, Michigan
Urinary Incontinence

DOUGLAS B. McKEAG, M.D.

Associate Professor of Family Practice, and Coordinator of Sports Medicine, Michigan State University, East Lansing, Michigan
Common Sports Injuries

ELI O. MELTZER, M.D.

Clinical Professor of Pediatrics, Division of Allergy and Immunology, University of California, San Diego, School of Medicine; Senior Staff, Children's Hospital and Health Center; Attending Staff, University Hospital and Mercy Hospital, San Diego, California
Allergic Rhinitis due to Inhalant Allergens

NANCY PRICE MENDENHALL, M.D.

Assistant Professor, Department of Radiation Oncology, University of Florida College of Medicine; Attending Physician, Radiation Oncology Department, Shands Teaching Hospital at the University of Florida, Gainesville, Florida
Hodgkin's Disease: Treatment with Radiation Therapy

JAMES. O. MENZOIAN, M.D.

Program Director, Surgical Training Program, Division of Surgery, and Co-Director, Vascular Fellowship Training Program, Boston University School of Medicine; Chief, Section of Vascular Surgery, and Associate Professor of Surgery, University Hospital; Attending Surgeon, Boston City Hospital, Boston, Massachusetts
Thrombophlebitis in Obstetrics and Gynecology

NICHOLAS H. E. MEZITIS, M.D.

Instructor, Columbia University College of Physicians and Surgeons; Medical Supervisor, Weight Control Unit, and Attending Physician, St. Luke's/Roosevelt Hospital Center, New York, New York
Parenteral Nutrition in Adults

J. PARKER MICKLE, M.D.

Associate Professor, Department of Neurological Surgery, University of Florida College of Medicine, Gainesville, Florida
Acute Head Injuries in Children

DON R. MILLER, M.D.

Professor of Surgery, University of California, Irvine, School of Medicine; Active Staff, University of California, Irvine, Medical Center, Irvine, California; Consulting Staff, Veterans Administration Medical Center, Long Beach, California
Pulmonary Effusion and Empyema Thoracis

RODNEY R. MILLION, M.D.

Professor and Chairman, Department of Radiation Oncology, University of Florida College of Medicine; Medical Director, Radiation Oncology Department, Shands Teaching Hospital at the University of Florida, Gainesville, Florida
Hodgkin's Disease: Treatment with Radiation Therapy

PAUL F. MILNER, M.D.

Professor of Pathology and Medicine, Medical College of Georgia; Medical Staff, Medical College of Georgia Hospitals and Clinics; Physician in Charge, Adult Sickle Cell Clinic, Augusta, Georgia
Sickle Cell Disease

SHERMAN A. MINTON, M.D.

Professor Emeritus, Department of Microbiology and Immunology, Indiana University School of Medicine, Indianapolis, Indiana
Snakebite

PAUL D. MINTZ, M.D.

Associate Professor of Pathology and Internal Medicine, University of Virginia Medical Center; Director, Blood Bank and Transfusion Services, University of Virginia Hospital, Charlottesville, Virginia
Therapeutic Use of Blood Components

DANIEL R. MISHELL, JR., M.D.

Professor and Chairman, Department of Obstetrics and Gynecology, University of Southern California School of Medicine; Chief of Professional Services, Women's Hospital, Los Angeles County/USC Medical Center, Los Angeles, California
Menopause

JOEL L. MOAKE, M.D.

Professor of Medicine, and Director, Medical Hematology Section, Baylor College of Medicine and Methodist Hospital; Associate Director, Biomedical Engineering Laboratory, Rice University, Houston, Texas
Disseminated Intravascular Coagulation; Thrombotic Thrombocytopenic Purpura and the Hemolytic Uremic Syndrome

HOWARD C. MOFENSON, M.D.

Professor of Clinical Pediatrics, State University of New York at Stony Brook, Stony Brook, New York; Adjunct Professor of Clinical Pharmacy, St. John's University College of Pharmacy, Jamaica, New York; Visiting Clinical Professor of

Pharmacy and Toxicology, New York College of Osteopathic Medicine, Old Westbury, New York; Director, Long Island Regional Poison Control Center, and Director of Pediatric Pharmacology, Department of Pediatrics, Nassau County Medical Center, East Meadow, New York; Attending Pediatrician, Winthrop-University Hospital, Mineola, New York
Acute Poisonings

BETTYLOU K. MOKRISKI, M.D.

Assistant Professor of Anesthesiology, University of Maryland Medical School; Attending Staff, University of Maryland Medical System, Baltimore, Maryland
Obstetric Anesthesia

A. MAJID MOLLA, M.D., PH.D.

Professor and Chairman, Department of Pediatrics, The Aga Khan University Hospital, Karachi, Pakistan; formerly Senior Scientist, International Centre for Diarrhoeal Disease Research, Dhaka, Bangladesh
Cholera

ALICIA B. MONROE, D.O.

Assistant Professor of Dermatology, University of New Mexico School of Medicine and Affiliated Hospitals, Albuquerque, New Mexico
Cutaneous Vasculitis

WILLIAM J. MORAN, D.M.D., M.D.

Assistant Professor, Head and Neck Surgery, University of Chicago Pritzker School of Medicine; Attending Staff, University of Chicago Medical Center, Chicago, Illinois
Diseases of the Mouth

LYNNE H. MORRISON, M.D.

Fellow in Immunodermatology, Johns Hopkins Hospital, Baltimore, Maryland
Bullous Diseases

GEORGE L. MORTON, M.D.

Clinical Assistant Professor, University of Vermont School of Medicine, Maine Medical Center; Attending Staff, Maine Medical Center and Mercy Hospital, Portland, Maine
Osteoarthritis

ROBERT R. MUDER, M.D.

Clinical Assistant Professor of Medicine, University of Pittsburgh School of Medicine; Associate Program Director, Department of Medicine, Mercy Hospital of Pittsburgh; Chief, Infection Control, Pittsburgh Veterans Administration Medical Center, Pittsburgh, Pennsylvania
Legionellosis (Legionnaires' Disease and Pontiac Fever)

J. PAUL MUIZELAAR, M.D., PH.D.

Associate Professor and Lind Lawrence Chair in Neurosurgery, Medical College of Virginia and MCV Hospitals, Richmond, Virginia
Acute Head Injuries in Adults

ONOFRE MUÑOZ-HERNANDEZ, M.D.

Professor of Infectious Diseases and Clinical Microbiology, Faculty of Medicine, National Autonomous University of Mexico; Director, Hospital de Pediatria, National Medical Center, Mexican Institute of Social Security, Mexico City, Mexico
Typhoid Fever

JOHN J. MURRAY, M.D.

Attending Staff, Lahey Clinic Medical Center, Burlington, Massachusetts
Hemorrhoids, Anal Fissure, and Anorectal Abscess and Fistula

THOMAS F. MYERS, M.D.

Associate Professor of Pediatrics and Associate Director, Newborn Medicine, Loyola University Stritch School of Medicine; Attending Staff, Foster G. McGaw Hospital–Loyola University Medical Center, Maywood, Illinois
Neonatal Resuscitation

GERALD V. NACCARELLI, M.D.

Associate Professor of Medicine, Director of Clinical Electrophysiology, and Acting Director of Cardiology, University of Texas Medical School at Houston and Hermann Hospital, Houston, Texas
Premature Beats

CHAU NGUYEN, M.D.

Fellow in Tropical Medicine, Faculty of Medicine, University of Toronto, Toronto, Ontario, Canada
Intestinal Parasites

G. ROBERT NUGENT, M.D.

Professor of Neurosurgery, West Virginia University Medical Center, Morgantown, West Virginia
Trigeminal Neuralgia

MICHAEL M. PAPARELLA, M.D.

Clinical Professor and Chairman Emeritus, Department of Otolaryngology, University of Minnesota; Secretary, International Hearing Foundation, Minneapolis, Minnesota
Meniere's Disease

LAWRENCE CHARLES PARISH, M.D.

Clinical Professor of Dermatology and Director, Jefferson Center for International Dermatology, Jefferson Medical College of Thomas Jefferson University; Chief of Dermatology, Frankford, St. Agnes, and Mt. Sinai Hospitals, Philadelphia, Pennsylvania
Decubitus Ulcers

SIMON C. PARISIER, M.D.

Clinical Professor and Chairman, Department of Otolaryngology–Head and Neck Surgery, Manhattan Eye, Ear and Throat Hospital, New York, New York
Tinnitus

JOHN E. PARKER, M.D.

Clinical Assistant Professor of Medicine, West Virginia University School of Medicine; Attending Physician, West Virginia University Health Sciences Center and Ruby Memorial Hospital; Medical Officer, National Institute for Occupational Safety and Health, Morgantown, West Virginia
Silicosis

ROBERT L. PENN, M.D.

Associate Professor of Medicine, Section of Infectious Disease, Louisiana State University School of Medicine in Shreveport; Chief, Infectious Disease Service, and Assistant Chief, Medical Service, Veterans Administration Medical Center, Shreveport, Louisiana
Toxoplasmosis

RICHARD F. PEPPARD, M.B., B.S.

Neurology Research Fellow, Department of Medicine, University Hospital, University of British Columbia, Vancouver, British Columbia, Canada
Parkinsonism

JAY I. PETERS, M.D.

Associate Professor of Medicine, University of Texas Health Science Center at San Antonio; Director of Medical Intensive Care Unit at Medical Center Hospital, San Antonio, Texas
Acute Respiratory Failure

JACK PICKELMAN, M.D.

Professor of Surgery and Chief, Division of General Surgery, Loyola University Medical Center; Attending Surgeon, Loyola University Hospital, Maywood, Illinois
Cholecystitis and Cholelithiasis

NEVILLE R. PIMSTONE, M.D.

Professor of Medicine and Chief, Division of Gastroenterology, University of California, Davis, School of Medicine, Davis, California; Division Chief and Program Director, Division of Gastroenterology, University of California, Davis, Medical Center, Sacramento, California
Porphyria

HAROLD PLOTNICK, M.D.

Clinical Professor of Dermatology, Wayne State University School of Medicine; Vice Chief, Department of Dermatology, Harper-Grace Hospital, Detroit Medical Center, Detroit, Michigan
Occupational Dermatitis

R. CRYSTAL POLATTY, M.D.

Assistant Professor of Medicine, Medical College of Virginia; Chief of Pulmonary Critical Care, McGuire Veterans Administration Medical Center, Richmond, Virginia
Chronic Obstructive Pulmonary Disease

HARRISON G. POPE, JR., M.D.

Associate Professor of Psychiatry, Harvard Medical School, Boston, Massachusetts; Staff Psychiatrist, McLean Hospital, Belmont, Massachusetts
Bulimia Nervosa

JOHN M. PORTER, M.D.

Professor of Surgery and Head, Division of Vascular Surgery, Oregon Health Sciences University, Portland, Oregon
Peripheral Arterial Disease

R. GERALD PRETORIUS, M.D.

Instructor, University of California, San Diego, School of Medicine; Attending Staff, Kaiser Permanente Medical Center, San Diego, California
Cancer of the Uterine Cervix

KANTI R. RAI, M.D.

Professor of Medicine, State University of New York at Stony Brook, Stony Brook, New York; Chief, Division of Hematology/Oncology, Long Island Jewish Medical Center, New Hyde Park, New York
The Chronic Leukemias

P. SYAMASUNDAR RAO, M.D.

Professor of Pediatrics and Director, Division of Pediatric Cardiology, University of Wisconsin School of Medicine; Attending Staff, University of Wisconsin Hospital and Clinics, Meriter/Madison General Hospital, Meriter/Methodist Hospital, and St. Mary's Hospital Medical Center, Madison, Wisconsin
Congenital Heart Disease

MARVIN RAPAPORT, M.D.

Clinical Professor of Medicine/Dermatology, University of California, Los Angeles, School of Medicine; Attending Staff, UCLA Medical Center and Cedars-Sinai Hospital, Los Angeles, California, and Santa Monica Hospital, Santa Monica, California
Pigmentary Disorders

ANTHONY T. REDER, M.D.

Assistant Professor of Neurology, University of Chicago Pritzker School of Medicine, Chicago, Illinois
Multiple Sclerosis

WILLIAM P. REED, M.D.

Professor of Medicine, University of New Mexico School of Medicine; Attending Staff, Albuquerque Veterans Administration Medical Center and University of New Mexico Hospital, Albuquerque, New Mexico
Plague

MICHAEL J. REITER, M.D., PH.D.

Associate Professor of Medicine (Cardiology), University of Colorado Health Sciences Center; Director, Cardiac Electrophysiology Laboratory, University Hospital, Denver, Colorado
Tachycardias

HERBERT Y. REYNOLDS, M.D.

Professor of Medicine and Head, Pulmonary Section, Yale University School of Medicine; Attending Physician, Yale–New Haven Hospital, New Haven, Connecticut
Hypersensitivity Pneumonitis

PHOEBE RICH, M.D.

Resident in Dermatology, Oregon Health Sciences University, Portland, Oregon
Herpes Simplex and Herpes Zoster

JOHN R. RICHARDSON, JR., M.D.

Associate Professor of Surgery (Urology), Dartmouth Medical School; Attending Staff, Mary Hitchcock Memorial Hospital, Hanover, New Hamshire, and White River Junction Veterans Administration Medical Center, Manchester, New Hampshire
Epididymitis

HARRIS D. RILEY, JR., M.D.

Distinguished Professor of Pediatrics, University of Oklahoma College of Medicine; Attending Physician, Children's Hospital of Oklahoma, University of Oklahoma Health Sciences Center, Oklahoma City, Oklahoma
Whooping Cough (Pertussis)

MICHEL E. RIVLIN, M.D.

Associate Professor of Obstetrics and Gynecology and Director of Ambulatory Care, Department of Obstetrics and Gynecology, University of Mississippi, Jackson, Mississippi
Pelvic Inflammatory Disease

W. NEAL ROBERTS, M.D.

Assistant Professor of Medicine, Medical College of Virginia; Attending Staff, Medical College of Virginia Hospitals, Richmond, Virginia
Hyperuricemia and Gout

JOHN A. ROCK, M.D.

Professor, Department of Gynecology and Obstetrics, and Director, Division of Reproductive Endocrinology, Johns Hopkins University School of Medicine and Johns Hopkins Medical Institutions, Baltimore, Maryland
Endometriosis

GEORGE T. RODEHEAVER, PH.D.

Research Associate Professor of Plastic Surgery, University of Virginia School of Medicine, Charlottesville, Virginia
Gas-Forming Infections

O. G. RODMAN, M.D.

Professor of Dermatology and Vice Chairman, Department of Dermatology, Henry Ford Hospital, Detroit, Michigan
Keloids

ALLAN R. RONALD, M.D.

Professor and Head, Department of Medicine, University of Manitoba; Physician-in-Chief, Department of Internal Medicine, Health Sciences Centre, Winnipeg, Manitoba, Canada
Chancroid

RAYMOND P. ROOS, M.D.

Professor of Neurology, University of Chicago, Chicago, Illinois
Multiple Sclerosis

MICHAEL A. ROSENBLUTH, M.D., D.T.M.&H. (London)

Assistant Professor of Clinical Medicine, Cornell Medical College; Adjunct Physician, Lenox Hill Hospital; Assistant Attending Physician, New York Hospital, New York, New York
Trichinellosis

DAVID S. ROSENTHAL, M.D.

Associate Professor of Medicine, Harvard Medical School; Clinical Director of Hematology, Brigham and Women's Hospital, Boston, Massachusetts
Acute Leukemia in Adults

HARLEY A. ROTBART, M.D.

Assistant Professor of Pediatrics (Infectious Diseases) and Microbiology/Immunology, University of Colorado School of Medicine, Denver, Colorado
Viral Meningoencephalitis

FREDERICK L. RUBEN, M.D.

Professor of Medicine, University of Pittsburgh School of Medicine; Associate Head, Infectious Diseases, Montefiore Hospital, Pittsburgh, Pennsylvania
Viral Respiratory Infections

H. GIL RUSHTON, M.D.

Assistant Professor of Urology and Child Health and Development, George Washington University School of Medicine; Vice Chairman, Department of Pediatric Urology, Children's Hospital National Medical Center, Washington, D.C.
Childhood Enuresis

LOUIS J. RUSIN, M.D.

Clinical Assistant Professor, Department of Dermatology, University of Minnesota; Attending Staff, Methodist Hospital, Minneapolis, Minnesota
Pruritus (Itching)

MARC J. SADOVNIC, M.D.

Fellow, Nephrology Division, University of Virginia School of Medicine, Charlottesville, Virginia; Faculty Member, Division of Nephrology, Allegheny General Hospital, Pittsburgh, Pennsylvania
Glomerular Disorders

ARTHUR B. SANDERS, M.D.

Associate Professor of Emergency Medicine, Department of Surgery, University of Arizona College of Medicine; Attending Physician, University Medical Center, Tucson, Arizona
Cardiac Arrest

JOEL R. SAPER, M.D., F.A.C.P.

Clinical Associate Professor of Medicine (Neurology), Michigan State University; Director, Michigan Headache and Neurological Institute, East Lansing, Michigan; Attending Staff, Chelsea Community Hospital, Chelsea, Michigan; St. Joseph Mercy Hospital, Pontiac, Michigan; Saline Community Hospital, Saline, Michigan; and Beyer Memoral Hospital, Ypsilanti, Michigan
Headaches

ARTHUR SAWITSKY, M.D.

Professor of Medicine, State University of New York at Stony Brook, Stony Brook, New York; Director Emeritus of Cancer Programs, Long Island Jewish Medical Center, New Hyde Park, New York
The Chronic Leukemias

ARTHUR B. SCHNEIDER, M.D., PH.D.

Professor of Medicine, University of Chicago Pritzker School of Medicine; Director, Division of Endocrinology and Metabolism, Michael Reese Hospital and Medical Center, Chicago, Illinois
Hyperthyroidism

ROBERT T. SCHOEN, M.D.

Assistant Clinical Professor, Yale University School of Medicine; Attending Physician, Yale–New Haven Hospital; Assistant Attending Physician, Hospital of St. Raphael, New Haven, Connecticut
Lyme Disease

DAVID E. SCHTEINGART, M.D.

Professor of Internal Medicine, University of Michigan Medical School; Staff Physician, University of Michigan Hospitals, Ann Arbor, Michigan
Cushing's Syndrome

ANTONIO SCOMMEGNA, M.D.

Professor of Obstetrics and Gynecology, University of Chicago Pritzker School of Medicine; Chairman, Department of Obstetrics and Gynecology, Michael Reese Hospital and Medical Center, Chicago, Illinois
Amenorrhea

NEIL J. SEVY, M.D.

Assistant Professor of Medicine, University of California, Los Angeles, School of Medicine; Director, Diagnostic and Therapeutic Endoscopy, Harbor-UCLA Medical Center, Los Angeles, California
Dysphagia and Esophageal Obstruction

RICHARD B. SEWELL, M.D.

Senior Lecturer and Deputy Director of Gastroenterology, Austin Hospital, University of Melbourne, Melbourne, Victoria, Australia
Acute and Chronic Viral Hepatitis

DANIEL J. SEXTON, M.D.

Clinical Associate Professor of Medicine, University of Oklahoma School of Medicine; Staff Physician, Oklahoma City Clinic; Medical Epidemiologist and Staff Physician, Presbyterian Hospital and St. Anthony Hospital, Oklahoma City, Oklahoma
Rocky Mountain Spotted Fever

CHARLES A. SHAMOIAN, M.D., PH.D.

Professor of Clinical Psychiatry, Cornell University Medical College, New York, New York; Director, Division of Geriatric Services, New York Hospital–Cornell Medical Center, Westchester Division, White Plains, New York
Alzheimer's Disease

THOMAS W. SHEEHY, M.D.

Professor, Department of Medicine, University of Alabama at Birmingham School of Medicine; Attending Staff, University of Alabama Medical Center, and Diabetes Hospital, Birmingham, Alabama
Disturbances due to Cold

JAMES C. SHEININ, M.D.

Clinical Associate Professor of Medicine, University of Chicago Pritzker School of Medicine; Attending Physician, Division of Endocrinology and Metabolism, Michael Reese Hospital and Medical Center, Chicago, Illinois
Hyperthyroidism

SHELDON G. SHEPS, M.D.

Professor of Medicine, Mayo Medical School; Consultant, Division of Cardiovascular Disease and Internal Medicine and Division of Hypertension and Internal Medicine, Mayo Clinic and Mayo Foundation, Rochester, Minnesota
Pheochromocytoma

DANIEL M. SIEGEL, M.D.

Assistant Professor of Dermatology and Director of Cutaneous Surgery, University of Texas Southwestern Medical Center at Dallas; Attending Physician in Dermatology, Parkland Memorial Hospital; Consulting Physician in Dermatology, St. Paul Medical Center; Consultant, Dallas Veterans Administration Medical Center, Dallas, Texas
Premalignant Lesions

TOBY L. SIMON, M.D.

Professor of Pathology and Associate Professor of Medicine, University of New Mexico School of Medicine; Medical Staff, University of New Mexico Hospital; Consulting Staff, Veterans Administration Hospital, Presbyterian Hospital, St. Joseph's Hospital, and Lovelace Medical Center, Albuquerque, New Mexico
Platelet-Mediated Bleeding Disorders

ANA ABAD SINDEN, M.S., R.D.

Clinical Instructor, Dietetic Internship Program, and Pediatric Clinical Nutritionist, Pediatric Units and Pediatric Intensive Care Unit, University of Virginia Hospital, Charlottesville, Virginia
Normal Infant Feeding

JOHN W. SIXBEY, M.D.

Associate Member, Department of Infectious Diseases and Department of Virology and Molecular Biology, St. Jude Children's Research Hospital, Memphis, Tennessee
Infectious Mononucleosis

ROBERT B. SKINNER, JR., M.D.

Associate Professor, Department of Medicine, Division of Dermatology, University of Tennessee–Memphis College of Medicine; Attending Staff, William F. Bowld Hospital, Baptist Memorial Hospital, Regional Medical Center at Memphis, Veterans Administration Medical Center, and Le Bonheur Children's Hospital, Memphis, Tennessee
Urticaria

IAN M. SMITH, M.D.

Professor, Department of Internal Medicine and Family Practice, and Director, Geriatrics Program, University of Iowa, Iowa City, Iowa
Bacterial Pneumonia

JOSEPH A. SMITH, JR., M.D.

Professor, Department of Surgery, Division of Urology, and Director, Urologic Oncology, University of Utah Health Sciences Center, Salt Lake City, Utah
Malignant Tumors of the Urogenital Tract

WILLIAM J. SNAPE, JR., M.D.

Professor of Medicine, University of California, Los Angeles, School of Medicine; Director, UCLA Inflammatory Bowel Disease Center, Los Angeles, California; Chief of Gastroenterology, Harbor-UCLA Medical Center, Torrance, California
Dysphagia and Esophageal Obstruction

MICHAEL I. SORKIN, M.D.

Associate Professor of Medicine and Director, Peritoneal Dialysis Program, University of Pittsburgh School of Medicine; Associate Chief, Renal Section, Veterans Administration Medical Center; Staff Physician, Presbyterian University Hospital, Pittsburgh, Pennsylvania
Acute Renal Failure

JAMES A. STANKIEWICZ, M.D.

Associate Professor and Vice Chairman, Department of Otolaryngology and Head and Neck Surgery, Loyola University of Chicago Stritch School of Medicine; Attending Staff, Loyola University Medical Center, Maywood, Illinois; Consultant, Hines Veterans Administration Medical Center, Hines, Illinois
Sinusitis

BARBARA W. STECHENBERG, M.D.

Assistant Professor of Pediatrics, University of Massachusetts Medical School, Worcester, Massachusetts; Director, Pediatric Infectious Diseases, Baystate Medical Center, Springfield, Massachusetts
Diphtheria

NEIL J. STONE, M.D.

Associate Professor of Medicine, Northwestern University School of Medicine, Chicago, Illinois
Hyperlipoproteinemia

ALAN STOUDEMIRE, M.D.

Associate Professor, Department of Psychiatry, Emory University School of Medicine; Director, Medical-Psychiatry Unit, Emory University Hospital, Atlanta, Georgia
Delirium

RICHARD A. STRICK, M.D.

Associate Professor of Medicine/Dermatology, University of California, Los Angeles, School of Medicine, Los Angeles, California
Nevi and Malignant Melanoma

JOHN G. SULLIVAN, M.D.

Clinical Professor of Surgery, Tufts University School of Medicine; Chairman, Department of Surgery, St. Elizabeth's Hospital of Boston, Boston, Massachusetts
Tularemia

SIMON B. SUTCLIFFE, M.B., B.S.

Associate Professor, University of Toronto; Staff Physician, Department of Radiation Oncology, Princess Margaret Hospital, Toronto, Ontario, Canada
Hodgkin's Disease: Chemotherapy

JAMES L. SUTPHEN, M.D., PH.D.

Associate Professor of Pediatrics, University of Virginia Children's Medical Center, Charlottesville, Virginia
Normal Infant Feeding

FRED M. SUTTON, M.D.

Assistant Professor of Medicine, Baylor College of Medicine; Chief of Gastroenterology, Ben Taub General Hospital; Attending Staff, Methodist Hospital, Houston, Texas
Irritable Bowel Syndrome

BAYU TEKLU, M.D.

Professor of Medicine, College of Medicine, King Saud University, Abha Branch; Consultant Physician, Assir Central Hospital, Abha, Saudi Arabia
Relapsing Fever

DAVID H. THOM, M.D.

Senior Fellow, Department of Epidemiology, School of Public Health and Community Medicine, University of Washington, Seattle, Washington
Psittacosis (Ornithosis)

COLIN G. THOMAS, JR., M.D.

Mr. and Mrs. Sanford S. Doxey Professor of Surgery and Chief, Division of General Surgery, Department of Surgery, University of North Carolina School of Medicine; Attending Surgeon, North Carolina Memorial Hospital, Chapel Hill, North Carolina
Thyroid Cancer

STEPHEN E. THURSTON, M.D.

Staff Neuro-Ophthalmologist, Departments of Neurology and Ophthalmology, and Director, Ocular Motor/Vestibular Laboratory, Geisenger Medical Center, Danville, Pennsylvania
Episodic Vertigo

THOMAS R. TODD, M.D.

Associate Professor of Surgery, University of Toronto; Attending Staff, Toronto General Hospital, Toronto, Ontario, Canada
Atelectasis

DORIS A. TRAUNER, M.D.

Professor, Department of Neurosciences, University of California, San Diego, School of Medicine; Chief, Pediatric Neurology, University of California, San Diego, Medical Center, San Diego, California
Reye's Syndrome

WILLIAM J. TREMAINE, M.D.

Assistant Professor of Medicine, Mayo Medical School; Consultant in Internal Medicine and Gastroenterology, Mayo Clinic, Medical School, and Foundation, Rochester, Minnesota
Crohn's Disease

EDUARDO TSCHEN, M.D.

Associate Professor of Dermatology, University of New Mexico School of Medicine and Affiliated Hospitals, Albuquerque, New Mexico
Cutaneous Vasculitis

LESLIE B. TYSON, R.N., B.S.N.

Clinical Research Nurse, Memoral Sloan-Kettering Cancer Center, New York, New York
Nausea and Vomiting

JOHN P. UTZ, M.D.

Professor of Medicine, Georgetown University School of Medicine; Attending Staff, Georgetown University Hospital, Washington, D.C.
Blastomycosis

JOSEPH G. VERBALIS, M.D.

Associate Professor of Medicine, University of Pittsburgh School of Medicine; Staff Physician, Presbyterian University Hospital and Veterans Administration Medical Center, Pittsburgh, Pennsylvania
Diabetes Insipidus

GREGORY RAY VEST, M.D.

Chief Resident Surgeon, Mt. Carmel Medical Center, Columbus, Ohio
Tetanus

EILEEN P. G. VINING, M.D.

Associate Professor of Neurology and Pediatrics, Johns Hopkins University School of Medicine; Attending Staff, Johns Hopkins Hospital, Baltimore, Maryland
Epilepsy in Infants and Children

WILLIAM D. WALDEN, M.D.

Clinical Associate Professor of Obstetrics and Gynecology, Cornell University Medical College; Associate Attending Obstetrician and Gynecologist, New York Hospital–Cornell Medical Center, New York, New York
Abortion

LESLIE A. WALTON, M.D.

Professor of Obstetrics and Gynecology, University of North Carolina School of Medicine; Attending Staff, Division of Gynecologic Oncology, North Carolina Memorial Hospital, Chapel Hill, North Carolina
Ectopic Pregnancy

RALPH E. WARREN, M.D.

Associate Professor of Medicine, University of Toronto; Staff Gastroenterologist, St. Michael's Hospital, Toronto, Ontario, Canada
Intestinal Parasites

ROBERT W. WARREN, M.D., PH.D.

Head, Section of Rheumatology, Department of Pediatrics, Baylor College of Medicine; Attending Staff, Texas Children's Hospital and Harris County Hospitals, Houston, Texas
Juvenile Rheumatoid Arthritis

DOTTIE L. WATSON, M.D.

Assistant Professor, Department of Obstetrics and Gynecology, Hutzel Hospital, Detroit Medical Center, Detroit, Michigan
Postpartum Care

ALAN J. WEIN, M.D.

Professor and Chairman, Division of Urology, Hospital of the University of Pennsylvania, Philadelphia, Pennsylvania
Trauma to the Genitourinary Tract

CARL P. WEINER, M.D.

Associate Professor and Director of Maternal-Fetal Medicine, Department of Obstetrics and Gynecology, University of Iowa, Iowa City, Iowa
Vaginal Bleeding in Late Pregnancy

ROBERT A. WEINSTEIN, M.D.

Associate Professor of Medicine, University of Chicago Pritzker School of Medicine; Associate Director, Infectious Diseases, and Hospital Epidemiologist, Michael Reese Hospital and Medical Center, Chicago, Illinois
Q Fever

NANETTE K. WENGER, M.D.

Professor of Medicine (Cardiology), Emory University School of Medicine; Director, Cardiac Clinics, Grady Memorial Hospital, Atlanta, Georgia
Rehabilitation after Myocardial Infarction

CLIFTON R. WHITE, JR., M.D.

Associate Professor of Dermatology and Pathology, and Staff Dermatopathologist, Oregon Health Sciences University; Chief of Dermatology Service, Portland Veterans Administration Medical Center, Portland, Oregon
Herpes Simplex and Herpes Zoster

JOHN L. WHITING, M.D.

Formerly Fellow in Division of Infectious Diseases, Department of Medicine, University of British Columbia, Vancouver, British Columbia; practicing Internist and Infectious Diseases Consultant, Brisbane, Queensland, Australia
Toxic Shock Syndrome

C. MELVIN WILCOX, M.D.

Instructor, Department of Medicine, University of Alabama at Birmingham School of Medicine, Birmingham, Alabama
Disturbance due to Cold

ROBERT L. WILLIAMS, M.D.

D. C. and Irene Ellwood Professor and Chairman, Department of Psychiatry, Baylor College of Medicine; Psychiatrist-in-Chief, Ben Taub General Hospital and Jefferson Davis Hospital; Chief of Psychiatric Service and Consulting Staff of Neurology Service, Methodist Hospital; Chief of Psychiatric Service, Texas Children's Hospital; Active Staff, Internal Medicine Service, St. Luke's Episcopal Hospital, Houston, Texas
Insomnia

FREDERICK A. WILSON, M.D.

Professor of Medicine, Chief of Division of Gastroenterology, and Attending Staff of University Hospital, Milton S. Hershey Medical Center of Pennsylvania State University, Hershey, Pennsylvania
The Malabsorption Syndromes

H. DAVID WILSON, M.D.

Professor of Pediatrics and Chief, Pediatric Infectious Diseases, University of Kentucky College of Medicine; Attending Pediatrician, University of Kentucky Medical Center, Lexington, Kentucky
Mumps

WILLIAM R. WILSON, M.D.

Professor of Surgery (Otolaryngology), George Washington University School of Medicine and Health Sciencies; Chief, Division of Otolaryngology and Head and Neck Surgery, George Washington University Hospital Medical Center, Washington, D.C.
Otitis Media

ROY WITHERINGTON, M.D.

Professor of Surgery and Chief of Urology Section, Medical College of Georgia School of Medicine; Active Staff, Medical College of Georgia Hospital; Consultant Staff, University Hospital, Veterans Administration Medical Center, and St. Joseph Hospital, Augusta, Georgia, and Dwight David Eisenhower Army Medical Center, Fort Gordon, Georgia
Urethral Stricture

JOSEPH A. WITKOWSKI, M.D.

Clinical Professor of Dermatology, University of Pennsylvania School of Medicine; Professor of Dermatology, Pennsylvania College of Podiatric Medicine, Philadelphia, Pennsylvania
Decubitus Ulcers

MARTIN S. WOLFE, M.D.

Clinical Professor of Medicine, George Washington University School of Medicine and Health Sciences; Clinical Associate Professor of Medicine, Georgetown University Medical School; Attending Physician, George Washington University Hospital and Georgetown University Hospital; Tropical Medicine Consultant, Office of Medical Services, Department of State, Washington, D.C.
Malaria

MICHAEL WORTHINGTON, M.D.

Associate Professor of Medicine, Tufts University School of Medicine; Chief, Division of Infectious Diseases, St. Elizabeth's Hospital of Boston, Boston, Massachusetts
Tularemia

YOHANNES W. YESUS, M.D.

Associate Professor of Pathology, University of Missouri–Columbia; Director, Blood Bank, University of Missouri Hospital and Clinics, Columbia, Missouri
Adverse Reactions to Blood Transfusion

EDWARD J. YOUNG, M.D.

Professor of Medicine and Professor of Microbiology and Immunology, Baylor College of Medicine; Attending Staff, Veterans Administration Medical Center, Houston, Texas
Brucellosis

KEITH P. YOUNG, M.D.

Associate in Medicine, Division of Pulmonary Disease and Critical Care, University of Alabama at Birmingham School of Medicine, Birmingham, Alabama
Tuberculosis and Nontuberculous Mycobacterial Diseases

RONALD L. YOUNG, M.D.

Assistant Professor, Department of Obstetrics and Gynecology, Baylor College of Medicine; Chief of Gynecology, Ben Taub General Hospital and Veterans Administration Hospital; Attending Staff, Methodist Hospital, St. Luke's Episcopal Hospital, and Texas Women's Hospital, Houston, Texas
Dysmenorrhea

STUART B. ZEILENDER, M.D.

Pulmonary Fellow, Medical College of Virginia, Richmond, Virginia
Chronic Obstructive Pulmonary Disease

CHARLES ZUGERMAN, M.D.

Associate Professor of Clinical Dermatology, Northwestern University Medical School; Attending Staff, Northwestern Memorial Hospital, Chicago, Illinois
Erythemas

NOTICE

Extraordinary efforts have been made by the authors, the editors, and the publisher of this book to ensure that dosage recommendations are precise and in agreement with standards officially accepted at the time of publication.

It does happen, however, that dosage schedules are changed from time to time in the light of accumulating clinical experience and continuing laboratory studies. This is most likely to occur in the case of recently introduced products.

It is urged, therefore, that you check the manufacturer's recommendations for dosage, *especially if the drug to be administered or prescribed is one that you use only infrequently or have not used for some time.*

THE PUBLISHER

Preface

The objective of this 41st edition is the same as that established by Howard Conn when he published the first edition in 1949. That is, to provide the practicing physician with concise, authoritative information regarding the most up-to-date treatment of problems frequently encountered in practice. Each year new material is presented that may approach the management of a problem in a different manner than the corresponding article published the previous year, often giving the reader a variety of options when the text is compared with earlier editions.

Although the majority of our contributors are authorities at leading medical schools in the United States, many authors have been selected from medical centers in other countries because of their wealth of experience with diseases infrequently encountered here.

It is difficult to meet the time schedule for an annual publication of this type as we solicit fresh material from new authors each year, but we feel this is essential if the information is to keep pace with the rapid advances being made in medicine today. We hope that this book provides a convenient, up-to-date source of information on medical therapy for the busy practitioner. A new topic added this year is the care of decubitus ulcers, a problem commonly encountered in the care of patients in nursing homes. Renewed interest in the care of the elderly has produced many advances in treating illnesses in that age group.

Once again, I want to express my gratitude to Peggy, my wife, and to the staff at the W. B. Saunders Company for their help with this edition. C. F. Robinson has, for many years, checked the accuracy of all drug names and dosages. My sincere appreciation is extended to him for his excellent work, along with my best wishes for a pleasant and rewarding retirement.

ROBERT E. RAKEL, M.D.

Table of Contents

SECTION 1. SYMPTOMATIC CARE PENDING DIAGNOSIS

SECTION 2. THE INFECTIOUS DISEASES

SECTION 3. THE RESPIRATORY SYSTEM

SECTION 4. THE CARDIOVASCULAR SYSTEM

SECTION 5. THE BLOOD AND SPLEEN

SECTION 6. THE DIGESTIVE SYSTEM

SECTION 7. METABOLIC DISORDERS

SECTION 8. THE ENDOCRINE SYSTEM

SECTION 9. THE UROGENITAL TRACT

SECTION 10. SEXUALLY TRANSMITTED DISEASES

SECTION 11. DISEASES OF ALLERGY

SECTION 12. DISEASES OF THE SKIN

SECTION 13. THE NERVOUS SYSTEM

SECTION 14. THE LOCOMOTOR SYSTEM

SECTION 15. OBSTETRICS AND GYNECOLOGY

SECTION 16. PSYCHIATRIC DISORDERS

SECTION 17. PHYSICAL AND CHEMICAL INJURIES

SECTION 18. APPENDICES AND INDEX

Section 1

Symptomatic Care Pending Diagnosis

PAIN

method of
STEVEN F. BRENA, M.D.
*Pain Control and Rehabilitation
Institute of Georgia
Atlanta, Georgia*

Neurophysiological Mechanisms

The experience of pain begins with the stimulation of specialized nerve endings, called nociceptors. Such stimulation is usually triggered by a large variety of stimuli of sufficient magnitude to effect tissue damage. The activation of nociceptors is encoded into a set of signals that are transmitted to the central nervous system. The encoding process is still not fully understood in its biochemical complexity.

Responses to the Perception of Pain

When nociceptive signals reach the brain, they are perceived as a pain message and trigger a cascade of physical, emotional, and cognitive responses.

Physical Responses. Sympathetic arousal and inactivity are among the typical physical responses to perceived pain. In turn, both these responses, when prolonged beyond healing time, may lead to various malfunctions, through altered blood flow to affected bodily parts, lack of musculoskeletal activity, and poor physical fitness, which may affect not only the injured part but almost every system of the body (Table 1).

Emotional Responses. Anxiety and depression are the best-documented emotional responses to a painful perception. In turn, both these psychologic malfunctions lead to sympathetic arousal and to profound changes in lifestyles and in activities of daily living.

Cognitive Responses. Individual values, attitudes, and thoughts may be deeply altered by a perception of pain, mostly in its chronic form, leading to a possible loss of

TABLE 1. **Consequences of Prolonged Inactivity**

Muscular weakness and deterioration
Circulatory impairment
Impairment in respiration
Digestive impairment
Obesity
Depression, cognitive dulling

self-esteem, with a resulting state of "learned helplessness."

The Taxonomy of Chronic Pain States

Chronic pain is usually described as a constant or intermittent pain lasting for long periods of time; 6 months is a common duration to establish a chronic pain state. Chronic pain may be associated with an ongoing structural defect, with chronic illness, or even with the natural process of aging. One special type of chronic pain is currently labeled as "chronic pain syndrome" (CPS). CPS as a diagnostic entity has been recognized by the Social Security Commission on Pain and Disability in its 1987 report to the Department of Health and Human Services. CPS presents six common diagnostic factors: (1) intractable pain of 6 months' or more duration; (2) marked alteration of behavior with depression or anxiety; (3) marked restriction in daily activities; (4) excessive use of medication and frequent use of medical services; (5) no clear relationship to organic disorder; and (6) history of multiple nonproductive tests, treatment, and surgery. A study performed by the Office of Disability of the Social Security Administration found that in patients meeting diagnostic criteria for CPS, malfunctions of the musculoskeletal system were involved in 56.7 per cent of individuals applying for disability benefits; diseases of the cardiovascular system in 16.6 per cent; neoplastic diseases in 13.6 per cent; and mental disorders in 4.1 per cent. One should be alerted to the possibility of a nondiagnosed chronic pain syndrome when confronted with a patient who complains of pain out of proportion anatomically, physiologically, and emotionally to any documented pathologic disorder.

The Social Security Commission on Pain and Disability has proposed a taxonomy of chronic pain patients, which is presented in Table 2. Persons in Group A present most of the symptoms of CPS. It must be clearly understood that although emotional and psychologic factors are important components of CPS, patients demonstrating CPS do not have "psychogenic, unreal, or imaginary pain." The Commission clearly stated that CPS is not a psychiatric diagnosis. By no means should malingering be associated with CPS. The essential feature of malingering is the voluntary production and presentation of false or grossly exaggerated physical or mental symptoms in pursuit of a goal. A clear consensus developed among members of

TABLE 2. **Classification of Chronic Pain States According to the Social Security Commission on Pain and Disability**

Group A	Chronic pain, inability to cope, insufficient documented impairment for lack of pertinent medical findings
Group B	Chronic pain, competent coping, insufficient documented impairment for lack of pertinent medical findings
Group C	Chronic pain, inability to cope, documented impairment from pertinent medical findings
Group D	Chronic pain, competent coping, documented impairment from pertinent medical findings

TABLE 3. **Goals of Pain Rehabilitation Programs**

1. Maximize physical function and activities within medical restrictions
2. Adjust medications to reduce use of habit-forming drugs
3. Increase ability to manage pain and related problems independently
4. Training in self-control of automatic functions
5. Decrease emotional distress associated with pain
6. Return patients to productivity and help settle disability claims
7. Reduce pain intensity levels while maintaining function
8. Educate support systems

the Social Security Pain Commission that malingering is not a significant problem in patients with CPS who apply for disability benefits.

Management of Patients with Chronic Pain

Clinical evidence in the medical literature as well as the report of the Social Security Pain Commission recognizes that it is currently possible to establish protocols for evaluation of individuals complaining of chronic pain and to establish an acceptable plan of management. Treatment in rehabilitation programs must be multimodal, structured, and time-restricted to be cost-effective. Minimum standards for a competent pain control program should include: interdisciplinary (team) evaluation to include medical, psychologic, functional, social, and vocational assessment; quantitative assessment of dysfunction and therapy-related improvements; specific rehabilitation goals; specification of treatment objectives in a format ensuring informed consent; measures of compliance with the rehabilitation goals by periodic reevaluation of medical, psychologic, and functional progress; and vocational and avocational counseling for patients with pending disability claims, in order to facilitate patients' return to work. At present, the Commission on Accreditation of Rehabilitation Facilities (CARF) has established criteria of excellence to provide certification for competent pain control programs in the United States, which are very similar to the standards recommended by the Social Security Pain Commission. Table 3 shows commonly accepted rehabilitation goals of competent pain control programs.

Treatment Modalities for Patients with Chronic Pain

At present, several treatment modalities have demonstrated various degrees of usefulness in the treatment of chronic pain patients. However, it must be clearly understood that each individual treatment modality should be structured within comprehensive, goal-oriented rehabilitation pro-

grams, monitored through the efforts of a competent pain care team. This structured approach has been recommended by both CARF and the Social Security Pain Commission.

Sympathetic Nerve Blocks. Historically, sympathetic nerve blocks have enjoyed a peculiar role of usefulness in managing patients with chronic pain. The recent advent of electronic thermography has provided a clinical explanation for such usefulness. In an overwhelming majority of chronic pain patients, thermographic studies have shown evidence of "cold" patterns in the painful body area, which demonstrate a sympathetic malfunction, leading to a diagnosis of "sympathetically mediated pain"; such "cold" thermographic patterns usually are corrected following proper sympathetic blockade within a structured pain rehabilitation program. If not properly corrected, sympathetically mediated pain is likely to lead to an overt syndrome of reflex sympathetic dystrophy. Therefore, early therapeutic intervention through nerve blocking may be one way to prevent the onset of a disabling painful syndrome.

Epidural Nerve Blocks. Most of the analgesic effects of an epidural block are similar to those obtained through sympathetic nerve blockade, mainly by blocking preganglionic sympathetic fibers as they leave the spinal cord and cross the epidural space. In the anesthesia literature, epidural blocks have been repeatedly advocated for pain control in recent-onset pain syndromes, with evidence of nerve root irritation following an acute back injury. However, such reports have never been validated by rigorous empirical evidence. Epidural blocks are highly invasive and their use should be restricted to selected cases of painful metastatic cancer syndromes involving the lumbosacral plexus.

Psychophysiologic Reactivation. Because psychosocial malfunctioning is a typical feature of a chronic pain patient, a program of psychophysiologic and social rehabilitation is often mandatory. Key modalities in such rehabilitation programs may include biofeedback and relaxation training, psychologic counseling, physical and occupational therapy, and work hardening programs for injured workers with a documented potential to resume work.

Drug Therapy. Drug therapy for pain is quite useful in acute and recurrently acute pain states. In chronic pain patients its value is questionable and it often leads to iatrogenic complications and physical dependence, which are the common features of CPS. The following are simple guidelines for prescription of drugs in patients with chronic pain.

PERIPHERAL ANALGESICS. These drugs (aspirin and the nonsteroidal anti-inflammatory drugs, NSAIDS) have four major pharmacologic properties: analgesic, antipyretic, antiplatelet, and anti-inflammatory action. They do not produce tolerance or physical dependence, and they influence nociceptive stimulation at the level of the peripheral nervous system. Acetaminophen is a peripheral analgesic also, roughly equipotent to aspirin in its analgesic potency, but with no known anti-inflammatory or antiplatelet effects. Use of peripheral analgesic drugs should be prescribed for patients with chronic pain from documented chronic inflammatory processes, but should be restricted in patients with CPS because of the well-known side effects from misuse of aspirin and NSAIDs.

CENTRAL ANALGESICS. Opiates and opioids are quite useful to manage severe acute pain and chronic pain from malignancy. Their use should be avoided in patients with chronic pain not related to malignancy, because of the obvious risk of physical dependence. When central analgesics are prescribed in cases of chronic cancer-related pain, the following principles should be followed. The central analgesic drug should be administered on a time contingency basis, not PRN. This should be done after establishing the optimal dose by titration. Once the dose requirement for a 24-hour period has been established, the analgesic can be administered on a round-the-clock basis with fewer side effects and enhanced analgesic protection. The route of administration to fit the patient's need should be carefully evaluated. The oral route is preferred because of its convenience and the relatively steady blood levels produced. The intramuscular route is most useful in postoperative patients, but has the disadvantage of wide fluctuations in absorption from muscle to muscle and rapid fall-off of action. The intravenous route provides the most rapid onset of effect but also leads to more rapid onset of physical dependence. Appropriate combinations with central and peripheral analgesics should be considered, with the purpose to enhance analgesia and decrease onset of physical dependence.

TRICYCLIC ANTIDEPRESSANTS. These drugs provide direct analgesic effect and may potentiate analgesia from central analgesic drugs, possibly through their serotonergic effects. Among the many tricyclic antidepressant drugs, when an analgesic effect is the primary pharmacologic target, preference should be given to drugs such as doxepin and amitriptyline, with higher affinities for serotonin receptors. Unfortunately, doxepin also demonstrates the highest affinity for histamine receptors, leading to drowsiness. On the other side, amitriptyline has less histamine affinity; for this reason, amitriptyline is probably the tricyclic antidepressant of choice whenever such medication is prescribed primarily for analgesia, which can be achieved long before the dosage reaches antidepressant levels. The tricyclics appear to have greatest usefulness in the management of pain from various forms of de-afferentation syndromes, such as postherpetic neuralgia. They also show clinical usefulness for the prophylaxis of chronic muscle contraction headaches. In patients with CPS and prominent symptoms of depression, carefully monitored use of tricyclic antidepressant may be of value.

ANTIHISTAMINES. Hydroxyzine (Atarax) has some analgesic and mild sedative activity in addition to its antihistamine effect. It may produce additive analgesia when combined with central analgesic drugs.

STEROIDS. These drugs have specific and nonspecific effects in the management of chronic cancer pain. They may directly affect some tumors (e.g., lymphoma) and provide relief of pain by reducing edema in the nervous tissue. In the dying patient, steroids may provide euphoria, increase in appetite, and relief of tumor-related pain. Steroids are also reported useful in the management of acute episodes of vascular headache syndromes. The well-known side effects of chronic use of steroids should be carefully weighed against their potential benefits.

ANTICONVULSANTS. These drugs (carbamazepine (Tegretol), phenytoin (Dilantin), clonazepam (Klonopin), and sodium valproate (Depakene) are particularly useful for the management of the lancinating pain associated with some neuralgias, mainly trigeminal and glossopharyngeal neuralgias.

DRUGS TO BE AVOIDED. Benzodiazepines, barbiturates, and other sedative drugs do not have analgesic properties and should be avoided in the management of pain. Many commonly used analgesic drugs are formulated in combination with barbiturates; this combination of drugs should be avoided if possible, or at least prescribed with extreme caution.

TABLE 4. **Structured Cancer Pain Control Program**

Stage One	Oncology management. Maintain activity and lifestyle. Increase coping skills through behavior management.
Stage Two	Oncology management. Drug management (peripheral analgesics first-choice drugs). Nerve blocks (sympathetic, epidural). Adjust activity to compensate for side effects of analgesic medication and nerve blocks. Maintain pleasurable daily activities.
Stage Three	Terminal phase. Oncology treatment discontinued. Drug management readjusted. Block therapy readjusted. Neuroablative procedures to be considered. Hospice-oriented support and respite programs.

Structured Management of Patients with Cancer-Related Pain

Estimates of the prevalence of pain associated with malignancy range from 60 to 80 per cent. Bone metastases are the most common cause of pain, followed by neural and visceral invasion. Despite the prevalence of pain in cancer patients, not enough attention has been given to structured pain control programs for cancer patients. With the exception of a few highly sophisticated cancer pain control centers in the United States, the overwhelming majority of cancer patients are still treated within an acute-care medical model, mostly with prescriptions of various drugs on a PRN basis. Even less attention is paid to the possibility of rehabilitation for nonterminal cancer patients, despite the fact that research data have indicated that over 40 per cent of patients with cancer in all sites do have physical and psychologic impairments that could be significantly improved through rehabilitative treatment. It is now well recognized that many painful cancer syndromes are actually caused by oncologic interventions. The common denominator in these syndromes is nerve damage and circulatory disturbances from damage to peripheral vessels. Both radiation therapy and extensive destructive surgery, such as radical nerve dissection, often result in extensive fibrosis of the connective tissue, with secondary entrapment of peripheral nerves and vascular structures. Several peripheral neuropathies, bony necrosis, and herpetic infections may follow extensive chemotherapy. Mostly in elderly people, the herpetic infection may result in painful postherpetic neuralgia. The nociceptive stimulation by both the malignant growths and the iatrogenic painful syndromes triggers the same psychophysiologic responses that were described for nonmalignant pain, and leads to inactivity, behavioral and interpersonal deterioriation, chronic stress, and mood disturbances. In other words, the physiologic and psy-chosocial factors associated with cancer pain are not significantly different from those associated with other chronic pain states. Therefore, the same basic philosophy of pain control programs as they are applied for nonmalignant pain states should be applied for cancer pain also; that is, to identify, address, and possibly correct all physical, behavioral, and psychosocial malfunctions present in each person in pain. Specifically, for the cancer patient, this multidimensional strategy should be diversified in three stages of intervention. Table 4 shows these three sequential stages and the various therapies appropriate for each stage.

NAUSEA AND VOMITING

method of
MARK G. KRIS, M.D.,
REBECCA A. CLARK, R.N., and
LESLIE B. TYSON, R.N.
Memorial Sloan Kettering Cancer Center
New York, New York

The brainstem emetic center controls the complex act of vomiting. This functional center near the floor of the fourth ventricle receives and processes input from the cerebral cortex, primary sensory centers, cranial nerves, the chemoreceptor trigger zone (a bloodstream chemosensor located in the medulla), and the gastrointestinal tract. Impulses from the emetic center are transmitted to the striated muscles of the thorax and abdomen and the smooth muscles of the gastrointestinal tract to initiate the vomiting reflex. The mechanisms causing (and controlling) nausea remain obscure. The emetic center and related sites in the gastrointestinal tract contain many neurotransmitters (and their receptors), including dopamine, histamine, acetylcholine, serotonin, and endorphins. To stop nausea and vomiting by pharmacologic means, the actions of one or more neurotransmitters in the central nervous system or gastrointestinal tract (or both) must be blocked. Emesis may be further reduced by the blockade of several different neurotransmitter receptors.

Causes of Nausea and Vomiting

Nausea and vomiting are caused by or complicate a number of illnesses and conditions, as outlined in Table 1. The most common etiologies of acute nausea and vomiting are infections (particularly "viral" gastroenteritis) and medications (especially narcotic analgesics, theophylline compounds, and anticancer chemotherapy). The recommended approach to the patient experiencing these symptoms is to generate a differential diagnosis, attempt to uncover the etiology, and then either remove or treat the underlying cause if possible. While this process is under way, it is important to

TABLE 1. **Common Causes of Nausea and Vomiting**

Infections, esp. gastroenteritis
Medications, esp. analgesics, theophylline, anesthesia
Anticancer chemotherapy and radiation
Peptic ulcer disease
Gastrointestinal tract obstruction and perforation
Pancreatitis
Cholecystitis
Disorders of gastrointestinal motility, e.g., gastroparesis, ileus
Intracranial causes, e.g., migraine, elevated intracranial pressure
Vestibular dysfunction
Motion sickness
Metabolic causes, e.g., ketoacidosis, uremia, hypercalcemia
Pregnancy
Adrenal insufficiency
Psychogenic

manage the patient with oral or intravenous hydration, to correct any electrolyte abnormalities, and to treat these symptoms with medications (Table 2).

DRUG THERAPY

Clinical studies have identified many safe and effective agents for controlling nausea and vomiting. At present, there is no firm evidence that a drug will control only those symptoms caused by a specific etiology. The recommendation of one drug over another for treating vomiting related to a specific cause usually occurs because not all drugs have been tested and doses and schedules of each agent have not been defined for all etiologies of emesis. In general, it is best to follow established dosages and schedules of these medications when treating any cause of vomiting. Phenothiazines, butyrophenones, substituted benzamides, corticosteroids, antihistamines, anticholinergics, cannabinoids, and benzodiazepines can control or lessen nausea and emesis. The selection of an antiemetic drug further depends on the type and severity of emesis, its expected duration, and the patient's size, preference, prior experience with emesis and antiemetics, and underlying medical condition.

Controlling Emesis Caused by Anticancer Chemotherapy

Vomiting remains a common complication of cancer and results from many causes (Table 3). The more widespread use of anticancer chemotherapy and the severity of nausea and vomiting it can produce has fostered a flurry of investigation into the control of these symptoms. This work has identified several potent single agents and defined drug combinations that not only further improve antiemetic control but also lessen the duration of therapy and treatment-related side effects. Vomiting can be prevented or lessened in most patients if the available agents are used according to the recommended doses and schedules.

Single Agents

Metoclopramide (Reglan), a substituted benzamide that blocks dopamine receptors and is related chemically to procainamide, is the most effective and widely studied antiemetic when used in high intravenous doses and is the only first-line drug approved by the Food and Drug Administration for controlling chemotherapy-induced emesis. In controlled trials, this agent proved more effective than placebo, intramuscular prochlorperazine, and dronabinol in controlling vomiting caused by high doses of cisplatin, the most common cause of severe vomiting due to chemotherapy. Common side effects include mild sedation, akathisia (restlessness), diarrhea, and acute dystonic reactions. Extrapyramidal symptoms can occur following treatment with any dopamine antagonist and occur more frequently in children and young adults. These symptoms can be quickly controlled by 50 mg of diphenhydramine (Benadryl), given orally or intravenously. The butyrophenones haloperidol and droperidol, which also block dopamine receptors, control cisplatin-induced emesis when used intravenously using investigational dosages and schedules. Side effects of these two drugs are similar to those of metoclopramide with the addition of mild hypotension. The corticosteroids dexamethasone and methylprednisolone are effective antiemetics when used at investigational high intravenous and oral dosages. Although their mechanism of action is not known, they can prevent vomiting caused by cisplatin and other anticancer agents at low cost. Their common side effects when used in this setting include insomnia, epigastric burning, and perineal sensations when given by rapid intravenous administration. The cannabinoids dronabinol (Marinol) and nabilone (Cesamet) are the only agents other than metoclopramide currently approved specifically for the control of chemotherapy-induced emesis. They are recommended for "patients who have failed to respond adequately to conventional antiemetic treatments." In controlled trials, they have been found to be superior to placebo and prochlorperazine in some trials and equivalent in others among patients receiving chemotherapy of mild to moderate emetic potential. Dronabinol is inferior to metoclopramide for adults receiving high-dose cisplatin. Common side effects of drowsiness, ataxia, orthostatic dizziness and hypotension, and dysphoria (particularly in older adults)

TABLE 2. **Dosages and Administration Schedules of Antiemetic Agents**

Metoclopramide (Reglan)	1–3 mg/kg, every 2 hours, 2–5 doses, intravenously, beginning 30 minutes before cancer chemotherapy 10 mg orally or intravenously 30 minutes before each meal and at bedtime
Butyrophenones Haloperidol (Haldol)	1–3 mg, every 2–6 hours, intravenously for cancer chemotherapy*
Droperidol (Inapsine)	1–2 mg orally or intramuscularly, 3 times daily; 0.5–2.5 mg intravenously, every 4 hours
Corticosteroids Dexamethasone (Decadron)	4–20 mg orally or intravenously, once only or every 4–6 hours*
Methylprednisolone (Solu-Medrol)	250–500 mg intravenously, once only or every 4–6 hours*
Cannabinoids Dronabinol (Marinol)	5–10 mg/M², orally, every 3 to 4 hours for patients who have failed to respond to conventional antiemetics following cancer chemotherapy
Nabilone (Casemet)	1–2 mg orally, every 12 hours for patients who have failed to respond to conventional antiemetics following cancer chemotherapy
Phenothiazines Prochlorperazine (Compazine)	5–10 mg orally 3 or 4 times daily; 5 to 10 mg intramuscularly every 3–4 hours (limit 40 mg/day); 25 mg suppository every 5 hours; 10–40 mg intravenously, every 3 hours, 3 doses, beginning 30 minutes before chemotherapy*
Chlorpromazine (Thorazine)	10–25 mg orally every 4–6 hours; 25 mg intravenously every 3 to 4 hours; 100 mg rectally every 6–8 hours
Thiethylperazine (Torecan)	10 mg orally, rectally, or intramuscularly, 1–3 times daily
Perphenazine (Trilafon)	8–16 mg orally, in divided dosages, 5 mg intravenously
Promethazine (Phenergan)	25 mg orally, rectally, or intramuscularly every 4–6 hours
Antihistamines Dimenhydrinate (Dramamine)	50 mg orally or intravenously every 4–6 hours
Meclizine (Antivert)	20–50 mg orally every 24 hours
Diphenhydramine (Benadryl)	25–50 mg orally or intravenously every 3–4 hours
Hydroxyzine (Vistaril)	25–100 mg orally or intravenously 3–4 times daily
Anticholinergic Scopolamine (Transderm-Scop)	1 patch behind the ear 4 hours before travel; change patch every 3 days
Miscellaneous Benzquinamide (Emete-Con)	50 mg intramuscularly, repeated in 1 hour and every 3–4 hours as needed; 25 mg intravenously (1 ml/minute), with later doses given intramuscularly
Lorazepam (Ativan)	1–1.5 mg/M² intravenously, 30 minutes prior to chemotherapy, repeated every 4–6 hours as needed*
Trimethobenzamide (Tigan)	200 mg orally, intramuscularly, or rectally, 3–4 times daily

*Investigational use, dose, or schedule.

limit its use. The phenothiazines, particularly prochlorperazine (Compazine), chlorpromazine (Thorazine), thiethylperazine (Torecan), and promethazine (Phenergan), are dopamine antagonists that are widely used for the treatment of chemotherapy-induced emesis. Few controlled trials document their effectiveness for this indication, and prochlorperazine has been found to be inferior to metoclopramide, dexamethasone, and dronabinol in randomized studies. The effectiveness of this class of agents may be increased

TABLE 3. **Vomiting in Cancer Patients**

Chemotherapy-related 　Acute emesis (0–24 hours after chemotherapy) 　Delayed (>24 hours after chemotherapy) 　Anticipatory (before chemotherapy) **Not chemotherapy-related** 　Radiation 　Metastases—brain and gastrointestinal tract **Other causes, esp. narcotic analgesics, see Table 1** **Multifactorial**

by their investigational use in high intravenous dosages. However, this method of administration exacerbates their tendency to cause orthostatic hypotension. Other side effects include sedation, akathisia, and acute dystonic reactions. The benzodiazepine lorazepam (Ativan) has limited antiemetic effectiveness but can be a useful adjunct to antiemetic therapies as described below. Scopolamine and antihistamines have not been extensively studied as single agents for this indication.

Combination Antiemetics

Several controlled trials have shown combinations of metoclopramide plus dexamethasone or methylprednisolone to be superior to the agents used alone in controlling cisplatin-induced emesis. These combinations have further been shown to lessen sedation and diarrhea and to shorten the duration of antiemetic treatment. The use of intravenous lorazepam with these two agents can further improve results by lessening treatment-related anxiety and restlessness.

TABLE 4. **Emetic Potential of Anticancer Chemotherapeutic Agents**

Most likely to cause vomiting	Cisplatin* (Platinol)
	Dacarbazine* (DTIC)
	Dactinomycin* (Cosmegen)
	Nitrogen mustard* (Mustargen)
	Cyclophosphamide* (Cytoxan)
	Doxorubicin* (Adriamycin)
	Lomustine (CCNU), Carmustine (BCNU)
	Cytarabine (Cytosar-U)
	Mitomycin (Mutamycin)
	Methotrexate (Mexate)
	Bleomycin (Blenoxane)
	5-Fluorouracil (Adrucil)
	Etoposide (Vepesid)
	Diethylstilbestrol
	Tamoxifen (Nolvidex)
Least likely to cause vomiting	Vinblastine (Velban)
	Vincristine (Oncovin)
	Chlorambucil (Leukeran)

*Pretreatment antiemetics required.

Management of Acute Chemotherapy-Induced Emesis

The emetic potential of commonly used anticancer drugs is presented in Table 4. In general, combination antiemetics should be given to all patients receiving cisplatin, actinomycin, dacarbazine, nitrogen mustard, or high doses of doxorubicin ($\geq$30 mg per M^2) or cyclophosphamide ($\geq$500 mg per M^2) before chemotherapy treatment in an effort to prevent emesis. Combination antiemetic programs for specific chemotherapeutic agents are presented in Table 5.

Other Emetic Problems in Cancer Patients

Delayed Emesis. This condition includes vomiting that begins or persists 24 or more hours following chemotherapy—generally with cisplatin. Although less severe than acute vomiting after cisplatin, delayed vomiting can begin abruptly up to 5 days after chemotherapy and occurs to some degree in the majority of patients 48 to 72 hours after cisplatin. Oral antiemetic combinations such as metoclopramide or prochlorperazine spansules plus dexamethasone, given routinely beginning the day after cisplatin, appear effective and safe in controlling this problem.

Anticipatory Emesis. This is a conditioned response in which individuals with poor control of emesis with prior chemotherapy vomit before chemotherapy is given. At present, prevention (through the control of emesis during initial treatments) is the best strategy. Behavior modification can lessen emesis in patients who develop this problem.

Postanesthesia Nausea and Vomiting

Nausea and vomiting experienced postoperatively, while generally temporary conditions, can lead to fluid and electrolyte imbalances and place strain on operative wounds. The incidence of postanesthesia nausea and vomiting has been reported to be as high as 82 per cent. Predisposing factors include type of preanesthetic and anesthetic, duration of anesthesia, age, sex, and site of operation. Prophylactic use of antiemetics may

TABLE 5. **Recommended Antiemetic Combinations for Specific Chemotherapeutic Agents**

Chemotherapy	Antiemetic Combinations	Dosage and Schedule
Cisplatin (Platinol)	Metoclopramide (Reglan) plus	1–3 mg/kg* intravenously, 30 min before and 90 min after chemotherapy
	Dexamethasone (Decadron) plus	20 mg intravenously, 40 min before chemotherapy
	Lorazepam (Ativan)	1.5 mg/M^2 intravenously 35 min before chemotherapy (3 mg maximum dose)
Cyclophosphamide-doxorubicin combinations (Cytoxan, Adriamycin)	Metoclopramide plus	2 or 3 mg/kg q 2 hr, 3 times, then q 4 hr, 3 times intravenously or 3 mg/kg intravenously q 2 hr twice, then 40 mg orally q 3 hr, 4 times
	Dexamethasone plus	20 mg intravenously 40 min before chemotherapy
	Lorazepam	1.5 mg/M^2 intravenously 35 min before chemotherapy (3 mg maximum dose)
Dacarbazine or dactinomycin (DTIC, Cosmegen)	Metoclopramide plus	3 mg/kg intravenously 30 min before and 90 min after chemotherapy
	Dexamethasone plus	20 mg intravenously 40 min before chemotherapy
	Lorazepam	1.5 mg/M^2 intravenously 35 min before chemotherapy (3 mg maximum dose)

*1 mg/kg intravenous metoclopramide: <40 mg/M^2 cisplatin
2 mg/kg intravenous metoclopramide: 40–70 mg/M^2 cisplatin
3 mg/kg intravenous metoclopramide: >70 mg/M^2 cisplatin

be indicated in patients with a history of postoperative vomiting, in those undergoing intraocular surgery, or to prevent Mallory-Weiss syndrome. General measures to eliminate or decrease the possibility of this problem include avoiding inflation of the stomach during induction of anesthesia and proper relief of pain, hypoxia, hypotension, and hypercarbia. Antiemetics used to manage this condition include phenothiazines or antihistamines. Prochlorperazine, chlorpromazine, and haloperidol are widely used and effective but may produce hypotension, extrapyramidal reactions, or sedation and may prolong emergence from general anesthesia. Benzquinamide (Emete-Con), a benzquinolizine derivative, has been reported to control nausea and vomiting in as many as 96 per cent of patients treated. However, when this drug is given intravenously, arrhythmias, hypertension, increased temperature, and flushing have been reported.

Vomiting and Nausea in Pregnancy

Fifty to 80 per cent of women experience some nausea or vomiting in the first trimester of pregnancy. Most of the symptoms are not severe and are controlled without the use of medications. Mild nausea and vomiting must be distinguished from hyperemesis gravidarum, a condition characterized by very serious symptoms that affects only a small number of women. It may lead to nutritional deficiencies, electrolyte imbalance, ketosis, and weight loss. This condition often requires hospitalization to maintain hydration and nutrition, and the use of antiemetics. Since hyperemesis gravidarum occurs more commonly with multiple gestations and in individuals with hydatidiform mole, a sonogram should be performed during the evaluation of these patients. In cases of significant vomiting during pregnancy, it should not be assumed that the emesis is caused by the pregnancy, since any other condition causing vomiting, especially pancreatitis and cholecystitis, can occur in pregnant women. At the present time, the cause of nausea and vomiting in pregnancy that is not related to other conditions is unknown.

The most commonly used drugs for this condition are phenothiazines and antihistamines. Cyclizine and meclizine were used widely in the 1950s. Studies have shown both drugs to be teratogenic in rats. Occasional congenital defects have been related to the use of these drugs, but retrospective studies are unable to support a relationship between human birth defects and meclizine or cyclizine use. These drugs, however, are not formally recommended for use by pregnant women. Little is known of the effectiveness of dimenhydrinate and trimethobenzamide; neither drug has been found to be teratogenic. Of the phenothiazines, prochlorperazine has been found to be superior to placebo for controlling emesis in pregnancy. Studies have shown no greater incidence of birth defects than normally expected when prochlorperazine is used. Prochlorperazine, however, reportedly has a greater incidence of side effects than either antihistamines or metoclopramide. Metoclopramide has been shown to be safe and useful in the treatment of hyperemesis gravidarum. No teratogenic effects or congenital malformations have been associated with metoclopramide. Currently, the Food and Drug Administration has not approved any drug for controlling nausea and vomiting in pregnancy.

Drug use in general should be discouraged in the first trimester of pregnancy unless absolutely necessary. For many women, the symptoms are mild and of limited duration and are best treated by supportive measures (small frequent meals, bland diet, avoidance of unpleasant odors, etc.). Drug therapy must be individualized and should be instituted only when the nausea and vomiting are severe enough that their effects outweigh the possible adverse reactions of the antinausea medications. If drugs must be used to control emesis, it appears that the risk to the fetus is very slight according to the trials reported to date.

Motion Sickness

The etiology of motion sickness still is not completely understood. It has been theorized that labyrinthine stimulation (repetitive pitching and rolling) as well as a possible imbalance between cholinergic receptors in the vestibular apparatus and subsequent stimulation of the chemoreceptor trigger zone and cerebral cortex may play a role in the development of this problem. Motion sickness can be prevented by decreasing visceral sensations of motion as well as visual stimulation. Reduction of anxiety related to an impending trip may also be helpful. Anticholinergics and antihistamines are most commonly used. These include scopolamine, dimenhydrinate, cyclizine, and meclizine. Patients have also reported relief when given the combination of promethazine, a phenothiazine, and ephedrine. Medications should be started 1 to 4 hours prior to travel. Symptoms of motion sickness always disappear with the cessation of motion.

FLATULENCE AND INDIGESTION

method of
BERNARD I. LEMAN, M.D., and
ANDREW F. IPPOLITI, M.D.
UCLA Division of Gastroenterology
Los Angeles, California

FLATULENCE

Flatulence is a common presenting complaint to both the primary care physician and the gastroenterologist. Care must be taken to distinguish between complaints of chronic eructation (which has little to do with gas production) and increased flatulence. A partial list of causes of increased flatulence includes excessive air or saliva swallowing, excessive use of carbonated beverages, gum chewing, irritative mouth lesions, excess smoking, xerostomia, use of antacids, rapid gastrointestinal transit, malabsorption, and disaccharidase (lactase) deficiency.

Most patients who complain of excessive flatulence actually produce gas equal in amount to that of individuals without complaints. Usual output is in the range of 200 to 1600 ml per day via a mean of 13 to 15 expulsions. A bean meal, containing oligosaccharides raffinose and stachyose, can increase gas output tenfold.

The composition of intestinal gas varies with its location in the gastrointestinal tract. Ninety-nine per cent of expelled flatus is accounted for by nitrogen and carbon dioxide, with variable contributions by oxygen and methane. About one third of the population are methane producers, a tendency which appears to have a familial component. Although quantitative data are lacking, the noticeable components of flatus probably include end products of anaerobic metabolism by colonic microflora, indole and skatole, as well as ammonia, volatile amines, short-chain fatty acids, mercaptans, methyl sulfides, methane thiol, hydrogen sulfide, dimethyl disulfide, and dimethyl trisulfide.

Treatment

Treatment of excessive flatulence most often involves reassurance that no serious problem exists and an earnest attempt at dietary manipulation. A low-flatulence diet is one low in wheat, oats, corn, fiber, lactose, and carbohydrates in general. This presumably allows for more complete small bowel carbohydrate absorption, which in turn decreases the availability of carbohydrates to act as substrates for carbon dioxide and hydrogen production by colonic bacterial fermentation reactions. If the patient wishes to include

TABLE 1. **Treatment of Excessive Flatulence and Indigestion**

Treatment	Dose	Assessment
Flatulence		
Dietary Modification		
Low-carbohydrate, low-fiber diet		Less substrate available for colonic fermentation reactions; less gas production
Low milk product intake		Essential in lactase-deficient individuals
Bulk-forming laxatives, psyllium seed–containing	Must be individualized	Increase stool bulk at expense of more gas production; may reduce crampy abdominal pain
Absorbing Agents		
Charcoal (Charcocaps)	1 capsule q 6 hours	No consistent efficacy in experimental trials; may retard absorption of other medications
Antibiotics		
Tetracycline	250–500 mg q 6 hr	Appropriate only in treatment of small bowel bacterial overgrowth. Never appropriate as empiric therapy
Indigestion		
Anticholinergics		
Dicyclomine (Bentyl)	10–20 mg q 6 hr	Nonspecific smooth muscle relaxation of the gastrointestinal tract
Antacids	30 ml orally prn	When given in large amounts, magnesium-containing antacids may cause diarrhea
H_2 Blockers		
Cimetidine	300 mg 4 times daily	If no response after 4 weeks of therapy, upper panendoscopy indicated
Ranitidine	150 mg twice daily	
Famotidine	20 mg twice daily	
Smooth Muscle Agents		
Metoclopramide	10 mg 4 times daily	Associated with CNS side effects in significant number of patients

fiber in the diet, psyllium seed supplementation should suffice. Anticholinergics, antibiotics, agents to quiet the gut, simethicone, charcoal, or antacids have never been shown to be of consistent benefit in controlled trials. Table 1 outlines current therapeutic alternatives.

INDIGESTION

Indigestion is also a common complaint of patients presenting in the primary care setting. It usually occurs postprandially and may be accompanied by pain and nausea or fullness. Just as flatulence has many potential causes, indigestion may be due to one or more of the following: esophagitis, gastrointestinal reflux, irritable bowel syndrome, biliary tract disease, peptic ulcer disease, or malignancy. Up to 20 per cent of patients with nonspecific functional dyspeptic symptoms will, after thorough investigation, have no identifiable organic cause for their complaints. These patients are given the diagnosis of essential dyspepsia. In some individuals with this diagnosis, delayed gastric emptying has been found. Of course, one cannot overemphasize the need to rule out treatable conditions prior to assigning a diagnosis of a functional illness.

Treatment

The use of antacids is appropriate as a first step in the treatment of idiopathic indigestion. Relief by antacids, on the other hand, is of little diagnostic value in the patient with indigestion and should not lead the clinician away from pursuing a specific treatable entity. Indeed, persistence of symptoms beyond 4 weeks of empiric therapy is an indication for further work-up which should include upper panendoscopy. If other entities can be ruled out a small number of patients with nonulcer dyspepsia or essential dyspepsia may benefit from therapy with an H_2 blocker. Cimetidine (Tagamet), ranitidine (Zantac), or famotidine (Pepcid) may be effective. As some patients have delayed gastric emptying, a trial of metoclopramide (Reglan) or urecholine (Bethanacol) may be worthwhile. Table 1 outlines current therapeutic regimens for the most common causes of indigestion.

ACUTE DIARRHEA

method of
JOSEPH L. BREAULT, M.S., M.D.,
    M.P.H.T.M.
Montefiore Family Health Center
Bronx, New York

Acute diarrhea (less than 3 weeks) can be classified as mild, moderate, or severe based on the number of unformed stools per 24 hours (1 to 3, 4 or 5, or 6 or more, respectively) and the intensity of other symptoms (fever, abdominal cramping, tenesmus, bloody stools). Grossly bloody stools should be considered indicative of severe illness even if stool volume is small. Treatment always involves fluids, with oral rehydration being sufficient in the vast majority. In mild cases nothing else is indicated. In moderate diarrhea nonantibiotic drug therapy may be used in addition to fluids. In severe cases a diagnostic work-up and antibiotic therapy are usually indicated. A thorough history will help distinguish infectious diarrhea from food poisoning (symptoms usually less than 24 hours), osmotic diarrhea (secondary to saline laxatives, antacids, or carbohydrate malabsorption), and the secretory diarrhea caused by irritative laxatives (castor oil, cascara). A broader differential diagnosis is needed in chronic diarrhea.

Oral Rehydration

Dehydration is potentially fatal, particularly in infants, the elderly, and those who are malnourished or in poor fluid balance. Vomiting is not a contraindication to oral rehydration therapy, and giving small amounts of fluid frequently will usually succeed. In infants, this may mean one or two teaspoons of fluid every 10 minutes. After each hour, the amount of fluid given should be doubled each time and the time between feedings should be gradually extended. If vomiting occurs the process should be repeated, with fluids increased more slowly. In the first 4 to 6 hours 40 to 100 ml per kg of oral rehydration solution (ORS) should be given for mild to moderate dehydration. Careful instructions should be given to the relatives of those at highest risk for severe dehydration and the patients should be observed to be receiving proper oral rehydration in the office for an hour or two prior to being sent home. They should also be seen the next day, with comparison of daily weights to ensure improvement. Breastfeeding should continue in infants along with additional properly balanced ORS. Formula feedings and food can be withheld 6 to 24 hours to avoid consequences of food-induced malabsorption (acidosis, fluid loss, depletion of bile acids, mucosal injury) while an ORS is administered. But adequate nutrients promote repair of the mucosal epithelium, prevent protein and energy deficits, and sustain breastfeeding, and studies show that early refeeding is both safe and perhaps better. Refeeding should be graded using no more than half-strength formula, and then three-quarter strength, so that 2 to 5 days (depending on the severity of the diarrhea) elapse before a return to full-strength formula is attempted. Opinions differ whether a low-lactose formula is better for the first week. Young children can advance from clear fluids to the BRAT (bananas, rice, applesauce, toast) diet, while older children and adults should have frequent small snacks, avoiding caffeine and lactose. Fasting is to be discouraged.

The fluids used for ORS are based on the realization that sodium and glucose transport are coupled in the small intestine and that glucose therefore accelerates absorption of solute and water. The electrolyte losses of diarrhea must be replaced, and normal household beverages are too low in sodium and potassium, while their osmolality is too high. Giving plain water is inappropriate. Gatorade is frequently used, but it contains 20 mEq of sodium per liter, which is too low. Household beverages have even less sodium. For minimally dehydrated persons this is not important and clear household liquids are satisfactory. The World Health Organization's (WHO) formula for ORS is shown in Table 1. *Rehydralyte* is a similar commercial preparation. Homemade solutions can be used, although mistakes in making them up may have serious consequences, such as hypernatremia or an iatrogenic osmotic diarrhea from too high a glucose load. Table 2 outlines how to make ORS. Sucrose is less effective than glucose but is more easily obtainable. It should be refrigerated or discarded after 4 to 6 hours. In older children and adults ORS can be approximated by making two drinks. One glass should contain 8 oz of fruit juice, a half teaspoon of honey, and a pinch of salt. In the second glass 1/4 teaspoon of baking soda should be mixed with 8 oz of water. The solutions in the two glasses should be sipped alternately. Once rehydration has occurred, maintenance solutions with smaller amounts of sodium (40 to 50 mEq per liter) should be used. This can be done by diluting ORS with equal amounts of water, alternating it with water, or using one of the commerical solutions listed in Table 1.

New super-ORS formulas may be available soon. These are based on sodium absorption being increased by a combination of glucose with an actively transported amino acid such as glycine. Substituting cooked rice powder for glucose in the WHO ORS has significantly decreased duration and amount of diarrhea as well as the total ORS requirement.

Traveler's Diarrhea

More than 8 million Americans will travel to developing countries this year, and about a third of these travelers will get diarrhea. Characterized by a twofold or greater increase in the frequency of unformed stools, it is commonly associated with abdominal cramps, nausea, bloating, urgency, fever, and malaise. It usually begins abruptly and is self-limited. Ten per cent of cases last more than a week. About 5 per cent of traveler's diarrhea (TD) is accompanied by fever or bloody stools or both. It is acquired through ingestion of fecally contaminated food or drink. The best prophylaxis is to "boil it, peel it, cook it, or forget it." Underlying health problems such as achlorhydria, gastric resection, dysgammaglobulinemia, or use of H_2 blockers or antacids increase susceptibility to diarrhea.

Chemoprophylaxis of TD is outlined in Table 3. The drug of choice is bismuth subsalicylate (Pepto-Bismol). Any prophylaxis should be continued for 2 days after the patient returns home. Antibiotics should be avoided for prophylaxis because of their side effects (skin rash is common,

TABLE 1. **Some Oral Electrolyte Solutions**

Product	Concentration When Diluted (mEq/l)				Glucose grams/l	Form	Cost/ Quart†	mOsm/l
	Na	K	Cl	Base*				
Rehydration								
WHO Oral Rehydration Salts	90	20	80	30	20	Powder	$0.35‡	333
Rehydralyte (Ross)	75	20	65	30	25	Liquid	4.08	305
Maintenance/Prevention								
Infalyte (Pennwalt)	50	20	40	30	20	Powder	2.88	251
Lytren (Mead Johnson)	50	25	45	30	20	Liquid	3.35	220
Pedialyte (Ross)	45	20	35	30	25	Liquid	2.81	250
Resol (Wyeth)	50	20	50	34	20	Liquid§	2.52	269
Household Beverages								
Coca-Cola	1.0	0.15						650
Pepsi-Cola	1.3	0.1						591
Gatorade	20	3						330

*HCO_3 or derived from citrate.
†Cost to the pharmacist, based on Average Wholesale Price, *Drug Topics Red Book* 1987 and June 1987 *Update*.
‡Available in the USA only from Jianas Brothers Packaging, 2533 SW Blvd., Kansas City, MO 64108.
§Also contains 4 mEq each of Ca and Mg, and 5 mEq of PO_4.
Modified with permission from *The Medical Letter* 29(743):64, July 3, 1987.

TABLE 2. **Ingredients for One Liter of the World Health Organization Oral Rehydration Solution**

Component	mEq/l	Source	Grams	Item	Amount
Base	30	$NaHCO_3$	2.5	Baking soda	½ teaspoon
Na	90	NaCl	3.5	Table salt	½ teaspoon
Cl	80				
K	20	KCl	1.5	Salt substitute (check label)	¼ teaspoon
Glucose	111	Glucose *or*	20.0		
		Sucrose	40.0	Table sugar	2 tablespoons
H_2O		Water	1000.0	Boiled water	1 liter

and rare but potentially fatal side effects can occur). Initial data do not support the theoretical concern that antibiotic prophylaxis increases the possibility of infection with drug-resistant enteric pathogens. Antibiotics are sometimes used on an individualized basis, particularly if the travel is only 2 to 5 days. They are not advised for more than 2 weeks, and are especially discouraged in children and during pregnancy. No specific group of travelers should be encouraged to use antibiotic prophylaxis. Contrary to common belief, lactobacilli are not protective, nor are antimotility drugs such as loperamide (Imodium) or diphenoxylate (Lomotil), which actually increase the chance of getting diarrhea and reduce the sense of well-being.

Treatment of TD depends on its intensity. Mild TD is self-limited and needs only attention to sufficient fluid intake and renewed enthusiasm for care in what one eats and drinks. Mild to moderate TD can be treated with bismuth subsalicylate (Pepto-Bismol) or loperamide. Bismuth subsalicylate can cut the rate of stooling by half. Loperamide has been shown to be more effective in decreasing the rate of stooling than bismuth subsalicylate. Diphenoxylate with atropine (Lomotil) has more side effects than loperamide and may not be as effective. Neither of these antimotility drugs should be used in children under 2 years old nor in anyone with bloody, mucoid

stools or high fever (dysentery). They should be stopped if no improvement occurs in 48 hours. Adsorbents such as kaolin and pectin (Kaopectate) treat the stool, not the patient. They are not effective in shortening diarrhea, decreasing stool frequency, or decreasing abdominal symptoms.

Those with severe diarrhea, especially if fever and bloody, mucoid stools are present, can be treated with an antibiotic. Empiric treatment with trimethoprim/sulfamethoxazole (Bactrim, Septra) is the drug of choice because 40 to 70 per cent of TD is due to enterotoxigenic *Escherichia coli* and another 15 per cent to *Shigella*, both of which are susceptible to this drug. Alternative antibiotics are listed in Table 4. The more severe the diarrhea, the more important proper oral rehydration therapy becomes.

Most people with TD will get it when they are in another country and medical care is less accessible. Prior to their trip, careful instructions should be reviewed and prescriptions given. The warning signs of bloody, mucoid stools, high fever, or lack of response to a 3-day course of antibiotics should prompt seeking out medical advice. In some circumstances a person can have the stools analyzed directly at a laboratory and, if they are positive for *Entamoeba histolytica* or *Giardia,* take metronidazole (Flagyl) according to Table 4. If a 3-day course of an initial antibiotic

TABLE 3. **Prophylaxis of Traveler's Diarrhea**

Drug	Adult Dose	Per Cent Protection	Comments
Bismuth subsalicylate (Pepto-Bismol)	262-mg tablets, one four times daily	40	Turns tongue and stool black Decreases bioavailability of doxycycline
	262-mg tablets, two four times daily	65	A tablet has 350 mg of calcium carbonate May be contraindicated if patient is on anticoagulants, aspirin, probenecid, methotrexate
	262 mg/15 ml liquid 60 ml four times daily	62	
Doxycycline (Vibramycin)	100 mg daily	58–86	Photosensitivity reactions Contraindicated if under 8 yr old or pregnant
Trimethoprim 160 mg/ sulfamethoxazole 800 mg (Bactrim DS, Septra DS)	One DS tablet daily	73–95	Can rarely cause hemolytic anemia, neutropenia, aplastic anemia, Stevens-Johnson syndrome Commonly causes skin rash
Trimethoprim (Proloprim)	200 mg daily	52	
Norfloxacin (Noroxin)	400 mg daily	88	Do not use in children or in pregnancy

TABLE 4. **Treatment of Traveler's Diarrhea**

Drug	Dose	Efficacy/Comments
For Mild to Moderate TD		
Bismuth subsalicylate (Pepto-Bismol)	Adults: 30 ml q 30 min for 8 doses 3–6 yr: 5 ml q 30 min for 8 doses 6–9 yr: 10 ml q 30 min for 8 doses 9–12 yr: 15 ml q 30 min for 8 doses If needed, repeat on second day	Cuts rate of stooling by half, length of diarrhea by 27 per cent Tablet form not as well studied for treatment, but substituting one tablet for each 15 ml of liquid is probably effective Do not use in febrile children (theoretical concern about Reye's syndrome) See other comments on this drug in Table 3
Loperamide (Imodium) 2 mg capsules 1 mg/5 ml liquid	Adults: 4 mg, then 2 mg after each loose stool to a maximum of 16 mg per day 2–5 yr: 1 mg three times the first day 5–8 yr: 2 mg two times the first day 8–12 yr: 2 mg three times the first day 2–12 yr: 1 mg per 10 kg after each loose stool starting the second day. Do not exceed total dosage of first day. Studies used 0.8 mg/kg daily in divided doses	38 per cent more effective than bismuth subsalicylate in decreasing the rate of stooling in 4–24 hours Dangerous in dysentery; never use if there is fever or stools are bloody
For Moderate to Severe TD		
Trimethoprim 160 mg/sulfamethoxazole 800 mg (Bactrim DS, Septra DS)	Adults: One DS tablet q 12 hr for 3 days Children over 2 months: 0.5 ml/kg q 12 hr for 3 days. Do not exceed adult dosage. (40 mg TMP/200 mg SMX per 5 ml)	Treatment of choice for moderate to severe TD. Five days only slightly more effective than 3, with increased side effects on days 4 and 5. Cuts length of diarrhea by 59 per cent. Skin rashes common (3 per cent). Rarely, Stevens-Johnson syndrome and blood dyscrasias. Contraindicated near term in pregnancy
Trimethoprim (Proloprim)	Adults: 200 mg q 12 hr for 3–5 days	As effective as trimethoprim/sulfamethoxazole (TMP/SMX)
Norfloxacin (Noroxin)	Adults: 400 mg q 12 hr for 3–5 days	As effective as TMP/SMX, covers *Campylobacter*, expensive, do not use in children or in pregnancy
Ciprofloxacin (Cipro)	Adults: 500 mg q 12 hr for 3–5 days	See comments about Norfloxacin
Doxycycline (Vibramycin)	Adults: 100 mg q 12 hr the first day, then 100 mg daily on days 2 and 3	Cuts length of diarrhea by 45 per cent
For Special Indications		
Furazolidone (Furoxone) 100 mg tablets 50 mg/15 ml liquid	Adults: 100 mg q 6 hr for 3–5 days Children: 5 mg/kg/day in 4 doses for 3–5 days for TD. For *Giardia* use 8 mg/kg/day in 3 doses for 7 days	Less effective than TMP/SMX, covers *Campylobacter* and *Giardia*, disulfiram effect, may tint urine brown, drug of choice for *Giardia* in children, may be useful if TMP/SMX fails and laboratory work-up is not possible, hypertensive reaction possible if given with adrenergic agents, tricyclic compounds, or tyramine-containing foods
Metronidazole (Flagyl)	*Giardia*: Adults: 2 grams daily for 3 days Children: Use furazolidone *Entamoeba histolytica:* Adults: 750 mg every 8 hours for 10 days Children: 50 mg/kg/day in 3 doses for 10 days *Clostridium difficile:* Adults: 500 mg three times a day for 7–15 days, or 250 mg four times a day for 10 days	Caution in pregnancy, especially in first trimester For *E. histolytica* follow metronidazole with iodoquinol (Yodoxin) 650 mg every 8 hours for 20 days. In children use 30–40 mg/kg/day in 2 or 3 divided doses for 20 days (maximum of 2 grams/day). Available in 210- or 650-mg tablets and as 25 grams of powder
Vancomycin (Vancocin) powder: 1 or 10 grams	Adults: 125–500 mg q 6 hr Children: 50 mg/kg/day in four doses	The traditional drug of choice for antibiotic-associated pseudomembranous colitis, but metronidazole is as effective, is much cheaper, and is becoming the drug of choice. Reconstituted oral solution is stable for 1 week if refrigerated

fails, and laboratory work-up is not feasible, furazolidone (Furoxone), which is effective for *Campylobacter* and *Giardia,* or metronidazole may be useful. The unusual case of antibiotic-associated pseudomembranous colitis due to *Clostridium difficile* can be treated as effectively, and far cheaper, with metronidazole than with vancomycin (Vancocin). If the patient with TD is seen after returning home and empiric treatment has not resolved it in a few days, a laboratory work-up is indicated.

Work-up and Treatment

Acute infectious diarrhea within the United States should not be treated empirically, because the etiology is different than that of TD. *E. coli* is the cause in only a minority of cases. Viruses play a major role. Noninfectious causes are also more likely, and a careful history (including recent drugs, food, travel, and sexual practices) is important. In any mild case of diarrhea, fluids alone are needed. Moderate to severe cases, and all cases with bloody stools and fever, require a laboratory work-up.

A positive office test for fecal leukocytes (using a thin layer on a slide, with a drop of methylene blue added, five or more per high-power field is positive), grossly bloody stools, fever higher than 37.8°C, rectal tenderness on exam, tenesmus, or severe diarrhea warrants a stool culture for *Campylobacter jejuni, Salmonella, Shigella, Yersinia enterocolitica,* and *Vibrio*-like organisms. Food handlers with diarrhea should always have their stools cultured. Diarrhea following recent antibiotics may require stool cultures for *Clostridium difficile;* a test for *C. difficile* toxin in stool may be better than a culture. If indicated by history or unexplained eosinophilia, a stool exam for ova and parasites should be done on a warm, freshly passed specimen by experienced laboratory technicians. The yield is improved if the specimen is obtained after a saline laxative is taken by mouth. This requires sending a patient to a parasitology laboratory where, if available and properly done, the traditional norm of 3 specimens does not apply. A 24-hour stool collection is occasionally useful to calculate the severity of diarrhea and the amount of fat in the stool. Colon disorders do not affect fat absorption.

Once results are available, standard treatment for identified organisms is given (if antibiotics are of use for the organism), and occasionally later sensitivities may modify this. Nontyphoidal salmonellosis is not helped by antibiotics except in the 5 to 8 per cent of cases in which bacteremia develops. Antibiotics may be helpful if the patient is at high risk for complications from bacteremia

(e.g., the patient with prosthetic valves). Treatment is one double-strength tablet of trimethoprim/sulfamethoxazole (Bactrim, Septra) every 12 hours for 2 weeks. However, antibiotics prolong the excretion of the organism and encourage the development of resistance. *Campylobacter jejuni* is a major cause of diarrhea and, in contrast to *E. coli* and *Shigella,* is not susceptible to trimethoprim/sulfamethoxazole. Erythromycin may be used, but unless it is started within the first few days of symptoms it will lead only to the elimination of *C. jejuni* from the stool and will not decrease the duration or the rate of diarrhea nor the symptoms. Either furazolidone (Furoxone), norfloxacin (Noroxin), or ciprofloxacin (Cipro) can cover both *Shigella* and *Campylobacter* if treatment should begin before stool culture results are available in severe diarrhea with fecal leukocytes. *Vibrio* can be treated with tetracycline.

Choosing drugs to use during pregnancy is a problem. About 90,000 births per year in the United States involve major birth defects. One to 5 per cent are attributed to environmental factors, including drug administration. Prescription drugs are labeled in FDA categories A, B, C, D, or X in increasing order of risk to fetus. In category A controlled studies in women demonstrate no risk, and in category X the risk of using the drug clearly outweighs any possible benefit and it is absolutely contraindicated. Categories B, C, and D are increasingly relatively contraindicated. Studies are inadequate, the dangers of using these drugs in pregnancy are uncertain, and they should be used only with caution for serious clinical indications when the benefits outweigh the risks. Metronidazole (Flagyl), loperamide (Imodium), and sulfonamides are in pregnancy class B. Ciprofloxacin (Cipro), furazolidone (Furoxone), iodoquinol (Yodoxin), norfloxacin (Noroxin), trimethoprim (Proloprim), and vancomycin (Vancocin) are in pregnancy category C. Tetracyclines are in category D. Of the drugs listed in Table 4, ciprofloxacin, doxycycline, norfloxacin, and vancomycin should be considered contraindicated during pregnancy. Furazolidone and sulfamethoxazole are contraindicated near term, but along with iodoquinol, metronidazole, and trimethoprim, can be used with caution if the benefits outweigh the risks. Metronidazole should be avoided in the first trimester of pregnancy if at all possible. If a serious clinical condition warrants the use of trimethoprim/sulfamethoxazole during pregnancy, it should be given in conjunction with folinic acid to prevent megaloblastic anemia (this will not interfere with the antibacterial action).

The American Academy of Pediatrics Committee on Drugs' 1983 statement recommended discontinuing breastfeeding for 12 to 24 hours after administration of metronidazole to allow for complete excretion. Maternal medications usually compatible with breastfeeding included trimethoprim, tetracycline (negligible absorption by infant), sulfonamides (avoid if infant has jaundice or G6PD deficiency, or is premature), salicylates (can cause dose-related metabolic acidosis, rash, or decreased platelet function in the infant), and diphenoxylate with atropine (Lomotil).

CONSTIPATION

method of
MARK S. FEDDER, M.D., and
JAY L. GOLDSTEIN, M.D.
University of Illinois at Chicago College of Medicine
Chicago, Illinois

The definition of constipation by clinicians and patients varies considerably. Patients equate constipation with such symptoms as infrequent passage of stool, passage of hard stools, passage of small stools, straining to defecate, or a sense of incomplete evacuation. For most physicians these parameters are difficult to quantitate. The range of "normal" bowel habits varies widely; approximately 95 per cent of subjects without bowel disease will have anywhere from three stools per day to three stools per week. Therefore, the deviation from an individual's regular pattern should be a more important consideration than the absolute frequency of bowel movements.

In evaluation of a patient with complaints of constipation it is important first to rule out organic causes; constipation often is a symptom of an underlying gastrointestinal or systemic disorder. In the initial evaluation a complete history and physical examination are emphasized, along with basic laboratory studies, including CBC, serum electrolytes, stool for occult blood, and proctosigmoidoscopy. Barium enema or colonoscopy is obtained in patients when there has been a recent change in bowel habits, when stools are positive for occult blood, or when malignancy is suspected. Special laboratory work is ordered as necessary to rule out disorders suspected based on clinical judgment. For example, patients may have constipation as a result of various metabolic, endocrine, or neurologic disorders (Table 1). The use of various medications also is an important factor that may predispose to alterations in bowel habits. In this regard, all medications that the patient is using are reviewed and those that may contribute to the patient's symptoms are discontinued or changed if possible (see Table 1). The use of laxatives should also be reviewed, as long-term use may be associated with the development of a laxative "requirement" as in the "cathartic colon syndrome."

Management

Education is an important first step to correct any misconceptions the patient might have about the frequency, consistency, and size of "normal" bowel movements. Next, patients should be instructed in "bowel training" habits and a regular, unhurried time to sit on the commode should be scheduled. This should take place whether or not the urge to defecate is present. Up to a half hour is not an unusual amount of time as an initial goal. It is preferable to schedule this time after breakfast to take advantage of the "gastrocolic reflex." Relaxation is important and many patients find a diversion such as reading material helpful. Patients should also be encouraged to maintain a regular schedule of exercise and activity commensurate with their age and ability.

After organic causes have been adequately ruled out and the above simple measures instituted, symptomatic medical therapy may be initiated. Our initial approach is to instruct the patient on a diet high in natural fiber (>30 grams per day) including bran cereals, whole wheat bread, fruits, and vegetables with adequate amount of fluid intake (six 8-oz glasses of water per day). Stool water content increases with these measures because of the water-holding capacity of the noncelluloid polysaccharide fraction in fiber. As a result, these manipulations will increase total softness, bulk, and weight and decrease colon transit time. Often this will be the only intervention required. In others, however, supplemental bulk-forming agents may also be needed. The commercially available fiber supplements contain either derivatives of psyllium seed or methylcellulose. A multiple number of products are available as powders, granules, tablets, candies, cookies, or wafers (e.g., Metamucil, Effersyllium, Hydrocil, Fiberall, Fibermed). The efficacy of these and equivalent generic products is primarily related to palatability and patient acceptance. Long-term and consistent patient compliance with these "bulk laxatives" must be stressed. The innovative use of juices, sweeteners, and other liquid vehicles may help to increase usage of the powdered products. Acute or intermittent use of bulk agents must be discouraged, as it usually takes several days before their desired effect is seen. It is important that patients are instructed to drink an adequate amount of fluid to prevent psyllium bezoar formation. When used over the long term (greater than 1 month) most patients will establish a more regular pattern of bowel movements. Generally, we do not advocate combination preparations of bulk and stimulant laxatives. If either or both are required, they should be used individually.

In patients with chronic complaints that fail to

TABLE 1. **Common Causes of Constipation**

Metabolic/Endocrine	Neurogenic	Drugs
Amyloidosis	Autonomic neuropathy	Analgesics
Diabetes	Cauda equina tumor	Antacids containing calcium or
Hypercalcemia	Cerebrovascular accident	aluminum
Hypokalemia	Chagas' disease	Anticholinergics
Hypopituitarism	Hirschsprung's disease	Antidepressants
Hypothyroidism	Multiple sclerosis	Antiparkinsonian agents
Pheochromocytoma	Parkinson's disease	Barium sulfate
Porphyria	Shy-Drager syndrome	Diuretics
Pregnancy	Spinal cord tumor or trauma	Heavy metal intoxication
Uremia	Tabes dorsalis	Iron sulfate
		Laxative abuse
Colonic		Opiates
Anal fissure		Psychotherapeutic agents
Diverticular disease		
Irritable bowel syndrome		**Miscellaneous**
Myotonic dystrophy		Dehydration
Obstruction		Immobility
Hernias		Lack of fiber
Rectal prolapse		
Strictures		
Tumors		
Volvulus		
Rectocele		
Scleroderma		

respond to the above measures, or for those with "acute" constipation, a variety of laxative agents are available for short-term use. These agents should be used with caution, as many are expensive and/or associated with potential side effects. Laxative agents including the above-mentioned bulk-forming agents are generally contraindicated in patients with abdominal pain of unknown etiology, intestinal obstruction, gastrointestinal bleeding, and fecal impaction.

Stool softeners, such as sodium docusate (Colace) or calcium docusate (Surfak), are useful for short-term use (1 to 2 weeks) when straining with stool passage is to be avoided. This is the case in patients with painful perianal disease, after abdominal or rectal surgery, after myocardial infarction, or during pregnancy. These agents are thought to act as dispersing agents, although recent data suggest they may also stimulate mucosal secretion.

Lubricant-type laxatives such as mineral oil act by coating fecal contents and allowing easier stool passage. These should be used with care in young or debilitated patients because aspiration may lead to lipoid pneumonia. Additionally, a potential detrimental effect may be the decreased absorption of fat-soluble vitamins (A, D, E, and K) if these laxatives are used chronically.

Saline laxatives (magnesium hydroxide, magnesium citrate, sodium phosphates, magnesium sulfate) can work by several mechanisms, including an osmotic effect. These agents should be used only in "acute" situations, such as for bowel preparation prior to diagnostic and endoscopic procedures, to remove toxins from the intestinal tract, or after barium studies. Indiscriminate use has been associated with sodium and magnesium overload, which may be especially pronounced in patients with chronic renal failure.

Stimulant laxatives include the anthraquinone derivatives (casara, senna, casanthrol, danthron) and the diphenylmethane derivatives (bisacodyl and phenolphthalein). These agents are thought to work by stimulating intestinal contraction, although some may work by altering fluid and electrolyte transport. Long-term use of these agents may lead to electrolyte imbalance and is believed to be related to the development of a "cathartic colon." The anthraquinone laxatives are also associated with the benign condition melanosis coli. Because of the potential for adverse effects, we do not often recommend these agents to our patients.

Lactulose (Chronulac, 15 to 60 ml per day) and sorbitol are alternative laxatives that appear to be safe for long-term use in chronic constipation. Lactulose has long been used in the treatment of hepatic encephalopathy. These agents are nonabsorbable, nondigestible disaccharides that work by an osmotic effect, and as such draw fluid into the colon, increasing intraluminal pressure and stimulating peristalsis. Intestinal degradation of lactulose lowers the pH of the colon, which may also stimulate peristalsis. Large doses of such agents may cause abdominal cramps, flatulence, and electrolyte imbalance.

Oral electrolyte preparations containing polyethylene glycol (Golytely, Colyte) are relatively new agents used for bowel preparation prior to various gastrointestinal or surgical procedures.

We have used these solutions effectively in the acute management of patients with chronic non-obstructive constipation. These solutions act by an osmotic effect, but are formulated so that there is minimal net electrolyte secretion or absorption. Owing to the large volume of oral fluid intake (3 liters) that is required over a short period of time (less than 90 min), patient compliance is a major disadvantage. These preparations are also associated with complaints of abdominal cramps and vomiting. In light of these disadvantages, these solutions should be used predominantly in hospitalized patients.

We reserve the use of enemas for bowel evacuation in preparation for a procedure or in situations associated with fecal impaction. Fecal impactions may be softened with 150 to 200 ml of a mineral oil retention enema followed by a tap-water enema and repeated as necessary. This is usually adequate, but manual disimpaction is occasionally necessary.

Surgical therapy of constipation is rarely, if ever, indicated except in patients with Hirschsprung's disease or anatomic abnormalities.

FEVER

method of
PAUL L. McCARTHY, M.D.
Yale University School of Medicine
New Haven, Connecticut

Fever is the response of warm-blooded animals to various inciting agents such as viruses, pathogenic bacteria, or circulating immune complexes. Oftentimes, as in juvenile rheumatoid arthritis, the specific inciting agent in a febrile illness may not be well defined. The febrile response is carefully regulated by a central temperature control mechanism located in the pre-optic region of the hypothalamus. In response to an inciting agent, polymorphonuclear leukocytes and other phagocytic bone marrow derived cells of the reticuloendothelial system release endogenous pyrogen, which acts on the thermoregulatory center through the mediation of prostaglandins. Usually, the thermoregulatory center is set at approximately 98.6° F (37.0° C). During a febrile response, the thermoregulatory center is set to maintain a higher level of body temperature. The center maintains this elevated temperature by increased heat production, especially through increased muscle activity such as shivering, by increased heat conservation, especially through peripheral vasoconstriction, by decreased sweating, and by behavioral measures such as covering oneself with blankets in response to chills even though the body temperature is elevated.

Fever should be differentiated from episodes of hyperpyrexia in which the thermoregulatory center has not been reset and is not operating in the precisely regulated fashion described above. For example, in episodes of heatstroke, which involve an insult to the central nervous system, the thermoregulatory center fails to balance heat production and heat loss. Body temperature may also be elevated because of super-heating by high ambient temperatures, and the physiologic responses recruited by the thermoregulatory center (e.g., sweating) are not able to compensate. An example of the latter type of temperature elevation is seen in an infant left in an automobile during warm summer months. Endogenous heat production occurring during anesthesia-related malignant hyperpyrexia can also overwhelm compensatory mechanisms.

Pathophysiology

The thermoregulatory center during febrile episodes has an upper physiologic limit of 106° F (41.1° C). Temperatures beyond this should be considered potentially harmful to the host because of the possibility of damage to the central nervous system. In ranges of fever from 100° to 105.8° F (37.8° to 41.0° C), there are conflicting data as to the value of the elevated temperature for the preservation of the host. Some types of microorganisms, for example, treponemas, are destroyed; others, such as selected types of *Streptococcus pneumoniae*, grow poorly at higher temperatures. Hence, one form of treatment for syphilis in the pre-antibiotic era was to induce fever. Other studies have documented enhancement of selected immune responses if elevated temperature is present. In certain cold-blooded animals, elevated body temperature, achieved by moving to an area of higher ambient temperature, increases survival during bacteremic episodes.

However, other studies utilizing different animal models have documented poorer survival during episodes of gram-negative sepsis when the body temperature is elevated. Other investigators have documented deterioration of selected immune responses when the temperature is greater than 104° F (40° C). Thus, the value of fever in host preservation during infectious episodes is far from resolved. Most of the studies that address this issue have been performed in vitro or in animals. Their applicability to humans is unclear.

That fever places increased metabolic demands on the host is clear. Fever also exaggerates the pulmonary vasoconstriction induced by hypoxemia. The patient who is febrile is often tachycardic, uncomfortable, and, because of irritability, difficult to assess for the underlying illness. Finally, there is a strong correlation between height of fever and the occurrence of febrile seizures in children with fevers of 104° to 106° F (40° to 41.1° C).

When fever places an undue stress on a patient who is compromised, such as patients with cardiac or pulmonary disease, fever control is warranted. If body temperature rises beyond the upper limit of physiologic thermoregulation—106° F (41.1° C), lowering the temperature is mandatory. In the more usual range of fever, the indications for temperature control are less clear. In the febrile patient who is uncomfortable and irritable because of the elevated temperature, antipyresis is warranted. If, in the physician's judgment, fever control will assist in evaluating the patient's state of well-being, antipyresis is warranted. Generally, it seems wise to treat temperatures above 103° F (39.4° C).

Treatment

Acetaminophen

The mainstay of antipyretic therapy is acetaminophen. Acetaminophen is an antiprostaglandin that acts to reset the thermoregulatory center toward normal by inhibiting prostaglandin synthesis and thus interfering with the action of endogenous pyrogen. Acetaminophen is well absorbed in the digestive tract, reaching peak plasma levels in 1 to 2 hours, and its antipyretic effect dissipates in 4 to 6 hours. Unlike other available antipyretics, acetaminophen is not a gastrointestinal irritant, nor does it have an antiplatelet effect. Unlike aspirin, it has not been associated with bronchoconstriction. The dosing schedule of acetaminophen for patients of various ages and weights is given in Table 1. Acetaminophen should be given every 4 hours, and in recommended dosages it is well tolerated. Generally, the dosage for children is approximately 10 to 15 mg per kg every 4 hours; for adults the upper limit is 640 mg, or 10 grains every 4 hours. Doses should not be given more than five times per 24 hours and should not exceed 4 grams per 24 hours in the adolescent or adult.

The major toxicity of acetaminophen is hepatic and occurs when the drug is given in an overdose. The parent compound is usually metabolized to the innocuous sulfated and glucuronidated compounds and excreted in the urine. In overdosages, these mechanisms are overwhelmed and acetaminophen is metabolized to toxic aryl interme-

TABLE 1. **Acetaminophen Dosage by Age and Weight**

Age	Weight (Pounds)	Dose (mg Every 4 Hours)*
0–3 mo	7–11	40†
4–11 mo	12–18	80
12–23 mo	19–27	120
2–3 yr	28–35	160
4–5 yr	36–47	240
6–8 yr	48–59	320
9–10 yr	60–71	400
11 yr	72–95	480
12 yr–adult	96 +	640

*Dose every 4 hours but not more than five doses in 24 hours.
†All dosages approximate 10 to 15 mg per kg per dose.
Usual dosage forms: drops, 80 mg = 0.8 ml; chewable tablets, 80 mg; elixir, 160 mg = 5 ml; junior tablets, 160 mg; and adult tablets, 325 or 500 mg.

diates by the P-450 mixed-function oxidase system. Initially, this intermediate is neutralized by sulfhydryl donors—especially glutathione—but when they are depleted, the metabolite binds to liver protein and cell damage ensues. One is more susceptible to liver damage if the mixed-function oxidase system has been induced by exposure to drugs, e.g., phenobarbital or alcohol, or if glutathiones are depleted, as in malnutrition. The treatment of overdoses is evacuation of gastric contents and therapy with a sulfhydryl donor, acetylcysteine.

Aspirin was previously a mainstay of antipyretic therapy but has several disadvantages when used in physiologic doses:

1. It is a gastric irritant and may occasionally cause hemorrhagic gastritis and ulcer formation.

2. It is an antiplatelet agent and may lead to increased bruising and bleeding.

3. Bronchospasm has been associated with aspirin usage.

4. In a substantial portion of young children, a noncholestatic hepatitis will develop that is usually reversible with discontinuation of the drug.

The use of aspirin has been especially curtailed because of its association with Reye's syndrome, which is manifested by encephalopathy, hyperammonemia, and microvesicular fat deposition in hepatocytes. The association is best documented following influenza or varicella infections. Although aspirin is an invaluable drug for certain inflammatory conditions—such as rheumatoid arthritis or Kawasaki's disease—the side effects associated with its use make acetaminophen the preferred antipyretic. Other nonsteroidal antiinflammatory agents, such as ibuprofen and naproxen, are available for treatment of fever and inflammation. These drugs are, like aspirin, gastric irritants and antiplatelet agents and are more valuable in treating inflammatory problems rather than fever alone.

Other Therapies

The efficiency of external cooling during fever has long been a subject of debate. One recent study found no advantage to antipyretics plus external cooling versus antipyretics alone. It is essential in fever that the thermoregulatory center be reset to normal by antipyretic use. Otherwise, the body would continue to produce and attempt to conserve heat even though external cooling is applied. If external cooling is applied in addition to antipyretics, it should be in the form of water at body temperature. As the water evaporates from the skin, calories are expended as the heat of evaporation, and thus heat is removed from the body. It is not usually necessary, because of these considerations, to use cold water, which may lead to shivering and increased heat production. A thin film of tepid water should be applied to the entire body, allowed to evaporate, and then reapplied. Since isopropyl alcohol may be absorbed through the skin and since appreciable blood levels may result, its use in sponging should be discouraged.

Sponging with tepid water should be reserved for the few patients in whom a higher grade of fever (103° to 106° F [39.4° to 41.1° C]) does not respond to acetaminophen. External cooling may also be used in those hyperthermic patients whose elevated temperature is due not to a reset of the thermoregulatory center but to increased heat production, as in malignant hyperpyrexia, or to high ambient temperatures. If the temperature is quite high in the latter circumstances, a more vigorous attempt at external cooling is warranted. Sponging with very cold water can lower temperature more quickly and can even dissipate the heat produced by shivering. The benefit of cooling in this circumstance outweighs the associated discomfort of very cold water. A cooling mattress can be used in tandem with sponging if necessary.

COUGH

method of
ROBERT G. LOUDON, M.B., Ch.B.
University of Cincinnati College of Medicine
Cincinnati, Ohio

Cough is one of the most common symptoms leading a patient to seek medical advice. It is a protective mechanism, and this must be kept in mind when symptomatic care pending diagnosis is considered. A patient's lungs should not be deprived of needed protection just to make him feel more comfortable. On the other hand, a protective mechanism can sometimes be more trouble than it is worth, like the suit of armor on a knight who has just fallen from his horse. A dry, irritable cough can sometimes be safely suppressed with benefit to the patient.

There are at least three ways in which cough can exercise a protective function. When solids or liquids are presented inappropriately at the larynx, a cough may be used to prevent them from entering the respiratory tract. Such a cough can be recognized by its explosive, choking character, and by the fact that the sudden expulsion of air is not preceded by an inspiration, as occurs with most coughs. A second protective function of cough is clearance of airways. When the mucociliary escalator is overloaded, or fails for other reasons, secretions pile up, and cough is called into service as a back-up clearance mechanism, an emergency high-speed elevator service propelling material rapidly mouthwards. A third protective function is as an early warning symptom that draws attention to the presence of pulmonary disease and thus contributes to its earlier diagnosis and treatment.

The input signal evoking cough can come from any one or more of several sites, and can be induced by any one of a multitude of diseases. The laryngeal and carinal areas are most richly endowed with sensory nerve endings evoking cough, but the latter are found also at sites ranging from the ear to stretch receptors in lung and pleura. Cough is a reflex act, but a complex one, tailored to meet various requirements and react to them flexibly. Perhaps the need for flexibility led to the organization of the cough response at a high level in the central nervous system, and the ability to influence or even suppress cough voluntarily or mimic it consciously. In some situations it is not clear that cough helps the patient. For example, the dry cough of interstitial lung disease may be quite troublesome, but does not seem to serve a useful function.

These considerations should be borne in mind while deciding whether to suppress a cough. Treatment of a cough resulting from laryngeal stimulation by post-nasal drip, for example, might involve giving an antihistaminic and decongestant preparation. This might not only alleviate the cough, but also help make a diagnosis by providing a therapeutic trial. In such a case suppression of cough by medications providing mild local anesthesia to the pharynx and larynx could increase the risk of aspiration, and should be avoided. A cough needed to clear copious secretions from the airways may be troublesome, but is important for the patient's survival and is better not suppressed until the underlying cause is controlled. A dry, hacking cough caused by inflammation of the tracheal or bronchial mucosa but not associated with secretions may be suppressed with advantage, as may a cough related to fibrosing alveolitis; in these cases the cough may perform no useful function, and may be harmful.

The discussion here is of symptomatic relief before a definitive diagnosis is reached, and the examples mentioned above are based not on having a complete diagnosis available, but on having sufficient preliminary information to allow an assessment of the safety of a particular approach. This information can almost always be obtained from a careful history; most patients can distinguish cough caused by postnasal drip from cough caused by secretions from below the larynx. And most patients can tell whether or not sputum is being produced. If the history leaves the matter in doubt, listening to a patient's cough (either spontaneous or requested) may tell whether the cough is moving secretions.

Physical examination provides additional information that may not lead to a definitive diagnosis, but may eliminate some possibilities or make others seem more likely. It may also influence the symptomatic care recommended in the meantime. Is the patient old or young? Coughing or not? Breathless? Cyanotic? Are there signs of heart failure? Listening to the chest may provide useful information. Wheezes suggest airflow obstruction, and crackles may suggest interstitial lung disease, congestive heart failure, or, if associated with signs of consolidation, pneumonia. Secretion sounds may provide a warning against cough suppression by antitussive drugs. Indications of fluid deprivation or overload may guide the approach to expectorant therapy.

History and physical examination are the most important steps in the assessment of a patient with cough. Further investigations will frequently be indicated before a complete diagnosis can be reached; they may include chest roentgenograms, pulmonary function testing, sputum examination, bronchial provocation to assess hyperreactivity of airways, or bronchoscopy. Which of these tests are needed, and when, will depend on the differential diagnosis formulated as a result of the history and physical examination.

Treatment

While other tests are pending, decisions about symptomatic treatment will also depend on the history and physical examination. There are only two categories of symptomatic treatment available: expectorants and antitussives (Table 1). Bronchodilators, useful in the treatment of cough due to airway hyperreactivity, do not come under the ground rules for this section, as they imply at least a tentative diagnosis, and are not really symptomatic treatment as much as treatment of the underlying cause. Although they may be used quite early in the work-up, particularly if wheezing is heard on physical examination, their use is better delayed until pulmonary function tests have been completed.

Expectorants

Coughing often disturbs a patient more when it is felt to be ineffective or unproductive. Expectorant medications are meant to help a patient cough something up, and thereby relieve his discomfort. In acute respiratory infections it is not unusual for a painful and unproductive cough to be succeeded after a day or two by a less disturbing cough that provides the satisfaction of sputum production, with temporary relief of the

need for further coughing until more secretions appear. In chronic lung diseases such as chronic bronchitis, thick, sticky sputum may be difficult to cough up, and increased ease in expectoration is appreciated. Expectorant drugs are designed to meet these needs. Objective evidence for their efficacy is not easy to obtain, as sputum collection is tedious and usually incomplete, and relevant sputum characteristics to be measured are not agreed upon. Although for this reason the majority of expectorant drugs lack enthusiastic professional endorsement, several of them maintain a high level of popularity as over-the-counter remedies. This may reflect the extent of the need rather than the extent to which the need is effectively met, but until better criteria and test methods are developed that will be a matter of opinion.

The best expectorant in most instances is water. Drinking plenty of water will help hydrate respiratory secretions; local or general dehydration can result from mouth breathing, tachypnea, or fever associated with a respiratory infection, and its correction will make expectoration easier and more effective. The history and physical examination are likely to give some feel for the patient's state of hydration, even when they do not allow a definitive diagnosis of the cause of a cough.

Many drugs have been recommended as expectorants, many of them being nauseant or emetic in larger than the expectorant dose. They include a saturated solution of potassium iodide, ammonium chloride, syrup of ipecac, and terpin hydrate. They are presumed to act by causing hypersecretion in airways reflexly associated with gastric irritation. A widely used expectorant, included in a large number of over-the-counter cough preparations, is guaifenesin. The mode of action of guaifenesin is unclear; evidence for any effect is subjective, but perhaps stronger than for other available expectorants. Oral mucolytic agents such as ambroxol have been widely used in Europe as expectorants in patients with chronic obstructive lung disease, but are less appropriate as a short-term symptomatic treatment prior to diagnosis.

Antitussives

If it is certain that a cough is doing little but irritating the throat of the cougher and the ears of bystanders, it may be suppressed while possible causes are investigated. A range of drugs are available, acting centrally to suppress the cough reflex or locally to reduce or abolish the input stimulus. They vary in their potency and in their side effects. Most narcotic and many sedative drugs have a central antitussive effect. Codeine

TABLE 1. **Symptomatic Treatment of Cough**

	Adult Dose	Side Effects
Expectorants		
Guaifenesin	200 mg every 4 hrs	Rarely, nausea
Potassium iodide oral solution	0.5–2 ml 4 times daily in water or milk	Bad taste, acne, salivary gland swelling
Antitussives		
Dextromethorphan	15–30 mg 4 times daily	Rarely, nausea
Codeine	10–20 mg 4 times daily	Constipation, nausea, rare addiction potential

is the most commonly used of the narcotic antitussives, as its addictive potential is a good deal less than that of morphine but its antitussive effect is almost as great. It also has analgesic and sedative effects, which may be useful in some situations. It can cause nausea and constipation, but does not suppress respiratory drive to the same extent as morphine. Codeine is included in a large number of cough preparations. The other major central antitussive is dextromethorphan. While it is almost as effective in suppressing cough as codeine, it has the great advantage of being non-narcotic. In effective antitussive doses it has virtually no sedative or analgesic properties, and it does not appear to depress respiration or to dry the respiratory secretions as narcotics may do.

Many opiates and other central nervous system depressants have been shown to have antitussive properties, and several are available in cough preparations alone or in combination. Some, for example hydrocodone and morphine, have antitussive effects equal to or greater than those of codeine, but may have a greater tendency to be addictive or produce unwanted side effects. For this reason they are better reserved for patients with limited life expectancy, for example those with terminal malignant disease. For most symptomatic cough suppression dextromethorphan is the drug of choice, with codeine as the alternative if sedation and analgesia are also required. Diphenhydramine also has some cough-suppressive action, in addition to sedative and antihistamine properties, and may have some advantages when allergic rhinitis is the cause of postnasal drip which in turn causes cough.

Antitussive effect can be exerted locally rather than centrally. Steam inhalation, aerosol inhalation, or simply crouching over a hot cup of tea or chicken soup and inhaling the vapors may prove comforting, perhaps in part by moistening secretions. Various volatile or demulcent substances may help soothe an irritating cough, especially if it arises at the larynx; sucking a cough drop, rubbing the chest with camphorated oil, or inhaling vapors from a steam kettle with added compound tincture of benzoin may prove comforting. It is *not* a good idea to put oily vapor rubs on the back of the tongue or into the nose; the mild local anesthetic action at the larynx can cause inhalation of oil into the lung and subsequent lipoid pneumonia.

HOARSENESS AND LARYNGITIS

method of
KEITH F. CLARK, M.D.
University of Oklahoma Health Sciences Center
Oklahoma City, Oklahoma

Hoarseness is a nonspecific symptom that can result from a variety of disease processes ranging from a short-lived viral laryngitis to a progressive and potentially life-threatening disease such as squamous cell carcinoma of the larynx. Furthermore, hoarseness can be a manifestation of systemic disease (e.g., hypothyroidism or rheumatoid arthritis) that may affect the larynx. A thorough history and physical examination of the patient complaining of hoarseness is required in addition to a proper visual inspection of the larynx. Recall the old adage that "any patient with hoarseness of 2 weeks, or longer duration must undergo a visualization of the vocal cords."

HOARSENESS IN CHILDREN

The most important consideration in the evaluation of children with hoarseness is whether there is airway compromise. Parents may confuse hoarseness with stridor, which is a wheezing sound produced by the flow of air through a partially obstructed airway during inspiration, expiration, or both. Using topical nasal anesthesia and the fiberoptic scope, the larynx can be examined with very little trauma in children of all ages. Congenital cysts, laryngeal stenosis, recurrent respiratory papillomatosis, and laryngeal hemangiomas are examples of lesions that may present with hoarseness that progresses to airway obstruction. Children, in contrast to adults, can experience airway distress with unilateral vocal cord paralysis. A foreign body in the larynx or in the esophagus may produce hoarseness with concomitant airway obstruction. Many times the parents are not aware of a foreign body ingestion, but the physician must always think of this possibility in a child with airway compromise.

Screamer's Nodes

Probably the most common cause of hoarseness in children is vocal nodules or "screamer's nodes." These are caused by vocal abuse and do not produce airway compromise. Speech therapy with behavior modification may be the only treatment needed. Surgical removal is not recommended unless the nodules are extremely large or persist despite adequate behavior modification.

Recurrent Respiratory Papillomatosis

Recurrent respiratory papillomatosis (RRP) is a potentially life-threatening disease characterized by the relentless growth of wart-like masses on the vocal cords. Although RRP is rare, it is the most common tumor of the larynx in children. Hoarseness is usually the initial symptom. Within several weeks or months the airway may become obstructed as these warty masses grow to completely fill the larynx. About 15 per cent of children with RRP will continue to experience the disease well into adulthood. RRP can occur primarily in adults, but it usually has a less aggressive course.

Treatment

Treatment consists of laser removal of the papillomas. Since they have a marked propensity for recurrence, it is not unusual for a child to require monthly excisions of the papillomas in order to keep the airway open and to avoid tracheotomy. Spread to the trachea and lungs occurs more commonly in those patients in whom a tracheotomy is performed. Adjuvant therapy with interferon has been very successful in many patients but is still experimental. Vaccines, vitamins, antibiotics, and antimetabolites are not helpful. Radiation therapy is to be condemned, since radiation is thought to cause malignant degeneration of the papillomas.

HOARSENESS AND LARYNGITIS IN ADULTS

Acute Laryngitis

Acute laryngitis is an inflammation of the mucosa of the larynx that usually occurs in association with an upper respiratory infection and is characterized by laryngeal and throat pain, hoarseness, and occasionally aphonia. Examination of the larynx reveals erythema and edema of the vocal cords. The infectious agent may be bacterial or viral. Acute laryngitis is usually self-limited; however, to assure the patient that there is no serious problem, the physician must perform a fiberoptic or indirect laryngoscopy.

Treatment

Symptomatic treatment with humidity, fluids, rest, and vocal care is helpful. Antibiotics should be given only in severe cases associated with fever and cervical lymphadenopathy.

Chronic Laryngitis

A chronic inflammation of the vocal cords can be caused by several factors, including allergy, chronic rhinitis, chronic sinusitis, voice abuse, reflux of gastric contents, and tobacco and alcohol abuse. Patients with chronic laryngitis usually do not have throat pain but simply complain of a long-standing abnormal voice that fatigues easily. The patient's occupation and personality are important etiologic considerations. An energetic, aggressive salesman may be prone to voice abuse, while a janitor breathing cleaning fluid fumes could experience a chemical or allergic laryngitis. Mild cases of chronic laryngitis may be caused by postnasal drainage from allergies, chronic rhinitis, or sinusitis, and treatment of these upper airway conditions will improve the laryngitis. Patients with hoarseness due to gastroesophageal reflux may have posterior laryngeal inflammation visible on laryngoscopy. These patients may respond to antireflux management. However, in a significant number of patients with reflux there will be no cervical symptoms and barium swallow, esophagoscopy, and esophageal biopsy will be normal. Acid reflux may be documented in these patients by 24-hour esophageal pH monitoring.

The appearance of the vocal cords in chronic laryngitis varies from mild erythema and edema to thick, red, and boggy with patches of leukoplakia. Leukoplakia is a descriptive term for white patches on the mucosal surfaces of the larynx and is considered a precancerous lesion that requires biopsy. In the more severe forms of chronic laryngitis, polyps can be seen focally or spread over the entire surface of the vocal cords.

Treatment

The offending agent or habit must be eliminated to produce a long-term cure. Abstinence from smoking is a particularly important goal but a difficult one to achieve for most patients. Symptomatic treatment with humidity is helpful and is accomplished by increasing fluid intake and by the use of a bedside humidifier. Voice therapy may also play a useful role. Antibiotics and steroids may relieve inflammation, but often the benefits are only temporary.

Vocal cord stripping of hyperplastic mucosa and areas of leukoplakia is effective as a means of biopsy and may produce a more normal-appearing vocal cord with an improved voice.

Contact Ulcers and Vocal Process Granulomas

Another form of chronic laryngitis is caused by trauma produced either by an endotracheal tube lying between the posterior portion of the vocal cords, or by prolonged abuse of the vocal cords presumably related to repeated throat clearing. Damage and breakdown of the mucosa covering the vocal process of the arytenoid cartilage results in ulceration with ensuing infection of the perichondrium and sometimes of the cartilage itself. Occasionally a large granuloma will grow out of the initial ulcer. These entities can produce throat pain or discomfort and sometimes cause referred pain in the ears. The quality of the voice is not primarily affected, since the vocal process portion of the vocal cords is not involved in phonation. However, voice changes can be caused by thickened tissue around a contact ulcer or by the mass of a granuloma itself, both of which can prevent proper closure of the vocal cords.

Treatment

Large granulomas should be removed surgically. Both granulomas and contact ulcers can be treated with antibiotics and steroids along with speech therapy. The course of treatment requires months and sometimes over a year with very slow resolution. Serial laryngoscopy in the office will confirm the response to therapy. Biopsy should be considered to rule out a neoplasm, especially if there is a history of tobacco abuse.

Laryngeal Stenosis

Serious laryngeal and tracheal scarring can be caused by endotracheal tubes left in place for long periods. The cricoid cartilage lies below the vocal cords and is the only circumferential skeletal structure in the laryngeal and tracheal passage. Necrosis of the thin mucosal lining of the cricoid cartilage occurs rapidly when the endotracheal tube compresses this lining against the rigid cartilage. Subsequent scarring may result in mild stenosis or complete closure of the airway. Laryngeal stenosis can be prevented by the use of small endotracheal tubes and early conversion to a tracheostomy tube. The advent of large-volume, low-pressure cuffs has greatly reduced the incidence of tracheal stenosis. Since after only 48 hours of intubation significant inflammation and ulceration can be seen in the larynx, a tracheotomy should be considered early. In the adult patient, if intubation is anticipated to last longer than 1 week, tracheotomy is indicated. Neonates can tolerate long-term intubation (i.e., 4 to 6 weeks) with a lower incidence of cicatricial complications, probably because of the elasticity of the cricoid cartilage in this age group.

Treatment

Treatment of laryngeal stenosis is often difficult, requiring multiple surgical procedures. Mild cases may be treated with laser excision and laryngeal dilation. Severe laryngeal stenosis may require laryngotracheal reconstruction with tracheotomy, cartilage implants, and internal stenting. The best form of treatment for laryngeal stenosis is prevention.

Vocal Nodules or Singer's Nodes

Vocal nodules do not cause airway obstruction or interfere with cord closure enough to cause aspiration. They are a form of chronic laryngitis caused by voice abuse and are a dreaded occupational hazard for singers. Acute nodules form during screaming when hemorrhage occurs beneath the mucosa of the free edge of the vocal cord. If this hemorrhagic injury organizes and becomes fibrotic, a chronic submucosal nodule is the result. Nodules can be quite small and almost invisible or so large that the vocal cords cannot close. They occur at the junction of the anterior and middle third of the vocal cords and seem to grow much like a callous, especially with continued heavy vocal abuse.

Treatment

Speech therapy, including behavior modification techniques, is frequently successful in curing vocal cord nodules. Surgical removal is not indicated unless the nodules are large or persistent despite adequate behavior modification. If behavior modification is not successful and poor vocal habits are not corrected, the nodules are sure to recur after surgical excision.

Laryngeal Trauma

Improper or difficult intubation can occasionally cause an anterior dislocation of the arytenoid cartilage with resulting hoarseness but usually no airway distress. If the arytenoid cartilage is not returned to its proper position within several days, the dislocation may become a permanent complication with an immobile vocal cord.

Foreign bodies lodged between the vocal cords, such as a piece of glass or denture plate aspirated during an automobile accident, will produce hoarseness and airway distress.

Injury to the larynx during motor vehicle accidents is common and is usually caused by compression of the larynx between the steering wheel or dashboard and the spine. Fractures of the cartilages of the larynx can greatly disturb laryngeal function. Hoarseness from laryngeal trauma can be minor when there is only submucosal hematoma. More serious laryngeal fractures can be recognized because of subcutaneous emphysema in the neck, point tenderness of the larynx on palpation, ecchymosis over the larynx or within the larynx, palpable deformity or crepitance of the laryngeal cartilages, voice change, and airway compromise. Computed tomography is very helpful for the recognition of these fractures.

Treatment

Early treatment will prevent the subsequent stenosis and hoarseness that occurs when treatment is delayed. Open reduction and fixation of the fractures, repair of mucosal lacerations, and short-term internal stenting is required for a satisfactory outcome in severe cases.

Laryngeal Carcinoma

All smokers with hoarseness need a careful laryngeal examination in order to rule out carcinoma, since the vast majority of patients with laryngeal carcinoma have a history of tobacco abuse. Hoarseness caused by a carcinoma of the vocal cords is constant and slowly progressive. As the tumor enlarges, it may invade deeper structures to cause vocal cord paralysis or metastatic lesions in the neck. Throat pain is unusual in the early stages.

Treatment

When identified early and treated properly, laryngeal carcinoma can be cured with a success rate of over 90 per cent. Moderate-sized tumors may be treated successfully with conservation laryngeal surgery, laser surgery, or radiation therapy without total laryngectomy. Larger lesions, however, may require laryngectomy combined with radiation therapy for cure. Fortunately, many techniques are available for the rehabilitation of a patient's speech after total laryngectomy.

Vocal Cord Paralysis

Injury of the recurrent laryngeal nerve during surgery of the thyroid gland and the aortic arch is the most common cause of vocal cord paralysis. In those patients in whom no apparent cause is found, a viral neuritis is thought to be the etiology. Neoplasms of the mediastinum, lungs, thyroid gland, base of skull, and vagus nerve can produce vocal cord paralysis. The patient with unilateral vocal cord paralysis presents with a breathy voice and may experience aspiration. The diagnostic work-up should consist of a thorough examination of the head and neck, a chest x-ray to identify a neoplasm of the lungs or mediastinum that may be affecting the left recurrent nerve as it loops under the arch of the aorta, and a barium swallow. Suspicious cases of neoplasia need computed tomography of the base of skull, neck, and/or mediastinum.

Treatment

Idiopathic vocal cord paralysis will usually resolve within 6 to 12 months after onset. Those who do not resolve may learn to compensate with the mobile cord and achieve good vocal cord closure despite a complete lack of motion of the involved vocal cord. Gelfoam can be injected lateral to the paralyzed vocal cord to displace it medially. This technique will allow the patient a good voice during the recovery period and is temporary since the Gelfoam is absorbed in several months. Gelfoam is used when it is critical to maintain voice or laryngeal competence while waiting for vocal cord movement to recover.

Those patients who have a vocal cord paralysis that persists a year after onset, without sufficient compensation by the mobile cord, are candidates for Teflon injection. This is a method of permanent vocal cord medialization that is very successful, is painless, and can be performed in an outpatient setting. More than one injection may be necessary to achieve optimal results.

Bilateral Vocal Cord Paralysis

Bilateral vocal cord paralysis is unusual. It may be caused by thyroid surgery, amyotrophic lateral sclerosis, traumatic laryngotracheal separation, and Shy-Drager syndrome. Paralysis of both vocal cords produces airway obstruction. An immediate tracheotomy and eventually a vocal cord lateralization procedure may be needed to establish the airway.

Neurologic Diseases

Cerebrovascular accident (CVA), amyotrophic lateral sclerosis (ALS), multiple sclerosis (MS), and myasthenia gravis are some of the neurologic disorders that can cause hoarseness.

Cerebrovascular Accident

The patient with a lateral brainstem CVA and a paralyzed vocal cord can be devastated by the resulting effects on communication and deglutition. The patient may literally drown in his own secretions, and tube feedings are often required to prevent aspiration and pneumonia. A Gelfoam or Teflon injection may be all that is needed to alleviate the aspiration and restore the voice. The addition of cricopharyngeal myotomy should be considered if a cine-esophagram demonstrates delayed passage of barium through the cricopharyngeus muscle.

Amyotrophic Lateral Sclerosis

Patients with ALS present with progressive weakness of cranial nerves. They have a prominent bilateral fasciculation of the tongue which is almost pathognomonic. At first the voice becomes weak. With progression, ALS patients may become aphonic and unable to swallow owing to hypopharyngeal muscle and tongue weakness, nasal regurgitation, and aspiration. Teflon injection is not an option for ALS patients, since progressive airway obstruction is the rule because of their inability to abduct the vocal cords. Cricopharyngeal myotomy may be helpful in the early stages, since it may improve swallowing and decrease aspiration temporarily.

Myasthenia Gravis

Myasthenia gravis is a readily treatable cause of hoarseness. As the problem lies with neurochemical transmission, improvement after the patient receives 1 mg of edrophonium (Tensilon) may be diagnostic. Ptosis and dysphagia also suggest the diagnosis of myasthenia gravis.

Spastic Dysphonia

Spastic dysphonia is a neurologic disorder characterized by a very choked, strangled speech pattern, with only a few words escaping before the sentence is ended prematurely by involuntary spasm of the cords. At one time patients with spastic dysphonia were labeled as malingerers or neurotics. The disorder is now thought to be due to a focal demyelinating process of the recurrent laryngeal nerve.

Treatment

Unfortunately, there is no successful medical or behavioral therapy for this debilitating disease. Unilateral recurrent nerve section may improve the voice in spastic dysphonia for several years, but reports of recurrence are common between 3 and 5 years after nerve section. The effectiveness of nerve section can be tested preoperatively by inducing a temporary recurrent laryngeal nerve paralysis with local anesthetic injection.

Systemic Disease

Myxedematous changes occur in the laryngeal mucosa in patients with hypothyroidism. The vocal cords become edematous and thickened with a corresponding drop in pitch. Thyroid replacement therapy will result in a normal voice.

Rheumatoid arthritis may affect the cricoarytenoid joint, a true synovial joint. Pain is often quite severe. Hoarseness is caused by inflammation surrounding the joint and by limitation of cord motion. Corticosteroid treatment is helpful; the drug is given systemically or, in severe cases, may be injected into the joint.

INSOMNIA

method of
ROBERT L. WILLIAMS, M.D.,
MURAT O. ARCASOY, M.D., and
ISMET KARACAN, M.D., D.Sc. (Med.)
Baylor College of Medicine
Houston, Texas

Insomnia, meaning "no sleep" in Latin, is actually a misnomer since the term represents a wide spectrum of sleep-related complaints. It is a symptom complex encompassing a range of subjective complaints of poor sleep and is characterized by difficulty initiating and/or maintaining adequate sleep. The subjective expression of the sleep complaint may represent the sleep-onset form of insomnia in which prolonged sleep latency is the prominent feature. In contrast, sleep-maintenance insomnia is inability to remain asleep. In this latter condition, sleep is disrupted by frequent nocturnal awakenings, early morning arousals with difficulty in getting back to sleep, or both. The complaints of patients with insomnia may be related to either the quality or the amount of their sleep. Among accompanying symptoms, these patients frequently report increased emotional tension, anxiety, fatigue, difficulties in concentration, and impaired daytime functioning.

Insomnia is by far the most common of the sleep disorders. Almost everyone will experience difficulty sleeping at some time. Based on nationwide and regional surveys in the United States, approximately one third of the adult population reports some form of sleep difficulty during the course of a year. Females have higher rates of insomnia in all age ranges. Although difficulty initiating sleep does not appear to be age-related, difficulty maintaining sleep and early morning awakenings increase with age. Complaints of insomnia are more prevalent among individuals of lower socioeconomic status and among those with psychologic disturbances.

Causes of Insomnia

The single most important step in the differential diagnosis of insomnia is the careful consideration of all possible causes. Medical dysfunctions, underlying psychopathology, use of certain drugs and alcohol, poor sleep hygiene, environmental factors, and some sleep-related disorders may contribute to poor sleep.

Insomnia may be associated with the use of alcohol and many drugs including central nervous system stimulants (amphetamines, methylphenidate, and caffeine), antihypertensives (beta-adrenergic blockers, reserpine), nicotine, MAO inhibitors, antiasthmatics (beta-adrenergic agonists, theophylline), oral contraceptives, and steroids. Chronic use of sedative-hypnotic medications may also result in sleep-maintenance problems with frequent awakenings. In addition, the development of tolerance to or dependence on these drugs leads to withdrawal symptoms following their discontinuation. Alcohol, although a sedative, causes disruption of the sleep architecture. Despite a decrease in sleep latency, alcohol causes decreased REM sleep and increased nocturnal and early morning awakenings.

Insomnia may be an accompanying feature of certain medical disorders. Any condition causing nocturnal pain or discomfort, neurologic disorders (e.g., neoplasms, cerebrovascular disease), and metabolic and endocrine disturbances (e.g., renal failure, hyper- or hypothyroidism) may lie at the root of many insomnias.

Insomnia associated with psychopathology constitutes the major differential diagnostic group. Among the most common psychiatric disorders that disrupt sleep architecture are the affective disorders, functional psychoses, and anxiety disorders. Sleep difficulty is a frequent vegetative complaint of depression. Although some patients with depression complain of hypersomnia, the more commonly seen sleep complaints are fragmented sleep, persistent restlessness at night, and early morning arousal. In manic and hypomanic patients, sleep latency is typically prolonged and total sleep time is decreased. Acute psychotic episodes usually cause a severe sleep-onset pattern of insomnia as a result of anxiety, suspiciousness, and concern over delusional and hallucinatory material.

In many cases, psychologic elements responsible for sleep disturbance are evident but a clear DSM-III diagnosis of a psychiatric disorder is not warranted. This psychophysiologic insomnia may be transient and situational, lasting less than 3 to 4 weeks and provoked by sudden emotional arousal associated with a period of increased anxiety. Examples for such situations are bereavement or anticipation of an important life event. Patients with this type of sleep disorder may not seek medical advice. Psychophysiologic insomnia may also have a persistent course characterized by maladaptive behavioral habits in which chronic somatized tension and anxiety have precipitated a negative conditioning to sleep. Such patients often have obsessional, introverted, and perfectionistic personality traits, with tendency to increased nonspecific internal arousal and high muscular tension. An important feature of this type of insomnia is development of a vicious circle resulting from increased cognitive arousal at bedtime leading to delayed sleep onset. The more these patients try to sleep, the more anxious and aroused they become and the less likely they will be able to fall asleep. Consequently, frustration becomes more intense and the arousal level continues to increase.

Insomnia may sometimes be associated with sleep-related disturbances. Breathing abnormalities that occur during sleep, such as sleep-induced central cessation of breathing and alveolar hypoventilation, may cause insomnia. Nocturnal myoclonus, which may also be a cause, is characterized by stereotyped leg muscle twitches resulting from brief contractions during sleep. Sleep-related disorders disturb sleep by causing frequent arousals. The restless legs syndrome, however, occurs while the patient is awake and relaxing and involves an irresistible urge to move the legs caused by an uncomfortable creeping sensation in the calves.

Disruption of the sleep-wake cycle and biologic rhythm may also result in insomnia. Jet lag is the daytime fatigue and sleep difficulty at night that occurs with air travel, especially following eastward flights, with rapid time-zone changes. Shift work may also cause a similar sleep-wake disturbance. In the delayed sleep-phase syndrome, individuals are unable to fall asleep until 2 to 6 a.m., but otherwise have normal sleep. Symptoms occur when the patients become sleep-deprived, as they sleep very little in their effort to go to work at conventional working hours.

Evaluation

The sleep problems of patients with insomnia require proper assessment and differential diagnosis, because the occurrence of the sleep disturbance is frequently a manifestation of an underlying primary medical dysfunction, psychiatric disorder, or both. The physician's task is to determine the cause and select the appropriate mode of treatment. The single most important diagnostic tool is the initial interview. Several factors should be carefully considered, including the patient's expression of the complaint, age-related sleep pattern changes, adverse effects of the problem on daytime functioning, and current physical and mental health status. Although patients with insomnia generally tend to exaggerate their sleep difficulties, subjective perception of the sleep disturbance by the patient gives some idea of the severity of the problem. Patients with insomnia generally tend to overestimate their sleep latency, but underestimate their nighttime awakenings and total sleep time.

In the elderly the incidence of disturbed-sleep complaints rises with age. Decreased total sleep time, frequent awakenings, and less refreshing sleep may be the norm for the elderly whereas similar changes might constitute sleep-maintenance insomnia in a younger adult.

The interview should focus on the onset, duration, and intensity of symptoms. The history should reveal any recent anxiety-promoting changes in the patient's waking life temporally related to the onset of the sleep problem. During the interview, the patient should be questioned regarding deterioration from a previous level of functioning in occupational or social life to determine the possible impact on current daily life.

Short-term insomnia lasting up to 3 to 4 weeks is usually triggered by acute psychic stress or sudden unexpected situational or environmental changes. In contrast, chronic insomnia is frequently a result of underlying medical or psychiatric dysfunctions and is an indication for further evaluation.

Other important issues concerning the initial approach are review of the past medical and psychiatric history, questioning about use of prescribed or nonprescribed medications, and evaluation of the current medical and mental health status. A history from the sleep partner may provide additional information about sleep habits, behavior patterns, and medication use. It could also suggest a possible sleep-related disorder such as sleep apnea or restless legs syndrome. In these cases, and also in patients with a history of sleep disturbance of more than several months' duration, polysomnographic evaluation is indicated.

Treatment

Effective treatment of insomnia is not a simple issue. It includes recommendations about sleep and waking environment modifications, regulation of diet and physical exercise, psychotherapy, behavioral approaches, and, finally, drug therapy.

As a general rule, treatment should be directed at the specific causes of insomnia. Mismanagement of the problem can be minimized by accurate identification of the etiologic factor(s), an understanding of the mechanisms that sustain the complaint, and the use of a multimodal approach in treatment which consists of a combination of pharmacologic and nonpharmacologic methods, as well as recommendations to improve sleep hygiene.

The patient with insomnia should be provided with extensive information on the principles and behavior patterns of good sleep hygiene. Improvement of the sleep environment can be achieved by regulation of the temperature and humidity and by preventing sleep disruption by external stimuli, such as excessive noise or light. Sleeping only as long as needed to feel refreshed, avoidance of naps, restriction of time in bed, and establishment of a regular time of arousal will improve the quality of sleep, regulate sleep-onset time, and strengthen the sleep-wake cycle. Other general measures include avoidance of cigarette smoking and of excessive consumption of caffeine and alcohol. When sustained use of alcohol or drugs is the cause of insomnia, a gradual withdrawal program should be initiated.

Nondrug treatment strategies for insomnia include psychotherapy and behavioral approaches. Supportive psychotherapy consists of reassuring the patient in an effort to overcome the fear of sleeplessness and a strengthening of the mechanisms for coping with stress. In difficult cases in which further evaluation seems necessary and more intensive psychotherapeutic approaches are indicated, psychiatric referral is appropriate. In patients with significant muscular tension, relaxation techniques and biofeedback may be helpful. Behavioral approaches, focused on the symptom of insomnia, aim at modifying the patient's conception of sleep. To extinguish the negative conditioning to sleep, the patient should be "taught" to associate the bed and bedroom only with sleep by limiting use of the bedroom to sleeping and sexual activity.

Pharmacologic Treatment

Among the available treatment modes for insomnia, pharmacologic treatment is the most commonly employed. However, insomnia should not be regarded as an insignificant complaint that can be easily handled by prescribing "sleeping pills." A variety of medications may be used in the management of insomnia, depending on the cause of the sleep disturbance. Drug treatment directed at the primary disease is indicated when insomnia is a result of an underlying medical or psychiatric disorder. The secondary sleep complaints of patients with major depression or psychotic disorders will generally respond to use of antidepressant and neuroleptic medications, respectively. Similarly, treatment of a medical disorder causing pain or discomfort will often relieve the accompanying sleep disturbance.

Sedative-hypnotic drugs may be used in the induction and maintenance of sleep for symptomatic relief. However, these compounds are not indicated in every patient with a complaint of insomnia. Before prescribing these medications, the physician should consider the duration and severity of the complaint and the age and general health status of the patient. Sedative-hypnotics are generally indicated for short-term use in transient and situational insomnia, especially for the patient with a decline in the level of daytime functioning. The purpose of drug treatment in this situation is improvement of sleep, which will in turn prevent the adverse effects of disturbed sleep on daily waking life. A trial of sedative-hypnotic medication may also be useful in patients with psychophysiologic insomnia by terminating the vicious circle of sleep disturbance and thus proving to the patient that sleeping is possible.

The goal of sedative-hypnotic drug treatment is depression of the waking function, promotion of sleep, and improvement of sleep maintenance. Desired properties of these drugs include a predictable onset of action, maintenance of physiologic sleep, a relatively low risk of the development of tolerance and dependence, and minimal rebound insomnia and hangover effects. However, the ideal drug does not exist. Use of sedative-hypnotic drugs should be limited to a short period of time (3 to 4 weeks), since prolonged use may lead to the development of tolerance, characterized by a need for increasing doses. Therapy initiated with small doses and continued with the lowest effective dose is ideal. Intermittent therapy should be encouraged. Decreasing efficacy of the drug preferably should be managed by brief periods of abstinence from the drug, instead of successive increments in dosage. Care should be taken in prescribing these drugs to the elderly and individuals with liver and kidney disease.

Currently the benzodiazepines are the sedative-hypnotic drugs of choice. They have a high therapeutic index and less cardiac and respiratory depressant effects compared with other hypnotics such as the barbiturates. Physicians prescribing a particular benzodiazepine should be familiar with its major pharmacokinetic properties: (1) the rate of absorption, which determines the rapidity of the onset of action, and (2) the half-life and rate of elimination, which determines the duration of effects.

In selecting the appropriate drug for a patient, the following should be considered: First, the nature of the sleep disturbance must be accurately determined. For the patient with delayed sleep onset a drug with a rapid initiation of action such as triazolam (Halcion) may be preferred, since drugs with slower action, such as temazepam (Restoril), will not decrease sleep latency. Second, the potential adverse effects of specific benzodiazepines must be kept in mind. These unwanted effects include daytime sedation, impaired psychomotor performance, attention and memory deficits, and anxiety following discontinuation of drug therapy. The residual sedative effects occur more often with long-acting drugs such as flurazepam (Dalmane), because long-acting metabolites accumulate. This accumulative property allows the intermittent use of these drugs. When used in high doses, short- or intermediate-acting drugs may also cause hangover effects. The rebound side effects are, however, more likely to occur following discontinuation of high doses of short-acting drugs. Tapering of treatment will minimize the possibility of recrudescence of symptoms.

PRURITUS
(Itching)

method of
LOUIS J. RUSIN, M.D.
Minneapolis, Minnesota

Pruritus, which is synonymous with itching, is the most common symptom encountered by dermatologists. This complex psychoneurodermatologic phenomenon, which involves CNS processes as well as peripheral mediators, has no one identifiable underlying cause. Itching can be associated with numerous skin diseases or underlying systemic diseases, or can be caused by neuropsychiatric disease.

Many dermatologic conditions are associated with pruritus (Table 1). The most common of these conditions is asteatosis (dry skin), which is seen most commonly in the winter months.

The systemic causes of pruritus are numerous (Table 2) and should be kept in mind particularly when

TABLE 1. Skin Conditions Associated with Pruritus

Asteatotic skin: senile, nutritional, hormonal
Scabies, pediculosis, insect bites
Contact dermatitis, atopic dermatitis
Urticaria
Miliaria
Pruritus vulvae
Lichen planus, dermatitis herpetiformis
Drug eruptions, pyogenic and fungal disease
Stasis dermatitis
Pityriasis rosea
Mastocytosis, bullous pemphigoid
Sunburn
Presence of fiberglass or other irritant topical chemicals

dealing with patients who have severe intractable pruritus.

Diagnosis

A careful history of pruritus must be taken specifically emphasizing the severity, periodic or seasonal nature, and time of day of the itching and a thorough review of systems. The history may indicate the type of disease present and suggest other focused laboratory tests or further diagnostic evaluation (for example, x-ray, ECG). If the history is not helpful, basic screening tests including complete blood count, liver and renal function tests, fasting blood sugar, thyroid function tests, routine urinalysis with microscopic examination,

TABLE 2. Systemic Conditions Associated with Pruritus

Endocrine and metabolic
  Diabetes mellitus
  Diabetes insipidus
  Myxedema
  Hyperthyroidism
  Hypoparathyroidism
  Gout
Hepatic, intrahepatic, and extrahepatic biliary obstruction
Chronic renal insufficiency
Blood disease and reticulosis
  Iron deficiency anemia
  Polycythemia
  Hodgkin's disease
  Lymphatic leukemia
  Mycosis fungoides
  Lymphosarcoma
  Mast cell disease
Internal malignancy
Tropical and intestinal parasites
Autoimmune disease
Neurologic disease
Psychoneurosis
  Anxiety
  Aggression
  Obsessional neuroses
Pregnancy
Allergic
  Subclinical urticaria
Drugs
  Cocaine
  Morphine

and examination of stool specimens for ova and parasites should be done.

Treatment

The ideal therapy is to eliminate the underlying causative disease or factors. When this is not possible, treatment consists of avoiding aggravating environmental and topical factors, establishing a good topical therapeutic program, and using systemic antipruritics.

General Measures

All aggravating factors to be avoided (Table 3) should be specifically discussed with the patient. Since many forms of pruritus are caused by asteatosis (dry skin), lubrication of the skin with emollients is very beneficial. It is preferable to bathe with warm showers at night using mildly lubricated soaps such as Dove, Basis, or Neutrogena. After bathing, the patient should dry off and immediately apply a moisturizing lotion such as Moisturel, Lubriderm, or Curél lotion, humectants (LactiCare), or oils (sesame seed oil, mineral oil). Applying emollients in this way traps water within the stratum corneum and helps eliminate dryness and microscopic fissuring of the skin more effectively than dry application. Ointments such as Vaseline or Aquaphor may be needed in elderly patients residing in colder or drier climates.

Topical Treatment

Application of lotions or creams with menthol or phenol following bathing and drying have proved particularly effective and soothing. Patients with severe dermatitis will benefit from tar bath oils (T-Derm, Balnetar), which can be applied to the skin following bathing and left on 30 to 60 minutes before rinsing off. Tar products can stain, and patient compliance is not good

TABLE 3. **Factors That Aggravate Pruritus**

Overheating
  Avoid electric blankets and heated waterbeds
  Keep room temperature at 68° F or lower
  Avoid vasodilators (alcohol, hot drinks, and spicy foods)
Dryness
  Bathe no more than once daily
  Have a working humidifier in the house
  Avoid Ivory, deodorant soaps, and liquid soaps
  Avoid urea-containing topical products
Topical sensitizers
  Avoid topical anesthetics, topical antihistamines
Friction
  Avoid tight-fitting clothing mode of synthetic fibers or
    tight elastic waistbands

unless the patient does have rather severe dermatitis.

Topical corticosteroid products should be used only in patients with actual visible dermatitis. In cold, dry climates the corticosteroid should be applied as an ointment following wetting and drying of the skin. In warm, dry climates, steroids should be used in lotions or light creams. It is most effective to apply these in the evening, and use once a day minimizes occlusive folliculitis and makes patient compliance easier. One per cent hydrocortisone is very effective, as are the intermediate-strength fluorinated topical steroids. Potent fluorinated steroids should be avoided, because prolonged use can result in permanent atrophy of the skin, telangiectasias, and striae. Nothing stronger than 1 per cent hydrocortisone should ever be applied to the face or intertriginous areas.

Systemic Therapy

It is very important to break the itch/scratch cycle or the scratching will perpetuate and exacerbate the itching. Pruritus is almost always worst for patients at night. The greater the sedative side effect of the antipruritic, the better it controls nighttime itching. Antihistamines such as hydroxyzine (Atarax, Vistaril), diphenhydramine (Benadryl), and cyproheptadine (Periactin) have been shown to be helpful in relieving pruritus. For maximum benefit, 10 to 25 mg hydroxyzine, 2 to 4 mg cyproheptadine, or 25 to 50 mg diphenhydramine should be administered 1½ to 2 hours before bedtime and repeated at bedtime if the patient is still itching. Trimeprazine (Temaril) and doxepin (Sinequan) have been used with good success in patients with associated anxiety, depression, or intractable pruritus. Trimeprazine and doxepin may take 4 to 8 weeks to reach maximum effectiveness and can be administered in evening doses of 2.5 to 5 mg of trimeprazine or one 5-mg spansule or 25 to 50 mg of doxepin.

All drugs must be used with a thorough understanding of potential side effects. This is particularly true with trimeprazine and doxepin, for which there are many contraindications.

Systemic corticosteroids are not indicated for treatment of pruritus unless there is severe dermatitis or they represent the treatment of choice for the underlying condition causing pruritus.

Systemic antibiotics are sometimes necessary for treatment and prevention of secondary impetigo caused by scratching. Nonsedating antihistamines such as Seldane and Hismanal have been shown to be ineffective in treating pruritus.

TINNITUS

method of
SIMON C. PARISIER, M.D.
Manhattan Eye, Ear & Throat Hospital
New York, New York

Tinnitus, a ringing, whistling, or clicking in the ears, is usually benign and often age-related. However, it also may be symptomatic of an acoustic neuroma or of underlying pathologies, such as diabetes, hypertension, thyroid dysfunction, or Meniere's disease. Therefore, it is imperative that the etiology be established, so that an appropriate therapy may be instituted. Successful treatment of the underlying condition has been found to result in the resolution of tinnitus in about 50 per cent of patients.

Tinnitus is categorized as either subjective or objective. Subjective tinnitus, the most common form, is thought to result from damage to the hair cells of the inner ear, and the resulting noise is heard only by the patient. Acute tinnitus may result from sinus congestion, exposure to loud noises, or a sharp change in altitude. Under such circumstances, the tinnitus is usually temporary. The cause of chronic tinnitus is generally related to an underlying neurosensory hearing loss frequently associated with either the aging process or prolonged exposure to noise.

Objective tinnitus is much rarer, and is usually caused by vascular neoplasms such as glomus tumors or arteriovascular abnormalities. Commonly, it is experienced by the patient as a loud pulsation that is audible to spouses, as well as to the examining clinician. However, because objective tinnitus does not involve the inner-ear hair cells and central auditory center, its prognosis is far more promising.

Diagnosis

A complete aural and general medical history and a thorough physical examination are critical in evaluating the pathophysiology of tinnitus. One of the more significant findings is that of unilateral tinnitus, which is suggestive of Meniere's disease, particularly when accompanied by episodic vertigo and variant hearing loss. The unilateral form may also indicate the presence of a cerebellopontine angle tumor; when tinnitus is pulsatile, one should suspect a vascular lesion, such as a glomus tumor.

The medications taken by patients should be reviewed. Sufferers of arthritis frequently take large doses of aspirin, which can cause tinnitus that is reversible with dose reduction or drug substitution. The diuretics furosemide and ethacrynic acid also produce reversible inner-ear hearing loss and tinnitus. However, the tinnitus caused by ototoxic drugs such as quinine, the aminoglycosides, and cisplatin may persist.

Treatment

Treatment should be directed at correcting any underlying pathology. Some measures that may be taken include removal of occlusive wax; administration of antibiotics in instances of otitis media; and institution or reevaluation of medications in order to facilitate better control of conditions such as diabetes or hypertension. A low-salt diet and a thiazide diuretic are helpful in treating Meniere's disease. Niacin in doses of 50 to 150 mg appears to lower blood cholesterol and has been used beneficially by tinnitus sufferers.

For those with benign subjective tinnitus, who will not benefit from such measures, it is important to provide reassurance, emotional support, and practical suggestions for ameliorating this condition. Distractive techniques have proved useful, particularly at bedtime. These include turning on a radio, wearing a "Walkman"-type cassette player to bed, and using devices that reproduce the sound of waves or rain. Biofeedback and behavior modification may help in reducing the anxiety and stress that often accompany and may be aggravated by chronic tinnitus. Finally, since tinnitus appears to be more pronounced in patients with significant hearing loss, restoration of some degree of hearing through the use of a hearing aid will activate the residual normal hair cells, thereby diminishing the oppressiveness of the tinnitus.

Section 2

The Infectious Diseases

ACQUIRED IMMUNODEFICIENCY SYNDROME (AIDS)

method of
SHELDON BROWN, M.D., and
DONALD ARMSTRONG, M.D.
Memorial Sloan-Kettering Cancer Center
New York, New York

A decade has passed since the human immunodeficiency virus (HIV) first infected sufficient numbers of people in this country to support its epidemic transmission. Since the unexpected appearance of *Pneumocystis carinii* pneumonia and Kaposi's sarcoma in previously healthy homosexual and bisexual young men in 1981, more than 60,000 new cases of the acquired immunodeficiency syndrome (AIDS) have been reported to the Centers for Disease Control. More than 23,000 of these people have died. In the United States, AIDS has been diagnosed in all 50 states, and the estimated prevalence of HIV, the etiologic agent, ranges between 1 and 2 million persons infected. The majority of people exposed to HIV continue to have readily identifiable risk factors associated with either intimate sexual contact with persons in high-risk groups or parenteral exposure to the virus (Table 1). Nonetheless, the magnitude of the epidemic and the documented existence of bidirectional heterosexual transmission make increased dissemination outside of risk groups highly possible if not likely.

Pathophysiology

Human immunodeficiency virus (HIV), formerly HTLV III/LAV, was shown to be the etiologic agent of AIDS in 1984. It is an RNA retrovirus with tropism for human T lymphocytes, especially of the T helper/inducer (T4) subset, as well as for cells of monocyte/macrophage lineage. While current evidence suggests that infection of the latter cells may account for its prolonged and variable latency and for primary central nervous system disease, it is infection and subsequent depletion of T4 lymphocytes that leads to the profound immunologic defects that are the hallmark of AIDS. Opportunistic infections that take advantage of this spectrum of immune defects constitute the majority of AIDS defining illnesses as reflected in the current case definition guidelines from the Centers for Disease Control (CDC) (Table 2). The details of HIV infection

Supported in part by NIH/NIAID Contract NO1-AI-62533.

are complex, and much remains to be learned. The time from infection to seroconversion averages 6 to 10 weeks but may be as long as a year. Kaposi's sarcoma, which has been a frequent finding in homosexual and bisexual men, has been rare in those infected parenterally or by heterosexual contact. Central nervous system involvement and the AIDS encephalopathy syndrome of primary HIV infection may be the only significant manifestation of disease in some patients, while others with recurrent opportunistic infections may have little or no cognitive dysfunction. This diversity of presentation is likely to have growing clinical significance in the timing and selection of treatment strategies directed against HIV and its secondary consequences.

General Considerations

Within the United States, HIV infection remains largely confined to identifiable risk groups. Reflecting the early epidemic spread of the virus among homosexual men, progression to AIDS still affects this group more than any other. However, with self-education and the voluntary adoption of behavior designed to limit the spread of HIV infection, the rate of seroconversion among this population is reportedly decreasing. The risk of further infection from contaminated Factor VIII concentrates has been virtually eliminated by the use of new processing techniques. With routine screening, the risk of transfusion-associated HIV infection has been vastly reduced but not eliminated owing to the prolonged latency that may occur between infection and seroconversion. It is hoped that a contamination-free blood pool will be assured by development of a practical test for antigen screening. Unfortunately, HIV infection among intravenous drug users and their sexual partners continues to spread at an alarming speed, and their rate of seropositivity may already exceed that of any other group. It is from this group

TABLE 1. Risk Groups for Transmission of HIV

I. Adults and adolescents
    Homosexual and bisexual males
    Intravenous drug abuser
    Hemophilia or other coagulation disorder
    Blood or blood component transfusion recipient
    Heterosexual partners of persons at high risk of HIV
      infection
II. Children
    Hemophilia or coagulation disorder
    Parent with or at high risk of HIV infection
    Blood or blood component transfusion recipient

TABLE 2. **Summary of CDC Surveillance Criteria for Diagnosis of AIDS**

I. Without laboratory evidence of HIV infection and with definitive evidence of:*
   Candidiasis of esophagus, trachea, bronchi, or lungs
   Extrapulmonary cryptococcosis
   Cryptosporidial diarrhea lasting < 1 month
   Invasive cytomegalovirus excluding liver, spleen, and lymph nodes
   Herpes simplex esophagitis, bronchitis, pneumonitis; or mucocutaneous disease > 1 month
   Kaposi's sarcoma, < 60 years old
   Primary brain lymphoma, < 60 years old
   Lymphoid interstitial pneumonia, < 13 years old
   Disseminated *M. avium-intracellulare*
   Pneumocystis carinii pneumonia
   Progressive multifocal leukoencephalopathy
   Toxoplasmosis > 1 month
II. With laboratory evidence of HIV infection and:†
   1. Definitive evidence of:
      Multiple infections with encapsulated or pyogenic bacterial in a child < 13 years old
      Disseminated coccidioidomycosis HIV encephalopathy
      Disseminated histoplasmosis
      Persistent diarrhea due to *Isospora*
      Kaposi's sarcoma
      Lymphoma of the brain
      Other lymphomas of B-cell or unknown phenotype
      Extrapulmonary *M. tuberculosis*
      Recurrent *Salmonella* septicemia
      HIV wasting syndrome
   2. Presumptive diagnosis of:
      Esophageal candidiasis
      Symptomatic cytomegalovirus chorioretinitis
      LIP < 13 years old
      Disseminated mycobacterial disease (no culture)
      Pneumocystis carinii pneumonia
      Cerebral toxoplasmosis > 1 month

*No test for HIV antibody performed.
†HIV antibody positive by ELISA, confirmed by Western blot.

that the largest number of heterosexual and congenital infections arise.

TREATMENT

The clinical approach to HIV has 3 principal components: (1) prevention of infection; (2) management of asymptomatic HIV infection and HIV-related disease; and (3) management of AIDS-associated opportunistic infections and neoplasms.

Prevention

HIV infection occurs predominantly if not exclusively through intimate sexual contact or parenteral exposure or their equivalent. There is no evidence for its transmissibility through casual contact, through use of shared household facilities, or via aerosolization. Once a person contracts HIV a lifelong carrier state ensues, and the individual is thereafter a potential source of infection to others. These observations have lead to the current guidelines recommending (1) the practice of safe sex, (2) no sharing of needles or syringes, and (3) for all health care and laboratory workers or other potentially exposed persons to observe precautions similar to those for hepatitis B infection.

Asymptomatic HIV Infection

Once HIV infection occurs, the progressive destruction of lymphocytes appears to be inevitable over a variable time course. When HIV infection has been determined, screening evaluation should include measures of the immune system with serial assays of T lymphocyte subsets and anergy testing. Testing for baseline exposure to potential opportunistic pathogens should include a tuberculin test and serology for toxoplasmosis, cytomegalovirus, syphilis, and, if indicated by history, histoplasmosis. As the absolute T4 count approaches 200 cells per microliter, there should be a heightened attention to nonspecific complaints of fever, fatigue, weight loss, night sweats, or malaise as possible manifestations of opportunistic infection requiring aggressive evaluation. It is also recommended that antiretroviral chemotherapy be considered at this time.

In the past year, zidovudine (Retrovir), previously azidothymidine (AZT), was licensed for treatment of AIDS and advanced HIV infection. This agent is a thymidine analogue which inhibits the in vitro replication of HIV by blocking the viral enzyme reverse transcriptase. Preliminary clinical trials in patients with AIDS and prior *Pneumocystis carinii* infection showed a decreased rate of opportunistic infections and an increase in survival for those taking zidovudine versus placebo. Subsequent beneficial effects that have been observed with zidovudine include stabilization or improvement in cognitive status in some patients with AIDS encephalopathy, and rapid reversal of thrombocytopenia in many with immune thrombocytopenic purpura. Treatment with zidovudine is recommended for patients with a history of opportunistic infection or with advanced immunodeficiency indicated by an absolute T4 count less than 200 cells per microliter. It should be started at a dose of 200 mg orally every 4 hours. Some patients experience headaches, malaise, gastrointestinal intolerance, or insomnia, but these are usually minor and often resolve with continued use. Up to 40 per cent of patients develop significant myelosuppression with anemia or neutropenia and require multiple transfusions. Both will usually reverse with cessation of the drug. If side effects continue to limit treatment after repeat challenge, a downward adjustment to 100 mg every 4 hours, followed by every 6 hours, and finally every 8 hours is recommended. Zidovudine is metabolized in the liver, and interactions with other hepatically handled medications should be watched for. It is recommended that simultaneous use of acetaminophen (Tylenol) and ganciclovir be avoided. The benefits and risks of long-term therapy with zidovudine in patients with less advanced HIV infection are unknown and await the outcome of clinical trials currently in progress. Similarly, there are numerous other medications being evaluated for efficacy in HIV infection, but none can be recommended at this time.

Opportunistic Infections

Infectious complications are the most important cause of morbidity and mortality in AIDS patients. Once a patient has developed, or is at risk for development of, an opportunistic infection, there must be a low threshold of sensitivity to relatively nonspecific signs and symptoms that may herald the onset of new acute illness. Clues to early diagnosis need to be vigorously pursued, and empiric therapy, when possible, should be avoided because of the high incidence of multiple infections and diverse etiologies of common syndromes (Table 3). While most infections are responsive to appropriate therapy, there is a high propensity for relapse, so chronic suppressive therapy and prophylaxis are becoming increasingly frequent treatment options.

TABLE 3. **Causes of Regional Disease Commonly Seen in Patients with AIDS**

Persistent or recurrent fever	Pulmonary
HIV	*P. carinii*
MAI	CMV
CMV	Kaposi's sarcoma
P. carinii (pneumonia)	MAI
Histoplasma capsulatum	*M. tuberculosis*
Listeria monocytogenes	*Cryptococcus neoformans*
Salmonella spp.	*H. capsulatum*
	T. gondii
Gastrointestinal	*Streptococcus pneumoniae*
MAI	*Haemophilus influenzae*
CMV	*Staphylococcus aureus*
Cryptosporidium spp.	
Salmonella spp.	Central nervous system
Herpes simplex virus	HIV
Campylobacter fetus	CMV
Adenoviruses	*T. gondii*
	C. neoformans
	JC papovavirus
	Syphilis
	Lymphoma

Adapted with permission, from: Armstrong D, et al: Treatment of infections in patients with acquired immunodeficiency syndrome. Ann Intern Med 1985; *103*:738–743.

Viral Infections

Human Immunodeficiency Virus. The cause of AIDS, human immunodeficiency virus (HIV), is reported to be responsible for a variety of clinical syndromes on its own. Both before and after the diagnosis of AIDS, HIV has been variously associated with a mononucleosis-like syndrome, acute aseptic meningitis, immune thrombocytopenic purpura, progressive generalized lymphadenopathy, subacute encephalitis, spinal vacuolar myopathy, and peripheral neuropathies. Up to now, the foregoing have been largely diagnoses of exclusion with treatment directed toward symptomatic relief. There is growing evidence that some of these syndromes may respond to specific antiretroviral treatment. Reversals of longstanding thrombocytopenia and improvement in cognitive function have been documented following treatment with zidovudine. It will become important to characterize these entities more fully with specific diagnostic markers as retroviral therapy evolves.

Cytomegalovirus. Cytomegalovirus (CMV) infections are among the most common in patients with AIDS. Neither positive serology nor culture is sufficient evidence that CMV is causing disease. Clinical syndromes that may be accepted as presumptive evidence of invasive CMV infection include (1) a characteristic chorioretinitis with hemorrhages, exudates, and vascular sheathing, and (2) adrenalitis in the presence of CMV viremia or uremia and without other explanation. Organ system involvement such as pneumonia, colitis, esophagitis, and hepatitis must be accompanied by histopathologic evidence of characteristic cytopathic changes before a diagnosis of cytomegalovirus disease can be made. Investigational therapy with intravenous ganciclovir has been shown to be effective in suppressing colitis and chorioretinitis. Therapeutic regimens have generally included 1 to 2 weeks of induction with 2.5 mg per kg, three times daily, followed by a maintenance schedule of one to three times per week with 5.0 mg per kg. Treatment is not curative, and lifelong maintenance therapy is required to prevent recurrence. Side effects may include azotemia, hepatotoxicity, and treatment-limiting granulocytopenia.

Herpes Simplex. Infections with herpes simplex virus are common in HIV-infected patients and may be unusually severe. Large persistent perianal erosions are frequently encountered. They may lack typical vesicle formation, and their appearance can be confused with cutaneous fungal disease. Ulcerative and erosive disease of the esophagus caused by herpes simplex is an important part of the differential diagnosis of dysphagia in AIDS patients. Endoscopy is often necessary to differentiate these lesions from those of candidiasis and CMV infection. Diagnosis of perianal as well as more typical oral and genital lesions is readily made by overnight culture of swabs of the lesions. Treatment with 5 to 7 days of oral acyclovir (Zovirax), 200 mg five times per day, is usually effective in milder cases. More severe disease may require intravenous therapy. Recurrence is common and may require suppressive medication.

Varicella-Zoster. Reactivation varicella-zoster virus infection is common in HIV infected individuals and may herald the onset of clinically significant immunodeficiency insofar as it frequently precedes the onset of AIDS-defining opportunistic infections by weeks to a few months. Herpes zoster may be severe and long-lasting, and, although usually dermatomal, it has an increased propensity toward dissemination. Acyclovir is the treatment of choice, with oral preparations recommended for early dermatomal disease and intravenous administration for disseminated disease. Intravenous vidarabine is also effective but is associated with increased gastrointestinal intolerance.

Epstein-Barr Virus. High titers of antibody to Epstein-Barr virus (EBV) are found in the majority of AIDS patients but have not been clearly associated with disease. There is evidence that B-cell lymphomas seen in AIDS are caused by EBV, and an association with lymphoid interstitial pneumonitis (LIP) has also been suggested.

Papovavirus. The JC papovavirus is the most common cause of progressive multifocal leukoencephalopathy (PML), a previously rare demyelinating disease of the central nervous system that is often seen in AIDS patients. Clinical presentation is generally insidious and may variously include a decline in cognitive function, visual impairment, or focal cranial, motor, or sensory nerve defects. Computed tomography typically demonstrates multiple nonenhancing hypodense areas with irregular borders in white matter without mass effect. Characteristically there is slowing on the electroencephalogram, and examination of the cerebral spinal fluid reveals nonspecific changes. These findings may overlap with features of granulomatous disease, astrocytoma, primary central nervous system lymphoma, and HIV encephalopathy. Definitive diagnosis is made by demonstration of viral particles with electron microscopy in biopsy specimens. No effective treatment is yet available.

Papilloma Virus. Papilloma virus is associated with oral hairy leukoplakia. It does not disseminate, and no specific therapy is presently recommended. Regression has been reported during therapy with zidovudine.

Fungal Infections

Candida albicans. Candidiasis is the most common opportunistic infection in HIV-infected patients and is often the first sign of a significant defect in cell-mediated immunity. Oropharyngeal disease is seen most commonly, but mucocutaneous, vaginal, and esophageal involvement is also very common. Disseminated disease has usually been associated with intravenous catheters. Diagnosis is best made by wet mount with potassium hydroxide or Gram stain of accessible lesions. Esophagitis clinically presents as a gradually progressive burning dysphagia, which is commonly but not always associated with oropharyngeal disease. With severe involvement, barium swallow may demonstrate feathering of the esophageal mucosa. Endoscopy may be necessary for definitive diagnosis of less severe cases and for differentiation from other causes of dysphagia. When the clinical suspicion of esophageal candidiasis is strong, symptomatic improvement with therapy is presumptive support for the diagnosis. Topical treatment of cutaneous and vaginal disease is usually effective. Oropharyngeal disease often clears with oral preparations of nystatin (Mycostatin) or clotrimazole (Mycelex). Patients generally express preference for the troche and pastille forms of these medications, and their effectiveness is at least equal to that of the suspensions and suppositories. Esophagitis and mucocutaneous disease may also respond to nonsystemic therapy, but treatment with oral ketoconazole (Nizoral), 100 to 200 mg twice daily for 10 to 14 days, is often required. Ketoconazole is usually well tolerated, although some patients develop nausea, vomiting, and abdominal pain. Other side effects have included intense pruritus and fulminant hepatic necrosis. Cross-reactivity with other medications metabolized in the liver occurs. Also, ketoconazole requires a normally low gastric pH to be absorbed. Refractory disease may require treatment with low-dose (20 mg per day) amphotericin B. Following response to systemic therapy, suppressive use of topical preparations can be employed as needed. Recurrence is common, and more severe disease is seen with progression of the underlying immune defect.

Cryptococcus neoformans. Cryptococcosis is the second most common fungal infection and the fourth most common life-threatening opportunistic infection in patients with AIDS. Meningoencephalitis is the most frequent manifestation, with fungemia and disseminated disease present in 50 per cent or more of cases. Presenting symptoms may be subtle and often include unexplained fever, progressive headache, and altered mental status lasting days to weeks.

Diagnosis is most readily established on examination of cerebrospinal fluid (CSF); pleocytosis may or may not be evident, but budding yeasts are nearly always found on India ink preparation, and culture is virtually always positive. Cryptococcal antigen may also be positive both in CSF and in blood, often in high titer, but false-negative results can occur because of a prozone effect at low dilutions. In the presence of rheumatoid factor, serum false-positive tests can occur. The amount of cryptococcal antigen is not predictive of response to therapy, but serial titers are useful in evaluating response to treatment.

Pulmonary infection also occurs and may present variously as lobar pneumonia, interstitial pneumonia, or pleural effusion. The most common parenchymal pattern is interstitial, but lung disease may range from peripheral granulomas to granulomatous pneumonia to massive alveolar infiltration. Other manifestations of cryptococcosis include adenopathy, mediastinitis, chorioretinitis, sinusitis, CNS cryptococcoma, arthritis, prostatitis, pustules, and molluscum-like skin lesions. As such, cryptococcal disease is an important part of the differential diagnosis of nearly every clinical syndrome associated with AIDS. It is therefore recommended that a serum test for cryptococcal antigen be routinely incorporated into the evaluation of unexplained symptoms in patients who are infected with HIV, although the test result is often negative with localized disease.

The cornerstone of therapy for systemic cryptococcosis is immediate treatment with amphotericin B (Fungizone) once the diagnosis has been established. Following a 1-mg test dose, escalation to 0.5 to 1.0 mg per kg per day within the first 24 hours is recommended with or without flucytosine (Ancobon) orally at 75 to 100 mg per kg per day in divided doses every 6 hours. Treatment of acute reactions to amphotericin B infusion such as fevers and rigors can be managed as needed with acetaminophen, diphenhydramine, and either meperidine or morphine, thereby avoiding the use of immunosuppressive steroids. The value of combination therapy with flucytosine in this population has not been established. Both amphotericin and flucytosine are nephrotoxic, necessitating frequent evaluations of renal function. Flucytosine usage may also be limited by myelosuppression or gastrointestinal intolerance. To minimize side effects, dosing should be adjusted according to serum peak and trough levels. Therapeutic efficacy should be monitored with serial sampling of blood and CSF for culture and cryptococcal antigen.

While response to treatment is to be expected, cryptococcal infection is rarely if ever cured in AIDS patients and chronic maintenance therapy with amphotericin is necessary to prevent relapse. Amphotericin three times weekly is usually adequate followed by a gradual taper to 1 mg per kg per week as long as antigen levels remain stable and low. Despite treatment, outcome for cryptococcal meningitis remains variable with from less than 10 per cent to as many as one third of patients succumbing to their initial infection, a relapse rate of 50 to 90 per cent, and average survival of only 5 months. Investigational regimens with a new oral imidazole, fluconazol, 100 mg per day, may be a promising alternative to maintenance with amphotericin.

***Histoplasma capsulatum* and *Coccidioides immitis*.** Disseminated histoplasmosis and coccidioidomycosis occur with increased frequency in AIDS patients who live in or give a history of prior travel to an endemic area. Both are presumed to represent reactivation of latent infections and are often accompanied by pulmonary involvement. Presenting symptoms are often nonspecific, with varying complaints of fever, cough, malaise, and weight loss, and sometimes mimic acute bacterial sepsis. Serology, which is more often positive with *Coccidioides* than with *Histoplasma*, may help to suggest the diagnosis for either one. A test for *Histoplasma* antigen in urine and in serum is also available that, when positive, correlates highly with active disease. Radiology may reveal perihilar calcification with histoplasmosis, and splenic calcifications may be seen in coccidioidal disease. Both diseases should be considered in any patient with unexplained fever and a history of potential exposure. The diagnosis must be confirmed by positive culture or demonstration of the organism in fungal stains of blood, bone marrow, or bronchoalveolar lavage or in biopsy specimens of lung, skin, liver, or lymph nodes. Treatment should include initial therapy with amphotericin B, 0.5 to 1.0 mg per kg per day up to a total of 2 to 2.5 grams. Because of frequent relapses, this should be followed by chronic suppressive therapy with either amphotericin B or ketoconazole, 400 mg per day. Another new azole, itraconazole, has shown promise where ketoconazole has failed.

Bacterial Infections

***Mycobacterium avium-intracellulare*.** Opportunistic infective bacteria in AIDS patients are typically intracellular parasites that proliferate with progressive decline in cell-mediated immunity. The most common of these are mycobacteria. *Mycobacterium avium-intracellulare* (MAI) is a group of closely related organisms that are ubiquitous inhabitants of soil and water; while previously a rare pathogen, MAI could frequently be isolated from respiratory and gastrointestinal tracts, where they were commensals in man. With the advent of AIDS, it has become the most frequent newly diagnosed mycobacterial infection in the United States. It may be found antemortem in about 20 per cent of AIDS patients, and has been found in greater than 50 per cent at autopsy. The typical presentation of pulmonary infection mimicking tuberculosis is rarely seen in AIDS patients, for whom progressive, disseminated infection is the rule. Diffuse involvement of bone marrow and structures of the reticuloendothelial system in the spleen, liver, lymph nodes, lungs, and gastrointestinal tract with massive bacterial loads and poorly formed granulomas is often seen along with a continuous high-grade bacillemia. Presenting symptoms typically include unexplained fever, night sweats, and weight loss. Signs of end-organ disease may include diarrhea, anemia, an elevated alkaline phosphatase, hypoalbuminemia, and progressive debilitation. While rarely the only direct cause of death, disseminated MAI is associated with a relentlessly deteriorating clinical course and an extremely poor prognosis. The diagnosis of disseminated MAI infection is suggested by positive smear and is established by culture of the organism from blood or bone marrow or from biopsies of affected organs other than lymph nodes. The yield from blood culture may be improved by lysis-centrifugation techniques. The finding of acid-fast bacilli (AFB) in direct smears of stool with positive cultures often correlates with disseminated disease and should prompt further investigation. Conversely, the finding of MAI in sputum or bronchoalveolar lavage specimens does not necessarily correlate with systemic infection.

Standard antituberculous therapy is ineffective for treatment of MAI. Despite the existence of in vitro susceptibility to a number of drugs, clinical experience has been disappointing and no effective treatment regimen has yet been found. Symptomatic improvement may occur following multiple-drug therapy with agents such as ansamycin, clofazimine (Lamprene), ethionamide (Trecator-SC), and ethambutol (Myambutol), but drug toxicity may outweigh these benefits.

Mycobacterium tuberculosis. Tuberculosis is also seen with increased frequency in HIV-infected patients, especially those living in inner cities or from Third World countries, and correlates with a history of prior exposure. In those in whom tuberculosis occurs preceding other AIDS-defining illness, the tuberculin test is often positive. Extrapulmonary disease is common, while miliary disease is rare. Pulmonary disease often lacks typical cavitation and may involve the lower lobes or present as diffuse interstitial disease.

Histopathology may show poorly formed granulomas without caseation necrosis. Since tuberculosis has occurred simultaneously with MAI infections, it is recommended that treatment with three drugs, including isoniazid and rifampin, be continued until *M. tuberculosis* has been excluded by culture whenever the clinical suspicion is high or when clinically significant AFB have been found. When tuberculosis is diagnosed there is generally a good response to traditional therapy, although treatment may need to be prolonged or indefinite. This, however, has not been documented.

Other Bacterial Infections

Other bacterial infections toward which HIV-infected patients are predisposed owing to defects in cell-mediated immunity include nontyphoidal salmonellosis, listeriosis, legionellosis, and nocardial infections. Of these, recurrent *Salmonella* bacteremia, usually with *S. typhimurium,* is the most important and often requires chronic suppressive therapy. The remainder generally respond well to conventional treatment. Secondary and tertiary syphilis have been described with increased frequency, may be seronegative, and may relapse following conventional therapy.

Functional B-cell defects and humoral immunodeficiency seen in HIV-infected patients account for increased infections, with encapsulated organisms up to 20 times the normal rate. *Streptococcus pneumoniae* and *Haemophilus influenzae* pneumonia are common presentations. Pneumococcal pneumonia is typically lobar and responds to conventional treatment. *Haemophilus* pneumonia may have a range of radiologic appearance from lobar consolidation to a diffuse pattern indistinguishable from that of other interstitial pneumonias. It is therefore recommended that treatment for *Haemophilus* be added to pentamidine when sensitivity to trimethoprim-sulfamethoxazole precludes its use in the early empiric therapy of presumed *Pneumocystis* pneumonia.

Pyogenic infections with such organisms as *Staphylococcus aureus* and *Pseudomonas aeruginosa* occur with increased frequency in AIDS patients, especially but not exclusively in those with granulocytopenia. The most common presentations are bronchitis, sinusitis, and pneumonia. Such infections can be expected to respond to conventional treatment, but relapse is common. The significance of neutropenia (absolute neutrophil count less than 500 cells per microliter) does not appear to be as foreboding as in patients with hematologic neoplasms or in those receiving chemotherapy. Localizing symptoms tend to be more reliable, and there is not the same need to continue empiric therapy long past the resolution of an acute febrile illness.

Other bacterial infections seen with increased frequency in patients with AIDS have been caused by *Campylobacter jejuni, C. fetus,* and *Shigella flexneri.* Both may be responsible for chronic diarrhea and occasionally bacteremia, both of which will usually but not always respond to conventional treatment. Increased antibiotic resistance has been observed, as has the development of a chronic carrier state despite appropriate and prolonged antibacterial therapy.

Protozoal and Parasitic Infections

Pneumocystis carinii. The most common life-threatening infection in AIDS patients is *Pneumocystis carinii* pneumonia (PCP). It is the AIDS-defining opportunistic infection in more than 50 per cent of patients and subsequently develops in many more. Although fulminant pneumonia similar to that seen in patients with lymphoma or leukemia and in those on immunosuppressive therapy may be seen in AIDS patients, it is often indolent, with symptoms evolving over weeks and sometimes months. Nonspecific complaints of easy fatiguability, fever, dry cough, and exertional dyspnea are present in most patients. Rales, wheezes, and rhonchi may be present on examination but frequently are absent. Radiologic changes do not correlate well with the severity of symptoms, and may be subtle despite significant hypoxia. Abnormalities are usually but not always diffuse and range from a mild interstitial pattern to dense alveolar infiltrates with or without cystic changes to a pattern resembling acute respiratory distress syndrome. Resting arterial blood gases may be normal, but oxygen desaturation with an increased arteriolar-alveolar gradient after 3 minutes of exercise can be an early and sensitive test of significant disease. When the clinical suspicion is very high, the radiologic picture is suggestive, or there is evidence of oxygen desaturation with exercise, empiric treatment with trimethoprim-sulfamethoxazole or pentamidine and ampicillin is recommended pending a microscopic diagnosis. A gallium scan is nonspecific but may help to exclude disease when negative or support a presumptive diagnosis if pulmonary function tests are unavailable or if diagnostic specimens cannot be obtained.

The diagnosis is established by microscopic demonstration of characteristic cysts or trophozoites in appropriate specimens. Biopsy is most sensitive, with a bronchoscopic approach being adequate greater than 90 per cent of the time. Bronchoalveolar lavage is almost as sensitive. Examination of induced sputum can be rewarding but requires experienced technical interpretation. Results may be improved by the recent development of immunofluorescent staining techniques for specimen analysis. We favor the continued use of bronchoscopy with transbronchial biopsy to establish the diagnosis with certainty and to detect simultaneous infections, such as cytomegalovirus infection, that may be present and require additional therapy.

Treatment of PCP is effective in the majority of cases with either trimethoprim-sulfamethoxazole (SXT) or pentamidine isethionate (Lomidine), and improved response correlates with early diagnosis. Treatment is often complicated by side effects of these medications. Pruritic rash and/or leukopenia occur in up to one half of patients receiving SXT, most commonly 7 to 10 days after initiation of therapy. Symptoms may improve with dose reduction, and there is some evidence that simultaneous use of folinic acid may reduce the myelosuppressive effects. Pentamidine may cause progressive azotemia and sterile abscesses at the injection site. Hypotension and hypoglycemic episodes have occurred during its intravenous infusion. The latter has been associated with increased serum amylase and occasionally the development of diabetes. Gastrointestinal intolerance, which at times limits treatment, can occur with both drugs but may be managed successfully with antiemetics. Because the side effects of SXT may occur late in treatment and are generally reversible, it is recommended for initial treatment of PCP; when reactions occur, completion of therapy with a reduced dose may be attempted. Successful alternative treatment with trimetrexate and leucovorin has recently been demonstrated, and several other alternatives, such as dapsone and trimethoprim, show promise for mild cases.

Prophylaxis against PCP has become an increasingly important issue. Recent studies have confirmed that treatment in AIDS patients and in HIV-infected individuals with low CD4 counts (less than 200 cells per microliter) using double-strength SXT twice daily is effective prophylaxis against PCP and improves survival. Fifty per cent of these patients experience side effects, and 17 per cent are unable to tolerate this regimen. The benefit versus toxicity of prophylactic SXT in combination with antiretroviral therapy with zidovudine has not been evaluated. Several alternative approaches to prophylaxis, such as aerosol pentamidine, are under investigation as well. As prophylaxis against PCP becomes more widespread, the observation that atypical presentations of PCP can result may further complicate present diagnostic strategies.

Toxoplasma gondii. The most common opportunistic infection of the central nervous system in AIDS is toxoplasmosis. Infection in most cases is due to reactivation of latent infection, so patients with elevated IgG titers are at increased risk. Neurologic manifestations include encephalitis, meningoencephalitis, and mass lesions which may present as altered mental status, seizures, focal motor and sensory defects, and coma. Computed tomography of the brain commonly reveals multiple bilateral contrast-enhancing lesions with or without edema, although single and non-enhancing defects have also been observed. Serology for IgM in acutely ill and convalescent patients is unreliable for diagnosis because of defects in humoral immunity. Definitive diagnosis is established by examination of brain biopsy specimens for tachyzoites, although false-negative results are not uncommon. Empiric therapy may be necessary for lesions that are inaccessible or when otherwise clinically warranted. Improvement with empiric therapy for a presumptive diagnosis of cerebral toxoplasmosis should be expected after 7 to 14 days of treatment. If there is no improvement or the patient deteriorates, further attempts at obtaining a biopsy should be considered. Pneumonia, pericarditis, chorioretinitis, and disseminated infection caused by *Toxoplasma gondii* have also been seen.

Treatment for toxoplasmosis consists of pyrimethamine (Daraprim), 100 mg oral loading dose followed by 25 mg daily, and sulfadiazine, 4 grams oral loading dose followed by 1 gram every 6 hours. Recurrence is common with cessation and also reduction of therapy, so indefinite treatment is usually required. Because of frequent bone marrow toxicity, adjunctive therapy with folinic acid (leucovorin), 5 mg daily, is indicated. Other side effects include rash, fever, anorexia, and gastrointestinal intolerance. Most reactions appear due to the sulfadiazine, but Stevens-Johnson syndrome has been reported with both therapeutic components. There is no alternative to pyrimethamine, but intolerance to sulfadiazine has been managed with some success by substituting with clindamycin (Cleocin), 900 mg orally three times daily, and increasing pyrimethamine up to 75 mg daily. Desensitization to sulfadiazine may also be effective.

Cryptosporidium and Isospora. Chronic diarrheal illness leading to weight loss, malabsorption, dehydration, and severe electrolyte disturbances caused by the protozoa *Cryptosporidium* and *Isospora belli* have been reported in AIDS patients. The diagnosis depends upon exclusion of other causes of diarrhea such as *Shigella, Salmonella, Yersinia, Campylobacter, Giardia,* herpes simplex, cytomegalovirus, and MAI. It is established by microscopic findings of characteristic oocysts of the respective species on acid-fast stain of stool smears. *I. belli* infection, seen most commonly in patients of Haitian origin, responds to treatment with trimethoprim-sulfamethoxazole (Bactrim, Septra), one double-strength tablet, four times daily for 10 to 14 days. Recurrence is common, and chronic suppressive therapy may be required, Metronidazole (Flagyl) and pyrimethamine-sulfadiazine (Fansidar) are also effective. No effective treatment has been established for cryptosporidial infections thus far, although spiramycin given early in the disease has resulted in clinical responses and decreases in the parasite load in some cases.

Consistent with the underlying immune defect, several cases of disseminated infection with *Strongyloides stercoralis* have been reported in patients with AIDS. Severe visceral leishmaniasis has been reported in other countries as well. As the epidemic of HIV infection becomes more international in scope, the variety and severity of infections with previously rare pathogens can be expected to increase. Careful attention to the extent of damage to the immune system and to each patient's history of exposure to potential pathogens will provide important clues to early diagnosis and treatment.

AMEBIASIS

method of
RICHARD A. DAVIDSON, M.D., M.P.H.
University of Florida
Gainesville, Florida

Worldwide, it is estimated that 480 million persons are infected with *Entamoeba histolytica* each year. Although only a small percentage (probably less than 10 per cent) will have mild clinical illness and a much smaller percentage will have dysentery or extraintestinal infection, approximately 40,000 deaths annually can be attributed to the infection. In the developed world, however, serious infection seems to be decreasing. Most new cases of amebic infection are found in immigrants or travelers from endemic areas. A new problem is the dramatic increase in infected homosexual men. The infection is transmitted through contaminated food or water or through person-to-person contact. Although treatment decisions are clear-cut in patients with invasive or symptomatic amebiasis, opinions differ as to the benefits of treating asymptomatic carriers.

Infection is divided into two categories: intestinal and extraintestinal. The diagnosis of intestinal disease requires demonstration of either cysts or trophozoites in the stool, but accurate recognition is difficult, even in experienced laboratories. Extraintestinal disease is most frequently diagnosed by serologic tests, such as the amebic indirect hemagglutination titer, which is positive in over 90 per cent of extraintestinal infections.

INTESTINAL INFECTION

Amebic Dysentery

Amebic trophozoites burrow into the intestinal mucosa, where they secrete lytic enzymes that form the characteristic flask-shaped ulcers. These ulcers may become contiguous, especially when organisms reach the submucosa, resulting in undermining and necrosis of the mucosa. Sloughing of varying amounts of mucosa results in bloody diarrhea. Tenesmus, prostration, and dehydration are common. If appropriate therapy is not undertaken promptly, progression to fulminant disease with fever, megacolon, and possible colonic rupture may occur. The characteristic trophozoites should be rapidly sought in fresh diarrheal stools.

Treatment

The mainstay of treatment in invasive colonic amebiasis is metronidazole (Flagyl), given either orally or intravenously, in a dosage of 750 mg three times daily for 10 days. (Pediatric dosages for all drugs are given in Table 1.) Metronidazole is a tissue amebicide, with good absorption; it also has some intraluminal activity. Major side effects are few, but include nausea and metallic taste. Patients taking metronidazole may have a disulfiram (Antabuse)-like reaction if they ingest alcohol, causing abdominal pain, nausea, and vomiting. Concern about carcinogenicity and mutagenicity of the drug exists, and it should not be given chronically or to pregnant women.

Alternatives to metronidazole include emetine and dehydroemetine; both are potent drugs that can cause cardiac toxicity, including arrhythmias and possibly ischemia. Patients given either drug should be monitored electrocardiographically and kept at bed rest throughout therapy. Both drugs are contraindicated in pregnancy. Emetine is given intramuscularly or subcutaneously in a dosage of 1 mg per kg per day (maximum 60 mg per day) for up to 5 days. Dehydroemetine, which may be less toxic, is also given subcutaneously or intramuscularly for 5 days. Doses of 1 to 1.5 mg per kg per day are used, with a maximum dose of 90 mg per day. Dehydroemetine is available only through the Centers for Disease Control (telephone number 404–329–3670).

The tissue amebicides are effective against invasive trophozoites but may not eradicate all luminal organisms. Therefore, a luminal amebicide that is poorly absorbed is usually given after the dysentery resolves. The most effective drug is diiodohydroxyquin (Yodoxin), also known as iodoquinol. It is given for 20 days, in a dosage of 650 mg three times daily. This dosage should not be exceeded because the drug may cause optic neuritis. A less toxic alternative, diloxanide furoate (Furamide), given 500 mg three times daily for 10 days, would be preferable; however, the drug is available only from the Centers for Disease Control.

Additional supportive care, including antibiotics, fluid and electrolyte management, hyperalimentation, and surgery may be necessary in severe amebic colitis.

Mild Intestinal Infection

Patients may present with mild diarrheal symptoms or with symptoms and x-ray findings mimicking colonic carcinoma due to amebic granulomas (amebomas). Metronidazole is the drug of choice, in the same dosage as in serious infections. Use of a luminal amebicide such as iodoquinol should be considered. An alternative approach, which has been studied recently, is the use of the nonabsorbable aminoglycoside paromomycin (Humatin) in a dosage of 25 to 30 mg per kg per day in three divided doses for a total of 7 days. Most frequent side effects include minor gastrointestinal complaints and change in stool frequency or consistency. This drug should not be used alone in cases of ameboma, which require multiple drug therapy.

Asymptomatic Carriers

Not all strains of *E. histolytica* are pathogenic, and there are no morphologic differences between pathogenic and nonpathogenic strains. Analysis of isoenzyme patterns, known as zymodemes, has suggested that there are differences between pathogenic and nonpathogenic strains when categorized by zymodeme. The permanence of these

TABLE 1. **Pediatric Dosages of Amebicidal Drugs**

Drug	Dose
Tissue Amebicides	
Metronidazole (Flagyl)	30–50 mg/kg/day for 10 days*
Emetine	1 mg/kg/day (maximum 60 mg/day) IM for 5 days†
Dehydroemetine‡	1–1.5 mg/kg/day (maximum 90 mg/day) IM for 5 days†
Luminal Amebicides	
Iodoquinol (Yodoxin)	30–40 mg/kg/day for 20 days*
Diloxanide furoate (Furamide)‡	20 mg/kg/day for 10 days*
Paromomycin (Humatin)	25–30 mg/kg/day for 7 days*
Hepatic Amebicide	
Chloroquine (Aralen)	15 mg/kg/day (maximum 480 mg/day) for 14 days

*Give in three divided daily doses.
†Give in two divided daily doses.
‡Available only from the Centers for Disease Control: telephone 404-329-3670; nights and weekends, 404-329-2888.

classifications, however, is unknown. There are suggestions that isolates may change their zymodemes (and their pathogenicity) upon exposure to certain bacteria or viruses or upon transmission to a different host. This question is becoming increasingly important because of the dramatic increase in infected homosexuals.

Screening of male homosexuals has revealed that 15 to 40 per cent have asymptomatic infections with *E. histolytica;* a variety of other protozoans and helminths have also been found in increased frequency. The overwhelming majority of these individuals have few, if any, symptoms, and isolates from their stools have been found to be among the nonpathogenic zymodemes. Some authorities have recommended not treating these individuals because they frequently become reinfected, and most of the therapeutic alternatives should not be used chronically. Nonetheless, the possibility of zymodeme alteration represents a potential public health risk if such patients are not treated. An unproven theoretical reason for treating such patients is that chronic infection may decrease the latency period of the human immunodeficiency virus (HIV) by mitogenic stimulation of infected T lymphocytes. Last, as many as 50 per cent of persons in whom extraintestinal infection develops have no history of intestinal symptoms; this suggests that these individuals were asymptomatic carriers. Long-term prospective studies are needed to demonstrate the true benign nature of chronic asymptomatic infection. A reasonable course of action is to treat asymptomatic carriers with nonabsorbed drugs such as paromomycin or drugs with low toxicity such as diloxanide furoate. Limiting sexual contacts and treating regular sexual partners may be useful.

EXTRAINTESTINAL DISEASE

The overwhelming majority of extraintestinal infections involve the liver; erosion into portal venules in the gut wall results in the migration of the trophozoites to the liver. Three-fourths of hepatic abscesses are solitary, right lobe lesions, easily localized by computer tomography (CT). Half of all abscesses involve the diaphragm and may rupture into the lung by direct extension. Other sites of infection include the skin, genitalia, brain, adrenals, kidney, bladder, and pericardium. Serologic tests, such as the indirect hemagglutination titer and the gel diffusion precipitin, are usually positive in extraintestinal disease. In general, aspiration of hepatic abscesses is not necessary for the diagnosis. Symptoms of infection depend on the site involved. In hepatic abscess, right upper quadrant pain, fever, and leukocytosis may make differentiation from

bacterial abscess difficult; in this setting, serologic tests are most useful.

Treatment

Patients with extraintestinal infection should be treated with metronidazole, either orally or intravenously, in a dosage of 750 mg three times daily for 10 days. Alternative tissue amebicides include emetine and dehydroemetine. An additional drug that is effective against hepatic amebiasis is chloroquine, given as a 1-gram loading dose per day for 2 days, followed by 500 mg per day for 14 days. Chloroquine is used only in combination with other tissue amebicides and is effective only in hepatic disease. Eradication of intestinal infection is usually recommended with a course of a luminal drug after specific tissue treatment.

Surgical intervention in hepatic amebiasis should generally be avoided. In cases of rupture or threatened rupture, lack of therapeutic response in a reasonable period of time, or a very large, slowly responding abscess, surgery may be performed. Drug therapy should be given for at least 48 to 72 hours prior to surgery if at all possible.

BACTEREMIA

method of
RICHARD E. BRYANT, M.D., and
JONATHAN JUI, M.D.
Oregon Health Sciences University
Portland, Oregon

Clinically significant bacteremia is associated with a substantial morbidity and mortality that can be reduced by rapid diagnosis and appropriate therapy. The symptoms and signs of bacteremia are neither sensitive nor specific and may be especially subtle in the very young, the elderly, and in patients with serious underlying disease (Table 1). Patients with

TABLE 1. **Clinical Clues Suggestive of Bacteremia**

Chills
Fever (one in six may be euthermic or hypothermic)
Shock
Confusion, stupor, lethargy
Tachypnea
Skin lesions (see Table 2)
Neutrophilia, immature forms, neutropenia
Thrombocytopenia
Disseminated intravascular coagulopathy
Organ failure
    Adult respiratory distress syndrome, cyanosis
    Oliguria, anuria
    Jaundice, hemolysis
    Congestive heart failure

TABLE 2. Dermatologic Clues to Bacteremia

1. **Petechiae**
   N. meningitidis, N. gonorrhoeae
   H. influenzae, S. aureus
   Streptococci
   Pustules surrounded by erythema—*N. gonorrhoeae, S. aureus*
   Purpura fulminans—Group A streptococci, *N. meningitidis*
2. **Boils, pustules**
   S. aureus
   Pustular petechiae (purpura with central pustules)—*S. aureus*
3. **Paronychia, felons**
   S. aureus, Group A streptococci
4. **Bullous lesions**
   Necrotizing fasciitis—Group A streptococcus
   Staphylococcal scalded skin syndrome
   Vibrio vulnificus
   Clostridia in compromised host
   Pseudomonas aeruginosa (early lesion)
5. **Necrotic lesions** (ecthyma gangrenosa)
   Pseudomonas aeruginosa (common)
   Aeromonas hydrophilia (rare)
6. **Sunburn-like rash**
   Toxic shock with wound or deep-seated sepsis, scarlet fever
7. **Infected Burns**
   Streptococci, *S. aureus*
   P. aeruginosa, Enterobacteriaceae
8. **Gangrene**
   Clostridium perfringens, bacteroides
   Other clostridia, peptococci, *Klebsiella*
   E. coli
9. **Animal bites**
   S. aureus, Group A streptococci, *P. multocida*
10. **Rose spots**
    Typhoid fever
    Similar lesions with *P. aeruginosa* (very rare)
11. **Cellulitis**
    S. aureus, S. pyogenes, H. influenzae
    a. With lymphangitic streaking—*S. aureus, S. pyogenes*
    b. Erysipelas—Group A streptococci, *S. aureus*
    c. Children ≤ 3 yrs—*H. influenzae* (lesion may have purple hue)
12. **Embolic lesions**
    Endocarditis, vascular graft infection

TABLE 3. Risk Factors That Provide Clues to the Cause of Bacteremia

1. **Sickle cell disease**
   S. pneumoniae, H. influenzae, salmonella
2. **Splenectomized or dysplenic states**
   Fulminant *S. pneumoniae, N. meningitidis,* or *H. influenzae* infection
3. **Recurrent neisserial infection**
   Late-acting complement component deficiency
4. **Sexually active female**
   Pelvic inflammatory disease, gonorrhea, *Chlamydia,* polymicrobic anaerobic infection, cystitis, or pyelonephritis
5. **Pregnancy**
   Listeriosis, urinary tract infection
6. **Psoriasis** (chronic dermatitis)
   S. aureus, Group A streptococcus
7. **Inherited or acquired disorder of lower extremity lymphatics**
   (Milroy's disease or saphenous bypass donor site)
   Group A streptococcal infection
8. **Dental work**—endocarditis
9. **Wound infection**
   S. aureus, gram-negative bacilli
10. **Venous access site infection**
    S. aureus, S. epidermidis, gram-negative bacilli, *Candida,* includes drug addiction
11. **Neutropenic patients**
    Gram-negative bacilli, venous access infection, bacteria above plus *Corynebacterium,* yeast
12. **Contaminated intravenous solutions**
    Gram-negative bacilli, *Candida*
13. **Elderly and/or infirm patients with silent cholangitis, empyema of the gallbladder, appendicitis, or diverticulitis**
    Gram-negative bacilli, anaerobic bacteria
14. **Infected abdominal aortic aneurysms**
    S. typhi, other salmonella
15. **Ascites**
    Streptococcus pneumoniae, Escherichia coli, gram-negative bacilli
16. **Rheumatoid arthritis**
    Staphylococcus aureus
17. **Nosocomial infection**
    With endemic strains of *Klebsiella, Enterobacter, Serratia,* or *Acinetobacter*
    a. Pneumonia in intensive care unit; gram-negative bacilli
    b. Adult respiratory distress syndrome with remote sepsis
18. Signs of **endocarditis** in patients with native heart valves
    Viridans streptococci, enterococci, or *S. aureus*
19. **No site suggested by history or physical examination**
    S. aureus (e.g., from epidural abscess, infected retroperitoneal hematoma, psoas abscesses), especially in diabetics

severe underlying disease or renal failure may be euthermic or hypothermic during bacteremia. Signs of dehydration, cyanosis, or hypotension are easily recognized as indicative of serious infection in all age groups, but in the elderly an altered mental state or tachypnea may be the first sign of bacteremia.

The probable source of infection and type of organism causing bacteremia usually can be identified from a careful history and physical examination. The dermatologic findings suggesting the cause of bacteremia are listed on Table 2. These are especially important because they may provide a site from which a rapid diagnosis can be made by smear and culture. Most patients with bacteremia are predisposed to their infection by underlying disease, trauma, or manipulative procedures or by exposure to infectious disease vectors that place them at increased risk of specific infection. Risk factors associated with specific causes of bacteremia are shown on Tables 3 and 4.

Treatment

Therapeutic assessment of bacteremic patients is based on knowledge of the probable site of infection; the organisms likely to cause infection in the involved tissues; the presumed antimicrobial sensitivity of the infecting bacteria; and the necessary doses, route, and duration of antibiotic therapy. It is imperative to determine whether

TABLE 4. **Occupation, Avocation, or Life Setting—Clues to the Diagnosis of Bacteremia**

1. Contact with imported leather, hair, wool, or elephant ivory—anthrax
2. Farmers, ranchers, veterinarians, abattoir workers
   a. Contact with cows, pigs—brucellosis
   b. Birthing cows, pigs, sheep—Q fever, *Campylobacter fetus*
3. Infected animal, animal skins, tick bites—tularemia
4. Rodent or animal contact in infected area—plague
5. Unpasteurized milk or poorly pasteurized cheese—*S. aureus*, streptococci, *Listeria, Brucella,* salmonellosis (especially if imported)
6. Domestic turtles—salmonellosis
7. Animal feeds—salmonellosis
8. Food handlers—salmonellosis, streptococci
9. Travel to endemic areas—achlorhydria/postgastrectomy—salmonella infections, *S. typhi*

surgical intervention or abscess drainage is required. Empiric therapy is replaced by specific therapy as soon as possible. The severity of the patient's infection and the presence of neutropenia or serious underlying disease modify the empiric regimen used. Delayed treatment is associated with a high mortality in patients with neutropenia. Although prognosis is multifactorial, survival is linked most clearly with the use of antibiotics active against the bacteria causing infection. The regimens of choice against specific bacteria causing bacteremia are shown on Table 5. In critically ill patients or those with compromised host defenses, it is customary to begin therapy with a combination of antibiotics that has synergistic activity against the bacteria likely to be causing infection. This approach has popularized the use of broadly active beta-lactam antibiotics combined with aminoglycosides to treat patients thought to have bacteremia. Combination therapy is continued for bacteremic infection caused by *Pseudomonas aeruginosa* or for deep tissue infections caused by *Serratia marcescens, Acinetobacter calcoaceticus,* and *Enterobacter cloacae.*

Bacteremic gram-negative pneumonia is associated with a high mortality and should be treated with antipseudomonal beta-lactams (APBL) or expanded-spectrum cephalosporins (ESC) plus an aminoglycoside until the patient responds and the infecting organism is known. Thereafter, an effective beta-lactam is sufficient except for infection caused by the organisms cited above.

Patients with bacteremia of gastrointestinal or pelvic origin require therapy effective against both aerobic and anaerobic bacteria. Patients with focal suppurative infection require urgent surgical evaluation and drainage procedures. Similarly, patients with empyemas, pericarditis, or perinephric or epidural abscesses require sur-

TABLE 5. **Empiric Selection of Antibiotic Therapy for Pathogens Causing Bacteremia**

Suspected Bacteria	Drugs of Choice	Alternatives
Gram-positive cocci		
Staphylococcus aureus		
Pencillin-sensitive	Penicillin	Cefazolin, vancomycin
Methicillin-sensitive	Nafcillin	Cephalothin, vancomycin
Methicillin-resistant	Vancomycin	Ciprofloxacin*, imipenem†
S. epidermidis		
Native heart valves	Vancomycin plus gentamicin or rifampin	Nafcillin or penicillin (if sensitive)
Prosthetic heart valve	Vancomycin plus gentamicin and rifampin	Nafcillin or penicillin (if sensitive)
Streptococcus pneumoniae	Penicillin G	ESC, vancomycin
S. pyogenes	Penicillin G	ESC, vancomycin
Enterococcus	Ampicillin plus gentamicin	Vancomycin plus gentamicin
Group D non-enterococcus	Penicillin G	Cefazolin, vancomycin
Peptostreptococcus	Penicillin G	Clindamycin, BEAS
S. viridans	Penicillin G	Cefazolin, vancomycin
Gram-positive bacilli		
Clostridium perfringens	Penicillin G	Clindamycin, metronidazole
Clostridium non-*perfringens*	Penicillin G	Metronidazole
Corynebacterium (JK)	Vancomycin	—
Listeria monocytogenes	Ampicillin plus gentamicin	SMX/TMP
Gram-negative cocci		
Neisseria gonorrhoeae	Ceftriaxone	Penicillin G (if sensitive)
Neisseria meningitidis	Penicillin G	Ceftriaxone
Gram-negative bacilli		
Acinetobacter calcoaceticus	Imipenem	Ceftazidime, APA, APBL, Amp-sulbactam
Bacteroides		
sp. *fragilis*	Metronidazole	Clindamycin, BEAS
non-*fragilis*	Clindamycin	Metronidazole, BEAS
Enterobacter cloacae	Imipenem†	Aztreonam or ESC +/− APA
Escherichia coli	ESC	Ampicillin (if sensitive), APBL
Haemophilus influenzae	ESC	Ampicillin (if sensitive), aztreonam
Klebsiella pneumoniae	ESC	Aztreonam
Proteus mirabilis	Ampicillin (if sensitive)	ESC, APS
Proteus (other)	ESC	Aztreonam
Providencia sp.	Amikacin or aztreonam	Moxalactam, SMX/TMP, imipenem†, ESC
Pseudomonas aeruginosa	Mezlocillin, or ticarcillin, or ceftazidime plus tobramycin	Other APBL plus tobramycin ciprofloxacin
Pseudomonas cepacia	SMX/TMP	Piperacillin, cefoperazone*
Pseudomonas maltophilia	SMX/TMP	Moxalactam*, chloramphenicol
Salmonella typhi		
a. blood stream only	Chloramphenicol	Ampicillin, SMX/TMP, ESC
b. infected aneurysm, fistula, or endocarditis	Ampicillin	ESC, SMX/TMP
c. acquired in Asia	Ceftriaxone or ESC	SMA/TMP, ampicillin (if sensitive), ciprofloxacin
Serratia	Amikacin plus APB or ESC	SMX/TMP, ciprofloxacin, aztreonam
Vibrio vulnificus	APA plus tetracycline	Chloramphenicol

*Some strains susceptible.
†Imipenem-cilastatin.
Abbreviations: APA = Antipseudomonal aminoglycoside; BEAS = beta-lactams with expanded anaerobic spectrum; ESC = expanded spectrum cephalosporins; APBL = anti-pseudomonal beta-lactam; SMX/TMP = sulfamethoxazole-trimethoprim.

TABLE 6. **Classification and Dosage of Current Drugs Preferred for Therapy of Adults with Bacteremia and Normal Renal Function**

Antibiotic*	Dosage	Frequency
Antipseudomonal beta-lactams (APBL)		
Mezlocillin/ticarcillin	75 mg/kg IV	q6h
Piperacillin/azlocillin	75 mg/kg IV	q6h
Ceftazidime	1–2 gm IV	q6–8h
Aztreonam	1–gm IV	q8h
Imipenem-cilastatin	0.5–1.0 gm IV	q6h
Antistaphylococcal beta-lactams (ASB)		
Nafcillin	1.5–2.0 gm IV	q4–6h
Cephalothin/cephapirin	1.5–2.0 gm IV	q4–6h
Cefazolin	1.5–2.0 gm IV	q6–8h
Ticarcillin-clavulanate	3.1 gm IV	q6h
Imipenem-cilastatin	0.5–1.0 gm IV	q6h
Ampicillin-sulbactam	2.0–3.0 gm IV	q6h
Penicillin G (if sensitive)	3 million units IV	q4h
Beta-lactams with expanded anaerobic spectrum (BEAS)		
Imipenem-cilastatin	0.5–1 gm IV	q6h
Ticarcillin-clavulanate	3.1 gm IV	q6h
Ampicillin-sulbactam	2.0–3.0 gm IV	q6h
Cefoxitin	2–3 gm IV	q6h
Cefotetan	2.0 gm IV	q12h
Expanded spectrum cephalosporins (ESC)		
Cefotaxime/ceftizoxime	2–3 gm IV	q8h
Ceftriaxone	1–2 gm IV	q24h
Ceftazidime	2 gm IV	q6–8h
Antipseudomonal aminoglycosides (APA)		
Gentamicin (1.7-2.0 mg/kg IV load [lean wt])	1.5–2.5 mg/kg IV	q12h
Tobramycin (1.7-2.0 mg/kg IV load [lean wt])	1.5–2.5 mg/kg IV	q12h
Amikacin (7.5 mg/kg IV load [lean wt])	7.5 mg/kg IV	q12h
Others		
Ampicillin	23–35 mg/kg IV	q4–6h
Chloramphenicol	0.5–1.0 gm IV	q6h
Ciprofloxacin	750 mg p.o.†	q12h
Clindamycin	800 mg IV	q8h
Metronidazole (1.5 mg/kg load)	0.5 gm IV	q8h
Sulfamethoxazole-trimethoprim (SMX/TMP)	3–5 mg/kg TMP IV	q8h
Vancomycin (15 mg/kg load)	15 mg/kg IV	q12h
Tetracycline	7.5 mg/kg p.o.	q6h
Rifampin	0.3–0.6 gm p.o.	q12h

*Antibiotics that are biologically equivalent are shown with a slash (/) between them (e.g., cephalothin/cephapirin) and can be used interchangeably and bid competitively for the hospital formulary. Generic prescriptions save the patient's money.

†Ciprofloxacin is relatively contraindicated in children or pregnant women. Parenteral ciprofloxacin is not yet approved by FDA. Dosage must be reduced in patients with renal function.

1. Chloramphenicol and metronidazole dosage does not have to be reduced in patients with decreased renal function. Nafcillin, chloramphenicol, clindamycin, rifampin, and metronidazole are retained in the presence of impaired hepatic function. Correction of drug dosage for renal failure should be guided by serum level determinations.

2. Nafcillin, mezlocillin, ticarcillin, ticarcillin clavulanate, piperacillin, azlocillin, and imipenem are penicillin congeners and carry an increased risk of allergic reactions in patients with penicillin allergies. Cephalosporins rarely cause allergic reactions in penicillin-allergic patients but should not be given to patients with a history of anaphylactic or necrotizing vasculitis reactions to penicillin. Aztreonam can be safely be given to patients with a history of penicillin or cephalosporin allergies unless they have had allergic reactions to cefoperazone.

3. Aminoglycoside dosages are calculated on the basis of lean body mass. For critically ill patients, peak serum levels of aminoglycoside should be determined 15 minutes after completion of infusion. Desired peak serum levels for gentamicin and tobramycin are 4 to 6 micrograms per ml for non-*Pseudomonas* infections and 6 to 8 micrograms per ml for *Pseudomonas* bacteremia. Peak amikacin levels should equal 15 to 30 micrograms per ml for non-*Pseudomonas* and 20 to 35 micrograms per ml for *Pseudomonas* bacteremia. Higher levels may be needed for *Pseudomonas* endocarditis. Dosages may need to be reduced to every 24 hours in patients with high serum levels and significant renal failure. All aminoglycosides including streptomycin should be used with caution in the elderly and in patients with prior auditory or renal impairment.

4. Patients in shock should receive antibiotics intravenously. Normotensive patients who are responding to therapy can receive chloramphenicol, metronidazole, or SMX/TMP orally as soon as bowel function is adequate. Patients receiving ticarcillin-clavulanate for non-*Pseudomonas* infections can be treated orally with amoxicillin clavulanate when oral therapy becomes possible.

5. Vancomycin dosage must be increased in obese patients. Serum levels must be monitored meticulously and dosage reduced in patients with renal failure. Desired peak serum vancomycin levels are 30 to 45 micrograms per ml 15 minutes after completion of infusion. Desired trough levels are 5 to 10 micrograms per ml 15 minutes prior to the next infusion. Oral vancomycin is not absorbed and cannot be used to treat systemic infection. Parenteral vancomycin does not enter the gut and cannot be used to treat gastrointestinal infection. Vancomycin infusions of 1.0 gram or more should be given over a 1-hour period so as not to put the patient at risk of the vancomycin-induced histamine release phenomenon termed the "red neck syndrome."

6. Clindamycin and gentamicin can be given in the same infusion bottle as a cost-saving measure. Aztreonam is compatible with most antibiotics.

7. Even the most potent antibiotics are inactive against certain classes of bacteria: aminoglycosides are inactive against anaerobes, metronidazole is inactive against aerobic bacilli and in an aerobic environment. Aztreonam is inactive against anaerobic and gram-positive bacteria.

8. Tetracycline dosage should not exceed 4.0 grams. Not recommended for pregnant women near term or for children < 8 yr of age. Rifampin dosage is usually limited to 300 mg twice daily for 35–50 kg patients, 300 mg three times daily for > 50 kg patients.

gery. Those with suppurative thrombophlebitis usually require antibiotic therapy and surgical resection of the involved vein. Valve ring abscesses are usually treated by surgery and placement of a prosthetic heart valve. *Salmonella* infections of aneurysms cannot be cured without excision, extra-anatomic shunting procedures, and vigorous antibiotic therapy. Those with vascular shunt infections may require resection of the involved areas, but most *S. epidermidis* infections of Hickman, Broviac, or similar catheters can be cured by intravenous vancomycin therapy. Patients with fulminant congestive heart failure and valvular insufficiency due to endocarditis require antibiotic therapy and urgent insertion of a heart valve prosthesis. Combination therapy is used to treat enterococcal group G streptococcal or tolerant viridans streptococcal endocarditis infection or shorten the course of therapy for endocarditis caused by viridans streptococci that are not tolerant to penicillin (Table 6). Combination therapy is not used to treat patients with staphylococcal endocarditis unless it is given in anticipation of urgent prosthetic valve placement or unless multiple pathogens are suspected.

Immunocompromised febrile neutropenic patients are initially treated with a combination of mezlocillin, ticarcillin, or ceftazidime plus an aminoglycoside. Those with sepsis of gastrointestinal or pelvic origin may be treated with ticarcillin-clavulanate and an aminoglycoside. Neutropenic patients with catheter-related sepsis due to *S. epidermidis* or *Corynebacterium* "JK bacillus" should receive vancomycin. Neutropenic patients who fail to respond to antibiotic therapy may require addition of amphotericin B to treat deep-seated fungal infection. Patients with profound neutropenia and apparent sepsis may need continuation of antibiotic therapy until neutrophil counts exceed 1000. Leukocyte transfusions may be indicated in the specific setting of persistent bacteremia despite appropriate antibiotic therapy.

The duration of therapy depends on the type and chronicity of the tissue infection. Those with staphylococcal or enterococcal endocarditis usually require 4 to 6 weeks of therapy. Patients with enterococcal endocarditis of more than 6 weeks' duration or with endocarditis caused by relatively resistant strains of streptococci should receive 6 weeks of therapy.

Most bacteremic infections that do not involve heart valves can be treated successfully with 10 to 14 days of therapy. Prolonged therapy may be necessary for those associated with abscesses or poorly drained suppurative disease. This occurs most often with staphylococcal, *Pseudomonas,* or polymicrobic anaerobic infections.

There is no convincing evidence that one effective antibiotic is better than another that has approximately equal activity against the organism causing disease. However, the expanded-spectrum cephalosporins imipenem-cilastatin, ticarcillin-clavulanate, and aztreonam may have a significant advantage over older beta-lactams because the new agents have greater resistance to bacterial beta-lactamase. Until clinical trials have defined optimal antibiotic therapy of bacteremia, antibiotic regimens should be selected on the basis of anticipated antimicrobial sensitivity plus adequacy of drug delivery to and stability in infected tissues. After the patient's course has stabilized and the identity and drug susceptibilities of the bacteria causing bacteremia are known, antibiotic therapy can be modified on the basis of both clinical efficacy and cost.

BRUCELLOSIS

method of
EDWARD J. YOUNG, M.D.
*Veterans Administration Medical Center and
Baylor College of Medicine*
Houston, Texas

Brucellosis is a disease of wild and domestic animals that is transmittable to humans (zoonosis). Man is always an accidental host, playing no role in maintaining the disease in nature. A relationship exists between the prevalence of brucellosis in animals and the incidence of human infection. Brucellosis exists worldwide but is especially prevalent in the Third World, where resources to control or eliminate the disease in animals are often inadequate.

Brucellosis is contracted by direct contact with diseased animals or from the ingestion of unpasteurized dairy products prepared from the milk of infected animals. The infection is transmitted through minor cuts and abrasions in the skin exposed to blood or other secretions. Other routes include infectious aerosols into the conjunctival sac or the upper respiratory tree and via the gastrointestinal mucosa. Individuals at greatest risk of infection are those whose occupations place them in close contact with animals (e.g., farmers, ranchers, veterinarians, abattoir workers, meat inspectors). Brucellosis associated with food is often not occupation-related and can involve persons who have no direct contact with animals.

The genus *Brucella* consists of six species, four of which (*B. abortus, B. melitensis, B. suis,* and *B. canis*) are pathogenic for man. Infection with *B. ovis* and *B. neotomae* appear to be limited to animals. The clinical manifestations of human brucellosis are protean, characterized by a multitude of nonspecific complaints (e.g., lethargy, malaise, anorexia, body aches, depressions) and a paucity of physical abnormalities (notably fever, sweats, and mild lymphadenopathy). The diagnosis is assured by isolation of the organism from blood, bone marrow, or other tissue. In the absence of bacteriologic confirmation, the diagnosis is suggested by a high (≥ 1:160) or rising titer of antibodies in the serum. The possibility of brucellosis is suggested by eliciting a history of animal exposure, travel to a brucellosis endemic area, or ingestion of raw milk or milk products.

A variety of arbitrary classifications of human brucellosis have been proposed (e.g., acute, bacteremic, serologic, subacute, recurrent, chronic). However, these often simply reflect the difficulties inherent in making the diagnosis or isolating the causative agent. Since more than half of the cases of acute brucellosis have an insidious onset, with symptoms extending over weeks to months, the term chronic brucellosis is best reserved for cases in which symptoms persist for more than a year.

Brucella are facultative intracellular pathogens that rapidly localize in tissues rich in elements of the reticuloendothelial system (lymph nodes, spleen, liver, bone marrow). Hence, involvement of these organs is common, especially in the vertebral column.

Treatment

Chemotherapy is useful for the relieving symptoms, shortening the course of illness, and decreasing the incidence of complications, some of which (meningitis, endocarditis) are life-threatening. This is especially important when infection is caused by *B. melitensis,* which tends to have particularly severe effects.

A variety of antimicrobial agents have in vitro activity against *Brucella,* including beta-lactam antibiotics, tetracyclines, aminoglycosides, chloramphenicol, trimethoprim/sulfamethoxazole, rifampin, and quinolones. Despite in vitro activity, the results of treatment with penicillins and first- or second-generation cephalosporins are disappointing. Some third-generation cephalosporins have been used (generally in combination with other drugs) to treat *Brucella* meningitis, in which their excellent penetration of the blood-brain barrier may preclude the requirement for intrathecal aminoglycoside.

The tetracyclines are the most effective antibiotics against *Brucella* and most strains are inhibited by less than 0.1 microgram per ml. Since tetracyclines are bacteriostatic, most authorities recommend combination therapy using tetracycline plus an aminoglycoside. Tetracycline HCl is used in a dose of 250 mg four times daily by mouth given for 4 to 6 weeks. Streptomycin (1 gram daily intramuscularly) is generally prescribed in addition to tetracycline for the first 1 to 2 weeks. I prefer doxycycline (100 mg twice daily by mouth) over tetracycline HCl because its greater lipid solubility permits better penetration into cells and its slower excretion rate allows

for less frequent dosing. Because of staining of teeth, tetracyclines should not be given to children younger than 8 years or to women after the sixth month of pregnancy.

Among the newer agents, trimethoprim/sulfamethoxazole (TMP/SMZ) (Bactrim, Septra) has proved to be an effective alternative, especially for treating childhood brucellosis. In the standard formulation (80 mg TMP/400 mg SMZ) the usual treatment for adults is 4 tablets daily by mouth administered for at least 6 weeks. Patients given TMP/SMZ should be monitored regularly for untoward effects with blood counts and liver cell function tests. Some authors have reported high relapse rates with TMP/SMZ compared with doxycycline and streptomycin, but this finding is not universal.

Rifampin is another drug that has been used in treating brucellosis. The minimal inhibitory concentration (MIC) against *Brucella* strains ranges from 0.15 to 2.5 micrograms per ml, and the drug is bactericidal at concentrations approximately four times the MIC. Unfortunately, the relapse rate is unacceptably high when rifampin is used alone; therefore, it is generally prescribed at a dose of 600 to 900 mg daily by mouth in combination with one or more other drugs, such as doxycycline or TMP/SMZ.

No clinical studies have yet appeared using quinolone compounds in brucellosis; however, the MIC of ciprofloxacin (Cipro) against *Brucella* ranges from 0.5 to 2.5 micrograms per ml, suggesting that it might be an effective alternative.

Treatment of Complications (Localized Infection)

Osteoarticular Complications. Complications affecting bones and joints occur in 25 to 50 per cent of patients with brucellosis, but rarely does this present special problems in treatment. The majority of patients respond to routine anti-*Brucella* therapy. Surgical intervention is rarely required except to drain septic joint effusions or large, symptomatic paraspinal abscesses. The indications for surgery of paraspinal abscess include neurologic dysfunction, continued pain and fever after adequate antibiotic therapy, or spinal instability due to vertebral body collapse.

Neurobrucellosis. Direct invasion of the central nervous system is fortunately rare, but when it occurs it poses special problems because of the need for bactericidal concentrations of drugs. Satisfactory results have been reported in *Brucella* meningitis using tetracycline and streptomycin. Equally good results have been reported with doxycycline and rifampin, but treatment is generally prolonged for periods of 2 to 7 months. In view of the generally poor penetration of aminoglycosides across the blood-brain barrier, many experts favor the use of rifampin and TMP/SMZ, both of which achieve good levels in the CSF. Because of the favorable MIC of doxycycline, which penetrates the CSF better than tetracycline HCl, this agent should be used in any treatment regimen for neurobrucellosis.

Endocarditis. Another complication requiring bactericidal concentrations of antibiotic is endocarditis. Various combinations of drugs have been used to treat *Brucella* infection of both native and prosthetic valves, including doxycycline or TMP/SMZ plus streptomycin or gentamicin. The addition of rifampin to these regimens may enhance the bactericidal effect, but this should be confined by *in vitro* tests. Even with prolonged antimicrobial therapy, valve replacement is often necessary to achieve a bacteriologic cure. Valve replacement is invariably necessary in the cure of *Brucella* prosthetic valve endocarditis, and antibiotics should be continued for weeks after the insertion of the prosthesis.

Relapse

The recurrence of symptoms is considered a relapse when cultures for *Brucella* again become positive, or when IgG antibodies rise or fail to decline as expected. The causes are not clear, but relapse does not appear to be due to the emergence of antibiotic-resistant strains. The role of patient compliance with prolonged antibiotic administration must always be considered in patients with relapse. Regardless, patients should be evaluated completely for the presence of localized complications (e.g., abscess) that may require surgical intervention. In most instances, a repeat course of antimicrobial therapy is sufficient.

Prophylaxis

A variety of live-attenuated *Brucella* vaccines are used to protect cattle, goats, and sheep, but immunization of humans is rarely practiced. Accidental self-inoculation with *B. abortus* strain-19 vaccine can result in brucellosis in persons with no prior exposure to *Brucella* or in "allergic" injection site reactions in those with pre-existing antibodies or hypersensitivity. Strain-19 brucellosis is treated the same as infection with field strains, while injection site reactions are generally self-limited and are treated with local wound care.

Adverse Reactions to Therapy

In rare instances the initiation of antimicrobial therapy of brucellosis is associated with a Herxheimer-like reaction characterized by elevated temperature and worsening of symptoms. This reaction is transient (usually less than 24 hours) and is rarely severe enough to warrant the use of corticosteroids. Herxheimer-like reactions are not a contraindication to continued therapy, but must be differentiated from adverse drug reactions. Steroids have also been used in patients with *Brucella* meningitis to control cerebral edema, but should not be administered without a definitive diagnosis and concomitant antibiotics.

Immunotherapy

Treatment with poorly defined *Brucella* antigens was once practiced, but there are no data to show that this was effective. Similarly, anecdotal reports of treating the symptoms of chronic brucellosis with the immunostimulant drug levamisole have not been confirmed by objective data of efficacy.

CHICKENPOX
(Varicella)

method of
ANN M. ARVIN, M.D.
Stanford University
Stanford, California

Varicella is a generalized vesicular exanthem caused by varicella-zoster virus, a DNA virus that belongs to the herpes virus group. The scattered cutaneous lesions of the primary infection with the virus result from a viremia that is associated with peripheral blood mononuclear cells. After primary infection, the virus produces latent infection of neuronal cells in the dorsal root ganglia that may reactivate to cause herpes zoster (shingles).

Epidemiology

Varicella is transmitted to a susceptible individual by contact with another person who has varicella or herpes zoster. Airborne transmission occurs via respiratory droplets from patients with varicella but not from those with herpes zoster; transmission from individuals with herpes zoster requires direct contact with the lesions. The incubation period of varicella is 10 to 21 days, and transmission can occur from patients 24 to 48 hours before the appearance of the exanthem. Varicella should be considered contagious until no new lesions have appeared for 24 to 48 hours and crusting of old lesions is noted. Children with varicella need not be isolated from other healthy children. However, exposure of adults and pregnant women who are susceptible and of immunocompromised patients should be avoided. More than 90 per cent of adults who are natives of the United States have had varicella, but only about 50 per cent have a clinical history of past infection; the percentage of immune adults is significantly lower among individuals from tropical areas.

Diagnosis and Management in the Normal Host

The diagnosis of varicella is usually made based upon the characteristic vesicular exanthem and does not require laboratory documentation. The management of varicella in healthy individuals is supportive. Discomfort caused by the rash can be decreased by application of calamine lotions, by cool compresses, and by bathing. Daily bathing is indicated to minimize risk of secondary bacterial infection of the lesions; use of medicated soaps is not necessary. The initial lesions appear on the face, scalp, and trunk and are followed by crops of new lesions for up to 7 days; in most cases, new lesions appear for 3 to 5 days. Mucous membrane lesions are common. Later lesions usually appear on the extremities and may be maculopapular rather than vesicular in appearance. Oral antihistamines may be helpful during the first few days if pruritus is severe and interferes with sleep, but care should be taken that their administration does not mask neurologic symptoms. Fever and malaise can be treated with acetaminophen; salicylates are contraindicated because of the association with Reye's syndrome. Discomfort of urethritis and vaginitis can be eased by bathing. Activity should be allowed as tolerated. Scabbed lesions may take several weeks to resolve. Areas of increased or decreased skin pigmentation may be prominent but will gradually resolve. A few of the larger lesions may produce scarring, but these scars become less obvious with time.

Complications of Varicella in the Normal Host

The most common problem in normal individuals with varicella is secondary bacterial infection of the skin lesions; however, significant pyoderma or cellulitis occurs in less than 5 per cent of patients. The usual organisms causing secondary infections are *Staphylococcus aureus* and Group A beta-hemolytic streptococci. Manifestations include rapidly progressive enlargement of skin lesions, impetigo, and cellulitis surrounding involved lesions; rarely, staphylococcal scalded skin syndrome or scarlet fever may develop. Bacteremia is rare, even in patients with infected skin lesions. After the lesions have been cultured, erythromycin or a semisynthetic penicillin (cloxacillin, dicloxacillin) should be given. If the organism is a streptococcus or penicillin-sensitive *S. aureus*, penicillin may be used.

Vesicular lesions of the conjunctivae can occur. These lesions usually resolve without residua, but if ocular infection is extensive ophthalmologic evaluation for keratitis and possible topical antiviral therapy is indicated.

The most common neurologic complications of varicella are cerebellar ataxia and encephalitis. Cerebellar ataxia is a self-limited syndrome that may occur in the acute phase of the illness or within 2 or 3 weeks after the exanthem appears. It resolves without treatment in 1 to 3 weeks and leaves no sequelae. Encephalitis in the normal host usually begins with symptoms of personality change: confusion, drowsiness, irritability, or seizures 5 to 7 days after the appearance of the rash. Symptoms may progress rapidly to obtundation and coma. Encephalitis is estimated to occur in 1 per 1000 cases of varicella. Lumbar puncture is indicated to rule out bacterial infection; the cerebrospinal fluid (CSF) usually shows a moderate increase in white blood cells, predominantly lymphocytes, with a normal glucose level and normal or moderately elevated protein. Lumbar puncture should be done only after careful assessment for signs of increased intracranial pressure. Management of these patients requires intensive supportive care with attention to maintaining the airway, fluid restriction, and monitoring vital signs. Seizures are treated with anticonvulsants. Patients who have increased intracranial pressure should be treated with dexamethasone, 1.5 mg per kg initially, with a maintenance dose of 1.5 mg per kg per day divided every 4 to 6 hours. Mannitol, 20 per cent solution, can be given at a dose of 0.25 gram per kg by intravenous push and increased to 1.0 gram per kg per dose if necessary. Mannitol should not be given if the serum osmolality is above 320 milliosmoles per liter. Steroid therapy for increased intracranial pressure should be tapered as soon as the problem has resolved. Symptoms of varicella encephalitis reverse rapidly after 24 to 48 hours, and sequelae are unusual. The fatalities that occur, estimated at 10 per cent, are attributed to increased intracranial pressure. The pathogenesis in healthy children is considered to be demyelination rather than viral infection of brain tissue. Antiviral therapy is not indicated unless encephalitis appears to be associated with visceral dissemination of the virus, as may occur in immunocompromised children.

Other neurologic manifestations that have been associated with varicella include Guillain-Barré syndrome, cranial nerve palsies, optic neuritis with transient blindness, and transverse myelitis. Reye's syndrome may follow varicella infection. Children with persistent vomiting should be evaluated for this complication, since repeated vomiting is unusual with varicella.

Varicella pneumonia is estimated to occur in about 15 per cent of healthy adults who acquire varicella. Its severity may range from asymptomatic pulmonary infiltrates on chest x-ray to life-threatening pneumonia. Respiratory symptoms develop within 2 to 5 days after the onset of the rash and are usually accompanied by continued formation of new skin lesions. Tachypnea is the initial sign; other findings on physical examination may be minimal. Chest x-ray shows diffuse infiltrates with multiple modular densities, often in the hilar and perihilar regions. This pattern is quite distinct from pneumonia caused by secondary bacterial infection, which produces a unilateral lobar infiltrate with effusion in most cases. Arterial Po_2 should be measured in patients with extensive pneumonia demonstrated by chest x-ray, even if respiratory symptoms appear mild. In severe cases, there is rapid progression with increased dyspnea, cyanosis, pleuritic pain, and tachycardia. Assisted high-pressure ventilation with 100 per cent oxygen may be required. Steroids are of no known benefit in this complication of varicella. Antiviral therapy is indicated because varicella pneumonia is caused by replication of the virus in lung tissue. Intravenous acyclovir (10 mg per kg per dose, given every 8 hours) should be given. Clinical recovery generally parallels the cessation of formation of new skin lesions. Antibiotics are not indicated unless there is evidence of secondary bacterial infection.

Although the virus appears to infect the liver (normal children with varicella have moderately abnormal liver function tests), severe hepatitis with varicella is rare.

Thrombocytopenia may occur during acute varicella as part of a generalized intravascular coagulopathy associated with purpura fulminans and hemorrhage into the skin lesions. Patients with these symptoms should be treated with broad-spectrum antibiotics until bacterial sepsis can be ruled out. Intensive supportive care is required, including platelet and blood transfusions. Some patients who develop transient thrombocytopenic purpura may actually have a postinfectious complication of varicella. These patients may require platelet support and steroid therapy. Henoch-Schönlein (anaphylactoid) purpura can occur after varicella; patients with this sequela should be observed for abnormalities of renal function and gastrointestinal symptoms.

Varicella can cause arthritis during or immediately after the acute infection. Patients with bone or joint symptoms should be evaluated carefully, since osteomyelitis caused by *Staphylococcus aureus* may follow varicella. Varicella arthritis is self-limited and does not require surgical management other than aspiration if necessary.

Other rare but important complications of varicella include glomerulonephritis, which may be caused by the virus or by intercurrent Group A streptococcal infection, and myocarditis.

Diagnosis and Management in Special Risk Populations

Pregnant Women and Infants. Varicella during pregnancy is unusual because most women of childbearing age are immune. Varicella is more likely to cause pneumonia in pregnant women, but whether the risk is age-related or associated with pregnancy is uncertain. Varicella-zoster virus can cause embryopathy, but the risk is estimated to be less than 5 per cent even after maternal varicella during the first trimester. Clinical findings reported with intrauterine varicella include microcephaly, cerebral atrophy, mental retardation, seizures, chorioretinitis, limb atrophy, and cicatricial skin scars. Spontaneous abortion may also occur. If an exposed pregnant woman is proved to be susceptible by a sensitive serologic assay for antibodies to varicella-zoster virus, such as enzyme immunoassay or the fluorescent antibody membrane antigen method, varicella-zoster immune globulin (VZIG) prophylaxis should be given to modify the severity of varicella. However, there is no evidence that its administration will prevent infection of the fetus or decrease the risk of sequelae. VZIG is available through the American Red Cross Blood Services.

If the mother develops varicella within 4 days before to 2 days after delivery, the infant is at risk for severe disseminated varicella, which may be fatal. These infants should be given varicella-zoster immune globulin (VZIG) as soon as possible after delivery. Infants who receive VZIG may develop varicella and should be treated with acyclovir if progression occurs. If varicella occurs in an infant born under these circumstances who was not given VZIG, antiviral therapy should be given. Varicella in infants born to mothers who develop the rash more than 4 days before delivery will be modified by transplacentally acquired antibody. Some of these infants have skin lesions at birth, but their prognosis for uncomplicated infection is good. In general, infants who are exposed to siblings or other contacts with varicella are usually protected from severe disease by transplacentally acquired maternal antibody. Although there is no definite evidence that varicella is more severe during the first few months of life, if an infant under 2 months of age whose mother is not immune to varicella has a close exposure it seems prudent to give prophylaxis.

Immunocompromised Children. Risk of visceral dissemination of varicella is increased in patients with congenital immunodeficiency, such as Wiskott-Aldrich syndrome and thymic dysplasia, or immunodeficiency due to treatment with immunosuppressive agents. Children with human immunodeficiency virus infection are also at risk, since severe varicella is associated with impaired cellular immunity. Corticosteroids, cytotoxic chemotherapy, antithymocyte globulin, and radiation diminish the immune response to varicella. Children who are receiving prednisone therapy for asthma, idiopathic thrombocytopenic purpura, juvenile rheumatoid arthritis, nephrotic syndrome, or other diseases at doses less than or equal to 0.25 mg per kg per day are not at significantly increased risk. Severe varicella may develop in children who are receiving more than 2.0 mg per kg per day of prednisone. Children with malignancies who are most likely to have life-threatening varicella are those whose absolute lymphocyte count is 500 cells per microliter or less and whose disease is in relapse. Bone marrow and organ transplant recipients are very likely to develop progressive varicella.

Parents of high-risk children should report any exposure to varicella or herpes zoster immediately. Prophylaxis with VZIG should be given for household contact or other close indoor exposure. Modification of varicella is optimal if passive antibody prophylaxis is administered within 3 days after the exposure and is not likely to modify the disease if given after 4 to 5 days. Parents should also be educated to recognize possible varicella lesions. The diagnosis of suspicious lesions should be pursued by scraping cells from the base of the lesion and staining with immunofluorescence reagents that detect varicella-zoster virus infected cells. If possible, children who are receiving high-dose steroids or chemotherapy should have the steroid dose decreased and chemotherapy interrupted for the duration of the incubation period. Although varicella is modified in most children who receive prophylaxis shortly after exposure, some children develop severe varicella despite its administration and may require intravenous acyclovir therapy.

Immunocompromised children who develop varicella may have fulminant infection with pneumonia, hepatic failure, and disseminated intravascular coagulation during the first few days of the illness. However, most children appear to do well initially but develop progressive varicella with new lesion formation for more than 5 to 6 days after the appearance of the exanthem. Progressive cutaneous infection may be accompanied by pneumonia, hepatitis, thrombocytopenia, encephalitis, and glomerulonephritis with severe hypertension. Severe abdominal or back pain is an ominous prognostic sign. Bacterial sepsis may also occur. To be effective, antiviral therapy should be initiated early in the clinical course, preferably within 3 days after the appearance of the rash. Acyclovir is preferred to vidarabine because it is more effective than vidarabine in high-risk patients with herpes zoster. Acyclovir

is given at a dose of 500 mg per M^2 per dose, every 8 hours. The drug must be given as a 1-hour infusion and the patient should be kept well hydrated. The dose must be decreased in patients with impaired renal function if the creatinine clearance is less than half of the normal rate. Some children develop severe varicella despite antiviral therapy, and intensive support is essential for the management of these patients. There is no evidence that passive antibody administration after the appearance of clinically apparent varicella will modify its severity. Immunosuppressive therapy can be resumed 1 week after skin lesions have crusted.

A live attenuated varicella vaccine is being evaluated for safety and efficacy in healthy children and adults and in selected immunocompromised children, but its use is investigational.

Nosocomial Transmission of Varicella

Nosocomial varicella can be a serious problem in pediatric wards. All patients being admitted should be questioned about recent exposures to varicella and herpes zoster; if an exposure has occurred, elective admissions should be delayed. If hospital exposure occurs, high-risk susceptible patients with close exposure should be given prophylaxis. Susceptible patients should be discharged during the incubation period if possible, and those who must remain in the hospital should be placed in strict isolation at the end of the incubation period. Hospital personnel who are susceptible to varicella should not care for these children. Isolation rooms for children with varicella should have negative air flow relative to the corridor and be vented to the outside. In implementing these measures, it is helpful to screen high-risk susceptible patients for antibody to varicella at the time the underlying disease is diagnosed.

Infants with nosocomial exposure to varicella or herpes zoster are rarely at risk, since most infants have maternally acquired antibodies to varicella. The maternal history should be determined; if there is doubt about the mother's immunity, the maternal varicella antibody titer should be measured. Infants with close exposure whose mothers have no antibodies to varicella should receive VZIG.

CHOLERA

method of
A. MAJID MOLLA, M.D., PH.D.
The Aga Khan University Hospital
Karachi, Pakistan

Cholera is one of the most devastating secretory diarrheas and is caused by *Vibrio cholerae,* which colonize the small intestine. Profuse diarrhea is caused by a toxin, protein in nature, that attaches to the specific receptor of the enterocytes. *V. cholerae* do not cause any structural changes in the intestinal mucosa. The toxin stimulates the cyclic nucleotide system inside the cells, resulting in the loss of profuse amounts of fluid and electrolytes. This produces dehydration, vascular collapse, and shock. Unless rehydration is done promptly, cholera can cause death in 40 per cent of the affected persons. With early and efficient rehydration therapy, mortality is reduced to less than 1 per cent. Cholera is spread by contaminated food and water. Good hygienic measures, such as drinking only pure water and washing hands after defecation or before handling food, can prevent cholera. This disorder affects all age groups, but young adults, particularly young women, are most susceptible.

V. cholerae responsible for causing clinical disease are of two serotypes, Inaba and Ogawa, and biotypes, El Tor and classical. Clinical features and severity in both types of *V. cholerae* are similar, although the carrier state is more prolonged in the El Tor variety. Cholera is a seasonal disease and occurs in epidemic and endemic forms. During nonepidemic seasons the whereabouts of *V. cholerae* is not definitely known.

Treatment

Assessment of Dehydration

The main effect of cholera is due to loss of fluid and electrolytes in the form of rice-water stools and vomiting, causing vascular collapse and dehydration. Correct assessment of dehydration is essential before starting therapy. Depending on the amount of fluid loss, the degree of dehydration may be mild, moderate, or severe. Table 1 presents some of the important signs of dehydration and the corresponding fluid deficit.

History, physical examination, and assessment of dehydration and fluid requirements should not take more than a few minutes. Rehydration therapy should be started promptly, as crucial time may be lost before instituting therapy.

The fluid requirement to correct the initial dehydration that the patient has already sustained can be calculated on the basis of the degree of dehydration and the body weight. For example, a patient weighing 45 kg and having severe dehydration is estimated to have lost 10 per cent of body weight, or 4.5 liters of fluid. Thus, 4.5 liters of fluid of appropriate electrolyte composition should be replaced through the intravenous route.

Treatment of Dehydration or Fluid Replacement Therapy

The basic principle of fluid therapy is to replace the fluid and electrolytes lost from the body in the stool and vomit. Fluid therapy can be best done in three phases:

1. Replacement of the already existing fluid and electrolyte deficit with which the patient presents.

2. Replacement of ongoing abnormal losses due to continuing diarrhea and/or vomiting in order to prevent recurrence of dehydration.

3. Provision of normal daily fluid requirements.

Oral Rehydration Solutions. Fluid therapy can be accomplished either by the intravenous route or by oral rehydration therapy. Before the development of oral rehydration solution (ORS) in 1967, intravenous therapy was the only treatment available. The composition of intravenous fluid was developed to match the electrolyte loss in the cholera stool. The composition of different commonly used intravenous solutions is shown in Table 2.

After the discovery of ORS, the treatment of cholera underwent a revolutionary change and has become very simple. The composition of ORS as recommended by UNICEF/WHO (United Nations Children's Fund/World Health Organization) is shown in Table 3.

A patient with severe dehydration should receive the initial rehydration intravenously within 3 to 4 hours after admission. Once dehydration is corrected, the general condition is im-

TABLE 1. **Assessment of Dehydration and Fluid Deficit in Cholera**

Signs and Symptoms	Mild Dehydration	Moderate Dehydration	Severe Dehydration
General appearance	Alert, thirsty, and restless	Thirsty, restless, irritable, giddiness with postural changes	Drowsy, cold and sweaty extremities, wrinkled, muscle cramps
Radial pulse	Normal rate and volume	Rapid and weak	Feeble, may not be palpable
Respiration	Normal	Deep, may be rapid	Deep and rapid
Anterior fontanelle	Normal	Sunken	Very sunken
Systolic blood pressure	Normal	Low	Very low, may be unrecordable
Skin elasticity	Retracts	Retracts slowly	Retracts very slowly (>2 sec)
Eyes	Normal	Sunken	Very sunken
Voice	Normal	Hoarse	Not audible
Loss of fluid	4–5% of body weight	6–9% of body weight	10% or more of body weight

TABLE 2. **Electrolyte Composition of Cholera Stool and Different Intravenous Fluids**

Concentration (mmol/liter)	Cholera Stool	Darrow's Solution	Ringer's Lactate	Dhaka Solution*
Na$^+$	135	122	131	133
K$^+$	15	35	4	13
Cl$^-$	100	104	111	98
HCO$^-_3$	45	53	26	48

*As used in the International Centre for Diarrhoeal Disease Research, Bangladesh.

proved, and the patient is able to take fluids orally, further rehydration therapy should be continued by means of ORS.

On the other hand, a patient with moderate to mild dehydration can be treated with ORS from the beginning. It is important to remember that oral rehydration therapy requires the patient's participation and cooperation. Hence, the patient should be conscious and able to drink ORS. Vomiting in cholera patients is mainly due to acidosis. Therefore, vomiting may persist initially, but on continuation of oral therapy the acidosis is corrected and vomiting disappears. Vomiting itself is not a contraindication to stopping oral therapy. Despite vomiting after starting oral rehydration therapy, patients retain a substantial portion of the consumed ORS. However, it is important to remember that there are certain situations in which ORS should not be pushed or should even be avoided. These include (1) convulsions, coma, or unconsciousness; (2) severe fatigue; (3) persistent vomiting; (4) severe dehydration with signs of shock; (5) prolonged oliguria or anuria (>24 hours); (6) associated complications, e.g., pneumonia; and (7) high purging rate (≥10 ml per kg per hour).

Replacement of ongoing losses by oral rehydration therapy can be carried out by recording the output (stool, urine, and vomit) accurately. When this is not possible, frequent weighing of the patient will be useful. Normal daily requirements of fluid intake can best be determined based on the daily allowance of food, including breast milk in infants and young children.

A standard packet of UNICEF/WHO formula contains 20 grams of glucose along with the

TABLE 3. **Composition of Oral Rehydration Solution***

Substance	Grams/Liter	Substance	mmol/Liter
Sodium chloride	3.5	Sodium	90
Sodium bicarbonate	2.5	Potassium	20
Potassium	1.5	Chloride	80
Glucose/sucrose	20/40	Bicarbonate	30
		Glucose	111

*One-liter packet.

electrolytes. Since ORS packets from WHO are not adequate to cover all of the diarrheal episodes, formula for homemade ORS using 50 grams (8 teaspoonfuls) of sugar and 3.5 grams (1 level teaspoonful) of salt has been found successful. During a further simplification, 2 tablespoonfuls of molasses with 1 level teaspoonful of salt have also been used successfully. More recently, a major improvement in ORS has been made by replacing the glucose or molasses by two fistfuls (50 grams) of rice flour and adding two three-finger pinches of salt in 1 liter of water. The composition of rice ORS is shown in Table 4. Rice-based ORS has been found to be highly effective, reducing stool output by 50 per cent, vomiting by 80 per cent, and ORS consumption by 50 per cent. The availability of these ingredients at home gives the mother an opportunity to treat her child early during diarrheal diseases. Glucose and sometimes even sugar are not available in many countries where cholera is endemic, and they must be imported. Rice ORS will eliminate this problem. The starch of the rice is digested by luminal enzymes and releases the glucose molecules slowly, thus avoiding osmotic problems even when large amounts are used.

If rice flour is not ready beforehand, two fistfuls of rice can be soaked in water and ground into a paste using the two grinding stones normally employed for grinding spices. These stones are available in every village home. A suspension should be made with this rice paste or two fistfuls of rice flour in slightly more than 1 liter of water. Boil the suspension for 5 to 7 minutes while stirring continuously until a uniform smooth solution is obtained. Add two pinches of salt, mix, and cool and the solution is ready for drinking.

Antisecretory and Antidiarrheal Agents. Theoretically, antisecretory agents hold promise for treating cholera. Clinical trials have shown that chlorpromazine has a substantial effect in reducing intestinal fluid secretion; however, it makes the patient too drowsy to take oral rehydration fluid. Berberine, nicotinic acid, aspirin, and GM$_1$ ganglioside have been tried (among other agents), but their effect was inadequate for clinical application.

Antidiarrheal agents, although commonly em-

TABLE 4. **Composition of Rice-Based Oral Rehydration Solution***

Substance	Grams/Liter
Sodium chloride	3.5
Sodium bicarbonate	2.5
Potassium	1.5
Rice flour	50 grams (8 to 10 teaspoonfuls)

*One-liter packet; osmolality = 288 mOsm.

ployed, are of no use in the treatment of dehydration and are not indicated in the routine treatment of acute cholera.

Absorbents. Absorbents such as kaolin, pectin, and bismuth have not been shown to be of any value in the treatment of acute cholera. Opiates and opiate derivatives have also not been found to be of any clinical value.

Antimicrobial Agents. Effective antibiotics shorten the duration of disease, reduce stool output, kill the vibrios rapidly, and hence are especially indicated in epidemic situations.

The choice of antibiotics is as follows:

Tetracycline:

Adults: 500 mg 4 times daily for 3 days.

Children: furazolidone (Furoxone), 5 to 6 mg per kg per day in divided doses for 3 days.

Pregnant women: Furoxone, 100 mg every 6 hours for 3 days.

Recently there have been reports of antibiotic-resistant *V. cholerae.* Hence, sensitivity tests are indicated in cases of clinical failure.

Associated Problems and Complications

The most common complications in cholera are electrolyte abnormalities such as *hyponatremia* or *hypernatremia, hypokalemia* or *hyperkalemia,* and severe *acidosis.* When ORS is used, these complications are infrequent. Hypoglycemia may be responsible for convulsions, especially in infants and young children. The cause of hypoglycemia is not definitely known, but with early therapy the outcome is quite satisfactory.

If dehydration is not corrected promptly and adequately, patients remain in a dehydrated state for a long time and may develop *renal failure* with oliguria, anuria, and high serum creatinine levels. With prompt diagnosis, biochemical tests, and close monitoring, the results of treatment of such cases are quite satisfactory. Early treatment with ORS has largely reduced these complications.

Pneumonia is quite common in severe cholera, especially in children. This may be due to severe vomiting and aspiration. Diagnosis should be made by chest x-ray and sputum culture after adequate hydration has been established, and treatment should be started with appropriate antibiotics.

TABLE 5. **Influence of Stooling Rate on the Rate of Absorption of Carbohydrate***

Stooling Rate (ml/kg/day)		Per Cent Absorption
Range	*Mean*	
0–15	82.2 ± 38.6	69.6 ± 14.6
>150	326 ± 292.6	65.8 ± 19.0

*Fifteen cholera patients in each group.

Dietary or Nutritional Management of Cholera

In countries where cholera is a health problem, malnutrition is also common, particularly in children. Unlike other invasive diarrheas, cholera exerts little nutritional effect on the body. When offered a normal diet, cholera patients are able to consume a substantial amount of food and digest most of it without influencing the volume of stool or duration of diarrhea. Hence, there is no justification for withholding or modifying the foods for cholera patients. Malnutrition is a common accompaniment of cholera, especially in the developing countries; therefore, simultaneous rehydration plus nutritional management is the cornerstone of treatment. Recent studies have shown that patients with acute severe cholera can consume about 80 to 90 kcal per kg per day and 70 per cent of the protein and fat are absorbed. Carbohydrate absorption is almost 90 to 95 per cent in the acute stage of cholera. Although the stooling rate is very high in cholera, it does not affect the absorption rate. Table 5 illustrates the relationship between stooling rate and carbohydrate absorption. Young breast-fed children should continue feeding. Recent studies from developing countries suggest that carbohydrate absorption remains most unaffected even during the acute phase of cholera.

Prevention

Prophylactic vaccination provides protection for a short time only. During an epidemic, attention to personal hygiene, such as hand washing, drinking boiled water, and other measures, seems to be rewarding.

DIPHTHERIA

method of
BARBARA W. STECHENBERG, M.D.
Baystate Medical Center
Springfield, Massachusetts

Diphtheria is an acute infectious disease caused by *Corynebacterium diphtheriae.* Generalized and localized symptoms follow production and elaboration of a toxin that is an extracellular protein metabolite of toxinogenic strains.

Diphtheria is acquired by contact with a carrier or a person with the disease. The bacteria may be transmitted via droplets or contact with skin lesions. The communicability in untreated individuals lasts about 2 weeks. The incubation period may range from 1 to 6 days.

C. diphtheriae initially enters the nose or mouth (or, occasionally, the eyes, skin, or genital mucosa), where the bacilli remain localized on the mucosal surfaces of the upper respiratory tract. A localized inflammatory response ensues with tissue necrosis and pseudomembrane formation. Toxin produced at the local site of infection is distributed via the bloodstream throughout the body and can damage any organ or tissue, but lesions of the heart, nervous system, and kidneys are most common. The signs and symptoms of diphtheria will depend upon the site of infection and the immunization status of the host and upon whether or not the toxin has entered the systemic circulation.

The diagnosis of diphtheria should be made on the basis of clinical findings because delay in therapy may pose a serious risk to the patient. An accurate diagnosis requires the isolation of *C. diphtheriae* on culture using appropriate selective media. Diphtheria bacilli isolated should be tested for toxigenicity.

Treatment

Antitoxic Therapy

Treatment of diphtheria is predicated upon neutralization of free toxin and eradication of the organism with antibiotics. The only specific treatment available is antitoxin of equine origin.

The antitoxin is delivered by the intravenous route in a single dose sufficient to neutralize all free toxin. One dose is given to avoid the risk of sensitization from repeated doses. A history of prior sensitization to horse serum should be sought, and testing for sensitivity to the horse serum must be performed prior to administration of the antitoxin. This can be accomplished with one drop of a 1:10 antitoxin dilution for conjunctival testing, or, more commonly, 0.1 ml of a 1:100 antitoxin dilution for intracutaneous testing; a positive reaction would be the development of tearing and conjunctivitis within 10 to 30 minutes, or wheal and/or erythema $\geq$ 10 mm within 20 minutes, respectively. If the patient is sensitive to the antitoxin, desensitization is necessary. Several regimens are available using slowly increasing dosage at 20-minute intervals. This procedure must be done by trained personnel familiar with the treatment of anaphylaxis. Aqueous epinephrine (1:1000) as well as resuscitative equipment should be at the bedside. One commonly employed regimen is as follows:

    0.05 ml of a 1:20 dilution subcutaneously
    0.1 ml of a 1:20 dilution subcutaneously
    0.1 ml of a 1:10 dilution subcutaneously
    0.1 ml undiluted subcutaneously
    0.3 ml undiluted intramuscularly
    0.5 ml undiluted intramuscularly
    0.1 ml undiluted intravenously

If no reaction occurs, the remaining dose is given by slow intravenous infusion. Intravenous administration results in more rapid excretion of antitoxin into saliva, rendering it atoxic and preventing further absorption of free toxin from the oropharynx.

The dosage of antitoxin is empiric. It depends on the site of the diphtheritic membrane, the degree of toxicity and swelling, and the duration of illness—but not on the age or size of the patient. Mild nasal or pharyngeal diphtheria can be treated with 40,000 units of antitoxin; 80,000 units should be used for moderately severe pharyngeal diphtheria. Severe pharyngeal or laryngeal diphtheria should be treated with 100,000 to 120,000 units. The latter dose also should be used in those patients with mixed clinical symptoms, brawny edema, or disease of greater than 48 hours' duration. The antitoxin is available from the Centers for Disease Control (CDC), Atlanta. An immediate allergic reaction to the infusion of antitoxin may be seen in approximately 16 per cent of patients. A serum sickness reaction characterized by rash, fever, and arthritis may develop in 20 to 30 per cent of older children and adults who receive equine antitoxin, usually at about 5 to 14 days after infusion. It may be treated symptomatically with aspirin, antihistamines, or, in severe cases, glucocorticosteroids.

Antibiotic Therapy

Antibiotics are not a substitute for antitoxin treatment, but are important for the eradication of the organism to prevent further toxin production and spread to other persons. Either erythromycin or penicillin constitutes effective therapy. Erythromycin may be given orally or intravenously at a dosage of 40 mg per kg per day in four divided doses (maximum: 1 gram per day) for 14 days. Penicillin may be given as aqueous procaine penicillin G intramuscularly at 300,000 units for those weighing less than 10 kg or as 600,000 units for those weighing greater than 10 kg once daily for 14 days. Each of these regimens is effective in eradicating Group A streptococci, which may complicate up to 30 per cent of cases. Elimination of the organism should be documented by three consecutive negative cultures after cessation of therapy.

In patients with cutaneous diphtheria, lesions should be cleansed vigorously with soap and water. Antimicrobial therapy, either oral erythromycin or penicillin, should be administered for 10 days. Antitoxic therapy is probably of no value in this form, but some authorities give 20,000 units of antitoxin if there is no sensitivity to the antitoxin.

Carriers of *C. diphtheriae* should be treated with antibiotics. Oral erythromycin, as noted above, is appropriate for a 7-day course. Alternative therapy includes oral penicillin or benzathine penicillin (Bicillin) at a dosage of 600,000 units for children weighing less than 30 kg and 1,200,000 units for those weighing greater than

30 kg. Two consecutive cultures should be obtained after treatment to prove elimination of the organism. If the result is positive, re-treatment may be necessary.

Supportive Therapy

Patients with diphtheria should be hospitalized. Bed rest is important and should be required for 2 to 3 weeks. Serial electrocardiograms should be obtained two or three times each week for 4 to 6 weeks to detect myocarditis as soon as possible. If myocarditis is present, absolute bed rest and cardiac monitoring should be enforced. The patient with diphtheria may be given digitalis carefully if congestive heart failure develops. In severe cases, prednisone 1 to 1.5 mg per kg per day for 2 weeks may lessen the severity.

Patients with respiratory tract diphtheria should be placed in strict isolation until two cultures from both nose and throat are negative for *C. diphtheriae*. Patients with cutaneous disease should be in contact isolation until two skin cultures are negative. These cultures should be obtained after cessation of therapy and at least 24 hours apart.

Maintenance of good hydration and nutrition is important. Parenteral nutritional support may be necessary. Risk of airway obstruction requires close observation. Secretions should be suctioned. Patients with laryngeal disease may require bronchoscopy and/or intubation for relief of obstruction. Careful observation for signs of other organ failure should be maintained. Neurologic complications such as palatal paralysis must be sought, since they may complicate nutritional or respiratory support.

Patients with diphtheria require immunization following recovery.

Care of Contacts

Care of exposed persons depends upon immunization status and likelihood of compliance with prophylaxis. Cultures should be done in contacts irrespective of immunization status. Those whose cultures are positive should be treated with antimicrobial agents.

Asymptomatic, previously immunized close contacts should receive a booster dose of an appropriate immunizing agent (DPT, DT, or dT) if they have not received a booster dose within 5 years.

Asymptomatic close contacts who are unimmunized, who are not fully immunized, or whose immunization status is unknown should have a culture done and should be started immediately on either oral erythromycin, 40 mg per kg per day for 7 days, or benzathine penicillin, 600,000 to 1,200,000 units intramuscularly as for carriers.

Cultures should be repeated after treatment. Active immunization with DPT, DT, or dT should be initiated depending on age.

Close contacts who cannot be kept under surveillance should be given benzathine penicillin as noted above (not erythromycin because of risk of noncompliance) and a dose of an appropriate immunizing agent depending on age and immunization status. I would not recommend the use of horse antitoxin at this point because of the risk of allergic reactions.

Prevention

Universal immunization with the diphtheria toxoid is the only effective control measure. Children up to age 7 should receive DPT (or DT) according to an appropriate schedule, usually at 2, 4, and 6 months with booster doses at 15 to 18 months and 4 to 6 years of age. After age 6, immunization should be carried out with adult-type toxoid, dT. Booster doses should be given at 10-year intervals.

FOOD-BORNE ILLNESS

method of
JOHN L. HO, M.D.
Cornell University Medical College
New York, New York

The gastrointestinal tract has a limited repertoire to register a complaint. Nausea, vomiting, diarrhea with bloating, and flatulence are the symptoms patients associate with gastrointestinal disturbance. The association between gastrointestinal pathology and systemic illness manifesting as fever, extraintestinal signs, or neurologic deficits with minimal or distant gastrointestinal symptoms usually requires diagnosis by an astute physician. Food-borne illness is produced by the ingestion of food contaminated with microbial pathogens or their toxins or toxic plants or chemicals.

Obtaining an epidemiologic history is crucial for excluding non-food-borne illness of the gastrointestinal tract as well as assisting in the diagnosis of food-borne illness. The diagnosis of an outbreak of food-borne illness usually requires illness in more than one person eating a common food. However, a single case of botulism or chemical poisoning constitutes an outbreak requiring investigation and institution of control measures. A complete epidemiologic history includes the following: the type and preparation of the suspected food, the place where the food was served, the time elapsed from ingestion to onset of symptoms, the time of year, recent travel, unusual food preferences or purchases (e.g., imported foods, raw milk, specialty cheeses, nondomesticated meat, wild mushrooms or plants, raw fish, honey) similar illness in family or friends, and ownership of or illness in pets (e.g., turtles, snakes). Although the majority of outbreaks of food-borne illness are contracted by eating restaurant food (45 per cent), 30 per cent of outbreaks reported to the Centers for Disease Control (CDC) in 1982 were from foods prepared at home. Although bacteria cause food-borne illness year round, peak incidence occurs during late spring to early fall. Hepatitis A and Norwalk virus occur mostly during summer to fall. Frequencies, cases, and etiologies of food-borne illnesses reported to the CDC and confirmed by identification are presented in Table 1. These diverse causes typically manifest as acute food poisoning syndrome, infectious diarrhea, and neurotoxic syndromes.

The majority of acute food poisoning syndromes are brief and self-limited. An etiologic diagnosis is useful in explaining the larger outbreak rather than for the individual patient. However, the etiologic diagnosis is important for infectious diarrhea and neurotoxic syndrome because it may affect treatment and patient outcome (see the first three footnotes at Table 1). Stool can be cultured for bacterial pathogens and examined for ova and parasites. Specific identification of *Campylobacter, Vibrio, Listeria,* and *Yersinia* requires special laboratory techniques not routinely employed. If these organisms are suspected, the laboratory (requisition) should be notified. Gastric contents, stool, and blood may be sent for examination for toxins (including botulinum toxin) as indicated by the epidemiologic history and clinical presentation.

TABLE 1. Confirmed Food-Borne Disease Outbreaks and Cases by Etiologic Agents, United States, 1982*

Etiologic Agent	Per Cent Outbreaks (No.)	Cases No.	Cases (%)
Bacterial			
Bacillus cereus	3.6	200	(1.8)
Brucella	0.5	3	(<0.1)
Campylobacter jejuni	0.9	31	(0.3)
Clostridium botulinum†	9.5	30	(0.3)
Clostridium perfringens	10.0	1,189	(10.8)
Escherichia coli	0.9	47	(0.4)
Salmonella‡	25.0	2,056	(18.6)
Shigella	1.8	116	(1.1)
Staphylococcus aureus	12.7	669	(6.0)
Streptococcus Group A	0.5	34	(0.3)
Vibrio cholerae 01§	0.5	892	(8.0)
Vibrio cholerae non-01	0.5	7	(0.1)
Vibrio parahaemolyticus	1.4	39	(0.4)
Yersinia enterocolitica	0.9	188	(1.7)
Total	68.7 (151)	5,501	(49.9)
Chemical			
Ciguatoxin	3.6	37	(0.3)
Heavy metals	2.3	26	(0.2)
Monosodium glutamate	1.4	10	(0.1)
Mushrooms	1.8	9	(0.1)
Scombrotoxin	8.2	58	(0.5)
Shellfish	0.5	5	(<0.1)
Other	3.6	75	(<0.1)
Total	21.4 (47)	220	(1.9)
Parasitic			
Trichinella spiralis	0.5	4	(<0.1)
Total	0.5 (1)	4	(<0.1)
Viral			
Hepatitis A	8.5	325	(2.9)
Norwalk virus	0.9	5,000	(45.2)
Total	9.4 (21)	5,325	(48.1)
Confirmed Total #	100.0 (220)	11,050	(100.0)

*Adapted from Foodborne Disease Outbreak, Annual Summary 1982. MMWR 35th (No. 1):7SS—16SS, 1986.

†The associated mortality was 16.7 per cent.

‡The associated mortality was 0.4 per cent.

§The associated mortality was 1.2 per cent.

#The confirmed total represent 40 per cent of all reported outbreaks. The prevalence of foodborne disease is estimated to be 10 to 100 times more frequent than reported. Of these diseases only botulism, typhoid fever, brucellosis, and cholera are notifiable diseases mandated by law. Thus, underreporting may be significant.

Treatment

The treatment of food poisoning is directed at (1) maintenance of hydration, (2) removal of the toxic agent, (3) symptomatic measures, and (4) specific therapy. Dehydration is not uncommon when vomiting and diarrhea occur concurrently, in the elderly or in the infant. Despite the induction of the gastrocolonic reflex, patients should be encouraged to increase their fluid intake. Avoidance of milk or milk products and fatty foods may decrease gastrointestinal distress. For rehydration, commercial or homemade oral rehydration solution (ORS) may be used. ORS is made with 16 ounces of water or juice plus table sugar (1 teaspoon), table salt (1 pinch), potassium (½ teaspoon, NoSalt), and baking soda (¼ teaspoon). Interspersed with plain juice or soda, ORS may prevent dehydration and hypernatremia (a concern in infants and children). Mild dehydration represented by loss of less than 5 per cent body weight (dry mucous membranes) can be managed with ORS. Intractable vomiting or 10 per cent dehydration (tenting of the skin, orthostatic hypotension) should be managed with intravenous fluids (isotonic solutions supplemented with potassium, lactate, or bicarbonate).

Removal of unabsorbed toxin is indicated in botulism, mushroom poisoning, and fish and shellfish poisoning. Gastric lavage (using a large oral tube) with or without the instillation of activated charcoal is indicated for patients with altered sensorium. For an alert cooperative patient, emesis may be induced by giving syrup of ipecac, 15 ml orally, or apomorphine, 6 mg subcutaneously (1 to 2 mg for children).

Symptomatic management of the patient with persistent vomiting includes (1) prochlorperazine (Compazine) given intramuscularly (5 to 10 mg), orally (5 to 10 mg) or rectally (25 mg); or (2) trimethobenzamide HCl (Tigan) given orally (250 mg) or rectally (200 mg). Both should be used with caution in young children and pregnant women.

No specific therapy is required for most mild diarrheal syndromes. Bismuth subsalicylate (Pepto-Bismol) has been shown to diminish symptoms for traveler's diarrhea. Pepto-Bismol should be avoided by patients with aspirin sensitivity, renal failure, or gout and in those taking warfarin (Coumadin) or oral hypoglycemic agents. For moderately to severely symptomatic patients without signs of inflammatory diarrhea (fever, gross blood, or microscopic leukocytes in stool), antimotility drugs may provide some relief. Loperamide (Imodium) is given orally as an initial dose of 4 mg, followed by 2 mg after each loose stool. The total daily dose must not exceed 16 mg. Alternatively, the combination diphenoxylate, 2.5 mg, with atropine (Lomotil), 0.025 mg, may be used: two tablets orally as an initial dose and one tablet after each loose stool (not to exceed eight tablets a day). Sedation is a side effect seen with all antimotility agents. Kaolin and pectin (Kaopectate) have no proven effect on symptoms of diarrhea.

Acute Food Poisoning

The acute food poisoning syndrome is caused by the ingestion of toxins of bacteria, plants, or man. Of the three bacterial species that cause acute food poisoning by elaboration of protein toxins, *Staphylococcus aureus* and *Bacillus cereus* produce clinical illness with a relatively short incubation period (2 to 9 hours), while *Clostridium perfringens* requires a slightly longer time (8 to 22 hours; Table 2). The distinction is due to the production of preformed toxins by *S. aureus* and *B. cereus*. Foods that have been associated with *S. aureus* acute food poisoning typically require a lot of handling during preparation, have a high salt or sugar content, and stand for at least several hours unrefrigerated (Table 2). These are selective conditions for *S. aureus* growth and elaboration of heat-resistant toxins (A to E). With the exception of milk (bovine mastitis), humans are the source of infection. The ingestion of *S. aureus* toxin(s) causes an upper gastrointestinal illness (Table 2).

B. cereus causes two distinct illnesses: a short incubation period (2 hours), predominantly upper gastrointestinal illness with diarrhea occurring in 30 per cent of cases; and a longer incubation period (9 hours) illness that is predominantly diarrheal (Table 2). The production by *B. cereus* of a heat-stable toxin causes the former illness, while a heat-sensitive toxin causes the latter illness. Foods associated with *B. cereus* acute food poisoning share the common features of being slowly cooled, rewarmed, or left warming for several hours (Table 2). The illnesses caused by *S. aureus* and *B. cereus* are self-limiting, and only supportive measures are necessary. Diagnosis of the etiology is made by isolation of the bacteria in food (*S. aureus*, *B. cereus*) or stool (*S. aureus*).

Eight to 12 hours after ingesting food contaminated with *C. perfringens* or its spores, lower gastrointestinal symptoms erupt, usually without vomiting or other signs (Table 2). The cause is usually cooked food in which the internal temperature was too low to kill spores of *C. perfringens*. The longer incubation period is due to the time required for intestinal germination and subsequent elaboration of toxin A by the vegetative form. This clinical illness is self-limiting, and only supportive measures are required. *C. perfringens* causes another distinct illness called enteritis necroticans, or pig-bel. Not seen in the United States, pig-bel has been documented in Germany and New Guinea as causing enteritis after ingestion of improperly cooked pork. This illness is associated with a 40 per cent mortality caused by intestinal perforation.

The remaining causes of acute food poisoning can be divided into illnesses that produce flushing and others that do not. Twenty or more minutes after ingestion of monosodium glutamate (used as a food additive in Chinese restaurants), symptoms of flushing, facial paresthesia, headache, and nausea may ensue, and with large doses, abdominal cramps. These symptoms are self-limiting and resolve after several hours. The ingestion of Coprinus mushrooms, which contain coprine, induces a disulfiram-like reaction with the intercurrent use of alcohol. Symptoms include flushing, nausea, vomiting, parasthesia, and a metallic taste. Treatment consists of avoidance of alcohol over the next 5 days and supportive therapy.

Scombroid fish poisoning is an illness that produces facial flushing, nausea, abdominal cramps, headache, and diarrhea within 30 minutes after contaminated fish is eaten. Clinical illness is caused by the contamination of dark-meat fish, such as tuna, bonito, mackerel, and mahi-mahi, by marine bacteria, *Proteus morganii,* which catabolize the fish meat to produce histamine-like substances (saurines). Severe forms are associated with bronchospasm. Antihistamines and bronchodilators provide relief while symptoms resolve over the next 4 hours.

The eating of wild mushrooms by novices can result in morbidity and fatalities. Mushrooms of the genus *Amanita* or *Galerina* contain cyclopeptides that cause an acute gastrointestinal illness 6 to 24 hours after ingestion. Within 1 to 2 days, renal and hepatic failure occur. Once acute illness

TABLE 2. Characteristics of Bacterial Food Poisoning*

Organism	Common Vehicles	Median Incubation Period (Hrs)	(Range)	Clinical Features	Median Days Duration (Range)	Secondary Attack Rates (%)
Salmonella sp.	Eggs, meat, poultry	24	(5–27)	D,C,N,V,H,B (rare), enteric fever	3 (0.5–14)	30–50
Shigella sp.	Milk, salads (potato, tuna, turkey)	24	(7–168)	C,F,D,B,H,N,V	3 (0.5–14)	40–60
B. cereus	Fried rice, cream, vanilla sauce, meatballs, boiled beef, barbecued chicken	2 9	(1–6) (1–14)	V,C,D (33%) D,C,V	4 (0.2–0.5) 1 (1–2)	— —
V. parahaemolyticus	Seafood, rarely salt water or salted vegetables	12	(2–48)	D,C,N,V,H,F (25%) B (rare)	3 (2–10)	—
C. perfringens	Beef, turkey, chicken	12	(8–22)	D,C (N,V,F rare)	1 (0.3–3)	—
S. aureus	Ham, pork, canned beef, cream-filled pastry	3	(1–6)	V,N,C,D (rare) F (rare)	1 (0.3–1.5)	—
Y. enterocolitica	Chocolate or raw milk, pork	72	(2–144)	F,C,D,V,S,† enteric fever	7 (2–30)	20
C. fetus ssp. *jejuni*	Milk, chicken, pet animals	72	(48–168)	D,F,C,B,H,M,N,V,S‡	7 (2–30)	25
E. coli	Salads, raw beef	24	(8–44)	B§,D,C,N,H,F,M	3 (1–14)	0§
Listeria	Milk, raw vegetables	?		D,C,N,F,V,S#	?	0

*Adapted from Snydman DR: Bacterial food poisoning. In SL Gorbach, ed: Boston, Blackwell Scientific Publications, pp 201–218.

†Pharyngitis, arthritis, mesenteric adenitis, skin rashes.

‡Bacteremia especially patients with cirrhosis (alcoholics).

§Vero-toxin producing *E. coli* 0157:H7 serotype causes hemorrhagic colitis, hemolytic uremic syndrome, and thrombotic thrombocytopenia purpura. Person-to-person transmission has been documented for hemorrhagic colitis.

#Bacteremia and meningitis predisposed by pregnancy, immunosuppression, and use of antacids.

Abbreviations: B = bloody diarrhea; C = crampy abdominal pain; D = diarrhea; F = fever; H = headache; M = myalgias; N = nausea; V = vomiting; S = systemic infection.

is recognized, elimination of stomach contents is essential and institution of supportive care is vital. Early use of charcoal hemofiltration aids toxin removal, while thioctic acid (50 to 150 mg) given intravenously every 6 hours with glucose infusion may be of benefit. Thioctic acid may be obtained from poison control centers.

A hemolytic syndrome is caused by the ingestion of mushrooms of the genus *Gyromitra*. This mushroom produces a toxin that is metabolized by humans to methylhydrazine, a potent competitive inhibitor of erythrocyte pyridoxal phosphate. Gastrointestinal symptoms ensue after an incubation period of 6 to 12 hours. Hemolysis with methemoglobinemia and hepatic failure follows. Without intervention, or in severe cases, seizure and coma may occur. In addition to supportive care, specific treatment includes the use of intravenous pyridoxine hydrochloride, 25 mg. A 40 per cent mortality is associated with severe intoxication.

Infectious Diarrhea Syndrome

Infectious diarrhea syndrome can be categorized by the locale of acquisition (domestic versus foreign) and by any signs of inflammation (absence or presence of fecal leukocytes and blood on methylene blue stain of a fresh specimen). *Salmonella* spp., *Escherichia coli*, and *Campylobacter fetus* ssp. *jejuni* are the most common pathogens acquired domestically (see Table 1), while *E. coli*, *Salmonella*, and *Shigella*, are the most prevalent enteric bacteria encountered in travels to the developing world. Acquisition of *Giardia lamblia*, *Vibrio cholerae*, *Vibrio parahaemolyticus*, and *Yersinia enterocolitica* occurs less frequently domestically than abroad. The highest prevalence of *Yersinia* infection occurs in Scandinavian countries. In Japan, *V. parahaemolyticus* is the most common cause of food-borne infection. Other intestinal pathogens include viruses (Norwalk, hepatitis A, and rotavirus), *Listeria monocytogenes*, *Entamoeba histolytica*, *Cryptosporidium*, and helminthic parasites. All can be contracted locally, but amebiasis, cryptosporidiosis, and helminthic infections are more common in developing countries.

The intestinal protestations from any one cause of noninflammatory diarrhea are indistinguishable from each other. For food-borne illnesses caused by viruses, no specific therapy other than maintenance of hydration is required. Of the bacterial causes of noninflammatory diarrhea, enterotoxogenic *E. coli* (producing a heat-stable and heat-labile toxin) is the cause of 40 to 70 per cent of traveler's diarrhea. Acute explosive diarrhea usually begins 1 to 7 days after arrival in a host country (see Table 2). Conservative treatment with oral hydration, Pepto-Bismol, and, in severe cases, an antimotility agent is adequate. Treatment of travel-acquired diarrhea with a 3- to 5-day course of antibiotics, such as twice daily trimethoprim-sulfamethoxazole (160 mg/800 mg; Bactrim-DS, Septra-DS, TMP-SMZ) or doxycycline, 100 mg, reduces the duration of clinical illness and may treat invasive pathogens of *Shigella* and *Salmonella* manifesting as watery diarrhea or occurring as a co-infection. However, the side effects of antibiotics and microbial resistance by enteric bacteria preclude their use prophylactically for all travelers.

V. cholerae typically causes an uncontrollable profuse rice-water diarrhea that may result in rapid development of dehydration. Prevalence of *V. cholerae* is low in the Gulf Coast of the United States and in Mediterranean regions; it is higher in the Indian subcontinent, Southeast Asia, and Africa. Oral rehydration is the cornerstone of therapy. In severe cases, four times daily doses of tetracycline, 250 mg, or ampicillin, 250 mg, shorten clinical illness. TMP-SMZ or furazolidone (Furoxone), 100 mg four times daily, is an alternative. Resistance by *V. cholerae* to these antibiotics has been reported.

Protozoans (*Giardia, Cryptosporidium*) produce a secretory diarrhea. However, intestinal bloating and malodorous flatulence are frequent complaints. The incubation period ranges from 7 to 14 days. Left untreated, *Giardia* may produce a chronic illness with malabsorption and weight loss. Effective treatments for Giardia include metronidazole (Flagyl),* 250 mg thrice daily for 5 days; quinacrine HCl (Atabrine), 100 mg thrice daily for 5 days; or furazolidone (Furoxone), 100 mg four times daily for 7 to 10 days. Metronidazole may be given as a single 2-gram dose. Treatment usually eradicates symptoms, but recurrence is not uncommon. Cryptosporidiosis is usually a self-limited illness in the immunocompetent host. However, chronic diarrhea and wasting are seen in malnourished children and immunosuppressed patients (e.g., those with acquired immunodeficiency syndrome). There is no currently available treatment.

Of the inflammatory diarrheas, three clinical illnesses can be discerned: systemic infection, enteric fever, and diarrhea-dysentery. Systemic infection may be characterized by a bacteremia

---

*This use is not listed by the manufacturer.

or, occasionally, by a vascular infection. Enteric fever is manifested as periodic fever, chills, and presence of mild or moderate intestinal symptoms. Inflammatory diarrhea may be grossly bloody (dysentery) or watery, mimicking a noninflammatory diarrhea. The clinical onset, features, duration of illness, and vehicles of transmission for bacterial food poisoning are reported in Table 2. *Salmonella typhi* and *S. paratyphi* cause all three clinical illnesses, whereas *S. enteritidis* usually causes diarrhea, sometimes dysentery, and infrequently systemic infection and enteric fever. Patients with cirrhosis are susceptible to systemic infection by *Campylobacter*. *Y. enterocolitica* may produce diarrhea and enteric fever as well as systemic signs, usually as a result of an autoimmune response. Recently, the vero toxin-producing *E. coli* serotype 0157:H7 has been demonstrated to cause hemorrhagic colitis, thrombotic thrombocytopenia purpura, and hemolytic uremic syndrome. Ingestion of contaminated hamburger meat was the cause of the epidemic cases, but the mode of acquisition in sporadic cases is unknown. Secondary transmission and acquisition from an asymptomatic household contact have been reported. *L. monocytogenes* has been recently recognized as a foodborne pathogen. Gastric neutralization, immunosuppression, or pregnancy predisposes patients to disease acquisition (bacteremia and/or meningitis). The acquisition and pattern of clinical illness produced by *Aeromonas* are similar to that produced by *Salmonella*.

The specific treatment of each infection requires identification of the pathogen by culture. Identification of *Yersinia* and *Listeria* is improved by cold enrichment; with *Vibrio*, thiosulfate-citrate-bile salt-sucrose (TCBS) agar is required. Mild diarrhea does not require antibiotic treatment. In fact, antibiotic use may prolong the fecal carriage of *Salmonella*. For dysentery, TMP-SMZ or ampicillin or ciprofloxacin (soon to be available, 500 mg twice daily) or norfloxacin (Noroxin), 400 mg twice daily (treatment for enteric infection is not an indication listed on the product information), is effective. TMP-SMZ and ampicillin are active against *Salmonella* and *Shigella*, while ciprofloxacin and norfloxacin are active against *Salmonella, Shigella, Campylobacter,* and *Yersinia*. Of concern is the evolution of plasmid-mediated resistance to most antibiotics (except ciprofloxacin and norfloxacin) by enteric pathogens. The drug of choice for *Campylobacter* infection is currently erythromycin. Tetracycline and TMP-SMZ are effective against *Y. enterocolitica*.

One protozoan parasite, *Entamoeba histolytica*, produces a spectrum of disease including asymptomatic cyst passing, diarrhea (colitis), hemorrhagic colitis, ameboma, and hepatic abscess. The incubation period may be 8 to 10 days. Diagnosis is by direct examination of a fresh stool demonstrating trophozoites or cysts, but examination of multiple stools may be necessary. The treatment of amebiasis is with metronidazole, 750 mg three times daily for 10 days. However, the cysts are insensitive and require treatment with iodoquinol (Yodoxin), 650 mg thrice daily for 20 days, or diloxanide furoate, 500 mg thrice daily for 10 days, available from Centers for Disease Control, Atlanta, Georgia; phone no.: 404/639–3670.

Neurotoxic Syndromes

The abrupt onset of neurologic symptoms should raise the clinician's suspicion of toxin-induced illnesses and primary infections of the central nervous system (for which fever is an accompanying sign). Several food poisoning syndromes present primarily with neurologic symptoms. Botulism (although a rare disease) is increasing in frequency and is caused by ingestion of foods contaminated by *Clostridium botulinum* or its heat-resistant spores. Symptoms usually begin 12 to 36 hours (range: 6 hours to 8 days) after eating contaminated food (which appears unspoiled). Vehicles for spores of *C. botulinum* include canned foods (homemade or commercial), preserved food, and honey (especially in infant botulism). *C. botulinum* produces neurotoxins (A, B, E in human disease) that block neural secretion of acetylcholine by autonomic nerves and at the neuromuscular junction. The blockage results in progressive flaccid paralysis. Nausea and vomiting may be present in less than one third of patients ingesting toxins A or B but more frequently for toxin E.

The clinical presentation of botulism includes complaints of weakness, lassitude, and dizziness. Subsequent involvement of autonomic transmission results in progressive dryness of the oropharynx (unrelieved by fluids) and dry eyes. Later motor involvement begins as ptosis and dilated pupils, progressing to symmetric descending weakness or flaccid paralysis. Diagnosis is made by identification of toxin in blood, gastric content, stool, or food. The local health department and CDC should be consulted for assistance. Treatment includes hospitalization; frequent checks for progressive paralysis; supportive measures, including ventilatory; administration of trivalent horse antitoxin (available through CDC, phone no.: 404/639–3753 [work hours] or 639–2888 [other times]—emergency telephone numbers for state and CDC are listed in MMWR 1988;36[January, No. 52]); and prevention of nosocomial infections. Guanidine HCl may enhance acetylcholine release from peripheral nerves, but

its use is still experimental. Prompt notification of public health officials will assist in identification of the source of the toxin and of other cases and in institution of measures to prevent further transmission.

Several seafood-borne poisons cause predominantly neurologic symptoms that manifest within 1 to 6 hours after ingestion. Scombroid, paralytic shellfish poisoning, and neurotoxic shellfish poisoning have an incubation period of less than 1 hour (5 minutes to 4 hours); the incubation period for ciguatera is 1 to 6 hours. Paralytic shellfish poisoning (PSP) is characterized by paresthesia of the mouth, face, and extremities. In severe cases dysphagia, dysphonia, dyspnea, muscle weakness, or frank paralysis with respiratory failure may develop. PSP is caused by consumption of bivalve mollusks (mussels, clams, oysters, scallops) that have ingested dinoflagellates that produce saxitoxin and other neurotoxins. These toxins are heat-stable. Saxitoxin blocks sodium channels, which are pivotal for nerve and muscle conduction. Shellfish from the New England coast, the West Coast of the United States, or other areas above 30° N latitude may be contaminated during the May through October season. Shellfish contamination in regions below 30° S latitude may occur from November to April. Neurotoxic shellfish poisoning (NSP) produces an illness similar to PSP but is without paralysis. Poorly characterized neurotoxins produced by dinoflagellates are the cause. Ingestion of shellfish from the Gulf and Atlantic coasts of Florida during spring and fall months may cause NSP. The treatment for both PSP and NSP is close observation and supportive care. Symptoms for each resolve over hours to a few days.

Ciguatera poisoning is differentiated from PSP and NSP by (1) the ingestion of large fish (barracuda, red snapper, grouper); (2) a slightly longer incubation period (1 to 6 hours); and (3) the complaints of abdominal cramps, nausea, vomiting, and diarrhea. These symptoms may precede or may be followed by numbness and paresthesia of the oropharynx. Other neurologic symptoms, including transient blindness, have been reported. In severe cases, sinus bradycardia, hypotension, cranial nerve palsy, and respiratory failure may occur. The illness is caused by ciguatoxin, which is produced by a dinoflagellate. Fish caught near Hawaii and Florida (between 35° N and 35° S latitudes) may contain saxitoxin-producing dinoflagellates. The mechanism of action of ciguatoxin appears similar to that of saxitoxin. The duration of illness ranges from days to a few months. Intermittent pains of the extremities may last for years.

Several mushrooms cause neurologic symptoms

within 2 hours of ingestion. Mushrooms containing muscarine (genus *Clitocybe* or *Inocybe*) cause parasympathetic hyperactivity: salivation, lacrimation, diaphoresis, blurred vision, abdominal cramps, and diarrhea. In severe cases, miosis, bradycardia, and bronchospasm may be present. Supportive therapy is supplemented with atropine, 1 to 2 mg intravenously every hour as needed, to titrate anticholinergic symptoms.

Eating mushrooms containing ibotenic acid or muscinol (*Amanita muscaria, A. panthernia*) causes an alcohol-like intoxicated state, followed by stupor, seizure, and coma. Physostigmine may improve severe symptoms, but sedatives or hypnotics are contraindicated. Symptoms resolve within 24 hours under supportive care. Lastly, the ingestion of mushrooms containing psilocybin or psilocin (genus *Psilocybe* or *Panaeolus*) causes hallucinations, hyperkinesis, and muscle weakness. Consumption may be intentional for these effects, but in some individuals psychosis develops. Symptoms resolve in 6 to 12 hours; supportive care and possible counseling are all that are indicated.

GAS-FORMING INFECTIONS

method of
RICHARD F. EDLICH, M.D., PH.D.,*
DAVID E. BERMAN, M.D.,* and
GEORGE T. RODEHEAVER, PH.D.*
University of Virginia
Charlottesville, Virginia

The presence of gas in infected tissue is an ominous clinical sign. Many facultative aerobic and obligate anaerobic bacteria have been reported to cause gas-forming infections, with production of insoluble gases occurring under anaerobic conditions in all cases. Three recognized but poorly defined anaerobic pathways—denitrification, fermentation, and deamination—produce insoluble gases, such as hydrogen and nitrogen, in these infections. The presence of these gases that are the products of anaerobic metabolism indicates tissue hypoxia extensive enough to support thriving anaerobic bacteria. Aerobic metabolism is not associated with gas in infected tissue, because the gas produced, carbon dioxide, diffuses rapidly and generally does not accumulate.

Cellulitis and myositis are the most common gas-forming infections caused by obligate anaerobic bacteria. Clinicians often confuse these distinct clinical entities, which can exist separately or coexist in the same patient. Anaerobic cellulitis usually results from a gas-producing infection of necrotic wounds with no

*Our clinical research has been supported by the Texaco Philanthropic Foundation, White Plains, NY.

progressive muscle involvement. The manifestations of this infection include a brownish "dishwater" seropurulent and foul-smelling discharge with crepitant tissue. Pain is not a prominent early feature, and the infection proceeds without significant systemic signs. These clinical findings should not be taken lightly, however, because the infection may progress to necrosis of skin and subcutaneous tissue ("necrotizing cellulitis").

The most lethal variety of anaerobic infection of soft tissue is myositis, which may progress to myonecrosis or true gas gangrene. It occurs in many cases of extensive tissue devitalization, and is particularly common in high-energy missile or shrapnel injuries that involve a great depth of muscle, as in the buttock, thigh, and shoulder. The presence of dirt (soil infection-potentiating fractions) in the devitalized muscle considerably increases the chance for a gas-forming infection. Anaerobic myositis frequently occurs in the limbs of diabetic patients with compromised vascular systems. Injection of illicit drugs into an extremity also is associated with increased risk of gas-forming infection in muscle. Myositis with necrosis of the abdominal wall due to obligate anaerobes can develop following emergency gastrointestinal surgery.

Anaerobic myositis is an infection of abrupt onset that may progress rapidly to death if untreated. In most cases, the time from wounding or surgery until the onset of gas gangrene is only 24 to 48 hours. The sudden onset of pain, sometimes rapid enough to suggest a vascular catastrophe, is the earliest and most important symptom of true gas gangrene. The pain then increases and spreads as the infection disseminates along the fascia. In these early stages of infection, the skin overlying the wound has a tense white appearance, and palpation usually elicits pain but no evidence of gas formation. Within the next few hours, systemic signs of toxemia (hypotension, tachycardia, and tachypnea) appear, along with an insignificant elevation of temperature. Toxic delirium (disorientation, obstreperousness) is another early systemic manifestation of this disease and may necessitate restraining the patient.

As the infection progresses, bullae filled with dark red fluid appear, causing a local bronzing of the skin. Gas is usually now visible on roentgenograms as it spreads along muscle and fascial planes. When gas appears in a feathery pattern, rather than large bubbles, on the roentgenograms, it indicates dissection along muscle fascicles with myonecrosis. The underlying muscle becomes reddened, often superimposed with a purple color, and eventually herniates into the wound. A putrid, seropurulent discharge appears. In clostridial infections, the alpha toxin, a C-lecithinase, is the major lethal toxin. It causes hemolysis that leads to anemia, hemoglobinuria, jaundice, oliguria, and often to renal failure.

Gas-forming infection of the uterus is less common than either myositis or cellulitis and is potentially fatal. The majority of cases result from inept attempts at abortion. Most patients with postabortal gas-forming infection complain of severe lower abdominal pain often associated with vomiting and diarrhea, and exhibit pulse rates disproportionately high in relation to their fever. As septicemia occurs, the patient develops hemolytic jaundice. Other patients with this uterine infection experience cardiovascular collapse with few local signs. Gas may be shown by radiography of the pelvic organs, and hemolysis may be evident in the serum. A late and startling feature of this condition is the appearance of bubbles at the external os during speculum examination.

Nonbacterial Causes of Gas in Tissue

Tissue gas does not necessarily signify life-threatening infection requiring extensive surgical debridement. A variety of nonbacterial mechanisms may produce gas in tissue and may be detectable by palpation or by radiography. Air may be introduced into tissue by severe trauma to an organ that contains air. For example, injury to the tracheobronchial tree and/or lung may result in subcutaneous emphysema. Perforation of the gastrointestinal tract occasionally is associated with air in the tissue (e.g., esophageal perforation following endoscopy). Injuries resulting from application of compressed air hoses to various orifices can result in gas in soft tissues. Irrigation of wounds with fluids delivered under high pressure (>10 psi) may also be associated with tissue crepitation. The use of hydrogen peroxide as a wound irrigant may encourage the formation of gas in tissues. The edges of a laceration may act as a one-way valve, trapping air and pumping it proximally by muscular action. Certain chemicals may generate gas, if they gain access to the wound. The injection of benzene, for example, can produce crepitant aseptic necrosis. As little as 10 mg of powdered magnesium alloys can generate crepitant soft tissue gas, considered to be hydrogen.

The clinical signs and symptoms of patients with tissue gas from nonbacterial causes are distinct from those of patients in whom the gas was generated by bacteria. The local signs of infection, erythema, local heat, and purulent discharge do not occur; systemic signs of infection (fever, tachycardia, leukocytosis) are also not evident. Roentgenograms also provide evidence against a bacterial origin of infection in such cases. Gas is limited to the loose soft tissues, without involving the muscles and deep fascia, and there is no suggestion of inflammatory edema, with well-preserved fat shadows and skin-fat differentiation.

Diagnosis

The diagnosis of gas-forming soft tissue infection is based on a constellation of clinical and bacteriologic findings. The essential clinical features include an injury or operation resulting in devitalized tissue; abrupt onset of severe localized pain; appearance of the wound; and signs of systemic toxicity. Radiographs will often *not* reveal gas consistently early in an infection, and the presence of gas is not pathognomonic for clostridial gas gangrene.

A decision regarding selection of the appropriate antimicrobial agent can be made quickly through bacteriologic monitoring of the wound microflora. Because some anaerobic bacteria may not tolerate exposure to oxygen, the tissue or fluid specimen should be obtained from the infected wound with minimum exposure to air prior to initiating antibiotic therapy. All fluids, including pus and exudates, should be collected in a sterile syringe and either transferred to an anaerobic vial or transported directly to the bacteriology laboratory. The specimens should be processed under anaerobic conditions, preferably in an anaerobic glove box. They should be weighed and then suspended in a measured amount of the prereduced salt solution that will be homogenized. The homogenate is then subjected to direct microscopic examination and qualitative and quantitative culture studies.

Direct microscopic examination of an aliquot of the bacterial suspension provides an estimate of the total number and morphology of the bacteria in the tissue. The suspension is spread uniformly over a glass slide, fixed with methanol, and then subjected to the modified Gram stain (Carr-Scarborough Microbiologicals, Inc., Stone Mountain, Georgia). These findings will suggest an appropriate antimicrobial therapy until the culture and antimicrobial susceptibility results are available, and also provide an important means of quality control. For example, if morphotypes observed in the smear do not appear in the culture, the collection, culturing, or subculturing procedures may have been defective. Results of the microscopic examination should be reported immediately to the clinician.

The Gram stain of the infected fluid or tissue usually will confirm gas gangrene as a polymicrobial infection with mixtures of obligate anaerobes and facultative organisms. Direct microscopic examination reveals clostridia as short, plump, gram-positive rods with squared ends. *Clostridium perfringens* has been implicated alone or in combination with other organisms in 50 to 100 per cent of all cases of gas gangrene. Other clostridial species reported as causative agents of gas gangrene are *C. septicum* and *C. novyi*. Clusters and chains of gram-positive cocci suggest the anaerobic *Peptococcus* and *Peptostreptococcus* as well as the facultative *Staphylococcus* and *Streptococcus*. Pale, irregular-staining, pleomorphic, gram-negative rods characterize *Bacteroides* or *Fusobacterium* as well as the facultative anaerobic bacteria in the families Enterobacteriaceae and Pseudomonadaceae.

Aliquots of the specimen fluid or tissue homogenate and their serial dilutions are incubated in air, in 10% carbon dioxide, and in the absence of oxygen to determine if the organisms are aerobic, microaerophilic, or anaerobic. Incubation at 37° C for 24 hours will usually reveal the facultative organisms; however, continued incubation may be necessary for microaerophilic bacteria and obligate anaerobes. Antibiotic susceptibility of the cultured isolates then can be determined and species identification made.

A major diagnostic problem in advanced postabortal clostridial sepsis is to differentiate colonization from evidence of life-threatening myonecrosis of the uterus. *C. perfringens* can be recovered from the vagina and cervix of 1 to 9 per cent of healthy pregnant and nonpregnant women, so the presence of gram-positive rods in a direct smear of the endocervix or uterine cavity must be evaluated in the context of the clinical presentation. A tender uterus and positive smear for clostridia in a patient presenting with septic abortion, for example, would likely confirm that diagnosis and warrant immediate surgery.

Treatment

Successful treatment of gas-forming infections is based on early diagnosis and rapid institution of therapy. Because these infections spread rapidly, a delay in diagnosis of 24 hours may be fatal. Initial therapy should be instituted immediately following clinical inspection of the patient and microscopic examination of the infected tissue or fluid.

Surgery and antibiotics remain the cornerstones of treatment. Hyperbaric oxygen has proved to be a beneficial adjunct. However, emergency operative treatment is the most important therapy. Its major objective is to excise all devitalized tissue, which may be identified from the distribution of intravenously administered fluorescein dye. After the dead skin is excised, the incision is extended through the fascia to expose the underlying muscle. Pale muscle that does not contract following stimulation is removed, and local excision of a single muscle group is attempted whenever possible to salvage a functional extremity. If the infection has caused irreversible changes in the muscle, guillotine-type open amputation will be necessary. If the diagnosis is made early, however, radical decompression of the underlying viable muscle may arrest the gas-forming infection and avert amputation. Uterine gas-forming infection usually requires immediate hysterectomy and bilateral salpingo-oophorectomy.

Following debridement, wounds should be left open and treated with a topical antimicrobial cream. The selection of the most effective agent is based on susceptibility of the prevailing pathogens to different creams. Once the wound bacterial count is suppressed below 10^6 bacteria per gram of tissue, and devitalized tissue has been replaced by granulating tissue, coverage of the wound with either an autogenous skin graft or flap is initiated.

Antimicrobial therapy is an important adjunctive measure that is dictated by microscopic examination of the infected tissue. Systemic antibiotics are indicated in all types of gas-forming infections. Penicillin G should be administered intravenously in large doses of 3 million units or more every 3 hours when clostridia or peptostreptococci are suspected. The sodium salt of penicillin is recommended rather than the potassium salt because the latter will increase the hyperkalemia that may be present secondary to hemolysis, tissue destruction, and renal failure. In patients with a history of an allergic reaction to penicillin, desensitization can be accomplished, but except in rare cases it is preferable to select an agent in another class, such as chloramphenicol. Metronidazole or clindamycin is indicated for putrid, gas-forming infections with gram-negative rods suggestive of *Bacteroides*. In nonputrid gas-forming infections with gram-negative rods, coliforms are likely and an aminoglycoside should be administered.

Patients with these gas-forming infections are often hypermetabolic and require considerable nutritional support to avoid weight loss and impaired resistance to infection. The nutritional needs of these patients must be determined and the nutrients supplied, enterally if possible. Intravenous feeding can be employed alternatively to achieve caloric and nitrogen balance.

Hyperbaric oxygen (HBO) appears to be a beneficial adjunct to surgery and antibiotics in the treatment of clostridial myonecrosis. Recommended therapy ranges from 100% oxygen at 3.0 atmospheres absolute (ATA) for 90 minutes to 2.0 ATA intermittently for 5 to 12 hours. HBO exposures at 3.0 ATA for 90 minutes three times a day during the active phase of the infection are well tolerated with few side effects. One of the major benefits of HBO is inhibition of toxin production by the clostridial species. Appropriate tetanus prophylaxis is mandatory.

INFLUENZA

method of
ROBERT F. BETTS, M.D.
University of Rochester School of Medicine and Dentistry
Rochester, New York

Influenza is caused by two types of influenza virus, Type A and Type B. The former occurs almost every year, whereas the latter occurs every 4 to 6 years. Influenza A has hemagglutinin and neuraminidase antigens on its surface. Three major hemagglutinins (H1, H2, and H3) and two major neuraminidase types are recognized. Combinations of these make up separate viruses. Over the last few years H1N1 and H3N2 subtypes have been recognized to circulate either in the same year together or separately in different years, oftentimes interspersed with Type B or concomitantly with Type B.

Three pieces of evidence make the diagnosis highly likely. Influenza almost always strikes in seasonal outbreaks, and the first type of evidence is virologic proof through laboratory means indicating that influenza is in the community. The second is epidemiologic evidence that influenza is present, i.e., excess absenteeism from work and school. The third is the presence of specific symptoms and signs in the patient, with myalgia, cough, and headache predominating.

Prevention

Prevention of influenza is the major means of control. The currently available vaccines, which should be administered in the fall, are safe and effective, and their widespread use for high-risk individuals can provide important protection. Vaccines will provide benefit as soon as 10 days after vaccine administration. Vaccine should also be given to health care workers, since nosocomial influenza is an important cause of increased mortality, and patients acquire infection from nurses and doctors who have not been immunized.

However, the use of vaccines falls short of the mark for control of influenza, for at least three reasons. First, and by far the most important, the majority of high-risk subjects either do not seek out or do not accept vaccine that is available. Second, not all subjects will develop protective immunity following vaccine administration. This is especially true when the circulating strain drifts away from the antigen that is contained in the vaccine. Third, in the years when a completely new surface antigen type (antigenic shift) appears, vaccine for the old type of virus is ineffective, and vaccine for the new type cannot be produced with sufficient speed to be available. Examples of this occurred in 1957 when H2N2 first appeared, and in 1968 when H3N2 appeared.

One other method of control of influenza is the use of daily prophylactic amantadine hydrochloride (Symmetrel) or the soon to be marketed rimantadine hydrochloride (Flumadine). One potential benefit of the use of these drugs is the prevention of acute influenza. Prophylaxis may be useful in two settings: first, for the family members of a patient with clinical influenza, preventive drug treatment could be used for the 5 to 7 days after onset of the index case; second, for the high-risk subject who is vaccinated when it is likely that influenza has already appeared locally and before protective immunity develops. In both of these instances duration of prophylaxis and therefore duration of risk can be shortened (Table 1). However, under most circumstances, in order to prevent influenza, drug must be taken each day during the duration of the influenza season, usually a period of 4 to 6 weeks. It has been assumed that since amantadine is effective in young people prophylactically, it will be useful in the high-risk elderly. There are no available data to confirm or deny that conclusion; the frequency of side effects in young subjects is similar to the maximum influenza attack rate that has been described in the vaccinated elderly.

TABLE 1. **Dosage Schedule for Antivirals in Patients by Age, Weight, and Renal Function**

	Dose in mg	
	Days 1–2	*Days 3–7**
Age ≥ 70	200	100
Age < 70	200	200
Weight < 50 kg	200	100
Creatinine		
≤ 1.4°†	200	200
1.5–3.0	200	100 on even days (4, 6)
≥ 3.1	200 day 1	100 day 3, 6, 9*, 12*

*Dosage schedule can be continued until day 14 for high-risk subjects after vaccination.
†Age or weight takes precedence.

Perhaps rimantadine, with its virtual absence of side effects in young subjects, will offer a lower risk/benefit ratio in the elderly. Carefully conducted studies of each of these compounds in the target population will be necessary to define their role.

Treatment

Although most of the studies showing the benefit of therapy have been conducted in young adults, the evidence that the duration of the influenza syndrome can be shortened by treatment is commanding. There is also evidence that small airways dysfunction, which occurs and progresses over 2 weeks in untreated influenza, can be blocked or at least shortened by such therapy. There is reason to believe that similar results would be achievable in the high-risk populations. It is important to recognize that with appropriate clinical symptoms and influenza in the community the clinician need not and should not wait for specific virologic proof in each patient to initiate therapy. Treatment is most beneficial if initiated early, so to wait for confirmation would render treatment much less effective.

Amantadine hydrochloride (Symmetrel) is the only approved specific anti-influenza agent, although rimantadine hydrochloride (Flumadine) will soon be available. These drugs probably impart their antiviral effect by blocking uncoating of the virus. Concentrations that are achievable in serum will, if used in vitro, inhibit synthesis of virus in tissue culture. Although the evidence is limited, it appears that 100 mg per day of either rimantadine or amantadine has less antiviral effect than 200 mg per day, but the meaning of this from a clinical standpoint is unknown. Based on the knowledge that both of these drugs are cleared by renal excretion and that therapy is necessary for only a few (5 to 7) days, dosage recommendation for treatment using either of these drugs can be made (Table 1).

If a young child is being treated, 6.6 mg per kg up to 200 mg per day is used (Table 1).

There is also limited but convincing evidence that fever is reduced within 10 to 12 hours of initiation of antipyretic therapy, compared with 24 hours if antiviral medication is used alone. In spite of the more rapid defervescence shown with aspirin and presumably acetaminophen, the overall feeling of well-being is improved more rapidly with antiviral than with antipyretic therapy. Pulmonary function is not improved by antipyretics. Logic, therefore, dictates that acetaminophen in an appropriate dose be taken along with the antiviral medication at the outset of symptoms. Thereafter, the antipyretic should be taken twice at 4-hour intervals and then discontinued while the antiviral is maintained. In addition, fluid intake should be increased appropriately to replace losses caused by temperature elevation. Bed rest should be prescribed as needed. "Prophylactic" antibiotics should not be used, because there is no evidence that they will prevent secondary bacterial infection.

Complications

Most cases of pneumonia following influenza virus infection are caused by bacteria as a secondary process. Some patients, however, will have pure viral pneumonia. The bacteriology of pneumonia following influenza is somewhat different from most cases of community-acquired pneumonia. Experience has demonstrated that in addition to pneumococcal disease, pneumonia due to *Staphylococcus aureus, Haemophilus influenzae,* and Enterobacteriaceae can follow influenza. Often these infections can be controlled only by parenteral antibiotic therapy, and hospitalization is required.

The spectrum of empiric therapy for secondary bacterial pneumonia following influenza needs to include all of these possible bacteria. A drug such as cefotaxime (Claforan), with appropriate spectrum to match the possible causes, should be considered. Otherwise, a combination of antibiotics is necessary. If the pneumonia has the characteristics of primary viral pneumonia, an antiviral should be used as well, although proof of its efficacy in this setting is lacking. Once sputum cultures are mature the antibiotic regimen should be narrowed to the specific agent that has been identified. The severe consequences of the infection, including fever and hypoxia, which may aggravate cardiac disease and produce heart failure and arrhythmias, probably contribute in a major way to the excess mortality seen in those individuals with heart or lung disease during influenza outbreaks. Administration of oxygen

and control of the heart failure and arrhythmias are essential in these cases.

In young children the major complication of influenza is Reye's syndrome, which occurs more commonly following influenza B than following influenza A. To reduce the incidence of Reye's syndrome, acetaminophen is recommended rather than aspirin.

LEISHMANIASIS

method of
EDGAR M. CARVALHO, M.D., and
ROBERTO BADARO, M.D.
University of Bahia, Salvador
Bahia, Brazil

Leishmania species are protozoa that cause a broad spectrum of clinical manifestations, including self-healing, chronic progressive, and acute fatal disease. The organisms are transmitted to humans by the bite of sandflies, in which they inhabit the intestine as flagellates (promastigotes) and from there enter macrophages and become nonflagellated, oval amastigotes. Parasite replication in man occurs only in the amastigote form, and only within mononuclear phagocytes. Four different species (*L. tropica, L. mexicana, L. braziliensis,* and *L. donovani*) are important as etiologic agents of human disease.

The classic manifestation of cutaneous leishmaniasis is a circular ulcer (*L. tropica*) with well-defined raised borders and a bed of granulation tissue. It is observed in Mediterranean areas, tropical Africa, China, India, the Soviet Union, and Iran. The lesion, called an oriental sore, spontaneously heals with scarring within several months to a year. In Central America and South America, similar lesions are also seen but the disease is caused by *L. mexicana* and *L. braziliensis.* In cutaneous leishmaniasis of the New World, however, vegetative skin lesions are prominent in some cases. Although the primary cutaneous ulcer may heal without therapy, treatment should be recommended for all patients, since metastatic lesions in the nose or mouth may appear weeks or years after cicatrization of the skin. This disease, called mucocutaneous leishmaniasis, is associated with severe tissue damage and is more difficult to treat. In a few patients with cutaneous leishmaniasis, there is no cellular immune response to leishmanial antigens, and uncontrolled parasite multiplication in multiple nodular lesions (diffuse cutaneous leishmaniasis) occurs. The diagnosis of cutaneous leishmaniasis can be made by culturing aspirates or biopsy material from the lesion. The intradermal skin test is positive in over 95 per cent of the patients. However, in the first 2 months of the disease, the test is positive in only 70 per cent of the patients.

Visceral leishmaniasis, or kala-azar, is most often caused by *L. donovani* and is characterized by fever, hepatosplenomegaly, hyperglobulinemia, anemia, and leukopenia. Patients with untreated visceral leishmaniasis die after months of this wasting disease, usually from bacterial infections or bleeding. Diagnosis of visceral leishmaniasis is made by culture or identification of leishmania in aspirated material from the spleen or bone marrow. The *Leishmania* skin test is negative in visceral leishmaniasis, but serum diagnosis may be done by ELISA or immunofluorescence.

Treatment

Pentavalent antimony (Sb^v) is the drug of choice for leishmaniasis. It is available either as sodium stibogluconate (Pentostam) or as *N*-methylglucamine antimonate (Glucantime). Pentostam is used in the Old World and is the only form available in the United States from the Centers for Disease Control. Glucantime is used in Central and South America and in some regions of Europe.

The parenteral route is the only safe and efficient way to use antimony. The drug is rapidly eliminated in the urine, and after 6 hours, more than 80 per cent has been excreted. About 12 per cent of the antimony dose is retained and has a half-life of 32.8 ± 3.8 hours. After repeated injections, a rise in the baseline level of retained antimony can be observed over the initial week of therapy. It takes 5 to 13 days to saturate the compartment. The antimony is concentrated in the liver and the spleen. It is not known, however, how much antimony is present in the skin and mucosal membranes.

For simple cutaneous leishmaniasis, pentavalent antimony (Sb^v) should be administered at a dose of 10 to 20 mg Sb^v per kg per day, for at least 21 days. For multiple cutaneous lesions or any lesion localized in the upper trunk or face, the maximum tolerated dose should be tried. Experience has shown that courses ranging from 20 to 30 mg Sb^v per kg per day for 30 consecutive days could be given (if no complications appear), or may be divided into two courses with an interval of at least a week. If after 30 days of therapy any sign of the disease persists, another course should be considered. Visceral leishmaniasis usually responds better to antimony than mucosal disease. Several therapeutic schedules have been tried with relative success. However, after well-controlled trials in Kenyan kala-azar, the dosage of 20 mg Sb^v per kg per day for 20 to 30 days is the recommended schedule.

Both Pentostam and Glucantime are best given by slow intravenous infusion, over at least 3 minutes. No diluent is usually necessary, unless the patient develops thrombosis at the venous inoculation site. In such cases, the drug is mixed in 50 ml of 5 per cent dextrose in water and given over a 10-minute period. Intramuscular injection is painful but may be used when small volumes are administered.

Pentostam is available as a 100-ml sterile solution containing 100 mg of antimony per ml. Glucantime is available in 5-ml ampules with 85 mg of Sb^v per ml. The maximum daily dose should not exceed 1700 mg of Sb^v for adults, or 850 mg for children. With the recommended dosage, the common side effects are arthralgia, myalgia, nausea, vomiting, and anorexia. Renal insufficiency and EKG abnormalities (nonspecific ST-T wave changes and arrhythmias) have been reported, as well as sudden death in patients under treatment for leishmaniasis. Therefore, renal function should be monitored and EKG should be performed during Sb^v therapy.

In cases of antimony unresponsiveness, the drugs of choice are pentamidine and amphotericin B. Both drugs are as effective as antimony, but the side effects are more serious. Pentamidine isothionate is used at 4 mg per kg per day for 10 days. Two or three courses may be necessary. Blood sugar levels should be monitored. Amphotericin B is given intravenously at 0.5 to 1.0 mg per kg per day for 30 to 60 days. Renal and cardiac toxicity should be monitored.

Cryotherapy (freezing of the lesions) or exposing the skin to elevated temperatures (39° to 41° C [102.5° to 106° F]) may improve the skin lesions. Other drugs such as rifampin, ketoconazole, itraconazole, and topically administered paromomycin or methylbenzethonium chloride have been effective in the treatment of cutaneous leishmaniasis in noncontrolled trials. Apparently cured skin lesions in New World leishmaniasis may recur as mucosal disease years later. These treatments currently cannot be recommended in treatment of cutaneous leishmaniasis caused by *L. mexicana* or *L. braziliensis*. Allopurinol and its derivatives have in vitro activity against leishmania, and controlled trials should be performed to determine the role of allopurinol in visceral leishmaniasis.

There is no chemoprophylaxis for leishmaniasis, but there is an increasing interest in the search for antigens capable of inducing a host immune response capable of destroying leishmania. This could lead to the development of a specific vaccine. The knowledge that gamma interferon is the lymphokine capable of activating macrophages to kill leishmania has increased the interest in the use of this cytokine, predominantly in visceral leishmaniasis and diffuse cutaneous leishmaniasis, in which there is a depression of the cellular immune response to leishmanial antigens. Gamma interferon is effective in leishmania infections in animals and could be valuable in the future treatment of leishmaniasis.

LEPROSY
(Hansen's Disease)

method of
JI BAOHONG, M.D.
Leprosy Unit, World Health Organization
Geneva, Switzerland

Leprosy is a chronic infectious disease caused by *Mycobacterium leprae*. Although the organism has not yet been cultivated in bacteriologic media or tissue cultures, it can be grown in the mouse footpad and in the armadillo. Humans are the only proven reservoir of *Mycobacterium leprae*. Naturally acquired leprosy has recently been detected in armadillos and nonhuman primates (chimpanzee and mangabey monkey), but the significance, in terms of reservoirs, of such observations is to be ascertained. The exact mode of transmission is not clear, but contacts of leprosy patients have a higher risk of contracting the disease. Millions of bacilli are released daily in the nasal discharges of untreated multibacillary leprosy patients, which then probably enter the body through the upper respiratory tract and possibly through broken skin. The World Health Organization (WHO) estimates that currently there are about 10 to 12 million cases of leprosy worldwide. High prevalences are found in the tropical and subtropical belt of Africa and southern Asia, and the disease is also endemic today in South and Central America. Although over 300 new leprosy cases are reported each year in certain areas of the United States, mainly southern Louisiana, Texas, southern California, and Hawaii, nearly 90 per cent of these new cases are in immigrants from endemic areas in Southeast Asia, Mexico, and the Philippines.

The manifestation of the disease varies from patient to patient in a continuous spectrum of types, and these depend mainly on the immune response of the hosts. Based on clinical, bacteriologic, histologic, and immunologic findings, Ridley and Jopling proposed a classification dividing leprosy patients into five groups. At one end of the spectrum, tuberculoid leprosy (TT), patients develop a high level of cell-mediated immunity, which results in the killing and clearing of bacilli in the tissue, and they present single or few skin lesions with sharply defined borders and localized but severe nerve involvement. At the other end, lepromatous leprosy (LL), patients exhibit a selective immunologic unresponsiveness to *Mycobacterium leprae* antigen, so that the organisms inexorably multiply in the body and cause nerve damage as well as numerous skin lesions which are diffused bilaterally and generally symmetrically distributed. The majority of patients are in the borderline categories between the two polar types and are further divided into three groups on an immunologic basis—borderline tuberculoid (BT, nearer the tuberculoid end), borderline lepromatous (BL, nearer the lepromatous end), and mid-borderline (BB, between BT and BL). Apart from the five groups, there is an indeterminate form (I) of leprosy, which presents single or few macular lesions with alterations of color and impairment of sensation, and a primary neuritic (pure neural) form of leprosy. These two forms have been established as definite clinical entities, but their frequency, significance, and prognosis still remain unclear. The relevance of classification to the present strategy for leprosy control mainly relates to the choice of appropriate chemotherapeutic regimens required for the treatment of individual patients and the identification of the more infectious patients as the principal targets for chemotherapy. Although the Ridley-Jopling classification is relatively more scientific, its general use is mostly limited to research purposes, and the majority of field workers are not able to apply the classification properly because of the limited facilities available under field conditions. In this context, the WHO Study Group on Chemotherapy of Leprosy for Control Programmes classified the disease as multibacillary and paucibacillary leprosy according to the degree of skin-smear positivity. This is essentially an operational definition to serve as a basis for chemotherapy for the two different categories. The WHO Expert Committee on Leprosy at its sixth meeting (1987) endorsed this classification with minor modifications. Paucibacillary leprosy refers to the initial skin smear–negative cases only and includes TT and the majority of I and BT cases, whereas multibacillary leprosy refers to the initial skin smear–positive cases and includes all BB, BL, and LL cases.

Since leprosy primarily affects the peripheral nerves and secondarily involves skin and certain other tissues, involvement and later destruction of peripheral nerves is a universal characteristic of the disease. Although leprosy mimics many dermatologic and neurologic disorders, the diagnosis can usually be made by careful clinical examination supported by skin smears. Occasionally histologic examination is necessary. The diagnosis is based on the presence of one or more of the following cardinal signs: (1) loss of cutaneous sensation, (2) thickening of nerves, and (3) presence of acid-fast bacilli in smears taken from the skin lesions as demonstrated by the Ziehl-Neelsen method of staining. The first two signs are present in the vast majority of paucibacillary cases; in early multibacillary cases these two signs may not be evident, but acid-fast bacilli are always present and therefore support the diagnosis. Since diagnosing leprosy is a serious matter, physicians in the United States who are relatively unfamiliar with the disease may contact the U.S. Public Health Service, Gillis W. Long, Hansen's Disease Center at Carville, Louisiana (Phone: 1-800-642-2477) or a regional Hansen's Disease Center. Physicians from other countries may also be able to contact similar referral facilities in their own countries.

Chemotherapy of Leprosy

Effective chemotherapy of leprosy became possible for the first time with the introduction of dapsone. Because it is an effective, cheap, and safe drug, since the late 1940s dapsone monotherapy has been widely used for the treatment of all types of leprosy. However, the bacterial population in multibacillary leprosy is very large, and therefore dapsone-resistant mutants and possibly mutants resistant to other drugs are present even before treatment. Although the majority of drug-susceptible organisms are killed during dapsone monotherapy, the dapsone-resistant mutants survive and selectively multiply. Finally, they replace the susceptible organisms in the bacterial population, which results in secondary dapsone-resistant leprosy. In the course of time, primary dapsone-resistant leprosy, i.e., that resistant to dapsone before treatment, also occurs as a result of infections with organisms from the secondary dapsone-resistant patients. Unlike secondary resistance, primary dapsone resistance probably occurs in at least as high a proportion of paucibacillary leprosy cases as of multibacillary cases, although one cannot demonstrate resistance in paucibacillary patients through inoculation of mice as they have too few bacilli in their skin biopsy specimens. Because of widespread dapsone resistance, a WHO Study Group recommended multidrug therapy (MDT) for both multibacillary and paucibacillary leprosy. For multibacillary leprosy, it is recommended that at least two additional drugs be combined with dapsone, whereas for paucibacillary leprosy, rifampicin should be administered along with dapsone.

Antileprotic Drugs

One of the basic concepts of MDT is that the treatment be administered for only a limited period and, by implication, that only bactericidal drugs be considered as candidates for MDT regimens. Only four types of bactericidal antileprotic drugs, which act by different mechanisms, are currently available—dapsone, rifampicin, clofazimine, and the thioamides (prothionamide/ethionamide).

Dapsone. Dapsone (DDS) is available as 25-, 50-, and 100-mg tablets. The routine dosage is 100 mg daily for adults and 1 to 2 mg per kg per day for children. It acts as a synthetase inhibitor in the folate synthesizing enzyme system of *Mycobacterium leprae,* and a dose of 100 mg daily is weakly bactericidal against *Mycobacterium leprae.* Dapsone is rapidly and nearly completely absorbed when taken orally, and its half-life is relatively long, with an average of about 28 hours. *Mycobacterium leprae* is extremely susceptible to dapsone in the sense that the minimal inhibitory concentration (MIC) of dapsone is extremely low, being on the order of 3 ng per ml as studied through the mouse footpad experiments. After ingestion of a single dose of 100 mg of dapsone, the peak blood level is 500 times the MIC and measurable amounts can be found in the blood even 10 days later. It is well distributed throughout the body and ultimately is excreted for the most part in the urine.

A variety of side effects have been attributed to dapsone, including hemolytic anemia and a reduced life span of red blood cells, various skin rashes, gastrointestinal complaints, agranulocytosis, hepatitis, psychosis, and peripheral neuropathies. Most of these effects are very rare. The so-called DDS syndrome, which is also rare, usually develops within the first 6 weeks after the start of therapy and consists of exfoliative dermatitis and/or other skin rashes, generalized lymphadenopathy, hepatosplenomegaly, fever, and hepatitis. When this syndrome does occur, dapsone should be discontinued immediately and corticosteroids should be given. The most common side effect with dapsone is anemia. However, this is usually very mild and well tolerated, unless the patient has a complete glucose-6-phosphate dehydrogenase (G6PD) deficiency. The safety of dapsone in pregnancy seems to be fairly well established, and no evidence of teratogenicity has been observed.

As mentioned earlier, dapsone resistance is a result of selective multiplication of resistant mutants during dapsone monotherapy, and it can be classified into three different levels of resistance: low degree (resistance equivalent to a dose of up to 1 mg daily), intermediate degree (resistance equivalent to a dose of up to 10 mg daily), and high degree (resistance equivalent to a dose of up to 100 mg daily). Until now, the vast majority of secondary dapsone-resistant leprosy cases have high-degree resistance, whereas most of the primary dapsone-resistant leprosy cases have low-degree resistance. The reason for this difference is still unclear. It is expected that in cases with low- and even intermediate-degree resistance the patient may respond to treatment with dapsone in full dosage. Therefore, there is justification for employing dapsone in the treatment of leprosy but in combination with other antileprotic drug(s) even without testing for drug susceptibility, as such testing is too time-consuming and too expensive to be applied as routine.

Rifampicin. Rifampicin (rifampin)* is a semisynthetic broad-spectrum antibiotic and is available as 150- and 300-mg capsules. It acts by inhibiting the DNA-dependent RNA polymerase of the organisms, thereby interfering with bacterial RNA synthesis. Rifampicin is rapidly absorbed from the gastrointestinal tract and distributed throughout the body. About two thirds of the absorbed drug is ultimately excreted via the gastrointestinal tract. It is much more rapidly bactericidal than other antileprotic drugs. *Mycobacterium leprae* recovered from biopsy specimens 3 to 4 days after a single 600- to 1500-mg dose of

---

*This use of rifampin is not listed by the manufacturer.

rifampicin failed to multiply in mice, indicating that at least 99 per cent of the bacilli are killed by the drug. It is because of this that rifampicin is the most important component of MDT for both paucibacillary and multibacillary leprosy patients. Based on the evidence that no difference in the bactericidal activity, as measured by serial mouse footpad inoculation, has been detected between the daily and the monthly administration of rifampicin, the WHO Study Group recommended the supervised administration of 600 mg of rifampicin at monthly intervals for adults. For children, the dose can be calculated at 10 mg per kg of body weight. The monthly rifampicin administration not only greatly reduces the costs but also reduces the frequency and severity of side effects as compared with daily administration of the drug.

The major side effect of rifampicin is hepatotoxicity, but this is extremely rare with monthly administration unless rifampicin is combined with other hepatotoxic drugs such as thioamides. Although "flu" syndrome and another syndrome combining shock, hemolytic anemia, and renal failure had been reported in the treatment of tuberculosis with once-weekly or twice-weekly rifampicin administration, very few "flu" syndrome occurrences have been reported in leprosy patients with monthly administration of 600 mg of rifampicin. Other side effects include skin rashes and mild gastrointestinal symptoms. Rifampicin can be safely used during pregnancy.

Secondary rifampicin-resistant leprosy has been detected after rifampicin monotherapy in multibacillary patients or after administration of rifampicin with dapsone for treatment in cases of relapse following initial dapsone monotherapy. A great majority of the latter cases end up with resistance to both dapsone and rifampicin if there is further relapse. Despite its extraordinary bactericidal effect, the development of secondary resistance to rifampicin, when used as monotherapy, occurs earlier than in the case of dapsone monotherapy. Rifampicin should therefore always be combined with other antileprotic drugs capable of preventing the development of rifampicin resistance.

Clofazimine. Clofazimine (Lamprene; B663) is an imino-phenazine dye and is available as 50- and 100-mg capsules. It is weakly bactericidal against *Mycobacterium leprae*. It also exhibits anti-inflammatory activity, but the mechanisms of action are unclear. The metabolism of clofazimine has been only partially elucidated. It is absorbed to the extent of about 70 per cent via the gastrointestinal tract and is deposited mostly in fatty tissues and cells of the reticuloendothelial system, including the skin. For treatment of mul-

tibacillary leprosy, the routine dosage recommended by the WHO Study Group is 50 mg daily plus 300 mg once monthly; for the treatment of erythema nodosum leprosum (ENL), higher doses, beginning with 100 mg two or three* times daily, are required (see below).

The most common side effect is a reddish-black pigmentation of the skin which normally develops within 4 to 8 weeks after the start of the therapy in patients with active lesions. The severity of pigmentation is dose-dependent and is intensified in the areas of the lesions. The pigmentation diminishes gradually in 6 to 24 months after discontinuation of the drug. Pigmentation may also be seen in the mucous membrane. Sebum, sweat, feces, and urine also show a reddish coloration. Because of the pigmentation, some light-skinned patients refuse to take the drug. Gastrointestinal symptoms, such as nausea, vomiting, crampy abdominal pain, and diarrhea, are common but mild in patients treated with 50 mg daily. However, in patients receiving higher doses (usually over 100 mg daily), these symptoms may appear more serious. Another common side effect is ichthyosis, resulting from the anticholinergic activity of the drug.

Ethionamide/Prothionamide. These thioamides are virtually interchangeable and give cross-resistance with each other. Both drugs are available as 250-mg tablets. Ethionamide† and prothionamide‡ are bactericidal against *Mycobacterium leprae* to about the same extent as are dapsone and clofazimine. The daily dose for adults is 250 to 375 mg daily, and 5 to 7.5 mg per kg of body weight daily for children. The peak blood concentration after a dose of 375 mg in adults is 60 times the MIC. The drugs are absorbed from the gastrointestinal tract and are excreted mainly in the urine.

Ethionamide and prothionamide were recommended by the WHO Study Group as alternatives to clofazimine in the MDT regimen for multibacillary cases in patients unable to take clofazimine. However, as it has been found that hepatotoxicity is quite common when ethionamide or prothionamide is combined with rifampicin, even with monthly administration, the WHO Expert Committee on Leprosy (1987) did not recommend the use of this substitute in the MDT regimen unless it was absolutely necessary. When used under exceptional situations, the drugs must be given with great caution and under close medical supervision. Liver function tests must be done

---

*300 mg per day exceeds manufacturer's recommendation of 200 mg per day maximum dose.
†This use is not listed by the manufacturer.
‡Investigational drug in the United States.

initially and periodically thereafter. Other gastrointestinal symptoms, such as nausea, vomiting, abdominal pain, and anorexia, are common and therefore the patients' compliance to self-administration is poor.

Treatment Regimens

Standard regimens were recommended by the WHO Study Group on Chemotherapy of Leprosy for Control Programmes in 1982 and endorsed by the WHO Expert Committee at its sixth meeting in 1987. The standard regimens are as follows:

Paucibacillary leprosy: Rifampicin, 600 mg once a month for 6 months, plus dapsone, 100 mg (1 to 2 mg per kg) daily for 6 months. The administration of rifampicin should invariably be fully supervised, but dapsone may be given unsupervised. If treatment is interrupted, the regimen should commence where it left off so as to complete the full course.

Multibacillary leprosy: Rifampicin,* 600 mg once monthly, supervised; plus dapsone, 100 mg daily, self-administered; plus clofazimine, 300 mg† once monthly, supervised, and 50 mg daily, self-administered. The combined therapy should be given for at least 2 years and should be continued, wherever possible, up to smear negativity. MDT should be given to all categories of skin smear–positive multibacillary patients. In order to prevent relapse caused by dapsone resistance, skin smear–negative multibacillary patients who are still taking dapsone monotherapy should also be brought into an MDT program.

The standard regimens have been widely accepted, and large numbers of patients have been treated with them. They have also proved to be effective and acceptable to patients, including those with dapsone-resistant cases. Compliance and regularity of treatment have been excellent, and side effects, including skin pigmentation due to clofazimine, have not been a serious problem. Operationally, the regimens have proved to be feasible in a variety of countries and in different types of programs.

Post-Treatment Surveillance

Patients who have completed the MDT course should be kept under surveillance, mainly to detect relapses and recognize reactional episodes. Clinical examination once a year for a minimum of 2 years is recommended in paucibacillary cases, and both clinical and bacteriologic examination should be carried out once a year for a minimum of 5 years in multibacillary cases.

---

*This use of rifampicin is not listed by the manufacturer.

†300 mg exceeds the manufacturer's recommendation of 200 mg per day maximum dose.

Relapse in multibacillary cases (including multibacillary cases erroneously classified as paucibacillary leprosy and treated for 6 months) is relatively easy to recognize clinically and must be confirmed bacteriologically by skin smear. Where facilities are available, biopsy and mouse footpad inoculation may be done to confirm the diagnosis. Relapse in paucibacillary cases can be difficult to distinguish clinically from late reversal reaction occurring after completion of therapy. Available data indicate that relapse in paucibacillary and multibacillary cases following the use of the WHO recommended MDT regimens is quite infrequent.

Management of Leprosy Reactions

Immunologically mediated episodes of acute or subacute inflammation known as "reaction" may occur in any type of leprosy except indeterminate, and unless promptly and adequately treated can result in permanent deformity. Most reactions belong to one of the two major types, erythema nodosum leprosum and reversal reaction.

Erythema Nodosum Leprosum (ENL or Jopling's Type II Reaction)

This type of reaction occurs in LL and BL leprosy. It appears to be less of a problem in programs using MDT than in schemes based on dapsone monotherapy, obviously owing to the anti-inflammatory activity of clofazimine in the MDT regimen.

Mild ENL consists of crops of ENL papules with low-degree fever and malaise, and can be treated with analgesics, either aspirin or acetaminophen, or antimonials.

ENL is graded severe when there is high fever along with severe general malaise; when even moderate fever lasts more than 4 weeks; when the papules become pustular and progress to ulceration or coalesce to form hard, tender sheets in the skin; when the lymph nodes become very tender and enlarged; when the nerves become painful or markedly tender or when there is any loss of nerve function; when there is iridocyclitis, orchitis, periostitis, or joint swelling; or when urine examinations reveal persistent albuminuria with red cells present under the microscope. Such severe ENL patients should be immediately hospitalized for treatment.

The treatment of choice for severe ENL is thalidomide,* because it is relatively inexpensive, acts rapidly in controlling ENL, and has fewer toxic effects than corticosteroids. Patients are given 200 mg twice daily, and with this dose

---

*Investigational drug in the United States.

the ENL reaction is usually controlled within 48 to 72 hours. The dose can then gradually be reduced to 50 mg daily. It must, however, be pointed out that because of its well-known teratogenicity, it should be given only to males and postmenopausal females. Women of child-bearing age should never be given thalidomide.

Prednisolone, the cheapest and most widely available corticosteroid, can also rapidly control ENL, but many severely ill patients require continuous and often high doses. For the treatment of severe ENL, the patients are given prednisolone, 30 to 60 mg daily, and in such doses ENL is generally controlled within 24 to 72 hours. The dose of prednisolone can then gradually be reduced. In general, the total duration of the steroid treatment for ENL should preferably not exceed 12 weeks.

If ENL recurs after thalidomide or prednisolone treatment has been stopped, a repeat course will be necessary. In steroid-dependent cases it may be useful to supplement the prednisolone therapy with higher doses of clofazimine. Since clofazimine often takes 4 to 6 weeks to develop its full effect, it may not be employed as the sole drug for the treatment of severe ENL. The patients may be put on clofazimine, 100 mg two or three times daily for 3 months, then gradually reduced to 100 mg daily. In the meantime, prednisolone can be gradually withdrawn. The major problems in the case of high doses of clofazimine therapy are the intolerance of the drug by some patients due to its gastrointestinal side effects and the nonacceptance by some patients due to skin pigmentation.

The antileprotic treatment should continue unchanged during ENL reaction.

Reversal Reaction (Jopling's Type I Reaction)

Reveral reaction occurs mostly in BT, BB, and BL leprosy and usually soon after the onset of successful chemotherapy, although it may also appear after the completion of MDT. During the reaction, some or all of the skin lesions may become raised and erythematous, there may be enlargement of pre-existing skin lesions, new skin lesions may appear, nerve thickening may increase, and nerve pain and nerve tenderness may occur accompanied by deterioration of nerve function. In some cases of paucibacillary leprosy, there may be difficulties in distinguishing between reversal reaction and relapse. However, in general, in the case of reversal reaction the onset is more acute, the skin lesions are considerably more raised and erythematous with severe edema, and the nerve involvement is more acute. A 1-month course of corticosteroid treatment as a trial may help in the differential diagnosis, as reversal reaction normally responds rapidly to corticosteroids but relapse will not respond satisfactorily.

For mild reversal reactions, i.e., slight swelling and redness of skin lesions with or without appearance of new lesions, or mild nerve tenderness without pain or deterioration of function, no specific treatment is required except analgesics. However, the patient must be seen at least once every 2 weeks and asked to return at once if the symptoms become more severe.

Reversal reactions are graded severe if there is marked fever and malaise; when there is edema of hands and feet; when the skin lesions ulcerate; when there is nerve pain and tenderness, with or without deterioration of nerve function; and whenever a mild reaction lasts more than 6 weeks. The patient with severe reversal reaction must be hospitalized, and corticosteroids, the most effective treatment for controlling reversal reaction, should be given immediately. The dose of corticosteroids must be determined according to the severity of the reaction, the body weight of the patient, and the response to treatment. The doses used should be sufficient to relieve both nerve pain and nerve tenderness. Patients usually start on higher doses of prednisolone, e.g., 20 to 30 mg twice daily. As the reaction becomes controlled, the dose of prednisolone can gradually decrease. A maintenance dose of prednisolone, e.g., 5 to 10 mg daily, lasting for several months may be necessary in some instances if there is a tendency for recurrence of reaction on complete stoppage of prednisolone.

If reversal reaction occurs during chemotherapy, the antileprotic treatment should not be stopped but should continue unchanged.

Quiet Nerve Paralysis (QNP; Silent Neuritis)

It is well known that neuritis in leprosy, identified by nerve thickening associated with acute or subacute nerve pain and tenderness, is frequently the precursor of irreversible nerve damage. However, nerves can become paralyzed in leprosy patients quietly, without pain or tenderness of the concerned nerve. This type of paralysis is referred to as "quiet nerve paralysis" (QNP) or "silent neuritis." The condition is usually missed in its early stages, when chances of recovery are high. This subject has not received sufficient attention, and therefore information regarding the factors or events that promote its occurrence is very limited. Although the frequency of QNP in leprosy is not well documented, it appears to be an important cause of nerve damage.

In order to detect QNP as early as possible, it is necessary not only to look for painful tender nerves but, more importantly, to look for signs of loss of motor and sensory function. Whenever the onset of QNP is confirmed, corticosteroid therapy should be instituted without delay. The use of corticosteroids in substantial doses (e.g., starting with prednisolone 60 mg daily) over a period of 3 to 6 months is reported to prevent permanent nerve damage in a high proportion of cases, particularly when the condition is identified and treated in time.

MALARIA
method of
MARTIN S. WOLFE, M.D.
George Washington University Medical School
Washington, D.C.

Malaria occurs worldwide, particularly in tropical areas, and is a serious potential threat to those living in or traveling to these areas. Malaria must be suspected in anyone living in or returning from a malaria endemic location who has fever, chills, and headache. It must be considered even if the patient claims to have taken malaria prophylactic drugs, since with the widespread occurrence of chloroquine-resistant *Plasmodium falciparum* (CRPF) malaria, no chemoprophylactic regimen can be assuredly protective. Even where *P. falciparum* remains sensitive to chloroquine, malaria can occur unless adequate suppressive medication is taken for at least 4 weeks after leaving the malaria endemic area. Less commonly, *P. vivax* and *P. ovale* malaria may occur for up to 3 years after the last exposure, unless primaquine is taken to eradicate the exoerythrocytic (liver) stage of these species.

Symptoms

The typical malaria paroxysm consists of shaking chills, high fever, and headache, followed by severe sweating. Attacks may recur at 48-hour intervals (or every 72 hours in *P. malariae* infection). Often, however, such periodicity is lacking, or typical paroxysms do not occur at all, especially in *P. falciparum* malaria, which characteristically causes an intermittent fever. Malaria mimics other infections and may cause malaise, myalgias, arthralgias, cough, or diarrhea, among other signs and symptoms. The liver and spleen are often enlarged. When severe, *P. falciparum* infections may cause cerebral malaria, renal failure, pulmonary edema, or hemolytic anemia, which can lead to a fatal outcome.

Diagnosis

In any febrile patient who may have been exposed to malaria, both thick and thin blood smears should be stained and examined promptly; a freshly prepared Giemsa solution is the preferred stain, but a Wright's stain may be used. A single negative result from a thin smear cannot rule out malaria; sometimes, thick and thin smears must be repeated every 6 hours to make the diagnosis. Malaria infection can also be partially suppressed or masked by subtherapeutic doses of antimalarial or certain antibiotic drugs. A technician experienced in diagnosing malaria should examine all smears. Once malaria is diagnosed, the species must be identified and the patient's travel history reviewed to determine if chloroquine-resistant *P. falciparum* malaria is likely.

Treatment (Table 1)

Chloroquine-Sensitive Plasmodium falciparum Infection—Uncomplicated

Plasmodium falciparum remains sensitive to chloroquine in Central America; Haiti and the Dominican Republic; northwest tropical Africa; and the Middle East. Malaria developing in someone while in or coming from these areas almost invariably occurs in those not on appropriate chloroquine or other drug prophylaxis. Sporadic chloroquine resistance occurs in South Asia, and if malaria develops in someone in or from this area who is on appropriate chloroquine suppression, treatment should be with other drugs used for CRPF malaria. Treatment with chloroquine in an uncomplicated case with low parasitemia (less than 3 per cent of red blood cells parasitized) is usually adequate. This is given with 25 mg per kg chloroquine base over a 48-hour period. Chloroquine comes as chloroquine phosphate, generically in 250 mg salt (equal to 150 mg base) tablets, or as Aralen in 500 mg salt (equal to 300 mg base tablets). An initial dose of 10 mg base per kg is followed at 6, 24, and 48 hours later with 5 mg base per kg. Chloroquine is generally well tolerated, but side effects in some patients may include headache, dizziness, blurred vision, gastrointestinal upset, or pruritus. The pruritus may be particularly severe in natives of Africa. Patients must be closely monitored during treatment with at least daily blood smears to assure that the drug is adequately absorbed and that possible CRPF is not present. If severe vomiting or diarrhea is present, parenteral chloroquine hydrochloride may be administered intramuscularly as 200 mg base every 6 hours until oral therapy can be taken. Caution must be exerted to avoid rapid intravenous infusion or excessively high doses, particularly in infants and young children. With adequate treatment of a chloroquine-susceptible, uncomplicated *P. falciparum* malaria episode, the patient should improve and parasitemia should clear in about 48 hours. The persistence of typical sausage-shaped *P. falciparum* gametocytes (sexual forms) after clinical improvement and clearance of asexual blood schi-

TABLE 1. **Treatment Regimens for Malaria**

Form	Drug	Dosage	
		Adults	*Children*

P. falciparum
  Acquired where chloro-
  quine resistance does
  not occur
    and
	Chloroquine phosphate*
	(Aralen)
		600 mg base orally stat; then 300 mg at 6 hr; then 300 mg daily for next 2 days (total of 1500 mg base)	10 mg base/kg orally stat, then 5 mg/kg as per adult doses

P. malariae	Chloroquine hydrochlo- ride intramuscularly	If patient is vomiting, give 200 mg IM q 6 hr until oral ingestion possible (maximum 800 mg/day)	IM chloroquine not recommended

P. falciparum
  Acquired in areas with
  chloroquine-resistant
  strains
	Quinine sulfate (salt)
	    plus
		650 mg tid for 3 days	25 mg/kg/day in 3 doses for 3 days

	Pyrimethamine-sulfadox- ine (Fansidar)	Single 3-tablet dose	See Table 3—same doses

P. falciparum—alterna-
  tive; or where resis-
  tance occurs to pyri-
  methamine-sulfadoxine
	Quinine sulfate (salt)
	    plus
		650 mg tid for 3 days	25 mg/kg/day in 3 doses for 3 days

	Tetracycline	250 mg qid for 7 days	5 mg/kg qid for 7 days

P. vivax and P. ovale
  (relapsing forms)
	Chloroquine phosphate
	    followed by
		As above—orally	As above—orally

	Primaquine phosphate (base)†	15 mg base daily for 14 days	0.3 mg/kg base daily for 14 days

Severe or complicated
  (usually P. falciparum)
	Quinine dihydrochloride‡
	(salt) intravenously
	(see text)
	    or
		10 mg/kg in 300 ml normal saline IV over 2–4 hours; repeat every 8 hours until oral therapy can be started (maximum 1800 mg/day)	25 mg/kg/day; give ⅓ of daily dose in normal saline or 5% dextrose over 2 to 4 hours; repeat every 8 hours until oral therapy can be started (maximum 1800 mg/day). See text

	Quinidine gluconate (IV)	See text	

*500 mg salt tablet contains 300 mg base; 250 mg salt tablet contains 150 mg base.
†Screen for G6PD deficiency before administration.
‡Available through the Centers for Disease Control, 404-639-2888.

zont forms does not indicate treatment failure or drug resistance. Gametocytes do not cause disease, and they will clear spontaneously in due course.

Chloroquine-Resistant Plasmodium falciparum Infection—Uncomplicated

Chloroquine-resistant *P. falciparum* malaria presently occurs in most of tropical Africa; Southeast Asia; Papua New Guinea and other malarious areas in the Southwest Pacific (Oceania); and the Para-Amazon region of South America (Table 2). As indicated above, CRPF occurs sporadically in South Asia (India, Pakistan, Sri Lanka), but the majority of cases appear to be with sensitive strains of *P. falciparum*. Many of those acquiring CRPF have been taking recommended chloroquine prophylaxis alone, though some others may be taking no or irregular chloroquine prophylaxis. Therefore, initial treatment of suspected CRPF must be with a drug other than chloroquine.

In areas where resistance has not developed to it, pyrimethamine-sulfadoxine (Fansidar) can be given in a single three-tablet dose for those over 45 kg in weight. Possible disadvantages of Fan-

sidar alone are that it acts more slowly than quinine and that Fansidar resistance is becoming more prevalent. Some experts therefore recommend that initial treatment be with oral quinine sulfate in an adult dose of 650 mg three times daily for 3 days, along with or followed by a three-tablet dose of Fansidar. Children's doses are given in Tables 1 and 3. Fansidar cannot be given to persons who are allergic to sulfa. Although Fansidar carries a significant risk of death from hypersensitivity reactions in weekly prophylactic doses, no deaths have as yet been recognized in those taking a single treatment dose. Fansidar resistance is widespread in Southeast Asia and Oceania, and this drug is not recommended for either treatment or prophylaxis in these areas. Reports of Fansidar resistance have also come from East Africa and South America.

Where Fansidar resistance occurs, or as an alternative in other CRPF areas, quinine plus a tetracycline can be used. For adults, quinine, 650 mg of salt, is given orally three times daily for 3 days, although some experts extend this to 7 to 10 days. These longer courses have not been proved to be any more effective but do have the

TABLE 2. **Areas with Reported Chloroquine-Resistant** *Plasmodium falciparum* **(CRPF)***

Africa†	South America	Oceania†
Angola	Bolivia	Papua New Guinea
Benin	Brazil‡	Solomon Islands
Burkina Faso	Colombia	Vanuatu
Burundi	Ecuador§	**Indian Subcontinent**†
Cameroon	French Guiana	Bangladesh (north and east)
Central African Republic	Guyana	India (isolated areas)
Comoros	Panama (east of the Canal Zone, in-	Pakistan (isolated areas)
Congo	cluding the San Blas Islands)	Sri Lanka (central)
Gabon	Peru (northern provinces)	
Ghana	Surinam	
Ivory Coast	Venezuela	
Kenya		
Liberia	**Asia**	
Madagascar	Burma	
Malawi	China (Hainan Island and southern	
Mali	provinces)	
Mozambique	Indonesia¶	
Namibia	Kampuchea†	
Niger	Laos‖	
Nigeria	Malaysia	
Rwanda	Philippines (Luzon, Basilan, Mindoro,	
Somalia	Palawan, and Mindano Islands;	
Sudan	Sulu Archipelago)	
Tanzania	Thailand	
Togo	Vietnam	
Uganda		
Zaire		
Zambia		
Zimbabwe		

Note: There is no malaria risk in urban areas unless otherwise indicated.
*Reports of CRPF as of May 1988.
†Malaria risk exists in most urban areas.
‡Malaria risk exists in urban areas of interior Amazon River Region.
§Malaria risk exists in urban areas of Esmeraldes, Manabi, El Oro, and Buayas provinces (including city of Guayaquil).
¶Malaria risk exists in urban areas of Timor and Kalimantan provinces. Irian Jaya should be considered as Oceania.
‖Malaria risk exists in all urban areas except Vientiane.

potential of increased side effects. Tetracycline, 250 mg four times daily, is given along with or after the quinine and continued for 7 days. The use of tetracycline in children below age 8 is controversial. It can be argued that the benefit of a virtually assured cure of a potentially life-threatening infection is worth any staining of teeth that might occur. However, some experts treat these children with quinine alone and monitor for recurrence of malaria, or substitute clindamycin for tetracycline.

Optimal treatment for all CRPF malaria is mefloquine (Lariam). This drug is still under review by the Food and Drug Administration in the United States and is not yet available. Mefloquine is currently marketed in Switzerland and France. The present recommended adult treatment dose is 1250 to 1500 mg, while children receive 25 mg per kg, which is administered in a single dose.

Plasmodium falciparum Infection—Complicated

Severe or complicated infection can occur with both chloroquine-sensitive and CRPF strains of *P. falciparum.* Patients with more than 3 per cent of their erythrocytes parasitized generally have more severe problems. Higher parasitemias are usually related to cases that are not readily recognized as malaria and in which diagnosis and initiation of treatment are delayed. An abnormal level of consciousness, shock, hemolytic anemia, hepatic dysfunction, renal insufficiency or failure, pulmonary or cardiac dysfunction, vomiting, and diarrhea are indications of severe malaria.

Patients with severe or complicated malaria should be managed with intensive care, immediate initiation of intravenous antimalarial drug treatment, and necessary supportive management. The initial therapy for these patients is intravenous quinine dihydrochloride by slow infusion. Quinine dihydrochloride is not commercially available in the United States, and for civilian use it can only be obtained through the Centers for Disease Control in Atlanta (24-hour emergency telephone number: 404-639-2888). If this product is not readily available, or until it can be obtained, intravenous quinidine gluconate should be used.

Some experts initiate intravenous quinine treatment with a loading dose of 20 mg salt per

TABLE 3. **Drug Prophylaxis for Malaria**

Condition	Drug	Dosage	
		Adults	*Children*
Areas with chloro-quine-sensitive strains	Chloroquine Po₄* (Aralen)	300 mg base (500 mg salt) weekly Take for at least 4 weeks after leaving malaria area	5 mg base kg weekly Same
Areas with chloro-quine-resistant strains	Chloroquine plus	As above	As above
	Proguanil† (Paludrine)	200 mg daily during and for 4 weeks after exposure	4–9 kg: 25 mg daily 10–14 kg: 50 mg daily 15–29 kg: 100 mg daily 30–50 kg: 150 mg daily >50 kg: 200 mg daily
	plus Pyrimethamine-sulfadoxine (Fansidar)	Carry a single (3 tablets) self-treatment dose	5–10 kg: ¼ tablet 11–20 kg: ½ tablet 21–30 kg: 1 tablet 31–45 kg: 2 tablets >45 kg: 3 tablets
	or Doxycycline	100 mg daily during and for 4 weeks after exposure	Contraindicated in children below 8 years >8 years: 2 mg/kg daily, up to 100 mg
Possibility of later re-lapsing malaria	Primaquine	15 mg base daily for 14 days Do not give to patients having deficiency of glucose-6-phosphate dehydrogenase	0.3 mg base/kg/day for 14 days

*Provided in 500 or 250 mg salt tablets, which equal 300 mg and 150 mg base, respectively.
†Not available in the United States.

kg, followed by doses of 10 mg salt per kg every 8 hours. Others, particularly in Africa, do not use the loading dose but begin with a dose of 10 mg salt per kg. Administration is in 300 ml normal saline or 5 per cent dextrose infused over 2 to 4 hours. Intravenous treatment is given at 8-hour intervals until parasitemia is considerably decreased and the patient is definitely improved. A 3- to 7-day total course of quinine can then be completed with oral quinine sulfate. If quinidine gluconate is used for initiation of treatment, the first dose should be 15 mg base per kg infused over 3 to 4 hours in 250 to 300 ml of normal saline or 5 per cent dextrose. Additional doses of 7.5 mg base per kg are similarly infused at 8-hour intervals for a total of 72 hours of treatment. If a patient's improved condition warrants it, treatment could also be completed with oral quinidine sulfate capsules in equivalent doses. Monitoring of both intravenous quinine and quinidine should be by measuring plasma levels, to achieve quinine levels of 5 to 15 micrograms per ml and quinidine levels of 5 to 10 micrograms per ml. The blood pressure and electrocardiogram should be followed closely for evidence of toxicity. When the patient is improved and able to tolerate oral therapy, tetracycline, 250 mg four times daily for 7 days, should be added to assure total cure.

The role of mefloquine, presently available only in oral dose form, in the treatment of severe and complicated malaria remains to be determined.

In patients with a parasitemia of over 10 per cent and/or marked deterioration of neurologic, renal, or hematologic function, or other grave prognostic sign, exchange transfusion may be life-saving. Advantages include much more rapid removal of parasites than with antimalarial drugs and the potential restoration of platelets and clotting factors from fresh whole blood.

Plasmodium malariae, Plasmodium vivax, and Plasmodium ovale *Infections*

These species give lower parasitemias than does *P. falciparum*, and pure infection with them is rarely severe. Treatment is with chloroquine, 25 mg base per kg over 3 days, as with uncomplicated chloroquine-sensitive *P. falciparum* infection. These three parasites have not developed resistance to chloroquine. Chloroquine alone is sufficient for *P. malariae*. However, *P. vivax* and *P. ovale* have persistent exoerythrocytic liver-stage parasites that can be eliminated only with primaquine. Following initial chloroquine treatment, primaquine, 15 mg base daily for 14 days, is given. Primaquine comes only in hard tablet form which cannot be put into solution. Young children should receive 0.3 mg base per kg daily for 14 days, which requires breaking the 15 mg base (equal to 26.3 mg primaquine phosphate salt) tablet into the approximate dose portion. Some strains of *P. vivax* from Southeast Asia and the Southwest Pacific (so-called Chesson strains) are relatively resistant to the usual dose of primaquine; these are usually responsive to 30 mg base primaquine daily for 14 days. Primaquine can cause hemolysis in persons with glucose-6-phosphate dehydrogenase (G6PD) deficiency. All persons receiving primaquine should be first tested to assure absence of G6PD deficiency. In those with the mild (African) variety of deficiency, primaquine can be tolerated in a weekly dose of 45 mg base for 8 weeks. In other varieties of G6PD deficiency, in which hemolysis can be so severe as to be life-threatening, primaquine must be avoided. If relapses occur, they can be treated with chloroquine.

General Supportive Care

Patients with pure *P. malaria, P. vivax,* and *P. ovale* infections rarely have heavy parasitemias or severe illness or complications. They can generally be treated as outpatients. Those infected with *P. falciparum* always have the potential for rapidly developing severe illness or complications and are best treated in the hospital. Chloroquine-sensitive *P. falciparum* infection recognized early should quickly respond to chloroquine. Patients with heavier *P. falciparum* infections or those with CRPF infection (some of whom may already have been unsuccessfully treated with chloroquine) are more likely to develop complications, and may require parenteral therapy, which must be closely monitored, and other intensive care. Treatment with analgesics, antiemetics, and antipyretics may be necessary. Thrombocytopenia, sometimes quite marked, commonly occurs with all forms of acute malaria, but this quickly reverts to normal with appropriate antimalarial chemotherapy.

Management of Complications

Cerebral malaria must be differentiated from other causes of coma; the airway must be carefully maintained. Adjuvant treatments such as corticosteroids, high-molecular-weight dextran, mannitol, heparin, and epinephrine have not been found useful and may be harmful; these should all be avoided.

Hyperpyrexia should be controlled with sponging, cooling blankets, and antipyretics.

Seizures are not uncommon, particularly with cerebral malaria, and should be treated with standard anticonvulsants. Status epilepticus may require diazepam therapy.

Severe anemia (hematocrit 20 per cent or less) should be treated with whole blood or packed red cell transfusions.

Hypoglycemia may occur with severe malaria and is especially common in pregnant women and patients with hyperparasitemia. Blood glucose levels must be carefully monitored. Treatment initially is with 50 per cent dextrose injection followed by a 10 per cent dextrose infusion.

Pulmonary edema can be a fatal complication of severe *P. falciparum* infection and can develop after clearance of blood parasitemia and apparent clinical improvement. It presents as adult respiratory distress syndrome (ARDS). Prevention is by careful attention to fluid intake monitored by central venous pressure. Treatment is with diuretics, fluid restriction, and other methods used for pulmonary edema and ARDS.

Renal failure is related to decreased renal capillary blood flow, most frequently caused by underhydration, but also associated with hyperparasitemia and intravascular hemolysis. In the absence of fluid overload and with a low central venous pressure and high urine specific gravity, the patient should be challenged with a normal saline infusion. Should this prove unsuccessful, a diuretic or vasopressor is given. Persistent oliguria may require renal dialysis.

Disseminated intravascular coagulation with bleeding is rarely a clinically important occurrence in the absence of hyperparasitemia or multiorgan failure. Treatment is with fresh whole blood transfusions. Heparin has not been found useful and is not recommended.

Prophylaxis

In choosing an appropriate chemoprophylactic regimen prior to travel, a number of factors must be considered (Table 3). The full itinerary should be carefully reviewed to determine whether the individual will be in specific areas where malaria actually occurs in a recognized malarious country. For example, most major cities of Asia and South America do not have endemic malaria; if only these cities are visited, chemoprophylaxis is not necessary. In tropical Africa, however, risk of acquiring malaria occurs in many cities as well as rural areas. If travel to rural areas where malaria occurs is only during daytime hours, prophylaxis may not be required. It should also be determined if the area to be visited is one with CRPF. Any previous allergic or other reaction to the antimalarials chosen should be determined. Duration of travel and availability of adequate medical care must also be weighed in the decision.

The continuing spread of CRPF malaria has created serious problems in protecting against infection. At this time there is no available drug or combination of drugs with proven efficacy or safety to prevent all malaria infections. A variety of recommendations made in different countries has resulted, which has led to confusion. The following recommendations are considered most appropriate at the present time, as offering the best combination of safety and relative effectiveness.

For areas with chloroquine-sensitive malaria species, or where only low-level or focal CRPF has been reported (South Asia), the drug of choice is chloroquine. This is taken in an adult dose of 300 mg base (equal to 500 mg salt) once weekly, beginning 2 weeks prior to arrival to assure tolerance, while in the malarious area, and for at least 4 weeks after leaving. Those unable to tolerate chloroquine should take proguanil (Paludrine) 200 mg daily for the same times.

For those going to areas where CRPF is endemic (see Table 2), chloroquine weekly (as above) is recommended. Proguanil 200 mg daily should also be taken. This latter drug is not yet approved in the United States by the Food and Drug Administration, but is available in England, France, and Kenya and many other places in Africa. Limited data suggest that it is effective in Africa, but not in Thailand or Papua New Guinea. A three-tablet treatment dose of Fansidar can also be carried by longer-term travelers or residents. They should be advised to take the Fansidar promptly in the event of a febrile illness while abroad, but only when professional medical care is not readily available; this is only a temporary measure, and prompt medical evaluation is imperative. A possible alternative for selected individuals who are at high risk of contracting CRPF where medical care is not available, and who have previously taken Fansidar without serious side effects, could be to add one tablet of Fansidar to weekly chloroquine. Fansidar should be taken prophylactically only after its potential benefit is weighed against its significant serious toxic potential.

In some malarious areas, particularly in Southeast Asia, Papua New Guinea, and the Amazon basin, multidrug resistance by *P. falciparum* parasites occurs. Doxycycline alone, 100 mg daily, can be considered in these areas for short-term travel, but users should be cautioned about side effects (see below). Doxycycline should be continued daily for 4 weeks after departure from the malarious area.

When mefloquine (Lariam) is licensed in the United States and definite recommendations for its use have been made, this drug will likely become the prophylactic drug of choice in all CRPF areas. It is expected that Lariam will be approved by the FDA by 1989. Mefloquine is currently available in France and Switzerland. It may be considered for use by travelers to areas where there is risk of CRPF infection and by travelers to areas where *P. falciparum* is resistant to both chloroquine and Fansidar. Current available information suggests an adult prophylactic dose of 250 mg weekly.

Amodiaquine and Maloprim (a combination of pyrimethamine and dapsone) are recommended by some experts. Neither is commercially available in the United States. Both have been associated with bone marrow problems and are not recommended.

Primaquine has no role in prophylaxis for individuals while in malarious areas. However, since persisting liver forms of *P. vivax* and *P. ovale* occur in most malarious areas (Haiti being a major exception), returnees from malarious areas run some risk of acquiring later relapsing malaria. This is more likely in those having prolonged exposure in malaria-endemic areas. As long as G6PD status is normal, primaquine is considered a safe and the only effective way of protecting against this risk. It is optimally desirable to take primaquine in an adult dose of 15 mg base daily (pediatric dose of 0.3 mg/kg base daily) for 14 days and it is best taken after completing the terminal 4-week prophylaxis with chloroquine and/or other drugs.

Personal Protection Measures

Exposure to malaria-carrying mosquitoes occurs from dusk to dawn only. Methods to reduce exposure include wearing long pants and shirts; using window screens; sleeping under mosquito nets; applying insect repellents containing DEET to exposed skin; and spraying indoors with pyrethrum-containing insecticides.

Contraindications and Side Effects of Antimalarials

Chloroquine. Chloroquine may exacerbate psoriasis and should not be taken by those with this condition. Chloroquine in higher doses used for rheumatoid arthritis or lupus, or in the 600 mg of base per week used in some French-speaking areas of Africa, has been associated with irreversible retinopathy and blindness. This is a virtually unheard of occurrence in those taking the recommended 300 mg base weekly dose. Temporary minor side effects, which are usually adequately tolerated, include headache, blurred vision, gastrointestinal disturbances, and skin rashes. Uncomfortable side effects may be alleviated by taking chloroquine with meals or in divided, twice-weekly doses.

Proguanil. This has been considered perhaps the best-tolerated of all antimalarial drugs. With the 200 mg daily dose, mouth ulcers have been rarely reported and there have been some minor gastrointestinal problems. There are no contraindications.

Fansidar. The long-acting sulfa component, sulfadoxine, has been associated with fatal cutaneous reactions with weekly Fansidar use. In Americans, the incidence of fatal reactions ranges from 1 in 11,000 to 1 in 25,000 users. These reactions have not yet been recognized with a three-tablet treatment dose. Fansidar has also caused serum-sickness reactions and hepatitis. If weekly Fansidar is prescribed, it must be discontinued immediately if the user develops skin or mucous membrane reactions including redness, itching rash, mouth or genital lesions, sore throat, or unexplained fever. Fansidar is contraindicated in those allergic to sulfa and in infants below age 2 months.

Quinine. Cinchonism (tinnitus, headache, nausea, abdominal pain, visual disturbance) is common. Drug fever rarely occurs.

Tetracyclines. Tetracyclines are contraindicated in children below age 8 years. Doxycycline may give a photosensitivity, usually manifested as an exaggerated sunburn reaction, to those using it in tropical climates; users should avoid direct and prolonged sun exposure. Tetracyclines may also lead to *Candida* vaginitis or gastrointestinal candidiasis or to gastrointestinal upset.

Mefloquine. Minor side effects have been reported rather frequently, including dizziness and gastrointestinal disturbances. Mefloquine has occasionally been associated with asymptomatic sinus bradycardia and prolonged QT interval and it should not be used by those receiving calcium channel antagonists or beta blockers.

Primaquine. Severe hemolysis may occur in G6PD-deficient individuals and it is generally contraindicated in this condition. Gastrointestinal symptoms rarely occur.

Malaria in Pregnant and Breast-Feeding Women. Malaria poses a serious threat to pregnant women and may cause abortion, premature labor, maternal anemia, and congenital infection. Under no circumstances should a pregnant woman go to a malarious area without taking appropriate malaria chemoprophylaxis. Chloroquine is considered safe for both prophylaxis and treatment. Proguanil has been very safe in pregnancy. The safety of Fansidar in pregnancy has not been completely established, and the safety of mefloquine is presently questionable. Tetracyclines and primaquine are contraindicated in pregnancy.

In treating severe CRPF malaria in pregnant women, any concern about side effects must necessarily be secondary to the potential life-saving value of quinine along with either tetracycline or Fansidar.

The small amounts of antimalarial drugs secreted in the breast milk of lactating women are not considered harmful to the nursing infant. Insufficient amounts of antimalarials are transferred in breast milk to protect infants, who require dosages of antimalarials recommended in Table 3.

BACTERIAL MENINGITIS
method of
WILLIAM R. BYRNE, M.D.
Letterman Army Medical Center
San Francisco, California

Acute bacterial meningitis is a real medical emergency requiring rapid initial evaluation followed immediately by initiation of therapy. In adults, the disease should be considered whenever fever, headache, and/or mental status changes (e.g., lethargy, confusion, delirium, stupor) are encountered. In elderly patients, a change in mental status may be the only clinical sign of meningitis. In children, the diagnosis of bacterial meningitis should be considered in the presence of fever plus mental status changes, neck stiffness or headache, focal neurologic signs, or seizures. In neonates, clinical manifestations may be limited to poor feeding, listlessness, irritability, diarrhea, or abdominal distention.

The incidence of bacterial meningitis is estimated to be approximately 10 per 100,000 population per year. It is predominantly a disease of children; the highest attack rates occur in infants less than 1 month old, followed by young children and then adults greater than 60 years of age. The lowest attack rates are seen in older children and young adults.

Initial evaluation, diagnostic procedures (including lumbar puncture and blood cultures), and administration of the first dose of antimicrobial therapy should all be completed within 30 to 60 minutes of presentation. Cerebrospinal fluid specimens should be cultured promptly. Rapid diagnostic tests for detection of bacterial antigens by latex particle agglutination are available for *Haemophilus influenzae* type b, *Neisseria meningitidis* types A, B, and C, *Streptococcus pneumoniae*, and group B *Streptococcus*. These tests may provide valuable information in the absence of a positive Gram stain or when prior antimicrobial therapy has caused bacterial cultures to be sterile.

X-ray films of the paranasal sinuses and the chest should also be done, but these tests should not delay the lumbar puncture, blood cultures, or first dose of antibiotic therapy. If focal neurologic signs are present, a computed tomographic scan of the head should be done before the lumbar puncture is performed, to exclude the possibility of an expanding mass lesion.

Antibiotic Therapy

Empiric therapy should be selected according to the patient's age (Table 1) or special clinical situation (Table 2). Appropriate antibiotic dos-

TABLE 1. **Presumptive Therapy for Bacterial Meningitis by Age Group**

Age Group	Likely Pathogens	Recommended Presumptive Therapy
Less than 1 month	Group B *Streptococcus* Gram-negative enteric bacilli *Listeria monocytogenes* *Haemophilus influenzae*[1] *Streptococcus pneumoniae* *Neisseria meningitidis* *Staphylococcus aureus*[2]	Ampicillin plus gentamicin *or* ampicillin plus cefotaxime
1 to 3 months	*H. influenzae*[1] *N. meningitidis* *S. pneumoniae* Group B *Streptococcus*	Ampicillin plus cefotaxime
3 months to 9 years	*H. influenzae*[1] *S. pneumoniae* *N. meningitidis*	Cefotaxime *or* ceftriaxone *or* ampicillin plus chloramphenicol
9 to 59 years	*N. meningitidis* *S. pneumoniae* *H. influenzae*[3]	Pencillin G, chloramphenicol, ceftriaxone, cefotaxime, or cefuroxime
60+ years	*S. pneumoniae* Gram-negative enteric bacilli[4] *N. meningitidis* *L. monocytogenes* *H. influenzae*[3] Group B *Streptococcus* *S. aureus*[5]	Ampicillin *plus* cefotaxime, ceftriaxone, or ceftizoxime

[1]Approximately 20 per cent of *H. influenzae* isolated from pediatric patients in the United States produce beta-lactamase, indicating resistance to ampicillin.

[2]Meningitis secondary to infection with *S. aureus* in this age group is seen predominantly in premature infants.

[3]*H. influenzae* meningitis in adults is seen in the setting of head trauma (either recent or remote), cerebrospinal fluid rhinorrhea, paranasal sinusitis, otitis media, pneumonia (particularly when associated with asthma or chronic obstructive pulmonary disease), or diabetes mellitus.

[4]Meningitis secondary to infection with gram-negative enteric bacilli is also seen in association with gram-negative bacillary septicemia from infection at a remote site, ruptured brain abscess, and disseminated strongyloidiasis.

[5]Meningitis secondary to infection with *S. aureus* is also seen in association with staphylococcal septicemia from infection at distant sites (endocarditis, infected vascular graft, soft tissue abscess, paranasal sinusitis, cellulitis, osteomyelitis, or mastitis), diabetes mellitus, chronic renal failure, alcoholism, or ruptured brain abscess.

ages are of critical importance (Table 3). Shortly after the first dose of antibiotic therapy, the coverage may be altered based on the results of the Gram stain of the cerebrospinal fluid, which will reveal a pathogen in 50 to 75 per cent of patients with bacterial meningitis. Further adjustments in antimicrobial coverage may be indicated when the results of cerebrospinal fluid culture and antimicrobial susceptibility testing are available (Table 4).

In neonates the ampicillin-gentamicin combination provides synergy against group B *Streptococcus*, while the ampicillin-cefotaxime combination is more effective against gram-negative

TABLE 2. **Presumptive Therapy for Bacterial Meningitis in Special Clinical Situations**

Situation	Likely Pathogens	Recommended Presumptive Therapy
Meningitis associated with cerebrospinal fluid shunt, neurosurgery, penetrating head trauma, cerebrospinal fluid rhinorrhea	Gram-negative enteric bacilli *Staphylococcus epidermidis* *Staphylococcus aureus* *Propionibacterium acnes* *Streptococcus pneumoniae*	Vancomycin *plus* ceftriaxone, cefotaxime, ceftizoxime, or ceftazidime[1]
Immunocompromised patient (organ transplant, cancer, antineoplastic chemotherapy, high-dose or prolonged steroid therapy)	*Listeria monocytogenes* Gram-negative enteric bacilli *S. aureus*	Ampicillin *plus* ceftriaxone, cefotaxime, ceftizoxime, or ceftazidime[1]

[1]Ceftazidime should be used if *Pseudomonas aeruginosa* is suspected.

TABLE 3. **Antibiotic Dosages for Bacterial Meningitis**

Antibiotic	Daily Adult Dose		Daily Child's Dose[1,2]	
	Total	*Interval*	*Total*	*Interval*
Ampicillin	12 gram/day	4 hr	200–300 mg/kg/day[3]	6 hr
Azlocillin (Azlin)	18–24 gram/day	4–6 hr	250–300 mg/kg/day	4–6 hr
Carbenicillin (Geocillin)	30–40 gram/day	4 hr	400–500 mg/kg/day	4 hr
Mezlocillin (Mezlin)	18–24 gram/day	4–6 hr	250–300 mg/kg/day	4–6 hr
Nafcillin (Nafcil)	12–18 gram/day[4]	4 hr	150–200 mg/kg/day	4–6 hr
Oxacillin (Prostaphlin)	12–18 gram/day	4 hr	150–200 mg/kg/day	4–6 hr
Penicillin G	20–24 million units/day	2–4 hr	200,000 to 300,000 units/kg/day	4–6 hr
Ticarcillin (Ticar)	18–24 gram/day	4–6 hr	250–300 mg/kg/day	4–6 hr
Pipercillin (Pipracil)	18–24 gram/day	4–6 hr	NA[5]	NA[5]
Cefotaxime (Claforan)	12 gram/day	4 hr	150–200 mg/kg/day	4–6 hr
Ceftriaxone (Rocephin)	4 gram/day	12 hr	100 mg/kg/day[6]	12 hr
Ceftizoxime (Cefizox)	9–12 gram/day	8 hr	150–200 mg/kg/day	8 hr
Ceftazidime (Tazicef)	6 gram/day	8 hr	100–150 mg/kg/day	8 hr
Cefuroxime[7] (Zinacef)	4.5–9 gram/day	8 hr	200–240 mg/kg/day	6 hr
Chloramphenicol	4 gram/day	6 hr	100 mg/kg/day	6 hr
Vancomycin (Vancocin)	2 gram/day	6–12 hr	40–50 mg/kg/day	6 hr
Amikacin (Amikin)				
Intravenous[8]	15 mg/kg/day[9,10]	8–12 hr[9]	15 mg/kg/day[9,10]	12 hr[9]
Intraventricular[11]	20–30 mg/day	24 hr	4–5 mg/day	24 hr
Gentamicin (Garamycin)				
Intravenous[8]	5 mg/kg/day[9,12]	8 hr[8]	5–7 mg/kg/day[9,12]	8 hr[8]
Intraventricular[11]	8–10 mg/day	24 hr	2–2.5 mg/day	24 hr
Tobramycin (Nebcin)				
Intravenous[8]	5 mg/kg/day[9,12]	8 hr[9]	5 mg/kg/day[9,12]	8 hr[9]
Intraventricular[11]	8–10 mg/day	24 hr	2–2.5 mg/day	24 hr
Trimethoprim-sulfamethoxazole (TMP-SMX) (Bactrim, Septra)	10 mg/kg/day TMP plus 50 mg/kg/day SMX	6 hr	10 mg/kg/day TMP plus 50 mg/kg/day SMX	6 hr

[1]Doses listed are for age more than 30 days. Different doses are required for infants during the first week after birth and the remainder of the first 30 days of life than for older children. Antibiotic therapy for children in this newborn period should involve appropriate consultation.

[2]Doses in children should not exceed the adult dose.

[3]After an initial dose of 100 mg per kg.

[4]After 5 to 7 days of nafcillin therapy, the dose should be reduced to 9 grams per day in order to avoid the development of neutropenia.

[5]NA = not available (dose recommendations for infants and children under age of 12 years are not available).

[6]After an initial dose of 75 mg per kg.

[7]Antibiotic failures have been reported with the use of cefuroxime in children with meningitis, and some authorities do not recommend its use in this situation.

[8]Peak and trough serum drug levels should be measured at least twice weekly along with tests of renal function.

[9]Adjustments to total daily dose and interval in the presence of abnormal renal function should be made with reference to standard nomograms and manufacturer's recommendations.

[10]After a loading dose of 7.5 mg per kg.

[11]A preservative-free preparation of gentamicin approved by the Food and Drug Administration for use in central nervous system infection is available. Since a similar preparation does not exist for amikacin and tobramycin, the use of this form of gentamicin for intraventricular aminoglycoside therapy is preferable, if the bacterial species involved is sensitive to gentamicin. Drug levels in the cerebrospinal fluid should be measured at least twice weekly. Dose is expressed as total daily dose, not in mg per kg per day.

[12]After a loading dose of 2 mg per kg.

enteric organisms. For children 1 to 3 months of age, the combination of ampicillin plus cefotaxime provides coverage for beta-lactamase–positive *H. influenzae* and avoids the theoretical possibility of antagonism between ampicillin and chloramphenicol if either *Listeria monocytogenes* or group B *Streptococcus* is present. For children older than 3 months of age, cefotaxime or ceftriaxone alone or ampicillin plus chloramphenicol is recommended. All three of these regimens provide initial coverage for beta-lactamase–pro-

ducing *H. influenzae*. Ampicillin may be substituted for chloramphenicol, ceftriaxone, or cefotaxime if *H. influenzae* is determined to be beta-lactamase–negative.

Pencillin or chloramphenicol should be used as initial presumptive therapy in adults less than 60 years old, except in the special situations listed in Table 2.

Initial presumptive therapy in the elderly should consist of ampicillin plus either cefotaxime, ceftriaxone, or ceftizoxime, since these pa-

TABLE 4. **Specific Antibiotic Coverage Based on Results of Cerebrospinal Fluid Culture**

Bacteria (Appearance on Gram Stain)	Antibiotics		Duration of Therapy
	First Choices	*Alternates*	
Gram-negative enteric bacilli[1] (Gram-negative rods)	—	—	At least 21 days, 10–14 days after CSF cultures have become negative
Escherichia coli and *Klebsiella-Enterobacter-Serratia*	Cefotaxime, ceftriaxone, ceftizoxime[2]	Trimethoprim-sulfamethoxazole	Same
Pseudomonas aeruginosa	Ceftiazidime plus intravenous aminoglycoside[3]	Azlocillin, mezlocillin, carbenicillin, or pipercillin plus intravenous aminoglycoside[3]	Same
Group B *Streptococcus* (Gram-positive cocci in chains)	Ampicillin or penicillin G plus gentamicin for 24–48 hr, then penicillin G alone	Chloramphenicol, ceftriaxone, cefotaxime	14–21 days
Haemophilus influenzae (Short gram-positive rods or coccobacilli, which may demonstrate bipolar staining resembling over-decolorized pneumococci)	—	—	7–10 days
Beta-lactamase–negative	Ampicillin	Chloramphenicol, cefotaxime, ceftriaxone, cefuroxime[4]	Same
Beta-lactamase–positive	Chloramphenicol, cefotaxime, ceftriaxone	Cefuroxime[4]	Same
Listeria monocytogenes (Gram-positive rods resembling diphtheroids; may appear coccoid or in pairs resembling pneumococci)	Ampicillin or penicillin G plus gentamicin	Trimethoprim-sulfamethoxazole	Usually, 14–21 days (4–6 weeks may be required if clinical response is slow)
Neisseria meningitidis (Gram-negative diplococci, biscuit- or kidney-bean-shaped, with flattened adjacent sides)	Penicillin G	Chloramphenicol[5]	7–10 days[6]
Propionibacterium acnes (Pleomorphic gram-positive bacilli; "diphtheroids")	Penicillin G	Chloramphenicol	14–21 days (4–6 weeks if osteomyelitis is present)
Staphylococcus aureus[7] and *S. epidermidis*[8] (Gram-positive cocci as singles, pairs, clusters, and short chains of up to five cocci)	—	—	21 days
Beta-lactamase–negative	Penicillin G	Vancomycin	Same
Beta-lactamase–positive	—		—
Methicillin-sensitive	Nafcillin, oxacillin	Vancomycin	Same
Methicillin-resistant	Vancomycin	Trimethoprim-sulfamethoxazole	Same
Streptococcus pneumoniae (Gram-positive cocci in singles and pairs; cocci are spherical, oval, or lancet-shaped)	—		—
Penicillin-sensitive	Penicillin G	Chloramphenicol[9]	10–14 days
Penicillin-resistant[10]	Cefotaxime, chloramphenicol[11]	Vancomycin	10–14 days

[1]Chloramphenicol is not considered to be an acceptable antibiotic for treatment of gram-negative bacillary meningitis, in spite of apparent in vitro activity, because it is bacteriostatic for most of these organisms at concentrations achievable in the cerebrospinal fluid (CSF).

[2]Plus intravenous and intraventricular aminoglycoside for difficult cases.

[3]Plus intraventricular aminoglycoside in difficult cases until cerebrospinal fluid cultures are negative. This usually occurs within 5 to 7 days.

[4]Caution should be exercised when using cefuroxime for children with meningitis, since some antibiotic failures have been reported.

[5]Cefotaxime, ceftriaxone, ceftazidime, ceftizoxime, and cefuroxime are also effective.

[6]A recent clinical study from Europe reported success with 4 days of intravenous penicillin therapy.

[7]The addition of rifampin, 600 mg orally twice daily, may improve outcome in difficult cases.

[8]About 60 per cent of *S. epidermidis* infections are methicillin-resistant, and initial presumptive therapy when this organism is suspected should be with vancomycin.

[9]Ampicillin, cefotaxime, ceftriaxone, cefuroxime, and ceftazidime are also effective.

[10]Penicillin-resistant pneumococci are rarely encountered in the United States.

[11]Because of the possibility of resistance to multiple antibiotics, including chloramphenicol, susceptibility of the patient's organisms to chloramphenicol should be checked.

tients have an increased incidence of infections with unusual organisms such as *L. monocytogenes*, enteric gram-negative bacilli (*Escherichia coli* and *Klebsiella-Enterobacter-Serratia*), and group B *Streptococcus*. The incidence of meningitis secondary to infections with *Staphylococcus aureus* and *Pseudomonas aeruginosa* is also increased in the elderly, usually in association with head trauma or neurosurgical procedures. Therapy specific for these pathogens should be initiated if they are suspected.

Follow-up Procedures

In routine cases of bacterial meningitis in which the patient responds to therapy, a follow-up lumbar puncture is not required after the diagnosis has been established by a positive cerebrospinal fluid culture. Repeat lumbar puncture is indicated when the patient with meningitis is not responding clinically to antibiotic therapy or when the patient has a bacterial pathogen known to be difficult to treat (e.g., enteric gram-negative bacilli, *S. aureus, L. monocytogenes*).

Adjunctive Therapy

Intravenous fluids should be administered with care during the first 24 to 48 hours of therapy to avoid the complication of hyponatremia resulting from the syndrome of inappropriate antidiuretic hormone secretion (SIADH), which occurs in approximately 8 per cent of cases. Seizures, which occur in up to 33 per cent of children with meningitis, usually respond to therapy with diazepam, phenytoin, or phenobarbital. The routine use of adrenal corticosteroids remains controversial except in the presence of acute adrenal insufficiency (Waterhouse-Friderichsen syndrome) associated with overwhelming septicemia. One clinical study in children, however, has demonstrated that dexamethasone 0.15 mg per kg every 6 hours for 4 days reduced the frequency of severe to profound hearing loss, although survival was not altered. A recommendation for routine use of dexamethasone in all children with meningitis must await the results of confirmatory trials, however. In adults, there are no published data that unequivocally support the use of dexamethasone therapy in bacterial meningitis; however,

it is reasonable to administer dexamethasone along with mannitol when there is evidence of increased intracranial pressure. The presence of persistent or recurrent fever, vomiting, seizures, focal neurologic findings, or signs of meningeal irritation should prompt consideration of subdural effusions or empyema, particularly in children. The diagnosis is established by computed tomographic scan of the head and/or by subdural paracentesis.

Chemoprophylaxis

Rifampin* is the recommended drug for chemoprophylaxis of contacts of patients with meningococcal and *H. influenzae* meningitis (Table 5). Minocycline is also effective for prophylaxis of meningococcal meningitis, but it is no longer recommended because of the high frequency of vestibular auditory toxicity. Sulfadiazine has also been used in the past with success, but widespread resistance of *N. meningitidis* to the drug precludes its routine use. Sulfadiazine may be useful, however, in an epidemic situation in which the organism is known to be sensitive.

Immunoprophylaxis

H. influenzae type b vaccine is recommended for all children at age 24 months. Children from

*This use of rifampin is not listed in the manufacturer's directive.

TABLE 5. Chemoprophylaxis with Rifampin[1, 2]

Bacterial Species	Indications for Prophylaxis	Daily Dose	
		Adult	*Child*[3]
Haemophilus influenzae type b[4]	All household and day care center contacts, when at least one of the contacts is 4 years of age or less. Index patient should also receive prophylaxis, since antibiotic therapy for meningitis may not eradicate the carrier state.	600 mg/day as a single dose for 4 days	20 mg/kg/day as a single dose for 4 days[5]
Neisseria meningitidis[6]	Close daily personal contacts of index patient (household, day-care, nursery school, roommates, girlfriend or boyfriend), particularly infants. Health care workers who have had intimate (e.g., mouth-to-mouth resuscitation) contact with an infected person should receive prophylaxis.[7]	600 mg every 12 hr for four doses	10 mg/kg every 12 hr for four doses[8]

[1]Pregnant women should not receive rifampin.

[2]Patients taking rifampin should be advised that this antibiotic is likely to cause a reddish-orange discoloration of urine, sweat, and tears.

[3]Dose for children should not exceed the adult dose.

[4]Contacts should be treated within 1 week of exposure, if possible, but there may be some benefit to prophylaxis administered as late as 2 to 4 weeks after exposure to the index case.

[5]Dose should not exceed a maximum of 600 mg. The dose for neonates (less than 1 month of age) is 10 mg per kg per day.

[6]Prophylaxis should be initiated as soon as possible after the index case is identified, preferably within 24 hours.

[7]Prophylaxis in the absence of intimate or regular close personal contact is not routinely indicated for medical personnel, classmates, or fellow office workers.

[8]Infants from 3 to 12 months of age should receive 5 mg per kg every 12 hours for four doses.

18 to 23 months of age should be immunized if they attend day care centers, are immunosuppressed, or have functional (e.g., in sickle cell disease) or anatomic asplenia. Pneumococcal vaccine is recommended for persons with chronic cardiac or pulmonary disease, illnesses that predispose to pneumococcal infection (sickle cell disease, nephrotic syndrome, Hodgkin's disease, asplenia, multiple myeloma, cirrhosis of the liver, alcoholism, renal failure, cerebrospinal fluid leaks), and conditions associated with compromised immune systems. The use of pneumococcal vaccine in all persons greater than 65 years of age has been recommended but remains controversial. Meningococcal vaccine is available for serogroups A, C, W135, and Y. Its use is recommended in epidemics of serogroups A and C disease, in military recruits, and in travelers to areas where disease is endemic.

Isolation

All patients with suspected bacterial meningitis should be placed initially in respiratory isolation. After a diagnosis has been established, continued isolation is necessary only for meningococcal meningitis, for the first 24 hours after initiation of effective therapy.

Recurrent Meningitis

Recurrent attacks of bacterial meningitis usually result from a congenital defect or traumatic event that causes a communication between the subarachnoid space and the paranasal sinuses, nasopharynx, middle ear, or skin. The occurrence of recurrent bacterial meningitis should prompt a search for such a defect. The most common offending pathogen is *S. pneumoniae*, and the clinical course is usually more benign than that of meningitis resulting from other causes. Noninfectious causes of recurrent meningitis include Mollaret's meningitis, sarcoidosis, systemic lupus erythematosis, Behçet's disease, and Vogt-Koyanagi-Harada syndrome.

INFECTIOUS MONONUCLEOSIS

method of
JOHN W. SIXBEY, M.D.
St. Jude Children's Research Hospital
Memphis, Tennessee

Infectious mononucleosis (IM) is a syndrome caused by primary infection with Epstein-Barr virus (EBV). It is most common in adolescents and young adults and is manifested as fever, sore throat, and lymphadenopathy. Hepatosplenomegaly is a frequent occurrence, and atypical lymphocytes (more than 10 per cent) are found in the peripheral blood. The spectrum of disease is highly variable and may present atypically in young children, in whom failure to thrive, hepatosplenomegaly, hypergammaglobulinemia, and pneumonitis may be presenting manifestations. Diagnosis of acute EBV infection is most often made with the nonspecific tests for heterophil antibody ("monospot," Paul-Bunnell test), although in infants and children under age 4 these tests are often negative. Serology for antibodies to EBV-specific antigens (viral capsid antigen, early antigen, and EB nuclear antigen) may be required for diagnosis in young children, although other viral agents, including cytomegalovirus, should be considered in heterophil antibody–negative mononucleosis. EBV-specific serologies may also be useful to differentiate IM from lymphoma, to identify neurologic manifestations of EBV infection, and in the workup of hepatitis and hematologic disorders of unknown origin. Intimate contact, such as exchange of saliva, is required for transmission, and EBV can be acquired by blood transfusion. As with other herpes group viruses, EBV persists for life after the primary infection. In adult populations worldwide, 95 per cent are EBV antibody–positive and 60 per cent of healthy adults are asymptomatic viral excretors. Therefore, the period of communicability after primary infection is indeterminate, isolation of patients with acute illness is not required, and normal social activities may be resumed at the patient's discretion on resolution of acute symptomatology.

Complications

Despite variability from patient to patient, acute IM is usually self-limiting, and most patients recover in 2 to 5 weeks. Rarely, the first manifestation of disease may be one of the complications discussed below.

Respiratory. Upper airway obstruction from tonsillar enlargement is a life-threatening complication of IM. Interstitial infiltrates have been reported in 3 to 5 per cent of cases of IM, and EBV-related lymphoid interstitial pneumonitis has been documented in children with acquired immunodeficiency syndrome.

Splenic Rupture. Splenic rupture must be considered whenever abdominal pain accompanies IM. A rare but life-threatening complication of IM, splenic rupture is most common in the second or third week of illness and may follow inapparent, mild trauma.

Neurologic. Encephalitis, aseptic meningitis, Guillain-Barré syndrome, optic neuritis, transverse myelitis, Bell's palsy, and psychosis have been reported. The majority of patients completely recover from neurologic complications, although they also represent the most frequent cause of death in IM.

Hepatic. Serum aminotransferases may be elevated two to five fold in almost all cases of IM. Mild elevations of bilirubin commonly occur, and frank jaundice may be seen in 5 per cent of cases.

Hematologic. Autoimmune hemolytic anemia, thrombocytopenia, and granulocytopenia may accompany acute EBV infection.

Chronic EBV Disease. Rarely, severe, chronic organ system dysfunction in association with serologic evidence of ongoing EBV infection may follow documented IM. Clinical manifestations include fever, hepatosplenomegaly, interstitial pneumonitis, pancytopenia, uveitis, and hepatitis. Antibodies to EBV replicative antigens (viral capsid antigen and early antigen) are extremely elevated, while a response to the EB nuclear antigen is low or absent. This illness is distinct from the chronic fatigue syndrome (previously called "chronic mononucleosis" or the "chronic Epstein-Barr virus syndrome"), which is characterized by a combination of nonspecific symptoms (severe fatigue, weakness, malaise, subjective fever, sore throat, painful lymph nodes, decreased memory, depression, cognitive dysfunction) in the absence of objective physical or laboratory findings. The latter symptom complex represents a syndrome of unknown cause in which positive EBV serologic results are of no diagnostic value. The lack of a proven correlation between EBV antibody titers and presence of chronic fatigue symptoms suggests diagnostic efforts should remain broad so that definable occult disease is not overlooked.

Malignant Complications. A familial, recessive, X-linked lymphoproliferative syndrome has been described that is characterized by fatal IM, aplastic anemia, agammaglobulinemia, or lymphoma. Patients with other immune deficiencies, particularly transplant recipients and those with acquired immunodeficiency syndrome, have been reported to develop fatal B-cell lymphoproliferative disease secondary to EBV-induced B lymphocyte proliferation.

Treatment

Treatment of IM is largely supportive, and recovery is usually uneventful. Strenuous exertion and contact sports should be avoided during the first weeks of illness, especially in the presence of splenomegaly. Prolonged bed rest has not been shown to be of benefit, and the patient's activity should be determined on an individual basis. Acetaminophen may provide relief from fever and sore throat. Corticosteroids and acyclovir have been used without proof of benefit and cannot be recommended for uncomplicated infectious mononucleosis. However, in the event of impending airway obstruction, severe thrombocytopenia, or hemolytic anemia, corticosteroids in doses equivalent to 60 to 80 mg of prednisone per day can be given with rapid tapering over a 1- to 2-week period. In patients with demonstrated organ system dysfunction that is progressive and associated with extreme elevation of EBV antibody titers, some rationale exists for specific antiviral therapy with acyclovir (Zovirax). Acyclovir has activity against EBV both in vitro and in vivo, but there has been no clear demonstration of clinical efficacy. Intravenous acyclovir can be given at a dose of 30 mg per kg per day (1500 mg per M^2 of body surface area per day) divided into three doses (every 8 hours). Therapeutic response should be measured in terms of objective parameters characterizing the patient's disease, and therapy should be discontinued in absence of a demonstrable beneficial effect.

MUMPS

method of
H. DAVID WILSON, M.D.
University of Kentucky College of Medicine
Lexington, Kentucky

Mumps is an acute generalized viral infection usually diagnosed by the sudden onset of painful swelling in one or both parotid glands. The mumps virus has a particular tropism for glandular and nervous tissues. The submandibular glands are principally involved in approximately 15 per cent of cases, and rarely are the sublingual glands alone affected. The illness is most common in the 5 to 10 year old age group, with 85 per cent of cases occuring before age 20. Subclinical infection occurs in 30 to 40 per cent of people, so many people who think they are susceptible are, in fact, immune.

Mumps is transmitted by salivary secretions and the disease is contagious from one day before parotid swelling until the swelling subsides, usually within a week. Following an incubation period of approximately 14 to 18 days, the child usually complains of earache, headache, and general malaise for a day before onset of parotid swelling. Both parotid glands are affected in two thirds to three fourths of cases. The overlying skin is warm and may be slightly pink, and the gland is tender when touched. Stensen's duct is usually identified easily because of redness and edema around its opening. Nervous system involvement is common, with 10 per cent of patients having symptoms of meningitis and 65 per cent of patients demonstrating cerebrospinal fluid (CSF) pleocytosis when cerebrospinal fluid is routinely examined.

Treatment

Mumps is generally a mild illness requiring only symptomatic treatment. Sour, spicy, or sweet foods and drinks may cause pain when ingested. A soft, bland diet is recommended. Fever can be treated with acetaminophen, 10 mg per kg every 4 to 6 hours for young children and 650 mg every 4 to 6 hours for adults. Cool or warm packs applied to the swollen glands may be soothing for some individuals. Strict bed rest is unnecessary.

Complications and Their Treatment

Meningitis occurs in about 10 per cent of patients, with onset before, during, following, or in the absence of salivary gland swelling. Mumps infection remains one of the causes of aseptic meningitis, albeit of lesser importance since widespread mumps immunization. The CSF usually shows 50 to 800 lymphocytes with a normal glucose and protein content, but up to 2000 or more cells with reduced sugar content can occur. Acetaminophen administered in the dosage listed for treatment of fever and headache is usually sufficient. The removal of CSF for diagnosis may result in improvement of the headache. Intravenous fluids may be needed for the patient with repeated vomiting. Recovery is usually complete within a week, and children can slowly resume their normal activities.

Mumps aseptic meningitis rarely simulates paralytic poliomyelitis with peripheral muscle weakness. Rare cases of aqueductal stenosis resulting in hydrocephalus are well documented following mumps infection.

True *encephalitis* caused by invasion of the brain by virus or as a postinfectious phenomenon is rare and occurs in about 2 individuals per 1000 cases of mumps. It is more common in adults and in males. Mortality of mumps encephalitis is reported to be 1 to 2 per cent, but neurologic sequelae occur in 10 to 20 per cent of those affected. Treatment of encephalitis is directed toward reducing increased intracranial pressure and general supportive care.

Deafness occurs in approximately 1 per 15,000 cases of mumps. It is usually unilateral but frequently results in permanent and complete nerve deafness.

Epididymo-orchitis is a frequent complication in postpubertal males and occurs in 15 to 40 per cent of men diagnosed as having mumps. Parotitis precedes the onset of orchitis by about a week in two thirds of cases. Bilateral testicular involvement is seen in 20 to 40 per cent of cases, with testicular atrophy resulting in half of affected testes. The condition results in high fever, nausea and vomiting, rapid testicular swelling, and erythema and edema of the scrotum. Most men are anxious about the loss of their masculinity. Sterility is seen in less than 2 per cent of cases even with bilateral disease, and impotence is not a complication. Treatment consists of pain medication with either codeine, 3.0 mg per kg per day in divided doses given every 4 to 6 hours by mouth or subcutaneously, or morphine sulfate, 0.1 to 0.2 mg per kg per dose given subcutaneously (maximum 15 mg) every 4 hours for relief of severe pain. The testis should be supported with a towel, and the use of ice packs may reduce discomfort. Pharmacologic doses of steroids such as prednisone, 2 mg per kg per day given by mouth in 3 to 4 divided doses for 3 to 4 days, then given in a tapering dosage for 1 week, usually results in fewer days of fever and a rapid decrease in pain and testicular swelling. After the first few days the prednisone should be given as a single daily dose to lessen adrenal suppression. Steroids do not reduce the incidence of testicular atrophy. Surgical decompression procedures and local infiltration of anesthetics into the spermatic cord are not advocated.

Other complications include pancreatitis (managed with IV fluids and nasogastric suction), oophoritis (seen in 5 to 7 per cent of postpubertal females and causing abdominal pain but not decreased fertility), and presternal edema in children (which may result from obstruction of lymphatic drainage of the upper chest from the enlarged submandibular glands). Thyroiditis, mastitis, myocarditis, nephritis, arthritis, Guillain-Barré syndrome, and transverse myelitis have all been reported in association with mumps.

Mumps Vaccine

Mumps vaccine is a live attenuated viral vaccine prepared in chick embryo cell cultures and usually given combined with measles and rubella vaccine (MMR). Mumps vaccine causes a noncommunicable subclinical infection and results in protective antibody in over 90 per cent of recipients. Over 70 million doses have been given in the United States since 1967 with almost no side effects. Protection against mumps has been demonstrated for at least 17 years. The vaccine should be given to susceptible children (after 14 months of age), adolescents, and adults unless there is a specific contraindication. Persons are considered susceptible unless there is laboratory evidence of mumps antibody, the individual has had mumps diagnosed by a physician, or the individual was immunized with live mumps vaccine after 12 months of age. Persons born in the United States before 1957 have probably been naturally infected and should be considered immune. When there is doubt, the vaccine should be administered since it can safely be given to immune as well as susceptible individuals.

The immediate administration of mumps vaccine to an exposed susceptible individual does not reliably provide protection from that exposure. However, if natural infection does not occur, the vaccine would protect from any subsequent exposure. The efficacy of immune serum globulin or mumps hyperimmune globulin for prevention of mumps is dubious and not recommended.

Contraindications

1. Mumps vaccination is contraindicated in pregnant women.

2. Mumps vaccination is contraindicated in people with immunodeficiency diseases or individuals immunocompromised and being treated for malignant disease or for organ transplantation.

3. Vaccine should not be administered to people for at least 3 months after they have received blood transfusions or immune serum globulin, which might interfere with vaccine effectiveness.

4. Patients with a history of anaphylactic reactions following egg ingestion or following neomycin administration should be vaccinated with extreme caution. Allergies to eggs, chickens, and feathers that do not result in anaphylactic symptoms are not contraindications.

One should recall that other agents such as parainfluenza virus, Coxsackie virus, and others may cause parotitis. Vaccine failures have been reported for a variety of reasons. When the immune status of an individual is in question or when clinical mumps occurs in a vaccinated individual one may obtain viral cultures of saliva, urine, or CSF and determine antibody status as a means of making a precise diagnosis. Complement-fixing antibody to soluble "S" antigen appears soon after infection and indicates recent mumps infection. Antibody to viral "V" antigen appears later and persists for a number of years. More sensitive tests, such as the enzyme-linked immunosorbent assay, are preferred for establishing the immune status of an individual.

PLAGUE

method of
WILLIAM P. REED, M.D.
University of New Mexico
Albuquerque, New Mexico

Plague is a worldwide disease, but only 10 to 40 cases have been reported annually in the United States in the last 10 to 15 years. The disease is thought to have been imported into the United States from Asia around 1900, and initially the cases occurred largely in California. At the present time most of the cases occur in New Mexico, but the disease has also been acquired in California, Colorado, Arizona, Utah, Oregon, and a few other locations. When the disease occurs in these locations it is frequently recognized and treated promptly and appropriately, but when patients acquire the disease in the western United States and travel to other areas before the manifestations have appeared, physicians may not recognize the possibility of plague, and treatment may be inappropriate or tardy. The seriousness of the disease is illustrated by the high mortality in Europe when the "Black Death" was estimated to have killed 25 million persons or about one quarter of the population in the mid 14th century. At that time plague occurred as a rat-flea-rat epidemic which was readily transmitted to human beings in an urban setting. The disease is now quite different, since it is largely expressed as a flea-transmitted epizootic involving rodents and other wild animals. Man and domestic pets may occasionally become infected. When domestic pets living in rural or semi-rural areas come into contact with dead or ill flea-infested animals infected with plague, the fleas may be brought home and subsequently infect humans. Currently it is considered that the majority of cases are acquired within about one mile of home. Other cases are acquired by people whose occupation brings them in contact with infected animals or through hunting and recreational activities. Males and females are presently about equally infected, and about 60 per cent of the cases occur in individuals who are less than 20 years of age. Major risk factors include contact with rodents or carnivores in a rural or semi-rural setting, harborage or food sources for rodents near the home, and possibly failure to control fleas on pets. Although plague has been sylvatic in this country since the 1920s, it remains possible that urban epidemics could still appear, especially in view of the fact that urban rat populations have occasionally been found to be infected with the organism.

Clinical Manifestations

A history of possible exposure is usually present, although in patients who have left endemic areas this history may not be sought. Usually the exposure occurs 2 to 7 days before the patient seeks medical attention. Fever is almost invariably present on presentation, and 85 to 90 per cent of the infected people have painful lymphadenopathy, often with an area of surrounding edema and erythema. Inguinal-femoral nodes are most commonly involved, but axillary, cervical, epitrochlear, and other nodes can also be involved. Even mediastinal node enlargement may be demonstrable by x-ray. Single node involvement is quite common but multiple nodes may be found, a situation that leads to a poorer prognosis. About 10 to 15 per cent of patients have septicemic plague, in which no lymphadenopathy is detected on initial examination but blood cultures are positive. These patients may present only with fever, malaise, nausea, vomiting, diarrhea, or even shock. Cough and/or pulmonary infiltrates occur in a small proportion of individuals, and this is usually considered to be pneumonia secondary to plague elsewhere in the body. Plague can be acquired from aerosol spread of the organism and be a primary infection in the lung, but fortunately this is extremely uncommon in this country. Primary pneumonic plague can have an extremely rapid course with death in 2 to 3 days. Pulmonary infiltrates or mediastinal adenopathy occur in approximately 10 per cent of patients with bubonic or septicemic plague.

The diagnosis of plague requires a high level of suspicion. A history of having been in a setting where exposure is possible is quite common, but the flea bite itself is usually unrecognized either by history or on physical examination. Fever and the usually characteristic bubo are readily recognizable, but at times there may be no bubo or it may simply be missed on physical examination. This is especially true when the patient has traveled to a distant area where physicians are not familiar with the disease. An initial rapid diagnosis may be made by aspirating the bubo under strict precautions with personnel wearing masks and avoiding aerosolization of the aspirate. Bacteriologic stains using the Gram or preferably the Wayson method may show organisms with characteristic bipolar staining resembling a safety pin. However, a fluorescent antibody stain is more satisfactory and can usually be arranged through state public health laboratories. Aspirated material should be cultured and at least two blood cultures should be obtained. The laboratory should be informed that plague is suspected. Blood cultures are positive in about 80 per cent of cases and may become positive only after 2 to 3 days of incubation. Occasionally the level of bacteremia is so high that organisms can be seen microscopically in the blood. Incorrect initial diagnoses include streptococcal or staphylococcal lymphadenitis, tularemia, incarcerated inguinal hernia, acute appendicitis, cat scratch fever, and sepsis of unknown origin. Some of these potential diagnoses could lead to therapy that is inappropriate for plague. Serologic diagnostic techniques are readily available and accurate, but the tests do not become positive until the second week of illness and thus are not useful as a guide for initial therapy.

Treatment

When plague is untreated the mortality rate is in the 50 to 60 per cent range. Thus, patients who are at risk and have a characteristic disease must be treated as rapidly as possible even in the absence of a definitive diagnosis. The patient should initially be strictly isolated even in the absence of a cough or pulmonary infiltrate. The isolation may be relaxed after 48 hours of treatment if there are no signs of pulmonary disease. No treatment has ever been shown to be superior to streptomycin given intramuscularly 30 mg per kg per day in divided doses. Other aminoglycosides are probably as effective, but in vivo studies are not available to prove this point. However, when the patient presents in shock and absorption of intramuscular drugs is questionable, it is probably preferable to use intravenous doses of another aminoglycoside such as gentamicin. Tetracycline, 15 mg per kg per day in divided doses, or chloramphenicol, 30 to 70 mg per kg per day in divided doses, is also effective, and these agents are commonly given in addition to the aminoglycoside. When meningitis is suspected or proved or when abscesses or unusual locations are involved, chloramphenicol should be given because of its excellent penetration into all tissue sites and abscesses. Trimethoprim-sulfamethoxazole may also be effective. Antibiotic treatment is customarily continued for approximately 10 days but may need to be extended in occasional cases. Relapse of plague meningitis has been reported. Superinfection of buboes with other organisms can occur and may require reaspiration for diagnostic purposes and subsequent change of antibiotics to treat the responsible organisms. Antibiotic sensitivity tests are not necessarily a good guide for antibiotic treatment with this organism. For instance, the organism is often reported as sensitive to ampicillin, but this drug as well as other penicillins and cephalosporins seems ineffective in vivo.

Prevention

The best way to prevent plague is to avoid situations where it may be acquired. Persons in endemic areas should avoid wild rodents, carnivores, and especially carcasses during summer. Particular attention should be given to teaching children to not handle such carcasses. Persons who have rural or semi-rural homes in such areas should take measures to remove potential rodent food and living places from around their homes. Appropriate measures should be taken to control fleas on household pets. A vaccine is available and has been shown to reduce the frequency and severity of plague, and may be indicated for individuals whose occupation places them at high risk for the disease.

A major problem exists when people have been exposed to a patient with proven plague. Household contacts are considered to have about a 5 per cent chance of developing plague, which is probably usually also flea-borne. Health care and laboratory workers may also be at risk, and others who might be at risk could include people who have been in a waiting room with a patient who has a cough and pulmonary infiltrates due to plague. A common practice is to treat such high-risk contacts with tetracycline (15 mg per kg per day) or a sulfonamide (40 mg per kg per day) for 5 to 7 days.

PSITTACOSIS
(Ornithosis)

method of
DAVID H. THOM, M.D., and
J. THOMAS GRAYSTON, M.D.
University of Washington
Seattle, Washington

Human psittacosis (also called ornithosis) is caused by *Chlamydia psittaci,* an obligate intracellular bacterium. The infection is typically manifested by fever, pneumonitis, and systemic symptoms, though subclinical infections are known to occur as well. Birds infected with *C. psittaci* have been implicated as the source of human psittacosis since 1879. Virtually all common pet birds and many species of wild birds can carry the organism, and often remain healthy while shedding organisms in their excreta and secretions. Human exposure occurs through inhalation of aerosolized particles containing *C. psittaci* or by direct contact with infected birds. Even brief exposure to birds or their excreta can cause infections. Turkey processing in the United States and duck processing in Europe account for the bulk of occupational psittacosis. Exposure to pet birds, including parakeets, parrots, and pigeons, account for the majority of the 150 to 200 cases of psittacosis reported annually in the United States.

Recently, a *Chlamydia* organism labeled TWAR, which is related to, but distinct from, *C. psittaci,* has been linked by culture and serology to human respiratory infections. No avian source of TWAR has been identified, suggesting that it is transmitted by human-to-human contact. Epidemics of TWAR in military and other populations have been documented. Several studies have found TWAR to be responsible for 6 to 12 per cent of community-acquired pneumonias, and a smaller percentage of bronchitis and pharyngitis, making TWAR infections much more common than infections with *C. psittaci*. In addition, it is likely that some of the sporadic cases and past outbreaks of respiratory disease diagnosed as psittacosis by complement fixation serology were actually TWAR infections.

Diagnosis

The clinical presentation of *C. psittaci* infection can range from mild upper respiratory symptoms to respiratory failure. Severe psittacosis typically presents with a moderate to high fever, headache, prominent cough, and a relative paucity of pulmonary findings on exam. The suspicion of psittacosis is usually raised only when a history of exposure to birds is obtained. Infections with TWAR tend to be milder than diagnosed *C. psittaci* infections, but can also range from a mild upper respiratory infection to severe pneumonia. Patients with TWAR infections may have a biphasic illness, with pharyngitis and upper respiratory symptoms followed in 1 to 3 weeks by pneumonia or bronchitis.

In a patient with pneumonia, a history of recent exposure to a new pet bird or to one that sickens and dies makes psittacosis a likely diagnosis. However, there are no features of the clinical presentation, common laboratory tests, or chest radiograph that are diagnostic of either *C. psittaci* or TWAR infections. *C. psittaci* is rarely isolated from the patient, and laboratory diagnosis depends on a four-fold rise in the *Chlamydia* complement fixation antibody titer between acute and convalescent sera drawn 2 to 4 weeks apart. Early treatment with tetracycline may blunt or prevent the antibody response to *C. psittaci* infections. The complement fixation test commonly used to diagnose psittacosis does not distinguish between *C. psittaci* and other systemic chlamydial infections, including

TWAR. Isolation techniques and TWAR specific antibody tests are not generally available.

Treatment

General treatment measures depend on clinical status. Patients with dyspnea, hypoxia, confusion, or other signs of severe disease should be hospitalized. Case fatality rates are generally less than 1 per cent with treatment, but can be higher in the elderly. Case fatality rates up to 40 per cent have been reported in untreated cases. Respiratory isolation to prevent human transmission is recommended. Patients should be observed for the reported nonrespiratory complications of psittacosis, which include endocarditis, pericarditis, myocarditis, encephalitis, meningitis, renal failure, spontaneous abortion, and reactive arthralgias. Health department authorities should be notified immediately.

The only widely accepted antibiotic therapy for psittacosis is tetracycline in doses of 2 to 3 grams per day, which usually results in a clinical response within 24 to 48 hours, though delayed responses have been reported. Alternatives have been less well studied. Doxycycline (Vibramycin), an oxytetracycline derivative, has been used successfully to treat *C. psittaci* endocarditis in doses of 200 mg per day. Rifampin* (Rifadin, Rimactane) and erythromycin have in vitro activity against *C. psittaci* and have been used alone or in combination in doses of 600 to 1200† mg per day for rifampin and 2 to 4 grams per day for erythromycin. Beta-lactam antibiotics such as penicillin are generally not recommended. If tetracycline or erythromycin is used, treatment with 2 grams per day should be continued for 14 days after defervescence, or for a total of 14 to 21 days, to prevent relapses.

Future immunity should not be assumed, as reinfections have been reported. A prolonged convalescence after successful treatment is not uncommon. TWAR infections should be treated using the same guidelines.

Prevention

There is no vaccine for psittacosis. The disease still occurs in turkeys, inadequately treated pet birds, and some wild birds. Appropriate surveillance of poultry flocks and pet shops and prompt investigation of outbreaks of psittacosis are needed to determine and eradicate sources of exposure. Only limited information is now avail-

---

*This use of rifampin is not listed by the manufacturer.
†Exceeds dosage recommended by manufacturer for listed use.

able on the *Chlamydia* TWAR organism, and no method of prevention has been found.

Q FEVER

method of
JOHN FLAHERTY, M.D., and
ROBERT A. WEINSTEIN, M.D.
Michael Reese Hospital and Medical Center
University of Chicago, Pritzker School of
*　Medicine*
Chicago, Illinois

Q fever, a zoonosis caused by the rickettsial organism *Coxiella burnetii,* is endemic worldwide. The primary reservoirs are cattle, sheep, and goats, but many species of mammals and birds may be infected. Man becomes infected by inhaling dust contaminated with infected products of animal conception, urine, or feces, or, less commonly, by ingestion of raw milk. Infection may be asymptomatic or produce an influenza-like illness, atypical pneumonia, granulomatous hepatitis, or "culture negative" endocarditis.

Unlike other rickettsiae, *C. burnetii* results in a negative Weil-Felix serum agglutination test, is only rarely tick-borne, and very infrequently produces a rash. Because of potential risk to laboratory personnel, serologic evaluation rather than culture is used for diagnostic testing. The specific serologic response can be correlated with the chronicity of infection. During acute disease, antibody to phase II antigen increases, while phase I antibody remains low; in chronic disease, phase I antibodies equal or exceed the titer of phase II antibodies.

Treatment

Nonspecific therapy includes bed rest, antipyretics, analgesics, and hydration.

Q fever is generally a self-limited illness; nevertheless, antibiotics (tetracycline, 500 mg every 6 hours, or doxycycline [Vibramycin], 100 mg every 12 hours) appear to shorten the clinical course and limit complications. In symptomatic patients with a diagnosis of or a clinical or epidemiologic setting that strongly suggests Q fever, therapy is indicated and is continued until the patient has been afebrile for 5 days. In patients with underlying cardiac valvular disease it may be prudent to complete a minimum 14-day antibiotic course despite a prompt clinical response. Chloramphenicol and trimethoprim are other rickettsiostatic agents reserved for patients in whom tetracyclines are contraindicated.

At times the diagnosis of Q fever either is not considered or is not established until after the patient has improved. The need to treat in this circumstance is unknown; however, the rarity of chronic infection, despite the probable underdiagnosis of acute disease, suggests that convalescent patients do not require antibiotics. Treatment in such cases may be reserved for the occasional patient with prolonged or recrudescent symptoms as well as patients with cardiac valvular abnormalities or prosthetic valves, who should be evaluated carefully for the development of endocarditis, including serial determinations of phase I and phase II antibodies.

The rare cases of Q fever endocarditis have been treated with some success with long-term tetracycline, generally in combination with rifampin, trimethoprim-sulfamethoxazole, or lincomycin. Recent evidence of the superior in-vitro activity of the quinolones suggests that one of these agents (for example, ciprofloxacin [Cipro] 750 mg twice a day), perhaps in combination with rifampin, may be considered for refractory cases. The optimal duration of therapy is unclear, although in general prolonged therapy (months to years) has been given. In a few cases, antibiotic therapy has been discontinued when the patient was clinically and hemodynamically improved and the phase I antibody titer had decreased to less than 1:200. Valve replacement has been recommended only when required by hemodynamic decompensation, recalcitrant infection, or recurrent emboli.

Prevention

The extensive enzootic distribution of Q fever makes it a potential problem for abattoir and tannery workers, farmers, ranchers, sheepherders, veterinarians, and medical researchers working with sheep or goats. Unfortunately, the resistance of *C. burnetii* to desiccation and disinfection makes its general elimination from the environment impractical.

Phase I vaccines have been shown to be protective but are not commercially available for human or veterinary use in the United States and must be obtained under investigational new drug (IND) protocol.

Putative person-to-person spread of Q fever has occurred rarely, primarily in relation to aerosols produced at postmortem examination. Nevertheless, infected patients are usually placed on "secretion precautions" if hospitalized. Although Q fever is not a reportable disease in many states, local health authorities should be notified of cases, since investigation may help identify specific high-risk situations amenable to control.

RABIES

method of
THOMAS R. ENG, V.M.D., M.P.H.
Centers for Disease Control
Atlanta, Georgia

Human rabies is extremely rare in the United States. From 1980 to 1987, inclusive, 11 cases of human rabies (0 to 3 cases per year) were reported to the Centers for Disease Control. Of these patients, 5 acquired the infection in the United States and 6 acquired it in another country.

No effective treatment is available for rabies once symptoms of the disease appear. Rabies postexposure prophylaxis (PEP) is administered to persons after exposure to the virus but before clinical manifestations of the infection. Rabies pre-exposure prophylaxis is recommended for persons who are at high risk of exposure to the disease (e.g., rabies laboratory workers, veterinarians, animal control officers).

During the 1980s, approximately 6000 cases of animal rabies were reported annually in the United States. Owing to the problem with animal rabies, approximately 18,000 people receive rabies PEP each year (in the United States). Since rabies is almost always a fatal disease in humans, some physicians may tend to give PEP liberally, even to patients who did not have a true exposure. Studies have found that the rate of PEP can be reduced five to seven fold when physicians consult with state health departments regarding a patient's exposure. Two reasons for limiting PEP only to patients who were likely to have been exposed to rabies are: (1) the PEP vaccines used, although much safer than previous rabies vaccines, cause some adverse reactions, and (2) the immune globulin and vaccine used are expensive.

Determining Whom to Treat

The process of deciding which individuals should be treated is complex and should be approached systematically. Physicians should consult with local and/or state health officials before making any decision about using PEP. Most state health departments have a health professional available for rabies consultations 24 hours a day. Generally, five major factors influence whether a patient should receive PEP: 1. Did a true exposure to rabies occur? 2. What type of animal was involved? 3. What is the current disposition of the animal? 4. What is the current epidemiology of animal rabies in the area? 5. What are the results of laboratory testing or quarantine?

The decision to give PEP to patients reporting a potential exposure (usually a bite) from a potentially rabid animal includes several factors (Fig. 1).

The first step is to determine if a true exposure occurred. Two types of exposures occur, bites and nonbites. A bite exposure is the penetration of the patient's skin by the teeth of the animal, with contamination of the wound with the animal's saliva. This is clearly the usual route of transmission for rabies. A nonbite exposure occurs when an open wound (e.g., scratches, abrasions, lacerations) or mucous membrane of the patient has been contaminated with saliva or other potentially infectious material, such as nervous tissue, from a rabid animal. An open wound is one that was bleeding within 24 hours of exposure. Rabies acquired from nonbite exposures to rabid animals is extremely rare. Seeing, petting, playing with, or any casual contact with a rabid animal is not an exposure.

Decisions regarding patients with potential exposures to rabid humans, laboratory rabies virus, bat-infested caves, or other unusual sources should be handled only with the assistance of local and state health authorities. In the United States, two patients have acquired rabies while working with the virus in laboratories, two patients acquired a probable airborne infection in heavily infested bat caves, and one patient acquired rabies after receiving a corneal transplant from an undiagnosed rabid donor.

After determining that a true exposure has occurred, the species of the exposing animal should be taken into account. Only mammals are susceptible to and capable of transmitting rabies. In the United States, approximately 89 per cent of all reported rabid animals are wild and 11 per cent are domestic. The wild animals that are the major reservoirs of rabies are wild carnivores (e.g., skunks, raccoons, foxes, coyotes, bobcats) and bats. These animals have accounted for the overwhelming majority of human rabies acquired in this country since 1960. In all states except Hawaii (the only state in which rabies is not endemic), exposures to wild carnivores and bats should be considered high-risk since these animals are likely to be rabid. Other wild mammals reported to be rabid with some frequency are various species of wild cats and badgers. Wild mammals that are commonly kept as pets (e.g., ferrets, skunks, raccoons) should be considered capable of transmitting rabies unless the animal's brain is examined and found negative for rabies. Exposures to other wild mammals such as hooved animals (e.g., deer, moose, antelope), rodents (e.g., mice, rats, gerbils, hamsters, guinea pigs), and lagomorphs (e.g., rabbits, hares) almost never call for administering PEP. An exception is exposure to the woodchuck (groundhog), which accounts for the majority of all rabid rodents. No case of human rabies associated with a rodent or lagomorph bite has ever been reported in the United States. However, exposure to unusually

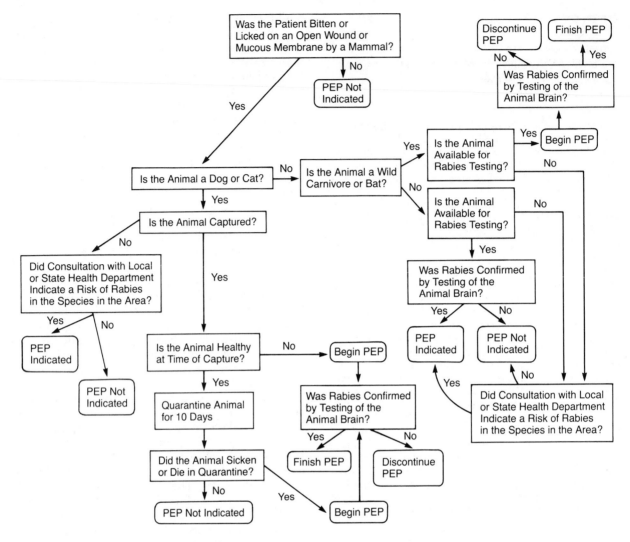

NOTE: CONSULT ACCOMPANYING TEXT BEFORE USING THIS ALGORITHM.

Figure 1. An algorithm for human rabies postexposure prophylaxis (PEP).

aggressive animals (e.g., a squirrel charges without provocation and inflicts severe bites) may be an indication for PEP.

Since 1970, only 2 cases of human rabies acquired in the United States were associated with rabid domestic animals (a dog and a cat). Although domestic animals account for only 11 per cent of animal rabies, they are responsible for the majority of PEP given in the United States. Among domestic animals, cattle, cats, dogs, and horses are most frequently reported to be rabid. Although dogs and cats are efficient transmitters of rabies, the majority of unnecessary PEP administered is associated with their bites. In states without significant wildlife rabies, dog and cat bites are usually not indications for PEP; therefore, consultation with local health officials is important. Although bites from cattle, horses,

and other livestock should be considered potential exposures to rabies, the risk of acquiring rabies from these animals is extremely low. Animals with current rabies vaccinations (approved vaccines are available for dogs, cats, cattle, horses, and sheep) are unlikely to be rabid, but vaccine failures are possible.

A patient who has been exposed to a mammal, wild or domestic, outside the United States should be evaluated in conjunction with state or federal health officials. During the 1980s, most human rabies cases diagnosed in the United States have been acquired following dog bites in developing countries.

After it has been determined that the patient was exposed to an animal likely to transmit rabies, the disposition of the animal should be determined. If a wild animal is involved and has been captured, the animal should be immediately and humanely killed without damaging its head, and its brain should be submitted for rabies testing; no safe quarantine periods exist for wild animals. Wild animals are almost impossible to identify and capture after they have escaped. Local animal control officers are helpful in handling these animals, and veterinarians are trained in safely removing the animal's brain. Local health officials will help coordinate the process and ensure that the brain is transported promptly to the rabies laboratory. Specimens should be refrigerated (not frozen) and should not be placed in a fixative. A direct fluorescent antibody test, which is virtually 100 per cent sensitive (no false negatives), is used to diagnose rabies in animals. The test is performed only at county or state health laboratories. Many state laboratories have the capability of performing the test within 24 hours of receipt. If a test result will be delayed for more than 48 hours or if the patient had a high-risk exposure, the course of PEP may be started while the results are awaited. If the animal is negative for rabies, the course of PEP can then be discontinued. In cases in which the exposing animal is not available for testing, the frequency and distribution of animal rabies in the area is considered. The likelihood of rabies in the animal is based on surveillance data in the area. If a skunk, raccoon, bat, fox, or other wild carnivore is involved and not available for testing, the patient should usually be given PEP. Since rabies in some wild carnivores and bats may be asymptomatic, the circumstances of the bite should not be used to evaluate the risk of human infection. Of rodent bites, only woodchuck bites may warrant PEP if the animal is not available for testing. Exposures to other wild animals that are not available for testing should be considered individually with local health officials.

If a dog or cat is involved and is determined to be healthy by a veterinarian or local health official, the animal should be placed in quarantine for 10 days. An animal that is not healthy should be immediately and humanely killed and tested for rabies. The quarantine period is based on the fact that a dog or cat will sicken or die within 10 days after the virus has invaded the salivary glands. If the animal sickens or dies within the quarantine period, its brain should be submitted for rabies testing. Although dogs and cats with current rabies vaccinations are seldom rabid, they should still be subject to quarantine. Physicians need not give or continue PEP if the animal remains healthy after 10 days. In situations where the dog or cat cannot be identified or has escaped, local health officials should be con-

sulted. Factors to consider in these cases include the circumstances of the incident (e.g., "provoked" bites usually do not call for PEP) and the epidemiology of domestic animal rabies in the area. Physicians may delay PEP for up to a week after an exposure to a low-risk animal if it is likely that the animal will be found. Other domestic animals, including livestock which are not healthy at the time of the incident, should be humanely killed and tested for rabies. Check with appropriate health officials regarding local quarantine regulations for these animals.

Treatment (Postexposure Prophylaxis)

PEP consists of three components: wound management, human rabies immune globulin (HRIG), and rabies vaccine.

Immediate, careful, and thorough washing of all bite and other contaminated wounds with soap and water for several minutes is one of the most important components of PEP. In animal studies, wound cleansing with soap and water markedly decreases the risk of rabies. Cleaning with water or saline alone is not as effective as cleaning with soap and water. All wounds inflicted by animals, regardless of the risk of rabies, should be thoroughly cleansed. The wound should also be evaluated for the risk of other infectious diseases (e.g., tetanus, pasteurellosis, rat bite fever).

HRIG is antirabies gamma globulin made from hyperimmunized human donors. The purpose of HRIG is to provide passive antirabies antibodies before active immunity develops (usually about 7 to 10 days after initial vaccination). HRIG is given once on the first day of treatment (designated as day 0). The dose is 20 international units (IU) per kg of body weight. HRIG is standardized to contain 150 IU per ml. It is supplied in 2-ml (300-IU) and 10-ml (1500-IU) vials. If anatomically possible, up to half of the HRIG dose should be infiltrated around the wound and the rest given intramuscularly in the gluteal area (which is really intragluteal fat). If it is not possible to infiltrate the wound, the entire dose of HRIG should be given intramuscularly. Adverse reactions to HRIG are rare. Although rabies immune globulin made from horse serum is still available, the associated risk of serum sickness is great and this product should be used only when HRIG is not available.

Two rabies vaccines are currently approved for use in the United States: human diploid cell vaccine (HDCV, manufactured by Merieux Institute) and rabies vaccine, adsorbed (RVA, manufactured by the Michigan Department of Public Health). HDCV has been licensed and widely used since 1982. RVA was licensed in 1988, and its availability outside of Michigan is limited. The recommendations for administering HDCV and RVA are identical, except that RVA should not be given intradermally. Persons who have not previously received PEP and have not received pre-exposure prophylaxis should receive 5 doses of vaccine. The first dose is given on the same day as HRIG, day 0. Subsequent doses are given on days 3, 7, 14, and 28. The vaccines are given intramuscularly in the deltoid; infants can be given the vaccine in the anterolateral upper thigh. Rabies vaccine should not be given in the gluteal area or in the same syringe or at the same site as HRIG. When the recommendations for proper wound management and for giving HDCV and HRIG have been strictly followed, PEP has never failed to protect a person against rabies. Adverse reactions to both vaccines are minor. Local reactions, such as pain, swelling, itching, and erythema at the site of injection, are common. Up to 50 per cent of patients who receive HRIG and HDCV experience mild systemic reactions such as headache, nausea, myalgias, abdominal pain, and dizziness. More serious side effects are extremely rare; however, two cases of neurologic illness similar to Guillain-Barré syndrome have been described. About 7 per cent of persons who have previously received HDCV experience an "immune complex–like" illness after receiving an HDCV booster. The illness is characterized by a pruritic rash or urticaria and may include arthralgias, arthritis, angioedema, nausea, vomiting, fever, and malaise. No life-threatening reactions have been reported with HDCV. Adverse reactions associated with RVA appear to be similar to those observed with HDCV. Adverse reactions to these vaccines should be reported to the manufacturer. Pregnancy, existing illness, and previous allergy to rabies vaccine are not contraindications for PEP if the patient has been exposed to rabies. Allergic reactions can be controlled with antihistamines, epinephrine, or corticosteroids. (Corticosteroids should be avoided if possible, since they may interfere with the production of rabies antibodies.)

Persons who have previously received pre-exposure immunization or have previously undergone PEP with HDCV or have an acceptable rabies antibody titer after receiving another vaccine should not receive HRIG. These individuals should receive proper wound management and two additional doses of rabies vaccine, one 1-ml dose IM on day 0 and one on day 3.

Pre-exposure Prophylaxis

Rabies pre-exposure immunization provides protection when an exposure may be unrecog-nized or when PEP may be delayed. Pre-exposure prophylaxis does not eliminate the need for PEP after an exposure but simplifies the regimen by eliminating the need for RIG and decreasing the number of vaccine doses required. Pre-exposure immunization is recommended for persons at high risk of rabies exposure such as rabies laboratory workers, veterinarians, wildlife workers, animal control officers, spelunkers, and travelers who spend over 30 days in a country where rabies is a constant threat. Highly endemic areas include most developing countries in Central and South America, Africa, and Asia. More country-specific information can be obtained from state health departments. For pre-exposure prophylaxis, HDCV can be administered intramuscularly or intradermally. RVA should not be used intradermally. For the intramuscular regimen, 3 doses (1 ml) are given in the deltoid, one each on days 0, 3, and 28. For the intradermal regimen, 3 doses (0.1 ml) are given in the skin over the deltoid area, one each on days 0, 3, and 21 or 28. If given intradermally, the three-dose series should be completed in travelers at least 30 days before departure. HDCV should not be given intradermally to travelers who are receiving chloroquine for malaria chemoprophylaxis, since the drug may interfere with the immune response to HDCV. Travelers who do not have sufficient time to complete the intradermal regimen at least 30 days before departure or those taking chloroquine should receive HDCV by the intramuscular route.

Diagnosis

Rabies should be suspected in any person with encephalitis or myelitis of unknown etiology, even in the absence of an exposure history, especially if the patient has traveled to a rabies-endemic area outside the United States. Human rabies often presents with protean manifestations, making early diagnosis difficult. Although the incubation period is usually between 20 and 90 days, well-documented cases have been reported in the United States with incubation periods from 12 to 701 days. The first symptoms of rabies are often nonspecific and include fever, malaise, headache, gastrointestinal and upper respiratory tract symptoms, and subtle changes in mental status. The first specific signs of rabies are paresthesias or pain at or near the site of exposure, but these appear in only about 50 per cent of patients. The course of the disease, characterized by a rapidly progressive encephalitis or myelitis, results in a coma 4 to 10 days after the onset of symptoms. In the United States, patients who did not receive intensive supportive care usually died about 7 days after the appearance of the first symptom. Routine laboratory tests are usually consistent with a viral encephalitis but are not helpful in establishing the diagnosis. An antemortem diagnosis can be made by a positive immunofluorescence antibody test on a neck skin biopsy, virus isolation from saliva, or demonstration of a positive antibody titer to rabies in serum (in persons who have never received rabies vaccines) or in cerebrospinal fluid. However, these tests are usually not positive until late in the course of the patient's illness. Postmortem diagnostic techniques include virus isolation, Seller's stain for detecting Negri bodies, and immunofluorescence antibody testing of brain tissue.

RAT-BITE FEVER

method of
FRANKLIN D. LOWY, M.D.
Montefiore Medical Center
Bronx, New York

Rat-bite fever is a single designation for two systemic febrile illnesses that are caused by two different bacterial species. Because of their clinical similarity, these two diseases are generally described together. Rat-bite fever has been recognized for over 2300 years in India. It is worldwide in distribution and most commonly affects individuals exposed to rats or other rodents. The two pathogens are *Streptobacillus moniliformis* and *Spirillum minor*. Both organisms are part of the normal oropharyngeal flora of many rodents. Infection is acquired through contact, usually bites or scratches, with rodents or, rarely, cats. In addition, *S. moniliformis* has been spread by contamination of food products with animal excreta. This disease is commonly called Haverhill fever. In a small percentage of patients, a history of antecedent exposure to rodents is not obtained.

Bacteriology

Streptobacillus moniliformis is a pleomorphic, gramnegative rod. It is a facultative anaerobe that grows best in medium supplemented with serum, although it can also be recovered from routine blood culture media. *Spirillum minor* is a gram-negative spiral rod that does not grow in standard culture media. It can be diagnosed by dark-field examination of blood or material obtained from skin lesions or draining nodes. Animal inoculation is usually required for a definitive diagnosis.

Clinical Manifestations

Following inoculation of the pathogen from the rat bite, two similar but distinct diseases may develop.

Their distinguishing features are summarized in Table 1. Both illnesses are associated with fever, chills, and constitutional symptoms, and both may be relapsing. Untreated, the disease may recur for several months. Complications, though rare, include chronic arthritis, endocarditis, and localized abscesses. Other diagnostic considerations usually include rickettsial diseases, leptospirosis, infective endocarditis, acute rheumatic fever, and septic arthritis.

Diagnosis

The diagnosis of rat-bite fever should be considered in individuals with fever, a history of animal exposure, elevated white cell count, and a false-positive test for syphilis. Confirmation of the diagnosis requires either isolation of the organism or, in the case of *S. minor*, visualization of the organism by dark-field techniques. Gas-liquid chromatographic analysis of the fatty acid profile of *S. moniliformis* has also recently been used as a means of diagnosis.

Therapy

The drug of choice for rat-bite fever caused by either pathogen remains penicillin. Patients requiring hospitalization should be given aqueous penicillin G, 400,000 to 600,000 units intravenously every 4 to 6 hours, or procaine penicillin, 600,000 units intramuscularly every 12 hours. Individuals who do not require hospitalization or who are clinically improved can be treated orally with penicillin V, 500 mg every 6 hours. Response to therapy is often prompt and dramatic. Although the length of therapy has not been definitively determined, a 10- to 14-day course is generally recommended. In individuals who develop complications of their infection, most notably endocarditis, therapy with penicillin, 12 to 24 million units per day for at least 4 weeks, is

TABLE 1. **Distinguishing Features of the Two Diseases Causing Rat-Bite Fever**

	Streptobacillus moniliformis	*Spirillum minor*
Incubation period	<10 days	≥7 days
Reaction at site of inoculation	Rare, prompt healing	Initial healing, but ulceration or eschar at onset of fever
Lymphadenopathy	Uncommon	Frequently regional
Rash	Morbilliform, petechial	Maculopapular beginning in the region of the bite
Joint involvement	Arthralgias, arthritis common	Arthralgias rare
False-positive test for syphilis	<25%	≥50 %

recommended. Alternative therapies include tetracycline, 500 mg orally or intravenously every 6 hours, or streptomycin, 500 mg intramuscularly every 12 hours.

Prevention of rat-bite fever primarily involves careful pest control, particularly in settings where exposure of children is likely. Because of the well-documented cases of rat-bite fever in laboratory workers, gloves should be worn to avoid accidental inoculation when handling rodents. All bites should be thoroughly cleansed with an antiseptic solution. It is unclear whether the prophylactic administration of an antibiotic, such as penicillin or tetracycline, is warranted. Therapy with one of these agents may be justified in individuals with underlying valvular heart disease. This has not, however, been subjected to clinical evaluation.

RELAPSING FEVER

method of
BAYU TEKLU, M.D.
King Saud University, Abha Branch
College of Medicine
Abha, Saudi Arabia

Relapsing fever is an acute infectious disease due to *Borrelia* spirochetes. There are two types of relapsing fever: the epidemic (louse-borne) caused by *Borrelia recurrentis* and the endemic (tick-borne) caused by several different species.

Epidemiology and Transmission

The louse-borne relapsing fever (LBRF) is most endemic in Ethiopia, occurring among the destitute and homeless, while the tick-borne relapsing fever (TBRF) has a worldwide distribution with sporadic cases occurring from the west coast of North America down to Central and South America, and in Africa and Asia.

The body louse takes a blood meal from an infected person and the spirochetes multiply in the hemolymph; transmission to man occurs when the louse is crushed and some of its contents get access to the bloodstream via an abraded skin. Man is the only reservoir of LBRF. In the TBRF, transmission occurs by a skin bite of an infected tick. Infection is transmitted to its progeny. Several rodents act as reservoirs for TBRF.

Clinical Manifestations

Both types of relapsing fever are characterized by febrile episodes with remissions and relapses occurring two to three times in LBRF and up to ten times in TBRF. The relapses are due to changing antigenicity of the spirochete. Patients develop fever, chills, headaches, and fatigue. Skin petechiae and splenomegaly are common. Serious complications include myocardi-

tis, renal and liver failure, coagulopathy, psychosis, shock, and coma.

The Jarisch-Herxheimer reaction occurs in all patients with LBRF and in one third of those with TBRF with or without treatment. The mortality in untreated LBRF may reach 30 to 70 per cent in epidemics, while it is only 4 per cent with antibiotic therapy. Poor prognostic signs include deep jaundice, gastrointestinal hemorrhage, pneumonia, and coma.

Diagnosis

Diagnosis is made by demonstrating spirochetes using dark-field microscopy or, more commonly, in a thin or thick peripheral blood smear stained with either Giemsa, Wright, or Leishman stain. If spirochetemia is light, smears may be negative.

Treatment

Antibiotics

The spirochete is exquisitely sensitive to antibiotics (Table 1). However, trimethoprim-sulfamethoxazole and aminoglycosides are not effective. The recommended regimen in moderately to severely ill patients is to administer procaine penicillin G, 400,000 units intramuscularly, followed by tetracycline, 250 mg orally, the next day. The rationale for this form of therapy is to avoid killing large numbers of spirochetes too quickly, which may precipitate a severe Jarisch-Herxheimer reaction. Spirochetes disappear within 3 hours of tetracycline administration, while it may take several hours with PAM (penicillin aluminum monostearate) or small-dose procaine penicillin G. In patients with negative smears but clinically suspected to have LBRF, tetracycline, 250 mg orally, can be administered and the patient carefully observed for the Jarisch-Herxheimer reaction. Occurrence of the crisis confirms the diagnosis, while its absence virtually rules out the disease.

Management of the Jarisch-Herxheimer Reaction

One of the serious and unavoidable complications of antibiotic therapy of LBRF is the Jarisch-

TABLE 1. **Single-Dose Antibiotic Treatment of LBRF**

	Dose	Relapse (%)
Procaine penicillin G	800,000 U IM/IV	0–15
Penicillin aluminum monostearate (PAM)	1,200,000 U IM	0
Ampicillin	500 mg PO	0–20
Tetracycline	250 mg PO/IV	0
Doxycycline	100 mg PO	0
Chloramphenicol	500 mg PO	0
Erythromycin	500 mg PO	0

TABLE 2. **The Jarisch-Herxheimer Reaction of Louse-Borne Relapsing Fever**

	"Chill Phase"	"Flush Phase"
Onset	30–60 min*	At end of "chill phase"
Duration	30–60 min	12 hr
Vital signs	Increase†	Fall‡
Rigors	Severe	None
Sweating	None	Profuse

*After IV tetracycline.
†Hyperpyrexia and hypertension may occur.
‡Severe peripheral vasodilation and shock may occur.

Herxheimer reaction, which by itself carries a mortality rate of up to 12 per cent. The characteristic findings are listed in Table 2.

Management of the Jarisch-Herxheimer reaction consists of very close monitoring of vital signs following antibiotic administration. Intravenous saline infusion must be started and central venous pressures or wedge pressures (if available) measured. In the event of cardiac failure, with rare cases of pulmonary edema, digoxin, 0.5 to 1.0 mg, should be administered slowly intravenously. Aspirin, acetaminophen, or even high-dose corticosteroids in the past have had no influence on the Jarisch-Herxheimer reaction. However, 300 to 500 mg of meptazinol,* an opioid antagonist with some agonist properties, intravenously, definitely ameliorates the Jarisch-Herxheimer reaction. The treatment of choice for TBRF is tetracycline, 500 mg orally every 6 hours for 10 days.

Prevention

LBRF is a disease of poverty. Improved personal hygiene and living conditions can eradicate the disease. As a temporary measure, all patients should have a thorough wash with soap and water and the scalp hair shaved, and 1 per cent lindane or Lysol solution, or even DDT, should be applied and the patient changed into new clothes. Family members or cohabitants of the index patient should be deloused in a similar manner.

It is suggested that special groups of people such as medical personnel, volunteer workers, and visitors who spend short periods in famine areas or feeding camps in Ethiopia or neighboring Sudan take doxycycline, 100 mg orally daily, for the duration of their stay. This regimen can cure both LBRF and typhus.

Spraying of buildings and walls with 2 per cent benzene hydrochloride is beneficial in controlling TBRF, but eradication of the disease is impossible. People camping outside should avoid tick-infested areas and apply insect repellent to the skin.

*Investigational drug in the United States.

RHEUMATIC FEVER

method of
EUGENIE F. DOYLE, M.D.
New York University Medical Center
New York, New York

The decline in incidence of acute rheumatic fever, starting early in this century, was dramatically accelerated with widespread use of penicillin for the treatment of streptococcal pharyngitis. However, many outbreaks recently reported from different sections of the United States demonstrate that rheumatic fever has not disappeared as a problem and that continued vigilance for streptococcal pharyngitis, and careful therapy when this disorder is present, are essential to prevent rheumatic fever.

The exact pathogenesis remains unknown, but rheumatic fever manifestations are thought to result from the production of immune complexes in genetically susceptible individuals upon exposure to Group A beta-hemolytic streptococcal infection in the pharynx. These complexes interact with the patient's heart, joints, caudate nucleus, and skin.

Diagnosis

Since no single manifestation is pathognomonic for rheumatic fever, the Jones criteria were devised to guide in diagnosis. The presence of two major or one major and two minor criteria, along with evidence of a recent streptococcal infection, permits a reliable basis for the diagnosis (Table 1).

Clinical manifestations of the criteria include:

Carditis: Tachycardia, impaired heart sounds, apical systolic and/or basal diastolic murmur, pericardial rub.

Polyarthritis: Migratory arthritis of large joints, especially knees, ankles, wrists, and elbows.

Chorea: Involuntary jerking movements of the extremities, incoordination, slurred speech, facial grimacing.

Erythema Marginatum: Pink, nonpruritic macular rash with distinct, wavy margin.

Subcutaneous Nodules: Hard, painless swellings over the extensor surfaces of the joints, notably elbows, knuckles, knees, dorsum of feet, and dorsal spine prominence.

TABLE 1. **Jones Criteria (Revised)**

Major Manifestations	Minor Manifestations
Carditis	Fever
Polyarthritis	Arthralgia
Chorea	Previous rheumatic fever
Erythema marginatum	Elevated ESR or + CRP
Subcutaneous nodules	Prolonged PR interval

plus

Supporting evidence of preceding streptococcal infection: history of recent scarlet fever; positive throat culture for group A *Streptococcus*; increased ASO titer or other streptococcal antibodies.

From Circulation 32:664, 1965. By permission of the American Heart Association, Inc.

TABLE 2. Recommended Anti-Inflammatory Agents for Acute Rheumatic Fever

Arthritis	Mild Carditis; No Cardiomegaly	Moderate, Severe Carditis; Congestive Failure
Salicylates 100 mg/kg/day (serum level 25–35 mg/dl) Continue for 2–4 weeks	Salicylates 100 mg/kg/day Continue for 6–8 weeks Change to prednisone if significant cardiomegaly develops	Prednisone 2 mg/kg/day for 1–2 weeks; taper during next 2–4 weeks Begin salicylates in final week of prednisone; continue for 6–8 weeks

Therapy

Salicylates and steroids remain the most effective anti-inflammatory drugs for therapy, although it is known that they are suppressive, not curative. For polyarthritis with mild or no carditis, aspirin alone is recommended. For moderate or more severe degrees of carditis, steroids have a greater anti-inflammatory effect. Dosage schedules are listed in Table 2. The duration of either salicylate or steroid therapy varies with the clinical course. Signs of recovery include subsidence of fever, resolution of clinical manifestations, and return to normal of the erythrocyte sedimentation rate and C-reactive protein.

Chorea, which frequently occurs weeks after other signs of rheumatic fever have subsided, may be mild, not warranting any sedation. For more severe chorea, haloperidol (Haldol), 0.25 mg orally twice daily, or chlorpromazine (Thorazine), 0.5 mg per kg per dose orally every 6 hours for 4 to 6 weeks, usually effects subsidence of the movements.

Congestive heart failure requires digoxin, diuretics, and sometimes oxygen. Surgery for repair or replacement of the mitral or aortic valve is usually not indicated during the acute phase of rheumatic fever. Only in rare cases may it be indicated during the acute phase if life-threatening valve dysfunction is present.

TABLE 3. Secondary Prevention of Rheumatic Fever

Preparation	Weight	
	60 lb or Less	Over 60 lb
Intramuscular		
Benzathine penicillin every 3–4 weeks	1,200,000 U	1,200,000 U
Oral		
Penicillin V	250 mg once daily	250 mg twice daily
Sulfadiazine	0.5 gm once daily	1 gm once daily
Erythromycin	250 mg once daily	250 mg twice daily

Bed Rest

Patients without carditis may be ambulated as soon as joint manifestation or chorea has subsided. Patients with carditis should be on bed rest until tachycardia has subsided and cardiomegaly is diminishing. Generally, the degree of cardiomegaly should act as a guide to resumption of activity. Subsidence of elevated CRP and ESR are supporting evidence of clearing of the infection.

Antibiotics during Acute Infection

With acute rheumatic fever, obliteration of any lingering forms of infection is needed. Intramuscular benzathine penicillin G is indicated: 600,000 units for patients 60 pounds or less, 1.2 million units for heavier patients. At the end of 21 days, the patient should be started on continuous prophylactic penicillin.

Prophylaxis against Recurrent Streptococcal Infection

Experience dating to the pre-prophylaxis era showed a high incidence of recurrent rheumatic fever, especially during the 5 years following the initial episode. Therefore, prevention of a second attack of rheumatic fever is an important part of patient management. The greatest protection is provided by *intramuscular* benzathine penicillin G, 1.2 million units every 3 to 4 weeks; it should be used for those with rheumatic heart disease who are most at risk if there is a recurrence or for those not compliant. *Oral* agents, to be prescribed for compliant patients, include penicillin V, sulfadiazine, and erythromycin. Dosage schedules are listed in Table 3.

ROCKY MOUNTAIN SPOTTED FEVER

method of
DANIEL J. SEXTON, M.D.
Oklahoma City Clinic
Oklahoma City, Oklahoma

Rocky Mountain spotted fever (RMSF) is caused by the bacterium *Rickettsia rickettsii*. It is the most prevalent and the most clinically important of the rickettsial diseases that occur in the United States. A variety of hard-shelled (ixodid) ticks are both the reservoir and vector for this disease. RMSF predominantly occurs in the Southeastern and Southern Plains regions of the United States but has been reported from 45 states. Because of the frequency of travel, physicians in nonendemic areas should be aware of the clinical features of this disease. RMSF occurs mainly in the spring and summer months, but in warm regions of the United States cases may occur even in late fall or early winter.

RMSF may range in severity from mild to fatal. The incubation period after a tick bite ranges from 3 to 14 days, but typically symptoms occur 4 to 8 days after tick exposure. Up to a third of patients with RMSF have no history of tick bite; therefore, the absence of a history of tick bite or exposure should not prevent the clinician from suspecting and treating this illness.

Clinical Features

The dominant clinical features of RMSF are headache, fever, and skin rash. However, many patients have atypical features such as nausea, vomiting, abdominal pain (which can occasionally be a dominant symptom), diarrhea, joint pain, stiff neck, or alteration of mental status. Typically the onset of symptoms is abrupt. Chills may precede or accompany the fever, and many patients have prominent myalgias. Headache may be severe enough to suggest a diagnosis of meningitis, particularly when alterations in mental status and vomiting are present. Occasionally, patients have splenomegaly, conjunctivitis, jaundice, seizures, or hallucinations.

The rash of RMSF classically begins on the ankles and wrists and spreads centrally. In the early stages a maculopapular rash is typical. In later stages, petechiae and frank purpura may be present. Some patients do not have a typical rash, and in others the rash does not progress from maculopapular to petechial. In dark-skinned individuals the rash may be overlooked, in some patients the rash may not be present until later in the illness, and rarely the rash may not appear at all. Withholding therapy until a rash appears may result in clinical catastrophe.

RMSF may be confused clinically with infectious mononucleosis, nonspecific viral illness, or drug eruptions (particularly if empiric antimicrobial therapy with sulfonamides, penicillins, or cephalosporins is given early in the course of the illness). Disseminated staphylococcal infection, viral meningitis, mononucleosis, meningococcemia, and ehrlichiosis may all clinically resemble RMSF. The latter disease is caused by *Ehrlichia canis*, a recently recognized rickettsial disease that may produce many of the features of RMSF with the exception of skin rash. Additionally, patients with *E. canis* infection often have leukopenia. Severe cases of ehrlichiosis may be difficult to distinguish from RMSF without specific serologic tests.

There are no diagnostic laboratory findings in RMSF. Many patients have hyponatremia, and occasionally the syndrome of inappropriate antidiuretic hormone secretion may occur. An elevated creatinine phosphokinase, azotemia, jaundice, hyperbilirubinemia, and abnormal results of liver function studies have all been described in severe cases of RMSF. Uncommon or late complications of the disease include pneumonitis; myocarditis with shock; rhabdomyolysis; renal failure; gangrene of the digits, scrotum, and ears; and encephalitis or encephalopathy. The cerebrospinal fluid in patients with RMSF may contain few or many leukocytes and an elevated level of protein. Thrombocytopenia may occur in some patients, and the laboratory findings of

disseminated intravascular coagulation are a well-known complication of this disease in its severe form. Rarely, patients may develop focal neurologic symptoms that persist after resolution of the acute illness.

Treatment

It is axiomatic that the diagnosis of RMSF must be made on clinical features alone. Delaying therapy until serologic proof of infection is available is a fundamental mistake. By necessity, therapy must be initiated in most patients on the basis of history and the clinical findings alone. The only two drugs effective against *R. rickettsii* are chloramphenicol and tetracycline. Both drugs are probably equally effective. Chloramphenicol has the potential for bone marrow toxicity. Tetracycline can cause dental staining in children and is potentially hepatotoxic in high intravenous doses and when given to pregnant women.

Chloramphenicol is particularly useful in patients with severe disease in whom meningococcemia cannot be clinically differentiated from RMSF. The recommended dose of chloramphenicol is 50 mg per kg per day in four divided doses for adults and 50 to 100 mg per kg per day in four divided doses for children. Chloramphenicol should not be administered intramuscularly, as absorption is erratic and unpredictable when this route is used. Patients receiving chloramphenicol should have frequent checks of their platelet count, hematocrit, and white blood count. It should be used with caution in patients with severe liver dysfunction. Chloramphenicol can produce two kinds of bone marrow toxicity; one is dose-related and reversible, whereas the other is idiosyncratic and rare and may result in irreversible aplastic anemia. Because of its potential hematopoietic toxicity, chloramphenicol is generally reserved for patients with more severe cases or for pregnant women. In the latter situation it can cause the gray baby syndrome if administered near the end of pregnancy.

Tetracycline hydrochloride should be given orally in a dose of 25 to 40 mg per kg per day for both adults and children up to a maximum dose of 2 grams per day. Lower doses are generally recommended when the intravenous route is used, since occasional severe hepatotoxicity may occur with intravenous tetracycline. If given orally, tetracycline should be taken between meals, and concomitant administration of milk, antacids, and food should be avoided. It should not be used in patients with severe renal dysfunction. Doxycycline (Vibramycin), 50 to 100 mg orally or intravenously twice daily, is especially useful if azotemia is present. Doxycycline by the oral route has better absorption than oral tetracycline hydrochloride but has the disadvantage of being more expensive. Although prolonged or repeated courses of tetracycline cause a gray dental discoloration of permanent teeth in children under age 8, a single course of therapy at a dose of 25 mg per kg per day is safe for children and may be life-saving. Sulfonamides should not be used in the treatment of Rocky Mountain spotted fever, not only because they are ineffective but also because they may actually aggravate rickettsial infections. Cephalosporins, penicillins, and aminoglycosides have no activity against *R. rickettsii.*

In addition to specific antimicrobial therapy, supportive care is extremely important. *R. rickettsii* produces a small vessel vasculitis that may damage most internal organs, including the nervous system. Late effects of this vasculitis may include hypoproteinemia, circulatory collapse, hypotension, metabolic acidosis, oliguria, edema, hyponatremia, seizures, and diffuse neurologic dysfunction. Dehydration is common in RMSF and should be corrected with appropriate fluid replacement. The maintenance of adequate intravascular volume is critical in severe cases, and fluid and electrolyte therapy must be carefully monitored. Diffuse vascular damage may result in marked edema in the face of inadequate intravascular volume, and occasionally colloid replacement using albumin or plasma may be helpful. Secondary bleeding complications due to disseminated intravascular coagulation (DIC) are best treated by specific antirickettsial antimicrobial therapy and judicious use of blood components. In severe cases measurement of pulmonary artery wedge pressure and monitoring of cardiac output may be necessary. Corticosteroid therapy has no proven value in RMSF, and experimentally corticosteroids may aggravate organ damage induced by rickettsiae.

Patients with mild RMSF may be safely managed as outpatients if careful follow-up is available. More severe cases require hospitalization. Most patients with mild disease will improve within 48 to 96 hours after the initiation of therapy. Improvement may take up to a week to 10 days in advanced or severe cases. Either chloramphenicol or tetracycline can be discontinued 48 to 96 hours after resolution of fever if the signs of active infection have abated. Isolation of infected patients is not necessary.

Early treatment may abolish or blunt diagnostic antibody rises in some infected patients. The Weil-Felix reaction (Proteus OX-2 and OX-19 agglutinins) is of little clinical use and has been replaced by more specific serologic studies. Weil-Felix agglutinins do not typically appear until the second week of illness, and antibody rises may occur in less than 75 per cent of infected patients. The complement fixation test is no longer recommended, since it is negative in up to half of all infected patients and antibody rises may take 14 to 21 days to appear. Both indirect fluorescent antibody (IFA) and latex agglutination (LA) tests are generally available and useful in the diagnosis of RMSF. In both tests antibodies appear late in the first week of infection and a marked rise in titer is usually detectable late in the second week of illness. Cultures for *R. rickettsii* are not generally available, as they require special equipment and safety precautions. It is important that therapy never be delayed awaiting serologic confirmation of infection. Skin biopsy and direct application of fluorescent immunologic reagents is occasionally useful in diagnosing RMSF but is not generally available outside of large medical centers.

Prevention

It is probably impossible to truly prevent the occurrence of this disease, since no vaccine is commercially available or practical and *R. rickettsii* cycles in nature among ticks and mammals independent of humans. Avoidance of ticks and their prompt removal after attachment are the best means of prevention. Ticks should be removed using care to avoid contamination of the fingers or mucous membranes with tick excretions or tick body contents. Paper or cloth should be used to protect the fingers if tweezers are not available at the time of tick removal. Crushing ticks with unprotected fingers may result in either aerosol or percutaneous transmission of disease to humans. Cleansing of the site of attachment with soap and water after removal is generally recommended. Prompt initiation of antirickettsial therapy is recommended if any clinical features of RMSF occur within 3 to 14 days following tick attachment. Prophylactic antirickettsial therapy after tick bite is of no proven benefit in preventing human disease.

Physicians in endemic areas should question all patients presenting with headache, rash, or unexplained febrile illness during the spring and summer months about ticks or tick exposure and should be highly suspicious of the diagnosis of RMSF when the clinical features of RMSF are present.

RUBELLA AND CONGENITAL RUBELLA

method of
MORVEN S. EDWARDS, M.D.
Baylor College of Medicine
Houston, Texas

POSTNATALLY ACQUIRED RUBELLA

Postnatally acquired rubella is usually a mild disease. During the 1 to 5 days preceding the exanthem, prodromal symptoms (which occur more frequently in adults than children), such as eye pain, fever, headache, malaise, sore throat, or mild coryza, may be observed. After an incubation period of 16 to 18 days (range 14 to 21 days), the maculopapular rash of rubella begins on the face and spreads downward and centrifugally. The pink-red lesions may coalesce on the trunk but remain discrete on the extremities. The rash clears from the face on the second day of illness and from the extremities by the end of the third day. Neither the rash nor the lymphadenopathy involving suboccipital, postauricular, and cervical nodes is sufficiently distinctive to be pathognomonic for rubella. It may be difficult clinically to distinguish rubella from infections such as erythema infectiosum, enteroviral illness, or infectious mononucleosis.

Postnatally acquired rubella generally is diagnosed serologically. Hemagglutination-inhibition (HAI) is the most commonly employed technique. Since HAI antibody is detectable by the third day of rash, reaches a peak by one month, and persists indefinitely, a single titer may not suffice for diagnosis of acute infection. A fourfold or greater increase in antibody titer *or* demonstration of rubella-specific IgM by an adaptation of the HAI is diagnostic of recent infection. Rubella-specific IgM tests are advantageous in that a diagnosis may be established from a single serum specimen; conversely, the extraction methods employed to separate IgM from IgG reduce the sensitivity of these assays. A number of tests equal to or exceeding the HAI in sensitivity, including the latex agglutination and enzyme immunoassay methods, are gradually replacing the HAI. Sera must be treated to prevent false-positive results when rheumatoid factor is present, but the newer methods are rapid and easy to perform.

Treatment

No specific therapy is required or indicated for uncomplicated postnatally acquired rubella.

Complications

The most common complications of rubella are arthralgias or arthritis. Arthritis is most common in adults, affecting up to 30 per cent of women with rubella, has its onset during recovery, and may persist for weeks to months. The treatment of choice, which usually results in dramatic improvement, is aspirin, 60 mg per kg per day for children and 2 grams daily for adults, given in four equal doses. Corticosteroids are not required and are contraindicated, since synovial fluid may contain live virus. Treatment of the infrequently observed complications of encephalitis (one per 5000 cases) and the hemorrhagic consequences of immune-mediated thrombocytopenia or vascular damage (one per 3000 cases) is primarily supportive, although blood replacement may occasionally be required for the latter.

Management of Pregnant Contacts

Ideally, the rubella immune status of women should be determined early in pregnancy. An HAI antibody titer greater than or equal to 1:8 or the presence of antibody by another properly performed test before or at the time of exposure indicates that the individual is immune and is not at risk. If antibody is not detectable, a second specimen should be obtained 2 weeks later. Infection can be assumed if seroconversion is documented. If the second specimen is negative, the test should be repeated 6 weeks after exposure; if it remains negative, infection did not occur. To document infection, detection of rubella-specific IgM or isolation of virus from the throat also can be useful.

The relative risk of congenital malformations as a consequence of maternal rubella during the first four weeks of gestation is 30 to 60 per cent. The risk declines to 25 per cent during the fifth to eighth weeks of gestation and to 8 per cent during the ninth to twelfth weeks. Occasionally, fetal damage occurs if rubella occurs up to the twentieth week of gestation. By the fifth month of gestation, some centers are able to obtain and process fetal blood for rubella-specific IgM to document the presence or absence of transmission to the fetus.

The relative risks to the fetus should be discussed in detail with the patient and a decision should be made regarding potential pregnancy termination if infection is documented. If termination of pregnancy is not an option, administration of immune globulin (IG) for post-exposure prophylaxis should be considered. While not uniformly efficacious, IG administered within 72 hours of exposure at a dosage of 0.55 ml per kg may prevent or modify infection in an exposed susceptible patient.

CONGENITAL RUBELLA

The classic manifestations of the congenital rubella syndrome include intrauterine growth retardation, microcephaly, cataracts and microphthalmia, congenital heart disease, and developmental retardation. Deafness, usually severe and bilateral, occurs frequently and may be the only manifestation of congenital rubella. As the result of intense investigation surrounding the epidemic of 1964, the late effects of congenital rubella syndrome have been elucidated. These include endocrinopathies (particularly diabetes), progressive hearing loss, and progressive rubella panencephalitis due to persistent and extending rubella infection of the brain.

The best method for the definitive diagnosis of congenital rubella syndrome is isolation of the virus. Specimens for viral culture should be obtained from the nasopharynx, throat, urine, and cerebrospinal fluid. The virus persists for many months in the urine and nasopharynx. An alternative method for establishing the diagnosis is the documentation in serum of rubella-specific IgM. For questionable cases, declining levels of maternally acquired IgG antibody may be a helpful adjunct for excluding the diagnosis.

Treatment

No drugs are available to curtail viral shedding or to prevent progressive symptoms. Multidisciplinary supportive care should be provided.

Isolation Procedures

Patients with postnatal rubella are most contagious when the rash is erupting. Viremia peaks just prior to the onset of exanthem and resolves shortly after the appearance of rash. Viral shedding in the nasopharynx occurs for approximately 1 week before and 1 week after the onset of rash. Patients should be isolated from susceptible pregnant contacts during this interval. Children with postnatal rubella should be excluded from school for 7 days after the onset of rash. In the hospital setting, contact isolation is required for 7 days after the onset of rash.

Infants with congenital rubella remain chronically infected for many months. The hospitalized patient and those in day care should be considered contagious for the first year of life, unless nasopharyngeal and urine cultures obtained after 3 months of age are negative for rubella virus. Contact isolation should be employed in the hospital setting. Severely affected infants may shed virus beyond the first year of life. Virus may persist in the eye for many years. Susceptible pregnant caretakers should be made aware of the potential hazard of exposure to these infants.

Prevention

Major rubella epidemics occurred at 6- to 9-year intervals before licensure of live attenuated rubella vaccine in 1969. Since then, more than 125 million doses of vaccine have been administered and the incidence of congenital rubella syndrome has declined by 97 per cent. However, 10 to 20 per cent of women in the childbearing years are susceptible to rubella. The low incidence of congenital rubella syndrome is attributed to reduced exposure of susceptible adults to acutely infected school-aged children.

The only rubella vaccine currently available in the United States is the RA 27/3 strain of virus grown in human diploid cell cultures. Serum antibody is induced in more than 95 per cent of recipients. Although antibody titers following vaccine are somewhat lower than those elicited from natural infection, they persist for at least 15 years after immunization, and are probably lifelong. The vaccine is administered as a single subcutaneous dose of 0.5 ml, alone or in a preparation containing mumps and/or measles components.

In children rubella vaccine is efficacious at or after 12 months of age. Currently, vaccine administration is recommended at 15 months of age in combination with measles and mumps vaccine. The vaccine may be given simultaneously at a different site from DTP and oral polio vaccine without reducing efficacy. Immunization is also indicated for susceptible prepubertal girls, day care personnel, college students, and military and health care personnel. Postpubertal seronegative women should be immunized if they are not pregnant and agree to avoid pregnancy for 3 months after receiving the vaccine.

The most common adverse reaction to rubella vaccine is arthralgia or arthritis. Involvement of joints tends to occur most commonly (10 to 20 per cent) in postpubertal females. Symptoms usually begin within 3 weeks after immunization and may persist for weeks or months. Less common reactions to vaccine include rash, lymphadenopathy, low-grade fever, or upper respiratory tract symptoms.

There are several specific contraindications to administration of rubella vaccine. It should be avoided in patients with primary or acquired immunodeficiency, such as leukemia, those with other malignancy, and those receiving steroid or cancer chemotherapy. After considering reports of severe measles (rubeola) in symptomatic children infected with human immunodeficiency virus (HIV) and in the absence of reports of serious or unusual adverse effects of measles, mumps, and rubella (MMR) vaccination, the Immunization Practices Advisory Committee suggests that administration of MMR vaccine should be considered for children with symptomatic HIV infection. The Immunization Practices Advisory Committee also recommends that children and young adults infected with HIV who have no overt clinical manifestations of immunosuppression may receive rubella vaccine. These patients should be monitored for possible adverse reactions, and it should be noted that immunization may be less effective in these individuals than in uninfected persons.

Pregnant women should not be given rubella vaccine. Although congenital rubella syndrome resulting from rubella vaccination in pregnancy has not been observed, the theoretical maximal risk for its occurrence may be as high as 2.6 per cent. This estimate is based upon the outcome of pregnancy in a cohort of 184 susceptible women reported to the Centers for Disease Control who received vaccine either 3 months before or 3 months after the estimated date of conception. All of the 144 living infants delivered to women susceptible to rubella were free of defects compatible with congenital rubella. Virus was isolated from the products of conception in 1 of 33 women who underwent abortion.

Rubella vaccine should be deferred for 3 months after the administration of blood transfusion or IG. It may be given to postpartum women who require blood products or Rho (D) immune globulin, but in that circumstance serum should be tested at 6 to 8 weeks after immunization to document seroconversion. Finally, vaccine administration should be deferred until resolution of acute febrile illnesses.

Since rubella vaccine virus is not transmitted from vaccinated individuals to others, there is no contraindication to immunization of susceptible children whose mothers are pregnant or to a child residing in the household of a patient with AIDS. Breastfeeding does not constitute a contraindication to immunization in the immediate postpartum period.

MEASLES
(Rubeola)

method of
JESS DIAMOND, M.D.
Kern Medical Center
Bakersfield, California

The goal to eradicate measles by 1982 has not been attained. There were more measles cases in 1986 (6273) than in any year since 1980. Highest incidence was in preschool-aged children, adolescents, and young adults. Infection of unvaccinated preschool-aged children and vaccine failures were the major causes.

Clinical Manifestations

After an incubation period of 10 to 12 days, the prodromal signs of fever, conjunctivitis, coryza, and a nonproductive cough appear. These are followed in 2 to 3 days by pathognomonic Koplik spots. Within 24 hours, a maculopapular eruption appears that starts on the head and spreads to the entire body, including the soles of the feet, within 2 or 3 more days. The temperature ranges from 38.8 to 40° C at the height of the rash, then returns to normal. The rash fades downward in the same manner as it appeared. In mild cases, the lesions remain discrete, but in severe cases, they completely cover the body and are followed by a copper discoloration of the skin. Individuals immunized prior to 1967 with the inactivated vaccine may develop a severe, atypical disease upon exposure to the wild virus. This form of measles is characterized by high fever and cough, followed in 40 to 72 hours by a maculopapular rash on the extremities, including palms and soles, which spreads centrally. The rash may become vesicular, purpuric, or petechial. The course is more severe and prolonged than that of the classic disease and usually lasts about 2 weeks.

Treatment of Uncomplicated Measles

Treatment is symptomatic. Antipyretics, acetaminophen, 15 mg per kg of body weight administered orally every 4 to 6 hours, are utilized for the elevated temperature. The diet should be light, should be rich in carbohydrates, and should provide an adequate fluid intake. Photophobia is managed by avoiding bright light and darkening of the room. When disturbing, cough may be suppressed by antitussives. Bed rest is advisable until the temperature returns to normal without antipyretics. Nothing specific is known to beneficially alter the course of the disease, although there is an assumption that failure to provide good supportive care may increase the likelihood of complications.

Treatment of Complications

The complications of measles are due to the virus or to secondary bacterial invaders. Otitis media is a common complication and is usually assumed to be bacterial in origin. The most frequent invaders are *Streptococcus pneumoniae*, *Branhamella catarrhalis*, and non-typable *Haemophilus influenzae*. The antibiotic of choice depends on the age of the patient and the likelihood of a specific causative organism. Erythromycin ethylsuccinate and sulfisoxazole acetyl (Pediazole), based on 50 mg per kg per day of erythromycin and 150 mg per kg per day of sulfisoxa-

TABLE 1. **Action for Individuals Exposed to Measles**

Age	Exposure Status	History of Previous Disease or Vaccine	Immediate Action	Eventual Action
6 to 11 months inclusive	I. Definite contact	None or in doubt	I. Immune serum globulin	I. Live virus vaccine at 15 months of age
	II. Increased risk of exposure		II. Live virus vaccine	II. Revaccination with live virus vaccine at 15 months of age
12 months or older	I. Definite contact A. 3 days or less B. 4 days or more	None or in doubt	I. A. Live virus vaccine B. Immune serum globulin	I. A. None B. Live virus vaccine 3 months later
	II. Increased risk of exposure		II. Live virus vaccine	II. None
All ages	Definite contact or Increased risk of exposure	No history of previous disease or live virus vaccine. Vaccination contraindicated	Immune serum globulin, 0.5 ml per kg of body weight intramuscularly	

From Edlich RF, Spyker D: Current Emergency Therapy '85. Reprinted with permission of Aspen Publishers, Inc., Rockville, Maryland. Copyright 1985.

zole orally in equally divided doses every 6 hours for 10 days or a combination of 8 mg per kg per day of trimethoprim and 40 mg per kg per day of sulfamethoxazole (Bactrim) orally in divided doses every 12 hours for 10 days, may be used. Other drugs seem equally effective, such as amoxicillin, 40 mg per kg per day orally in divided doses every 8 hours.

Pneumonia caused by the rubeola virus is interstitial, and there is no specific treatment for this complication. Supportive measures are all that are required. Pneumonia caused by secondary bacterial invaders, such as *Streptococcus pneumoniae, Haemophilus influenzae,* or *Staphylococcus aureus,* is a bronchopneumonia. Proper antimicrobial therapy of the bacterial pneumonia is based on blood cultures, if positive, or lung puncture if required.

Encephalitis is a rare complication; only one or two in 1000 patients develop clinical signs of central nervous system involvement. The severity of involvement and the degree of permanent neurologic damage, if any, vary. Management is supportive and symptomatic. Adequate nutrition must be maintained. Seizures are controlled with anticonvulsants. Dawson's subacute sclerosing panencephalitis is a late complication. The incidence is five to ten cases per 1 million cases of measles.

Active Immunization

To eradicate measles, susceptible individuals should be identified and immunized or reimmunized. All healthy children should be immunized with the live virus vaccine at 15 months of age. All persons infected with the human immunodeficiency virus, regardless of symptoms, and individuals with leukemia in remission whose chemotherapy has been terminated for 3 months, may receive the measles vaccine. There is no risk in vaccinating a previously immunized person. The combined measles, mumps, rubella (MMR) vaccine is recommended. The vaccine viruses are easily destroyed by heat and light. Therefore, to preserve potency, the material should be stored at 4° C in a closed container and administered subcutaneously as soon as reconstituted. When properly handled, it will provide an adequate antibody response for 95 per cent of the persons immunized.

Side effects of the live vaccine occur 7 to 10 days after immunization, and may include an elevated fever or rash, or both, for 1 to 2 days. Adverse reactions to the vaccine are not more common in adolescents and adults than in young children. The incidence of encephalitis following measles immunization is about one per 1 million vaccinations. The risk of subacute sclerosing panencephalitis following measles vaccine is 10 to 100 times less than that following natural measles. Among individuals previously immunized with the inactivated vaccine, the reaction to vaccine may be most severe, characterized by fever, malaise, local erythema, induration, and regional lymphadenopathy.

Contraindications

Live measles vaccine is contraindicated for pregnant women, for individuals taking immunosuppressive drugs, and for those with leukemia and immunodeficiency diseases. Administration should be delayed for 3 months in persons who have received immune serum globulin or any blood products because of the possible presence of antibodies that may neutralize the vaccine. Minor afebrile illness is not a contraindication to the administration of the vaccine. However, it should not be administered during an acute febrile illness. Neither neomycin nor egg allergy is a contraindication unless there is a history of an anaphylactic reaction to these substances. Measles vaccine does not contain penicillin.

Management of Exposed Individuals

Measles is a highly contagious disease, and any case may generate an epidemic. Therefore, prompt identification of all contacts and determination of susceptibility to infection are essential (Table 1). When measles occurs in a school, students without documented proof of immunity should be excluded until they provide proof of immunity or 2 weeks have elapsed since the onset of the rash in the last case. During outbreaks of measles, in junior and senior high schools, individuals vaccinated at 12 to 14 months of age should be revaccinated.

Infants 6 to 11 months old with definite measles contact should be given immune serum globulin within 5 days of exposure. When given later, it may modify the severity of the disease, or it may have no effect. The dose is 0.25 ml per kg of body weight intramuscularly. Subsequently, at 15 months of age, vaccination with live vaccine should be accomplished. At least 3 months must elapse between the last dose of immune globulin and administration of the live vaccine. Individuals 1 year of age or older should be given live vaccine; when given within 3 days of exposure, it will prevent the disease. Four days or more after exposure, immune serum globulin should be given and, subsequently, live vaccine.

Infants 6 to 11 months old in whom a definite contact with a case of measles is not confirmed, but who are at increased risk of exposure, may be given live vaccine. They should be revaccinated when they are 15 months of age. Children 1 year of age or older at increased risk of exposure should be immunized with live virus vaccine. They should not be reimmunized at 15 months of age. If live vaccine is contraindicated, immune serum globulin, 0.5 mg per kg of body weight, is given intramuscularly for protection.

TETANUS

method of
WESLEY FURSTE, M.D.,
Ohio State University,

GREGORY RAY VEST, M.D.,
Mt. Carmel Medical Center,

and

AUGUSTO AQUIRRE, M.D.,
Riverside Methodist Hospitals
Columbus, Ohio

Tetanus (lockjaw) is a severe and dreaded infectious complication of wounds and is caused by the toxin-producing *Clostridium tetani*. This disease is characterized by tonic spasms of the voluntary muscles, by a tendency toward episodes of respiratory arrest, and, over the entire world, by a mortality rate of approximately 50 per cent.

Prophylaxis

Adequate tetanus prophylaxis is based on (1) proper use of tetanus toxoid, (2) immediate surgical care of all wounds of violence, (3) proper employment of antitoxin (heterologous equine antitoxin, and more recently tetanus immune globulin [human]), and (4) proper use of emergency medical identification devices.

Tetanus can be prevented by proper immunization. For normal infants and children younger than 7 years, tetanus toxoid is administered along with diphtheria and pertussis vaccines using DTP (diphtheria and tetanus toxoids and pertussis vaccine adsorbed). Primary vaccination is given at age 2 months or older; the second dose, 2 months after the first dose; the third dose, 2 months after the second dose; and the fourth dose, approximately 15 months after the third dose. A DTP booster is given at 4 to 6 years of age, before the child enters school. Additional boosters using Td (tetanus and diphtheria toxoids adsorbed) are given every 10 years after the last dose. For those persons 7 years or older who have not had a complete immunization series for tetanus, this can be accomplished using Td, in the following sequence: primary vaccination, first visit; second dose, 4 to 8 weeks after the first dose; third dose, 6 to 12 months after the second; and subsequent Td boosters, every 10 years.

Prophylaxis against tetanus in wound management requires an adequate history and very careful wound evaluation in accordance with the principles outlined in Tables 1, 2, and 3.

TABLE 1. General Principles for Tetanus Prophylaxis

1. Active immunization against tetanus with tetanus toxoid plays a major role in markedly reducing the incidence of cases of this disease, and the resulting deaths.

2. Recommendations for tetanus prophylaxis are based on 1) the condition of the wound, especially as related to its susceptibility to tetanus, and 2) the patient's immunization history.

3. Regardless of the active immunization status of the patient, all wounds should receive immediate surgical treatment, using meticulous aseptic technique, to remove all devitalized tissue and foreign bodies. Such care is an essential part of prophylaxis against tetanus. (See *A Guide to Initial Therapy of Soft-Tissue Wounds,* American College of Surgeons.)

4. **Warning:** The only contraindication to tetanus and diphtheria toxoids for the wounded patient is a history of neurologic or severe hypersensitivity reaction to a previous dose. Local side effects alone do not preclude continued use. If a systemic reaction is suspected to represent allergic hypersensitivity, postpone immunization until appropriate skin testing is performed later. If a contraindication to a tetanus toxoid–containing preparation exists, consider passive immunization against tetanus for a tetanus-prone wound.

Contraindications to pertussis vaccination in infants and children less than seven years old include: a previous adverse reaction after diphtheria and tetanus toxoids and pertussis vaccine adsorbed (for pediatric use) (DTP), or single antigen pertussis vaccination; and/or the presence of a neurologic condition characterized by changing developmental or neurologic findings. If such a contraindication to using pertussis vaccine adsorbed (P) exists, diphtheria and tetanus toxoids adsorbed (for pediatric use) (DT) are recommended. Neither a static neurologic condition, such as cerebral palsy, nor a family history of convulsions or other central nervous system disorders is a contraindication to giving vaccines containing the pertussis antigen.

Disposition: Give each patient an appropriate written record describing treatment rendered and providing instructions for follow-up that outline wound care, drug therapy, immunization status, and potential complications. Arrange for completion of active immunization.

Give every wounded patient a wallet-sized card documenting immunization dosage and date received.

From American College of Surgeons, Committee on Trauma: Prophylaxis against Tetanus in Wound Management. Chicago, American College of Surgeons, 1987.

Treatment

The following recommendations for management are given in order of chronologic priority.

Complete History and Physical Examination

A complete medical and surgical history of the patient should be obtained and a complete physical examination performed. In particular, the information obtained should include the date of injury, the circumstances of injury, the depth of the injury below the skin, and allergies. Such information forms a baseline for the recognition of such complications as atelectasis, pneumonia, traumatic glossitis, muscle injuries, fractures of the vertebrae, decubital ulcers, and fecal impaction.

TABLE 2. Wound Classification

Clinical Features	Tetanus-Prone Wounds	Non–Tetanus-Prone Wounds
Age of wound	> 6 hours	≤ 6 hours
Configuration	Stellate wound, avulsion, abrasion	Linear wound
Depth	> 1 cm	≤ 1 cm
Mechanism of injury	Missile, crush, burn, frostbite	Sharp surface (e.g., knife, glass)
Signs of infection	Present	Absent
Devitalized tissue	Present	Absent
Contaminants (dirt, feces, soil, saliva, etc.)	Present	Absent
Denervated and/or ischemic tissue	Present	Absent

From American College of Surgeons, Committee on Trauma: Prophylaxis against Tetanus in Wound Management. Chicago, American College of Surgeons, 1987.

Antitoxin

Intramuscular Injection. As soon as the diagnosis of tetanus is made, deep intramuscular injection of 500 to 10,000 units of tetanus immune globulin (TIG) should be given. Five hundred units may be as effective as the dose of 3000 to 10,000 units that has been recommended in the past.

Since TIG causes no hypersensitivity phenomena when injected intramuscularly and since it appears to be at least equal in efficacy to equine antitoxin, TIG should be given instead of the heterologous tetanus antitoxin (equine).

TIG is to be given intramuscularly in the prox-

TABLE 3. Immunization Schedule

Verify a history of tetanus immunization from medical records so that appropriate tetanus prophylaxis can be accomplished.

Td: Tetanus and diphtheria toxoids adsorbed (for adult use)
TIG: Tetanus immune globulin (human)

History of Adsorbed Tetanus Toxoid (Doses)	Tetanus-Prone Wounds		Non–Tetanus-Prone Wounds	
	Td[1]	TIG	Td[1]	TIG
Unknown or fewer than 3	Yes	Yes	Yes	No
3 or more[2]	No[4]	No	No[3]	No

[1]For children less than seven years old: DTP (DT, if pertussis vaccine is contraindicated) is preferable to tetanus toxoid alone. For persons seven years old and older, Td is preferable to tetanus toxoid alone.

[2]If only three doses of fluid toxoid have been received, a fourth dose of toxoid, preferably an adsorbed toxoid, should be given.

[3]Yes, if more than 10 years since last dose.

[4]Yes, if more than 5 years since last dose. (More frequent boosters are not needed and can accentuate side effects.)

From American College of Surgeons, Committee on Trauma: Prophylaxis against Tetanus in Wound Management. Chicago, American College of Surgeons, 1987.

imal portion of the extremity in which is the wound responsible for tetanus, or in the gluteal muscles when the wound is not in an extremity or when the causative wound cannot be found.

In the United States, where there are now adequate supplies of TIG, there are no indications for the administration of heterologous tetanus antitoxin (equine), which has been responsible for serum sickness, myocardial infarctions, peripheral neuritis, and anaphylactic shock with death. Moreover, in the human being, the life span of the heterologous antitoxin cannot be predicted with certainty.

In countries in which TIG is not available, heterologous tetanus antitoxin (equine) is still being used. A dosage of 10,000 units is considered adequate. No significant lowering of the mortality rate has been found for doses ranging from 5000 to 60,000 units of equine antitoxin in adults. Fifteen hundred units of heterologous tetanus antitoxin (equine) appears to be as effective as a larger dose in neonates.

Intrathecal Injection of a Mixture of Antitoxin and Prednisolone. Serious consideration should be given to simultaneous single injections of TIG and prednisolone intrathecally and of TIG intramuscularly. For neonatal tetanus, 250 units of TIG and 12.5 mg of prednisolone are administered intrathecally, and 250 units of TIG is given intramuscularly. For adults, the dose of TIG for the intrathecal route is increased to 1000 units and for the intramuscular route to 1000 units. Complications of intrathecal administration are believed to be due to the preservatives rather than to the antitoxin itself.

Laboratory Tests

The following tests are recommended:
1. Complete blood cell count with differential white blood cell count.
2. Urinalysis.
3. Serologic test for syphilis.
4. Prothrombin time and partial thromboplastin time.
5. Blood chemistry tests: urea nitrogen, creatinine, electrolytes, serum protein electrophoresis, bilirubin, calcium, glucose.
6. Arterial blood gases.
7. Chest roentgenogram.
8. Electrocardiogram.
9. Electroencephalogram.
10. Wound and, if the patient is febrile, blood cultures.
11. If necessary for diagnosis, cerebrospinal fluid for culture, smear, cells, and chemistry tests.
12. Diazepam levels of serum.
13. Tetanus antitoxin levels of serum if the diagnosis is questionable.

Nursing Care

Provide 24-hour constant nursing care. Having a resident or intern immediately available to treat complications, particularly respiratory problems such as respiratory arrest, will greatly increase the patient's chance for recovery from tetanus.

Analgesics

Analgesics should be administered that will relieve the pain associated with the tonic contractions of tetanus but will not cause respiratory depression. Codeine, meperidine (Demerol), meperidine with promethazine (Phenergan), and morphine are acceptable analgesic drugs.

Sedatives and Muscle Relaxants

Sedatives and muscle relaxants must be used correctly. A most important consideration is that the physician know how to use safely the sedatives and muscle relaxants that he orders for the patient with tetanus and that he use those with which he obtains the best results.

Patients with the mildest cases of tetanus can be sedated adequately with phenobarbital, pentobarbital, secobarbital, paraldehyde, diazepam (Valium), and midazolam (Versed).

In the more severe cases, thiopental sodium (Pentothal) may be administered intravenously in a very dilute solution (0.5 to 1.0 gram per 1000 ml) at a rate of 20 to 25 drops per minute in an effort to lower the patient's threshold of irritability to external stimuli and to reduce the number and severity of seizures and respiratory arrests. Care is taken to avoid overdosage. The optimal level of continuous sedation is obtained when the patient remains sleepy but still can be aroused by moderate external stimuli sufficiently to obey commands. Objectively, the best indication of this level is that the rectus muscles of the abdomen lose their hypertonic states and have only a normal degree of resistance to palpation. When a severe convulsive seizure occurs, with respiratory arrest, 2 to 8 ml of a 2.5 per cent solution of thiopental sodium is injected intravenously immediately and as necessary. This usually produces muscle relaxation within 30 to 45 seconds, and permits spontaneous re-establishment of the respiratory cycle.

Some centers have been enthusiastic about the use of muscle-relaxant drugs to control convulsive seizures. Such drugs are difficult to manage and have not prevented death from respiratory arrest. Drugs more commonly suggested for such use are d-tubocurarine, succinylcholine (Anectine), pancuronium (Pavulon), atracurium (Tracrium), and vecuronium (Norcuron). The margin of safety with these drugs is narrow; they seem best designed for patients excessively difficult to manage—and then only under careful observation of an experienced anesthesiologist and with endotracheal intubation.

Surgical Wound Care

Optimal surgical care of wounds should be carried out in accordance with the following concepts:

1. The wounds are taken care of at the earliest possible moment.

2. Aseptic technique is observed, with the use of gloves, gowns, masks, and sterile instruments and the application of proper solutions to prepare the skin before the necessary operative procedures at the injured site.

3. During skin preparation, the wound should be covered with gauze to prevent further contamination.

4. Proper lighting is provided so that the surgeon can exactly identify and protect vital structures such as nerves and vessels.

5. Adequate instruments and adequate help should be available so that there is the best and gentlest possible retraction of structures in wounds.

6. Hemostasis is effected with delicate instruments and with fine suture material so that there is a minimum of necrotic tissue left in wounds.

7. Tissues are handled gently at all times so that necrotic tissue is not produced.

8. Complete debridement is carried out with scalpel excision of necrotic tissue and with removal of foreign bodies so that no pabulum is left on which any unremoved bacteria can propagate.

9. The wound is irrigated copiously with large amounts of physiologic salt solution to wash out minute avascular fragments of tissue and to eliminate foreign bodies.

10. If there is any doubt concerning a wound providing anaerobic conditions so that the tetanus bacillus can grow and produce its lethal toxin in it, the wound is left wide open. Drainage is instituted when necessary.

Antibiotics

Antibiotics may be administered for the treatment of the infectious complications of tetanus.

In vitro, penicillin is effective against the tetanus bacillus. It is not surprising, however, that antibiotic therapy is clinically disappointing insofar as it is directed against the tetanus disease itself. Tetanus is not a bacteremia, for the bacillus remains at the place of its entry. By the time antibiotic therapy is begun, the wound often has been excised, and the toxins often are already spread in the circulation. When the site of infection is not known and the antibiotic effect would be particularly desired, there is little probability that the bacteria are reached by parenteral administration of an antibiotic owing to avascular conditions in a concealed, closed puncture wound. Despite the in vitro effects of penicillin, a noticeable, specific therapeutic reaction cannot be expected.

On the other hand, the antibiotics given according to sensitivity tests do play their part in the therapy plan. They are irreplaceable in the care of infectious complications of tetanus, especially in combating pneumonia or secondary, invasive wound infections. A combination of clindamycin phosphate injection, 600 mg every 6 hours, and gentamicin sulfate injection, 80 mg every eight hours, may be given intravenously. A broad-spectrum antibiotic, such as a cephalosporin, may be administered intravenously.

The possible complications that may develop with antibiotic therapy must be given particular attention in the case of tetanus patients. Especially in the more severe cases, in which nourishment is accomplished through less than ideal methods, there will be a tendency toward gastrointestinal disturbances.

Tracheostomy

Tracheostomy is performed when indicated if personnel and facilities are available to care adequately for the tracheostomy.

If the incubation period has been only a few days, so that the patient may have very severe tetanus, a tracheostomy probably will be necessary, and can be performed with general anesthesia when extensive wound debridement is necessary, with local anesthesia, or with a combination of local and general anesthesia.

Tetanus patients in whom a tracheostomy is necessary also will need, in most cases, continuous artificial respiration. Such respiration is facilitated by attaching, with a gas-tight adapter, a tracheostomy tube with double inflatable cuffs to a volume-controlled respiration unit.

Nursing care of the seriously ill tracheostomy patient is not easy. Inspired air must be moist. If the patient can breathe spontaneously, moisturizing apparatus is set up in the patient's hospital room; if, however, the patient is being given artificial respiration, the respirator used must be one that continuously moistens the gas mixture. Dehydration of the respiratory tract can lead to severe hemorrhagic tracheobronchitis, which can be fatal. Even with absolutely correct conditioning of the inspired air, secretions can collect in the airway. A suction machine always must be at the patient's bedside. Patients with paralyzed respiratory muscles must be suctioned every hour. Also of extreme importance is the cleanliness of the tracheostomy tube; dehydrated secretions, pseudomembranes, and crusts can form on the inner margin of the cannula, and may lead to narrowing of the respiratory airway. The tracheostomy tube should be changed whenever it cannot be made to function correctly by cleaning and manipulation.

A tracheostomy that is improperly cared for may be worse than none.

Tracheostomy may be poorly tolerated in the newborn infant, and decannulation may be quite difficult. In infants, particularly those with neonatal tetanus, endotracheal intubation by insertion of an endotracheal tube through the nose, or, less preferably, through the mouth, should be considered prior to tracheostomy.

Iatrogenic Problems

Constant alertness is required to avoid iatrogenic problems. For example, if rectal probes are left in place for constant recording of temperature, they must be checked carefully to prevent trauma to the rectal mucosa and anorectal veins during convulsions.

Private, Dark, Quiet Room

The patient should be placed in a private, dark, quiet room. Efforts should be made to reduce as much as possible all external stimuli. Visitors should be limited to the absolute minimum. It should be pointed out that, with adequate sedation and muscle relaxation, some patients no longer require the dark, quiet room. Conversations with patients who have recovered from tetanus indicate that the constant attention to them 24 hours a day is most unpleasant and annoying for them.

Proper Environment for Infants

Place infants with neonatal tetanus in an incubator in which the oxygen partial pressure, the environmental temperature, and a nebulized atmosphere of distilled water can be monitored and maintained.

Roentgenograms

Roentgenograms may be indicated for (1) fractures associated with the initial injury, (2) determination of pulmonary problems such as atelectasis and pneumonia, (3) fractures or avulsions of muscle insertions produced by the tonic muscle contractions of tetanus, and (4) evaluation of resulting osteoarthropathies. Compression fractures of the vertebrae may be the result of the intense paroxysms that characterize the disease, and their diagnosis may be easily missed without roentgenograms.

Padded Tongue Depressor

Insertion of a padded tongue depressor can protect the tongue from being bitten during tonic contractions.

Oral Hygiene

The lips, teeth, tongue, and oral cavity should be cleaned daily to lessen the possibility of growth of pathologic bacteria and viruses. Remove all loose debris from the oral and nasal cavities.

Nutrition

Correct amounts of nourishment should be given by oral, nasogastric tube, gastrostomy tube, or intravenous routes. The relaxed patient is totally dependent on artificial nourishment. Initially, tube feedings through a soft nasogastric or nasojejunal tube are indicated. Aspiration pneumonia is a common complication of such feedings, and care must be taken that the stomach empties. Frequent, *small* feedings are indicated. If difficulties are encountered with the tube feedings, it may be necessary to resort to intravenous supplements. Central venous pressure systems using the subclavian vein provide an excellent route for feeding, including hyperalimentation. Transfusions of blood, plasma, and human albumin can be supplemented with electrolyte solutions of glucose, alcohol, fructose, and protein hydrolysates. The infusions can be further supplemented with high doses of vitamins C and B complex. Serum protein and electrolytes should be checked repeatedly. Nothing is given by mouth until improvement begins. In choosing a diet, the fact that the patient on occasion may feel pain when he eats and endeavors to open his mouth should be taken into consideration.

Alimentary Tract Elimination

Adequate gastrointestinal elimination must be maintained. Spontaneous defecation usually is absent. Defecation can be controlled by saline laxatives given orally or into the nasogastric tube and by enemas as required.

Urine Elimination

When necessary, elimination of urine can be facilitated by the insertion of a Foley catheter into the bladder. The catheter should be removed at the earliest possible time to reduce the possibility of urinary tract infections.

Intake and Output Records

Record intake and total output, and alter intake as indicated.

Protection of the Eyes

In protecting the eyes, particular attention must be given to incomplete closure of the eyelids.

Without prophylactic measures, exsiccation, keratitis, and corneal ulcer can develop. An ophthalmic ointment may be applied, and the eyes may be covered with a moist gauze sponge.

Prevention of Decubital Ulcers

Keeping the patient's skin dry and cushioning pressure points can reduce the chance that the patient will develop decubital ulcers.

Blood Dyscrasias and Bleeding Problems

If there is a possibility of blood problems, complete blood cell counts should be obtained, clotting mechanisms promptly investigated, and any indicated treatment promptly rendered.

Prevention of Pulmonary Emboli

Indicated procedures, including ordering of heparin, must be carried out to avoid the risk of pulmonary embolization.

Prevention of Cardiac Exhaustion and Circulatory Disruption

Advances during the past decade have indicated the importance of proper use of alpha and beta blockers for sympathetic overactivity, which may be manifested by tachyarrhythmias and hemodynamic instability.

Temporary Endocardial Pacemaker

A temporary endocardial pacemaker may be indicated in cases with severe, medically refractory bradycardia of unknown cause.

Prevention of Muscle Contractures

As the patient improves, muscle contractures with resulting deformities, such as foot drop, must be prevented. Use of foam-rubber padding, pillows, sandbags, and splints may be indicated. When necessary for muscle imbalance, physiotherapy should be instituted as soon as possible.

Electroencephalograms

Electroencephalograms should be ordered when it is technically possible to obtain them and when their procurement will not interfere with the patient's recovery. Such records may be of considerable importance in the long-range evaluation and care of the patient, particularly as regards the possibility of brain damage.

Steroid Therapy

Steroid therapy should be considered if there is a possibility of adrenal gland exhaustion. Although not used routinely, steroid therapy has been employed in a few severe cases of tetanus in which the prolonged course of the disease was thought to exhaust the adrenal glands. Prior to administration of corticosteroids for adrenal insufficiency, cortisol levels should be checked and an ACTH stimulation test should be performed to assess the need for supplemental steroids.

Tetanus Toxoid

At the end of the hospital treatment of tetanus, 0.5 ml of adsorbed tetanus toxoid intramuscularly should be given for active immunization, 1 month later another dose, and 6 months from this latter dose one more dose to complete the basic active immunization. Then, routine tetanus toxoid boosters are given every 10 years. Such immunization is necessary because *an attack of tetanus does not produce antibodies to prevent another attack.*

Emergency Medical Identification Devices

At the time of discharge from the hospital, the cured patient should be given a completed emergency medical identification device (EMID) and should be instructed to complete the course of active immunization with tetanus toxoid to prevent recurrent tetanus.

Hyperbaric Oxygen

Hyperbaric oxygen is not recommended in view of its minimal good effects, if any, and the complications of such treatment. Tetanus is a toxemic state, and is not due to bacteria that are spreading throughout the body and that might be acted on by oxygen in the circulating blood.

Control of Body Temperature

Necessary procedures to lower excessively high body temperatures should be carried out. Tetanus per se does not cause fever, but the complications of tetanus cause fever. Hence, tetanus and its complications should be treated, not the fever itself.

Recording of Data

In view of professional liability problems, the progress and treatment, and especially significant reasons for giving or not giving drugs, should be recorded completely and accurately.

TOXOPLASMOSIS

method of
ROBERT L. PENN, M.D.
Louisiana State University School of Medicine
Shreveport, Louisiana

Toxoplasmosis is a systemic infection caused by the coccidian parasite *Toxoplasma gondii.* Although the parasite's life cycle is completed to produce oocysts only in cats, most mammals may become infected to produce tissue cysts. Infection is acquired by people through ingestion of oocysts excreted in cat feces, through ingestion of viable cysts in raw or undercooked meats, transplacentally to the fetus of a mother acquiring toxoplasmosis during pregnancy, through blood or white cell transfusions, or by organ transplantation. After entry into the host, the organism frequently spreads to infect many sites, including retina, brain, muscles, and lung. As immunity develops, tissue cysts may form in any of these organs. However, the encysted parasite may remain viable and reactivate anytime during the life of the host. Thus, toxoplasmosis may result either from an acute infection or from reactivation of a chronic infection.

Treatment

Treatment is required in certain circumstances determined by the status of the host and the organs involved (Table 1).

Normal Adults. In patients with a normal humoral and cell-mediated immune response, most acute *T. gondii* infections remain subclinical and do not require therapy. The most common manifestation is lymphadenopathy, which also does not usually require treatment. Therapy of acute toxoplasmosis is indicated for those rare patients with persistent or severe systemic symptoms, or with vital organ dysfunction (e.g., myocarditis, encephalitis, pneumonitis, hepatitis). Some investigators feel that laboratory-acquired infections and those acquired through transfusions may be more severe, so that therapy may be given to all patients who contract toxoplasmosis by these means. The therapy of choice is pyrimethamine (Daraprim) plus either sulfadiazine or trisulfapyrimidine (Terfonyl) for 4 to 6 weeks. The pyrimethamine may be given daily to very ill patients.

TABLE 1. **Therapy of Toxoplasmosis**

Host Status	Therapy Indicated
Normal Patients	
Asymptomatic	No
Congenital infection (all forms)	Yes
Lymphadenopathy	Rarely
Ocular infection	Yes
Vital organ dysfunction	Yes
Pregnant Patients	
Asymptomatic acute infection	Yes
Symptomatic acute infection	Yes
Immunosuppressed Patients	
Ocular infection	Yes
Encephalitis	Yes
Disseminated infection	Yes

Ocular toxoplasmosis is usually the result of reactivated chronic infection, and takes the form of retinochoroiditis. It should be managed in conjunction with an ophthalmologist to monitor response to therapy and the need for photocoagulation or surgical intervention. Multiple symptomatic recurrences are common, and each requires treatment. Drugs of choice are pyrimethamine plus either sulfadiazine or trisulfapyrimidine daily for 4 weeks. Prednisone (60 to 100 mg per day) is often added to reduce inflammation, especially if vision is threatened by papillitis or macular involvement. Uncontrolled reports suggest that clindamycin (Cleocin) (about 2400 mg per day), which is concentrated in the choroid, may be a useful alternative to the sulfonamide.

Congenital Infection. Transplacental transmission of *T. gondii* to the fetus can occur only if the mother acquires a primary infection during pregnancy; congenital infection may result if the mother's infection is symptomatic or asymptomatic. The risk of congenital infection is greatest if maternal infection is acquired in the last trimester, but most infants are asymptomatic. Congenital infections are less frequent if maternal infection is acquired earlier in pregnancy, but infants are more likely to be severely involved.

Symptomatic neonates should be treated in the hope of preventing ongoing damage from new lesions. Pyrimethamine is given as a loading dose of 2 mg per kg daily for 2 days, followed by 1 mg per kg every 2 to 3 days.* Sulfadiazine or trisulfapyrimidine is given simultaneously in a loading dose of 75 mg per kg, followed by 100 mg per kg per day in divided doses. Folinic acid, 5 to 10 mg every other day, should be administered while pyrimethamine is given. Pyrimethamine plus the sulfonamide may be continued for a minimum of 6 months, but most authorities suggest a 12-month course. An alternative treatment regimen for the symptomatic infant is pyrimethamine plus either sulfadiazine or trisulfapyrimidine given for 21 days, followed by spiramycin, 100 mg per kg per day for 4 to 6 weeks. These cycles are continued, alternating pyrimethamine plus the sulfonamide with spiramycin alone, for 6 to 12 months.

Asymptomatic infants born to mothers acquiring toxoplasmosis during pregnancy must be suspected of having subclinical congenital infection. Treatment in these cases has been shown to reduce the incidence of later reactivation. Pyrimethamine plus either sulfadiazine or trisulfapyrimidine should be given for 3 weeks, followed by spiramycin alone until the diagnosis can be established. If serologic studies confirm the presence of congenital toxoplasmosis, then treatment

---

*These doses exceed the doses recommended by the manufacturer for pediatric use

should be given for 6 to 12 months using one of the regimens described for symptomatic infection.

Pregnant Patients. Treatment of toxoplasmosis acquired during pregnancy can reduce the incidence of subsequent fetal infection. However, if treatment is given after the fetus has already been infected, there is little evidence that treating the mother will arrest the disease in the fetus. Thus, infants born with evidence of congenital toxoplasmosis should be treated even if the mother was treated during pregnancy.

The teratogenic potential of pyrimethamine precludes its use during at least the first trimester of pregnancy. The safest effective regimen consists of cycles of spiramycin, 2 to 3 grams per day for 21 days, followed by 14 days without spiramycin. Therapy is begun at the time toxoplasmosis is diagnosed, and cycles are repeated until term. Another regimen consists of sulfadiazine or trisulfapyrimidine alone for 2 weeks followed by no drug for 3 to 4 weeks, repeating the cycles until term. After the sixteenth week of gestation, some investigators add pyrimethamine to the sulfonamide and continue cycles until term. However, the efficacy of sulfonamide alone, and the safety of pyrimethamine in the later stages of pregnancy, have yet to be established.

Immunosuppressed Patients. Any form of toxoplasmosis is potentially dangerous during immunosuppression. The absence of an effective immune response may predispose to reactivation of chronic infection in vital organs, or to overwhelming acute infections. Patients at highest risk are those with lymphomas, cardiac or renal transplants from a seropositive donor into a seronegative recipient, and acquired immunodeficiency syndrome (AIDS). In fact, toxoplasmic encephalitis is now one of the most frequent neurologic complications of AIDS, occurring in up to 40 per cent of patients.

Daily therapy with pyrimethamine plus sulfadiazine or trisulfapyrimidine should begin as soon as toxoplasmosis is suspected in an immunosuppressed patient. With life-threatening infections, the dose of pyrimethamine should be 50 mg per day. Most patients will show some improvement within 10 to 14 days. Therapy should be continued for about 1 month after signs and symptoms of the infection have completely resolved. Corticosteroids may be given to patients with significant intracranial edema accompanying toxoplasmic encephalitis without apparent adverse effect on outcome. AIDS patients with toxoplasmic encephalitis have up to an 80 per cent chance of recurrence, in part because cysts remain viable even after therapy. For this reason twice-weekly maintenance doses of pyrimethamine plus the sulfonamide have been given to prevent recurrences, and are felt to be indicated for the life of the patient.

Toxicity from this regimen in AIDS patients is high. Severe neutropenia or thrombocytopenia is an indication to interrupt therapy. Serious allergic reactions to the sulfonamides may preclude their use. In this circumstance, clindamycin, 2400 mg per day, may be substituted for the sulfonamide. Treatment failures are common if pyrimethamine is used alone; perhaps higher doses will prove to be more effective as a single agent, but this may increase the risk for toxicity. Spiramycin is not effective in immunosuppressed patients. Newer drugs are being tested, but are currently experimental and of unknown benefit.

Drugs. The drugs most commonly used to treat toxoplasmosis are listed in Table 2. Pyrimethamine is available only for oral use. In adults, it is usually given as 25 mg every 2 to 4 days after loading with 25 mg twice daily for the first 2 days. In children, the usual maintenance dosage is 1 mg per kg every 2 to 4 days after loading with 2 mg per kg daily for the first two days. The major toxicities of pyrimethamine relate to its anti-folate activity, and include thrombocytopenia, anemia, and leukopenia. Blood cell counts should be checked twice weekly to monitor for bone marrow suppression. Folinic acid, 5 to 10 mg orally or parenterally once a day, should be given to all patients receiving daily pyrimethamine and to all children receiving pyrimethamine, in order to limit hematologic toxicity. For most other patients being treated for toxoplasmosis with pyrimethamine, folinic acid also is often recommended. Less commonly, pyrimethamine may cause gastrointestinal reactions or headache.

Sulfadiazine and trisulfapyrimidine act synergistically with pyrimethamine against *T. gondii.* Other sulfonamides, including trimethoprim-sul-

TABLE 2. **Drugs Used to Treat Toxoplasmosis**

Drug	Usual Pediatric Dosage	Maximum Adult Dosage
Pyrimethamine* (Daraprim)	1–2 mg/kg	50 mg/day
Sulfadiazine†	100 mg/kg/day	6–8 grams/day
Spiramycin	50–100 mg/kg/day	4 grams/day

*Folinic acid 5 to 10 mg per day is given with pyrimethamine.
†Trisulfapyrimidine may be substituted.

famethoxazole, are less active and have no proven role in the therapy of toxoplasmosis. Sulfadiazine or trisulfapyrimidine is given in a loading dose of 75 mg per kg (maximum of 4 grams), followed by 100 mg per kg per day (maximum of 6 grams) in four divided doses. In seriously ill adults, the maximum daily dose may be raised to 8 grams. Solid and liquid forms for oral use, and intravenous preparations are available. Nephrotoxicity and hypersensitivity reactions are the most severe adverse effects of the sulfonamides, with the latter a common problem in AIDS patients.

Spiramycin is a macrolide widely used outside the United States to treat toxoplasmosis acquired during pregnancy and congenital infections. It is given in divided oral doses as 2 to 4 grams per day to adults, or as 50 to 100 mg per kg per day to children. Permission for use of spiramycin (Rhone-Poulenc Pharmaceuticals, Montreal, Quebec, Canada) in an appropriate patient in the United States may be obtained through the Division of Antiviral Drug Products, Food and Drug Administration, Rockville, Maryland.

TRICHINELLOSIS

method of
MICHAEL A. ROSENBLUTH, M.D.
New York, New York

Trichinellosis (trichinosis) is an uncommon disease produced by the nematode *Trichinella spiralis*. Although fewer than 100 cases are reported annually to the Centers for Disease Control, more than 200,000 new cases are estimated to occur annually, but are apparently subclinical in the majority or so mild in nature that the diagnosis is missed; 2 per cent of all autopsies reveal *Trichinella* cysts, suggesting a high incidence of subclinical infection.

Ninety to 95 per cent of infections are caused by eating undercooked or raw pork obtained from commercial sources; rare cases occur from eating bear or seal meat. When striated meat containing the encysted *Trichinella* larvae is eaten, the cyst wall is digested by gastric acid and pepsin. Liberated larvae are then passively carried by peristalsis to the upper two thirds of the small intestine, where they penetrate the columnar epithelium at the base of a villus, and after several molts over the next 30 hours become adult worms. After copulation, the females each give birth to approximately 1000 live larvae, which migrate through the lamina propria and lymphatics, passing through the thoracic duct, the right side of the heart, the lungs, and the left side of the heart into the arterial circulation, from which they are carried throughout the body. They are capable of penetrating any cell of the body. While most cells die after invasion, the skeletal muscle supports the growth of these larvae in what are called

"nurse cells." Inside these nurse cell complexes, the larvae are protected and receive nutrients, and may survive for years, eventually dying and undergoing calcification.

Clinical Picture

The clinical manifestations arise more from the immune response to helminthic invasion than from direct helminthic injury. The time for reproduction and dissemination is so short, as noted above, that the larvae are safely inside skeletal muscle cells before the host's immune defenses have been fully activated. However, the initial, nonspecific signs usually include a brief enteritis occurring between the second and seventh day after ingestion of infected meat. Following this, chills, fever, myalgias, rash, malaise, periorbital edema, and eosinophilia signal the intravascular migration of larvae and the resultant tissue reactions when they reach their final destination. This secondary stage may occur from 5 to 50 days after ingestion of infected meat, although it most commonly occurs within 7 days. The diagnostic clue is the history of having eaten pork or pork products; it should be remembered that occasionally hamburgers are mixed with pork.

Laboratory Data

Since larval entry into muscle cells permits the release of various muscle enzymes, including creatine kinase, these may be elevated in the blood, along with hypoalbuminemia. Eosinophilia occurs in approximately 90 per cent of infected patients and occurs concomitantly with the systemic manifestations, constituting between 10 and 50 per cent of the total white blood count. Immunologic tests may begin to show positive results within 2 weeks, but do not begin to become significant until 3 weeks or later. These include immunodiffusion, counterimmunoelectrophoresis, immunofluorescence, ELISA, latex fixation, and bentonite flocculation tests.

Treatment

The disease, though worldwide, is generally benign, with a mortality rate of less than 1 per cent even in those infected patients who receive no therapy at all. Basically, the therapy will depend on the intensity of infection, the strain of the infecting *Trichinella spiralis,* the duration and stage of the infection (i.e., early acute or late stage of the disease), and most particularly the character of the host response to the infection. No drug currently available can alter the course of the disease once the migratory phase has begun. Usually antipyretics and analgesics (aspirin, acetaminophen) are sufficient to relieve the acute-stage symptoms of fever, myalgias, and generalized fatigue. Allergic manifestations resulting from host immune responses include periorbital edema, conjunctival hemorrhages, and high eosinophilia. These effects usually respond to corticosteroids in a dose of 40 to 60 mg of prednisone per day, which are given until the fever and allergic manifestations have subsided and then tapered off over one week. Since corticosteroids suppress the natural inflammatory and immune responses of the host, they prolong the intestinal phase of the infection and increase the number of larvae born to fecund adults. It is for this reason that mebendazole (Vermox), 5 mg per kg per day (maximum 400 mg) divided into two doses, for 7 to 10 days, should reasonably be given to all patients who are seriously ill.* This includes those patients who develop myocarditis (about one in five patients), neurologic effects (lassitude), or pulmonary complications (nonproductive cough). Mebendazole and thiabendazole will stop further dissemination from the intestinal tract but have little effect on already encysted larvae. Furthermore, since an acute systemic allergic reaction may occur secondary to a hypersensitivity to antigenic substances liberated from dying or disintegrating T. spiralis larvae, the physician should always combine an antihelminthic drug treatment with corticosteroids. During the late stages of this disease, the hypoalbuminemia may require replacement with human albumin, and the hypokalemia must be monitored in order to prevent cardiac arrhythmias.

TULAREMIA

method of
MICHAEL WORTHINGTON, M.D., and
JOHN G. SULLIVAN, M.D.
St. Elizabeth's Hospital
Tufts University School of Medicine
Boston, Massachusetts

Tularemia is caused by *Francisella tularensis,* a small, nonmotile, aerobic, nonencapsulated, gram-negative coccobacillus. *F. tularensis* is distributed throughout the Northern Hemisphere between 30 and 71° north latitudes. In the United States the organism has caused human disease in all 50 states and has been recovered from approximately 100 types of wild animals, as well as birds, amphibians, fish, and some insects and domestic animals. In the United States, the most important vectors are ticks, rabbits, and hares. Humans usually acquire infection following contact with the tissues or body fluid of an infected mammal, such as a rabbit, or following the bite of an infected arthropod.

Almost all patients have abrupt onset of fever, chills,

malaise, and fatigue, followed by one of the following six clinical syndromes related to the site of entry: ulceroglandular, glandular, oculoglandular, typhoidal, oropharyngeal, or pneumonic.

The ulceroglandular form (75 to 85 per cent of cases) is characterized by an ulcerated skin lesion and painful regional lymphadenopathy. The diagnosis is generally made on clinical grounds and confirmed serologically. A fourfold rise in the tularemia agglutination titer is strongly suggestive of infection. The organism will grow in thioglycolate broth, glucose blood agar, or glucose cysteine agar. Growth may also be detected using automated blood culture sampling devices (BACTEC). Laboratory isolation of the organism is not recommended because of the exceptionally high risk of infection in laboratory personnel.

Treatment

Drug Regimens

Streptomycin remains the drug of choice for all forms of tularemia. In severely ill patients, up to 30 mg per kg per day can be administered for the first 2 to 3 days; the dose should then be reduced to the more standard 15 to 20 mg per kg per day twice daily.

Streptomycin is bactericidal to the organism, and clinical response is usually prompt. Relapse after streptomycin therapy is unusual, as is the development of resistance to streptomycin. Therapy should be continued for at least 10 to 14 days. Serum levels of streptomycin should be measured to minimize the potential vestibular and renal toxicity of streptomycin.

Gentamicin in standard doses appears to be effective, but there is considerably less clinical experience with this drug. Tetracycline and chloramphenicol (both 30 mg per kg per day in four divided doses) have been used and appear to be effective; relapses occur more frequently with these agents, particularly when they are administered for less than 2 weeks.

Prevention

Tularemia is transmitted to humans largely from infected animals and insect vectors. Therefore, hunters and trappers should wear gloves and work carefully while skinning, dressing, or handling animals, particularly rabbits. Efforts should be made to avoid and repel ticks, mosquitoes, and deer flies in regions with a high incidence of the disease. All tick-infested areas should be avoided if possible; clothing and body should be frequently inspected, and ticks should be promptly removed when found.

A live, attenuated vaccine is available. This vaccine does not provide complete protection, but it is effective and the severity of the disease is modified in vaccinated individuals who acquire clinical illness. The vaccine should be particu-

---

*Note: The manufacturer's official directive states that mebendazole is contraindicated in pregnant women.

larly considered for laboratory workers who handle *F. tularensis* and individuals who will be repeatedly exposed to wild mammals or infected vectors. The vaccine is available from the Centers for Disease Control, Atlanta, Georgia.

SALMONELLOSIS

method of
CLARE L. CHERNEY, M.D., and
MATTHEW E. LEVISON, M.D.
The Medical College of Pennsylvania
Philadelphia, Pennsylvania

Salmonellosis refers to a group of diseases caused by *Salmonella*. These organisms are motile, non–spore-forming, non–lactose-fermenting gram-negative rods of the family Enterobacteriaceae. *Salmonella* has three primary species, *S. typhi*, *S. choleraesuis*, and *S. enteritidis*, the last of which contains over 2000 serotypes. The most common serotype isolated at the Centers for Disease Control is *S. enteritidis*, serotype *typhimurium*. Although humans are the only known reservoir for *S. typhi*, the non-*typhi Salmonella* colonize the majority of the animal kingdom, including man. Humans become infected by ingesting large numbers of salmonellae in contaminated food or water. *Salmonella* is the most common etiologic agent identified in outbreaks of foodborne illness. Improperly cooked poultry (chicken, turkey, and duck) and poultry products (eggs) have been implicated as the source of non-*typhi Salmonella* in most investigated outbreaks, although beef, pork, dairy products, frozen pasta, water, marijuana, biologic extracts, and pet turtles are also known vectors. Direct human-to-human transmission can occur, but usually only in impaired hosts, such as infants or the very old and debilitated.

Host characteristics play an important role in susceptibility to salmonellosis. Altered humoral or cellular immunity increases the risk of infection. Patients with HIV infection, diabetes mellitus, malignancy, splenectomy, or malnutrition as well as infants and patients receiving immunosuppressive drugs (e.g., organ transplant recipients or those receiving steroids) are known to have an increased risk of salmonellosis. Impaired gastric acidity, whether surgically or medically induced, also enhances the risk of salmonellosis. This is probably a result of diminished killing of these acid-sensitive organisms in the gastric lumen, allowing for a low inoculum of ingested salmonellae to colonize the bowel. Patients with hemolysis (e.g., due to malaria, sickle cell disease,

or bartonellosis) also are at increased risk of infection because of an impaired ability to clear salmonellae from the blood. Areas of anatomic abnormalities such as infarcted tissue, tumors, atherosclerotic plaques, and renal or biliary stones are especially prone to focal infection following *Salmonella* bacteremia.

ENTEROCOLITIS (GASTROENTERITIS)

Acute enterocolitis is the most common form of salmonellosis and accounts for 70 per cent of documented clinical disease. *S. typhimurium* is the usual pathogen in the United States. The majority of patients have an acute, self-limited illness consisting of fever, myalgia, headache, nausea, abdominal cramping, and diarrhea, which occurs 6 to 48 hours after the ingestion of contaminated food or water. Diarrhea may be either watery and profuse or dysenteric (containing blood and mucus). Stools will often reveal white blood cells on Wright's stain. Fever may last 2 to 3 days and diarrhea may last 7 to 10 days. Early in the course of *Salmonella* enterocolitis transient bacteremia has been estimated to occur in less than 5 per cent of adults, in 8 to 15 per cent of children, and in up to 40 per cent of infants (less than 3 months of age). Complications, such as intravascular infection or a localized extraintestinal infection, should be suspected if the patient has persistently positive blood cultures or a prolonged febrile illness.

Most episodes of *Salmonella* enterocolitis can be managed conservatively with attention to hydration and electrolyte replacement. Intravenous fluids may be necessary, especially in the infant or young child, when adequate intravascular volume cannot be maintained orally. Drugs that slow intestinal motility (e.g., diphenoxylate hydrochloride with atropine sulfate [Lomotil] or loperamide hydrochloride [Imodium]) are not recommended because they may decrease clearance of salmonellae or bacterial toxic products from the bowel.

Antimicrobial therapy is not indicated for this self-limited disease because it neither shortens the length of illness nor decreases the time of stool carriage of the organism, and may select for resistant organisms. Antimicrobial therapy has been recommended in patients with sickle cell disease, infants less than 3 months of age, and patients greater than 50 years of age, and perhaps HIV-positive patients as well, since these groups have been shown to be at increased risk of developing complications from bacteremia; however, there is no evidence to support the hypothesis that antimicrobial therapy for *Salmonella* enterocolitis in these groups can actually prevent these complications. In one study of *Salmonella* enterocolitis in children, the occurrence of bacteremia was unpredictable and did not worsen the prognosis.

ENTERIC (TYPHOID) FEVER

Enteric fever is a prolonged, febrile illness caused by any serotye of *Salmonella*, although the usual pathogen is *S. typhi*. Enteric fever begins insidiously with progressively worsening systemic symptoms that include fever, headache, anorexia, myalgia, and generalized weakness. Nausea, vomiting, and diarrhea are not strikingly characteristic of this disease. In fact, constipation, cough, sore throat, and/or abnormal mentation may dominate the clinical picture at the time of presentation. A pulse that is slower than expected for the height of the body temperature, rose spots on the lower chest and upper abdomen, hepatosplenomegaly, and rales may be noted on physical examination. Blood and stool cultures are positive in the majority of cases. If untreated, enteric fever may last 3 to 4 weeks and may have a 10 to 30 per cent mortality.

Complications, including intestinal hemorrhage, bowel perforation, localized infections, and relapse, occur in up to 10 to 20 per cent of patients, even among treated individuals. Therapeutic measures important in the care of patients with enteric fever include antibiotics, rehydration, and nutritional supplementation. In the severely ill patient a short course of high-dose corticosteroids (e.g., prednisone, 60 mg orally per day for 3 days, or dexamethasone, 10 mg intravenously every 6 hours for 3 days) has been shown to decrease morbidity and mortality. Steroids, as well as nonsteroidal anti-inflammatory drugs, should be given with extreme caution, since they can lead to a precipitous fall in temperature and blood pressure.

Chloramphenicol (Chloromycetin) has traditionally been the antimicrobial of choice for enteric fever since its first documented success in 1948. There are well-known problems with this drug, including idiosyncratic aplastic anemia and dose-related marrow suppression, but it generally can be used safely. Resistance to chloramphenicol has been documented in Mexico, Great Britain, Vietnam, India, and parts of the United States, although the frequency is low (less than 1 per cent).

Ampicillin is a therapeutic alternative for enteric fever if the organism is sensitive to this drug. Ampicillin resistance is common among non-*typhi Salmonella* in this country, although most strains of *S. typhi* are susceptible. Ampicillin should not be used alone as first-line therapy for enteric fever, when the pathogen or its sensitivities are not as yet known. Trimethoprim-sulfamethoxazole also can be used as alternative treatment for enteric fever, especially when strains are resistant to both ampicillin and chloramphenicol, but in one study this agent was associated with an unacceptably high failure rate.

There is a growing, albeit small, amount of literature attesting to the efficacy of ciprofloxacin (Cipro) in the treatment of enteric fever. This drug has not been recommended for children less than 18 years of age (because of cartilage malformations reported in certain animals) or pregnant females (because of reported teratogenicity). Advantages include no known resistance, excellent intracellular penetration and rapid bactericidal action.

Table 1 lists dosages of the aforementioned drugs.

BACTEREMIA

Patients with *Salmonella* bacteremia present with spiking fever, sometimes persisting for

TABLE 1. **Therapeutic Alternatives for Enteric Fever and *Salmonella* Bacteremia**

Drugs	Dosage*	Comments
Chloramphenicol (Chloromycetin)	12.5 mg/kg IV or PO q 6 hr for 14 days	Still considered drug of choice Do not use alone as initial therapy when resistance suspected Attention to side effects
Ciprofloxacin (Cipro)	500–750 mg PO q 12 hr for 14 days	Only to be used in the nonpregnant adult Must have adequate oral absorption
Ampicillin	25 mg/kg IV or PO q 6 hr for 14 days	Use alone only if sensitivity is confirmed
Ceftriaxone (Rocephin)	25–50 mg/kg IV or IM q 12 hr	Largest clinical experience for the cephalosporins
Trimethoprim-sulfamethoxazole (Bactrim, Septra)	4 mg/kg of trimethoprim component IV or PO q 12 hr	An alternative agent, but may have significant hematologic, hepatic, and dermal toxicity, especially in HIV-positive patients

*In older children and adults with normal renal function.

weeks, and no localizing signs of infection. Gastrointestinal symptoms usually do not occur. Blood cultures are positive, but stool cultures are usually negative. *S. choleraesuis* is the most common species that causes this disease. Complications include focal suppurative infections and a high relapse rate, especially in the immunocompromised patient.

It has recently become evident that patients with HIV infection are at an increased risk for *Salmonella* bacteremia and, in fact, this may commonly be their first manifestation of the acquired immunodeficiency syndrome (AIDS). These patients appear to have a high rate of relapse, and some experts have advocated chronic suppressive therapy in this group.

Treatment of *Salmonella* bacteremia is similar to that of enteric fever. Chloramphenicol and extended-spectrum cephalosporins, as outlined in Table 1, are alternative agents. In the nonpregnant adult with adequate oral absorption, ciprofloxacin is efficacious. Duration of therapy is 14 days unless a complication requiring more prolonged therapy is discovered. Because more than 40 per cent of non-*typhi Salmonella* are ampicillin-resistant, ampicillin should be used only if the in vitro sensitivity to this antibiotic is confirmed.

Hepatosplenic schistosomiasis is known to predispose to persistent *Salmonella* bacteremia and to relapse after therapy. Treatment of the salmonellosis may be facilitated in these patients by treatment of schistosomiasis.

CHRONIC CARRIER STATE

Most patients will continue to carry salmonellae in their stool for up to 8 weeks after enterocolitis or enteric fever. Patients who continue to excrete salmonellae for greater than 1 year are considered chronic carriers. In adults, chronic stool carriage after infection with *S. typhi* occurs in 1 to 3 per cent of patients. Chronic carriage after infection with non-*typhi Salmonella* is rare in the adult and probably occurs in less than 1 per cent of patients.

It is difficult to eradicate the chronic carrier state, especially when cholelithiasis is present. Chronic carriers should be counseled as to the practice of strict personal hygiene. If eradication is felt to be necessary, prolonged courses of ampicillin or trimethoprim-sulfamethoxazole (Bactrim, Septra) may be tried (Table 2). Some studies have noted success with trimethoprim-sulfamethoxazole along with rifampin (Rifadin) when gallbladder disease is present. A preliminary report suggests that ciprofloxacin may also be effective. In only the unusual chronic carrier who is unresponsive to medical therapy and in whom eradication of the carrier state is mandatory should cholecystectomy be considered. However, the chronic carrier state may persist even following cholecystectomy in some patients.

LOCALIZED INFECTION

Focal suppurative infections caused by *Salmonella* can occur anywhere, especially at sites of previously damaged tissue. Abnormalities such as atherosclerotic plaques, scars, infarcts, tumors, or stones are often predisposing lesions. Clinical manifestations include those of osteomyelitis, infected arterial aneurysms, endocarditis, pericarditis, meningitis, pyelonephritis, pneumonia, empyema, abscesses in the liver or spleen, and soft tissue infections. Most of these complications require prolonged antimicrobial therapy and consideration of surgical drainage. Individualized therapeutic regimens are obviously needed but are beyond the scope of this review.

TABLE 2. **Therapeutic Alternatives for Chronic Carriage of Salmonella**

Therapy	Dosage*	Comments
Ampicillin plus probenecid	1.5 gm PO q 6 hr with 500 mg PO q 6 hr for 6 weeks	May need to repeat 2–3 times but often is ineffective in patients with gallbladder disease
Ciprofloxacin (Cipro)	500–750 mg PO q 12 hr for 3–6 weeks	Only in the nonpregnant adult
Trimethoprim-sulfamethoxazole (Bactrim, Septra) plus rifampin (Rifadin)	1 DS (160 mg trimethoprim/400 mg sulfamethoxazole) q 12 hr with 600 mg PO daily	For 3 months
Cholecystectomy	—	Consider only if: 1. Cholelithiasis is present 2. Eradication of the carrier state is mandatory 3. Benefits outweigh risks, and 4. Multiple medical trials have failed

*In adults with normal renal function.

TYPHOID FEVER

method of
ONOFRE MUÑOZ-HERNÁNDEZ, M.D.

Mexican Institute of Social Security
Mexico City, Mexico

Typhoid fever is a systemic disease caused by *Salmonella typhi*. Man is the only reservoir and natural host of *S. typhi*. Typhoid fever is an endemic-epidemic disease in developing countries related to the lack of potable water and to ineffective environmental sanitation. Infection is acquired through fecally contaminated food and water. Bacteria penetrate the intestinal mucosa and produce a disseminated infection characterized by fever, malaise, diffuse abdominal pain, loss of appetite, and ulcerative lesions in intestinal mucosa. Nutritional status is seriously affected owing to negative nitrogen balance. Relapses, hemorrhage, perforation of the terminal ileum, and prolonged fecal elimination of the organism constitute remarkable characteristics of the disease. Isolation of *S. typhi* from blood and bone marrow culture is the most reliable diagnostic method.

Treatment

Antimicrobial Agents. Chloramphenicol remains the drug of choice for typhoid fever produced by susceptible strains. It has been used successfully since 1948, when its introduction caused the mortality of typhoid fever to decrease from 10 to 15 per cent to 1 to 3 per cent. The recommended dosage in adults is 3.0 grams per day divided into four doses, and in children 100 mg per kg per day. Treatment must be maintained for 10 to 12 days, and reduction of fever generally occurs between the third and fifth days. Chloramphenicol should usually be given orally, with the intravenous route reserved for unconscious or incompetent patients. The intramuscular route should be avoided because it is painful and irregular blood levels are achieved.

It should be stressed that chloramphenicol does not change the rate of convalescent or chronic carriers, and relapses occur in 2 to 5 per cent of well-treated patients. Medullary aplasia with fatal pancytopenia occurs once in every 40,000 to 50,000 courses of therapy. The widespread resistance of *S. typhi* to chloramphenicol in different areas of the world (Mexico, Vietnam, Thailand, India, Indonesia, Algeria, Egypt, and the United States) and the undesirable dose-related bone marrow suppression in patients with acquired immunodeficiency syndrome (AIDS), malignancy, hemolytic anemias, malaria, and collagen-vascular disease emphasize the need for a reliable, alternative oral drug.

If chloramphenicol-resistant strains are identified, the patient is immunosuppressed, or it is undesirable to induce more hematopoietic depression, alternative oral drugs should be used, such as amoxicillin, trimethoprim-sulfamethoxazole, or furazolidone.

Amoxicillin is closely related to ampicillin but with better intestinal absorption and higher blood levels. It is an effective alternative when chloramphenicol-resistant strains are identified. Adults are given 4.0 grams per day in four divided doses, and children are given 100 mg per kg per day by the oral route. Therapy should be continued for 14 days, with fever control response occurring between 5 and 7 days. Drug rashes and gastrointestinal upsets occur as frequently as with ampicillin. Certain endemic strains may also carry resistance to ampicillin, and infections caused by these strains can be treated with trimethoprim-sulfamethoxazole or furazolidone.

Trimethoprim-sulfamethoxazole (Bactrim, Septra) is an acceptable choice for the treatment of cases resistant to the aforementioned drugs. This drug combination is given in doses of 160 mg of trimethoprim and 800 mg of sulfamethoxazole orally every 12 hours in adults and 8 mg of trimethoprim and 40 mg of sulfamethoxazole per kg per day in children, also in two doses, continued for 14 days. Fever is usually controlled between the fifth and seventh days. The most frequent side effects are nausea, vomiting, and rash. Indian and Mexican experiences have shown that chloramphenicol-resistant strains can be treated successfully with furazolidone (Furoxone). This drug is available orally only; 800 mg is given daily in four divided doses for adults and 10 to 15 mg per kg per day for children, for 12 to 14 days. Side effects are generally related to the gastrointestinal tract and include nausea, vomiting, and heartburn.

The quinolone antibiotics (norfloxacin and ciprofloxacin) also offer promise as oral agents; the in vitro activity against *S. typhi* is impressive, but it will be necessary to demonstrate its clinical usefulness.

Supportive Measures. Bed rest is important even in mild attacks. Attention should be given to the maintenance of nutrition and an unrestricted diet is probably better, although a low-residue diet is well tolerated. Fluids should be drunk liberally. Intravenous fluid infusions are necessary when dehydration, vomiting, and low intakes are present, and also in case of gastrointestinal complications. Antipyretics, even in therapeutic dosage, induce severe hypothermia with risk of vascular collapse. Fever must be controlled by physical means (exposure and sponging with tepid water). Laxatives and enemas must be avoided because of danger of precipitating intestinal hemorrhage.

Lactulose may be useful when constipation becomes a problem.

Treatment of Complications. Because typhoid fever is a septicemic condition, extraintestinal focalization is possible, but this has been markedly reduced since the advent of antimicrobial agents. Some of the extraintestinal complications include meningitis, arthritis, neuropsychiatric alterations, osteomyelitis, pneumonia, pleural effusion, myocarditis, primary peritonitis, disseminated intravascular coagulation, nephritis, otitis, parotitis, orchitis, hepatitis, and empyema of the gallbladder. Corticosteroids have been reserved for the rare patient with severe toxicity who is given a 2-day course of high-dose dexamethasone. The main hazards of their use are that they may induce bleeding from gastrointestinal ulcers or obscure the initial signs of an acute abdomen. Intestinal complications such as hemorrhage and perforation are most common. Intestinal hemorrhage most often occurs late in the second week, and its major clinical signs are melena and fresh blood evacuations, depending on intestinal transit; hypovolemic shock due to acute anemia can occur. Treatment includes close surveillance of the patient and repeated transfusions in order to restore blood losses.

Intestinal perforation occurs in less than 3 per cent of patients and is more common during the second and third week of disease. Treatment includes medical and surgical measures:

1. Management of shock is necessary before surgery.

2. Surgical treatment depends on the extent of the damage; simple closure of the perforation with excision of surrounding devitalized tissues or resection of affected ileum with enteroanastomosis and temporary ileostomy or derivative colostomy if necessary.

3. Surgery must be accompanied by the use of additional antibiotics, such as amikacin and cefoxitin or intravenous metronidazole, against peritoneal infection caused by enteric flora, including anaerobes.

Relapse is a peculiar feature of typhoid and occurs despite adequate antimicrobial therapy. The frequency of relapse as reported in a large number of studies varies between 5 and 20 per cent; in our experience it is less than 5 per cent. The afebrile interval between the end of the primary attack and the relapse is 1 or 2 weeks. The course is usually milder and shorter, and treatment is the same as for the initial episode, unless chloramphenicol was used at the maximum dose, in which case it is preferable to prescribe an alternative antibiotic.

Carrier State

The chronic carrier state is poorly understood; consequently, it is difficult to achieve a successful treatment. Women and older adults with cholecystitis and gallstones have an increased risk of becoming chronic carriers. Treatment with amoxicillin, 2 grams by mouth, three times per day for 4 to 6 weeks, achieves a 90 per cent cure rate; its main limitation is the gastrointestinal intolerance to large doses. In chronic carriers with cholecystitis and gallstones, cholecystectomy may be necessary, followed by oral amoxicillin. Preliminary results with quinolone antibiotics suggest potential efficacy in eliminating the carrier state.

Prevention

Typhoid fever should be controllable by the application of the principles of hygiene and public health, as has been proved in developed countries, but it is still highly endemic in less developed areas of the world.

The acetone-killed *S. typhi* vaccine has shown 40 to 90 per cent protective efficacy in endemic areas. Its application is recommended for persons living or traveling in highly endemic areas, with two doses of 0.5 ml 1 month apart. Side effects are fever, which occurs in 20 per cent of subjects, and malaise and lethargy for 1 or 2 days. Local reactions include edema and erythema.

A live oral attenuated vaccine (*S. typhi* strain Ty21a) is now available, but several field trials have not indicated that this vaccine provides satisfactory protection.

TYPHUS FEVERS

method of
DAVID T. DENNIS, M.D., M.P.H.
Centers for Disease Control
Atlanta, Georgia

Typhus fevers are caused by any of the nine species of *Rickettsia* known to be pathogenic to humans. These obligate intracellular parasites are carried in nature by various insects (lice, fleas, ticks, mites) and transmitted to humans by bites, by the rubbing of infected insect feces into the skin, or by inhalation of infective material. Mammalian reservoirs other than humans are found for all species, and with the exception of infection with *Rickettsia prowazekii*, the cause of epidemic typhus, humans are incidental hosts. Typhus fevers have a wide geographic distribution, but some (e.g., mite- and tick-borne forms) have discrete foci of transmission determined by the ecologic requirements of vectors and reservoir hosts. Worldwide, most typhus fevers are caused by *Rickettsia prowazekii* (epidemic, louse-borne typhus), *Rickettsia typhi* (endemic, flea-borne typhus), and *Rickettsia tsutsugamushi* (scrub, mite-borne typhus). The most frequent causes of typhus fevers in the United States are *Rickettsia rickettsiae* (Rocky Mountain spotted fever), *Rickettsia typhi,* and *Coxiella burnetii* (Q fever). Classic louse-borne typhus, Brill-Zinsser disease, and rickettsialpox occur rarely in this country.

Typhus infections encompass a broad spectrum of clinical entities that are generally characterized by incubation periods ranging from 3 days to 3 weeks; onset periods of rising fever and chills lasting about 2 days; and acute, toxic illness with continuous fever, severe headache, muscle and joint pains, and malaise leading to prostration. Cutaneous manifestations are common, including morbilliform and maculopapular exanthems, petechiae and ecchymoses, and discrete eschars at the sites of mite or tick attachment. *Rickettsia* proliferate in endothelial cells of small vessels, causing increased permeability and extravasation of plasma into the interstitium. The result can be a decreased effective circulating blood volume, electrolyte imbalance, prerenal azotemia, and shock. Delirium, stupor and coma, myocarditis, hepatitis, and consumptive coagulopathy with bleeding sometimes occur in severe forms. Complications include bronchopneumonia, pyogenic otitis, neurologic deafness, thrombosis, and gangrene. A working diagnosis of typhus is made on the basis of epidemiologic and clinical findings; laboratory confirmation is obtained by testing paired serum specimens for group- and type-specific antibodies and by observing Weil-Felix reactions, which become positive on the seventh to tenth days.

Rocky Mountain spotted fever (RMSF), a disease limited to the Americas, occurs most frequently in the south Atlantic and Gulf states, especially during late spring and summer, the season of greatest tick activity. More than 50 per cent of patients give a history of recent tick attachment. Dog owners living in rural and suburban areas are at highest risk of exposure. The characteristic macular rash of RMSF begins on the distal extremities on the third to fifth days of illness. The disease may be fulminant and fatal, and treatment should not be delayed to await serologic results. Forms of tick-borne typhus other than RMSF occur in persons newly returned from foreign travel and are distinguished by the presence of eschars and local lymphadenopathy. If a rash is present, it is more central and less prominent than in RMSF.

Endemic typhus in the United States occurs most often in southern states, in urban settings, and in late summer and fall months. The illness is generally mild, and the rash is less prominent than that of RMSF. Q fever occurs most commonly in persons exposed to the placenta and birth fluids of infected livestock, such as abattoir workers, veterinarians, and ranchers. The infection may present as a nonspecific febrile illness or as a hepatitis, pneumonitis, or endocarditis. The Weil-Felix test is nonreactive, and serologic diagnosis is based on specific immunofluorescent testing.

Treatment

The management of typhus fevers must consider the duration of illness at the time of treatment, the degree of toxicity and physiologic disturbance, and complications. Antibiotics, although highly effective in bringing about cure of typhus fevers, suppress but do not kill rickettsial organisms. Patient management is directed toward suppressing the infection with antibiotics until immunity develops; physiologic supportive measures; and prevention, early recognition, and treatment of complications. Disease is rarely life-threatening during the first week of symptoms even with the more severe forms. A patient's condition, however, may rapidly deteriorate in the second week and later if appropriate antibiotic treatment is delayed.

Tetracyclines and chloramphenicol are the drugs of choice in the treatment of typhus fevers and have been successfully used against rickettsial illness worldwide for 30 years. Although rickettsiostatic, their clinical effect is almost always rapid and reliable. Tetracyclines are preferred because they do not cause bone marrow suppression or aplastic anemia. Chloramphenicol is useful in circumstances in which differentiation between typhus and typhoid fever is not possible and in children too young to be treated with tetracycline. Doxycycline has the advantage of ease of administration and has been successfully used as a prophylactic against scrub typhus. The response of rickettsial infections to antibiotics is so rapid and clear that a lack of symptomatic improvement and defervescence of fever within 36 to 48 hours of the initiation of treatment implies misdiagnosis, superimposed bacterial infection, or a complication such as infarction or thrombophlebitis. Relapses, however, are not infrequent if antibiotics are begun within the first 5 to 7 days of illness and discontinued before the development of protective levels of antibodies in the second week of illness (see below); this occurs most frequently in scrub typhus.

Tetracycline

Tetracycline is given orally in an initial loading dose of 25 mg per kg of body weight. Subsequent doses are given in four equal portions at 6-hour intervals for a total of 25 to 50 mg per kg of body weight daily. If a patient is unable to swallow, retain, or adequately absorb medication, tetracycline can be administered intravenously at a dose of 0.5 gram every 12 hours, diluted in 100 ml of isotonic saline or dextrose solution, and infused over a 30-minute period. The dose provided above should be revised downward if renal or hepatic function is significantly impaired. Tetracycline may be given by nasogastric tube if parenteral preparations are not available. It is best to continue treatment for at least 48 hours after the patient's temperature has returned to normal.

Chloramphenicol

Chloramphenicol is given orally in an initial loading dose of 50 mg per kg of body weight. Subsequent doses are given in four equal portions at 6-hour intervals for a total of 50 to 75 mg per kg of body weight daily. When necessary, 1.0 gram of chloramphenicol sodium succinate, diluted to a 10 per cent solution, is given intravenously every 8 to 12 hours until the patient is able to take oral medications. Chloramphenicol can be given by nasogastric tube if parenteral preparations are not available. Treatment should be continued for at least 48 hours after the patient has become afebrile.

Doxycycline

This long-acting methacycline derivative is effective in treating all typhus fevers. It has the advantage of being easy to administer and is safe to use in the presence of diminished renal function. The standard daily adult dose is 100 or 200 mg orally. Single oral doses have been used to successfully treat patients with louse-borne typhus, and this is considered to be the method of choice where medical services are limited, such as in refugee camps. Although single-dose regimens cure most cases of scrub and murine typhus, relapses do occur, especially if treatment is given in the first week of illness. Relapses can be prevented by continuing treatment over several days. Single oral doses of doxycycline do not cure all cases of RMSF, and if used in this disease, the drug should be given once or twice daily and continued for at least 48 hours after the patient has become afebrile.

Duration of Antibiotic Treatment

Cure of typhus is dependent in part on immune response, which is not well developed until about the twelfth day of illness. Treatment started early, especially before the fifth day of symptoms, should be continued until the twelfth day after the onset of symptoms to prevent relapse. Relapses that do occur can be treated with the same drug used in the initial course, since there is no evidence of the emergence of antimicrobial resistance.

Corticosteroids

Controlled clinical trials have not been carried out on the efficacy of steroids in typhus fevers. High-dose, short-term adrenocortical steroids have been used to supplement antibiotics in patients who are first treated late in the course of illness, who are toxic and demonstrate symptoms of encephalitis, or who have other severe conditions such as vascular collapse.

Supportive Care

Patients suspected of having typhus fever should be hospitalized until it becomes clear that the illness is responding to antibiotics and that complications have not arisen. When the patient is treated early, the response in the uncomplicated case is rapid and straightforward and the patient is often ready to be discharged within 72 hours. However, patients treated late in the course of illness, persons with RMSF and scrub typhus, and patients with complications need a longer period of care to ensure optimum recovery.

The most critical need in severe cases is to preserve adequate perfusion of vital organs; this is achieved by closely monitoring the vital signs, central venous pressure, and urinary output and by administering blood volume expanders as needed. Volume expansion must be carefully titrated in the presence of myocarditis, pulmonary congestion, and peripheral edema. Unless renal shutdown has occurred, diuresis takes place rapidly as rickettsiae are suppressed, perfusion improves, and vascular permeability returns to normal.

Thrombocytopenia, bleeding, and shock present difficult therapeutic choices, since administration of heparin in the presence of vasculitis can promote bleeding, and the giving of platelets and associated clotting factors may aggravate intravascular coagulation. Fluids should be given to ensure a urine output of at least 1500 ml per day. Persons unable to take oral fluids should have daily needs supplied by nasogastric tube or intravenous drip. Attention needs to be given to meeting the excessive protein and caloric demands of a toxic, febrile patient. Special nursing procedures are required to manage persons who are confused, delirious, or obtunded, and to prevent complications such as pneumonia and skin ulceration in the critically ill. No special isolation procedures are required, although blood precautions should be observed. Prevention is best achieved by avoiding known habitats of vectors and by taking measures against being bitten by ticks and mites. Protective clothing and insect repellents can prevent bites by ticks and mites. Doxycycline, in an oral dose of 200 mg once a week, has been shown to provide protection to persons exposed under field conditions to scrub typhus.

WHOOPING COUGH
(Pertussis)

method of
HARRIS D. RILEY, JR., M.D.
University of Oklahoma Health Sciences Center
Oklahoma City, Oklahoma

Pertussis is an acute infection that affects children predominantly, but no age group is exempt. It is caused by *Bordetella pertussis*, a small, gram-negative, nonmotile bacillus with rather fastidious growth requirements. *B. pertussis* shares certain antigenic components with *Bordetella parapertussis* and *Bordetella bronchiseptica*, both of which (as well as adenoviruses) may cause respiratory disease resembling pertussis, but there is no evidence of cross-immunity with *B. pertussis*. After an incubation period of 2 to 10 days, pertussis classically presents in three distinct clinical stages. The initial or catarrhal stage is characterized by the nonspecific manifestations of an upper respiratory infection. This progresses to the paroxysmal stage, which is characterized by violent paroxysms of cough followed by a distinctive inspiratory whooping sound. This stage may last only a few days but in some cases it may linger for up to 2 or 3 weeks. In the convalescent stage the patient gradually improves and the paroxysms are replaced by a chronic cough. Symptoms may last only 3 to 4 weeks, but in some cases the cough may last for months. In infants less than 6 months of age and in adults the whoop may be absent.

Pertussis is highly contagious and more dangerous than is usually believed, especially for infants and for children debilitated by underlying disease. The young infant is not protected by transplacental antibodies. Approximately 70 per cent of all deaths from pertussis occur in the first year of life. Pertussis is highly communicable, with secondary attack rates of 80 to 90 per cent in susceptible family members and 30 to 80 per cent in those with less intimate exposure. As a rule, one attack confers solid immunity, but the duration of immunity is likely not as long as it is generally thought to be. Fifteen to 25 per cent of immunized children will contract the disease on exposure, but in these patients the disease is usually milder. In recent years 6.5 per cent of the cases occurred in individuals who were 15 years of age or older. Laboratory confirmation (by culture or by fluorescent antibody techniques) is particularly important in atypical cases. Control of pertussis depends chiefly on immunization.

Treatment

General Measures. The patient should be isolated during the first 4 weeks of illness, which is the usual accepted period of communicability, or for 3 weeks from onset of paroxysms, as this date usually can be set with more accuracy. Isolation serves not only as a protection for the patient from other infectious agents but also as a prophylactic measure for susceptible contacts. In partic-ular, patients with active or potentially active cases of tuberculosis should be rigidly guarded against contact with pertussis. Nonimmunized children should be quarantined for 14 days following intimate exposure.

Hospitalization is usually indicated for children less than 2 years of age and always for patients with severe paroxysms or apnea. Intensive care management with constant and resourceful nursing care cannot be overemphasized; in few other diseases is it as crucial, and it may spell the difference between life and death. Nursing attendants should be equipped to institute mechanical lifesaving procedures such as suctioning, insertion of an airway, and other measures. Choking attacks should be relieved by gentle suctioning at frequent intervals. Avoidance of factors that precipitate attacks of coughing, such as activity, excitement, and inhalant irritants, is important. Environmental temperature should be constant to reduce the paroxysm of coughing produced by sudden fluctuations in temperature, and humidification is often helpful. Oxygen is indicated for patients with respiratory complications or convulsions. Cough suppressants, expectorants, and sedatives should not be used.

It is important to maintain adequate nutrition and hydration. Small frequent feedings should be provided, and refeeding is important if vomiting is associated with the paroxysms. Parenteral supplementation is necessary if hydration or nutrition cannot be maintained by the oral route.

Strict respiratory isolation of infected patients is necessary to control the spread of pertussis. Uncomplicated pertussis is usually not accompanied by significant fever; the occurrence of significant fever suggests the development of a secondary bacterial complication, usually of the respiratory tract.

Specific Therapy. Pertussis immune globulin (human) has been widely recommended both for treatment of patients with active cases and for prevention of pertussis in exposed susceptible individuals. However, its efficacy has not been scientifically established, and the results of controlled studies show little or no therapeutic benefit attributable to it. It is no longer recommended.

No antimicrobial agent has been established to be effective in modifying the severity or shortening the course of the pertussis, and the role of antimicrobial therapy is difficult to evaluate. *B. pertussis* is usually susceptible in vitro to a wide variety of antibacterial agents. Erythromycin, tetracycline, and chloramphenicol have been used on the thesis that they produce bacteriologic conversion of cultures to negative and render the child noncontagious. Erythromycin estolate in a dose of 40 to 50 mg per kg per day in four divided doses administered for 5 days is the regimen of choice. When given in the preparoxysmal stage, it may abort and eliminate the disease. Antibiotics may be useful in the face of complicating bacterial infections, and the choice of drug should be guided by microbiologic test results.

Because of the difficulty in diagnosis and the generally unsatisfactory therapy for the established disease, the control of pertussis lies in its prevention by means of active immunization. Vaccines are of no benefit, however, once clinical manifestations have begun.

Favorable claims for the use of corticosteroids in pertussis have been advanced, but additional and controlled studies are needed before such can be recommended.

Complications

Respiratory Tract. The most common and usually the most severe complication is pneumonia, which usually takes the form of an interstitial bronchopneumonia. It is usually caused by secondary invaders, most commonly *Haemophilus influenzae, Streptococcus pneumoniae,* and Group A streptococci. *B. pertussis* has been shown on occasion to be the predominating microorganism. Although every attempt should be made to identify the causative organism, this is only infrequently productive, and antibacterial therapy must be based on clinical grounds. Ampicillin or erythromycin may be used, because they are effective to varying degrees against the most common causative pathogens. If the causative organism is isolated, antimicrobial therapy may be guided by the results of in vitro susceptibility tests.

Atelectasis may occur and is often recognized only by radiographic examination. If it does not subside spontaneously, bronchoscopic aspiration may be necessary to prevent the development of bronchiectasis. No child with pertussis should be released from medical surveillance until the lungs have been shown to be clear roentgenographically.

Otitis media is a frequent complication, particularly in infants. Emphysema usually resolves spontaneously after the acute illness but may lead to interstitial emphysema or pneumothorax.

Central Nervous System. Convulsions are relatively common and represent a serious complication of pertussis. There are probably several different causes, including asphyxia from severe paroxysms, petechial hemorrhages, subarachnoid bleeding, or the development of a diffuse encephalopathy. Convulsions should be treated with sedatives, establishment of an adequate airway, oxygen, and lumbar puncture to relieve increased pressure. Phenobarbital, 3 to 5 mg per kg per dose intramuscularly, is recommended because it does not ordinarily result in depression of the cough reflex.

Other Complications. Hemorrhages, which are mechanical in origin and result from increased venous pressure and congestion associated with paroxysms, occur relatively frequently. Epistaxis and subconjunctival hemorrhages are particularly common; intracranial bleeding may also occur.

Other complications include hernia and prolapsed rectum associated with severe paroxysms and nutritional disturbances. Alkalotic tetany resulting from loss of acid gastric contents secondary to excessive vomiting should be treated with calcium gluconate intravenously. Digitalization should be done for the rare case of secondary cardiac failure.

Management of Contacts

The dissemination of pertussis can be limited by decreasing the infectivity of the case and by protecting close contacts of the patient. The use of oral erythromycin for infected patients shortens the period of infectivity. Close contacts may be protected by active immunization and antibiotics. Those less than 7 years of age who have not received all four doses of diphtheria-tetanus-pertussis (DTP) or who have not received DTP within 3 years of exposure should be given a dose of vaccine. The value of chemoprophylaxis with erythromycin administered orally has never been conclusively demonstrated. It is usually recommended, however, that a 14-day course of erythromycin be provided to close contacts who are less than 1 year of age and to unimmunized close contacts less than 7 years of age. Passive immunization with human pertussis immune globulin of susceptible, exposed contacts is no longer recommended because there is no evidence that it alters the incidence or severity of the disease.

Section 3

The Respiratory System

ACUTE RESPIRATORY FAILURE

method of
JAY I. PETERS, M.D., and
J. MICHAEL JORDAN, M.D.
The University of Texas
San Antonio, Texas

The term respiratory failure implies the inability to maintain the normal delivery of oxygen to the tissues or removal of carbon dioxide from the tissues. Thus, there are actually three processes involved: transfer of oxygen across the alveolus, transport to the tissues (by cardiac output), and removal of carbon dioxide from the blood into the alveolus with exhalation into the environment. Failure of any part of this system can lead to respiratory failure or worsen pre-existing respiratory failure. Clinically, most physicians define "respiratory failure" by analysis of arterial blood gases. Although levels of Pa_{O_2} and Pa_{CO_2} that are said to constitute "respiratory failure" are obviously somewhat arbitrary, an arterial P_{O_2} of less than 60 mm Hg or a P_{CO_2} of greater than 45 mm Hg generally indicates serious respiratory compromise.

CLASSIFICATION

Respiratory failure may be usefully classified by distinguishing between "ventilatory failure" and "oxygenation failure."

Ventilatory Failure

Ventilatory failure is diagnosed when the Pa_{CO_2} exceeds 45 mm Hg and may be due to defective respiratory control mechanisms, impaired function of the respiratory muscles, or mechanical abnormalities of the lungs or chest wall. Thus, ventilatory failure may occur in patients with normal lungs, although mechanical impairment of the lungs—usually caused by chronic airways obstruction—is the most frequent cause. In addition to an elevated Pa_{CO_2}, ventilatory failure is always associated with hypoxemia if the patient is breathing room air because of the effect of an increased Pa_{CO_2} on the alveolar oxygen tension. This effect is defined by the alveolar air equation, which relates alveolar oxygen tension (PA_{O_2}) to Pa_{CO_2}:

$$PA_{O_2} = FI_{O_2} \times (P_B - P_{H_2O}) - Pa_{CO_2}/R.Q.$$

where P_B is barometric pressure, P_{H_2O} is water vapor pressure at 37°C (usually assumed to be 47 mm Hg),

and R.Q. is the respiratory quotient (generally taken to be 0.8). From this equation, it can be seen that at a constant FI_{O_2} (fraction of O_2 in inspired air) and P_B, PA_{O_2} (and thus Pa_{O_2}) decreases as Pa_{CO_2} rises. As a general rule, the Pa_{O_2} decreases by 5 mm Hg for every increase of P_{CO_2} of 3. Thus, in hypoventilation states reflected by an elevated PA_{CO_2}, ventilatory failure leads to oxygenation failure as well.

Oxygenation Failure

In addition to alveolar hypoventilation, failure of oxygenation may be caused by shunting, $\dot{V}/\dot{Q}$ (ventilation-perfusion ratio) mismatching, and impaired diffusion. Of these, impaired diffusion is a rare cause of arterial hypoxemia, except during exercise in patients with interstitial lung disease or at extreme altitude. To distinguish the remaining three causes, the magnitude of the difference between alveolar and arterial oxygen tensions, $P(A-a)O_2$, is useful.

The measured arterial P_{O_2} is always somewhat lower than the ideal alveolar oxygen tension calculated by the alveolar air equation, owing to the presence of $\dot{V}/\dot{Q}$ mismatching and normal anatomic shunts. The normal $P(A-a)O_2$ is about 10 mm Hg in young persons, but increases with age to about 30 mm Hg in healthy people by age 70. Oxygenation failure due to shunting and $\dot{V}/\dot{Q}$ mismatching causes increases in $P(A-a)O_2$ above normal, while alveolar hypoventilation causes hypoxemia with a normal $P(A-a)O_2$ gradient.

Physiologic shunting is defined as the persistence of an increased $P(A-a)O_2$ during O_2 breathing and is due to anatomic right-to-left shunts or to continued perfusion of lung units that receive no ventilation ($\dot{V}/\dot{Q} = 0$). The latter abnormality is usually associated with alveolar filling processes such as pneumonia, atelectasis, or severe pulmonary edema, which are readily apparent on radiographs of the chest. Hypoxemia that is not relieved by breathing oxygen in the presence of clear lung fields radiographically suggests the presence of an intracardiac shunt, pulmonary arteriovenous fistula, or microatelectasis (most often seen in postoperative patients). Arterial hypoxemia due to shunting is worsened by conditions that reduce the oxygen content of the mixed venous blood, such as a low cardiac output.

Mismatching of ventilation ($\dot{V}$) and perfusion ($\dot{Q}$) is the most common cause of arterial hypoxemia in hypoxemic patients. Lung units that have low $\dot{V}/\dot{Q}$ ratios contribute to arterial hypoxemia in a fashion similar to shunt units; this effect is termed "venous admixture." However, in contrast to true shunts, the effect of low $\dot{V}/\dot{Q}$ units is eliminated by O_2 breathing. Hypoxemia due to $\dot{V}/\dot{Q}$ mismatching is thus improved by small increases in FIO_2, whereas hypoxemia due to shunting requires a high FIO_2 and often other measures as well.

Respiratory failure due to pure hypoventilation (as seen most commonly following strokes, head trauma, central nervous system infections, or ingestion of CNS-depressant drugs) is characterized by CO_2 retention as well as hypoxemia. The degree of hypoxemia is directly related to the rise in $PaCO_2$, resulting in a normal $P(A-a)O_2$. Calculation of the $P(A-a)O_2$ can thus distinguish hypoventilation from other causes of oxygenation failure.

Treatment

When approaching the patient in acute respiratory failure, whatever the underlying cause, we must remember the ABCs of resuscitation: airway, breathing, and circulation. A patent airway is the first priority. Upper airway obstruction may be manifested by stridor in awake patients or by inability to elevate the chest with inspiratory efforts applied at the nose or mouth in unconscious patients (via mouth-to-mouth or face mask and self-inflating bag). Obstruction must be rapidly dealt with by manually clearing the obstruction or instrumenting the airway. Important information may be gained by a quick assessment of the presence or absence, as well as the apparent adequacy, of the patient's spontaneous breathing as well as its rate, pattern, and laboredness. Similarly, rapid assessment of the patient's circulatory status—pulse, jugular venous pressure, and blood pressure—provides useful clues to the patient's status. Once these initial observations are made and any necessary emergency support measures are instituted, decisions regarding specific therapies may be made based on arterial blood gas determinations.

Oxygen Therapy

Two primary considerations are involved in deciding on the method of oxygen administration for a hypoxemic patient: How much O_2 will be required? Is it important to know the FIO_2? For many patients, "some" O_2 is sufficient, whereas for others each of these is an important issue.

Administration of O_2 via nasal cannulas at flow rates of 1 to 5 liters per minute provides some augmentation of the FIO_2 and is the best tolerated means of O_2 therapy. However, the magnitude of increase in FIO_2 is unknown, being determined primarily by the patient's ventilatory pattern. On average, provision of low-flow O_2 increases FIO_2 by 3 per cent per liter per minute O_2 flow, but the increase is greater in patients with low minute ventilation and smaller in patients with large minute ventilation. In general,

low-flow nasal O_2 provides adequate O_2 supplementation for patients whose hypoxemia is due to $\dot{V}/\dot{Q}$ mismatching (in contrast to shunting), who are not excessively tachypneic, and whose O_2 requirement is not large. These criteria would include patients with airway obstruction, mild heart failure, mild pneumonias, or pulmonary embolism, for example, but would not include patients with extensive pneumonias, severe pulmonary edema, or any of the above associated with cardiogenic shock.

In the latter conditions, provision of a known, high concentration of O_2 is often necessary to correct hypoxemia. High-flow O_2 devices generally incorporate a dilution apparatus that reduces the final concentration of O_2 by entraining and adding air to the stream of O_2, usually using the Venturi principle. Because of entrainment characteristics, fixed O_2 concentration devices can provide O_2-enriched gas at flow rates that are likely to exceed the patient's inspired flow at low O_2 concentrations ($FIO_2 \leq 0.40$). However, delivery of high O_2 concentrations requires less air entrainment and results in lower flow rates. Patients often "overbreathe" these systems, resulting in lowering of the effective FIO_2. This may explain why in some tachypneic patients increasing the FIO_2 fails to improve the patient's oxygenation. To provide high FIO_2 levels, tight-fitting masks with reservoir bags and unidirectional valves must be used; with these devices, FIO_2 in the range of 0.8 to 0.95 is achievable.

Mechanical Ventilation

Absolute indications for initiation of mechanical ventilation include apnea and the need for administration of paralyzing agents. Mechanical ventilation is also usually required in patients who exhibit ineffectual respiratory efforts, inspiratory muscle fatigue, refractory hypoxemia, or progressive hypercapnea with acidosis. More specific indications are advocated by some, and these include a vital capacity less than 15 ml per kg, FEV_1 less than 10 ml per kg, PaO_2 less than 60 mm Hg on supplemental O_2, and PCO_2 greater than 55 mm Hg.

Although a number of types of ventilators exist, volume-cycled ventilators (i.e., ventilators that deliver a preset tidal volume) are by far the most common. When mechanical ventilation is instituted with such a ventilator, tidal volumes in the range of 10 to 15 ml per kg are reasonable. Tidal volumes of this size minimize atelectasis but at the upper end of this range may generate high peak airway pressures. In general, if peak pressures exceed 40 cm Hg at higher tidal volumes, the tidal volume should be lowered to the range of 10 to 12 ml per kg to minimize the risk of barotrauma.

When the respiratory rate of a patient on mechanical ventilation is to be determined, a crucial decision concerns which ventilator "mode" is most appropriate. In the assist-control mode, the ventilator delivers a full preset tidal volume each time the patient initiates an inspiration. This mode is preferred by most conscious patients and should be used in patients with cardiogenic or other forms of shock. This decreases the blood flow to the diaphragm and allows blood to be diverted to more critical organs. Additionally, patients with diffuse lung disease and metabolic acidosis should be placed on assist-control to allow them to reduce their level of carbon dioxide to compensate for the acidosis. However, problems may arise with patients who "fight the ventilator" and with hyperventilation. The former situation arises when the patient perceives that the ventilator settings as determined by the physician are inadequate for his needs and breathes out of synchronization with the ventilator. This can be corrected by changing the settings, by sedating the patient, or by switching to another mode. Hyperventilation results when the patient's drive to breathe is not diminished by correction of hypoxemia or the provision of large tidal volumes, as often occurs with diffuse pulmonary processes and in patients with altered sensorium and increased central drive. This can most readily be corrected by changing modes to intermittent mandatory ventilation.

Intermittent mandatory ventilation (IMV) is a mode of ventilation in which the patient draws spontaneous tidal volumes from a reservoir and receives intermittent breaths from the ventilator at mandatory intervals. Thus, IMV combines assisted and unassisted ventilation. IMV should always be used in patients intubated for chronic CO_2 retention. Rapid reduction of CO_2 leads to CNS alkalosis and results in seizures. IMV may be useful in patients with central hyperventilation by avoiding the delivery of large tidal volumes each time the patient inspires. Also, IMV may be useful in weaning patients from mechanical ventilation, as it provides a method for gradually reducing the amount of mechanical assistance to ventilation. IMV is obviously not well suited to the patient with respiratory muscle fatigue in whom rest is required; indeed, if the spontaneous circuit is not properly adjusted, the work of breathing with IMV may be substantially greater than with unassisted breathing.

One other newer mode is available on some ventilators, namely "pressure support." A preset inspiratory pressure is maintained throughout inspiration, whereas tidal volume depends on patient effort. This mode helps to overcome the systemic resistance during spontaneous ventilation, thereby decreasing the work of breathing. Pressure support may prove helpful in weaning patients who have difficulty coming off the ventilator.

To select the initial FIO_2 when instituting mechanical ventilation, there are two reasonable approaches. With many patients, previous blood gas determinations will be of help in knowing what O_2 concentrations were previously inadequate, and a somewhat higher FIO_2 should be selected initially. With other patients, a level around 0.80 is a good place to start. If an acceptable PaO_2 (approximately 60 mm Hg) is not obtained with an FIO_2 of greater than 0.6, positive end-expiratory pressure (PEEP) should be instituted and invasive hemodynamic monitoring considered.

The principal value of PEEP is that it often allows a reduction in the FIO_2 required to achieve adequate oxygenation of the arterial blood, and it should be used in most patients who require an FIO_2 of 0.6 or more without it. The beneficial effects of PEEP derive from a number of factors, including improved lung compliance, increased FRC, and diminished shunting. The use of PEEP may be associated with deleterious effects as well. The incidence of barotrauma is greater among patients ventilated with PEEP than without, although it is uncommon when less than 15 cm H_2O PEEP is used. Since PEEP tends to decrease cardiac output, the usual increase in PaO_2 and arterial O_2 content with PEEP may be offset, resulting in an actual reduction in O_2 delivery (the product of cardiac output and O_2 content).

Weaning from Mechanical Ventilation

Minimal criteria for discontinuing mechanical ventilation include (1) awake and cooperative mental status; (2) FIO_2 of 0.40 or less; (3) ventilatory capacity sufficient to support unassisted breathing for 30 to 60 minutes while intubated; and (4) ability to control secretions through spontaneous coughing. More objective measures of ventilatory capacity have been suggested: Successful weaning is unlikely if FVC is less than 15 mg per kg, maximal inspiratory pressure is less than -25 cm H_2O, or maximal voluntary ventilation (MVV) is less than twice the patient's minute ventilation while being assisted. Weaning in most patients may be accomplished by "T-tube trials," which involve connecting the endotracheal tube to a high flow gas source delivered via tubing that connects at a right angle to the endotracheal tube. The critical determinations are based on clinical observation rather than blood gas analysis. If heart rate, respiratory rate, and blood pressure remain stable for 30 to 60 minutes on the T-tube, blood gases should then be checked. If the patient becomes obviously dyspneic or tachycardic, blood gases are not necessary to confirm failure. Patients who fail an extended T-tube trial may be weaned by progressive T-tube trials, gradually increasing the length of time on the T-tube until it is clear that the patient no longer requires ventilatory support. Alternatively, IMV may be used in weaning by gradually reducing the mandatory rate until the patient is essentially breathing without assistance. This latter technique is especially useful in chronically ventilated or debilitated patients and in those with severe lung disease. Finally, some patients with severe underlying lung disease may fail weaning attempts because the added resistance of an endotracheal tube precludes adequate spontaneous ventilation. In these patients, it may be necessary to proceed with a trial extubation once all reversible components of the patient's disease have been corrected, with the knowledge that reintubation may be necessary.

Chronic Obstructive Pulmonary Disease (COPD)

The hallmark of respiratory failure in patients with COPD is worsening dyspnea. Most often, respiratory failure is precipitated by infection. Sputum becomes discolored, yellow or green, and is more difficult to raise than usual. The pattern of breathing may have important prognostic implications. A slow respiratory pattern, with expiratory flow rates controlled by pursed-lip breathing, is a favorable sign, whereas rapid panting respirations are usually ineffectual and signify rapid deterioration. Asking the patient to cough is a useful test; ineffectual efforts indicate that intubation may be required. Heart rates in excess of 130 per minute and pulsus paradoxus of 15 mm Hg or more correlate with severe obstruction.

Relief of hypoxemia is the first goal in the treatment of respiratory failure. Hypoxemia in COPD patients is due principally to $\dot{V}/\dot{Q}$ mismatching, and thus only a small increment in FIO_2 is usually required. This may be accomplished by either low-flow O_2 by nasal cannulae or high-flow O_2 delivering fixed O_2 concentrations by face mask. On average, the PaO_2 increases by 10 mm Hg in acutely ill COPD patients when the FIO_2 is increased from 0.21 (air) to 0.24, equal to about 1 to 2 liters per minute by nasal prongs, and by 20 mm Hg when the FIO_2 is increased to 0.28. In about 10 per cent of acutely ill COPD patients, relief of severe hypoxemia is followed by respiratory depression, respiratory acidosis, and mental obtundation. In general, such patients cannot be accurately identified beforehand, although they are more likely to have

a high $PaCO_2$ and to be acidemic on presentation. In managing such patients, if the initial FIO_2 was high (> 0.30) and the PaO_2 exceeds 60 mm Hg, it may be reasonable to attempt to lower the FIO_2. However, it must be remembered that the patient may become profoundly hypoxemic at the lower FIO_2 because of the time required to "blow off" the accumulated stores of CO_2. Prompt intubation is often required. This problem can best be avoided by starting with a low FIO_2 and increasing it incrementally until an acceptable PaO_2 is reached.

Pharmacologic management of respiratory failure in COPD is important. Intravenous aminophylline is usually given. The loading dose for a patient who has not taken a theophylline preparation in the last 24 hours is 5 to 6 mg per kg given over 20 minutes; this dose is reduced by 50 per cent if the patient is taking oral theophylline. Following this, an infusion of aminophylline is maintained at a rate of 0.5 to 0.6 mg per kg per hour. Inhaled beta-agonists such as isoetharine or metaproteranol are administered by hand-held nebulizer. Epinephrine should be avoided in COPD patients because of its cardiac effects and because it may induce bronchospasm in patients on beta-blockers. Intravenous corticosteroids in doses of 4 mg per kg of hydrocortisone or 0.5 mg per kg of methylprednisolone should be given every 6 hours initially to most COPD patients with severe respiratory failure. Antimicrobial agents have not been clearly shown to have a role in management of acute respiratory failure in COPD and should be reserved for patients whose sputum shows a single predominant organism on Gram stain or for those with concomitant pneumonia.

Adult Respiratory Distress Syndrome

Patients who present with respiratory failure requiring high FIO_2 in the presence of diffuse radiographic infiltrates may be divided into two categories based on results of Swan-Ganz catheterization: those with high wedge pressure are defined in terms of cardiac failure, and those with a normal or low wedge pressure are said to have adult respiratory distress syndrome (ARDS). In ARDS, hypoxemia is the patient's major threat to life. This hypoxemia is due mainly to shunting and thus responds poorly to increments in FIO_2. These patients almost always require intubation and mechanical ventilation, although high-flow O_2 delivery by mask may be attempted initially. Frequently, patients will remain hypoxemic even after intubation, despite increasing FIO_2. PEEP is usually initiated at 5 to 10 cm H_2O when FIO_2 requirements reach the 0.60 to 0.80 range, in an effort to increase PaO_2 while minimizing the toxic effects of high oxygen concentrations. With the initiation of PEEP, most patients should undergo Swan-Ganz catheterization to ensure rapid identification of untoward hemodynamic effects. It should be remembered that although PEEP increases Pao_2, it also tends to decrease cardiac output; it is the amount of O_2 delivered to tissues that is the important end-point in ARDS, and O_2 delivery (the product of O_2 content and cardiac output) may actually decrease with increasing PEEP. This situation can be rapidly identified with a Swan-Ganz catheter in place. Daily chest x-rays should be obtained of patients with ARDS requiring mechanical ventilation and PEEP as a result of the increased incidence of barotrauma (tension pneumothorax, pneumomediastinum). In all patients with ARDS, vigorous measures should be undertaken to maintain the lowest possible wedge pressure without inducing hypotension; this minimizes the transudation of fluid from the vasculature into the alveoli, thus minimizing shunt.

Neuromuscular Diseases

Patients with neuromuscular disorders affecting the respiratory system characteristically breathe with rapid, shallow tidal volumes. They often complain of dyspnea before deterioration of arterial blood gases is evident. Tachypnea usually maintains normal blood gases until respiratory reserve is markedly diminished. The onset of frank respiratory failure is often initiated by the development of a complication, such as aspiration, atelectasis, or a minor respiratory infection.

In acute neuropathies, such as Guillain-Barré syndrome, serial measurements of respiratory muscle function are useful in determining the timing of intervention with ventilatory support. In previously normal patients, a reduction of FVC to less than 40 per cent of predicted, or a maximum inspiratory pressure of less than -20 cm H_2O, identifies a high-risk patient who is likely to require intubation in the near future. When mechanical ventilation is required, most patients are best managed in an assist mode, allowing the patient to set the ventilator rate. Weaning of patients with neuromuscular diseases from ventilatory support is more difficult if the respiratory muscles are "loaded" by breathing through the added resistance of an endotracheal tube, and early tracheostomy may allow for earlier weaning.

The question of whether or not to provide long-term ventilation support for patients with progressive neuromuscular disease is difficult to answer. If the nature of the disease is known beforehand, the prognosis and likely outcome should be discussed with the patient and the family. Faced with the prospect of relentless loss of body function plus the limitations imposed by continuous ventilatory support, many patients decide that intubation should not be performed. Alternatively, the physician may decide that the patient's sudden deterioration is due to a reversible process, such as pneumonia, and that only short-term ventilatory support will be required.

ATELECTASIS

method of
THOMAS R. TODD, M.D.
Toronto General Hospital
Toronto, Ontario, Canada

The importance of atelectasis rests in the fact that it leads to impaired gas exchange and potentiates the onset of bacterial pneumonitis. Although it may be accompanied by compensatory hypoxic vasoconstriction, the latter is never complete and hence ventilation perfusion mismatch is ubiquitous. Stagnation of secretions within the atelectatic segment or lobe may at times lead to pneumonitis if the lower respiratory tract has already been colonized with pathogenic organisms, as is frequently the case in the postoperative or intensive care unit patient.

Diagnosis involves the assessment of chest radiographs. However, clinical acumen is a necessary adjunct, in that atelectasis may involve multiple areas to a degree not apparent on standard chest films. The accumulative physiologic effects may be just as significant as the development of lobar or even pneumonic atelectasis. Therapy depends on the etiology and the degree of physiologic compromise.

Treatment

Airway Obstruction

Nonoperative patients who present with radiographically apparent atelectasis should undergo visual examination of the tracheal bronchial tree to determine the cause. In such situations, therapy will depend on the cause of the airway obstruction, be it neoplastic, foreign body, or inflammatory. Biopsies of intraluminal masses are readily performed. When extraluminal obstruction is present, it is suggested that bronchial brushings be obtained for cytologic and bacteriologic examination. Postoperative patients may forgo bronchoscopy for diagnosis unless hemoptysis suggests unrelated pathology and not simply sputum retention.

Decreased Ventilation

In the absence of proximal airway obstruction, this is by far the commonest cause of atelectasis.

Failure to expand the lung appropriately is secondary to the inability to generate sufficiently negative pleural pressure.

Pain is one of the major causes of this problem. Narcotic analgesia is the commonest method of pain relief. The intravenous route is far superior to the parenteral form, in that it can be frequently repeated and avoids the possibility of tissue accumulation and resultant respiratory depression. Following operative or nonoperative trauma, intercostal blocks or strapping the chest is also useful. The former depends on the availability of staff. Although one would suppose that strapping might potentiate hypoventilation, this is not the case if strapping is applied only to the affected hemothorax. Under such circumstances, pain is relieved and we have demonstrated remarkable improvement in vital capacity, negative inspiratory force, and arterial blood gases. When the above methods fail, the optimal means of pain relief is the administration of morphine or lidocaine via epidural catheters inserted in the lumbar disc space. The former is particularly efficacious, as specific opiate receptors on the dorsal columns allow for significant analgesia without neuromuscular impairment.

Too often we overlook neuromuscular problems in the pathogenesis of pulmonary atelectasis. Diaphragmatic paralysis, whether neoplastic or idiopathic, may result in lobar atelectasis. Similarly, neuromuscular disorders may have their presentation as ventilatory failure and atelectasis. Chest wall incoordination may occur in patients who have required mechanical ventilatory support for periods of time. The therapy is directed at respiratory muscle training, largely accomplished by repeated short intervals of spontaneous ventilation with positive end-expiratory pressure. Another cause of chest wall incoordination is the instability of the chest wall generated by traumatic flail segments and resultant decreased pleural pressure. Relief of pain and chest wall strapping are important, and operative stabilization is reserved for those patients without pulmonary contusion in whom respiratory failure is imminent.

Pleural Space Problems

Pneumothorax or hemothorax may be readily apparent, and tube thoracostomy is required. Chronic pleural disease from infection (bacterial or mycobacterial) or trauma may result in thickening of the visceral and/or parietal pleura that results in pulmonary entrapment and atelectasis of major portions of the lung. Elected decortication should follow careful evaluation of the etiology, possible pleural sepsis, and regional pulmonary function. It is important to remember that complete lung collapse from pleural entrapment may be persistent for many years and that success may yet be realized with decortication.

Adjunctive Measures

Chest Physiotherapy. This is the mainstay of all therapeutic regimens. In the absence of an undiagnosed airway obstruction and progressive hypoxemia, chest physiotherapy should initially preclude bronchoscopy. At the outset, postural drainage and vibration are important further adjuncts.

Bronchoscopy. As noted above, bronchoscopy is important in the non-postoperative patient as a diagnostic as well as a therapeutic tool. In the postoperative period, it is indicated if atelectasis is accompanied by pulmonary sepsis, hypoxemia, or the inability to expand radiographically apparent collapse within 24 hours. In most circumstances, bronchoscopy with flexible instruments will be adequate, but occasionally inspissated sputum or blood fibrin and clots may be tenacious enough to warrant a rigid, open-tubed instrument. It is important to remember that hypoxemia will worsen during the procedure and thus high-flow supplemental oxygen is essential. Patients with precarious conditions who are already receiving supplemental oxygen greater than 50 per cent should be considered for elective oral tracheal intubation to enable a safe therapeutic bronchoscopy via the endotracheal tube. Constant monitoring of oxygen saturation via pulse oximetry is a valuable adjunct in such patients. Adequate analgesia is essential for bronchoscopy and can best be achieved by the injection of 5 to 10 ml of 1 per cent lidocaine through the cricothyroid membrane, employing a 22- to 23-gauge needle.

Inhalations. Intermittent positive pressure breathing is of little or no use and has been abandoned by most centers. However, inhalations of medications via ultrasonic nebulization have proved to be efficacious.

1. With accompanying bronchospasm, albuterol (Ventolin), applied every 4 to 6 hours, is helpful. Bronchospasm is alleviated, and effective coughing and clearing of secretions are potentiated.

2. Acetylcysteine (Mucomyst), administered via nebulization, is a bronchial irritant. However, if administered in a dose of 1 ml of a 10 per cent solution usually mixed with 2.5 mg of albuterol two to three times per day it will break up tenacious secretions and make physiotherapy more productive. It is a most useful adjunct in the patient with thick, mucoid secretions who produces a strong cough.

3. Racemic epinephrine inhalations have classically been reserved for epiglottitis and other

forms of glottic obstruction. However, it is a bronchodilator and will shrink inflammatory or neoplastic strictures of the trachea or main stem bronchi. Even apparently rigid fibrous strictures and obstructing tumors have an inflammatory component and surrounding edema augmenting the degree of airways obstruction. We routinely employ it in obstructions at these levels.

CHRONIC OBSTRUCTIVE PULMONARY DISEASE

method of
STUART B. ZEILENDER, M.D., and
R. CRYSTAL POLATTY, M.D.
Medical College of Virginia
Richmond, Virginia

Chronic obstructive pulmonary disease (COPD) is characterized by prolonged expiratory flow rates (Table 1) that remain unchanged over a period of several months. The major disorders included are chronic bronchitis and emphysema. These entities may present distinctly, but features of both are usually present in an individual patient. Either of these diseases may be associated with a reversible bronchospastic component. Chronic bronchitis is characterized by excessive mucus secretion manifested by chronic or recurrent productive cough on most days for a minimum of 3 months in the year for not less then 2 successive years and not caused by diseases such as bronchiectasis and tuberculosis.

Emphysema is defined as permanent air space distention distal to the terminal bronchioles, and alveolar septal destruction without obvious fibrosis. Centriacinar emphysema, which involves the respiratory bronchioles and alveolar ducts, is classically associated with cigarette smoking. In contrast, panacinar emphysema involves all acinar components and is commonly associated with $alpha_1$-antitrypsin deficiency.

Prevalence, incidence, and mortality rates increase with age, are higher in men than in women, and are higher in whites than in nonwhites. Risk factors include cigarette smoking, increased age, male sex, occupational exposure, air pollution, and $alpha_1$-antitrypsin-deficient phenotypes (PiZZ, PiSZ). Presenting symptoms include cough, wheezing, sputum production, recurrent pulmonary infections, and dyspnea. Physical findings depend on the predominant disease process. For example, emphysema patients, often termed "pink puffers," are usually asthenic and have evidence of weight loss. Hypoxemia is uncommon, as ventilation and perfusion ($\dot{V}/\dot{Q}$) are well matched. Tachypnea, prolonged expiration through pursed lips, and accessory inspiratory muscle use are common findings. Patients tend to sit leaning forward with extended arms to optimize respiratory muscle mechanics. Chest wall percussion yields a hyperresonant note, and diminished breath sounds are found on auscultation. In contrast, chronic bronchitic patients are usually overweight, cyanotic, and edematous ("blue bloater"). Patients may be hypoxemic owing to perfusion of nonventilated or poorly ventilated alveoli ($\dot{V}/\dot{Q}$ mismatching). Coarse rhonchi and wheezes may be present on auscultation. Right ventricular enlargement and right heart failure are occasionally found on physical examination.

A flattened diaphragm, an enlarged retrosternal air space, hyperlucency, and vascular attenuation are present on the roentgenogram in patients with emphysema. Increased lung markings and enlarged right ventricular and pulmonary artery shadows may be found in patients with chronic bronchitis.

Pulmonary function tests confirm the diagnosis of COPD and include a diminished forced expiratory volume at one second (FEV_1) and a reduced FEV_1 to forced vital capacity (FVC) ratio ($FEV_1\%$). There is frequently an increase in total lung capacity (TLC) and residual volume (RV) secondary to air trapping. A 15 per cent or greater increase from baseline in either FEV_1 or FVC after inhaled bronchodilator therapy is considered significant (Table 1).

Prevention

Smoking

Cigarette smoking, the major preventable cause of death and disease in the United States each year, is the major risk factor for COPD. Almost one third of the adult American population continues to use tobacco products. These patients have a greater rate of FEV_1 decline per year than is found in the general population (Table 2). Ten to 15 per cent of smokers will develop COPD, which may be detected early by noting excessive yearly declines in serial FEV_1 measurements. Smoking cessation halts this accelerated decline.

The physician's role in cessation of smoking cannot be overemphasized. Successful quitters on the average have tried and failed two to three times prior to succeeding. Through brief and

TABLE 1. **Spirometry in Chronic Obstructive Pulmonary Disease**

$FEV_1\%$	Degree of Impairment
>70	Normal
61–69	Mild
45–60	Moderate
<45	Severe

TABLE 2. **Yearly Change in FEV_1**

Age (yrs)	Decline of FEV_1 per ml per Year
Normal nonsmokers	
30–70	20–30
>70	45
Smokers (all ages)	55–100

frequent counseling physicians can help the majority of their patients become nonsmokers. Smoking cessation clinics achieve approximately a 30 per cent maintained abstinence rate. Leaflets such as "Freedom from Smoking" (American Lung Association) provide helpful hints. Nicotine gum is a useful adjunct in the nicotine-dependent smoker (2 packs per day). Since the nicotine is absorbed slowly through the buccal mucosa, patients should start chewing the gum as soon as they anticipate the urge to smoke. The dose of nicotine gum dose depends on the patient; it is determined by the severity of addiction, and should be tapered over weeks to months as tolerated. Relapse is common, usually related to increased life stresses, and the patient is encouraged to try to quit again.

Exposure to Toxins

Environmental and occupational air pollution may cause an increased death rate in COPD patients. Patients should remain indoors during periods of heightened air pollution. If exposure in the workplace cannot be minimized, a change of job may be warranted.

Alpha₁-Antitrypsin Deficiency

Among all cases of emphysema 2.5 to 3.5 per cent (20,000 to 35,000 cases) are due to alpha$_1$-antitrypsin deficiency. PiZZ is the most severe phenotypic variant. Individuals with alpha$_1$-antitrypsin levels of $\leq$ 50 mg per dl have an 80 per cent chance of developing significant emphysema. Alpha$_1$-antitrypsin enzyme prepared from pooled human plasma is available for replacement therapy and is given intravenously once weekly to maintain serum levels above 80 mg per dl. However, no long-term studies are available that document cessation of deterioration in pulmonary function. Treatment does not reverse existing disease and is costly, $30,000 per year per patient. Patients should be immunized with hepatitis B vaccine. Now that a treatment is available, screening mechanisms to detect susceptible individuals while pulmonary function is still normal must be developed.

Treatment

Bronchodilators

Aerosol therapy is the treatment modality of choice in most patients with COPD. Metered dose inhalers (MDI) are more efficacious than nebulizer therapy. Proper MDI technique includes holding the device 4 cm in front of the mouth, slowly inhaling to TLC while activating the canister, and breath holding for 10 seconds. MDIs with an extension device or valved aerosol hold-ing chamber, or nebulizer therapy is recommended for patients who are unable to perform these maneuvers. These devices allow the medication to be inhaled without the need for accurate timing between actuation and inhalation. Additionally, they can eliminate the dysphonia and laryngeal candidiasis experienced by some patients who use steroid inhalers.

Beta-Adrenergic Agonists. Airway tone is controlled by neurohumoral (cholinergic) mechanisms and sympathetic receptors. Alpha-adrenergic receptors mediate bronchoconstriction, while beta$_2$-adrenergic receptors cause smooth muscle relaxation and bronchodilation. Sympathomimetic agents stimulate these beta$_2$ receptors. Clinically useful groups include catecholamines (epinephrine, isoproterenol, isoetharine), resorcinols (metaproterenol, terbutaline), and saligenins (albuterol) (Table 3). Metaproterenol, terbutaline, and albuterol possess predominantly beta$_2$ effects, have a slower onset of action and a longer half-life than the catecholamines, and achieve peak bronchodilator effects within 60 minutes. Inhalation produces more bronchodilation and fewer systemic side effects than oral administration. Oral administration may be useful in patients unable to use inhalation devices. These selective beta$_2$ adrenergic agents have some cardiac stimulatory properties, and heart rate rises with increased plasma drug levels. The major side effect is tremor due to skeletal muscle stimulation. Some studies have shown synergy between beta$_2$ agonists and theophylline.

Theophylline. Theophylline is the most widely used bronchodilator in patients with COPD. In addition to being a smooth muscle relaxant, other potential benefits include enhanced mucociliary clearance, increased ventilatory response to hypoxemia, delayed onset and reversal of inspiratory muscle fatigue, an increase in cardiac output and right ventricular ejection fraction, and lowering of pulmonary artery pressures. Serum concentrations of 10 to 20 micrograms per ml are associated with a therapeutic response and few side effects. Multiple factors affect the clearance of the drug (Table 4).

For patients not taking theophylline, the intravenous dose of aminophylline (80 per cent theophylline solubilized by the addition of ethylenediamine) needed to achieve a blood level of approximately 10 micrograms per ml is 6 mg per kg over 20 minutes via peripheral vein. If the patient is already taking theophylline, a 3 mg per kg loading dose is administered over 20 minutes. The maintenance dose is 0.8 mg per kg per hr in smokers and 0.5 mg per kg per hr (lean body weight) in nonsmokers and critically ill patients. In patients with acute pulmonary

TABLE 3. **Adrenergic Agents**

Agent	Route	Dose	Length of Action (Hours)
Isoetharine	MDI*	340 mcg puff; 2 puffs, every 4–6 hr	1–4
(Bronkometer)	Nebulizer	1.25–5 mg; every 4–6 hrs	1–4
Metaproterenol	MDI	650 mcg/puff; 2 puffs, every 4–6 hr	1–5
(Alupent, Metaprel)	Nebulizer	15 mg; every 4–6 hr	2–6
	Oral	10–20 mg; every 6–8 hr	3–4
Terbutaline	MDI	250 mcg/puff; 2 puffs, every 4–6 hr	3–4
(Brethaire)	Subcutaneous	0.25 mg every 4–6 hr initially; may be given twice separated by 15–30 min.	
	Oral	2.5–5 mg; every 6–8 hrs	4–6
Albuterol	MDI	90 mcg/puff; 2 puffs, every 4–6 hr	3–6
(Ventolin, Proventil)	Oral	2–4 mg; every 6–8 hr	4–6
Bitolterol	MDI	370 mcg/puff; 2 puffs, every 4–6 hr	5–8
(Tornalate)			

*MDI = Metered dose inhaler.

edema or severe liver disease, 0.1 to 0.2 mg per kg per hr is recommended. To convert to an oral dose, the daily intravenous dose in milligrams is multiplied by 1.2 to give the daily oral theophylline dose. This dose is divided by two or three to determine doses to be given at 12-hour or 8-hour intervals, respectively.

Oral dosing is usually begun with a long-acting preparation, 200 mg twice a day. In smokers the dose is increased to 500 to 600 mg per 24 hours after 5 to 7 days. The serum theophylline level should be measured after 48 hours of treatment.

Theophylline side effects, including nausea, cramps, insomnia, and headaches, may be seen at therapeutic levels. At higher blood levels (15 to 35 micrograms per ml) persistent nausea and vomiting, diarrhea, tremor, sinus tachycardia, and atrial and ventricular ectopic beats have been reported. More serious reactions ($\geq$ 35 micrograms per ml) include confusion, agitation, seizures, and ventricular arrhythmias. Seizures do not usually occur unless the serum theophylline level is greater than 40 micrograms per ml.

TABLE 4. **Factors Influencing Theophylline Clearance**

Decreased Clearance	Increased Clearance
Severe (70–90%)*	
Congestive heart failure	
Liver failure	
Considerable (50–70%)	*Considerable (>50%)*
Acute critical illness	Tobacco and marijuana
Cimetidine	Phenytoin
Increased age	Young age
Moderate (25–50%)	*Moderate*
Mild cirrhosis	Charcoal-broiled beef
Erythromycin	Young age
Cor pulmonale	High-protein, low-carbohy-
Viral infection	drate diet
Oral contraception	
Allopurinol	
Phenobarbital	

*Approximate percentage of decrease of clearance.

Treatment of severe toxicity requires intensive care monitoring, cessation of drug therapy, oral charcoal administration, and, rarely, charcoal hemoperfusion.

Anticholinergic Agents. Inhibition of the parasympathetic (cholinergic) pathway with anticholinergic agents produces bronchodilation. Atropine, the prototype anticholinergic drug, although an effective bronchodilator when inhaled, is systemically absorbed, crosses the blood-brain barrier, has a long half-life, and frequently causes systemic toxicity. Dryness of the mouth and skin, tachycardia, blurred vision, precipitation of narrow-angle glaucoma, and skin flushing occur at doses of 0.5 to 2 mg. Speech problems, swallowing, micturition, and mental changes are seen at 5 mg doses. The usual effective bronchodilator dose is 1.0 to 2.5 mg, allowing little if any margin between therapeutic and toxic doses.

Ipratropium bromide, a quaternary ammonium compound available as an MDI, is poorly absorbed from the bronchial and gastrointestinal mucosa, and much of the absorbed drug is rapidly re-excreted in the gastrointestinal tract. Ipratropium does not cross into the central nervous system, has a longer half-life than atropine, and is relatively free of side effects. It does not significantly affect mucus production, viscosity, or clearance and can be used safely in patients with glaucoma and urinary bladder neck obstruction. It is a more potent bronchodilator than beta$_2$-adrenergic agonists and is rapidly becoming a first-line agent in patients with chronic bronchitis and emphysema. The dose is 2 to 4 actuations (20 micrograms per actuation) every 4 to 6 hours.

Corticosteroids. Corticosteroids increase airflow in patients with COPD and acute respiratory failure. Intravenous methylprednisolone can be used in doses from 40 to 125 mg every 6 hours. Once the patient's condition has stabilized, the drug may be tapered.

Although some patients with *severe* COPD benefit from corticosteroids, multiple clinical studies have not defined a subset of stable patients who will predictably respond. A greater than 15 per cent increase in either the FVC or the FEV_1 after a 2 to 3 week trial of oral prednisone 40 mg daily indicates a favorable response. The drug should then be tapered to the lowest effective dose. Alternative-day treatment is preferable to daily dosing. A trial of inhaled corticosteroids can be undertaken when a minimal oral dose is reached. Few steroid-dependent patients can be maintained solely on inhaled corticosteroids for any length of time.

Anti-Infective Modalities

Antibiotics. Although patients with COPD are often colonized by *Haemophilus influenzae* and *Streptococcus pneumoniae*, empiric antibiotic treatment has not proved beneficial and is controversial. However, antibiotics may shorten exacerbations of dyspnea, sputum production, and purulence. Broad-spectrum oral antibiotics such as trimethoprim-sulfamethoxazole, ampicillin, amoxicillin-clavulanate, erythromycin, and tetracycline may all be effective. Treatment of pneumonia should be based on a sputum Gram stain, since sputum cultures alone are of little value.

Antiviral Agents. Amantadine should be considered for prophylactic use in patients during influenza epidemics or as primary treatment if instituted during the first 24 to 48 hours of an influenza-like illness.

Vaccination. Patients with COPD are at greater risk than other persons both to develop and to die from infections. They should receive influenza vaccination yearly and the 23-valent pneumococcal vaccine once. It is unclear whether the pneumococcal vaccine is beneficial, as antibody titers decrease rapidly and pneumonia deaths are generally not due to *Streptococcus pneumoniae*.

Clearance of Tracheal Bronchial Secretions

Patient with chronic bronchitis, bronchiectasis, and cystic fibrosis are prone to increased mucus production. Excessive sputum production increases dyspnea, airway resistance, and discomfort. Mucus plugging may worsen $\dot{V}/\dot{Q}$ relationships, causing hypoxemia.

Mechanical removal, enhancing ciliary motility, and physically altering the mucus are all helpful in controlling secretions.

Chest physiotherapy aids in removal of secretions, particularly in hospitalized patients with acute infections, but is not helpful in stable COPD outpatients producing less than 30 ml of sputum in 24 hours. Beta agonists and theoph-

ylline enhance ciliary motility and may improve mucus clearance.

Mucus viscosity may be lowered by increasing the water content of sputum. However, moderate dehydration or overhydration has no significant effect on sputum volume or pulmonary function. Numerous agents, including guaifenesin, ammonium chloride, and ipecac, decrease mucus production, possibly through vagal mechanisms. Iodides (e.g., Organidin) are purported to improve tracheobronchial clearance in some patients.

Mucolytic agents, such as *N*-acetylcysteine (Mucomyst) if placed directly on a mucus plug (such as during bronchoscopy), liquefy thick sputum by disrupting sulfide bonds. Since it is probably ineffective in nebulized form and is associated with bronchospasm, *N*-acetylcysteine should be used judiciously and not as a routine measure. Corticosteroids decrease sputum production in patients with chronic bronchitis, but are not first-line agents. Respiratory infection, if present, is treated as discussed above. Cessation of smoking is imperative.

Oxygen Therapy

Both the Medical Research Council (MRC) Study and the Nocturnal Oxygen Therapy Trial (NOTT) showed that supplemental oxygen improves survival in COPD patients with hypoxemia, pulmonary hypertension, and cor pulmonale. In the NOTT study, survival was greater in patients using oxygen more than 19 hours per day than in those using it less than 19 hours per day. Correcting hypoxemia with supplemental oxygen can also reverse or halt progression of pulmonary hypertension and erythrocytosis. Patients who respond to oxygen by decreasing their pulmonary artery pressures have a better survival than patients who do not respond to oxygen. The 3-year mortality rate is 30 per cent in responders versus 92 per cent in nonresponders.

COPD patients who are candidates for long-term oxygen therapy should have optimal medical treatment and be at baseline with stable oxygenation for 4 weeks. A PaO_2 less than 55 torr or an O_2 saturation (SaO_2) less than 85 per cent must be demonstrated to verify need. Patients with a PaO_2 between 56 and 59 torr or an SaO_2 of 86 to 89 per cent are candidates for oxygen therapy if polycythemia and/or cor pulmonale is also present.

In patients without significant resting daytime hypoxemia, desaturation may occur with exercise and/or sleep. In one fourth of COPD patients with awake PaO_2 greater than 60 torr, desaturation occurs at night. Arterial blood gases and/or oxygen saturations measured during exercise or sleep determine need for oxygen therapy. In general, the lower the awake Pa_{O_2} the more likely nocturnal desaturation is to occur. To avoid a precipitous rise in arterial carbon dioxide (Pa_{CO_2}), oxygen must be carefully prescribed.

Patients should discontinue smoking prior to initiation of long-term continuous oxygen. Oxygen-conserving devices prolong the life of portable tanks. Oxygen wastage can be lessened by storing oxygen in reservoirs during expiration or delivering oxygen only during inspiration. A recent development in which oxygen is delivered directly into the trachea (transtracheal oxygenation) bypasses upper-airway dead space and decreases the flow of oxygen needed. This method is more comfortable for the patient and can adequately oxygenate some patients who cannot be oxygenated by nasal cannula or mask.

Pulmonary Rehabilitation

Patients with any limitation from COPD are candidates for inclusion in a pulmonary rehabilitation program. A well-coordinated program should involve a physician; a nurse; respiratory, physical, and occupational therapists; and a professional with skills in psychosocial and vocational rehabilitation. Goals include an increase in exercise endurance and a decrease in the number of days hospitalized. Although pulmonary function does not improve with rehabilitation, there is a trend toward improved survival.

Exercise. Six weeks of exercise training pedaling a stationary bicycle or walking on a treadmill for 30 minutes three times a week is an integral part of a rehabilitation program. Training permits the COPD patient to perform the same amount of exercise at a lower heart rate, minute ventilation, and oxygen consumption. In addition, appetite and sleep are improved, endurance is increased, and dyspnea is lessened.

Respiratory muscle training using inspiratory resistance breathing may have beneficial physiologic effects similar to overall exercise conditioning. However, this technique must be used with caution to avoid respiratory muscle fatigue.

Miscellaneous Treatment

Drugs

VASODILATORS. Selected individuals with cor pulmonale may benefit from vasodilators, which may reduce pulmonary artery pressures and increase cardiac output. However, vasodilators may worsen $\dot{V}/\dot{Q}$ matching and cause hypoxemia. The best therapy for pulmonary hypertension is the administration of supplemental oxygen.

DIURETICS. Diuretics should be used only in patients with volume overload, such as may be present with left ventricular failure. In cor pulmonale, aggressive preload reduction may reduce

TABLE 5. **Indications for Hospitalization of the Patient with COPD**

Exacerbation of symptoms (e.g., dyspnea, wheezing, cough) that are not responding to outpatient care
Acute respiratory failure characterized by hypercapnia with worsening acidosis, or worsening hypoxemia
Pneumonia
Acute right heart failure with worsening hypoxemia or decreasing exercise capacity
Surgery requiring general anesthesia
Pulmonary invasive diagnostic procedures (i.e., bronchoscopy, transbronchial biopsy, or transthoracic needle aspiration)

cardiac output. Diuretic-induced metabolic alkalosis can exacerbate CO_2 retention. A carbonic anhydrase inhibitor, such as acetazolamide, is a rational alternative to loop diuretics, if diuresis is desired in patients with a metabolic alkalosis.

RESPIRATORY STIMULANTS. Respiratory stimulants, such as progesterone or doxapram, are contraindicated in COPD patients, as the etiology of CO_2 retention is not central hypoventilation but $\dot{V}/\dot{Q}$ mismatch and increased dead space. Almitrine may be an exception to this rule but is not presently available in the United States. Almitrine increases the ventilatory response to hypoxemia and hypercapnia, and improves $\dot{V}/\dot{Q}$ matching by enhancing hypoxic pulmonary vasoconstriction. Significant increases in Pa_{O_2} have been reported, but potential side effects have delayed release of this drug in this country.

DIGOXIN. Cardiac glycosides such as digoxin do not alter the course of cor pulmonale or right ventricular failure and have no place in the treatment of COPD.

Mechanical Ventilation. Ideally the physician should discuss the possibility of long-term mechanical ventilation with the patient and family to ascertain whether or not this aggressive measure should be undertaken if and when circumstances arise. Some COPD patients with chronic respiratory failure will require mechanical ventilation 24 hours per day. Others will require ventilation only at night to allow the respiratory muscles to rest. Positive or negative ventilation may be used. Long-term ventilator beds are available in a variety of centers—skilled nursing homes, chronic care facilities, and hospitals. Home ventilation is another alternative for selected patients with stable disease and an adequate support system, that is, a coordinated health care team and a competent, caring family. Requirements for home ventilation include clinical and psychologic stability, fractional inspired oxygen (FI_{O_2}) of 0.40 or less, a tracheostomy, and enough manpower to give and maintain adequate care.

Nutrition. Proper nutrition is an important,

often overlooked, facet in the treatment of the COPD patient. Mortality is markedly increased in patients who weigh 10 per cent less than ideal body weight, regardless of the FEV_1 value. These patients tend to eat poorly and are hypermetabolic, possibly from expending excess calories for breathing. They may require up to 15 to 30 per cent more calories than are calculated for maintenance. There is some evidence that the type of calories (i.e., carbohydrate versus fat) may affect respiratory function. Excessive carbohydrates increase CO_2 production and may aggravate CO_2 retention. Pulmocare, a nutritional supplement with 28 per cent carbohydrates and 55 per cent fat, is designed to avoid this problem. Usually the carbohydrate: fat ratio is unimportant as long as the patient receives adequate calories. Caloric supplementation may improve respiratory muscle strength and exercise endurance.

Hospitalization and Elective Surgery. Indications for hospitalization are listed in Table 5. Patients should discontinue smoking for at least 3 to 4 weeks prior to elective or nonemergent surgery. Respiratory infections should be treated with a course of antibiotics. Maximal bronchodilator therapy is indicated. Baseline spirometry is helpful in determining risk of surgery, as the FEV_1 will be affected by certain procedures. Thoracic and abdominal procedures lead to the greatest postoperative impairment in pulmonary function and may cause the FEV_1 to decrease by 50 per cent. Patients with a baseline FEV_1 less than 2 liters per second may require short-term mechanical ventilation postoperatively. Early ambulation, coughing, chest physiotherapy, and incentive spirometry may prevent complications. Pain control helps prevent splinting and atelectasis. Narcotic-induced CO_2 retention should be anticipated.

CARCINOMA OF THE LUNG

method of
JACOB D. BITRAN, M.D.
Pritzker School of Medicine
Michael Reese Hospital & Medical Center
Chicago, Illinois

Last year carcinoma of the lung accounted for 125,000 cancer-related deaths in the United States. It is the leading cause of cancer-related deaths in both men and women. While the incidence of lung cancer has plateaued in men, it continues to increase steadily in women. Lung cancer can be prevented; all that it takes is for people to *stop smoking* cigarettes. As physicians, we must preach the risks of smoking cigarettes and the benefits of stopping, and continue to

nag and cajole smokers into quitting. The most common histologic type of lung cancer is squamous cell carcinoma, which accounts for approximately 35 per cent of all lung cancers; adenocarcinoma accounts for 25 to 30 per cent; small cell carcinoma accounts for 25 per cent, and large cell carcinoma accounts for the remaining 10 per cent. The incidence of adenocarcinoma has been steadily increasing over the past 10 years.

Diagnostic Methods and Staging of Lung Cancer

The chest radiograph is the cornerstone of detection of lung cancer; however, chest radiography when used as a screening procedure in asymptomatic cigarette smokers has not significantly lowered the death rate from lung cancer as compared with the rate in unscreened populations. If a suspicious lesion is found on chest radiography, obtaining old chest radiographs for comparative purposes is essential. If a lesion has been stable for 2 years, further work-up is not necessary. New lesions obviously need to be investigated.

A thorough history and physical examination are central to the investigation of a pulmonary nodule or hilar mass. Particular attention should be paid to the lymph nodal exam (cervical or supraclavicular lymph nodal involvement), the chest exam (localized rales or rhonchi, absence of breath sounds), the abdominal exam (organomegaly), and the neurologic exam. The presence of lymphadenopathy or organomegaly will provide staging information and indicate an area for biopsy so that a histologic diagnosis can be rendered. Sputum cytology examination and bronchoscopy (for centrally located lesions) are useful noninvasive procedures in making a histologic diagnosis. A transthoracic ("skinny") needle aspiration can yield a cytologic diagnosis for peripherally located lesions.

Computed tomography (CT) of the chest to the level of the adrenals should be performed while the physician attempts to make a histologic diagnosis of lung cancer. The CT scan of the chest can confirm the presence and extent of a lung mass suspected on chest radiography, confirm or exclude the presence of additional pulmonary nodules, and demonstrate the presence of enlarged mediastinal or hilar lymph nodes likely to contain metastases. A CT scan of the chest to the level of the adrenals can also detect intra-abdominal metastases to the liver or adrenal glands. Magnetic resonance imaging (MRI) of the chest does not yield additional information beyond that revealed by chest CT scans.

Once a histologic diagnosis of lung cancer has been made, further clinical staging is based on symptoms and signs. A complaint of bone pain or back pain mandates a technetium-99m bone scan. If the patient complains of a headache or has any neurologic symptoms or signs, an MRI scan or CT scan of the brain should be obtained. With the completion of the aforementioned staging procedures, patients are placed into the clinical stage categories shown in Table 1.

Patients with clinical Stage IIIB or IV have incurable lung cancer and require no further staging procedures, whereas patients with clinical Stages I to IIIA adenocarcinoma, large cell carcinoma, or squamous

TABLE 1. **International Staging for Lung Cancer**

TNM

Tumor size (T)

TX = Occult carcinoma (cytologically positive; bronchoscopically and radiographically nondetectable)

T1 = Tumor 3 cm or less surrounded by lung or visceral pleura

T2 = Tumor greater than 3 cm

T3 = Tumor of any size with direct extension into chest wall; or with 2 cm of the carina, or associated with atelectasis or obstructive pneumonia of the entire lung

T4 = Tumor of any size invading into the mediastinal structures or vertebral body, or presence of malignant pleural effusion

Nodal Status (N)

N0 = No hilar or mediastinal nodal involvement

N1 = Ipsilateral hilar nodal involvement

N2 = Ipsilateral mediastinal nodal or subcarinal nodal involvement

N3 = Contralateral hilar or mediastinal nodal involvement, supraclavicular nodal involvement (ipsilateral or contralateral)

Metastases (M)

M0 = No distant metastases

M1 = Distant visceral metastases present

Stage

Occult carcinoma	TXN0M0
Stage I	T1–2N0M0
Stage II	T1–2N1M0
Stage IIIA	T3N0–1M0
	T1–3N2M0
Stage IIIB	T4N1–3M0
	T1–3N3M0
Stage IV	Any T Any N M1

Adapted from Mountain CF: Chest (Suppl) *89*:2255, 1986.

cell carcinoma have potentially resectable and thus curable lung cancer and require pathologic staging. Patients with small cell lung cancer of any stage (with the exception of Stage I) are treated with chemotherapy (see section on Small Cell Lung Cancer).

Pathologic Staging. Fiberoptic bronchoscopy is an accurate and safe technique for rendering a definitive diagnosis of lung cancer. It provides direct visualization of the trachea and bronchial tree and can be used for brush biopsy of a centrally located tumor. The carina can be inspected and sampled by biopsy for staging purposes.

Clinical evaluation of the mediastinum is provided by the CT scan of the chest. The CT scan yields accurate information regarding size and location of abnormal mediastinal lymph nodes. Unfortunately, although enlarged mediastinal nodes (>2 cm) are likely to contain tumor metastases and normal-sized nodes (<1.0 cm) usually are uninvolved, exceptions to this rule occur with sufficient frequency that biopsy is usually required. Using 1 cm as the upper limit for "negative nodes" and 2 cm as the lower limit for "positive nodes," one can obtain a high degree of predictive accuracy from chest CT scans, 86 per cent; however, this is achieved at the expense of relegating a portion of patients into an intermediate category (nodes 1 to 2 cm in size).

Mediastinoscopy or a parasternal mediastinal exploration provides an opportunity to take tissue for biopsy directly from mediastinal lymph nodes and to determine whether the nodes are involved or uninvolved by metastatic lung cancer. Mediastinoscopy is a surgical procedure performed with the patient under general anesthesia. A mediastinoscope, a hollow, rigid instrument, is introduced through a small incision in the superpsternal notch and advanced along the pretracheal plane to the level of the carina. Enlarged lymph nodes can be visualized and sampled for biopsy. On the right side the upper margin of the hilum may be reached, whereas on the left side the aortic arch prevents access to the hilum. Contraindications to mediastinoscopy include superior vena caval obstruction, mediastinal surgery, and previous radiotherapy.

A limited parasternal mediastinoscopy can be performed for pathologic or diagnostic staging. This procedure provides access to areas of the mediastinum that are beyond the mediastinoscope, particularly the left hilum and the aortopulmonary window.

The pathologic staging procedures outlined above are necessary in patients with clinical Stage I to IIIA adenocarcinoma, squamous cell carcinoma, and large cell lung cancer (non–small cell lung cancer). With completion of these studies, the physician can then decide whether the patient is a candidate for a thoracotomy and an attempt at a curative resection.

Therapeutic Approaches

Surgical resection is the treatment of choice in patients with non–small cell lung cancer (NSCLC) Stage I to IIIA. Preoperative elevations should include the aforementioned clinical and pathologic staging studies and pulmonary function tests. Specific attention should be given to the preoperative FEV_1, as the postresection FEV_1 should be at least 0.5 to 0.8 liter. If the planned resection is apt to reduce the FEV_1 to below 0.5 liter, the patient should have quantitative pulmonary ventilation and perfusion lung scans to assess the contribution of that portion of the lung to be resected to the overall pulmonary function. In smokers and patients with chronic obstructive airway disease who have marginally resectable lesions, intensive preoperative respiratory therapy may dramatically improve pulmonary function to permit lung resection. Contraindications to surgical resection of the lung include FEV_1 of less than 0.5 liter postresection and the presence of cardiac disease and an ejection fraction of less than 0.40. Chronologic age is not a contraindication to lung resection. At the time of thoracotomy, particular attention is paid to the mediastinal and hilar lymph nodes. If there is extensive involvement of the mediastinal lymph nodes or parietal pleura, the patient has unresectable disease and requires alternative therapy. If there is hilar or limited mediastinal nodal involvement (microscopic involvement of low paratracheal nodes) on frozen section, a pneumonectomy is advisable. Those patients with limited mediastinal involvement should have mediastinal dissection. A lobectomy is the procedure of choice for patients with no hilar involvement (on frozen section) if the tumor is small (less than 4 cm) or peripheral. A pneumonectomy is the procedure of choice for a central tumor or for tumors greater than 4 cm. The cure rate for patients with unresectable lung cancer is shown in Table 2.

Adjuvant Therapies. Radiotherapy has been utilized as an adjuvant therapy in Stage II and III NSCLC; however, the only subset of patients in whom preoperative radiotherapy (30 Gy/10 fractions) appears indicated are those with T3 lesions of the upper lobe (superior sulcus tumors or Pancoast tumors). The use of radiotherapy in other subsets of Stage II and III patients with NSCLC confers no benefit.

Adjuvant chemotherapy with cyclophosphamide, Adriamycin (doxorubicin), and Platinol (cisplatin) (CAP) has been tested in a prospective randomized clinical trial of patients with Stage II and III adenocarcinoma and large cell lung cancer by the Lung Cancer Study Group (LCSG). The use of adjuvant CAP chemotherapy led to a statistically significant survival advantage at 1 and 2 years (p = 0.013); however, beyond the first 24 months, the survival curves for the CAP-treated patients and controls converged. Thus, the use of CAP chemotherapy delayed the onset of recurrent disease, but did not eradicate it. Nonetheless, the LCSG study now provides momentum for additional trials employing other chemotherapeutic combinations. The use of preoperative adjuvant chemotherapy in Stage IIIA patients is under investigation. There is no role for adjuvant chemotherapy in Stage I NSCLC.

Palliative Therapies. Standard therapy in patients with advanced NSCLC (Stage IIIB and IV) has consisted of radiotherapy for the palliation of respiratory symptoms (hemoptysis, obstructive pneumonia) or pain. The radiotherapeutic approach is 55 to 60 Gy, in 20 cGy fractions, to a portal that includes the primary lung lesion and the ipsilateral hilus and mediastinum. The use of CT scans in radiotherapy treatment planning is useful. A very small subset of Stage IIIB and inoperable Stage IIIA cancers may be cured with radiotherapy; at best, 10 to 15 per cent of *good performance status* patients with Stage IIIA and IIIB NSCLC will be alive at 5 years. The median survival for patients with Stage IIIA and IIIB NSCLC is 10 to 11 months. Given this poor cure rate, clinical trials have focused on combined modality approaches (chemotherapy and radiotherapy) in patients with inoperable Stage IIIA and IIIB NSCLC. To date, no published comparative trial has shown the superiority of chemotherapy and radiotherapy over radiotherapy alone.

The role of chemotherapy in the treatment of patients with Stage IV NSCLC has been extremely controversial. There has been little evidence that chemotherapy impacts on the natural history of Stage IV NSCLC. Many single agents and combinations have been tested over the past 10 to 15 years. The most important prognostic factor is the performance status of the patient. Performance status (graded on a 0 to 100 scale or a 0 to 4 scale), denotes the ability of patients to carry out daily activities (100 per cent or 0, implying a normally functioning individual; 50 per cent or 2, an individual who spends more than 50 per cent of the time in bed; 10 per cent or 4, a bedridden patient). Most recently, a large Canadian clinical trial has compared supportive care alone with two types of combination chemotherapy, CAP or vindesine and Platinol (V-P), in the treatment of patients with Stage IV NSCLC. The patients randomly assigned to either chemotherapy regimen had a longer median survival than those receiving only supportive care. The patients assigned to receive V-P treatment had a statistically significant longer survival than those who received only supportive care, 22 weeks versus 10 weeks, respectively. While these results are far from satisfactory, they represent a starting point for further comparative trials with chemotherapy in patients with Stage IV NSCLC. Future chemotherapy trials in these patients should be restricted to patients with good performance status (PS 0, 1, 2). Patients with a poor performance status (PS 3, 4) never derive any benefit from chemotherapy and experience only the toxic side effects.

Small Cell Lung Cancer

Small cell lung cancer (SCLC) is a distinct clinicopathologic entity. SCLC arises from basal reserve cells that have neuroendocrine proper-

TABLE 2. **5-Year Disease-Free Survival Rates for Surgical Resection in Patients with Non–Small Cell Lung Cancer**

Stage		5 Years Disease-Free (%)
I	T1N0M0	70–85
	T2N0M0	55–65
II	T1N1M0	30–50
	T1N2M0	25–30
IIIA	T3N0M0	25–35
	T3N1M0	15–20
	T1–2N2M0	9–24
	T3N2	0–5

ties, and thus SCLC has distinct histologic and biologic characteristics. The histologic features detectable by electron microscopy are the presence of dense core neurosecretory granules. The biologic features of SCLC include the presence of: L-dopa decarboxylase (a key amine-handling enzyme), high levels of neuron-specific enolase (a glycolytic isoenzyme characteristic of the endocrine system), high levels of creatine kinase brain isoenzyme, and the production of peptide hormones (ACTH, arginine vasopressin, oxytocin, calcitonin, beta-endorphin, lipotropin). A peptide immunologically related to the amphibian neuropeptide bombesin or its mammalian homologue gastrin-releasing peptide is present in almost all SCLC tumors. SCLC has at least two distinct genetic abnormalities: amplification of the members of the myc gene family of proto-oncogenes (C-myc, N-myc, L-myc) and the loss of the short arm of chromosome No. 3 (3p14–p23). The 3p deletion is a consistent and specific abnormality for small cell lung cancer.

Clinically, SCLC is usually a hilar or central lesion, has a rapid growth rate, and metastasizes widely. SCLC is a rapidly progressive carcinoma if untreated. The median survival of untreated patients is 3 to 4 months. Rarely, SCLC may present as a peripheral lesion (coin lesion) on chest radiography.

Once a histologic or cytologic diagnosis of SCLC is made, the stage of the disease is determined (see Diagnostic Methods and Staging). In addition to the routine clinical and pathologic staging procedures, bone marrow aspiration and core biopsy are performed in patients with SCLC, as it frequently metastasizes to the bone marrow (15 to 20 per cent incidence). Unlike the staging system used for NSCLC, patients with SCLC are placed into two staging categories, "limited stage" (disease confined to the hemithorax and supraclavicular nodal region) and "extensive stage" (disease beyond the hemithorax and supraclavicular nodal regions). While the stage of patients with SCLC does not alter the therapeutic approach, again it carries prognostic information.

The treatment of patients with small cell lung cancer, either limited or extensive stage, is combination chemotherapy. The most widely used chemotherapeutic regimens are cyclophosphamide, Adriamycin, and vinblastine; cyclophosphamide, Adriamycin, and etoposide; and etoposide and Platinol. With the use of these chemotherapeutic regimens, objective responses (remissions) are expected in 80 to 100 per cent of patients with limited disease and 50 to 60 per cent with extensive disease. Recent prospective randomized clinical trials have shown a beneficial effect of chest radiotherapy when combined with chemotherapy in the treatment of patients with limited stage SCLC as compared with chemotherapy alone. A combined modality approach is indicated for patients with limited stage SCLC. The median survival that can be anticipated for patients with limited stage SCLC is 18 to 22 months, and at 2 to 3 years 20 to 30 per cent are alive and disease-free; however, the 5-year survival rate for limited stage SCLC patients is only 10 per cent. Late recurrences of SCLC and second non–small cell primary lung cancers are increasingly being reported in 2-year survivors of limited stage SCLC. The use of chest radiotherapy to the lung primary tumor confers no survival benefit in patients with extensive disease SCLC and is not warranted. The median survival for patients with extensive SCLC treated with combination chemotherapy is 9 to 12 months. For patients with limited or extensive SCLC who achieve a complete response (complete remission), the use of prophylactic cranial irradiation (20 Gy/10 fractions) is indicated; prophylactic cranial irradiation decreases the morbidity and mortality of CNS relapse.

If a patient with SCLC presents with a peripheral lesion (a coin lesion), evaluation of the mediastinal region is carried out, since it will alter therapy. If no mediastinal involvement is found, resection of the lung is carried out similar to the approach used in patients with NSCLC. Patients with Stage I SCLC can be cured surgically.

There are a number of areas being explored at the current time in the management of patients with SCLC; however, these areas of investigation are experimental. Surgical resection after combination chemotherapy in patients with limited SCLC is being examined by some groups. Use of interferons as "cytostatic" agents after combination chemotherapy is currently under investigation. Autologous bone marrow transplantation following conventional chemotherapy or chemoradiotherapy is also under investigation.

COCCIDIOIDOMYCOSIS

method of
EDUARDO G. ARATHOON, M.D.
Francisco Marroquin University
Guatemala City, Guatemala

Coccidioidomycosis is an infection caused by the dimorphic fungus *Coccidioides immitis*. It is endemic in certain areas of North, Central, and South America, where the organism is harbored in soil foci. Skin test surveys suggest 100,000 new cases annually in the United States, where it is endemic in certain areas of

California, Arizona, New Mexico, Texas, Nevada, and Utah.

Infection usually results from inhalation of arthroconidia. In the host tissue the fungus grows as endosporulating structures called spherules. The incubation time from exposure is usually 1 to 3 weeks. The initial infection is asymptomatic or inconspicuous in approximately 60 per cent of persons, as detected by coccidioidin skin test surveys. Of the 40 per cent with symptoms, most develop a benign disease, though 5 to 10 per cent may be left with pulmonary sequelae (e.g., cavity or granuloma) as a result of a subacute, self-limited pneumonia. In a few patients pulmonary involvement may progress to chronic lung disease, and in about 0.5 per cent disseminated (extrapulmonary) coccidioidomycosis develops. The most common sites of dissemination are skin, bones, joints, and meninges, but almost any organ in the body can be affected. Pregnancy and deficiencies of cell-mediated immunity have been found to predispose to dissemination.

The diagnosis of coccidioidomycosis is confirmed by isolating *C. immitis* or microscopically identifying spherules from respiratory secretions, urine, cerebrospinal fluid, or tissue specimens. Serology testing, when performed by laboratories familiar with detecting coccidioidal antibodies, is highly specific and useful in the diagnosis and management of coccidioidomycosis.

Treatment

Different management strategies are recommended for individuals on the basis of their immunologic status, underlying diseases, and the location and severity of their infections.

Amphotericin B. Amphotericin B (Fungizone) has been the standard drug of therapy for nearly 3 decades. Its mechanism of action involves binding to ergosterol, which results in enhanced permeability of the fungal cell membrane, with loss of critical intracellular constituents. The drug is administered intravenously, and clearance from tissue is slow. Because it is extremely protein bound, relatively little appears in urine and cerebrospinal fluid. A major problem of amphotericin B is its high toxicity. Common side effects include phlebitis, fever, chills, nausea, vomiting, hypokalemia, renal tubular acidosis, hypomagnesemia, shock, and anemia. Transient azotemia is frequent during therapy. Permanent renal impairment has been reported in some patients who received a total of 3 grams or more. Other less common side effects are anaphylactic reactions, arrhythmias, coagulopathy, hemorrhagic enteritis, tinnitus, vertigo, pruritus, seizures, neuropathy, leukopenia, and thrombocytopenia. To monitor some of these side effects, the following laboratory analyses should be performed on a weekly basis during therapy: serum creatinine concentration tests, hemograms with leukocyte, erythrocyte, and platelet count, and measurements of potassium and other electrolytes. Modifiers can reduce some of the symptoms associated with the administration of amphotericin B, such as nausea, chills, and fever. These modifiers include antipyretics, antihistamines given 30 minutes before the infusion, and low-dose steroids (e.g., 20 mg of hydrocortisone succinate) mixed with the infusion.

Ketoconazole. Ketoconazole (Nizoral) is an oral imidazole. Its intestinal absorption is enhanced by an acid gastric pH, and achlorhydria may result in lower serum levels. The usual dose is 400 mg per day given on an empty stomach. At this dose nausea and vomiting, the most common side effects, are seen in approximately 20 per cent of patients, but in only 5 per cent are they severe enough to lead to discontinuation of the drug. Mild elevations of liver enzymes are frequent, but clinical hepatitis is rare. With larger doses, ketoconazole can produce gynecomastia and azoospermia by a reversible blockage of testosterone production, which can be treated with testosterone replacement. Relapse rates may be as high as 25 per cent, even after 12 months of therapy.

Selection of Antifungal Drugs. Although amphotericin B and ketoconazole are both effective in the treatment of coccidioidomycosis, they have never been compared in a clinical trial. As a general rule, amphotericin B should be used in patients who are acutely ill with fulminant disease. Ketoconazole, on the other hand, is preferred for indolent infections because of its ease of administration and relative safety.

Therapy of Specific Clinical Manifestations

Primary Pulmonary Coccidioidomycosis. Although most patients with symptomatic primary infections recover without therapy, a patient with severe primary infection should receive chemotherapy. Because of the possibility of incipient or occult dissemination, patients with rising titers of coccidioidal antibodies should be treated. Other criteria used to determine the need for treatment are symptoms lasting more than 6 weeks; prostration; extensive, enlarging, or persistent pulmonary involvement; continued elevation of the precipitins; negative skin test; infancy; debilitation; pregnancy; concurrent diseases affected by coccidioidal infection; and immune impairment. A short course of amphotericin B (total dose, 0.5 to 1 grams) has been used for such patients. Clinical trials have not yet established that oral drugs such as ketoconazole are efficacious for the therapy of primary coccidioidomycosis.

Pulmonary Nodules. Pulmonary nodules are formed when a coccidioidal pneumonia undergoes a characteristic evolution from the typical soft infiltrate to a spherical, dense nodule (coccidioidoma) without surrounding infiltration. They tend to occur in the midlung field, within 5 cm of the hilum; they vary from 1 to 4 cm in diameter. Because it is impossible to distinguish them from malignancies by skin testing alone, a nodule resection is necessary to establish the diagnosis. No drug therapy is necessary before or after resection.

Pulmonary Cavities. The pneumonic process in primary coccidioidal infection may produce necrosis with pulmonary cavitation. Coccidioidal cavities are benign, and from a radiographic point of view, they usually are thin-walled, and measure 2 to 4 cm in diameter. Ninety per cent of cavities are single, and 70 per cent are in the upper lung fields. If the cavities are small and the patient is asymptomatic, they require no treatment, and the majority close within 2 years of their detection. Surgical removal of the cavity is indicated if there is recurrent or severe hemoptysis, an enlarging cavity despite chemotherapy, or intrapleural rupture. Controversial indications for surgery include subpleural locations (because of danger of rupture), a cavity with a symptomatic mycetoma, persistent positive sputum culture for *C. immitis*, secondary infection of a previous cavity, and recurrent disease. Chemotherapy with amphotericin B (total dose, 500 to 1000 mg) or ketoconazole is indicated if the cavity has thick walls, produces symptoms, or enlarges rapidly. Amphotericin B (total dose, 500 mg) is indicated before and after resection of a coccidioidal cavity to avoid dissemination. Such procedures carry no assurance of cure.

Chronic Pulmonary Coccidioidomycosis. In some patients the acute pneumonia progresses to chronic pulmonary disease, usually with cavitary lesions as part of the syndrome. In these patients the disease may wax and wane over many years; it may never be cured. Treatment limits the symptoms of exacerbations. Amphotericin B (total dose, 500 to 1000 mg) or a course of ketoconazole generally results in improvement of constitutional symptoms (malaise, sputum production, weight loss, and low-grade fevers), and the sputum may become negative for *C. immitis*. Relapses have been frequent when either drug has been discontinued.

Miliary Coccidioidomycosis. This presentation, which is seen most frequently in immunosuppressed patients, is common in patients with acquired immunodeficiency syndrome (AIDS). Because meningitis can go undetected in these patients, spinal fluid analysis is recommended early in the disease. Treatment with amphotericin B should be rapidly increased to a dose of approximately 0.4 mg per kg per day.

Disseminated Coccidioidomycosis. Once the disease has disseminated outside the lungs, chemotherapy is always indicated. Except for meningeal and miliary coccidioidomycosis, disseminated infections are often chronic. Patients can be appropriately treated as outpatients with oral drugs such as ketoconazole. If the patient improves, oral therapy should be given for a minimum of 1 year, at which time the drug can be discontinued if no further improvement has occurred in the previous 6 months. If relapse occurs, the drug can be reinstituted for an indefinite period of time. If amphotericin B is necessary, a total dose of 1.0 to 3.0 grams may be administered, depending on the patient's response. A good response to therapy is evidenced by negative fungal cultures, decrease in antibody titers, and return of skin test reactivity.

Coccidioidal Meningitis. Because neither amphotericin B nor ketoconazole penetrates into the cerebrospinal fluid, patients are treated with intrathecal amphotericin B. Miconazole (Monistat I.V.) has been reported to be an effective alternative when amphotericin B cannot be used.

Investigational Drugs. Itraconazole, an oral triazole, is effective for the treatment of coccidioidomycosis. Its efficacy is at least comparable to that of ketoconazole, and it is less toxic.

Fluconazole has the potential to be a useful drug in the treatment of coccidioidal meningitis, because of the significant levels found in cerebrospinal fluid. Efficacy studies are still under way.

HISTOPLASMOSIS

method of
ROBERT H. ALFORD, M.D.
Nashville, Tennessee

Clinical Manifestations

Initial Infection. Initial infections caused by *Histoplasma capsulatum*, although usually asymptomatic, may cause a variety of clinical manifestations. Recognized infections may cause a flu-like illness. Areas of patchy, granulomatous pneumonitis sometimes develop with associated regional hilar or paratracheal adenopathy that subsequently calcifies. Self-limited dissemination is the rule, judging from the high prevalence of healed *Histoplasma* granulomas in spleens from the endemic area examined at autopsy. Heavy inocula can produce multiple areas of pneumonitis that sometimes eventually calcify, resulting in classic "buckshot" calcification radiographically. After a 10- to 18-day incubation period, very large inocula can cause acute pulmonary illness with fever, nonproductive cough, chest pain, dyspnea, and infrequently pulmonary insufficiency with features of adult respiratory distress syndrome (ARDS). Most symptomatic cases are self-limited, not requiring antifungal chemotherapy. However, extremely heavy inocula, immunologic immaturity (infants), or immunologic incompetence (e.g., AIDS) may permit rapidly progressive primary infection with dissemination and a fatal outcome without therapy.

Complications of histoplasmosis that result from inflammatory or desmoplastic reactions to infection include pericarditis, sclerosing mediastinitis, and pulmonary histoplasmomas. Pericarditis usually occurs in young, immunocompetent persons following a bout of acute pulmonary infection. Apparently a hypersensitivity-mediated response to infectious antigen, it is usually self-limited but may produce severe pain and rarely tamponade.

Reinfection. Reinfection with *Histoplasma* causes disease modified by persisting antifungal immunity. Illness resembling initial infection may result after a shorter incubation period of 7 to 10 days. Heavy inocula still cause pneumonitis that is usually self-limited over days to weeks, having an acute onset of nonproductive cough, fever, malaise, dyspnea, and, rarely, impaired oxygen diffusion. Large inocula in the fully immune person may produce patchy pneumonitis with less hilar adenopathy than in initial infections, occasionally with small, discrete granulomatous foci that may give a miliary appearance on x-ray.

Progressive Histoplasmosis. Progressive histoplasmosis is usually chronic, except as noted above. Chronic pulmonary histoplasmosis, the most frequently encountered symptomatic manifestation, uncommonly develops almost exclusively in middle-aged white men with underlying chronic obstructive pulmonary disease with bullous changes. Episodes of necrotizing segmental or lobar (usually upper) granulomatous pneumonitis having a tendency to cavity formation, contraction, fibrosis, and compensatory emphysema tend to recur often in subjacent pulmonary segments. Rarely, chronic progressive disseminated histoplasmosis evolves in adults of either sex and any race who have no immune disorder. It presents with fever, weakness, weight loss, hepatosplenomegaly, leukopenia, mucous membrane ulceration involving the oropharynx, tongue, or larynx; and adrenal insufficiency that eventually evolves in up to 50 per cent of patients.

Treatment

Amphotericin B. Amphotericin B (Fungizone, intravenous) has long been the standard agent used for histoplasmosis needing therapy.

PATIENT SELECTION AND DOSAGE. Total amphotericin B dosage varies according to likelihood of relapse. Forms of histoplasmosis requiring therapy and suggested dosages are as follows:

1. Serious acute pulmonary disease on initial infection or reinfection, especially when symptomatic beyond 2 weeks or associated with progressive diffusion abnormalities, requires 500 mg of amphotericin B over 2 to 3 weeks.

2. Significant exacerbations of chronic pulmonary histoplasmosis should be treated with 1.5 to 2.0 grams of amphotericin B over a period of 2 months.

3. Acute or chronic disseminated infection requires 2.0 to 3.0 grams of amphotericin B over 2 to 3 months.

4. *Histoplasma* endocarditis or meningitis should be treated with 3.0 to 4.0 grams of amphotericin B.

TOXICITY. Amphotericin B, a toxic colloidal polyene, is solubilized with sodium desoxycholate for intravenous injection. Its common toxicities are local phlebitis and systemic reactions including chills, fever, aching, nausea or vomiting, reversible renal toxicity, hypokalemia, and anemia. Infrequently, anaphylaxis, marrow suppression, and cardiovascular or hepatic toxicity develop.

The drug is provided in vials containing 50 mg. Dilutions are made only in 5 per cent dextrose in water because sodium chloride and various other salts cause precipitation of the colloidal suspension. The final volume for infusion is usually 500 to 1000 ml but can be limited to 50 ml per 5 mg if fluids must be restricted. Infusions should be administered over 1 to 4 hours according to patient tolerance; usually 2 hours is satisfactory. Diluted amphotericin B should be shielded from direct sunlight. It can be infused through small bore (20 or 22 gauge) butterfly-type cannulas that are removed after each infusion. Daily infusions in differing sites, beginning with the most peripheral hand veins, will preserve venous access. If a total dose of greater than 500 mg is anticipated, administration through an indwelling central venous line (Hickman type) may be advantageous.

A 1 mg test dose is strongly advised, as anaphylactoid reactions can occur. If that dose is well tolerated, the next (usually 5 mg) may be administered immediately. Usually, increments of 5 to 10 mg daily are given as tolerated until a daily dose of 40 to 50 mg is reached. Nausea, vomiting, chills, fever, and aching frequently occur but tend to diminish as patients appear to become tolerant despite a steady dose or even gradually increasing dosage. In my opinion, there is no advantage in exceeding 50 mg daily. Usually this dose is administered daily for 2 to 4 weeks, and then an every other day or 3 times weekly regimen is initiated. Intermittent regimens usually are better tolerated late in therapy and are rational because amphotericin B remains in the body for relatively long periods.

Systemic toxicity usually can be lessened by premedication with 600 mg of aspirin, acetaminophen, or ibuprofen (Motrin), and with 25 mg of diphenhydramine (Benadryl) or promethazine

(Phenergan) orally, and hydrocortisone succinate (Solu-Cortef), 20 to 50 mg, added to the infusion. To minimize phlebitis, heparin, 10 mg (1200 units), can be added to the infusing fluid when administered through a peripheral vein. If systemic intolerance becomes excessive, the daily dosage should be decreased, or suspended and then restarted at a lower dose.

Azotemia, which is generally reversible, occurs upon amphotericin B administration. The level of azotemia should be monitored by biweekly blood urea nitrogen (BUN) or serum creatinine determinations. A BUN of greater than 40 or creatinine nearing 3.0 indicates a need for temporary reduction or omission of drug administration to allow improvement of azotemia and continuation of therapy. The dose does not necessarily have to be modified in persons with *pre-existing* renal disease, because amphotericin B is cleared chiefly by extrarenal means. Zidovudine (Retrovir), because of its renal clearance, should not be administered to patients receiving amphotericin B. Serum potassium concentration should also be determined at least twice weekly, and hypokalemia should be treated with oral or parenteral potassium supplementation. Anemia is frequent usually stabilizing at a hematocrit of 25 to 35 per cent. Transfusion with packed red blood cells should be reserved for patients with anemia-aggravated congestive heart failure or angina pectoris. In an attempt to reduce toxicity, lipid-microencapsulated suspensions of amphotericin B are under investigation.

Ketoconazole. Ketoconazole (Nizoral), an antifungal substituted imidazole that is well absorbed orally, is quite active in vitro against *H. capsulatum* and has produced gratifying therapeutic results in chronic disseminated and other forms of histoplasmosis. Patients having immune deficiencies with progressive disseminated histoplasmosis should still receive amphotericin B at least initially. The role of ketoconazole for therapy of chronic pulmonary histoplasmosis is promising, but is problematic because of the unpredictable course of that form of the disease. Chronic pulmonary disease has responded to ketoconazole with symptomatic improvement and sterilization of cultures in some cases, but culture-positive relapse has occurred after completion of 1 year of therapy in others. Chronic suppression of incurable cases should be considered. The currently recommended dose of ketoconazole is 400 mg (2 tablets) daily to be continued for a minimum of 6 months. Higher doses of ketoconazole are not known to be of greater benefit than conventional doses in histoplasmosis but result in more toxicity, including increased risk of pruritis, headache, gastrointestinal intolerance, and toxic hepatitis.

To avoid producing toxic levels of cyclosporine (Sandimmune), ketoconazole should not be administered to persons receiving cyclosporine.

Other Therapeutic Modalities. Convalescence is prolonged in some persons with histoplasmosis and requires limitation of activity for control of symptoms. Some authorities have advocated moderate-dosage prednisone (60 mg) in addition to amphotericin B for severe acute disease with respiratory insufficiency. However, too rapid tapering of prednisone in this situation may lead to precipitous exacerbation of respiratory insufficiency.

Resection pulmonary surgery is rarely needed. It is reserved for patients with adequate pulmonary reserve and cavities that progress despite amphotericin B.

In *Histoplasma* endocarditis, affected valves usually must be surgically replaced. In those patients, at least 1.5 grams of the total dose of amphotericin B should be given after surgery.

Pericarditis will usually respond to nonsteroidal anti-inflammatory drugs, but tamponade can require surgical placement of a pericardial "window" for drainage. Surgical therapy or corticosteroids for desmoplastic complications of histoplasmosis are usually not beneficial.

BLASTOMYCOSIS

method of
JOHN P. UTZ, M.D.
School of Medicine, Georgetown University
Washington, D.C.

Blastomycosis is a chronic disease, caused by the dimorphic fungus *Blastomyces dermatitidis*, to which the tissue reaction is both suppurative and granulomatous. The fungus is acquired by the respiratory route, from a still uncertain source in nature, and the primary focus of infection is the lung. Hematogenous dissemination characteristically occurs. The infection may also spread, in declining order of frequency, to cutaneous tissue, subcutaneous tissue, the male genitourinary tract, bone, mucous membranes, and reticuloendothelial tissue; other organs are affected in about 10 per cent or less of patients.

The diagnosis is established unequivocally by the culture and identification of *B. dermatitidis* from any specimen. The diagnosis is more quickly arrived at by the finding of appropriately sized, budding yeast forms in direct preparations, especially KOH, of fresh specimens, including sputum, pus, skin lesions, and prostatic massage secretions. Histopathologic studies using periodic acid–Schiff staining or other methods showing microscopic forms that, in the eyes of any experienced mycologist or pathologist, are consistent in size and form with *B. dermatitidis* also establish the diagnosis.

However, histopathologic study does not establish activity of disease. Such activity is established by culture of the fungus (or seeing it on direct examination of specimens as just described). Laboratory values that support the presence of inflammation include leukocyte count, erythrocyte sedimentation rate, lactic dehydrogenase (and other enzymes), hemoglobin, changes in roentgenographic findings, and ventilatory measurements. These tests assess activity and also serve to document response to therapy.

Serologic studies are not generally available, since they have not been helpful to physicians. A negative test does not rule out disease, and a positive test is inadequate proof of diagnosis or activity.

No skin testing material is available.

Determination of status of immune competence (cellular, serologic, or phagocytic) seems important, though less relevant than in other infections, such as cryptococcosis, candidiasis, aspergillosis, or zygomycosis (mucormycosis), that are more frequently opportunistic.

There are no symptoms, signs, or laboratory or chest film findings that are specific to this disease. Cough, chest pain, sputum production, and hemoptysis are only slightly more suggestive of one etiology than of another. For example, generalized signs of inflammation such as fever, chills, night sweats, anorexia, weight loss, depression, and malaise may be more frequent than in bronchogenic carcinoma, but are usually less frequent than in bacterial pneumonia.

Treatment

Once the diagnosis and evidence of disease activity have been established, there is no reason to delay onset of therapy. Chemotherapy for blastomycosis is summarized in Table 1.

Amphotericin B

Amphotericin B (Fungizone), remains the "gold standard" against which all older and more recent agents must be measured. Experience with it covers almost 30 years. Although new aspects of the drug (e.g., immunostimulatory and immunosuppressive effects) continue to come to light, knowledge of its effects seems stable and well established. At present Amphotericin B is the preferred agent for immunocompromised patients and those with more serious diseases such as meningitis.

The mode of action of the drug is its binding to steroids, chiefly ergosterol, in the fungal cell membrane. That binding is irreversible and renders the cell permeable, so that small molecules, notably potassium, leak out. (Ketoconazole, which also interferes with ergosterol synthesis and thus reduces binding sites on the membrane, interferes with and reduces amphotericin B activity, in vitro and in experimental infections in animals.)

Amphotericin B is administered intravenously. To a vial containing 50 mg, 10 ml of sterile water is added. (Carrying the vial in a pocket after mixing for an hour or so during walking rounds is one method that allows maximal suspension.) The dose to be given is then added to 5 per cent glucose in water, at a concentration not to exceed 10 mg of amphotericin B per 100 ml of infusion. A Y-tube assembly and infusion pump are important. I prefer an initial dose of only 1 mg. Subsequent doses can be increased daily by increments of 5 or 10 mg depending on the reaction to the previous day's dose. Since the work of Bind-

TABLE 1. **Chemotherapy of Blastomycosis**

Drug	Indications	Route	Dosage (mg)			Duration* (weeks)	Side Effects	Remarks
			Initial	Optimal	Total			
Amphotericin B	All forms	IV	1.0	1.0/kg (not to exceed 50)	2000	6	Azotemia, hypokalemia, anemia, fever, chills, nausea, vomiting	"Gold standard"
Ketoconazole	Except for central nervous system disease, more serious disease, and disease in immunocompromised patient	Oral	400	400	100,000	26–52	Hepatotoxicity, depression of testosterone and adrenal corticoids, gastrointestinal	Role being defined
Hydroxystilbamidine†	Nonprogressive noncavitary pulmonary and cutaneous disease	IV	25	225	8000	6	Dizziness, flushing, dyspnea	Used after other drug failures (rare); hepatic disease a relative contraindication
Miconazole‡	Pulmonary	IV	600	3000–3600	120,000	6	Nausea, vomiting, pruritus	Role may never be defined

*Various authorities may recommend different total dosage and duration of therapy (see text).
†Discontinued by the manufacturer in June 1988.
‡This use of miconazole is not listed in the manufacturer's directive.

schadler and Bennett, I have not given a daily dose greater than 50 mg (approximately 0.7 mg per kg of patient's body weight). Although various authors recommend total dosages up to 2.5 grams and continuation of therapy up to 10 weeks, I aim for 2.0 grams given in approximately 6 weeks. Despite the impressive experience of a few others, the predictable and quantifiable cardiotoxicity in our dog experiments has kept me from giving the infusion over a period shorter than 2 to 4 hours, again depending on the patient's tolerance and preference. As an additional precaution the patient's pulse, temperature, blood pressure, and state of well-being are measured every half hour during the infusion and thereafter as indicated by the values found during the infusion. Potassium or sodium salt solutions should never be mixed with the contents of the vial, as they precipitate the already precarious colloid suspension. I do not use a membrane filter with a pore size less than 0.45 micrometer. Studies in our lab show that the infusion need not be protected from light. I have rarely given the drug outside of a hospital setting, although it need not be restricted to use on an inpatient basis. When reactions have been severe, 50 mg of hydrocortisone sodium succinate given into the tubing or bag at the beginning may reduce or lessen severity of reactions. Aspirin (1200 to 1500 mg), diphenhydramine (25 to 50 mg), and prochlorperazine (5 to 10 mg) orally 15 to 30 minutes before the infusion are other premedications that are slightly less effective. I do not use heparin (final concentration 50 units per liter) routinely, although it is recommended by a few others.

There is no antimicrobial drug I know of that has such severe side effects as amphotericin B. Chills, fever, nausea, vomiting, anorexia, headache, and shortness of breath are clearly perceptible and unpleasant for the patient. Paradoxically, these usually occur more often and to a greater degree with the earlier infusions and lower doses (a phenomenon that has led me to use a more conservative initial dose than that recommended in the package insert). These side effects are not predictable, and a few patients escape almost completely. Hypotension is less symptomatic, but if severe it can be relieved by elevation of the foot of the bed, by 15 to 50 mg ephedrine intramuscularly, or by infusion of normal saline by the alternate Y arm after clamping off the arm delivering amphotericin B.

With daily infusions of any drug, but especially one suspended in glucose solution (pH 3.5 to 5.0), phlebitis is a problem. This is reduced by using a pediatric 23-gauge butterfly needle. Poor veins should never be an excuse for discontinuing a course of therapy; a Broviac or Hickman catheter solves the problem of access immediately.

With the 50-mg daily dose impaired glomerular filtration, as measured by blood urea nitrogen or serum creatinine, occurs in approximately 85 per cent of patients. If this occurs, temporary interruption of therapy is indicated. The indications are arbitrary, but values of 50 and 3.0 mg per dl, respectively, are useful cutoff points. Salt depletion, either intentional, asymptomatic, or accidental, increases azotemia.

Anemia occurs in approximately 75 per cent of patients and complicates a subtle hemolytic process that is usually present as a result of the infection. The anemia from treatment seems to be a function of suppression of erythropoietin. The hemoglobin or hematocrit stabilizes as the infection is controlled. Transfusions are not necessary, and oral iron is useless. Thrombocytopenia rarely occurs and is not severe.

Hypokalemia is a threat to virtually all patients, and serum values should be monitored at least twice weekly. Unrecognized hypokalemia has led to frightening muscle weakness and electrocardiographic changes. Foods rich in potassium help, but 20 to 40 mEq of potassium intravenously—not through the infusion bottle—is more immediately helpful. The mechanisms of loss are from cells and from excretion in the urine. Anorexia, diarrhea, and vomiting may also contribute.

Deterioration in respiratory function when amphotericin B is given shortly after leukocyte transfusion has been reported by some and denied by others. Such reactions have been found in experimental studies, and caution is recommended. Fortunately, blastomycosis is rarely an opportunistic infection, and agranulocytopenia or even leukopenia is rarely encountered.

Regular monitoring during treatment of abnormalities present before treatment—in addition to tests necessary by virtue of the drug itself—documents response. Patients usually report symptomatic improvement within a week, providing they can distinguish this from counterbalancing ill effects of the drug itself. Repeat chest films, ventilatory studies, culture of sputum or other specimens, blood tests, and, occasionally radionuclide studies are appropriate. For reasons cited earlier we do not monitor serology, and determinations of either peak or trough levels of amphotericin B are not routine.

Relapse after treatment has occurred with increasing frequency. In contrast to cryptococcosis, in which relapse almost invariably occurs within 12 months, in blastomycosis it may occur many years later.

Hydroxystilbamidine

Hydroxystilbamidine* was almost abandoned when amphotericin B appeared, because relapse seemed to occur so frequently after therapy with hydroxystilbamidine. When the side effects of amphotericin B were appreciated, interest in the older drug revived. At present it is reserved for patients in whom amphotericin B treatment fails (rarely encountered) and for nonprogressive, noncavitary pulmonary or cutaneous disease.

Ketoconazole

Ketoconazole has a better (oral) route of administration than amphotericin B, hydroxystilbamidine, or miconazole, and in non-immunocompromised patients it may be the preferable agent. In two published studies this drug was effective in 79 and 81 per cent of patients. My beginning regimen is 400 mg in one or two doses daily. A higher dose of 800 mg, in my experience, has usually resulted in nausea, vomiting, anorexia, and diarrhea. I monitor the serum bilirubin, alkaline phosphatase, alanine aminotransferase (SGOT, SGPT), and lactic acid dehydrogenase, at first weekly and thereafter at monthly intervals. The side effects of ketoconazole are almost as severe as those of amphotericin B. Adrenal cortical suppression is a recognized side effect that requires occasional serum cortisol levels. However, this side effect has not been symptomatic in my patients. Suppression of testicular function with impotence and azoospermia has been symptomatic and can be documented by testosterone levels, though the results of these are not helpful in management. I continue the drug for at least 6 months, and longer as indicated by response using the tests cited before.

Miconazole

Miconazole† (Monistat), like ketoconazole, has demonstrated in vitro and in vivo activity and has been used successfully in a few patients. The intravenous route of administration with miconazole is a disadvantage as compared with the oral route used for ketoconazole. Pruritus is a sufficiently severe side effect to lessen interest, and thus there is no defined role of this drug in the treatment of blastomycosis.

Surgery

Surgery is often of initial importance in the management of blastomycosis, but it is never definitive. Biopsy of skin lesions provides good

---

*Hydroxystilbamidine has been discontinued by the manufacturer as of June, 1988.

†The use of miconazole in blastomycosis is not listed in the manufacturer's directive.

material for histopathologic study. Open lung biopsy is only rarely needed for diagnostic purposes. Drainage of abscesses is most helpful in both diagnosis and treatment. Excision of a sequestrum in a bone lesion or repair of bronchopleural fistula is rarely necessary. As in the case of tuberculosis, thoracic surgery for cavitary or other pulmonary disease is rarely necessary.

Remaining Considerations

Should every patient with acute, primary pulmonary blastomycosis receive treatment? It is clear that some patients, especially those in whom the disease is recognized after a single site infection, have recovered without treatment. Initial recovery in other series has been tarnished by subsequent relapses. Even so, the relapses seem to occur in a minority of patients. But how does one distinguish the patient with active disease who does not need treatment or the one who will relapse later? These are both unanswered questions at the moment.

Should every patient in whom blastomycosis is encountered unexpectedly after thoracotomy and histopathologic study be treated? A well-organized, complete protocol to establish (or exclude) activity is helpful for the individual patient. Even so, activation of dormant disease has occurred frequently enough that some thoughtful physicians have recommended chemotherapy "routinely" in such patients.

PLEURAL EFFUSION AND EMPYEMA THORACIS

method of
DON R. MILLER, M.D.
*University of California Irvine Medical Center
Orange, California*

Pleural effusion is a common clinical feature of many local and systemic diseases, the most frequent being congestive heart failure, bacterial pneumonia, malignancy, pulmonary embolism, and viral infections. Less frequent causes include cirrhosis, gastrointestinal problems, collagen diseases, tuberculosis, and others.

Although normally there is a large continuous fluid exchange across the pleural surfaces, little fluid collects in the pleural space because of the balance between oncotic pressure of plasma proteins and the hydrostatic pressure in parietal and visceral pleural vessels. Alterations in this delicate balance result in pleural effusion.

Clinical features of dyspnea and at times chest discomfort result as the increasing fluid volume displaces functioning lung. The physical examination of the chest shows dullness or flatness to percussion, and reduction or absence of breath sounds and vocal and tactile fremitus over the unilateral or bilateral collections. The complete history and physical examination may also indicate the precise cause of the effusion, or provide a rational differential diagnosis.

Routine posterior-anterior radiologic examinations of the chest characteristically show obliteration of lateral or posterior sulci. The lateral decubitus film defines the layered fluid more accurately. Ultrasound and the CT scan permit precise localization of even small accumulations and are increasingly helpful in needle or catheter drainage of small fluid collections and in the diagnosis of thoracic diseases in critically ill patients.

Pleural effusions are commonly classified as transudates or exudates based upon the protein or LDH concentrations and their relationship to the respective serum concentrations. Exudates have at least one of the following characteristics, while transudates have none:

1. Pleural fluid protein concentration or serum protein concentration is greater than 0.5.

2. Pleural fluid LDH or serum LDH is greater than 0.6.

3. Pleural fluid LDH is greater than two thirds of the upper limits of normal for the serum LDH.

Any significant pleural effusion should be sampled for study by needle aspiration. Once the fluid is established as an exudate or transudate, further diagnostic determinations will be necessary for exudates, while transudates are usually related to congestive heart failure, cirrhosis, and nephrotic syndrome and require no further diagnostic tests. Exudates result from local pleural alterations from a large number of causes, and careful selection of tests for further analysis of the fluid should be made depending upon the differential diagnosis. The gross and microscopic appearance may be diagnostic. Additional tests of value are the specific gravity, pH, glucose concentration, white cell count and differential, red cell count, bacterial culture and Gram stain, cytology, and lipid and amylase measurements. The pH may be less than 7.20 in tuberculous, parapneumonic, and malignant effusions and in rheumatoid arthritis. The glucose level may be below 60 mg per dl in tuberculosis and rheumatoid arthritis. Amylase may be present with esophageal rupture and pancreatitis. The culture for tubercle bacilli is positive in less than 20 per cent of the cases of tuberculous pleurisy. Lymphocytes predominate in the cell counts of tuberculosis and rheumatoid arthritis, while red cells are associated with trauma, pulmonary embolism, and malignancy. In chylothorax the effusion has a milky appearance and lipid content greater than that of the plasma. While the fluid analysis is diagnostic in 60 to 88 per cent of patients, results of specific tests may be variable in patients with the same diagnosis, and in unrelated conditions test results may be similar. In some cases the cause of the effusion cannot be established.

The diagnostic tap should be made below the upper level of percussion dullness and referenced to the chest x-ray, avoiding the diaphragm, the heart shadow, and the internal mammary, axillary, and intercostal vessels. A test aspiration with the anesthetizing needle assures the correct placement. Pneumothorax is the most common complication of thoracentesis (10 per cent) and is usually associated with malignancy, cough during the procedure, or therapeutic thoracentesis. Use of a blunt needle, termination of the procedure if cough ensues, and use of a plastic cannula may reduce this complication. If selected studies of the exudative pleural fluid are not diagnostic, closed pleural biopsy, thoracoscopy, or open pleural biopsy may be indicated.

Treatment

Empyema

Empyema is a purulent infection of the pleural space that accompanies or follows pneumonia, lung abscess, thoracic surgery, trauma, or chest tube insertion. Its bacterial source may also be hematogenous. The overall mortality rate of this complication is reportedly as high as 20 per cent. The organisms involved frequently are *Staphylococcus aureus*, *Streptococcus pneumoniae*, or multiple organisms, including anaerobes. *Haemophilus influenzae* is frequent in the pediatric age group. Gram-negative organisms often originate from infections below the diaphragm. As an example, a subphrenic abscess subsequent to a hepatic abscess or pancreatitis may be an underlying cause.

Multiple trauma with thoracic injury and hemopneumothorax commonly requires chest tube insertion and prolonged tracheal intubation with respiratory support. Pleural sepsis is a complication in patients with such injuries in whom systemic infection is frequent. Appropriate antibiotic therapy of pulmonary infection based upon sputum culture, or prophylactic antibiotics and careful aseptic management of tubes is important in prevention of empyema.

Pleural effusion is common in association with pneumonia (parapneumonic effusion). Fluid should be aspirated. If serous, it may resolve on repeated aspiration and antibiotics alone. Analysis of a fluid sample for pH and glucose has been helpful in predicting the need for early placement of tube drainage. When the pH is below 7.0 and the glucose is below 40 mg per dl, the effusion is unlikely to clear without tube drainage, which should be promptly instituted. Purulent collections or the presence of bacteria on Gram stain requires prompt tube thoracostomy drainage and the use of appropriate antibiotics. When steady improvement does not follow tube thoracostomy, open surgical drainage with segmental costal removal is often needed. Purulent loculations that interfere with successful tube management may require additional tubes or open drainage. It is important that complete pulmonary expansion be maintained throughout the course to assure adequate respiratory function and avoidance of trapped lung. A persistent space or unexpanded lung with or without bronchopleural fistula sets the stage for fluid collection leading to chronic empyema, thickened pleura, and consideration of open thoracotomy and decortication. Early operative drainage is advocated for empyema in the immunocompromised patient or for postoperative empyema, instances in which the response to tube drainage only may be poor. The use and timing of decortication during open surgical drainage is controversial in the early management of empyema. A large series in a recent report showed the inadequacy of tube drainage and greater success with earlier rib resection and open drainage. While children with empyema usually respond well with the use of tube drainage and antibiotics, failure in response can be reversed by decortication with good results and a shortened hospital stay.

Empyema necessitatis occurs when neglected or undiagnosed empyema seeks spontaneous drainage pathways which may extend to involve subdiaphragmatic structures, the lung and bronchi, or the chest wall.

Pleural Effusion Caused by Neoplasm

The most frequent causes of malignant pleural effusions are adenocarcinoma of the lung, breast carcinoma, and the lymphomas. The primary site of origin may be unknown, and may remain so in 10 per cent of cases. The effusion may be bloody or clear, unilateral or bilateral. Cytologic study of pleural fluid is usually diagnostic, and when positive is a contraindication to definitive curative surgical treatment of the primary neoplasm. If the primary tumor has not been located, a search should be made for it.

Systemic chemotherapy will usually be the initial treatment. Pleural biopsy using special needles or thoracotomy may be indicated when cytology is negative. When systemic therapy does not control the effusion, local treatment of pleurodesis is aimed at palliation by preventing recurrent effusion in the symptomatic patient. While many substances, including talc, nitrogen mustard, and chemotherapeutic agents, have been used to accomplish adherence of pleural surfaces, intrapleural tetracycline has many advantages and has been effective in over 90 per cent of cases reported by Sherman and associates. Strict attention to technical details is necessary. A No. 28 French chest tube is inserted and all fluid is removed. If the mediastinum is shifted ipsilaterally or the underlying lung remains collapsed or trapped after fluid withdrawal, sclerosants will not be effective and should not be used.

Rapid removal of large volumes in fluid-depleted patients should be avoided. Pain is reduced by analgesia and intrapleural lidocaine. Tetracycline, 1.5 grams diluted in 30 ml of sterile water, is introduced into the pleural space, followed by an equal amount of water to flush the tubing, which is then clamped. The patient is then promptly positioned to promote gravitational distribution of the drug to all pleural surfaces (i.e., anterior, posterior, lateral, superior, inferior). The position is changed frequently, since the inflammatory action of the drug, which induces symphysis, dissipates rapidly over a period as short as 60 minutes. The tube remains clamped, and the positions are repeatedly changed over a 2- to 4-hour period. The tube then is unclamped, and is left overnight for suction at a pressure of −20 cm of water and then removed. Full expansion of the lung is maintained to assure synechia.

The morbidity of open surgical methods to effect pleurodesis has often outweighed the palliative effect. Early reports of the use of pleuroperitoneal shunts similar to peritoneovenous shunts for ascites have shown acceptable results in small series of patients, and further experience may prove their effectiveness. This technique has also been used in chylothorax.

Tuberculosis and Other Effusions

The effusion of tuberculosis is often seen in younger individuals without apparent cause for the effusion. The fluid is thin and nonpurulent and may not show tubercle bacilli on smear or culture. The use of needle biopsy may be of help in the diagnosis of chronic pleural disease in tuberculosis or malignancy. Thoracoscopy and open biopsy procedures may be indicated when other measures have failed to resolve the diagnostic problem. With a positive PPD skin test for tuberculosis and no other cause for the effusion, treatment for tuberculosis using isoniazid (INH) and rifampin should be instituted. Spontaneous resolution of the fluid may be supplemented by thoracentesis if required. The use of chest tubes, which may become secondarily infected, should be avoided. Some patients may later be candidates for decortication for residual pleural disease.

Patients who have empyema in which the culture is negative and who do not respond to treatment should be suspected of having tuberculosis or fungal infection.

A recent review of 24 patients with tuberculous effusion by Epstein and others showed an older population with a mean age of 56 years. Lymphocytosis of fluid was not uniform, and 4 patients had greater than 90 per cent polymorphonuclear leukocytes in the fluid.

Pulmonary embolus is commonly overlooked as a cause of pleural effusion. Although the effusion is classically bloody and has a predominance of polymorphonuclear leukocytes, either or both of these characteristics may be absent. One fourth of the effusions are transudates. Ventilation-perfusion scanning and pulmonary arteriography are helpful in establishing the diagnosis of the underlying embolus. No characteristic pattern is seen in tests on the exudate. The effusions resolve on anticoagulant therapy, which is administered as for emboli without effusion.

Rheumatoid pleural effusion is associated with a granular parietal pleural surface with lesions histologically characteristic of the disease. Resolution of the effusion occurs spontaneously over several months. Diagnosis can be made by thoracoscopy and pleural biopsy.

Transudates are managed by control of the primary disease, but tetracycline pleurodesis has been used effectively in refractory patients.

Intra-abdominal subdiaphragmatic conditions may result in communication of hepatic, pancreatic, or subphrenic abscess with the pleural space. CT scanning and endoscopic retrograde pancreatography are of considerable value in the diagnosis and in selection of the surgical approach for correction of the pancreatopleural fistula.

PRIMARY LUNG ABSCESS

method of
JOHN G. BARTLETT, M.D.
Johns Hopkins University School of Medicine
Baltimore, Maryland

The term lung abscess traditionally refers to pulmonary necrosis caused by bacteria other than mycobacteria. The usual method of detection is a chest x-ray showing a parenchymal infiltrate accompanied by a cavity, usually with an air-fluid level. The usual associated findings are cough, fever, and leukocytosis. Lung abscesses are often classified as "primary" or "secondary," based on associated conditions that also dictate microbiologic probabilities, prognosis, and management decisions. Primary lung abscesses are most commonly found in patients who are prone to aspiration as a result of compromised consciousness or dysphasia. Secondary lung abscesses represent a complication of bronchial obstruction, as with a malignancy or foreign body, or a systemic disease in which immunologic defenses are compromised, such as neutropenia, cancer chemotherapy, steroid administration, or acquired immunodeficiency syndrome (AIDS). The most frequent microbiologic pathogens in primary lung abscess are anaerobic bacteria that normally reside in the gingival crevice, such as *Bacteroides melaninogen-*

icus, Fusobacterium nucleatum, and anaerobic streptococci. The usual patient has disease of the gingival crevice, such as pyorrhea or gingivitis, and a condition that predisposes to aspiration, such as alcoholism, general anesthesia, seizure disorder, or drug abuse. Other bacteria that occasionally cause pulmonary suppuration include *Staphylococcus aureus,* gram-negative bacilli (especially *Klebsiella pneumoniae*), *Streptococcus pneumoniae, Haemophilus influenzae, Legionella,* Group A beta-hemolytic streptococci, *Actinomyces,* and *Nocardia.*

Diagnostic Evaluation

Diagnostic considerations in patients who present with a cavitating lesion on chest x-ray include an infected pulmonary cyst or bullae, a loculated empyema with an air-fluid level, infection due to mycobacteria or fungi, a cavitating neoplasm, a cavitating pulmonary infarction, or Wegener's granulomatosis. Diagnostic tests that are often useful in patients with atypical presentations are bronchoscopy, sputum cytology, and computer tomography. The usual method of identifying bacterial pathogens of lung infections is culture of expectorated sputum. However, the most frequent pathogens in lung abscess are anaerobic bacteria that normally reside in the upper airways, and the expectorated specimen is invariably contaminated with these organisms so that they are not valid for meaningful anaerobic culture. The primary use of expectorated sputum is for detection of mycobacteria, fungi, *Nocardia,* and the other aerobic pathogens noted above, such as *S. aureus* and gram-negative bacilli. Specimen sources that are valid for detecting anaerobic bacteria include pleural fluid, transtracheal aspirates, transthoracic aspirates, and bronchoscopy using quantitative culture of specimens collected with the protected catheter device. Pleural fluid should always be obtained for microbiologic studies, including Gram stain as well as both aerobic and anaerobic culture. With this exception, most authorities feel that invasive diagnostic tests to identify anaerobic bacterial pathogens are not necessary in patients with the typical findings of an anaerobic lung abscess. This especially applies to patients with putrid sputum, since this is diagnostic of anaerobic infection. Once antibiotics are given, the diagnostic yield of anaerobes as well as other fastidious bacteria is notably reduced, so that cultures even of uncontaminated specimens are commonly negative.

Treatment

Antimicrobial Selection for Anaerobic Lung Abscess

The three regimens that are frequently advocated for empiric use are penicillin G, clindamycin, or penicillin plus metronidazole. The initial penicillin regimen in hospitalized patients is aqueous penicillin G, given intravenously in a dose of 8 to 10 million units daily, until the patient is afebrile and there is definite evidence of clinical improvement. At that time, penicillin may be given intramuscularly or orally as penicillin V, penicillin G, amoxicillin, or ampicillin in doses of 500 to 750 mg four times daily. Oral treatment is continued on an outpatient basis until the chest x-ray shows either complete resolution of the infiltrate, a cyst, or a small stable scar. The initial regimen of clindamycin (Cleocin) is 600 mg, given intravenously every 8 hours until the patient is afebrile and clinically improved. Subsequent treatment is with oral clindamycin, in a dose of 300 mg four times daily, until the x-ray criteria noted above are achieved. With the metronidazole plus penicillin regimen, the initial dose of penicillin may be the high intravenous dose noted above or it could be the oral regimen with one of the four penicillin derivatives noted; either oral or parenteral penicillin is combined with metronidazole (Flagyl), 500 mg orally every 6 hours for the duration of therapy. The advantage of the penicillin regimen is that it is relatively cheap, is well tolerated, and has been regarded as the preferred drug for nearly three decades by many authorities. Clindamycin is a more recently introduced drug that is substantially more active against the anaerobic organisms involved in lung abscess and has proved superior to penicillin in a controlled clinical trial. Most authorities view this to be the drug of choice for patients who are seriously ill with a lung abscess or in whom penicillin is contraindicated. The potential advantages of the metronidazole plus penicillin regimen are that it is substantially less expensive than clindamycin, and the addition of metronidazole provides enhanced activity versus anaerobic bacteria that are penicillin-resistant. Experience with this latter regimen is somewhat limited, and extreme care must be exercised in alcoholic patients because of the possibility of a disulfiram (Antabuse)-like reaction due to metronidazole.

Drainage

Adequate drainage is considered crucial for any empyema that accompanies a lung abscess. Antimicrobial agents represent the mainstay of treatment for lung abscess, although some authorities feel that postural drainage or bronchoscopy is an important ancillary measure.

Failure to Respond

The expected response is subjective improvement within 3 to 5 days and elimination of fever within 7 to 14 days. Improvement on chest x-ray is delayed, and, in fact, there may be extension of the infiltrate with new cavity formation during the first 1 or 2 weeks. Considerations in patients who fail to respond include bronchoscopy to detect an underlying lesion or to facilitate drainage,

evaluation for alternative diagnostic possibilities, changes in the antimicrobial regimen, or surgery. With regard to antibiotics, patients with anaerobic lung abscesses treated with penicillin will often respond when clindamycin is substituted or metronidazole is added. Pleural effusions must be carefully assessed, since an inadequately drained empyema is an important cause of persistent fever. Surgery is rarely required. The major indications are an abscess that is totally unresponsive to antibiotics, severe or life-threatening hemoptysis, or an obstructing lesion. The usual procedure is a lobectomy. An alternative option for patients with an inadequate pulmonary reserve is external drainage with percutaneous catheter insertion, usually under fluoroscopic control. When this is done, there must be care to avoid contamination of the pleural space so that patients without adhesions should have pleural synthesis or stay sutures prior to catheter insertion.

OTITIS MEDIA

method of
A. JULIANNA GULYA, M.D., and
WILLIAM R. WILSON, M.D.
The George Washington University
Washington, D.C.

Despite a wealth of experience with otitis media (OM), a firm consensus regarding appropriate management is lacking. Some confusion may be related to the differing terminology used to describe the various forms of OM. "Otitis media" refers to an inflammation of the middle ear; a distinction is generally drawn between "suppurative" (bacterial, purulent) otitis media, in which a purulent effusion accompanies the middle ear inflammation, and "nonsuppurative" (OM with effusion, secretory OM, serous OM, glue ear), which lacks the features of acute inflammation. An "acute" episode has a rapid onset and generally clears by 10 to 21 days; OM lasting 21 to 90 days is considered "subacute," and the term "chronic" implies duration of greater than 90 days. "Myringitis" is OM without effusion.

Epidemiology

Both extrinsic and intrinsic factors play a role in the occurrence of OM.

Infants older than 6 months and children up to approximately age 7 years compose the population at highest risk for OM, with the peak incidence occurring in the 1-year-old population; after the age of 7 years, OM gradually becomes less common. Another intrinsic factor that accentuates the incidence of OM is race; American Indians and Eskimos have great problems with OM, more so than Hispanics and Caucasians. The black population tends to have a lower incidence of OM. Craniofacial anomalies, such as those of Down's syndrome and cleft palate, tend to be associated with a higher incidence of OM. Sex may also play a role; there is some suggestion that boys may have more problems with OM than girls.

The incidence of OM in the winter months is quadruple that of the summer months. Low socioeconomic status, exposure to other young infants and children, and exposure to tobacco smoke in the home also seem to predispose to OM.

ACUTE SUPPURATIVE OTITIS MEDIA

A typical episode of acute suppurative otitis media (ASOM) occurs in the setting of an upper respiratory tract infection. Irritability, otalgia (tugging at the ear), hearing loss, and fever quickly develop. Sanguinopurulent otorrhea may follow, with diminution of pain. Even untreated, the condition is self-limiting, with spontaneous resolution usually occurring within 10 days.

Early examination may show decreased mobility and hyperemia of the posterior superior quadrant of the tympanic membrane only. As the purulent effusion accumulates, the tympanic membrane becomes increasingly opaque, immobile, and erythematous and bulges laterally. The usual landmarks disappear. With perforation, a pinpoint hole may be visualized posterosuperiorly. An adequate examination demands removal of cerumen and debris followed by careful evaluation with pneumatic otoscopy.

Pathogenesis

Eustachian tube dysfunction has an important role in the pathogenesis of OM; the dysfunction may be obstructive, owing to an intrinsic failure of the normal opening mechanisms (as seen in cleft palate) or to an extrinsic compression by an enlarged adenoidal mass. Upper respiratory viral infections (especially RSV, influenza virus, and adenovirus) and nasopharyngeal bacterial colonization also contribute to the development of OM. Abnormal patency of the eustachian tube allows for reflux of infected nasopharyngeal debris into the middle ear.

Etiology

ASOM is predominantly an aerobic bacterial infection, with *Streptococcus pneumoniae* (30 per cent), *Haemophilus influenzae* (25 per cent), and *Branhamella catarrhalis* (19 to 24 per cent) being the predominant pathogens. *Streptococcus pyogenes, Staphylococcus aureus,* anaerobes, and viruses are detected in less than 10 per cent of the cases. In infants younger than 6 weeks, *Staphylococcus aureus,* group B streptococci, and gram-negative enteric bacteria are found in 20 per cent of the cases. *Mycoplasma pneumoniae* does not appear to be an important cause of ASOM.

Management

Although most cases of ASOM can be expected to resolve spontaneously, antibiotic therapy is recommended to speed resolution and avoid complications. Oral amoxicillin (20 to 40 mg per kg per day in 3 divided doses) for 10 days constitutes the initial therapy of choice; in penicillin-allergic patients, trimethoprim-sulfamethoxazole (Bactrim, Septra) (8 and 40 mg per kg per day in two divided doses) or erythromycin and sulfisoxazole, (Pediazole) (50 and 150 mg per kg per day in four divided doses) can be substituted. Analgesics, antipyretics, antihistamines, and nasal sprays may be helpful in relieving some of the associated symptoms.

Evaluation at 72 hours should find significant improvement in fever and/or otalgia. Failure of resolution calls for a change of antibiotic therapy, preferably based upon culture results obtained by tympanocentesis. Myringotomy may also be considered at this point.

The new antimicrobial agents should be effective against the bacteria known to be associated with treatment failures in the community and be resistant to the effects of beta-lactamases; 10 to 35 per cent of *H. influenzae,* 75 per cent of *B. catarrhalis,* and many *Staphylococcus aureus* organisms are beta-lactamase producers. If not given as initial therapy, erythromycin-sulfisoxazole or trimethoprim-sulfamethoxazole can be effective; however, if *Streptococcus pyogenes* or *Staphylococcus aureus* are etiologic, the latter combination is not effective. Cefaclor (Ceclor) (40 mg per kg per day in three divided doses) is resistant to the beta-lactamase, as is a combination of amoxicillin and clavulanate sodium (Augmentin).

The patient should be re-evaluated at 10 days and again at 30 days after initiation of therapy. Even with successful antibiotic therapy, 40 per cent of children will have persisting effusions 4 weeks after the acute episode, dropping to 10 per cent after 3 months of treatment.

Tympanocentesis as an initial diagnostic step should be considered in those who are immunocompromised, are critically ill, are neonates, experience the onset of ASOM while on antibiotic therapy, or experience the onset of complications (for example, mastoiditis).

Recurrent Otitis Media

Sporadic episodes of ASOM can be treated as the need arises; however, for the patient who experiences three or more episodes of ASOM over a 6-month period, the morbidity of repeated infections mandates their elimination. In addition to evaluation to identify any allergies, adenoidal hypertrophy, palatal cleft, sinus infection, or immunodeficiency that may predispose to the recurrences, prophylactic antibiotics, either amoxicillin (20 to 50 mg per kg per day at bedtime) or sulfisoxazole (50 to 75 mg per kg per day in one or two doses daily) should be administered. Trimethoprim-sulfamethoxazole can also be used, but both the physician and parents (or the adult patient) should be aware of the potential risks of vasculitis (Stevens-Johnson syndrome). Immunotherapy may be helpful in selected allergic patients, but the pneumococcal vaccine has proved a disappointment thus far.

If the patient "breaks through" to two or more episodes of ASOM or otorrhea in less than 3 months, tympanostomy tube insertion should then be considered, generally allowing the tubes to remain in place until spontaneously extruded. Custom-fitted ear plugs are recommended for bathing, while sulfacetamide sodium and prednisolone sodium phosphate ophthalmic drops (Vasocidin) are used to treat otorrhea.

NONSUPPURATIVE OTITIS MEDIA

An effusion will persist for a variable time period after an episode of ASOM, but a nonpurulent middle ear effusion may also appear without an antecedent acute infection. Such nonsuppurative otitis media represents the major cause of hearing loss in children.

The populations at greatest risk and the pathophysiologic features are essentially those described for ASOM. A major exception is the onset of unilateral nonsuppurative otitis media in the adult, which demands evaluation for the possibility of a nasopharyngeal mass.

The symptoms of nonsuppurative otitis media are hearing loss, delayed speech, inattentiveness, and occasionally vertigo. A careful examination with the pneumatic otoscope will reveal an amber, relatively immobile tympanic membrane, occasionally with an unusually white malleus handle. In some patients, air bubbles or an airfluid level may be visualized, and occasionally the tympanic membrane may appear blue (the so-called idiopathic blue eardrum). Tympanometry is a useful diagnostic agent in children older than 6 months, revealing a characteristic nonpeaking curve with the effusion-filled middle ear.

Antibiotic therapy (either erythromycin-sulfisoxazole or trimethoprim-sulfamethoxazole) can be successful in resolving some cases. The role of steroids and/or decongestants/antihistamines is not clear. Autoinsufflation or politzerization may be beneficial in cooperative patients. If the effusion persists for more than 2 to 3 months, tympanostomy tube insertion should be performed. If the effusion recurs after extrusion of the tube, strong consideration should be given to concomitant adenoidectomy with tube replacement. In fact, recent evidence suggests that adenoidectomy with myringotomy should be considered as the initial surgical therapy after medical treatment has failed. Tympanostomy tube insertion would then be reserved for those cases in which recurrent effusion occurs and fails to respond to treatment.

Complications and Sequelae

The sequelae of OM relate to uncontrolled suppuration; fortunately, such dreaded complications as mastoiditis, petrous apicitis, labyrinthitis, and intracranial complications such as brain abscess have been greatly reduced with antibiotic therapy. Other problems, such as chronic suppurative OM with tympanic membrane perforation, middle ear atelectasis, tympanosclerosis, adhesive OM, cholesteatoma, ossicular discontinuity or fixation, and facial nerve paralysis still occur. Sensorineural hearing loss is believed to develop as a consequence of the penetration of toxic inflammatory substances through the round window in particular. "Silent" OM, in which pathologic changes occur behind an intact tympanic membrane, also continues to be a therapeutic challenge.

The hearing loss of OM is associated with sequelae of a different nature. Not infrequently, problems with speech and language development, inattentiveness, or suspected hearing loss are the presenting symptoms of OM. Whether the auditory deprivation of OM is sufficient to cause deficits in academic performance, cognitive development, or speech and language development continues to be a focus of debate, but certainly is a great concern of those treating the pediatric population.

BACTERIAL PNEUMONIA

method of
IAN M. SMITH, M.D.
The University of Iowa Hospitals
Iowa City, Iowa

Bacterial pneumonia is caused by the aspiration of organisms from an area of pharyngeal carriage of organisms, as in a pneumococcal or gram-negative rod pneumonia, or by inhalation of an environmental contaminant, such as *Staphylococcus aureus* or *Pseudomonas aeruginosa*. In some 25 to 35 per cent of cases, the lung is damaged immediately prior to the pneumonia by a viral infection, frequently influenza and sometimes respiratory syncytial virus. The type of organism causing pneumonia differs according to whether the infection was acquired in the community or shortly after institutionalization in a hospital or nursing home (nosocomial infection). Some organisms are typically community acquired, such as *Streptococcus pneumoniae* (which can also be acquired in an institution), and certain organisms are usually acquired in an institution, such as *Klebsiella-Enterobacter* species (which can also be acquired in the community). Most pneumonias are acquired in the fall or winter. An exception to this is Legionnaires' pneumonia, which is acquired primarily in the summer. Infections can spread person-to-person under crowded conditions. Until recently, many pneumonias have remained undiagnosed. Studies in England have shown that the majority of these undiagnosed pneumonias are due to *S. pneumoniae* as shown by counterimmunoelectrophoresis of sputum, blood, and urine. A convenient classification of pneumonia by incidence rates and case fatality rates is shown in Table 1.

The typical clinical picture is the onset of a fever, often associated with an initial shaking chill or rigor, quickly reaching 102° F or higher. The patient develops a cough productive of bloody-colored or rusty-colored sputum associated with pleurisy (a deep stabbing pain on coughing or deep inspiration). The respiratory rate is usually 24 per minute or higher. Physical examination of the lung may be negative or may show localized rales with or without consolidation. About 15 to 35 per cent of patients have an associated bacteremia. In young adults, underlying diseases are present in approximately 15 to 30 per cent, and in patients over 70 years of age such diseases are present in 85 per cent or more. In Legionnaires' disease all the signs and symptoms of pneumonia occur and in addition are associated with signs and symptoms in the central nervous system, gastrointestinal tract, or genitourinary system, such as headache, confusion, diarrhea, or albuminuria.

Diagnosis

It is essential to make an exact diagnosis of the cause of pneumonia and any complicating bacteremia. Treatment must often be started before the results of this investigation are available. It is essential to obtain a proper specimen of sputum, which should be obtained by the physician. This should contain 25 or more pus cells and less than 10 epithelial cells per high-power microscopic field. Pleural fluid should be obtained if present. A single blood culture should be taken. X-rays are useful primarily to show the presence of pneumonia and to indicate whether one, two, or more lobes are involved. Associated cardiac disease may also be made evident. In certain immunocompromised or otherwise seriously ill patients, bronchoscopy with biopsy may be necessary.

Prognosis

Certain patients do poorly, such as those with two or more lobes involved, bacteremic patients, and patients with a complicating underlying disease that may be exacerbated by the diversion of energy to make new white cells and other proteins necessary to combat the infection. The elderly do less well than the young. Patients with pneumonia acquired in the hospital or nursing home have a poorer prognosis than those who acquired their pneumonia in the community. These factors will influence the intensity of treatment.

Treatment

Patients with a single-lobe pneumococcal pneumonia without a significant underlying disease can be treated in the office or at home. Patients with two or more lobes involved should be admitted to the hospital. Patients with severe involvement of the lungs may need blood gases checked for hypoxemia or hypercapnia. Patients are frequently dehydrated and require fluids. Some patients will require mechanical ventilation and intensive care. If patients are confused, they should have a lumbar puncture to exclude meningitis. Pleural effusions should be aspirated to exclude empyema, which if present may require chest tube drainage. Patients with reduced serum albumin, particularly the elderly, may require nutritional support, and hyperalimentation may be necessary.

Prompt early treatment with the appropriate antibiotic is essential in the treatment of pneumonia (Table 2). An early high level of antibiotic should be established as soon as possible by intramuscular or intravenous injection. This can be done in the office after the appropriate cultures are drawn and before hospital admission to avoid a 2- to 4-hour delay. Since approximately 75 per

TABLE 1. **Community-Acquired Pneumonias**

Etiology	Incidence (%)	Case Fatality Rate (%)
Streptococcus pneumoniae	76	10
Gram-negative rods	17	70
Legionella species	5	10
All others	2	2

TABLE 2. **Antimicrobial Therapy of Bacterial Pneumonia**

Pathogen/Syndrome	Drug	Dose	Route
Gram-positive cocci			
Streptococcus pneumoniae	Aqueous penicillin G (VK)	400,000 U q 4 hr	IV or IM, then oral
	Erythromycin	250–500 mg q 6 hr	PO or IV
	(Cephalosporin or vancomycin)		
Staphylococcus aureus	Oxacillin or nafcillin	1–3 grams q 4 hr	IV
	Vancomycin[1]	500 mg q 6 hr	IV
Mixed anaerobic organisms (Aspiration pneumonia)			
Community-acquired	Aqueous penicillin G	2 million U q 4 hr	IV
	Clindamycin	600 mg q 6–8 hr	IV
Hospital-acquired or nursing home–acquired	Aqueous penicillin G or clinda- mycin	As above	IV
	plus		
	Gentamicin[2] or tobramycin[2]	1–1.5 mg/kg q 8 hr	IM or IV
	(Cefoxitin)		
Mycoplasma pneumoniae	Erythromycin	250 mg q 6 hr	PO (or IV)
	Tetracycline	250 mg q 6 hr	PO (or IV)
Gram-negative bacilli			
Klebsiella pneumoniae	Cephalosporin[3, 5]	Depends on cephalosporin chosen	
	plus		
	Gentamicin[2] or tobramycin[2]	1–1.5 mg/kg q 8 hr	IM or IV
	Ampicillin or cephalosporin[3, 4, 5]	1 gram q 4 hr	IV
	plus		
	Gentamicin[2] or tobramycin[2]	1–1.5 mg/kg q 8 hr	IM or IV
Pseudomonas aeruginosa (ICU/CCU-acquired)	Ticarcillin, piperacillin (or carbenicillin)	3 grams q 4 hr	IV
	plus tobramycin[2,4]	1–1.5 mg/kg q 8 hr	IM or IV
	Ampicillin plus gentamicin or tobramycin[2]	1–1.5 mg/kg q 8 hr	IM or IV
	(Cephalosporin[3])	Depends on cephalosporin chosen	IV
Proteus species	Same as for *Pseudomonas*		
Enterobacteriaceae	Same as for *Pseudomonas*		
	(Cephalosporin[3])	Depends on cephalosporin chosen	
	or		
	Trimethoprim/sulfamethoxazole[4]	2.5–5.0 mg/kg q 6 hr based on trimethoprim compo- nents	PO or IV
Serratia marcescens	Gentamicin[2]	1–1.5 mg/kg q 8 hr	IM or IV
	Cephalosporin[3, 4]	Depends on cephalosporin chosen	
	(Ticarcillin)		
	(Trimethoprim/sulfamethoxazole)		
Haemophilus influenzae	Ampicillin	1 gram q 4–6 hr	IV
	(Cephalosporin[3])		
	(Chloramphenicol)		
Legionella pneumophila	Erythromycin	500 mg–1 gram q 6 hr	PO or IV
	(± Rifampin)		

[1]Vancomycin is indicated for treatment of resistant strains.

[2]Dosage must be adjusted for renal disease.

[3]Newer cephalosporins are indicated only in case of an organism resistant to first- or second-generation cephalosporin (cefotaxime, 2 grams q 2 hr; ceftizoxime 2 grams q 8 hr; ceftriozine 2 grams q 12 hr; ceftazidime 1–2 grams q 8 hr).

[4]Imipenem 0.25 to 1 gram q 6 hr, adjust dose in presence of renal disease.

[5]Aztreonam 1 gram q 8 hr.

Drugs for alternative therapy are listed in parentheses.

cent of pneumonias are due to pneumococci, the majority will respond to penicillin G (or erythromycin, vancomycin, or a first-generation cephalosporin if the patient is allergic to penicillin). If gram-negative rod pneumonia can be excluded on staining of the sputum but the exact etiology is uncertain, erythromycin is the treatment of choice because it will control the *Mycoplasma*, pneumococcus, and *Legionella* organisms. Having chosen the indicated antibiotic, it is essential on the second or third day to check all cultures to make sure that the right antibiotic is being used. The patient's temperature should also be decreasing. Around 6 to 8 p.m. the temperature should fall like a bouncing ball. If it does not fall, the diagnosis or treatment or both are wrong and should be re-evaluated. The temperature falls more slowly with gram-negative rod pneumonia and Legionnaires' pneumonia than with pneumococcal pneumonia. There is evidence in the literature to show that pneumococcal pneumonia can be treated with 1 to 3 days of treatment, but most physicians treat for 1 week. The same duration is appropriate for *Mycoplasma* pneumonia. Other pneumonias should be treated for 2 weeks. In all cases, the treatment can be changed from parenteral to oral therapy in the presence of a good response on the third or fourth day. If the response is good, no new cultures are necessary and no further chest x-rays are needed.

VIRAL RESPIRATORY INFECTIONS
method of
FREDERICK L. RUBEN, M.D.
University of Pittsburgh
Pittsburgh, Pennsylvania

Viral respiratory infections affect all age groups and are the most common type of acute illness seen by physicians in the United States. The principal virus families responsible for these illnesses are rhinovirus, coronavirus, respiratory syncytial virus, adenovirus, parainfluenza virus, and influenza virus. Other less common virus groups are herpes simplex type 1, Coxsackie virus, Epstein-Barr virus, echovirus, and poliovirus. Syndromes caused by these agents range from the common cold to severe pneumonia. Different viruses can cause the same clinical picture. Cultures or viral serology can identify the specific virus responsible, but until these diagnostic tests are more widely available, management is usually empiric. In many instances it is necessary to exclude the group A hemolytic streptococci, which can mimic a viral respiratory infection and should be treated with antibiotics.

Symptomatic Treatment

Rhinorrhea and Nasal Stuffiness

Nasal congestion can be adequately treated with topically applied sympathomimetic amines. Drops or sprays of 0.05 per cent oxymetazoline or of 0.1 per cent xylometazoline (each marketed under a variety of brand names) are available, with half-strength preparations also available for use in children. Prolonged or excessive use should be avoided to prevent rebound congestion with chronic swelling of nasal mucosa. These medications should not be used in patients who are taking monoamine oxidase (MAO) inhibitors or tricyclic antidepressants.

Oral sympathomimetic amines are generally less effective than the topical ones and may cause systemic side effects such as excessive nervousness or transient increases in blood pressure.

Antihistamines, although widely used for symptomatic relief of nasal congestion, are not conclusively effective.

Sore Throat

As indicated above, infection with group A streptococci can mimic viral respiratory disease. Sore throat is a symptom that is common with these bacteria. Although sore throat associated with viruses may be milder than that with the streptococci, it may require therapy. Either aspirin or acetaminophen is effective with viral sore throat; however, aspirin should not be used in children 16 years of age or younger because of the danger of inducing Reye's syndrome. If the sore throat is unusually severe, some relief may be obtained with Xylocaine viscous, usually 2 per cent. For adults 15 ml is a single dose as a gargle that may, if necessary, be swallowed. The pediatric dose must be individualized by the physician. Dosages should not exceed eight in 24 hours.

Cough

Cough suppression is generally not needed in patients with uncomplicated viral respiratory infection. Moderate to severe cough can be treated with either codeine or dextromethorphan hydrobromide. Codeine can be given orally every 4 hours at a dose of 10 mg in adults and 0.25 mg per kg in children. Dextromethorphan is given orally every 6 to 8 hours, 15 to 30 mg in adults and 0.25 mg per kg in children. Neither medication should be used in patients taking MAO inhibitors.

Headache and Myalgia

Headache and myalgia are not prominent except in patients with influenza, for which specific antiviral therapy is available. Mild analgesics as described above for sore throat will usually be effective.

Croup

In managing croup it is essential to rule out the presence of epiglottitis. The latter usually has a sudden onset and rapid progression in conjunction with high fever and dysphagia.

Most viral croup can be managed in the outpatient setting without therapeutic intervention. Signs of significant respiratory compromise such as restlessness, severe retractions, or cyanosis require that the patient be hospitalized for observation and for any necessary intervention to ensure adequate ventilation.

Symptomatic treatment of viral croup is directed at reducing airway edema. The most effective medication is racemic epinephrine as an aerosol. The aerosol solution is made by mixing 0.5 ml of racemic epinephrine with 3.5 ml of saline, and the mixture is given via aerosolization in a face mask. Use of IPPB, although more effective, is more difficult for giving the aerosol. The effect of therapy may last from 1 to 3 hours, and aerosols are usually given every 3 to 4 hours or more frequently if needed. Tachycardia is the most common side effect. These aerosols provide only temporary relief and do not alter the natural course of the disease. In general they should only be used in the hospitalized patient.

Croup tents and corticosteroids are probably not helpful. Cool mist does seem to be beneficial for acute spasmodic croup.

Specific Antiviral Therapy

Respiratory Syncytial Virus

Ribavirin (Virazole) as an aerosol has been approved for the treatment of RSV infection. Previously healthy patients with uncomplicated disease are not candidates for ribavirin aerosol. Patient populations with high morbidity and mortality from RSV disease such as patients with underlying cardiac or pulmonary disease, neonates, and immunocompromised patients may benefit from therapy. The drug is given as an aerosol via tent, head box, or face mask for 12 to 18 hours daily for 3 to 7 days. A small-particle aerosolizer is available from ICN Pharmaceuticals. Ribavirin is not administered through a ventilator.

Influenza Virus, Type A

Amantadine hydrochloride (Symmetrel) is effective for both prophylaxis and treatment of influenza A infections in adults and children. The use of amantadine in children less than 1 year of age has not been adequately evaluated. Amantadine dosage for prophylaxis and treatment should be based on age and renal function. For children 1 to 9 years of age 4.4 to 8.8 mg per kg per day, not to exceed 150 mg per day, is recommended, with the lower range of dose preferable to avoid toxicity. For adults 200 mg daily is suggested, but studies have shown efficacy at 100 mg daily, and this author prefers the lower dosage. For patients with reduced renal function the package insert gives the reduced dosages. Prophylaxis is generally needed for up to 6 weeks after the influenza outbreak is noted. Therapy with amantadine should begin within 24 to 48 hours of the onset of symptoms for maximum

benefit, and should continue for 5 to 7 days. A derivative of amantadine, rimantadine, may be available by 1989. It has the advantage of not needing dosage adjustments for renal function, but is otherwise comparable. Neither drug is effective against type B influenza viruses.

The toxicity and side effects of amantadine and rimantadine mainly affect the central nervous system (e.g., insomnia, drowsiness) or the gastrointestinal tract. Lower dosages reduce the likelihood of side effects.

It should be noted that both drugs have been more efficacious against influenza A than aspirin or placebo in controlled trials.

VIRAL AND MYCOPLASMAL PNEUMONIA

method of
STARKEY D. DAVIS, M.D.
Medical College of Wisconsin
Milwaukee, Wisconsin

For purposes of this discussion, pneumonia will be defined as including signs and symptoms of lower respiratory tract disease and pulmonary infiltrates on chest radiograph.

VIRAL PNEUMONIA

Viruses are unusual causes of pneumonia in healthy adults. Most pneumonias in adults are caused by *Streptococcus pneumoniae, Legionella pneumophila,* and other organisms.

Among the viruses, influenza A is the most common cause of pneumonia in adults. Influenza epidemics occur almost every winter. Large outbreaks often begin in December, reach a peak in January or February, and then may continue into the spring. Patients present with an abrupt onset of coryza, sore throat, fever, myalgia, headache, cough, and malaise. Pneumonia should be suspected as a complication of influenza when the patient becomes more acutely ill and develops signs of pulmonary disease. In those patients who develop viral pneumonia symptoms include dyspnea, hyperpnea, cyanosis, consolidation on chest radiograph, and a cough productive of scanty sputum. Some patients develop secondary pneumonia due to bacteria, most often *Streptococcus pneumoniae, Staphylococcus aureus,* or *Haemophilus influenzae.* These patients become more acutely ill and develop a cough productive of purulent sputum. Gram stain of sputum is helpful in identifying the organism. These patients require therapy with antibiotics.

Patients with influenza who develop pneumonia often have a severe, underlying cardiac disease such as mitral stenosis.

Uncommon causes of viral pneumonia in adults include varicella, measles, and adenovirus.

The most common causes of viral pneumonia in children include respiratory syncytial virus, parainfluenza virus, influenza A, and adenoviruses. Other rare causes include measles, varicella, and cytomegalovirus.

Respiratory syncytial virus causes severe pulmonary disease in infants. Patients have fever, cough, rhinitis, dyspnea, wheezing, rales, retractions, and hyperinflation visible on a chest radiograph. Most communities have annual winter epidemics of respiratory syncytial virus infection.

Treatment

A presumptive diagnosis of influenza can often be made with some confidence during annual influenza epidemics. Most patients require nothing more than general supportive care, good hydration, rest, and relief of fever and malaise with aspirin in adults or acetaminophen in children.

Amantadine (Symmetrel) can reduce fever and other signs and symptoms of influenza A infection if therapy is begin within 24 to 48 hours after the onset of the illness. Adults are given 100 mg twice a day for 5 to 7 days. Patients over 65 years of age should be given no more than 100 mg once daily. Dosage should be reduced in patients with renal disease or seizure disorders. Dosage in children aged 1 to 9 years is 5 to 8 mg per kg per day in one or two divided doses, with no more than 150 mg per day being given. Children 9 to 12 years of age are treated with 200 mg per day in one or two divided doses. Toxic effects include central nervous system irritability, such as nervousness, insomnia, and difficulty in concentration. Symptoms usually appear in the first 2 days of treatment. These reactions may be more severe in older patients.

Ribavirin (Virazole) has been shown to be efficacious in some trials for treatment of respiratory syncytial virus infection. The drug is given by aerosol for 3 to 5 days. Consideration can be given to using ribavirin in some infants who have severe respiratory syncytial virus infections and underlying cardiac or pulmonary disease. Ribavirin is not recommended for general use in patients with respiratory syncytial virus infection.

MYCOPLASMAL PNEUMONIA

Mycoplasma pneumoniae is the most common cause of pneumonia among school-age children and young adults. It is rare in adults over 40 years of age. Other common clinical presentations include tracheal bronchitis and pharyngitis. Infections are endemic and occur throughout the year. Epidemics among members of a household are common. Patients with pneumonia present with fever, cough, malaise, and rales. A few patients have ear involvement. A skin rash is common among children, most often an erythematous maculopapular rash. Patients with mycoplasmal pneumonia are seldom acutely ill, and few require hospitalization. About half the patients have a rise in cold agglutinin titer.

A diagnosis is most often made on clinical grounds because laboratory confirmation cannot be obtained soon enough. *Mycoplasma* should be suspected as the cause of pneumonia in a patient between 5 and 40 years of age who is not acutely ill.

Treatment

Both tetracycline and erythromycin are effective by the oral route. Adults are treated with 0.5 gram of erythromycin orally every 8 hours for 10 to 14 days. Children are treated with erythromycin 40 mg per kg per day for 10 to 14 days. The frequency of dosing depends on the formulation. Tetracycline may be given to adolescents or adults in the dosage of 250 mg orally every 6 hours for 10 to 14 days. Tetracycline is not the antibiotic of choice for children under 12 years of age.

LEGIONELLOSIS
(Legionnaires' Disease and Pontiac Fever)

method of
ROBERT R. MUDER, M.D.
The Mercy Hospital of Pittsburgh
Pittsburgh, Pennsylvania

The family Legionellaceae includes some two dozen species of gram-negative bacilli. The majority (approximately 90 per cent) of human infections are caused by a single species, *Legionella pneumophila*. The Legionellaceae are unusual among the common etiologic agents of human pneumonia in that they are aquatic organisms. They are common in natural and manmade aquatic habitats, and can be readily isolated from cooling towers and the hot-water systems of buildings. Epidemics of disease have been linked to environmental sources of the organism; the source in sporadic cases is frequently uncertain. Although inhalation of contaminated aerosols and aspiration of contaminated water are postulated mechanisms of infection, in most reported outbreaks of disease the means of transmission has not been convincingly demonstrated.

Recognized risk factors for legionellosis include advanced age, male sex, and cigarette smoking. In addition, immunosuppressive therapy with corticosteroids and/or cytotoxic agents poses a major risk. Hospital-acquired pneumonia in the general inpatient population has been increasingly recognized. In addition to the aforementioned factors, tracheal intubation and surgery may be associated with an increased risk of nosocomial legionellosis.

Diagnosis

Two distinct forms of legionellosis exist. Nonpneumonic legionellosis (Pontiac fever) is a self-limited flu-like illness that results from intense exposure to contaminated aerosols containing *Legionella*. Twelve to 36 hours after exposure, the patient develops fever, chills, headache, and myalgia; upper respiratory symptoms may also occur. Neither physical nor radiographic signs of pneumonia are present, and the symptoms resolve over several days without specific therapy. Diagnosis is by demonstration of seroconversion to the responsible *Legionella* species. It is uncertain whether this syndrome is due to infection or to a hypersensitivity response.

Pneumonic legionellosis (Legionnaires' disease) was originally described as a distinctive clinical syndrome. Multisystem involvement was reported to be a typical feature, with a high incidence of complications such as renal failure, central nervous system symptoms, diarrhea, and abnormalities of hepatic function. However, subsequent comparative studies indicate that the signs and symptoms of Legionnaires' disease are not sufficiently distinctive to permit a differentiation from other pneumonias on clinical grounds alone. As the organism is not readily visualized by Gram stain and is fastidious in its growth requirements, definitive diagnosis depends on the use of specialized diagnostic tests.

Culture of sputum or tracheal aspirate using special media, such as buffered charcoal yeast extract (BCYE) agar with added antibiotics, will detect the organism in 80 to 90 per cent of cases; specificity approaches 100 per cent. When clinical circumstances warrant, bronchoscopy or lung biopsy may yield a diagnostic specimen. Although *Legionella* organisms are not detectable when blood is cultured by the usual methods, special techniques may detect bacteremia in up to 40 per cent of cases. The most rapid means of diagnosis is the direct demonstration of organisms in respiratory secretions, pleural fluid, or lung tissue by direct fluorescent antibody (DFA) staining. The test, which can be performed in one hour, is highly specific when used in the diagnosis of *L. pneumophila* infection. It has a sensitivity of only 40 to 70 per cent when applied to sputum or tracheal aspirate. Its reliability in the diagnosis of infection caused by other *Legionella* species is not precisely known. Seroconversion occurs in 80 to 90 per cent of patients, and usually requires 2 to 6 weeks. Specificity is high for *L. pneumophila* serogroup 1, the most common etiologic agent of Legionnaires' disease.

Sensitivity and specificity are less certain for other *Legionella* species. Promising diagnostic techniques that are not yet widely available include the detection of *Legionella* in clinical specimens using a radiolabeled DNA probe and immunologic detection of *Legionella* antigens in urine.

Treatment

Legionella are intracellular parasites that are capable of multiplying within phagocytic cells. Although they are sensitive in vitro to a wide variety of antibiotics, agents that fail to reach adequate intracellular levels, such as cephalosporins and aminoglycosides, have poor in vivo activity. Agents that penetrate intracellularly, such as erythromycin, rifampin, and the newer quinolone derivatives, have demonstrable in vivo activity against intracellular *Legionella* in experimental models.

There are no controlled trials of therapy in human legionellosis; most clinical experience is with use of erythromycin. In patients hospitalized with Legionnaires' disease, erythromycin 1 gram intravenously every 6 hours is recommended as initial therapy. The dosage should be reduced in patients with advanced renal or hepatic failue to avoid ototoxicity. Once the patient has clearly responded clinically, oral therapy at a dose of 500 mg every 6 hours may be substituted. The duration of antibiotic therapy should be at least 3 weeks; shorter courses may be associated with relapse, especially in immunocompromised patients. Erythromycin inhibits but does not kill intracellular *Legionella*. Therefore, in patients who are receiving corticosteroid or other immunosuppressive therapy, or who have extensive or multilobar pulmonary involvement, oral rifampin* should be added in a dose of 600 mg twice daily. Rifampin should not be used as sole therapy because of the possibility of emergence of resistant organisms.

Tetracycline has been reported to be effective in human legionellosis, but clinical experience is less extensive than with erythromycin. The combination of trimethoprim-sulfamethoxazole and rifampin has been reported to be effective when erythromycin has failed. The newer quinolones, such as ciprofloxacin, are promising agents that require further evaluation in human legionellosis.

Legionnaires' disease is notable in that the radiographic findings may initially worsen in the face of appropriate therapy and a good clinical response. Thus, extension of the radiographic infiltrates early in the course is not in and of

---

*This use of rifampin is not listed in the manufacturer's directive.

itself a reason to alter therapy if the patient is otherwise responding. Cavitation of infiltrates is commonly seen in patients receiving corticosteroids; these cavities do not ordinarily require specific intervention. Small to moderate pleural effusions are frequent, and usually resolve spontaneously. Empyema ocurs occasionally, and requires prompt tube drainage.

Patients may undergo deterioration in pulmonary function even after institution of appropriate therapy, especially in the presence of immunocompromise or pre-existing pulmonary disease. Careful attention to oxygenation is needed; mechanical ventilation may be required.

Nonpneumonic legionellosis (Pontiac fever) resolves spontaneously in several days and does not require specific antibiotic therapy.

Prognosis

Mortality in previously healthy, treated patients is low. Patients who are immunocompromised or who have serious underlying illnesses are at higher risk; mortality in hospital-acquired Legionnaires' disease may exceed 25 per cent. Delay in diagnosis and in institution of specific therapy may result in increased mortality.

Prevention

The most effective means of prevention is the avoidance of exposure of susceptible persons to potentially infectious environmental sources of *Legionella*. This is problematic for several reasons. *Legionella* are ubiquitous in the environment, and the risk posed by a given reservoir of organisms is uncertain. In addition, the source of infection is frequently not determined, especially in sporadic cases. If cases of Legionnaires' disease are epidemiologically linked to an environmental source of the organism, an attempt should be made to eliminate the source. Studies suggest that the presence of *Legionella* in a hospital water system is a risk factor for nosocomial legionellosis. Eradication measures may be warranted, and should be strongly considered if cases of nosocomial legionellosis are documented.

Erythromycin prophylaxis has been used to prevent infection among highly immunosuppressed patients in a hospital with a high incidence of Legionnaires' disease. This approach may be useful when such patients are exposed to a known source of infection that cannot be eliminated. Prophylactic therapy is not recommended in most circumstances, however.

PULMONARY EMBOLISM

method of
PETER F. FEDULLO, M.D.
Veterans Administration Medical Center,
University of California Medical Center
San Diego, California

Retrospective analysis suggests that pulmonary thromboembolism is responsible for approximately 200,000 deaths in the United States annually. The incidence of fatal plus nonfatal emboli probably exceeds 600,000. The majority of deaths due to pulmonary embolic disease occur either within 1 hour of the acute event or in those in whom the diagnosis is not considered until autopsy.

Diagnosis

It is important to recognize that the clinical presentation of pulmonary embolism, with the exception of massive pulmonary embolic events, is often nonspecific. This is especially true in the elderly and in those with underlying cardiopulmonary disease, in which the manifestations of pulmonary embolism are often obscured. This lack of specificity of clinical symptoms and signs is a major contributing factor in the unnecessary mortality of the disease. Pulmonary ventilation/perfusion scanning, often interpreted in terms of "probabilities," can provide only two meaningful pieces of information: (1) a normal perfusion scan excludes the diagnosis of pulmonary embolism; (2) a scan characterized by multiple, mismatched, segmental or larger defects suggests the diagnosis with a high degree (90 per cent) of certainty. Other ventilation/perfusion scan patterns (single defects, matched defects, subsegmental defects, defects associated with corresponding radiographic abnormalities) can neither suggest nor exclude the diagnosis with reasonable certainty. Recent evidence suggests that scan patterns once considered "low or intermediate probability" are associated with a clinically unacceptable incidence of angiographically documented pulmonary embolism.

Additional diagnostic procedures, when clinically indicated, must be pursued. Pulmonary angiography remains the "gold standard" for the diagnosis of pulmonary embolism. The diagnosis of acute venous thrombosis, although not confirming that a pulmonary embolic event has occurred, has the same therapeutic implications as a positive pulmonary angiogram. Negative lower extremity studies, however, cannot exclude the diagnosis of pulmonary embolism. Approximately 30 per cent of patients with angiographically documented pulmonary emboli will have negative venographic results.

Treatment

Prophylaxis

Over the past decade, a number of prophylactic methods have been introduced into clinical practice. In order to apply these methods optimally, the relative risk of thromboembolism must be determined for the individual patient and appropriate prophylaxis applied based on the degree of risk. Factors that increase risk include (1) general surgical procedures lasting longer than 30 minutes, (2) general surgical procedures in patients over the age of 40, (3) lower extremity orthopedic procedures, (4) transabdominal prostatectomy, (5) a prior history of venous thromboembolism, (6) malignancy, (7) obesity, (8) prolonged immobilization, and (9) chronic congestive heart failure.

Low-dose heparin, 5000 units subcutaneously every 12 hours, has proved effective in reducing the incidence of venous thrombosis, pulmonary embolism, and fatal pulmonary embolism in patients undergoing abdominal and thoracic surgical procedures. Low-dose heparin should be started 2 hours prior to surgery and continued until the patient is fully ambulatory. Low-dose heparin prophylaxis is also effective in reducing the incidence of venous thrombosis in the following nonsurgical patients: (1) patients admitted with myocardial infarction, respiratory failure, or a prior history of venous thromboembolism; (2) those with obesity, congestive heart failure, or malignancy; and (3) patients who are immobilized for extended periods of time. Low-dose heparin, by accelerating the inhibitory activity of antithrombin III on factor X, is able to inhibit thrombus formation without inducing a systemic anticoagulant effect. Although bleeding complications with low-dose heparin are unusual, populations exist in which even this low risk is unacceptable. These include patients undergoing ophthalmic, spinal, or neurosurgical procedures; trauma victims; patients with an underlying bleeding diathesis; and patients with a hemorrhagic stroke. In these patients, the use of intermittent pneumatic compression stockings (IPC) serves as an essentially risk-free and effective alternative. Intermittent pneumatic compression devices also appear to be the prophylactic method of choice in patients undergoing elective knee surgery and in those undergoing urologic procedures. Prior to placement of IPC, noninvasive evaluation of the lower extremities should be performed to exclude the possibility of asymptomatic venous thrombi, which could be dislodged and embolized by the squeezing action of the stockings. The use of IPC is also contraindicated by advanced peripheral arterial disease.

Patients undergoing neurosurgical or genitourinary procedures are considered to be at moderate risk. Patients with multiple medical risk factors are also considered to be at moderate risk. Available studies indicate that the risk of venous thrombosis and its sequelae escalates as risk factors accumulate. Unfortunately, quantitative data about the additive effect of risk factors in specific populations are not available. In these patients, the frequency of subcutaneous heparin can be increased to an every-8-hour schedule or intermittent compression stockings can be added to subcutaneous heparin administered every 12 hours. The combination of heparin-dihydroxyergotamine appears to have an increased prophylactic effect when compared with heparin alone in patients with multiple risk factors. Vasospastic reactions to dihydroxyergotamine can occur but are rare.

High-risk patients include (1) those with a recent history of venous thromboembolic disease who require surgery, (2) those undergoing lower extremity orthopedic surgery, and (3) those undergoing extensive abdominal or pelvic surgery for malignant disease. In these patients, low-dose heparin administered every 8 to 12 hours in addition to intermittent pneumatic compression should be used. In the high-risk orthopedic population, subcutaneous heparin, administered every 8 hours and adjusted to maintain the activated partial thromboplastin time (aPTT), 6 hours after the subcutaneous dose, between 32 and 36 seconds, has also proved effective. A strategy of "two-step" warfarin therapy has proved effective in patients undergoing elective hip or knee surgery. Warfarin is administered for 2 weeks prior to surgery in a dose sufficient to prolong the prothrombin time 1.5 to 3.0 seconds longer than control and then to 1.5 times control value immediately after surgery. Aspirin has not proved effective as a prophylactic agent. Other prophylactic options include low-molecular-weight dextran, alone or in combination with intermittent compression stockings, and oral anticoagulation.

The "intensity" of any prophylactic regimen must be based on the degree of risk in the individual patient. The higher the thromboembolic risk, the more urgent the need for prophylaxis and the higher the acceptable risk of the prophylactic choice. Selection of any regimen depends on one's view of safety and efficacy data.

General Measures

Heparin remains the mainstay of therapy for pulmonary embolism not associated with hemodynamic compromise. With a strong suspicion of embolism based on clinical findings and routine laboratory tests, therapy should be instituted immediately, without awaiting diagnostic confirmation, unless anticoagulation places the patient at clear risk.

Three methods of heparin administration have

been advocated: continuous intravenous, intermittent intravenous, and subcutaneous. Continuous intravenous administration has become the method of choice despite lack of definitive evidence that it is safer or more effective than the alternative methods. This method maintains more consistent blood levels, allows for simpler monitoring, and makes dosage adjustments easier. In the adult patient, a 10,000-unit bolus should be administered, followed by a continuous infusion of 1000 units per hour; dose adjustments are determined by subsequent aPTT results. It is currently uncertain whether the risk of hemorrhage (the principal complication of heparin therapy) is related to the degree of anticoagulation as reflected by the results of any monitoring assay. Rather, bleeding appears to be principally related to factors such as the coexistence of a focal (duodenal ulcer disease) or systemic (uremia) bleeding predisposition. Current recommendations, although based on incomplete and potentially misleading data, suggest that the aPTT be prolonged to 1.5 to 2.5 times the control value. Since maintenance of the aPTT within a rigidly defined range does not appear to improve either efficacy or safety of the drug, frequent dosage adjustments are not necessary. The need for daily aPTTs beyond the first 3 or 4 days of therapy remains unclear. Heparin requirements tend to decrease during the course of therapy with a resultant increase in aPTT levels. Platelet counts should be monitored during heparin prophylaxis and full-dose heparin therapy. Therapy is maintained for 7 to 10 days to allow dissolution and/or organization of the embolus to occur. Bed rest is recommended for at least 3 to 5 days to avoid the potential of dislodging and embolizing residual lower extremity thrombi.

The decision to utilize thrombolytic agents must be weighed against the potential complications associated with their use. Despite extensive study and a clear demonstration that these agents can enhance the rate but not the total extent of thrombolysis, it has not been clearly established that their use alters short- or long-term morbidity and mortality associated with pulmonary embolism.

It is in patients with pulmonary embolism associated with hemodynamic compromise that thrombolytic agents may offer a therapeutic advantage. It is essential that the diagnosis of pulmonary embolism be angiographically confirmed. It is also essential that any contraindications to the use of thrombolytic agents be excluded. These agents increase bleeding risk through the induction of a systemic thrombolytic state. Recent surgery or organ biopsy, trauma (including cardiopulmonary resuscitation), recent stroke, severe hypertension, advanced renal or hepatic disease, and diabetic retinopathy are contraindications to their use.

Two agents are currently available: streptokinase and urokinase. The potential role of newer thrombolytic agents, such as tissue plasminogen activator, which may pose less hemorrhagic risk, remains to be established. If the decision to use thrombolytic agents is made, it is essential that there be a clear understanding of the details of therapy. Ideally, the patient should be monitored in an intensive care setting during the period of infusion. Care should be taken to minimize arterial and venous punctures; pressure should be applied to recent puncture sites. A carefully dressed indwelling arterial catheter can be used for pressure measurements and to obtain blood samples. Central venous catheters, if necessary, should be inserted via a brachial approach. Support with other therapeutic modalities, including supplemental oxygen, intravenous fluids, pressor agents, and antiarrhythmics, should not be neglected.

Heparin is discontinued prior to initiating thrombolytic therapy. Streptokinase, 250,000 units, is infused over 30 minutes. This is followed by 100,000 units per hour for 24 hours using a constant infusion pump. Prior to delivery of the loading dose, 100 mg of hydrocortisone and 50 mg of diphenhydramine (Benadryl) can be administered intravenously to reduce the febrile and allergic responses to the streptococcal antigens. Urokinase, 4400 units per kg of body weight, is infused over 10 minutes. This is followed by a maintenance dose of 4400 units per kg per hour for 12 hours. Unlike monitoring during heparin therapy, there is no discrete therapeutic "range" to attain. It is only necessary to determine that a systemic thrombolytic state has been reached. This can be determined by measurement of the thrombin time, euglobulin lysis time, or aPTT. Following the infusion, heparin should be restarted when the aPTT falls to 1.5 times the control value. Thrombolytic therapy does not replace heparin therapy; it is used as an adjunct to it. When used, thrombolytic agents must be followed by a standard course of intravenous heparin therapy.

Emergency pulmonary embolectomy should be considered only if evidence of severe hemodynamic compromise due to embolism is present that is not responsive to supportive measures and thrombolytic agents. The mortality with the procedure is high; it should be attempted only if the equipment and expert personnel required for cardiopulmonary bypass and emergency embolectomy are available.

Postembolic Prophylaxis

The rationale for providing long-term protection is clear: to prevent recurrence of venous thrombosis and, therefore, potential recurrence of embolism. Early recurrence rates are sufficiently high to justify a 6-week course of outpatient anticoagulation in all who have experienced an embolic episode. The only possible exception includes a situation in which the predisposition to venous thrombosis has been identified and eliminated, lower extremity venous studies and perfusion scan are normal, and the risk with outpatient anticoagulation is high.

Outpatient anticoagulation should be continued for a minimum of 6 weeks. Since persistence of venous outflow obstruction and pulmonary vascular obstruction represent new risk factors, the patient is re-evaluated at 6 weeks with a perfusion scan and impedance plethysmography (IPG). In those with negative IPG and normal or near-normal perfusion scan, anticoagulation is discontinued. If venous outflow obstruction persists or if the perfusion scan remains abnormal, anticoagulation is continued for an additional 6 to 12 weeks, at which time the patient is re-evaluated. Although persistently abnormal results suggest some risk of recurrence, small but unknown, a patient-interactive decision is made, usually resulting in discontinuation of anticoagulation. There are no firm data to suggest that the benefits of prolonging anticoagulation beyond this time period justify the potential risks.

In patients with an irreversible predisposition to venous thrombosis and in those who have had documented recurrent episodes, indefinite anticoagulation is recommended.

Once the decision to provide postembolic prophylaxis is made, two options are available: oral anticoagulation with warfarin sodium or "adjusted" subcutaneous heparin. On the basis of currently available information, the two options appear equally effective and safe if administered and monitored properly. In order to be effective, the dose of subcutaneous heparin must be adjusted to maintain the mid-interval (6 hours after injection) aPTT at 1.5 times control value. In most patients, the dose of heparin approximates 10,000 units every 12 hours. "Standard" doses of heparin (5000 units every 12 hours) have not proved effective as a means of postembolic prophylaxis. The use of subcutaneous heparin provides a simpler inhospital transition and does not require frequent outpatient monitoring. Available studies do not indicate that osteoporosis is a significant risk. Heparin effect can be interrupted more promptly than warfarin effect. This method, however, does require the inconvenience of twice-daily injections. The individual patient, and practical considerations, will determine whether this option is a realistic one.

Oral anticoagulation with warfarin sodium should be started 5 days prior to discontinuing intravenous heparin therapy. The decision to use warfarin should be made early, so that the prothrombin time (PT) is in a therapeutic range for several days before heparin is discontinued. An early decision avoids unnecessary prolongation of the hospital stay as well as the need for large "loading doses" of warfarin. Therapy is usually started with 10 mg of warfarin per day for several days and then adjusted based on PT results. Recent evidence suggests that maintaining the PT at 1.3 to 1.5 times control value is as effective in reducing recurrence rates as maintaining the PT at two times control value as previously recommended. This lower therapeutic target is also associated with a substantially reduced rate of bleeding complications, approaching that attained with the adjusted subcutaneous heparin option.

Interruption of the Inferior Vena Cava

Inferior vena caval interruption is considered for patients with proven embolism if clinical and perfusion scan assessments suggest that an immediate recurrence may be fatal. It is also indicated when significant bleeding, or the risk of bleeding, contraindicates anticoagulant use. Embolic recurrence is not an absolute indication for interruption as long as a substantial unobstructed pulmonary vascular bed is present and there is no evidence of cardiopulmonary compromise. Heparin, although capable of preventing thrombus propagation, cannot guarantee against early embolic recurrence from residual lower extremity thrombotic material. Recurrent symptoms during the course of therapy may represent fragmentation and distal migration of the original embolic material as organization and lysis occur. "Heparin failure" should not occur if adequate anticoagulation with heparin has been maintained.

Ligation and plication procedures should be avoided. Anesthesia and surgery pose a significant risk. Recurrence rates through collateral channels are high, and substantial morbidity ensues from subsequent venous stasis. Ligation procedures can result in acute, life-threatening hypotension from the sudden decrease in circulating blood volume. Transvenous intracaval devices (Mobin-Uddin umbrella and Greenfield filter) can be placed with the use of local anesthesia and guided into position under fluoroscopic monitoring. The Greenfield filter appears to have a higher patency rate than the Mobin-Uddin umbrella and seems to be technically easier to insert.

The procedure employed, however, should be that with which the vascular surgeon is most familiar. The Greenfield filter can be placed via a percutaneous femoral approach. Prior to placement, venography must be performed to exclude the presence of asymptomatic femoral or inferior vena caval thrombosis.

Chronic Thromboembolic Pulmonary Hypertension

The prognosis of the patient with pulmonary embolism in whom therapy is properly instituted is excellent. Morbidity following embolism is uncommon, since embolic resolution is the rule. On rare occasions, however, resolution of emboli does not occur. If residual pulmonary vascular obstruction is substantial, the patient may present, months or years later, with evidence of pulmonary hypertension or right ventricular failure.

Many of these patients are unable to provide a history of a discrete thromboembolic event. Many are misdiagnosed as having primary pulmonary hypertension or interstitial lung disease. Chest x-ray and electrocardiographic findings are consistent with right ventricular hypertrophy. Pulmonary function tests may be normal, or they reveal a restricted pattern. Ventilation/perfusion scanning appears to offer a means of differentiating primary pulmonary hypertension (PPH) from large-vessel, thromboembolic pulmonary hypertension (TEPH). In PPH, perfusion scans are normal or demonstrate a "mottled" pattern; in TEPH, multiple, mismatched, or segmental or larger defects are invariably present. Pulmonary angiography is indicated in those patients with perfusion scans consistent with TEPH, since perfusion scanning cannot provide information concerning anatomic extent of disease and frequently underestimates the true angiographic extent of pulmonary vascular obstruction.

Although these patients should receive chronic anticoagulation and an inferior vena caval filter should be placed to prevent repeat embolization, thrombolytic therapy is not indicated because of the chronic, fibrotic nature of the thrombi. Patients with main or lobar pulmonary artery involvement, documented by angiography or angioscopy, may be candidates for pulmonary thromboendarterectomy. Patients with suspected TEPH should be evaluated at an institution where the staff is familiar with this form of pulmonary hypertension. Unique difficulties complicate the preoperative evaluation and postoperative care of these patients. Surgical intervention involves a true thromboendarterectomy of chronic, endothelialized thrombus rather than an embolectomy. Results in patients with surgically accessible disease (main or lobar pulmonary arteries) have been excellent, allowing cure of this otherwise fatal form of pulmonary hypertension.

SARCOIDOSIS

method of
ROBERT P. BAUGHMAN, M.D.
University of Cincinnati
Cincinnati, Ohio

Sarcoidosis is a multisystem disease that can present to the physician in several different ways. The most common manifestations are pulmonary, but other organs can be involved. Treatment for sarcoidosis is determined by the level of involvement of the various organs after complete evaluation. There are some absolute indications for therapy, but in most manifestations of the disease, treatment depends on the level of disease activity (Table 1). In addition, therapy if instituted is for acute disease, although some manifestations of the disease will need chronic suppressive therapy after acute treatment.

Treatment

Acute Disease

For acute disease to be treated with systemic steroids, I start with prednisone 40 mg daily for 2 months followed by 20 mg of prednisone for an additional 4 months. After that point, I try to taper the patient off the steroids. Most patients are treated for a total of 18 to 24 months with some dose of prednisone. After tapering of steroids, the patient is closely watched for signs of recurrence of disease. Relapse, if it occurs, is usually seen between 3 and 6 months of stopping steroids. However, patients may have a delayed relapse, and I follow patients with inactive sarcoidosis every 6 months over the next few years.

Other doses of prednisone have been used, especially the use of alternate-day steroids. This regimen is most successful for the more sensitive manifestations of sarcoidosis, especially hypercalcemia.

Chloroquine has been successfully used in some

TABLE 1. **Manifestations of Sarcoidosis and Requirement for Treatment**

Manifestation	Treatment
Asymptomatic	None
Pulmonary	None to chronic
Skin	None to chronic
Hypercalcemia	Acute
Eye	Acute
Cardiac	Chronic
Central nervous system	Chronic

TABLE 2. **Proposed Treatment Decisions for Patients with Pulmonary Sarcoidosis**

Pulmonary Function Tests	Symptoms	Gallium Scan	Treatment
Normal	Absent	Positive	Watch
Mildly reduced	Absent	Negative	Watch
Mildly reduced	Present	Positive	Treat
Moderately reduced	Present	Positive	Treat
Moderately reduced	Present	Negative	Treat

forms of sarcoid (not listed in manufacturers' directives). It is often used in patients with only skin sarcoid, since the drug has fewer side effects than prednisone. The dose ranges from 250 mg twice a day to 200 mg on alternate days. If a patient is on chloroquine, eye examinations should be performed on a regular basis to watch for the irreversible retinopathy and blindness that is occasionally seen with chloroquine use.

Chronic Disease

For chronic sarcoidosis, once the disease is under control with higher dosage of prednisone, patients are treated with some dose of corticosteroids, usually 5 to 10 mg every other day for years.

Immunosuppressive drugs have been used in some patients with sarcoidosis in an attempt to avoid steroids, although the use of these agents is not listed in the manufacturers' directives. Several drugs have been used, with the largest experience reported to date being for chlorambucil (Leukeran). Methotrexate (Folex, Mexate), in dosages similar to those used for rheumatoid arthritis, has also been used with success. The drug can be given orally at a dose of 5 to 10 mg weekly to biweekly. It does not appear necessary to achieve neutropenia. Its major drawback seems to be its slow onset of action; it appears to take over a month of therapy before the symptoms of sarcoidosis are significantly relieved.

In patients who are diagnosed incidentally on biopsy, there is no indication for treatment. These patients should be followed for possible disease activity, usually pulmonary symptoms. Patients should be followed by serial examinations and chest roentgenograms for 2 years after initial diagnosis.

Pulmonary Involvement

The lungs are involved in about 90 per cent of patients with sarcoidosis. The extent of disease can vary, ranging from an asymptomatic state to irreversible pulmonary fibrosis and cor pulmonale. In assessing patients with pulmonary sarcoidosis, the use of gallium scan and bronchoalveolar lavage (BAL) fluid obtained during flexible fiberoptic bronchoscopy has recently been studied as a means of assessing patients' need for ther-

apy. Table 2 summarizes a few possible presentations of pulmonary sarcoidosis and how gallium scan and BAL can be useful in deciding about therapy. Gallium uptake in the lung or an increased percentage of T-helper lymphocytes in the BAL fluid appears to tell us the same thing, that the patient has active inflammation in the lung. However, the patient's symptoms and pulmonary function tests (especially the lung volume) are a major factor in deciding whether to treat.

Acute pulmonary disease is usually treated with systemic steroids. The use of aerosol steroids has been suggested, but more information is necessary. If patients show evidence of deterioration of pulmonary function more than 2 years after their initial presentation, or evidence of cor pulmonale, I assume they have chronic sarcoidosis. I therefore would treat them for chronic disease as outlined above.

Skin Involvement

Erythema nodosum is not disfiguring, but the associated arthralgias can be bothersome. These often respond to nonsteroidals such as ibuprofen or aspirin. Skin lesions of the face, especially lupus pernio, require specific therapy. If areas of disease are small, creams or intradermal injections may control disease. Chloroquine is useful for skin sarcoidosis, mainly because it is easy to evaluate this drug's efficacy. Some aggressive forms of skin sarcoid, especially lupus pernio, require systemic steroids. Lupus pernio has a high frequency of relapse and can be a troublesome, lifetime manifestation of disease. Methotrexate appears to be a useful drug for this problem.

Hypercalcemia

This unusual but specific problem of sarcoidosis is due to alteration in vitamin D metabolism by the granulomas themselves. In patients with hypercalcemia, increased calcium or vitamin D in the diet or increased sunshine may make the hypercalcemia worse and should be avoided. Steroids are quite effective in treating the hypercalcemia. A recent report suggests chloroquine can also be useful.

Ocular Involvement

Patients with eye symptoms are best treated in consultation with an ophthalmologist. Slit-lamp examination is crucial in determining whether a posterior uveitis is present. If not, and if the patient has only conjunctivitis or anterior uveitis, optic drops of steroids may lead to a good response. However, if posterior uveitis or retinitis is present, the patient will probably require systemic steroids.

Cardiac Involvement

Documentation of cardiac disease is often difficult. Patients may present with cardiac arrhythmias or heart failure. In patients with known sarcoidosis, clinical symptoms including palpitations and congestive heart failure may require further work-up. In patients with documented or strongly suspected cardiac sarcoid, the treatment of choice is long-term steroids.

Central Nervous System Involvement

Involvement of the central nervous system usually manifests itself as a cranial nerve palsy; however, diabetes insipidus and seizures can also be manifestations. Treatment here is usually steroid therapy. It may take several months before any response is noted. In cases in which disease is entirely limited to the brain, radiation therapy has been tried with limited success.

SILICOSIS

method of
JOHN E. PARKER, M.D.
Morgantown, West Virginia

Silicosis is a fibrotic disease of the lungs caused by inhalation, retention, and pulmonary reaction to crystalline silica. Silica, or silicon dioxide, is the predominant component of the earth's crust. The three important crystalline forms of silica are quartz, tridymite, and cristobalite. These forms are also called "free silica" to distinguish them from the silicates. The silica content in different rock formations, such as sandstone, granite, and slate, varies from 20 to nearly 100 per cent. Occupational exposure to silica particles of respirable size (0.5 to 5 microns) is associated with mining, quarrying, drilling, and tunneling operations. Silica exposure is also a potential hazard to sandblasters, stonecutters, and pottery, foundry, and refractory workers. The true prevalence of the disease is unknown, but more than one million workers in the United States are employed in trades at risk for the development of silicosis.

The precise pathogenic mechanism for the development of silicosis remains uncertain. Abundant evidence implicates an interaction of the pulmonary alveolar macrophage and silica particles deposited in the lung. These cells mobilize and ingest the silica particles into an intracellular phagosome. It is proposed that surface properties of the silica particle cause disruption of the membrane around the phagocytic vacuole. This releases cytotoxic lysosomal enzymes within the macrophage, resulting in cell death and leaving extracellular crystalline silica particles still free to repeat the cycle. Macrophages also release chemotactic factors that result in further cellular response by polymorphonuclear leukocytes, lymphocytes, and additional macrophages. Fibroblast-stimulating factors are released that promote hyalinization and collagen deposition. The resulting pathologic silicotic lesion is the hyaline nodule, containing a central acellular zone with free silica surrounded by whorls of collagen and fibroblasts, and an active peripheral zone composed of macrophages, fibroblasts, plasma cells, and additional free silica. Impaired macrophage function also plays a role in susceptibility to infectious organisms such as *Mycobacterium tuberculosis* and *Nocardia asteroides*.

Forms of Disease

Simple silicosis is often asymptomatic and presents as a radiographic abnormality with small (<10 mm), rounded opacities predominantly in the upper lobes. A history of 20 years or more since onset of exposure is common. Pulmonary function testing may be normal or may show mild restriction. Less commonly, mild obstruction to airflow or reduced diffusing capacity may be present. Simple silicosis progresses to complicated disease in 20 to 30 per cent of cases.

Complicated silicosis, also called progressive massive fibrosis, is more likely to present with exertional dyspnea. This form of disease is characterized by nodular opacities greater than 1 cm on chest radiograph and commonly will involve reduced carbon monoxide diffusing capacity, reduced arterial oxygen tension at rest or with exercise, and marked restriction on spirometry or lung volume measurement. Distortion of the bronchial tree may also lead to airway obstruction and productive cough. Recurrent bacterial infection not unlike that seen in bronchiectasis may occur. Weight loss and cavitation of the large opacities should prompt concern for tuberculosis or other mycobacterial infection. Pneumothorax may be a life-threatening complication, since the fibrotic lung may be difficult to re-expand. Hypoxemic respiratory failure with cor pulmonale is a common terminal event.

Accelerated silicosis may appear after more intense exposure of shorter (5 to 15 years) duration. Symptoms, radiographic findings, and physiologic measurements are similar to those seen in the chronic form. Deterioration in lung function is more rapid, and as many as 25 per cent of patients with accelerated disease may develop mycobacterial infection. Autoimmune disease, including scleroderma and rheumatoid arthritis, is seen with silicosis, often of the accelerated type. The progression of radiographic abnormalities and functional impairment can be very rapid when autoimmune disease is associated with silicosis.

Acute silicosis may develop within 6 months to 2

years of massive silica exposure. Dramatic dyspnea, weakness, and weight loss are often presenting symptoms. The radiographic findings of diffuse alveolar filling differ from those in the more chronic forms of silicosis. Histologic findings similar to pulmonary alveolar proteinosis have been described, and extrapulmonary (renal and hepatic) abnormalities are reported. Rapid progression to severe hypoxemic ventilatory failure is the usual course. Mycobacterial infection in acute silicosis is even more likely than in chronic or accelerated disease.

Prevention

There is no specific therapy for silicosis. Prevention remains the cornerstone of eliminating this occupational lung disease. The education of workers and employers regarding the hazards of silica dust exposure and measures to control exposure are important. The use of improved ventilation and local exhaust, process enclosure, wet techniques, air-supplied personal protection respirators, and, where possible, industrial substitution of agents less hazardous than silica all reduce exposure.

Silicosis is a reportable disease in many states. If silicosis is recognized in a worker, removal from continuing exposure is advisable. Unfortunately, the disease may progress even without further silica exposure. Additionally, finding a case of acute or accelerated silicosis should prompt notification of state or federal agencies, such as the Occupational Safety and Health Administration (OSHA), Mine Safety and Health Administration (MSHA), or the National Institute for Occupational Safety and Health (NIOSH) to obtain workplace evaluation to protect other workers also at risk.

Treatment

When prevention has been unsuccessful and silicosis has developed, therapy is directed largely at complications of the disease. Therapeutic measures are similar to those commonly used in the management of airway obstruction, infection, pneumothorax, hypoxemia, and respiratory failure complicating other pulmonary disease. Historically, the inhalation of aerosolized aluminum has been unsuccessful as a specific therapy for silicosis. Polyvinyl pyridine-N-oxide, a polymer that has protected experiment animals, is not available for use in humans. Search for a specific therapy for silicosis has to date been unrewarding.

If obstructive airway disease with bronchospasm develops, bronchodilator therapy is indicated. Inhaled selective beta$_2$-adrenergic agents, such as albuterol (Ventolin, Proventil), two inhalations every 4 to 6 hours, may be helpful. Oral long-acting theophylline preparations, given twice daily, to achieve a blood level of 10 to 20 micrograms per ml are also beneficial alone or in combination with inhaled beta agonists.

Episodes of acute bronchitis, commonly caused by *Streptococcus pneumoniae* or *Haemophilus influenzae,* can be treated with ampicillin 250 to 500 mg every 6 hours for a 10-day course. Tetracycline, erythromycin, and trimethoprim-sulfamethoxazole are also useful for treatment of initial or recurrent episodes of infectious bronchitis. If infection does not improve on empiric therapy, re-evaluation with sputum Gram stain, culture, and sensitivity tests should be performed. Pneumococcal and influenza vaccinations are recommended.

Airway secretions causing copious, tenacious sputum production and occasionally disabling cough should be managed with time-honored methods of adequate hydration, humidification, and postural drainage. Cessation of smoking is clearly important and must be strongly encouraged.

Tuberculosis is a common and serious complication, especially in complicated, accelerated, and acute silicosis. Patients with silicosis who have a significant tuberculin reaction but no clinical, bacteriologic, or radiographic evidence of active disease should be treated with isoniazid (INH) preventive therapy. Oral INH, 300 mg daily, should be given for a minimum of 1 year. Some physicians recommend lifelong preventive therapy. Silicotic patients receiving glucocorticoids should also be given INH preventive therapy.

The diagnosis of active tuberculous infection in patients with silicosis can be difficult. Clinical symptoms of weight loss, fever, sweats, and malaise should prompt radiographic evaluation and sputum acid-fast bacilli stains and cultures. Radiographic changes, including enlargement or cavitation in conglomerate lesions or nodular opacities, are of particular concern. Bacteriologic studies on expectorated sputum may not always be reliable in silicotuberculosis. Fiberoptic bronchoscopy for additional specimens for culture and study may often be helpful in establishing a diagnosis of active disease.

Proven active tuberculosis and clinically suspected disease should be treated with INH, 300 mg, and rifampin (Rifadin, Rimactane), 600 mg, daily for a minimum of 9 months. Many authorities recommend a third drug such as ethambutol (Myambutol), 15 mg per kg, as well as more prolonged courses. Initiation of therapy prior to bacteriologic confirmation is prudent in silicotic patients with clinical signs compatible with active tuberculosis. Careful long-term follow-up with chest radiographs, bacteriologic cultures, and clinical symptoms is imperative in view of numerous reports of recurrent pulmonary tuberculosis in silicotic patients after discontinuation of apparently adequate therapy.

Hypoxemia should be treated with supplemental oxygen to prevent the development of polycythemia, to delay or prevent development of pulmonary hypertension and cor pulmonale, and to improve exercise tolerance. The goal of oxygen therapy should be to elevate the Po_2 above 60 torr. Two to 4 liters per minute of oxygen by nasal cannula will often achieve this level of arterial oxygenation. Measurement of arterial blood gases should guide the selection of flow rate. Portable and home oxygen systems are widely available for managing these patients.

Ventilatory support for respiratory failure is indicated when precipitated by a treatable complication. Pneumothorax, spontaneous and ventilator-related, is usually treated by chest tube insertion. Bronchopleural fistula may develop and surgical consultation and management should be considered.

Acute silicosis may rapidly progress to respiratory failure. When this disease resembles pulmonary alveolar proteinosis and severe hypoxemia is present, aggressive therapy would include massive whole-lung lavage with the patient under general anesthesia in an attempt to improve gas exchange and remove alveolar debris. Although not proven effective, glucocorticoid therapy has been used for acute silicosis. Prednisone, 40 to 60 mg per day, for 1 to 2 months if accompanied by evidence of clinical improvement can be tapered to 15 to 20 mg per day and continued for 6 months to 1 year. Early, rigorous initial evaluation for tuberculosis and other mycobacterial infection is necessary. INH given as above while steroids are administered is recommended. Empiric therapy with two or three antituberculous drugs pending results of cultures for 6 weeks may be appropriate in the life-threatening acute form of disease.

Some young patients with end-stage silicosis may be considered candidates for lung or heart-lung transplantation by centers experienced with this technology. Early referral and evaluation for this intervention may be offered to selected patients.

HYPERSENSITIVITY PNEUMONITIS

method of
HERBERT Y. REYNOLDS, M.D.
Yale University School of Medicine
New Haven, Connecticut

Repeated inhalation of a variety of organic dusts or simple chemicals can cause hypersensitivity pneumonitis, also known as extrinsic allergic alveolitis (Table 1). Colorful, descriptive names for the diseases underscore the frequent occupational nature of exposure. This diagnosis implies that the affected subject has acquired a heightened reactivity to the inciting agent and the inflammatory response is located in the alveolar and interstitial portions of the lung and not in the larger conducting airways, which are usually involved in asthmatic diseases. The distinction is important, for extrinsic, IgE antibody-mediated allergic asthma is also a form of hypersensitivity lung disease and can be caused by airborne organic antigens. Exposure to chemicals such as trimellitic anhydride may also cause asthma.

Although many people can be exposed to these common antigens and many will develop specific serum antibodies to them (precipitins are present in 5 per cent of exposed office workers and 30 to >50 per cent of grain handlers, dairy workers, and pigeon or bird handlers), relatively few manifest symptoms of respiratory disease. Sensitization to an organic dust is often insidious, but repeated exposure can produce lung changes of a lymphocytic alveolitis, yet the subject remains asymptomatic. An alveolitis that persists for several years may not cause detrimental lung function, so physicians must weigh this fact before recommending that a change in job or relocation is necessary. Obviously, unique host susceptibility or resistance influences the individual response; this is especially true for younger subjects. Chronic exposure, however, can result in an interstitial, granulomatous, and fibrotic lung disease that is debilitating.

Clinically, two distinct syndromes can occur:

1. An acute reaction, occurring 2 to 6 hours after heavy exposure, consisting of dyspnea, cough, chills, fever (up to 40° C), transient restrictive impairment of pulmonary function, and leukocytosis. In the absence of a repeat exposure, spontaneous recovery occurs in 12 to 24 hours.

2. With chronic exposure, persistent dyspnea, cough, anorexia, weight loss, and progressive pneumonitis can lead to hypoxemia and restrictive lung function. With time the chest radiograph reveals diffuse reticular shadows in the lung fields, but there is no evidence of adenopathy. In the latter chronic form, the diagnosis can be very difficult and considerable detective work may be necessary. Often a visit to the patient's workplace or home is needed. Positive serum precipitins give a clue to the cause but in themselves do not constitute a diagnosis. Airway challenge with the putative antigen may be required for a cause and effect relationship, especially if occupational exposure and possible compensation or litigation are issues.

Therapeutic Approach

In the isolated or sporadic case, establishing a firm diagnosis and a putative cause is difficult. Therapy can be simple by comparison. Avoidance is the best treatment if precipitating circumstances are identified. A perceptive subject may do this instinctively and the disease process ends. Problems develop if exposure persists either by the patient's choice or by necessity. For example,

TABLE 1. **Some Etiologic Agents in Hypersensitivity Pneumonitis**

Major Antigens	Exposure or Source	Disease
Thermophilic bacteria		
Micropolyspora faeni	Moldy hay	Farmer's lung
Thermoactinomyces vulgaris	Moldy grain	Grain handler's lung
M. faeni, T. vulgaris	Mushroom compost	Mushroom worker's lung
Thermoactinomyces sacchari	Moldy sugar cane (bagasse)	Bagassosis
T. vulgaris, M. faeni	Heated water reservoirs	Humidifier or air conditioner lung
Aureobasidium pullulans		
Other bacteria		
Bacillus subtilis	Water	Detergent worker's lung
Bacillus cereus	Water reservoir	Humidifier lung
True fungi		
Cryptostroma corticale	Moldy bark	Maple bark stripper's lung
Aspergillus clavatus	Moldy malt, barley	Malt worker's lung
Aureobasidium pullulans and	Moldy redwood dust	Sequoiosis
Graphium sp.		
Mucor stolonifer	Moldy paprika pods	Paprika splitter's lung
Penicillium caseii	Cheese mold	Cheese worker's lung
Penicillium frequentans	Moldy cork dust	Suberosis
Aspergillus spores	Water reservoir	Aspergillosis
Animal proteins		
Avian proteins (serum and excreta)	Pigeons, parakeets	Bird breeder's lung
Chicken feathers, serum	Chickens	Chicken plucker's lung
Turkey feathers, serum	Turkeys	Turkey handler's lung
Duck feathers	Ducks	Duck fever
Rat urine, serum	Rats	Rodent handler's disease
Porcine and bovine pituitary protein	Pituitary snuff	Pituitary snuff-taker's lung
Amebae		
Acanthamoeba castellani	Water	Humidifier lung
Naegleria gruberi	Water	Humidifier lung
Bacterial products		
Lipopolysaccharide	Cotton brac	Byssinosis
Streptomyces verticillus glycopeptides	Bleomycin	Bleomycin hypersensitivity lung (in contrast to fibrosis)
Insect products		
Sitophilus granarius	Contaminated grain	Miller's lung (wheat weevil disease)
Chemicals		
Trimellitic anhydride	Plastics	Chemical worker's lung
Toluene diisocyanate	Polyurethane foam *or* rubber manufacture	
Methylene diisocyanate		

pigeon breeders are often so dedicated to their avocation that they will accept the respiratory symptoms rather than forgo the hobby of racing birds. This problem is not unlike the asthmatic who is allergic to animal dander but refuses to get rid of the household dog or cat. People in agricultural jobs, such as dairy farming and grain handling, may not have a ready option of changing employment. Wearing protective face masks has limited usefulness, so environmental reduction of dust in the workplace is a better solution for workers. Prophylactic use of inhaled bronchodilator drugs or corticosteroids is not efficacious. As respiratory symptoms following acute exposure are self-limited and subside in a day or two, no special treatment, including corticosteroids, is necessary.

With repeated exposures, the acute symptoms gradually diminish with succeeding episodes but are then replaced by chronic and persistent ones that may be more subtle to recognize, such as fatigue, poor appetite, dyspnea, and nonproductive cough. Since this subacute progressive phase of illness can be associated with restrictive lung function, decreased diffusion capacity, radiologic shadowing, and interstitial fibrosis, patient management is similar to that for other forms of diffuse, interstitial lung disease. After establishment of a good baseline of pulmonary function parameters, and perhaps an analysis of cells in bronchoalveolar lavage fluid (characteristically, a lymphocytic alveolitis is present, featuring an increased percentage of T-suppressor cells over T-helper cells, alveolar macrophages with foamy-appearing cytoplasm, and slight elevation of the number of mast cells), a trial of corticosteroid therapy is indicated. Prednisone, 60 mg daily (or 1 mg per kg) given as a single oral dose, is begun and continued for 2 to 3 weeks, then tapered over a 2-week interval to a daily dose of 15 to 20 mg. After an interval of 6 to 8 weeks of therapy, pulmonary function should be reassessed along with patient symptoms, and a judgment made about continuing therapy for several more months or reducing it unless a relapse occurs. With avoidance of the antigen and corticosteroid therapy most patients with chronic disease are improved in 6 to 12 months. Other medications, including bronchodilators, are not indicated.

SINUSITIS

method of
JAMES A. STANKIEWICZ, M.D.
Loyola University Medical Center
Maywood (Chicago), Illinois

The nose maintains its own normal flora and depends on proper nasal physiology to prevent disease. Foremost physiologically are mucus drainage and ciliary clearance of debris. Any etiologic entity that causes mucosal congestion may lead to cilial dysfunction, mucus inspissation, bacterial colonization, and infection. Marked nasal congestion and nose blowing leads to increased positive pressure in the nasal cavity that contributes to bacterial invasion through the small sinus drainage tracts or openings (ostia) into the sinus. The most frequent cause of sinusitis is the common cold, whereby marked congestion can be apparent and the cilia are affected primarily by the virus. Other causes are allergy, nasal polyps, environmental pollution, septal deviation, and indwelling nasotracheal or nasogastric tubes. The main anatomic area from which all sinuses can become infected is the anterior ethmoid.

Diagnosis

Acute sinusitis can be distinguished from the common cold by upper molar tooth pain, marked pressure when bending over, nasal purulence, and high fever (present in one half of patients). Using nasal spray to decongest the nose can often produce purulence that was not apparent because of marked congestion. Headache, particularly that located over a particular sinus and accentuated with firm finger palpation, can be a helpful diagnostic sign. Periorbital swelling, especially in children, may be related to sinusitis, but many patients are not this acutely ill. Most of them present with a cold that does not resolve after 4 to 6 weeks. A child with nasal drainage, bad breath, and cold-like symptoms persisting for 4 weeks has sinusitis until proven otherwise.

Chronic sinusitis is related to improperly treated or untreated acute sinusitis. Symptoms and signs are nasal obstruction and congestion, postnasal drainage, and headache. Radiographs after age 2 are the "gold standard" for making a diagnosis. Most hospitals or clinics offer a standard sinus series. Total opacification, mucosal thickening greater than 5 mm, air-fluid levels, and retention cysts all indicate sinusitis. Multiple sinuses are often involved. In an immunosuppressed patient, involvement of one sinus may be indicative of a fungal or opportunistic bacterial infection.

The microbiology of sinusitis is variable, but *Streptococcus pneumoniae, Haemophilus influenzae* (not type B), and *Branhamella catarrhalis* are the most commonly cultured organisms in acute sinusitis. *Staphylococcus aureus* (non-coagulase-positive) and *Streptococcus pyogenes* are also seen. *Staphylococcus aureus* (coagulase-positive) often is seen in fulminant sinusitis, especially frontal. The flora in chronic sinusitis are the same in acute sinusitis with the addition of anaerobic organisms, including *Peptostreptococcus, Fusobacterium,* and *Bacteroides*.

Treatment

Amoxicillin, 500 mg orally three times a day in adults and 40 mg per kg per day in the child, is the antibiotic of choice for acute and chronic sinusitis. Alternatives if the patient is allergic, resistant, or unresponsive to penicillin are trimethoprim-sulfamethoxazole (Bactrim, Septra), erythromycin, and sulfisoxazole (Pediazole for children) and cefaclor (Ceclor). Amoxicillin/potassium clavulanate (Augmentin) is another good alternative. The patient's symptoms and signs usually begin to respond within 48 to 72 hours. If the patient is still symptomatic without signs of orbital complications (periorbital swelling, decreased vision, cellulitis, extraocular movement fixation, forehead swelling), the antibiotic should be changed. If the patient continues to be unresponsive after 4 to 5 days, consultation is recommended. Nasal cultures are not helpful, since they rarely identify the organism. Supportive therapy to reduce intranasal edema and to promote sinus drainage and aeration includes decongestant nasal sprays, oral decongestants, and cool vapor humidity. Antihistamines are not helpful and should not be used since they interfere with cilial function and lead to further mucus inspissation, unless an allergic etiology is certain.

Hospitalization and intravenous antibiotics are necessary for patients with severe sinusitis in whom there is often involvement of orbital or intracranial structures. If possible, a culture should be obtained by sinus aspiration prior to initiating therapy. Otherwise, antibiotics should be directed toward treating both resistant *Staphylococcus aureus* and *H. influenzae*. Surgical drainage involving sinus puncture, nasoantral windows, ethmoidectomy, and frontal sinus trephination may be necessary in the unresponsive patient. Nasal decongestion with 5 per cent cocaine pledgets, nasal sprays, and high humidity (croup tent) may be helpful. Immunosuppressed patients require culture of nasal exudate prior to treatment because of the multitude of organisms that can cause disease.

Chronic sinusitis therapy requires 4 to 6 weeks of amoxicillin. The sinuses are relatively avascular and have limited drainage, thus requiring an extended period of time to heal. It is often helpful if an organism can be aspirated from the sinus prior to treatment. Patients with nasal polyps or severe mechanical obstruction (septal deviation), or whose symptoms, signs, and x-rays do not clear, may require surgical intervention. Sinus x-rays should be obtained 1 to 2 weeks after treatment is completed to assess the degree of improvement. There is a lag time of 1 to 2 weeks between actual resolution of sinusitis and clearing on x-ray.

STREPTOCOCCAL PHARYNGITIS

method of
JAMES W. BASS, M.D., M.P.H.
Tripler Army Medical Center
Honolulu, Hawaii

Numerous clinical studies have shown that experienced physicians are able to clinically differentiate patients who have streptococcal pharyngitis from those who have nonstreptococcal pharyngitis with little more than 50 per cent accuracy. Accordingly, throat culture has been considered the "gold standard" for laboratory confirmation of this diagnosis for the past four decades. Since a delay in treatment of up to several days does not incur the risk of rheumatic fever and many authorities have taught that early treatment does not significantly alter the acute clinical course of the disease, delay in treatment for 24 to 72 hours until results of the throat culture may be known has been considered acceptable.

Recent well-controlled clinical studies have shown that early antibiotic treatment of children with streptococcal pharyngitis does significantly alter the acute clinical course of the disease. Also, tests that permit rapid laboratory-confirmed diagnosis of streptococcal pharyngitis by detecting group A carbohydrate-specific antigen directly on the throat swab have recently become available. These tests, called rapid strep tests (RST), require only minutes to perform, and in most studies results correlate well with the throat culture. A throat culture taken at the same time as the RST could serve as a check to identify the rare individual who may have a false negative RST.

Most individuals with streptococcal pharyngitis who receive early antibiotic treatment are afebrile and have marked symptomatic improvement within 24 hours. Early treatment decreases the incidence of suppurative complications and limits spread of the disease in the family and community. Throat cultures from patients who have received antibiotic treatment are usually negative within 24 hours after initiation of treatment, so they can be presumed to be noncontagious and can return to school or work. With both parents in many households in the United States currently working outside the home early antibiotic treatment of children with streptococcal pharyngitis clearly offers significant clinical, public health, social, educational, and economic benefits.

Antimicrobial Treatment

Penicillin remains the drug of choice for treatment of streptococcal infections. All strains of group A beta-hemolytic streptococci (GABHS) remain exquisitely sensitive to penicillin, and there has been no indication of emerging resistance to this drug. The optimal preparation and route of administration varies with clinical circumstances.

Oral Penicillin. In private practice settings good compliance with oral treatment and results equal to those with intramuscular penicillin G benzathine can be achieved with counseling of the patient and/or parents that emphasizes the need for the medication to be given for a full 10 days to eliminate the infecting organisms and prevent rheumatic fever. Oral penicillin G and penicillin V are equally effective, but the latter is preferred as it is acid-stable, is better absorbed, and produces predictably higher blood levels of penicillin. For children under 12 years of age optimal oral penicillin treatment of streptococcal pharyngitis is achieved with a dose of 250 mg given twice daily for 10 days. For children over 12 years of age, adolescents, and adults a dose of 500 mg twice daily for 10 days (an FDA-approved treatment regimen) is optimal. Higher doses or dosages more often than twice daily or for longer than 10 days do not produce greater cure rates. Because compliance in taking oral medications decreases with frequency of dosing and duration of treatment, dose intervals of more than twice daily and treatment periods longer than 10 days should probably not be prescribed. In addition, twice-daily treatment can be more realistically achieved in school children with working parents. A rational exception might be in the first 24 to 48 hours of treatment, when doses may be given every 6 to 8 hours while the child remains sick and at home in an effort to assure an early bacteriologic cure and render the child noncontagious as early as possible.

Intramuscular Penicillin Preparations. In contrast to the circumstances outlined in which oral penicillin treatment is preferred, intramuscular benzathine G should be given to patients with streptococcal pharyngitis in areas where rheumatic

The opinions or assertions contained herein are the private views of the author and are not to be construed as official or as reflecting the views of the Department of the Army or the Department of Defense.

fever is prevalent, particularly in poor and crowded inner-city populations where medical care is episodic and where compliance in taking oral penicillin cannot be relied on. These conditions apply in many pediatric populations in the United States and for most children in developing or Third World countries. In these circumstances intramuscular penicillin G benzathine in a dose of 600,000 units for children weighing less than 27 kg (60 pounds) and 900,000 to 1,200,000 units for those weighing more than 27 kg provides optimal treatment. A significantly less painful and better-accepted intramuscular preparation that contains 900,000 units of penicillin G benzathine and 300,000 units of penicillin G procaine within a 2-ml volume has been shown to be effective for children. In addition to reducing the pain at the injection site, the procaine component produces higher initial blood levels of penicillin; although this does not effect a more rapid clinical response than is seen with straight penicillin G benzathine, it produces an earlier bacterial cure rate approaching 100 per cent after 24 hours, presumably rendering the patient noncontagious and able to return to school. For adults optimal parenteral therapy is best achieved with 1,200,00 units of penicillin G benzathine.

Extended-spectrum oral penicillins, including ampicillin and ampicillin-like penicillins (amoxicillin, cyclacillin, and bacampicillin), and oral penicillinase-resistant penicillins (cloxacillin, dicloxacillin, oxacillin, and nafcillin) are all effective for treatment of streptococcal pharyngitis. Their use should be reserved for situations where they afford added benefit. They are generally more expensive and are associated with more untoward reactions, including skin rashes, gastrointestinal disturbances, and emergence of organisms resistant to antimicrobial drugs.

Alternatives to Penicillin. For individuals who cannot take penicillin, erythromycin is considered the first alternative for oral treatment of streptococcal pharyngitis. The recommended dosage for erythromycin estolate is 20 to 40 mg per kg per day in two to four divided doses, and for erythromycin ethylsuccinate it is 40 mg per kg per day in two to four doses, both for 10 days. Erythromycin estolate given at 20 mg per kg per day in two divided doses has been shown to be well tolerated and equally effective as 250 mg of penicillin V given three or four times daily. Erythromycin ethylsuccinate must be given in a dosage of 40 to 50 mg per kg per day to be equally effective, and at this dosage range it is better tolerated when given in four divided doses daily. Unlike most other oral antimicrobial agents, both of these oral erythromycin preparations are better absorbed and better tolerated when given

with food rather than fasting. Although the incidence of resistance of GABHS to erythromycin has been reported to be as high as 60 per cent in Japan, only 16 (2.8 per cent) of 578 isolates from several areas across the United States were shown to be erythromycin-resistant in a recent report.

Oral first-generation cephalosporins have been shown to be equally effective alternatives for individuals who cannot take penicillin or erythromycin. Cephalexin (Keflex), 25 to 50 mg per kg per day in two divided doses for children and 500 mg twice daily for adolescents and adults; cephradine (Velosef), 25 to 50 mg per kg per day in two to three divided doses; and cefadroxil (Duricef), 30 mg per kg per day in two divided doses, are equally effective as penicillin V for treatment of streptococcal pharyngitis. Some studies have even shown these drugs to produce greater cure rates than penicillin, allegedly owing to their resistance to penicillinase-producing anaerobes and staphylococci in the tonsillopharyngeal flora which may inactivate penicillin. Cefaclor (Ceclor), an oral second-generation cephalothin, 40 mg per kg per day in three divided doses, may be used to treat individuals with streptococcal pharyngitis who also have otitis media (because of its additional activity against *Haemophilus influenzae*) who cannot take penicillin drugs. Erythromycin-sulfisoxazole (Pediazole), 40 mg per kg per day of the erythromycin component, in four divided doses is an alternate under these circumstances, but trimethoprim-sulfamethoxazole is not since it is inadequate for the treatment of GABHS infections. Although oral cephalosporins are generally more expensive than oral penicillins, cephalosporin suspensions taste better and are significantly better accepted. Clindamycin (Cleocin), 25 to 40 mg per kg per day in three to four divided doses, is an acceptable alternative for individuals who cannot take penicillins, cephalosporins, or erythromycin.

As with penicillin V treatment regimens using twice-daily dosage schedules, the alternative antimicrobial treatment regimens listed above with twice-daily dosage schedules appear optimal as they employ the lowest dose of drug given least often and for the shortest duration of time that achieves the best results. These regimens also reduce cost and untoward reactions to a minimum and enhance compliance to a maximum.

Response to Treatment

Clinical response of children with streptococcal pharyngitis to appropriate antimicrobial treatment is nearly always evident within 24 hours. Most children are fully recovered and have become culture-negative within 1 to 2 days after initiation of treatment and can be returned to school. Persistence of high fever and severe symptoms beyond this period suggests the development of a suppurative complication or some other underlying disease.

Follow-up

Post-treatment follow-up throat cultures are not recommended for individuals who remain asymptomatic. Exception to this policy should be made for patients who have had rheumatic fever or where other family members in the household have had rheumatic fever. Every attempt should be made to eradicate GABHS from these patients and other household members in a effort to prevent further episodes of rheumatic fever.

Chronic Carriers

Nearly all treated individuals remain culture-negative during the 10 days of treatment. However, if follow-up cultures are obtained during the 6-week period after treatment is completed, about 10 to 15 per cent will again develop positive cultures for GABHS regardless of the type of treatment given. Most of these isolates are the same serotype as the initial isolate made before treatment was given, and they represent the "asymptomatic chronic convalescent carrier state." This chronic carrier state usually persists for several months or more regardless of whether the patient is re-treated or not, although cultures usually become negative during re-treatment. In children who have classic streptococcal pharyngitis, throat cultures grow a heavy or almost pure culture of GABHS, and these patients are highly contagious and are at significant risk of developing rheumatic fever if left untreated; in contrast, throat cultures of chronic carriers usually yield only a scant growth or a few colonies of GABHS, and there is general agreement that chronic carriers are not a significant source of spread of infection and are not at risk of developing rheumatic fever. Therefore, there is no need or reason to seek detection of individuals who manifest only the asymptomatic chronic convalescent carrier state of GABHS.

Relapses and Reinfections

Patients who develop symptomatic illnesses suggestive of streptococcal pharyngitis during the first 2 to 3 months after treatment and whose throat cultures are again positive for GABHS should be considered to have relapses or reinfections. Those with GABHS of the same serotype as the initial isolate before treatment should be considered to have relapses, and they should be re-treated. Those with a different serotype from the initial isolate should be considered to have reinfections; they should also be re-treated. Serotype information on GABHS isolates is difficult to obtain, expensive, time-consuming, and not practical for use in making decisions for management of these patients. It is not possible to clinically differentiate patients who are symptomatic after treatment because of treatment failures or reinfections from those who may be chronic convalescent carriers of GABHS who are symptomatic owing to coincidental nonstreptococcal pharyngitis. Accordingly, all individuals who have symptomatic illnesses suggestive of streptococcal pharyngitis whose throat culture yields any growth of GABHS should probably be treated.

Contacts

Household members of index cases have a high incidence of secondary infection. From 30 to 50 per cent of siblings and 10 to 20 per cent of parents or adult household contacts are culture positive for GABHS, and up to half of the siblings with positive cultures develop symptoms of streptococcal pharyngitis within several weeks. These observations have led some treating physicians in the past to take samples for culture from all household members of index cases at the onset and to treat those who are culture positive in order to prevent "ping-pong" infection and reinfection in the household during and after the index case is treated. Most primary care physicians today, however, prefer to take culture samples only from symptomatic household contacts and treat only those whose cultures are positive.

Recurrent Streptococcal Pharyngitis

Children who have frequent and recurrent bouts of culture-proven streptococcal pharyngitis are sometimes encountered as special management problems in pediatric clinic settings. If oral antibiotics were prescribed, compliance may be questioned, and consideration should be given to the use of intramuscular benzathine penicillin G for treatment. If other family members (usually siblings) are involved, intrafamily spread of infection in a "ping-pong" fashion may be suspected and consideration should be given to performing culture studies for all household members and treating those with positive cultures for GABHS simultaneously in an effort to eradicate the organism from the household.

Recent studies present convincing evidence that the presence of beta-lactamase–producing organisms in tonsillar tissue may inactivate penicillin drugs and promote survival and persistence of GABHS in these tissues, leading to recurrent infection. If this is suspected, a trial of treatment with antimicrobial drugs that are not inactivated by penicillin–beta-lactamases such as erythromycin, a cephalosporin, or clindamycin should be considered. Preliminary studies suggest that clindamycin may be most effective in this regard, and this drug is the most active against beta-lactamase–producing anaerobic organisms that are commonly found in tonsillar tissues. Recent reports claim that "tolerance" to penicillin by some strains of GABHS may be implicated in some cases of penicillin treatment failure for streptococcal pharyngitis. These claims require further verification. Meanwhile, the use of nonpenicillin treatment regimens including erythromycin and clindamycin should obviate this possibility.

Non–Group A Streptococcal Pharyngitis

Individuals who have symptoms of streptococcal pharyngitis whose throat cultures yield a significant growth of non–group A streptococci (usually group C or G) pose a problem to the treating physician. Although it is agreed that these patients are not at risk of developing rheumatic fever if they do not receive antimicrobial treatment, there is controversy as to whether these organisms actually cause symptomatic streptococcal pharyngitis. There is also controversy as to whether the clinical illness in these patients is responsive to antimicrobial therapy. Over 80 per cent of responding physicians in a recent survey of 500 pediatricians, 500 internists, and 500 family practitioners indicated that they considered that non–group A streptococci were a significant cause of streptococcal-like pharyngitis and that the clinical illness in these individuals was responsive to penicillin treatment. Although clinical data specifically substantiating these claims are lacking, antimicrobial treatment is recommended for individuals with symptoms of streptococcal pharyngitis whose throat culture yields a significant growth of non–group A streptococci. Since these organisms are usually sensitive to the same antimicrobial drugs that are effective against group A streptococci, the same treatment regimens recommended for streptococcal pharyngitis caused by group A organisms are recommended.

TUBERCULOSIS AND NONTUBERCULOUS MYCOBACTERIAL DISEASES

method of
KEITH P. YOUNG, M.D., and
WILLIAM C. BAILEY, M.D.
University of Alabama
Birmingham, Alabama

Tuberculosis remains an important infectious disease in the United States and abroad. After several years of steady decline in incidence, achieved primarily through improvement in socioeconomic conditions and secondarily through public health measures and chemotherapy, new cases of tuberculosis are again on the increase. Atypical presentations are becoming more frequently recognized, and extrapulmonary tuberculosis represents a larger proportion of illness than before.

Many factors have recently influenced the traditional management of tuberculosis. Although the chemotherapeutic agents available have changed little over the past decade, new combinations and dosing have allowed the duration of treatment to be shortened considerably.

Diagnosis

Correctly diagnosing tuberculosis requires adequate comprehension of disease presentations and available diagnostic tests. Strong clinical suspicion of tuberculosis must be maintained when encountering a potential patient. Staining of aseptically collected body secretions or tissue should be the initial procedure to support the diagnosis.

The tuberculin skin test is useful in supporting the diagnosis of tuberculosis. A positive reaction of 10 mm of cutaneous induration to 0.1 ml of 5 tuberculin units of purified protein derivative (PPD) at 48 to 72 hours after intradermal injection is diagnostic of tuberculous infection, but does not determine the presence of disease. Several factors may contribute to a falsely negative PPD test, including age, coexistent diseases associated with impaired cellular immunity, malnutrition, and immunosuppressive drug therapy. Therefore, a negative PPD skin test cannot exclude tuberculosis.

Diagnosis of tuberculosis is established by culturing the organism on laboratory media from appropriately collected clinical specimens. Specimens are cultured on Löwenstein-Jensen or Middlebrook 7H10 media or several variations of these media. When present, *Mycobacterium tuberculosis* is always considered pathogenic. Cultures should be established for sensitivity testing when the likelihood of drug resistance is high, such as when the patient has been previously treated or is an immigrant from an area with high resistance states.

Rapid diagnostic testing for *M. tuberculosis* and some nontuberculous mycobacteria is now available in many labs. A radioactive iodinated DNA probe has been developed (Gen-Probe) that can identify organisms in culture as early as 2 to 4 weeks. This diagnostic test, when fully utilized, should dramatically decrease diagnostic delays.

Treatment of Tuberculosis

Until a diagnosis of tuberculosis is secured by the above methods, a presumed diagnosis of tuberculosis should be made. The rationale of this approach centers on the communicable nature of tuberculosis. The duration of sputum positivity for acid-fast organisms is variable after treatment is instituted, but it is not necessary to maintain respiratory isolation until sputum is clear of acid-fast bacilli (AFB). The exact duration of infectivity is variable; however, it is generally accepted that patients newly diagnosed should be considered infectious until 2 weeks of effective chemotherapy. Reporting of newly diagnosed tuberculosis cases to local public health officials is important in management to allow possible contacts to be screened for infection. Concurrent therapy of other medical illnesses (e.g., COPD, alcoholism) and nutritional support are important ancillary measures that can improve the outcome of treatment.

Chemotherapy of tuberculosis requires consideration of several factors related to both the tuberculosis organism and the drugs involved in therapy. The bacterial population in various disease states needs to be considered with reference to number, size, location, metabolic activity, and possible drug resistance. Active disease will have a large population of organisms consisting of metabolically active extracellular organisms, active organisms inside macrophages, and metabolically dormant organisms in caseous material. The intracellular organisms will require drugs active at low pH and capable of macrophage penetration. The dormant organisms will require prolonged therapy in order to achieve microbial killing. Large populations of organisms also increase the likelihood of drug resistance by spontaneous mutation. It has been estimated that spontaneous mutation resulting in isoniazid (INH) resistance occurs once in every 10^6 organisms, an organism population easily achieved in active disease. Multiple-drug therapy of active disease has been established as a means of avoiding drug resistance, allowing shorter duration of therapy, and reducing treatment failures.

The choice of antituberculous drugs also should be considered according to the bactericidal activity of the agents used in therapy. Bactericidal agents decrease treatment time. Common bactericidal agents include isoniazid, rifampin, pyrazinamide, streptomycin, and ethionamide (Table 1). Agents with adequate intracellular penetration include isoniazid, rifampin, ethambutol, pyrazinamide, and ethionamide. Rifampin has an unusual ability to kill dormant organisms during very brief growth spurts.

Specific Antituberculous Drugs

Isoniazid. Isoniazid (INH) is an essential drug in the management of tuberculosis. It exhibits several characteristics favorable for therapy, including bactericidal activity, oral administration, intracellular penetration, and low cost. It is metabolized in the liver, and its principal toxic effects are hepatitis and a peripheral neuropathy. INH hepatitis is increased in persons over age 35 years and in those with alcohol intake during drug therapy. Neuropathy may occur from INH therapy due to interference with pyridoxine metabolism, particularly in alcoholics and pregnant women, but is prevented by the daily administration of 25 mg of oral pyridoxine. The usual dose of INH is 5 mg per kg per day orally (usually about 300 mg).

Rifampin. Rifampin is an extremely potent antituberculous agent. Similar to INH, it is bactericidal; in addition, it has an important impact when dormant organisms grow transiently, has good intracellular penetration, is administered orally, and is useful in combination with INH. Rifampin is generally well tolerated, with its principal adverse effects being hepatitis and thrombocytopenia. Rifampin is metabolized partially by the kidneys. Dosage is 10 mg per kg orally per day, usually about 600 mg per day. Rifampin will turn the urine orange, a side effect surprising to some patients.

Ethambutol. Ethambutol is bacteriostatic with penetration into phagocytic cells. It has been used with INH and rifampin in combination therapy. Ethambutol is excreted renally, and the dosage must be reduced in patients with renal failure. The principal toxicity is optic neuritis, which should be screened for by periodic ophthalmologic exams. The dosage is 15 mg per kg per day.

Pyrazinamide. Pyrazinamide is a bactericidal oral agent given in oral doses of 20 to 30 mg per kg per day, usually about 1.5 grams. It is excreted by the kidneys and has a principal toxic side effect of hepatitis. Its use is important early in therapy to decrease the length of chemotherapy by eliminating persistent organisms.

Streptomycin. Streptomycin is an aminoglycoside that is bactericidal. It is administered parenterally in doses of 10 to 15 mg per kg per day, usually 0.75 to 1.0 gram intramuscularly per day. It is excreted renally and has principal toxic effects of renal failure and eighth cranial nerve toxicity.

TABLE 1. **Characteristics of Antituberculous Drugs**

Drug	Bactericidal	Dosage	Metabolism	Toxicity
Isoniazid (INH)	Yes	5 mg/kg/day (usually about 300 mg/day)	Hepatic	Hepatitis Neuropathy
Rifampin (RIF) (Rifadin, Rimactane)	Yes	10 mg/kg/day (usually about 600 mg/day)	Hepatic	Hepatitis GI distress Thrombocytopenia
Ethambutol (EMB) (Myambutol)	No	15 mg/kg/day	Renal	Optic neuritis
Pyrazinamide (PZA)	Yes	25 mg/kg/day	Renal	Hepatitis Hyperuricemia Arthralgia
Streptomycin	Yes	10–15 mg/kg/day (usually about 0.75–1.0 gm) intramuscularly	Renal	Eighth cranial nerve toxicity Renal failure
Ethionamide (ETH) (Trecator-SC)	No	10–15 mg/kg/day		GI distress Hepatitis Neuropathy

Ethionamide. Ethionamide is a bacteriostatic agent, but it penetrates into phagocytic cells well. It is given in doses of 10 to 15 mg per kg per day orally, and the principal toxic effects are gastrointestinal disturbances, peripheral neuropathy, hepatitis, and allergic reactions.

Therapy of Specific Tuberculosis Situations

Preventive Treatment (Table 2). Active tuberculosis is usually a result of previous infection that has occurred months to years before. Consequently a substantial portion of tuberculosis exists in a dormant or inactive state for a period of time. Detection of these cases might be found through PPD skin testing, and if effective treatment is instituted, active tuberculosis might be prevented and transmission reduced.

Isoniazid has proved effective in preventing active disease. Single-drug therapy with isoniazid for 1 year has been shown to reduce disease activity by 70 to 80 per cent during the year of treatment and to lead to a long-term reduction in disease activity by 50 per cent. Identifying

TABLE 2. **Indications for Isoniazid**

Documented PPD conversion within 2 years regardless of age
Positive PPD of any duration in individual less than 35 years old
Household contacts of active tuberculosis developing positive PPD
Children less than 5 years old with positive sputum regardless of skin test status
PPD positivity regardless of duration associated with:
  Diabetes mellitus
  Silicosis
  Corticosteroid or immunosuppressive drug therapy
  Postgastrectomy states
  Reticuloendothelial malignancy
  AIDS
  Dialysis patient

individual patients appropriate for preventive therapy obviously has major benefits.

Identification of patients who might benefit from preventive therapy requires understanding of the epidemiology of tuberculosis and of underlying potential diseases. Certain persons with positive skin tests will benefit from isoniazid preventive therapy, regardless of age, including any new skin test converter; contacts of an active case; and patients with reticuloendothelial malignancy, silicosis, renal insufficiency, diabetes mellitus, heroin addiction, or AIDS. Any patient with a positive skin test who is less than 35 years old or any child with positive sputum smears but negative skin tests should also be treated with INH.

Isoniazid in an oral daily dose of 10 mg per kg per day, usually 300 mg per day, for 1 year is standard treatment. The course of treatment may be shortened to 9 months if 1 year of therapy is impractical. Completion of therapy is important in assuring cure. Lapses of therapy of less than 1 month can be ignored. Lapses of greater than a month require that therapy be started over, if less than 6 months of treatment has occurred. If more than 6 months of therapy has been completed by the time of a lapse of greater than a month, most clinicians discontinue treatment if there is no evidence of active disease. Supervised therapy twice weekly may be considered on occasion. Rifampin in usual doses may be used as an alternative agent for preventive therapy if isoniazid resistance is likely; no data on efficacy are available, but theoretically this agent should be effective.

Chemotherapy of Active Pulmonary Disease. Effective chemotherapy exists for active pulmonary disease, and several strategies of therapy consider organism numbers, potential for resistance, and potential for noncompliance. The most widely used therapy for active tuberculosis today is a combination of isoniazid and rifampin given daily by mouth for 9 months. This short-course chemotherapy is administered as isoniazid 300 mg and rifampin 600 mg orally per day. With successful completion of this regimen, the relapse rate is extremely low. Combination chemotherapy serves to decrease the likelihood of drug resistance, reduce treatment time, and reduce relapse potential. Other combinations, which include such drugs as streptomycin or ethambutol, have to be given for up to 18 months.

Occasionally it will be necessary to supervise therapy in noncompliant individuals. When this situation occurs, intermittent chemotherapy becomes desirable. Again combination therapy with isoniazid 300 mg per day and rifampin 600 mg per day is instituted daily for the first month. After the initial month of therapy, the isoniazid dose becomes 15 mg per kg given twice weekly and rifampin is given 600 mg twice weekly. Intermittent therapy is continued for 9 months and has relapse rates comparable to those occurring after cessation of daily therapy.

Extrathoracic Tuberculosis. Extrathoracic tuberculosis requires consideration of several details that may modify therapy. Central nervous system tuberculosis should be treated with isoniazid and rifampin in doses mentioned previously. Both drugs penetrate the CNS well. There is no proven benefit of a third drug, and corticosteroids should be given only if there is evidence of increased intracranial pressure. Pericardial tuberculosis is also treated with isoniazid and rifampin, but corticosteroids should be given to reduce the chance of constrictive pericarditis and arrhythmias. Pericardiectomy might be necessary initially if tamponade is likely. Genitourinary tuberculosis is usually well managed by isoniazid and rifampin alone. Spinal tuberculosis is medically managed with isoniazid and rifampin, but neurologic complications of nerve root or cord compression may require immediate surgical intervention.

Re-Treatment and Drug Resistance. Therapy of patients who have had treatment failure or partial treatment or of patients with a high likelihood of resistance is best directed by sensitivity testing. Patients highly likely to be resistant are immigrants from areas with endemic resistant tuberculosis or those with previously unsuccessful therapy. Two bactericidal drugs should be used. When resistance is possible, therapy should be instituted with a combination including at least two drugs to which the patient has not been exposed, while sensitivity tests are in process. If failure occurs on therapy, resistance should be identified by sensitivity testing, and a new regimen should be started that should include two drugs never before used. Never add a single new agent, in order to avoid the development of resistance to that drug.

Treatment of Nontuberculous Mycobacterial Infections (Table 3)

Nontuberculous mycobacterial (NTM) infections have been of increasing importance over the last decade. Previously seen as unusual infections in patients with structural lung disease, nontuberculous mycobacteria are gaining recognition as causes of infection in immunocompromised patients and patients with prosthetic devices. The therapeutic options for nontuberculous mycobacterial infections are also changing. Increased utility of antimicrobial sensitivity testing is leading to more specific therapy of NTM infections using antituberculous agents as well as general antimicrobial agents. NTM may be viewed most simply in two categories. First, there are a group of NTM infections that are easily treated with standard antituberculous drugs. Second, there are NTM infections that are difficult to treat because of drug resistance. NTM are stained by acid-fast preparations and can initially be confused with tuberculous infections. Therefore, initial therapy of an undiagnosed NTM infection should include consideration that the process might represent tuberculosis. Reporting and appropriate chemotherapy are necessary because of the potential communicability of tuberculosis. NTM infections have not been shown to be transmitted from person to person. Skin testing is not specific for these infections and does not add diagnostic information. Cultures and sensitivity testing should be relied on for diagnosis and selection of drug therapy.

Mycobacterium kansasii is usually a chronic

TABLE 3. **Nontuberculous Mycobacteria and Disease Associations**

Site	Organisms
Pulmonary	*Mycobacterium kansasii, M. avium-intracellulare, M. fortuitum, M. chelonei*
Lymphadenopathy	*M. kansasii, M. fortuitum, M. chelonei, M. avium-intracellulare, M. serofulaceum*
Postoperative infections Prosthetic device	*M. fortuitum, M. chelonei, M. avium-intracellulare*
Skin	*M. marinum, M. ulcerans, M. fortuitum, M. chelonei*
Disseminated disease	*M. avium-intracellulare, M. kansasii, M. fortuitum, M. chelonei*

pulmonary infection which can closely simulate tuberculosis both clinically and radiographically. Response to chemotherapy is also similar to that seen in tuberculosis, and standard doses of INH, rifampin, and ethambutol for 18 months is suggested management. *M. kansasii* may disseminate and is often seen in patients with acquired immunodeficiency syndrome (AIDS). *M. avium-intracellulare* (MAI) usually presents as an insidious pulmonary infection in persons with structural lung disease, causing chronic cough and upper lobe disease. Multiple-drug regimens of isoniazid, rifampin, ethambutol, streptomycin, pyrazinamide, and ethionamide, in combinations of three to five drugs, are used with variable success. All combinations should incorporate ethambutol because of its efficacy. MAI is also becoming a frequently isolated pulmonary or disseminated pathogen in AIDS patients. The same multiple-drug regimens are used in treatment of these individuals, frequently including ansamycin or clofazimine in the combinations. Prognosis for survival is not improved by therapy in these patients, however.

Other NTM less frequently cause pulmonary infection and may cause disease in other organs. *M. fortuitum* and *M. cheloni* can cause infections of prosthetic devices, including implants for augmentation mammoplasty, orthopedic devices, and prosthetic cardiac valves. These infections are best treated with standard antimicrobial agents. In severe or deep tissue infections, treatment is started with intravenous cefoxitin and amikacin for approximately 10 to 12 weeks, then switched to oral sulfonamides, rifampin, or erythromycin based on sensitivity testing. *M. marinum* and *M. ulcerans* are associated with infection of the skin and subcutaneus tissues. *M. marinum* usually responds well to oral rifampin, ethambutol, or trimethoprim-sulfamethoxazole. *M. ulcerans* is responsive to trimethoprim-sulfamethoxazole, rifampin, or ethambutol. Mycobacterial lymphadenopathy now more commonly occurs as a nontuberculous mycobacterial infection, usually in children. *M. scrofulaceum, M. kansasii, M. fortuitum, M. chelonei,* and *M. avium-intracellulare* are the most common causes, and therapy is surgical excision.

The Cardiovascular System

ACQUIRED AORTIC DISEASE

method of
JOHN J. BERGAN, M.D., and
WALTER J. McCARTHY, M.D.
Northwestern University Medical School
Chicago, Illinois

AORTIC OCCLUSIVE DISEASE

Although chronic aortoiliac occlusive disease can be called the Leriche syndrome, in fact there are a number of distinct syndromes composing this group of conditions. Among these are isolated aortoiliac thrombosis, multilevel aortic and distal occlusive disease, the small aortic syndrome, and mid-aortic occlusions involving renal and visceral vessels.

Isolated aortoiliac occlusion is the condition that René Leriche described in patients in their 20s, 30s, and early 40s. He observed, and others have also reported, that such patients have a high aortic bifurcation, a narrow angle between the iliac arterial limbs, and relatively long common iliac arteries. Now it is known that these anatomic variations produce areas of ambient low sheer stress which decrease endothelial oxygenation and increase surface platelet aggregation. These in turn contribute to early atheromatous change. Such patients do not have generalized atherosclerosis, although traditional risk factors may contribute to an acceleration of this aortoiliac occlusive process. In the absence of generalized atherosclerosis, such patients may be severely disabled by claudication and yet expect normal longevity and total rehabilitation by aortoiliac reconstructive surgery. An important condition in the differential diagnosis of aortoiliac occlusive disease—induced claudication and other causes of exercise intolerance is pseudoclaudication of neurospinal origin. This is caused by spinal stenosis. In patients with aortoiliac occlusion, femoral pulsations are notably decreased. In patients with central spinal stenosis of developmental or degenerative origin, the femoral pul-

sations may be normal. Careful extremity blood flow and pressure studies as well as conventional studies to assess spinal disease will result in an accurate differentiation between these conditions.

In contrast to younger patients with isolated aortoiliac occlusion is the population of individuals with aortoiliac, femoro-popliteal, and tibioperoneal occlusive disease occurring in disparate segments concomitantly and coincidentally. In such patients, severe ischemia predominates over claudication. Although limb salvage can be achieved in greater than 95 per cent of such patients by proximal reconstruction utilizing the aortofemoral bypass principle, life expectancy is impaired. Patients with single aortoiliac occlusions can be expected to have a 10-year life expectancy of greater than 60 per cent, whereas those with multilevel occlusive disease will be expected to have a 10-year life expectancy of 40 per cent or less. Part of the explanation for this is the older age of the multilevel group and the prevalence of coincidental cardiovascular disease, complicated by diabetes.

A third distinct aortoiliac occlusive syndrome is seen in patients with a small aorta and iliac arteries. This has been entitled the hypoplastic aortoiliac syndrome. It has been noted that many patients suffering this abnormality are young women of short stature, frequently with red hair, who have an excessive habitual smoking history and who frequently present with elevated triglyceride levels and a type IV hyperlipoproteinemia. Such a syndrome suggests a genetic predisposition. This is not sex-linked, as hypoplasia of the abdominal aorta distal to the renal arteries is found in men as well as in women. This isolated group of patients is important clinically as well as intellectually. They present technical problems of arterial reconstruction, and their postoperative course is characterized by surgical failure. The contributions of early menopause and excessive smoking combined with hypertriglyceridemias are additive or synergistic.

Another variation on the aortoiliac occlusive

theme is an extremely rare condition that causes aortic occlusion at the level of the renal arteries and splanchnic vessel origins but that spares the distal aorta. These assumedly developmental narrowings of the abdominal aorta have been termed segmental hypoplasia or abdominal aortic coarctation. They are not inflammatory or atherosclerotic, but the affliction compromises blood flow to the renal arteries and mesenteric bed. The etiology of such abdominal coarctation and segmental hypoplasia appears related to other congenital developmental abnormalities. For example, some patients have an inordinately large number of renal arteries and a bicuspid aortic valve. While this condition is unusual, it must be recognized and treated. It is associated with premature death from ravages of secondary hypertension.

While developmental segmental stenosis of the mid-abdominal aorta is rare, atherosclerotic occlusive disease at this level is not. Treatment of the atherosclerotic variant implies use of conventional aortic reconstructive techniques.

ACUTE AORTIC OCCLUSION

Acute occlusion of the abdominal aorta is a catastrophic condition that may result from thrombosis of aortic atheroma or embolization from a cardiac source. When thrombosis is the primary problem, manifestations of severe distal ischemia caused by smaller emboli of aortic origin may be the chief manifestation. When the cause of the aortic occlusion is a cardiac embolus, the manifestations of severe ischemia may include bilateral lower extremity paralysis or paresis as well as the other cardinal finding of arterial occlusion. Despite prompt surgical intervention, the mortality rate of such patients is high because of renal failure, distal compartment syndromes, and adult respiratory distress syndromes. When the condition follows an acute myocardial infarction or disseminated intravascular coagulation, the clinical problems become most challenging. In patients demonstrating the cutaneous manifestations of peripheral atheromatous embolization, an aortic source should be searched for. Mural thrombosis occurring on an ulcerated atheroma is commonly found and should be considered a malignant condition demanding prompt therapy. Exclusion of the affected aortic segment is the goal of intervention.

AORTIC INFLAMMATORY DISEASE

Although in Western civilization inflammatory conditions affecting the aorta are rare, they do occur and are difficult to diagnose and manifestly difficult to treat. They can be divided into non-bacterial inflammatory disease, (e.g., the aortoarteritis of Takayasu), and the bacterial inflammations caused by salmonella, Gram-positive cocci, and Gram-negative organisms such as *Escherichia coli.*

Nonbacterial inflammatory aortoarteritis may affect the aortic arch and its branches or the descending thoracic and abdominal aorta without arch manifestations. It may produce late occlusive lesions or localized aneurysms. The pulmonary artery may be affected. Clinical manifestations are divided into acute and late phases. During the acute phase, nonspecific symptoms include fever, myalgia, malaise, arthralgia, chest and abdominal pain, night sweats, vomiting, pleurisy, and skin rash. Many of the patients are between 10 and 20 years of age, and three out of four patients are women. The late phase is characterized by marked fibrosis and thickening of the vessels affected. At this time, saccular aneurysms may also form. The time division between acute and late phases may vary from months to years, and during the interval period, intermittent exacerbations of systemic symptoms may occur. Late phase symptoms include severe hypertension, lower extremity claudication, chest pain, angina pectoris, and pulmonary arteritis with hypertension.

BACTERIAL AORTITIS

It was Osler who coined the term *mycotic aneurysms.* The normal aorta is resistant to infection, but bacteria may implant in the wall through the lumen with implantation at sites of atherosclerotic disease or may reach the aorta as spread from contiguous adjacent structures. As in syphilis, bacteria may reach the aortic lumen through the vasa vasorum located in the media. When bacteria are found in the thrombi of aortic aneurysms, clinical invasive infection is rare. However, when systemic manifestations of invasive infection are present, suppurative aortic aortitis is fearsome. Fever is the most common initial symptom, and the triad of fever, back pain, and pulsating abdominal mass is strongly suggestive. When leukocytosis of greater than 10,000 is present, blood cultures may be positive in the majority of cases. Diagnosis is made by computed tomography (CT) of the aorta. Frank rupture of the aorta is to be expected whenever bacterial contamination has occurred.

AORTIC ANEURYSMS

Aortic aneurysms are common in an adult population. Untreated, they are lethal. When treated, longevity of patients is similar to that of normal individuals. The incidence of abdominal aortic aneurysms in adults varies from 2 to 4 per cent and in community screening studies has been established at 2.7 per cent. If screening is confined to patients above age 50, the incidence is 5 per cent. Although aortic aneurysms appear to be atherosclerotic, many factors are not recognized that cast doubt on such a simplistic view. In family studies, it is clear that fathers may transmit to sons the tendency toward aortic aneurysms, and when husband and wife are both afflicted, all offspring are affected. The genetic marker for aneurysms may contain other defects that predispose the patient to malignancy and/or chronic obstructive pulmonary disease.

An exploration into a defective copper metabolism, which leads to reduced activity of lysyl oxidase in cross-linking collagen, has not been fruitful. In contrast, studies of proteolytic enzymes have shown that high serum elastolytic activity is found in patients with aortic aneurysms, especially those who smoke. When the aneurysmal tissue itself is studied, this demonstrates a significantly greater collagenase and elastase activity than arteriosclerotic aorta used as control. Patients with ruptured abdominal aortic aneurysms have the highest aortic tissue elastase activity. It is felt that a homeostatic balance between elastase and antiprotease activity may be altered in the aortic wall at the time of aneurysm rupture. An increase in proteolytic activity unchecked by low antiprotease activity causes elastin breakdown, which may be the inciting event for rupture of an otherwise compromised and thin aortic aneurysmal wall. It is intriguing to note that an imbalance between elastase and alpha-1-antitripsin occurs as a direct toxic effect of smoking and results in emphysema and chronic obstructive pulmonary disease. Chronic obstructive pulmonary disease is a known risk factor in predicting rupture of small aortic aneurysms.

ANEURYSMOSIS

Observations of dilated and elongated arteries fascinated Leriche in the 1940s. Now, it is known that such generalized arterial giving-way predisposes patients to aneurysms of the aorta, iliac arteries, femoropopliteal, and distal segments. Clinically, the importance of recognizing such aneurysmosis is that patients under treatment for single aneurysm may be expected to develop other aneurysms proximal or distal to the first manifestation. Histologically, in such patients, the aortic media is markedly thinned with a striking loss of elastic tissue. In fact, elastic fibers are scant, fragmentary, and in many areas, almost entirely absent.

Unfortunately, the natural history of every aneurysm is that of enlargement progressive to rupture. Rate of enlargement of abdominal aortic aneurysms has been the focus of several studies, all of which conclude that the average rate of enlargement is 4 millimeters per year. Rapid expansion occurs and is unpredictable. Similarly, acute rupture is unpredictable. Computed tomography of the aorta has allowed identification of a subpopulation of patients with chronic contained rupture of such aneurysms. This is manifested as a periaortic soft tissue mass presenting to the left or right of the aortic axis. Such patients may be totally asymptomatic or may exhibit nonspecific symptomatology, including chest pain. The mortality of surgery after aortic rupture has occurred remains between 30 and 50 per cent, while the mortality of elective surgical procedures is now approaching 1 per cent. Chronic, contained rupture as seen on CT allows elective surgical repair.

Included in the natural history of abdominal aortic aneurysms is the occasional acute thrombosis that develops in these lesions. The clinical presentation of such patients is identical to that of patients with acute aortic thrombosis without aneurysm. This requires urgent care.

Rupture of abdominal aortic aneurysms may occur into four different structures. The most common presentation is retroperitoneal rupture of the aneurysm with tamponade and stability of the patient's condition which allows urgent surgery to proceed. In contrast is the intraperitoneal rupture which occurs in 15 per cent of patients and in which intractable hypotension occurs. This is associated with the highest mortality. A more favorable form of aortic aneurysm rupture is that which occurs in some 5 per cent of patients, when the hemorrhage is into the adjacent vena cava. When this happens, the patient is autotransfused as the aortic aneurysm ruptures. Such patients are salvageable by urgent surgery. The rarest form of aneurysm rupture is that which occurs into the duodenum, frequently heralded by minor gastrointestinal hemorrhages that allow immediate evaluation by endoscopy, CT scanning, and direct transport of the patient to the operating theater for cure.

THORACIC ANEURYSMS

The thoracic aorta is subject to a particular type of traumatic injury. This is traumatic tear of the aorta distal to the origin of the left subclavian artery at the site of attachment to the ligamentum arteriosum. Here, the free-swinging aortic arch and attached heart meet the fixed descending aorta pinioned against the spine by intercostal vessels. In acute deceleration, the aortic wall is disrupted and escaping blood tamponades as the pseudoaneurysm develops. This is first suspected in the multi-trauma patient by widening of the mediastinum as seen on chest X-rays. A CT scan and/or aortogram confirms the diagnosis and allows orderly surgery to proceed.

TREATMENT

Therapy of acquired aortic conditions has become well standardized. Occlusive conditions are relieved by intervention. Balloon angioplasty may be used effectively in treating stenosis. By-pass grafts, usually from the aorta to femoral arteries, are used in treating occlusion. Endarterectomy is virtually obsolete.

In treating aneurysms, the affected tissue is seldom resected. An inlay prosthetic graft has been found to be eminently satisfactory.

Alternative, non-anatomic reconstructions such as axillary-femoral grafts are used as temporary solutions to problems that are life (or limb) threatening; these grafts are not expected to maintain permanent patency.

ANGINA PECTORIS

method of
JAMES R. HIGGINS, M.D.
Tulsa, Oklahoma

Angina was initially described as a form of chest discomfort imparting a sense of "strangling and anxiety." Today, "squeezing," "crushing," "heavy," or "constricting" retrosternal discomfort is the most common clinical description of angina pectoris. Other primary or radiating sites include the arms, neck, jaw, throat, and subxiphoid area. Anginal equivalents represent symptoms of myocardial ischemia and include breathlessness, faintness, fatigue, and belching.

The symptoms of angina result from an imbalance between myocardial oxygen supply and demand. *Typical* or *fixed-threshold angina* is characterized by a precise amount of physical activity that causes angina and is the result of oxygen demands that exceed the supply provided by critically stenosed coronary arteries. *Rest angina* occurs without physical exertion and is the result of a primary decrease in oxygen supply without an associated increase in demand. This type of anginal syndrome implies some degree of coronary artery spasm. Most patients fall between these two extremes, and the term *mixed angina* has been applied to this large group. Thus, a change in vascular tone (spasm) superimposed upon a fixed stenosis may explain the occurrence of rest and exertional angina in the same patient.

Specific therapies aimed at each of these subclasses of angina may differ. With the availability of medications with somewhat specific actions, a careful history must be obtained in each patient before starting medical therapy.

General Management

Exercise electrocardiography is usually indicated in patients with chest discomfort suggestive of angina. This test is not only helpful in confirming the diagnosis of coronary artery disease but is also useful in defining its severity. Exercise test variables that are associated with multivessel coronary artery disease and increased risk for myocardial infarction include (1) ≥ 2 mm horizontal ST depression at a heart rate ≤ 120 beats per minute, (2) a decrease in systolic blood pressure with exercise, and (3) inability to complete Stage II of a Bruce protocol. In general, patients with these exercise test abnormalities should undergo coronary angiography to determine the location and severity of their coronary artery disease. Baseline electrocardiographic abnormalities (e.g., left ventricular hypertrophy, left bundle branch block, baseline ST abnormalities), digitalis therapy, and hypokalemia are common causes of a false-positive exercise test. Stress thallium-201 myocardial perfusion imaging may be helpful in these patients.

Conditions exacerbating angina should be sought in all patients. Thus, therapy directed at thyrotoxicosis, anemia, arrhythmias, congestive heart failure, or hypertension may be all that is needed to prevent angina. Medications including sympathomimetic amines and amphetamine should be used with caution. Educating the patient about the disease is important, especially concerning precipitating factors such as emotional stress, overeating, cold weather, physical exertion, smoking (active or passive), smog, and high altitudes.

Aerobic exercise such as walking, swimming, or biking is important. The conditioning effect of exercise on skeletal and cardiac muscle allows a decrease in the heart rate at any level of exercise. Thus, physical conditioning reduces the amount of oxygen needed by the heart for any given amount of total body work and improves the duration of exercise before angina occurs. Regular exercise also gives the patient a sense of well-being and self-confidence, both important in managing patients with coronary artery disease.

Major risk factors for coronary artery disease are hypertension, hyperlipoproteinemia, smoking, diabetes mellitus, and a family history of coronary artery disease. Therapy for hypertension and hyperlipoproteinemia should be instituted with diet, medications, or both, and vigorous attempts at eliminating smoking are imperative. Aggressive control of blood sugar levels has not been shown to prevent or delay the development of atherosclerosis but may prevent other secondary manifestations of diabetes mellitus. Counseling of family members concerning risk management is necessary. Although obesity has not been established as an *independent* risk factor for coronary artery disease, it is important, since weight reduction reduces blood pressure, lowers cholesterol, improves glucose utilization, and improves exercise performance.

Drug Therapy

Pharmacologic therapy for the treatment of angina consists of three classes of medications: (1) nitrates, (2) beta-adrenergic blockers, and (3) calcium channel blockers. Within each class several different preparations are available with differences in action and side effects. Thus, in order to maximize the therapeutic effectiveness of each class, a clear understanding of each medication is desirable, especially when combination therapy is contemplated.

Nitrates

The clinical effectiveness of nitroglycerin has been recognized since the 1800s. The mechanism of nitrate antianginal action is complex, but the basic pharmacologic action is to relax vascular smooth muscle. Thus, vasodilation of arteries and veins occurs, resulting in diminished myocardial ischemia by several mechanisms. First, vasodilation of systemic vascular beds decreases systemic vascular resistance (afterload) and venous return (preload), leading to decreased myocardial oxygen demand. Second, epicardial coronary blood flow is augmented by dilation of normal and diseased arterial lumina. Third, nitroglycerin causes redistribution of coronary blood flow to the subendocardium, thereby enhancing oxygen delivery to ischemic areas (Table 1).

Sublingual Nitroglycerin. Nitroglycerin (Nitrostat) given sublingually is the treatment of choice for an acute anginal attack. Sublingual isosorbide dinitrate (Isordil) has a slightly slower onset but a longer duration of action and is recommended for prophylaxis shortly before beginning activities that are likely to cause angina.

Oral Nitroglycerin. Sustained-release nitroglycerin (Nitro-Bid) and long-acting nitrate esters (Isordil, Peritrate) are available for oral administration. Although oral nitrate preparations undergo extensive first-pass hepatic degradation, beneficial hemodynamic and clinical effects have been established. However, the effective dose in an individual patient must be titrated to symptomatic improvement or side effects. Dosages higher than those recommended by the pharmaceutical company are commonly needed.

Topical Nitroglycerin. Nitroglycerin ointment (15 mg per inch) is efficacious and has a duration as long as 6 hours. This form of administration is useful in patients who are hospitalized with severe angina and are confined to bed or for prophylactic bedtime application in patients with nocturnal angina. However, many ambulatory patients find the ointment cosmetically unacceptable, and sustained-release transdermal patches (Transderm-Nitro, Nitro-Dur, Nitrodisc) offer an alternative. In these preparations, nitroglycerin is impregnated into a polymer with a semipermeable inner and an impermeable outer surface. The unit is then attached to the skin via an adhesive. The dose depends upon the unit size, but 25 to 150 mg of nitroglycerin can be delivered over a 24-hour period. The patches are applied once daily and are a convenient form of therapy, especially in noncompliant patients. Initial reports were encouraging, but recently measured serum nitroglycerin concentrations have raised questions concerning claims of sustained 24-hour release. The patch delivery systems are much more expensive than the ointment. Recent reports of tolerance to the chronic administration of long-acting nitroglycerin, regardless of the

TABLE 1. **Dosage and Pharmacokinetics of Nitrate Preparations**

Preparation	Onset of Action (min)	Peak Action (min)	Duration of Action	Usual Dosage (mg)	Dosing Interval
Sublingual NTG	1–3	4–8	10–30 min	0.3–0.6	As needed
Sublingual ISO	2–5	15–60	90–120 min	2.5–10	As needed
Buccal NTG	2–5	4–10	0.5–5 hr	1–3	q 4–6 hr
Oral NTG	20–45	45–120	4–6 hr	6.5–18.0	q 4–6 hr
Oral ISO	15–45	45–120	4–6 hr	10–60	q 4–6 hr
Oral PENT	60	60–120	3–5 hr	40–80	q 4–6 hr
NTG ointment	15–60	30–120	3–6 hr	0.5–2 inches	q 4–6 hr
NTG disks	30–60	60–180	24 hr	5–20	Once daily

Abbreviations: NTG = nitroglycerin; ISO = isosorbide dinitrate; PENT = pentaerythritol tetranitrate.

formulation, may decrease the use of these medications as "first line" therapy in the future.

Intravenous Nitroglycerin. Intravenous nitroglycerin (Tridil) administration is common in the intensive care unit setting; caution must be taken to use special tubing that does not absorb the medication. This drug has become useful in the treatment of certain patients with acute myocardial infarction, pulmonary edema, and unstable angina. If used in large doses, intravenous nitroglycerin is effective in the treatment of severe hypertension. It is preferred over sodium nitroprusside, a more potent antihypertensive agent, in patients with associated ischemia. In general, 50 mg of nitroglycerin is mixed in 250 ml of D_5W (200 micrograms per ml). Starting at 10 micrograms per minute, the infusion is titrated to a desired hemodynamic response. Determination of pulmonary capillary wedge and intra-arterial pressures during intravenous infusion is almost always essential for safe administration.

Side Effects. Headache is an expected side effect of initial nitroglycerin therapy. The patient should therefore be warned and counseled that the headaches will usually diminish and disappear during the first weeks of therapy. Although pretreatment with mild analgesics (acetaminophen or aspirin) can be helpful, an occasional patient cannot tolerate nitrate therapy because of this side effect. Other side effects include dizziness, nausea, flushing, and, rarely, syncope or hypotension. An allergic dermatitis may develop with topical administration, usually secondary to a reaction to the adhesive; thus, changing to another preparation can be successful. Methemoglobinemia, caused by intoxication from the ethanol diluent have been reported in patients receiving high doses (> 1000 micrograms per minute) of intravenous nitroglycerin.

Beta-Adrenergic Blockers

These medications represent a cornerstone of therapy for typical or fixed-threshold angina. In doses that are generally well tolerated, these medications substantially reduce anginal episodes and increase the anginal threshold by competitive inhibition of the effects of catecholamines on beta-adrenergic receptors. There are two types of beta-adrenergic receptors: $beta_1$-receptors are found in the heart, whereas $beta_2$-receptors are located primarily within the smooth muscle of the bronchial tree and peripheral arteries. Although beta blockade decreases the resting heart rate, the principal antianginal action is the profound attenuation of sympathetic effects during periods of activity. Thus, by blunting adrenergic stimulation, exercise heart rate and contractility are reduced significantly, thereby decreasing myocardial oxygen demands. Even nonselective beta blockers lower systemic blood pressure (possibly by a central mechanism), which further lowers myocardial oxygen requirements.

There are currently seven different beta blockers available in the United States. Although all prevent angina by similar mechanisms, differences in individual properties make each drug somewhat unique. Pharmacologically, these drugs differ with respect to absorption, protein binding, and bioavailability. These variables assure a considerable interpatient disparity in plasma drug levels, and thus there may be marked differences in the dosage requirements among patients. For example, some patients have adequate beta blockade while taking 80 mg per day of propranolol (Inderal), whereas others may require 480 mg per day to achieve the same clinical effect. Because of these variables, it is important to objectively document effective beta blockade. The decrease in resting heart rate should not be used as a therapeutic end point; rather, a controlled heart rate response to exercise should be determined. Exercise electrocardiography is useful in this regard and has the added benefit of assessing the degree of protection from ischemia.

Probably the three most important differences in the beta blockers that affect their clinical use are *cardioselectivity, lipid solubility,* and *intrinsic sympathomimetic activity.* At low to moderate plasma levels, atenolol (Tenormin), metoprolol (Lopressor), and acebutolol (Sectral) are "cardioselective"—that is, they preferentially block $beta_1$-receptors. These drugs may be preferable in patients with reactive airway disease, peripheral vascular disease, and diabetes mellitus. However, at higher dosages the selective beta-blocking effect is lost, and they behave like other nonselective drugs.

The least lipid-soluble beta blockers, nadolol (Corgard) and atenolol (Tenormin), have two advantages: (1) less hepatic uptake and metabolism, and (2) less central nervous system penetration. These two properties translate into longer plasma half lives and fewer central nervous system side effects, respectively. However, because of renal excretion, these drugs must be used with caution in patients with renal insufficiency. On the other hand, non–lipid-soluble beta blockers must be dose adjusted in patients with hepatic insufficiency.

Intrinsic sympathomimetic activity refers to the ability of a drug not only to block intrinsic catecholamine stimulation but also to act as a weak beta-adrenergic agonist. Pindolol (Visken) and acebutolol (Sectral) have this property. Theoretically, this results in less slowing of sinus node activity and atrioventricular conduction; however, the response to exercise remains blunted. It is not entirely clear whether partial agonist activity is an advantage or a disadvantage in angina therapy, although most studies have shown an excellent clinical response to these medications.

Dosage guidelines are listed in Table 2; however, therapy must be individualized per the previous discussion. Several clinical trials have now demonstrated that certain beta-blocking drugs can substantially reduce the number of deaths during the first 2 years after myocardial infarction. These data suggest that such therapy should be considered for all patients after myocardial infarction, even in the absence of angina.

Side Effects. Most of the side effects of these medications are related to their major pharmacologic action, the blockage of beta receptors. Direct adverse effects on the heart include the potential for severe bradycardia, atrioventricular block, or congestive heart failure. Severe complications can be treated by careful infusion of a beta agonist. Precipitation or worsening of bronchospasm, claudication, or variant angina may occur secondary to beta$_2$-receptor blockade. Central nervous system side effects, including insomnia, depression, and hallucinations, seem to be dose dependent. Gastrointestinal adverse effects and impotence are uncommon. Some degree of caution must be taken when prescribing these medications for patients with insulin-dependent diabetes, as these agents may abolish the warning signs of hypoglycemia.

Sudden withdrawal of beta-blocker therapy in ambulatory patients has been associated with acute ischemic episodes and death. Because of this possible "rebound phenomenon," patients must be instructed not to stop taking these medications abruptly, and beta blockers should not be discontinued prior to major surgery.

Calcium Channel Blockers

Calcium ions play a critical role in normal contraction of cardiac and vascular smooth muscle and in the action potential of various myocardial tissues, including the sinoatrial and atrioventricular nodes. With decreasing intracellular calcium concentrations, cardiac contractility and vascular tone are diminished, as is the slow current phase of the cardiac action potential. Thus, calcium channel blockers have several potential beneficial cardiovascular effects: (1) arterial vasodilatation, (2) negative inotropic effects, and (3) slowing of sinoatrial and atrioventricular conduction. These drugs have the potential of increasing myocardial oxygen supply (by coronary artery dilatation) while decreasing myocardial oxygen demand (decreased heart rate, contractility, and afterload).

There are currently three calcium channel blockers approved for clinical use in the United States: nifedipine (Procardia), verapamil (Isoptin, Calan), and diltiazem (Cardizem). There is substantial variation in the chemical structure of these drugs, and each inhibits calcium flux by a different mechanism. Therefore, it is not surprising that there are major differences in the pharmacologic effects between the three drugs (Table 3). In general, the net in vivo effects of each medication depend upon direct cardiovascular actions (as discussed above) and secondary baroreceptor sympathetic stimulation.

Nifedipine. Nifedipine (Procardia), the most potent vasodilator of the three, is capable of causing a profound fall in systemic and coronary vascular resistance. Its in vitro actions on depression of myocardial contractility and impulse conduction are significant. Clincally, however, those direct effects are offset by an intense sympathetic output secondary to intense peripheral dilatation. This results in a positive inotropic response and sinus tachycardia. In most clinical situations the net myocardial oxygen consumption is reduced because the decrease in oxygen demand from the reduced afterload and the increase in oxygen supply from coronary vasodilatation exceed the increase in oxygen demand caused by the reflex responses.

TABLE 2. **Dosage and Pharmacokinetics of Beta-Adrenergic Blocking Drugs**

	Relative Beta$_1$ Selectivity	Lipid Solubility	Intrinsic Sympathomimetic Activity	Route of Elimination	Usual Dose
Atenolol (Tenormin)	+	Low	0	Renal	50–100 mg q day
Metoprolol (Lopressor)	+	Moderate	0	Hepatic	50–200 mg q 12 hr
Acebutolol (Sectral)	+	Moderate	+	Renal and hepatic	200–400 mg q 8 hr
Nadolol (Corgard)	0	Low	0	Renal	40–320 mg q day
Pindolol (Visken)	0	Moderate	+	Renal and hepatic	10–30 mg q 12 hr
Propranolol (Inderal)	0	High	0	Hepatic	10–120 mg q 6 hr; Inderal LA = 80–480 mg day
Timolol (Blocadren)	0	Low	0	Renal and hepatic	10–30 mg q 12 hr

Abbreviations: + = Present; 0 = Absent.

TABLE 3. **Dosages and Properties of Calcium Channel Blockers**

	Arterial and Coronary Vasodilatation	Contractility	Atrio-ventricular Conduction	Resting Heart Rate	Onset of Action (Oral)	Excretion (%Renal/Fecal)	Usual Dose
Nifedipine (Procardia)	↑ ↑ ↑	0 (net)	0	↑ (Reflex)	<20 min 2–3 min SL	80/15	10–40 mg q 6–8 hr
Verapamil (Isoptin, Calan)	↑	↓ ↓	↓ ↓ ↓	↓	<30 min	70/15	80–120 mg q 6–8 hr (5–15 mg IV)*
Diltiazem (Cardizem)	↑ †	↓	↓	↓ or 0	<30 min	35/65	30–90 mg q 6–8 hr

*Given over 1 to 2 minutes for the control of certain dysrhythmias.

†May be more potent as a coronary vasodilator.

Abbreviations: ↑ = increases; ↓ = decreases; 0 = no effect; SL = sublingual. *Note:* The number of arrows reflects the intensity of effect.

In general, nifedipine is used as a supplemental antianginal agent and not as first-line therapy. It is especially useful in combination with beta blockers, which tend to block the reflex sinus tachycardia. Nifedipine should be considered as initial therapy in patients with a history suggesting coronary vasospasm or when potential adverse side effects limit the use of other medications (i.e., beta blockers in asthmatic patients) and in patients with significant hypertension.

The side effects of nifedipine mainly result from its potent vasodilating properties. Common adverse reactions include headache, dizziness, flushing, nausea, and leg edema (not related to heart failure). Rarely, a paradoxical increase in angina can result, presumably from excessive sinus tachycardia or hypotension. In 5 to 10 per cent of patients, intolerable side effects necessitate discontinuation of therapy. If necessary, nifedipine can be given sublingually by cutting the capsule and placing the liquid contents under the tongue.

Verapamil. Verapamil (Isoptin, Calan) dilates peripheral and coronary arteries but is less potent than nifedipine. During clinical use, verapamil decreases myocardial contractility much more than nifedipine, probably because verapamil causes less secondary sympathetic stimulation. This negative inotropic action does decrease myocardial oxygen consumption; however, it may trigger an exacerbation of congestive heart failure in patients with significant underlying systolic ventricular dysfunction.

Although verapamil decreases sinoatrial node automaticity slightly, its main effect is a significant reduction in atrioventricular nodal conductivity. This property is exceedingly useful in treating paroxysmal atrial tachyarrhythmias involving atrioventricular nodal tissue and in slowing the ventricular response to atrial fibrillation and flutter. Because of these effects on atrioventricular conduction, verapamil administration can cause high-degree heart block in patients with underlying conduction disorders. Particular

caution must be used in patients taking beta blockers or digitalis.

Side effects associated with verapamil administration include those listed for nifedipine, although they occur less often with verapamil. Constipation is common but rarely limits therapy. As discussed earlier, exacerbation of congestive heart failure and high-degree atrioventricular block can occur in some patients.

Diltiazem. Although diltiazem (Cardizem) dilates peripheral arteries, there is evidence that its action on the coronary vasculature is relatively selective. In general, as can be seen from Table 3, the cardiovascular effects of this drug are intermediate between nifedipine and verapamil. However, one must still exercise caution when using it in patients with significant left ventricular dysfunction or advanced degrees of atrioventricular block.

Adverse side effects are similar to those of the other calcium channel blockers, although initial reports suggest that they are much less frequent.

Combination Drug Therapy

In patients with more severe angina, a combination of two or even three classes of medications can be employed. With each class containing several specific agents, numerous possibilities for combination therapy exist. While many studies have shown the added effectiveness of blockage of calcium entry and beta blocker receptors, this combination must be approached with caution in patients with ventricular dysfunction and in those with impaired sinoatrial or atrioventricular conduction. In general, the combination of nifedipine and a beta blocker is well tolerated, with the latter drug blocking the reflex tachycardia induced by the former. The combination of nifedipine and nitrates is less ideal, since profound vasodilatation with significant hypotension, tachycardia, or both can occur. In general, additional antianginal medications should be added in low dosages and gradually raised to tolerance.

If the patient's life style is limited by persistent angina despite combination therapy, angioplasty or surgical therapy should be considered.

Other Antianginal Drugs

Digitalis is not of benefit in the treatment of angina unless used to treat coexistent congestive heart failure. Anticoagulant therapy with warfarin (Coumadin) is not recommended in patients with angina unless there are other predisposing factors for thrombosis. There is evidence that antiplatelet therapy with aspirin may decrease the incidence of acute myocardial infarction in patients with unstable angina. Whether antiplatelet medications are useful in the therapy of stable angina is still controversial.

Percutaneous Transluminal Coronary Angioplasty

Percutaneous transluminal coronary angioplasty is a technique employing standard cardiac catheterization methods to place a balloon across a stenotic segment and inflating the balloon to relieve the stenosis. The most appropriate candidates for this procedure are patients with significant angina who are on medical therapy and who are otherwise being considered for surgical revascularization. Anatomic variations such as proximal discrete stenosis in a major epicardial coronary artery must also be considered. The procedure is rarely performed for left main coronary artery disease. Its role in patients with multivessel disease or prior coronary bypass grafting is expanding.

Depending upon operator experience, successful angioplasty can be performed in 95 per cent of patients. Because coronary occlusion occurs in 1 to 3 per cent of patients, a cardiac surgical team may need to be on standby for emergency coronary bypass grafting. Stenosis recurs, usually within 6 months, in 25 to 30 per cent of patients with an initially successful angioplasty. In about two thirds of these patients, a second angioplasty will be successful. Exercise electrocardiography and thallium perfusion imaging are useful in following patients after angioplasty.

Coronary Artery Surgery

Despite the large numbers of coronary artery bypass operations performed each year, arguments persist over the indications for surgery. Two indications are supported universally: (1) left main coronary artery stenosis (greater than 60 per cent), (2) severe angina on maximal medical therapy. There is some evidence that symptomatic patients with three-vessel disease and those with two-vessel disease involving the proximal left anterior descending artery benefit from surgery, especially if associated with impaired left ventricular function. There is no evidence that surgical therapy prolongs survival in patients with any form of single vessel disease, including isolated left anterior descending obstructions.

Unfortunately, there is no simple formula for recommending surgery, and the decision must be individualized. Factors to be considered in addition to coronary anatomy and symptoms include the patient's lifestyle, age, and general health; disease in other organs and disease in other vascular beds; and the experience of the cardiovascular surgical team.

SPECIFIC ANGINAL SYNDROMES

Unstable Angina

Unstable angina is also known as crescendo or preinfarction angina. Clinical features include either (1) angina that has become more severe, prolonged, or frequent and is superimposed upon stable angina; or (2) new onset of angina that is brought on by minimal exertion. In addition to a typical history, many studies have required transient electrocardiographic changes (ST and/or T wave changes) during episodes of pain to establish the diagnosis, although the absence of changes does not exclude the diagnosis.

Management

Since unstable angina is a potentially life-threatening condition, its management must be aggressive. The patient should be admitted to an intensive care setting and placed at bed rest. A vigorous effort to diagnose and treat underlying conditions that increase the cardiac workload must be undertaken. Treatment for fever, thyrotoxicosis, anemia, exacerbations of congestive heart failure, infections, and arrhythmias can relieve symptoms in up to 15 per cent of patients. In certain patients, the reverse Trendelenburg position and oxygen inhalation may be helpful.

Nitrate administration is the mainstay of therapy of unstable angina. Although these agents may be given by any of the routes previously discussed, intravenous nitroglycerin offers more consistent control of ischemia. The dose of nitrates should be sufficient to lower arterial systolic pressure by 15 mmHg or to 100 to 110 mmHg, whichever is smaller. Beta blockers play a key role in the pharmacologic treatment of unstable angina. Unless contraindications exist initially or develop during therapy, the dosage should be titrated to decrease the resting rate to 50 to 60 beats per minute. This usually requires the equivalent of 240 mg of propranolol per day. Calcium channel blockers are also helpful in the treatment of unstable angina. Although usually added to nitrate and beta-blocker therapy, they are also effective as initial therapy. Recent studies have suggested a significant reduction in mortality and nonfatal myocardial infarctions in patients with unstable angina treated with one aspirin tablet (325 mg) daily.

There is controversy concerning the role of coronary arteriography and coronary artery bypass grafting in the management of unstable angina. Many recommend coronary arteriography for all patients with unstable angina because of the higher incidence of "surgical" coronary artery disease (left main or triple-vessel disease) or critical proximal single-vessel disease amenable to percutaneous transluminal coronary angioplasty.

Variant (Prinzmetal's) Angina

Rest angina is the principal historical finding in patients with variant angina. In contrast to unstable angina, the rest pain does not represent an "evolution" from a stable exertional pattern. Patients with this syndrome are typically younger than those with classic exertion-induced angina, and up to 25 per cent have evidence of a generalized vasospastic disorder (migraine or Raynaud's phenomenon). Electrocardiographic changes are the key to the diagnosis of variant angina. The development of ST segment elevation during rest pain is characteristic. Ventricular arrhythmias and conduction disturbances are common and can cause syncope and sudden death. When anginal attacks are infrequent, the administration of ergonovine maleate during coronary arteriography can be useful in making the diagnosis.

The medical management of variant angina differs in some important aspects from that of stable angina pectoris. Both forms of angina respond to nitrates, although the mechanism of action of the drugs may differ. In variant angina, the direct vasodilating effect of the nitrates on the coronary arterial bed prevents spasm, whereas in exertion-induced angina the reduction in preload secondary to venodilation may predominate. The response of patients with Prinzmetal's angina to beta blockade is variable. Nonselective beta blockade allows the occurrence of unopposed alpha-receptor–mediated coronary artery vasoconstriction. The duration and frequency of variant angina have been reported to be prolonged by propranolol. The calcium channel blockers are extremely effective in preventing the coronary artery spasm of variant angina. Many consider these medications as first-line agents in the treatment of variant angina, with sublingual nitroglycerin used as a supplement. Coronary artery bypass surgery is not indicated for patients with pure coronary artery spasm.

CARDIAC ARREST

method of
ARTHUR B. SANDERS, M.D., and
GORDON A. EWY, M.D.
University of Arizona Health Sciences Center
Tucson, Arizona

Over the past 20 years there has been a steady decline in deaths due to cardiovascular disease. Multiple factors are thought to play a role in this decline, including decreased cigarette smoking by high-risk populations, improved awareness and treatment of hypertension and hyperlipidemia, improved diet and exercise programs by the general population, and advances in medical and surgical care of patients with cardiovascular disease. Despite these impressive advances, cardiovascular disease remains far and away the leading cause of death in the United States today. Almost half of the deaths in the United States in any given year are due to cardiovascular disease, and many patients die of cardiac arrest.

Prevention

Most patients who suffer cardiac arrest have significant arteriosclerotic coronary artery disease. However, not all patients are aware of their heart disease. Up to 20 per cent of patients suffering cardiac arrest collapse from arrhythmias as their first sign of coronary artery disease. An important effort of primary care physicians should be directed toward prevention of atherosclerosis in young patients. Screening programs to detect and treat patients with hypertension and hyperlipidemia are important for decreasing the risk for cardiac arrest. Patients need to be educated regarding cigarette smoking, prudent diets, and exercise programs. In those patients who have developed coronary artery disease, treatment with beta-adrenergic blocking agents or anti-arrhythmic drugs may be appropriate to prevent sudden death. Finally, it is crucial that all patients be educated regarding actions to be taken to ensure emergency treatment of patients in cardiac arrest. This involves knowledge of how to access the emergency medical services (EMS) system in their community. Older individuals and patients with risk factors should be educated as to the early warning signs of an acute myocardial infarction and encouraged to be evaluated early if symptoms develop. Spouses of high-risk patients should be encouraged to learn basic cardiopulmonary resuscitation (CPR) techniques.

Concepts of Emergency Medical Services (EMS) Systems

Most out-of-hospital cardiac arrest is due to ventricular fibrillation, a dysrhythmia that is potentially curable if treated early by basic and advanced cardiac life support systems. In order to speed treatment of patients suffering cardiac arrest, two new concepts in our health care delivery system had to be developed. The first extended treatment from the hospital coronary care unit and emergency departments into the community. This was done with mobile coronary care units capable of providing advanced life support to patients in the community. These efforts, pioneered in Belfast, New York, Seattle, and Miami have now become a standard part of our medical care system. The second concept was the realization that in order to provide emergency care in the community, an entire system of emergency medical care would have to be developed. The emergency medical services system varies somewhat from community to community, but basically revolves around three levels of care.

1. Citizens should be trained to access the EMS system and, if possible, deliver basic life support or CPR. Ideally, all citizens should know how to access the EMS system in their community. Many but not all communities have adopted 911 as the emergency telephone number. In addition, 20 to 30 per cent of the community should be trained in CPR, with emphasis on family or spouses of patients with known coronary artery disease. If the recently pioneered telephone assistance CPR proves to be effective, some people may be able to learn and provide CPR at the time they call for help.

2. A second level of the EMS system is provided by emergency medical technicians (EMTs). EMTs are trained in first aid and CPR. In most communities, ambulance attendants, fire fighters, and police officers are trained EMTs and can deliver basic life support until advanced life support is available. Recent studies have shown that many EMTs can be trained to defibrillate patients with the use of automatic external defibrillators. Studies have shown improved survival for patients suffering cardiac arrest with the use of EMTs trained in defibrillation in areas where paramedics are not available or have delayed response times.

3. Paramedics provide the highest level of prehospital care treatment in most communities. Paramedics have received approximately 1000 hours of training and have passed stringent oral and written examinations. They are able to provide the full gamut of advanced cardiac life support in the field, including intubation, defibrillation, and administration of cardiovascular drugs. Data from Seattle have demonstrated that if basic life support can be provided in less than 4 minutes and advanced life support within 8 minutes, 43 per cent of patients suffering from ventricular fibrillation in the community can be resuscitated and survive to leave the hospital. If either CPR or defibrillation is delayed, survival falls off drastically. Thus, time is a crucial element. Many systems are designed so that CPR can be initiated by either trained citizens or EMTs within a few minutes of cardiac arrest and advanced life support provided by trained paramedics within 8 minutes. Physicians should be aware of the EMS system in their community and educate their patients regarding its utilization.

Basic Life Support

Cardiopulmonary resuscitation (CPR) and defibrillation are the cornerstones for the treatment of patients in cardiac arrest. It is important to remember that CPR itself does not resuscitate patients with cardiac arrest. It merely slows the process of dying so that effective advanced life support (defibrillation) may be instituted to resuscitate patients. Standards for basic life support are set through a consensus conference sponsored by the American Heart Association every 5 to 6 years. The last consensus conference was held in 1985 and published in the *Journal of The American Medical Association* (JAMA) (255: 2905, 1986). In this review we will briefly outline important aspects of CPR with emphasis on areas of controversy.

Airway

The head-tilt/chin-lift maneuver is recommended for opening the airway. Backward pressure on the victim's forehead is provided by one hand while the fingers of the other hand lift the chin upward. If neck injury is suspected for any reason, the jaw-thrust maneuver should be utilized to open the airway. The rescuer moves the mandible forward with pressure applied at the angles of the victim's lower jaw.

Breathing

Once the airway is open the rescuer looks, listens, and feels for the free flow of air. If no spontaneous breathing is observed, the rescuer should give mouth-to-mouth respirations while pinching the victim's nostrils. Initially, the rescuer should apply two slow ventilations (1 to 1½ seconds per breath) while watching for chest expansion and exchange of air. These initial two slow breaths represent a change in CPR standards from the four quick "stair-step" breaths previously recommended. Two slow breaths provide adequate ventilation and decrease the possibility of producing pharyngeal pressure so high that gastric distention and aspiration may occur. The recommendations emphasize the importance of adequate ventilation for providing oxygenation and removal of carbon dioxide. Throughout CPR a "ventilatory pause" is recommended, taking a full 1 to 1½ seconds for each ventilation after 15 compressions (one-person CPR). Once the patient is intubated and adequate ventilation assured, chest compressions need not be interrupted for the ventilatory pause. If adequate air exchange is not detected, one should be concerned about an obstructed airway.

Obstructed Airway

If the victim presents with an obstructed airway and air exchange cannot be obtained, the Heimlich maneuver, or "subdiaphragmatic abdominal thrust," is recommended. The hand should be positioned above the navel but below the xiphoid process and several quick thrusts provided in an attempt to relieve the foreign body obstruction. In the unconscious victim, the Heimlich maneuver may be followed by a visualized finger sweep to remove the foreign body. Regurgitation and trauma to abdominal viscera may result if the Heimlich maneuver is used inappropriately.

Circulation

Pulselessness should be determined through palpation of the carotid. If no pulse is detected, external chest compression should be instituted. The patient must be placed on a firm surface and the heel of one hand positioned two finger breadths above the xiphoid. In the average adult, the sternum is depressed 1.5 to 2 inches. Compressions are given 80 to 100 times per minute (60 compressions per minute were previously recommended). If the patient is not intubated, compressions are interrupted to allow for two ventilations after every 15 compressions for one-rescuer CPR. When two rescuers are present, a 5:1 compression ventilation ratio should be used.

Physiologically, closed-chest CPR delivers between 10 and 30 per cent of normal cardiac output. Several investigators over the past 5 years have suggested alterations in the technique of CPR to improve cardiac output and organ perfusion. These methods have included simultaneous compression and ventilation, chest compression with intermittent or simultaneous abdominal compression, high-frequency CPR, and the application of the MAST suit. While some initial studies of these techniques were encouraging, and research in this area is continuing, no alternative technique has consistently shown improved resuscitation and survival. Thus, until an alternative technique is clearly shown to be superior to the presently recommended form of CPR (JAMA 255:2905, 1985), they should not be used for treatment of patients in cardiac arrest.

Advanced Cardiac Life Support

Advanced cardiac life support (ACLS) involves the institution of sophisticated therapeutic procedures including defibrillation and arrhythmia treatment. Advanced life support, like basic life support, involves the learning and practice of manual skills and sequences of events. These are best learned through the formal ACLS course for health care providers sponsored by the American Heart Association.

In cardiac arrest, the patient's prognosis depends upon his underlying rhythm. While ventricular tachycardia and ventricular fibrillation have relatively good prognoses if defibrillation is instituted early, electromechanical dissociation and asystole are poor prognostic indicators. Thus, the first ACLS concern is to determine the patient's underlying rhythm by placing either monitor leads or defibrillator monitoring paddles on the chest. As soon as time permits, the patient should be endotracheally intubated and ventilated with 100 per cent oxygen. In addition, an intravenous line should be started for administration of medications. Most commonly, a peripheral vein in the antecubital area may be used. Alternatively, and depending on the rescuer's capability, a central venous line may be started using the internal/external jugular vein. Intravenous lines below the diaphragm are generally discouraged because there is poor venous return from the lower half of the body. Small distal veins of the wrist and hand are not as good as antecubital or central veins because of diminished blood flow to the distal extremities during cardiac arrest. Intracardiac injections are discouraged. If intravenous access cannot be readily attained, intratracheal administration of some medications is acceptable (see below).

Drug Therapy

Epinephrine. Epinephrine is the pressor agent of choice for use in patients in cardiac arrest, primarily because of its alpha adrenergic stimulating properties. Epinephrine raises the aortic diastolic pressure, which increases coronary blood flow and myocardial perfusion. It has also been shown to increase central nervous system blood flow during cardiac arrest in animal models. The recommended dose of epinephrine in adults is 1 mg (10 ml of a 1:10,000 solution) every 5 minutes during the resuscitation effort. If an intravenous line is not present, epinephrine may be given through the endotracheal tube.

Atropine. Atropine is a parasympatholytic agent that is indicated in asystole and symptomatic bradycardias. It is thought that some patients in asystolic cardiac arrest have an excess of parasympathetic stimulation. For these patients, 1 mg of atropine may be given intravenously and repeated in 5 minutes for a total dose of 2 mg. If an intravenous line is not established, atropine may be given through the endotracheal tube.

Isoproterenol. Isoproterenol is a pure beta-adrenergic stimulator and is not useful in patients in ventricular fibrillation or asystole. Isoproterenol may lower the fibrillation threshold and will increase myocardial oxygen consumption of the fibrillating heart. Isoproterenol is not indicated if the patient is in arrest without a pulse. Until a pacemaker can be initiated, isoproterenol (2 to 10 micrograms per minute) may be indicated for patients with symptomatic bradycardia (pulse present) that is refractory to atropine.

Calcium. Recent studies have shown no beneficial effects from the use of calcium for most patients in cardiac arrest. Thus, calcium should not be used routinely in the setting of cardiac arrest except when hyperkalemia, hypocalcemia, or calcium channel–blocker toxicity is suspected.

Bicarbonate. There is much confusion as to the role of alkali treatment for patients in cardiac arrest. Although theoretically the correcting of lactic acidemia from tissue hypoperfusion is important, the administration of bicarbonate may produce other problems, including alkalosis and hyperosmolarity. In addition, there is concern that the administration of bicarbonate will increase CO_2 levels, which can worsen intracellular and central nervous system acidosis. Therefore bicarbonate therapy is not recommended in the first 10 minutes of cardiac arrest treatment. After 10 minutes, the potential beneficial and harmful effects of bicarbonate treatment must be individually weighed. If used, 1 mEq per kg intravenously should be given initially. One exception is the patient with suspected hyperkalemia, who should be vigorously treated with bicarbonate.

Lidocaine. Lidocaine raises the fibrillation threshold and is useful for patients who have been successfully defibrillated to prevent recurrent ventricular fibrillation. Lidocaine itself will not chemically defibrillate the heart. Lidocaine should be given in bolus injections to patients in cardiac arrest. An initial bolus of 1 mg per kg should be administered slowly, with additional boluses of 0.5 mg per kg at 15-minute intervals (total bolus dose not to exceed 3 mg per kg). A lidocaine drip of 2 to 4 mg per minute is used following resuscitation.

Bretylium. Bretylium is the second-line antiarrhythmic drug that may be useful for patients in ventricular fibrillation. Bretylium is given initially in doses of 5 mg per kg intravenously and may be increased to 10 mg per kg fifteen minutes later if needed. A theoretical disadvantage of bretylium is that it lowers peripheral vascular resistance, an undesirable effect during cardiac arrest and resuscitation.

Pacemaker Therapy

With the advent of transcutaneous pacemakers a number of studies have looked at the usefulness of pacemaker therapy for the treatment of patients in asystolic arrest. Outside of isolated case reports, no study has demonstrated the effectiveness of pacemakers for the routine patient in cardiac arrest.

Precordial Thump

The precordial thump theoretically delivers about 0.5 to 1 joule of energy to the myocardium. It has been reported that 2 per cent of patients immediately going into ventricular fibrillation may respond to a precordial thump with cardioversion. Once ventricular fibrillation is established for a few minutes, however, a precordial thump will not be effective, and immediate cardioversion with 200 joules should be instituted. A precordial thump may also be useful for patients in ventricular tachycardia. However, while some patients in ventricular tachycardia will convert to superventricular rhythms with the thump, others will convert to a more malignant dysrhythmia, ventricular fibrillation. Thus, a precordial thump is not recommended for ventricular tachycardia unless the patient is pulseless or one is prepared to defibrillate immediately.

Treatment of Cardiac Arrest Sequences

Ventricular Fibrillation and Pulseless Ventricular Tachycardia. It is crucial to remember that patients in ventricular fibrillation must be cardioverted in order to resuscitate them successfully. All other treatment is an attempt to better prepare the patient for electrical defibrillation. The longer the patient remains in fibrillation, the more difficult it will be to cardiovert him or her. Thus, as soon as the diagnosis is made the patient should be defibrillated with up to 3 shocks of 200 to 360 joules even before basic CPR is instituted or the patient is intubated. If a defibrillator is not immediately available, basic CPR should proceed until its arrival. Following three attempts at defibrillation, 1 mg of epinephrine may be given intravenously or endotracheally in attempts to produce selective vasoconstriction to increase myocardial and cerebral blood flow. This should be followed by another defibrillation attempt with 360 joules. Following the fourth defibrillation attempt, antiarrhythmic drugs may be used. Lidocaine, 1 mg per kg, is the initial drug recommended. Lidocaine administration may be followed by repeat cardioversion attempts with 360 joules. If therapy is still unsuccessful, a second-line antiarrhythmic drug, bretylium at 5 mg per kg intravenously, may be used followed by repeat defibrillation with 360 joules. Administration of 1 mg of epinephrine intravenously or endotracheally should be repeated every 5 minutes until the patient is resuscitated or attempts terminated. As discussed above, 1 mEq per kg of bicarbonate may be given at 10 minutes of arrest. If one suspects hyperkalemia, the patient should be treated vigorously with bicarbonate and calcium until a potassium level can be determined.

Asystole. Asystole must be distinguished from fine ventricular fibrillation. The diagnosis can be confirmed by switching monitor leads to assure that fibrillation is not present. If there is any question that fibrillation is present, proceed with defibrillation attempts as described previously. If asystole is present, one should begin CPR and establish intravenous access. Epinephrine (1 mg intravenously or endotracheally) should be given to improve myocardial and cerebral blood flow and repeated every five minutes. Atropine (1 mg intravenously) may be given and repeated to a total dose of 2 mg. The prognosis for patients in true asystole is poor.

Electromechanical Dissociation. One must distinguish myocardial from extramyocardial causes of electromechanical dissociation. Extramyocardial causes include hypovolemia, cardiac tamponade, tension pneumothorax, hypoxemia, and severe acidosis. Therefore, when monitor electrical activity is present without pulses or pressure, one must always evaluate the patient's airway, breath sounds, and volume status. A pericardiocentesis may be done in attempts to relieve a tamponade. If correctable causes of electromechanical dissociation are ruled out, the prognosis for resuscitation is poor. Epinephrine (1 mg intravenously or endotracheally) is indicated every 5 minutes to improve myocardial and cerebral perfusion.

Coordination of ACLS Team

An efficient advanced life support resuscitation effort involves a highly coordinated, well-run team. The physician in charge should be the only person to give orders. A second team member should be assigned the documentation of all drugs and procedures used during the resuscitation effort. Appropriate training drills and coordination of the team process are essential for efficient resuscitation efforts. Each hospital and all EMS system personnel should evaluate their success rate against data reported in the literature to determine if resuscitation efforts are of optimal quality.

Termination of ACLS

Studies have repeatedly demonstrated that the longer the patient remains in cardiac arrest, the more difficult it will be to resuscitate him. Thus, after 30 minutes of arrest and unsuccessful advanced life support, the prognosis is very poor. Currently, there are no early indicators the clinician can use to determine if there is irreversible neurologic or cardiovascular damage. Therefore one must continue the resuscitation efforts until there is cardiovascular unresponsiveness to the advanced life support protocols previously outlined.

ATRIAL FIBRILLATION

method of
MICHAEL E. ASSEY, M.D.
Medical University of South Carolina
Charleston, South Carolina

Atrial fibrillation is a commonly encountered arrhythmia that occurs in 1 per cent of the general population. Its frequency rises sharply with age and generally follows the development of overt cardiovascular disease. It can, however, be seen in the absence of underlying heart disease, as with thyrotoxicosis or in a paroxysmal form secondary to excessive alcohol ingestion ("holiday heart syndrome"). Patients with atrial fibrillation have a higher than normal mortality rate, but the increased risk is most closely associated with the underlying etiology. Paroxysmal atrial fibrillation without underlying heart disease has not been shown to have an increased mortality.

Etiology

Table 1 lists cardiac and noncardiac disorders associated with atrial fibrillation. A high percentage of patients with rheumatic mitral insufficiency or mitral stenosis will have atrial fibrillation, the onset of which

TABLE 1. **Causes of Atrial Fibrillation**

Cardiac Causes
  Rheumatic heart disease
  Hypertensive heart disease
  Arteriosclerotic coronary artery disease
  Primary myocardial disease
  Primary conduction system disease
  Lone atrial fibrillation
  Pericardial disease

Extracardiac Causes
  Thyrotoxicosis
  Pulmonary disease
  Toxins

is frequently associated with clinical deterioration. Ten to 25 per cent of hypertensive patients will have atrial fibrillation during the course of their disease, and this may be poorly tolerated if concentric left ventricular hypertrophy is present. When patients with atherosclerotic risk factors present with atrial fibrillation, underlying coronary artery disease should be suspected, since this arrhythmia may be due to otherwise silent myocardial ischemia. Alcoholic and other types of dilated cardiomyopathies are frequently complicated by atrial fibrillation. This usually occurs late in the course of the disease as the left atrium enlarges, and it is associated with a high risk of systemic embolization.

Primary conduction system disease may be congenital (e.g., Wolff-Parkinson-White and other pre-excitation syndromes) or acquired (e.g., sick sinus syndrome). Often, the ventricular rate is a clue to the etiology. A young patient presenting with atrial fibrillation and a very fast ventricular response (above 170 beats per minute ventricular rate) might have an anomalous atrioventricular (AV) pathway, in which case the normal path through the AV node which has a delaying effect on conduction is bypassed. Alternatively, a patient who is not taking medications but who has a slow ventricular response (below 90 beats per minute ventricular rate) should be suspected of having underlying AV node disease. In elderly patients, this slow ventricular response to atrial fibrillation suggests the presence of sick sinus syndrome manifested as disease of the SA node (resulting in atrial fibrillation) and of the AV node (manifested as an unexpectedly slow ventricular rate).

Lone atrial fibrillation may represent 10 per cent of the total number of cases. Patients are usually men with relatively small left atria; the resting ventricular rate never rises above 100 beats per minute, but the rate increases with exertion. The prognosis is excellent, and generally no specific therapy is needed. Atrial fibrillation occurs infrequently in patients with acute pericarditis. It can, however, be a chronic rhythm in patients with pericardial constriction.

Extracardiac causes of atrial fibrillation include thyrotoxicosis, which can occur without other signs of hyperthyroidism (apathetic hyperthyroidism) in elderly patients. Atrial fibrillation is rare in pulmonary embolism but does occur in chronic obstructive pulmonary disease, often in combination with atrial flutter and multifocal atrial tachycardia when triggered by acute pneumonitis. Toxins such as ethanol and excessive caffeine ingestion can induce atrial fibrillation but this is usually short-lived.

Hemodynamic Changes and Clinical Presentation

Atrial fibrillation may be asymptomatic, but most patients complain of palpitations or a combination of low output and congestive symptoms. The rapid ventricular rate and loss of coordinated atrioventricular contraction decrease ventricular filling, resulting in a lower forward stroke volume and symptoms of fatigue, dizziness, or syncope. Higher left atrial and pulmonary pressures resulting from the rate-induced limitation of ventricular filling may cause dyspnea—a common mode of presentation in patients with mitral stenosis. Patients with noncompliant left ventricles, such as occur in concentric left ventricular hypertrophy due to aortic stenosis or hypertension, are dependent on the atrial contribution to ventricular filling and may remain symptomatic even after the ventricular rate is slowed until sinus rhythm is restored. The rapid ventricular response to atrial fibrillation increases myocardial oxygen consumption and may cause angina in patients with underlying coronary artery disease. Systemic embolization, including embolic stroke, can be the initial presentation. The fibrillating atria develop thrombi, which can expel emboli during atrial fibrillation or when sinus rhythm is spontaneously or iatrogenically restored.

Treatment

Initially, one aims at controlling the rapid ventricular response with drugs that slow atrioventricular conduction. These include digitalis, beta blockers, and certain calcium channel blockers. I usually start with digoxin at a dose of 0.25 mg intravenously every 2 hours (up to 1.5 mg total) or until the ventricular response is controlled. Because of the specific electrophysiologic effects of digitalis, the adequacy of therapy can be assessed by the ventricular response. Determination of the level of digitalis in the blood is rarely useful, and may be misleading. Atrial fibrillation does not often result from digitalis toxicity. When it does, the patient will usually have a slow ventricular response (less than 50 beats per minute) and multiform premature ventricular beats. The classic digitalis toxic arrhythmia is accelerated junctional tachycardia with atrioventricular dissociation. The physician should be suspicious when a patient who was given large amounts of digoxin to convert an arrhythmia suddenly develops a regular rhythm with physical findings suggesting AV dissociation. An electrocardiogram should be performed to validate that the regular rhythm is in fact normal sinus rather than a junctional tachycardia secondary to digitalis toxicity.

Beta blockers are particularly useful in controlling atrial fibrillation secondary to thyrotoxicosis. I use propranolol (Inderal) 1 mg intravenously or 10 to 40 mg orally, every 6 hours, or metoprolol (Lopressor) 5 mg intravenously or 50 mg orally every 6 to 12 hours. When verapamil (Calan, Isoptin) is used, the dose is 5 to 10 mg intravenously or 80 mg orally every 6 to 8 hours. This dose of verapamil will usually control the ventricular rate but only rarely converts the patient to sinus rhythm. Verapamil, like quinidine, will increase the digoxin level.

After controlling the ventricular rate, one considers whether or not to restore normal sinus rhythm. Cardioversion should be used in symptomatic patients. Asymptomatic patients who are unlikely to convert or to maintain sinus rhythm following initial conversion should be left alone. Such patients include those with long-standing atrial fibrillation (greater than 1 year's duration), patients with large left atria (greater than 50 mm determined by echocardiography), or those whose atrial fibrillation is due to an active disease process (pneumonitis, thyrotoxicosis).

In preparation for conversion, I generally administer the anticoagulant warfarin (Coumadin) and maintain the patient's prothrombin time at twice control for 7 to 14 days prior to attempted cardioversion. This is done to minimize the chances of systemic embolization. With this approach, the risk of embolism is only 1 per cent following direct current cardioversion, while it may be four to five times greater if the patient has not received anticoagulant medication. Embolism can occur immediately following conversion or several days later, indicating that there is a delay in recovery of atrial contractility after successful electrical cardioversion. For this reason, anticoagulation is continued 1 to 4 weeks after cardioversion. Even if cardioversion is not attempted, I generally administer anticoagulants to patients with atrial fibrillation who have a high risk of systemic embolism. This includes patients with large left atria and those in whom atrial fibrillation is secondary to rheumatic heart disease, congestive cardiomyopathy, idiopathic hypertrophic subaortic stenosis, or recent myocardial infarction with a low output state.

Chemical cardioversion is usually attempted with one of the Type IA antiarrhythmic drugs. I generally use quinidine, starting at 300 mg orally every 6 hours. For those who cannot tolerate quinidine, disopyramide (Norpace) or procainamide (Pronestyl) is used. Other antiarrhythmic agents used to convert atrial fibrillation include amiodarone (Cordarone), which may be successful when type IA agents fail and in patients with large left atria. The usefulness of amiodarone is limited by its numerous side effects (pulmonary fibrosis, thyroid disease, visual disturbances, and photosensitivity).

If chemical cardioversion fails, direct current (DC) shock is used. Ideally, an anesthesiologist or an individual skilled in endotracheal intubation should be present. Popular regimens for providing the light anesthesia desired for DC cardioversion include intravenous diazepam (Valium), thiopental (Pentothal), and methohexital (Brevital). Cardioversion should be performed in the Coronary Care Unit or equivalent where cardiopulmonary resuscitative equipment is available. An intravenous line should be started, and after appropriate anesthesia has been obtained, DC shock is applied at 100 joules. The use of anterior-posterior paddles is associated with the lowest energy needed for cardioversion. Rarely, a patient with a thick chest wall will require 300 or even 400 joules of energy to restore sinus rhythm. When DC cardioversion is used, the cardioverter should be synchronized so that the shock is applied during the QRS segment of the electrocardiogram. Failure to synchronize the DC shock could result in ventricular fibrillation. Following conversion to sinus rhythm, the patient is monitored for 6 hours at which time he or she should be fully alert and allowed to return to a regular hospital room or be discharged.

One of the frustrating aspects of treating atrial fibrillation by this method is that up to 50 per cent of patients who are successfully converted to sinus rhythm will revert to atrial fibrillation within 6 months. Most of these patients will redevelop atrial fibrillation within the first month, a large minority within the first week, and many will fail to hold sinus rhythm for even 24 hours. Conversely, those who do maintain normal sinus rhythm for the first month have an excellent chance of maintaining sinus rhythm chronically.

Special Considerations

Atrial fibrillation secondary to Wolff-Parkinson-White syndrome should probably not be treated with digitalis, since this drug decreases the refractory period of the anomalous pathway and may accelerate the ventricular response, possibly causing ventricular fibrillation. This is particularly true if the R to R intervals are less than 300 milliseconds apart. If atrial fibrillation is secondary to the sick sinus syndrome, cardioversion is generally contraindicated. When these patients undergo electrical or pharmacologic cardioversion, serious bradyarrhythmias and even asystole may develop. Often these patients need a permanent pacemaker to prevent bradyarrhythmias before the atrial fibrillation can be safely treated with drugs like digitalis that depress atrioventricular conduction.

PREMATURE BEATS

method of
GERALD V. NACCARELLI, M.D.
University of Texas Medical School at Houston
Houston, Texas

Ectopic beats may occur from the atrium (premature atrial complexes), the atrioventricular (AV) junction (premature junctional complexes), or from the ventricles (premature ventricular complexes). Junctional premature complexes are very rare.

PREMATURE ATRIAL COMPLEXES

Premature atrial complexes (PACs) are common but usually asymptomatic. The cause of PACs is not completely understood, although they seem to occur most commonly secondary to enhanced automaticity. PACs occur frequently in patients with organic heart disease, especially if atrial enlargement or intra-atrial conduction abnormalities are present. However, PACs may also occur in patients with normal hearts and can be caused by stimulants such as sympathomimetic drugs, caffeine, or alcohol and by anxiety. PACs often cause significant symptoms if they trigger atrial tachyarrhythmias such as atrial fibrillation, atrial flutter, ectopic atrial tachycardia, and paroxysmal re-entrant supraventricular tachycardia.

PREMATURE VENTRICULAR COMPLEXES

Ventricular arrhythmias have been classified as benign, potentially lethal or lethal based on severity of the arrhythmia, underlying heart disease, hemodynamic consequences of the arrhythmia, and estimated risk of sudden death.

Benign ventricular arrhythmias primarily include frequent premature ventricular complexes (PVCs), couplets, and sometimes nonsustained ventricular tachycardia (VT) associated with no to minimal heart disease, normal left ventricular function, and no hemodynamic compromise from the arrhythmia. Patients with disorders in this group have minimal risk of sudden death, and thus treatment is primarily aimed at the elimination of symptoms such as palpitations and dizziness. Evaluation of efficacy is based upon symptom relief and a marked reduction of ventricular ectopic activity as assessed by noninvasive measures such as Holter monitoring.

Potentially lethal ventricular arrhythmias pri-

TABLE 1. Vaughn-Williams Classification of Antiarrhythmic Drugs

Class	Action	Drugs
I	Sodium channel blockers	
IA	Moderate phase O depression Moderate conduction slowing ($\uparrow$ QRS)	Quinidine Procainimide
	Prolongs repolarization ($\uparrow\uparrow$ QT)	Disopyramide
IB	Minimal phase O depression Shortness repolarization ($\downarrow$ QT)	Lidocaine (IV) Tocainide Mexiletine
IC	Marked phase O depression Marked conduction slowing ($\uparrow\uparrow$ QRS) Slight effect on repolarization	Flecainide Encainide
II	Beta-adrenergic blockers ($\uparrow$ PR)	Propranolol Acebutolol Esmolol (IV)
III	Prolongs repolarization ($\uparrow$ QT)	Bretylium (IV) Amiodarone
IV	Calcium channel blockers ($\uparrow$ PR)	Verapamil (IV)

marily include frequent PVCs and nonsustained VT associated with organic heart disease and left ventricular dysfunction. Affected patients have a moderate risk of sudden death. However, few data exist demonstrating that antiarrhythmic therapy prevents sudden death in this group of patients. Therefore, treatment is aimed at both symptom relief and, hopefully, prevention of sudden cardiac death. Evaluation of efficacy is based on symptom relief and reduction of ventricular ectopic activity during continuous electrocardiographic monitoring.

Lethal ventricular arrhythmias include sustained VT and/or ventricular fibrillation. These arrhythmias are usually associated with organic heart disease and left ventricular dysfunction and often cause significant hemodynamic compromise. Affected patients are at high risk for sudden death, and the goal of therapy is not only relief of symptoms but also prevention of sudden cardiac death. Evaluation of efficacy in this group of patients is based on symptom relief and survival in addition to objective improvement assessed by both Holter monitoring and electrophysiologic testing.

In addition to the above classes of ventricular arrhythmias a separate class of acute ventricular arrhythmias is seen in patients with acute myocardial infarction or following open-heart surgery.

TREATMENT

Evaluation, Testing, and Monitoring

Regardless of the arrhythmia treated or the antiarrhythmic drug selected, proper evaluation

TABLE 2. **Oral Antiarrhythmic Agents**

Generic Name	Trade Name	Dose Forms (mg)	Usual Dosage in mg
Quinidine sulfate	Quinora	200, 300	200–400 q 6 hr
Quinidine polygalacturonate	Cardioquin	275	275 q 8–12 hr
Quinidine gluconate	Quinaglute	324	324–648 q 8–12 hr
Quinidine sulfate—long-acting	Quinidex	300	300–600 q 8–12 hr
Procainamide	Pronestyl	250, 375, 500	200–1000 q 3 hr
Procainamide—sustained release	Pronestyl SR	500	250–1000 q 6 hr
	Procan SR	250, 500, 750	
Disopyramide	Norpace	100, 150	100–200 q 6 hr
Disopyramide—sustained release	Norpace CR	100, 150	200–300 q 12 hr
Tocainide	Tonocard	400, 600	400–600 q 8 hr
Mexiletine	Mexitil	150, 200, 250	200–300 q 8 hr
Flecainide	Tambocor	100	100–200 bid
Encainide	Enkaid	25, 35, 50	25–50 tid
Propranolol	Inderal	10, 20, 40, 60, 80	10–80 qid
Acebutolol	Sectral	200, 400	200–600 bid
Amiodarone	Cordarone	200	200–400 per day

and appropriate testing needs to be performed in control and treated states. During therapy, appropriate monitoring of electrocardiographic intervals, blood levels, and subjective toxicity and laboratory monitoring of end-organ toxicity has to be tailored to the specific patient and the antiarrhythmic drug selected. Electrocardiographic monitoring is necessary to type and quantitate the arrhythmia. Long-term Holter recordings may document coexisting or more complex arrhythmias that were not initially appreciated. A baseline EKG may give clues to the type of arrhythmia in addition to screening for chamber enlargement, conductive defects, and old myocardial infarctions. Owing to spontaneous variability, symptomatic arrhythmias may be difficult to document electrocardiographically. Event recorders ("cardiobeepers") may be useful if routine EKGs or Holter monitors are not helpful. Stress testing may be useful to rule out exercise aggravation of the arrhythmia or latent coronary artery disease. Electrophysiologic testing is primarily reserved for patients with sus-

tained re-entrant supraventricular tachycardia and sustained VT and/or ventricular fibrillation.

Antiarrhythmic Therapy

Antiarrhythmic drugs are often used to suppress premature beats and also to treat more serious arrhythmias. A classification of antiarrhythmic drugs is listed in Table 1. Table 2 lists trade names and usual doses of the currently available oral antiarrhythmics; Table 3 lists the comparative efficacy of these drugs to suppress PACs and PVCs; and Tables 4 and 5 list comparative hemodynamics and toxicities. A priori, no antiarrhythmic drug will be effective all of the time. However, certain drugs make better first choices in certain situations. The type of arrhythmia, previous drug failures, coexisting arrhythmias and disease states, and left ventricular function all affect the choice of a drug for an individual patient. Type IA and IC drugs are often useful in coexisting atrial and ventricular arrhythmias, whereas type IB drugs are not useful in suppressing PACs. In patients with congestive heart failure, drugs with significant negative inotropic activity (disopyramide, flecainide, beta-blockers) should be used cautiously. The recommendations outlined below should be used as guidelines. Exceptions to these guidelines can occur.

Treatment of PACs

PACs are primarily treated in an attempt to relieve symptoms such as palpitations. In patients with atrial tachyarrhythmias, drug therapy may be used to suppress PACs that can trigger the atrial tachycardia. Our first treatment approach consists of conservative measures such as avoidance of alcohol and caffeine. This ap-

TABLE 3. **Comparative Antiarrhythmic Efficacy of the Antiarrhythmic Drugs**

	PAC Suppression	PVC Suppression
Quinidine	+ +	+ +
Procainamide	+ +	+ +
Disopyramide	+ +	+ +
Lidocaine	0	+ +
Tocainide	0	+ +
Mexiletine	0	+ +
Flecainide	+ +	+ + +
Encainide	+ +	+ + +
Beta-blockers	+	+
Amiodarone	+ +	+ + +
Digoxin	0	0
Verapamil	0	0

TABLE 4. **Comparative Hemodynamics, Digoxin Interaction, Proarrhythmic Potential**

	Negative Inotropy	Digoxin Interaction	Proarrhythmia Nonsustained VT Patients	Proarrhythmia Sustained VT Patients	TDP
Quinidine	±	+	+	+ +	+ + +
Procainamide	±	0	+	+ +	+ + +
Disopyramide	+ +	0	+	+ +	+ + +
Tocainide	±	0	+	+	0
Mexiletine	±	0	+	+	0
Flecainide	+	0	+	+ + +	±
Encainide	±	0	+	+ + +	±
Propafenone	+	+	+	+ +	±
Beta-blockers	+ +	0	+	+	0
Amiodarone	±	+	+	+	+

Abbreviations: VT = ventricular tachycardia; TDP = torsades de pointes.

proach is more likely to work if historically these agents seem to aggravate the patient's symptoms. If these measures do not improve the patient's symptoms, we will treat the patient with antiarrhythmic drugs. Beta-blockers, type IA (quinidine, procainamide, disopyramide) and type IC sodium channel blockers (encainide, flecainide) can all be useful in suppressing an irritable atrial focus. However, type IB agents (mexiletine, tocainide), which are lidocaine-like, are not useful in treating these patients. As with treatment of patients with benign PVCs, we try to avoid drugs that cause end-organ toxicity.

Treatment of PVCs

Acute ventricular arrhythmias in the myocardial infarction setting are typically treated and controlled with intravenous lidocaine (1 to 4 mg per minute). We avoid high doses of lidocaine (3 to 4 mg per minute) in patients who are elderly and more sensitive to neurologic side effects and in patients with known left ventricular dysfunction. The latter group has a decreased cardiac output and thus a diminished perfusion of the liver; because of this, lidocaine is not as efficiently metabolized, resulting in toxic levels.

If lidocaine is not effective, our second drug of

choice is intravenous procainamide (1 to 4 mg per minute). Once the patient has survived the acute high-risk period, long-term oral therapy should be decided according to symptoms and risk. The risk of a more serious arrhythmia causing sudden death can be judged by quantitative and qualitative evaluation of the arrhythmia with electrocardiographic monitoring and assessment of left ventricular function.

If the physician notes PVCs in a patient, a Holter monitor is useful to quantitate the frequency and screen for more complex forms or coexisting atrial dysrhythmias. We attempt to find an antiarrhythmic agent that will suppress PVCs by 75 per cent and couplets by 90 per cent and that will completely eliminate runs of VT.

For patients who are being treated for benign, symptomatic PVCs, we prefer to use drugs with a minimal potential for end-organ toxicity and a low incidence of causing proarrhythmia (Tables 4 and 5). If beta-blockers or mexiletine are ineffective, we preferentially use flecainide or encainide before resorting to type IA antiarrhythmic agents. We avoid the use of amiodarone in this group of patients because of its end-organ toxicity.

We prefer beta-blockers or mexiletine for patients with potentially lethal ventricular arrhythmias, especially in the outpatient setting, as first-line agents, because of their lack of end-organ toxicity and low proarrhythmic potential. Our other front-line choices are type IC agents, given their high efficacy and low toxicity and proarrhythmic potential in this group of patients. Our next choice would be type IA agents alone or in combination with a type IB agent. In refractory cases, we might consider amiodarone therapy if the patient had refractory, nonsustained VT, especially with coexisting left ventricular dysfunction or hemodynamically compromising atrial fibrillation.

When a patient has a lethal ventricular arrhythmia, we use type IA agents and mexiletine

TABLE 5. **Comparative Toxicity of Antiarrhythmic Drugs**

	Subjective Toxicity	Cardiovascular Adverse Effects*	End-Organ Toxicity
Quinidine	+ +	+	+ +
Procainamide	+	+	+ +
Disopyramide	+	+ +	±
Tocainide	+ +	±	+
Mexiletine	+ +	±	±
Flecainide	±	+ +	0
Encainide	±	+	0
Beta-blockers	+	+	0
Amiodarone	+	+	+ + +

*Summary of conduction changes, negative inotropy, and proarrhythmia.

alone or in combination as front-line agents. We prefer these drugs despite efficacy rates of less than 25 per cent because of the high incidence (greater than 10 per cent) of drug-induced incessant VT with type IC drugs in this group of patients. We reserve amiodarone for sustained ventricular tachyarrhythmias that are refractory to treatment with types IA, IB, and IC drugs (at least one failure with each type).

HEART BLOCK

method of
PAUL G. COLAVITA, M.D.
The Carolinas Heart Institute
Charlotte, North Carolina

Heart block, a transient or permanent disturbance of electrical impulse conduction, has been classified into three categories. In first-degree block conduction time is prolonged but all impulses are conducted. Second-degree block is classified as Mobitz Type I (Wenckebach) and Type II. Mobitz Type I occurs when there is a progressive increase in the conduction time until an impulse fails to conduct. In Type II there is a sudden block of impulse conduction without prior increase in conduction time. Third-degree, or complete block occurs when no impulses are conducted. Heart block can occur between the sinus node and atria (sinoatrial), between the atria and ventricles (atrioventricular), or within the atria (intra-atrial) or ventricles (intraventricular). Therapy is based on the location of block, the severity of symptoms, and the presence of underlying heart disease or precipitating factors.

ACUTE HEART BLOCK

Acute Sinoatrial Block

Sinoatrial block is due to conduction delay within the sinus node that may result from enhanced vagal tone, myocarditis, drug therapy, or metabolic abnormalities. It may also occur as a complication of a myocardial infarction.

Therapy is indicated for symptomatic bradycardia and sinus pauses several seconds in duration. Intravenous atropine (0.5 to 1 mg) or isoproterenol (1 to 2 micrograms per minute) is effective in suppressing sinus pauses, although better results are obtained with a temporary pacemaker. Treatment is maintained for several days or until the block resolves.

Acute Atrioventricular Block

First-degree atrioventricular block may result from conduction delay within the atrium, atrioventricular node, His bundle, or bundle branches.

Acute first-degree atrioventricular block is a benign condition and does not require therapy.

Mobitz Type I atrioventricular block with a narrow QRS complex almost always occurs in the atrioventricular node; however, a wide QRS complex may represent block in the atrioventricular node or His-Purkinje system. Type II atrioventricular block is located in the His-Purkinje system. Third-degree atrioventricular block occurs in the atrioventricular node when associated with a narrow QRS complex but is located in the His-Purkinje system when associated with a wide QRS complex.

Acute Mobitz Type I atrioventricular block is frequently a complication of drug intoxication, electrolyte imbalance, or myocardial ischemia. When atrioventricular nodal block (Type I or third-degree) is associated with a narrow escape complex, therapy is indicated only if there is evidence of compromise due to a slow heart rate (e.g., presyncope, heart failure, or angina). Atropine should be used initially to treat atrioventricular nodal block when associated with mild hemodynamic compromise. If symptomatic block persists, temporary ventricular pacing should be employed. Pacing should be continued until atrioventricular conduction returns to normal. Isoproterenol can also be used to enhance atrioventricular conduction but is associated with adverse side effects that limit its usefulness. When the block is located in the His-Purkinje system (Type II or third-degree), the QRS complexes are wide and the escape rate is inadequate to maintain hemodynamic stability. A temporary pacemaker should be inserted in any patient who develops a block in the His-Purkinje system, even if the patient remains asymptomatic. Isoproterenol, 2 to 4 micrograms per minute, is useful in maintaining an adequate escape rhythm until a temporary pacemaker can be inserted. The temporary pacemaker should be left in place until the block resolves.

Acute Bundle Branch Block

Acute bundle branch block usually occurs during myocardial infarction and is associated with an increased risk of developing second- or third-degree (high-degree) atrioventricular block. The need for temporary pacing is determined by the risk of developing high-degree block. High-degree block is most likely in patients with the new onset of bifascicular block with and without PR interval prolongation. There is also a good chance of developing high-degree block with first-degree atrioventricular block in the presence of bifascicular block or a new bundle branch block. A temporary pacemaker should therefore be inserted in these patients. The progression to high-degree block is infrequent in patients with newly isolated bundle branch block or pre-existing bifascicular block, and close monitoring of these patients is probably all that is necessary.

Permanent cardiac pacing is probably indicated in patients with acute myocardial infarction, bundle branch block, and transient complete atrioventricular block, as there is a high incidence of sudden death reported in this group. There are no data to support permanent pacemaker implantation in patients who have resolution of transient atrioventricular block following myocardial infarction or those with new bundle branch block who did not have high-degree block during the acute event.

CHRONIC HEART BLOCK

Chronic Sinoatrial Block

Sinoatrial block is frequently found in asymptomatic healthy individuals. It is also noted in patients with sick sinus syndrome due to a variety of causes. When abnormal sinus node activity produces cerebral dysfunction or hemodynamic compromise, permanent pacing is justified.

Chronic Atrioventricular Block

Chronic first-degree atrioventricular block, whether caused by delay in the atrioventricular node or the His-Purkinje system, does not require therapy. Type I second-degree atrioventricular nodal block and third-degree block associated with a narrow QRS complex is usually a benign process in the absence of organic heart disease. It is frequently seen in physically trained individuals and other normal people, especially during sleep. In the presence of organic heart disease, the prognosis is poor owing to the underlying heart disease. Therapy for chronic atrioventricular nodal block associated with a narrow QRS complex consists of permanent pacemaker implantation. Treatment is indicated for symptoms such as transient cerebral dysfunction, syncope, or congestive heart failure. Pacemaker implantation may also be necessary when essential drug therapy for underlying heart disease aggravates heart block. Patients with second- or third-degree atrioventricular block associated with a slow, wide complex escape rhythm require permanent pacemakers. Congenital complete heart block does not usually require therapy, although pacemakers are indicated for recurrent syncope or congestive heart failure.

Chronic Bundle Branch Block

There is a strong correlation between the presence of bundle branch block and an underlying cardiovascular disease. Although the risk of progression to complete heart block is low, the 5-year survival in patients with acquired bundle branch block is high owing to the underlying heart disease.

No specific treatment is required for chronic bundle branch block. Permanent cardiac pacing should be reserved for patients with symptoms caused by transient atrioventricular block. There is considerable controversy regarding the proper therapeutic approach to the patient with bundle branch block and recurrent neurologic symptoms in whom no high-degree atrioventricular block has been documented. These patients should probably undergo detailed electrophysiologic studies to assess nodal function and inducibility of ventricular arrhythmias. Permanent pacing would be indicated if distal His-Purkinje block is induced by atrial pacing. Although pacemaker insertion can be expected to relieve symptoms in this group of patients, it will not necessarily prolong life.

TREATMENT

Drug Therapy

Atropine increases the rate of functional pacemakers and improves atrioventricular conduction. Intravenous atropine (0.5 to 1 mg) is the treatment of choice for symptomatic Type I second-degree block associated with a narrow QRS complex. This can be repeated two or three times, as necessary, although temporary pacing is indicated if the block persists. Long-term therapy with atropine is limited by side effects that include mental confusion, blurred vision, and drying of secretions. Intravenous isoproterenol infused at a rate of 1 to 4 micrograms per minute can also be used. This agent is the drug of choice for atrioventricular block associated with a wide QRS complex. Adverse effects of isoproterenol include sinus tachycardia, increased myocardial contractility (which may aggravate ischemia), and ventricular arrhythmias.

The use of anticholinergic or sympathomimetic agents such as propantheline bromide, ephedrine, and sublingual isoproterenol is effective in chronic second- and third-degree atrioventricular block but is associated with a high incidence of side effects.

Cardiac Pacing Therapies

Temporary Pacing. The simplest and easiest way of applying temporary pacing is the external transthoracic method. This method is useful in emergency rooms and ambulances until a transvenous pacing catheter can be inserted.

Although a transvenous pacing catheter can be inserted through most large veins, the subclavian and internal jugular veins are preferred. A 5- or 6-Fr bipolar catheter can be positioned under fluoroscopic or electrocardiographic control. An adequate threshold to pace is ensured and the electrode secured. With proper care, this electrode can be left in place for 5 to 7 days.

Permanent Pacing. A permanent pacemaker lead is usually inserted through the cephalic or subclavian vein and advanced to the right ventricular apex. Adequate thresholds to sense and pace are ensured. A second lead can also be inserted through the subclavian vein and advanced into the right atrium for dual chamber pacing if an atrial contribution for hemodynamic benefit is necessary.

TACHYCARDIAS

method of
MICHAEL J. REITER, M.D., PH.D.
University of Colorado
Denver, Colorado

Strictly speaking, tachycardia is present whenever the heart rate exceeds 100 beats per minute. This definition includes physiologic sinus tachycardia. Pathologic tachycardias imply, in addition, abnormalities of mechanism or origin, or both. Clinical tachycardias generally result from one of two mechanisms: automaticity, which is an acceleration of the rate of cells that normally exhibit a slow, spontaneous rate of firing; or reentry, a continuous and repetitive circuit of myocardial activation.

Intelligent management of tachycardias requires (1) understanding of the mechanism of the tachycardia, (2) appreciation of the clinical setting in which the tachycardia occurs, and (3) examination of the need and specific goals of therapy.

Diagnosis of a specific tachycardia should start with careful analysis of the electrocardiogram for information about rate, regularity, morphology, and atrioventricular (A-V) relationship. Tachycardias can be classified as supraventricular (origin above the His bundle) or ventricular (origin below the His bundle). Distinction between them may be difficult if a supraventricular tachycardia is associated with bundle branch block. Features suggesting ventricular origin include a QRS duration of 140 msec or greater, atypical bundle branch block morphology, and evidence of A-V dissociation. Occasionally a particular arrhythmia may be difficult to interpret. In this instance, intracardiac electrophysiologic evaluation can usually clarify the nature and mechanism of the tachycardia. Patients with spontaneous and episodic tachycardia are difficult to assess. Holter monitoring or event recording during symptoms may be useful in these patients.

Tachycardias cause symptoms because of decreased cardiac output as a consequence of both the increased heart rate and the abnormal sequence of myocardial activation. Symptoms may be minor and merely troublesome (e.g., palpitations, lightheadedness) or more severe (near or frank syncope). The severity and frequency of symptoms determines the need and urgency of therapy. Since all antiarrhythmic agents are associated with significant side effects, toxicity, uncertain efficacy, and potential for worsening arrhythmias, it is important to determine whether therapy is warranted. Goals of therapy may include termination of an acute tachycardia, chronic therapy to prevent recurrent tachycardia, or amelioration of a chronic arrhythmia or one likely to recur.

Treatment

Sinus Tachycardia

Sinus tachycardia is most frequently a physiologic response to hypotension, hypovolemia, hypoxia, anemia, cardiac failure, pain, fever, or anxiety. This tachycardia is generally benign and therapy should be directed at the underlying cause.

Ectopic Atrial Tachycardia

This tachycardia results when atrial cells develop a more rapid rate of firing than sinus rhythm. Electrocardiographic features include a P wave morphology that is different than sinus, usually a normal QRS morphology, and rate variability over time. It is frequently associated with 1:1 A-V conduction but can occur with A-V block (2:1 or higher). Multifocal atrial tachycardia is a form of ectopic atrial tachycardia in which at least three different atrial foci appear to be involved. Multifocal atrial tachycardia frequently occurs in patients with severe chronic obstructive pulmonary disease or cardiac failure. Both these tachycardias are most effectively terminated and prevented by quinidine, procainamide, or disopyramide (Tables 1 and 2). Therapy of multifocal atrial tachycardia should be directed toward improving the condition of the underlying disease. Both tachycardias do not respond to cardioversion and are frequently refractory to pharmacologic therapy. In this situation, therapy to slow the ventricular rate (with verapamil, digoxin, or propranolol) is appropriate. Since digoxin at high levels may exacerbate ectopic atrial tachycardia and propranolol may worsen bronchospasm in patients with chronic lung disease, verapamil may be the best choice in many patients with these arrhythmias.

Paroxysmal Supraventricular Tachycardia

This tachycardia frequently occurs in otherwise healthy young individuals. Paroxysmal supraventricular tachycardia is regular, is usually as-

TABLE 1. **Commonly Used Antiarrhythmic Drugs**

Drug	Available Routes	Effective Plasma Concentration	Primary Means of Metabolism	Elimination Half-life (hr)	Important Side-Effects	Predominant Effect
Digoxin	IV, po	1–2 ng/ml	Hepatic	36–38	GI, arrhythmias	Depresses AV node conduction
Procainamide	IV, po	4–10 mcg/ml	Hepatic/renal	2½–5	Allergic (LE), GI	Slows conduction and prolongs refractoriness of atrial, ventricular, and accessory pathway tissue
Quinidine	po	2–5 mcg/ml	Hepatic	5–7	Allergic, GI	
Disopyramide	po	2–5 mcg/ml	Renal	7	Anticholinergic, negative inotropy	
Lidocaine	IV	1.2–6 mcg/ml	Hepatic	1½	CNS (confusion, seizures)	Shortens refractoriness of ventricular tissue
Tocainide	po	3.5–10 mcg/ml	Hepatic/renal	11–16	CNS, rash, GI	
Mexiletine	po	0.5–2 mcg/ml	Hepatic	10–12	GI	
Flecainide	po	0.2–1 mcg/ml	Hepatic/renal	13–20	Negative inotropy	Slows ventricular conduction
Verapamil	IV, po	Not established	Hepatic	4–6	Bradycardia, edema, negative inotropy	Depresses AV node conduction
Propranolol	IV, po	40–100 ng/ml	Hepatic	2–6	Bradycardia, bronchospasm, negative inotropy	Depresses AV node conduction
					All antiarrhythmic agents have a significant potential of worsening existing or causing new arrhythmias	

Abbreviations: CNS = central nervous system; GI = gastrointestinal; IV = intravenous; LE = drug-induced lupus erythematosus; po = per os (oral).

TABLE 2. **Characteristics of Commonly Used Oral Antiarrhythmic Agents**

Drug/Preparation	% Bioavailability	Time to Peak Concentration (hr)	% Bound	Usual Dose (mg)
Quinidine			80	
Quinidine sulfate	80	1½		200–600 q 6 hr
Quindine sulfate—sustained release	80	2–6		600–900 q 8–12 hr
Quinidine gluconate	60–70	4		324–972 q 6–8 hr
Polygalacturonate	75	2–4		275–825 q 8–12 hr
Procainamide	85	1	15	250–1000 q 3–4 hr
Sustained release	85	2–3		500–2000 q 6 hr
Disopyramide	90	2–3	40	100–300 q 6 hr
Sustained release	90	5		200–400 q 12 hr
Tocainide	100	1	50	150–600 q 6–8 hr
Mexiletine	90	2–4	50	200–400 q 8 hr
Flecainide	95	3–4	40	100–200 q 12 hr
Propranolol	10–40	1–2	95	10–80 q 6 hr
Verapamil	20	2	90	40–120 q 6–8 hr

sociated with a narrow QRS morphology, and has an abrupt onset and termination. The A-V relationship is always 1:1, although at times the A-V relationship cannot be discerned because the P wave is hidden within the QRS.

Episodes of tachycardia frequently terminate spontaneously or with patient-induced yawning, gagging, or Valsalva maneuvers. If persistent, these tachycardias can frequently be terminated by vagal maneuvers, which should be attempted before pharmacologic therapy. Intravenous verapamil (Table 3) is the drug of choice if vagal maneuvers fail. Elective cardioversion may be used in patients refractory to pharmacologic therapy or if the tachycardia is associated with significant hemodynamic compromise.

In some patients with paroxysmal supraventricular tachycardia, symptoms are too infrequent or mild to warrant chronic therapy. Avoidance of caffeine, nicotine, or fatigue may limit the frequency of recurrence. Chronic pharmacologic prophylaxis should be reserved for patients with frequent or debilitating symptoms. Digoxin has the advantages of once-a-day administration, low cost, and relative safety and is modestly effective in preventing recurrent tachycardia. Chronic therapy with verapamil or propranolol is effective and is indicated if patients have recurrent tachycardia.

Atrial Fibrillation/Flutter

Both these arrhythmias are characterized by a rapidly circulating wave of depolarization limited to the atrium. In the case of atrial flutter, the atrial rhythm has a regular rate of about 300 beats per minute and a sawtooth appearance on the electrocardiogram. This atrial rhythm is usually conducted to the ventricle with 2:1 A-V block in the untreated patient. Atrial fibrillation is a chaotic and disorganized atrial rhythm. No atrial activity can be appreciated on the electrocardiogram and the ventricular response rate is irregular. Paroxysmal atrial fibrillation or flutter can usually be converted to sinus rhythm by quinidine-like antiarrhythmic agents or cardioversion. Chronic atrial fibrillation generally tends to be resistant to termination. The frequency of acute episodes can frequently be reduced or sinus rhythm maintained by chronic therapy with quinidine, procainamide, or disopyramide. However, in many patients (especially if atrial fibrillation has been chronic or the atria are enlarged) this approach is ineffective and therapy to decrease the ventricular response is the goal of chronic therapy. Digoxin is the drug of choice. If additional slowing is required, oral verapamil or propranolol may be added. However, digoxin and verapamil are contraindicated in patients with

the Wolff-Parkinson-White syndrome and atrial fibrillation or flutter (see below).

Atrial fibrillation in patients with mitral valve disease or in patients who have experienced a previous thromboembolic event is associated with an increased risk of thromboembolism. Anticoagulation should be considered in these patients.

Wolff-Parkinson-White Syndrome

In the Wolff-Parkinson-White syndrome, an accessory pathway provides an additional connection between the atrium and ventricle. The electrocardiogram in sinus rhythm is the result of fusion over both the normal (A-V node–His-Purkinje) conducting system and the accessory pathway and shows a short PR interval and a wide QRS complex with anomalous early ventricular activation (delta wave). Affected patients most commonly have typical paroxysmal supraventricular tachycardia or may have a variety of wide QRS tachycardias that are often difficult to diagnose.

During atrial fibrillation or flutter in patients with the Wolff-Parkinson-White syndrome, conduction from the atrium to the ventricle can occur over both pathways. The QRS complex is wide when conduction takes place predominantly over the accessory pathway. The presence of the accessory pathway may permit very rapid ventricular rates and a potentially dangerous arrhythmia. Atrial fibrillation or flutter in patients with the Wolff-Parkinson-White syndrome, if poorly tolerated, should be terminated by cardioversion. The drug of choice is intravenous procainamide to slow accessory pathway conduction. The use of digoxin and verapamil in patients with the Wolff-Parkinson-White syndrome is problematic because both drugs can facilitate accessory pathway conduction and increase the ventricular rate during atrial fibrillation. Chronic therapy is probably most effective with quinidine, procainamide, or disopyramide.

TABLE 3. **Characteristics of Commonly Used Intravenous (IV) Antiarrhythmic Agents**

Drug	Loading	Maintenance
Procainamide	500–1000 mg (<50 mg/min)	2–4 mg/min
Lidocaine	1–2 mg/kg— suggested: 75 mg, then 50 mg q 5 min × 2	1–4 mg/min
Propranolol	2–10 mg (<1 mg/min)	Not established
Bretylium	5–10 mg/kg	1–2 mg/min
Verapamil	0.075 mg/kg— 0.150 mg/kg in 30 min if necessary	0.125 mg/min— after rapid loading infusion of 0.375 mg/min × 30 min

Some patients with the Wolff-Parkinson-White syndrome have potentially lethal tachycardias or are refractory or intolerant to pharmacologic therapy. Some of these patients may be candidates for surgical interruption of the accessory pathway.

Ventricular Tachycardia

Ventricular tachycardia, which almost always occurs in the setting of significant ventricular dysfunction, is a potentially lethal tachycardia. It is characterized by a regular, wide QRS with rates generally between 140 and 180 beats per minute. Evidence of A-V dissociation can frequently be found.

Cardioversion is the treatment of choice if there is significant hemodynamic compromise. If the tachycardia is well tolerated, intravenous lidocaine or procainamide (see Table 3) may be effective in restoring sinus rhythm. Ventricular tachycardia is frequently recurrent and prophylactic therapy is, for the most part, empiric. Chronic therapy with an oral lidocaine analogue (mexiletine or tocainide) (see Table 2), a quinidine-like drug, or one of the newer antiarrhythmic agents may be effective in individual patients. Assessment of therapeutic efficacy by either repeated electrophysiologic evaluation or suppression of spontaneous arrhythmias is generally considered necessary and is best performed in centers specializing in these problems. It is important to emphasize that in 10 to 15 per cent of patients, ventricular arrhythmias may be worsened by antiarrhythmic therapy.

Ventricular Fibrillation

Ventricular fibrillation is a chaotic and ineffective tachycardia and is a medical emergency. Immediate cardioversion is the treatment of choice. Cardioversion should be repeated as necessary and may be more effective after the administration of lidocaine or bretylium (see Table 3).

Torsades de pointes

This is a unique, potentially lethal ventricular arrhythmia with a distinct morphology in which the amplitude of the QRS complexes vary and the polarity appears to spiral around the baseline. This arrhythmia is always seen in association with QT interval prolongation and may be caused by antiarrhythmic drugs that can prolong the QT interval (e.g., quinidine, procainamide, disopyramide). Treatment consists of stopping administration of the causal agent.

CONGENITAL HEART DISEASE
method of
P. SYAMASUNDAR RAO, M.D.
University of Wisconsin School of Medicine
Madison, Wisconsin

The incidence of congenital heart defects is approximately 8 per 1000 live births. Thus each year about 25,000 infants with cardiac defects are born in the United States. Twenty per cent of these infants will present with symptoms in the early neonatal period.

MANAGEMENT OF NEONATE WITH HEART DISEASE

Neonates with distress caused by a cardiac malformation may die if not treated appropriately and rapidly. Prompt identification and initial management of these infants is the responsibility of the primary physician caring for the newborn. Rapid and safe transportation to a *regional pediatric cardiology center* equipped with facilities for diagnosis and treatment is the next logical step. Accurate anatomic diagnosis and appropriate medical and/or surgical treatment are in the realm of the pediatric cardiologist and cardiovascular surgeon.

Transportation to Pediatric Cardiology Center

Selection of Infants for Transfer. As soon as congenital heart disease is suspected in a distressed infant, immediate transfer to a regional pediatric cardiology center is mandatory. Virtually all neonates with cyanosis appearing soon after birth, with or without heart failure, should be promptly investigated. Infants with minimal or no cyanosis but with signs of left or right heart failure are also candidates for further study, as are infants with respiratory distress.

Infants with murmurs of small ventricular septal defect, patent ductus arteriosus, or peripheral pulmonary stenosis, decreased femoral pulses, an abnormal electrocardiogram, or an abnormal x-ray finding, but without signs of impaired cardiac function, are not candidates for immediate transfer. These infants should be referred to a pediatric cardiologist between 2 and 6 weeks of age. In addition to these guidelines, early and frequent use of telephone consultation with a pediatric cardiologist at the referral center should help clarify problem cases and result in the appropriate timing of cardiac evaluation.

Transportation. If there are no adequate facilities for immediate and safe transportation of the sick neonate from the community hospital to a regional medical center, transportation can generally be arranged through the pediatric cardiology center, which is on "round-the-clock" call 365 days a year. The type of transportation used, helicopter or ambulance, is dependent upon the distance and the type of transportation available in a given area. The vehicle used should have adequate facilities for monitoring vital signs and for resuscitation. A sick infant should *never* be transferred by a private automobile in the arms of a distressed parent or other relative. The infant should be accompanied by a nurse, paramedic, or physician.

Care of Infant Before and During Transfer. Upon identification of an infant with cardiac distress, the primary physician should have a telephone consultation with his or her pediatric cardiologist and make arrangements for referral. A summary as well as copies of all infant's and mother's records and the infant's chest x-rays should be sent with the baby. Most of the infants are likely to require blood transfusion; therefore, 5 ml of clotted maternal blood should also accompany the infant. A thorough explanation to the parents of the need for the transfer and the procedures that the infant is likely to undergo at the medical center is the responsibility of the referring physician. The primary physician should also allow the parents to see and touch the baby, and any appropriate religious rites should be performed before the transfer.

Before and during the transfer, monitoring the infant's temperature and maintenance of a neutral thermal environment are extremely important. Metabolic acidosis (pH less than 7.25) should be corrected with sodium bicarbonate (usually 1 mEq per kg diluted half and half with 5 per cent dextrose solution) immediately. Respiratory acidosis should be cared for by appropriate suctioning, intubation, and assisted ventilation. In hypoxemic infants, ambient oxygen (less than 40 per cent) should be administered. Hypoglycemia is a significant problem; therefore, the infant's serum glucose (Dextrostix) should be monitored and the infant should receive 10 per cent glucose in water intravenously. If there is hypoglycemia (less than 30 mg per 100 ml), 15 per cent dextrose solution should be administered. Monitoring of serum calcium and correction of hypocalcemia if present is also recommended. Any other medications (e.g., digitalis, dopamine, and diuretics) should be administered after consultation with the pediatric cardiologist under whose care the infant is to be transferred. With ductal dependent lesions, intravenous prostaglandin E_1 (Prostin VR), 0.05 to 0.1 microgram per kg per minute, may be administered while closely monitoring for apnea and hyperpyrexia.

During transport, facilities for monitoring the temperature of the incubator and the infant's heart rate, temperature, and inspired oxygen concentration should be available, as well as facilities for suction, cardiorespiratory resuscitation including intubation, and intravenous medication. Meticulous care must be given to the neonate prior to and during the transfer to ensure optimal conditions for successful diagnostic and therapeutic procedures.

Common Problems Requiring Immediate Treatment

Cyanosis

In infants with cyanotic heart disease, no more than 40 per cent humidified oxygen is necessary. Metabolic acidosis (pH less than 7.25) should be corrected, as well as hypoglycemia, hypocalcemia, and anemia, if present.

In infants with severe right ventricular outflow tract obstruction, the pulmonary flow is ductal dependent. The ductus arteriosus may be kept patent by an infusion of prostaglandin E_1 or E_2 (PGE_1, PGE_2). The current recommendations are for intravenous infusion of PGE_1, 0.05 to 0.1 microgram per kg per minute. We usually start a dose of 0.05 microgram per kg per minute and reduce the rate of infusion, provided desired Po_2 levels are maintained. The PGE_1 infusion rate may be increased if there is no response. If PGE_1 is not available, PGE_2* may be used, but at a much lower dose (0.002 to 0.006 microgram per kg per minute). Although prostaglandins have been used in infants from 1 day to 99 days of age, they are more likely to be effective the earlier in life they are begun, because a small ductus may be made to dilate but an already closed ductus cannot be reopened. Side effects include apnea (in 10 per cent), elevation of temperature (in 10 per cent), muscular twitching, and severe flushing. The side effects can be minimized by keeping the infusion rate of PGE_1 at the lowest level at which an acceptable arterial Po_2 can be maintained.

The major benefits of prostaglandin therapy are the higher Po_2 and corrected metabolic acidosis, so that well-planned specialized cardiac studies as well as palliative or corrective surgery can be performed with relative safety. Also, the infusion of PGE_1 can be maintained during and immediately after the shunt operation so that the blood flow across the ductus may be beneficial while the surgical shunt is being established.

If the cause of cyanosis is transposition of the great arteries, balloon septostomy should be performed. Alternatively, an arterial switch procedure (Jetane operation) should be considered; in some centers, this is the procedure of choice.

---

*This use of PGE_2 is not listed by the manufacturer.

Prostaglandins are helpful in increasing arterial oxygenation while awaiting the above procedures.

Heart failure, if present, should be treated. If there is marked hypercarbia ($PaCO_2 > 60$ mm Hg) or respiratory depression, then intubation and mechanical ventilation are indicated. If the cause of cyanosis is persistent fetal circulation, see discussion under that heading. Other types of treatment are dependent upon the specific cause of the cyanosis and may require palliative or corrective surgery.

Congestive Heart Failure

The treatment of congestive heart failure is discussed at length in this chapter. Of particular importance is the use of PGE_1 in the neonate with heart failure in conditions in which the systemic perfusion to the lower part of the body is ductal dependent, as in severe coarctation of the aorta or interruption of the aortic arch. The dosage and method of administration of PGE_1 are the same as described above (0.05 to 0.1 microgram per kg per minute intravenously).

Persistent Fetal Circulation

In some neonates, markedly increased pulmonary vascular resistance causes severe right-to-left shunting across the patent foramen ovale and/or patent ductus arteriosus, with resultant severe hypoxemia. This may be secondary to pulmonary disease or to a variety of other causes. In many infants, a specific cause cannot be determined.

Diagnosis. The diagnosis must first be established. This can be done with the usual history, physical examination, and laboratory studies. Simultaneous right radial (temporal) artery and umbilical artery PO_2 in 100 per cent inspired oxygen will reveal a lower umbilical artery (descending aorta) PO_2. However, such a difference may not be seen if a major right-to-left atrial shunt exists. Echocardiography is helpful in identifying all cardiac chambers and valves, thus assuring that there is no structural heart disease. It is also helpful in estimating pulmonary artery pressure; increased right-sided pre-ejection period to ejection time ratio (PEP/RVET) and shortened time to peak velocity in the Doppler flow tracing of the pulmonary artery suggest elevated pulmonary pressures. These parameters are also useful to monitor the effectiveness of the treatment. If doubt remains regarding the diagnosis, cardiac catheterization is indicated.

Treatment. Ambient humidified oxygen is necessary to maintain $PaO_2 \geq 50$ mm Hg. Hypothermia, hypoglycemia, acidosis, polycythemia, and hypocalcemia should be corrected promptly. Treatment with digoxin and diuretics is indicated if heart failure is present.

Intubation and mechanical ventilation may

sometimes be beneficial. Paralyzing the infant with pancuronium (Pavulon), 0.1 mg per kg intravenously, and controlling ventilation may be helpful. Hyperventilation to decrease arterial PCO_2 to 25 to 30 mm Hg also has been helpful in some infants. Occasionally the use of positive end expiratory pressure (PEEP), 6 to 10 cm H_2O, may improve oxygenation; however, caution should be exerted because it may cause clinical deterioration.

Tolazoline (Priscoline) is a potent vasodilator; 1 to 2 mg per kg may be infused over a 10-minute period with a beneficial effect in many infants. The drug also produces systemic vasodilatation and may cause systemic hypotension. Therefore, it should be given intravenously in an arm or neck vein to encourage delivery of the drug into the pulmonary circuit, taking advantage of the fetal circulatory pathways. Administration of tolazoline into the pulmonary artery is most effective; however, even from this site of administration, right-to-left shunting across the ductus arteriosus or via intrapulmonary shunts may make it ineffective. If effective by either route, it should be continued as an infusion at a rate of 1 to 2 mg per kg per hour. If no improvement occurs or hypotension develops, tolazoline should be discontinued. Some workers have added systemic vasoconstrictors (e.g., dopamine) to the regimen to counter the hypotension. Recent reports suggest that dopamine, 2 to 5 micrograms per kg per minute, is effective in the treatment of persistent fetal circulation. Further experience with this modality of treatment is necessary before it can be recommended for routine use.

Theoretically PGE_1 and PGE_2 should be effective by acting as pulmonary vasodilators, but limited experience thus far has not shown any consistent benefit. Currently, studies with other prostaglandin analogues (e.g., PGI_2, PGD_2) are evaluating their effect on dilating pulmonary arterioles.

Extremely severe cases without response to the treatment regimen described above may be candidates for extracorporeal membrane oxygenation (ECMO).

Patent Ductus Arteriosus in the Premature Infant

Premature infants with hyaline membrane disease may have an open ductus arteriosus with a large left-to-right shunt, which can cause further deterioration of respiratory function and delay the expected timely recovery from hyaline membrane disease.

In premature infants with hyaline membrane disease with a patent ductus arteriosus, instead of the expected recovery there will be a greater requirement for inspired oxygen concentration and a greater need for ventilatory support. A cardiac murmur may appear; hyperdynamic precordium and bounding pulses may also be observed. Chest x-ray may reveal cardiomegaly. Echocardiograms may show enlarged left atrium and left ventricle, increased left atrium to aortic root (LA/Ao) ratio, and normal or increased left ventricular shortening fraction. These findings are indicative of a significant ductus. Recording of main pulmonary artery Doppler flow velocity signal in a precordial short axis view shows positive diastolic flow with wide spectral dispersion in addition to normal negative systolic flow deflection. At this time a trial of fluid restriction (<70 ml per kg per day) and diuretics (furosemide, 1 mg per kg per dose intravenously) is indicated. Digitalis preparations are not usually necessary.

Further measures to close the ductus should be undertaken if (1) there is no improvement in 24 to 48 hours, (2) worsening of the signs described above occurs, and (3) on a repeat echocardiogram further enlargement of left atrium and ventricle occurs and left ventricular shortening fraction diminishes.

Pharmacologic Closure. Since prostaglandins are necessary to keep the ductus open, administration of prostaglandin synthesis inhibitors may result in constriction of the ductus arteriosus. This concept has been applied by several groups of workers, and it is now clearly shown that indomethacin, a potent inhibitor of prostaglandin synthesis, can cause constriction and closure of the ductus and result in abatement of the symptoms caused by the patent ductus.

Indomethacin may be administered via a gastric tube,* by retention enema,* or intravenously in a dose of 0.2 mg per kg. If no clinical improvement occurs, the dose may be repeated in 6 to 8 hours, and again in 6 to 12 hours if no improvement occurs after the second dose. The beneficial effect of indomethacin appears to be age related. It is most effective when the infant's actual age (gestational plus chronologic) is less than 36 weeks. Indomethacin seems to be less effective when the infant is more than 10 days postpartum.

Potential complications of indomethacin therapy include impairment of renal function (oliguria, increase in blood urea nitrogen [BUN] and creatinine, and reduction in urinary sodium concentration), altered platelet function, and necrotizing enterocolitis. Therefore, renal and coagulation functions should be normal in these infants prior to indomethacin administration.

Surgical Closure. Surgical ligation of the patent ductus arteriosus may be performed in infants who are unresponsive to pharmacologic closure and in those in whom indomethacin is contraindicated.

Polycythemia

Significant degrees of polycythemia may cause cyanosis, heart failure, or respiratory distress. Polycythemia is considered to be present if the central hematocrit is greater than 65 per cent. Specific treatment of polycythemia is exchange plasma transfusion. The exchange transfusion should not be performed unless the polycythemic infant is symptomatic.

Methemoglobinemia

When severe cyanosis is seen in the absence of distress, methemoglobinemia should be suspected. Affected infants appear ruddy and have a peculiar lavender color. The blood from heel stick is chocolate colored and does not become pink when exposed to room air. The Po_2 may be normal, but the O_2 saturation by direct oxymetry will be markedly reduced. Methemoglobinemia may be either hereditary in origin or acquired from exposure to agents such as nitrites in contaminated well water or from aniline derivatives.

Before beginning treatment, it is important to exclude other causes of cyanosis and to confirm the diagnosis by spectrophotometric analysis of blood for methemoglobin; it has a characteristic absorption peak at 634μ. Methylene blue, 1 to 2 mg per kg intravenously, should promptly eliminate the cyanosis. This should be followed by either 3 to 5 mg per kg of methylene blue orally or 200 to 500 mg of ascorbic acid orally.

Cardiomyopathy in Infants of Diabetic Mothers

Infants of diabetic mothers (IDM) have been known to have a high incidence of postnatal complications. These include macrosomia, hypoglycemia, hypocalcemia, hyperbilirubinemia, polycythemia, hyperviscosity syndrome, transient tachypnea of the newborn, hyaline membrane disease, persistent fetal circulation, cardiomyopathy, renal vein thrombosis, and an increased incidence of congenital anomalies. The incidence of cardiac involvement may be as high as 50 per cent. Two basic forms of cardiomyopathy have been recognized in IDM: a congestive cardiomyopathy and an obstructive cardiomyopathy.

Congestive Cardiomyopathy. This may be related to (or secondary to) the hematologic, metabolic, or respiratory problems listed above, or it may occur independent of them. Treatment includes correction of hypoglycemia, hypocalcemia, polycythemia, or other problems listed above, and

---

*Administration of indomethacin by nasogastric tube or by retention enema is not listed by the manufacturer.

administration of digitalis, and diuretics (see the section on Congestive Heart Failure below).

Obstructive Cardiomyopathy. The findings in this group of infants have been described as similar to those of patients classified as having hypertrophic obstructive cardiomyopathy (HOCM). On the echocardiogram there is a thickened interventricular septum, increased septal to left ventricular free wall ratio (>1.3), and systolic anterior motion of the anterior leaflet of the mitral valve. Cardiac catheterization data reveal a systolic pressure gradient across the subaortic region. Left ventricular angiography shows a thickened interventricular septum bulging into the left ventricular outflow tract, a finding similar to that characteristically observed in HOCM.

Administration of digitalis and diuretics, the standard treatment in most cases of congestive heart failure, is contraindicated in HOCM. Digitalis may accentuate the left ventricular outflow obstruction and cause clinical deterioration.

Metabolic, hematologic, and respiratory problems, if present, should be corrected. Propranolol is administered orally, 1 to 4 mg per kg per day, in 3 or 4 divided doses, beginning with 1 mg per kg per day and increasing until clinical response.*

The HOCM of IDM improves with time; echocardiographic findings may revert to normal within 6 months. Propranolol may be discontinued once the echographic abnormalities revert to normal.

Congestive Heart Failure

About 20 per cent of children born with congenital heart defects will develop congestive heart failure (CHF). Ninety per cent of those who develop CHF are likely to do so within the first year of life.

The cardiac function is regulated by four principal factors: (1) contractile state of the heart, which is the inherent force of the ventricular contraction and independent of the load on the ventricle; (2) preload or ventricular end-diastolic volume; (3) afterload, which is the load or force imposed on the myocardial fibers after the onset of ventricular contraction; and (4) heart rate. In the medical management of CHF, manipulation of the contractile state of the heart and preload have long been known. Recently efforts to manipulate afterload in the treatment of CHF have also been made. Each of these will be discussed in the ensuing pages.

---

*This use of propranolol is not listed in the manufacturer's official directive.

TABLE 1. **Digoxin Preparations**

Oral	Digoxin (Lanoxin) elixir	0.05 mg/ml
	Digoxin (Lanoxin) tablets	0.125 mg (yellow)
		0.25 mg (white)
		0.5 mg (green)
Injectable	Digoxin (Lanoxin)	0.1 mg/ml (pediatric)
		0.25 mg/ml (adult)

Digitalis (Digoxin) Therapy

Digitalis is a positive inotropic agent that enhances myocardial contractility. The mechanism of action of digitalis is not clearly understood; it is presumed to act by inhibiting sodium-potassium ATPase. Of the two major preparations of digitalis, namely digitoxin and digoxin, digoxin is almost exclusively used in pediatric patients. Commonly used digoxin forms are listed in Table 1. A loading dose is followed by maintenance doses. These doses are calculated on the basis of age and weight and are listed in Table 2. From this table, the oral total loading dose (TLD) for initial digitalization can be calculated. One half of the TLD should be administered immediately. Infants with CHF should receive the first dose intravenously; in infants with moderate to severe CHF, the absorption of oral or intramuscular digoxin may be markedly delayed because of edema and diminished cardiac output. When given intravenously, three fourths of the calculated oral dose should be given. The second and third doses (one fourth of the TLD each) may be administered at 6- to 8-hour intervals (Table 3). However, when treating severe CHF, one or both intervals may be reduced to 1 or 2 hours. Prior to the third dose, the cardiac rhythm and rate should be evaluated, preferably by an electrocardiographic (ECG) rhythm strip. Twelve hours following the TLD, maintenance digoxin should be started. The maintenance dose is one fourth of the TLD per day. This is usually administered orally in 2 equally divided doses (one eighth of the TLD, 2 times a day). It should be noted that the maintenance dose is arbitrary and can be increased gradually until full therapeutic effect is attained or toxicity symptoms appear.

TABLE 2. **Total Loading Dose (TLD) of Oral Digoxin***

Preterm infants	0.03 mg/kg
Newborn infants, 0–6 weeks	0.04 mg/kg
6 weeks–2 years	0.06–0.08 mg/kg
2–5 years	0.04–0.06 mg/kg
5 years and older	0.03–0.04 mg/kg†

*This dose is for oral digitalization only. If digitalis is administered parenterally, give three fourths of the oral dose.

†If the total calculated dose exceeds the average adult dose (1.0 mg), give only the average adult dose.

Most, perhaps all, infants with CHF are treated in the manner described above. However, a few infants and children who have minimal signs of CHF may not need hospitalization and rapid digitalization. These babies can be started on maintenance doses of digoxin (one eighth of the TLD, twice a day). By this method, the infant is completely digitalized within 5 to 7 days.

Contraindications. Digitalis is contraindicated in children with paroxysmal hypoxemic spell syndrome seen in patients with tetralogy of Fallot or similar lesions, idiopathic hypertrophic subaortic stenosis (hypertrophic cardiomyopathy), and ventricular tachycardia. Overzealous administration of digoxin in patients with cor pulmonale or myocarditis may result in toxicity, and therefore one should be cautious with these patients.

Digoxin Toxicity. There is a narrow margin between therapeutic and toxic effects of digoxin; the therapeutic dose represents 65 per cent of the toxic dose. Furthermore, there is considerable individual variation in tolerance to digoxin. The most common manifestations of digoxin toxicity are premature ventricular contractions and varying degrees of atrioventricular block, including prolongation of the PR interval. Any arrhythmia beginning after the institution of digoxin therapy must be attributed to it until proved otherwise. Other rhythm disturbances associated with digoxin toxicity are marked sinus arrhythmia and wandering atrial pacemaker, severe sinus bradycardia (excessive vagal tone), supraventricular or ventricular tachycardia, and atrial flutter or fibrillation. Anorexia, nausea, and vomiting may accompany digoxin toxicity. Central nervous system signs of toxicity such as headache, fatigue, malaise, drowsiness, mental confusion, and blurred vision are not common in pediatric patients. Depression of the ST segment and inversion of the T wave (the so-called digitalis effect on the ECG) do not necessarily imply digoxin toxicity nor do they indicate adequacy of digitalization.

DIGOXIN LEVELS. Radioimmunoassay of serum digoxin levels is now readily available. The theoretic basis for clinical use of serum digoxin levels rests on the constant relationship between tissue and serum levels and the fairly uniform serum concentration over several hours of the postabsorptive phase. It is now known that the ratio of digoxin concentration in the heart and serum is rather constant (about 30:1); however, there is a wide range (Table 4) of digoxin levels in patients receiving digoxin, and routine digoxin levels cannot separate toxic from nontoxic patients. Therefore, we do not recommend obtaining routine digoxin levels on all patients on digoxin therapy. There are four major indications for obtaining digoxin levels: (1) if clinical signs of toxicity are present (then, even if the digoxin level is in the borderline range, one might consider the patient to be digoxin intoxicated and reduce the dosage); (2) if there is a strong suspicion that the infant or child has not been receiving the prescribed digoxin; (3) accidental poisoning; and (4) patients with renal failure. Finally, it should be remembered that the digoxin level should be obtained about 6 hours after the last dose was given to avoid determining the serum level prior to its equilibration with the issue level.

TREATMENT OF DIGOXIN TOXICITY. Administration of digoxin should be discontinued immediately whenever digitalis toxicity is suspected. If an excessive amount was administered by mouth, it is desirable to induce vomiting or to attempt gastric lavage. Serum potassium levels should be determined. If the serum potassium level is normal or decreased, potassium may be administered intravenously, 40 to 60 mEq per liter of 5 per cent dextrose in water. Rate of administration should not exceed 0.5 mEq per kg per hour, and the total daily dose should not be greater than 2 to 3 mEq per kg. The favorable effect of potassium is nonspecific, and it has relatively little influence on the toxic and inotropic actions of digitalis when it is administered after binding of the glycoside to the myocardium. This is the usual situation encountered in clinical practice. Potassium pretreatment with increased serum levels reduces the uptake of digitalis by the heart, thus diminishing electrical toxicity of subsequently administered digitalis. It should be remembered that when digitalis toxicity inhibits the potassium uptake by skeletal muscle, a significant rise

TABLE 3. **Schedule of Initial Digitalization**

First dose	½ TLD* stat, intravenous (¾ of oral dose)
Second dose†	¼ TLD in 6–8 h, intravenous or oral
Third dose‡	¼ TLD in 6–8 h, usually given orally

*TLD = Total loading dose (see Table 2).

†The time interval between the first and second as well as the second and third doses can be reduced to 2 hours or even 1 hour if severe heart failure or pulmonary edema is present.

‡Prior to the third dose, the patient's cardiac rhythm and rate should be evaluated, preferably by an ECG rhythm strip.

TABLE 4. **Toxic and Nontoxic Levels of Serum Digoxin (ng/ml) in Infants and Children**

Level	Less than 2 Years of Age	Above 2 Years of Age
Nontoxic	<2.0	<1.0
Borderline	2.0–4.0	1.0–2.0
Toxic	>4.0	>2.0

in serum potassium may result from the administration of small amounts of this cation. Potassium depresses atrioventricular conduction and therefore is contraindicated in patients with atrioventricular block secondary to digitalis intoxication.

For severe digoxin toxicity, Fab fragments of digoxin-specific antibodies should be used. These are available at some medical centers.

DIGOXIN-INDUCED ARRHYTHMIAS. Minor arrhythmias will resolve with simple discontinuation of the digoxin. Severe arrhythmias need further treatment. Phenytoin (Dilantin) has been shown to be capable of reversing digitalis-induced tachyrhythmias. This drug depresses the enhanced ventricular automaticity without any significant depression of conduction. It may be given intravenously in a dose of 3 to 5 mg per kg over a 5 minute period. If necessary, it may be repeated in 10 to 15 minutes.* Phenytoin is contraindicated in bradyrhythmias or atrioventricular block. It should be mentioned that it is a short-acting agent, and thus it is not suitable in treating the sustained and recurrent tachyrhythmia.

Propranolol is useful in the treatment of both supraventricular and ventricular arrhythmias secondary to digitalis toxicity, and it has been most successful in terminating premature ventricular extrasystoles. Propranolol, 0.1 mg per kg, may be given intravenously over a period of 10 minutes with great caution and constant ECG monitoring, since this potent adrenergic blocking agent could suppress all pacemaker activity and depress cardiac contractility, resulting in either cardiac standstill or sudden cardiocirculatory collapse with hypotension. (See manufacturer's official directive.) This drug should not be used in the presence of significant congestive heart failure. If effective, propranolol may later be continued orally, 1 to 4 mg per kg per day in three to four divided doses. Other drugs such as lidocaine, quinidine, and procainamide may be useful. Dosages of these drugs are listed on Table 5.

Electrical conversion for the treatment of digitalis-induced arrhythmias may be hazardous, since serious ventricular arrhythmias have occurred after countershock even with nontoxic doses of digitalis. Cardioversion should be used only when all other measures have failed to control sustained arrhythmias induced by digitalis. Pretreatment with phenytoin prior to cardioversion may reduce postconversion ventricular arrhythmias. In newborns and infants, low energy levels of countershock should be used (1 to 2 watt-seconds per kg).

*This use of phenytoin is not listed in the manufacturer's official directive.

TABLE 5. Drugs Commonly Used in Management of Arrhythmias

Drug	Dose and Route of Administration
Phenytoin* (Dilantin)	3–5 mg/kg/dose IV given over a 5-minute period 3–5 mg/kg/day, PO in 2 divided doses
Lidocaine (Xylocaine)	1 mg/kg IV as a bolus May be repeated in 20–60 minutes; or start continuous IV infusion, 20–50 µg/kg/min
Quinidine	6 mg/kg PO or IM qid (loading dose, 3–6 mg/kg q 2–3 h, five doses, and 12 mg/kg q 2–3 h, five additional doses)
Procainamide (Pronestyl)	6 mg/kg IM qid 15 mg/kg PO qid
Propranolol†	0.05–0.1 mg/kg IV: dilute in 50 ml of D5W; infuse slowly while monitoring ECG 1 mg/kg/day PO in 3 to 4 divided doses; then increase as needed (2–4 mg/kg/day)

*This use is not listed in the manufacturer's official directive.

†Should not be used in the presence of significant congestive heart failure.

DIGOXIN-INDUCED CONDUCTION DISTURBANCES. Impending heart block or symptomatic complete heart block should be immediately treated. Atropine, 0.01 to 0.03 mg per kg intravenously, may be given, with a maximum of 0.4 mg per dose, in treating conduction disturbances induced by digitalis. Atropine may be effective in atrioventricular block produced by the excessive vagal action of the digitalis if the ventricular pacemaker is junctional or in the high His bundle. However, the therapeutic success is unpredictable.

Isoproterenol, 0.1 to 0.5 microgram per kg per minute in 5 per cent dextrose in water, may be given in complete heart block (while preparing for pacemaker insertion) and the dose adjusted to the response. However, the drug may have certain disadvantages in digitalis-induced conduction disturbances because of increased incidence of ventricular ectopic rhythms associated with its use in the presence of toxic levels of digitalis. Transvenous pacemaker insertion may be necessary in patients with a high degree of atrioventricular block; this may be particularly useful in patients who have accidentally ingested large doses of digoxin.

Diuretic Therapy

Manipulation of the preload includes restriction of fluid and salt intake and administration of diuretics. Diuretics are a useful pharmacologic adjunct in the management of infants with CHF. Digitalis and rest may be all that is necessary in order to treat mild or even moderate CHF. Severe forms of CHF require diuretic therapy. Sodium and water retention, increased blood volume, increased preload, and augmented cardiac output occur in sequence in patients with CHF and are significant compensatory mechanisms. Therefore, we feel that diuretics should not be used as the first drugs in the treatment of CHF unless pulmonary edema is evident; with this exception, digitalis should precede the administration of diuretics. The adequacy of diuresis is often estimated better by daily weights than by urine outputs, since the latter values are notoriously inaccurate owing to inadequate collection methods in infants and children.

Furosemide (Lasix), 1 mg per kg intravenously, is our first choice. Ethacrynic acid (Edecrin) has similar actions and may also be used (see manufacturer's official directive before using). Furosemide may be given one or more times a day, depending upon the patient's response. Once the infant is stable, furosemide may be given orally, 2 to 4 mg per kg per day as a single dose. We usually give furosemide three times a week (Monday, Wednesday, and Friday). This intermittent therapy usually does not produce the electrolyte imbalance that is often observed with continuous diuretic therapy, and therefore there is no need for potassium supplement.

In patients who do not respond to these diuretics, a diagnosis of secondary hyperaldosteronism should be considered, and the aldosterone antagonist spironolactone (Aldactone) should be added. The recommended dose is 3 mg per kg per day in 2 to 3 divided doses. We have had little success with thiazide diuretics.

In cases in which there is no response to diuretics (e.g., severe chronic CHF; nephrotic syndrome with severe edema), we have been able to induce diuresis by administration of aminophylline, 5 mg per kg diluted in 5 per cent dextrose in water infused intravenously over a 30-minute period, immediately followed by intravenous furosemide, 1 mg per kg.

Techniques and procedures such as rotating tourniquets and venisection are rarely necessary now because of the availability of potent diuretic drugs.

Other Therapeutic Measures

Position. Propping up the patient to elevate the head and shoulders to 45 degrees may be beneficial. This position probably encourages peripheral pooling in the inferior portion of the body rather than in the lungs.

Rest and Sedation. Exercise and activity require an increase in cardiac output. Therefore, this extra burden on the compromised heart should be avoided. In older children, bed rest is recommended during the acute phase. Thereafter, the patient should be slowly allowed to resume nor-

mal activity as the cardiac function improves with treatment. Parenteral feeding of infants will conserve the energy normally expended in sucking. Intravenous fluids should be adjusted to replace insensible and other losses (approximately 50 to 60 ml per kg per day) and should contain 10 per cent dextrose because of possible hypoglycemia. Potassium maintenance should be given, but sodium chloride should not be added because of the elevated total body sodium.

If the patient is restless and agitated, sedation with morphine sulfate, 0.1 mg per kg, should be given subcutaneously. Apart from sedation, morphine has other beneficial effects, the nature and mechanism of which are not clearly defined. However, one should observe the patient for signs of respiratory depression.

Oxygen. Increasing the ambient oxygen concentration overcomes the pulmonary component of hypoxia and enables systemic arterial Po_2 to rise. Initially 40 per cent humidified oxygen should be given to all infants and children with acute CHF. The oxygen should be discontinued after improvement with CHF.

Diet. In a sick infant, feeding should be withheld to avoid aspiration. As the infant improves, start feeding with 10 per cent dextrose in water. Formula and solid foods can then be added to provide adequate calories. For infants and children who continue to be in chronic CHF, salt restriction may be necessary. In young babies, low-salt formulas such as Similac PM 60-40 or Lonalac may be used. In children, avoiding salt-containing snacks (e.g., chips, pretzels) and restricting added salt to food may be necessary.

Treatment of Underlying Conditions

Treatment of associated and/or underlying abnormalities is beneficial in management of CHF and may include packed red blood cells for anemia, glucose for hypoglycemia, calcium for hypocalcemia, substitution therapy for other metabolic disorders, antihypertensive medications for hypertension, countershock or antiarrhythmic drugs for arrhythmias, steroids for severe carditis, respiratory toilet for cystic fibrosis, and tonsillectomy with adenoidectomy for chronic upper airway obstruction syndrome. Specific palliative or corrective surgery for underlying cardiac defects should also be considered.

Other Drugs Used in Refractory Failure

In patients with severe CHF not responding to conventional treatment, additional drugs may be used. These can be subdivided into other inotropic agents and afterload reducing agents.

Inotropic Agents

ISOPROTERENOL. Infuse 0.1 to 0.5 microgram per kg per minute intravenously or mix 0.2 to

0.4 mg of isoproterenol in 250 ml of 5 per cent dextrose in water and adjust the rate to the desired effect. The drug markedly increases the heart rate and may also produce arrhythmias. The severely distressed infant who is a candidate for catheterization and/or surgery and who is deteriorating rapidly can sometimes be transiently assisted by an infusion of isoproterenol in 30 ml of 20 per cent dextrose and 20 ml of sodium bicarbonate. Isoproterenol should be added, 0.2 microgram per kg per minute, delivered by infusion pump.

EPINEPHRINE. Infuse 0.25 to 1.0 microgram per kg per minute intravenously in 5 per cent dextrose in water. Adjust the rate according to response.

DOPAMINE. This drug is preferable to isoproterenol and epinephrine because it does not have a chronotropic effect when used at low doses. Additionally, it selectively dilates the renal vessels (see manufacturer's official directive). When only oliguria is present, infuse 2 to 5 micrograms per kg per minute in 5 per cent dextrose in water intravenously. When both oliguria and hypotension are present, a dosage of 5 to 20 micrograms per kg per minute may be given. Since dopamine is inactivated by sodium bicarbonate, do not add it to an infusion containing dopamine.

DOBUTAMINE. This is a catecholamine derivative that can be given intravenously without the occasionally deleterious chronotropic effects of catecholamines. Hemodynamic studies in adults with coronary artery disease and in children with heart failure during continuous infusion of dobutamine have revealed a persistent increase in left ventricular contractility. Dobutamine appears to be a better drug than dopamine with regard to increasing stroke volume and cardiac output and to decreasing systemic and pulmonary vascular resistance and pulmonary arterial wedge pressure. Furthermore, dobutamine has less chronotropic effect and produces no significant premature ventricular contractions. The recommended dose is 5 to 8 micrograms per kg per minute by continuous intravenous infusion.

AMRINONE. This is another inotropic agent; it is a bipyridine derivative and its subcellular mechanism of action appears to be inhibition of the phosphodiesterase isoenzyme PDE III. It is believed that amrinone exerts its effect directly on the contractile mechanism of the heart muscle. It increases cardiac output and decreases left ventricular end-diastolic pressure without altering the heart rate in patients with severe CHF that is refractory to conventional digitalis and diuretic therapy. In addition, amrinone decreases systemic vascular resistance, thereby reducing the afterload. No significant side effects have been observed with short-term administration of amrinone. However, several adverse effects, namely thrombocytopenia, life-threatening ventricular tachyarrhythmias, and long-term detrimental effects on the myocardium, have been reported following long-term use of this drug in adult patients. No controlled studies of this drug in children are available.

MILRINONE. This bipyridine derivative, closely related to amrinone, increases indices of left ventricular systolic and diastolic function. Preliminary studies on its effectiveness in long-term oral therapy have been encouraging, without detectable adverse effects.

Afterload-Reducing Agents. Conventional treatment regimens of congestive heart failure have relied on manipulation of the preload (diuretics, salt restriction) and contractile state (digoxin and other inotropic agents) of the heart. Over the past several years significant advances in the understanding of afterload manipulation have occurred.

In both acute and chronic heart failure, near normal blood pressure is maintained in spite of decreased cardiac output. This is accomplished by reflex vasoconstriction, and therefore increased peripheral resistance, which increases the afterload on the ventricle and further impairs the cardiac output. The larger cardiac size in heart failure also increases afterload on the left ventricle. If the afterload is reduced by administration of vasodilator agents in acute or chronic heart failure, the cardiac output and myocardial function will improve.

A variety of vasodilators are available that can be given intravenously, orally, sublingually, or cutaneously. In addition to lowering the ventricular afterload, some vasodilators decrease the venous tone and thereby reduce the venous return (preload). Thus, vasodilator drugs produce their effect on cardiac functions by modifying the preload and afterload. Because there is a decrease in the afterload and the wall tension, there is a concomitant decrease in the myocardial oxygen consumption.

SODIUM NITROPRUSSIDE. This is a direct peripheral vasodilator with balanced effect on systemic venous (capacitance) and arteriolar (resistance) vessels. It has been used in infants and children with low cardiac output following open heart surgery. A dosage of 1 to 8 micrograms per kg per minute may be given intravenously. It is important to maintain left atrial pressure at an acceptable level by transfusion of blood and volume expanders during nitroprusside administration. This drug can be used in any acute heart failure that cannot be controlled by conventional management regimes. It has been effective in patients with severe acute cardiac failure secondary to myocarditis and cardiomyopathy. Continuous measurement of blood pressure and central venous pressure and, when possible, pulmonary arterial wedge pressure or left atrial pressure and intermittent determinations of the cardiac index and systemic vascular resistance are necessary for accurately adjusting the dosage of intravenous vasodilator agents.

PRAZOSIN. This piperazine derivative exerts its hypotensive action by reducing peripheral vascular resistance by blocking vascular alpha-adrenergic receptors. Prazosin causes a prolonged dilatation of both systemic arteriolar bed and venous capacitance vessels and therefore improves congestive heart failure by reducing the preload and afterload. It does not significantly alter the heart rate. Because of the development of severe orthostatic hypotension, the so-called first-dose phenomenon, and tachyphylaxis following chronic use, we have restricted its use.

HYDRALAZINE. This phthalazine derivative has a direct relaxing effect on vascular smooth muscle. It has a greater effect on arteriolar smooth muscle than it does on the veins. In patients with chronic CHF, hydralazine increases stroke volume and cardiac output. The pulmonary and systemic vascular resistances fall while pulmonary and systemic venous pressures do not change. Hydralazine can produce tachycardia in hypertensive patients as their blood pressure falls, but such tachycardia is not seen in patients with chronic heart failure. Hydralazine appears to improve cardiac function primarily by reducing the afterload. The mean arterial pressure does not change significantly; it is presumed that decreased systemic vascular resistance is offset by an increase in cardiac index. This drug has been used in infants and children with severe myocardial disease (cardiomyopathy, endocardial fibroelastosis, and adriamycin cardiomyopathy) and severe chronic CHF. We start with a small dose (1.0 mg per kg per day in 4 divided doses given orally every 6 hours), while monitoring the blood pressure, and increase the dose gradually to 4 to 5 mg per kg per day. Hydralazine therapy is begun after adequate treatment with digoxin, furosemide, and spironolactone.

CAPTOPRIL. This angiotensin-converting enzyme inhibitor is useful in the situations described above for hydralazine. It is given orally at a dose of 1 to 4 mg per kg per day in 3 to 4 divided doses.

Several other vasodilator agents, parenteral and oral, are currently available. These include nitroglycerin, phentolamine, trimethaphan, phenoxybenzamine, sublingual or topical nitroglycerin, thymoxamine, and sublingual or oral isosorbide dinitrate. These drugs have been used in adults with various types of cardiac problems, and there is gradually accumulating experience in their use in pediatric patients.

It should be understood that vasodilator therapy does not change basic cardiac pathology, but it is helpful in temporarily improving cardiac output. If the natural history of the disease process is such that the cardiac function improves spontaneously, the vasodilators are of great benefit.

Pulmonary Edema

If signs of pulmonary edema are present, the following immediate treatment should be instituted:

1. Prop the patient at approximately 45 degrees.
2. Morphine sulfate, 0.1 mg per kg intravenously.
3. Furosemide (Lasix), 1 mg per kg intravenously.
4. Rapid digitalization by the intravenous route over a 2- to 4-hour period.
5. Humidified oxygen in high concentration may be administered via a face mask or a hood. Continuous positive airway pressure (CPAP), 6 to 8 cm H_2O with oxygen, may be instituted in severe cases. Severely ill infants with pulmonary edema and elevated $PaCO_2$ (>60 mm Hg) require endotracheal intubation and mechanical ventilation. PEEP (6 to 8 cm H_2O) on the ventilator may beneficial.
6. In severe pulmonary edema, rotating tourniquets may be beneficial, especially when other methods are not effective. Blood pressure cuffs may be placed around three extremities and cuffs inflated with a pressure midway between systolic and diastolic blood pressure. Rotate the tourniquets every 15 to 20 minutes.
7. If significant improvement is not observed with the aforementioned measures, treatment listed under Other Drugs Used in Refractory Failure, above, should be instituted, particularly dopamine or nitroprusside.

Paroxysmal Hypoxemic Spells (Hypercyanotic Spells)

The spell syndrome has variously been described by several names, including anoxic spells, hypoxic spells, paroxysmal hyperpnea, blue spells, tetralogy spells, paroxysmal hypoxic attacks, and hypercyanotic spells. These spells are most common in patients with tetralogy of Fallot, although they can also occur in patients with tricuspid atresia or any lesion with severe pulmonary outflow tract obstruction and a systemic-to-pulmonary communication. The spells are most commonly seen between 1 and 12 months of age, with a peak frequency in infants 2 to 3 months old. They can occur at any time of the day but are most common in the morning after awakening from sleep; defecation, crying, and feeding are common precipitating factors. The spells are characterized by increased rate and depth of respiration and increased cyanosis progressing to limpness and syncope but usually with subsequent recovery. Occasionally, the spells terminate with convulsions, cerebrovascular accident, or rarely death. During the spell, the previously heard murmur either disappears or markedly diminishes in intensity. The exact cause of the spell syndrome is not known, but numerous hypotheses have been advanced. The two most plausible mechanisms are hypercontraction of the right ventricular outflow tract, precipitated by acute increase in catecholamines, and any stimulus producing hyperpnea. Treatment should be as follows.

Treatment of Milder Spells

The infant should be placed in the knee-chest position. The reason for its effectiveness appears to be related to its effect in increasing the systemic vascular resistance and thus decreasing the right-to-left shunt and improving the pulmonary blood flow. Humidified oxygen via a face mask should be administered. Since the major defect in the spell syndrome is pulmonary oligemia rather than alveolar oxygenation, the oxygen administration has limited usefulness. If the infant is unduly disturbed by the face mask, oxygen therapy should be discontinued.

Morphine sulfate, 0.1 ml per kg subcutaneously, may be effective in aborting the spell. The mechanism of action is not clearly delineated, but its effect on the central nervous system respiratory drive (thus reducing hyperpnea) and sedation of the infant may be important in its favorable effect. Once the physical examination is completed (and the limited but important laboratory studies are obtained), the infant should be undisturbed and allowed to rest; this in itself may improve the infant's condition. Metabolic acidosis should be corrected (with sodium bicarbonate or THAM), as well as anemia (by blood transfusion) and dehydration, if present.

Treatment of More Severe Spells

If the spell continues, vasopressors to increase the systemic vascular resistance and thus increase the pulmonary blood flow may be tried. In our experience, methoxamine (Vasoxyl), an alpha agonist, has been most helpful. Administer 20 to 40 mg in 250 ml of 5 per cent dextrose in water intravenously and adjust the rate of infusion to increase the systolic blood pressure by 15 to 20 per cent. Beta blockade with propranolol, 0.1 mg per kg body weight, diluted in 50 ml of 5 per cent dextrose in water, may be administered intravenously while monitoring the heart rate (by ECG if possible). Should there be any marked bradycardia, the propranolol should be stopped. Once it is found to be effective, the infant may be switched to 1 to 4 mg per kg per day orally in 3 to 4 divided doses. Infrequently, general anesthesia may be necessary to break the spell.

If the infant improves with the management outlined above, total surgical correction of the cardiac defect, if anatomically feasible, or a systemic-to-pulmonary shunt to improve the pulmonary blood flow on an elective basis within the next several days may be performed. An alternative to surgery is oral propranolol (dose as above), which may help postpone surgery by several months to years. If the infant does not improve with any of the aforementioned measures, an emergency systemic-to-pulmonary artery shunt (we prefer Blalock-Taussig anastomosis) should be performed. Occasionally, total correction, if the anatomy is adequate, may be performed on an emergency basis. The important principle is that the infant requires more pulmonary blood flow.

Transcatheter and Surgical Therapy

Palliative Procedures

The palliative procedures are designed to improve physiologic abnormalities, including (1) decreased pulmonary blood flow, (2) increased pulmonary blood flow, and (3) inadequate interatrial mixing.

Decreased Pulmonary Blood Flow. Since the original description of subclavian artery to ipsilateral pulmonary artery anastomosis by Blalock and Taussig in 1945, several types of these shunt operations have been devised. These include other types of systemic artery to pulmonary artery shunts—namely Potts anastomosis (descending aorta to left pulmonary artery shunt), Waterston-Cooley shunt (ascending aorta to right pulmonary artery anastomosis), ascending aorta to main pulmonary artery anastomosis (creation of aortopulmonary window), aorta to pulmonary artery Gore-Tex shunt, and modified Blalock-Taussig shunt (subclavian artery to ipsilateral pulmonary artery shunt with an interposition Gore-Tex graft)—and the Glenn procedure (superior vena cava to right pulmonary artery anastomosis). Maintenance of ductal patency by formalin infiltration of the ductus arteriosus and blind pulmonary valvotomy (Brock procedure) have also been used to palliate pulmonary oligemia. Systemic artery to pulmonary artery shunt operations are commonly used in surgical palliation. Because of the small size of the subclavian artery in the neonate and young infant, some surgeons have preferred central aortopulmonary (Potts and Waterston) shunts. However, because of the complications associated with these shunts, most pediatric cardiologists recommend and most cardiovascular surgeons perform the Blalock-Taussig shunt or its modification. The recent modifications of the procedure and the use of microsurgical techniques make it feasible to perform the Blalock-Taussig shunt in very small infants, and at present we use the Blalock-Taussig anastomosis exclusively in infants with cyanotic heart disease and pulmonary oligemia. The cardiac defects for which this shunt is performed include pulmonary atresia with an intact ventricular septum, pulmonary atresia with ventricular septal defect, severe tetralogy of Fallot, tricuspid atresia, and complex congenital heart defects with severe pulmonary stenosis or atresia.

In some patients who are not candidates for total surgical correction either because of their size or because of complexity of their cardiac defects, balloon pulmonary valvuloplasty may be used as an alternative to palliative shunt to augment pulmonary blood flow. Hopefully this will make the patients better-risk candidates for total surgical correction at a later date and avoid immediate palliative shunt surgery.

Increased Pulmonary Blood Flow. In infants with increased pulmonary blood flow and increased pulmonary arterial pressures (most of these infants will be in heart failure), surgical constriction or banding of the main pulmonary artery was recommended in the past. However, because of improvements in open heart surgical techniques in younger infants, most of these infants, particularly those with large ventricular septal defects, will have primary surgical correction. Defects that cannot be completely corrected in small infants may require pulmonary artery banding. These defects include the muscular (Swiss cheese) type of ventricular septal defect, single ventricle, double outlet right ventricle, transposition of the great arteries with a large ventricular septal defect, and rare types of tricuspid atresia (all without associated pulmonic stenosis).

Inadequate Interatrial Mixing. There are several congenital heart defects in which an interatrial septal defect with shunting across it is highly beneficial. Most important of these lesions is transposition of the great arteries with intact ventricular septum. In this cyanotic cardiac anomaly, the aorta arises from the right ventricle and the pulmonary artery from the left ventricle. Here the circulation is parallel instead of "in series." The systemic venous blood does not pass through the lungs to become oxygenated. Some intracardiac admixture is essential for patient survival. These infants will usually present in the first few days of life with severe cyanosis. The treatment of choice is atrial septostomy performed at cardiac catheterization. A deflated balloon catheter is advanced into the left atrium from the right atrium via a patent foramen ovale, and the balloon is inflated with diluted radiopaque liquid and rapidly pulled back across the patent foramen ovale, rupturing the lower margin of the atrial wall below the patent foramen ovale. Balloon septostomy is palliative in most infants until the age of 6 months to 1 year, when the defect can be corrected surgically with much less risk. Septostomy may also be performed in other cardiac defects in which a better mixing at the atrial level and/or relief of high right or left atrial pressure (as the case may be) are required. These defects include pulmonary atresia with intact ventricular septum, tricuspid atresia, mitral atresia, and total anomalous pulmonary venous connection.

Beyond the neonatal period, balloon atrial septostomy is technically difficult because the lower margin of the foramen ovale is thick and cannot be ruptured by balloon. However, a catheter with a retractable knife can be used to cut the septum and a balloon septostomy can then be performed. If this technique is not successful or not readily available, atrial septostomy may be performed surgically either by the Blalock-Hanlon technique or by an open method.

Corrective Procedures

Since the introduction of cardiopulmonary bypass for open heart surgery in the 1950s and the introduction of these techniques in small infants in the 1960s and deep hypothermia technique in the early 1970s, there have been considerable advances in the surgical management of congenital heart disease. Almost every congenital heart defect can be "corrected," and the few that cannot be completely repaired can be effectively palliated. The term corrective surgery is used when defects of the heart or great vessels are anatomically repaired or the circulation is restored to a normal physiologic state. This does not necessarily mean that the cardiovascular system is restored to normal and that the patients are not without any residual cardiac defect; corrective surgery in the purest sense is possible in only a few defects. Table 6 lists the lesions that can be

TABLE 6. Lesions That Can Be Primarily Repaired Without Prior Palliative Procedures

Acyanotic Lesions
  Left to right shunt
    Atrial septal defect
    Common atrioventricular canal
    Endocardial cushion defect
    Partial anomalous pulmonary venous connection
    Patent ductus arteriosus
    Ventricular septal defect

  Obstructive Lesions
    Aortic stenosis
    Coarctation of the aorta
    Interrupted aortic arch
    Pulmonic stenosis

Cyanotic Lesions
  Double outlet right ventricle
  Single atrium
  Tetralogy of Fallot
  Total anomalous pulmonary venous connection
  Transposition of the great arteries
  Truncus arteriosus

completely repaired without prior palliative procedures, and Table 7 lists lesions that may require palliation before total correction several years later. This classification, of course, is arbitrary and with considerable overlap.

The conventional treatment of choice for structural abnormalities of the heart and blood vessels, whether congenital or acquired, is surgical correction. However, during the last decade there has been an enormous increase in the use of transcatheter techniques to improve or correct structural defects in the cardiovascular system.

Balloon dilatation of valvular stenotic lesions by a pullback or dynamic technique was first described in 1954; the technique of static dilatation, as it is used now, originated in 1982. This technique has been used successfully in infants, children, and adults to relieve congenital, acquired, and postoperative stenotic lesions of the pulmonary valve, peripheral or main pulmonary artery, pulmonary vein, aortic valve, mitral valve, descending aorta (coarctation of the aorta), interatrial baffle after Mustard's operation for transposition of the great arteries, and superior

TABLE 7. Lesions That May Require Prior Palliation

  Double outlet right ventricle
  Pulmonary atresia
  Single ventricle
  Transposition of the great arteries
  Tricuspid atresia

vena cava. The indications for this procedure are essentially those for surgical correction.

The technique consists of introducing a guidewire across the stenotic lesion (usually through an end-hole catheter already in place), advancing a balloon dilatation catheter over the guidewire so that the stenotic lesion is located in the middle of the balloon, and rapidly inflating the balloon with diluted contrast material. The recommended size of the balloon varies with type of stenotic lesion to be dilated. Pressure used during inflation of the balloon varies between 4 and 8 atmospheres, depending upon the lesions to be dilated. The recommended duration of balloon inflation is 5 seconds; 3 to 4 balloon inflations at least 5 minutes apart are also recommended.

The relief of obstruction is seen by sudden disappearance of "waisting" of the balloon, fall in trans-stenotic pressure gradient, and increase in the size of the stenotic area by angiography. In general, valvular stenotic lesions can be relieved by balloon dilatation, central arterial (pulmonary artery and aorta) stenotic lesions have variable results, and venous (pulmonary or systemic venous) stenotic lesions have least favorable results.

The risks of surgical relief of most of the stenotic lesions are low, but open-heart operations still have many disadvantages, including prolonged hospitalization, scars of the operation, and greater cost. For these reasons alone, catheter techniques may be more attractive. Successful immediate results in pulmonary valve stenosis with indications that relief persists on follow-up suggest that percutaneous balloon dilatation is the treatment of choice for moderate to severe pulmonary valve stenosis. In light of the high risk of surgical resection of coarction of the aorta in neonates and small infants (especially when other intracardiac anomalies are present), a high incidence of recurrence (10–30 per cent), and difficulties encountered during reoperation, balloon dilatation of coarctation of the aorta offers a safer and effective alternative.

Several types of devices (plugs and umbrellas) have been developed for transcatheter closure of patent ductus arteriosus and atrial septal defect. Because of the bulky size of the catheter delivery system and the extreme low mortality and morbidity rates of surgical closure of these defects, the technique has not gained wide popularity. Further refinement and miniaturization of these devices and additional clinical trials are necessary prior to general use.

MITRAL VALVE BILLOWING AND PROLAPSE

method of
JOHN B. BARLOW, M.D.
University of the Witwatersrand
Johannesburg, South Africa

For nearly three decades an "information explosion" relating to mitral valve prolapse (MVP) and billowing mitral leaflets (BML) has resulted essentially from two observations: the first, in 1963, confirmed a mitral valve origin of an apical late systolic murmur and mid (non-ejection) systolic click; the second, probably of wider interest, was the subsequent correlation of symptoms, clinical signs, and other features associated with the mitral valve anomaly that justify the recognition of a specific syndrome.

The word "prolapse" was introduced in 1966, based on the cineangiocardiographic appearance of the valve. MVP has ominous connotations because some patients draw an analogy to prolapse of the rectum or uterus. Prolapse entails "the slipping out of place or falling of some internal organ," which implies abnormality. It is thus regrettable that the term is used even when the valve anomaly is anatomically mild, clinically silent, and functionally normal. The definition of billowing, prolapse, floppy, and flail is more than a matter of semantics. Such definitions should depend on the functional anatomy or pathology of the mitral valve mechanism. Echocardiographic, cineangiocardiographic, auscultatory, and other clinical features must then be correlated with the probable functional anatomy in order to formulate policies of management.

Normal mitral leaflets bulge slightly, after closure, into the left atrial cavity. When this physiologic billowing is exaggerated, the term "BML" is appropriate. The valve remains competent during systole and is a "normal variant." A constant or intermittent nonejection systolic click may be audible, and the billowing leaflet bodies are marginally prominent on echocardiography. When a BML is more advanced, with voluminous leaflets and elongated chordae, the term "floppy" is often used. Because the BML is severe, partial loss of leaflet edge apposition may ensue and mitral regurgitation, albeit mild or even minimal, inevitably results. A cardiac valve is competent only while there is sustained coaptation of the leaflets. The floppy, or voluminous, bodies of the leaflets are clearly demonstrated by M-mode or 2-dimensional (2-D) echocardiography, but not the failure of leaflet edge coaptation. The term MVP should be confined to the failure of the leaflet edges to appose normally, and the resultant mitral insufficiency is detected clinically by a regurgitant systolic murmur. Progression to severe MVP and consequent hemodynamically important mitral regurgitation, with grossly elongated or ruptured chordae, allows part of a leaflet edge to be "flail." Two-D echocardiography will demonstrate the incomplete leaflet edge apposition.

Many pathologic conditions affecting the papillary muscles, chordae tendineae, anulus, leaflets, or the size of the left ventricular cavity may result in BML or MVP. When BML or MVP is a secondary or an associated entity, the prognosis is determined as much or more by the underlying or coexistent condition. This is well exemplified by a BML or MVP secondary to hypertrophic cardiomyopathy or occlusive coronary artery disease.

Primary Billowing Mitral Leaflets and Prolapse

Primary BML or MVP is a degenerative process of leaflets and chordae which has been described as a "dyscollagenosis." The redundancy of leaflet tissue may be mild and focal, involving only a portion of one scallop, or it may be severe and diffuse, involving both leaflets. The valve is functionally abnormal only when mitral regurgitation, and therefore true MVP, is substantiated. Clinical or echocardiographic features of BML alone are prevalent and have been detected in approximately 15 per cent of the normal population.

The Syndrome

The syndrome associated with this anomaly variously called primary MVP, floppy valve, myxomatous leaflet, click-murmur, or Barlow's syndrome, but the term BML syndrome is preferred. Idiopathic or primary MVP syndrome is a misnomer in the large number of patients who have no evidence, principally on auscultation, of mitral insufficiency. A distinction between BML syndrome alone and that with MVP is crucial in formulating a management policy. The physician has to decide whether repeated auscultation, vasoactive maneuvers, echocardiography, or Doppler ultrasound will be contributory in determining whether regurgitation is present. As already intimated, echocardiographic criteria for BML are suspect but the demonstration of advanced billowing, or floppy, bodies of leaflets would be compatible with clinically suspected mitral regurgitation and MVP. The Doppler criteria for mild mitral insufficiency that is pathologically significant currently require clarification.

In addition to the auscultatory, electrocardiographic, and anatomic features of the syndrome described in 1965, other components include skeletal abnormalities, arrhythmias, conduction defects, systemic emboli, hereditary factors, and possibly autonomic disorders. The importance of making the diagnosis of primary BML syndrome, particularly in symptomatic patients, lies in the knowledge that in the large majority of cases reassurance can be given that serious heart disease is not present and that the prognosis for life is excellent. Many symptomatic patients are anxious. Reasons for anxiety in patients with primary BML are not always apparent and the role of a causally related autonomic disorder requires confirmation. Anxiety supervenes in some patients after an incorrect diagnosis of occlusive coronary artery disease has been made. An explanation that there is "a very mild but also very common anomaly of a heart valve, which sometimes causes ill-understood symptoms of nuisance value only" is a comprehensible explanation from which the patient can derive reassurance. Excessively anxious patients who do not respond to reassurance often improve on a small dose of a beta-adrenergic blocking drug, such as propranolol (Inderal). Because chest pain and an abnormal ECG reading are prominent features of both the primary BML syndrome and occlusive coronary artery disease, the differentiation of these two conditions is a prevalent problem in clinical practice. This differentiation is clearly more difficult in a middle-aged man than in a young woman, but careful history-taking and stress electrocardiography should resolve the problem in most instances. The widely held belief that the post-exercise ST segment and T wave changes of MVP are indistinguishable from those of myocardial ischemia, and hence are a cause of a "false-positive" stress test, is no longer valid. These electrocardiographic abnormalities can be reliably differentiated on their different time-course patterns after cessation of exercise. Radionuclide studies or selective coronary arteriography should seldom be necessary.

Although most patients with the BML syndrome follow a benign course, complications may supervene in a few that cause morbidity and even mortality and that require attention.

Treatment of Complications

Infective Endocarditis and Progression of Mitral Regurgitation

Whether symptomatic or not, patients with mitral regurgitation will generally have a more marked BML, and both prophylaxis against infective endocarditis and observation for progression of the MVP are required. Most nonpansystolic murmurs, whether confined to early or late systole, do not change over many years. Nonetheless, rapid progression of MVP, even in the absence of infective endocarditis, may unpredictably occur. Unequivocal billowing on echocardiography does not imply that severe MVP will inevitably ensue.

Systemic Emboli

Bland emboli manifested as transient ischemic attacks or partial strokes are a recognized but rare complication. Deposits of fibrin and platelet thrombi on the atrial surface of a floppy posterior leaflet may be the site of origin. Coronary emboli with coronary artery spasm have been suggested as a possible mechanism for otherwise unexplained myocardial infarction. A purported association of MVP and migraine requires confirmation, but increased platelet aggregability may be a common pathophysiologic mechanism relating to platelet emboli from the valve and migraine. Antithrombotic therapy is recommended in patients who have had emboli. We have had good results with aspirin (160 to 320 mg daily) plus dipyridamole (Persantine) (100 mg 3 times daily) although the effectiveness of dipyridamole as an anti-thrombotic has recently been challenged. If

systemic emboli are recurrent or large or if an underlying supraventricular tachyarrhythmia is suspected, warfarin (Coumadin) therapy should be added.

Arrhythmias and Sudden Death

Palpitations, lightheadedness, or dizziness suggest the presence of arrhythmias, but exercise electrocardiography or ambulatory monitoring is advisable for evaluation. Arrhythmias may occur without symptoms and, conversely, dizziness and palpitations have been prominent complaints at times when electrocardiographic monitoring and clinical examination provide no objective confirmation. Orthostatic hypotension should be excluded in all patients with these symptoms. A wide variety of arrhythmias have been encountered with the primary BML syndrome and includes supraventricular tachycardia, atrial fibrillation and flutter, atrial ectopic beats, ventricular tachycardia, and ventricular fibrillation. Ventricular extrasystoles are the most prevalent rhythm disturbance, may be unifocal or multifocal, may occur with or without an abnormal resting electrocardiogram, and rarely display the R-on-T phenomenon. They are often precipitated or aggravated by emotion and exercise. If symptoms are troublesome, even if the arrhythmias are not potentially dangerous, patients should be given the benefit of treatment with anti-arrhythmic drugs, preferably verapamil (Isoptin) (if supraventricular) or beta-blocking agents.

A reliable history of syncope, provided that it occurs outside of a context of probable vasovagal syncope, is of major importance. In such instances, ambulatory monitoring and stress testing are indicated in order to detect multiform ventricular extrasystoles, the R-on-T phenomenon, or ventricular tachycardia. Although any anti-arrhythmic drug or beta-receptor blocking agent may contribute to therapy, we have had favorable experience with the unique beta-receptor blocking agent sotalol (Sotalex)* (usual dose range 80 to 320 mg daily). Because of its important class III activity, sotalol has the potential to precipitate ventricular tachycardias of the torsade de pointes variety and should be used with caution in high dosage or in the presence of hypokalemia.

Amiodarone (Cordarone), 200 to 400 mg daily after a loading dose, is extremely effective in the treatment of refractory ventricular tachyarrhythmias but serious side effects mitigate against its long-term use, especially in young subjects. Further study is required of management of potentially lethal arrhythmias, in accordance with

---

*Not yet approved for use in the United States.

electrophysiologic drug testing, by overdrive pacing or with implantable defibrillator devices.

Fewer than 100 patients with the BML syndrome and unexplained sudden death have been reported, and clinical or necropsy details are often lacking. Identification of the patients at higher risk is crucial. A prominent BML, readily demonstrated on M-mode or 2-D echocardiography, and indisputable MVP, evaluated clinically by a constant apical late systolic murmur that becomes louder and longer on standing, are pertinent features especially if detected at an early age. Abnormal T waves, ventricular ectopy on the resting ECG, multiform ventricular ectopy on exercise or ambulatory monitoring and, most importantly, a history of unexpected syncope are other risk factors. Should patients continue to exhibit dangerous arrhythmias despite therapy with sotalol, amiodarone, other anti-arrhythmic agents, or overdrive pacing, the question of mitral valve surgery arises.

A policy of surgical treatment for ventricular arrhythmias in patients with the BML syndrome without hemodynamically significant mitral regurgitation may seem unduly aggressive. On the other hand, there are several mechanisms by which floppy leaflets and elongated chordae could predispose to ventricular ectopy. Technically more difficult valvuloplastic procedures for severe mitral regurgitation are highly successful and a similar operation in a patient with mild mitral regurgitation is relatively easy. Provided that a surgeon experienced in valvuloplastic procedures is available, the combination of an advanced BML demonstrated echocardiographically, a reliable history of syncope, and potentially lethal ventricular arrhythmias unresponsive to anti-arrhythmic therapy is an indication for mitral valve repair. Mitral valve replacement, however, is probably not justified.

CONGESTIVE HEART FAILURE

method of
JONATHAN ABRAMS, M.D.
University of New Mexico
Albuquerque, New Mexico

Congestive heart failure (CHF) is a common cardiac condition in which the heart is unable to meet the blood flow needs of the major organs and body tissues during exertion and, in severe cases, at rest. CHF is usually accompanied by pulmonary and/or systemic venous congestion. Classic hemodynamic abnormalities include elevated left and right heart filling pressures, a subnormal cardiac output, and a depressed left ventricular ejection fraction (less than 40 per cent).

The cardinal signs and symptoms of heart failure are dyspnea on exertion (DOE), orthopnea, paroxysmal nocturnal dyspnea (PND), fatigue, weakness, and swelling of the feet. Pulmonary congestion results in shortness of breath that occurs only during exertion in mild heart failure but may be present at rest in severe CHF; patients are often unable to lie flat (orthopnea, PND). These symptoms result from "backward failure" due to elevation of left heart filling pressure that is transmitted to the pulmonary capillary bed and right heart. "Forward failure" is manifest by decreased stroke volume and cardiac output; related symptoms are weakness and easy fatigue.

In patients who have biventricular failure or dominant right heart failure, signs of an elevated right ventricular filling pressure are present, including elevated jugular venous pressure, peripheral edema, hepatomegaly, and, in advanced cases, abdominal ascites.

Some subjects with heart disease can have a hypertrophied and/or noncompliant left ventricle (LV) with a relatively normal LV ejection fraction (diastolic dysfunction with intact systolic function). These patients may present with signs and symptoms of CHF solely due to an elevated LV filling pressure. It is thus essential to document abnormal ventricular contractile performance in all patients diagnosed with CHF; an ejection fraction determination by echo, radionuclear angiography, or cardiac catheterization should be obtained on all such patients.

Treatment of Chronic Congestive Heart Failure

Mild Congestive Heart Failure

General Measures. Patients with mild CHF or those seen early in their illness usually respond very well to conventional measures such as salt restriction, weight reduction, and intermittent or daily diuretic therapy. It is important to counsel individuals regarding sources of salt in the diet; sodium intake should be less than 3 grams per day. In this era of potent diuretics, it is usually not necessary to severely limit sodium intake in mild CHF. Older patients with a diagnosis of heart failure should have thyroid function studies and a hemogram obtained if the etiology of CHF is not clear. Electrolytes and renal function should be measured.

Diuretic and Digitalis Therapy. Many individuals who present with mild CHF will have peripheral edema, at least at the end of the day, and may have breathlessness at night. Such patients respond well to initial diuretic therapy. One should begin with a thiazide diuretic, giving hydrochlorothiazide 25 to 50 mg orally daily or every other day. In mild heart failure it is better to use the less potent but longer-acting thiazide diuretics as opposed to the loop diuretics. Occasional electrolyte monitoring and potassium replacement is usually indicated, even in individuals who eat foods with a high potassium content. The relationship of hypokalemia and hypomagnesemia to ventricular arrhythmias and sudden death remains speculative but is sufficiently suggestive such that the serum potassium should be maintained at a level of 3.8 mEq per liter or higher.

The role of digitalis in heart failure remains the subject of considerable controversy. Digitalis glycosides are not as potent therapy as previously believed in CHF and even when used with a diuretic may not be sufficient treatment for many patients. Nevertheless, I believe that digitalis should be given to *all* such individuals with rare exceptions. Oral digoxin is the most widely prescribed glycoside; digitoxin therapy is effective and probably should be used more often, especially in patients with changing renal function. Unless one is dealing with an urgent situation, one can safely "load" a patient with digoxin over a period of several days. Thus, for a middle-aged subject with normal renal function, the recommended dosage is 0.25 mg orally 2 to 3 times daily for 2 to 3 days, followed by a maintenance dose of 0.25 mg per day. In stable patients one can simply begin dixogin therapy with a once-daily maintenance dose. Remember that in older subjects, small-sized individuals, or those with azotemia, the risk of digitalis toxicity is increased and the digoxin dose must be reduced. In patients over 70, I give a daily maintenance dose of 0.125 mg of digoxin.

Recent data suggest that a patient with mild heart failure can be treated with angiotensin-converting enzyme (ACE) inhibitor therapy instead of digitalis. Thus, the use of captopril (Capoten) or enalapril (Vasotec) (Table 1) is considered by some physicians as preferential to digitalis. Because of cost and safety factors, I prefer to use ACE inhibitors only after a patient has remained symptomatic on digitalis and diuretic therapy.

I do not recommend frequent assessments of electrolytes, BUN, and serum digoxin levels. The latter should be used only when one is suspicious that a patient may have too much or too little digoxin in his or her system; it is not necessary to obtain digoxin levels on patients who are doing well while taking a conventional dose of digoxin. Remember that at least 6 to 8 hours should elapse after the last oral digoxin dose before obtaining the blood sample.

Moderate Heart Failure

Most patients with moderately severe CHF remain symptomatic on digoxin and diuretics. As the goal of therapy is to render a patient as functional as possible, the physician must determine what symptoms are most bothersome to the patient.

Diuretic and Digitalis Therapy. In a subject who continues to have end-day edema, a more potent diuretic regimen is necessary. Patients with heart failure should weigh themselves daily and be instructed that a weight gain of several pounds over 1 to 2 days usually means the body is retaining salt and water and that diuretic requirements need to be increased. Most patients with moderate heart failure will require an oral loop diuretic such as furosemide (Lasix), 40 to 80 mg daily, or bumetanide (Bumex), 1 to 2 mg daily. Depending on renal function and other factors, effective diuretic dosage varies considerably in different patients who appear to have the same clinical severity of heart failure. It is useful to ask the patient to carefully note the urine volume response after a dose of diuretic. The diuresis stimulated by a potent loop diuretic occurs within the first 60 to 90 minutes; therefore, a patient can guide his diuretic needs by the amount of urine output occurring in the first several hours after the diuretic is taken.

Patients who remain edematous on what appears to be adequate doses of diuretic should be

TABLE 1. **Dosage Recommendations for Oral Vasodilator Therapy of Congestive Heart Failure**

	Initial	Maintenance
Nitrates		
2% nitroglycerin ointment	½–1 inch tid	1–2 inch tid–qid
Transdermal nitroglycerin patch (remove for 8–12 hours daily)	10 mg/24 hr	20–60 mg/24 hr
Buccal nitroglycerin	1 mg tid	2–5 mg tid
Oral isosorbide dinitrate	20 mg tid	40–80 mg tid
Angiotensin-Converting Enzyme (ACE) Inhibitors		
Captopril (Capoten)	12.5 mg tid first few doses (6.25 mg high-risk patients*)	12.5–50 mg tid
Enalapril (Vasotec)	5 mg bid first few doses (2.5 mg for high-risk patients)	10–20 mg bid
Lisinopril (Prinivil)	5 mg first few doses (2.5 mg for high-risk patients)	10–40 mg once daily

*High-risk patients are those with hyponatremia, low blood pressure, or azotemia, or on diuretic therapy, especially high-dose (hold diuretics for 1 to 2 days if possible).

carefully questioned about dietary habits, inadvertent use of excessive salt, and medication compliance.

All subjects with moderate heart failure should receive an appropriate amount of digitalis; if there is a question as to the efficacy of the digoxin dose, a serum level may be obtained. Remember that patients who have atrial fibrillation and CHF often require larger than usual maintenance doses of digoxin to control their ventricular rate; in this setting serum digoxin levels may be in the "toxic" range (over 2.0 ng per ml) without necessarily indicating digitalis toxicity.

Vasodilator Therapy. Since the early 1970s, potent vasodilators have been available for the therapy of moderate to severe CHF. The rationale is the reduction in impedance or afterload that the left ventricle "sees" after the aortic valve opens. Arterial vasodilators reduce systemic resistance and allow the left ventricle to empty its contents more efficiently and more rapidly, resulting in an increased stroke volume and cardiac output. In addition, vasodilators that induce venodilatation directly (nitrates) or indirectly (alpha antagonists, prazosin, ACE inhibitors) improve the heart failure syndrome and the concomitant sequela of "backwards failure" by reducing right and left heart filling pressures. Vasodilators are indicated in CHF patients on digitalis and diuretic therapy who remain significantly symptomatic. When signs and symptoms of congestive or backward failure dominate, a vasodilator with venodilating capability is imperative.

Nitrate Therapy. Long-acting nitrates are safe and effective drugs to use in patients who are not controlled on digitalis and diuretic therapy alone. The dominant effect of nitrates in heart failure is to lower left and right ventricular filling pressures. In spite of a nitrate-induced decrease in cardiac preload, cardiac output does not decline and usually increases modestly because of the arterial dilating actions of nitrates. Nitrates should be used in considerably higher dosage in CHF therapy than in angina. Side effects of nitroglycerin such as headache and dizziness are relatively infrequent in patients with heart failure, even with large doses.

Nitrates produce sustained reductions in left ventricular filling pressure and, with the ACE inhibitors, are the only drugs that have been shown to improve long-term exercise performance in patients with CHF. The combination of oral isosorbide dinitrate and hydralazine decreases mortality in patients with CHF. Recommended nitrate dosage is listed in Table 1. The nitroglycerin patches should be used in large amounts, with a minimum of 20 to 30 mg per 24 hours.

Nitrate tolerance is a definite problem that can adversely affect the therapeutic response. Physicians should be careful to incorporate a nitrate-free interval of 8 to 12 hours into the drug regimen. Intermittent therapy with the nitroglycerin patches (12 to 14 hours on, 10 to 12 hours off) appears to prevent tolerance development. For oral isosorbide dinitrate and nitroglycerin ointment, it is best to use no more than a 3-times daily dosage regimen. Thus, in patients with marked nocturnal symptoms of orthopnea and PND, the nitrate-free interval should be scheduled during the day.

ACE Inhibitor Therapy. The advent of drugs that act by interruption of the renin-angiotensin-aldosterone system has proved to be extraordinarily important. Activation of the renin-angiotensin axis contributes to increased systemic resistance and afterload as well as salt and water retention in CHF. ACE inhibitors have been documented to produce improvements in general well-being and an increase in exercise tolerance. A recent trial with enalapril (Vasotec) in severe (Class IV) CHF patients resulted in an impressive improvement in one year mortality compared with placebo.

Physicians are often reluctant to utilize these agents because of concern of precipitating renal insufficiency, hypotension, rash, or neutropenia. In fact, when used carefully, these drugs are reasonably safe in CHF. The major danger is excessive hypotension. Patients who are relatively over-diuresed or hyponatremic or who run a low blood pressure are at particular risk for a fall in blood pressure following ACE inhibitor administration. Such individuals may develop worsening renal function as a result of the sustained hypotension. Thus, in high-risk individuals, ACE inhibitors should be initiated very cautiously, utilizing extremely low doses (see Table 1). Patients do not need to be hospitalized to begin ACE inhibitor therapy if the first dose is given under careful observation with frequent blood pressure measurements for several hours. Thereafter, upward dosage adjustments can be made every 3 to 7 days. One should aim for a final dose of 25 to 50 mg of captopril (Capoten) 3 times daily, 10 to 20 mg of enalapril (Vasotec) twice daily, and 10 to 20 mg once daily of lisinopril (Prinivil), stopping at a lower dosage if the subject is clinically improved.

The physician must monitor for hyperkalemia and avoid the concomitant use of potassium supplements or potassium-sparing drugs, as the ACE inhibitors tend to conserve potassium. Serum BUN may rise or fall but usually does not change significantly. Occasional white blood cell counts are advisable for detection of neutropenia.

Other Vasodilators. Hydralazine (Apresoline) and prazosin (Minipress) have been used in CHF. These drugs have not been uniformly effective during chronic therapy and cannot be recommended except in unusual cases. Prazosin commonly produces tachyphylaxis. Hydralazine is a potent arterial vasodilator and predictably increases cardiac output. In patients who demonstrate marked "forward failure" or who have CHF associated with significant aortic or mitral regurgitation, hydralazine should be employed. The usual dosage is 75 to 100 mg 4 times a day. Side effects of hydralazine (Apresoline) include palpitations, angina, arthralgia, and a serum sickness–like illness.

Some physicians prefer to use an ACE inhibitor before a nitrate as the initial vasodilator in CHF. For reasons of safety, cost, ease of dosing, and the variety of available formulations, I believe a nitrate is an appropriate first choice.

For refractory patients, or those in whom a nitrate or an ACE inhibitor alone does not produce optimal improvement, the drugs may be combined. Hydralazine has been used with captopril to maximize the rise in cardiac output. Because of the potential for serious hypotension related to the use of potent vasoactive agents alone or in combination, one must be particularly cautious in patients with coronary artery disease or those with a borderline low blood pressure.

Severe Heart Failure

In general, aggressive use of vasodilators, often with the help of an indwelling Swan-Ganz catheter, is required in severe CHF. Intravenous nitroglycerin or nitroprusside will rapidly lower left and right heart filling pressure and improve cardiac output (Table 2). Diuresis is often difficult in such patients. Remember that the loop diuretics act only when a specific "threshold" dose is achieved in a given patient; this dose may be higher as CHF worsens. A trial of intravenous loop diuretics may be very useful, using far lower dosage than the patient's current oral requirements (e.g., 20 mg of intravenous furosemide or 0.5 to 1 mg of bumetanide). The use of oral

metolazine (Zaroxolyn) (5 to 10 mg) combined with furosemide (Lasix) is a potent regimen that works in all but truly refractory cases.

Acute Congestive Heart Failure

Patients who have recent onset of acute heart failure or who have severe CHF or pulmonary edema require a higher level of care than relatively stable outpatients with CHF. Such individuals are invariably hospitalized, usually in an intensive care unit. Initial treatment of severe heart failure should include measures that reduce salt and water retention; lower intracardiac filling pressures; provide control of hypertension, tachyarrhythmias, fever, and other precipitating or exacerbating factors; and, in rare instances, provide inotropic support of the heart. The traditional use of small doses of intravenous morphine may be useful in patients who are severely apprehensive and dyspneic, although one must be careful not to use such drugs in individuals who have chronic lung disease. While limb tourniquets have been a long-standing adjunct in the therapy of pulmonary edema, a recent study indicates that they are not beneficial in heart failure.

Reduction of cardiac preload can be readily accompanied by an intravenous infusion of sodium nitroprusside or nitroglycerin, potent venous and arterial vasodilators (see Table 2). These drugs rapidly lower elevated pulmonary capillary wedge, pulmonary artery, and right atrial pressures. If the blood pressure is normal to high and there is no question that the patient is in a congestive state, these drugs can be given safely without a pulmonary artery (Swan-Ganz) catheter. If the diagnosis of acute heart failure is correct, the pulmonary capillary wedge or pulmonary artery diastolic pressure will be 20 mm Hg or greater. The therapeutic goal should be to reduce the left ventricular filling pressure to 12 to 16 mm Hg. It is not usually necessary to drive the wedge pressure to excessively low levels (e.g., less than 12 to 15 mm Hg).

Concomitant with the infusion of a potent intravenous vasodilator, diuretics should be insti-

TABLE 2. **Dosage Recommendations for Intravenous Drug Therapy of Congestive Heart Failure**

	Initial	Maintenance
Sodium nitroprusside (Nipride)	20 µg/min	40–250 µg/min
Nitroglycerin	10–20 µg/min*	40–300 µg/min
Dopamine (Dopastat)	2–5 µg/kg/min†	3–10 µg/kg/min†
Dobutamine (Dobutrex)	3–5 µg/kg/min	5–10 µg/kg/min
Amrinone (Inocor)	0.75 mg/kg/min bolus over 2–3 min; may repeat in 30–60 min	5–10 µg/kg/min

*Use lower initial infusion rates with specialized nonadsorbent tubing.
†Normotensive—use 3–8 micrograms/kg/min; hypotensive—use >8 micrograms/kg/min.

tuted. The immediate early response to intravenous furosemide is systemic vasoconstriction, which may be detrimental and therefore should be accompanied by concomitant administration of intravenous nitroprusside or nitroglycerin. Oxygen by mask or nasal cannula should be used at the outset. For patients who are extremely ill and unable to keep up with the work of breathing or whose lungs are "wet" with intra-alveolar congestion and/or pleural effusions, intubation and respiratory support may be necessary and indeed can be life-saving.

If the acute heart failure is related to acute myocardial ischemia (either infarction or severe ischemic pain), nitroglycerin should be used preferentially over nitroprusside. If mitral regurgitation is present, nitroprusside is a more effective drug. Either drug should be administered with great caution to patients who are relatively hypotensive; care must be used when starting these agents, beginning at very low infusion rates. The initial and maintenance doses of intravenous nitroglycerin and nitroprusside are shown in Table 2. The dosage should be increased every 3 to 10 minutes as the clinical situation demands. Close attention should be paid to the systolic pressure and heart rate and the patient's clinical condition. If an excessive hypotensive response occurs owing to the vasodilator, heart rate will usually increase. If the stroke volume is substantially augmented by the unloading agent, blood pressure may not fall very much or at all.

Tachyarrhythmias in patients with severe CHF should be treated quickly and vigorously. Atrial fibrillation with a rapid ventricular response is a common associated dysrhythmia. Careful use of a rapid-acting intravenous beta blocker (e.g., esmolol or propranolol) may dramatically improve the clinical situation. This is particularly true in the setting of an acute anterior wall infarction and rapid atrial fibrillation. The negative inotropic properties of these drugs present a true therapeutic dilemma in such situations, and use of a beta blocker demands meticulous clinical care.

For patients with acute CHF and significant ventricular ectopy, intravenous lidocaine is the drug of choice, beginning with a bolus infusion of 75 to 100 mg given over 1 minute. The normal lidocaine maintenance infusion rate of 2 to 4 mg per minute should be reduced by one third to one half because of decreased lidocaine clearance in CHF.

Inotropic or Pressor Agents. Inotropic agents are indicated in extreme or refractory cases of severe CHF. Heart failure with marked hypotension (shock) requires pressors. Drugs that act directly on $beta_1$ receptors in the heart (dobutamine, iso-

proteronel, dopamine) are rarely needed in acute CHF except when there is coexisting profound bradycardia or low blood pressure. Isoproteronel tends to induce marked sinus tachycardia and ventricular arrhythmias and also lowers blood pressure; however, in the setting of heart block or sinus node dysfunction, it is the drug of choice. Dopamine should be used only when there is inadequate central aortic blood pressure or to augment renal perfusion independent of cardiac output. In the setting of acute myocardial ischemia, CHF, and hypotension (cardiogenic shock), dopamine is the drug of choice. This agent should be started at low concentrations (3 to 5 micrograms per kg per min) and increased as needed (see Table 2). Remember that at high infusion rates, dopamine takes on dominant alpha-adrenergic properties and induces peripheral vasoconstriction. Dopamine usually drives the pulmonary wedge pressure higher, an unwanted sequela. Low-dose dopamine can be used with great effectiveness in patients who have oliguria; stimulation of the renal dopaminergic receptors can enhance urine output with no effect on blood pressure or stroke volume.

The best inotropic drug for acute left ventricular dysfunction is dobutamine, a drug that does not usually increase blood pressure. Dobutamine at low to moderate concentrations (see Table 2) will enhance myocardial contractility and should be used in refractory patients with CHF who have normal or somewhat subnormal blood pressure and who are not responding to conventional therapy. Some individuals who are overtly hypotensive will have a beneficial response to dobutamine with an increase in blood pressure if a marked increase in stroke volume occurs. Dobutamine is not nearly as effective as dopamine for elevating central aortic pressure in severe hypotensive states. Both drugs are beta agonists and may cause sinus tachycardia and ventricular arrhythmias at higher doses. Table 2 lists the initial and maintenance infusion rates for intravenous agents used for acute heart failure and/or pulmonary edema. Amrinone is a non-glycoside, non-sympathomimetic intravenous drug that may acutely augment cardiac output but is generally not recommended as initial therapy for severe CHF.

Cardiogenic Shock

Patients with massive myocardial infarction may present with heart failure as well as marked hypotension. This combination is cardiogenic shock, an extremely dangerous clinical syndrome often resulting in death. In such cases, urgent attention should be given first to elevating coronary (central aortic) perfusion pressure. When heart failure is a prominent feature, a terrible dilemma is present in that the best drugs for reducing pulmonary congestion (nitroprusside, nitroglycerin) also lower systemic blood pressure. Combinations of intravenous dopamine with nitroprusside have been used with occasional success. Intravenous amrinone can be tried on a short-term basis. This drug should be employed only in patients who are extremely ill. Amrinone has indications for use similar to those of dobutamine and in general is not beneficial as a pressor agent.

INFECTIVE ENDOCARDITIS

method of
CLAUDIA R. LIBERTIN, M.D.
Loyola University Medical Center
Maywood, Illinois

Infective endocarditis is a microbial infection of the cardiac valves and endocardium. In the preantibiotic era, infective endocarditis was considered a uniformly fatal disease. Surgical advances and aggressive antibiotic therapy have reduced its mortality, although the mortality rate is still 14 to 21 per cent.

Infective endocarditis has been classified two ways. One method of classification is based on the divisions of acute, subacute, and chronic time relationships determined by the onset of symptoms. The acute form of endocarditis traditionally progressed in days or weeks, the subacute form evolved in weeks to months, and the chronic form existed for greater than 6 months. However, since the use of antibiotic therapy the chronic form is extremely rare. The other classification arranges divisions by the infecting microorganism. Each organism has specific implications for the rapidity of the infectious process and for the presence or absence of underlying heart disease. Infections caused by *Staphylococcus aureus*, *Streptococcus pneumoniae*, *Neisseria gonorrheae*, and group A streptococci most frequently have a fulminant course. Often there is severe destruction of the cardiac valves, which were normal prior to the infection. Infections caused by the viridans group of streptococci or *Staphylococcus epidermidis* run a more indolent course and occur on deformed heart valves or prostheses, and valvular damage evolves more slowly. Since classification by the infecting organism can be useful in therapy, suggesting the antibiotic regimen to be used, it is the scheme most commonly adopted.

Infective endocarditis tends to originate at areas of turbulence, such as on deformed valves or at sites of damaged endocardium. Endocarditis tends to occur in areas of high pressure. For example, endocarditis is more frequent on the left side of the heart. Approximately 70 per cent of patients with endocarditis have evidence of pre-existing structural cardiac abnormalities. High-risk patients are those with prosthetic cardiac valves, aortic stenosis or insufficiency, patent ductus arteriosus, mitral insufficiency, or ventricular septal defect. Patients undergoing hyperalimentation with a right heart indwelling catheter are similarly at risk. Those at intermediate risk for infection are patients with mitral stenosis and prolapse, tricuspid valve disease, hypertrophic obstructive cardiomyopathy, tetralogy of Fallot, and calcific aortic sclerosis. In the remaining 30 per cent of patients, no underlying heart disease may be found or known.

The spectrum of infective endocarditis has changed significantly within the past 30 years. This is explained by the increasing number of patients with prosthetic heart valves, the problem of intravenous drug abuse, the occurrence of antibiotic-resistant, nosocomial infections, and the widespread use of antibiotics that replace normal host flora with unusual organisms. Prosthetic valve endocarditis occurs in approximately 1 to 5 per cent of patients who receive such prostheses. With the advent of this procedure, early-onset prosthetic valve endocarditis (occurring within 2 months of surgery) was frequent and often fatal. Mortality associated with it was reported to be as high as 50 per cent and often resulted from intraoperative contamination with nosocomial bacteria, especially *Staphylococcus epidermidis*. Now, with the use of prophylactic antibiotic therapy and improvement in surgical techniques, early-onset prosthetic valve endocarditis has become less common. The incidence of late-onset prosthetic valve endocarditis (occurring at least 2 months after surgery) has remained constant. Late-onset prosthetic valve endocarditis is caused by the same microorganisms that cause native valve endocarditis.

Diagnosis

The presence of endocarditis is often difficult to identify and should be based on careful physical examination and the general clinical presentation of the patient rather than on individual symptoms and signs. Any organ system can first manifest symptoms or signs of endocarditis. A non-specific history such as a fever, anorexia, and weight loss may suggest endocarditis. Therefore, careful serial physical examinations are necessary to detect the development of a new organic murmur, embolization, or cardiac compromise. Rarely are peripheral cutaneous manifestations such as petechiae and splinter hemorrhages seen. Osler's nodes and Janeway's lesions are seen in only 20 to 40 per cent of cases. Splenomegaly is found in as few as 5 to 15 per cent of all endocarditis patients. Consequently, suspicion of the disease process must be high to make the diagnosis. The most helpful laboratory tests include those revealing anemia, increased erythrocyte sedimentation rate, and red blood cells on urinalysis.

The definitive diagnosis of infective endocarditis is made by isolating the infecting microorganism. Three separate blood cultures should be collected within a 24-hour interval from patients who have not received antimicrobial therapy within the prior 2 weeks. This number of blood cultures is adequate for isolation of the etiologic agent in at least 96 per cent of previously untreated patients with infective endocarditis. Collection of an additional two or three separate blood cultures may be necessary in previously treated patients or in those with endocarditis due to fastidious microorganisms. Blood cultures need to be repeated during therapy to document clearance of the microorganism as well as 1 and 2 months after the cessation of therapy because of the possibility of relapse.

Determinations of minimum inhibitory concentrations as well as minimum bactericidal concentrations need to be done on the infecting microorganism. The role of the serum bactericidal titer (SBT) to guide the choice and dosage of antibiotics for patients with infective endocarditis is uncertain. The principal problem has been the lack of a standard method for determining the SBT. It is suggested that a peak SBT equal to or greater than 1:64 correlates with cure. However, lower titers do not correlate with treatment failures. Consequently, concerns remain about the reliability of SBT monitoring in infective endocarditis patients, and this technique is seldom used.

Although echocardiography is a relatively nonspecific and insensitive method of diagnosing infective endocarditis, it is an important part of the patient assessment, particularly in surgical candidates. A combined M-mode and two-dimensional echocardiogram (with Doppler evaluation) is useful for detecting valvular incompetence, fistulas, annular ring abscesses, ruptured chordae tendinae, and prosthetic valve dehiscence. However, the absence of a vegetation does not exclude the diagnosis of infective endocarditis.

Treatment

General Principles

No single regimen exists for the management and treatment for all patients with infective endocarditis. However, the following general principles will be helpful.

Establish the microbiologic diagnosis. Before starting antimicrobial therapy, the microbiologic diagnosis should be established by obtaining 3 separate blood cultures drawn approximately 10 to 15 minutes apart. Since the majority of patients with infective endocarditis have a subacute course, antimicrobial therapy does not need to be expeditious. Once the microorganism has been cultured in the laboratory, antimicrobial therapy can be started before the *in vitro* susceptibility data are available. Failure to secure the diagnosis may prolong hospitalization, increase cost, result in iatrogenic complications related to inappropriate therapy, and lead to possible recurrence of the infection. On the other hand, if the patient presents acutely or if the microbiologic diagnosis has been established, therapy should be initiated promptly.

Empiric antimicrobial regimens should be used in acute cases. This therapy should be initiated only after three separate sets of blood cultures have been obtained. The antimicrobial regimen should definitely include a combination of antibiotics effective against streptococci, staphylococci, and enterococci in native valve endocarditis. Penicillin, a semi-synthetic penicillin (such as nafcillin), and gentamicin or vancomycin and gentamicin (in penicillin-allergic patients) are reasonable choices. In individuals with acute prosthetic valve endocarditis, the regimen should include antibiotics effective against coagulase-negative staphylococci, *S. aureus*, streptococci, and gram-negative nosocomial pathogens. A combination of vancomycin and gentamicin is adequate empiric therapy in early-onset prosthetic valve endocarditis. These regimens should be adjusted when the microorganism is identified and when *in vitro* susceptibilities are known.

Obtain early consultation from cardiovascular surgery. Patients with infective endocarditis may require emergency cardiac valve replacement. In particular, patients with aortic valve infective endocarditis or prosthetic valve endocarditis may have acute insufficiency or valve dehiscence in association with cardiac decompensation. Immediate surgical intervention may be necessary.

Daily physical examination should be performed. Subtle changes in findings, such as the blood pressure and cardiac auscultation, may precede cardiac decompensation. The hemodynamic status is important in determining the need for and the timing of cardiac valve replacement.

Portal of entry should be identified. The microorganism causing endocarditis may suggest the portal of entry. For example, viridans streptococci commonly arise from the oral cavity; dental roentgenograms are appropriate for identification of an abscess. *Streptococcus bovis* is associated with colonic lesions; consequently, proctoscopy and a colon roentgenogram are warranted. These procedures should be conducted while the patient is receiving antibiotics for endocarditis.

Repeat blood cultures during and after therapy. Blood cultures should be repeated 48 to 72 hours after the initiation of therapy to establish clearance of the microorganism. Persistent bacteremia is suggestive of a myocardial or peripheral abscess, inappropriate antimicrobial therapy, or an error in the choice of the parenteral antibiotic. Since most relapses occur within the first 2 months after the completion of therapy, repeat blood cultures at that time are also warranted.

Instruct patient in prophylaxis for infective endocarditis prior to dismissal. Transient bacteremia occurs after a variety of different invasive procedures. Even though the effectiveness of antibiotic prophylaxis has not been fully documented, proposed recommendations by the American Heart Association have been made.

Therapy of Specific Types of Endocarditis

Approximately 75 per cent of cases of native valve infective endocarditis are caused by gram-positive microorganisms. Recently, relatively uncommon causes of endocarditis have been identified because of improved microbiologic techniques. The incidence of culture-negative endocarditis is generally less than 1 to 4 per cent. Common causes of culture negativity are the previous use of antibiotics, fastidious organisms, right-sided endocarditis, and noninfective endocarditis. In general, parenteral administration of antibiotics by either intravenous or intramuscular routes will give good bactericidal drug levels in the blood. Drug doses may need to be adjusted for renal function; the following recommendations assume normal renal function.

Streptococcal Endocarditis. Penicillin G or ampicillin, often combined with an aminoglycoside, such as streptomycin or gentamicin, remains the cornerstone of therapy for endocarditis caused by streptococci (Table 1). *S. viridans* and *S. bovis* are very sensitive to penicillin in minimum inhibitory concentrations of less than 0.1 micrograms per ml. Most viridans streptococci are susceptible at this level. Dosage recommendations vary, but penicillin G, 12 million units per day intravenously as a continuous drip or given in divided doses every 4 hours, is adequate. Four weeks of therapy with appropriate doses of penicillin should be effective. Because the combination of an aminoglycoside with penicillin results in synergistic killing of streptococci, streptomycin (0.5 gram every 12 hours) or low-dose gentamicin

(1 mg per kg every 8 hours) for 2 weeks has been successful in the treatment of streptococcal endocarditis. This regimen is as curative as penicillin alone, with relapse rates of approximately 1 per cent. Contraindications for aminoglycoside use include renal insufficiency and auditory or vestibular disorders. Patients not able to be identified or evaluated for eighth nerve toxicity also should be excluded from the short-course regimen. Some viridans streptococci have minimum inhibitory concentrations to penicillin between 0.1 and 0.4 microgram per ml. For these organisms no definitive guidelines exist. However, higher levels of penicillin G or vancomycin are advisable, combined with an aminoglycoside for the first 2 weeks of a 4-week antibiotic regimen. For patients with prosthetic valve endocarditis due to these same organisms, 6-week therapy with penicillin or vancomycin is recommended, combined with an aminoglycoside for the first 2 weeks if feasible. Penicillin-allergic patients may be treated with vancomycin or a cephalosporin, provided a history of allergy does not include anaphylaxis.

Enterococcal Endocarditis. Enterococci are relatively resistant to penicillin G in minimum inhibitory concentrations of 1.0 to 4.0 micrograms per ml. The source of infection is often the genitourinary tract. Because of the relative resistance, penicillin G or ampicillin must be combined with an aminoglycoside for the duration of therapy. Until recently, low-dose gentamicin (1 mg per kg every 8 hours) would have been synergistic in all cases of endocarditis. During this

TABLE 1. **Treatment Regimens for Infective Endocarditis Caused by Gram-Positive Cocci**

Organism	Regimen
Viridans streptococci, *Streptococcus bovis* (MIC ≤ 0.1 mcgm/ml)	1. Penicillin G, 12 million units total/day, given as continuous drip or divided into 4-hr doses, for 4 weeks 2. Penicillin G, as above; plus streptomycin, 20 mg/kg/day IM, divided into 2 equal doses, every 12 hr for 4 weeks 3. For penicillin-allergic patients: cefazolin, 1–2 gm every 8 hr for 4 weeks; or vancomycin, 25 mg/kg/day IV every 8 hr for 4 weeks
Streptococcus fecalis and other penicillin-resistant streptococci (MIC > 0.1 mcgm/ml)	1. Ampicillin, 1–2 gm every 4 hr for 4–6 weeks; plus gentamicin, 3 mg/kg/day, in 3 equal doses, every 8 hr for 4–6 weeks; or streptomycin 20 mg/kg/day in 2 equal doses, every 12 hr for 4–6 weeks 2. For penicillin-allergic patients: vancomycin, 25 mg/kg/day IV, in 3 equal doses, every 8 hr for 4–6 weeks; plus gentamicin or streptomycin, as above.
Staphylococcus aureus	1. Nafcillin (Nafcil) or oxacillin (Prostaphlin), 1–2 gm IV, every 4 hr for 4 weeks after defervescence; plus gentamicin (Garamycin). 3–5 mg/kg/day IV, in 3 equal doses, every 8 hr for first 3 days 2. Cefazolin (Ancef, Kefzol), 1–2 gm IV, every 8 hr for 4 weeks following defervescence; plus gentamicin, as above 3. Vancomyin (Vancocin), 25 mg/kg/day IV in 3 equal doses, every 8 hr for 4 weeks after defervescence; plus gentamicin, as above.

MIC, minimum inhibitory concentration.

decade, however, high-level gentamicin- and streptomycin-resistant strains have been found sensitive to MICs $\geq$ 500 micrograms per ml and > 2000 micrograms per ml, respectively. The presence of this high-level aminoglycoside resistance implies the absence of synergy when combined with penicillin. Resistance to streptomycin does not confer resistance to gentamicin, and vice versa. However, high-level resistance to gentamicin does negate the synergistic benefits of tobramycin, netilmicin, amikacin, kanamycin, and sisomicin. Therefore, high-level susceptibility testing of gentamicin and streptomycin is warranted to select the aminoglycoside for therapy. A 6-week course of combination therapy is ideal. Patients allergic to penicillin should be treated with the combination of vancomycin and gentamicin.

Staphylococcal Endocarditis. Because patients infected with *S. aureus* are often acutely ill, urgent initiation of antibiotics is appropriate. The antibiotics of choice are the semisynthetic penicillins, nafcillin and oxacillin, in a dose of 2 gm every 4 hours. If the minimum inhibitory concentration of penicillin G is less than 0.1 microgram per ml, then penicillin G will be equally effective. On the other hand, if the bacterial strain is found to be resistant to methicillin (and consequently to all other semisynthetic penicillins and cephalosporins), vancomycin therapy is indicated. A 6-week course of antibiotics is recommended and may have to be longer if an initial delay in clinical response occurs or complications arise. Because low-dose gentamicin in combination with a semisynthetic penicillin may lead to more rapid killing of staphylococci, gentamicin for the first 3 days may be beneficial; evidence of increased efficacy beyond this time is lacking. The benefits of such use of aminoglycosides must be weighed against their potential toxicities. Cases of native valve, prosthetic valve, and addict-associated endocarditis should be considered individually because of differences in their prognosis and approach.

Gram-negative Endocarditis. Endocarditis caused by gram-negative bacteria is relatively rare. Appropriate therapy depends on the in vitro susceptibility of each organism. *Pseudomonas aeruginosa*, most commonly seen in intravenous drug addicts, requires combination therapy with an anti-pseudomonal penicillin or cephalosporin combined with tobramycin for a duration of 6 weeks.

Fastidious Organisms. The HACEK group of organisms, which includes *Haemophilus* species, *Actinobacillus actinomycetemcomitans, Cardiobacterium hominis, Eikenella corrodens,* and *Kingella kingii*, rarely cause endocarditis. In general, these organisms are sensitive to ampicillin, which may be combined with an aminoglycoside for 6 weeks of therapy. Nutritionally deficient streptococci are fastidious organisms that require pyridoxal supplementation for growth. Blood culture gram stains show gram-positive cocci, but the organisms fail to grow on agar plates without addition of a *staphylococcal* streak or pyridoxal supplementation. Penicillin or vancomycin combined with an aminoglycoside is recommended for 4 to 6 weeks of therapy. If the strain is penicillin resistant, vancomycin should be used.

Prosthetic Valve Endocarditis. Coagulase-negative staphylococci and *S. aureus* together account for approximately half of the total cases of prosthetic valve endocarditis. The microbiology of early-onset prosthetic valve endocarditis (less than 2 months postoperatively) differs from that of late-onset prosthetic valve endocarditis. In the former type, resistant organisms such as gram-negative rods, fungi, and staphylococci are more common. As in any case of endocarditis, antibiotic therapy is guided by the susceptibility of the infecting organism.

Management of Complications

Congestive heart failure is the most common serious complication of infective endocarditis and is a leading cause of death. In patients with hemodynamic compromise, prompt valve replacement should be considered, regardless of the duration of preoperative antibiotic therapy. Simi-

TABLE 2. **Prophylactic Therapy for Infective Endocarditis**

Indication	Low-Risk Patients	High-Risk Patients	Low-Risk Penicillin-Allergic Patients
Procedures involving the oral cavity, respiratory tract, and endoscopies	2 gm oral penicillin V 60 min before procedure followed by 1 gm penicillin V 6 hr later	1–2 gm ampicillin plus 1.5 mg/kg gentamicin IV or IM 30 min before procedure, followed by 1 gm oral penicillin V 6 hr later	1 gm oral erythromycin 60 min before procedure, followed by 500-mg dose 6 hr later
Procedures involving genitourinary or gastrointestinal tract	3 gm oral amoxicillin 60 min before procedure followed by 1.5-gm dose 6 hr later	1–2 gm ampicillin plus 1.5 mg/kg gentamicin IV or IM 30 min before procedure; repeat regimen 8 hr later	Substitute 1 gm vancomycin IV for ampicillin; no following dose needed

larly, most patients with multiple major emboli should undergo valve replacement or débridement. However, in the absence of severe congestive heart failure or major embolic events, a complete course of antibiotics should be attempted before cardiac valve replacement is considered.

Other complications of infective endocarditis include arrhythmias, renal failure, mycotic aneurysms, neurologic complications, and splenic abscesses. Medical management for each of these situations should be tailored to the individual situation. For example, a patient with atrioventricular block may require transvenous pacemaker insertion for the extravalvular extension of the infection. The development of *S. aureus* pericarditis may need prompt surgical drainage or pericardiectomy. A patient with a splenic abscess will need splenectomy. The recurrence or persistence of fever, which may complicate management, may be related to intravenous administration–related phlebitis, metastatic abscess formation, drug fever, uncontrolled valvular infection, or nosocomial infections at other sites.

Prophylactic Therapy

Conclusive proof of the efficacy of chemoprophylaxis for endocarditis is lacking and the choice of an optimal prophylactic regimen is controversial. Nevertheless, the recently revised recommendations by the *Medical Letter*, British Society, and American Heart Association are basically similar. Standard prophylaxis is 2 grams of oral penicillin V 60 minutes before the procedure, with 1 gram 6 hours later (Table 2). Patients with prosthetic valves are given a combination of ampicillin and gentamicin parenterally 30 minutes before the procedure. A second dose of 1 gram of penicillin V should be given orally. Penicillin-allergic patients are given 1 gram of oral erythromycin or intravenous vancomycin. For gastrointestinal or genitourinary procedure, parenteral ampicillin and gentamicin are given 30 minutes before the procedure and a repeat dose is given 8 hours later. Vancomycin and gentamicin are used in penicillin-allergic patients. In low-risk patients, an oral regimen of amoxicillin (3 grams) is given orally 60 minutes before the procedure, followed by 1.5 grams 6 hours later. Continued antibiotic therapy beyond the second dose is unnecessary because the bacteremia is transient.

HYPERTENSION

method of
EDWARD D. FROHLICH, M.D.
Ochsner Clinic
New Orleans, Louisiana

At present, almost 60 million Americans are known to have an abnormally elevated arterial pressure. As a result of public and physician awareness most Americans have had their blood pressures taken in the past 5 years; more people are aware of their elevated pressures, and more are receiving therapy and are obtaining an effective antihypertensive treatment program. We certainly have come a long way since the first Joint National Committee Report on the Detection, Evaluation, and Treatment of High Blood Pressure was issued. In May, 1988, the fourth report was published, and its scope and message have evolved and kept pace with our increasing knowledge and improved diagnostic and therapeutic skills. Nevertheless, we have a long way still to go. While we have seen a 50 per cent decline in deaths from strokes and 35 per cent reduction in coronary deaths, the number of cardiovascular deaths still is equal to the sum of all other causes of death in this country.

Following dramatic therapeutic advances, there have been remarkable gains in the sophistication of antihypertensive medications and in our understanding of the epidemiology and pathophysiologic mechanisms of hypertension. Nevertheless, several points must still be underscored.

First, we know that the higher the systolic or diastolic pressure, the greater will be the cardiovascular mortality and morbidity rates. For example, a 35 year old man with an arterial pressure of 130/90 mm Hg, will die 4 years earlier than another 35-year-old man with the same medical background except for a "normal" pressure. If his pressure was 140/90 mm Hg, he would die 9 years earlier (all things being equal); and if it was 150/100 mm Hg he would die 17 years earlier.

Second, we must continue to be aware that effective reduction of abnormally elevated arterial pressure will significantly reverse these horrifying mortality and morbidity rates. Recent national health statistics have demonstrated this with abundant clarity. Even suboptimal antihypertensive therapy will improve these high complication rates from the hypertensive vascular disease process; it is better than no treatment at all. Thus, our initial findings attesting to the value of antihypertensive therapy were derived from studies that demonstrated the efficacy of therapy in patients with malignant hypertension and hypertensive emergencies. In the days when these patients received no treatment at all, less than 3 per cent lived for a year; these data have been dramatically reversed so that now 75 per cent or more will live for 5 years. And now we know that patients whose pressures had been elevated, but were without target organ involvement, may not ever be rated on their insurance policies if they can document effective blood pressure control over a specified number of years.

A third point concerns the finding that the effectiveness of therapy will be maintained for only as long as the patient continues to receive antihypertensive treatment. Even though antihypertensive therapy has controlled a patient's arterial pressure in the past, discontinuance of the treatment will shift the prognosis back to the position when the patient was untreated.

One final word must be added to relate these findings to patients with coronary heart disease. It still is frequently asserted that although antihypertensive therapy has been shown to reduce the developmental rates of congestive heart failure, dissecting aortic aneurysm, hypertensive encephalopathy, malignant hypertension, and hemorrhagic and thrombotic strokes, the available data from prospective studies have failed to demonstrate the efficacy of therapy in preventing heart attacks, angina pectoris, and sudden death. In my opinion, this argument only simplifies the issue. First, we know that hypertension is one of the major risk factors predicting eventual development of atherosclerotic cardiac disease and its complications. However, hypertension is only one of these factors of risk; the other treatable factors include cigarette smoking, hyperlipidemia, exogenous obesity, excessive alcohol consumption, and diabetes mellitus. Moreover, we know that the average age of the patients entering the Veterans Administration Cooperative Study (and most other multicenter studies) was about 50 years, an age at which most Americans already have developed significant atherosclerotic changes in their coronary arteries. (Autopsy findings of Americans killed in Korea and Vietnam showed that by age 18 significant coronary arterial atherosclerotic changes had taken place.) Also, in earlier years, higher doses of diuretics were employed, doses that may have been associated with hypokalemia. This could be of particular significance in patients with a symptomatic coronary disease or with left ventricular hypertrophy, predisposing such patients to the development of cardiac dysrhythmias and sudden death.

Nevertheless, clinical experience and a fundamental understanding of cardiovascular physiologic principles indicate that with effective reduction of ventricular systolic pressure (and also reduced cardiac size) myocardial tension, which is the major determinant of myocardial oxygen consumption, will be decreased proportionately. With this tension reduction, myocardial oxygen demand will diminish and improvement in functional coronary insufficiency will result.

Evaluation of the Hypertensive Patient

It is beyond the scope of this article to discuss in detail considerations for an adequate work-up of the patient with an elevated arterial pressure. Some physicians believe that because hypertension is such a significant problem today in so many patients, we must expeditiously obtain a minimal cost-effective evaluation—enough "screening" to exclude other diseases and risk factors in order to anticipate potential complications of disease and to plan antihypertensive therapy (Table 1). Others believe that the hypertensive evaluation should be more comprehensive in order to provide a complete evaluation of the patient and to permit the physician to select more specific, individualized ther-

TABLE 1. Basic Information Necessary Prior to Institution of Antihypertensive Therapy

1. At least three confirmatory pressures in the supine or sitting and standing positions, obtained on separate occasions, in order to document an elevated arterial pressure. (Obviously, if a "hypertensive emergency" exists, more rapid institution of therapy and perhaps even hospitalization are indicated.)
2. Complete history and physical examination. Most important (in addition to symptoms of cardiac, renal, and neurologic involvement) is a family history of hypertension and/or premature death. Examination should include particularly retinal fundoscopy, careful cardiac auscultation (for extra sounds and murmurs), and vascular auscultation for bruits and absent or reduced pulsations.
3. Chest x-ray and electrocardiogram. Remember, the electrocardiographic (ECG) evidence of left atrial abnormality (enlargement) can presage x-ray or ECG evidence of ventricular hypertrophy. Only in special circumstances should an echocardiogram be necessary.
4. Laboratory studies:
   a. Hemogram, including hematocrit or hemoglobin, white cell count
   b. Blood chemistries*
      i. For hypertension: Serum potassium, calcium, and creatinine and uric acid concentrations.
      ii. For other risk factors: Plasma glucose (fasting, if possible or 2-hr postprandial), lipid and lipoprotein concentrations.
5. Urinalysis

*In my opinion an automated battery of blood chemistry tests is more cost effective and provides the clinician with additional, often important, clinical information.

apy (Table 2). Tables 1 and 2 provide a rationale for the selection of studies and the vast array of diagnostic aids available. It is necessary in the basic evaluation to ascertain the extent of target organ involvement and of complications from hypertension (e.g., renal function tests, extent of proteinuria, cardiac enlargement, presence of aortic enlargement).

TREATMENT

Nonpharmacologic Therapy

Weight Reduction. Exogenous obesity may reflect itself at times in erroneous blood pressure measurements in some obese patients with hypertension. However, obesity and hypertension are frequently correlated, and a highly significant relationship exists between body weight and blood pressure levels, even in children and adolescents. Weight control not only may result in a reduction of arterial pressure in overweight (i.e., greater than 15 per cent over ideal body weight) patients with hypertension but also may make possible a reduction of dosages of antihypertensive drugs in patients receiving pharmacotherapy. Thus, weight control is recommended in all overweight hypertensive patients.

Moderation in Alcohol Intake. Excessive alcoholic intake has now been clearly related to the extent of arterial pressure elevation. It also is associated

TABLE 2. **Studies Useful in Diagnosis of Hypertension and Selection of Antihypertensive Therapy**

Test	Value
Urine culture (and sensitivity)	Urinary tract infections frequently coexist with or antedate hypertension
Serum electrolytes (including Ca^{++}, PO_4, Na, K, Cl, CO_2) and urinary (24-hr) electrolyte excretion studies	Hypercalcemic diseases (70%) coexist with hypertension, and correction of increased calcium is associated with restoration of normotension; several secondary forms (or complications) of hypertension are associated with hypokalemic alkalosis (e.g., renal arterial disease, hyperaldosteronism, and other adrenal steroidopathies); but diuretic therapy and laxative abuse and chronic diuretic use must be excluded.
Plasma renin activity	May help in selection of antihypertensive therapy as well as detect secondary forms of hypertension
Plasma (or urinary) aldosteronism	Diagnosis of hyperaldosteronism (primary or secondary to diuretic therapy or renal arterial disease)
Other hormone assays (bioassay or immunoassay)	Thyrotoxicosis, Cushing's disease or syndrome, and other adrenal steroidal diseases
Differential renal venous collections or adrenal venographic studies	For collection of blood lateralizing renal arterial stenosis or adrenal tumors producing steroids
Renal arteriography	Diagnosis of renal arterial disease, renal and adrenal (medullary and cortical) tumors
CT scan of adrenals	May define adrenal cortical and medullary tumors without need for hospitalization
Serum catecholamines	Particularly with CT scan of adrenals (and possibly with clonidine suppression), may permit or exclude diagnosis of pheochromocytoma
Blood volume studies	Define vasoconstrictor and volume-dependent hypertensions
Hemodynamic studies	Establish forms of hypertension associated with hyperkinetic circulation and cardiac functional impairment

with poor adherence to a workable antihypertensive treatment program and long-term control of hypertension and with subsequent development of so-called "refractory" hypertension. For this reason the recent Joint National Committee report recommends moderation of alcohol intake, defined as no more than 1 ounce of ethanol (i.e., 2 ounces of 100-proof whiskey, 8 ounces of wine, or 24 ounces of beer) daily.

Sodium Restriction. This, like other nonpharmacologic treatment modalities, continues to be the subject of much controversy. Nevertheless, it is clear that excessive sodium intake (i.e., greater than 70 to 100 mEq per day) plays a critical role in elevating arterial pressure at least in some patients with hypertension and in limiting the effectiveness of pharmacologic therapy in other patients. A sodium intake of no more than 70 to 100 mEq per day is a reasonable means to obviate these effects. It should be kept in mind that almost half of the daily sodium intake exists in the form of food additives and the addition of salt to processed foods.

Smoking Cessation. Nicotine raises arterial pressure transiently but is not associated with a persistently increased pressure. Nevertheless, it should be emphasized that chronic cigarette smoking increases the risk of cancer and pulmonary diseases and doubles the risk for the development of coronary heart disease and sudden death. Moreover, such individuals also have a much higher chance of developing malignant hypertension and hemorrhagic stroke. Smoking may also interfere with the antihypertensive benefits of certain forms of pharmacotherapy (e.g., propranolol).

Stress Reduction. A commonly employed general therapeutic measure is the "glib" instruction to the patient to relax and to avoid emotionally tense situations. Many physicians even prescribe antianxiety agents to help achieve this end. Although relaxation and elimination of tension-related events and activities are desirable for one's overall good health, this is hardly practical advice. Furthermore, improvement of extraneous and environmentally produced circumstances will not be associated with remission of the hypertensive vascular disease problem. It is unfortunate that the last seven letters of hyper*tension* is a word that characterizes our society. *Tension* should be considered to be related to the increased tone of the arteriolar smooth muscle that is reflected in increased vascular resistance—the hemodynamic hallmark of hypertensive disease. Studies demonstrate that anxiety-relieving measures—whether drug therapy, psychotherapy, or restructuring of life style—are not significantly associated with adequate control of arterial pressure.

Exercise. Although sensible isotonic (e.g., walking, "jogging," bicycling, swimming) exercise habits are good general health measures, to date there is no evidence that long-term regular exercise programs alone can control abnormally elevated arterial pressure. In contrast, isometric exercises (e.g., weightlifting) only adds to the increased total peripheral resistance and afterload imposed on the left ventricle.

Pharmacologic Therapy

Diuretics

This group of antihypertensive drugs has been available for over 30 years, and they continue to be a mainstay of most antihypertensive therapeutic programs. Inherent in their use are the concept and rationale for low-sodium diet therapy. Various studies demonstrated the value and efficacy of marked restriction of dietary sodium in reversing severe hypertensive disease and in enhancing the effectiveness of other antihypertensive drugs. However, these studies demonstrated that in order to be effective as the sole therapy, dietary sodium restriction must be on the order of 200 mg per day. Since this form of diet therapy is highly impractical (for reasons discussed above), we must depend upon oral diuretics to achieve this end. There are three classes of oral diuretic agents: the thiazides and their congeners, "loop" diuretics, and the potassium-retaining agents spironolactone, triamterene, and amiloride.

Thiazide Congeners. These agents, including chlorothiazide and hydrochlorothiazide, are similar in action, side effects, and dosages (Table 3). One tablet of any one agent is equivalent to another in its antihypertensive and natriuretic potency, hypokalemic potential, and frequency of side effects. This class of diuretic agents should be considered first (as opposed to the other types of diuretics) for the treatment of the patient with "uncomplicated," essential hypertension—either alone or in combination with other antihypertensive drugs. Further, inherent in understanding this generalization is the fact that the thiazide congeners produce the same degree of natriuresis and diuresis as other diuretics, *providing* that the renal excretory function of the hypertensive patient is normal. Thus, with increasing diuretic dosages (up to 500 to 1000 mg of chlorothiazide or 50 to 100 mg of hydrochlorothiazide), there will be an increasing diuretic effect; with larger doses little more in the way of sodium and water excretion will occur. In contrast, the dosage of loop diuretics may be increased progressively in patients with renal functional impairment until, eventually, adequate diuresis may be expected to be achieved.

Arterial pressure is reduced by thiazide diuretics in patients with hypertension primarily as a result of the contraction of extracellular (plasma and interstitial) fluid volume. Thus, initially after the administration of the diuretic, there is a fall in plasma volume and cardiac output associated with a reduction in total body sodium and water. Shortly thereafter, arterial pressure falls (by approximately 10 to 15 per cent), associated with further natriuresis and diuresis. In time, however, the plasma volume and cardiac output return toward pretreatment levels, and the reduced arterial pressure is then related to a reduction in total peripheral resistance. The precise mechanism for this decreased arteriolar resistance is still poorly understood.

In addition to this effect in controlling pressure,

TABLE 3. **The Diuretics**

Generic Name	Proprietary Name	Daily Dosage (mg)
Thiazides and Congeners		
Bendroflumethiazide	Metahydrin, Naturetin	2.5–5
Benzthiazide	Aquatag, Exna, Hydrex, Marazide, Proaqua	12.5–50
Chlorothiazide	Hydro-Diuril, Esidrix, Oretic	125–500
Chlorthalidone	Saluron	12.5–50
Cyclothiazide	Lozol	1–2
Hydrochlorothiazide	Aquatensen, Enduron	12.5–50
Hydroflumethiazide	Zaroxolyn	12.5–50
Indapamide	Renese	2.5–5.0
Methyclothiazide	Hydromox	2.5–5.0
Metolazone	Naqua, Metahydrin	1.25–10
Polythiazide		2–4
Quinethazone		25–100
Trichlormethiazide		1–4
Loop Diuretics		
Bumetanide	Bumex	0.5–10
Ethacrynic acid	Edecrin	50–200
Furosemide	Lasix	20–480 (or more)
Potassium-Sparing Agents		
Amiloride	Midamor	5–10
Spironolactone	Aldactone	25–100
Triamterene	Dyrenium	50–150

there is an additional hemodynamic effect that seems to be related to the volume contraction. Thus, if one were to infuse (intravenously) into a patient an amount of pressor or depressor agent, before and during diuretic therapy, he would find that with the associated volume contraction there would be an attentuated response of the pressor agent and an enhancement of the effect of the infused depressor substance. This mechanism provides, in part, one explanation for the hypotensive action of the oral diuretics (attenuation of the effects of naturally occurring circulating pressor substances in the patient) and the enhancing effect of diuretics when used in conjunction with other antihypertensive drugs (e.g., vasodilators, beta blockers, other antiadrenergic compounds, and the angiotensin-converting enzyme inhibitors). Other mechanisms to explain the antihypertensive action of diuretics are as follows: an altered transmembrane ionic potential across vascular smooth muscle; an altered responsiveness to naturally occurring neural stimuli (this may be related to the altered responsiveness to pressor substances described above); and a reduced "waterlogging" of the hypertensive arteriolar wall. It is logical to assume that no one mechanism is totally operative and that all may participate in the antihypertensive effect.

The thiazide diuretics promote natriuresis at various nephron levels: inhibition of carbonic anhydrase and of sodium reabsorption in the proximal and distal tubules. Associated with the natriuresis is a loss of potassium and chloride ion. The net result of this renal action is the production of hypokalemic alkalosis and an alkaline urine (i.e., secondary hyperaldosteronism), which may be confused with other causes of hypokalemic alkalosis (e.g., renal arterial disease, primary aldosteronism). It should be kept in mind that in the presence of an excessive sodium intake, this induced state of hyperaldosteronism will result in a further augmentation of the hypokalemic effect of the diuretic.

Because these agents increase the tubular reabsorption of urate, the plasma uric acid level will increase; if this is severe enough, *hyperuricemia* develops that may be associated with symptomatic gout. This is another reason for routinely obtaining serum uric acid levels prior to initiation of diuretic therapy; if the uric acid level is borderline or elevated, it should be rechecked intermittently to anticipate the potential problem of gout. If the hyperuricemia approaches levels of 10.0 to 11.0 mg per 100 ml or more, we may then prescribe therapy to reduce the blood level of uric acid. This can be achieved with the uricosuric agent probenecid or with the inhibitor of the enzyme xanthine oxidase allopurinol, which will prevent the formation of excessive amounts of circulating uric acid. Alternatively, other antihypertensive agents that are effective as initial therapy may be substituted for the diuretic agent.

The thiazides will also produce *hyperglycemia* of varying degrees. This, for the most part, may be explained by the diuretic's ability to inhibit the release of insulin from the beta-cell pancreatic islets. Another factor that may also participate in this "diabetogenic" propensity is the hypokalemic milieu, although this concept still remains controversial. In any event, it is my experience that overt insulin-dependent diabetes mellitus will not result in those hypertensive patients who do not already have an abnormality of carbohydrate tolerance prior to initiation of diuretic therapy. Should overt diabetes mellitus develop, this does not mean that the thiazide diuretic need be discontinued. It may be possible to control the problem with diet therapy and weight reduction alone or coincident with an oral hypoglycemic agent or, if necessary, insulin. Alternatively, as indicated above, another agent may be substituted as initial therapy.

Hypokalemia had been minimized in the earlier years of thiazide therapy, especially in the United States. In recent years we have learned that lower doses of the thiazides may result in equal control of arterial pressure and less degrees of hypokalemia. Spironolactone and amiloride may further reduce arterial pressure, but triamterene has little, if any, antihypertensive effect. Symptoms of hypokalemia (polyuria and nocturia, muscle weakness, and ectopia cardiac activity) should be corrected by adding potassium or the use of a potassium-retaining agent. If primary hyperaldosteronism is considered a feature of this problem, the diuretic should be discontinued prior to further evaluation. If the diagnosis is established, the disease should be treated more specifically. If the patient is receiving digitalis or there are other explanations for aggravating hypokalemia (e.g., chronic diarrhea), potassium levels should be corrected as indicated above. An alternative antihypertensive agent should be considered; the angiotensin-converting enzyme inhibitors should be used with extreme caution (if at all) in patients receiving potassium supplementation or potassium-retaining agents (e.g., spironolactone, triamterene, or amiloride).

Other side effects that have been related to the use of thiazide diuretics include hyperlipidemia, occasional maculopapular rashes, reduction in the circulating number of any or all of the blood-formed elements, hypercalcemia, and transient reduction in renal function as a consequence of reduced renal blood flow (this may be more persistent in patients with impaired renal function). Although it is necessary for the physician to recognize the last-mentioned side effect, its occurrence should not deter him from persistence in maintenance of antihypertensive therapy; should he "ease up" on therapy, the consequences may be even more disastrous. In this regard, one should consider therapeutic alternatives to the use of diuretics (with or without smaller doses of the natriuretic agent).

The issue of *hyperlipidemia* has engendered great controversy in recent years. Some deny this possibility; others feel that an elevated lipid level will return to pretreatment levels in time. It is my feeling that should hyperlipidemia be induced, other therapeutic options may be equally efficacious.

The thiazide diuretics, as indicated, have been found to be effective in initial treatment of selected patients with hypertension. These are patients who are more volume-dependent and with lower plasma renin activity. They may have a history of renal parenchymal infections (even if renal excretory function is normal); essential hypertension and low plasma renin activity (e.g., blacks, obese individuals); or steroid-dependent forms of hypertension (e.g., primary aldosteronism, Cushing's disease or syndrome, and perhaps oral-contraceptive associated); and they may be elderly.

Loop Diuretics. Bumetanide, ethacrynic acid, and furosemide, which are the most potent diuretic agents in clinical use today, exert their natriuretic action by inhibition of sodium transport from the ascending limb of the loop of Henle (see Table 3). As a result, more sodium is available for exchange at the distal nephron and a greater degree of potassium loss is achieved. Unlike the thiazides and their congeners, the onset of action with the loop diuretics is immediate and abrupt, with a dramatic diuresis noted not infrequently within 15 to 20 minutes. As a result, the persistence of diuresis is more evident than with the thiazides, rebound retention may be more noticeable, and there may be a greater degree of potassium loss. Hence, it is recommended that these compounds be reserved for patients who cannot take a thiazide or in whom a more prompt onset of diuretic action is desired, for patients with renal functional impairment, and when the use of an intravenous diuretic is necessary. With respect to considerations about their use in patients with renal functional impairment, it should be emphasized that, unlike the thiazides, the dose-response curve of the loop agents is linear. For example, if an effect is not achieved with a daily dosage of 40 or 80 mg of furosemide, the dosage may be increased (e.g., to 160 mg or

more) until diuresis is achieved. Indeed, some nephrologists have reported that diuresis may eventually be achieved at daily doses of 2000 mg.

In general, the loop diuretics are not recommended for the patient with uncomplicated, essential hypertension unless a significant degree of renal functional impairment exists. Another important, but occasionally overlooked, indication for the use of these diuretics may be in the hypertensive patient who already is receiving antihypertensive drug therapy, including maximum daily doses of a thiazide diuretic. This patient may develop a so-called pseudotolerance as a consequence of intravascular volume expansion secondary to thiazide therapy. This pseudotolerance may be overcome by switching to the loop-acting diuretic. The net effect of this therapeutic maneuver is to promote a more vigorous depletion of retained water.

Potassium-Sparing Agents

Spironolactone. This diuretic is discussed separately because it promotes diuresis by a distinctive mechanism—inhibition of the action of aldosterone at the distal tubule. Thus, by interfering with this sodium-for-potassium ion exchange mechanism, natriuresis and diuresis are effected and retention of the potassium ion is achieved. Since much of the obligate sodium ion transport occurs at the proximal tubule level, the order of potency of spironolactone is not as great as with the thiazide congeners. Nevertheless, spironolactone is useful, either alone or in combination with a thiazide compound. This agent has been used for treatment of patients with primary aldosteronism, and its success was no different than with the use of the thiazides; however, total body potassium was protected with the spironolactone. Hence, in patients with aldosterone excess, the major value of spironolactone is that it achieves a significant loss of sodium and water without wasting further potassium stores.

Spironolactone is also effective in secondary hyperaldosteronism or with other diuretic therapy, and it may be used in patients receiving digitalis or with cardiac failure to correct or prevent further hypokalemia that predisposes the patient to cardiac dysrhythmias. Since spironolactone resembles progesterone in its chemical configuration, side effects that may occur in male patients include gynecomastia and mastodynia. The physician should also be aware of the potential for developing hyperkalemia in patients with impaired renal function; thus, especially in patients with chronic renal diseases, supplemental potassium should be considered with great caution.

Amiloride and Triamterene. These agents act on a non–aldosterone-dependent sodium-for-potassium active transport mechanism. Therefore, their action is different from that of spironolactone. They effectively reduce arterial pressure and may also be used with a thiazide diuretic to pressure potassium. Triamterene has an amiloride-like potassium-sparing action; it also has minimal diuretic and antihypertensive properties. Like spironolactone, these agents should be used with extreme caution in patients with renal functional impairment and probably not at all in patients who are receiving angiotensin-converting enzyme inhibitors, since hyperkalemia is possible.

Beta-Adrenergic Blocking Agents

The beta blockers have been considered as alternative agents for the initial (i.e., first step) therapy of hypertension for some years. These agents inhibit the stimulation of beta-adrenergic receptor sites by those adrenergic neurohumoral agents (norepinephrine, epinephrine) that are circulating or are released from the postganglionic adrenergic nerve endings. By inhibiting beta-receptor stimulation, the effects of peripheral arteriolar (beta-mediated) dilation and of increased heart rate, myocardial contractility, and myocardial metabolism are reduced. Moreover, because beta-adrenergic receptor sites in the kidney are also inhibited, the renal renin release is inhibited. The result is a reduction of arterial pressure that is associated with a reduced cardiac output, and calculated total peripheral resistance increases. It should be kept in mind, however, that the cardiac output may be reduced by as much as 20 to 25 per cent without a proportionate reduction in organ blood flows. In fact, renal blood flow and excretory function may not be reduced at all with beta-blocking therapy. Another important feature of these agents is the lack of expansion of intravascular volume as arterial pressure is reduced.

At present, eight beta blocking agents are available for antihypertensive therapy; a ninth agent (labetalol) possesses in a single molecule both alpha- and beta-adrenergic receptor inhibiting properties (Table 4). Two agents (acebutolol and pindolol) possess cardiostimulatory (intrinsic sympathomimetic) properties; because of this, they do not reduce heart rate and cardiac output as much as the other agents and therefore have some value in patients with pre-existing bradycardia or low cardiac output syndromes. The so-called cardioselective beta$_1$ blockers (acebutolol, atenolol, metoprolol) probably exceed this property in the doses used for the treatment of hypertension and angina pectoris. Nevertheless, they

may be of value in patients with Raynaud's phenomenon and some peripheral arterial insufficiency.

Because of the foregoing physiologic and pharmacologic actions, these agents may be more effective in initial treatment of certain patients with hypertension. Patients with hyperdynamic circulatory states having faster heart rates, symptoms of cardiac awareness, palpitations related with enhanced cardiac contractility, and extrasystoles may be more responsive to beta blockers. Studies indicate that young patients may be more responsive to beta blockers than older individuals; similarly, that patients who are lean, male, and/or white are more responsive than those who are obese, female, and/or black, respectively.

Since beta-blocking therapy is effective for other clinical conditions, it may be wise to utilize this therapy for the initial treatment of hypertension. This may include patients with angina pectoris, previous history of myocardial infarction, cardiac dysrhythmias responsive to beta blockers, and patients with migraine headaches, muscle tremors, and glaucoma who already receive timolol eyedrops without having systemic side effects.

Because of its systemic inhibitors of beta-receptors, this form of initial antihypertensive therapy should not be used in patients with a history of asthma, chronic obstructive lung disease, cardiac failure, heart block of second degree or more, or severe peripheral arterial insufficiency.

If full doses of the selected beta-blocking agent do not control arterial pressure, the addition of a diuretic or even a calcium antagonist may be effective. Finally, if side effects such as fatigue, depression, hallucination, or nightmares preclude further use of the selected beta blocker, it might be worthwhile to switch to another beta-blocking drug before switching to another class of antihypertensive agents.

Adrenergic Inhibiting Compounds

With the present array of sympathetic-depressant drugs, it is possible for the clinician to dissect pharmacologically the autonomic nervous system (Table 5). The earliest available of these drugs were the ganglion-blocking drugs; later came the agents that selectively inhibit sympathetic nervous activity (in the brain or at the postganglionic neuronal terminal). Among this latter group are the neurohumoral (norepinephrine) nerve-ending depleting drugs, and the centrally acting agents that stimulate alpha receptors in the hindbrain and ultimately reduce adrenergic outflow to the cardiovascular system and kidney.

TABLE 4. **Beta-Adrenergic Receptor Blocking Drugs**

Agent	Proprietary Name	Cardioselective	Intrinsic Sympathomimetic Activity	Dose Range (mg/day)
Acebutolol	Sectral	+	+	100–800
Atenolol	Tenormin	+	−	25–200
Metoprolol	Lopressor	+	−	50–300
Nadolol	Corgard	−	−	40–300
Penbutolol*	Levatol	−	−	10–80
Pindolol	Visken	−	−	10–80
Propranolol	Inderal	−	−	40–480
Timolol	Blocadren	−	−	20–80
Labetalol†	Normodyne, Trandate	−	−	200–1200

*Not yet available in the United States.
†A single compound with both alpha and beta blocking action.

Ganglion Blockers. The ganglion-blocking agents decrease arterial pressure through reduction in autonomic outflow to the heart and vascular smooth muscle from the thoracodorsal autonomic ganglia. The result is a decrease in vascular smooth muscle tone that produces venular and arteriolar dilation. Venodilation promotes venous pooling and diminishes venous return of blood to the heart, thereby producing a greater antihypertensive effect in the upright position as a consequence of venous blood pooling in the dependent parts of the body; the arteriolar dilation results in a fall in total peripheral resistance. Inhibition of autonomic control of cardiac function results primarily in attenuation of cardiac reflexes. Thus, with upright posture, as hypotension results from reduced venous return of blood to the heart, the normally expected reflexive increase in heart rate and reflexive arteriolar vasoconstriction is not observed. Other examples of inhibited compensatory reflexes are documented by the abolition of the overshoot phase of the Valsalva maneuver, augmentation of postural hypotension and the "tilt-back" overshoot

of arterial pressure when returning to the supine position. These same hemodynamic effects may be observed after administration of postganglionic inhibitors that deplete the sympathetic nerve endings of norepinephrine; however, in this instance one does not generally encounter the additional action of inhibition of parasympathetically mediated neural function that is observed with ganglion-blocking drugs.

Although this class of autonomic depressants was the mainstay of treatment for the very severe hypertensive patient a number of years ago, they are now used almost exclusively in the intravenous form for treatment of certain severe hypertensive emergencies and for control of pressure during certain operative procedures. In this circumstance the agent (trimethaphan camsylate) is infused intravenously (1 mg per ml) to achieve the desired reduced level of arterial pressure. The hypotensive effect is immediate, and the pressure will increase promptly upon reduction (or cessation) of the infusion. Antihypertensive effectiveness is enhanced by upright posture (elevating the head of the bed) or with the concomitant use

TABLE 5. **Adrenergic Inhibiting Drugs (Exclusive of Beta-Adrenergic Blocking Agents)**

Site of Action (Class)	Generic Name	Proprietary Name	Daily Dosage (mg)
Ganglion blockers	Trimethaphan	Arfonad	1 mg/ml (IV infusion)
Postganglionic (catecholamine-depleting compounds)	Reserpine	Serpasil	0.25–0.50
	Rauwolfia serpentina	Raudixin	50–100
	Alseroxylon fraction	Rauwiloid	2–4
	Rescinnamine	Moderil	0.25–0.50
	Deserpidine	Harmonyl	0.25–0.50
	Syrosingopine	Singoserp	1–2
	Guanethidine	Ismelin	12.5–50
	Guanadrel	Hylorel	10–150
Centrally acting alpha blockers (at vascular smooth muscle, alpha receptors in brain; or by inhibition of renin release)	Methyldopa	Aldomet	200–2000
	Clonidine	Catapres	0.1–1.2
	Guanabenz	Wytensin	4–32
	Guanfacine	Tenex	1–3
Alpha-adrenergic receptor inhibitors	Phentolamine	Regitine	5–10 (IV injection)
	Phenoxybenzamine	Dibenzyline	10–40

of diuretics. With this and all other antiadrenergic and vasodilating drugs, pseudotolerance (development of fluid retention after initial control of pressure is achieved) will frequently occur unless diuretics are given simultaneously. Furthermore, the hypotensive action is enhanced by diuretics. Because the ganglion-blocking drugs also inhibit parasympathetic nerve activity, intestinal and urinary bladder smooth muscle activity is also inhibited, thereby predisposing the patient to paralytic ileus and urinary retention. These drugs are most valuable for control of pressure in certain hypertensive emergencies, during angiographic procedures, and for control of arterial pressure during certain operative procedures.

Rauwolfia Alkaloids. Included in this group are a number of agents having varying potencies and abilities to deplete neuronal tissue (brain, adrenal, and postganglionic sympathetic nerve endings) of the biogenic amines. These compounds were used with greater frequency in earlier years of antihypertensive drug therapy. When administered by injection (e.g., reserpine, 1.0 to 5.0 mg), they have been effective in treatment of hypertensive emergencies and for thyrotoxicosis. A test injection of 0.25 or 0.5 mg is wise to avoid excessive pressure reduction with greater amounts. However, more recently other agents with less bothersome side effects (e.g., obtunded sensorium) have been used for these purposes. When administered orally, these agents serve as mild antihypertensives and should be used in conjunction with diuretics and/or vasodilating drugs. The rauwolfia compounds reduce arterial pressure through a fall in total peripheral resistance, with decreased heart rate and relatively unchanged cardiac output. One of their major side effects is nasal stuffiness relating to the vasodilating action. Other side effects include postural hypotension and bradycardia, overriding parasympathetic gastrointestinal tract stimulation (increased acid production, peptic ulcerations, increased frequency of bowel movements), mental depression, and sexual dysfunction. The mental depression may be most subtle and should be considered when evaluating any patient who has been receiving these agents over a prolonged time if there is concern about behavioral changes.

Postganglionic Neuronal Depletors. Included among this class of drugs are guanethidine and guanadrel. The former compound has been available for patients with more severe hypertension for over 30 years; the latter has been used for the past several years for patients with mild hypertension. Both compounds have similar pharmacologic actions, although in the relatively lower doses used with guanadrel, its side effects appear to be less bothersome. Guanethidine has a prolonged delay in onset of action (frequently over 24 to 48 hours); but once its hypotensive action has been achieved, its action may persist for days or weeks (up to 1 month) after it has been discontinued. Both agents demonstrate hemodynamic effects similar to those of the ganglion-blocking drugs, although they do not demonstrate the additional effects of parasympathetic inhibition of neural function. There is a slight fall in vascular resistance, venodilation, with decreased venous return of blood to the heart and a consequent decrease in cardiac output, attenuated cardiovascular reflexive adjustments, and a reduced renal blood flow that may impair excretory function. This reduced renal function will adjust itself in the patient with good pretreatment renal functional reserve, and less completely in the patient with already compromised function. Additional side effects associated with sympathetic neuronal inhibition include: bradycardia, orthostatic hypotension, increased frequency of bowel movements and diarrhea (from unopposed parasympathetic function), and retrograde ejaculation.

These adrenolytic compounds are taken up by the postganglionic nerve endings, thereby inhibiting the re-uptake mechanism of norepinephrine. As a result, the nerve endings become depleted of the neurohumoral substance. This concept is important to grasp, because certain commonly used tricyclic antidepressant drugs, such as imipramine (Tofranil), desipramine (Pertofrane), amitriptyline (Elavil), and protriptyline (Vivactil), inhibit this ability of the nerve ending to incorporate guanethidine and guanadrel. Thus, the tricyclic antidepressants will antagonize the antihypertensive actions of these potent antihypertensive drugs; conversely, when the antidepressant drug is discontinued, arterial pressure may fall rather suddenly and precipitously.

Centrally Acting Postsynaptic Alpha-Adrenergic Agonists. Methyldopa has been widely used for almost 30 years. Although originally thought to reduce arterial pressure through an inhibition of the enzyme dopa decarboxylase, it was later postulated to work by false neural transmission. This action implies the conversion of the drug alpha methyldopa to the less biologically active amine alpha methylnorepinephrine, which then binds to alpha-adrenergic vascular smooth muscle receptor sites in competition with the norepinephrine. More recently, however, the major antihypertensive action has been shown to be mediated by its false neurohumoral substance, alpha methylnorepinephrine, which stimulates postsynaptic alpha receptor sites in the brain (i.e., nucleus tractus solitarii) resulting in a reduced adrenergic outflow from the brain to the cardiovascular system and kidney, resulting in decreased arterial pressure. This is achieved through a fall in arteriolar resistance and a lesser fall in venous tone than is observed with the above-described agents. Cardiac output and renal blood flow are not reduced as much and, therefore, postural hypotension is not observed as frequently as with those compounds which deplete the nerve ending of norepinephrine (e.g., guanethidine) or block the ganglion (trimethaphan).

The most common side effects include dry mouth, lethargy, easy fatigability and somnolence, and sexual dysfunction. These complaints may be attributed to methyldopa's central action and may disappear shortly after therapy is begun. Other less common side effects include Coombs' test–positive reactions (and still less frequently, hemolytic anemia), high fever after initial drug doses, and hepatotoxicity, all of which remit with cessation of therapy.

Clonidine, guanabenz, and guanfacine, although different from methyldopa, share certain pharmacologic actions with that agent. They, too, have little direct peripheral arteriolar dilating properties but reduce arterial pressure primarily through a decreased vascular resistance as a result of central stimulation of alpha postsynaptic receptor sites. In addition, as with methyldopa, the reduced adrenergic outflow from the brain also reduces renin production by the kidney.

These agents share many of the side effects of other adrenergic inhibiting compounds, including bradycardia, orthostatic hypotension, somnolence, and sexual dysfunction, which can be ascribed to their adrenolytic action. One particular additional effect of clonidine that merits attention is the possibility of a precipitous rebound of arterial pressure after abrupt withdrawal. When this does occur, the symptoms of palpitations and tachycardia can be treated with a beta-adrenergic blocking drug (e.g., propranolol). The pressor phenomenon may be counteracted by injection of an alpha-adrenergic blocking drug (e.g., phentolamine) and reinstitution of the clonidine or another adrenergic inhibitor. In recent years, clonidine has been made available as a transdermal patch medication, thereby making therapy less frequent and the rebound perhaps less likely. As with the other adrenergic inhibitors, these agents when used alone are associated with intravascular volume expansion and pseudotolerance.

Pre- and Postsynaptic (Alpha₁ and Alpha₂) Receptor Antagonists. The alpha₁ and alpha₂ receptor blocking drugs developed earlier have very limited usefulness in the treatment of most hypertensive patients; they may be used whenever an unexplained pressor episode suggests excessive release of catecholamines (e.g., phentolamine, 5 to 10 mg intravenously). They may also be used by continuous intravenous infusion in a patient with a pheochromocytoma crisis or in a patient with pressor crisis–associated clonidine withdrawal. Since pargyline hydrochloride and other monoamine oxidase inhibitors are still marketed as antihypertensive and antidepressant agents, they also may be associated with hypertensive crisis. This state may occur after ingestion of certain foodstuffs (e.g., Chianti wine, marinated foods, certain cheeses) containing tyramine; alpha-adrenergic blocking compounds are valuable in treating these pressor crisis episodes. In brief, the pressor episode occurs because the tyramine contained in the food releases stored norepinephrine from the nerve endings, and the released norepinephrine is less able to be degraded in the presence of monoamine oxidase inhibitors.

Postsynaptic (Peripheral) Alpha₁ Antagonists. There are two general classes of alpha-adrenergic receptors in the periphery. When the postsynaptic alpha₁ receptors are stimulated by the catecholamines released from the postganglionic nerve ending, the response is arteriolar and venular constriction. In contrast, when the presynaptic alpha₂ receptors are stimulated, further release of the norepinephrine from the nerve ending is inhibited. Thus, in contradistinction to the alpha₁ and alpha₂ receptor inhibiting compounds (i.e., phentolamine and phenoxybenzamine), agents that selectively block the postsynaptic alpha₁ receptors (prazosin and terazosin) do not prevent alpha₂ receptor stimulation. Hemodynamically, the alpha₁ receptor antagonists reduce arterial pressure associated with a fall in total peripheral resistance; there seems to be no associated reflex increase in heart rate, cardiac output, or myocardial contractility.

These agents may produce a rather disturbing postural hypotension, often after the first dose. As a result, treatment is frequently begun with a dose of 1 mg at bedtime, with instructions to the patient not to arise for 4 to 6 hours; symptomatic hypotension more usually would be expected 1 to 3 hours after the initial dose. With more prolonged treatment, higher doses of up to 10 to 20 mg per day may be required. In this regard, two common problems may occur with pressure control: dose titration may be associated with symptomatic orthostatic hypotension, and pseudotolerance may develop. This latter problem can be offset by the addition of a diuretic; however, this may only exacerbate the first problem. Other agents belonging to this class of drugs* include indoramin, trimazosin, doxazosin, and tiodazosin.

---

*None of these drugs has been approved for this use by the Food and Drug Administration.

Vasodilators

With the introduction of beta-adrenergic–blocking therapy there was a resurgence in interest in direct-acting smooth muscle vasodilating drugs for hypertension. These agents (e.g., hydralazine [Apresoline] and minoxidil [Loniten]) act by decreasing vascular smooth muscle tone and decreasing arteriolar resistance. With the fall in total peripheral resistance and arterial pressure, there is a reflex stimulation of the heart so that tachycardia and palpitations (from increased myocardial contractility) frequently result. For this reason, these agents should not be administered to the hypertensive patient with myocardial infarction, angina pectoris, cardiac failure, or dissecting aortic aneurysm, because these reflexive cardiac effects will aggravate the underlying cardiac conditions. Other side effects are headaches and nasal stuffiness, attributable to the local vasodilation; fluid retention and edema, even in the presence of adequate thiazide therapy, can occur (more frequently with minoxidil). An unusual side effect of hydralazine is the precipitation of a syndrome manifested by a positive lupus erythematosus (LE) test, skin rash, leukopenia, thrombocytopenia, and arthralgias. The syndrome is more apt to occur in patients receiving in excess of 400 mg (the usual daily dosage of hydralazine is 100 mg, in divided doses, although as much as 200 mg may be prescribed). A not infrequent side effect of prolonged therapy with minoxidil 2.5 to 5.0 mg two or three times a day is facial hair growth, of major concern to female patients.

Hydralazine may be administered by injection (10 to 15 mg intravenously). Its associated hemodynamic effects are the same as for the oral route. Another parenteral vasodilator, diazoxide, is a thiazide congener which is not natriuretic; on the contrary, diazoxide causes sodium retention. In order to be an effective antihypertensive, diazoxide must be injected in a rapid, single-bolus dose of 300 mg or in successive pulsed boluses of the divided dose. If injected slowly, some of the administered agent would bind with circulating albumin in the blood and thereby lose much of the hypotensive and vasodilating effectiveness. It should not be administered to the hypertensive patient with cardiac failure, angina pectoris, myocardial infarction, or an actively dissecting aortic aneurysm, for the reasons given above. Diazoxide is of extreme value in the patient with hypertensive encephalopathy, intracranial hemorrhage, and severe malignant or accelerated hypertension (without cardiac failure), in whom rapid and immediate reduction in arterial pressure is mandatory.

Sodium nitroprusside, also an injectable vasodilator, is useful in hypertensive emergencies. This agent, infused by microdrip (60 micrograms per ml), produces an immediate reduction in arterial pressure. When the infusion rate is decreased, there is a rapid return of arterial pressure to pretreatment levels. Since the agent produces venular as well as arteriolar dilation, there is less venous return to the heart and less increase in heart rate and cardiac output. Thus this compound, like trimethaphan (a ganglion-blocking drug), decreases ventricular preload as well as arterial pressure and total peripheral resistance (ventricular afterload). This drug therefore has particular pertinence in treating the severely hypertensive patient having a myocardial infarction, cardiac failure, or dissecting aneurysm. Since the nitroprusside is metabolized to thiocyanate and thiocyanate toxicity may become manifest with prolonged infusion, it is advisable to monitor blood thiocyanate levels in these severely sick and hypertensive patients.

Angiotensin-Converting Enzyme Inhibitors

This relatively new class of antihypertensive agents (Table 6) has proved to be effective as monotherapy for controlling arterial pressure in patients with mild to moderately severe hypertension as well as in patients who have severe and/or refractory hypertension. These agents reduce arterial pressure by preventing the generation of the hemodynamically active octapeptide angiotensin II from its inactive decapeptide angiotensin I. Inhibition of the angiotensin-converting enzyme (ACE) inhibits the formation of angiotensin II and the degradation of the active, naturally recurring vasodilator bradykinin. In addition, since angiotensin II interacts with the adrenergic neurohormone norepinephrine in the

TABLE 6. **Alpha$_1$-Adrenergic Receptor Inhibitors, Angiotensin-Converting Enzyme Inhibitors, and Calcium Antagonists**

	Proprietary Name	Daily Dosage (mg/kg)
Alpha-Adrenergic Receptor Inhibitors		
Prazosin	Minipress	1–20
Terazosin	Hytrin	1–20
Angiotensin-Converting Enzyme Inhibitors		
Captopril	Capoten	12.5–300
Enalapril	Vasotec	2.5–40
Lisinopril	Zestril, Prinivil	5–40
Calcium Antagonists		
Diltiazem	Cardizem	60–360
Nifedipine	Procardia, Adalat	20–180
Nitrendipine*	Baypress	5–40
Verapamil	Calan, Isoptin	120–480

*Not yet approved for use in the United States.

brain as well as at peripheral neurones, less angiotensin II may be available for that action. Several investigators have also suggested that there is an increased availability of prostacyclin as converting enzyme inhibition. Finally, recent studies have demonstrated that the entire renin-angiotensin system (in all of its components) exists in the vascular and cardiac myocytes; this might explain the effectiveness of these compounds in patients with normal (or even low) plasma renin activity. These agents reduce arterial pressure as a result of arteriolar dilation and a reduced total peripheral resistance. Heart rate and cardiac output do not reflexively increase, and renal blood flow may even increase, in association with the reduced renal vascular resistance. Glomerular filtration rate usually remains stable and the renal filtration fraction may even diminish, suggesting that the fall in glomerular hydrostatic pressure results primarily from efferent arteriolar dilation, a finding not associated with the direct-acting smooth muscle vasodilators.

Because of its effects on other intrarenal homeostatic mechanisms (e.g., prostaglandins and kinins), treatment with ACE inhibitors has been shown to exacerbate renal functional impairment and elevate arterial pressure in patients with bilateral renal arterial disease and in patients with a solitary kidney who have unilateral renal arterial disease. Moreover, these agents should not be used in conjunction with supplemental potassium therapy.

ACE inhibitors, as suggested, have been found to be effective in patients with low and normal plasma renin activity as well as in patients with renin-dependent forms of hypertension. In this regard, they are of great value in hypertensive patients with unilateral renal arterial disease and one normally functioning kidney, with congestive heart failure, or with high-renin essential hypertension. They are useful as monotherapeutic agents and their effectiveness is enhanced with the addition of a diuretic. Recent reports also suggest their effectiveness with calcium antagonists.

The ACE inhibitors have a low incidence of side effects. Initial studies with captopril suggested that neutropenia and proteinuria should be sought for during the first few months of therapy, but long-term studies suggest that these effects would be more likely to occur in patients with impaired renal function prior to therapy, or those who were receiving immunosuppressive agents. Other side effects include a rash and cough (ascribed to the inhibited degradation of the kinins), which disappear following cessation of therapy.

Because metabolic effects related to electrolytes and carbohydrate and lipid metabolism have not been reported with these agents, patients having these problems related to other antihypertensive therapy are likely beneficiaries of this class of drugs. Other problems less frequently encountered with the ACE inhibitors include sexual dysfunction and gastrointestinal side effects. As a result, an improved "quality of life" has been ascribed to these agents; and this has even been ascribed to a postulated central effect of the agents.

Calcium Antagonists

Calcium antagonists (see Table 6), the newest class of antihypertensive agents, have been available for study and clinical use for at least 25 years; however, in the United States they have been introduced for the treatment of hypertension only relatively recently. These compounds are quite heterogeneous in chemical structure, action, and indications—more so than the beta-adrenergic receptor blocking agents the actions of which are more homogeneous. Nevertheless, the calcium antagonists have a certain commonality of action: inhibition of the movement of calcium ions into cardiac and vascular smooth muscle cells, thereby inhibiting the contractility of the myocyte. As a result, arteriolar resistance is diminished, thereby decreasing the total peripheral resistance and, hence, arterial pressure.

Three calcium antagonists—verapamil, diltiazem, and nifedipine—are available in the United States; a fourth agent, nitrendipine, is marketed elsewhere and its approval by the FDA is imminent. Verapamil, in addition to its vasodilating property, has a cardiac inhibitory action to diminish conduction transmission. As a result, it has been used initially for the treatment of cardiac tachyarrhythmias. In contrast, nifedipine has an exclusive peripheral action to dilate arterioles; its cardiac effects are secondary to reflex stimulation of the heart as a result of the arterial pressure induction. Diltiazem's action is in between, having little cardioinhibitory effects although there is little reflex stimulation. All calcium antagonists reduce pressure without a consequent expansion of intravascular volume; therefore, they also may be used alone for the treatment of hypertension. Some of these compounds (primarily nifedipine) have been associated with pedal edema related to the pressure reduction. The alteration in fluid distribution is probably related to postcapillary reflex venoconstriction, an increased hydrostatic pressure that favors transcapillary migration of fluid into extravascular tissue. Indeed, fluid retention is a highly unlikely explanation for the edema; the natriuretic effect of these agents has been well documented.

In general, all four agents are similar in their antihypertensive action, which is related to a decreased total peripheral resistance. The reduction in vascular resistance seems to be distributed throughout the vasculature, with the target organs of hypertension—heart, brain, and kidney—sharing in this effect. The reduced vascular resistances in these organs may also be associated with increased organ flow. All agents appear to increase coronary blood flow, but diltiazem increases renal blood flow without increasing glomerular filtration rate. Most calcium antagonists reduce cardiac mass; however, as indicated earlier, the significance of this effect remains to be shown. The calcium antagonists are reported to be more efficacious in volume-dependent hypertensive patients with lower plasma renin activity; consequently, they have been recommended for older patients and black patients with hypertension. Other investigators stress that these agents are equally useful in young and white patients. Because there are no metabolic side effects (e.g., hypokalemia, carbohydrate intolerance, hyperlipidemia, hyperuricemia) associated with these compounds, they may be used in patients who have had these biochemical alterations with other antihypertensive agents (e.g., diuretics). Moreover, their actions have not been associated with sexual dysfunction. However, other side effects related to these drugs have been constipation (primarily with verapamil) and flushing and headaches (with the other compounds).

An Approach to Therapy

Stepped Care

Over the past 15 years, and throughout successive publications of the Joint National Committee's recommendations on the detection, evaluation, and treatment of the hypertensive patient, a very useful concept of the stepped-care approach to treatment has emerged and evolved. However, in recent years its use has become controversial because of its seeming "empiricism."

To be sure, the stepped-care approach does have some empirical attributes: clearly, it has worked. However, the rationale for this course of therapy has a true physiologic and pharmacologic basis. About a decade ago, there were only three classes of antihypertensive agents: diuretics, adrenergic inhibitors, and smooth muscle vasodilators. Without a first-step initiation of the diuretic, the hypotensive action of either of the other two classes of agents would be markedly attenuated.

Since then, three new groups of antihypertensive agents have become available. The beta blockers were included as a first-step alternative as stepped care evolved. And, now, in the most recent edition (1988) of the Joint National Committee report there are two additional classes of agents: the angiotensin-converting enzyme inhibitors and the calcium antagonists. The other two classes of agents—the centrally and peripherally adrenergic inhibitors and the direct-acting smooth muscle vasodilators still fall short of an ideal first-step agent: they are associated with pseudotolerance and reflex cardiac stimulation, and they must usually be given two or more times daily. The other groups of agents include many alternatives that can be given only once daily, as well as a few requiring twice-daily dosing.

Individualized Stepped Care. Clearly, the basis of any pharmacologic program is a sound patient education program keyed to the applicability of any (or all) of the nonpharmacologic alternatives: weight control, sodium restriction, alcohol moderation, and cessation of cigarette smoking. Selection of the first-step pharmacologic agent then depends on the following clinical criteria: (1) the patient's medical history and physical findings (which may exclude certain agents and include others); (2) demographic criteria (e.g., age, race, gender, body habitus); (3) laboratory findings, including the presence of biochemical risk factors; (4) coexisting diseases, such as coronary arterial disease, previous myocardial infarction, hyperlipidemia, diabetes mellitus, gout, and migraine headaches; (5) previous experience with other antihypertensive drugs; and (6) the mechanism of action of the classes of antihypertensive agents.

Once selection of an agent is made it should be prescribed initially in less than full doses. Then only one of two effects can occur: the drug may be completely effective and without unwanted effects or the drug may not be effective. Clearly, if the first alternative occurs then therapy is maintained. If the initial option is found to be ineffective, there are three alternatives: (1) the drug can be prescribed at full doses; (2) a second agent may be added; or (3) the initial dosage can be discontinued and an alternative first-step option prescribed (Figure 1).

In the preceding discussion of the different classes of antihypertensive agents, I have suggested likely hypertensive patient populations and clinical indications for the selection of a first-step option for each class of drugs. If a diuretic agent is not selected first, it may be added to any of the alternative agents. Beta blockers have been used with the vasodilators, but consideration should be given to the patient's cardiac status. The calcium antagonists and ACE inhibitors can be used with one another, and clearly any of the

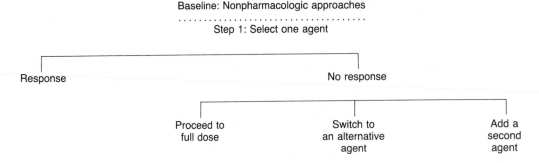

Figure 1. Individualized stepped-care approach. The agent may be chosen from a thiazide diuretic, a beta-adrenergic receptor blocking agent, an angiotensin-converting enzyme inhibitor, or a calcium antagonist.

adrenergic inhibitors (alpha blockers or centrally active) have a long track record of efficacy with the dilators. In any event, at least 1 to 3 months should be allowed before proceeding to other therapeutic options.

If necessary, a vasodilator (direct-acting smooth muscle relaxant, ACE inhibitor, calcium antagonist, or even guanethidine) can be added as a third agent, although few patients with hypertension require more than two antihypertensive drugs. Once the therapeutic goal is achieved (I usually aim for diastolic pressure less than 90 mm Hg), it is wise to consider "stepping down" in therapy. This can be achieved by reducing the dose of the least desired agent first and eventually discontinuing its use or maintaining therapy at the lowest possible dosage of the agent(s) employed.

Antihypertensive Compounds and the Surgical Patient

In general, there is little concern about the use of antihypertensive agents in the hypertensive patient who anticipates anesthesia and surgery. If the patient is receiving diuretic therapy, it is important to check the serum potassium and the

TABLE 7. **Hypertensive Emergencies**

Hypertensive encephalopathy
Hypertension and intracranial hemorrhage
Malignant (and accelerated) hypertension
Hypertensive cardiac failure
Hypertension and dissecting aortic aneurysm
Severe hypertension associated with myocardial infarction
Hypertension (systolic pressure >160–170 mm Hg) following vascular surgery and/or vessel grafting
Pheochromocytoma crisis
Hypertensive crisis during cardiovascular catheterization procedure
Clonidine-withdrawal hypertension
Foodstuff-related hypertension associated with monoamine oxidase (MAO) inhibiting drugs
Hypertension (in child) with acute glomerulonephritis
Eclampsia

electrolyte concentrations and blood sugar prior to surgery. Hypokalemia should be corrected to safe levels. Not all therapeutic agents need be discontinued prior to surgery, but the anesthesiologist should be made aware of the treatment and dosage schedule. Medications for that day may be administered with a small amount of water on the day of surgery. Both anesthesiologist and surgeon should realize that any blood loss or fluid volume contraction or intra-abdominal pressure on (or retraction of) the inferior vena cava will be associated with a greater fall in blood pressure in these patients receiving sympatholytic drugs. These patients will demonstrate a greater responsiveness to exogenously administered sympathomimetic pressor agents (e.g., norepinephrine, phenylephrine, methoxamine) than the patient not receiving sympathetic blocking drugs.

Hypertensive Emergencies

Listed in Tables 7 and 8 are specific hypertensive emergencies and the agents and dosages best suited for each problem. From the myriad of agents with varying antihypertensive actions that are presently on the market, it is wisest to choose the agent that best "fits the bill" of the disease. Inherent in the concept is the point that no one antihypertensive drug should be selected as the "first choice" for a specific hypertensive emergency. Thus in the absence of heart failure or angina pectoris, diazoxide might be the first choice for hypertensive encephalopathy because it rapidly reduces arterial pressure without the need for maintaining a continuous intravenous infusion. Further, the response of remission of nausea, vomiting, coma, and neurologic signs should occur coincident with and after the fall in arterial pressure. In contrast, if congestive heart failure, coronary arterial insufficiency, or aortic dissection is a feature of the patient's problem, the associated reflexive stimulation of the heart

TABLE 8. **Drugs Useful for Treatment of Hypertensive Emergencies**

Agent	Proprietary Name	Dosage	Prime Indication Emergencies
Parenteral Agents			
Cryptenamine	Unitensen	2 mg in 1000 ml isotonic saline infusion (IV)	Eclampsia
Diazoxide	Hyperstat	300 mg (IV), bolus	Hypertensive encephalopathy Intracranial hemorrhage Malignant hypertension
Furosemide	Lasix	40 mg (IV) or higher q 4, 6, or 8 hr (as necessary)	Hypertensive heart failure Hypertension with acute glomerulonephritis
Guanethidine or Bethanidine	Ismelin	25–50 mg (PO) initially, 1 dose daily 0.25–0.50 mg/kg (PO), q 6–8 hr (Repeat to achieve effects eventually)	Malignant (and accelerated) hypertension Oral therapy to replace IV drugs (for emergency)
Hydralazine	Apresoline	10–20 (IV or IM) q 4–6 hr	Eclampsia Malignant (and accelerated) hypertension Hypertension with glomerulonephritis
Labetalol	Normodyne, Trandate	20–80 mg IV bolus 10 min and then 2 mg/min IV infusion	Eclampsia Malignant (and accelerated) hypertension Hypertension with glomerulonephritis
Methyldopa	Aldomet	250–500 mg (IV or IM) q 6 hr	Malignant (and accelerated) hypertension Hypertension with glomerulonephritis
Nitroprusside or Trimethaphan or Nitroglycerin	Nipride or Arfonad or Tridil	50–100 mg/L IV infusion 1000 mg/L IV infusion 5–100 μg/min infusion	Hypertensive encephalopathy Hypertensive heart failure Hypertension and aortic dissection Hypertension and intracranial hemorrhage Hypertensive crisis during catheterization Malignant (and accelerated) hypertension Hypertension after vascular reconstructive surgery
Phentolamine	Regitine	5–10 mg (IV) bolus or 5–10 mg (IV), then infusion	Pheochromocytoma crisis Pressor crisis during catheterization Clonidine-withdrawal hypertension Foodstuff-related hypertension associated with monoamine oxidase (MAO) inhibiting drugs
Reserpine	Serpasil	1.0–5.0 mg (IM) q 6 hr	Malignant (and accelerated) hypertension
Orally Administered Agents			
Captopril	Capoten	12.5–25.0 mg (repeat as necessary)	Congestive heart failure; hypertensive pressor urgencies
Clonidine	Catapres	0.1–0.2 mg hourly as necessary	Clonidine withdrawal, hypertensive pressor urgencies, for diagnostic tests that suppress excessive circulating catecholamines in patients without pheochromocytoma
Minoxidil	Loniten	2.5–5.0 mg q 2–3 hr	Hypertensive pressor urgencies
Nifedipine	Procardia, Adalat	10 mg q 30 min as necessary	Hypertensive pressor urgencies

and ventricular ejection may only aggravate the primary problem.

A discussion of most of the agents listed in Table 8 may be found elsewhere in this article. The following section elaborates on these considerations, particularly as these agents concern the patient with hypertensive crisis.

Captopril. Captopril (as well as enalapril and lisinopril) is an angiotensin-converting enzyme inhibitor whose oral administration may be as-

sociated with a rather striking reduction of arterial pressure. Hypertensive emergencies or severe pressor urgencies that may be particularly worthy of ACE inhibitor therapy include congestive heart failure and unilateral renal arterial disease associated with hypertension. These agents are contraindicated if renal failure is present or if there is bilaterally occlusive renal arterial disease (or unilateral disease of a solitary kidney). The patient with hyperkalemia or who is receiving potassium or potassium-retaining agents should also not receive these drugs.

Clonidine. This orally administered centrally active alpha blocking agent has been used in hypertensive urgencies not requiring controlled intravenous medication. When given hourly in doses of 0.1 to 0.2 mg, pressure is reduced. In patients who do not have pheochromocytoma but whose circulatory catecholamine levels are elevated, clonidine will reduce these levels to the normal range. In patients with elevated circulatory cathecholamine levels, clonidine will reduce these levels to the normal range seen in individuals without pheochromocytoma.

Cryptenamine. This drug belongs to the class of compounds termed veratrum alkaloids and was one of the earliest adrenergic inhibiting agents. It reduces arterial pressure through inhibition of cardiovascular centers in the brain and modification of reflexive responses to reduction of arterial pressure. The oral form is used rather infrequently now because of the narrow therapeutic threshold between the antihypertensive dose and the dose that stimulates vomiting centers in the brain. Nevertheless, this agent has been very useful in the patient with eclampsia and convulsions, when infused intravenously (2 mg in 1000 ml isotonic saline with 0.5 per cent chlorobutanol, and adjustment of pH with sodium bicarbonate). It will not arrest labor, and its effect is dissipated rapidly without producing a hypotensive effect after delivery of the baby.

Diazoxide. This intravenous agent is a valuable antihypertensive compound when used appropriately. It belongs to the thiazide class of compounds chemically, although it does not produce diuresis. Its action is achieved by producing an immediate reduction in smooth muscle tone after its rapid administration as an intravenous bolus (300 mg, or 5 mg per kg). Slow administration will be associated with an attenuated or little effect, owing to the affinity of the drug for circulating plasma proteins. As a result of the abrupt reduction in arterial pressure, brought about through a fall in vascular resistance, there is a marked increase in cardiac rate, output, contractility, and metabolism. Hence, this drug should be used with extreme caution in congestive heart failure (even if borderline), coronary arterial insufficiency with angina pectoris or myocardial infarction, and acute aortic dissection. Other efficacious antihypertensive drugs are available for use in these circumstances (see Table 8). In the patient with hypertensive encephalopathy, intracranial hemorrhage, or severe hypertension associated with renal disease, diazoxide is most useful. Remember, as discussed above, that vasodilator-induced hypotension will be associated with sodium retention and eventual pseudotolerance. Thus, it is advisable with these cases to administer a diuretic agent. Under the circumstances of most hypertensive crises, an intravenous diuretic such as furosemide is wise.

Furosemide. An intravenous diuretic such as furosemide is definitely indicated under those circumstances when the hypertensive emergency is associated with intravascular volume expansion. These circumstances include the use of vasodilator and antiadrenergic therapy, in which pseudotolerance is a concern, and in renal failure (often associated with a congested circulation) and congestive heart failure.

Hydralazine. Although the oral form of this compound is most commonly used with a diuretic and beta blocker in patients with moderate hypertension, it is a potent antihypertensive agent for emergencies when administered by injection. After intravenous injection (10 to 20 mg), pressure will be reduced within 30 minutes to 1 hour; injection must be repeated every 6 to 8 hours. Since it acts through arteriolar dilation and reduction of vascular resistance, its hypertensive action is associated with reflexive cardiac stimulation. As a result (as with diazoxide), hydralazine should not be used alone in patients with cardiac failure, angina pectoris, myocardial infarction, and aortic dissection. Some obstetricians have found this agent of particular value in patients with toxemia of pregnancy.

Methyldopa. Like hydralazine, methyldopa may be administered by injection or by mouth. As a result, this centrally active alpha blocker is useful in hypertensive emergencies that do not demand hypotensive action within moments. Its advantage is that once its antihypertensive effect is achieved (in conjunction with a diuretic), the physician may switch over to the oral route without need for introducing another antihypertensive compound. This agent, then, may be indicated for the patient with malignant (and accelerated) hypertension and in hypertension associated with acute or chronic renal parenchymal disease.

Nifedipine. Nifedipine, like most calcium antagonists, reduces arterial pressure promptly, particularly in patients with markedly elevated arterial pressure. Most notably, many reports have indicated a prompt reduction of arterial pressure within 20 to 30 minutes of oral ingestion of a 10 or 20 mg capsule. The 10 mg dose should be used first and then repeated in approximately 30 minutes if there is a suboptimal effect. Some have suggested the sublingual administration of the capsule contents; other studies also indicate that the onset of action is just as rapid after swallowing the capsule.

Nitroglycerin. The intravenous administration of this vasodilator (0.5 to 100 micrograms per minute) is of particular value in the severely hypertensive patient with coronary arterial disease (unstable angina pectoris, acute myocardial infarction, or following coronary arterial bypass grafting). Flushing, headaches, and vomiting are frequent disturbing side effects, and methemoglobinemia may be a complication of prolonged administration of the drug.

Nitroprusside. This vasodilating agent is most useful in patients with hypertensive emergencies complicated by cardiac and aortic disease. Because the drug produces a relaxation of arteriolar *and* venular smooth muscle, the fall in pressure is associated with a reduced total peripheral resistance and little reflexive increase in cardiac output. Nitroprusside will immediately reduce pressure and remit symptoms and signs in hypertensive encephalopathy; it is also useful in severely hypertensive patients with cardiac failure, angina pectoris, or myocardial infarction. In these patients, cardiac work and performance are improved not only through a reduction in left ventricular afterload but also in preload. Further, this concept is also useful in hypertensive emergent situations associated with aortic dissection, in intracranial hemorrhage, and in situations in which there is an unexpected rise in pressure during cardiovascular catheterization or after cardiovascular reconstructive surgery (when a rise in pressure may threaten the integrity of suture sites).

Trimethaphan. Like nitroprusside, trimethaphan when infused intravenously reduces arterial pressure instantly. However, its action is not that of a vasodilator but of a ganglion-blocking agent; as such, it reduces pressures with the patient in the supine position primarily through a decreased venous return to the heart and reduced cardiac output, and less through a fall in vascular resistance. Its indications are similar to those for nitroprusside, but it may be considered first in the patient with acute aortic dissection, because its hemodynamic action is associated with less chance for increasing the shear rates of aortic flow and for reflexive increases in ventricular ejection.

Phentolamine. This compound is an alpha-adrenergic receptor blocking drug and therefore is indicated in any situation associated with excessive circulating amounts of catecholamines. These situations include a hypertensive crisis associated with pheochromocytoma; exogenously administered catecholamines; the pressor crisis associated with certain ingested foodstuffs containing tyramine (e.g., Chianti wine, marinated herring, cheeses) in patients receiving mono-

amine oxidase–inhibiting drugs (e.g., pargyline); and the sudden withdrawal of clonidine antihypertensive therapy. In addition, an acute pressor crisis may occur after injection of radiopaque contrast material in cardiovascular catheterization procedures. This has been explained by a provoked release of catecholamines from a pheochromocytoma. As such, then, the intravenous administration of 5 to 10 mg of phentolamine may be not only therapeutic but also diagnostic, and the cardiologist or radiologist so engaged would do well to keep an ampule of the alpha-blocking compound available just for such rare occasions.

Reserpine. This antihypertensive agent, although extremely valuable in years past, has been of lesser value in recent years—especially since the introduction of the aforementioned newer agents. When injected intramuscularly (1.0 to 5.0 mg), reserpine reduces arterial pressure within 30 minutes to 2 hours; repeated injection is required every 4 to 6 hours. Injection of a 0.5 mg test dose is wise to avoid an unusual but excessive response. Because many of the emergencies described may already be associated with obtunded sensorium, I feel that introduction of reserpine may only further complicate an already complicated condition.

Oral Agents for Urgencies. Not all hypertensive crises or emergencies demand immediate reduction of arterial pressure with intravenously administered drugs. Some patients, although acutely ill, may do just as well (or even better) with prompt reduction of arterial pressure with oral compounds (see Table 8). For example, in the patient with malignant (or accelerated) hypertension who has had severe pressure elevation for days prior to presentation, it may be wise to administer an oral drug such as nifedipine, captopril, guanethidine, minoxidil, or clonidine—and then observe for the fall in pressure over the ensuing hours or days.

ACUTE MYOCARDIAL INFARCTION

method of
PIRZADA A. MAJID, M.B.B.S., Ph.D.
Baylor College of Medicine
Houston, Texas

In the United States, fewer people are dying of coronary artery disease compared to two decades ago. Despite this welcome trend, ischemic heart disease remains at the forefront of causes of death, accounting for approximately one third of all deaths of the middle-aged and the elderly. Over one million Americans succumb to acute myocardial infarction each year, and half of them die before reaching the hospital.

Extensive laboratory and clinical studies over the past 20 years have contributed largely to our present concepts of treatment of acute myocardial infarction (AMI). A wait-and-see attitude has given way to a number of aggressive interventional strategies at various stages during the clinical course of patients with AMI that have resulted in a steady decline in the mortality rates. The salient features of modern management include (1) a vigorous treatment of early malignant arrhythmias and hemodynamic disturbances; (2) an active effort to restore patency of obstructed coronary arteries with the help of thrombolytic agents in order to limit the size of infarction; (3) maintenance of patency of infarct-related vessels with use of percutaneous transluminal coronary angioplasty (PTCA) or coronary artery bypass grafts (CABG); (4) use of potent pharmacologic agents (nitrates, beta-adrenergic blockers, slow calcium channel blockers) and mechanical assistance devices (intra-aortic balloon pump [IABP]) to maintain a balance between myocaroxygen supply and demand in the acute phase; (5) recognition of differences in the clinical course and prognosis of patients with Q wave and non–Q wave infarction; (6) frequent utilization of CABG as a complete revascularization procedure in patients with multiple vessel disease who exhibit symptoms and signs of recurrent ischemia; (7) identification of risk factors for reinfarction, angina, and death during the convalescent phase of AMI and application of appropriate treatment, medical or surgical, for patients showing signs of ischemia (spontaneous or provocable), ventricular arrhythmias, and left ventricular dysfunction; (8) modification of risk factors for development of atherosclerosis and progression of coronary artery disease (smoking, hypertension, hyperlipidemia, obesity, glucose intolerance); (9) development of newer diagnostic and therapeutic modalities for patients with very poor prognosis, such as electrophysiologic testing with programmed ventricular stimulation, electrical ablation or surgical removal of arrhythmogenic foci, and introduction of new generation antitachycardia pacemakers and automatic internal defibrillators.

Approximately 30 to 50 per cent of deaths after an AMI occur within 1 hour of onset of symptoms, and most are due to ventricular fibrillation. The high incidence of sudden death within minutes of an acute ischemic event has put a spotlight on educating the public to recognize the symptoms promptly. Increased awareness of the nature of symptoms on the part of the patient hastens delivery of thrombolytic therapy and treatment to correct arrhythmias and hemodynamic disturbances, allowing improvement of myocardial oxygenation surrounding the area of infarction. Expeditious treatment reduces the incidence of cardiogenic shock and improves survival.

Early hospitalization of patients also permits prompt initiation of continuous monitoring and care for the first 48 to 72 hours in the coronary care unit setting. The value of coronary care units in the management of patients with AMI has been fully established. A unit staffed by highly trained nurses with the authority to administer treatment and prophylaxis of arrhythmias and to use defibrillation equipment has reduced the mortality from approximately 30 per cent to less than 15 per cent. Very few deaths result from in-hospital arrhythmias, and these are usually associated with severely compromised left ventricular function secondary to large infarctions. A trend toward increased survival is also due to emphasis on invasive monitoring to detect and treat the hemodynamic abnormalities caused by right ventricular infarction, acute mitral insufficiency, ventricular septal rupture, acute left ventricular failure due to loss of muscle or compliance, cardiogenic shock, and so forth, using such treatment modalities as volume expansion, afterload reduction, inotropic therapy, and IABP. Invasive monitoring also helps in selecting patients for angiographic studies with a view to early revascularization by PTCA or CABG.

The arrival of patients in the hospital within the first few hours of onset of symptoms is critical. Development of a thrombus as a final event occupies prime place in the pathogenesis of AMI; over 90 per cent of patients with transmural infarction and perhaps a similar number with other acute ischemic syndromes have a thrombus obstructing the infarct-related artery. Since the ultimate size of the infarction is directly related to the duration of ischemia, restoration of patency of the infarct-related vessel, whether mechanically or by pharmacologic means, becomes a matter of urgency. Thrombolytic therapy is becoming an integral part of the management of patients with AMI. Thrombolytic therapy administered within 6 hours of the onset of pain reopens the infarct-related vessel in 60 to 80 per cent of cases, improves left ventricular function and, by implication, reduces myocardial infarction size. Hospital mortality is also reduced.

The infarct size is a primary determinant of morbidity and mortality after myocardial infarction. Patients exhibiting signs of significant left ventricular impairment or cardiogenic shock have larger infarcts than those with uncomplicated infarctions. Data derived from animal experiments and clinical studies are consistent with the concept that AMI is a dynamic process and that measures designed to aid in the survival of ischemic yet viable myocardium may provide sufficient time for the development of physical and anatomic compensatory mechanisms that limit the ultimate size of infarction. The principles of treatment of AMI thus depend upon maintaining a balance between myocardial oxygen supply and demand so that jeopardized myocardium is allowed to survive. Besides abrupt cessation of antegrade flow due to occlusion of infarct-related artery, the early limitation to perfusion is compounded by a number of other factors including coronary arterial spasm, local release of catecholamines from ischemic tissue, and the accumulation of metabolites. Treatment required to limit the size of infarction consists, in the first place, of prompt partial or complete restoration of blood flow to the peri-infarction zone. Use of thrombolytic therapy in this respect has already been alluded to. Oxygen supply can be further augmented by relief of coronary arterial spasm and improvement of hemodynamics (increase coronary perfusion pressure, reduce left ventricular filling pressure). Nitrates, calcium channel blockers, and IABP help in achieving this goal. Equal attention is focused on reducing the oxygen demands of the myocardium. Approximately two thirds of patients sustaining AMI have multivessel coronary artery disease. It is not unusual for patients to demonstrate signs of ischemia in territory remote from that of the infarction. If the infarct-related coronary artery had been perfusing the noninfarcted myocardium through collateral vessels, sudden disruption of flow due to occlusion by thrombus would compromise perfusion of the unaffected myocardium. Moreover, the area of myocardium perfused by the occluded coronary artery loses its pumping ability. In order to maintain forward output, the noninfarcted myocardium compensates by increasing contractility. However, its demands for oxygen easily outstrip the supply available from the diseased coronary arteries. Measures designed to reduce myocardial oxygen demands include bed rest, effective treatment of pain, sedation to relieve anxiety, rapid correction of brady- or tachyarrhythmias, and judicious use of beta-adrenergic blockers.

Traditionally, the classification of AMI has been based on the location of the infarct, namely anterior (anterolateral) and inferior (inferoposterior or inferolateral). Anterior infarction is associated with a larger volume of cell death, more left ventricular impairment, and higher mortality than inferior infarction. While this is generally true, it is important to point out that approximately 60 per cent of patients with acute inferior infarction show significant disease of the left anterior descending artery angiographically and thus may be at high risk for future cardiac events. Acute myocardial infarction has also been classified as transmural (electrocardiographically showing Q waves with ST segment elevation) and nontransmural or subendocardial (electrocardiographically showing no Q waves and only ST and T wave changes). However, pathologic studies have demonstrated that necrosis may extend across the entire width of the ventricular wall in patients presenting with subendocardial infarction. Furthermore, many patients with subendocardial infarction have ST segment elevation (25 to 30 per cent) on the electrocardiogram. It has been, therefore, proposed to redefine the two by presence or absence of Q waves on the electrocardiogram. Based on the latter classification, a number of studies have determined that non–Q wave infarction is associated with less myocardial injury and a lower in-hospital mortality than Q wave infarction. However, patients with non–Q wave infarction are prone to reinfarction that repeatedly occurs in the area of the original injury. Extensive damage from recurrent infarction is reflected in a mortality rate that approaches that of the Q wave infarction in the long term. These observations have put emphasis on careful monitoring of all patients with non–Q wave infarction for longer periods of up to 2 weeks with regular creatine kinase MB (CKMB) determinations, noninvasive and invasive assessment of myocardium at risk, and, finally, aggressive medical management and possibly early surgical intervention. There are indications that with increasing use of thrombolytic therapy and rapid restoration of coronary flow, we may see more patients with non–Q wave infarction with an attendant unstable clinical course.

An acute heart attack has catastrophic physical, psychological, and emotional impact on patients, who are usually in the prime of their economic life and who, up to time of admission, had probably been leading the type of lifestyle conducive to impending trouble. Their first confrontation with the reality begins in the high-tech environs of a coronary care unit. Although coronary care units are designed primarily to serve medical needs, a concept of total cardiac rehabilitation has evolved over the years that begins with the premise that the majority of patients with AMI are ultimately going to recover and lead normal lives. The attending physician plays a central role in this process by supervising the medical management as well as providing psychological support and reassurance to the patients and their families. A frank discussion of the nature and severity of the illness, together with the implications for future recovery, provides the framework on which to build the confidence and expectations of the patient. Considerable help in this objective is extended by the nursing staff in the coronary care unit, which has increasingly taken over the mantle of "friend, philosopher, and guide" for the patient. In addition, services of diverse paramedical personnel (psychologists, physiotherapists, occupational therapists, social workers) are sought to reinforce the groundwork laid by the medical and nursing staffs. The overall goal is to provide the patient and the family with a clear understanding of the physical, social, and occupational consequences of the illness and prepare him or her for a fresh start on discharge from the hospital.

In addition to overall psychological and emotional support, cardiac rehabilitation encompasses many other factors. Early assessment of risk factors that may have contributed to the heart attack (smoking, uncontrolled hypertension, hyperlipidemias, obesity, stressful lifestyle) and also those risk factors that have implications for future cardiac events, such as angina, reinfarction, and death, is essential. Ventricular arrhythmias 3 to 6 weeks after acute infarction, left ventricular dysfunction, and ischemia (provocable or spontaneous) are independent predictors of future cardiac events: angina, reinfarction, and death within the first 12 months after acute myocardial infarction. Patients are classified into high-risk, intermediate-risk, and low-risk categories, depending on the presence of one or more of these risk factors. The mortality of patients with all three risk factors is between 30 and 50 per cent during the first year after AMI and only 1 to 2 per cent in patients without any risk factors. Exercise testing, with or without thallium-201 scintigraphy, echocardiography, rest and exercise radionuclide ventriculography, and ambulatory cardiography are carried out to identify those patients who are at high risk. Coronary angiography is undertaken before discharge in patients at high risk. Advice concerning modification of risk factors is given, encouraging the patient to actively participate in controlling his or her own disease. These include cessation of smoking, dietary changes, weight loss, compliance with drug therapy for hypertension, and learning ways to cope with stress.

An in-hospital exercise program should begin on day

1 of admission, preferably supervised by a qualified physiotherapist. Graded exercise is an essential component of rehabilitation. Regular exercise allows early return of a sense of well-being and a number of beneficial systemic effects, which include a reduction in heart rate, blood pressure, peripheral resistance, and lactate production at any given workload. There are also increases in exercise capacity, endurance, and maximum oxygen uptake. However, the patient should be informed about a lack of evidence that exercise prevents future heart attacks or death. Regular follow-up of the patient during the first year after myocardial infarction when morbidity and mortality are directly related to the acute event is necessary.

Advice concerning returning to work, resuming sexual activity, and driving motor vehicles should be given. The majority of patients with uncomplicated AMI should be able to return to their original occupations in 6 to 8 weeks after discharge. The decision to return to work should take into account the physical and emotional stress associated with the job and the degree of physical incapacity at that stage. Objective information may be obtained by maximal exercise stress testing.

CONVENTIONAL THERAPY

Prehospital Care

Systems of prehospital care are of utmost importance in the management of AMI if any impression is to be made on the high mortality rate (usually due to ventricular fibrillation or tachycardia) within the first hour of onset of symptoms. Studies have shown that bystander-initiated resuscitation results in a doubling of the survival rate compared with no resuscitation effort. Of the patients resuscitated, 40 to 50 per cent leave the hospital. With confirmation of the safety and tolerance of recently introduced thrombolytic agents, such as tissue plasminogen activator (rt-PA), this therapy may be given in the ambulance or even at the patient's home.

The following steps should be taken in all patients who are suspected of having or proved to have AMI, irrespective of whether they are seen at home, in the ambulance, in the emergency room, or in the coronary care unit.

1. The patient should be made comfortable with the head end of the bed raised to prevent gravity-induced pulmonary congestion.

2. Administer 100 per cent oxygen at a rate of 2 to 4 liters per minute by mask or nasal prongs. Hypoxemia in patients with AMI is common and usually secondary to ventilation-perfusion abnormalities resulting from incipient left ventricular failure. Increased oxygen in the inspired air protects ischemic myocardium. Oxygen is commonly continued for 24 to 48 hours in all patients. It should be pointed out, however, that additional oxygen does not increase oxygen delivery to tissues in patients who are not hypoxemic. Oxygen-enriched inspired air may also increase systemic vascular resistance and arterial pressure and thus increase left ventricular afterload. It is recommended that continuation of oxygen therapy should be constantly reviewed with serial arterial blood gas estimations. In patients with pulmonary edema and cardiogenic shock, endotracheal intubation and controlled ventilation at positive pressure may be necessary.

3. An intravenous line should be established as soon as possible, using an 18- to 21-gauge plastic cannula. If thrombolytic therapy is planned, at least two intravenous lines should be established. Blood samples should be drawn for laboratory investigations, which should include a complete blood count, blood urea nitrogen, creatinine, glucose, electrolytes, and cardiac enzyme tests. Intravascular access is maintained with 5 per cent dextrose at the rate of 10 ml per hour or by a heparin lock.

4. The patient should be connected to a battery-operated electrocardiographic oscilloscope, allowing continuous display of heart rhythm. A 12-lead-electrocardiogram (ECG) should be obtained at the same time.

5. For relief of pain, morphine should be administered intravenously in a dose of 4 to 8 mg at intervals of 5 to 15 minutes until the pain is relieved. Alternative agents may be used if there is a well documented history of morphine hypersensitivity. The alleviation of pain and reduction of anxiety resulting from morphine diminish the patient's restlessness and the activity of the autonomic nervous system as well as myocardial oxygen needs. Judicious administration of morphine is usually uncomplicated; however, hypotension, respiratory depression, and nausea and vomiting may ensue if the patient requires large doses to achieve analgesia. Hypotension can be minimized by maintaining the patient in the supine position. When hypotension and bradycardia are present together as an indication of the excessive vagomimetic effect of morphine, atropine 0.5 to 1 mg intravenously may be useful. Impairment of ventilation can be treated with naloxone (Narcan) in doses of 0.4 mg intravenously at 5-minute intervals to a maximum of 1.2 mg. Nausea and vomiting may be troublesome side effects and should be treated with a phenothiazine derivative. Nalbuphine (Nubain), a narcotic analgesic agent similar in its action to morphine, may be used if large doses are required to achieve satisfactory relief of pain. Nalbuphine is given in a dose of 5 mg intravenously and repeated at 3- to 5-minute intervals until an adequate response is obtained. The respiratory depression induced by nalbuphine is similar to

morphine at lower doses; however, with increasing dosage, the agonist action of nalbuphine stimulates respiratory drive. Doses up to 50 mg intravenously have been used with impunity. Meperidine (Demerol) is another narcotic analgesic agent similar in its action to but less effective than morphine. It has the advantage of producing fewer vagotonic effects and thus has been recommended for use in patients with inferior wall myocardial infarction. It may be given in a dose of 25 to 50 mg intravenously, and the dose may be repeated at 5- to 15-minute intervals until satisfactory relief of pain is obtained. A rebreathing mask with 20 to 50 per cent nitrous oxide in combination with 50 to 80 per cent oxygen can be used to supplement the analgesic effect of morphine or a related group of drugs in patients with recurrent episodes of prolonged pain. The nitrous oxide–oxygen mixture may provide effective analgesia in patients with milder episodes of pain, obviating the need for morphine. Nitrous oxide inhalation should not be continued for more than 12 to 24 hours. Bone marrow depression has been observed in patients inhaling nitrous oxide for more than 48 hours. There is no effect on left ventricular function, and concomitant oxygen inhalation may be beneficial, since an increase in arterial oxygen tension has been observed in patients with acute myocardial infarction.

6. A posteroanterior chest x-ray film should be obtained as soon as possible. Radiologic signs of early left ventricular failure often precede the clinical signs in patients with acute myocardial infarction. A good chest x-ray film also helps in the diagnosis of a dissecting aneurysm if it is suspected as a cause of chest pain.

7. Blood pressure and respiratory rate should be measured at least every 15 minutes for the first 8 to 10 hours, and further frequent measurements are dictated by the clinical course of the patient.

8. At the time of presentation, many patients may be taking medications for heart disease. Beta blockers should be continued in the same dosage as prior to the admission, unless contraindications exist such as heart failure, conduction abnormalities, or severe bradycardia. Calcium channel blockers and nitrates should also be continued. Digoxin should be discontinued in most patients unless there is evidence of congestive heart failure or atrial fibrillation. Digoxin should be discontinued temporarily if the serum potassium level is low or if there is evidence of atrioventricular block. Antiarrhythmic agents such as quinidine, procainamide, or disopyramide, used for suppression of premature ventricular beats, may be continued with the knowledge that all these agents have negative inotropic properties. Amiodarone, if used for treatment of malignant ventricular arrhythmias, should also be continued. The decision about any other agents should be made on a drug-to-drug basis. Generally, agents that promote salt and water retention such as nonsteroidal anti-inflammatory agents may be discontinued temporarily.

9. Ventricular ectopic beats (VPBs) occur in 90 per cent of all patients within the first hour of infarction. If VPBs are seen frequently (more than 5 per minute) in multiform configuration or closely coupled to a previous normal beat, lidocaine should be administered intravenously, starting with a bolus of 75 to 100 mg followed by an intravenous infusion of 2 mg per minute. Evidence of parasympathetic overactivity (bradycardia with or without hypotension) is seen in almost half of the patients. Atropine in aliquots of 0.5 or 0.6 mg is given slowly intravenously every 3 to 10 minutes to increase the heart rate to approximately 60 beats per minute if bradycardia is associated with hypotension.

10. If there is electrocardiographic evidence of acute subepicardial injury (ST segment elevation in more than two anterior or inferior leads of the ECG) and if the hospital offers facilities for intracoronary administration of thrombolytic therapy, the catheterization laboratory should be notified. If intravenous thrombolytic therapy is planned, the coronary care unit staff should be notified of the patient's admission as soon as possible.

In-Hospital Care

In the absence of complications, the coronary care unit stay for patients with acute myocardial infarction is usually limited to 24 to 48 hours. Patients need not be confined to bed for more than 24 to 36 hours; they may use a bedside commode from the time of admission, and they may be allowed to sit in a chair for short periods on the second and third day. The physiotherapy department is notified, and an exercise program is started with the help of qualified physiotherapists. Other general measures should be taken.

1. A liquid diet should be given for the first 24 hours because of the possibility of nausea and vomiting or cardiac arrest early after infarction and the need to reduce the risk of aspiration. From the second day, patients should be allowed a 1200- to 1500-calorie soft diet with no added salt, divided into multiple small feedings for several days. Patients who are obese should be started on a 1000 calorie diet. At the end of the first week, the patient should have a regular diet that is low in cholesterol and saturated fats.

2. A stool softener to prevent constipation and straining is given.

3. A mild sedative, diazepam, 2 to 5 mg orally four times a day, or lorazepam, 2 to 3 mg two to three times a day, to allay anxiety and a sleep medication such as flurazepam, 15 to 30 mg, or an equivalent narcotic are used.

4. Aspirin or acetaminophen (Tylenol, Panadol), given 0.5 to 1 gram every 6 hours, is used to maintain normal body temperature in patients with high fever. AMI is frequently accompanied by fever during the first few days of hospitalization and is presumably secondary to myocardial necrosis and inflammation. Appropriate investigations should be undertaken to exclude infection of respiratory or urinary tract. Hyperpyrexia causes increases in heart rate and cardiac output that may be deleterious by increasing myocardial oxygen consumption.

5. Heparin, 5000 units, is administered subcutaneously every 8 to 12 hours in the absence of specific contraindications. Subcutaneous heparin should be discontinued as soon as the patient is transferred out of the coronary care unit and resumes physical activity. Low-dose heparin substantially lowers the incidence of deep vein thrombosis without affecting the partial thromboplastin time. Its action is due to activation of factor X. Full-dose anticoagulation is not needed routinely. However, full-dose heparinization (intravenous administration of a bolus of 10,000 units followed by continuous infusion of 800 to 1000 units per hour) sufficient to raise the partial thromboplastin time to 1.5 to 2.5 times normal is indicated in patients who have undergone thrombolytic therapy, in patients developing large ventricular aneurysms with echocardiographically documented intramural thrombus, in patients with a present or past history of thrombophlebitis or arterial or pulmonary embolism, and in patients with extensive anterior wall infarction with cardiogenic shock. Oral anticoagulants are started immediately, and heparinization is discontinued once prothrombin time is prolonged to adequate levels (16 to 19 seconds). The duration of oral anticoagulant therapy is dictated by the clinical course of the patient.

6. Beta blockers reduce mortality after myocardial infarction. The effects on sudden cardiac death are more pronounced. The mechanisms by which they produce these effects are not clear at present. Some authorities recommend using these drugs only in patients who are at high risk for future cardiac events. However, most studies have shown benefit in patients in all risk groups who can tolerate beta blockers. The reduction in cardiac morbidity or mortality is probably related to beta-adrenergic receptor antagonism and is not due to a specific action of individual drugs that have been used in large studies (such as timolol, propranolol, metoprolol, and atenolol). However, beta blockers with intrinsic sympathetic activity such as oxprenolol (Trasicor*) and pindolol (Visken) have failed to show a long-term benefit after infarction. Approximately 25 per cent of patients will not be able to take beta blockers because of the following contraindications: congestive heart failure secondary to left ventricular dysfunction, obstructive airways disease, sick sinus syndrome, conduction abnormalities, reactive airways disease, severe intermittent claudication, insulin-dependent diabetes with recurrent attacks of hypoglycemia, severe fatigue, or symptomatic bradycardia. Patients with compensated and well controlled heart failure with ejection fractions between 25 and 35 per cent may be considered for the therapy. In the absence of contraindications, beta-blocker therapy should be started soon after the patient's clinical condition is stabilized (see Table 5). This is usually 3 to 4 days after admission. Present evidence does not favor earlier initiation of therapy. The therapy should be continued for at least 2 years after acute myocardial infarction.

Although beta blockers are of proven value in patients with Q wave infarction, their effectiveness in non–Q wave infarction is less certain. Only one study has demonstrated a reduction in mortality in patients with non–Q wave infarction. As pointed out previously, the early course of non–Q wave infarction is characterized by a benign course associated with relatively small infarct size. Because these patients have an increased incidence of reinfarction as well as a higher frequency of complex ventricular arrhythmias, the long-term mortality is almost certainly due to cumulative myocardial damage due to recurrent episodes of infarction. A calcium channel blocker, diltiazem (Cardizem), has been shown to significantly reduce the incidence of reinfarction during the hospital stay when compared to a placebo. Diltiazem is recommended in a dose of 60 to 90 mg four times daily soon after non–Q wave infarction is diagnosed (see Table 6).

7. In an effort to further decrease the incidence of future cardiac events, several studies have been performed using drugs that inhibit platelet function. Pooled results of several large studies on aspirin suggest a significant benefit in decreasing mortality and reinfarction within the first month. In view of the relative safety of aspirin therapy at a dose of 325 mg or less daily, the drug should be started within the first 24 hours

---

*Investigational agent.

of acute myocardial infarction and continued on a long-term basis.

Following discharge from the coronary care unit, which is usually 2 to 3 days in cases of uncomplicated myocardial infarction, the in-hospital exercise program is continued under supervision of a physiotherapist. During progressive mobilization, special attention is given to the development of shortness of breath, chest pain, or palpitations. The time of discharge from the hospital may be variable, but is usually 10 to 14 days following infarction, at a time when patients are fully ambulatory. Prior to discharge from the hospital, the patients should undergo a submaximal treadmill exercise test to a heart rate of approximately 120 beats per minute. The purpose of this test is (1) to assess patient's exercise tolerance and to provide a future exercise regimen; (2) to detect signs of ischemia, arrhythmia, or hypotension; and (3) to show to the patient how far he or she can go without untoward effects. If there is subjective and objective evidence of myocardial ischemia, early cardiac catheterization is recommended, followed possibly by PTCA or CABG. The patient should also undergo monitoring by 24-hour ambulatory ECG to detect the presence of any arrhythmias. An echocardiogram or a radionuclide ventriculogram at rest and during exercise is carried out to assess left ventricular function.

Patients should also receive detailed instructions concerning physical activity. Frequently, they are asked to come back to the hospital once or twice a week to participate in group exercise sessions under supervision of the physiotherapist. They should be advised to avoid any isometric activity such as lifting and have several rest periods during the day. They should be given nitroglycerin tablets for use if they develop angina at home. Patients should be followed for 4 to 6 weeks after discharge, at which time a maximal exercise test should be carried out. If the test turns out to be positive for myocardial ischemia, cardiac catheterization is recommended to delineate coronary artery disease. If the results are normal, the medically supervised formal rehabilitation program is continued. Sexual activity can be resumed 3 to 4 weeks after acute myocardial infarction if the discharge exercise test and the 6-week exercise test results are negative. The peak heart rate obtained by men during sexual intercourse is in the range of 110 to 120 beats per minute. The principal indications for formalized exercise rehabilitation programs are the reduction of symptoms and the feeling of self-confidence gained by the patient. No significant differences have been demonstrated in the incidence of reinfarction or overall mortality during 2-year follow-up, nor is there objective evidence that myocardial perfusion or contractility is modified favorably by exercise. In the absence of complications, the patient should be followed at 3-month intervals for the first year.

Advice to discontinue smoking should be given repeatedly, particularly to younger patients. At 6 weeks after infarction the lipid profile of the patient should be obtained, and dietary modifications should be made if necessary. The patient should be encouraged to eat a balanced diet that is low in cholesterol and fats. Overweight patients should be referred to dietitians for prescription of a low-calorie balanced diet. Alcohol is allowed in moderation, mainly because of its sedative effect and its ability to mildly elevate the HDL cholesterol level. Most patients under the age of 65 are advised to return to work between 6 and 8 weeks after discharge. The return to work depends upon the patient's vocation and financial resources. Return to work is earlier in sedentary occupations as compared to work involving strenuous physical exertion. The physical and emotional stress associated with the job should be fully assessed.

AGGRESSIVE THERAPY

Many centers now offer a number of aggressive therapies (thrombolytic therapy, PTCA, and CABG) designed to restore patency of infarct-related vessels and reperfuse the area of infarction, on the assumption that such maneuvers will limit the eventual amount of irreversible injury, preserve left ventricular function, and, possibly, improve survival. Indeed, large randomized studies comparing the use of intravenous streptokinase with a placebo have shown that there is improvement in left ventricular function and survival after thrombolytic therapy. Although not proved helpful by randomized studies, it is anticipated that PTCA or CABG will be routinely employed after thrombolytic therapy. After successful thrombolysis, a residual high-grade obstruction often persists at the site of previous occlusion and is usually responsible for continued ischemia and re-occlusion of the vessel. In this situation, PTCA or CABG is indicated if the patient shows signs of either spontaneous or provocable ischemia. It is universally agreed that the success of therapy is severely restricted by a time window that usually is not much longer than 3 hours after the onset of symptoms. In other words, the majority of patients with acute myocardial infarction must receive treatment quite early to gain maximum benefit.

Thrombolytic Therapy

Several thrombolytic agents are available, and these can be administered by intracoronary or intravenous routes. Streptokinase or urokinase, administered directly into the infarct-related coronary artery, causes reperfusion 60 to 80 per cent of the time. Intravenous streptokinase or urokinase restores patency of the infarct-related artery in approximately 35 to 65 per cent of patients. Successful reperfusion is associated with rapid relief of pain; decrease in or abolition of ST segment elevation on the electrocardiogram; frequent appearance of ventricular arrhythmias within 30 to 60 minutes after the start of the infusion (late coupled ventricular premature beats or accelerated ventricular rhythm); a rapid increase in the concentration of creatine phosphokinase (CPK) and creatine kinase MB enzymes, with the peak values reached in less than 12 hours associated with an equally accelerated fall; improved uptake of thallium-201 by infarcted myocardium in the equilibrium phase; and improvement in the regional wall motion and the global ejection fraction, which is best demonstrated at 7 to 10 days after the acute event. Successful reperfusion also commonly results in substantial hemodynamic improvement in patients with heart failure or cardiogenic shock.

Intracoronary administration of streptokinase carries the advantage of delivering a small dose of the drug at the target thrombus, implying fewer hemorrhagic complications. In addition, establishment of reperfusion under direct vision, evaluation of residual stenosis, and delineation of coronary anatomy aid in planning a more rational management of the patient. However, there are a number of drawbacks to intracoronary administration of streptokinase. For the therapy to be successful, patients must present within 1 to 2 hours of the onset of pain. Under most favorable circumstances, it requires a minimum of 100 minutes to mobilize a skilled catheterization team and a catheterization-angiographic laboratory to carry out the procedure. This means that the team must be available 24 hours a day, 7 days a week. Despite considerable media attention, fewer than half the patients with acute myocardial infarction present within 1 to 2 hours after the onset of symptoms. At present, fewer than 15 per cent of hospitals within the health care system can offer facilities for catheterization. Even in hospitals that offer their patients intracoronary thrombolytic therapy, logistic difficulties frequently prevent optimal delivery of the therapy. The cost of developing facilities to offer therapy to most patients is so prohibitive that intracoronary thrombolytic therapy presently remains limited to only a small number of patients.

Intravenous administration of thrombolytic agents (large doses of streptokinase or urokinase) overcomes some of the problems associated with the intracoronary route. The treatment can be started much earlier, for example in the ambulance or in the emergency room, saving considerable time in a situation when timing is critical. Perhaps the most significant advantage is that a catheterization team and laboratory are not required, making the treatment suitable for use in most medical care facilities. Intravenous administration also avoids a small risk associated with an invasive procedure and, of course, is much cheaper. The intravenous route offers these advantages at a cost of slightly lower efficacy and, perhaps, greater risk of hemorrhage from the larger dose of streptokinase or urokinase employed in comparison to the smaller doses required for intracoronary administration.

Tissue plasminogen activator (t-PA), a serine protease manufactured largely by recombinant technique (rt-PA), and two other drugs, acyl derivatives or equimolar streptokinase plasminogen complex and prourokinase, may be capable of successful thrombolysis without inducing a severe systemic lytic state. These drugs are under active clinical investigation at present. When administered intravenously to patients with acute myocardial infarction, rt-PA reopens the occluded artery in 65 to 75 per cent of cases. It is more effective and faster than streptokinase administered by the same route. This fact, together with the knowledge that rt-PA may have less potential for hemorrhagic complications, makes is feasible for administration to the majority of patients.

Streptokinase

Streptokinase is a nonenzymatic protein isolated from beta-hemolytic streptococci (Lancefield Group C). Streptokinase forms a complex with plasminogen, and the streptokinase-plasminogen complex behaves as plasminogen activator, converting plasminogen to plasmin. Human plasma contains antibodies against streptokinase formed from previous streptococcal infections. Sufficient amounts of streptokinase must be infused to neutralize the antibodies before fibrinolytic action can take place. A high loading dose is associated with rapid and profound reduction in the levels of circulating plasminogen, antiplasmin, and fibrinogen. Injection of iodine[131]-labeled streptokinase demonstrates a rapid clearance phase with a half-life of approximately 20 minutes followed by a slow disappearance phase with a half-life of 83 minutes. However, the effect on the blood coagulation components lasts for approximately 24 hours. There is no sensitive test for monitoring safe levels of streptokinase. The magnitude of systemic fibrinolysis and its laboratory derangements do not strictly correlate with bleeding manifestations. Studies of streptokinase administered by intracoronary injection have shown that the drug recanalizes the occluded coronary artery in up to 80 per cent of patients. When streptokinase is given intravenously, recanalization rates of 35 to 65 per cent are obtained. Streptokinase administered by the intracoronary and intravenous routes has been approved by the FDA for general clinical use.

Intracoronary Administration. Following identification of an occluded coronary artery at cardiac catheterization, the patient should receive 100 mg of hydrocortisone together with a bolus of 10,000 units of heparin intravenously. Heparin should be continued by infusion at the rate of 800 to 1000 units per hour. Infusion of streptokinase is begun at a rate of 4000 to 6000 units per minute directly into the infarct-related artery. The artery is opacified with a contrast agent at 5- to 10-minute intervals to detect recanalization. The infusion is continued for approximately an hour, up to a maximum dose of 250,000 units of streptokinase.

Intravenous Administration. Once an indication for thrombolytic therapy is established for a patient with evolving infarction, a minimum of two intravenous lines should be established. The patient should receive hydrocortisone, 100 mg and heparin 10,000 units intravenously. The heparin infusion is continued at the rate of 800 to 1000 units per hour. Partial thromboplastin time should be adjusted between 1.5 and 2 times normal. The infusion of streptokinase (1.5 million units dissolved in approximately 150 ml of a suitable vehicle) is started, and the total dose is given over a period of 1 hour. In order to minimize bleeding complications, the patient should be disturbed as little as possible. Blood for creatine kinase MB enzyme levels should be drawn every 4 hours for 36 to 48 hours. Clinical indications of successful recanalization are a rapid relief of chest pain, hemodynamic stability, speedy resolution of ST segment elevation on the electrocardiogram, appearance of ventricular arrhythmias during infusion (idioventricular rhythm, late-coupled VPBs), and early peaking of CKMB values (usually within the first 12 hours).

Hemorrhagic diathesis, active peptic ulcer during the past 6 months, colitis, esophageal varices, aortic aneurysm, hypertension resistant to treatment with systolic blood pressure higher than 200 mmHg and diastolic blood pressure higher than 120 mmHg, resuscitation with cardiac massage, trauma, surgery during the past 10 days, history of stroke, history of headaches or visual disorders, and history of epilepsy are contraindications to the use of streptokinase.

Adverse effects are (1) bleeding complications in 5 per cent of patients, including serious bleeding, particularly intracranial, in 0.5 per cent; (2) nausea and vomiting; (3) bradycardia and hypotension; (4) minor skin rashes; (5) rigors; and (6) rarely, anaphylactic shock.

Urokinase

Urokinase is a trypsin-like serine protease derived from human urine and cultured human and embryonic kidney cells. Gene coding for urokinase has been cloned and expressed in *Escherichia coli*. Urokinase is a direct activator of plasminogen. Urokinase, in contrast to streptokinase, is not antigenic in humans. The mean clearance half-life of urokinase in humans is 14 ± 6 minutes. It is degraded by the liver. Doses in the range of two million units over a period of 15 to 20 minutes produce effects similar to intravenous streptokinase. Urokinase has also been administered by the intracoronary route as an infusion at a rate of 4000 to 6000 units per minute, up to a maximum dose of 250,000 to 500,000 units.

Tissue Type Plasminogen Activator (t-PA)

Tissue type plasminogen activator (t-PA) (Activase) is a serine protease isolated and purified from human uterine tissue and human melanoma cell line; more recently the gene for human t-PA has been cloned and recombinant t-PA expressed. Recombinant t-PA (rt-PA) binds specifically to fibrin and plasminogen and is activated only after this binding. Pharmacokinetic studies have revealed an alpha phase half-life of 5.7 minutes and a half-life of 1.3 hours. A decrease in fibrinogen concentration to about 50 per cent of the pretreatment values has been observed in patients with acute myocardial infarction when 80 mg of rt-PA was infused. Studies also showed that rt-PA was twice as effective as streptokinase (1.5 million units intravenously) in restoring patency of infarct-related arteries. Pooled results have shown that rt-PA produces lysis of the clot in 71 per cent of patients treated within 6 hours of the onset of symptoms. The drug has been approved by the FDA for general clinical use. rt-PA is administered by intravenous infusion following a bolus of 6 to 10 mg given over 1 to 2 minutes. A total of 60 mg should be administered over the first hour, 20 mg over the second hour, and 20 mg over the third hour. For smaller patients (less than 65 kg) a dose of 1.25 mg per kg administered over 3 hours may be used. Doses in excess of 100 mg should be avoided because of demonstrated increase in intracranial bleeding. Contraindications to use of rt-PA are similar to the contraindications to use of streptokinase.

Acyl Derivatives of Equimolar Streptokinase– Plasminogen Complex

Stable acyl derivatives of an equimolar strep-tokinase–plasminogen complex have been pre-pared that can circulate in the vascular system without reaction with the plasmin inhibitors or plasminogen, yet bind to fibrin. The *p*-anisoyl derivative (BRL26921-ASPAC) has a half-life of approximately 40 minutes. With an intracoro-nary injection of a 10-mg bolus of BRL26921, recanalization rates of 75 per cent were obtained in patients with acute myocardial infarction. After intravenous injection of a 30-mg bolus, reperfusion rates of 80 per cent were achieved. Fibrinogen levels were reduced up to 80 per cent of the preinjection values with the larger dose. The drug is undergoing investigation at present and is not available for clinical use.

Single Chain Urokinase–Type Plasminogen Activator (Prourokinase)

Single chain urokinase–type plasminogen ac-tivator (SCU-PA) directly activates the conver-sion of plasminogen to plasmin. The generated plasmin then converts SCU-PA to urokinase, which, in turn, activates the conversion of plas-minogen to plasmin. The gene coding for prou-rokinase has recently been cloned and expressed in *E. coli*. The drug is in the very early phase of investigation and appears to be an effective thrombolytic agent when administered by the intravenous route. Early indications are that it may be usefully employed in combination with rt-PA.

Further Management

Following administration of thrombolytic ther-apy, irrespective of the agent or the route utilized, further management is dictated by the patient's clinical course. In the case of intracoronary ther-apy, the success of the procedure is confirmed immediately, and further steps are undertaken, depending upon the type of lesion and severity of coronary artery disease. In the case of intrave-nous therapy, fair assumption of the success of the perfusion is obtained by following serial CKMB determinations during first 24 to 48 hours. As previously indicated, peak CKMB con-centrations attained within the first 12 hours are a reasonably sensitive confirmation of recanali-zation of the infarct-related artery. To safeguard against reocclusion, systemic anticoagulation, in-itially with heparin, followed by oral anticoagu-lants, is carried out. If the patient remains asymptomatic, approximately 1 week after ther-apy noninvasive methods (exercise testing with thallium-201 scintigraphy) are used to detect ischemia and evaluate the area of myocardium at risk. Coronary angiography is carried out if ischemia is provoked, followed by revasculariza-tion procedures (PTCA or CABG). In clinically unstable patients, a revascularization procedure is carried out immediately.

Primary Angioplasty or Surgical Revascularization

The logistic difficulties that apply to intra-coronary thrombolytic therapy are magnified appreciably in cases of angioplasty or surgical revascularization. In cases of PTCA, a catheteri-zation team possessing technical skill and expe-rience to perform emergency angioplasty at low risk to patients with acute myocardial infarction that can be available around-the-clock is an ex-pensive proposition. It is even more expensive to have operating rooms, cardiovascular surgeons, anesthetists, nurses, and technicians standing by around-the-clock. Primary angioplasty and sur-gical options are going to remain in the domain of a handful of hospitals. Nevertheless, if per-formed early, both procedures offer a number of potential advantages. With PTCA, they are defin-itive treatment of the residual stenosis, absence of hemorrhagic complications, lower incidence of reocclusion, and, if needed, CABG without risk of hemorrhagic complications. With CABG, they are definitive treatment of the obstructed vessel with a success rate much higher than PTCA and a more complete revascularization that can be carried out in case of multiple vessel disease.

TREATMENT OF COMPLICATIONS

Arrhythmias

Acutely ischemic myocardium is highly vulner-able to electrical instability and has a tendency to develop re-entrant and automatic arrhythmias originating in the atria or the ventricles. Ven-tricular arrhythmias are also common after re-perfusion (spontaneous or after thrombolytic therapy). Arrhythmias following myocardial in-farction need treatment because they frequently cause

1. *Hemodynamic impairment.* Cardiac output in patients with significant left ventricular dys-function is heart-rate dependent, since stroke volume is relatively fixed. Extreme slowing or acceleration of the heart rate can depress cardiac output. The optimal heart rate in a patient with AMI is probably between 80 to 90 beats per minute.

2. *Elevated heart rate.* Heart rate is one of the primary determinants of myocardial oxygen con-sumption. Tachycardias may increase myocardial oxygen consumption to levels that may have

a deleterious effect on jeopardized myocardium, further compounding left ventricular dysfunction.

3. *Atrioventricular asynchrony.* Atrial contraction plays a minor role in sustaining forward stroke volume (less than 20 per cent) in patients with normal ventricular function; however, atrial contribution to cardiac output is substantial in patients with compromised left ventricular function, particularly in the setting of acute myocardial infarction.

4. *A predisposition to malignant arrhythmias.* Arrhythmias following myocardial infarction can be broadly classified as tachyarrhythmias and bradyarrhythmias. The prognosis and treatment of arrhythmias may differ according to the time they appear during the course of acute myocardial infarction. It is, therefore, useful to subdivide arrhythmias into early (less than 6 hours and 6 to 72 hours) and late (72 hours to 6 weeks).

Early Arrhythmias (less than 6 hours)

Bradyarrhythmias. More than 50 per cent of patients show sinus or junctional bradycardia, and approximately 6 per cent show varying degrees of first- or second-degree atrioventricular block. The arrhythmias are particularly common in patients with inferior or posterior wall infarcts. Bradycardia with or without hypotension reflects intense vagal stimulation, presumably due to stimulation of cardiac vagal afferent receptors residing in the inferoposterior wall of the heart with resultant efferent cholinergic stimulation. Hypotension is deleterious to patients because it limits perfusion to jeopardized yet viable myocardium and intensifies ischemia. In the first 4 to 6 hours after infarction if slow heart rate (less than 60 beats per minute) is associated with hypotension, atropine in a dose of 0.6 mg every 3 to 5 minutes (total dose 2 mg), sufficient to bring heart rate up to 60 to 70 beats per minute often increases blood pressure and abolishes premature beats. In early hours of infarction, excessive vagotonia may be protective, and sometimes relief of parasympathetic tone with atropine will unmask sympathetic overactivity, resulting in sinus tachycardia and even ventricular arrhythmias. Caution should, therefore, be exercised in titrating the dose of atropine to the heart rate response. Atropine also helps in first-degree heart block if it is caused by excessive vagal activity and accompanied by bradycardia and hypotension.

Tachyarrhythmias. *Sinus tachycardia* occurs in one third of patients with acute myocardial infarction and is commonly associated with anterior wall infarction. Acceleration of the heart rate is due to sympathetic overactivity brought on by activation of cardiac receptors by local release of catecholamines and by an increase in circulating catecholamines. Catecholamines are also arrhythmogenic for ischemic myocardium. Pain and anxiety at this stage contribute to an increase in heart rate. Ventricular premature beats are frequently observed in association with sinus tachycardia in the early hours after infarction. Beta-adrenergic receptor antagonists are the drugs of choice in this situation. They relieve pain, slow the heart rate, diminish blood pressure, reduce electrocardiographic ST segment elevation, and increase the threshold for fibrillation. Propranolol (Inderal) is given by slow intravenous injection at the rate of 1 mg per minute (maximum 0.1 mg per kg), or metoprolol is given at the rate of 1 mg per minute (maximum 15 mg). Contraindications to use of beta blockers have already been described (see Table 5). Particular attention should be given to the presence or absence of left ventricular failure, because it is an important cause of sinus tachycardia in the setting of acute infarction.

Frequent *premature ventricular contractions* are common after the onset of AMI, particularly during the first hour. The arrhythmias in the early phase are strictly rate-related and under the influence of the autonomic nervous system. Sympathetic stimulation during the early hours contributes to premature ventricular contractions and malignant ventricular arrhythmias. Work from animal models suggests that a re-entry mechanism is responsible for arrhythmias soon after the onset of AMI. Vagal stimulation leads to slowing of the heart rhythm and may protect against ectopic ventricular activity.

Lidocaine, which impairs conduction and diminishes automaticity, may be less effective in these circumstances. Beta-adrenergic blockers, on the other hand, are the treatment of choice when ventricular ectopic beats are encountered soon after the onset of MI and when the ventricular ectopic beats are accompanied by sinus tachycardia. As previously indicated, caution should be exercised when administering atropine to patients with bradycardia and hypotension. Rapid parasympatholysis may unmask ventricular ectopic activity and even provoke malignant ventricular arrhythmias.

Malignant ventricular arrhythmias are the prime cause of death in patients with out-of-hospital sudden cardiac death syndrome. In the majority of the survivors, symptoms do not evolve into acute myocardial infarction. A portion of patients develop symptoms of chest pain followed by *ventricular fibrillation* and show evidence of acute myocardial infarction. Treatment involves immediate initiation of cardiopulmonary resuscitation and delivery of electrical direct current countershock. To prevent the recurrence of ventricular fibrillation, lidocaine is given intravenously by a bolus injection of 75 to 100 mg, and an infusion of lidocaine is begun at a rate of 2 to 3 mg per minute.

Early Arrhythmias (6 to 72 hours)

Arrhythmias that occur up to 3 days after acute myocardial infarction are extremely common and involve practically all patients. The types of arrhythmias encountered in the coronary care unit are discussed below.

Bradyarrhythmias. *Sinus bradycardia* is less common (20 per cent) as compared to that occurring soon after the onset of an inferoposterior wall myocardial infarction and is often transitory. It is usually caused by sinus node dysfunction or atrial ischemia. Hypotension is a rare accompaniment, and bradycardia rarely predisposes to ventricular arrhythmias. Unless the bradycardia is accompanied by hypotension, treatment is not required.

Atrioventricular (AV) *block* commonly occurs in patients with inferoposterior wall infarction and is due to ischemia and edema of the conduction tissue. AV block associated with anterior wall infarction denotes extensive damage and carries a very poor prognosis.

First-degree AV block is seen in 10 per cent of patients with AMI admitted to the coronary care unit. In over 90 per cent of patients, the conduction abnormality is located above the bundle of His and almost never progresses to higher degrees of block. Complete heart block or ventricular asystole is confined to a small number of patients who have a conduction abnormality located below the bundle of His that is commonly associated with bundle branch block and anterior wall infarction. No treatment is required other than continued observation for development of higher degrees of block.

Second-degree AV block is of two types. *Mobitz Type I (Wenckebach) block* is seen in 5 to 10 per cent of patients with AMI, usually involving the inferior wall. The conduction abnormality is transient, rarely lasting more than 3 to 4 days. No treatment is required if the heart rate is adequate and there is no hemodynamic impairment. In case of excessive slowing of the heart, heart failure, or shock, a temporary pacemaker should be inserted intravenously. *Mobitz Type II block* occurs in less than 1 per cent of patients with AMI. The conduction abnormality is usually located below the bundle of His and is associated with a wide QRS complex and often progresses suddenly to complete AV block. The patient requires a temporary transvenous pacemaker electrode because of the high chance of progression to complete AV block.

Complete heart block occurs in 5 to 10 per cent of patients with AMI. In patients with inferior wall infarction, the conduction defect is presumably due to hypoperfusion of the AV node, and the His-Purkinje system usually escapes injury. The escape rhythm is often junctional with narrow QRS complexes. Hemodynamic impairment is usually mild. In patients with anterior wall infarction, the lesion is located more often below the bundle of His; the block occurs abruptly and escape rhythm shows wide QRS complexes. Ventricular asystole may occur suddenly in this group of patients. The mortality is much higher in patients with anterior wall MI (50 to 60 per cent) than in patients with inferior wall MI (20 to 25 per cent). A temporary transvenous pacemaker should be inserted in all patients with complete AV block.

Transthoracic pacemakers or intravenous pacemakers are indicated urgently if it is established that the rhythm is truly ventricular asystole. In many cases, fine ventricular fibrillation may be mistaken for asystole and electrical countershock should be carried out routinely as a first step.

Intraventricular block such as complete right (R) or left (L) bundle branch block (BBB), RBBB with left anterior or posterior hemiblock (LAHB or LPHB), or trifascicular blocks are commonly associated with anterior wall infarctions (10 to 20 per cent) and reflect substantial myocardial damage. Poor prognosis is related to the extent of infarction rather than the conduction defect. The appearance of intraventricular block during the evolution of the infarction is an indication for use of a temporary transvenous pacemaker, since these conduction abnormalities may progress to complete heart block. The prophylactic transvenous pacemaker should be left in place for up to a week, and, depending upon the clinical course, may be removed or replaced by a permanent pacemaker if there is progression to higher degrees of block. Pacing in survivors of acute myocardial infarction associated with conduction defects (LBBB, RBBB, RBBB with LAHB or LPHB) is a subject of debate at present. Permanent pacemakers should be inserted in patients with bundle branch block who progress to transient high-degree AV block. However, it should be remembered that sudden deaths in this patient population are not always due to recurrent AV block. There is a high incidence of late in-hospital ventricular fibrillation in patients with anterior wall infarction and either RBBB or LBBB.

A number of *drugs* prescribed to patients prior to or during recovery from acute myocardial infarction may have adverse effects on AV conduction and may accentuate AV or intraventricular block. These include digoxin, beta-adrenergic blocking agents, calcium channel blockers (verapamil, diltiazem), and Type I antiarrhythmic agents (quinidine, procainamide, disopyramide). Unless there is clinical evidence of congestive heart failure or atrial fibrillation, digoxin should be discontinued in all patients with evolving infarction. Digoxin is usually not indicated in acute myocardial infarction unless accompanied by onset of atrial fibrillation or congestive heart failure due to systolic dysfunction. Caution should also be exercised in the continuation of digoxin therapy in the presence of significant renal insufficiency and electrolyte abnormalities. Beta blockers and Type I antiarrhythmic agents may cause conduction abnormalities. If it is essential to use beta blockers or Type I antiarrhythmic agents for other clinical indications, electrical pacing may provide easy control of cardiac rhythm in the presence of conduction abnormalities.

Tachyarrhythmias

SINUS TACHYCARDIA. As previously indicated, *sinus tachycardia* may be due to heightened sympathetic drive at the onset of myocardial infarction. About 30 per cent of patients develop sinus tachycardia within the first few days of admission to the coronary care unit. A number of mechanisms may be operative, including anxiety associated with recurrent chest pain, left ventricular failure, pericarditis, hypovolemia, fever, pulmonary infection or embolism, and administration of vasodilators, particularly nifedipine. Treatment should be directed to correcting the cause and includes analgesics, anti-inflammatory agents, antifailure treatment, and volume expansion. Sinus tachycardia in the presence of left ventricular failure is a poor prognostic sign. Cardiac acceleration is deleterious in any circumstance, and if all causes are excluded, beta blockers may be helpful in controlling the heart rate.

VENTRICULAR ARRHYTHMIAS. *Ventricular premature beats* (VPBs) are extremely common (more than 90 per cent) in the setting of AMI. They occur in single or multiform configurations with early ("R-on-T" phenomena) or late coupling and in repetitive forms as couplets or triplets. The ectopic activity reflects the electrical instability of the injured ventricular myocardium and is traditionally considered to be a harbinger of malignant arrhythmias. However, a substantial debate over the association between VPBs and development of ventricular arrhythmias exists. (1) In over 50 per cent of patients with primary ventricular fibrillation following AMI, no warning arrhythmias can be demonstrated; (2) despite adequate suppression of VPBs with lidocaine, ventricular fibrillation continues to occur in a significant number of patients; (3) primary ventricular fibrillation is a rare event (±5 per cent) when compared to the number of patients seen with VPBs; (4) other factors such as release of catecholamines in the infarcted area, cellular hypoxemia, acidosis, tachycardia, and electrolyte abnormalities may be closely related to the development of ventricular fibrillation.

Treatment of VPBs is equally fraught with controversy. Advocates of prophylactic treatment for all patients with acute myocardial infarction argue that when lidocaine is administered prophylactically at the onset of AMI, a reduction in the frequency of spontaneous ventricular fibrillation is observed; since 50 per cent of patients with ventricular fibrillation do not show warning arrhythmias, premature ventricular beats are not good predictors of ventricular fibrillation. Proponents of no treatment have several counter-arguments. (1) Ventricular fibrillation occurring in the coronary care unit can be efficiently managed by a well-trained nursing and medical staff. (2) The administration of the prophylactic lidocaine does not reduce overall mortality. (3) Drugs commonly used as prophylactic agents such as lidocaine do not uniformly elevate the ventricular fibrillation threshold, and ventricular fibrillation may occur despite treatment with lidocaine. (4) The condition of the majority of patients admitted to the coronary care unit with chest pain (greater than 60 per cent) does not evolve into acute myocardial infarction. Even in those with established infarction, ventricular fibrillation occurs in less than 5 per cent of cases. Prophylactic lidocaine would be given to many patients who are not at risk. (5) Ventricular arrhythmias occurring early in the course of acute myocardial infarction may be caused by reentrant mechanisms and may be less susceptible to suppression by lidocaine.

The author follows a middle approach adopted by many others and administers lidocaine to (1) patients with complex forms of ventricular premature beats or with beats at a frequency that is more than 5 per minute after acute myocardial infarction, (2) patients with early or late coupled ventricular premature beats, (3) patients following an episode of ventricular fibrillation or tachycardia, and (4) patients with accelerated idioventricular rhythm causing hemodynamic impairment. If lidocaine therapy is ineffective, other Class I antiarrhythmic agents may be employed (Tables 1 through 3).

ACCELERATED IDIOVENTRICULAR RHYTHMS. Ventricular rhythms with a rate of 60 to 110 beats per minute are commonly seen on the second or third day after myocardial infarction. They sometimes result from reperfusion of the infarct zone, either spontaneously or after throm-

TABLE 1. **Class Ia Antiarrhythmic Agents***

Characteristic	Quinidine	Procainamide (Proestyl)	Disopyramide (Norpace)
Dose	oral: 200–400 mg q 6 hr After 200 mg test dose Sustained release 250–500 mg q 8 hr IV: Loading dose 600 mg 1–2 mg/min by infusion	oral: 500–1000 mg q 4 hr Sustained release 500–1000 mg q 6 hr (Procan SR) IV: Loading dose 1000 mg (100 mg every 5 min); 1.5–5.5 mg/min by infusion	oral: Loading dose 300 mg, 100–150 mg q 6 hr Sustained release 300 mg q 12 hr IV: Loading dose 300 mg/hr Maintenance dose 0.4 mg/kg/hr (not approved by FDA)
Peak plasma level	oral: 1.5–2 hr (sulfate) 3–4 hr (gluconate) IV: 15–20 min	1.0–1.5 hr ?	1.5–2.0 hr ?
Half-life	7–9 hr ($\uparrow$ Hepatic, renal disease)	3–4 hr	6–8 hr ($\uparrow$ Renal disease)
Absorption from GI tract (%)	70	85	80
Bioavailability (%)	80	80	80
Protein binding (%)	80–90	20	30
Elimination	Hepatic 85%; renal 15%; metabolites active	Hepatic 40–50%; active metabolites (NAPA); renal 40–50%	Renal 50%; metabolites active; anticholinergic
Therapeutic plasma concentration	2.3–5 µg/ml	4–10 µg/ml	2–5 µg/ml
Indications	Atrial fibrillation Conversion + + Prophylaxis + + + + SVT + + + APBs + + + VPBs + + + VT + +	Atrial fibrillation Conversion + + Prophylaxis + + + + SVT + + + APBs + + + VPBs + + + VT + + + + Most commonly used if lidocaine fails	Atrial fibrillation Conversion + Prophylaxis + + + + SVT + + + APBs + + + VPBs + + + VT + + +
Drug interaction	Serum digoxin level $\uparrow$, oral anticoagulants (PT $\uparrow$)	Relatively free	None
VF threshold	Decreased	Decreased	Decreased
Other effects	Vagolytic, mild alpha-adrenergic blocker, increase AV conduction	Mild to moderate; negative inotropic effect	Moderate to severe negative inotropic effect
Adverse effects	Proarrhythmogenic (VT/VF), sinus arrest, SA block, AV block asystole, hypotension, cinchonism, nausea, vomiting, diarrhea, fever, thrombocytopenia	Acute: hypotension AV block (IV) QRS duration $\uparrow$, VT/VF Chronic: giddiness, psychosis, hallucinations, fever, agranulocytosis, skin rashes, digital vasculitis, Raynaud's disease, drug-induced lupus	Dry mouth, urinary hesitancy, constipation, blurred vision, GI symptoms Relative contraindications: glaucoma, hypotension, hypertrophy of prostate, heart failure; VT/VF, AV block asystole

*Membrane stabilizing, $\downarrow$ fast Na channel, $\uparrow$ action potential; slows phase 0 of action potential; sinus node automaticity unchanged, $\downarrow$ Purkinje system automaticity; $\uparrow$ ERP of Purkinje fibers and ventricular muscle; sinus rate and PR interval unchanged; $\uparrow$ QRS duration, $\uparrow$ QT.

Abbreviations: ERP = effective refractory period; SVT = supraventricular tachycardia; VT = ventricular tachycardia; VF = ventricular fibrillation; VPB = ventricular premature beat; APB = atrial premature beat; GI = gastrointestinal; IV = intravenous; SA = sinoatrial; $\uparrow$ = increased or prolonged; $\downarrow$ = decreased or shortened; + + + + = strongly effective; + + + and + + = moderately effective; + = weakly effective.

bolytic therapy. The arrhythmias are seen with equal frequency in anterior and inferior infarction. About half of the episodes occur as escape rhythm during slowing of the basic cardiac rhythm, and half of the episodes follow an ectopic beat. The arrhythmia is usually self-limiting and does not carry an adverse prognosis. No treatment is usually necessary, except when associated with hemodynamic impairment.

VENTRICULAR TACHYCARDIA. Ventricular tachycardia is defined as three or more consecutive ventricular premature beats occurring at a rate of under 200 beats per minute. Ventricular tachycardia occurs in 10 to 30 per cent of patients with AMI; it is more common in transmural infarction and is associated with significant left ventricular dysfunction. Urgent treatment of sustained ventricular tachycardia is essential. If the

TABLE 2. **Class Ib Antiarrhythmic Agents***

Characteristic	Lidocaine	Tocainide (Tonocard)	Mexiletine (Mexitil)	Phenytoin (Dilantin)
Dose	*IV only*: Bolus 1–2 mg/kg (75–150 mg) followed by second bolus 0.5–1 mg/kg (50–75 mg) in 20–40 min; simultaneous IV infusion 2–4 mg/min, maximum dose in 1 hr 300 mg; halve dose in severe heart failure, shock, hepatic disease, patients over 65 years, correct hypokalemia	Oral loading dose 400–600 mg; repeat in 4–6 hr, then 800 mg q 8 hr. IV not approved by FDA	Initial dose 200–400 mg followed after 2 hr by 200–500 mg q 8 hr. IV not approved by FDA	Oral: 15 mg/kg 1st day, 7.5 mg/kg 2nd and 3rd day, 4–6 mg/kg maintenance; IV 100 mg q 5 min up to maximum of 1000 mg; flush after each dose to prevent phlebitis
Peak plasma level	30–45 min	60–90 min	2–4 hr	4–12 hr
Half-life	1–2 hr	11–15 hr	9–12 hr (prolonged in heart failure and AMI 19–30 hr)	18–36 hr
Absorption from GI tract (%)	NA	100	80	50–70
Bioavailability (%)	NA	100	80	90
Protein binding (%)	20–40	50	80	90
Elimination	Metabolism 90% hepatic active metabolites, renal 10%	Renal 40% (half-life in renal insufficiency 25–30 hr); 60% hepatic	Renal 20%; 80% hepatic	Renal 5%; 95% metabolized; metabolites not active
Therapeutic concentration	1.5–6 µg/ml	6–12 µg/ml	1–2 µg/ml	10–20 µg/ml
Indications	VBPs + + + + VT + + + + VT/VFib (prophylaxis) + + +	VPBs + + + VT + + +	VPBs + + + VT (maintenance) + + +	VPBs + + + VT + + +
Drug interactions	Blood level ↑ in presence of beta-blockers	?	?	?
VF threshold	Increased	Increased	Increased	?
Other effects	No negative inotropic effects	Minimal negative inotropic effects	Minimal negative inotropic effects	Minimal negative inotropic effects
Adverse effects	At plasma levels of 50 µg/ml parasthesias, drowsiness; mild agitation, muscle twitching, seizures (particularly in elderly), nausea, vomiting, AV block in patients with depressed conduction, sinus arrest	Anorexia, nausea, vomiting, constipation, rashes, ataxia, light-headedness, rarely pulmonary intestinal alveolitis	Proarrhythmias, tremors, diplopia, paresthesias, ataxia, nystagmus, confusion	Drowsiness, nystagmus ataxia (usually over 20 µg/ml), nausea, anorexia, hyperglycemia, hypocalcemia, osteomalacia, skin rashes, megaloblastic anemia, malignant lymphoma
Contraindications	Grade 2 or 3 AV block, nodal or idioventricular escape rhythms	AV block; severe hepatic disease	Severe LVF, shock, hypotension, sinus node disease	Heart failure, AV block

*Membrane stabilizing, ↓ fast Na channel; ↑ outward currents; sinus node automaticity unchanged; ↓ Purkinje fiber automaticity; ↓ action potential duration of Purkinje fibers and ventricular muscle; ↓ ERP of Purkinje and ventricular muscle; sinus rate, PR interval QRS duration, QT interval unchanged.

Abbreviations: ERP = effective refractory period; VPB = ventricular premature beats; VT = ventricular tachycardia; VFib = ventricular fibrillation; LVF = left ventricular failure; AV = atrioventricular; IV = intravenous; ↓ = inhibit or reduce; ↑ = stimulate or increase; + + + + = strongly recommended; + + + and + + = moderately recommended; + = weakly recommended.

TABLE 3. **Class Ic Antiarrhythmic Agents***

Characteristic	Flecainide (Tambocor)	Encainide (Enkaid)	Propafenone (Rytmonorm)
Dose	100 mg bid increased by 50 mg at 4-day intervals to a maximum of 300 mg/day	25 mg tid increasing at 4- to 8-day intervals to a maximum of 200 mg/day	75 mg tid increasing at 4- to 7-day intervals to a maximum of 900 mg/day
Half-life (hr)	20	2.3; increased in poor metabolizers (11), hepatic disease (4)	2.5–12
Absorption (%)	90	90	50
Bioavailability (%)	30–40	30 (85 in poor metabolizers, renal and hepatic disease)	50
Elimination	Hepatic metabolism	Extensively metabolized metabolites active (2 distinct phenotypes for metabolism—extensive, 92%; nonextensive, 8%)	Hepatic metabolism, renal excretion 1%
Therapeutic concentration	450–500 ng/ml	Not known	0.5–2 ng/ml
Drug interaction	Should not be used with verapamil or disopyramide	None known	None known
Ventricular fibrillation threshold	?	?	?
Other effects	Negative inotropic effect can cause or worsen CHF (5%)	Minimal negative inotropic effect	Weak beta blocking and calcium channel blocking effects
Indications	Documented life-threatening ventricular arrhythmias, symptomatic VPBs or non-sustained VT	Same as for Flecainide	Same as for Flecainide
Contraindications	AV conduction abnormalities	AV conduction abnormalities	AV conduction abnormalities
Adverse effects	Proarrhythmogenic 7%, can be fatal; dizziness, blurred vision	Proarrhythmogenic 5–10% blurred vision, ataxia, dizziness	Proarrhythmogenic, elevation of serum transaminases, cholestatic hepatitis, GI upset

*Inhibits fast sodium channel, slows rate of rise of action potential, membrane stabilizing effect; action potential duration unaffected or decreased.

rhythm is well tolerated (normal mentation, blood pressure greater than 80 mmHg systolic), a brief trial with lidocaine or procainamide may be undertaken. In case of hypotension or rapid deterioration in mentation, electric direct current (DC) countershock at a low energy level (10 to 50 watts per second) is used. Occasionally, a sharp precordial thump may cause ventricular tachycardia to revert to sinus rhythm. In order to prevent recurrence of arrhythmia, lidocaine or procainamide infusion is started immediately. In a conscious patient, diazepam (Valium), 10 mg intravenously, is given before delivering DC shock. Particular attention should be given to the airway, and the patient should be ventilated with 100 per cent oxygen via a mask or a bag.

VENTRICULAR FIBRILLATION. Two forms of ventricular fibrillation are seen between 6 and 72 hours after onset of infarction. Primary ventricular fibrillation is most common within first 6 to 8 hours in absence of cardiac failure or shock and represents 80 per cent of all cases of in-hospital ventricular fibrillation. If treated promptly, it does not affect prognosis adversely. Secondary ventricular fibrillation occurs most commonly be-

tween 12 and 72 hours after infarction and develops in patients presenting with hypotension, heart failure, or shock. Secondary ventricular fibrillation is associated with a high mortality rate and reflects the underlying severity of the heart disease. Ventricular fibrillation is treated with DC countershock at high energy levels (commencing at 200 watts per second) accompanied by measures designed to protect the airway, maintaining adequate ventilation by bag, mask, or endotracheal intubation, and to prevent recurrence with simultaneous commencement of antiarrhythmic therapy with infusion of lidocaine (see Table 1). Prompt electrical DC countershock generally interrupts fibrillation and restores an effective cardic rhythm in patients under continuous medical observation. Failure to restore an effective rhythm is almost always caused by rapid recurrent malignant ventricular tachycardia or fibrillation in the setting of persistent ischemia, acidosis, and electrolyte abnormalities. Patients require prompt treatment of metabolic and electrolyte abnormalities and repeated electrical countershocks. Intracardiac administration of epinephrine (10 ml of 0.1 per cent solution) sometimes facilitates successful electrical defibrillation. Bretylium tosylate, 5 mg per kg intravenously repeated in 15 to 20 minutes, may also help in successful interruption of ventricular fibrillation.

SUPRAVENTRICULAR ARRHYTHMIAS. *Atrial premature contractions* are common after acute myocardial infarction, occurring in up to 50 per cent of patients. They usually herald the onset of atrial fibrillation or flutter. Atrial premature contractions may be due to left atrial dilatation, overt or occult heart failure, early pericarditis or ischemia, and injury to atria or sinus node. Occasionally an atrial premature beat may initiate ventricular tachycardia or fibrillation in patients with large myocardial infarctions. No treatment is usually indicated, except for continued observation.

In 10 to 15 per cent of patients *atrial fibrillation* develops within the first 24 hours after infarction. Atrial fibrillation is more frequent in patients with large infarctions and carries a poor prognosis. Left atrial dilatation following left ventricular failure, pericarditis, atrial infarctions, and pulmonary embolism can also trigger atrial fibrillation in the setting of acute myocardial infarction. Because of loss of atrial transport function, particularly in the presence of a rapid ventricular response, the patient may show progressive hemodynamic deterioration, and prompt treatment is mandatory. Synchronized electrical cardioversion at an energy level of 50 to 200 watts per second is indicated if patients with atrial fibrillation develop hypotension, chest pain, or acute left ventricular failure. In the absence of hemodynamic impairment, digoxin is effective in reducing ventricular rate and should be administered in the initial dose of 0.5 mg intravenously followed by 0.25 mg intravenously every 6 hours, for a total dose of 1.0 to 1.5 mg in 24 hours. In a small percentage of patients, adequate digitalization fails to achieve satisfactory slowing of the heart rate, and in order to further depress AV conduction and slow ventricular response, metoprolol (Lopressor), a cardioselective beta blocker, may be prescribed in the dose of 25 to 50 mg orally every 12 hours. Atrial fibrillation is usually a transient arrhythmia with spontaneous reversion to sinus rhythm in 24 to 48 hours. If atrial fibrillation persists after 24 hours, quinidine, 300 mg every 6 hours orally, may be started to induce pharmacologic cardioversion. Continued presence of atrial fibrillation for a few days necessitates full anticoagulation with elective cardioversion before discharge from the hospital. The associated clinical conditions, such as left ventricular failure and pericarditis, should be treated appropriately and may help in restoring sinus rhythm in many cases.

Atrial flutter is an uncommon arrhythmia associated with acute myocardial infarction, occurring in only 1 to 2 per cent of patients. In addition to clinical conditions described under atrial fibrillation, atrial flutter may be associated with pulmonary disease such as pneumonia, obstructive airways disease, atelectasis, and so forth. Atrial flutter is commonly accompanied by hemodynamic impairment and is best managed by synchronized DC cardioversion at low energy levels of 10 to 50 watts per second. An additional option for the treatment of atrial flutter is the use of rapid atrial pacing through a transvenous intra-atrial electrode. Direct atrial stimulation is a logical approach to treat atrial flutter when large doses of digoxin have failed to provide adequate slowing of ventricular response. Stimulation of the lower right atrium, usually with a rapid burst of stimuli, is frequently effective in converting atrial flutter to sinus rhythm.

Paroxysmal supraventricular tachycardia is seen in about 5 per cent of patients with acute myocardial infarction admitted to the coronary care unit. The rapid ventricular rate (usually faster than 150 beats per minute) leads to considerable hemodynamic disturbance, and prompt treatment is required to restore sinus rhythm, which is best achieved by synchronized DC cardioversion using low energy levels of 25 to 50 watts per second. However, prior to using DC cardioversion, carotid massage is often successful in breaking the re-entrant circuit by increasing vagal tone and should be routinely tried. Intravenous verapamil (Isoptin, Calan) is also highly effective in converting AV nodal re-entrant tachycardia to sinus rhythm (success rate greater than 90 per cent) and may be tried if the patient is tolerating the arrhythmia well. Verapamil is given by a slow intravenous injection of 5 mg and repeated once or twice up to a maximum dose of 20 mg. Verapamil should not be given intravenously to patients who are receiving beta-blocker therapy for fear of inducing cardiovascular collapse. This is particularly true in elderly patients and in those with significant left ventricular dysfunction. In order to prevent recurrence of arrhythmia, patients should be started on quinidine, 300 mg every 6 hours. In patients with recurrent arrhythmias that are refractory to pharmacologic maneuvers, rapid atrial stimulation through a transvenous intra-atrial electrode may be used just as for atrial flutter.

Accelerated junctional rhythm occurs at rates of up to 120 beats per minute. At slow rates, it is usually a benign escape rhythm commonly seen among patients with slow sinus rates and associated with inferior wall infarction. Retrograde P waves may be seen, or there may be AV dissociation with junctional rates slightly faster than sinus rates. Loss of atrial transport function may be tolerated poorly by patients. In selected patients, AV sequential pacing may be required to improve hemodynamics.

Paroxysmal junctional tachycardia is seen in 1 to 2 per cent of patients with acute myocardial infarction at rates of 120 to 220 beats per minute. It starts and ends abruptly. It often occurs in patients with left ventricular failure, ischemia of the conduction system, or as a manifestation of digoxin toxicity. Treatment follows the same principles as described under supraventricular tachycardia.

Late Arrhythmias

Complicated ventricular arrhythmias developing after the first 3 days of onset of acute myocardial infarction usually reflect an advanced degree of left ventricular dysfunction consequent to substantial myocardial damage. Three to 8 per cent of patients recovering from acute myocardial infarction die suddenly during the first year. Both left ventricular dysfunction and complex ventricular arrhythmias are independent predictors of total mortality as well as of sudden cardiac death. The peak of complex ectopy is 3 to 6 weeks after infarction. Recent data suggest that arrhythmias may be more potent predictors of sudden death in non–Q wave infarctions than in Q wave infarctions. Although it is a common clinical practice to treat asymptomatic ventricular arrhythmias detected in the post-infarction period, considerable controversy exists regarding the rationale for subjecting the patients to long-term antiarrhythmic agents because no cause-and-effect relationship has been demonstrated between the complex ventricular ectopy and future sudden death, and the sensitivity and specificity of asymptomatic ventricular arrhythmias to predict sudden death is very low. Predischarge Holter monitoring has a sensitivity of only 25 to 64 per cent and a positive predictive accuracy of less than 20 per cent for identifying patients who are at risk of dying. Thus far, long-term trials of antiarrhythmic agents have failed to reduce the number of patients dying suddenly. Practically all available antiarrhythmic agents produce adverse effects when administered on a long-term basis. Proarrhythmogenic effects of these drugs may also contribute to significant morbidity and mortality.

Major clinical trials are underway, including one funded by the National Institutes of Health, to answer some of these questions. Until the role of asymptomatic ventricular arrhythmias in the development of ventricular fibrillation is better elucidated and the effect of therapy or a combination of therapy is better assessed, skeptics will continue to question the wisdom of treating all patients. Nonetheless, a common consensus to give benefit of doubt and treat complex asymptomatic arrhythmias continues to prevail. There is, however, no argument over treating symptomatic arrhythmias.

The aim of the antiarrhythmic therapy is to prevent nonsustained ventricular tachycardia and suppress ventricular premature beats. The list of antiarrhythmic agents to achieve this goal is large, but there is very little to choose among various drugs available at the present time (see Tables 1 through 4). The selection of a particular agent at this stage depends upon personal preference and experience. In patients with symptomatic arrhythmias that are not life-threatening, empiric therapy with one of the antiarrhythmic agents is initiated mainly to relieve symptoms, regardless of the effect on ectopic activity. Holter monitoring may be used for objective documentation.

Ventricular Tachycardia/Fibrillation. Sustained ventricular tachycardia/fibrillation occurs in 2 to 4 per cent of patients, with a peak incidence at 2 to 4 weeks after AMI. No frequency or morphologic characteristics of ventricular arrhythmia in the early phase predicts this event. Patients with intraventricular conduction defects (particularly RBBB), persistent sinus tachycardia, congestive heart failure, extensive anterior wall infarction, atrial flutter or fibrillation, or ventricular fibrillation during the earlier course of the illness are at high risk for developing late in-hospital malignant arrhythmias. Such patients should be monitored for longer periods of time in intermediate coronary care units or by telemetry. When episodes of nonsustained ventricular tachycardia occur in this setting, they may lead to more malignant forms including ventricular fibrillation. Syncope or presyncope may be the presenting symptom in this group. For those patients who have very frequent nonsustained episodes of tachycardia, the aim of treatment is to abolish prolonged symptomatic episodes. Holter monitoring can be used for objective evaluation of such therapy. Marked spontaneous variability of simple or complex arrhythmia in coronary artery disease does not permit use of Holter monitoring for evaluation of therapy in patients with low frequency of arrhythmias. In this group, electrophysiologic testing (programmed ventricular stimulation) is appropriate to select antiarrhythmic therapy. Electrophysiologic testing should also be undertaken in patients who have sustained ventricular tachycardia and in patients who are survivors of sudden cardiac arrest (ventricular fibrillation). Programmed ventricular

TABLE 4. **Class III Antiarrhythmic Agents***

Characteristic	Amiodarone (Cordarone)	Bretylium Tosylate (Bretylol)	L-Sotalol† (Sotacor)
Dose	Oral 200 mg q 6 hr for 2 weeks, followed by 200–400 mg daily IV 5 mg/kg over 5 min. followed by infusion 50 mg/kg not approved by FDA	*IV only* 5 mg/kg by bolus repeated if necessary; 10 mg/kg; 5–10 mg/kg every 6–8 hr or continuous infusion 1–2 mg/min, maximum dose 30 mg/kg	See Table 5 (Beta-adrenergic receptor antagonists) L-Sotalol has beta blocking potency D-Sotalol has no beta blocking effect; however, antiarrhythmic (Class III) action is present
Half-life	30–60 days	7.8 hr	
Absorption from GI tract (%)	50	NA	
Protein binding (%)	NA	NA	
Bioavailability	Action depends on tissue stores built up over prolonged period	NA	
Elimination	Not fully worked out; activity persists up to 45 days after stopping the drug Therapeutic concentration 0.5–3 μg/ml	Renal 77%	
Ventricular fibrillation threshold	↑ ↑ ↑ ↑	↑ ↑ ↑ ↑	
Indications	Atrial fibrillation to control rate; malignant ventricular arrhythmia unresponsive to other antiarrhythmic agents	Recurrent ventricular fibrillation; refractory to lidocaine and DC shock; sometimes malignant ventricular tachycardia, unresponsive to other agents	
Drug interaction	Digoxin level ↑, warfarin ↑, quinidine ↑		
Other effects	No negative inotropic effect; coronary and peripheral vasodilatation	Increased sensitivity to other sympathomimetic agents, epinephrine and norepinephrine	
Adverse effects	Corneal deposits (50–100%) during long-term therapy; vision unaffected, reversible after stopping the drug; ophthalmic exam every 3 months; photosensitivity rashes—sometimes permanent, grayish blue hue; pulmonary infiltration, 2–5%, sometimes fatal; hypo- or hyperthyroidism (each 200 g tablet contains 77 mg iodine), T4 ↑, reverse T3 ↑ ↑, T3 ↑; increase in transaminases (10–20%); proximal muscle weakness 1%; bradycardia; proarrhythmias		

* ↑ Duration of action potential, ↑ ERP of ventricular myocardium and Purkinje system.
†Investigational agent.
Abbreviations: ↑ = increased; ↑ ↑ ↑ ↑ = markedly increased; NA = not applicable.

stimulation also allows mapping of the tachycardia and, possibly, localization of arrhythmogenic foci. Patients with only one or two episodes of ventricular tachycardia and a moderate-sized infarction do reasonably well on antiarrhythmic therapy. However, a small group of patients presenting with repeated episodes of sustained ventricular tachycardia, congestive heart failure, and intraventricular conduction defects do poorly on antiarrhythmic agents, and without further intervention, 80 to 90 per cent of these patients are dead within the first year. Aggressive medical and surgical treatment of severe left ventricular dysfunction and coronary artery disease and removal of the arrhythmogenic focus are the only options available for these patients. Surgical therapy includes aneurysmectomy, endocardial resection, or coronary artery bypass surgery. Several uncontrolled studies have confirmed the beneficial outcome of the aggressive approach in this very high-risk group.

Hemodynamic Disturbances

By definition, all patients with acute myocardial infarction have varying degrees of left ventricular dysfunction compounded frequently by associated autonomic disturbances and myocardial ischemia in the border zone between the normal and the infarcted region. The severity of hemodynamic abnormalities produced by depressed left ventricular function depends upon the extent and location (anterior more than interior) of the infarction, the presence or absence of mechanical complications (acute mitral regurgitation, ventricular septal rupture, or free wall rupture), and the presence or absence of left ventricular dysfunction prior to the AMI. Objective hemodynamic evaluation with disposable pulmonary artery catheters in patients with AMI has allowed several entities with characteristic hemodynamic profiles to be recognized (Fig. 1).

Invasive monitoring is not indicated in patients with clinically uncomplicated acute myocardial infarction. Fairly accurate estimation of the gross abnormalities in cardiac output and left ventricular filling pressure can be obtained by careful clinical examination (heart rate and rhythm, systemic arterial pressure by cuff, assessment of jugular venous pressure, repeated auscultation of lung fields for crackles, auscultation of the heart for third and fourth heart sounds, adequacy of peripheral perfusion by examination of skin and mucous membranes, and measurement of urine flow), a chest x-ray film taken in posteroanterior view, and systemic arterial blood sampling for P_{O_2}, P_{CO_2}, and pH. In most clinical circumstances, therapy is guided by frequent clinical assessment. Nonetheless, invasive hemodynamic monitoring is required for a number of diagnostic and therapeutic indications.

Hemodynamic monitoring is used *to assist in the diagnosis of patients with* (1) mechanical complications such as acute mitral regurgitation, ventricular septal rupture, or pericardial effusion; (2) hypotension unresponsive to simple measures such as elevation of lower limbs and administration of atropine; (3) discrepancy be-

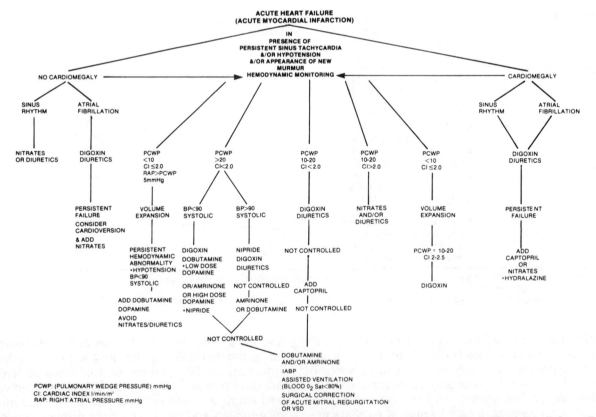

Figure 1. A scheme for treatment of heart failure following acute myocardial infarction. (From Majid PA, Roberts R: Treatment of heart failure. *In* Civetta JM, Kirby RR, Taylor RW (eds.): Intensive and Critical Care. Philadelphia, J. B. Lippincott, 1987.)

tween clinical and radiographic signs of pulmonary congestion; (4) noncardiac causes of hypotension, particularly hypovolemia; (5) extensive right ventricular infarction presenting with hypotension; (6) unexplained or severe cyanosis, hypoxemia, metabolic acidosis, or tachypnea; or (7) unexplained or refractory sinus tachycardia.

Hemodynamic monitoring is also helpful in the treatment of patients with (1) severe left ventricular failure and shock due to loss of muscle or mechanical complications, (2) persistent or recurrent chest pain refractory to conventional doses of analgesics, (3) hemodynamic impairment due to left ventricular stiffness requiring judicious infusion of fluids to optimize left ventricular filling pressure, or (4) right ventricular infarction requiring volume expansion for increasing left ventricular filling pressure and cardiac output.

Hemodynamic abnormalities may be encountered in patients after AMI during the pre-hospital phase, or in the coronary care unit.

Pre-hospital Phase

Hypotension associated with bradycardia most commonly occurs in patients with inferoposterior wall infarctions and responds to intravenous atropine and elevation of lower extremities as previously described. Hypotension associated with normal or rapid heart rates that worsen when the patient assumes an upright posture may be due to hypovolemia, which is common in patients with previous diuretic therapy for hypertension, nausea and vomiting or reduction of fluid intake at the time of onset of pain, and reduced ventricular compliance requiring high filling pressures (usually 18 to 20 mmHg) to maintain forward output. In the absence of crackles at lung bases, patients should be given a bolus of 50 ml of 5 per cent dextrose/half normal saline, and the infusion should be continued at 100 to 200 ml per hour. If atropine and volume expansion fail, dopamine should be started at 5 micrograms per kg per minute, and the rate of infusion tailored to the blood pressure response.

Coronary Care Unit

A number of mechanisms are responsible for producing hemodynamic impairment in patients with acute myocardial infarction. It is extremely important to recognize *hypovolemia* as a cause of reduced cardiac function, since improvement can be effected readily by use of fluids administered intravenously. Very often, hypovolemia can only be detected by invasive hemodynamic monitoring. Because of the reduction in left ventricular compliance that occurs with acute ischemia and infarction, left ventricular filling pressures above 18 mmHg are usually needed to maintain optimal stroke output. If, during hemodynamic monitoring, left ventricular filling pressure below 18 mmHg is associated with low cardiac output, fluid challenge with 50 ml of isotonic normal saline or 5 per cent dextrose/half normal saline should be given to assess the effect on the filling pressure and cardiac output. An increase in the pulmonary capillary wedge pressure to between 18 to 20 mmHg with normalization of cardiac output indicates hypovolemia. Fluids should then be replaced to equal the volume lost.

Some patients presenting with AMI have systemic arterial pressure consistently about 150 mmHg systolic. Hemodynamic monitoring in this group of patients has shown that *hypertensive* response is usually accompanied by sinus tachycardia and increased cardiac output in the presence of normal or low left ventricular filling pressures. The hypertension is most likely due to excessive circulating catecholamines in response to the acute myocardial injury. Immediate treatment of hypertension is essential to reduce myocardial oxygen demands and, it is hoped, myocardial infarct size. In the majority of patients, satisfactory lowering of blood pressure can be obtained by judicious use of analgesics, particularly morphine, which also has a central sympatholytic effect. However, hypertension may persist, and treatment with hypotensive agents should be started. In the absence of contraindications and after exclusion of other causes of sinus tachycardia, beta-adrenergic blockers are the treatment of choice (Table 5). Recent evidence suggests that calcium channel blockers may also be equally effective and should be preferred to the use of diuretics. In the case of resistant hypertension, nitroglycerin should be administered intravenously at the rate of 5 to 10 micrograms per minute and the dose titrated to the blood pressure response in combination with beta blockers or calcium channel blockers.

Heart Failure. Mechanisms responsible for heart failure in AMI are diverse.

Acute mechanisms include:

1. Loss of muscle, as occurs in acute myocardial infarction
2. Acute mitral regurgitation following myocardial infarction due to rupture, infarction, or dysfunction of papillary muscles
3. Ventricular septal rupture
4. Acute aneurysm formation with paradoxical systolic bulging
5. Right ventricular infarction
6. Recurrent acute ischemia that produces significant diastolic dysfunction

Chronic mechanisms include:

1. Ischemic cardiomyopathy due to severe three-vessel disease and multiple infarctions

TABLE 5. Beta-adrenergic Receptor Antagonists*

Characteristic	Propranolol (Inderal)	Metoprolol (Lopressor)	Timolol (Blocadren)	Atenolol (Tenormin)	Oxprenolol† (Trasicor)	Nadolol (Corgard)	Sotalol† (Sotacor)	Acebutalol (Sectral)	Pindolol (Visken)
Dose									
Oral	Start 60–120 mg in divided doses maximum 320 mg/day	Start 50–100 mg in divided doses, maximum 400 mg/day	Start 5–10 mg in divided doses, maximum 30 mg	50 mg once daily, maximum 200 mg‡	Start 60–120 mg in divided doses, maximum 320 mg	Start 40–50 mg; maximum 160 mg, once daily	Start 80–160 mg in divided doses, maximum 450 mg	Start 100–400 mg, maximum 1200 mg	5–10 mg in divided doses, maximum 15 mg
IV	1 mg/min, maximum 0.1 mg/kg	1 mg/min, maximum 15 mg	No	No	No	No	No	No	No
Approved for myocardial infarction	IV: Yes; Oral: Yes	Yes							
Angina	Yes	Yes	No	No	No	No	No	No	No
Cardioselective	No	Yes	No	Yes	No	No	No	No	No
ISA	No	No	No	No	Yes	No	No	Yes	Yes
MSA	Yes	No	No	No	Yes	No	No	Yes	No
Lipophilic	+ + +	+ +	+	+	+ +	+	+	+ +	+ +
Water soluble	No	No	No	Yes	No	Yes	Yes	?	?
Half-life (hr)	2–6	2–6	2–6	6–9	1–4	14–24	7–20	2–6	2–6
Absorption (%)	90	95	90	50	75	30	90	75	90
Bioavailability (%)	30	50	75	50	40	30	90	40	90
Elimination									
Hepatic metabolism	Yes	50%	50%	5–10%	Yes	No	No	10–20%	60%
Renal	Small	50%	20%	90%	10–20%	90%	90%	60%	40%
Active metabolites	Yes	?	No	Yes	No	No	No	?	No
Indications	1. AMI, sinus tachycardia, hyperdynamic state, pain 2. Post-infarction	Same as propranolol	Postinfarction angina	Postinfarction angina	Angina	Angina	1. Angina 2. Has Class Ib antiarrhythmic effect	Angina	Angina
Adverse effects	Severe bradycardia, sinus arrest, AV block, hypotension, cold extremities, fatigue, depression, nightmares, impotence, bronchospasm, insomnia, intermittent claudication	Adverse effects and contraindications described under propranolol (Inderal) are common to all beta blockers. Drugs possessing significant ISA (pindolol, oxprenolol, acebutalol) produce less bradycardia at rest. Cardioselective agents (atenolol, metoprolol) produce less bronchospastic effect at low doses. Lipophilic drugs cross blood-brain barrier and may produce CNS effect. Atenolol and nadolol can be given in once daily dose. Sotalol has unique Class Ib antiarrhythmic activity. Propranolol, metoprolol, timolol, and atenolol are the only agents shown to have reduced mortality (total and sudden) after AMI							
Contraindications	Heart failure, bronchial asthma, 3rd-degree AV block, severe bradycardia, insulin-dependent diabetes, severe peripheral vascular disease								

*Competitive antagonism of catecholamines at beta-receptor site. Decrease heart rate, myocardial contractility and reduce systemic blood pressure. Class II antiarrhythmics: depress Phase 4 diastolic depolarization, reduce sinus node automaticity, increase AV node effective refractory period, ventricular and Purkinje system automaticity and effective refractory period reduced. Increase ventricular fibrillation threshold.

†Investigational agent.

‡Manufacturer states: Doses over 100 mg/day are unlikely to produce further benefit.

Abbreviations: ISA = intrinsic sympathomimetic activity; MSA = membrane stabilizing effect; IV = intravenous; AV = atrioventricular; AMI = acute myocardial infarction; + + + = marked; + + = moderate; + = weak.

2. Ventricular aneurysm

Acute Myocardial Infarction. A linear correlation exists between the extent of left ventricular damage after acute myocardial infarction and systolic dysfunction. Clinical heart failure develops when 20 to 25 per cent of ventricular myocardium shows contractile abnormalities (hypokinesis, akinesis, or dyskinesis). Loss of more than 40 per cent of ventricular myocardium results in cardiogenic shock.

Myocardial ischemia or injury affects not only the pumping function but also the diastolic properties of the left ventricle. The diastolic pressure rises at any given volume. Depressed contractility, however, increases end-diastolic volume and the elevation of end-diastolic pressure is the result of reduction of both left ventricular diastolic compliance and systolic function.

In early stages of myocardial infarction, compliance of the infarcted myocardium may be normal or even increased, although the muscle itself cannot contract. There is passive bulging during each systole. Paradoxical systolic expansion of a ventricular segment decreases stroke output. With time, however, edema and cellular infiltration in the infarct zone lead to a decrease in the ventricular compliance, which may actually improve systolic function by preventing expansion of the ventricular wall during systole.

Acute diminution in stroke output is accompanied by a fall in blood pressure, which leads to a reflex increase in heart rate and systemic vascular resistance as well as stimulation of sympathetic nerve activity. Increased adrenergic activity not only sustains the increase in heart rate and peripheral vascular tone, but also increases contractility of the noninfarcted muscle. In acute heart failure, thus, compensatory response is limited to tachycardia, ventricular dilatation, and increased sympathetic activity.

Patients respond well to diuretics if heart failure is mild. Intravenous administration of furosemide reduces pulmonary vascular pressure before the onset of diuresis. Recent evidence suggests that nitrates may be preferable to diuretics in this setting.

Moderate or severe congestive heart failure requires more extensive therapy, including diuretics, inotropic agents, and vasodilators. In more severe cases, mechanical support may be needed. A scheme for management of acute heart failure following myocardial infarction is suggested in Figure 1.

Meticulous attention to ventilation is also necessary. Excessive doses of narcotic-analgesics may have an added effect by depressing respiration, diminishing lung compliance, and increasing vascular congestion. Assisted ventilation should be considered if, despite adequate oxygen therapy, arterial blood gas saturation cannot be maintained above 75 per cent. Assisted ventilation also reduces work for breathing, hence helping to conserve already compromised cardiac output.

Acute Mitral Regurgitation. Approximately 25 to 50 per cent of patients develop mild to moderate mitral regurgitation following acute myocardial infarction. However, sudden development of a loud murmur accompanied by significant hemodynamic deterioration in a patient recovering from acute myocardial infarction usually indicates either complete rupture of the papillary muscle or rupture of one or more chordal heads. In two thirds of patients, acute mitral regurgitation is associated with inferior wall infarction and involves the posteromedial papillary muscle. It usually occurs within the first week of infarction. Development of mitral regurgitation later in the course of myocardial infarction suggests either reinfarction or extension of the myocardial injury. The onset of heart failure is usually catastrophic. If heart failure is accompanied by shock, 70 per cent of the patients die within 24 hours and 90 per cent die within 2 weeks. It may be difficult on clinical grounds to distinguish between acute mitral regurgitation and ventricular septal rupture in patients with myocardial infarction. Insertion of a pulmonary artery catheter not only helps to differentiate between the two conditions but also allows administration of therapy on the basis of hemodynamic response (see Fig. 1). Patients with rupture of the ventricular septum demonstrate a "step-up" in oxygen saturation in blood samples drawn from the right ventricle or pulmonary artery compared to those taken from the right atrium. Patients also need urgent assessment with cardiac catheterization and angiography. Particularly, coronary angiography is desirable since revascularization appears to help in a successful outcome. Prognosis is improved appreciably with replacement of the mitral valve.

Mitral regurgitation may also be due to annular dilation associated with progressive left ventricular failure in patients with extensive myocardial infarction. This type of regurgitation rarely needs surgical correction.

Ventricular Septal Defect. Rupture of the ventricular septum is seen in approximately 2 per cent of hospitalized patients with acute myocardial infarction. It accounts for 5 per cent of postinfarction deaths. Development of a communication between the left and right ventricles carries a very high mortality. Ninety per cent of patients die within the first year if reconstruction of the defect is not undertaken. It commonly occurs within the first week of myocardial infarction, and in 85 per cent of patients it is associated with a first infarction. Ventricular septal rupture is accompanied by sudden hemodynamic deterioration and cardiogenic shock in 50 per cent of patients. Up to one third of patients have some degree of associated mitral regurgitation. Patients require immediate diagnosis with pulmonary artery catheterization and ventricular angiography. Management is based on inotropic and vasodilator therapy supported by intra-aortic balloon counterpulsation (see Fig. 1). Traditionally, patients were stabilized on medical therapy, and reconstruction was attempted 2 to 3 weeks after acute myocardial infarction. However, a significant mortality within the first 2 weeks has necessitated a review of the timing of surgical intervention. It appears that patients with ventricular septal defect, despite initial stabilization by pharmacologic and mechanical support, should undergo surgical repair soon after rupture. Survival depends upon the presence or absence of shock. Only 28 per cent of patients survive if rupture is accompanied by shock; however, 80 per cent of patients survive if there are no signs or symptoms of shock.

Left Ventricular Aneurysm. Depending upon the type of study, clinical or autopsy, left ventricular aneurysm has been shown to develop in 4 to 38 per cent of patients who have sustained a substantial infarction. The functional abnormalities produced by the aneurysm depend upon its size, location, and compliance characteristics. If more than a quarter of the left ventricular area is involved in the aneurysm, the compensatory increase in the contractility of the residual myocardium as well as ventricular dilation fails to maintain forward output, and clinical heart failure sets in. Stroke volume is further depressed if a portion of the output is dissipated into a compliant, noncontractile area during systole.

In the majority of the patients, the symptoms produced by an aneurysm can be controlled by conventional measures. However, patients with severe hemodynamic impairment benefit considerably from surgical reconstruction of the left ventricle. Follow-up studies have confirmed that there is usually a dramatic improvement in the functional capacity. Careful preoperative assessment of left ventricular functional reserve is desirable, since it appears that successful operative outcome is dependent on the function of the residual contractile segment of the ventricle. Impaired ejection fraction of the contractile segment (less than 38 per cent) predicts a poor functional result. Patients with a large left ventricular aneurysm and echocardiographically documented clot should be started on long-term anticoagulant therapy.

Recurrent Ischemia with Diastolic Dysfunction. Coronary artery disease alters the diastolic properties of the left ventricle by increasing stiffness of the ventricular wall, resulting in elevated end-diastolic pressures at a relatively normal volume with maintenance of normal pumping performance. During active ischemia, compliance may be reduced further, because of additional stiffening of the heart. Acute changes are likely caused in part by impaired relaxation of the myocardium.

The symptoms and signs resulting from abnormally high left ventricular end-diastolic pressure include shortness of breath due to a rise in pulmonary venous pressure. In severe cases, dyspnea may be present at rest or may result in pulmonary edema. Physical examination is usually normal, although a fourth heart sound may be heard. A third heart sound is heard in rare cases. Chest x-ray films show a normal heart size even in the presence of pulmonary edema. The left atrium may be enlarged. An echocardiogram will show normal or relatively normal left ventricular size and systolic function. Cardiac catheterization reveals elevated left ventricular end-diastolic pressure with normal end-diastolic volume. Left ventricular angiography shows near normal ejection fraction with mild degree of global hypokinesis.

Systolic heart failure, chronic pulmonary disease, and restrictive heart diseases (cardiomyopathy, constrictive pericarditis) should be considered in the differential diagnosis in patients complaining of dyspnea. In patients presenting with pulmonary edema, other causes of pulmonary edema should be excluded.

Since small changes in volume can either cause pulmonary congestion or edema or decrease stroke volume, meticulous attention should be given to the fluid status. Sodium restriction, diuretics, and nitrates are useful to reduce volume. Volume expansion may be required in volume-depleted patients.

Atrial transport function is critical in patients with a stiff left ventricle. Onset of atrial fibrillation is associated with a catastrophic fall in stroke volume. Restoration to sinus rhythm should be considered a priority. Depending upon the urgency, this may be done with quinidine or electrical cardioversion.

Therapy should also be directed toward preventing or improving ischemia through the use of nitrates, beta-adrenergic receptor antagonists and calcium channel blockers (Tables 5 through 7). Transluminal coronary angioplasty and surgical revascularization should also be considered. Left ventricular compliance has been shown to normalize after coronary artery bypass surgery for symptomatic coronary artery disease.

Right Ventricular Infarction. A characteristic clin-

TABLE 6. **Slow Calcium Channel Blockers***

Characteristic	Nifedipine (Procardia)	Diltiazem (Cardizem)	Verapamil (Calan, Isoptin)
Dose	Oral start 10 mg q 8 hr, maximum 30 mg q 8 hr Sublingual 10–20 mg	Oral start 30–60 mg q 6 hr, maximum 90 mg q 6 hr	Oral start 80 mg q 8 hr, maximum 160 mg q 8 hr IV 2.5 mg/min, maximum 20 mg
Coronary blood flow	↑ ↑ ↑	↑ ↑	↑
Peripheral dilatation	↑ ↑ ↑	↑ ↑	↑
A-V conduction	0	↓	↓ ↓
Contractility	0	0	↓ (Especially in patients with pre-existent LV dysfunction)
Sinus automaticity	0 or ↓	↓	↓
GI tract absorption (%)	>90	>90	>90
Bioavailability (%)	65–85	<30	<30
Onset of action (min.)	<20 (sublingual 3–5)	<30	<30
Therapeutic concentration (ng/ml)	25–100	15–100	30–130
Half-life			
Alpha (min)	150	15–30	20
Beta (hr)	5	3–7	4
Protein binding (%)	90	90	90
Metabolism	Inert, free acid, lactone	Extensive first pass liver extraction, 70%	Deacetylation
Elimination			
Renal	80	70	35
Fecal	<15	<15	65
Indications	Angina: stable, unstable, vasospastic	Angina: stable, unstable, vasospastic	SVT: drug of choice (IV), angina
Adverse effects	Headaches, flushing, hypotension, dizziness, peripheral edema, GI upset, accentuation of angina, hypokalemia	Headaches, dizziness, occasionally elevation of transaminases	Dizziness, peripheral edema, flushing, bradycardia, AV conduction, heart failure, hypotension, constipation
Drug interaction	Avoid combining with vasodilators	Beta blockers (watch for conduction abnormalities)	Beta blockers, never give IV to patients taking beta blockers
Contraindications	Relative: severe heart failure, hypotension	Severe bradycardia, AV block, sick sinus syndrome, heart failure (relative), hypotension	Same as for diltiazem

* ↓ Transmembrane calcium influx during plateau phase of myocardial action potential; individual drugs may act at different membrane sites; Class IV antiarrhythmic agents; ineffective in ventricular arrhythmias.

Abbreviations: ↑ = increased or prolonged; ↓ = decreased or shortened; LV = left ventricular; GI = gastrointestinal; AV = atrioventricular; IV = intravenous.

ical and hemodynamic picture accompanies right ventricular involvement in patients with inferoposterior wall infarction. Clinical features include a positive Kussmaul sign (inspiratory rise in jugular venous pressure), elevation of jugular venous pressure, right ventricular gallop sounds, and pulsus paradoxus (fall of greater than 10 mmHg in systemic systolic pressure on inspiration) with or without hypotension. Increased pressure in the vena cava may lead to pulsatile liver. Hemodynamic measurements demonstrate elevated mean right atrial pressure with preserved Y descent, reduced systolic and elevated diastolic pressure in the right ventricle with diastolic pressure showing an early dip followed by a plateau (square-root sign), normal or near normal pulmonary wedge pressure, reduced mean systemic arterial pressure, inspiratory fall of greater than 10 mmHg in systemic arterial pressure, and depressed cardiac output. Chest x-ray films show clear lung fields. Radionuclide angiography reveals a markedly reduced right ventricular ejection fraction. Differential diagnosis includes pulmonary embolism and cor pulmonale identified by clinical features and elevated pulmonary artery pressure. Pericardial tamponade is excluded by echocardiography and also by normal pulmonary wedge pressure in the case of right ventricular infarction.

Patients with extensive right ventricular infarction can present with symptoms and signs of shock. Volume expansion and judicious use of inotropes (dobutamine) have greatly improved the prognosis, with a 60 per cent survival rate. Nitrates and diuretics should be avoided at all costs.

TABLE 7. Pharmacologic Agents Used in Treatment of Heart Failure

Route of Administration	Hemodynamic Effects CI	PWP	SVR	Dose	Onset of Action	Duration of Action	Indications	Remarks and Adverse Effects
Direct Smooth Muscle Relaxants								
Nitrates								
Sublingual	→↓	↓	↓	0.4–0.8 mg	2–5 min	10–30 min	TO REDUCE PRELOAD	Headaches sometimes debilitating, dizziness, nausea, syncope, occasionally paradoxical bradycardia & hypotension in acute myocardial infarction (empty-heart syndrome)
Buccal	—	↓	↓	3–5 mg	1–5 min	4–6 hr	Acute myocardial infarction: Nitrates may be preferable to diuretics	Methemoglobinemia
Topical 2%	—	↓	—	½–2"	35–60 min	4–8 hr	Chronic heart failure with pulmonary congestion in combination with hydralazine	Tolerance can develop
Inhalation	—	↓	↓	0.4 mg/puff	1–5 min	10–30 min		*Avoid in:* Right ventricular infarction, in significant diastolic dysfunction, hypertrophic cardiomyopathy, hypovolemia
Oral (isosorbide dinitrate)	↑→	↓		10–40 mg qid	15–30 min	120–180 min		Pericardial effusion or constriction, glaucoma
Intravenous	→↑	↓	↓	3–10 mg/hr by infusion	1 min	Continuous titration		Increased intracranial pressure
Nitro discs	↓	↓	↓	10–20 mg	30–60	Up to 24 hr		*Give IV NTG* by infusion pump using polyethylene tubing. Polyvinyl chloride tubing adsorbs up to 80% of NTG
								Skin irritation with topical prep
Nitroprusside								
Intravenous	↑↑	↓	↓	50 mg in 500 ml 5% dextrose = 100 µg/ml; 0.05–5 µg/kg/min; 0.005–0.05 ml/kg/min. Wrap in aluminum foil (protect from light). Avoid extravasation	1–2 min	Continuous titration	Acute myocardial infarction with pulmonary edema and normal BP; Chronic heart failure (Acute exacerbation)	Accumulation of thiosulfates, increase in renal insufficiency. Blood thiosulfate level should not exceed 6 mg/100 ml. *Thiosulfate toxicity:* Psychosis, convulsions, hypothyroidism, muscle twitching, abdominal pain, dizziness. Methemoglobinemia, Vitamin B$_{12}$ deficiency
Hydralazine								
Oral	↑→	↓	↓↓	100–300 mg	15–30 min	4–6 hr	Afterload reducing agent In low cardiac output states with normal blood pressure may combine with nitrates	Vascular headaches, flushing, nausea, vomiting, drug fever, skin rash, positive ANF. Drug-induced SLE (usually over 400 mg/day, slow acetylators). Pyridoxin deficiency
Intravenous	↑→	↑	↓	10–20 mg	10–15 min	3–4 hr		
Alpha-Adrenergic Blocking Agents								
Phentolamine								
Intravenous	↑↑	↓	↓	0.3–2 mg/min by IV infusion	1 min	Titrated	Refractory congestive heart failure *Pulmonary edema*	Hypotension, tachycardia, nausea, vomiting, abdominal pain

Drug	Route	CI	SVR	PWP	Dose	Onset	Duration	Indications	Side Effects
Prazosin	Oral	↑↑	↓↓	↓↓	1–10 mg bid	30 min	6 hr	Chronic congestive heart failure requiring balanced dilation. May have acute arrhythmic effect	"First dose phenomenon"—faintness, dizziness, palpitation, and, rarely, syncope after first dose. Transient rashes, dry mouth, mental depression, polyarthralgia. Salt and water retention with chronic treatment due to activation of renin-angiotensin axis requires increase in diuretic dose

Beta-Adrenergic Receptor Agonists

Drug	Route	CI	SVR	PWP	Dose	Onset	Duration	Indications	Side Effects
Dopamine	Intravenous infusion low dose	↑↑	—	↓	2.5–5 µg/kg/min	1 min	Titrated	Normotensive cardiac failure combined with dobutamine	Cardiac arrhythmias, gangrene of digits in patients with peripheral vascular disease (seen on high-dose dopamine)
	high dose	↑↑	↑↑	—	5–15 µg/kg/min	1 min	Titrated	Hypotension combined with nitroprusside	
Dobutamine	Intravenous	↑↑	↓	↓	5–15 µg/kg/min	Immediate 30–45 min	Titrated	Dilated cardiomyopathy	Cardiac arrhythmias, hypokalemia (from B₂ stimulation)
Salbutamol	Oral	↑↑	↓	↓	2–4 mg tid		6 hr		
Pirbuterol*	Oral	↑↑	↓	↓	20 mg tid			Associated with CPOD	Tachycardia, tremor, rarely diabetic ketoacidosis

Converting Enzyme Inhibitors

Drug	Route	CI	SVR	PWP	Dose	Onset	Duration	Indications	Side Effects
Captopril	Oral	↑↑	↓	↓	12.5–50 mg tid	30–45 min	4–6 hr	Low output chronic failure	Hypotension, proteinuria, skin rashes, loss of taste, rarely worsening of renal function in preexisting renal disease, pancytopenia (in patients with collagen vascular disease)
Enalapril	Oral	↑↑	↓	↓	2.5–20 mg/day	60 min	24 hr	Low output chronic failure	Hypotension, hyperkalemia, angioedema, syncope, palpitations. Insomnia, nervousness, abdominal pain, dyspepsia

Phosphodiesterase III Inhibitors

Drug	Route	CI	SVR	PWP	Dose	Onset	Duration	Indications	Side Effects
Amrinone	Intravenous	↑↑	↓	↓	0.75–1.5 mg/kg bolus in 3–5 min. 0.75 mg/kg 2nd bolus in 15–30 min. Maintenance infusion 5–10 µg/kg/min	5–10 min	Continuous titration	Low output chronic failure. Acute myocardial infarction	Nausea, vomiting, diarrhea, anorexia 0.5–2%. Thrombocytopenia 2.4%, hypotension. Liver function abnormalities. Increase in ventricular ectopic activity. Can be used in combination with dobutamine, nitrates, and nitroprusside

*Investigational drug.

Abbreviations: CI = cardiac index; PWP = pulmonary wedge pressure; SVR = systemic vascular resistance; ↓ = reduced; ↓↓ = markedly reduced; ↑ = increased; ↑↑ = markedly increased; — = no effect.

Reprinted by permission from Majid PA, Roberts R: Treatment of heart failure. *In* Civetta JM, Kirby RR, Taylor RW (eds.): Intensive and Critical Care. Philadelphia, J. B. Lippincott, 1987.

Cardiogenic Shock. Cardiogenic shock results directly from severely impaired left ventricular function due to loss of a critical muscle mass or following development of mechanical complications (acute mitral regurgitation, ventricular septal rupture, rupture of the free wall of the left ventricle, ventricular aneurysm with systolic bulging) in patients with AMI. The severity of the hemodynamic impairment is directly related to the total amount of myocardial damage, and the development of shock syndrome has been correlated with the loss of 40 per cent or more of left ventricular myocardium. The amount of ventricular damage associated with shock represents a cumulative loss of myocardium. The syndrome may be precipitated by a small infarction in patients with prior myocardial infarction or by a single massive infarction. Repeated extension of a previously uncomplicated infarction may also lead to cardiogenic shock.

The primary problem of shock syndrome is inadequate tissue blood flow. Blood flow depends not only on pressure, but also on vascular resistance. The blood flow may be diminished to below critical levels required for viability of the tissues at a time when arterial pressure is maintained by an increase in total systemic resistance. Thus, shock syndrome can be seen without severe hypotension. Shock syndrome is clinically recognized by a peak systolic blood pressure of less than 90 mmHg or 30 to 40 mmHg below the previous baseline level; a urine output of less than 20 ml per hour; cool, clammy skin; obtunded mentation, confusion, agitation, or coma; and persistence of shock after correction of nonmyocardial factors contributing to hypotension and low cardiac output (acidosis, hypoxemia, tachyarrhythmias, bradyarrhythmias, conduction disorders, AV asynchrony, hypovolemia, severe pain with vasovagal reaction, cardiac tamponade due to insertion of a pacemaker catheter, acute pulmonary embolism in bedridden patients, cardiovascular drugs such as antiarrhythmic agents with negative inotropic properties, beta-adrenergic blockers, vasodilators, anesthetic agents, and barbiturates). A detailed discussion of the pathogenesis of shock is beyond the scope of this chapter. Cardiogenic shock is a rapidly progressive syndrome of left ventricular dysfunction and peripheral circulatory failure. It is the leading cause of death in patients admitted with AMI. Despite aggressive medical therapy combined with mechanical circulatory support, the mortality remains high (greater than 70 per cent) even in patients with mechanical lesions that are amenable to correction by surgery.

Management of cardiogenic shock is as follows.

1. The patient should be placed in a horizontal position with his or her legs slightly elevated to increase venous return.

2. In the presence of severe hypotension, inotropic vasoconstrictive drugs, dopamine or norepinephrine, should be administered intravenously while the patient is being clinically evaluated and the arterial and pulmonary artery catheters are inserted. Continuous infusion of a minimal dose required to maintain a palpable pulse should be given until intra-arterial blood pressure measurements are obtained.

3. A 12-lead electrocardiogram should be done immediately followed by continuous electrocardiographic monitoring. Arrhythmias contributing significantly to shock syndrome, such as ventricular tachycardia, atrial fibrillation, and supraventricular tachycardia, should be treated with immediate cardioversion. Severe bradycardias due to vagotonia may be treated by intravenous atropine at the first instance. Transvenous ventricular pacing or, preferably, AV sequential pacing should be established in patients wtih persistent bradycardia, AV block, or AV asynchrony.

4. An adequate airway should be established with efficient ventilation and oxygenation; 100 per cent oxygen is given by nasal prongs or mask to maintain arterial P_{O_2} at about 70 mmHg. In a significant number of patients, endotracheal intubation and mechanical ventilation are required to maintain adequate oxygenation and reduce the work of breathing.

5. Morphine, 2 to 4 mg intravenously every 3 to 5 minutes, should be used to maintain effective analgesia.

6. After insertion of an intra-arterial line and pulmonary artery catheter, both pharmacologic and mechanical maneuvers are used in an attempt to optimize hemodynamics. Mechanical support is provided by intra-aortic balloon counterpulsation (IABP). Drugs that raise systemic vascular resistance and augment contractility are usually necessary to maintain adequate coronary perfusion pressure. Norepinephrine and dopamine are used for this purpose. Norepinephrine increases cardiac contractility and constricts arteriolar and venous beds. At low doses, the central effect predominates and cardiac output and blood pressure are increased. At high doses, severe peripheral vasoconstriction leads to a fall in cardiac output due to increase in afterload. Norepinephrine, in a dose of 2 to 10 micrograms per minute, should be administered through an indwelling catheter to avoid extravasation into the subcutaneous tissues; 4 mg of norepinephrine are added to a liter of 5 per cent dextrose. The use of dopamine has been described elsewhere (see Table 7). The possible role of dobutamine (Dobutrex)

and amrinone (Inocor) in the treatment of cardiogenic shock is not clear and needs further investigation.

7. The exact role of vasodilators in the management of cardiogenic shock remains controversial. Some reports have demonstrated hemodynamic improvement in cardiogenic shock in the absence of severe hypotension and when systemic vascular resistance and left ventricular filling pressures are elevated. In addition, afterload reduction has been of benefit in treating cardiogenic shock associated with severe mitral regurgitation or ventricular septal rupture when regurgitation or shunt are reduced respectively with attendant enhancement of cardiac output. Sodium nitroprusside (Nipride) or phentolamine infusion is utilized to reduce systemic vascular resistance. The dose is titrated so that systemic blood pressure does not fall more than 10 mmHg or below 80 to 90 mmHg systolic. Vasodilators are contraindicated in the presence of severe hypotension.

8. Nonmyocardial factors contributing to the impairment of cardiac function already enumerated should be actively sought for. These factors are important because they are usually amenable to therapy, and prompt correction may prevent further progression of shock syndrome. The most important factors in this respect are hypovolemia and arrhythmias. It should be remembered that optimal left ventricular filling pressure to maintain forward output in AMI is between 18 to 20 mmHg. Minor changes in filling pressures may profoundly affect the cardiac output.

9. Disruption of the ventricular septum or acute mitral valve regurgitation may be responsible for precipitating the shock state. Early diagnosis is important since the patient may respond to aggressive medical and surgical intervention. Cardiac catheterization and coronary angiography should be carried out in practically all cases of cardiogenic shock to exclude potentially correctable lesions and, possibly, for surgical revascularization.

10. As indicated previously, the mortality associated with cardiogenic shock is exceedingly high (greater than 90 per cent). It would appear that any reduction in mortality associated with acute myocardial infarction will require therapy that limits infarct size and prevents development of cardiogenic shock. Myocardial reperfusion can be rapidly and safely achieved by thrombolytic therapy. Coronary angioplasty may also contribute to reperfusion of ischemic myocardium and prevent reocclusion. Experience with these forms of therapy has indicated a beneficial effect on left ventricular function and survival. Indeed, there are anecdotal reports of reversion of shock state in some patients treated with thrombolytic therapy within the first few hours after onset of AMI. The impact of early reperfusion on the incidence of cardiogenic shock remains to be established.

11. When predominantly right ventricular infarction occurs in the setting of acute inferior myocardial infarction, the ability of the right ventricle to maintain adequate filling pressure is impaired. Recognition of this entity contributing to cardiogenic shock is important, since careful volume expansion to enhance left ventricular filling leads to improvement in left ventricular performance and survival.

12. The rupture of the ventricular free wall is usually fatal unless recognized immediately. It occurs in up to 10 per cent of patients dying in the hospital from acute myocardial infarction. It occurs four times more frequently in women than men, seven times more frequently in the left ventricle than in the right ventricle, and is associated with large transmural infarctions. Peak incidence is 3 to 5 days after infarction (range, 1 day to 3 weeks) and is more common in hypertensive patients. The clinical picture is usually characterized by a sudden onset of pain, hypotension, signs of pericardial tamponade, a new ST segment elevation on electrocardiogram, and rapid development of electromechanical dissociation. Urgent periocardiocentesis followed by surgical correction has resulted in salvage of a few patients with rupture of ventricular free wall.

Therapeutic approaches designed to *treat heart failure* are based on improving the four determinants of cardiac performance (preload, afterload, contractility, and heart rate) in a manner so as to allow the failing heart to deliver a normal or near normal cardiac output (see Fig. 1 and Tables 5 through 8).

SPECIFIC THERAPY

Inotropic Drugs

Digitalis Glycosides

Current evidence supports the view that digitalis glycosides have no well-defined role in the management of acute myocardial infarction, except in cases of congestive heart failure or supraventricular rhythm disturbances.

Digoxin, derived from the *Digitalis lanata* leaf, is the most commonly used preparation clinically. For adults, in the absence of conditions that may increase sensitivity to digoxin (hypokalemia; renal insufficiency; concomitant antiarrhythmic medication with quinidine, amiodarone, or calcium channel blockers; cardiogenic shock; hypothyroidism; advanced age; hypoxemia associated with pulmonary disease), the total loading dose should not exceed 0.5 to 1 mg. It may be given rapidly; 0.75 to 1 mg is given by slow intravenous injections, for example, in cases of atrial fibrillation with fast ventricular response. Additional doses up to 0.25 to 0.50 mg may be needed, or 0.75 to 1.5 mg of digoxin in 250 ml of 5 per cent dextrose may be given by infusion over a period of 2 hours. The loading dose may also be given slowly; 0.5 to 1 mg of digoxin is administered orally followed by 0.25 mg twice daily or 0.25 mg twice daily for 1 week. Serum digoxin levels are routinely obtained. Normal levels are 1 to 2 ng per ml determined 6 hours after the last dose of digoxin was given. Values greater than 2 ng per ml are normally associated with toxic manifestations, although lower levels do not exclude toxicity in the presence of conditions that increase sensitivity to digoxin. Particular attention should be paid to hypokalemia. Irrespective of the serum digoxin levels, digoxin should be discontinued temporarily if potassium levels are less than 2.5 mEq per liter. There is no correlation between serum digoxin levels and the therapeutic response to the drug.

A close therapeutic to toxic ratio renders patients sensitive to the development of adverse manifestations. Toxic symptoms include anorexia; nausea and vomiting; disorientation; confusion; delirium; insomnia, particularly in the elderly; seizures; and visual symptoms such as scotomas, blue-green-yellow vision, and halos. Toxic effects of digoxin can present with every known form of arrhythmia. These include ventricular bigeminy or trigeminy, paroxysmal atrial tachycardia with variable block, multifocal ventricular premature beats, AV junctional escape rhythms, ventricular tachycardia and fibrillation, or AV block. Digitalis toxicity should be treated by discontinuation of the drug, specific therapy for hypokalemia and life-threatening arrhythmias, and identification of factors that may increase sensitivity to Digoxin. Cardiac glycoside-specific antibodies may prove to be the most specific treatment for advanced life-threatening digitalis toxicity in patients who fail to respond to conventional measures. Purified digoxin-specific Fab fragments have recently been approved for clinical use.

Other Inotropic Agents

In an effort to develop new inotropic agents, a number of drugs have been introduced clinically or are under investigation at present. However, none of the tested drugs has achieved universal acceptance except for two sympathomimetic amines, dopamine and dobutamine, and a phosphodiesterase inhibitor, amrinone. All three can be used by the intravenous route only.

Dopamine. Dopamine is a catecholamine that stimulates myocardial contractility by acting directly on beta$_1$-adrenergic receptors of the myocardium and indirectly by releasing norepinephrine from sympathetic nerve terminals. Dopaminergic receptor stimulation causes renal, mesenteric, coronary, and cerebral vasodilation. Vasodilation is also observed in innervated skeletal muscle vascular beds. Peripheral vasodilation is only observed at low dose levels (2 to 5 micrograms per kg per minute). At high doses (5 to 10 micrograms per kg per minute), dopamine causes vasoconstriction of arteries and veins of all vascular beds probably through a combined action on alpha-adrenergic, serotonin, and tryptamine sensitive receptors. At low doses, dopamine causes increase in cardiac output and renal blood flow with little change in heart rate or systemic vascular resistance. At high doses arterial pressure, systemic vascular resistance, and heart rate increase. Renal blood flow may fall.

Dobutamine (Dobutrex). Dobutamine is a synthetic sympathomimetic amine that has high affinity for beta$_1$- and alpha$_1$-receptors and a weak affinity for alpha$_2$- and beta$_2$-receptors. Dobutamine increases contractility without causing tachycardia or an increase in peripheral vascular resistance. It does not alter renal blood flow but does cause a redistribution of cardiac output in favor of coronary and skeletal muscle beds over the mesenteric and renal vascular beds. In patients with heart failure, dobutamine increases cardiac output and decreases left ventricular filling pressure without a major change in heart rate or blood pressure. Several studies have demonstrated the superior value of dobutamine over dopamine in the treatment of patients with severe congestive heart failure.

In normotensive patients with severe congestive heart failure, dobutamine in a dose of 5 to 15 micrograms per kg per minute may be given by infusion under hemodynamic monitoring.

Dopamine at low dose levels (2.5 to 5 micrograms per kg per minute) may be added to improve renal blood flow and increase diuresis. Dopamine at high doses is not needed in patients with heart failure unless it is accompanied by shock.

Adverse effects of dopamine and dobutamine include ventricular arrhythmias and precipitation of angina pectoris in patients with coronary artery disease. Intense vasoconstriction by dopamine may cause gangrene of the digits in the patients with pre-existing peripheral vascular disease. Rapid development of tolerance, usually within the first 72 hours, occurs after dobutamine infusion.

Amrinone (Inocor). Amrinone is a bipyridine

that, through its inhibition of phosphodiesterase fraction III, augments myocardial contractility and smooth muscle relaxation in vitro and vivo. It increases cardiac output and reduces filling pressure and systemic vascular resistance in patients with severe heart failure. Heart rate and blood pressure usually do not change.

Amrinone is used in severe congestive heart failure refractory to conventional treatment with Digoxin, diuretics, and oral vasodilators in patients requiring temporary inotropic support and in acute heart failure associated with myocardial infarction to reduce pulmonary vascular pressure and improve cardiac output.

Amrinone, although available in oral formulation, is approved only for intravenous use. A bolus of 0.75 to 1.5 mg per kg is given over 3 to 5 minutes followed by an additional bolus of 0.75 mg per kg in 15 to 30 minutes and a maintenance infusion of 5 to 10 micrograms per kg per minute. A maximum dose of 18 mg per 24 hours is recommended. Alternatively, 40 micrograms per kg per minute for 1 hour followed by 10 micrograms per kg per minute as maintenance infusion may be used.

Adverse effects of amrinone include nausea and vomiting in 0.5 to 2 per cent of patients and thrombocytopenia in 2.4 per cent; hypotension and fever rarely occur. Ventricular arrhythmogenicity may increase.

Diuretics

Diuretic drugs are by far the most commonly used agents in acute and chronic heart failure (Table 8). Diuretics reduce venous return that appears to be closely related to associated diuresis, although venodilatation has been suggested as an additional mechanism influencing acute administration of potent diuretics such as furosemide (Lasix). The overall hemodynamic effect is a reduction in filling pressure without any improvement in cardiac output. In fact, the latter may decline in patients with acute heart failure. The most commonly used diuretic drugs in heart failure are the so-called loop diuretics (furosemide and ethacrynic acid) because of their rapid onset of action, high potency, ability to induce diuresis in clinical situations when renal blood flow is markedly reduced, and ability to reverse shunting of blood from cortical to juxtamedullary nephrons that is seen commonly in heart failure. Furosemide (Lasix) and ethacrynic acid (Edecrin) inhibit active chloride reabsorption in the ascending limb of the loop of Henle. Drugs with mechanisms of action different from loop diuretics can have synergistic effects with furosemide and ethacrynic acid. For example, addition of

thiazide diuretics such as metolazone (Zaroxolyn), which inhibits sodium and chloride reabsorption in the distal tubule, greatly enhances diuresis in patients with congestive heart failure. Similarly, potassium-sparing diuretics such as spironolactone (Aldactone), triamterene (Dyrenium), or amiloride (Midamor), ordinarily possessing a weak diuretic action, greatly augment diuresis when combined with thiazide or loop diuretics.

Vasodilators

The introduction of vasodilators has been a major advance in the treatment of severe heart failure. Systemic vasodilator drugs reduce left ventricular afterload, thereby improving cardiac output and decreasing pulmonary venous pressure. Augmentation of pump performance is achieved concomitantly with reduction in myocardial oxygen consumption. A variety of intravenous, oral, sublingual, and topical vasodilator agents are now available, which provide a broad range of hemodynamic effects. They are classified mainly into three groups: those that predominantly dilate veins and hence reduce preload, those that predominantly dilate arterioles and reduce systemic vascular resistance, and those that have a balanced effect on both systemic vascular resistance and venous return (see Table 7).

Direct Smooth Muscle Relaxants

Nitrates. Nitrates are potent dilators of smooth muscle in the walls of veins and arteries. They produce their effects directly, but the exact mechanism is not known. On systemic administration, blood vessels throughout the body take up organic nitrates rapidly. Veins appear to be more selective in their affinity for nitrates, with venodilatation occurring at much lower plasma concentration than arteriolar vasodilatation. The latter is seen only at high plasma concentrations. Nitrates are effective in congestive heart failure, particularly in patients with very high filling pressure and low cardiac output. They lower left ventricular filling pressure without reducing cardiac output. Depending on the preparation used, they may also increase cardiac output in selected cases. There is no significant alteration in nitrate kinetics in patients with heart failure. Tolerance to nitrates has been demonstrated repeatedly in patients with angina pectoris and may also occur in congestive heart failure.

Sodium Nitroprusside. Sodium nitroprusside is probably the most commonly used vasodilator in acute heart failure and in acute exacerbations of chronic heart failure. Sodium nitroprusside re-

TABLE 8. **Diuretics in Heart Failure**

Diuretic	Dose Oral (mg)	Dose IV (mg)	Duration Onset of Action (hr)	Duration Peak Effect (hr)	Site of Action	Adverse Effects
Thiazides						
Chlorothiazide	50–1000	—	1	4 (6–12)†	Distal con- voluted tubule	Hypokalemia, metabolic acidosis, hyperuricemia, hyponatremia Carbohydrate intolerance, hyper- calcemia
Hydrochloro- thiazide	50–100	—	2	4 (>12)	"	Agranulocytosis, thrombocytopenia Pancreatitis, hepatic coma in liver insufficiency
Chlorthalidone	50	—	2	6 (>24)	"	
Metolazone	2.5–5	—	1	2–4 (24–48)	"	
Cyclopenthiazide*	0.5–1	—	1	2–4 (>12)	"	May have synergistic effects with loop diuretics. Metolazone does not reduce renal blood flow and glomerular filtration rate, hence may be particularly suitable
Loop						
Furosemide	40—80	20–80	Oral 1 IV 5 min	Oral 1–2 (6) IV 30 min (1–2)	Loop and ascend- ing limb of Henle	Glucose intolerance, deafness, thrombocytopenia
Ethacrynic acid	50–100	50 in 50 u 5% dextrose or saline	Oral 30 min IV 15 min	Oral 2 hr (6–8) IV 45 min (3)		Synergistic effects with thiazide or potassium-sparing diuretics
Bumetanide	0.5–4	1–2				
Potassium-sparing						
Spironolactone	50–100		2	1–2 days (2–3 days)	Distal con- voluted tubule, collect- ing duct system	Hyperkalemia, gynecomastia, im- potence, diminished libido, do not use in acute or chronic renal failure
Triamterene	50–100		2	6–8 (12–16)	"	Azotemia, muscle cramps, renal calculi, do not combine with in- domethacin
Amiloride	5–10		2	6–8 (12–16)	"	Potassium-sparing diuretics should always be combined with loop diuretics
Carbonic Anhydrase Inhibitor						
Acetazolamide	250 tid for 2–4 days		1	2–4 (8)	Proximal tubule	Metabolic acidosis, hyperchlore- mia, renal calculi Weak diuretic action lasts for 3–4 days. Useful in patients with heart failure who have devel- oped hypochloremic metabolic alkalosis in presence of normal serum potassium

*Not available in the United States.
†Figures in parentheses indicate total duration of action.
Reprinted by permission Majid PA, Roberts R: Treatment of heart failure. *In* Civetta JM, Kirby RR, Taylor RW (eds.): Intensive and Critical Care. Philadelphia, J. B. Lippincott Co., 1987.

laxes vascular smooth muscle both in arteries and veins, producing a balanced arteriolar and venous dilatation. It has no direct action on heart muscle. The mechanism of action is not known. The drug must be given intravenously, and the effects should be carefully monitored with he-modynamic measurements to assess reduction in afterload and to avoid excessive systemic hypotension and reduction of ventricular filling pressure. In experimental animals, nitroprusside infusion with modest reduction in blood pressure produces beneficial effects on regional ischemia.

However, if blood pressure is lowered below normal, poststenotic coronary blood flow is reduced, thereby aggravating myocardial ischemia. Myocardial ischemia may also be produced by coronary arteriolar dilatation in nonischemic areas "stealing" flow from ischemic areas. Coronary arteriolar dilatation is more potent with nitroprusside infusion than with nitroglycerin, which preferentially dilates epicardial arteries.

Tolerance to nitroprusside is not a clinical problem over the relatively short time for which it is used. Nitroprusside infusion is particularly useful in severe heart failure secondary to acute myocardial infarction when associated with acute mitral regurgitation (due to chordal or papillary muscle rupture) or ventricular septal rupture.

Hydralazine. Hydralazine is predominantly an arteriolar vasodilator that can be given orally or intravenously. It increases cardiac output with a relatively mild reduction in left ventricular filling pressure and systemic arterial pressure or increases in heart rate in patients with heart failure. The relatively specific afterload reducing effect may be useful in patients with mitral regurgitation.

Alpha-Adrenergic Agents

Phentolamine. Phentolamine was the first vasodilator used to increase cardiac output in patients with heart failure following myocardial infarction. The drug is an alpha-adrenergic blocking agent that dilates arterioles and veins and acts as a direct relaxant of vascular smooth muscle. It releases cardiac norepinephrine stores and may exert a mild positive inotropic effect. Phentolamine produces less dilatation of the venous capacitance bed, resulting in a smaller reduction in left ventricular preload for a given reduction in afterload.

Prazosin. Prazosin is a potent alpha$_1$-adrenergic receptor antagonist; it also possesses direct smooth muscle relaxing properties due to phosphodiesterase inhibition. It is an orally effective vasodilator, relaxing both veins and arterioles. Tolerance to the drug has been reported and is most likely related to sodium and water retention from activation of the renin-angiotensin system. With appropriate increases in diuretic dose or the addition of an aldosterone antagonist, the patient's sensitivity to prazosin is regained. Care should be taken to initiate the therapy with a low dose, since *first dose phenomenon* may result in symptoms from excessive postural hypotension.

Converting Enzyme Inhibitors

Captopril is the first angiotensin converting enzyme inhibitor for oral administration. The drug acts by blocking the converting enzyme that catalyzes the conversion of inactive angiotensin I to angiotensin II. Other mechanisms, such as increased levels of kinin and prostaglandins, may also contribute to its vasodilator activity. Captopril improves cardiac output and reduces pulmonary vascular pressures in patients with severe heart failure, even if the condition is refractory to other vasodilators. Captopril has become the drug of choice for long-term treatment of severe heart failure. A closely related drug, enalapril, also an angiotensin converting enzyme inhibitor, has been approved for clinical use. Enalapril has a long half-life and is clinically effective in a once-daily dose.

Combination Therapy

Appreciation of the basic pathophysiologic mechanisms involved in the development of heart failure and the broad range of disparate hemodynamic actions offered by vasodilator and inotropic agents allows one to tailor therapy in a particular clinical situation. There is also evidence that various combinations of inotropic and vasodilator agents may have synergistic effects. Drugs with predominantly arteriolar dilator effects may be combined usefully with those that have venodilator effects. Thus, oral administration of hydralazine with isosorbide dinitrate produces a hemodynamic response almost identical to that observed during infusion of sodium nitroprusside. Combined, nitroprusside and dopamine or dobutamine synergistically enhance low cardiac output and decrease raised left ventricular end-diastolic pressure. Amrinone may be combined with hydralazine. A comparison study showed that when given separately, amrinone increased cardiac output by 47 per cent, and hydralazine increased it by 37 per cent. Combining the two resulted in a 65 per cent rise in cardiac output. Similarly, a combination of nitrates and amrinone produced greater diminution of preload than either drug alone. An intriguing synergism may be provided by a combination of the sympathomimetic amine dobutamine and amrinone. Sympathomimetic amines stimulate synthesis of cyclic AMP, and amrinone prevents degradation of cyclic AMP. The increased cyclic AMP concentration catalyzes the reaction that makes calcium available to the contractile elements. Furthermore, dobutamine shunts large quantities of blood to skin and far less to kidneys and the skeletal muscle. On the other hand, amrinone increases flow to the skeletal muscle and to a lesser extent to the kidneys. Thus, vasodilatation seen with the two drugs may be complementary. Preliminary data suggest that two agents may be combined to provide an increased cardiac output without compromising flow to any of the peripheral vascular beds.

Intra-aortic Balloon Counterpulsation

Intra-aortic balloon counterpulsation (IABP) involves passing a catheter-balloon system via one of the femoral arteries and positioning it in the descending aorta just distal to the left subclavian artery. Until recently, the procedure consisted of inserting a graft prosthesis in the femoral artery by direct surgical technique and advancing the balloon through the sidearm of the graft into the aorta. The introduction of a catheter-balloon system suitable for percutaneous insertion by the Seldinger technique has greatly facilitated the insertion of the balloon and appreciably widened the clinical application of the procedure.

The balloon is connected externally to a pneumatic pump, which produces phasic volume changes in the balloon synchronized with the patient's electrocardiogram. Rapid inflation of the balloon during ventricular diastole increases aortic diastolic pressure and augments coronary perfusion pressure. Sudden deflation of the balloon in systole reduces resistance to left ventricular emptying, thereby enhancing cardiac output and reducing myocardial oxygen consumption. Hemodynamic changes generally include a 10 to 20 per cent increase in cardiac output, an unchanged mean aortic pressure (systolic pressure decreased and diastolic pressure increased), a fall in heart rate, and a reduction in myocardial oxygen consumption and ischemia.

The major application of this technique has been in patients with acute left ventricular failure due to acute myocardial infarction (cardiogenic shock). The benefits are seen mostly in patients who have developed surgically correctable mechanical lesions such as ventricular septal defect or acute mitral regurgitation. After the balloon is inserted, the duration of counterpulsation requires constant review, since, in the absence of surgically correctable lesions, it may be impossible to wean the patient off the machine. Application of the technique in the setting of cardiogenic shock also allows use of vasodilator and inotropic agents to aid in improving the hemodynamic status. Counterpulsation is also used in the presence of persistent ischemic pain during the postinfarction state. Favorable effects are reflected in prompt relief of chest pain. Relatively safe performance of cardiac catheterization and angiography is also possible with IABP, so that patients may be evaluated for possible surgical intervention. The IABP has been frequently employed during the perioperative period in patients undergoing cardiac surgery and developing heart failure. The counterpulsation is usually discontinued 24 to 48 hours after operation; in some instances it may be continued for as long as 4 weeks.

Contraindications to IABP include aortic regurgitation, aortic aneurysm, and severe peripheral vascular disease. Tachyarrhythmias or irregular heart rhythms are also relative contraindications. Complications of IABP are infrequent. They include damage or perforation of the aortic wall, ischemia distal to the insertion of the catheter in femoral artery, peripheral arterial embolization, thrombocytopenia, and hemolysis.

POSTINFARCTION CHEST PAIN

Patients with acute myocardial infarction present with the onset of severe retrosternal chest pain at rest described variously as vicelike, oppressive, or burning in character; radiating to one or both arms, neck, jaws, and the back; accompanied frequently by diaphoresis, nausea, or vomiting; unresponsive usually to sublingual nitroglycerin; and needing intravenous morphine or substitutes for complete relief. The pain is due to inflammation and necrosis of the infarcted myocardium and commonly lasts for 12 to 24 hours. In a small number of patients, a mild background discomfort may last for a little longer.

The onset of chest pain after the first 12 to 24 hours should alert the physician to look for other causes of chest pain associated with AMI: pericarditis, postinfarction angina, extension of the infarction, and, rarely, hyperventilation, acute peptic ulcer (stress), and pulmonary embolism.

Pericarditis

Approximately 30 per cent of patients with transmural AMI have evidence of pericarditis, and up to 20 per cent present with pericardial friction rub. The friction rub appears within the first 4 days of infarction in 90 per cent of patients. In rare instances, a rub may be heard up to 2 weeks after infarction. The patient complains of pain, which is characteristically of a constant dull, aching type, worse upon inspiration, motion, and on lying flat or in the lateral position. The pain typically lasts for a number of days. Frequent auscultation is necessary to hear a friction rub, which may be transitory. A pericardial effusion can often be demonstrated by echocardiography. Occasionally pericardial effusion may be large enough to produce a hemodynamic embarrassment. In patients with mild symptoms, no treatment is required. Severe pain commonly responds to aspirin (650 mg every 6 hours) or indomethacin (Indocin, 25 to 50 mg 3 times a day). In rare instances, a rapid response may be obtained to parenteral dexamethasone, 4 to 6 mg given every 12 hours for 48 hours, or methylprednisolone, 40 to 60 mg every 8 hours for 48 hours, followed by indomethacin (Indocin), 25 to 50 mg every 8 hours.

Postmyocardial infarction syndrome (Dressler's syndrome) is an autoimmune pericarditis that occurs in up to 4 per cent of patients, with peak incidence between 2 and 4 weeks after infarction. The patient presents with chest pain, fever, and pericardial friction rub. Chest x-ray films show cardiomegaly and pleural effusions in up to 70 per cent of patients. Electrocardiographic changes consistent with pericarditis are seen. The syndrome is usually self-limited, but corticosteroid therapy hastens resolution. Aspirin and indomethacin are also effective. Rarely, recurrent effusion leads to marked accumulation of fluid and may need tapping. Occasionally a pericardial window may be needed.

Postinfarction Angina

Anginal attacks are common in patients recovering from acute myocardial infarction and usually become apparent within the first 3 months after discharge. However, onset of recurrent, spontaneous attacks while the patient is at rest within 10 days of an AMI require special consideration. There is evidence to suggest that recurrent angina at rest soon after infarction may precede infarct extension and is associated with a poor prognosis. This is particularly common in patients with non–Q wave infarction. In Q wave infarction, two types of angina have been described. One is angina caused by ischemia originating in the infarct region and the other is angina caused by ischemia in areas remote from the initial infarct, which correlates with the presence of severe multivessel coronary artery disease. Mortality after follow-up of about 6 months was 33 per cent in patients with ischemia in the infarct zone and 72 per cent in patients with ischemia at a distance. Survivors had a high incidence of recurrent infarction and unstable angina and an increased need for surgical revascularization. In a small number of patients, recurrent angina may be due to coronary artery spasm.

Ischemic chest pain resembles that of initial infarction but may be less intense. In all patients, a 12-lead electrocardiogram is obtained immediately, followed by administration of sublingual nitroglycerin, 0.4 mg at 5-minute intervals up to a maximum of 3 tablets. If the pain is not re-lieved, 2 to 4 mg of morphine should be administered intravenously and the patient should be transferred (if not already in the CCU) to the coronary care unit for continuous monitoring and management. The patient should receive 100 per cent oxygen at a rate of 2 to 4 liters per minute by mask or nasal prongs. An intravenous line should be established as soon as possible using an 18- to 21-gauge plastic cannula. Blood samples should be drawn for cardiac enzyme studies. A posteroanterior chest x-ray examination should be done as soon as possible. Radiologic signs of mild left heart failure often precede clinical signs and may be responsible for angina at rest. Vital signs (pulse rate, blood pressure, and respiratory rate) should be determined frequently.

If the electrocardiogram shows transient ST segment elevation during episodes of pain, suggesting coronary artery spasm, the patient should be started on one of the calcium blockers (see Table 6), and the dose is rapidly increased until a satisfactory clinical response is obtained. Calcium channel blockers (except verapamil) should also be the drugs of choice in patients with significant left ventricular dysfunction and clinical evidence of left ventricular failure.

It is a common clinical practice to add long-acting nitrates to the therapeutic regimen at this stage (see Table 7). Isosorbide dinitrate (Isordil) is given orally in a dose of 10 to 40 mg every 6 hours. The author prefers not to use nitrates as the first line of treatment. There is abundant evidence that tolerance to nitrates develops rapidly, particularly when large doses of isosorbide dinitrate or other long-acting nitrate preparations are used in treatment of angina pectoris or congestive heart failure. The response to sublingual nitroglycerin is substantially attenuated in patients who are on long-term nitrate therapy. Since sublingual nitroglycerin is a powerful agent to abort an episode of anginal attack, it seems appropriate not to lessen its potency in patients who inevitably are going to experience a few episodes of angina on maximal medical treatment. There is evidence that when isosorbide dinitrate is used intermittently by the sublingual route, one can avoid development of tolerance to a significant degree. It is the author's preference to prescribe isosorbide dinitrate in a dose of 10 to 20 mg sublingually every 6 hours when indicated.

If the electrocardiogram shows varying degrees of ST segment depression, beta-adrenergic blockers (if not already begun after infarction) may be the first line of treatment (see Table 5). These drugs may be combined with calcium channel blockers. Several studies have shown that calcium channel blockers can be safely combined with beta blockers; however, patients on the combination of diltiazem (Cardizem) and beta blockers should be carefully followed for development of conduction abnormalities. It also appears that diltiazem and nifedipine, when combined, have synergistic effects and produce a favorable clinical response when individual therapy fails.

Experimental and clinical studies have shown that platelets may have a significant role to play in the pathogenesis of unstable angina. The interaction between platelets and injured vascular endothelium encourages aggregation of platelets and release of vasoconstrictive substances. Aspirin, a cyclo-oxygenase enzyme inhibitor, reduces platelet adhesion and release of vasoconstrictive substances. Large-scale clinical trials have demonstrated the beneficial effect of aspirin in reducing the incidence of infarction in patients presenting with unstable angina. The dose of aspirin that may be used in unstable angina is a subject of considerable debate. Doses of 80 mg once daily to 325 mg 4 times daily have been suggested. It is probably not necessary to use more than 325 mg of aspirin taken once a day. With this dose, the effects on platelets can be demonstrated up to a period of 10 days. In an occasional patient with variant angina, aspirin may precipitate coronary artery spasm and should be avoided. In all other cases, aspirin should be routinely prescribed.

The status of systemic anticoagulation in the treatment of unstable angina is not clear at present. A few uncontrolled trials have shown a beneficial effect of therapeutic heparinization in unstable angina. Heparin is administered intravenously as a 10,000 unit bolus followed by an infusion of 800 to 1000 units per hour. Partial thromboplastin time is adjusted at 1.5 to 2 times the normal. Heparin is continued until there is relief of symptoms. Cardiac catheterization is carried out at this stage to delineate the coronary anatomy.

Over half the patients respond to medical treatment and become asymptomatic. It is the author's preference to persist with medical treatment in asymptomatic patients with electrocardiographic evidence of ischemia confined to the infarct zone and a negative predischarge submaximal exercise test. However, coronary angiography is recommended in asymptomatic patients with electrocardiographic evidence of ischemia in leads remote from the infarction (suggesting multiple vessel disease) and in those with positive predischarge submaximal exercise test results. The decision to perform coronary artery bypass surgery or coronary angioplasty is made after characterization of coronary anatomy.

In the initial assessment of patients with post-infarction angina, it is important to look for other factors that may be responsible for precipitation of ischemic chest pain, such as unsuspected anemia, tachyarrhythmias, undiagnosed hyperthyroidism, or excessive use of bronchodilators containing isoproterenol. These factors should be identified and speedily corrected.

If, in spite of treatment with maximally tolerated doses of beta blockers, calcium channel blockers, or both, symptoms persist, nitroglycerin is administered intravenously, starting at a dose of 3 mg per hour, and the dose is increased until symptoms subside or until the maximal tolerated dose is reached. An arterial line is inserted to monitor blood pressure if it is less than 90 mmHg systolic. Intravenous nitroglycerin is a potent vasodilator of venous capacitance vessels at low doses, and it also dilates peripheral arterioles if high doses are used. Contraindications to the use of intravenous nitroglycerin include hypovolemia, cardiac tamponade or constrictive pericarditis, obstructive cardiomyopathy, aortic stenosis, glaucoma, and increased intracranial pressure. Polyethylene tubing should be used for infusing intravenous nitroglycerin, since up to 80 per cent of the drug binds to polyvinyl chloride sets. The use of infusion pumps is recommended to deliver accurate doses of the drug (see Table 7).

Invasive monitoring is also necessary in case of hemodynamic instability or in the presence of persistent chest pain. Measurement of pressures and cardiac output allows optimization of factors responsible for myocardial oxygen consumption (heart rate, systolic blood pressure, filling pressures) and coronary perfusion pressure (diastolic systemic pressure). The author has also been impressed by the support of circulation provided by utilization of intra-aortic balloon counterpulsation in patients with severe postinfarction angina. Counterpulsation decreases afterload and preload, increases coronary perfusion pressure and blood flow, and improves cardiac performance. It also minimizes the high risk of cardiac catheterization and angiography in this setting. It is recommended that IABP should be used if available.

Cardiac catheterization and angiography are carried out to delineate the coronary anatomy. Recent evidence suggests that approximately one third of patients catheterized within a week or two after infarction have an in situ coronary thrombus that may be operative in sustaining the symptomatic state. Dissolution of the thrombus with intracoronary streptokinase (4000 to 6000 units per minute) leads to the relief of symptoms in a significant number of patients. Indeed, the author has used intracoronary streptokinase in selected patients with excellent results. In patients who have suitable coronary anatomy, revascularization is carried out immediately either by aortocoronary bypass surgery or by coronary angioplasty. Even with an experienced surgeon, surgical risks are slightly higher in this group of patients.

Angina occurring after discharge and up to 3 months after infarction is an independent risk factor for future coronary events. Patients with recurring episodes should be readmitted to the hospital for evaluation and management. The principles follow those described previously.

Infarct Extension

Infarct extension occurs in 10 to 15 per cent of patients admitted with AMI to the coronary care unit; it is indicated by recurrence of severe chest pain at rest that is unresponsive to nitrates and requires narcotic analgesics for complete relief, new electrocardiographic changes superimposed on previous abnormalities, and a second distinct rise in the level of cardiac enzymes in the blood. Infarct extension is frequently preceded by episodes of postinfarction angina. It is possible that aggressive management of postinfarction angina may prevent infarct extension in many cases.

Management of patients with infarct extension follows the principles already enunciated. Infarct extension is common in patients developing cardiogenic shock. In view of the serious prognostic import, patients showing substantial electrocardiographic current of injury should undergo immediate cardiac catheterization and angiography for purposes of intracoronary thrombolytic therapy followed by percutaneous transluminal coronary angioplasty or coronary artery bypass surgery.

Non–Q Wave Myocardial Infarction

Approximately one third of patients admitted to the coronary care unit have non–Q wave myocardial infarction. The incidence is likely to increase with frequent use of thrombolytic therapy, which may result in non–Q wave infarction in the majority of patients treated within the first few hours after onset of pain. Multiple studies have shown that patients with non–Q wave infarction have a better short-term prognosis. However, due to a predilection for recurrent angina and infarction, the morbidity and mortality increases over the long term. The clinical course is complicated by arrhythmias, congestive heart failure, and sudden death. Recent evidence suggests that malignant arrhythmias are more frequent in non–Q wave infarction than in Q wave

infarction. A detailed discussion of the subject is beyond the scope of this chapter. Suffice it to say that patients with non–Q wave infarction represent an unstable group and qualify for an aggressive evaluation and management. Previous studies have highlighted the increased incidence of reinfarction during the initial 2 weeks (peak incidence 10th day) of hospitalization, emphasizing the need for extending clinical observations and monitoring of rhythm, preferably in an intermediate care setting. Because the problems of patients with early reinfarction are significantly worse than those in patients without reinfarction, serial CKMB sampling every 12 hours should be carried out throughout the hospital stay. Patients should receive antianginal therapy, beta blockers, and calcium channel blockers singly or in combination if they suffer from recurrent episodes of angina. Recent evidence indicates that diltiazem (Cardizem) administered orally in a dose up to 90 mg 4 times a day significantly reduces incidence of reinfarction within the first 2 weeks after initial infarction. Whether the cardioprotective effect is unique to diltiazem or applicable to all available calcium channel blockers is not clear at present. Until such time that other calcium channel blockers are evaluated in patients with non–Q wave infarction, diltiazem should be prescribed in the dose described. Patients who have recurrent episodes of postinfarction angina should undergo coronary angiography. In asymptomatic patients, radionuclide ventriculography (to assess ventricular function), submaximal treadmill exercise test with or without thallium scintigraphy (to assess myocardium at risk), and ambulatory electrocardiography (to assess presence or absence of frequent or multiform ventricular ectopic beats and episodes of nonsustained ventricular tachycardia) should be carried out. Patients with mild to moderate left ventricular dysfunction or positive treadmill exercise test for ischemia or both should undergo coronary angiography. Although there are no long-term studies of diltiazem, it is suggested that asymptomatic patients with normal left ventricular function and no provocable ischemia may be discharged on diltiazem (Cardizem), up to 360 mg in divided doses daily either in combination with or without nitrates. If invasive investigations reveal significant left main coronary artery disease or triple-vessel disease with or without depressed left ventricular function, coronary artery bypass surgery should be undertaken. In patients with one- or two-vessel disease, medical therapy may be given as a brief trial. Alternatively, angioplasty of the diseased vessel may be attempted followed by maintenance medical therapy with nitrates and calcium channel blockers.

REHABILITATION AFTER MYOCARDIAL INFARCTION

method of
NANETTE K. WENGER, M.D.
Emory University School of Medicine
Atlanta, Georgia

Conventional medical and surgical therapies for the patient with myocardial infarction are designed to decrease symptoms, enhance functional status, and, at times, improve prognosis. A combination of medical, psychosocial, and behavioral factors appears to determine the extent of recovery. The rehabilitative approach is increasingly incorporated into traditional medical care; interventions are aimed at limiting the adverse physiologic and psychologic consequences of the acute illness and improving long-term physical, emotional, and vocational status. About 20 per cent of the 850,000 annual survivors of myocardial infarction in the United States have some physiologic, psychosocial, or vocational disability. The major components of rehabilitative care include physical activity (early ambulation during the hospital stay and prescriptive exercise training in the ambulatory care phase of the illness) and the provision of information and counseling designed to enhance resumption of a productive, active, and satisfying lifestyle.

Rehabilitative care ideally begins at the onset of illness and remains a component of the long-term management of the patient. This concept highlights the responsibility of the primary physician to initiate, coordinate, and encourage the rehabilitation of patients with myocardial infarction.

The rehabilitative approach to care is designed to reduce the physical and psychosocial invalidism associated with coronary disease. Important aspects of rehabilitation for patients with myocardial infarction involve the behaviors and capacities to favorably alter lifestyles. The acquisition of personal skills, techniques, attitudes, and knowledge derived from participation in physical activity and educational and counseling regimens may enhance the patient's realistic adaptation to illness and ability to cope with challenges and problems in the family, workplace, and community.

THE ACUTE PHASE: REHABILITATIVE CARE

The current shortened hospital stay, particularly for patients with uncomplicated myocardial infarction, has accentuated the need for early ambulation but limited the provision of adequate information and counseling to the coronary patient and interested family members.

Early Ambulation

A goal of early ambulation is to avert the deleterious consequences of protracted bed rest, the most prominent of which is a decrease of up to 25 per cent in physical work capacity after two to three weeks of immobilization, owing to a decrease in maximal cardiac output. Orthostatic hypotension and reflex tachycardia are manifestations of the hypovolemia (a decrease of 700 to 800 ml in circulating blood volume) that can occur after seven to ten days at bed rest. Blood viscosity increases, owing to a greater contraction of plasma volume than of red blood cell mass. This, coupled with circulatory stasis, predisposes to thromboembolic complications. Pulmonary ventilation decreases, as do systemic muscle mass and muscular contractile strength. Inefficient muscular contraction increases the oxygen requirement for any submaximal task.

Most patients who do not have complications of myocardial infarction (recurrent chest pain, serious cardiac rhythm disturbances, congestive heart failure, or cardiogenic shock) can safely perform low-intensity physical activity as early as the first day after infarction. Personal care activities, use of a bedside commode, and sitting in a bedside chair are within the 1 to 2 met level appropriate for coronary care unit activities (1 met = approximately 3.5 ml O_2 per kg body weight per minute). Sitting in a chair two or three times daily is within the physical capability of most patients; the orthostatic challenge seems adequate to prevent the hypovolemia, deterioration of oxygen transport capacity, and effort intolerance. Patients with complications of infarction should have their physical activity delayed until the complications are controlled and their clinical status is stable.

The current early intensive management of myocardial infarction with combinations of thrombolytic therapy, coronary angioplasty, or coronary bypass surgery is designed to salvage myocardium. The relative immobilization attendant on these procedures may evoke the unwanted manifestations of bed rest.

During the remainder of the hospital stay, progressive physical activity is designed to attain a functional level that permits usual household activities (an energy expenditure of 2 to 3 mets) by the time of discharge from the hospital. To accomplish this, patients perform dynamic range of motion warm-up exercises and progressively increase the pace and distance of walking. If stair-climbing is required at home, patients should practice this before leaving the hospital. Electrocardiographic monitoring or telemetry during early ambulation activities is required only for selected patients, such as those with significant cardiac rhythm disturbances or symptomless myocardial ischemia. However, supervision of early ambulation activities is desirable to detect any adverse responses. These may include the development of chest pain, dyspnea, undue fatigue, or palpitations; a heart rate in excess of 120 or below 50 beats per minute (for patients receiving beta blocking drugs, heart rate should increase less than 20 beats per minute above resting level); the occurrence of arrhythmias; ST segment displacement compatible with ischemia; or a fall in systolic blood pressure, which usually reflects ischemic ventricular dysfunction with inadequacy of the cardiac output to meet the demand. Antihypertensive therapy should be considered for an increase in systolic blood pressure above 180 mm Hg. Abnormal responses indicate the need for activity reduction and clinical reassessment. Appropriate responses permit serial progression of activity intensity.

The safety of supervised early ambulation after myocardial infarction is well-documented; complications are not increased. Benefits include limitation of the deconditioning effects of immobilization, as well as decrease in the common emotional responses, anxiety and depression. Early ambulation permits medically determined early discharge because of the improved functional status of the patient, allows for predischarge exercise testing, and is associated in some studies with an earlier return to work.

Predischarge exercise testing can document the functional impact of the episode of myocardial infarction on the patient. An abnormal response to low-level exercise, either sign- or symptom-limited testing or testing to a predefined heart rate, helps identify patients at increased risk of proximate coronary events who require additional or more prompt diagnostic procedures and increased medical or surgical interventions. Patients at increased risk include those with a low exercise capacity (below 4 to 6 mets) and those with angina, ischemic ST segment abnormalities, or hypotension induced at low levels of exercise. Predischarge exercise testing more precisely defines safe activity levels for the minimally impaired patient and may permit earlier return to pre-illness activities, including return to work. Further, it may lessen the common fear of physical exertion after infarction.

Education and Counseling

The goal of this rehabilitative component is to provide the information, motivation, and skills that can help patients assume responsibility for personal health care. Many psychosocial outcomes after infarction appear related to the patient's perception of his or her health status; this may be favorably altered by education and counseling.

The information presented in the coronary care unit is typically a brief explanation of the diagnosis and what is to be anticipated. Orientation to the procedures and equipment, with emphasis on the temporary nature of most restrictions, helps patients adjust to a life-threatening situation.

More detailed information provided during the remainder of the hospitalization enhances the patients' ability to cope with the problems of illness as they begin to plan for returning home. Normal cardiac function, the development of atherosclerotic lesions, and changes of myocardial infarction (emphasizing healing) should be presented as a background for subsequent therapeutic recommendations. Advice is given about resumption of activity (including sexual activity and return to work), smoking cessation, dietary modifications (of fat, sodium, and calories as needed), and control of other coronary risk factors. Recommendations for reduction of conventional coronary risk factors are designed to prevent or retard the progression of atherosclerosis; a multifactorial approach has been reported to reduce the risk of reinfarction. The American Heart Association Step 1 Diet is a reasonable recommendation, with caloric adjustment designed to attain near-ideal body weight. Control of hypertension decreases the risk of cerebrovascular complications as well as decreasing myocardial oxygen demand. Continued cigarette smoking following myocardial infarction increases the risk of reinfarction and coronary death in patients of all ages and decreases their ability to achieve physical fitness.

Since many components of care after infarction entail long-term modifications of lifestyle, education should provide insight into behaviors that may increase the risk of reinfarction and into the value of altering these habits. Acquisition of knowledge appears to favorably affect health-related behaviors. The role of behavior modification as an adjunct to effecting habit change is uncertain, but promising results are described. Similarly, the concept of stress management requires validation before this can be generally recommended. Counseling about return to sexual activity should involve both the patient and spouse, using the guideline that sexual intercourse can be safely resumed when other activities of daily living are reinstituted. In general, asymptomatic post-infarction patients report resumption of sexual activity within eight weeks after infarction, although many symptomatic patients do not resume sexual activity until several months after the acute illness. Patients should be informed about their prescribed medications; purpose, dosage, and potential adverse effects.

Included in the teaching should be the recommended response to recurrent symptoms and how to gain access to emergency medical care; the identification of community resources that may be helpful, such as home-care agencies, counseling and guidance services, vocational rehabilitation organizations, services for financial aid, and post-coronary groups or clubs, should also be provided. Counseling of family members should address the adjustments in lifestyle to be anticipated during convalescence, while emphasizing the importance of averting unnecessary invaliding of the patient.

Inadequate or ambiguous information about coronary disease and its management (including symptoms, prognosis, planned tests or procedures, allowable activities, return to work, and similar factors) has been documented to cause major concern for patients recovering from myocardial infarction. These features should be discussed before discharge from the hospital, as adequate time to address problems and receive information is often not available during subsequent office visits.

The teaching format must be flexible. A group approach often decreases anxiety, aids learning, is economical of professional time, and offers peer support. Involving the patient in planning for recovery helps return control and responsibility to the patient and enhances self-esteem. Audiovisual presentations can also facilitate learning. Written directions and take-home pamphlets and instruction sheets provide a convenient reference for the patient and family and avoid problems related to vague or ambiguous instructions for post-hospital care. Increasingly, technological advances such as home videocassettes and interactive computer educational programs will be used to facilitate the provision of information and guidance to the patient and family.

THE CONVALESCENT OR RECOVERY PHASE

Exercise Regimens

Guidelines for Exercise Prescription and Surveillance

Physical activity during convalescence is designed to improve endurance to a level that permits return to work or appropriate preinfarction activities. Activity regimens may be supervised or unsupervised. Supervised exercise currently is recommended for patients with a low exercise capacity; significantly depressed ventricular function; angina, ischemia, or hypotension that is induced at low levels of exercise; or complex ventricular arrhythmias; or for those who are unable to monitor their heart rate responses to activity. Ideally, even unsupervised exercise should follow a brief period of supervised training during which exercise guidance can be provided. Supervision may increase motivation and reassurance and enables emergency care to be given if needed. As exercise performance and fitness improve, medical supervision can be decreased. Supervised and unsupervised exercise training equally improved the functional capacity of a low-risk patient group after myocardial infarction.

Although fewer complications of exercise had been described in supervised exercise programs with continuous ECG monitoring, it is not known whether ECG monitoring per se, closer medical supervision, or lesser exercise intensity was the major determinant. A more recent survey did not document a significant safety advantage of continuous ECG monitoring; the greater current safety of exercise for coronary patients at least in part relates to risk stratification and newer therapies. In supervised exercise programs without continuous electrocardiographic monitoring, intermittent pulse counting is advised to ascertain that the heart rate response remains within the target heart rate range. Electrocardiographic monitoring need not be an all-or-none phenomenon. An ECG rhythm strip can be intermittently recorded in supervised exercise programs, using the paddles of a defibrillator as ECG leads. Patients exercising without supervision, even at a distance from a rehabilitation program, may use periodic transtelephonic ECG transmission.

Individualized prescriptive exercise is the hallmark of rehabilitative physical activity, whether supervised or unsupervised. The dosage of exercise, determined by its frequency, intensity, and duration, is defined for each patient, as is the type of predominantly dynamic exercise recommended. Exercise test data provide the basis for the prescription of exercise intensity. Age-predicted target heart rates are inappropriate, because heart rate response may be modified by coronary disease, its therapy, the prior state of fitness, or all of these features. During exercise training, patients were previously recommended to attain 70 to 85 per cent of the highest heart rate safely achieved at exercise testing. This corresponds to 57 to 78 per cent of the peak oxygen uptake, a safe yet effective range to stimulate aerobic metabolism and develop endurance. Previously sedentary patients can improve their functional status with activity of lesser intensity.

More recent data show an adequate training effect with a lesser exercise intensity and compensatory increase in exercise duration. The increased comfort of exercise at 60 to 75 per cent of the highest heart rate safely achieved at exercise testing may encourage adherence to the exercise regimen. The lower heart rate ranges offer greater safety with unsupervised exercise. Coronary patients should exercise only within the intensity documented at exercise testing to maintain an acceptable cardiovascular response. Exercise testing performed for exercise prescription requires that patients be tested on an optimal medical regimen, taking all drugs that will be used during training. Exercise training can be accomplished in patients receiving antianginal drugs. Two or three exercise sessions each week are recommended, preferably on nonsuccessive days. Although unfit, sedentary, or older patients may improve their exercise capacity with as few as one or two exercise sessions weekly, more than four exercise periods each week do not significantly increase maximal oxygen uptake. Exercise sessions should be 30 to 40 minutes in duration, including warm-up and cool-down periods. Although a modest increase in the frequency or duration of exercise can compensate for decreased exercise intensity, excessively long or inappropriately frequent exercise sessions engender poorer adherence to training and excessive musculoskeletal complications.

Interval training, alternating periods of high- and low-intensity exercise, is recommended for symptomatic coronary patients to avoid an excessive oxygen debt, an approach that also permits imposition of a greater workload at each session before the occurrence of symptoms. Because the benefits of arm and leg exercise are only moderately interchangeable, both arm and leg training are required. One study identified only 50 to 70 per cent improvement in the untrained as compared with the trained extremity, suggesting that about half of the increase in trained limb performance is due to a generalized training effect and half is due to specific changes in trained skeletal muscle.

Serial exercise testing is recommended with both supervised and unsupervised exercise training to ascertain the effects of training and to revise the exercise prescription as needed to incorporate activities of greater intensity. Documentation of functional improvement also encourages adherence to exercise training.

Supervised Exercise Training

Although the design of a supervised exercise program varies with the number of patients involved, the available space and equipment, and the pattern of electrocardiographic monitoring, certain common features can be recommended.

The initial 5 to 10 minutes of exercise, the warm-up period, includes stretching and range of motion exercises that provide musculoskeletal and cardiorespiratory readiness for exercise. The target heart rate should be attained during the 15- to 20-minute aerobic or endurance component of exercise. This may consist of walk-run sequences or exercise on a stationary bicycle or treadmill. Since these exercises train primarily the leg muscles, arm training exercises using selected calisthenics, rowing machines, and shoulder wheels should be added. In the early weeks of training, the recommended activities are those in which skill contributes little to the intensity of work demand, making the energy costs of exercise more predictable. The final component is a 5- to 10-minute cool-down period during which the gradual decrease in exercise intensity allows the heat load to be dissipated, the heart rate to slow, and the peripheral vasodilation of exercise to subside.

Because long-term supervision of activity is neither necessary nor feasible, most patients who attain a 7 to 8 met level can progress to unsupervised or minimally supervised exercise, usually within three to six months after infarction.

Unsupervised Exercise

Appropriately selected patients can exercise without supervision, but they require detailed instructions to do so safely. Since both economic and logistic problems limit the availability of supervised exercise, the safety and cost-effectiveness of unsupervised exercise are currently under evaluation. Written directions for each patient should include the type of exercise; exercise intensity, duration, and frequency; the target heart rate range and the method of checking it; signs and symptoms of excessive exercise; appropriate clothing and footwear; and other particulars.

Initially, most patients use walking as their major activity, with gradual increases in pace and distance; warm-up exercises should precede the period of walking. Predischarge exercise test results can more precisely guide activity recommendations. For patients whose exercise testing is deferred to several weeks after the hospitalization, the in-hospital guidelines can be used for pulse-monitoring, i.e., a heart rate response below 120 beats per minute or not exceeding 20 beats above resting level for patients taking beta blocking drugs.

Initial home exercise regimens, based on exercise testing, often involve progressive walk-jog sequences or progressive increases in the intensity and duration of exercise on a stationary bicycle.

Appropriate Expectations: Exercise Training

The goal of prescriptive physical activity for the patient recovering from myocardial infarction is an improvement in cardiovascular function. This occurs in addition to the "spontaneous" functional improvement in the early weeks after infarction. Aerobic capacity improves with training, with maximal oxygen uptake increasing by as much as 20 per cent. The enhanced peripheral arteriovenous oxygen extraction by trained muscle and the improved redistribution of cardiac output decrease the demand for oxygen and thus for blood flow. Systemic vascular resistance decreases, and skeletal muscle and autonomic nervous system adaptations decrease the rate-pressure product. These peripheral adaptations appear to be the major factor in improved performance. The training-induced decrease in the heart rate and blood pressure response to submaximal work decreases myocardial oxygen demand. This explains the absent or lessened angina and ischemic ST electrocardiographic changes at any level of submaximal work that increase the patient's ability to perform submaximal tasks before the onset of myocardial ischemia and angina. This allows them to function farther from their ischemic threshold when performing daily activities. Training reduces the myocardial oxygen demand for any body oxygen demand, i.e., it allows a higher level of exercise at a lessened myocardial energy cost. It increases the exercise threshold for angina. Because usual activities require a lesser percentage of the improved physical work capacity, patients describe improved stamina or endurance. Further, the number and dosage of antianginal medications needed may decrease.

In addition to the effect of exercise training in improving physical work capacity, permitting an increased intensity and duration of work, exercise also aids in weight control and favorably affects psychologic status. Serum triglyceride levels decrease with exercise training, and although the effect on total cholesterol level is inconclusive, HDL cholesterol levels increase with training. Glucose utilization improves. Effects on fibrinolysis and platelet function remain controversial. However, participation in an exercise regimen often encourages patients to modify other more powerful coronary risk factors and aids patients in renouncing the sick role and in resuming their pre-illness lifestyle, including return to work.

There is no evidence that exercise training of moderate intensity and duration improves the coronary collateral circulation, alters coronary obstructive lesions, or increases myocardial oxygen supply or intrinsic myocardial performance; nor do the results of clinical trials of exercise training show that exercise significantly alters the outcome (despite the 20 to 30 per cent trend favoring survival in exercising patients in most intervention studies).

Education and Counseling

If the benefits of hospital-based education are to be maintained, the recommendations for care must be reinforced after the patient returns home. The patient's attitudes and beliefs about the importance of therapy influence compliance.

The current decreased length of the hospital stay limits the ability to address many of the patient's and family's needs for information and advice. Continuity of in-hospital and ambulatory education and counseling is requisite in that needs not apparent in the hospital become evident when patients must make decisions about long-term care. Participation in community heart clubs or comparable organizations for coronary patients may encourage modification of risk-related behaviors and aid in reinforcing recommendations for care. Technological advances such as computer-assisted education and counseling and interactive video systems may enable teaching, reinforcement of education, and tracking of accomplishments to be performed at sites distant from a rehabilitation or hospital center—for example, at work, in the home, or in a senior citizen facility.

Recommendations should be made for progressive resumption of occupational, social, recreational, and retirement activities.

THE MAINTENANCE PHASE

For exercise to become a long-term component of lifestyle, a feature necessary to maintain fitness, the activities must be enjoyable, convenient, and typically social. The ultimate goal for most patients is independence in exercising.

Exercise recommendations vary with the patient's needs and goals, general health status and musculoskeletal competence, desired occupational and recreational activities, skills, and likes and dislikes, as well as the accessibility of exercise facilities and availability of exercise equipment.

In supervised or group exercise programs, aerobic games such as volleyball, basketball, handball, and tennis are limited early in exercise training because variations in skill, excitement, and competitiveness vary the oxygen cost of these activities. However, they add variety to an exercise program and improve adherence, as well as providing arm and torso exercise. Alternatively, the initial walk-jog-run sequences in unsupervised or supervised programs can be replaced by endurance activities such as swimming, bicycle riding, skating, rope jumping, rowing, and aerobic dancing.

Serial exercise testing at longer intervals can

document maintenance of improved function and encourage adherence.

As exercise supervision decreases, alternate ways to encourage and monitor risk reduction must be devised, so that necessary reinforcement can be provided to adhere to healthy lifestyles.

PERICARDITIS

method of
NOBLE O. FOWLER, M.D.
Univ. of Cincinnati College of Medicine
Cincinnati, Ohio

Evaluation

The treatment of pericarditis depends upon its symptoms, underlying cause, complications, and anticipated clinical course.

In acute pericarditis, it is important to carry out an etiologic evaluation. The cause may be obvious: for example, septicemia, renal failure, infective endocarditis, metastatic neoplasm, acute myocardial infarction, surgical operation, or trauma. On the other hand, in many cases the cause is not obvious and certain diagnostic evaluations should be carried out. These include evaluation of the history for the use of certain drugs that may cause pericarditis, such as procainamide, phenytoin, hydralazine, anti-coagulants, and anti-neoplastic agents. Evidence of connective tissue disease and of rheumatoid arthritis should be sought. Electrocardiograms should be studied for evidence of myocardial infarction. When clinically indicated, studies for mycoplasmal and antecedent viral disease, especially Coxsackie B virus, should be made. Serological tests for histoplasmosis and skin tests for tuberculosis may be indicated. When rheumatic fever is a possibility, antistreptolysin titer or streptozyme serologic titer evaluation should be carried out. The patient should be evaluated for the possibility of a neoplasm, lymphoma, or leukemia.

Treatment

Acute Nonspecific Pericarditis

Many patients will be found to have nonspecific pericarditis, perhaps the commonest variety of acute pericarditis. In this case, and also for Dressler's postmyocardial infarction syndrome or postpericardiotomy syndrome, treatment is usually limited to hospital observation for possible cardiac tamponade and to relief of pain and fever. Aspirin in doses of 1.0 gram every 4 to 6 hours may be used but is often unsuccessful. Indomethacin (Indocin) in doses of 25 to 50 mg 3 times a day or Ibuprofen (Motrin) 400 to 800 mg 4 times a day may be more successful. Adrenal corticosteroids may be required to treat continued pain

and fever and pericardial effusion that does not respond to the foregoing. We begin with 20 mg prednisone 3 times daily for a few days, gradually decrease the dosage to 20 mg twice daily for a few days, reduce the dosage to 10 mg twice daily for a few days, then to 5 mg twice daily for a few days, and then discontinue the agent. Unfortunately in some patients symptoms recur when the dosage is reduced below 15 mg a day; in these patients, adrenal corticosteroid therapy must be continued for a longer period of time. We try to maintain the long-term dosage of prednisone below 15 mg and preferably below 7.5 mg a day, since complications are unlikely at this dosage.

Pericardiocentesis should not be carried out routinely when there is no cardiac tamponade. Pericardiocentesis is indicated for diagnostic purposes when there is evidence of pericardial effusion with fever and other systemic symptoms for 2 to 3 weeks and no definite etiologic diagnosis has been made. In addition, pericardiocentesis is carried out when there is persistent fever suggesting purulent pericarditis or to relieve cardiac tamponade. Unless there is an emergency, limited pericardial resection with biopsy is probably safer and is to be preferred if thoracic surgeons are available.

Pericarditis with Specific Causes

Drug-related pericarditis is treated by withdrawing the offending agent. If there are persistent symptoms, treatment is as recommended for nonspecific pericarditis.

Infectious pericarditis is treated with appropriate antibiotics. Tuberculous pericarditis is treated with isonicotinic acid hydrazide (Isoniazide), 300 mg daily, and pyridoxine, 50 mg daily for 9 months. Rifampin (Rifadin), 600 mg daily, is the preferred second drug. Some authorities recommend a third drug, e.g., ethambutol (Myambutol), 15 mg per kg daily. If there is purulent pericarditis, additional open pericardial drainage and at times pericardial resection is required. Purulent pericarditis is especially likely following burns and in immunocompromised patients. Uremic pericarditis is treated by more frequent hemodialysis or the substitution of peritoneal dialysis. Adrenal steroid therapy may be indicated, as described in the section on Nonspecific Pericarditis. At times triamcinolone (Aristocort) instillation into the pericardial sac is helpful in the treatment of uremic pericarditis. Pericardial resection may be indicated when there is continuing reaccumulation of pericardial fluid with cardiac tamponade.

Pericarditis associated with connective tissue disease, such as systemic lupus erythematosus, rheumatoid arthritis, and acute rheumatic fever, is treated with adrenal steroids as described in the section on Nonspecific Pericarditis. The rheumatic fever patient additionally is treated with penicillin (e.g., oral Penicillin V, 250 mg 4 times daily for 10 days). Recurrent pericarditis in patients with idiopathic pericarditis, Dressler's postinfarction syndrome, or postpericardiotomy or post-traumatic syndrome is treated as described in the section on Nonspecific Pericarditis. Pericardial resection is reserved for the occasional intractable case.

Pericardiocentesis should be carried out under cardiac monitoring by either an experienced cardiologist or thoracic surgeon, preferably in a hemodynamic laboratory unless there is a life-threatening emergency.

Patients treated for cardiac tamponade are monitored for recurrence of tamponade in a critical care unit or cardiac monitoring unit and are observed for the development of elevated venous pressure and paradoxical arterial pulse. Invasive monitoring is used when available. Recurrence of cardiac tamponade after aspiration and treatment of the cause may be an indication for pericardial resection.

Chronic pericarditis characterized only by pericardial thickening or calcification without symptoms does not require surgical treatment. If an underlying cause can be identified, that cause should be treated. Chronic pericarditis characterized by chronic effusion should be managed by a search for the etiologic agent, including hypothyroidism. If no specific cause can be found and there is no hemodynamic compromise, pericardial resection is not required.

Constrictive pericarditis is ordinarily treated by pericardial resection. Some improvement can often be obtained by digitalis and diuretic therapy. Patients with constrictive pericarditis who are in New York Heart Association functional class 1 or 2 can be observed without pericardial resection if their quality of life is satisfactory. In some patients with subacute constrictive pericarditis, treatment of the underlying disease combined with adrenal steroid therapy may relieve the cardiac compression and obviate the need for cardiac surgery. This is uncommon, however.

PERIPHERAL ARTERIAL DISEASE

method of
JAMES M. EDWARDS, M.D., and
JOHN M. PORTER, M.D.
Portland, Oregon

INTERMITTENT CLAUDICATION

Intermittent claudication is ischemic muscle pain of the lower extremities brought on by exercise and relieved by rest. It is caused by inadequate blood flow to meet the metabolic demands of exercising muscle of the involved limb. The condition is almost always caused by atherosclerotic stenosis or occlusion of the aorta or iliac, femoral, or popliteal arteries. In a small percentage of young patients it may result from unusual causes of arterial stenosis such as fibromuscular dysplasia, arterial entrapment syndromes, and cystic adventitial disease. The claudicating muscle group is always one level distal to the site of arterial stenosis; thus, iliac stenosis causes thigh claudication, femoral stenosis causes calf claudication, and so forth. It is important to note that true claudication is always relieved by a few minutes of rest. Limb pain requiring considerably longer periods of rest for relief is probably not arterial claudication but probably due to such conditions as arthritis or nerve compression syndrome.

The incidence of claudication increases with age, as shown in Table 1. The most important risk factors are smoking ($9\times$ increase), diabetes mellitus ($5\times$ increase), and coronary artery disease ($4\times$ increase). Surveys of elderly patients suggest that as many as 75 per cent of patients with claudication do not complain of it to their physicians because they view limb pain when walking as a part of normal aging. Thus it is important that every examination of patients beyond age 50 years include the question "How many blocks can you walk on level ground at normal speed?" Claudication is usually classified as mild (less than three city blocks), moderate (one to three blocks) and severe (less than one block) (a city block is nominally 70 to 90 meters). It is most important to assess the femoral, popliteal, and pedal pulses. Claudication may, however, occur even if normal pulses are present at rest.

Noninvasive vascular laboratory studies should be used to confirm the diagnosis and quantitate the amount of disease present. Laboratory testing, using the multi-cuff non-invasive determination of leg blood pressure and treadmill walking is virtually 100 per cent sensitive in the diagnosis of intermittent claudication. Additionally, the actual site of arterial blockage can be accurately localized in more than 90 per cent of patients.

TABLE 1. **Incidence of Intermittent Claudication**

Age (years)	Incidence (per cent)
>50	0.3
50–59	1
60–69	3–5
>69	10 plus

Selection of optimal treatment for the individual patient requires detailed knowledge of the natural history of untreated claudication. Numerous studies have shown that at least 75 per cent of patients with claudication will stabilize or improve slightly without specific treatment. The remaining 25 per cent, almost always those with the more severe initial symptoms, will develop progressive disease and require surgical intervention. Only 3 to 5 per cent of claudicating patients ever require amputation. While claudication has a benign limb prognosis, it is a marker for systemic atherosclerotic disease. Ninety per cent of patients with claudication have coronary artery disease, which is significant in 30 to 50 per cent, and amenable to bypass grafting in 25 per cent. The 5-, 10-, and 15-year mortality rates of patients after the diagnosis of claudication are 30, 50, and 70 per cent, respectively, all of which are two to three times greater than in age-matched controls. The excess deaths are almost all due to coronary disease.

Treatment

Treatment options for intermittent claudication include operative and non-operative therapy. Patients who can walk more than one block and who have ankle blood pressures greater than one half their arm pressure should be treated with non-operative therapy initially. Patients with shorter walking distances and lower ankle blood pressure should be considered for surgery if their general health and life expectancy is reasonably good. Another group of patients that may be considered for therapy are those patients with mild to moderate claudication who cannot perform the tasks required by their employment.

Non-operative therapy consists of a daily walking program (one mile or more) and, if the patient is a smoker, cessation of smoking. The patient should be instructed to walk to the point of claudication, rest a few minutes, and walk on again. Indoor shopping malls are a convenient place for this activity. This regimen will often double or triple walking distance over several months. The only drug approved in the United States for the treatment of claudication is pentoxifylline (Trental), 400 mg 3 times daily. While the overall response in pentoxifylline studies was 30 to 40 per cent, there was a great deal of interpatient variability, with a 50 per cent improvement in one half of treated patients. Pentoxifylline may be useful in a program of cessation of smoking and exercise, as well as for selected patients who are not operative candidates. We feel pentoxifylline should not be used alone, but as part of a program of exercise, smoking cessation, and weight loss if needed.

Although we will not discuss specific surgical therapy here, it is important to note that well-performed surgical revascularization is associated with an operative mortality of well under 5 per cent. In the best series, the patency of revascularization repairs is greater than 80 per cent five years postoperatively. Unfortunately, the five-year mortality rate in this patient group exceeds 30 per cent, almost all due to cardiac disease. Because of this, many physicians in recent years are pursuing vigorous cardiac evaluation of claudicants prior to any treatment. In our center we increasingly rely on thallium cardiac scans as part of the pre-treatment evaluation. A markedly abnormal scan frequently indicates coronary arteriography and even coronary bypass prior to treatment of the claudication.

CAROTID ARTERY DISEASE

Although the incidence of stroke has fallen dramatically during the last decade, it remains the third leading cause of death in the U.S. It has been estimated that one half of patients over the age of 50 years with thromboembolic strokes have surgically accessible carotid artery disease, but the percentage of strokes resulting from cervical carotid artery stenosis is unknown, although the number is probably about 30 per cent.

In recent years, duplex carotid artery scanning has allowed the accurate assessment of cervical carotid artery atherosclerotic disease with a sensitivity and specificity approaching 95 per cent, and in many cases has proven more accurate than carotid arteriography.

All patients at risk should be screened with a carotid duplex scan. The "at risk" category includes patients with transient ischemic attacks (TIA), prior stroke, asymptomatic cervical bruits, and other peripheral vascular diseases such as claudication and coronary artery disease. Table 2 is a simple risk assessment of patients with carotid artery disease. Patients with normal scans are restudied every other year and those with abnormal scans are studied every 6 months to check for progression.

Treatment

The benefit in stroke reduction from carotid endarterectomy in patients with TIA is widely but not universally accepted. The treatment of asymptomatic lesions remains controversial. Available evidence persuasively demonstrates that good-risk patients with an asymptomatic carotid stenosis of greater than 80 per cent di-

TABLE 2. **Risk Assessment of Patients with Carotid Artery Disease**

Category	Annual Risk (per cent)	
	Stroke	Death
Unselected U.S. population (ages 65–74)	0.8–1	3
Asymptomatic carotid bruit	2.3	6.6
Asymptomatic carotid stenosis (>80%)*	8	5
Symptomatic carotid stenosis (TIA)	8.5	5.8
After uncomplicated carotid surgery for:		
Asymptomatic stenosis	1	6.5
TIA	2.3	5.2

*Greater than 80 per cent diameter reduction.

TABLE 3. **Incidence of Abdominal Aortic Aneurysm (AAA) in High-Risk Subgroups**

Subgroup	Incidence (per cent)
Males over age 60 years	2–4
Males with coronary disease	5
Patients with peripheral atherosclerosis	9

ameter reduction (as determined by duplex scanning or arteriography) have an annual stroke rate approximating 8 per cent, which is similar to patients with TIA and carotid stenosis. The combined stroke and mortality rate of carotid endarterectomy for asymptomatic stenosis should not exceed 2 per cent, with the annual stroke rate after surgery being 1 to 2 per cent. Based on these figures, we recommend that asymptomatic carotid stenosis with a diameter reduction of 80 per cent or greater be treated surgically. It is important to note that operative complications of stroke and death vary widely, with complication rates as high as 10 to 20 per cent reported from some hospitals. Thus, carotid surgery in certain communities is clearly of no benefit.

The role of antiplatelet drugs in the prevention of stroke remains unclear. Aspirin therapy appears to convey a moderate benefit in both symptomatic and asymptomatic carotid stenosis. We believe that the benefits of aspirin in patients with TIA are marginal and that this drug does not eliminate the need for surgery in selected patients. It is important to remember that one third to one half of patients selected for carotid surgery will have severe coronary artery disease that places them at increased risk for cardiac death in the postoperative period. Appropriate cardiac evaluation should be obtained as needed in this patient group.

ABDOMINAL AORTIC ANEURYSM

Abdominal aortic aneurysm (AAA) is a frequent manifestations of systemic atherosclerosis and all too often goes undiagnosed until rupture occurs, with an associated overall mortality rate in the best of hands of over 80 per cent. Table 3 reviews the incidence of AAA in the high-risk subgroups of males over 60 years of age, males with coronary disease, and patients with periph-

eral atherosclerosis. The incidence of AAA in the general population is not known with certainty.

The major and most catastrophic complication of AAA is rupture, which is associated with an overall mortality rate in excess of 80 per cent in spite of the advances in critical care. The risk of rupture is related to the size of the aneurysm. Small aneurysms (<5 cm) have a rupture rate of about 5 per cent per year; larger aneurysms (>6 cm) have a rupture rate of 10 per cent per year or more. Patients with chronic obstructive pulmonary disease and/or hypertension appear to have a higher incidence of aneurysmal rupture than patients without these risk factors.

The likelihood of a routine physical examination detecting any but the largest AAA is notoriously low. Two thirds of unruptured AAAs are discovered incidentally during the performance of unrelated abdominal diagnostic procedures. Therefore, to decrease the mortality from ruptured aneurysms, we must become much more efficient at detection. Ultrasonography is a highly accurate, safe, and inexpensive diagnostic test for AAA. We recommend that all patients over sixty years, especially men, smokers, and patients with peripheral atherosclerosis, have abdominal ultrasonography every two years to rule out AAA.

Treatment

While it is clear that the rupture potential of large aneurysms is greater than that of small aneurysms, there is a definite risk of rupture of small aneurysms, which is obviously unpredictable for the individual patient. Serial ultrasonography every six months is an alternative. Patients with large (>6 cm) or rapidly enlarging aneurysms (>1 cm per year) should be considered for surgery in spite of severe medical problems if their life expectancy is more than two years.

One third to one half of patients with AAA have associated severe coronary artery disease (CAD). Since the nationwide elective operative mortality rate of AAA repair remains at 5 to 10 per cent, and much of this is cardiac related, we feel detailed preoperative cardiac evaluation should be obtained in those patients as described above. Patients without significant coronary disease who have a successful AAA repair have a relatively normal life expectancy.

DEEP VENOUS THROMBOSIS OF THE LOWER EXTREMITIES

method of
ANTHONY J. COMEROTA, M.D.
Temple University Hospital
Philadelphia, Pennsylvania

It has long been established that the clinical diagnosis of deep venous thrombosis (DVT) is grossly unreliable. Additionally, it is instructive to realize that in the majority of patients presenting with pulmonary embolism, DVT has not been diagnosed prior to or at the time of the pulmonary embolic event. The need for an objective diagnosis is further emphasized by the many studies utilizing ascending phlebography in patients with suspected DVT. These data show that the commonly accepted signs and symptoms of acute DVT are present just as frequently in patients with phlebographically normal veins as in those with phlebographically proven DVT.

Diagnosis

Noninvasive diagnostic tests are highly reliable when performed by experienced personnel from established vascular laboratories. Venous duplex imaging, impedance plethysmography (or any of the many maximal venous outflow techniques), and phleborheography are physiologic studies that indicate abnormalities in venous hemodynamics.

Ascending phlebography is generally considered the definitive diagnostic study, although it is being challenged by venous duplex imaging, which appears to be the most accurate noninvasive study and actually rivals the accuracy of ascending phlebography in some centers. Nonetheless ascending phlebography is performed in most hospitals with reliable results and a low complication rate.

Patients who have thrombi located in the popliteal or more proximal veins are said to have "proximal vein thrombosis." Clotting that is limited to the infrapopliteal veins is termed "calf clot."

It is agreed that most patients with proximal vein thrombosis should be treated, since they run a high risk of suffering acute complications of pulmonary embolism and long-term complications of the postthrombotic syndrome. Patients with calf vein thrombosis are not routinely treated because the risk of pulmonary embolism is thought to be low, although when carefully evaluated it has been reported to be 10 to 40 per cent. There is controversy over whether calf thrombi need to be treated. There is always the risk of extension of the infrapopliteal thrombi to the larger veins, which has been reported to occur approximately 20 per cent of the time.

Superficial venous thrombosis usually can be diagnosed clinically. The obviously thrombosed veins lying beneath the skin can be seen and easily palpated. Commonly they are tender, with overlying erythema and associated cutaneous and subcutaneous edema. When this process extends above the level of the knee, it should be treated with surgical excision, since the risk of recurrence persists long after anticoagulants are discontinued. This vein is of no further use as a potential bypass conduit; therefore there is little justification for leaving it in place when acutely thrombosed. It is also important to realize that the thrombus generally extends several inches higher than can be clinically appreciated. In all patients with superficial venous thrombosis, the entire deep venous system must be evaluated to be sure a silent DVT does not exist.

Management: Therapeutic Goals

When managing patients with DVT, three therapeutic goals should be considered: (1) elimination of the thrombus; (2) stopping additional thrombosis and preventing embolism; and (3) preventing embolism. Theoretically, elimination of the thrombus is the optimal result and can be achieved pharmacologically with thrombolytic therapy or surgically with operative venous thrombectomy. If patients are not candidates for either of these alternatives, preventing extension of thrombosis and embolism is the therapeutic goal and is usually accomplished with anticoagulant therapy. If contraindications to anticoagulation exist or the patient is a failure of anticoagulant therapy, mechanical interruption (filtration) of the vena cava is indicated to prevent potentially large pulmonary emboli.

To assist in making the appropriate therapeutic decision, the natural history of patients treated with anticoagulation should be compared with patients treated with thrombolytic therapy. There are now 14 published studies evaluating patients randomized to thrombolytic therapy or standard anticoagulation with pre- and post-therapy ascending phlebography. A total of 593 patients have been evaluated. In those patients treated with heparin anticoagulation, 6 per cent regained significant or complete patency of their occluded deep venous system and 12 per cent regained partial recanalization. Eighty-two per cent of the patients remained occluded or extended their thrombus. In patients treated with thrombolytic therapy, 47 per cent regained significant or complete patency of their deep venous system, 21 per cent achieved partial clot lysis, and 32 per cent failed to respond. These data indicate that patency can be restored to acutely thrombosed veins significantly better in patients treated with lytic agents than in patients treated with standard anticoagulation.

Several studies evaluating patients over the long term indicated that the signs and symptoms of the post-thrombotic syndrome were reduced in patients treated with a lytic agent compared to those treated with heparin. More important, it was shown that venous function 5 to 10 years following therapy was significantly better when lysis occurred compared with function of veins that were persistently obstructed.

Treatment

Thrombolytic Therapy

Streptokinase and urokinase are the two currently available thrombolytic agents for the treatment of acute DVT. Recombinant tissue plasminogen activator has recently been approved by the FDA, but has been infrequently used for acute DVT.

Streptokinase is administered as an intravenous bolus of 250,000 IU, followed by a continuous infusion of 100,000 IU per hour. Because streptokinase is antigenic, I prefer to administer hydrocortisone, 100 mg intravenously prior to the streptokinase infusion and 100 mg every 8 hours during the first 24 hours of therapy. Because a pyretic response is common, acetaminophen, 650 mg every 6 hours, is also administered.

Urokinase is the preferred lytic agent because its efficacy is similar to that of the other lytic agents and, compared with streptokinase, the duration of therapy is shorter and bleeding complications are significantly decreased. Urokinase is administered intravenously as a bolus of 4000 IU per kg over 10 minutes, followed by a continuous infusion of 4000 IU per kg per hour. Since urokinase is a human protein derivative, allergic reactions are unlikely, and pretreatment with hydrocortisone is not necessary.

The appropriate duration of infusion of the fibrinolytic agent should be monitored with noninvasive studies. It has been our experience that all patients who respond to lytic agents begin to show that response within the first 24 hours. If the patient fails to respond in the first 24 hours, as documented by noninvasive studies, lytic therapy should be discontinued. If the patient is improving but has not normalized, the infusion is continued. Treatment should be continued until the patient normalizes or reaches a plateau such that there has been no change in clot resolution over a 24-hour period. Monitoring of thrombolytic therapy with noninvasive studies eliminates the needless prolongation of infusion after a thrombus has been lysed and appropriately terminates the infusion when it is obviously ineffective.

Anticoagulant Therapy

Anticoagulation with heparin followed by warfarin sodium (Coumadin) is the most common form of treatment for DVT. If heparin is chosen as primary therapy, rapid anticoagulation should be accomplished. Preliminary data suggest that the incidence of recurrent DVT is higher among those patients requiring 1 to 2 days to achieve therapeutic anticoagulation compared with those rapidly anticoagulated.

Heparin

Heparin is given as a bolus of 100 IU per kg, followed by a continuous infusion of 10 to 15 IU per kg per hour. The partial thromboplastin time (PTT) is checked 6 to 8 hours following the bolus administration to ensure that the rate of heparin infusion is adequate to maintain an anticoagulated state. Opinions differ as to how much heparin should be given. Some suggest maintaining the PTT above 100 seconds while others maintain the PTT at 2 to 3 times the control value. The critical factor is the successful anticoagulation of the patient, and one should err on the side of infusing more rather than less heparin. Since bleeding complications in patients therapeutically anticoagulated do not correlate with the PTT value, it is our policy to give higher doses of heparin early and adjust the PTT values downward during the second and third days of therapy.

If there is difficulty maintaining an anticoagulated state with heparin, one must consider either anti-thrombin III deficiency or the presence of a heparin antibody. Anti-thrombin III levels assayed prior to heparin infusion will indicate whether there is an adequate level of this heparin co-factor. Platelet counts should always be monitored during heparin therapy daily or at least every other day. If the platelet counts drop during heparin infusion, heparin-induced thrombocytopenia should be suspected. If the platelet count drops by more than 30 per cent of the baseline value, heparin should be discontinued and alternative forms of antithrombotic therapy initiated.

After a minimum of 3 days of Coumadin therapy, and when the prothrombin time (PT) is 1.2 to 1.4 times the control value, heparin therapy is discontinued.

Warfarin Sodium (Coumadin)

After 6 to 12 hours of heparin therapy, when the patient is anticoagulated, a dose of 10 mg of Coumadin is given and repeated daily for the first 2 to 3 days of anticoagulant therapy. Once the PT is at therapeutic levels and the patient has received Coumadin for 3 to 4 days, as discussed above, heparin is discontinued. The PT must be followed carefully, since concurrent heparin will have an effect. We often stop the continuous heparin infusion on the second or third day of anticoagulation and give the patient heparin as an intravenous bolus of 5000 IU every 6 hours, checking the PT immediately before the next heparin bolus is given. This will accurately reflect the effect of the Coumadin on anticoagulation, minimizing the effect of heparin.

Once the patient is anticoagulated on Coumadin therapy noninvasive studies are repeated and plans for discharge made.

PTs are determined twice a week for the first week after discharge, weekly for 2 weeks, and then every other week during anticoagulation therapy. The Coumadin dose should be adjusted according to the patient's requirements. All patients are given 5-mg tablets because the majority of patients require 5 to 7.5 mg daily. If multiple-size tablets are given, overdosage and underdosage occur more frequently.

Coumadin affects the vitamin K–dependent clotting factors (VII, IX, X, and II). The half-life of Factor VII is quite short. Early and high doses of Coumadin will rapidly deplete Factor VII concentration and affect the PT. The half-lives of Factors X and II are much longer, and therefore true therapeutic anticoagulation does not occur for 3 to 4 days with Coumadin therapy, despite a prolonged PT. A "therapeutic prothrombin time" on the first day of therapy may reflect only a drop in Factor VII but not true anticoagulation in the therapeutic sense.

Protein-C and protein-S are naturally occurring anticoagulants that are also vitamin K dependent. These proteins serve to inactivate Factors V and VIII. Coumadin decreases the functional level of protein-C and protein-S. If the patient has a heterozygous protein-C deficiency, he may actually become hypercoagulable with initial doses of Coumadin, thus precipitating thrombosis. The complication of Coumadin-induced skin necrosis is generally attributed to protein-C deficiency. For this reason, patients should be fully anticoagulated with heparin prior to initiating Coumadin therapy.

Patients are maintained on Coumadin for a minimum of 3 months; however, our policy is to continue therapy for 6 to 12 months or possibly longer, depending upon the predisposition of the patient to develop recurrent thromboses compared with the risk of bleeding problems with the anticoagulant. Since we maintain the patient's PT at 1.2 to 1.4 times control values, the bleeding complications have been minimized.

Venous Thrombectomy

Venous thrombectomy is an important consideration in patients presenting with acute iliofemoral venous thrombosis, phlegmasia cerulea dolens, and phlegmasia alba dolens. In these patients there is a high likelihood of a severe post-thrombotic syndrome, and the obstructing thrombus should be removed whenever possible. Therefore, surgical thrombectomy and pharmacologic thrombectomy are the two major considerations in these patients.

In surgical thrombectomy, using local or general anesthesia an incision is made over the femoral vein and a balloon catheter is used to remove the thrombus from the iliofemoral venous segment. The leg is raised and the lower leg and thigh are "milked" and/or compressed to remove the thrombus from the lower leg. Since a large amount of blood can be lost by this procedure, a cell saver is employed to return non-clotted blood to the patient. Operative phlebography is performed to ensure that all of the thrombus is removed from the iliofemoral venous segment.

A distal arteriovenous fistula is created to increase the blood flow velocity through the thrombectomized venous segment. This fistula is electively closed approximately 6 weeks postoperatively.

Patients are maintained on anticoagulation with heparin infusion during the postoperative period, which is converted to Coumadin therapy as described previously. Additionally, external pneumatic compression boots are placed on all patients to further accelerate venous return and to stimulate increases in regional fibrinolysis. It is preferable to maintain the patient's hemoglobin level at 10 to 12 to decrease viscosity.

Venous thrombectomy has fallen into disfavor because of early reports documenting a high incidence of postoperative thrombosis with no particular long-term benefit. With recent improved techniques of operative phlebography that ensure complete thrombectomy, continued anticoagulation, distal arteriovenous fistula, and external pneumatic compression, results are significantly improved, especially when compared to heparin anticoagulation alone.

Patients who have pulmonary embolism while on anticoagulant therapy or who have proximal vein thrombosis and cannot be treated with lytic agents or anticoagulants must be protected from further embolic episodes. The most effective method of preventing significant pulmonary emboli while maintaining a patent vena cava is the use of a Greenfield filter.

These can be inserted in the operating room under fluoroscopy, generally using local anesthesia. More recently, radiologists are able to insert these filters percutaneously through large-bore introducers from the non-involved iliofemoral venous segment. These filters prevent additional large emboli; also, trapped emboli frequently lyse because blood flow continues around the clot. With the introduction of the guide-wire technique, placement is facilitated and the complications of improper placement and filter migration have been minimized.

Post-Thrombotic Syndrome

Many patients with proximal vein thrombosis and some with calf vein thrombosis have significant problems with the post-thrombotic syndrome. If venous function can be evaluated sufficiently to ensure that the superficial and deep veins are functioning normally, the incidence of long-term post-thrombotic problems should be low. However, abnormalities of venous function place the patient at a high risk for chronic signs and symptoms.

External compression from the metatarsal head to the anterior tibial tubercle is uniformly recommended. The degree of compression must be of sufficient force to prevent swelling. Generally, if swelling can be prevented, the severe sequelae of the post-thrombotic syndrome are prevented. Ankle gradient compressions of 30 to 50 mm Hg are recommended, depending upon the needs of the patient and the degree of residual obstruction of the deep venous system. Patients with significant unresolved deep venous obstruction generally require 40 to 50 mm Hg ankle gradient compression stockings to control their problems. Stockings are put on in the morning before the patient arises and should not be removed until bedtime.

Acute symptoms during the long term may represent acute episodes of venous thrombosis or exacerbations of the post-thrombotic syndrome.

If noninvasive studies have normalized prior to these acute symptoms, they can be used to evaluate the patient during the acute presentation. If they have not normalized, additional studies such as the radiofibrinogen-uptake test or repeat phlebography are indicated. If acute DVT is diagnosed, appropriate therapy for the acute episode is re-instituted.

The Blood and Spleen

APLASTIC ANEMIA

method of
JAN JANSEN, M.D., PH.D.
Indiana University School of Medicine
Indianapolis, Indiana

Aplastic anemia usually represents a failure of all bone marrow cell lines and therefore presents as pancytopenia. In some cases isolated thrombocytopenia or anemia is initially present. Mild and moderate forms of the disease occur, but progression to severe aplastic anemia is often observed. According to generally accepted criteria, severe aplastic anemia is defined by at least two of the following characteristics: granulocytes less than 500 per cubic mm, platelets less than 20,000 per cubic mm, and reticulocytes less than 20,000 per cubic mm. In addition, a bone marrow biopsy must show a hypoplastic bone marrow with predominance of lymphoid elements.

In two thirds of cases of acquired aplastic anemia, no causative mechanism can be identified, and the disease is therefore scored as idiopathic. About 10 per cent of the cases are associated with toxic substances, such as drugs or chemicals, and about the same percentage is associated with viral infections. Occasional cases occur during or shortly after a pregnancy.

Chloramphenicol is the drug that is classically known for its association with aplastic anemia. Now that chloramphenicol is used much less frequently, other drugs have become more important. Among these are the butazones (pyrazole drugs), gold compounds, anticonvulsants, chlorpromazine, and quinacrine. More rarely, antimicrobial agents (such as tetracyclines, penicillins, sulfonamides, and antifungal agents), antithyroid drugs, oral antidiabetic drugs, analgesics, and cimetidine have been implicated in the pathogenesis of aplastic anemia. Cytotoxic drugs and ionizing radiation induce pancytopenia in a dose-related fashion. Among the chemicals that can lead to aplastic anemia, benzene and insecticides should be mentioned.

Several viral infections have been implicated in the pathogenesis of aplastic anemia. The most common is posthepatitis aplastic anemia. This syndrome, which is probably associated with non-A, non-B hepatitis, most often occurs several months after the clinical signs of hepatitis have subsided. Aplastic anemia has also been associated with Epstein-Barr virus (infectious mononucleosis), cytomegalovirus, herpesvirus, rubella virus, dengue virus, and the human parvovirus. Sometimes the diagnosis of aplastic anemia is diffi-

cult, and other disorders should be ruled out. One should be hesitant to make the diagnosis of aplastic anemia in a patient with splenomegaly because patients with pancytopenia and splenomegaly may have a lymphoproliferative disorder, such as hairy-cell leukemia. These diseases can occasionally present with a hypocellular bone marrow. Careful analysis of bone marrow cytology and histology is mandatory to rule out these entities. Cytogenetic examination of the bone marrow is very important for the differential diagnosis with a leukemic disorder or myelodysplastic syndrome. In particular, if the bone marrow is not completely aplastic, a myelodysplastic syndrome (preleukemia) should be considered. The cytologic and histologic analysis of the bone marrow usually leads to the correct diagnosis. Occasionally, the in vitro culture of hematopoietic progenitor cells can be important; commonly only in aplastic anemia, no growth at all is observed, whereas in leukemic disorders many small aggregates (clusters) are observed.

THERAPY

Optimal supportive care is the cornerstone of treatment in all patients with severe aplastic anemia. Patients may well have pancytopenia for a prolonged time, and, therefore, antibiotic prophylaxis and support with blood products must be carefully planned. As for specific therapy, a treatment plan will have to be made as soon as possible after diagnosis. The two major therapy options are allogeneic bone marrow transplantation and immunosuppressive therapy. The choice between the two should be made on the basis of the age of the patient and the availability of an HLA-matched sibling donor.

Supportive Care

Supportive care should be directed toward the prevention of infection and the prevention of hemorrhagic complications.

Red Cell Transfusions

The aim of red cell transfusions is to control the symptoms of anemia. The clinical symptoms of the patient are much more important than the absolute hemoglobin level, but we generally try to keep the hemoglobin level above 9 grams per dl. In elderly people, it may be necessary to keep the hemoglobin at a much higher level, e.g., 11 grams per dl. There is no indication for the use of whole blood, and therefore packed cells should be used. Packed red cell transfusions contain a considerable number of leukocytes, which can easily induce sensitization against HLA antigens. Since the induction of such HLA antibodies in the long run will jeopardize the supportive care with platelet transfusions, it is definitely worthwhile to try to transfuse red cells that are depleted of leukocyte contamination. The following four techniques are available.

Washed Red Blood Cells. Repeated washings of the red cells in physiologic saline remove about 75 per cent of the leukocytes. This is sufficient to prevent febrile nonhemolytic transfusion reactions but probably not sufficient to prevent sensitization to HLA antigens.

Transfusion Through Microaggregate Filters. Microaggregate filters (e.g., the Pall filter) remove 75 to 85 per cent of the white cells; again, this is sufficient to prevent febrile nonhemolytic transfusion reactions but not sufficient to prevent HLA sensitization.

Transfusion Through Leukocyte Filters. Leukocyte-poor red cells can be obtained by filtration through cotton wool filters (e.g., Erypur) in the blood bank, or through cellulose acetate filters (Sepacel R-500A) at the bedside. These filters are highly effective in removing more than 95 per cent of the leukocytes and thus probably prevent HLA sensitization.

Cryopreserved Red Cells. The cryopreservation of red cells in the presence of glycerol, followed by thawing and deglycerolization, leads to a nearly complete removal of leukocytes and leukocyte fragments. Therefore, deglycerolized red cells are basically leukocyte free.

For aplastic anemia patients we routinely use leukocyte-poor red cell transfusions, obtained either through leukocyte filters or by freezing/thawing. The latter technique, however, is logistically more difficult and definitely more expensive.

Platelet Transfusions

The decision of when to give patients with severe aplastic anemia platelet transfusions is always very delicate. On the one hand is the risk of hemorrhagic complications if the platelet count drops below 15,000 to 20,000 per cubic mm. On the other hand, repeated platelet transfusions can easily lead to HLA sensitization, which would jeopardize future transfusions. Particularly in the early stage of aplastic anemia, it is wise to keep the platelet count above 15,000 per cubic mm. This can be accomplished primarily by transfusing platelets two to three times per week. The platelet dose should be approximately 1 unit per 10 kg body weight of the patient.

The larger the number of platelet donors the patient is exposed to, the higher the risk of HLA sensitization. Therefore, we do not use pooled platelets from random donors for these patients, but platelets obtained by pheresis of single donors. Thus, volunteer donors are subjected to pheresis on a blood cell separator, such as the FENWAL CS-3000. Number of platelets comparable to approximately 6 units of random platelets can be obtained in about 2 hours. In order to further decrease the risk of alloimmunization, we centrifuge the platelets prior to transfusion in the Leukotrap platelet bag to remove leukocytes as completely as possible.

When the aplastic anemia becomes more chronic, it is often possible to decrease the frequency of platelet transfusions. Many such patients will have no hemorrhagic diathesis at all, although their platelet count is only 10,000 per cubic mm, or less. Recurrence of symptoms of easy bruisability, and in particular retinal hemorrhages, should lead to reinstitution of aggressive supportive care with platelets. Such episodes are often triggered by bacterial and/or viral infections.

Granulocyte Transfusions

The indications for granulocyte transfusions are extremely limited. These should never be given prophylactically, since they necessarily lead to HLA sensitization. The only remaining indication is in patients with granulocyte counts of less than 100 per cubic mm who have persistent severe infections with gram-negative bacteria (*Pseudomonas, Klebsiella, E. coli*) after at least 48 hours of adequate antibacterial treatment. If granulocyte transfusions are started for this indication, they probably should be continued for at least 4 days.

Transfusions From Family Members

For patients who are still candidates for allogeneic bone marrow transplantation, blood products should not be obtained from family members because of the high risk of sensitization against family-specific antigens, which increases the risk of marrow rejection. From the day of bone marrow transplantation on, however, family members can be valuable transfusion donors.

Infection Prophylaxis

Patients with a granulocyte count of less than 500 per cubic mm are at an increased risk for infection. Most of these infections originate from colonization of the gastrointestinal tract. Therefore, antibiotic prophylaxis directed at selectively modulating the flora of the gastrointestinal tract is worthwhile. A relatively simple way of achieving this is with trimethoprim/sulfamethoxazole (Septra, Bactrim), one double-strength (DS) tablet twice a day. A new, attractive, alternative may be norfloxacin (Noroxin), 400 mg 3 times a day.* For prophylaxis against *Candida* infections, we use ketoconazole (Nizoral), 2 to 3 200 mg tablets per day.

If a patient nevertheless develops a suspected infection as documented by fever of over 38.5° C, empirical antibiotic therapy should be started. In granulocytopenic patients, systemic infections can progress very rapidly; therefore, antibiotic treatment should be started immediately after cultures of blood, urine, and sputum have been obtained. At present we believe that a combination of a cephalosporin (e.g., Cefoperazone, 2 grams every 8 hours intravenously) in combination with an aminoglycoside (e.g., Amikacin, 5 mg per kg every 8 hours intravenously) is optimal. Obviously, as soon as positive cultures become available, the antibiotics are changed according to the antibiogram.

Androgens

In severe aplastic anemia, no value of androgens has been demonstrated. Nevertheless, in many centers, androgens are routinely given to patients with aplastic anemia. These hormones are probably active in only a small minority of patients, and their main effect is on the red cell series. The potential beneficial effect should be weighed against the risk of side effects. Hepatotoxicity, which can range from mildly elevated liver function tests to peliosis hepatis and hepatomas, is the most prominent. However, virilization, impotence, amenorrhea, and growth retardation in children can also occur. Among the androgens, oxymetholone (Anadrol) has been most widely used. The drug is usually given orally in a dose of 2 to 3 mg per kg per day. Androgens act relatively slowly, and hematopoietic improvement can take several months.

Antilymphocyte Globulin (ALG)/ Antithymocyte Globulin (ATG)

The value of immunosuppressive therapy with ALG or ATG in severe aplastic anemia has now been documented by several groups. At present it is by far the best available treatment for patients with severe aplastic anemia who are not eligible for bone marrow transplantation. Although originally ALG/ATG was believed to act

through the removal of lymphocytes that suppress hematopoiesis, the exact mechanism of action of this therapy is still unknown. Immunosuppression is the most likely mechanism of action, but direct stimulation of hematopoietic stem cells cannot be excluded. In the United States, ALG/ATG treatment for severe aplastic anemia is still considered investigational.

We use ATG manufactured by Upjohn (ATGAM) in a dose of 20 mg per kg per day intravenously for 5 days. We infuse the ATG over 4 to 6 hours and premedicate with antihistaminics. Other horse ATG preparations are manufactured by Merieux, and a horse ALG is produced by the Swiss Serum Institute. In addition to these horse preparations, ATGs from rabbits and goats are available. The side effects of infusion of these xenogeneic sera can be severe and can include anaphylaxis. Hyper- and hypotension are relatively frequent, making careful cardiovascular monitoring mandatory. High spiking fevers can also occur. Most patients need extensive platelet transfusions because of the marked thrombocytopenic action of ALG/ATG with sequestration of platelets in the liver. We routinely give a platelet transfusion before and 2 to 3 hours after the ATG infusion. Many patients develop serum sickness about 10 days after the start of ATG therapy. This serum sickness can lead to severe arthralgias, vasculitis, and fever. Renal complications are uncommon. We usually treat the serum sickness with prednisone, 1 to 2 mg per kg per day orally, until the symptoms subside.

Recently, we have been combining the ATG treatment with high-dose corticosteroids. We believe that the potential side effects of the corticosteroids, such as increased risk of infection, hyperglycemia, and hypertension, are more than offset by the improved tolerance of ATG infusion and the decreased need for platelet transfusions. Furthermore, there are some indications that the combined therapy may result in faster bone marrow recovery than with ATG alone. We administer methylprednisolone–sodium succinate (Solu-Medrol) 20 mg per kg per day intravenously for 3 days followed by 10 mg per kg per day for 3 days and then 5 mg per kg per day for 3 days. Subsequently, we switch to prednisone 2.5 mg per kg per day orally for 3 days, with halving of the dose every fourth day. This way, serum sickness becomes very rare because the patient still has sufficient steroid therapy around that time to suppress the symptoms nearly completely.

The effect of ALG/ATG on bone marrow function is rather slow. Few patients respond within the first couple of weeks after treatment, and on average, 3 months are required until the patient is independent of transfusions. Overall, 40 to 70

---

*This dose of norfloxacin exceeds the manufacturer's recommended maximum dosage.

per cent of patients can be expected to respond to this therapy and will become independent of transfusions. Complete recovery of the peripheral blood counts is far less frequent than partial recovery with persistent thrombocytopenia. Even in patients with normal peripheral blood counts, the bone marrow often continues to be severely hypocellular, suggesting persistent disease. Occasional patients relapse with pancytopenia after an initial response. Less than 10 per cent of the patients with severe aplastic anemia treated with ALG/ATG will ultimately develop a clonal disease, such as paroxysmal nocturnal hemoglobinuria or acute leukemia.

Bone Marrow Transplantation

Bone marrow transplantation is possible if a syngeneic or HLA-identical sibling is available as a marrow donor. The results are excellent in children and young adults; in untransfused young patients, it is possible to achieve 80 per cent cure rates. However, with increased age, the results rapidly become much poorer. Therefore, we currently use bone marrow transplantation as first therapeutic option only in patients under 25 to 30 years of age. In older patients, treatment with ATG is used first. Patients under the age of 45 who do not respond to ATG, and who have a suitable donor, undergo transplantation as second-line therapy.

The major risks of allogeneic bone marrow transplantation include marrow rejection in polytransfused patients, acute and chronic graft-versus-host disease, and interstitial pneumonitis.

To condition the patient for allogeneic bone marrow transplantation, we use cyclophosphamide (Cytoxan), 50 mg per kg intravenously on each of 4 successive days. To prevent graft rejection, we add total lymphoid irradiation (mantle field and inverted Y) of 500 rad (cGy) in a single dose on the day before transplantation. On that day, bone marrow is collected from the donor through multiple punctures from the posterior iliac crests. We aim to obtain at least 2×10^8 nucleated marrow cells per kg body weight of the recipient; the marrow is infused intravenously through the central line.

The patient is nursed in a laminar air-flow room to prevent bacterial and fungal infections and receives prophylaxis against herpes infections with acyclovir. For prophylaxis against graft-versus-host disease, we use cyclosporin A, starting the day before transplantation with 5 mg per kg as an 18-hour continuous intravenous infusion. The dose is adjusted to the renal function as measured by serum creatinine, and to the cyclosporin A trough level. Prior to discharge, the cyclosporin A is switched to an oral dose of approximately 5 mg per kg every 12 hours. Again, the dose is adjusted to renal function and cyclosporin A trough levels. After 6 months, the cyclosporin A is gradually tapered.

The advantages of bone marrow transplantation are the more complete recovery of hematopoiesis and the absence of development of clonal diseases. The disadvantages are the prolonged hospitalization, the risks of acute and chronic graft-versus-host disease, and the protracted immunosuppression with the attendant high risk of infection.

Prognosis

Severe aplastic anemia has a poor prognosis. With conventional therapy, approximately half the patients die within 6 months, and spontaneous hematopoietic recovery is relatively rare. With bone marrow transplantation or ATG therapy, much better survival rates can be obtained, and probably at least half the patients can be alive at 2 years after diagnosis.

IRON DEFICIENCY
method of
SEAN R. LYNCH, M.D.
University of Kansas
Kansas City, Kansas

Iron deficiency is usually recognized when it causes anemia. However, several nonhematologic consequences of iron lack may also occur. They include atrophic changes in the endothelium of the gastrointestinal tract, with resultant stomatitis, glossitis, and chronic gastritis; impaired exercise tolerance, especially for endurance tasks; abnormalities in the function of the immune system and neurologic dysfunction associated with deficits in attention span and cognitive function in children; and perversions of taste in both children and adults.

Chronic iron deficiency anemia is characterized by the presence of microcytosis and hypochromia with an increased red cell volume distribution width. More specific laboratory evidence of a discrepancy between the iron supply and the rate of erythropoiesis may be provided by the finding of a transferrin saturation of less than 15 per cent in association with a raised total iron-binding capacity, or an increase in the free erythrocyte protoporphyrin concentration. However, confirmation of the presence of true iron deficiency requires the demonstration of significantly diminished iron stores. The most specific indicators are a serum ferritin level below 12 micrograms per liter or the absence of stainable iron in the bone marrow. The serum ferritin assay is the most convenient test. Unfortunately, patients who have iron deficiency complicated by inflammatory disorders, neoplasms, or liver disease may have serum ferritin levels in the normal range. Bone marrow examination is then necessary for a definitive evaluation of iron stores to be made.

The improved living standard in Western societies has been associated with a marked fall in the prevalence of nutritional iron deficiency anemia. Nevertheless, an analysis of the results of the Second National Health and Nutrition Examination Survey carried out in the United States between 1976 and 1980 demonstrated that approximately 6 per cent of infants, teenage girls, and young women have laboratory evidence of iron deficiency anemia. This indicates that the quantity of bioavailable iron in the diet may still be insufficient for some individuals with increased physiologic requirements. Extensive investigation of iron deficiency may therefore not be warranted in children and menstruating women when the clinical features and peripheral blood smear support the diagnosis of iron deficiency. A therapeutic trial of iron is generally appropriate. On the other hand, a positive identification of iron deficiency must be made when there is failure to respond to iron, when anemia is discovered in a clinical situation in which iron deficiency is uncommon or in a population group in which thalassemia is prevalent, or when the clinical and laboratory features are not completely characteristic of iron lack. The choice of test depends on the clinical situation. Serum iron, iron-binding capacity, and serum ferritin will usually suffice in uncomplicated iron deficiency, whereas a bone marrow examination may be necessary in patients with more complicated illnesses.

Once the presence of iron deficiency has been established, the extent of further evaluation again depends on the clinical assessment. Vigorous investigation may not be warranted in young children and menstruating or pregnant women, but a diligent search for a site of blood loss should always be instituted in men and older women. Malabsorption of iron is rarely the sole cause of anemia, although it may be a contributing factor after gastric surgery or in patients with celiac disease.

Treatment

Oral Iron Therapy

Iron therapy should both repair the deficit in functional iron by correcting the anemia and tissue iron lack and restore the normal body iron reserve. Most patients will respond promptly to oral iron preparations. Even patients with impaired food iron absorption following gastric surgery usually absorb sufficient medicinal iron to correct the deficiency. Ferrous salts are absorbed approximately three times as well as ferric salts. Iron deficiency is therefore best treated with a simple ferrous salt, such as the sulfate, gluconate, or fumarate. The usual approach in an adult is to prescribe a ferrous sulfate tablet containing about 60 mg of elemental iron 3 times daily. In children, a dose of 2 to 3 mg of elemental iron per kg per day, usually in the form of an elixir, is recommended. Optimal absorption is achieved if the doses are taken between meals, since food will usually reduce absorption by 50 to 60 per cent. Iron preparations should not be taken with tea or coffee. Both beverages inhibit absorption.

The side effects of oral iron therapy are largely confined to the gastrointestinal tract. Lower bowel symptoms, such as mild diarrhea or constipation, are common but unrelated to iron dose. On the other hand, nausea, epigastric discomfort, and abdominal cramps appear to be a function of the quantity of available iron taken. Side effects are uncommon in children, although iron solutions can produce temporary staining of the teeth. This can be minimized by placing the medication on the back of the tongue, brushing the teeth, or encouraging the child to drink liberal quantities of liquid following iron administration. The rapid correction of iron deficiency is seldom important. Therefore, when patients complain of untoward upper gastrointestinal symptoms, the dose should be reduced or the patient advised to take the iron with meals.

Some iron preparations contain vitamins as well as other so-called hematinics. There is no evidence to indicate that they significantly improve the therapeutic response to iron. Large quantities of ascorbic acid increase the absorption of ferrous sulfate by 30 to 40 per cent. However, there is a parallel rise in side effects and no therapeutic advantage over an equivalent increase in iron dosage.

Attempts have been made to design iron preparations with fewer side effects. Enteric coating is effective but reduces availability appreciably. However, some delayed-release iron preparations are absorbed to an extent comparable with that of ferrous sulfate when taken without food, and significantly better when taken with meals. Side effects may be reduced. Delayed-release preparations cannot be advocated for all patients because of their higher cost, but they should be considered as an alternative to parenteral iron in patients who continue to be intolerant of simple iron salts despite the use of the simple maneuvers outlined above.

Finally, it is important to stress the serious toxicity that occurs as a consequence of accidental iron ingestion in children. It is very important to warn parents of the need to keep all iron preparations out of the reach of young children.

Response to Iron Therapy

It is important to monitor the therapeutic response to iron therapy both to confirm the diagnosis and to ensure that complete correction of the anemia occurs. This is done most easily by following the change in hemoglobin or hematocrit. A rise in hemoglobin concentration of less than 2 grams per dl over a 3-week period or failure to correct the hemoglobin level in 2 months should be considered a therapeutic failure, unless the dose of iron has been reduced severely to avoid gastrointestinal side effects. It is generally recommended that iron therapy be continued for 6 months to replenish iron stores in patients who demonstrate a satisfactory response.

Poor compliance is the most common cause of a suboptimal response to oral iron therapy. Other causes are relatively infrequent. An incorrect diagnosis can be excluded by demonstration of the continued presence of iron deficiency on the basis of a serum ferritin level or a bone marrow examination. Combined iron and folic acid deficiency may limit the response to iron alone. Continued blood loss at a rate that matches the increased red cell production during therapy should be detected easily. Malabsorption, although often considered, is uncommon if a soluble ferrous salt is prescribed. Patients who have had upper gastrointestinal surgery may absorb suboptimal quantities of food iron but will usually absorb therapeutic iron adequately if it is given between meals. Extensive involvement of the upper small bowel in severe celiac disease may cause true malabsorption.

If malabsorption is suspected, the serum iron level should be measured before, and again at 60 and 120 minutes after, the administration of 100 to 130 mg of iron as ferrous sulfate in the fasting state. In an iron-deficient patient with a baseline serum iron level below 50 micrograms per dl, a rise of less than 100 micrograms per dl in the serum iron concentration is suggestive evidence of malabsorption and an indication for more detailed investigation.

When iron deficiency is attributed to a specific remediable cause, such as bleeding, there should be no recurrence after body iron stores have been repleted. In many patients, however, iron deficiency reflects an imbalance between available iron in the diet and physiologic requirements. Recurrence can then be expected unless measures are taken to improve the dietary iron supply. This is particularly important in children with high physiologic requirements. In infants the high bioavailability of iron in breast milk offers some protection against iron deficiency. Iron-fortified formula is also effective. Excessive consumption of cow's milk should be avoided because it is a poor source of iron and may cause intestinal blood loss in some infants. When solid foods are first offered at 4 to 6 months of age, the early introduction of meat and ascorbic acid–rich foods with meals will ensure an adequate supply of bioavailable iron. The dietary supply of iron for adults can be optimized by encouraging the consumption of meat or fish and ascorbic acid–containing foods or drinks with the major meal of the day. It is also helpful to avoid drinking tea or coffee with meals, since they inhibit iron absorption. Occasionally women who fall at the upper end of the normal range for menstrual loss will require a small supplement until the menopause unless their diets contain large quantities of meat. Continued iron supplementation may also be essential to prevent the recurrence of iron deficiency in individuals who have had upper gastrointestinal surgery. Unfortunately, the risks of iron overload are very real, and although conclusive evidence is not yet available, it is possible that individuals who are heterozygous for the gene responsible for idiopathic (hereditary) hemochromatosis may develop iron overload if exposed to sufficient supplemental iron. Since this gene appears to be common in some population groups, continued administration of an iron supplement, particularly to men or women after menopause, cannot be recommended in Western societies unless the size of the iron store is monitored by measuring the serum ferritin concentration.

Parenteral Iron Therapy

Parenteral iron therapy is rarely justified, since most patients respond rapidly to oral preparations. Moreover, oral iron is usually adequately tolerated even by patients with gastrointestinal diseases, such as peptic ulceration, regional ileitis, and ulcerative colitis. Specific indications for parenteral iron administration include extensive small bowel disease in patients who fail to absorb oral iron adequately, and situations in which the rate of iron loss through bleeding exceeds the rate of iron absorption. In addition, occasional patients cannot tolerate oral iron despite dosage reduction and the trial of different preparations and regimens. Parenteral iron should be recommended only after every attempt has been made to improve their tolerance to oral preparations.

Iron dextran is the form of injectable iron available in the United States. It is a complex of ferric hydroxide with dextran in a 0.9 per cent sodium chloride solution and contains 50 mg elemental iron per ml. The drug may be administered intramuscularly or intravenously after a 0.5 ml dose to test for anaphylaxis. Intravenous administration is preferable in adults. The total dose given is based on the iron deficit calculated as follows:

$$\text{Total iron required (mg)} = \frac{\text{Hgb deficit (grams/dl)}}{100} \times \text{estimated blood volume} \times 3.4$$

An additional 500 mg is usually added to replenish stores. The approved method for intravenous use in adults in the United States is to give 0.5 ml on the first day to test for anaphylaxis. If no reaction has occurred within an hour, a further 1.5 ml is given. Individual daily doses of 2 ml (100 mg iron) are administered until the total calculated amount is reached. All injections must be given slowly (1 ml or less per minute). An alternative method that is more convenient and widely accepted elsewhere is total-dose infusion. The total quantity of iron required to replace the deficit is diluted in isotonic saline to a concentration of 5 per cent or less. The infusion is started at less than 10 drops per minute, and the patient is monitored closely for the first 10 minutes. If no untoward side effects occur, the infusion is completed over 4 to 6 hours.

The most serious adverse reaction to iron dextran is anaphylaxis. Although it is rare, it may occur with both intramuscular and intravenous use. The drug should therefore be administered only in situations in which full resuscitative measures are available. Other adverse reactions include urticaria, rashes, fever, arthralgia and myalgia, phlebitis at the injection site, and peripheral vascular flushing with intravenous infusions that are given too rapidly. Reactivation of arthritis may occur in patients with quiescent rheumatoid arthritis.

AUTOIMMUNE HEMOLYTIC ANEMIA

method of
RICHARD J. DAVEY, M.D.
National Institutes of Health
Bethesda, Maryland

Autoimmune hemolytic anemia (AIHA) is the accelerated destruction of red cells caused by pathologic autoantibody. This accelerated destruction may be rapid and profound, with severe and life-threatening symptoms, or it may be more modest, with only a nominal decrease in the normal red cell life span of 110 to 120 days.

Modest reductions in red cell life span may not be noticed by the patient or clinician. The normal bone marrow is capable of a tenfold increase in the production of red cells in response to anemic stress. Therefore, low-grade immune hemolysis may be fully compensated by an increased production of red cells, with an elevated reticulocyte count being the primary indicator that increased red cell turnover is occurring.

Symptomatic anemia develops when the rate of hemolysis exceeds the ability of the marrow to respond, or when the marrow becomes depleted of the necessary substrates to sustain the accelerated rate of red cell production. If immune hemolysis is suspected, the most helpful confirmatory test is the direct antiglobulin test (DAT), also known as the direct Coombs test. The presence of immunoglobulin or complement components on the red cell membrane in combination with anemia and an elevated reticulocyte count is strong evidence of an immune hemolytic process. The major varieties of immune hemolysis are primary and secondary autoimmune hemolytic anemia (AIHA), immune hemolytic anemia secondary to drugs, cold agglutinin disease (CAD), and paroxysmal cold hemoglobinuria (PCH). A more detailed classification of these disorders is shown in Table 1.

PRIMARY AND SECONDARY AUTOIMMUNE HEMOLYTIC ANEMIA

Autoimmune hemolytic anemia mediated by warm-reacting autoantibodies can be either primary (idiopathic) or secondary to diseases such as chronic lymphocytic leukemia, lymphocytic and histiocytic lymphomas, systemic lupus erythematosus, and AIDS. AIHA is an uncommon disorder, with an incidence of about 1 in 80,000. Idiopathic AIHA is seen in all age groups, with women being affected more than men (about 60 to 40). Secondary AIHA parallels the age and sex distribution of the underlying disorder.

The etiology of AIHA is unclear. The observation that the disease is often seen in association with disorders of the immune system suggests a

TABLE 1. **Classification of Autoimmune Hemolytic Anemias**

Autoimmune Hemolytic Anemia—Warm-Reactive Antibody
  Primary (idiopathic)
  Secondary
    Lymphoproliferative disorders (chronic lymphocytic leukemia, lymphomas)
    Connective tissue disorders (systemic lupus erythematosus)

Drug-Induced Immune Hemolytic Anemia
  Red cell autoantibody type (methyldopa)
  Immune complex type (quinidine)
  Drug absorption (hapten) type (penicillin)
  Membrane modification type (cephalosporin)

Cold Agglutinin Disease
  Primary (idiopathic)
  Secondary
    Lymphoproliferative disorders
    Infections (infectious mononucleosis, *Mycoplasma pneumoniae*, postviral syndrome)

Paroxysmal Cold Hemoglobinuria
  Primary (idiopathic)
  Secondary
    Syphilis
    Postviral syndrome

defect in normal immune function—a loss of the ability to differentiate "self" from "non-self." There is evidence that AIHA may be related to an impairment in normal T-suppressor lymphocyte function, thus allowing unrestrained B-cell activity and the production of abnormal antibodies.

A small number of IgG molecules (<50) are found on the red cells of normal individuals. This number increases as the cell ages, leading to speculation that membrane-bound IgG plays a role in the removal of senescent red cells from the circulation. As the number of cell-bound IgG molecules increases (>200), the likelihood of immune hemolysis correspondingly increases. In the typical case of AIHA, large numbers of IgG molecules are found on the red cell surface, usually of the IgG subclasses IgG1 and IgG3. There are well-documented cases, however, when no hemolysis is seen, although many thousands of molecules are on the red cell and the DAT is strongly positive. There is evidence that anti-idiotype antibodies against the red cell autoantibody may block or otherwise modify the events that lead to immune hemolysis of the cell. This phenomenon may also be related to the subclass of the IgG autoantibody that is being produced. Subclasses IgG2 and IgG4 are not associated with severe hemolysis. Conversely, hemolysis is almost always found when IgG3 is present. Immune hemolysis cannot be predicted with as much certainty when the most common subclass, IgG1, is present.

Although the immunoglobulin class of autoantibody in warm AIHA is almost always IgG, examples of warm-reactive IgM and IgA autoantibodies have been reported and should be considered when "DAT-negative" immune hemolytic anemia is encountered.

Diagnosis

Patients with AIHA present with weakness, dizziness, pallor, jaundice and moderate splenomegaly. If the anemia is severe, hemoglobinuria, fever, palpitations, chest pain and syncope may be prominent. If AIHA is suspected, it is imperative that a thorough search be made for an implicated drug or for a potentially treatable underlying disorder.

Laboratory findings that support the diagnosis are spherocytes on the peripheral blood smear, reticulocytosis, hyperbilirubinemia (indirect), low or absent serum haptoglobin and elevated serum lactic dehydrogenase (LDH). Thrombocytopenia may indicate that immune destruction of platelets is also occurring, an association known as Evans's syndrome. The direct antiglobulin test detects IgG and complement components on the red cell and is positive in the vast majority of patients with AIHA; however, this test is not diagnostic. The DAT can be positive in other disorders and in normal individuals. Conversely, AIHA can be DAT negative under unusual circumstances (e.g., IgA autoantibodies). The indirect antiglobulin test (IAT), if positive, indicates the presence of red cell auto- or alloantibodies in the serum of the patient. This usually indicates that sufficient red cell autoantibody is being produced to maximally coat the red cells, with additional autoantibody being present in the serum.

Treatment

Treatment of AIHA is effective in the majority of patients: however, various published series have reported a mortality rate between 14 and 38 per cent. The initial steps in the treatment of AIHA are well established. If the disease is not controlled after these efforts, then one or more of several secondary treatments may be considered.

Initial treatment of the disease is with a corticosteroid, usually prednisone. The starting dose of prednisone should be in the range of 1.0 mg to 1.5 mg per kg per day. Larger doses are not more effective. About 80 per cent of patients will respond to this regimen with a decrease in hemolysis, a rise in hemoglobin, and an improvement in symptoms. If no response is seen after 3 weeks of high-dose prednisone, the treatment should be considered a failure. The mechanism of action of prednisone is not known. Steroids may interfere with the binding of antibody to the red cell surface, may delay the clearance of antibody-coated red cells, or may reduce the rate of synthesis of the abnormal autoantibody.

In patients who have responded to prednisone with a stabilization of hematocrit, a schedule of tapering the drug should be initiated. The dose should be reduced over 4 to 6 weeks to 30 mg per day, then reduced by 5 mg every 4 weeks until a level of 10 to 15 mg per day is reached. At that point either a very slow tapering of the dose or alternate-day therapy should be considered. If a relapse occurs, the dose should be increased to the previous dose and tapering should be reinstituted after the hemolysis stabilizes. If the prednisone dose cannot be lowered to below 15 mg per day without relapse, splenectomy should be considered. Although some patients can be maintained on low-dose, alternate-day prednisone for several years, most will eventually require splenectomy.

Splenectomy will result in improvement in symptoms in a majority of patients (about 60 per cent) who have failed with prednisone. Splenectomy not only eliminates the primary site of red cell destruction but also removes a major organ where antibodies are produced. It may permit the lowering of an unacceptably high maintenance dose of prednisone to one that is within tolerable limits. Relapses after splenectomy are common, however, and may occur months to years after the procedure.

As initial treatment of AIHA, all patients should be given a trial of steroids, followed by splenectomy if necessary. Failure of this initial regimen leads to a consideration of secondary treatments. Intravenous gamma globulin* (IVIgG) is effective in some patients if it is given in a sufficient dose. Initial studies with this therapy were disappointing, but more recent work has shown that large doses (0.5 to 1.0 gram per kg per day for 5 days)† often result in a sustained response. It is thought that IVIgG blocks the Fc gamma receptor on reticuloendothelial system (RES) macrophages, thus blocking RES removal of sensitized red cells.

Immunosuppressive drugs such as azathioprine* (Imuran) (125 mg per day) and cyclophosphamide (Cytoxan) (100 mg per day) given for up to 6 months will result in improvement in 40 to 50 per cent of patients, but side effects (e.g., marrow suppression) must be carefully monitored. Splenic irradiation has been advocated for those in whom splenectomy is contraindicated. Platelets coated with vinca alkaloids have been used as an experimental treatment in patients with AIHA. These platelets are ingested by RES macrophages, thus reducing the number and activity of these phagocytic cells. Plasma exchange is generally not useful, although it may temporarily lower plasma antibody levels. A summary of treatment modalities of AIHA is found in Table 2.

Transfusion

Transfusing patients with AIHA poses difficult challenges for both the clinician and the blood bank. The autoantibodies formed by these patients are directed against red cell membrane structures that are common to almost all human red cells, often being serologically identified as reacting with basic components of the Rh red cell antigen system. All donor red cells are usually incompatible with the patient's serum in the cross match. Minor variations in the serologic strength of the incompatibility among units are usually of no consequence and should not be used as a primary guide in selecting units for transfusion. Red cells transfused to these patients can be

---

*This use is not listed in the manufacturer's directive.

†This dose exceeds that recommended by the manufacturer for approved uses.

TABLE 2. **Treatment of Autoimmune Hemolytic Anemia—Warm Antibody Type**

Primary Treatments
1. Prednisone: Starting dose of 1.0 to 1.5 mg per kg per day (60 to 100 mg) with slow taper to 10 to 15 mg per day depending on response*
2. Splenectomy: For relapses or failures on prednisone
3. Transfusion: Do not withhold incompatible transfusions if necessary for life-threatening anemia*

Secondary Treatments
1. Immunosuppressive drugs†—azathioprine, cyclophosphamide
2. Intravenous gamma globulin† (IVIgG)—0.5 to 1.0 grams per kg per day for 5 days
3. Plasma exchange—temporary benefit only
4. Vinca-loaded platelets—experimental

---

*See text.
†This use is not listed in the manufacturer's directive.

expected to survive no better but also *no worse* than the patient's own red cells. The transfusion of red cells incompatible with the patient's autoantibody should not be withheld in the case of severe symptomatic anemia, especially if there has been insufficient time for the effect of other therapies to be fully evaluated.

The major risk of transfusion in these patients is that one or more red cell alloantibodies may be masked by the stronger autoantibody. Blood bank reference laboratories are usually able to identify these alloantibodies through the use of sophisticated serologic techniques, but the clinician should be especially cautious in transfusing patients with AIHA who have been exposed to red cell products in the past. Some transfusion medicine specialists recommend transfusing patients with red cells that are phenotypically matched with those of the patient for antigens in the Rh, Kell, and Kidd systems to prevent the development of dangerous alloantibodies in these systems.

Drug-Related Immune Hemolytic Anemia

Many drugs have been etiologically associated with warm-antibody AIHA. The patient with the onset of AIHA should be questioned closely for a history of prescription or over-the-counter drug ingestion. The mechanisms of drug-induced immune hemolysis fall into the following categories:

1. *Drug-induced red cell autoantibody (e.g., alpha-methyldopa [Aldomet]).* The antibody that is produced in response to the drug is not directed against the drug but against red cell membrane components. The antibody is identical in its characteristics to the autoantibodies seen in idiopathic warm AIHA. About 15 per cent of patients receiving alpha-methyldopa will develop a positive DAT, whereas about 1 per cent will have hemolytic anemia. It has been suggested that

alpha-methyldopa may alter the function of T-suppressor lymphocytes, thus allowing B-lymphocytes to elaborate pathologic antibody.

2. *Immune-complex mechanism (e.g., quinidine).* An immune complex of drug and anti-drug antibody is formed in the plasma. This immune complex activates complement on the surface of the otherwise uninvolved red cells, leading to accelerated destruction of the sensitized cells.

3. *Drug absorption (hapten) mechanism (e.g., penicillin).* The drug or drug components bind directly to the red cell surface. Therefore, anti-drug IgG antibody that binds to the drug is also bound to the red cell, leading to the cell's immune destruction.

4. *Membrane modification mechanism (e.g., cephalosporins).* The drug alters the red cell membrane so that other proteins are nonspecifically absorbed. Although the DAT is positive, immune hemolysis is rarely seen with this mechanism.

A given drug can cause a positive DAT and red cell hemolysis by more than one of these mechanisms. If a patient is on a drug that has been implicated in causing AIHA, the drug should, of course, be stopped. This will usually result in prompt improvement in the hemolysis and stabilization of the hematocrit. In some cases, such as the immune hemolysis associated with alpha-methyldopa, reversion of the DAT to normal may take several months.

COLD AGGLUTININ DISEASE

Hemolytic anemia upon exposure to cold, and symptomatology related to intermittent occlusion of the microvasculature, compose the syndrome of cold agglutinin disease (CAD). The primary (idiopathic) form of CAD is a disease found primarily in the elderly. CAD can also be secondary to several infectious diseases (e.g., infectious mononucleosis) and to lymphoproliferative disorders.

Cold-reactive red cell autoantibodies can be detected in the plasma of most individuals if serologic reactions are conducted at 4° C. These IgM antibodies usually have anti-H, anti-I, or anti-i specificity and are of no clinical importance. On occasion, however, these autoantibodies can be active over a wide thermal range, with agglutination of red cells occurring at temperatures approaching 37° C.

The pathologic IgM cold agglutinins of CAD usually have anti-I specificity. The antibodies activate complement, resulting in the deposition of C3b molecules on the red cell surface. These red cells adhere to the C3b receptors on RES macrophages and are removed from the circulation. The chronic hemolytic anemia of CAD is usually not as severe as that seen in warm AIHA, but acute exacerbations with hemoglobinuria can occur, usually associated with exposure to cold temperatures.

Patients with CAD also have symptoms (aside from those of anemia) related to ischemia of areas of the body exposed to cold. Pallor and acrocyanosis of the fingers, toes, nose, and ears are common and are thought to be secondary to red cell agglutination in the microvasculature of these areas. Raynaud's phenomenon is often seen. The spleen is only slightly enlarged in most cases.

Laboratory findings include autoagglutination of blood samples that are allowed to cool after being drawn, a cold agglutinin of high titer reacting at a temperature of at least 30° C or higher in serologic tests, and red cells that are coated with C3 but not IgG. Compatible cross matches can usually be obtained if all serologic tests are conducted at 37° C or if a cold autoabsorption procedure is carried out prior to cross matching.

Treatment of cold agglutinin disease consists primarily of avoidance of the cold. Patients should be advised to protect exposed areas and, in more severe cases, to consider changing their residence to a warmer climate. Other treatments are generally unsatisfactory. Steroids, immunosuppressive drugs, and splenectomy are less effective than in warm-antibody AIHA and should be used only with considerable caution. Plasma exchange has been used with some success as a temporary measure to lower plasma IgM levels during an acute hemolytic episode.

PAROXYSMAL COLD HEMOGLOBINURIA

This unusual disorder is caused by a biphasic hemolytic antibody that reacts with the patient's red cells at low temperatures, with subsequent complement fixation and cell lysis when the cells are returned to physiologic temperatures. Paroxysmal cold hemoglobinuria (PCH) was originally thought to be related to syphilis, but it is now recognized that it also follows many types of viral infections. Often PCH cannot be related to any distinct antecedent event. Patients experience acute paroxysms characterized by fever, chills, abdominal and back pain, and hemoglobinuria. Exposure to cold often precipitates an acute attack, but symptoms can develop in the absence of such an exposure.

The bithermic hemolysis test (Donath-Landsteiner test) is essential for the diagnosis of PCH. The patient's serum is incubated with test red cells in ice for 30 minutes, incubated at 37° C for 30 minutes, and then observed for the presence of hemolysis. The pathologic red cell antibody that is responsible for this bithermic hemolysis is anti-P.

Treatment of PCH is generally supportive. The patient should be instructed to avoid the cold and should be screened for syphilis and treated if necessary. Acute postinfectious PCH often resolves spontaneously. Short courses of steroids may be beneficial during acute attacks of the illness but are not recommended for long-term therapy. Transfusion of either the P or P^k blood types avoids the offending antibody, but these blood types are very rare. In the absence of these types, transfusions of cross match–compatible, P-positive units can be given through a blood warmer.

NONIMMUNE HEMOLYTIC ANEMIA

method of
JAMES P. CROWLEY, M.D.
Brown University
Providence, Rhode Island

A patient with anemia in whom there is a reticulocytosis and a negative Coombs direct antiglobulin test suggests the diagnosis of a chronic nonimmune hemolytic anemia (NHA). The major differential diagnosis is recent blood loss. Because of the comparatively rapid delivery of iron from red cells recently destroyed within the reticuloendothelial system (RES) to the marrow, anemia that results from hemorrhage does not reach the level of reticulocytosis that is commonly seen in NHA. In following the progress of NHA, it is more useful to express the reticulocyte count as an absolute value (that is, multiplying the percent of reticulocytes by the red count) than by simply enumerating a percent value.

Hemolysis is both intravascular and extravascular in most NHA and a reduced haptoglobin content of serum is the most specific test to differentiate NHA from blood loss. The presence of infection, malignancy, or steroid therapy may increase the production of haptoglobins making it difficult to interpret changes in haptoglobin levels in relation to hemolysis. Increases in plasma unconjugated bilirubin concentration are a sensitive indicator of hemolysis; however, if liver function is abnormal, bilirubin estimates may be misleading. Similarly, determination of lactate dehydrogenase (LDH) is useful in many situations, because a normal value excludes excessive hemolysis in most cases. However, elevated values may be difficult to interpret because of the multiple potential sources for increases in lactate dehydrogenase (LDH). Urinary hemosiderinuria, if done properly, may assist in a late diagnosis of an earlier, abrupt, self-limited hemolytic anemia. Measurement of plasma-free hemoglobin is widely used but is often misleading, since slight traumatic hemolysis when the blood is drawn can artifactually release hemoglobin. [51]Chromium and red blood cell survival, hemopexin levels, and estimations of fecal urobilinogen may be difficult to obtain but occasionally have value in documenting mild or intermittent hemolysis. As will be discussed later, simple examination of the peripheral blood smear often provides the most valuable clues to the specific etiology of NHA. Once the diagnosis is established, serial observation of LDH levels and the absolute reticulocyte count have proven the most useful means of following the progress of NHA and response to therapy.

Treatment

Transfusion Therapy

Red cell transfusions for patients with severe NHA are effective therapy but need to be held to a minimum to reduce complications and iron overload. In general, transfusions are only indicated for patients with hemolysis who exhibit signs of hypoxia or whose hemoglobin is falling rapidly. Transfusions to correct hemoglobin levels above 8.0 grams per dl in clinically stable patients are rarely justified. Some patients may adapt to hemoglobin levels even lower than this if cardiopulmonary function is adequate.

Compensatory reticulocytosis may fail because of reduced total body iron stores or factors that result in a reduced iron transport from the reticuloendothelial system such as infection. Parvovirus infection produces a transient erythroblastopenia and an aplastic crisis may result. The usual signs of hemolysis may decrease or even become absent and obscure the diagnosis of an underlying hemolytic anemia. Immediate transfusions are indicated in this situation.

Folic Acid and Iron

Chronic hemolysis is associated with accelerated folate utilization. Accordingly, all patients with hemolysis should receive folic acid, 1 mg per day orally. Doses of 2 to 3 mg per day may be indicated if patients are folate deficient or recovering from an aplastic crisis. Iron therapy for patients with chronic hemolytic anemia is usually contraindicated. Exceptions to this rule are patients with a coexistent iron-deficient state such as may occur in patients with cardiac hemolysis, paroxymal nocturnal hemoglobinuria, or with concomitant sources of significant blood loss.

Splenectomy and Cholecystectomy

The spleen is a major site of destruction of abnormal red cells. Removing the spleen cures some NHA when the defect in the red cells is minimal, as in hereditary spherocytosis. Hereditary hemolytic diseases associated with splenomegaly generally will also be ameliorated by splenectomy. Splenectomy should be performed *only* on patients with chronic nonimmune anemia who require frequent blood transfusions. The risks associated with splenectomy are usually less than the cumulative risks over a lifetime of repeated blood transfusions.

Asplenic patients are susceptible to overwhelming pneumococcal bacteremia. The magnitude of the risk is low (<0.1%), but the mortality of these infections is high (60 to 70 per cent), and this risk is clearly greater in children under the age of 10. The longest reported interval between splenectomy and overwhelming bacteremia has been 25 years. All patients should receive pneumococcal vaccination (Pneumovax, 0.5 ml), ideally two weeks before splenectomy. Vaccination has a reduced efficacy in children under the age of 10. For this reason, children should be given daily oral prophylactic penicillin, 125 to 250 mg orally twice a day. The gallbladders of all patients subjected to splenectomy should be removed if there is concomitant evidence of cholelithiasis.

Iron Overload

The removal of iron deposition associated with chronic blood transfusions (about 250 mg per unit) should be considered early but deemed urgent in any patient who has received 100 transfusions, since significant endocrine, hepatic, and cardiac damage is likely. Constant, subcutaneous delivery of desferoxamine (1 gram per 24 hours) with small portable pumps will often achieve negative iron balance in frequently transfused patients. Ascorbic acid (250 mg per day) enhances iron excretion by desferoxamine, but there is a small risk of enhancing cardiac iron toxicity. Ascorbic acid should always be taken an hour or two after desferoxamine has been started to ensure that adequate levels of iron chelation have been achieved before superimposing the mobilizing effects of ascorbic acid on iron deposits.

HEMOLYSIS CAUSED BY INFECTIONS, TOXINS, AND NEOPLASIA

Of acquired infectious, neoplastic, and toxic (AINT) etiologies (Table 1), malaria is undoubtedly the most common worldwide cause of hemolytic anemia. The anemia is due to the rupture

TABLE 1. **Infections and Toxins Causing Hemolysis***

Malaria and babesiosis
Volatile nitrites
Transitional elements and heavy metals
Hypophosphatemia
Clostridial infection
Snake and spider venoms

*Modified from Jandl, JH. *Blood: Textbook of Hematology.* Boston, Little, Brown and Co., 1987 (with permission from the author and publisher).

of infected cells at the end of the asexual development cycle. The extent of hemolysis is greatest in *Plasmodium falciparum* malaria. Fulminant intravascular hemolysis (Blackwater fever) has a mortality of 20 to 30 per cent. Intravascular volume, replacement iron, and folic acid supplements are the mainstays of therapy. Transfusion in some countries is a frequent cause of human immunodeficiency virus (HIV) transmission; therefore, transfusion therapy should be reserved only for fulminant cases of malaria-induced hemolysis if HIV testing is not available.

Babesiosis is an uncommon, parasitic hemolytic disorder of the northeastern United States that superficially resembles *P. falciparum* malaria. In North America most infections are transmitted from animals to humans by ticks of the *Ixodes* genera. These ticks are also the vector for the spirochete responsible for Lyme disease, and both babesiosis and Lyme disease have occurred in the same patient. Splenectomized patients are especially susceptible to infection via transfusions from an asymptomatic carrier. Transfusion therapy usually resolves the hemolysis. Chemotherapeutic treatment of malaria and babesiosis are treated in another section.

Amyl nitrite and other volatile nitrites are used for their mood-altering effects by some homosexuals and occasionally by heterosexuals. Hemolysis may follow their use. The ingestion or inhalation of several transitional elements or heavy metals also may cause hemolysis. Arsine vapor (AsH_3) may cause severe intravascular hemolysis and is a hazard of the acid processing of tin and the manufacture of certain fertilizers. Occupational exposure to compounds containing copper, arsenic, mercury, silver, gold, and lead also can produce hemolysis because they are highly reactive with red blood cell membrane thiols. Hemolysis during hemodialysis has been traced to the high copper content of some tap water. Hemolytic crises occasionally occur in the early stages of Wilson's disease because of high levels of copper. In general, mild cases of heavy metal– or transitional element–induced hemolysis will be corrected following occupational withdrawal. In severe cases, emergency measures may be needed to ensure oxygenation and adequate volume. If plasma Hb rises above 400 to 500 mg per dl, exchange transfusions should be performed daily.

Hemolysis may develop as a consequence of severe hypophosphatemia due to diabetic ketoacidosis or anorexia nervosa, since depletion of intracellular phosphate blocks ATP production. Oral and parenteral phosphate supplementation may be required when severe symptomatic hypophosphatemia is complicated by hemolysis.

Hemolysis due to clostridial infection may occur in patients with septic abortion, gangrenous cholecystitis, or any deep-seated infection and is a hazard in cancer patients receiving aggressive chemotherapy. In these cases, the hemolysis is caused by a toxic phospholipase. Therapy includes vigorous transfusions, antibiotics and immediate surgery.

Pit viper venoms also cause hemolysis by a phospholipase. Also, a relative of the black widow spider, the brown recluse spider, may cause hemolysis that may become evident only several days after the bite. Treatment of hemolysis due to spider and snake bites consists of local wound management, prophylactic antibiotics, and transfusions.

Paroxysmal nocturnal hemoglobinuria (PNH) is a rare neoplastic disease that causes hemolysis. An acquired membrane abnormality results in the fixation of complement by the alternative pathway to red blood cells that produce lysis. The clinical course of PNH is highly variable and may be exacerbated by iron or folate deficiencies or by intercurrent infections. Patients with PNH are prone to venous thrombosis due to enhanced platelet adhesiveness. These thrombi form in unusual parts of the body such as the hepatic, portal, or cerebral veins. Aplastic crisis or frank aplastic anemia frequently occurs and may precede the development of acute myelogenous leukemia.

The diagnosis of PNH is made by the Ham test, or its more recent technically simpler modification, the sugar water test. Sensitive tests for the detection of complement have been recently developed using monoclonal antibodies to activated forms of complement, which in some cases allow a diagnosis when other studies are equivocal.

Daily oral iron therapy (ferrous sulfate, 325 mg three times daily) should be given to all affected patients. Some patients will require intermittent intravenous iron therapy. Iron administration may result in the sudden production of large numbers of cells susceptible to complement lysis. To avoid this, patients should be given transfusions of washed red blood cells to transiently suppress hematopoiesis. Some patients respond to corticosteroids (prednisone, 60 mg per day). Patients who have thrombosis can be treated with heparin and coumadin, but they should also be transfused with washed red blood cells. Some patients require chronic, low-dose oral anticoagulants to avoid repeated thrombosis.

Leukoerythroblastic anemia is characterized by bizarre fragments, teardrop red cells, and nucleated erythroid precursors, together with immature leukocytes and giant platelets due to marrow involvement with leukemia or to fibrosis. Some patients with leukoerythroblastic anemia exhibit a PNH-like hemolysis. Management depends on the underlying etiology. In severely affected patients, splenectomy is effective.

HEREDITARY SPHEROCYTOSIS AND RELATED MEMBRANE DISORDERS

Hereditary spherocytosis (HS) is a dominant hemolytic disorder with variable penetrance. The abnormal red blood cells have increased mechanical and osmotic fragility. Elliptocytosis closely resembles HS in inheritance, but hemolysis is usually much milder. Many patients are free of anemia as a result of complete compensation by the bone marrow. The red cell membrane in HS is progressively lost during red cell aging and, as the surface area decreases, the red cells become more spheroidal and are destroyed in the spleen. Osmotic fragility is increased and has long been used to confirm the diagnosis. Some patients with HS have a marked reduction in spectrin and these cases tend to be more severe. Abnormalities of spectrin or a reduction in its amount may also be associated with morphologic consequences other than spherocytosis.

Hereditary pyropoikilocytosis (HPP) is a rare, moderate-to-severe congenital hemolytic anemia that is usually seen in blacks and is characterized by striking micropoikilocytosis and microspherocytosis, autosomal recessive inheritance, and thermal instability of red cells. HS, HPP, and related disorders almost invariably benefit from splenectomy and cholecystectomy when cholelithiasis is present.

Some patients with severe alcoholic cirrhosis acquire a hemolytic anemia associated with splenomegaly and acanthocytosis (spur cell anemia). This acanthocytosis closely resembles the acanthocytosis of hereditary abetalipoproteinemia. Since the defect is induced by the patient's plasma, transfusions are of only temporary value. Splenectomy has increased risk in these end-stage liver disease patients but is occasionally indicated. Hemolytic anemia with erythrocyte spicule formation and hyperlipidemia (Zieve's syndrome) may also be observed in severe alcoholic hepatitis. Treatment is supportive and based upon management of the liver disease. A rare form of x-linked acanthocytosis affects red cells deficient in the K_x antigen (McLeod phenotype). McLeod red cells react poorly with Kell antisera. For unknown reasons this unusual phenotype results in acanthocytosis and a mild compensated hemolysis. The McLeod phenotype is seen in some patients with chronic granulomatous disease. If these patients have developed a high-titer isoimmune anti-Kell antibody, there may be difficulties in cross matching and procurement when they require blood transfusion.

Stomatocytosis, or a cup-shaped deformity of the red cell, may be present in a small number of patients with hemolytic anemia due to abnormalities in red cell cation transport. The anemia is usually an autosomal pattern of inheritance, and approximately 20 to 30 per cent of red cells in peripheral smears are stomatocytes. Osmotic and mechanical fragility is increased, and marked red cell membrane hyperpermeability to monovalent cations but not to divalent cations or to anions has been demonstrated.

Stomatocytosis accompanied by transient moderate hemolysis has also been observed in a few patients with acute alcoholism. Alterations in cation permeability without stomatocytosis have also been reported in association with a variety of rare, inherited, hemolytic anemias due to either primary metabolic or hemoglobin abnormalities. Hemolysis is due to sodium permeability and the consequent cell water increase resulting in large osmotically fragile cells. The severity of the anemia varies greatly in the red cell cation transplant abnormalities and severe cases are only partially corrected by splenectomy.

HEREDITARY NONSPHEROCYTIC ANEMIAS

Glucose-6-phosphate dehydrogenase (G6PD) deficiency is the most common cause of episodic nonspherocytic hemolytic anemia and probably the most common genetic abnormality known in man. G6PD regenerates reduced nicotinamide adenine dinucleotide phosphate (NADPH), which reduces glutathione (GSH) which detoxifies oxidative substances in the RBC. When G6PD is deficient, hemoglobin may be irreversibly oxidized and denatured to form precipitated globin called Heinz bodies, leading to removal of the red blood cells by the spleen and liver. Transmission occurs from mother to child, with full expression developing primarily in hemizygous males.

The two most important clinical variants of G6PD occur in American blacks and some individuals of Mediterranean descent. The American black variant is a less severe form than the Mediterranean type. G6PD activity in affected blacks is almost normal in the youngest cells but declines rapidly as the cells age. The activity of the Mediterranean variant deficient enzyme is greatly diminished even in the youngest cells. Because there is a more selective destruction of the older red blood cells by oxidant degradation, residual enzyme activity present after hemolysis tends to limit hemolysis. This makes the diagnosis difficult, since G6PD assays may be normal once all the older cells have been destroyed.

Oxidant drugs are the most common precipitating factor in G6PD-related hemolysis, and the ability of a given drug to induce hemolysis in a G6PD-deficient individual correlates with the drug's oxidizing potential. Commonly used drugs that may precipitate hemolysis are shown in Table 2. Offending drugs can sometimes be continued in blacks if necessary, since the increased production of new cells will compensate for the anemia; higher than usual doses of folic acid are then recommended (2 to 3 mg per day). In contrast, the anemia produced by the Mediterranean variant will persist in the presence of the offending agent because of the high degree of enzyme deficiency even in young red blood cells. In these patients all possible offending drugs should be immediately discontinued.

Other factors often predispose a G6PD-deficient person to hemolysis and viral infections, especially hepatitis, bacterial infections such as pneumococcal pneumonia, uremia, and diabetic ketoacidosis. Even mild oxidants may aggravate or precipitate hemolysis in these settings (Table 2). Chronic hemolysis in G6PD deficiency is unusual in blacks but common in patients of Mediterranean origin. Vitamin E, 800 units per day orally, will reduce chronic hemolysis in patients with the Mediterranean type of G6PD deficiency.

Sickle cell disease is the most common form of chronic nonspherocytic hemolytic anemia. Sickle cell disease and thalassemia are discussed in detail in articles later in this section. Sickle cells interact abnormally with endothelium and obstruct blood flow, resulting in organ damage. Periodic painful crisis with no precipitating cause is the hallmark of sickle cell disease and occurs in at least 75 per cent of patients. Dehydration occurs in many patients because of their inability

TABLE 2. **Some Agents Producing a Hemolytic Process in G6PD-Deficient Individuals**

Independently

Aqua Mephyton (vitamin K)	Pentaquine
Dapsone	Primaquine
Furazolidine	Sulfanilamide
Nalidixic acid	Sulfapyridine
Nitrofurantoin	Sulfasalazine
Pamaquine	

Usually Only in Presence of Other Factors

Ascorbic acid	Procainamide
Aspirin	Pyrimethamine
Chloramphenicol	Quinacrine
Chloroquine	Quinidine
Dimercaprol	Quinine
Diphenhydramine	Sulfadiazine
Menadione	Sulfamerazine
Methylene blue	Sulfathiazole
Phenacetin	Sulfisoxazole
Probenecid	Tripelennamine

to conserve water due to poor renal concentrating function.

The mainstay of therapy for the sickle cell crisis is hydration and analgesics given in judicious but sufficient amounts. Aspirin may aggravate acidosis and, if taken in large amounts, may cause hypercapnia predisposing the patient to cerebral edema. Transfusions are generally indicated to maintain the hemoglobin above 7.0 grams per dl. Patients not responding to this therapy should be considered for exchange transfusions that will dilute circulating HbS and suppress its production. Neocytes if available by cytopheresis represent the youngest cell population in the donor and are preferred for the small number of patients requiring regular transfusions. Five or six unit exchange procedures will result in the reduction of hemoglobin S concentration to approximately 50 per cent in the majority of patients, at which point the refractory crisis will usually stop. Exchange transfusions are also indicated in the treatment of cerebral vascular occlusion, some intractable cases of ankle ulcers, and priapism. Oxygen therapy should be given to hypoxic patients, but continuous oxygen therapy results in a decline in erythropoietin levels, which may exacerbate hemolysis when oxygen is stopped because of a rebound reticulocytosis. Nifedipine, 10 mg three times a day, is a calcium channel blocking antihypertensive agent which is effective in resolving vaso-occlusive retinopathy. Experimental approaches to sickle cell disease are discussed elsewhere.

More than 30 abnormal hemoglobins that lead to hemolysis because of intrinsic instability of the hemoglobin molecule have been described. Of these, the most frequently encountered are hemoglobin H which occurs predominantly in people of Southeast Asia, and hemoglobin Köln, which is usually encountered in non-Asians. Hemolytic anemia and aplastic crisis are the predominant clinical manifestations of these unstable hemoglobins. Approximately one third of the unstable hemoglobins represent spontaneous mutations; therefore, the abnormality may not be present in other members of the family.

Routine electrophoresis methodology for defining hemoglobin variants may be misleading, since many of the unstable hemoglobins represent neutral substitutions. More dependable information is obtained from the application of techniques that demonstrate the unstable solubility of hemoglobin. Of these tests, the isopropanol technique is the most useful and should be a part of the workup for any obscure hemolytic disorder.

Splenomegaly is often present but splenectomy is indicated only in severe cases. Parodoxically, erythrocytosis may follow splenectomy in some patients with some unstable hemoglobins, due to strongly left-shifted oxyhemoglobin dissociation curves.

Enzyme deficiencies of the Embden-Meyerhof pathway constitute the least common congenital nonspherocytic hemolytic anemias. In most cases there is an inherited enzyme deficiency of pyruvate kinase (PK) that results in mild hemolysis in patients with autosomally recessive inherited disease. In families in which the inheritance is dominant, severe hemolysis occurs. In patients with PK deficiency there is a higher than usual content of 2,3-DPG.

A strongly right-shifted oxyhemoglobin dissociation curve may suggest the disorder. Splenectomy will not completely stop the hemolytic process, but it will usually reduce the need for transfusions. A remarkable reticulocytosis often follows splenectomy in PK-deficient patients.

ANGIOPATHIC HEMOLYTIC ANEMIAS

Cardiac hemolysis is the most common cause of macroangiopathic hemolysis. If the hemolysis is mild, folic acid with or without oral iron supplementation may be sufficient in the management of these patients. Sulfinpyrazone (up to 250 mg four times a day) may decrease hemolysis in some patients, but periodic transfusions may still be required when the patient's activity level increases. Transfusions in severe hemolysis are often ineffective, in which case replacement of the pathologic valve will be required, the only alternative being for the patient to limit activity consistent with the degree of anemia. Episodic hemolysis of this type may also be noted in runners, martial artists, bongo drummers, and marching soldiers.

Microangiopathic hemolytic anemia results from red cell fragmentation by fibrin strands in the arterioles and is seen in a variety of clinical settings. Malignant hypertension is a prototypic example, and treatment of severely elevated blood pressure dramatically controls hemolysis. Similar changes are seen in patients with meningococcemia with fulminant intravascular coagulation. Plasma exchange, although rarely employed, may be life-saving in this setting.

Giant cavernous hemangiomas (Kasabach-Merritt syndrome) may shear erythrocytes as they move through the capillary network of the hemangioma, and treatment is by surgical excision or radiation.

Thrombotic thrombocytopenic purpura (TTP) is a relatively uncommon syndrome of thrombocytopenia, microangiopathic hemolytic anemia, fluctuating neurologic abnormalities, fever, and renal dysfunction. An infectious cause has been long suspected, but immunologic disturbances and abnormally high amounts of high molecular weight Factor VIII have been observed.

Aspirin, persantine, steroids, and immunosuppressive drugs may produce a transient beneficial response but are unreliable when used alone. The addition of plasma transfusions and continuous plasma exchange have recently improved the outlook dramatically. Plasma exchange must be vigorously applied to first reduce LDH levels and then keep them below 1000 units. In the past, splenectomy was done on an emergency basis for TTP, but this operation is now rarely performed unless plasma exchange has proved ineffective.

A new form of TTP has recently been described in cancer patients treated with mitomycin C even when the tumor is in complete remission or when there is only minimal residual or recurrent disease. Plasma perfusion over filters containing staphylococcal protein A (SPA) has been used successfully to treat patients with adenocarcinoma who have developed this complication.

Eclampsia also is often accompanied by microangiopathic hemolysis and thrombocytopenia. Hemolysis usually resolves spontaneously with delivery. Hemolysis and thrombocytopenia persisting after delivery are treated as for TTP, with antiplatelet agents, steroids, and plasma. Some patients experience severe renal failure that may completely resolve with short-term hemodialysis or that may lead to progressive renal insufficiency requiring long-term dialysis treatment.

PERNICIOUS ANEMIA AND OTHER MEGALOBLASTIC ANEMIAS

method of
NEVILLE COLMAN, M.D., Ph.D
Mount Sinai School of Medicine
Bronx VA Medical Center
New York, New York

The megaloblastic anemias are disorders of DNA synthesis characterized by changes in morphology of bone marrow and other rapidly dividing cells. More than 90 per cent are caused by folate or vitamin B_{12} deficiency, but increasing numbers are attributable to DNA-active drugs such as hydroxyurea.

Pernicious anemia, the best-known megaloblastic anemia, is caused by idiopathic deficiency of gastric intrinsic factor, which is necessary for receptor-mediated vitamin B_{12} absorption in the ileum. It is associated with antibodies against intrinsic factor, gastric parietal cells, and the thyroid. It is also a cause of neurologic changes, as are other causes of vitamin B_{12}

deficiency. The term "pernicious anemia" is sometimes erroneously applied to megaloblastic anemias of other types.

Management before Replacement Therapy

Management of megaloblastic anemia involves three phases, each as essential as appropriate replacement therapy: (1) diagnosis of the megaloblastosis, (2) characterization of the deficient vitamin or other mechanism, and (3) identification of the underlying disease.

These critical evaluations are often neglected because acute care of megaloblastic anemia can be effectively handled by "shotgun" treatment with folic acid and vitamin B_{12}. The hazard of this approach lies in the trap it creates for long-term care, because it is frequently extremely difficult to prove whether megaloblastosis was present, or which deficiency caused it, once treatment has begun. The physician is then left with the choice of either instituting life-long vitamin B_{12} replacement, a significant burden if unnecessary, or foregoing treatment and risking irreversible neurologic damage if vitamin B_{12} deficiency develops. Fortunately, most cases with shotgun therapy still allow subsequent testing for vitamin B_{12} malabsorption.

Phase 1 of management is diagnosis of megaloblastic anemia. This requires examination of the bone marrow aspirate, since all the peripheral blood features of these disorders may be seen in other conditions such as the myelodysplastic syndromes and hematologic malignancies. The bone marrow typically shows red cell precursors with cytonuclear dissociation, usually accompanied by giant granulocytic precursors and neutrophil hypersegmentation.

In the peripheral blood, erythroid macrocytosis has become extremely easy to recognize because the mean corpuscular volume (MCV) is measured with great accuracy in the routine complete blood count (CBC) provided by most automated blood counters, irrespective of whether they are based on electronic or laser technology. There are important pitfalls in the use of macrocytosis as a marker for megaloblastosis. Firstly, in most locations, the majority of patients with elevated MCV do *not* have megaloblastic anemia but rather a poorly defined mild macrocytosis of alcoholism that is unrelated to megaloblastosis. Through its separate effects on folate metabolism, alcohol is also one of the prominent causes of megaloblastosis. Secondly, a significant minority of megaloblastic patients do *not* have macrocytosis; common factors responsible for this paradox are superimposed iron deficiency, alpha thalassemia, and perhaps the anemia of chronic disease.

In my experience, megaloblastosis is almost universally present if the MCV is over 115 fl, whereas this is no more likely with an MCV of 100 to 110 fl than with an MCV less than 100 fl.

The red cell distribution width (RDW), an automated measure of variation in red cell size (anisocytosis), is a useful tool in distinguishing the megaloblastic anemias (abnormal RDW elevation) from nonmegaloblastic macrocytic anemias (normal RDW). Another valuable indicator is the fact that leukopenia and/or thrombocytopenia are common in megaloblastosis, reflecting the involvement of all rapidly dividing cells in the pathologic process.

It is important to remember that neurologic damage in vitamin B_{12} deficiency may present without severe anemia. However, virtually all subjects with vitamin B_{12} neuropathy have abnormalities of the peripheral blood and bone marrow, even if these do not cause flagging on the automated CBC.

Phase 2 of management is to evaluate whether the deficiency is of folate or of vitamin B_{12}, which together account for almost all cases. This can usually be done by assays for serum B_{12} and for serum and red cell folate. Two new important experimental tools are becoming increasingly available at this stage. The deoxyuridine suppression test was described in 1968 as a diagnostic test for both defining the presence of biochemical megaloblastosis and diagnosing its cause, and has been the gold standard in research laboratories. It recently became more available for routine diagnostic use because the technologist time required for incubation and washing has been halved.

The second tool, available for even more rapid introduction into routine laboratories, is assay for elevated serum methylmalonate (in vitamin B_{12} deficiency) and homocysteine (in both vitamin B_{12} and folate deficiency), precursors for enzymes which require vitamin B_{12} or folate.

All of the tests used in phases 1 and 2 of management must be performed before treatment because they normalize within hours of appropriate treatment. Reversion in the deoxyuridine suppression test is almost instantaneous; morphologic marrow megaloblastosis reverts to normoblastosis in 18 to 48 hours; and peripheral blood retains evidence of neutrophil hypersegmentation for 10 to 14 days and of red cell changes for 4 to 8 weeks.

Phase 3 of management is definition of the underlying causes of vitamin deficiency. A limited number of specific tests may assist this process; these mainly identify features of pernicious anemia and, unlike other tests, remain valid after treatment. The first is analysis of gastric volume

and pH for the definition of achlorhydria, which precedes pernicious anemia. Direct measurement of intrinsic factor is possible in many institutions; this involves careful attention to detail during stimulated gastric analysis to prevent peptic hydrolysis of any intrinsic factor that may be present. This provides the only direct test for absent intrinsic factor, the hallmark of pernicious anemia. Intrinsic factor antibody assay is a valuable ancillary test, providing a highly specific finding in more than two thirds of subjects with pernicious anemia. It is also positive in 7 to 10 per cent of patients with autoimmune thyroid diseases associated with pernicious anemia, and virtually never positive in other subjects. Intrinsic factor antibodies are now widely available in clinical laboratories.

The two-part Schilling test for vitamin B_{12} absorption is another important assessment and can partly replace intrinsic factor assay. This is an excellent method of documenting vitamin B_{12} malabsorption and defining whether it is corrected by intrinsic factor. This test should not be conducted until the rest of the assessment is completed, because it involves administration of a flushing dose of vitamin B_{12} (1000 micrograms intramuscularly), which is itself therapeutic and thus masks the signs of deficiency. In addition, in about 20 per cent of pernicious anemia patients, correction of malabsorption (in Part I of the test) by intrinsic factor (in part 2) is masked by gastrointestinal megaloblastosis until there have been approximately 6 weeks of appropriate replacement therapy. For this reason, I routinely wait until after 6 or more weeks of replacement therapy before using the Schilling test.

If Part II of the Schilling test shows no correction with intrinsic factor, it is presumed that the cause of vitamin B_{12} malabsorption is located at intrinsic factor receptors in the ileum. If the history and physical examination give cause for suspicion of tropical sprue or a blind loop syndrome, it may be prudent to administer a trial of antibiotics (tetracycline, 250 mg 4 times daily for 3 weeks) and repeat the Schilling test without intrinsic factor; this is sometimes referred to as the Part III Schilling Test.

A recent modification of the Schilling test was designed to detect malabsorption of food vitamin B_{12} when crystalline vitamin B_{12} is absorbed normally. The tracer B_{12} isotope is cooked into an egg, and absorption from this bound ovalbumin source is assessed. It finds its application primarily in elderly patients with low serum vitamin B_{12} levels who have achlorhydria but a normal Part I Schilling test. Significant numbers of these patients show abnormalities of the ovalbumin Schilling test despite the normal Part I test.

Phase 3 requires a careful clinical history and physical examination. Vitamin B_{12} deficiency is virtually always due to malabsorption based on inadequate intrinsic factor or on interference with ileal receptor uptake. The former results from pernicious anemia or gastrectomy, whereas the latter is most commonly secondary to ileal inflammation (Crohn's disease), damage (tropical or celiac sprue), or removal. It has recently become evident from studies in Great Britain of subjects of Indian origin that a significant proportion of strict vegans (who ingest no dairy products or eggs) have nutritional deficiency of vitamin B_{12}.

In contrast, folate deficiency can be caused by a gamut of conditions, ranging from inadequate intake, absorption, and utilization, to excess requirement, destruction, and loss. In the United States, the commonest cause of folate deficient megaloblastic anemia is alcohol, which has multiple effects on hematopoiesis in general and on folate metabolism in particular. It is now believed to exert its effect mainly through altering folate utilization; the mechanism for this has not yet been elucidated. Other important causes of folate deficiency include pregnancy and lactation; malabsorption, especially due to tropical sprue and celiac sprue; and two main classes of drugs, namely anticonvulsants such as Dilantin and folate antagonists such as methotrexate.

Treatment of Vitamin B_{12} Deficiency Anemia

Initial Therapy

Definitive therapy of vitamin B_{12} deficiency is accomplished with parenteral administration of vitamin B_{12}, usually as cyanocobalamin. Although hydroxocobalamin may be a more physiologic form of vitamin B_{12}, the lack of demonstrated toxicity of either form and the high cost of the hydroxo compound have prevented many from switching to the "more physiologic form." In specific clinical circumstances when cyanocobalamin may be harmful, however, hydroxocobalamin is preferable despite its cost; these include nitroprusside reactions, tobacco amblyopia, and perhaps sulfite sensitivity.

The established method of parenteral administration is by intramuscular or deep subcutaneous injection. I have recently evaluated a new preparation of cyanocobalamin prepared as a nasal gel and find that it is an effective method for treating vitamin B_{12} deficiency (discussed in more detail below).

The therapeutic dose of injected cyanocobalamin is usually 1000 micrograms daily for a week and then weekly for a month. Pharmacokinetic curves indicate that urinary excretion is complete within 8 hours, and I have seen no evidence to support the idea that initial therapy should be given on alternate days to minimize urinary losses. There is ample evidence that most of the dose provided in these 1000-microgram injections is lost in the urine, but it is also true that more is retained from these than from lower doses, thus justifying their use.

Several workers believe that this initial dosing combination (1000 micrograms daily for a week and then weekly for a month) is necessary to provide an adequate safety net of sufficient stores to sustain DNA synthesis and nerve integrity between subsequent monthly treatments, despite that fact that initial therapy with as little as 0.5 to 1 microgram daily is sufficient to induce optimal hematologic response in vitamin B_{12} deficiency. When severe neurologic damage is present, it is common to prolong the administration of these frequent doses to ensure adequate therapy, partly because the neurologic response can not be monitored in the way that the hematologic response can.

It is far preferable to manage initial therapy on an inpatient rather than outpatient basis, even if the anemia is only moderate in severity. This allows for better regulation of laboratory testing and of treatment and is the only way to ensure that reticulocyte counts are performed frequently enough (ideally daily) for adequate monitoring of the hematologic response to therapy. It is also important because the crucial period of initial replacement therapy can be associated with deaths in patients with megaloblastic anemia.

Most vitamin B_{12} deficient patients experience subjective euphoria within hours to days of initial therapy and progressively recover from fatigue and anorexia. In both folate and vitamin B_{12} deficiency, reticulocyte responses peak 5 to 10 days after the commencement of therapy, at levels inversely related to the hemoglobin (the higher reticulocyte counts being seen with more severe anemias). Bone marrow begins its normoblastic transformation within hours of treatment, whereas neutrophil hypersegmentation persists for 10 to 14 days and abnormal peripheral blood erythrocytes persist for much longer (4 to 8 weeks).

Once the hemoglobin has risen significantly, usually for at least 2 weeks after the reticulocytosis, it is reasonable to consider discharge. By this time, most patients have stabilized and are no longer at high risk.

Deaths seen in megaloblastic anemia were thought to be due to tremendous electrolyte shifts following massive red cell recruitment early in treatment. Careful study revealed that significant hypokalemia was quite rare and that it conferred no increased risk of sudden death. Despite this data, some workers administer potassium replacement therapy if serum potassium is low, even though these lower levels are almost invariably mild, short-lived, and uneventful.

Maintenance Therapy

After initial therapy, a dose of 1000 micrograms of cyanocobalamin monthly is recommended. It is clear that this exceeds the requirement for most patients, but it is also clear that the ideal dosage frequency varies considerably.

When initial treatment is completed, the most important role of the physician is to convey the necessity of continuing vitamin therapy for the rest of the patient's life. Analysis of 333 patients presenting with pernicious anemia in New York City over 14 years indicated that 11 per cent had presented previously and had been appropriately diagnosed and treated but were then lost to follow-up until their disease relapsed 2 to 10 years later. About 30 per cent of those relapses could be attributed to the failure of the treating physician to plan adequate follow-up.

In my experience, the most effective management is accomplished by having a nurse administer the monthly injections, with CBC and physical examination by a physician at intervals of 3, 6, or 12 months, depending on clinical need. This allows for rapid detection of patient noncompliance, the major risk during maintenance therapy. Without this detection, recidivism is frequent owing to patients' aversion to regular injections and the unfortunate belief that they are risking little if they feel and look well.

The increase in relative risk of gastric carcinoma for patients with pernicious anemia is nonexistent or so small that one can expect no clinical yield from routine investigation for this disorder.

I recommend that all causes of vitamin B_{12} malabsorption be treated in the same way for the duration of the malabsorption. Permanent vitamin B_{12} therapy is necessary in Crohn's disease, but no maintenance therapy is necessary if the intestinal defect can be corrected, such as in celiac disease, tropical sprue, and blind loop syndrome. Chronic pancreatitis frequently presents with low serum vitamin B_{12} levels without clinical deficiency, and maintenance vitamin B_{12} therapy is not recommended. Strict vegans who consume no animal foods, including dairy products and eggs, may benefit from vitamin B_{12} replacement by oral or other routes.

Nasal Cyanocobalamin Gel

A recent development has been the use of nasal cyanocobalamin gel in patients with gastrointes-

tinal vitamin B_{12} malabsorption. F.D.A. approval for clinical use is pending, but I have evaluated hundreds of doses of the gel in FDA-regulated clinical trials that I have conducted.

The nasal gel delivers vitamin B_{12} to the blood stream efficiently, achieving far higher blood levels in normals than oral tablets of like dosage. Initial monitoring may be necessary to establish an optimal dose, but the medication efficiently maintains blood levels in the therapeutic range. Patients adapt to the medication well, self-administer it with efficiency once appropriately instructed, and have reported no significant side effects.

It is useful to monitor compliance by having emtpy gel containers returned at follow-up visits. I believe that the relative convenience of administration has significantly improved compliance. It is extremely unusual for patients to request a return to injections once therapy with nasal gel has been instituted.

Treatment of Folate Deficiency Anemia

Although much more common, folate deficiency is far less ominous than vitamin B_{12} deficiency, primarily because of the absence of neuropathy. The most common underlying causes (alcohol, pregnancy, malabsorption syndromes, and drugs) are frequently associated with multifactorial anemias. While a patient is in the hospital, reticulocyte responses without specific therapy are common, presumably due to alcohol withdrawal and/or folate in the hospital diet. As a result, the underlying cause in folate deficient patients is often incompletely investigated.

Treatment consists of initial replacement therapy and correction of the underlying cause, if possible. Oral folic acid, 1 mg per day, is an effective remedy in virtually all patients, even those with intestinal malabsorption of dietary folates. When necessary, it is permissible to administer 1 mg, 5 mg, or even 15 mg of folic acid by intramuscular or intravenous injection.

Unfortunately, if oral folic acid is given when the vitamin deficiency is in doubt, even doses as small as 1 mg daily effectively correct megaloblastosis in vitamin B_{12} deficiency as well as folate deficiency; as a result, the nervous system may be unprotected from the hazards of vitamin B_{12} deficiency. Despite reports that blood smears retain some abnormality when folic acid is given in vitamin B_{12} deficiency, this subtlety is lost on all but the experts and it can be anticipated that the problem will remain undetected.

For this reason, if there is any residual doubt concerning the nature of the vitamin deficiency responsible for the anemia, patients should be managed more cautiously, using lower doses. One can give 0.1 mg of folic acid daily and expect to correct hematologic changes due to folate deficiency but not vitamin B_{12} deficiency.

Folinic acid (citrovorum factor) is a metabolically active form of folic acid that is administered by oral, intravenous, and intramuscular routes. It is approved for "rescue" from toxicity of methotrexate, which inhibits the enzyme dihydrofolate reductase. However, I have also used this analogue to achieve higher cerebrospinal fluid (CSF) folate levels in infants with congenital folate malabsorption, supposedly associated with poor CSF folate transport and mental retardation. Folinic acid was used because it crosses the blood-CSF barrier much more effectively than folic acid, and there is a possibility that these children may have had less developmental delay than those treated with folic acid.

Treatment of Coexistent Iron Deficiency

It is extremely common for iron deficiency to coexist with folate or vitamin B_{12} deficiency because of the common causes (e.g., pregnancy, gastrectomy, other achlorhydria, alcoholism). If megaloblastosis predominates, the only clue to iron deficiency may be a suboptimal hematologic response to folic acid or vitamin B_{12} therapy. If iron deficiency predominates, red cell precursors may be normoblastic and the only evidence of megaloblastosis may be in white cells, with giant precursors in the bone marrow and neutrophil hypersegmentation in the peripheral blood. If patients with the latter finding are treated with iron alone, they become megaloblastic and demonstrate the true range of their disease. Iron deficiency responds well to oral iron (ferrous sulfate, 325 mg 3 times daily).

Treatment of the Critically Ill Patient

Most patients develop megaloblastic anemia so gradually that they compensate well and demonstrate remarkably few hemodynamic disturbances. The most common problem in treatment of these subjects is the inability of physicians to proceed cautiously. Far more harm can ensue, and does ensue, from immediate and precipitous transfusion and fluid overload than from excessive caution.

Patients with severe anemia can be confined to bed and carefully monitored while undergoing diagnostic tests. Even if some dyspnea and circulatory distress are reported, decreased physical demands during bed rest may allow transfusion to be avoided. Even relatively severe thrombocytopenias usually respond promptly to vitamin

replacement, rarely requiring platelet therapy. It is almost never necessary to immediately start these patients on both vitamin B_{12} and folic acid or to consider transfusion therapy. Within a few days, the specific deficiency is identified and the therapy can begin.

An occasional, rare patient can cause concern because of an extremely severe anemia, with a hematocrit of, for example, 15 per cent and with circulatory distress such as cardiac failure or angina pectoris, and it may not be possible to wait the 4 to 5 days required for the reticulocyte response to specific therapy. After collecting diagnostic samples, it may be justified to institute cautious transfusion with diuretics, under the direction of an experienced physician prepared to respond to the development of hemodynamic difficulty. Simultaneously, replacement vitamin therapy should be instituted, since this is one of the extremely rare occasions when shotgun therapy is justified.

If the patient is unconscious, is unable to take oral folate supplements, or has malabsorption, intravenous folic acid is given in doses of 1 to 5 mg daily.

Prophylactic Supplementation with Folic Acid

There are several conditions in which prophylactic supplementation with folic acid has been recommended. Pregnancy is the best documented, and virtually all authorities agree that a supplement approximating the recommended dietary allowance (RDA) for folate in pregnancy (800 micrograms daily) is reasonable. In fact, this dose is much higher than that needed and should probably be halved.

An increased need for folic acid has been described in chronic hemolytic anemias such as hereditary spherocytosis; the aplastic crises associated with that condition have led to the use of folic acid supplements. Another group which apparently benefits from prophylactic supplements is patients on hemodialysis, who clearly become folate depleted without supplements. However, a more complex picture is seen in sickle cell anemia and thalassemia, for which many physicians still recommend supplements despite little or no evidence of their benefit.

Patients who have developed folate deficiency while taking anticonvulsants (particularly Dilantin) can be continued on the drugs if they take 1 mg of folic acid daily. A similar approach may be used with oral contraceptives, although there is much less evidence for an association of these drugs with folate deficiency. In patients with malabsorption syndromes, folic acid in daily doses of 2 to 5 mg should be administered. Megaloblastic anemia in patients with tropical sprue is treated with both folic acid and vitamin B_{12}, and if the malabsorption syndrome cannot be corrected, patients may be maintained indefinitely on folic acid/vitamin B_{12} replacement.

THALASSEMIA

method of
TIMOTHY J. LEY, M.D.
Washington University Medical Center
St. Louis, Missouri

The thalassemia syndromes are among the world's most common genetic disorders. Hundreds of thousands of individuals of Mediterranean, Middle Eastern, Indian, Chinese, and Southeast Asian descent are affected by alpha- or beta-thalassemias. In the past several years, globin genes from a large number of individuals with thalassemia have been cloned and characterized, leading to a nearly complete understanding of the molecular defects responsible for these disorders. With this knowledge, investigators are developing new strategies for diagnosis and treatment, which, it is hoped, will provide a means for rational genetic cures by the end of the century. Until then, conservative therapy with transfusions, appropriately timed splenectomy, and chelation will lead to improved life expectancy for most patients.

Pathophysiology

Normal hemoglobins are tetrameric proteins composed of two alpha and two betalike globin chains. During normal development, embryonic globins are produced during the first 8 to 10 weeks of gestation, and then fetal hemoglobin (hemoglobin F, $alpha_2$ $gamma_2$) is produced during fetal life. Just before birth, the adult betalike globin genes (delta and beta) are activated, and produce adult hemoglobins for the rest of life ($alpha_2$ $delta_2$ produces hemoglobin A_2; $alpha_2$ $beta_2$ produces hemoglobin A).

There are two identical alpha globin genes on each chromosome 16, and therefore four alpha genes per diploid cell. The inherited alpha-thalassemia syndromes are usually due to deletions of one or more of these genes. Deletion of one or two of the four alpha globin genes leads to a disorder (alpha-thalassemia trait) characterized by a mild hypochromic microcytic anemia that requires no therapy. Deletion of three of the four alpha globin genes leads to a more serious syndrome (hemoglobin H disease) characterized by a moderately severe hypochromic microcytic anemia. Deletion of all four alpha globin genes leads to the production of *hemoglobin Bart's* ($gamma_4$ tetramers) and intrauterine death (hydrops fetalis). Acquired hemoglobin H disease sometimes develops in elderly patients with preleukemic or myelodysplastic disorders. Acquired hemoglobin H disease occurs not because of alpha globin gene deletions but because of suppression of alpha globin production by unknown mechanisms.

Each normal chromosome 11 contains a single beta globin gene, and therefore normal diploid cells contain two of these genes. Clinical disease results only when both beta globin genes are defective: that is, the patient is homozygous for beta-thalassemia. Beta gene defects are classified into two general types: a beta° thalassemia gene is completely disabled and therefore produces no beta globin chains. A beta⁺ thalassemia defect only partially disables a beta globin gene, so that it produces reduced amounts of normal beta globin chains. A large number (> 30) of thalassemic beta globin genes have been cloned and characterized. Studies of these abnormal beta globin genes have greatly aided our knowledge of normal gene anatomy and physiology and have increased our understanding of how different genetic defects produce clinical disorders of varying severity.

Most individuals with homozygous beta-thalassemia have different defects in each of their beta globin genes. Individuals who are homozygous for beta° thalassemia mutations, heterozygous for beta° and beta⁺ mutations, or who have severe beta⁺ thalassemia mutations on both chromosomes generally have a severe disorder known as *thalassemia major*. These individuals usually present at age 3 to 6 months of age with a severe hypochromic microcytic anemia (hemoglobin 2 to 5 grams per dl). Patients who are homozygous for milder beta⁺ globin gene lesions have a syndrome of intermediate clinical severity, known as *thalassemia intermedia*. These individuals present at age 3 to 6 months with moderate anemia (hemoglobin 5 to 8 grams per dl), and may not require transfusions to sustain life. Individuals with one beta-thalassemia gene and a normal beta globin gene on the other chromosome have *beta-thalassemia trait*. These individuals generally have hemoglobin levels over 10 grams per dl, and have no manifestations of disease.

In patients with thalassemia intermedia or thalassemia major, reduced production of beta globin chains is not accompanied by any reduction in alpha globin synthesis. The excess alpha globin chains combine to form $alpha_4$ tetramers, which are relatively insoluble and precipitate inside forming red cells and reticulocytes. These precipitates damage the red cell membrane, leading to ineffective erythropoiesis and hemolytic anemia. As a result, erythropoiesis expands drastically, and bone marrow examination reveals severe erythroid hyperplasia. The medullary cavities of long bones can be eroded by the enormous mass of erythroid tissue, leading to severe skeletal deformities and osteoporosis. Damaged red cells released into the circulation are rapidly trapped by the spleen, causing splenic hypertrophy and hypersplenism at an early age.

In patients with three deleted alpha globin genes, continued beta globin production results in the production of $beta_4$ hemoglobin tetramers (hemoglobin H). Since $beta_4$ tetramers are more soluble than $alpha_4$ tetramers, less red cell damage occurs, and the clinical severity of hemoglobin H disease is therefore less than that of beta-thalassemia major.

Diagnosis

In most cases, a diagnosis of thalassemia can be established with knowledge of the patient's ethnic background, family history, and a few laboratory tests (complete blood count, hemoglobin electrophoresis, quantitative hemoglobin F, serum iron and total iron binding capacity, serum ferritin). Patients with beta-thalassemia trait have a mild hypochromic microcytic anemia, elevated hemoglobin A$_2$ levels, and no evidence of iron deficiency. Establishing the diagnosis of thalassemia trait is important for family planning and so that iron therapy is not mistakenly given to these individuals. Patients with alpha-thalassemia trait are clinically similar to those with beta-thalassemia trait, but do not have elevated hemoglobin A$_2$ values. Patients with beta-thalassemia intermedia or major usually develop a severe hypochromic microcytic anemia during the first 6 months of life. The peripheral blood smear reveals marked anisopoikilocytosis and target cells, and may also contain nucleated red cells. The reticulocyte count is relatively low for the degree of anemia because of ineffective erythropoiesis. The percentages of circulating hemoglobin A$_2$ and hemoglobin F are usually markedly elevated, with reduced or absent hemoglobin A. Hematologic parameters from both parents should be consistent with thalassemia trait. If these studies do not establish a diagnosis, then more sophisticated analyses (e.g., quantitation of globin chain production and direct DNA analysis of the beta globin genes) will reveal the exact nature of the molecular defects. Patients with hemoglobin H disease present with a moderately severe hypochromic microcytic anemia and a peripheral smear similar to that of beta-thalassemia. Hemoglobin H (beta$_4$ tetramers) can be identified by brilliant cresyl blue staining of red cells, or by a characteristic hemoglobin H band on hemoglobin electrophoresis.

Antenatal diagnosis of the thalassemia syndromes can be accomplished by direct examination of fetal DNA from cells obtained from amniocentesis or chorionic villus biopsy. The genotype of the fetus can usually be determined by mapping specialized chromosomal markers near the beta globin genes of both parents, and by linking these markers to the beta globin genes inherited by the infant at risk. Chorionic villus biopsy allows earlier (first trimester) sampling of fetal tissue; therefore, affected pregnancies may be terminated earlier. However, this procedure may carry a higher risk of fetal wastage than amniocentesis.

Natural History

Infants with severe beta-thalassemia require regular transfusions beginning at age 6 to 12 months in order to sustain life and provide normal exercise tolerance. If transfusions are given in quantities sufficient only to sustain life, erythroid expansion in the bone marrow may cause severe bony abnormalities, osteoporosis, pathologic fractures, and growth retardation. Chronic hemolysis causes the spleen to enlarge, and eventually hypersplenism (accompanied by leukopenia and thrombocytopenia) will develop, further increasing transfusion requirements.

The most serious complication that develops in the thalassemic child is that of iron overload. Each unit of transfused blood contains approximately 200 to 250 mg of iron, which is metabolized and deposited in the reticuloendothelial and parenchymal cells of vital organs. In addition, ineffective erythropoiesis and erythroid hyperplasia in the bone marrow cause the gastrointestinal tract to absorb excess iron. Humans have no normal mechanism to eliminate this excess iron, and it therefore accumulates in all tissues, where it can damage cells by causing peroxidation of lipid membranes.

Endocrine abnormalities caused by iron loading are common. Iron deposition in the hypothalamus and pituitary frequently leads to impaired gonadotropin release, delayed sexual maturation, delayed menarche and abnormal menses, and sexual dysfunction. Panhypopituitarism is uncommon, but other minor abnormalities of pituitary reserve can frequently be seen. Heavy deposition of iron in the pancreas leads to abnormal glucose tolerance tests in most patients, and to insulin-dependent diabetes in a smaller number. Exocrine pancreatic insufficiency is rare, however. Adrenal deposition of iron generally occurs in the zona glomerulosa, but clinical deficiencies of adrenocortical hormones are unusual. Diminished adrenocorticotropic hormone reserve may frequently be present in iron-loaded patients, so corticosteroid coverage should be given to affected patients during periods of surgical or physiologic stress. Although the thyroid and parathyroid glands are often heavily laden with iron, overt hypothyroidism and hypoparathyroidism are uncommon.

Heavy deposition of iron in the parenchymal cells of the liver frequently leads to hepatic fibrosis, mild hepatomegaly, and mild increases in the levels of transaminases. Ultimately, patients may develop progressive hepatic fibrosis and nodular cirrhosis. Although the liver disease of thalassemic patients is similar to that of patients with hereditary hemochromatosis, hepatomas and death due to hepatic failure are rarely seen.

The most serious consequence of iron overload is that of cardiac hemochromatosis. During the first decade of life, patients generally have no overt cardiac dysfunction, but during the early teens, subclinical dysfunction of the left ventricle with exercise is frequently found. During the next several years, the patient may develop intermittent episodes of pericarditis, atrial arrhythmias, and ventricular ectopic beats. In the late teens, the patient may develop intractable ventricular arrhythmias or progressive congestive heart failure unresponsive to diuretic and digitalis therapy. Congestive heart failure is a very poor prognostic sign; most patients die within 2 years of the onset of clinical symptoms. Almost all nonchelated, transfused patients with severe beta-thalassemia die of cardiac disease by the age of 20.

Patients with hemoglobin H disease have moderate anemia and usually do not require transfusions. Erythropoiesis is more effective than in patients with homozygous beta-thalassemia, and therefore bony abnormalities and hypersplenism are mild, if present at all. Some patients may develop hypersplenism and worsening anemia later in life; splenectomy may be advisable under these circumstances.

Conventional Therapy

Transfusions

The goals of transfusion therapy include the sustenance of life, prevention of skeletal deformities, and maintenance of adequate exercise tolerance, using the smallest possible amount of blood to minimize iron loading. A variety of strategies have been developed to meet these goals. Hypertransfusion regimens (maintenance of minimal hemoglobin > 10 grams per dl) were instituted to suppress erythropoiesis, limit skeletal deformities, and reduce iron hyperabsorption by the gut. More recently, "supertransfusion" (maintenance of minimal hemoglobin > 12 grams per dl) has been explored. The goal of this regimen is to completely suppress erythropoiesis in the marrow, thereby reducing the blood volume and eventually reducing transfusion requirements. Although this strategy has been successful in some trials, others have not found it to reduce transfusion requirements. At this time, many investigators feel that maintaining a minimum hemoglobin of 8 to 9 grams per dl is adequate to prevent skeletal deformities during development, and utilizes a minimum number of transfusions. Most patients can achieve this goal by receiving 2 units of packed red cells at approximately monthly intervals; if possible, the author recommends that patients receive 1 unit of packed red cells every 2 to 3 weeks, which tends to ameliorate exercise intolerance at the end of a transfusion cycle. Smaller, more frequent transfusions may also tend to reduce transfusion requirements by maintaining the average hemoglobin at a slightly higher level.

The blood product of choice is packed red blood cells, since these units deliver the greatest number of viable red cells. However, since many patients experience febrile white cell reactions, the use of in-line white cell filters may be required. If white cell filtration fails to eliminate febrile reactions, frozen washed packed blood cells may be given, although these units are generally smaller and more expensive than similar units of packed red blood cells.

Accurate records of transfusions should be kept for all patients. In children who have not been splenectomized, increasing transfusion requirements generally indicate developing hypersplenism and help to determine the timing of splenectomy (see later discussion). In patients who have already been splenectomized, increasing transfusion requirements may indicate alloimmunization to minor red cell determinants, or the presence of an accessory spleen. Appropriate workup and treatment of these disorders should be undertaken if necessary.

Recently, the technologies of automated cell sorting and apheresis have made it possible to harvest units of relatively young red blood cells (neocytes). These young cells have a prolonged half-life in vivo compared with routinely prepared red blood cells, and could potentially reduce transfusion requirements. However, these units are still expensive to prepare and must be considered experimental, since large controlled trials demonstrating their efficacy have not yet been performed.

Splenectomy

Appropriately timed splenectomy is an important adjunct to the management of children with beta-thalassemia. Splenectomy should be avoided during the first 5 years of life because of an increased risk of overwhelming sepsis in young asplenic children. Between the ages of 5 and 15, transfusion requirements should be carefully evaluated on a yearly basis, and splenectomy should be performed if the transfusion requirement reaches a level greater than 250 ml of packed red blood cells per kg per year, or if other evidence of hypersplenism (leukopenia, thrombocytopenia) develops. The need for splenectomy should be anticipated so that a prophylactic polyvalent pneumococcal vaccine can be administered at least 1 month prior to surgery and so that surgery can be performed during the summer months when the child is not in school.

It is not unreasonable to administer oral prophylactic penicillin G (125 to 250 mg per day) to asplenic children who are less than 10 years of age, especially in light of recent data that children with sickle cell anemia who receive prophylaxis have fewer episodes of serious bacterial infections. Trimethoprim-sulfamethoxazole can be substituted in individuals who are allergic to penicillin. Post splenectomy, all patients should be advised to seek immediate medical attention for unexplained fever. In addition, patients should have a small supply of ampicillin tablets available at home in the event that fever develops and medical attention cannot be immediately rendered. Asplenic patients who present to the hospital with unexplained fever should be treated with intravenously administered, broad-spectrum antibiotics until the results of cultures are obtained.

Iron Chelation Therapy

The only currently available iron chelator is deferoxamine mesylate (Desferal). This compound is essentially ineffective when given orally, and has a very short half-life when given parenterally. Intramuscular injections of Desferal given once daily are therefore relatively ineffective as a means of preventing the complications of iron overload. Desferal must be given as a continuous infusion, either subcutaneously by infusion pump, or by an intravenous route.

Thus far, Desferal's efficacy has been demonstrated only for the *prevention* of the complications of iron overload; one study suggests that Desferal may not prevent cardiac disease in transfused thalassemic children if it is started after the age of 5 years. Therefore, the author recommends that children begin on a regular program of nightly subcutaneous Desferal (given 5 to 6 nights per week) at the age of 4 or 5 years. Iron overload (serum ferritin greater than 1000 ng per ml) and increased urinary iron excretion in response to Desferal infusion should be documented prior to initiating therapy. A dose of 40 to 50 mg per kg per day is administered into the subcutaneous fat of the abdomen over a period of 8 to 12 hours via a 27-gauge butterfly needle connected to a portable infusion pump. As the child grows, the dose is gradually increased to a maximum level of 2 grams per day. On this regimen, almost all patients achieve net negative iron balance, with 20 to 40 mg of iron excreted daily in the urine, and at least equal amounts excreted in the stool. The regular use of this regimen almost certainly forestalls the consequences of iron overload and prevents early cardiac mortality. However, problems with compliance generally appear during adolescence, and these should be sensitively addressed with appropriate psychosocial and family counseling.

The most common complications of Desferal therapy include local pruritus and burning at the site of injection. Generally, patients cannot tolerate infusions of more than 2 grams per day at a single injection site. These symptoms can be ameliorated by adding 5 to 10 mg of hydrocortisone to the infusion mixture or by the topical use of cold packs or diphenhydramine (Benadryl) at the infusion site. Rotation of infusion sites on the abdominal wall and the anterior thigh is recommended. Recently, one group has noted serious, partially reversible neurotoxicity manifested as optic neuropathy or acute sensorineural hearing loss in young patients receiving high-dose Desferal (> 50 mg per kg per day). Although other groups have not noted these complications, yearly audiovisual monitoring is advised for all patients.

Because of the high cost and cumbersome administration of Desferal, the search for an orally effective iron chelator continues. Several agents are at different stages of experimental trials, and some, in animal experiments, appear to be as effective as parenterally administered Desferal. Clinical trials are in progress, but approval for general use remains several years away.

Nutritional Therapy

Most patients with transfusional hemochromatosis are deficient in several vitamins. Vitamin C deficiency produces a partial blockage of iron release from the reticuloendothelial stores. Administration of vitamin C therefore can lead to increased iron excretion in many patients. However, large doses of vitamin C can cause massive release of iron from reticuloendothelial stores, causing cardiac toxicity and congestive heart failure. We recommend that vitamin C be administered at a dose of 100 mg by mouth on days when Desferal is administered. The vitamin C dose should be taken at least 30 minutes after the Desferal infusion has begun, so that circulating levels of Desferal are high when the iron stores are released. Patients should be advised that high-dose vitamin C intake can cause serious toxicity and that they should not self-medicate with this vitamin for colds or influenza. Thalassemic patients are also frequently deficient in vitamin E. Although vitamin E deficiency is associated with abnormal hematopoiesis and a decreased survival of circulating red blood cells, replenishment of vitamin E does not alter transfusion requirements. Nonetheless, it is reasonable to administer 200 International Units of vitamin E daily to all transfused thalassemic patients. Finally, all patients with accelerated hematopoiesis have increased folate requirements, and should be supplemented daily with 1 mg of folate by mouth.

Several reports have indicated that the drinking of tea may reduce iron absorption in patients with accelerated erythropoiesis. Since this practice is innocuous and may provide benefit, the author recommends that all patients drink at least two cups or glasses of tea daily with meals.

Treatment of Cardiac Hemochromatosis

Almost all patients with beta-thalassemia and iron overload die because of cardiac hemochromatosis. If prophylactic chelation therapy is started too late, or if the patient has not complied with chelation therapy, the consequences of myocardial iron deposition will appear in the second or third decade. Episodes of pericarditis may occur, and they are best treated with bedrest and nonsteroidal anti-inflammatory agents. Atrial and ventricular arrhythmias frequently develop and should be managed in the same fashion as those associated with other congestive cardiomyopathies. Ventricular arrhythmias may be particularly refractory to therapy, and may, in fact, be impossible to eliminate. Therapy should be individualized with the help of a cardiologist, and the patient's response to therapy should be carefully followed with Holter monitoring and appropriate drug level monitoring. Since some patients have mild to moderate liver dysfunction due to hepatic iron overload, particular attention must be paid to the levels of drugs metabolized by the liver.

The onset of congestive heart failure in patients with cardiac hemochromatosis is a very poor prognostic sign, and most patients die within 2 to 3 years of the onset of overt clinical symptomatology. Occasionally, patients may have reversible congestive heart failure due to ingestion of massive quantities of vitamin C, or to an episode of viral myocarditis. However, most patients who present with signs of left-sided heart failure will gradually progress to biventricular heart failure that is refractory to all forms of treatment. The management of patients with congestive heart failure should include standard medical therapy, including salt restriction, diuretics, digoxin, and afterload reduction for those with congestive cardiomyopathy.

Recently, several investigators have attempted to alter the course of advanced cardiac disease by giving continuous high-dose intravenous infusions of Desferal (4 to 8 grams daily) via chronic indwelling catheters. Massive excretion of iron can be achieved (> 200 mg iron per day via the urinary route, and unknown amounts via the fecal route). In some patients, improvement in the cardiomyopathy has been seen, but in others, progression of disease and death have ensued. This approach must still be considered experimental, and its ultimate efficacy must be established in controlled clinical trials. However, since cardiac hemochromatosis can be effectively reversed by phlebotomy in many patients with hereditary hemochromatosis, aggressive chelation may ultimately prove effective for some transfused patients with severe cardiac iron overload.

Experimental Therapy

Bone Marrow Transplantation

During the past several years, several groups have explored the use of allogeneic bone marrow transplantation for cure of children with homozygous beta-thalassemia. The most satisfying results have come from transplantation of minimally transfused children with HLA identical, nonthalassemic siblings as donors. Although about 75 per cent of children transplanted thus far appear to be cured of their disease, 10 to 20 per cent die of transplant-related complications (infection or graft-versus-host disease). Because of significant transplant-related mortality, this procedure must still be considered experimental, especially in view of the possibility of a genetic cure of beta-thalassemia in the next 10 to 20 years.

Activation of Fetal Hemoglobin Synthesis

Since beta-thalassemia is essentially caused by the activation of two defective beta globin genes at birth, this disease could presumably be cured by preventing the switch from fetal to adult hemoglobin synthesis, or by reversing this switch during adult life. Knowledge of the molecular organization and physiology of the globin genes has led to attempts to reactivate fetal hemoglobin synthesis in thalassemic patients with 5-azacytidine. Although this drug can temporarily increase fetal hemoglobin synthesis, the increase in hemoglobin production is moderate and has not eliminated the need for transfusions. Also, 5-azacytidine must be considered carcinogenic, and, therefore, it is not suitable for chronic administration to thalassemic children. Nonetheless, these studies have demonstrated that it may someday be possible to safely reactivate fetal hemoglobin production in adults with beta-thalassemia or sickle cell disease. Other strategies to achieve the same end will undoubtedly be tested in the years to come.

Gene Transfer

The cure of beta-thalassemia may someday be realized with transfer of a normal beta globin gene into the hematopoietic stem cells of a thalassemic patient, and subsequent expression of that normal beta globin gene in the developing red cells. Gene transfer to murine hematopoietic stem cells has already been achieved, and correction of a murine model of beta-thalassemia has been accomplished by transferring normal mouse or human beta globin genes into the germline of affected animals. The DNA sequences that will be required to reliably correct the globin gene defects are beginning to be understood. These encouraging experiments indicate that correction of beta-thalassemia by gene transfer may occur in the not too distant future. Until then, regimens of transfusions, splenectomy, and chelation will, it is hoped, delay the consequences of iron overload in patients who will be candidates for a genetic cure at a later time.

SICKLE CELL DISEASE

method of
PAUL F. MILNER, M.D.
Medical College of Georgia
Augusta, Georgia

The sickle cell mutation occurs in about one in 12 American blacks. Subjects who carry this sickle trait (A/S) have about 30 to 45 per cent sickle hemoglobin (Hb S) in each of their red cells; under normal conditions this does not cause hemolysis, anemia, or symptoms. However, symptoms may develop at high altitudes (above 10,000 feet), and about 3 per cent of such individuals have episodes of painless hematuria. When both parents have sickle trait there is a 1:4 chance of having an offspring with the homozygous disease, sickle cell anemia (SS). The trait for Hb C is carried by about one in 40 American blacks. Much less common are traits for β^+ and β^0 thalassemia. These traits can occur in double heterozygotes with the sickle cell trait to cause Hb SC and Hb S/β thalassemia. Even rarer are combinations with traits for Hb D, Hb O, and Hb E. In the red cells of subjects with SC disease there are equal amounts of Hb S and Hb C but anemia is usually mild and symptoms are infrequent. However, all the complications that affect patients with sickle cell anemia can occur in these subjects, and they are particularly prone to proliferative retinopathy, which can cause blindness if left untreated. Patients with Hb S/β$^+$ thalassemia have the mildest form of sickle cell disease because there is about 30 per cent Hb A in every red cell; anemia is very slight and symptoms are mild, although typical pain crises and bone infarcts can occur. In Hb S/β^0 thalassemia no Hb A is present and the condition is clinically indistinguishable from sickle cell anemia. Distinguishing laboratory features are marked microcytosis, expressed as a low mean corpuscular volume (MCV), and an increase in the minor hemoglobin A$_2$. These features, however, are common to SS patients with concomitant alpha thalassemia.

At birth the SS infant's red cells contain mainly fetal hemoglobin (Hb F), but sufficient Hb S is present to make a diagnosis by hemoglobin electrophoresis, which ideally should be done at birth. Within a few months, red cells containing Hb F (F cells) are mostly replaced by cells containing Hb S which, because of their reduced flexibility and deformability, can block the microcirculation, causing typical attacks of pain frequently accompanied by fever. Pneumonia is a common presenting symptom. The spleen is palpable, but may not be visible on a liver spleen scan because it is blocked by sickled cells, causing hypofunction or asplenia. This makes the infant very vulnerable to pneumococcal bacteremia, which has been responsible for a high mortality rate (about 15 per cent). Acute sequestration of blood in the spleen is a medical emergency, because death occurs rapidly from acute anemia and hypovolemia. Bone infarcts at this age frequently involve the hands and feet, causing pain and swelling, the so-called "hand-foot syndrome."

About 30 per cent of SS patients in America also have one alpha-thalassemia gene, and about 5 per cent are homozygous. This causes microcytosis and a reduced mean corpuscular hemoglobin concentration (MCHC), which decreases Hb S polymerization, thus increasing red cell survival. Some SS patients have many F cells, which also increases the red cell survival. When there is more than 15 per cent Hb F the result is clinically noticeable. Because these additional genetically controlled factors are not linked, and segregate independently, very few SS patients have both alpha thalassemia and a high Hb F level. These patients have a relatively benign disease which may not be diagnosed until their late teens or early adult life. Sickle cell anemia of this type is common in eastern Saudi Arabia and India. However, it seems that alpha thalassemia alone does not protect against pain crises or the incidence of bone infarction, which may actually be higher in this group, probably because of their higher hematocrits and blood viscosity.

In considering the treatment of patients with sickle cell anemia at any age, it is important not only to consider all these factors but also to approach each case individually rather than to apply preconceived notions as to the expected course of the disease. Some patients are now living beyond the sixth decade.

Treatment

Management in Office or Clinic

As with any chronic, life-long progressive disease for which there is no cure, regular checkups should be carried out at intervals that will depend, to some extent, on the course of the disease and the frequency of symptoms. To prevent pneumococcal infection, infants should be given oral prophylactic penicillin, 125 mg twice daily, from the age of 3 months until after age 3 years, at which time they should be immunized with a polyvalent pneumococcal vaccine. Immunization against childhood illnesses should be given.

The adult responsible for the child should be educated as to the nature of the disease, instructed on how to take the temperature and feel for the spleen, and told to report any illness immediately. The National Association for Sickle Cell Disease, Inc.* publishes a useful pamphlet on sickle cell disease in childhood entitled "How to help your child to take it in stride."

From about age 8 years through the teens, the frequency of crises and symptoms may decrease, only to recur with greater intensity after puberty. The bone age may be delayed as much as 5 years in some cases, and the onset of puberty and the adolescent growth spurt also are often delayed. When the growth spurt occurs, the child may

---

*3460 Wilshire Boulevard, Suite 1012, Los Angeles, California 90010-2273.

return to the same height percentile, or a slightly higher one. Although a decreased weight for height is the rule, some teenage SS children may become obese.

At the routine visit, the hemoglobin, hematocrit level, reticulocyte count, and white cell count should be checked. In SS patients the hemoglobin may range from 6.5 to 10.5 grams per dl but in most cases will be around 7.5, or slightly higher in men. Iron deficiency is uncommon, but it can occur in young women and children. If the hemoglobin is unusually low the ferritin level should be checked before giving iron. Folate deficiency can occur but is prevented by giving folic acid, 1 mg daily. Rarely the spleen may enlarge and become firm, causing hypersplenism with increasing anemia and mild thrombocytopenia. Splenectomy is indicated if this persists.

Abdominal pain is quite common in children and may mimic an acute abdomen; pigment gallstones, which are common in older patients, also occur in about 27 per cent of children under 18 years and may cause symptoms. Cholecystectomy is not indicated in the asymptomatic patient. Duodenal ulceration is not uncommon in young men, and should be considered in the differential diagnosis of abdominal pain and indigestion. Recurrent attacks of priapism of short duration (1 to 2 hours) may wake the patient at night. Treatment with 10 mg of nifedipine, repeated as necessary, is often effective.

All SC and S/β$^+$ thalassemia patients over 20 years of age, and SS patients with unusually high hematocrits, should be referred for a retinal examination by an experienced ophthalmologist when first seen. The hip and shoulder joints should be examined for limitation of range of movement or pain, which would indicate avascular necrosis of the femoral or humeral heads. Early referral to an orthopedic surgeon is important if hip pain is present. Examination of the cardiovascular system will usually reveal a slightly enlarged heart and a functional systolic ejection murmur, which is of no particular significance. As the more anemic adults approach middle age, congestive cardiac failure may set in, requiring treatment.

Bone Infarcts

Sometimes a child or young adult presents with a painful, swollen, and very tender extremity. This is caused by an infarct in a long bone; the tibia and humerus are common sites. An adjacent joint may be involved secondarily, causing an effusion. If the lower limb is involved, weight-bearing on it may be impossible because of pain. While the most severe cases may have to be hospitalized, many may be treated in the office.

These lesions respond to immobilization and indomethacin, 25 mg 3 times a day orally for about a week. Close follow-up is advisable in case osteomyelitis develops, but this is rare. An x-ray will not show anything. Joint effusions need not be tapped unless the condition worsens, and then only in the operating room.

Pain Control

In children, attacks of mild pain can usually be managed at home with aspirin or acetaminophen, but older children may need a stronger pain reliever for a few days, such as 15 to 30 mg of codeine every 4 to 6 hours. If this is insufficient, oxycodone in the form of Percodan Demi is justified, and similar tablets containing 5 mg of oxycodone can be used for adults. Only small amounts should be prescribed at one time. Fluid intake should be increased. Confidence improves when parent and child (or the adult patient) know that pain can be dealt with effectively. A few patients will claim that they have chronic pain, and this is best treated with nonsteroidal analgesics. Narcotic dependence can become a problem and must be avoided.

Children should be encouraged to lead a normal life and attend school. Teachers should be aware that the child is physically handicapped because of anemia and attacks of pain and needs to urinate frequently. Home-bound teaching should be arranged when necessary. Competitive sports should be avoided, but regular exercise should be encouraged. Swimming seems to precipitate pain crises and is best avoided. It is important to encourage a healthy lifestyle with an optimistic outlook, particularly in the adolescent. Few adult patients are unable to work if their occupation is sedentary. Manual work, if it requires physical exertion, is not suitable for most SS patients.

Ankle Ulcers

Ankle ulcers occur in about 25 per cent of young adults and older patients and can be very resistant to treatment. It is essential to eradicate infection, and this can be achieved by instructing the patient to bathe the ulcerated area with dilute hypochlorite solution (one tablespoon of Clorox added to a quart of water) twice a day and cover the ulcer with a gauze pad soaked in the same solution. Ointments containing proteolytic enzymes (Elase or Travase) are useful for dissolving thick sloughs, but these are very expensive. Other ointments and topical antibiotics, except chloramphenicol, are best avoided. When the area is clean, zinc cream or Una boots can be applied to encourage healing. Blood transfusions given over several months, to raise the hemoglobin level and reduce sickling, may induce healing.

As a last resort, skin grafting may be needed. Recurrence is often a problem and should be handled in the same way, with attention to patient compliance and morale.

Pregnancy

Sickle cell anemia is not a thrombotic disease, and there is no evidence that the risks associated with oral contraceptives are any greater than in the rest of the female population. Teenage pregnancy should be prevented; an open attitude to sex education and contraceptive advice is helpful.

Preceding conception, genetic counseling should explain clearly the chances of an offspring inheriting sickle cell disease. This counseling should also include information about prenatal diagnosis, which is now widely available at a relatively early stage in pregnancy. Most women with SS disease will opt for a tubal ligation after one or two pregnancies if these have been complicated, but it is not justifiable in the nulliparous female unless symptoms are so frequent and severe that pregnancy is best avoided. Data from a large clinical study of sickle cell disease recently conducted by the National Heart, Lung, and Blood Institute indicates that maternal mortality is now less than 0.5 per cent. There is an increased incidence of spontaneous abortion, but late fetal wastage has been greatly reduced by modern methods of fetal-maternal care. However, it is necessary to warn patients that pain crises may be more frequent and that intensive prenatal care will be necessary, preferably in a high-risk clinic where obstetricians are familiar with the effect of sickle cell disease on pregnancy.

Management of Acute Events

Acute Pain Crises

ETIOLOGY. The acute pain crisis is the commonest acute event in sickle cell disease, although only about 25 per cent of SS patients experience frequent attacks and they are uncommon in the other genotypes. Precipitating factors include dehydration, infection, change in climate, muscular exertion (especially swimming), and emotional upset. Dehydration from decreased fluid intake, in the face of continued polyuria caused by the kidney concentrating defect, is probably the most important factor, and a slight decrease in blood pH during sleep may be another. Crises frequently start during the hours of sleep. Recent studies have shown that the most significant indicator of pain crises is the level of the hematocrit. The higher the hematocrit, in the absence of a high fetal hemoglobin, the greater the blood viscosity and the greater the likelihood of a vasoocclusive episode. In trying to prevent crises, all these factors should be discussed with the patient, particularly the importance of a high fluid intake (at least 2 quarts daily).

SIGNS AND SYMPTOMS. Prior to admission the patient may have tried to combat the pain with oral fluid and analgesics. Pain is located commonly in the back, the ribs, and one or more limbs. Pulmonary infiltrates may develop. Mild fever is common in children but is initially unusual in adults, although a swinging fever may develop later. An increase in the white cell count (up to 25,000 per cu mm) is common. The sclera may become more icteric and the urine darker, and serum liver enzymes, particularly lactate dehydrogenase, may be greatly increased. In severe crises the hemoglobin may fall by 1 to 2 grams per dl, but the so-called hemolytic crisis is a very uncommon occurrence.

TREATMENT. The main aim of treatment is to correct dehydration. There is some controversy as to whether the plasma volume is reduced, but reductions in tissue fluid and total body water have been demonstrated, and the red cells are dehydrated. This is the rationale for giving intravenous fluid, which should initially be 5 per cent dextrose (D5W) at a rate of about 5 ml per kg per hour (250 to 300 ml per hour for the average adult). After diuresis has occurred, 0.45 per cent NaCl in D5W can be used. There is no defect in water excretion, so large infusions can be quickly excreted. Continued infusion of 0.9 per cent NaCl can produce circulatory overload because of impaired excretion of sodium. If serum potassium falls, supplements can be given, but mild hyponatremia is beneficial. There has been some controversy about the continued use of oxygen because it inhibits erythropoietin formation, leading to a fall in reticulocytes and hemoglobin. It is, however, logical to provide a high alveolar and arterial PO_2, and a slight fall in hemoglobin and hematocrit may be beneficial because it reduces blood viscosity.

Most acute pain crises will resolve in a few days if treated conservatively with intravenous fluid and analgesics. If the condition of the patient deteriorates, a partial exchange transfusion (see below) may be necessary, but it should not be part of routine treatment. Analgesics should be used in adequate doses, preferably by the intravenous route to avoid repeated painful injections and unpredictable absorption from intramuscular, often fibrotic, sites. Although meperidine is a widely used analgesic, it is not ideal for use in sickle cell crises because its analgesic effect is too short-lived and its sedative effect too strong; its metabolite, normeperidine, has a long half-life and toxic side effects that include seizures. In children, morphine is the drug of choice (0.15 mg per kg every 3 hours). Long-acting preparations such as buprenorphine (Buprenex) (0.3 mg per dose), which has a built-in antagonist, are useful in adults, and are advantageous when pain is prolonged over several days. Pain medication should be given on a strict time schedule compatible with the pharmacokinetics of the drug used. As comfort is restored and the patient improves, the dose is gradually reduced, keeping the interval between doses the same. It is very important to conserve veins by using small (21 or 23 gauge) needles in peripheral veins rather than catheter needles, and to ensure that all drug injections are well diluted. Last, a caring, supportive, and optimistic rapport with the patient will go a long way toward allaying the anxiety that all patients feel when they go into crisis.

Aplastic Crises

Viral infections, particularly parvovirus infection, which tends to occur in epidemics, can cause a temporary arrest of the erythroid bone marrow, resulting in a rapid decrease in the hematocrit because of the continued hemolysis. The patient, usually a child under 18 years old, presents because of the profound anemia, having usually recovered from the infection. The reticulocyte count falls to less than 1 per cent at the nadir, and may not recover for several days. Blood transfusion, up to a hemoglobin of about 10 grams per dl, is usually indicated, but not as an emergency. A bone marrow aspiration confirms the diagnosis but is not essential. Recovery occurs spontaneously within 10 to 14 days.

Hepatic Crises

Hepatic crises are uncommon and have a varied etiology. Sequestration of red cells in the liver may cause abdominal pain with right upper quadrant tenderness. Nausea and vomiting may occur, and the serum bilirubin and liver enzymes are increased. The differential diagnosis from acute cholecystitis may be difficult, especially if stones are present, but an ultrasound examination may be helpful if it shows that the gallbladder wall and duct system appear normal. Cholecystitis should be treated with ampicillin, and elective cholecystectomy performed when the patient has recovered from the acute attack. Infarction of liver lobes is extremely rare. Viral hepatitis must also be considered.

Occasionally, the main feature is a dramatic increase in the total bilirubin, up to as much as 100 mg per dl, with few or no symptoms, and only a modest change in the level of liver enzymes. Recovery is spontaneous in a few days. This is contrasted with a much more serious condition in which cirrhosis has occurred, perhaps on the basis of alcohol abuse, leading to progressive liver failure, with rising liver enzymes and decreasing coagulation factors, and death, usually from uncontrollable internal hemorrhage.

The Acute Chest Syndrome

Pain crises are often complicated by pulmonary infiltrates, but sometimes cough, fever, and pleuritic pain are the main presenting symptoms. Pneumonia has to be considered, particularly in children, and antibiotic therapy should be started. In the older patient there is usually no sputum production, and a sickle cell infarct is the cause of the problem. With good supportive care appropriate to a crisis, most patients recover in about a week. Others may deteriorate, with increasing dyspnea and falling arterial Po_2, and require an exchange blood transfusion (see below).

Stroke

About 6 per cent of children with sickle cell anemia suffer a stroke, and without treatment the recurrence rate is about 60 per cent. The most common cause is cerebral infarction as a result of narrowing or complete occlusion of the internal carotid artery or one of its branches. Treatment of the acute event may involve intensive care to combat the effects of cerebral edema. Consultation with a neurologist is essential. Seizures require anticonvulsant therapy. Although some strokes may be mild and recovery quite rapid, the risk of another episode, which may be crippling, mandates starting a transfusion program as soon as possible. Because this has to be continued for at least 3 years, iron overload may be a problem and should be prevented by a program of iron chelation cherapy.

Subarachnoid hemorrhage can occur in adults, probably related to subclinical cerebral pathology which occurred in childhood. Computed tomography and magnetic resonance imaging are useful in diagnosis and follow-up of these problems. In certain cases arteriography may be indicated, and for this procedure prior exchange transfusion is advisable.

Hematuria

Gross, painless hematuria is a complication most often encountered in patients with either Hb SC or sickle cell trait. It is caused by necrosis of the tip of a renal papilla and prolonged by the action of urokinase. Although the hematuria may continue for several weeks, it is not usually a serious event and may cease spontaneously. It is important to rule out more serious causes of hematuria. Treatment with epsilon amino caproic acid (EACA), 5 grams 3 times a day, combined with rest in a horizontal position, is usually effective. EACA should not be given parenterally or in a higher oral dose because of the risk of a blood clot in the renal pelvis.

Blood Transfusion

Because of the differing frequency of blood group antigens between blood donors (mostly Caucasians) and sickle cell patients (mostly of African descent), about 18 per cent of transfused patients will develop alloantibodies that can cause serious blood transfusion reactions. Patients should be typed for Rhesus antigens C and E as well as D and, if possible, for Kell, Jka, and Jkb. Many patients will be negative for some or all of these antigens, in which case regional blood banks should be asked to provide negative blood. The antibody screen test cannot be relied on to detect prior sensitization by previous transfusions. The following formulas are useful for children. Blood volume (BV) = 75 × body weight in kg, and the hemoglobin of the average packed cell unit = 22 grams per 100 ml.

Simple transfusion:

$$\text{packed cell required, ml} = \frac{\text{BV} \times \text{desired increase in Hb in grams}}{22}$$

Exchange transfusion:

$$\text{ml of exchange with packed cells} = \frac{\text{BV} \times \text{desired increase in hemoglobin}}{22 - \frac{(\text{starting Hb} + \text{desired Hb})}{2}}$$

Surgery and Anesthesia

Patients should be admitted 24 hours before surgery. Intravenous fluids should be started at 1.5 × maintenance requirements. At least 50 per cent oxygen should be given with the anesthetic agent and should be continued until the patient is fully conscious. If the patient's hemoglobin is 8.0 grams per dl or more, transfusion is not indicated for minor surgical procedures or when blood loss will be minimal. An exchange transfusion should be performed if such patients require major surgery. The commonest postoperative complication is atelectasis or pulmonary infarct, which may be prevented by physiotherapy and use of an incentive spirometer.

NEUTROPENIA

method of
HARRY L. MALECH, M.D., and
JOHN I. GALLIN, M.D.
*National Institute of Allergy and
    Infectious Diseases*
Bethesda, Maryland

Clinically relevant neutropenia may be defined as a substantial decrease in the absolute number of circulating neutrophils from a normal steady state level to a lower number, even if that lower number is still in the normal range. A falling neutrophil count may be important as a sign of an underlying disease process and as a harbinger of further decreases in neutrophil counts. Normal neutrophil counts are quite variable between individuals, but constant in a particular healthy individual followed over several years. The normal range of peripheral blood neutrophil counts is from 1500 to 8000 per microliter, though the count can be as low as 1000 per microliter in some normal black persons.

Because of the widespread use of potent cytotoxic agents, iatrogenic neutropenia is often encountered in clinical practice. Determination of the risk of infection associated with particular levels of circulating blood neutrophils has been derived from studies of such patients. In these patients there is severe limitation of marrow reserve with a markedly impaired marrow response to infection. In this clinical setting neutrophil counts between 1000 and 1500 neutrophils per microliter are associated with a slightly increased risk of infection, with significant risk of infection below 1000 per microliter. At neutrophil counts below 500 per microliter there is a more marked risk of infection, which correlates inversely with the neutrophil count. A falling neutrophil count is associated with a greater risk of infection than the same count in a patient in whom neutrophil numbers are increasing or in whom there is a substantial increase in response to infection.

The bone marrow of a normal healthy adult produces more than 100 billion neutrophils per day, and this number may increase to more than one trillion cells per day with serious bacterial infection. The half-time in circulation for the neutrophil is 6 to 10 hours and is shorter in the setting of infection. A third to a half of the neutrophils in the peripheral circulation are adherent to the endothelial cells of postcapillary venules, and do not contribute to the measured peripheral blood neutrophil count. Marginated neutrophils may return to the circulation or in the presence of local inflammation exit into tissues. In a healthy individual a significant proportion of neutrophils are lost to the gingival crevices and other portions of the gastrointestinal tract. The spleen is probably the site of destruction of senescent neutrophils not lost to other tissue sites.

Etiology

Hereditary neutropenia may be autosomal dominant or recessive, cyclic or noncyclic. In chronic, noncyclic inherited neutropenias, marrow myeloid cells are decreased, although there may be variable marrow reserve available for response to infection. The infection risk may be less than the steady-state peripheral blood neutrophil counts would suggest in cases in which there is adequate marrow reserve. A few individuals who appear to have a steady-state neutropenia actually have a larger than normal proportion of their peripheral blood neutrophils in the marginated pool, retain a normal response to infection, and are not at increased risk of infection.

Inherited cyclic neutropenia of childhood is an autosomal dominant disorder characterized by extremely regular changes in peripheral blood neutrophil counts from profoundly neutropenic levels to the high neutropenic or low normal range and back to very neutropenic levels with a 21-day cycle. While other, less well-defined disorders may be associated with some cycling of neutrophil counts, the regularity of the cycling over many years distinguishes this disorder. During the decrease from the peak, the bone marrow pattern suggests marrow arrest at the early precursor stage, while during recovery from the nadir the marrow may appear qualitatively normal. The nadirs of the cycle are often associated with fevers, gingivitis, aphthous stomatitis, rectal abscesses, malaise, and leg pains, which improve as counts recover. Occasionally more severe problems such as pneumonia, lymphadenitis, or other soft tissue infections may occur. A sometimes missed, and potentially fatal infection is gangrene of the small intestine or colon, which may be seen in adolescents with inherited cyclic neutropenia.

Acquired forms of cyclic neutropenia can begin at any age. The pattern of cycling and degree of neutropenia at nadir may be indistinguishable from the inherited disease, or the cycle period may be much longer and less regular. Acquired cyclic neutropenia may be associated with an increased number of NK-type large granular lymphocytes, suggesting an autoimmune etiology. In some individuals acquired cyclic neutropenia may be a premalignant condition evolving to frank leukemia.

A severe neutropenia of the newborn can occur as a result of maternal antibody response to neutrophil-specific antigens on the child's neutrophils. This is a self-limited process resolving over several weeks as maternal antibodies are cleared. However, the risk of infection is significant during the neutropenic period. Similar neutrophil-specific antibodies may occur in autoimmune neutropenias as a primary disorder or in association with other immune disorders such as lupus erythematosus. Marrow stores of neutrophils in such individuals may appear normal or may be depleted of mature forms. A few individuals have been seen with acquired hypogammaglobulinemia and neutropenia. There may be relative sparing of IgM production with presence of anti-neutrophil IgM antibody.

Neutropenia may be associated with diseases in which there is splenomegaly with trapping and destruction of neutrophils. For example, this may be seen in Felty's syndrome (rheumatoid arthritis with splenomegaly), portal hypertension, and lipid storage diseases. The bone marrow is characteristically hyperplastic.

A transient neutropenia may be seen acutely in gram-negative bacteremia, as circulating neutrophils abruptly marginate in response to circulating bacterial endotoxin. Occasionally, severe infection in the premature infant or the elderly may be associated with a more gradual decline in neutrophil counts to neutropenic levels in a setting in which large numbers of circulating early neutrophil precursors also are seen. This may be evidence of a poorly understood process of bone marrow failure in the setting of severe infection in these two patient groups and is a grave prognostic sign.

Drugs and toxins may cause neutropenia by a number of mechanisms. First, drugs or toxins may cause neutropenia because they are intrinsically toxic to rapidly growing cells. Cytotoxic chemotherapeutic agents fall into this category, but certain antibiotics such as chloramphenicol, trimethoprim-sulfa, 5-fluorocytosine, adenine arabinoside, and the anti-retroviral drug AZT also may cause neutropenia by inhibiting myeloid precursor proliferation. The marrow suppression is generally dose related and dependent upon continued administration of the offending agent.

Secondly, drugs or toxins may cause neutropenia by serving as a haptenic group in an immune response that results in the sensitization of neutrophils or neutrophil precursors to immune-mediated destruction. Bone marrow may appear to be arrested at any stage. This type of drug-dependent immune neutropenia may appear as early as seven days after exposure to a drug; however, in a setting in which the drug has been recently administered, the neutropenia may occur after only a few days of drug administration. Almost any drug can cause this type of immune neutropenia. While there can be associated fever or eosinophilia, these signs are often not present. Most commonly, the penicillin or cephalosporin group of antibiotics are a cause of this type of neutropenia, but commonly used antipyretics, antihistamines, and pain medications can cause this syndrome. It is important to suspect all medications, including ordinary self-remedies, as possible causes of acute idiopathic neutropenia. While this form of drug-induced neutropenia can be severe, the disease is generally self-limited if the offending agent is discontinued. Often the neutrophil counts may show signs of increasing within five to seven days and not longer than ten days after the drug is stopped. Readministration of the sensitizing drug is usually associated with abrupt decreases in neutrophil counts and should not be done deliberately as a specific diagnostic challenge, since even short periods of neutropenia entail some risk of infection.

Drugs, toxins, and certain viruses (e.g., hepatitis) can be associated with aplastic anemia affecting all formed blood elements or with agranulocytosis. This third type of marrow response to drug, toxin, or viral injury results in a prolonged neutropenia that may remit spontaneously, but may be permanent. In many cases, no drug, toxin, or viral cause of the marrow failure can be identified. An immune mechanism may be responsible for some forms of these types of severe marrow failure. The neutropenia characteristically occurs from two to six weeks after exposure to the causative agent, does not appear to be dependent upon the dose or duration of exposure, and may occur long after the last exposure to the agent. Some substances such as aromatic hydrocarbons, phenothiazines, and chloramphenicol have been specifically connected with idiosyncratic reactions resulting in neutropenia.

Certain infections with bacteria (e.g., typhoid fever), viruses (e.g., echo, coxsackie, measles, hepatitis), and rickettsial agents may be associated with mild to moderate neutropenia that generally responds to resolution of the infectious process. In addition, metabolic abnormalities, such as Vitamin B_{12} or folate deficiency, or heavy metal poisoning may be associated with neutropenia.

Diagnostic Studies

A family history of unexplained deaths of other siblings may indicate familial neutropenia. The history of fatigue, malaise, gingivitis, or poorly healing infections may indicate the duration of the neutropenia before diagnosis or may hint at a cyclic pattern. All current and recent past medications, including over-the-counter preparations, must be noted. Potential exposures to toxins in the home or work place must be documented. At physical examination it is important to note fever, gingivitis, lymphadenitis, rectal abscess or fistula, splenomegaly, liver tenderness, and cutaneous infections. Because of the lack of pus formation in the presence of neutropenia, the degree of swelling and redness may be muted. Signs of cutaneous or deep tissue infection may be limited to pain, heat, and only slight redness.

Idiopathic acute neutropenia should prompt a workup for acute infection, even when other signs of infection are lacking. Blood cultures, urine culture, and complete blood count should be obtained, as well as chest x-ray. Other studies should be dictated by history and physical findings. In cases of chronic neutropenia, laboratory studies should include chest x-ray, possibly liver-spleen scan, complete blood count with differential, blood folate, B_{12}, copper, serum protein electrophoresis, immunoglobulin levels, and renal and liver function. When appropriate, a white blood cell count and differential should be done at least 3 days a week over an 8-week period to determine any cyclic pattern. A bone marrow aspirate and biopsy for histology and culture are an essential part of the workup of chronic neutropenias but may be delayed in some cases of acute neutropenia in which the cause is clear and recovery likely.

Patients with chronic neutropenia should be screened for autoimmune diseases, and this should include evaluation of lymphocyte subtypes with assessment of NK cell number. Detection of antineutrophil antibodies should be done. Several methods for determining the presence of circulating antineutrophil antibodies have been published. No one type of test appears to be capable of detecting all cases of immune neutropenia. Fluorescence-activated cell sorting to detect antineutrophil antibodies should be done using patient serum with both patient neutrophils and a panel of control neutrophils. Another useful test examines the ability of patient serum to induce motile leukoagglutination with a panel of normal control neutrophils.

The workup of chronic neutropenia includes assessment of the size of the marginated pool of neutrophils, which is done by evaluating the change in neutrophil count 5 minutes after administration of epinephrine. For a normal adult, the dose is 0.1 mg epinephrine in 100 ml of normal saline infused intravenously over 5 minutes, which results in an increase in the peripheral blood neutrophil count of from one half to two and one half fold as the marginated pool of neutrophils is mobilized. The marrow reserve pool can be evaluated by determining the increase in neutrophil count 4 to 6 hours after administration of steroids. For an adult, a single oral dose of 80 mg of prednisone, or equivalent, results in an increase of two- to threefold in the peripheral neutrophil count at 4 to 6 hours. Evaluation of peripheral destruction of neutrophils can be assessed using Indium-111 radiolabeling of patient or donor neutrophils.

Treatment

In the setting of acute idiopathic neutropenia, it is essential to stop or change all medications if possible. Limiting the length of therapy or dose of antibiotics or other drugs with known bone marrow suppressive effects may be effective in limiting associated neutropenia. The neutropenia associated with trimethoprim-sulfa may be controlled by periodic administration of leucovorin without compromising the antimicrobial activity. There is no role for the use of steroids in acute nonimmune-mediated neutropenias resulting from cytotoxic therapy. Lithium carbonate will increase the myeloid cell mass and neutrophil counts in normal and some neutropenic individuals, but has not proved to be an effective long-term therapy in treatment of any of the neutropenias.

A trial of steroids is indicated in the setting of autoimmune neutropenia and has been effective in eliminating cycling in some patients with acquired cyclic neutropenia. A trial of high-dose gamma globulin has been variably successful in increasing counts in some patients with chronic neutropenias. There is some evidence that a subset of patients with acquired severe chronic agranulocytosis or aplastic anemia may respond to anti-thymocyte globulin treatment, though this therapy is not generally available. A number of myeloid cell growth factors (granulocyte-macrophage colony stimulating factor, granulocyte colony stimulating factor, interleukin-3) have been cloned, and some are now in clinical trials and appear promising as agents to enhance myeloid cell recovery from cytotoxic therapy or in the treatment of some congenital or acquired chronic neutropenias. These factors, alone or in combination, are likely to become important treatment modalities for many types of nonimmune-mediated neutropenias.

For neutropenias associated with increased peripheral destruction of neutrophils with an autoimmune component, steroids or other immunosuppressive therapy have been helpful. In situations in which significant splenomegaly is associated with severe neutropenia, splenectomy may increase the circulating neutrophil count, but this response is variable and unpredictable. Because splenectomy is itself a factor adding to the infection risk of such patients, splenectomy should not be performed specifically as a treatment of neutropenia unless severe noncyclic chronic neutropenia with significant peripheral destruction can be documented.

Treatment of Infections Associated with Neutropenia

In cases of chronic neutropenia, management of infection risk should be dictated by the patient's medical history, although any infections, no matter how minor, should receive prompt medical attention. Patients with neutrophil counts that generally remain above 500 per microliter, or those who show a significant marrow reserve in the setting of infection (or by steroid challenge) and who by history do not appear to have problems with recurrent infections, should not receive prophylactic antibiotics and should not limit their activities. Patients with constant or cyclic neutrophil counts below 300 per microliter and who show little marrow reserve response to infection are generally at more risk of infection, although infection history may differ significantly between individuals with similar degrees of chronic neutropenia. These patients may benefit from prophylactic antibiotics. Oral trimethoprim-sulfa, single strength, twice daily is a commonly used regimen. These patients should try to avoid situations with heavy exposure to airborne soil dust or decaying organic matter in order to decrease the exposure to aspergillus spores. Restriction of other types of activities or social contacts probably makes little difference in infection risk. Good oral hygiene is essential for neutropenic patients. In addition to routine professional dental care, patients can decrease gingivitis by use of chlorhexidine mouthwash and by routine brushing with hydrogen peroxide–sodium bicarbonate paste.

Many of the principles of infection prevention indicated in the care of severe chronic neutropenia also apply to acute-onset neutropenia. There is some evidence that in the setting of cytotoxic therapy–induced severe acute neutropenia, a simple reverse isolation regimen can be helpful in reducing infection during the neutropenic period. This regimen consists of use of face masks and careful hand washing by staff and visitors. More stringent isolation probably is unnecessary and only serves to impede patient contact with family and medical personnel. Prophylactic trimethoprim-sulfa is useful in this setting, as is the use of mouthwash and swallow of a nonabsorbable antifungal agent such as nystatin to reduce colonization with *Candida* species.

As noted previously, signs of inflammation with severe neutropenia are muted, such that fever and/or hypotension and occasionally pain at the site of infection may be the only sign of life-threatening infection. Very slight infiltrates on chest x-ray may be the only sign of severe pneumonia. Bacteremia without an obvious source of infection is common. When a site of infection can be documented, it is usually the mouth, sinuses, gastrointestinal tract, rectum, lungs, or skin. Bowel wall cellulitis and necrosis can present insidiously with fever and abdominal pain and is a surgical emergency. Urinary tract infection occurs but in the absence of instrumentation or anatomic abnormality is less common. With neutropenic patients, it is essential that in the presence of fever or other potential sign of infection, including hypotension in the absence of fever, the patient is evaluated rapidly; that blood, sputum, urine, and other cultures are obtained; and that the patient is given broad-spectrum antibiotics intravenously. The prompt institution of intravenous antibiotics markedly reduces mortality from infection and must take precedence over complete evaluation.

The major bacterial pathogens causing infection in neutropenic patients are often those commonly colonizing the skin, oropharynx, and gastrointestinal tract. These include gram-negative coliforms such as *Escherichia coli, Klebsiella pneumonia, Enterobacter* species, and *Proteus* species, as well as aerophilic organisms such as *Pseudomonas aeruginosa,* and *Serratia* species. Common gram-positive pathogens include *Staphylococcus aureus* (which in some institutions may include a high incidence of methicillin-resistant isolates), *Staphylococcus epidermidis,* and streptococcal species. Survey cultures before infection have not proved to be very useful in predicting the infectious agent. Many studies have been done to demonstrate that any of a number of combination or single antibiotic choices are similarly effective. It is important to cover a broad spectrum that will provide bactericidal activity against the organisms listed above. A combination of broad-spectrum penicillin with activity against both *Pseudomonas* and *Klebsiella* species (mezlocillin or piperacillin) and an aminoglycoside (gentamicin, tobramycin, or amikacin) is a good choice. Blood aminoglycoside levels should be obtained after 48 hours and then periodically to guide dose and schedule in order to achieve optimum bactericidal blood levels and minimize renal toxicity. Imipenem or any of a number of very broad-spectrum third-generation cephalosporins may be substituted for the penicillin. Some studies have indicated that an extended spectrum third-generation cephalosporin alone may be equally effective. These combinations are only moderately effective against staphylococcus and it has been suggested that vancomycin be added to this regimen for the short period until cultures have ruled out staphylococcus. In the hospital setting, organism prevalence and susceptibility patterns are important in choosing initial antibiotic coverage.

Antibiotic changes should be dictated by culture results. In the absence of the isolation of a specific organism and when fever persists for more than seven days, amphotericin B should be added to the antibiotic regimen because of the high risk of fungal infection with *Candida* or *Aspergillus* species in these patients. For the same reason, the persistence of fever and infiltrate on chest x-ray requires bronchoscopy and often open lung biopsy to rule out fungal infection. In the absence of a known etiology for the fever, patients should be continued on antibiotics until afebrile for three days or until the neutropenia resolves; others have suggested continuing antibiotics until resolution of the neutropenia regardless of the febrile response.

Granulocyte transfusions should not be used prophylactically in neutropenic patients, and controversy continues regarding any role for granulocyte transfusions in infected, severely neutropenic patients. In a severely neutropenic patient in whom bacterial or fungal infection is clearly documented and a trial of appropriate antibiotic therapy is not controlling the infection, granulocyte transfusions may be helpful. Transfused granulocytes should be obtained by centrifugation leukapheresis, be ABO and Rh matched, and consist of a minimum of 10^{10} granulocytes. In the setting of chemotherapy for leukemia, the transfused granulocytes should be irradiated to prevent graft-versus-host disease, even though irradiation may suppress the capacity of neutrophils to produce toxic oxygen products. Granulocytes should be given daily for at least a week or until resolution of the infection or of the neutropenia. A cautionary note is that an increased incidence of severe pulmonary decompensation has been seen in some patients receiving both amphotericin B and granulocyte transfusions.

HEMOLYTIC DISEASE OF THE NEWBORN

method of
GARY R. GUTCHER, M.D.
Medical College of Virginia
Richmond, Virginia

The term *Hemolytic disease of the newborn* (HDN) is generally used as if it were synonymous with only isoimmune hemolytic diseases. Although isoimmune hemolytic diseases do account for the majority of cases of HDN, the relative decrease in the severe manifestations of problems related to the Rh blood group requires a heightened awareness on the part of physicians of the other causes outlined in Table 1. All of these conditions are characterized by the production of bilirubin from red cell destruction to a degree that overwhelms the excretory system. This is in contrast to those causes of neonatal hyperbilirubinemia that result from delayed or blunted excretion.

TABLE 1. **Causes of HDN and Overproduction of Bilirubin**

1. **Isoimmunization**
   Rh, ABO, anti-c, anti-E, anti-Kell, anti-Duffy, anti-M

2. **Spherocytic Diseases (Membrane Defects)**
   Spherocytosis, elliptocytosis, stomatocytosis, pyknocytosis

3. **Nonspherocytic Diseases (Enzyme Defects and Hemoglobinopathy)**
   G-6-PD, pyruvate kinase deficiency, alpha-thalassemia trait

4. **Drug-Induced**
   High-dose water-soluble vitamin K

5. **Infection**
   Bacterial sepsis
   Viral (especially intrauterine): cytomegalovirus, rubella, coxsackie B, and herpes
   Syphilis
   Protozoan (toxoplasmosis, malaria)

6. **Inborn Errors of Metabolism**
   Galactosemia

7. **Microangiopathic**
   Disseminated intravascular hemolysis, hemangioma (Kasabach-Merritt syndrome), severe arterial stenosis (renal, aortic)

As the classic example of HDN, the Rh antibody system provides the model for other forms of isoimmune disease. The Rh blood group has three antigenic groupings (Cc, Dd, Ee) on the surface of the erythrocyte. Rh "positivity" is conferred by the presence of D, and Rh "negativity" by its absence. Although modified by the closely aligned Cc-Ee antigens, an individual's Rh status is predominantly determined by the presence or absence of a "big" D from at least one parent. Approximately 15 per cent of the Caucasian population but only 5 per cent of American blacks are Rh-negative.

Throughout the pregnancy of an Rh-negative mother who is carrying an Rh-positive fetus, fetomaternal transplacental transfusions will initiate a response of both an anti-D IgM (saline, or complete) antibody and an anti-D IgG (incomplete) antibody. IgG is capable of crossing the placenta, sensitizing the fetal Rh-positive cells, and initiating destruction and clearance of erythrocytes by the fetal reticuloendothelial system (RES). The severity of the ensuing disease is in large part, then, determined by the degree of sensitization (leak) and the ability of the fetal RES to process the erythrocytes. To the extent that subsequent sensitizations are "primed," each succeeding Rh-positive fetus in an Rh-negative woman will be more severely affected. Table 2 delineates the manifestations and mechanisms involved in producing this process.

Unlike the Rh system, which is limited to primate erythrocytes, the ABO blood group antigens are also present in foods and bacteria. Thus, previous exposure to blood products is not the prerequisite that it is in Rh disease. A maternal blood group O sets the stage for an isoimmune response to fetal A or B antigen. Fetal antigen A is more sparsely distributed on erythrocytes than is fetal B. This may account for the relatively less severe manifestations of O-A incompat-

TABLE 2. **Clinical Features of HDN**

Manifestation	Mechanism
1. Hemolysis	Erythrophagocytosis in RES
	Induction of enzymes degrading heme and globin
	Hyperbilirubinemia (in infant)
2. Erythropoiesis—peripheral blood reticulocytosis and normoblastemia	Enhanced in response to ongoing hemolysis
	Extramedullary hematopoiesis in liver, spleen, and skin ("blueberry muffin")
3. Anemia	Exhausted erythropoiesis
4. Hydrops fetalis—edema, anasarca	Anemia
	Decreased oncotic pressure
	Increased portal venous pressure
	Heart failure
5. Other (e.g., hypoglycemia)	Pancreatic cell hyperplasia secondary to in utero amino acid (alanine) stimulation

TABLE 3. **Utilization of Liley Graph Plot of Delta OD^{450}**

Delta OD^{450}	Action
Zone I	Repeat every 2 to 3 weeks
Zone II, falling	Repeat every week
Zone II, rising/ Zone III	Intervene
	≤33 weeks: intrauterine transfusion
	>33 weeks: assess pulmonary maturity and consider delivery

ibility when compared with O-B. Though generally not associated with erythroblastosis fetalis, ABO isoimmune hemolytic disease can produce unpredictable and severe degrees of hyperbilirubinemia.

As indicated above, the decline in Rh disease as a result of prophylactic immune therapy (see below) has resulted in the relative increase in isoimmune diseases secondary to other blood group antigen incompatibilities: anti-c, anti-E, anti-Kell, anti-M, and anti-Duffy. The diagnosis and nonimmune therapy of these diseases are identical to those of the Rh model.

Antenatal Management

All pregnant women should be screened early (first visit) with blood group typing and antibody screening (indirect Coombs' test). The diagnosis should be suspected in a set-up (maternal Rh-negative or O-type) and confirmed when specific antibody titers exceed 1:8. When the titers are ≤1:8, monthly retesting is indicated. When >1:8, closer evaluation by amniocentesis is required.

Amniocentesis is performed with ultrasonographic guidance. The fluid (free of meconium or blood) may be scanned in a recording spectrophotometer and the peak optical density (above baseline) at 450 nanometers (nm), called the delta-OD^{450}, is plotted against gestational age on semilogarithm paper. The normative reference zones of Liley classify patients into Zone I (normal, no action); Zone II, declining (abnormal, no action without other compromising data); and Zone II, rising/Zone III (abnormal, intervene). The general scheme is depicted in Table 3. Once the need for amniocentesis is determined, referral to fetomaternal specialists is indicated, as the management becomes quite complex, involving intrauterine transfusion and/or early, premature induction of delivery.

For those infants requiring intrauterine transfusion, ultrasonographic guidance of a radiopaque catheter permits the intraperitoneal infusion of cytomegalovirus-negative, O-negative, washed, packed erythrocytes. The volume of blood infused is empirically calculated as

$$[\text{Gestational age (in weeks)} - 20] \times 10 \text{ ml}$$

Close fetal monitoring is used in decisions to slow or terminate the infusion as indicated. Peritoneal lymphatics will assimilate >90 per cent of the cells. The procedure will need to be repeated every two to three weeks. Failure to assimilate is an ominous sign. Because of the development of high-resolution sonography and enhanced operative skills, the intraperitoneal technique is being replaced by the direct intravascular infusion technique.

Other forms of therapy purported to alter the maternal immune response have been proposed, using a variety of agents. None have worked consistently. On the other hand, anti-D globulin (RhoGam), which was introduced nearly 20 years ago, has proved to be an effective prophylactic immunotherapy. In documented maternal Rh-negative/neonatal Rh-positive situations, 300 micrograms are given intramuscularly within 72 hours of delivery. If there is some question or delay in defining the neonatal blood type, the Rh-negative mother should receive RhoGam anyway, since nearly two thirds of the infants will be Rh-positive. Furthermore, while less effective, administration of RhoGam up to four weeks later may be helpful and should *not* be withheld. These generous recommendations are made despite a reported persistent, disappointing so-called failure rate of RhoGam. These failures are typically the result of errors in the accurate diagnosis of blood type (maternal or infant) or errors of omission (failure to administer at all times when sensitization may occur, such as amniocentesis, placenta previa or abruptio placentae, ectopic pregnancy, or spontaneous abortion). Furthermore, sensitization may occur early in pregnancy, so that current recommendations are for a prophylactic dose at 28 weeks gestation in all unsensitized women. The recommendations for RhoGam administration are outlined in Table 4.

Neonatal Management

The mainstay of neonatal management remains the exchange transfusion. Exchange transfusions are advocated for three general reasons:

Anemia. When present at birth, there should be a partial exchange with packed erythrocytes for hematocrits less than 30 per cent.

Rapidly Rising Serum Bilirubin. When this occurs at any time, whole blood should be utilized to remove sensitized cells from the circulation in an effort to blunt the peak bilirubin attained.

Elevated Bilirubin. An exchange transfusion using whole blood should be given at any time when the bilirubin exceeds some threshold level above which the risk of bilirubin encephalopathy is unacceptable.

A body of evidence suggests that the first and third types of exchange transfusions described above are beneficial; no such supportive data exists for the second indication. In any event, as the accurate measurement of bilirubin is fraught with problems, any assessment of the rate of rise should be based on several bilirubin determinations, not just two.

The exchange transfusion is conducted under the same clean/sterile conditions as for the insertion of umbilical catheters. For all infants, approximately twice the calculated blood volume (80 to 100 ml per kg) is projected to exchange about 85 per cent of circulating blood. When the removal of bilirubin (especially at high levels) is the object, then "priming" the patient with 1 gram per kg of 25 per cent salt-poor albumin will help scavenge tissue-bound bilirubin into the circulation if given 30 minutes to 1 hour prior to

TABLE 4. **Recommendations for Rh Immune Globulin (RhoGam)**

Status	Action
Every Rh-negative unimmunized woman with:	
Rh-positive baby delivered	240–300 µg
Abortion*	50 µg
Amniocentesis*	240–300 µg
28 weeks completed gestation*	240–300 µg
Massive transplacental hemorrhage (known Rh-positive fetus)	240–300 µg/25 ml estimated bleed
Every Rh-negative, weakly immunized† pregnant woman with Rh-positive baby delivered (Rh antibody by Autoanalyzer only)	240–300 µg

*Unless father is known to be Rh-negative.
†May not be effective.

the exchange. When a longer time elapses, the effect may not be as good, as the albumin will rapidly re-equilibrate to the extravascular space. When cardiorespiratory status is precarious, the potential for decompensation with a rapid volume expansion may argue against this practice. For infants with HDN weighing 2500 grams or more at birth, any with a bilirubin $\geq$ 20 mg/dl (or $\geq$ 15 mg/dl if over 72 hours) should be exchanged. For those under 2500 grams, the birthweight in 100-gram increments may serve as a guide (e.g. 15 mg/dl at 1500 grams). Sepsis, hypoxia, and acidemia require exchange at lower levels, but good guidelines are lacking. In infants weighing more than 1500 grams, exchange transfusion utilizing specially designed kits, catheters, and stopcocks can be accomplished via a single umbilical vein catheter, alternately removing and infusing blood. Because this causes rapid fluctuations in blood volume and pressure, for infants weighing less than 1500 grams simultaneous infusion and withdrawal from two sites (so-called isovolemic transfusion) may be less traumatic when the risk of pressure-dependent hemorrhage (intracranial) is of real concern. The current relatively infrequent need for exchange transfusions suggests referral of the patient to units and/or physicians familiar with the technique.

Phototherapy with blue or white lamps producing 6 to 13 microwatts per cm² from irradiance at 420 to 480 nanometers bandpass is effective in producing photoproducts more rapidly excreted than native bilirubin. However, in the face of severe hemolysis, the impact on serum bilirubin may not be easily discernible. Here, phototherapy is an *adjunctive* therapy only.

Not only the irradiance per area listed above is important but also the total area of bilirubin-rich skin exposed. Thus the infant should have a *minimally* sized diaper to shield gonads and collect excreta. Periodically "rolling" the infant to expose new skin to the lamps is helpful.

In mild cases, phototherapy alone may be sufficient. Complications of the treatment include increased insensible water loss and dehydration, loose stools, photosensitized rash, and tanning. In order to prevent retinal damage, some form of eye patches are used. These are occasionally dislodged, with the potentially severe complications of airway occlusion (nares) or corneal abrasion. When used in severe cases, phototherapy may produce the bronzed baby syndrome, resulting from the complex photodegradation of bilirubin in the presence of the cholestasis caused by hepatic extramedullary hematopoiesis and hepatocellular damage.

Even if the disease is mild with respect to hyperbilirubinemia, hemolysis may be brisk.

Moreover, in severe cases, exchange transfusions may mask the underlying destruction of erythrocytes and erythrocyte precursors outside the circulation. Consequently, late anemia may result at 4 to 6 weeks of age. Sequential assessment is necessary to decide on the need for simple transfusion. Hematocrits may fall below 20 per cent and treatment should largely be based on symptoms. The earliest is generally poor feeding, followed by resting tachypnea and tachycardia and diaphoresis.

HEMOPHILIA AND RELATED CONDITIONS

method of
W. KEITH HOOTS, M.D.
University of Texas Health Science Center
Houston, Texas

Comprehensive Care

Special treatment centers have been established in the U.S.A. and many other countries to provide multidisciplinary care of hemophilia and related disorders. Patients who have been chronically infused with plasma derived factor concentrates prior to 1984–1985 are at high risk for infection with the human immunodeficiency virus (HIV) or one of the hepatitis viruses. The comprehensive hemophilia centers are mandated to provide voluntary testing for these viruses and counseling of patients found seropositive for previous infection. Since seropositive individuals have a high risk for transmission of HIV to their sexual partners, counseling and prevention education are essential. In addition, screening for clinical and biochemical evidence of hepatitis infection should be a routine facet of comprehensive hemophilia management.

Information about hemophilia care, hemophilia centers, and HIV risk reduction and counseling is available through the National Hemophilia Foundation, The Soho Building, 110 Greene Street, Room 106, New York, New York 10012 (telephone 212-219-8180) or from its local chapters.

Inheritance and Prenatal Diagnosis

Chromosome localization of the genes for hemophilia A and hemophilia B on the X-chromosome and von Willebrand's disease on autosome 12 has now been determined. In addition, the nucleotide sequences for both the Factor VIII and Factor IX genes are known, including characterizations of several genetic variants for hemophilia A. Utilizing a DNA restriction fragment length polymorphism (RFLP) technique, definitive carrier testing is possible among selected pedigrees for the first time. For those pedigrees in whom restriction mapping proves inconclusive, classic carrier testing techniques utilizing the determination of the ratio of Factor VIII coagulant (Factor VIIIc) to Factor VIII von Willebrand activity (Factor VIII$_{\text{VWF}}$) in the candidate female can estimate a probability of her being a carrier of hemophilia A. Comparable predictability for hemophilia B awaits more complete application of the DNA recombinant technology.

Antenatal diagnosis of hemophilia A utilizes chronic villus sampling of a determined hemophilia carrier mother during the tenth to twelfth week of gestation. Restriction mapping of the fetal cells so definitively ascertains whether the male fetus has hemophilia A. As with carrier testing, some mothers will not be candidates for such antenatal diagnosis because of a non-illustrative RFLP pattern. For such individuals, fetal blood sampling by fetoscopy following amniocentesis for sex determination is an option to define a Factor VIIIc:Factor VIII$_{\text{VWF}}$ ratio in candidate male fetuses. Comparable technology for antenatal diagnosis of hemophilia B is being developed at the present time.

Preventive Care

Male infants born to known or suspected hemophilic carrier mothers should not be circumcised until hemophilia in the infant has been excluded by laboratory testing. Blood for assay for APTT and Factor VIII or Factor IX assay (or both if family history is uncertain) should be drawn from a superficial limb vein in order to lessen the likelihood of producing a hematoma that might then require replacement therapy. Certainly, femoral and jugular sites *must be avoided.*

Routine immunizations requiring injection such as DPT or MMR may be given in the deep subcutaneous tissue (rather than deep intramuscular as is the usual practice), using the smallest gauge needle that is feasible. Hepatitis B vaccine should be given as soon after birth as possible to all infants with confirmed diagnosis of hemophilia. The oral polio live attenuated viral vaccine should not be given to an infant whose hemophilic older brother (or grandfather in the household) is known to be HIV immune–suppressed from previous HIV exposure, because of the risk to the latter of intrahousehold spread poliomyelitis. Salk vaccine may be substituted.

Early infant dental examination is recommended to teach proper tooth brushing and to ensure adequate household water fluoridation. In addition to education about hemophilia, both genetic and psychosocial counseling are important for the mother of a newborn with hemophilia. This is particularly true for the approximately 30 per cent for whom the hemophilia represents a new mutation and for whom there is no previous family experience with the disease. Reluctance to clean the teeth routinely should be dispelled early and anticipated problem areas for causing bleeding should be discussed.

Both parents should be encouraged to participate intensively in every part of the infant's care. Further, normal socialization opportunities must not be limited because of the hemophilia. Experienced personnel should discuss specifically what minimum limitations are reasonable versus what constitutes over-protection and, therefore, may jeopardize the child's normal development.

An appropriate exercise regimen that excludes "contact" sports (e.g., tackle football) should be encouraged as a daily routine. Further, the role of such a program for the child and adult following episodes of hemarthrosis is best discussed before the child has a joint bleed.

Impact of Hemophilia on Other Illnesses

Hemophilia A and B do not protect against atherosclerotic heart disease, stroke, and other common diseases that are initiated or exacerbated by thrombosis. The risks for hepatitis and HIV are noted above, and these have been undergoing a reduction recently as newly available purification measures for plasma products have become available (see under Infusion Therapy). For older patients who have received the earlier generations of plasma clotting concentrates, clinical surveillance for chronic viral effects by the managing physician is necessary.

Self-Infusion

Intravenous infusion of Factor VIII or Factor IX concentrates, cryoprecipitate, or desmopressin (see under Other Therapies for Inherited Coagulopathies) by the patient, his parents, or some other household member has become an important mainstay of bleeding management over the last 20 years.

Such a program, which requires vigilant supervision by the physician and the staff of the hemophilia center, begins with training and certification of the patient or family member for home infusion. Such education goes beyond instruction on venipuncture procedures. Appropriate candidates should be proficient in bleed recognition, have proper knowledge of dosing for different anatomic sites, and be committed to strict record keeping. Since this regimen represents a direct extension of the treating physician's care, close contact between the person giving the home infusion and the treating physician is essential. This regular dialogue protects against overtreatment and incomplete clinical assessment. In addition to the obvious convenience for the family that home infusion offers, it allows for the earliest possible therapy for hemarthroses (and other evolving hemorrhagic events). This early inter-

vention has been shown to reduce long-term morbidity from chronic joint disease.

Treatment

Infusion Therapy: An Evolving Phenomenon

The exigency of the HIV epidemic among hemophiliacs has profoundly influenced and continues to impact the choice of clotting replacement for the hemophiliac population. Viral attenuation procedures using heating, detergents, and monoclonal technology began in earnest in 1983 in response to the AIDS and hepatitis risks for hemophiliacs. By early 1985, all products for both hemophilia A and B were being heated to alleviate HIV and secondarily hepatitis risk. More efficacious methodology for viral attenuation continues to be developed. The indication for applying any or all technological advances to the therapy of bleeding in an individual patient will be discussed below in the context of present knowledge. Since this is far from a static process at this time, careful assessment of these options must be made within the context of new data regarding safety and efficacy. Discussion will begin with the most elemental of therapies and continue to the more recently available.

Fresh Frozen Plasma. Fresh frozen plasma (FFP) is derived from either individual units of whole blood or by plasmapheresis. One unit typically is 200 to 275 ml in volume. Since clotting factor activity for both Factor VIII and Factor IX is defined in units, a calculation of expected clotting replacement capability can be calculated for either deficient factor. Specifically, one unit of either factor activity is defined as the amount present in one unit of fresh, average, normal human plasma anticoagulated with one tenth part sodium citrate. Therefore, a fresh unit of frozen plasma from a typical donor has approximately 80 to 110 units per dl or from 160 to 300 units of Factor VIII and Factor IX, respectively. In addition FFP contains 2.5 to 4.5 mg per dl of fibrinogen; approximately 80 to 110 units per dl of procoagulant Factors II, V, VII, X, and IX; and similar functional quantities of the naturally occurring inhibitors protein C, protein S, and antithrombin III and the fibrinolytic agent plasminogen. FFP is the treatment of choice for deficiencies of these clotting or inhibitory proteins for which specific component therapy is not available and for which cryoprecipitate cannot serve as an enriched source (see below).

The use of FFP to treat severe deficiencies of Factors VIII or IX that require restoration of the missing factor to normal levels (i.e., 50 per cent in vivo activity) is often limited by the amount of intravascular volume expansion the individual can tolerate. Naturally, the volume constraint is influenced by factors such as age, blood pressure, cardiac output, and respiratory function. An individual in whom these parameters are normal can usually tolerate volumes of 18 ml per kg per hour; however, older patients or compromised neonates with less than optimal parameters usually will tolerate less. Volume constraints may be overcome utilizing plasmapheresis carried out with careful cardiovascular and nephrologic monitoring. Allergic reactions from repeated exposure to plasma are not uncommon.

Cryoprecipitate. Cryoprecipitate is the cold-insoluble protein matrix that remains when FFP is slowly thawed. When re-dissolved, this precipitate usually has a volume of 10 to 30 ml and contains approximately 80 to 100 units of Factor VIIIc and Factor VIII$_{VWF}$ activity, 200 to 300 mg of fibrinogen, and approximately one third to two thirds of both the fibronectin and Factor XIII in the original unit of FFP. Cryoprecipitate requires frozen storage to maintain factor activity.

Because there is wide individual variation in clotting factor activity, the minimum expected activity per bag of cryoprecipitate should probably be used for dosage calculation. Accordingly, at least two bags should be utilized to treat an infant, because of this variability from bag to bag and the fact that 100 units (a single bag) is scarcely adequate dosing for any type of infant hemorrhage. The Factor VIII activity of a single bag of cryoprecipitate can be augmented if the donor is pretreated with 0.3 microgram per kg of desmopressin 30 minutes prior to donation. This is not done routinely; however, it has been effectively utilized to augment supply from directed family plasmapheresis donations when risk for viral infection from pooled concentrates is considered unacceptable.

Cryoprecipitate has long served as the major source of Factor VIII$_{VWF}$. When requirements for Factor VIII$_{VWF}$ exceed the amount that DDAVP infusion can provide or when an individual has severe Type I von Willebrand's disease (VWD) or Type II VWD, cryoprecipitate is an appropriate source of this activity. The relative risks, benefit, and cost of cryoprecipitate versus pasteurized Factor VIII, VIII$_{VWF}$ (Humate P) must be weighed for such patients. In the United States, cryoprecipitate is still the most available and enriched product for treating deficiency of or defects in both fibrinogen and Factor VIII.

Types of Factor VIII Concentrate. Lyophilized human Factor XIII concentrates are made from pooling and fractionation of large batches of donated plasma. Typically, 10,000 to 25,000 donor units are pooled for preparations into a single lot of Factor VIII concentrates. The final preparation

of lyophilized human Factor VIII preparations has been undergoing rapid alterations in recent months in order to effect better virus attenuation. The following products are available at this time.

DRY-HEATED, LYOPHILIZED FACTOR VIII CONCENTRATE. Until very recently, this was the primary type of viral attenuated Factor VIII preparation. Certain of these products that were heated for less than 36 hours have been implicated in the HIV infection of a very small number of hemophilia A patients among thousands of such individuals who have received millions of units of this generic product since its introduction in 1983. Donor screening of all dry-heated products has been the norm since early 1987. This has resulted in even further reduction in HIV risk, although non-A, non-B hepatitis continues to contaminate these dry preparations. As of early 1988, only one dry-heated Factor VIII preparation remained on the United States market (heated at 68° C for 72 hours), since many of the manufacturers had opted for the newer attenuation procedures discussed below.

WET-HEATED, LYOPHILIZED FACTOR VIII PREPARATIONS. These preparations were first available in the United States in 1987. They are made from large pools as described above but are processed in varying techniques analogous to a pasteurization process. There is a significant loss of Factor VIII activity during this heating; hence, these products are expensive. The first of these products marketed in the United States appears remarkedly more purified from both HIV and non-A, non-B hepatitis, based on data from longer use in Europe. Variations of this wet treatment process are now available from several manufacturers. Those treating patients with hemophilia are urged to continually reassess the safety and efficacy of any or all products prescribed, particularly in this dynamic treatment milieu.

DETERGENT/SOLVENT-TREATED FACTOR VIII PREPARATIONS. These preparations utilize organic solvents to destroy viruses in pooled Factor VIII preparations prepared from large-donor pools. Lipid-envelope viruses, including HIV and at least some of the hepatitis viruses, appear to be effectively removed by this procedure. Cost of this material is intermediate between dry heat-treated and wet-heated preparations.

MONOCLONALLY PREPARED FACTOR VIII PREPARATIONS. This type of Factor VIII preparation, first available in 1987, utilizes monoclonal antibody affinity columns to prepare highly purified Factor VIIIc. A second viral attenuation step of either heat or detergent is usually combined to maximize viral safety. To date, such preparations have been free of HIV and non-A, non-B hepatitis. Additionally, the high purity resulting from this process gives an additional advantage of very low-infusion volume and a preparation virtually free of Factor VIIIc protein antigen. Like the wet preparations, the cost of such specially purified preparations is much greater than that of dry-heated Factor VIII concentrates.

RECOMBINANT FACTOR VIII PREPARATION. A recombinant Factor VIII preparation is presently being tested. A target date for availability has not yet been determined.

Hemophilia B Therapy

The therapeutic diversity described for Factor VIII does not exist at the present time for Factor IX preparations, since dry-heated preparations are the only kind presently available. This is likely to change as the technologies described above are applied to Factor IX and perhaps other procoagulant proteins. Several purified Factor IX preparations free of the other serine proteases and, therefore, less likely to be thrombogenic (see below) have recently been tested in a therapeutic trial phase and will soon be available.

Prothrombin Complex Concentrates. Presently available Factor IX preparations are prothrombin complex concentrates (PCCs) containing Factors II, VII, IX, and X. There is some slight activation of these proteases that occurs during preparation which makes them potentially thrombogenic. Clinical thrombosis has been seen most often in hemophilia B patients following high-dose, frequent infusion regimens, although single infusions have occasionally been implicated. For this reason the International Committee on Thrombosis and Hemostasis recommends that 5 to 10 units of heparin per ml of infusate be added prior to infusion, particularly in adult patients or in children receiving frequent dosing. In addition to being the mainstay of therapy for hemophilia B, PCC preparations are often utilized to treat mild to moderate bleeding in patients with Factor VIII inhibitors when activated prothrombin complex concentrates (APCCs) are not available or are too costly (see below). Although rare, thrombotic complications from PCC therapy in the latter patients has been described with very high-dosage regimens.

Other Therapy For Patients With Inhibitors

Activated Prothrombin Complex Concentrates. Activated prothrombin complex concentrates (APCC) have been deliberately activated to produce an active prothrombinase that will "by-pass" the activation step of Factor VIIIc in the intrinsic clotting pathway. The two available APCC products are Autoplex (Hyland Laboratories) and FEIBA (Immuno Laboratories). These were developed specifically for treating patients with

Factor VIIIc antibodies whose antibody titers were so high that saturation therapy with Factor VIII concentrates was not feasible. Calculation of unit size is somewhat variable for these products and their mode of preparation is somewhat different. Therefore, correlation between improved in vitro coagulation and successful achievement of hemostasis in vivo is variable at best and efficacy with one product does not assure efficacy with the other. Hence, an empiric trial constitutes the only reliable therapeutic assessment of efficacy.

Porcine Factor VIII Concentrate. Porcine Factor VIII concentrate can be used to treat patients with acquired inhibitors (antibodies) to Factor VIII. Inhibitors develop in approximately 10 per cent of all hemophilia A patients. Patients with high antibody titers (measured as Bethesda units) that behave anamnestically with antigen (i.e., Factor VIIIc) challenge often cannot be treated with enough human Factor VIII concentrates to achieve adequate in vivo Factor VIII levels for hemostasis. In these cases, the avid antibody quickly neutralizes the administered human Factor VIIIc. However, in many cases, the specific antibody to human Factor VIIIc does not bind to porcine Factor VIII as avidly; therefore, a sustainable circulating Factor VIII level can be achieved using the porcine preparation when it is not feasible with the human preparation. Although porcine Factor VIII preparations have not transmitted hepatitis or other viruses, they do have a greater propensity to cause allergic reactions because of the presence of small amounts of porcine antigen. However, recent technological advances have remarkably diminished this xenogeneic problem. The functional analogy between human and porcine Factor VIII does make it possible for the patient to have an anamnestic rise in the Bethesda unit titer (antibody level) following infusion of porcine Factor VIII.

Other Therapy for Inherited Coagulopathies

Desmopressin (DDAVP) (Rohrer Pharmaceutical) is a synthetically modified analogue of vasopressin that has scant vasoconstrictive properties. In addition to its antidiuretic effect, it induces the immediate release of Factor VIIIc, Factor VIII$_{VWF}$, and plasminogen activator from storage sites in endothelial cells. Typically, infusion of 0.3 microgram per kg of desmopressin intravenously over 15 to 20 minutes results in a 2.5- to 3-fold increase in Factor VIIIc and a 2- to 2.5-fold increase in Factor VIII$_{VWF}$ within approximately 30 minutes. Both activities decay at a rate comparable to infused Factor VIIIc or Factor VIII$_{VWF}$. Since tachyphylaxis quickly occurs with repeated administration of this drug, a 48-hour interval between doses is recommended, presumably to allow endothelial stores to be repleted. The desmopressin dose should be diluted in 50 ml of sterile saline for infusion. Side effects of flushing and headaches are usually mild. Advantages include moderate cost, product sterility, and exceedingly long shelf life. Desmopressin is the treatment of choice for mild to moderate bleeding or even minor surgery in patients with hemophilia and von Willebrand's disease (Type I). In more severe bleeding, peak levels following infusion may be insufficient for sustained hemostasis. It is therefore important to observe the desmopressin response of different types of bleeding in an individual before determining long-term therapeutic management. Desmopressin is ineffective for treatment of patients with moderate or severe hemophilia A and of all patients with hemophilia B, and it is contraindicated in Type IIB von Willebrand's disease, in which there is a defect in the highest molecular weight forms of von Willebrand factor multimers, and administration may trigger massive platelet aggregation.

Antifibrinolytic agents such as epsilon aminocaproic acid (EACA, Amicar) or tranexamic acid (Cyklokapron) are specific inhibitors of plasminogen activation and help to preserve clots. The usual dosage for EACA is up to 100 mg per kg every 6 hours in infants and small children and a maximum of approximately 40 mg per kg in an adult. Tranexamic acid dosage is 25 mg per kg every 6 hours. These agents are particularly effective in obviating the need for any or further infusion therapy for oral bleeds, epistaxis, or menorrhagia. Use is contraindicated when hematuria is present. Caution must be exercised in the concomitant use of these agents with PCC or APCC because of an increase in thrombogenic potential.

Analgesics are frequently necessary to treat pain accompanying bleeding, particularly when the bleeding is intra-articular or intramuscular. Moderate pain can often be mediated with acetaminophen; aspirin must be avoided because of its adverse effect on platelet cyclooxygenase. More severe pain may require the addition of narcotic or narcotic-like drugs such as codeine, meperidine, and hydroxymorphone. Although careful prescribing practices reduce the risk of chronic narcotic abuse, continued vigilance is needed, since the infusion therapy and related treatment frequently occur at home or outside the clinic.

Corticosteroids may prove beneficial in treating edema associated with hemorrhage, although long-term therapy is rarely indicated. Nonsteroidal anti-inflammatory agents may relieve arthritis pain and inflammation associated with chronic hemarthroses, although great care must be taken because these aspirin-like drugs may exacerbate bleeding in these patients.

Treatment Principles

Hemophilia A

Traditionally, hematologists have attempted to attain a circulating Factor VIIIc level of 40 to 50 units per dl of plasma to achieve hemostasis in common bleeding episodes such as hemarthroses. This typically requires 20 to 25 units per kg of body weight, since plasma volume is approximately 50 ml per kg. Stated another way, one unit of Factor VIII concentrate per kg of body weight typically elevates the plasma Factor VIII level 2 per cent. In older children and adults who have learned early recognition of bleeding before the classical signs of inflammation are evident (usually a twinge of pain at the site), levels of 25 to 30 units per dl (12 to 15 units per kg per dose) are frequently sufficient to abort an evolving hemarthrosis or other mild to moderate bleeding episode. In younger children for whom such early recognition may be difficult, the higher dosage may often be required to alleviate the necessity for a follow-up infusion. For mucous membrane hemorrhage (e.g., gingival or oral bleeding) a slightly higher circulating Factor VIIIc, 60 to 75 units per dl (30 to 35 units per kg), may obviate the need for subsequent infusions if EACA (see above) is begun immediately and continued for 5 to 7 days. Treatment of urinary tract bleeding may remit with a single infusion or multiple infusions, depending on severity of bleeding, and concomitant administration of oral corticosteroids at moderate doses for 3 days. Prophylaxis for dental extraction or for injection of lidocaine as a mandibular block can be routinely achieved with a single infusion of Factor VIII concentrate at a dose of 15 to 25 units per kg to attain levels of 30 to 50 units per dl. Some patients may also benefit from a prophylactic infusion of 10 to 20 units per kg before a physically strenuous activity such as physical therapy.

Gastrointestinal hemorrhage, hemorrhage into the retropharyngeal space with the potential for airway compromise, and central nervous system hemorrhage (intracranial, intracerebral, or paravertebral) constitute life-threatening or major hemorrhage. These conditions require aggressive replacement with Factor VIII concentrates at a dose of 50 units per kg every 12 hours (or comparable total dose by continuous infusion) for an extended period of time based on the organ of involvement. This will usually maintain a normal Factor VIIIc level in the patient at all times.

However, frequently performed Factor VIIIc assays are required to ensure adequate circulatory levels. For documented central nervous system hemorrhage, this dosing scheme with laboratory corroboration of Factor VIIIc levels should be maintained for a minimum of 14 days.

Prior to elective surgery, a Factor VIIIc in vivo survival determination should be considered to ascertain the peak Factor VIIIc level and decay pattern for that patient following infusion of a specified dose of Factor VIII concentrate. This is often helpful, since the half-life for infused Factor VIII can vary from 8 to 15 hours (median 12 hours) in non-inhibitor patients. Factor VIIIc survival characteristics for the surgical patient allow more accurate determination of dosing schedules and may obviate the need to overinfuse to ensure adequate hemostasis following the procedure. Although trivial overdosage of Factor VIII is not a problem, the increased cost of the newer preparations may more than justify the fine-tuning of dosing that a well-done survival study makes feasible. Desmopressin may be utilized to treat non–life-threatening bleeding in mild hemophiliacs, as mentioned previously. In other hemophilia A patients, the choice of Factor VIII concentrate preparation for treatment should be based on individual needs as discussed above.

Management of Patients With Inhibitors

Patients with inhibitors usually have their treatment regimen defined by whether they are a "low" or a "high" responder. A high responder is an individual whose antibody behaves as a typical IgG antibody directed against Factor VIIIc. These individuals predictably have an anamnestic rise in their antibody titer when infused with any Factor VIII concentrate. Individuals who are low responders, on the other hand, have a nonspecific type of inhibition to Factor VIIIc activity that does not exhibit anamnesis in response to infusion of the Factor VIIIc antigen. Low responders may be treated by giving greater amounts of Factor VIII concentrate in doses sufficient to achieve the desired circulating Factor VIIIc level by assay.

High responders represent a more difficult therapeutic problem. When their antibody level (measured in Bethesda units) falls, they may be treated like low responders. However, this inevitably results in markedly elevating their antibody titer within days. This effectively eliminates the possibility for sustained therapy with Factor VIII preparations. Therefore, many hematologists reserve this option for life-threatening hemorrhage. The remainder of bleeding episodes in such patients, and bleeding in patients whose antibody titer does not fall, can be treated with any or all of the following: PCC, APCC, porcine Factor VIII, or combination therapy with these preparations used in conjunction with procedures designed to lower the antibody level. For hemarthroses and other non–life-threatening bleeding episodes, it is important that prolonged therapy with PCC or APCC be avoided because of the risk of thrombosis. Additionally, although PCC has only trace amounts of Factor VIIIc antigen and rarely induces an anamnestic rise in the Bethesda unit titer, continuous prolonged therapy may increase this likelihood.

Methods to reduce the antibody or Bethesda unit titer have had variable benefits. Immune suppression with corticosteroids or chemotherapeutic agents such as cyclophosphamide or cyclosporine have been variably effective in suppressing antibody production of this Factor VIII–specific immune globulin, even at toxic doses. Plasmapheresis or plasma exchange can be beneficial in acute life- or limb-threatening situations in an effort to lower the specific IgG anti–Factor VIIIc enough so that a large dose of Factor VIII concentrate may temporarily saturate the remaining unbound antibody. This may permit short-term maintenance of a measurable plasma Factor VIIIc level during a critical period of acute hemorrhage or emergency surgery.

Recently, specialized staphylococcal protein A affinity columns that nonspecifically bind large amounts of plasma immunoglobulins (thus reducing the specific anti–Factor VIII proportionately) have become available in a few hemophilia centers in the United States. Their use may open new opportunities for rehabilitative surgery in hemophilia A patients with high responsive inhibitors, a practice that has usually been considered excessively risky. Emergency surgery in such patients, on the other hand, may require a combination of the above modalities in order to achieve and maintain hemostasis.

Long-term management options for inhibitor patients now include immune tolerance induction utilizing daily infusions of Factor VIII (50 units per kg) for several months. In many cases, the Bethesda unit titer will, after a period of anamnestic rise, fall gradually in subsequent months until it eventually disappears. Reliable reduction and removal of a Factor VIIIc inhibitor by this means requires rigid compliance with the daily regimen. Although exceedingly expensive in the short term because of the large amounts of factor required, the long-term advantages of clinical management without fear of antibody complications may well justify this regimen in problem inhibitor patients. This is particularly true for inhibitor patients who already have a maximal anamnestic rise in their Bethesda unit titer following infusions of Factor VIII concentrate.

As the above discussion indicates, management of hemorrhage in patients with inhibitors can be very complicated. Therefore, close liaison with the regional comprehensive hemophilia center in managing such patients in both the acute and chronic situation should be considered.

Hemophilia B

The clinical management of hemorrhage in patients with hemophilia B is similar to that of hemophilia A except that the physiologic behavior of infused Factor IX is somewhat different than that of Factor VIIIc. Specifically, the peak plasma level achieved following the infusion of a defined number of units of Factor IX is only one half that of Factor VIIIc. Hence, 1 unit per kg of Factor IX raises the plasma level approximately 1 unit to 1½ units per dl (as compared with 2 units per dl with 1 unit per kg of Factor VIIIc). On the other hand, the half-life of infused Factor IX concentrate is 24 hours to 32 hours, twice that of Factor VIIIc. Following are specific recommendations for therapy based on this biologic behavior:

1. For early and minor bleeding episodes, 15 to 20 units per kg (plasma level of 15 to 30 units per dl plasma concentration) may suffice in a single dose. For young children in whom early detection is difficult, 25 to 40 units per kg (plasma level of 25 to 60 units per dl) is typically required.

2. For more severe but non–life-threatening bleeding, 25 to 45 units per kg (plasma level of 25 to 65 units per dl) is usually required. This is the recommended dosing scheme for prophylaxis prior to dental procedures such as extractions.

3. For life-threatening bleeding and major surgery, every effort should be made to maintain minimum normal physiologic levels at all times (i.e., plasma levels equal to or in excess of 50 units per dl). Daily dosing of 50 to 75 units per kg will usually achieve this maintenance; however, careful monitoring of plasma Factor IX to ensure adequate but not excessive levels (because of the higher risk for thrombosis with these preparations) is essential. In surgical situations, the higher plasma level (50 units per dl) may be required only during the 2- to 3-day perioperative period. Thereafter, the dose may be reduced gradually to 20 to 30 units per kg (20 to 30 units per dl plasma level) for the remainder of the postoperative period, the duration of which is dependent on the procedure. The newer, soon-to-be available single component Factor IX preparation (as opposed to PCC) may well become the treatment of choice for surgery to alleviate risk of untoward clotting complications.

von Willebrand's Disease

There are many laboratory and clinical variants of von Willebrand's disease (VWD). For effective therapy, each of the respective types requires repleting with normal VWD factor (VWF) multimers, either exogenously or endogenously. For individuals who have a relative deficiency of normal VWF multimers, recommended therapy begins with desmopressin (DDAVP), 0.3 microgram per kg intravenously, to induce increased release of the VWF molecules from the endothelial cells of the circulation. In most individuals with mild or moderate Type I VWD, this will result in an approximate 2.5-fold increase in the circulating levels. This is often adequate to treat mild to moderate bleeding or to provide prophylactic hemostatic coverage for many surgical procedures. Unfortunately, tachyphylaxis occurs predictably following administration of desmopressin, so that repeated administrations are less effective in achieving the increase in circulating VWF multimers. On most occasions, approximately 24 to 36 hours between dosing is required to achieve maximal response; presumably the endothelial stores require this period for repletion of the VWF multimers.

In patients with severe Type I VWD who are markedly deficient in endothelial VWF multimers, desmopressin is ineffective. Further, patients with Type IIB VWF, who have a genetic defect in their capacity to polymerize the highest molecular weight forms of VWF, should not receive desmopressin under any circumstances because of the propensity to induce significant in vivo platelet aggregation. The latter may predispose to microthrombosis in the circulation. Hence, for these individuals and for mild to moderate Type I VWD patients requiring sustained increases of their VWF levels, alternative therapy has to be utilized. Traditionally, cryoprecipitate has been the therapy of choice in both of these types of patients. For significant bleeding, dosing with cryoprecipitate should achieve 30 to 50 Factor VIIIc units per dl of plasma. Since one bag of cryoprecipitate contains on the average 80 to 100 units of Factor VIIIc, in most cases one bag per 10 kg of body weight will achieve the desired increment in Factor VIIIc level and the concomitant increase in Factor VIII$_{VWF}$ activity. Similarly, in most cases this will correct the abnormality in the bleeding time and sustain the correction for at least 12 hours. Repetition of dosing will depend on severity of the bleeding source and type and the duration of the bleeding time normalization.

Mucous membrane bleeding (particularly oral, nasal, or vaginal mucosal bleeding) often will ameliorate or cease with antifibrinolytic therapy with EACA (Amicar) or tranexamic acid (Cyklokapron) alone; further, protracted therapy with cryoprecipitate or desmopressin may be obviated in episodes of mucous membrane bleeding by combining oral antifibrinolytic therapy.

Other Plasma Clotting Deficiencies

For most inherited bleeding or thrombotic deficiencies, FFP infusion will replete the missing protein. In those instances in which the missing protein is concentrated in cryoprecipitate (e.g., Factor VIII, fibrinogen, and Factor XIII), this may serve as another source. In hypofibrinogenemia, cryoprecipitate is the preferred source because 50 to 60 per cent of the clottable fibrinogen in a unit of FFP is concentrated in the cryoprecipitate fraction; by estimating the patient's blood volume and using this parameter along with the determined plasma fibrinogen level, the total vascular deficit is approximately calculated. Since a typical 20- to 30-ml bag of cryoprecipitate contains 12 to 15 mg per ml of fibrinogen, the appropriate number of bags can be calculated to restore the plasma fibrinogen to the desired level.

Besides the hemophilic factor concentrates, few specific purified clotting or clotting inhibition protein concentrates are available at present. Certain types of Factor IX concentrates contain relatively greater concentrations of other proteins in the prothrombin complex (e.g., Factor VII) and may be utilized to treat a deficiency more effectively than with FFP. Pharmaceutical firms usually will provide data on specific assays of Factor VII in various lots of PCC. Deficiencies of Factors X and II can usually be treated adequately with FFP. In addition, antithrombin III concentrate is available on an investigative basis for those children born with antithrombin III deficiency. Deficiencies of Factor V, Factor IX, prekallikrein, protein C, protein S, and antiplasmin require replacement therapy with FFP; a usual starting dose is 10 ml per kg body weight.

Special Considerations for Hemophilic Bleeding

It should be emphasized that early treatment is not only necessary but in many cases may diminish the ultimate duration of therapy. For example, infusion for an acute hemarthrosis with an appropriate dose of factor concentrate immediately on recognition of pain may often obviate the need for a second infusion by forestalling the inflammatory response in the joint. This likely curtails the predisposition for re-bleeding. Appropriate dosage is discussed above.

For life-threatening bleeding in a hemophiliac, the exigency for immediate infusion is superseded only by resuscitative requirements. Further, an acutely hemorrhaging hemophiliac should be transported, if at all possible, to an emergency center that stocks *appropriate plasma products.* All head injuries must be considered nontrivial unless proved otherwise by observation and computed tomography or magnetic resonance imaging scan. Late bleeding after head trauma can occur as long as 3 to 4 weeks following the injury. Hence, patients with head and neck injuries should be infused immediately unless one is totally convinced that the injury is insignificant. Additionally, if the patient is not hospitalized, the patient and his or her family should be instructed in the neurologic signs and symptoms of central nervous system bleeding so that the patient will return for reinfusion, clinical and radiologic reassessment, and hospitalization at the earliest manifestation of bleeding.

Bleeding from the floor of the mouth or the pharyngeal or epiglottic region frequently results in partial or complete airway obstruction. Therefore, such bleeding should be treated with an aggressive infusion program with extended clinical follow-up to ensure resolution. Such bleeding may be precipitated by coughing, tonsillitis, oral or otolaryngologic surgery (e.g., extraction of wisdom teeth, tonsillectomy, adenoidectomy), or regional block anesthesia. For the surgical and anesthetic etiologies, prophylaxis with appropriate infusion therapy prior to the procedure usually obviates the need for treatment.

Patients with hemophilia who have gastrointestinal lesions, such as ulcers, varices, or hemorrhoids, must be managed with an appropriate continuous infusion regimen that maintains nearly normal circulating levels of Factor VIIIc or IX until some healing has been achieved. Concomitant transfusions with packed red blood cells may also be required.

Selected types of hemarthroses may be particularly problematic. Hip joint or acetabular hemorrhages can be dangerous because the increased intra-articular pressure from bleeding and the associated inflammation may lead to aseptic necrosis of the femoral head. Twice-daily infusion therapy designed to sustain a factor level above 10 units per dl for at least 3 days should be given, along with enforced bed rest that includes Buck's traction for immobilization.

A hemarthrosis of the hip joint may, at first appearance, be difficult to differentiate from a bleed in the iliopsoas muscle. The latter limits primarily hip extension, whereas a bleed in the joint makes any motion of the hip excruciatingly painful. Further, an iliopsoas bleed may decrease sensation over the ipsilateral thigh because of compression of the sacral plexus root of the femoral nerve. Ultrasonography may demonstrate a hematoma in the iliopsoas region. Treatment of the two is similar, although rehabilitation from the hip bleed is more protracted. Both will benefit from a physical therapy regimen that strengthens the supporting musculature while slowly mobilizing the affected area. Closed compartment muscle and soft-tissue hemorrhages are dangerous because they frequently impinge on the neurovascular bundle. These can occur in the upper arm, forearm, wrist, and volar aspect of the hand as well as in the anterior or posterior tibial compartments. Swelling and pain precede tingling, numbness, and loss of distal arterial pulses. Infusion must maintain an adequate hemostatic level of Factor VIIIc or IX. Other possible therapeutic maneuvers include elevation to enhance venous return and, as a last resort, surgical decompression if medical therapy fails to forestall progression.

PLATELET-MEDIATED BLEEDING DISORDERS

method of
TOBY L. SIMON, M.D.
*University of New Mexico School of Medicine
and United Blood Services
Albuquerque, New Mexico*

Diagnosis of Platelet-Mediated Bleeding Defect

Platelet-mediated bleeding defect may be treated with specific replacement therapy with concentrates of platelets or with pharmacologic agents that may improve platelet function or stimulate platelet numbers. The aim of the diagnostic approach is to determine incompetence of platelet plug formation. Platelet plug formation may be defective because of diminished platelet number (thrombocytopenia) or inadequate function of circulating platelets. Thrombocytopenia is diagnosed on the basis of history and physical examination, with particular attention to mucosal and small vessel bleeding, which is typically related to defective platelet plug formation. Platelet count and blood cell evaluation, bleeding time, bone marrow examination and, when appropriate, other platelet function tests are the principal laboratory tests utilized. Testing of the coagulation system may also be needed to determine if it is involved along with the platelets in the defect.

Decreased platelet numbers are classified as (1) disorders of production, which can be congenital or acquired (radiation, chemicals, drugs, alcohol, idiopathic aplasia, neoplastic or fibrotic replacement); (2) ineffective production, which can be hereditary or acquired (vitamin B_{12} or folate deficiency or myeloproliferative, myelodysplastic, or preleukemia syndrome); (3) disorders of distribution or dilution, which are seen with

splenomegaly and pooling of platelets in the spleen, hypothermia, and massive transfusion; and (4) disorders of destruction, seen with combined consumption (e.g., disseminated intravascular coagulation), isolated platelet consumption (e.g., thrombotic thrombocytopenic purpura, vasculitis, prosthetic valvular or vascular devices), or immune platelet destruction. Multiple causation is also seen. Qualitative platelet defects can involve defects in (1) adhesion, as in von Willebrand's disease, Bernard Soulier syndrome on a hereditary basis, or uremia on an acquired basis; (2) aggregation, as seen in hereditary thrombasthenia or in acquired diseases with increased fibrin degradation products; and (3) defects in release of granular constituents such as in storage pool deficiencies seen in autosomal recessive disorders or with cardiopulmonary bypass.

THROMBOCYTOPENIA

In thrombocytopenia, there is a relationship between the number of platelets and the likelihood of bleeding. In patients with reduced production of platelets as the cause of the thrombocytopenia, the platelet count is a relatively reliable predictor of the likelihood of bleeding. No prolongation of bleeding time or increase in bleeding risk is seen until the platelet count falls below 100,000 per microliter (μl) even though the mean platelet count in normal populations is approximately 250,000 per μl. Hemorrhagic manifestations are very uncommon with the moderate increase in bleeding propensity seen with counts between 50,000 and 100,000 per μl. Below 50,000, bleeding may be seen with major hemostatic challenges such as surgery, highly invasive procedures, or trauma. Between 10,000 and 30,000 there may be some increased bleeding in patients, but the most significant increase in bleeding is below 10,000. Stool blood loss studies have shown that between 5000 and 10,000 platelet count there is some increased likelihood of bleeding, whereas below 5000 it is virtually certain that clinically significant bleeding will occur. The clinically significant bleeding apparently relates to the loss of red cells between endothelial cells that require a minimum count of 5000 platelets to preserve vessel integrity. This blood loss into the gastrointestinal tract and the brain can cause life-threatening hemorrhage.

The situation is different in syndromes of increased platelet destruction. Platelet production typically increases owing to the marrow response. The younger platelets appear to be more functional. Therefore, bleeding is less likely to be seen at a low platelet count when increased destruction is the cause of the thrombocytopenia than with decreased production. Hemostasis may be adequate even with a very low platelet count below 5000, particularly in immune thrombocytopenia.

It should be noted that in clinical situations, patients often have multiple causation for their thrombocytopenia; for example, a patient with acute leukemia ordinarily has reduced production due to leukemic involvement of the bone marrow and chemotherapeutic drugs, and at the same time may have increased destruction due to superimposed infections, as well as the increased platelet consumption seen with any neoplastic disorder. Certain antibiotic drugs may then also superimpose platelet dysfunction on the thrombocytopenia.

Platelet Concentrate Transfusion

The goal of platelet concentrate transfusion is to correct the hemostatic defect. Such a transfusion should be used only when a clinical problem has resulted or is very likely to result from the thrombocytopenia or qualitative defect.

Indications for Platelet Concentrate Transfusion

In these complex situations, the physician must examine both clinical and laboratory data to determine when a platelet transfusion should be given. Platelet transfusions should be given in the presence of thrombocytopenia and clinical bleeding that can reasonably be explained by the thrombocytopenia. Platelet transfusions should be given prophylactically (i.e., to prevent bleeding) in patients with platelet counts below 5000 per μl whose thrombocytopenia is due to decreased platelet production. In cases in which surgery is necessary and platelet counts are below 50,000 because of decreased production, platelet concentrates may also be given prophylactically. In syndromes of increased platelet destruction and platelet dysfunction, platelet concentrates should ordinarily be given only when there is clinical bleeding or in association with an invasive procedure. Studies have now shown that in cardiopulmonary bypass there is thrombocytopenia and platelet dysfunction due to the reaction between platelets and the artificial surface of the bypass material. Platelet transfusions will correct this but are not usually required, since the problem is typically transient. Thus, platelet transfusions should be used only when unexpected bleeding occurs in the face of continuing thrombocytopenia and/or platelet dysfunction. Similarly, in trauma, prophylactic platelet transfusions have not been shown to prevent microvascular bleeding. Here, too, the clinician should be selective in his use of platelet transfusions.

Ordering a Platelet Transfusion

Platelet concentrate transfusions currently come in two forms: random donor platelets or single donor platelets. Random donor platelets are obtained from whole blood donations by centrifuging the unit of whole blood to obtain platelet-rich plasma followed by a concentration of the platelets in approximately 50 ml of plasma. Each unit is then stored at 20 to 24°C, with gentle agitation for up to 5 days using currently approved blood bags. The units have some diminution of viability with storage, but not so much that the clinical efficacy is compromised. These units are ordinarily pooled for administration to the patient.

Platelet concentrates may also be obtained on a cell separator from a single donor. By processing several liters of the donor's blood, and returning to the donor his red blood cells and plasma, platelets can be obtained in a moderately concentrated form in a blood bag. If an open system cell separator is used, storage is ordinarily limited to 24 hours. When a closed system is used, platelet concentrates can be stored for 5 days.

Dosage

Each unit of platelet concentrates obtained from random donors ordinarily has 5 to 7 × 10^{10} platelets. As a general rule, one unit will raise the platelet count immediately after transfusion in a 70-kg individual by between 5000 to 10,000 per μl. Another approach is to figure 10,000 to 15,000 per μl platelet increment per meter squared of body surface area (M^2). The greater the body surface area, the less the increment. Cell separators typically produce 3 to 5 × 10^{11} platelets in approximately 300 ml of plasma. They thus equal 6 to 8 of the individual platelet concentrates.

In general, thrombocytopenia or platelet dysfunction can be adequately treated with approximately 6 units of platelet concentrates or 1 unit per 10 kg body weight. If platelets obtained from a cell separator are used, 3 to 4 × 10^{11} platelets usually are adequate as a single dose for an average size individual.

Platelets circulate 9.5 days in a normal individual; however, in patients with thrombocytopenia, platelet survival is almost always reduced, owing to increased utilization related to thrombocytopenia. Typically, the circulating time is reduced to about 3 days. As a matter of practicality, then, platelets are given on a daily basis, with determination made each day of the need for platelets.

Platelets will have improved survival in the patient if they are ABO matched. However, ABO identity is not absolutely necessary. The plasma in the platelet concentrate, if incompatible with the patient's blood, can result in a positive direct antiglobulin test.

Platelets should be given by a slow drip over approximately 1 to 4 hours. An ordinary blood filter or a special platelet filter may be used. Microfilters may trap some of the platelets. Platelets should not be mixed with any diluent.

Risks and Adverse Sequelae of Platelet Concentrate Transfusion

Platelet concentrate transfusions involve the transfusion of human blood products and cannot be treated for removal of infectious agents. The safety of the product is dependent on careful screening of donors, exclusive use of volunteer donors, and testing for possible transmissible diseases. Platelet concentrates, therefore, must be used with the knowledge that transmission of disease is possible. Although the units are tested routinely for antibodies to human immunodeficiency virus (HIV), hepatitis B surface antigen, and rapid plasma reagin (RPR), and surrogate tests are made for non-A and non-B hepatitis, transmission of any of the aforementioned diseases is possible. Transmission of cytomegalovirus and Epstein-Barr virus is also possible. For immunocompromised CMV seronegative recipients, the use of units tested serologically negative for cytomegalovirus may be advisable. Malaria has rarely been found to be transmitted by platelet concentrates; presumably this is related to the small number of red cells contaminating the unit.

White cells typically are present in the platelet concentrate unit, although their numbers may be small with some of the new cell separators. There are also methods for rendering platelet concentrates leukocyte poor. Nevertheless, any viable lymphocytes remaining can cause graft-versus-host disease. Irradiation of the unit can prevent this. This is only necessary in patients with Hodgkin's disease or those who are severely immunocompromised.

Of greater frequency are two other effects of white cells in the unit. First, a febrile transfusion reaction may be caused by remaining granulocytes. This reaction, characterized by fever and chills, typically occurs during or shortly after the transfusion and may be prevented by anti-pyretics. The second effect, of greater concern, is leukocyte-lymphocyte mediated alloimmunization. In this situation, the recipient may form platelet-specific antibodies. These typically cross-react with HLA antibodies. These antibodies not only promote the previously mentioned febrile reactions but also cause immediate platelet destruction, with the resultant lack of benefit from the platelet transfusion. Alloimmunization can be diagnosed empirically by a poor increment to the platelet concentrate 1 hour after the platelet transfusion. If patients do not have an acceptable increment the day following platelet transfusion, a 1-hour count may be helpful in determining if alloimmunization is taking place. Various specially designed antibody tests specific for platelet-related antibodies can also be used to make the diagnosis.

In order to restore increments to platelet concentrate transfusions in patients who continue to need platelets, it is necessary to give platelets matched beyond ABO. The most common method for doing this is to use HLA-matched platelets. These platelets can be of varying degrees of matches (A, B, or C), depending on the patient's response. Since this matching method is not always effective, investigators have sought various platelet compatibility tests. Unfortunately, these tests have not become sufficiently standardized to routinely recommend them, although they are used in some institutions to select more compatible donors.

Alternative Methods for Improving Platelet Plug Formation

Several alternative methods have been tested to improve platelet plug formation. Some of these methods preclude the necessity for the human blood transfusion of concentrated platelets, and most of them are based on augmenting the function of existing platelets. Observations in the treatment of patients with uremia-induced platelet dysfunction revealed that cryoprecipitate improved platelet function. The presumption was that cryoprecipitate provided the von Willebrand factor to improve platelet adhesion. Subsequently this was also documented in patients with inherited platelet disorders.

With the observation that desmopressin could improve hemostasis in patients with hemophilia and von Willebrand's disease, investigators have tested the hypothesis that desmopressin could correct platelet dysfunction, and there have been many reports of clinical experience using desmopressin for this purpose. Desmopressin has also been used in cardiopulmonary bypass surgery and major orthopedic surgery to diminish blood loss. Presumably, the method of achieving clinical success is the increase in von Willebrand factor, with the consequent improvement in platelet function. Dosage of desmopressin (DDAVP) is 0.3 to 0.4 microgram per kg. This produces a two- to fivefold increase in von Willebrand factor in normal individuals. It must be administered diluted in a solution such as normal saline and given over an approximately 30-minute period to prevent inordinate hypertension or flushing.

The efficacy of anti-fibrinolytic agents such as aminocaproic acid (Amicar) for platelet plug formation to prevent bleeding has not been well established.

While less reliable than platelet concentrate transfusions in these situations, desmopressin as a pharmacologic agent, without the adverse effects of disease transmission or alloimmunization, may be used in a variety of clinical situations. Its use can now be recommended in complicated cardiac surgery, which carries a high likelihood of platelet dysfunction and bleeding.

DISSEMINATED INTRAVASCULAR COAGULATION

method of
JOEL L. MOAKE, M.D.
Baylor College of Medicine
Houston, Texas

Disseminated intravascular coagulation (DIC) and associated secondary fibrinolysis result from excessive activation of either the extrinsic or intrinsic coagulation pathway. Excessive extrinsic pathway activation occurs whenever cellular destruction is extensive and surface and organelle membranes intrude into the circulation. These whole phospholipoprotein membranes bind and activate Factor VII and initiate activation of the extrinsic coagulation pathway. Common clinical problems associated with excessive extrinsic pathway activation include sepsis, with phagocytosis of microbes and consequent white cell disruption; necrosis of neoplastic tissue by ischemia, cytotoxic drugs, or irradiation; premature separation of the placenta; hypertonic saline-induced abortion; retained dead fetus; heat stroke with associated hypovolemia and tissue ischemia; and severe injuries, especially those involving membrane-rich brain tissue. Leakage into the blood stream of an unusual Factor X–activating protease that has cysteine (instead of serine) as a critical amino acid component of the active enzyme site may also occur in some neoplastic disorders.

Excessive activation of the intrinsic pathway is less common than excessive extrinsic pathway activation. It occurs in patients with endothelial abnormalities, as in the giant hemangioma of the Kasabach-Merritt syndrome, or extensive endothelial cell damage, with dissecting aneurysm a prominent clinical example.

The most frequent complications of DIC are venous thromboembolism and bleeding from sites of injury, surgery, or vascular invasion (including sites of venipuncture or catheter placement). If the natural plasma anticoagulant proteins antithrombin III, protein C, and protein S are used at rates exceeding their production by liver cells, the patient is at risk for venous thromboembolism. In contrast, if severe thrombocytopenia and coagulation factor depletion develop in DIC, bleeding is more likely than thromboembolism. Thrombo-cytopenia occurs when the rate of intravascular thrombin-induced aggregation of platelets exceeds the rate of platelet production. Coagulation factor depletion evolves as consumption of these factors exceeds their rate of synthesis and secretion by liver cells.

Fibrinolysis is inevitably associated with DIC because plasminogen activator is liberated from thrombin-stimulated endothelial cells and from disrupted endothelial and tissue cells. Plasminogen activator binds, along with plasminogen, to fibrin polymers. On fibrin, plasminogen activator converts plasminogen to the active proteolytic enzyme, plasmin. Plasmin proteolytically degrades the fibrin polymers, usually within a matter of hours of fibrin formation. For this reason, occlusive vascular symptoms and signs occur less frequently than bleeding in DIC. Nevertheless, in a seriously ill or injured nonambulatory patient with DIC, the risk of venous thromboembolism is enhanced.

Diagnosis

The diagnosis of DIC, with the associated fibrinolysis, is suspected whenever fibrin degradation products (FDP), also known as fibrin split products (FSP), are found in the patient's plasma and serum samples. Increased levels of fibrin degradation products in the patient's plasma impair the interaction of fibrinogen molecules with thrombin, impede fibrin monomer polymerization, and prolong the thrombin time (i.e., the time to fibrin formation after the addition of a small quantity of thrombin to citrated platelet-poor plasma). When abnormally increased quantities of fibrin degradation products are present in the patient's serum, the degradation products attach to latex particles coated with antibodies that have been raised against the D and E regions of fibrinogen. The attachment causes the latex particles to agglutinate as the positive end-point of this commercially available, frequently used test.

In a minority of patients, perhaps about 20 per cent, fibrin remains in the microcirculation long enough to damage red cells flowing through the fibrin polymeric mesh. This results in the fragmentation of erythrocytes. These *schistocytes* ("cut" red cells) are then seen on the peripheral blood smear.

In the early stage of DIC, the partial thromboplastin time (a measure of the intrinsic coagulation pathway) may be *shortened* in association with a normal prothrombin time (a measure of the extrinsic coagulation pathway) and a platelet count that is normal or only mildly decreased. The shortened partial thromboplastin time probably indicates that the patient's plasma contains decreased levels of the natural anticoagulant proteins, antithrombin III, heparin cofactor II, protein C, and protein S, because these molecules are being utilized during early DIC at rates exceeding their hepatic production.

Treatment

Patients with DIC who are *bleeding* usually have increased serum levels of fibrin degradation products, thrombocytopenia (platelets less than

100,000 per µl), a prolonged prothrombin time and partial thromboplastin time, and decreased fibrinogen levels (often below 100 mg per dl). Medical or surgical treatment of the underlying disorder is the most effective therapy. Until the underlying disease can be controlled, fresh frozen plasma (containing all coagulation factors), platelet concentrates, and cryoprecipitate (containing fibrinogen, as well as the coagulant and von Willebrand factor components of the factor VIII complex) are used as necessary to control bleeding.

Patients with DIC who are *not bleeding* and in whom overt *venous thromboembolism* develops are treated with full-dose intravenous heparin (i.e., 5000 to 10,000 units loading dose, followed either by about 1000 to 2000 units per hour via continuous infusion or by the intermittent injection of 5000 to 10,000 units every 6 hours). This cannot be done if anticoagulation is contraindicated, as it is in head injury, central nervous system surgery, or when the patient has an open wound. If heparin is contraindicated, a prosthetic filter may have to be placed in the inferior vena cava to prevent the passage of emboli from veins in the pelvis or the lower extremities to pulmonary vessels.

In patients with DIC who are *not bleeding* and have not developed overt venous thromboembolism, *risk of thromboembolism* is often sufficiently great to justify the administration of prophylactic subcutaneous heparin in doses of 5000 units every 8 to 12 hours.

The antifibrinolytic agent epsilon-aminocaproic acid (Amicar), which inhibits the binding of plasminogen to fibrin, is contraindicated in patients with DIC.

Occasionally, arterial thromboses occur in association with DIC. A dramatic example in children is purpura fulminans (widespread skin infarction and hemorrhage caused by thrombotic occlusion of dermal arterioles and capillaries). Purpura fulminans has been associated with underlying congenital deficiencies of the natural anticoagulant molecules, proteins C and S. It is treated acutely with heparin and replacement of protein C or S by the administration of normal fresh frozen plasma.

Excessive Local Fibrinolysis: A Syndrome Distinct From DIC

Following open suprapubic prostatectomy, there may be extensive local release of plasminogen activator from prostatic cells. The plasminogen activator binds, along with plasminogen from the blood stream, to local fibrin polymers that form at the operative site. Fibrin-bound plasminogen is then converted by this plasminogen activator to plasmin at an excessive rate. The local lysis of fibrin polymers is so rapid that hemostasis is ineffective. Excessive local fibrinolysis is likely to be the problem in a patient who passes blood devoid of clots from a urethral catheter placed after surgery. On the other hand, if clots are present, defective surgical hemostasis is the more likely cause of excessive postoperative bleeding. Relatively excessive rates of local fibrinolysis also follow dental procedures in patients with hemophilia A or B or other congenital defects of coagulation in whom there is scanty fibrin polymer production. Excessive local fibrinolysis can be treated effectively by the intravenous administration of large doses of epsilon-aminocaproic acid (1 gram per hour following a 5 gram loading dose). When epsilon-aminocaproic acid is used after prostatectomy, it first must be ascertained that the patient does not have DIC (with secondary fibrinolysis), a situation in which epsilon-aminocaproic acid is contraindicated.

THROMBOTIC THROMBOCYTOPENIC PURPURA AND THE HEMOLYTIC UREMIC SYNDROME

method of
JOEL L. MOAKE, M.D.
Baylor College of Medicine
Houston, Texas

Thrombotic thrombocytopenic purpura (TTP) and the hemolytic uremic syndrome (HUS) are rare disorders. They are extraordinary examples of the thrombotic process in the arterial circulation. TTP is a combination of thrombocytopenia, hemolytic anemia, and fluctuating ischemic vascular signs, including neurologic abnormalities. A similar syndrome, HUS, is a constellation of thrombocytopenia, hemolytic anemia, and acute renal failure, but it does not usually include neurologic symptoms. In TTP, the formation of platelet occlusive lesions, along with some fibrin, occurs in arterioles and capillaries throughout the arterial microcirculation. The intravascular platelet thrombi probably form and disperse repeatedly, causing the characteristic intermittent symptoms and signs of ischemia in many organs. In HUS, the intravascular platelet clumping and accompanying fibrin formation are confined almost exclusively to the renal vessels.

When TTP episodes occur, they are often associated with tissue necrosis (infection, vaccinations, injury, or surgery) or pregnancy. Some patients have single episodes of TTP that never recur after successful treatment. A chronic form of the disorder, characterized by relatively frequent periodic relapses, has also been recognized now that many patients survive the initial TTP episode. An intermittent form of TTP, characterized by occasional (infrequent) relapses, has also been described. In contrast, it is extremely rare for a patient to suffer more than a single attack of HUS.

It has been suggested that episodes of TTP may be caused by (1) inadequate endothelial cell production of prostaglandin I$_2$ (PGI$_2$) or excessive lability of PGI$_2$, due to a deficiency of either an endothelial cell stimulating or a stabilizing factor present in normal plasma; (2) deficient plasminogen activator in endothelial cells and, consequently, inadequate fibrinolysis; (3) deficient production of IgG molecules that may normally interfere with platelet aggregation, perhaps by combining with an as yet unidentified microbe (or microbial product) capable of aggregating platelets; or (4) presence in the circulation of a substance or substances capable of inducing intravascular platelet aggregation. The first three hypotheses do not have convincing support as possible explanations for TTP because infusions of PGI$_2$, streptokinase, or concentrated IgG have not been demonstrated to be effective modes of therapy. The fourth explanation is most likely. The aggregating substance in the blood stream may be unusually large von Willebrand factor (vWF) multimeric forms derived from injured or immunologically altered endothelial cells. Unusually large vWF multimers have been demonstrated to be present between episodes in patients with the chronic relapsing type of TTP, and they disappear along with platelets (into the platelet clumps that form in the microcirculation) during TTP episodes. There is evidence to suggest that large vWF multimers, perhaps derived from renal endothelial cells damaged by the products of enteropathogenic *Escherichia coli*, may be involved in the pathophysiology of HUS in children and adults. The platelet aggregating substance, or substances, in the blood of individuals with single, nonrecurring episodes of TTP or in patients with intermittent and infrequent TTP episodes may also include large vWF forms.

Diagnosis

In both TTP and HUS, the extent of intravascular clumping is related to the degree of thrombocytopenia. The platelet clumping is systemic in TTP and predominantly renal in HUS. Platelet counts are, therefore, usually lower (often less than 10,000 per μl) in TTP. In HUS, in contrast, platelet counts are often below 100,000 per μl but seldom less than 20,000 per μl. Erythrocyte fragmentation occurs in both TTP and HUS because red blood cells are injured as they move through the partially occluded arterioles and capillaries. This results in microangiopathic hemolytic anemia and the characteristic schistocytes ("cut" red cells) on peripheral blood smears. The hemolysis is intravascular and, along with tissue damage, results in elevated serum lactate dehydrogenase (LDH) levels. Intravascular hemolysis, as well as thrombocytopenia, is usually more profound in TTP than in HUS. In TTP, ischemic arterial signs and symptoms can involve any organ; however, for the diagnosis to be made, ischemia must involve the central nervous system. Clinical manifestations range from behavioral changes to sensory-motor dysfunction to coma. In TTP, renal failure is often not a part of the presentation. In HUS, in contrast, renal failure is a predominant part of the clinical problem, usually unaccompanied by neurologic dysfunction. Fever may or may not be present in TTP or HUS. TTP and HUS are clinical diagnoses. Tissue obtained from biopsy of bone marrow, gingiva, or kidney may not contain arterial thrombi, and thus biopsy is not considered necessary (or even, in some circumstances, safe).

Treatment

Thrombotic Thrombocytopenic Purpura

In many patients with TTP episodes, perhaps 50 per cent or more, the process can be reversed by intensive plasma manipulation. This is best done using the combination of plasmapheresis and plasma exchange with normal fresh frozen plasma (60 ml per kilogram). It is presumed that a platelet aggregating agent (unusually large vWF multimers ± other cofactors?) is being removed by plasmapheresis, and that normal plasma is providing some antiaggregating agent that is present in the patient's plasma in inadequate amounts (unusually large vWF "depolymerase"?). If exchange plasmapheresis is not immediately available, infusion of normal fresh frozen plasma at the rate of about 30 ml per kg daily can be used initially until plasmapheresis and plasma exchange can be arranged. (This should be within 24 to 48 hours in most circumstances). Patients with TTP who are in a coma or have cardiac failure or renal dysfunction should receive exchange plasmapheresis commencing immediately after diagnosis, if possible.

Relapses in some chronic relapsing TTP patients may respond to, or be prevented by, transfusions of normal fresh frozen plasma alone (in quantities varying from one to many units), without the need for concurrent plasmapheresis.

Glucocorticoids may be helpful; the reasons for this are not yet clear, but possibly relate to an underlying autoimmune pathogenesis (production by the patient of antiendothelial cell antibodies?). Methylprednisolone should be started immediately following diagnosis, in a dosage of about 0.75 mg per kg intravenously every 12 hours, and continued until the patient recovers.

Depending on the hemoglobin level and intensity of hemolysis, red blood cell transfusions may be required. Platelet transfusions should be avoided, if possible, as they may exacerbate the microcirculatory thrombotic process. If the platelet count is very low and bleeding is a primary problem, then platelet transfusions may be necessary.

Plasmapheresis and plasma exchange should be continued for a minimum of about 5 days in patients who respond completely (i.e., attain a normal neurologic status, platelet count greater than 150,000 per μl, rising hemoglobin and normal serum lactate dehydrogenase levels). If there is subsequent relapse, the same treatment protocol should be repeated. In patients who achieve a partial response without deterioration in clinical condition, plasmapheresis and plasma exchange should be continued for a period of a few to many days in an effort to achieve a complete remission.

If a patient does not respond within the first 5 days of therapy or deteriorates within the first 3 days, other forms of therapy should be tried. Options include: addition of vincristine (1.4 mg per square meter, but not exceeding 2 mg total dosage, given by intravenous push on day 1, followed by 1 mg on days 4, 7, and 10); substitution of cryosupernatant (plasma from which the vWF-rich cryoprecipitate portion has been removed) for fresh frozen plasma in plasma exchange; splenectomy (removal of immunologic cells involved in antiendothelial cell autoimmune response?); and addition of other immunosuppressive agents (e.g., azathioprine [Imuran] or cyclophosphamide [Cytoxan]).

The use of aspirin and dipyridamole is controversial. Aspirin may exacerbate hemorrhagic complications. Neither drug has been unequivocally demonstrated to be useful in TTP. The same comments pertain to intravenous prostacyclin (PGI₂) and dextran. Transfusions or exchange transfusions with fluids other than plasma or its cryosupernatant fraction are ineffective.

When the patient is in remission and the plasma exchanges (or infusions) have been discontinued for about one week, the platelet count should be monitored regularly. Patients with a protracted initial episode, as well as patients with the chronic relapsing form of TTP, usually relapse within a few weeks of discontinuation of therapy. In some patients the disorder may not recur for months to years. Analysis of the patient's plasma for the continued presence of unusually large vWF multimers has been a useful indicator that the patient has the chronic relapsing type of TTP.

Hemolytic Uremic Syndrome

There has been considerable controversy concerning the management of patients with HUS. The variability of the disorder explains the difficulty in determining the effectiveness of any specific form of therapy. The severity of renal involvement, reflected by the duration of oliguria, generally correlates with the rate of recovery in both adults and children. In mildly affected children in whom anuria is present for less than 24 hours, careful attention to fluid and electrolyte status may be sufficient. In more severely affected children, dialysis is frequently required, and its early institution has resulted in improved survival. However, HUS in children is associated with some mortality and often residual renal dysfunction. There is no consensus on the therapeutic value, if any, of heparin, fibrinolytic therapy, or agents that impair platelet function. In adults with HUS, renal impairment is often more severe than in children, and hemodialysis is generally necessary.

Based upon the utility of plasma manipulation in TTP, plasma infusion has been used in HUS (initial transfusion of 30 to 40 ml per kg of normal fresh frozen plasma, followed by 15 to 20 ml per kg daily). Volume control is by hemodialysis. Plasmapheresis with plasma exchange can be employed if a patient fails to respond to plasma infusion and hemodialysis.

HEMOCHROMATOSIS

method of
KENNETH R. BRIDGES, M.D.
Harvard Medical School
Boston, Massachusetts

Iron overload results either from increased iron absorption from the gastrointestinal tract (idiopathic hemochromatosis [IHC]) or from parenteral iron loading (e.g., chronic transfusion therapy for thalassemia major or sideroblastic anemia). Although it was once a dictum that patients with transfusional iron overload (termed "hemosiderosis") had less frequent and less severe clinical consequences than individuals with IHC, more recent data indicate that iron deposition in and injury to vital organs is virtually identical in the two categories. The sequelae of iron overload are often insidious and include hepatomegaly, secondary fibrosis and cirrhosis, cardiac failure and arrhythmias due to sarcoplasmic iron deposition, arthralgias, diabetes mellitus, pituitary dysfunction, hypogonadism, and hyperpigmentation.

Idiopathic Hemochromatosis

Diagnosis

Diagnosis of IHC requires the demonstration of an elevation in total body iron stores. Factors favoring this diagnosis are listed in Table 1. The liver biopsy is the "gold standard" in this regard and should be performed whenever feasible for information on both iron content and liver histology. The triad of "bronze diabetes," hepatomegaly, hyperpigmentation, and diabetes, is uncommon in early cases of IHC. The gene coding for IHC is linked to the A-locus of the human lymphocyte antigen (HLA) system, and once the diagnosis has been established in the proband, family

TABLE 1. **Diagnosis of Idiopathic Hemochromatosis**

Clinical Features	Laboratory Features
Arthralgias	Transferrin saturation of greater than 70 per cent
Hepatomegaly	
Splenomegaly	Elevated serum ferritin levels
Hyperpigmentation	
Abdominal pain	(Mildly) elevated transaminases
Impotence (usually must be specifically elicited)	(Mildly) elevated serum bilirubin
	Diabetes or glucose intolerance
	Urinary iron excretion of greater than 4 mg per 24 hr with deferoxamine challenge
	Moderate to heavy hepatic parenchymal iron deposition

screening should be performed to identify other homozygotes. Heterozygotes have increased body iron stores, but fall short of injurious levels unless there are concomitant factors such as chronic alcohol abuse.

Treatment

Phlebotomy is the treatment of choice for patients with IHC, and Table 2 is an example of the typical schedule used. Patients are bled to the point that early signs of iron-deficiency (microcytosis and mild anemia) are manifested. The number of phlebotomies needed to remove excessive iron stores may range from 25 to 100. A net even iron balance can be then maintained with 3 or 4 phlebotomies per year. A serum transferrin saturation of under 50 per cent should be maintained during the chronic phase of treatment since this is one of the first parameters to rise with iron loading and one of the last to decline with phlebotomy. Early phlebotomy prevents the development of cirrhosis and the 30 per cent chance of hepatocellular carcinoma that accompanies this complication in patients with IHC.

Transfusional Iron Overload

Treatment

Chelation therapy is the only modality available for individuals in this category. The most widely used agent at present is deferoxamine

TABLE 2. **Phlebotomy Schedule for Idiopathic Hemochromatosis**

1. Initial phase—2 units per week for 10 weeks

2. Median phase—1 unit per week until evidence of iron deficiency

3. Chronic phase—1 unit every 3 to 4 months

(Desferal), a siderophore with a very high affinity for iron. The drug is not effectively absorbed when administered orally, and the best results are obtained with a 24-hour continuous intravenous infusion. Intravenous bolus administration is ineffective, since deferoxamine is excreted into the urine with a half life of only about 15 minutes. Continuous subcutaneous infusion of the drug produces results that are nearly as good as those obtained with intravenous administration and is more practical. Infusion times of 12 to 16 hours result in levels of iron excretion of about 80 per cent of that obtained over 24 hours and are better tolerated by patients. Most adults require 2 grams of deferoxamine to obtain a reasonable iron output: greater than about 30 milligrams per 24 hours. A 24-hour urine collection with iron determination should be done initially in all patients to ensure that a negative iron balance is reached (calculated from the transfusion requirement, which represents 225 milligrams of iron per unit). Following dissolution in 5 to 10 ml of sterile water, the deferoxamine is infused by a portable syringe pump via a 12-inch catheter tubing with a 25- or 27-gauge needle implanted just beneath the skin of the abdomen. Since there is a small chance of an anaphylactic or urticarial reaction with the first administration, a physician should be present. The most common problem with deferoxamine administration is the development of local pain and erythema and swelling at the infusion site due to chemical irritation of the subcutaneous tissue. The location of the infusion should, therefore, be rotated daily. The inclusion of 2 to 3 milligrams of cortisol in the deferoxamine infusion mixture or the application of cortisol ointment to the skin following the infusion will usually lessen this problem. Skin irritation effectively limits subcutaneous administration of deferoxamine to 2.5 grams in adults. For patients in whom higher doses of deferoxamine are needed, an indwelling central venous line, such as a Hickman catheter, may be used. Ascorbic acid will boost iron output in patients on deferoxamine therapy, with marginal iron excretion. Chelator administration should be ongoing prior to the addition of ascorbate to the treatment regimen to avoid vitamin-induced cardiac iron toxicity. Ascorbate administration should be limited to 250 to 500 milligrams per day.

Recent data indicate that a new orally active iron chelator, 1,2-dimethyl-3-hydroxypyrid-4-one, may be effective in iron mobilization in patients with transfusional hemochromatosis. In early trials this agent has been relatively nontoxic, and should the initial results be sustained, a major improvement in the treatment of transfusional iron overload will have been attained.

HODGKIN'S DISEASE: CHEMOTHERAPY

method of
SIMON B. SUTCLIFFE, M.D.
*Princess Margaret Hospital/Ontario Cancer
Institute, University of Toronto, Toronto,
Ontario, Canada*

Hodgkin's disease is a malignant lymphoma with an incidence of approximately 3.5 per 100,000 person years. It has a bimodal incidence curve with modes in early adult years and late mid-life. It affects males and females equally and is uncommon in childhood in developed countries. The etiology is unknown. Comparison of annual incidence and mortality figures indicates that approximately 75 per cent of patients may anticipate cure with current management programs. The key features of successful management are a secure histologic diagnosis, accurate assessment of disease extent and distribution, and the application of extended-field radical radiation or combination chemotherapy, according to the determination of disease extent.

Diagnosis and Staging

Hodgkin's disease commonly presents as lymph node enlargement, most frequently in cervical nodes and less commonly in axillary or inguinal regions. Mediastinal adenopathy is common but frequently asymptomatic. Presentation in extranodal sites may occur in patients with advanced disease but is unusual in the absence of clinical adenopathy. Similarly, presentation in the tonsil or nodal sites such as the epitrochlear, occipital, submental, or preauricular regions is unusual. Unusual presentations should invoke careful consideration of the diagnosis, as non-Hodgkin's lymphomas more commonly present in this manner.

The diagnosis of Hodgkin's disease is by examination of appropriately prepared biopsy material, usually lymph node (Table 1). Histologic subtyping is of prognostic significance inasmuch as the process of lymphocyte depletion relative to other cellular elements characterizes the progress of the natural history of the disease (Table 2). Biopsy of an extranodal site for diagnosis is less satisfactory and is secure only if all histologic criteria can be met or in the circumstance of an existing unequivocal diagnosis from a lymph node biopsy.

TABLE 1. Histologic Features of Hodgkin's Disease

Effacement of normal lymph node architecture

Pleomorphic cellular infiltrate (lymphocytes, eosinophils, plasma cells, large mononuclear cells)

Reed-Sternberg cells or variants (e.g., lacunar cells)

Coarse bands of fibrous tissue in the presence of the cytologic features noted above (nodular sclerosing type)

TABLE 2. Histologic Subtypes of Hodgkin's Disease

Subtype	Incidence (%)	Associated Features
Lymphocytes predominant	10	Early disease, commonly localized; more common in young incidence mode
Nodular sclerosis	60	Mediastinal adenopathy common
Mixed cellularity	25	Greater tendency for disseminated peripheral nodal disease
Lymphocyte depletion	<10	Seen in previously treated patients; rare as de novo presentation—usually advanced and symptomatic; requires careful distinction from non-Hodgkin's lymphoma (particularly peripheral T-cell type)

The majority of patients with Hodgkin's disease present with no symptoms other than a palpable mass. Although disease may be symptomatic by virtue of space occupation, the presence or absence of specific disease-related symptomatology should be actively elicited (Table 3). The presence or absence of such symptoms influences stage, management, and prognosis.

The purpose of staging is to define the anatomic extent and distribution of disease. In principle, the process will define whether the disease is (1) localized in a manner that will be compatible with radiation treatment, (2) apparently localized but unfavorable for treatment with irradiation alone because of disease bulk or systemic symptoms, or (3) generalized such that chemotherapy will be the treatment of choice. The Ann Arbor staging classification is shown in Table 4 and the recommended staging procedures are shown in Table 5.

In addition to a chest x-ray, computed tomography (CT) examination of the thorax is valuable when mediastinal adenopathy is present. Extension of an anterior mediastinal mass into the chest wall, hilar adenopathy, pulmonary extension, pericardial thick-

TABLE 3. Prognostically Relevant Symptomatology of Hodgkin's Disease*

Symptom	Characteristics
Fever	>38.4° C; repeat episodes; no documented infectious cause
Night sweats	Repeated episodes, sufficient to moisten night attire or bed linens
Weight loss	>10% body weight in 6 months prior to diagnosis, in absence of other identifiable cause

*If any or all symptoms are present, disease is classified "B"; if all symptoms are absent, disease is classified "A." Other relevant symptoms/history include lassitude, anorexia, alcohol-induced pain, and immunodeficiency state (congenital or acquired—e.g., human immunodeficiency virus disease or predisposition; therapeutic immunosuppression).

TABLE 4. **Ann Arbor Staging of Hodgkin's Disease***

Stage	Involvement
I	Single lymph node region
II	Two or more lymph node regions on the same side of the diaphragm
III	Lymph nodes on both sides of diaphragm (the spleen is considered a lymph node in the classification)
IV	Disseminated involvement of one or more extralymphatic organs or tissue, with or without associated lymph node involvement

*All stages can be A (asymptomatic) or B (symptomatic); Stage III can be subdivided into III_1 (involvement of upper abdomen—i.e., spleen, splenic hilar, celiac, or porta hepatis nodes) or III_2 (involvement of lower abdomen—i.e., paraaortic, mesenteric, pelvic, or inguinofemoral nodes); Stage IV, disseminated involvement, is distinguished from "E" disease (applicable to Stages I to III), in which extension into an extranodal site occurs contiguous with adjacent nodal disease. Both nodal disease and extranodal extension can be treated with radical irradiation, with equivalent prognosis to that of the nodal stage of disease.

ening, and pericardial effusion are all relevant factors in treatment planning and these findings may remain unidentified on a plain chest x-ray. Bipedal lymphography remains a valuable procedure for description of external and common iliac nodes and paraaortic nodes to the level of the superior mesenteric artery, providing information on nodal size, internal architecture, collateral flow, and lymphatic obstruction. CT examination of the abdomen can provide information on liver and spleen size and homogeneity and on the distribution of adenopathy and is complementary to lymphography in the definition of pelvic and paraaortic nodes. Ultrasonography and magnetic resonance imaging (MRI) may also provide information on visceral and nodal involvement by Hodgkin's disease. Gallium scanning may also be useful in the assessment of initial disease extent and in the determination of remission. Despite such exhaustive clinical staging, laparotomy series in untreated patients with disease apparently confined to supradiaphragmatic sites have consistently demonstrated occult disease in the spleen, splenic hilar nodes, and celiac axis region in approximately 30 per cent of patients. In many centers the procedure of

TABLE 5. **Staging Procedures in Hodgkin's Disease**

1. History—special attention to fever, nocturnal sweats, weight loss
2. Complete physical examination—distribution and size of peripheral nodal disease, presence of hepatosplenomegaly, evidence of extranodal disease
3. Laboratory examination—complete blood count, sedimentation rate, liver and renal function studies
4. Chest x-ray—PA and lateral
5. CT of thorax
6. Lymphangiogram
7. CT of abdomen
8. Bone marrow biopsy
9. Staging laparotomy and splenectomy, if indicated

PA = posteroanterior; CT = computed tomography.

staging laparotomy with splenectomy, liver biopsy, and lymph node mapping is undertaken in patients with clinically localized disease to determine the surgico-pathologic extent of disease. Patients with no demonstrable abdominal disease benefit most from surgical staging, as radiation fields may be restricted to nodal regions. In patients with clinical evidence of nodal disease above and below the diaphragm (Stage III), extranodal disease (Stage IV), or unfavorable presentations of localized disease (bulky mediastinum, extranodal extension, or florid symptomatology), the requirement for chemotherapy or combined modality therapy renders laparotomy of no value in management. Thus the decision for surgical staging should acknowledge the ability of the findings to influence management, and of the appropriate surgical and pathology expertise to yield optimal information. The value of metal clip placement at laparotomy as an adjunct to radiation therapy planning should be weighed against their interference with subsequent CT and MRI studies. Oophoropexy should be considered for women undergoing staging laparotomy in their reproductive years.

Other than the procedures of diagnostic lymph node biopsy, staging laparotomy with splenectomy and lymph node mapping, and oophoropexy, surgery plays no part in the actual treatment of Hodgkin's disease.

Chemotherapy for Primary Treatment

Indications

Patient groups who benefit most by initial treatment with combination chemotherapy are shown in Table 6. Chemotherapy is an effective therapy for all patients irrespective of stage; however, the adverse side effects of chemotherapy in the context of high remission rates with irradiation for patients with localized disease usually preclude routine administration of chemotherapy to untreated patients other than as indicated in Table 6. Although radiation has not shown survival advantage when used as an adjuvant to

TABLE 6. **Indications for Chemotherapy as Initial Treatment of Hodgkin's Disease**

Stage of Disease	Indication(s)
I	Massive mediastinal adenopathy
II	Symptoms present (B classification) and/or massive mediastinal disease (>10 cm transverse diameter on PA radiograph or >1:3 transthoracic ratio); extranodal extension into chest wall, lung, or pericardium
IIIA	Clinical stage usually lymphogram- or CT-positive and pathologic stage $IIIA_2$; or pathologic stage $IIIA_1$ with extensive splenic involvement
IIIB	Clinical or pathologic stage
IV	Asymptomatic (A classification) or symptoms present (B classification)

PA = posteroanterior; CT = computed tomography.

TABLE 7. **MOPP Regimen**[*]

Agents	Route	Dose (mg/m²)	Days
Nitrogen mustard (*M*ustargen)	IV	6	1 and 8
Vincristine (*O*ncovin)	IV	1.4	1 and 8
*P*rocarbazine (Matulane)	PO	100	1–15
*P*rednisone (Deltasone)	PO	40	1–15

[*]Cycle repeats every 4 weeks; prednisone is used in cycles 1 and 4 only.

chemotherapy, its adjuvant use in patients with initially localized disease or in patients with bulky presentation sites may be beneficial in terms of increased local disease eradication.

Multiple-Drug Induction Regimens

Although chemotherapy agents used singly may produce good responses, the basis of curative chemotherapy for Hodgkin's disease derives from the use of multiple agents given in combination according to set schedules.

The principal regimen, MOPP [nitrogen mustard (Mustargen), vincristine (Oncovin), procarbazine (Natulan), and prednisone (Deltrasone)], has been in common usage for over 20 years (Table 7). In patients with advanced (Stages IIB to IV), previously untreated disease or in those whose condition had relapsed following initial irradiation, the original MOPP study yielded a complete response rate of 80 per cent, a median survival in excess of 7 years, and a median duration of complete response in excess of 10 years. In approximately 35 per cent of patients the disease recurred, usually within a 5-year period of completing initial therapy.

Several modifications have been made to the original MOPP program in an attempt to improve results, increase patient tolerance, diminish side effects, and facilitate administration (Table 8). To date, no modification of the primary regimen has yielded superior results.

Two non–cross-resistant combination regimens have been introduced in primary therapy, based on their established role in salvage of patients failing after MOPP therapy (Table 9). The complete response rates, relapse rates, and median

survival durations of both regimens are similar to those of the MOPP program. They differ in their acute and long-term morbidity characteristics, ease of administration, and reliance on oral medication compliance.

Overall, approximately 70 per cent of patients achieve complete remission with a multiple-drug program, and 35 per cent relapse from a state of complete remission. Thus approximately 50 per cent require therapy in addition to their initial multiple-drug program. The median survival for those failing to achieve remission is approximately 18 months, and for those achieving complete remission it exceeds 10 years, thus yielding an overall median survival of approximately 7 years. The factors predicting for an adverse outcome are shown in Table 10.

Alternating-Sequence Chemotherapy Induction Regimens

The utility of ABVD (Table 9) as a salvage regimen for patients failing to respond on the MOPP regimen and the demonstration of equal efficacy in previously untreated patients with advanced disease prompted the introduction of a program of alternation of MOPP and ABVD each month over a 12-month period for induction of remission in patients with advanced Hodgkin's disease (Table 11). In a randomized comparison with MOPP in patients with stage IV disease, there was significant improvement in complete response rate, freedom from first disease progression, relapse rate, and overall survival for patients achieving complete remission in the MOPP/ABVD program (Table 12). The results of this study are being re-examined by other groups in randomized trials to establish the superiority of alternating-sequence regimens.

At present, although results of confirmatory studies are not available, alternating-sequence induction chemotherapy is considered by many to be optimal treatment for patients with advanced Hodgkin's disease with prognostic factors predictive of lower control rates with the MOPP regimen alone (see Table 10).

TABLE 8. **Modifications of MOPP Regimen**

Agent	Substitution or Addition	Route	Dose (mg/m²)	Day(s)	Principal Benefit
Cyclophosphamide (Cytoxan)	substitution for nitrogen mustard	IV	300	1 and 8	Less nausea and vomiting
Chlorambucil (Leukeran)	substitution for nitrogen mustard	PO	6	1–15	Ease of administration Less nausea and vomiting
Vinblastine (Velban)	substitution for vincristine	IV	6	1 and 8	Less neurotoxicity
Bleomycin (Blenoxane)	addition	IV	2	1 and 8	—
Carmustine (BiCNU)	addition	IV	100	1	—
Cyclophosphamide (Cytoxan)	substitution for nitrogen mustard	IV	600	1	—
Vinblastine (Velban)	substitution for vincristine	IV	5	1	—

TABLE 9. **Primary Regimens Alternative to MOPP Regimen***

Agent	Route	Dose (mg/m²)	Day(s)
ABVD Regimen			
doxorubicin (Adriamycin)	IV	25	1 and 15
bleomycin (Blenoxane)	IV	10	1 and 15
vinblastine (Velban)	IV	6	1 and 15
dacarbazine (DTIC)	IV	375	1 and 15
SCAB regimen			
streptozotocin (Zanosar)	IV	500	1–5
lomustine (CeeNU)	PO	100	1
doxorubicin (Adriamycin)	IV	45	1
bleomycin (Blenoxane)	IM	15	1–8

*Cycle repeats every 28 days; 6 cycles recommended for responding patients.

Assessment of Remission Status

The decision to stop therapy is almost as important as the decision to initiate therapy. Only those patients whose disease is eradicated are considered cured. The assessment of disease eradication (complete remission) is based on the absence of symptoms, and on a normal physical examination and the return of all investigative parameters to normal. Tests that were abnormal initially should be monitored throughout therapy and determined to be normal at the end of the program. When extranodal tissue biopsies revealed disease initially, these nodes should, within the limits of practicality, be determined to be free of disease after therapy. Great caution should be exercised in the attribution of abnormalities to post-treatment "scarring" or "inactive disease," and every attempt should be made to establish total disease eradication before considering treatment to be complete. Failure to secure complete remission may result in a reduction in treatment options and have a prejudicial effect on long-term disease control.

Maintenance Chemotherapy Following Chemotherapy-Induced Remission

The role of maintenance chemotherapy following MOPP-induced remission has been studied by several groups, with a consensus that there is no demonstrable benefit; therefore continuation of chemotherapy is not recommended beyond documentation of remission upon completion of the prescribed induction regimen.

TABLE 10. **Adverse Prognostic Factors in Multiple-Drug Chemotherapy Regimens**

Age greater than 40 years
Symptoms present (B classification)
Stage IV disease
More than 1 extranodal site
Large tumor bulk
Deviation from schedule of dose intensity

TABLE 11. **MOPP/ABVD Alternating-Sequence Regimen***

Agents	Route	Dose (mg/m²)	Day(s)
MOPP Regimen			
nitrogen mustard (Mustargen)	IV	6	1 and 8
vincristine (Oncovin)	IV	1.4	1 and 8
procarbazine (Matulane)	PO	100	1–15
prednisone (Deltasone)	PO	40	1–15

After 14-day treatment-free period, then:

ABVD Regimen			
doxorubicin (Adriamycin)	IV	25	1 and 15
bleomycin (Blenoxane)	IV	10	1 and 15
vinblastine (Velban)	IV	6	1 and 15
dacarbazine (DTIC)	IV	375	1 and 15

After 14-day treatment-free period, then repeat MOPP.

*For MOPP cycle, prednisone is given in cycles 1, 4, 7, and 10; cycle repeats cycle 28 days; 12 cycles (months) of therapy complete program.

Irradiation Following Chemotherapy-Induced Remission

Several studies have demonstrated that recurrence occurs most commonly in sites of disease bulk at initial presentation. Randomized studies of combined chemotherapy and radiotherapy versus chemotherapy alone for patients with advanced disease have demonstrated a lower recurrence rate in the irradiated volume. Higher recurrence rates beyond the radiation field have resulted in no overall survival advantage.

There appears to be no indication of synergy between radiation and chemotherapy applied as combined modality therapy. The benefits of radiation are improved disease control within the irradiated volume; the benefits of chemotherapy are control of systemic disease (either overt or occult) and reduction of disease bulk as an adjunct to radiation field planning. Although there is no strong indication of benefit of combined modality therapy for those with advanced disease, such an approach may be particularly beneficial for those patients with adverse presentations of apparently localized disease.

Treatment for Patients Failing Multiple-Drug Induction

Approximately 50 per cent of patients with advanced Hodgkin's disease will require additional chemotherapy as a result of either non-remission or recurrence following 4-drug chemotherapy. Those patients whose disease worsens despite 4-drug (or alternating-sequence) chemotherapy must be distinguished from those whose disease recurs after an initial period of complete remission. The former group has a lesser likeli-

TABLE 12. **Results of Randomized Comparison of MOPP and Alternating MOPP/ABVD Regimens in Treatment of Advanced Hodgkin's Disease**

	Complete Response Rate (%)	Actuarial Freedom from First Progression Rate at 5 Yr (%)	Actuarial Relapse-free Rate at 5 Yr (%)	Median Duration of Complete Response (Months)	Overall Actuarial Survival Rate at 5 Yr (%)
MOPP	71	36.6	47.3	20	54.3
MOPP/ABVD	92	70.1	77.4	>31	84.2

hood of chemotherapy response and a more adverse prognosis.

The role of radiation for patients with localized disease progression or recurrence must be considered following appropriate demonstration of limited disease extent. This situation is, however, relatively uncommon. The more usual circumstance is progression of disease not amenable to localized therapy.

Patients whose disease recurs, particularly after a period of complete remission of disease, commonly respond to an alternative chemotherapy regimen. The use of MOPP for recurrent disease that was treated initially with MOPP was associated with a 59 per cent complete remission rate, a median duration of remission of 21 months, and a median survival of >60 months for "remitters" and 31 months for "non-remitters." When the period of initial complete remission is short (<1 year), the use of a 4-drug alternative regimen is often preferred (e.g., ABVD; SCAB) (see Table 9). Patients who never achieve remission with MOPP are commonly switched to an alternative regimen. From series to series, complete response rates vary from 10 to 60 per cent; however, median duration of response is commonly 12 to 60 months, thus implying that complete response is less durable in the "salvage" situation. This variability in reported outcome probably reflects differences in patient selection parameters (e.g., presence of symptoms, nodal versus extranodal disease progression, number of extranodal sites, prior response to MOPP, performance status).

Patients who fail to achieve remission or whose disease recurs following an alternating-sequence regimen have fewer options for alternative "salvage" chemotherapy. Two alternative regimens are CEP and CAD (Table 13), with complete response rates of 35 per cent and 13 per cent, respectively, and a median duration of response for CEP-treated patients of 17 months. The limited success of standard "alternative" chemotherapy regimens in this situation has resulted in the evolution of programs of massive chemotherapy with autologous bone marrow transplantation. Preliminary reports indicate complete response rates up to 70 per cent, even with inclusion of patients who have not previously achieved complete remission with standard regimens.

The attractiveness of this approach is the ability to deliver very intensive therapy, the high probability of engraftment of autologous bone marrow, the absence of graft-versus-host disease, and the reported success in patients "refractory" to standard chemotherapy. The limitations include the necessity for referral to specialized treatment units, the acute mortality rate of approximately 5 to 15 per cent, inapplicability to patients with bone marrow involvement at the time of transplantation, and the lack of follow-up data beyond 3 to 4 years to indicate the long-term results. At present, it must be considered an experimental therapy, applied in the context of clinical trial following full informed consent and justified by a well-established poor prognosis with other standard therapies given for patients failing alternative or alternating-sequence chemotherapy programs.

Complications of Treatment

Combination chemotherapy programs are associated with both acute and delayed side effects. The acute side effects reflect individual toxicities specific to the agent(s) in question and also the combined toxicity on organ systems with a significant cell-renewal compartment (e.g., the bone

TABLE 13. **CEP and CAD Regimens for Patients Failing After Alternative or Alternating-Sequence Regimens**

Agents	Route	Dose (mg/m²)	Day(s)
CEP Regimen*			
lomustine (CeeNU)	PO	80	1
VP-16 (Etoposide)	PO	100	1–5
prednimustine†	PO	60	1–5
CAD Regimen‡			
lomustine (CeeNU)	PO	100	1
melphalan (Alkeran)	PO	6	1–4
vindesine§ (DVA)	IV	3	1 and 8

*Cycle repeats every 28 days; 6 cycles recommended for responding patients.

†Orphan drug available from the National Information Center for Orphan Drugs and Rare Diseases, 800-336-4797.

‡Cycle repeats every 35–42 days; 6 cycles recommended for responding patients.

§Investigational drug produced by Lilly.

TABLE 14. **Major Acute Side Effects of Chemotherapy and Their Management**

Side Effect	Drug	Precautionary Measures	Treatment
Cytopenias	Most cytotoxics	Blood count supervision	Blood component support; antibiotics
Alopecia	Doxorubicin	Ice pack on scalp; tourniquet	Wig
Nausea and vomiting	Nitrogen mustard		Prochlorperazine (Stemetil)
	Doxorubicin		Metoclopramide (Maxeran)
	Dacarbazine		Domperidone (Motilium)
	CCNU; BCNU		Dexamethasone (Decadron)
	Streptozotocin		Nabilone (Cesamet)
Constipation	Vincristine; vinblastine	Regular laxative use	Suppository/enema
Peripheral neuropathy	Vincristine; vinblastine		Omit agents
Indigestion	Prednisone	Diet control; antacids	Ranitidine (Zantac); cimetidine (Tagamet)
Diabetes mellitus	Prednisone	Urinalysis (Ketodiastix)	Insulin
Phlebitis	Nitrogen mustard; doxorubicin; dacarbazine; BCNU; vinca alkaloids	Good IV access IV access device	
Hyperuricemia	All cytotoxics	Uric acid measurement	Allopurinol (Zyloric)
Monoamine oxidase inhibitor effects	Procarbazine	Diet control; no alcohol	
Skin rash	Procarbazine	—	Chlorpheniramine (Chlor-Tripolon)
	Allopurinol	—	Diphenhydramine (Benadryl)
			Hydroxyzine (Atarax)
			Hydrocortisone (Solucortef)
Pulmonary fibrosis	Bleomycin	Lung function surveillance	Omit agent
Cardiotoxicity	Doxorubicin	Cardiac function surveillance	Omit agent
Febrile reaction	Bleomycin	—	Hydrocortisone (Solucortef)

marrow, gastrointestinal tract). In general, toxicity is dose-related, although wide variation exists in terms of individual threshold or tolerance to drug-induced side effects. Although the incidence or severity of acute toxicity may be diminished by dose reduction or prolongation of cycle frequency, such reduction in dose intensity may have adverse implications in terms of disease control. The principal acute side effects and the strategies for their minimization are shown in Table 14.

The two principal delayed or long-term complications of chemotherapy in adults are gonadal dysfunction and the induction of second malignancies. Gonadal dysfunction is expressed in men as infertility. A hormonal basis for impotence is unusual. In women, menstrual irregularity, premature ovarian failure (menopause), and consequent infertility characterize gonadal damage. The effects of chemotherapy on the testes are independent of age; in women, however, chemotherapy effect is characterized by reduction of functioning ovarian life span (i.e., the probability of dysfunction increases with increasing age within the reproductive years). Chemotherapy regimens employing alkylating agents and chronic oral cytotoxic agents (MOPP or derivatives) are more gonadotoxic than regimens employing intravenous agents only (e.g., ABVD). Following MOPP chemotherapy, recovery of spermatogenesis occurs in less than 10 per cent of males. Recovery from ovarian failure is unlikely. Thus, for the patient who is to receive combination chemotherapy the following issues should be considered:

1. Is the chemotherapy really necessary?
2. Have the gonadal side effects been discussed with the patient?
3. Has semen cryopreservation been considered?
4. Has a regimen such as ABVD been considered to minimize gonadotoxic effects?
5. In follow-up, will hormonal therapy be necessary?

If reproductive issues are of high priority, appropriate referral should be made to reproductive endocrinologists at the time of initial assessment.

Second malignancies following treatment of Hodgkin's disease reflect the success of therapy in achieving prolonged survival. There is an actuarial probability of developing acute leukemia (usually non-lymphocytic type) of about 5 to 8 per cent over a 10-year follow-up period. The risk does not appear to increase thereafter. Chemotherapy, either adjuvant to irradiation or as sole treatment, is strongly associated with the risk of leukemia. Some investigators believe the risk to be greater in patients first treated after the age of 40 years. A similar level of risk also exists for the development of non-Hodgkin's lymphoma, although both irradiation and chemotherapy are causally associated. Other solid tumors continue to occur following therapy with an actuarial risk of approximately 10 to 15 per cent over a 15-year follow-up period. These tumors (lung carcinoma, squamous carcinoma of the skin, stomach cancer, soft-tissue sarcoma, melanoma) are strongly associated with radiation therapy and may also reflect pre-existing immunosuppression resulting from initial therapy or continuing immunologic abnormalities that characterize both treated and untreated Hodgkin's disease.

HODGKIN'S DISEASE: TREATMENT WITH RADIATION THERAPY

method of
NANCY PRICE MENDENHALL, M.D., and
RODNEY R. MILLION, M.D.
University of Florida College of Medicine
Gainesville, Florida

Radiation is the single most effective agent available in the treatment of Hodgkin's disease. The success of radiation treatment depends on three factors: the relative radiosensitivity of Hodgkin's disease in comparison with the radiation tolerance of associated normal tissues, a predictable pattern of tumor spread, and technical advances in the field of radiation therapy that allow comprehensive treatment of all areas involved or at risk for tumor involvement. Cure is achieved in at least two thirds of patients treated for Hodgkin's disease, and attention must be paid to sequelae of successful treatment. Treatment goals are not only relapse-free survival and survival but also survival without complications of treatment. Treatment alternatives include radiation therapy alone, chemotherapy alone, and a combination of the two modalities. Because of the effectiveness of combination chemotherapy in the salvage setting, a treatment plan resulting in lower relapse-free survival rates may be selected in order to avoid adverse complications of chemotherapy or combined-modality therapy without compromising a patient's overall chance of survival. In addition to Ann Arbor staging, other factors including bulk of disease (more or less than one third of the maximum intrathoracic diameter for mediastinal lesions), number of sites of involvement (more or less than four), and degree of splenic involvement (more or less than five nodules) may be used to define three general risk groups. The low-risk group includes Ann Arbor stages IA, IB, and IIA without other risk factors and is treated with radiation therapy alone with a high degree of success (Table 1). The intermediate group includes Ann Arbor stages IA, IB, and IIA with bulky mediastinal disease, IIA with more than four sites of involvement, IIB, and IIIA$_1$ with minimal (less than five nodules) or no spleen involvement. The in-

termediate group may be treated with combined modality therapy or with radiation therapy alone with chemotherapy reserved for salvage with equal changes of overall survival. The high-risk group includes stages IIIA$_1$ with extensive spleen involvement, IIIA$_2$, IIIB, IVA, and IVB and should be treated with combined-modality therapy or occasionally with chemotherapy alone, when the bone marrow is extensively involved.

Treatment Recommendations and Results

Treatment for all patients is individualized, but basic guidelines are shown in Table 1 along with expected 10-year relapse-free, absolute, and determinate disease-free survival rates.

Special Considerations

Older patients tolerate laparotomy and combination chemotherapy less well than younger patients. Consequently, there is a tendency to rely on clinical rather than pathologic staging in patients 60 years of age or older and to rely on radiation therapy except in advanced disease, when chemotherapy is mandated. Musculoskeletal defects from the use of radiation therapy in children have led to increased reliance on combination chemotherapy in children and the use of lower doses and more limited radiation treatment volumes.

Technical Aspects of Radiation Therapy for Hodgkin's Disease

Successful radiation therapy requires treatment of all clinically involved lymph nodes and all nodal and extranodal regions at risk for subclinical involvement. The anatomic position and extent of the lymphatic regions at risk in most patients necessitate treatment of very large fields and large volumes of normal tissues. Potential acute complications in normal tissues incidentally treated necessitate sequential irradiation of segments of the entire treatment volume; fractionation, protraction, and limitation of the radiation dose; careful tailoring of the radiation portals with individualized blocks made of Lipowitz's metal; and careful matching of the treatment portals to avoid overdosage through overlapping fields or underdosage in areas between fields.

Treatment Volumes

Involved-field irradiation refers to the treatment of only the site of clinical involvement. *Extended-field irradiation* refers to treatment of the site of clinical involvement plus elective treatment of contiguous, clinically uninvolved lymph node areas. *Total nodal irradiation* refers to treatment of all nodal and extranodal areas commonly involved in Hodgkin's disease, including the mantle, para-aortic, spleen, and pelvic fields; in some clinical settings, the liver is also treated. *Modified* or *subtotal nodal irradiation* differs from total

TABLE 1. **Hodgkin's Disease: Treatment Recommendations and Results Achieved at the University of Florida**

Stage	Treatment	10-Year Survival Rate* (%)		
		Relapse-Free	*Absolute*	*Cause-Specific*
Low-risk				
IA, IB, IIA, IIB–no poor prognostic factors	MTNI or TNI	90	82	93
Intermediate-risk				
IA, IB, IIA, IIB–large mediastinal mass or >4 sites involved	MTNI or TNI	60	86	83
	CB	80	78	78
IIIA1	TNI	80	80	80
IIIA$_{1_s}$–minimal	TNI	50	90	80
	CB	100	75	75
High-risk				
IIIA$_{1_s}$–extensive	CB	67	63	60
IIIB	CB	40	40	40
IV	CH	20	29	32
III, IV†	alt. CB or alt. CH	67–85	77–100	nd

Abbreviations: MTNI = modified total nodal irradiation; TNI = total nodal irradiation; CB = combined modality with radiation therapy and chemotherapy; CH = chemotherapy alone; alt. CB = chemotherapy alternating with segments of irradiation; alt. CH = alternating chemotherapy regimens; nd = no data.

*In relapse-free survival, only disease relapse was counted as an event. For absolute survival, death from any cause counted as an event. For cause-specific survival, deaths due to Hodgkin's disease or treatment-related causes (i.e., complications of treatment or secondary leukemia) were counted as events.

†3-year results from Stanford University trials (SA Rosenberg and HS Kaplan, *Int J Radiat Oncol Biol Phys* 11:5–22, 1985).

nodal irradiation only in that the pelvic volume is not treated. *Comprehensive lymphatic irradiation* refers to treatment of Waldeyer's ring, mantle, and whole abdomen and is used more often in the treatment of non-Hodgkin's lymphoma, in which mesenteric node involvement is common.

The *Waldeyer's ring* treatment volume includes not only the lymphoid tissue in the tonsil, base of tongue, and nasopharynx, which is rarely involved in Hodgkin's disease but also, more important, the preauricular, postauricular, occipital, submaxillary, submental, upper jugular, and spinal accessory lymph nodes, which are not optimally treated in the mantle field. Waldeyer's ring fields are treated through opposed lateral portals when clinically involved or when subclinical involvement is suspected because of upper cervical lymphadenopathy or bulky involvement of midneck nodes.

The *mantle* is an irregularly shaped volume that includes the cervical, supraclavicular, infraclavicular, axillary, mediastinal, and hilar lymph nodes. When indicated, treatment of the whole lung, hemilung, or whole heart is incorporated into the mantle. Opposed anterior and posterior fields are used. The lower border of the mantle is approximately at the bottom of T10 when there is either minimal or no mediastinal disease. Custom blocks made of Lipowitz's metal shield the lung parenchyma, larynx, humeral heads, and portions of the mandible and parotid glands. When there is extensive mediastinal involvement with masses greater than one third of the maximum intrathoracic diameter, subcarinal or hilar node involvement, or pleural effusion, consideration must be given to an *extended mantle field* including the hemilung or

whole lung; if there is gross pericardial involvement or pericardial effusion, consideration must be given to treatment of the whole heart.

The *para-aortic volume* includes all para-aortic and paracaval lymph nodes between the aortic bifurcation and the bottom of the mantle field. The celiac axis nodes are incidentally covered. The para-aortic volume is treated through opposed anterior and posterior fields, matched (with an appropriate gap) to the mantle fields superiorly, the pelvic fields at the bottom of L4 inferiorly, and the spleen field(s) laterally.

The *spleen treatment volume* includes the spleen and the splenic hilar nodes. When the spleen has been removed, a small field may be treated for coverage of the splenic hilum, which can be identified by clips placed at laparotomy. When the spleen is extensively involved or there is known liver involvement, the liver may be treated in a separate field.

The *pelvic volume* includes the femoral nodes and the common, external, and internal iliac nodes. The pelvic volume is treated through opposed anterior and posterior fields. The superior border is at the bottom of L4, matched, with an appropriate gap, to the bottom of the para-aortic fields. A customized block made of Lipowitz's metal shields the midline structures not at risk, including the ovaries after oophoropexy and the iliac wings. In males, special anterior and posterior testicular shields are used to decrease the dose of internally scattered radiation to the testicles from the pelvic fields. An *inverted Y treatment volume* combines the para-aortic and pelvic volumes. A *spade volume* is an abbreviated inverted Y that does not treat the femoral or pelvic lymphatics below the common iliac nodes.

Special Technical Features

The mantle is technically one of the most difficult treatment volumes used in radiation therapy and should be undertaken only by an experienced radiotherapist. Because doses are modest and the set-up for the large, irregularly shaped mantle fields is quite difficult, a physician checks the set-up each day in the treatment room, and daily port films are taken to verify adequate coverage of all target areas. If an area is missed, the dose is made up with a boost. Because of the potential for overdosage from overlapping of the sequential matched segmental fields, visually verifiable gaps on the skin between the adjacent fields are maintained.

Attention must be given to the position of the left kidney when treating the spleen and to para-aortic treatment volumes. If more than two thirds of the left kidney must be included in these fields, consideration should be given to laparotomy with splenectomy. When the liver or whole abdomen must be treated, special kidney blocks are placed at 1500 cGy.

Time-Dose Factors

When radiation therapy alone is used, the dose delivered at the University of Florida is 3500 cGy to clinically involved areas and 3000 cGy to clinically uninvolved areas. Many institutions use doses 15 per cent to 25 per cent higher. The overall time required for total nodal irradiation, including a planned break prior to pelvic irradiation, is 4 months; for modified total nodal irradiation the time is approximately 2 months. For particularly bulky disease treated with radiation therapy alone, an additional 250 cGy may be delivered. Doses in patients receiving 6 courses of chemotherapy are usually reduced to 3000 cGy for clinically involved sites and 2500 cGy for uninvolved sites. No dose reduction is made in adults receiving only 3 courses of chemotherapy. In children receiving 4 to 6 courses of chemotherapy, doses may be limited to 2500 cGy for clinically involved sites and 1500 cGy to 2000 cGy for uninvolved sites.

Patients are treated 5 days a week and all fields are treated each day. The daily dose depends on the site and treatment volume. The standard mantle receives 160 to 170 cGy per day; the daily dose is reduced to 150 cGy when the whole heart is incorporated into the mantle volume and to 100 cGy when a hemilung or whole lung is included. The Waldeyer's ring, spleen, para-aortic, and pelvic fields receive 160 to 170 cGy per day. When the liver is treated, the daily dose is 150 cGy per day. When the whole abdomen is treated, the daily dose is 100 cGy per day.

To decrease acute normal-tissue toxicity and to allow for field reduction after tumor shrinkage, particularly in patients with large mediastinal masses, a split-course technique is used, in which the mantle and upper abdominal segments are each divided into two parts and treated in alternating, ping-pong fashion. As opposed to split-course techniques in carcinomas, this approach has not been associated with decreased control rates.

Sequencing and Modifications of Radiation Therapy in Combined-Modality Therapy

Three courses of chemotherapy may be used prior to definitive radiation therapy to shrink bulky mediastinal disease or reduce failure rates in stage II patients with more than four sites of involvement. In this setting, radiation doses are not decreased, but the mantle treatment volume is usually significantly reduced so that more lung parenchyma may be shielded. In stage III patients (excluding A_1 with minimal or no spleen disease) there is a high risk of failure in an extranodal site with total nodal irradiation, so six courses of chemotherapy are given. The radiation therapy may be sandwiched between the third and fourth courses of chemotherapy, delivered after completion of chemotherapy, or delivered in an alternating fashion with two courses of chemotherapy followed by mantle irradiation, two more courses of chemotherapy followed by upper abdominal irradiation, and a final two courses of chemotherapy followed by pelvic irradiation. The disadvantage of sandwich therapy is the relatively long period of time during completion of modified or total nodal irradiation after three courses of chemotherapy when some clinically involved areas receive neither chemotherapy nor radiation therapy. When total nodal irradiation is attempted after delivery of six courses of chemotherapy, it is often not possible to complete the sequential segments of irradiation because of marrow compromise, and there are often long treatment delays during the irradiation. The alternating approach has the advantages of induction chemotherapy prior to consolidative irradiation of all commonly involved areas. During the planned two-month splits between the segments of irradiation, the patient is continuously treated with chemotherapy.

Potential Side Effects and Complications

Acute Side Effects

Expected side effects of treatment include transient hair loss, xerostomia, and skin reaction associated with the mantle and Waldeyer's ring fields, and nausea associated with the upper abdominal fields. Hair loss is particularly noticeable in the occipital region and preauricular regions in all patients and in the beard and anterior chest of men. Partial regrowth is usually observed within 2 to 4 months of treatment. Transient xerostomia occurs in all patients because of incidental parotid irradiation. The degree of recovery of normal salivary function is related to the patient's pretherapy salivary output, with complete resolution of symptoms of xerostomia usually observed in young patients and partial resolution in older patients. The skin reaction observed in the supradiaphragmatic fields is usually limited to mild erythema and occasional patchy, dry desquamation along tangentially irradiated surfaces; after completion of radiation therapy, a lanolin, vitamin-E, or aloe-based lotion will provide symptomatic relief. The nausea and vomiting associated with para-aortic and splenic irradiation can be controlled with standard antiemetics such as prochlorperazine maleate (Compazine), promethazine HCl (Phenergan), metoclopramide HCl (Reglan), or chlorpromazine HCl (Thorazine) capsules or suppositories. Nausea and vomiting occasionally are observed with mantle irradiation, when the inferior mantle border is lowered to accommodate whole lung or heart irradiation. Because of the extensive bone marrow treated with total nodal irradiation, hemograms and platelet counts should be monitored weekly throughout the course of treatment, and more often when counts begin to fall. When radiation therapy alone is given, the sequential treatment of segments of the irradiation volume allows for sufficient recovery so that few patients require treatment interruptions for bone marrow recovery. When combined-modality therapy is used, treatment interruptions are frequently required. Generally, radiation therapy is withheld until the white blood cell count is greater than 2000 and the platelet count is greater than 50,000.

Subacute Side Effects

Fatigue and loss of energy are common complaints during and after irradiation. Although most patients are able to continue their routine activities during treatment, it is often 4 to 6 months after completion of treatment before the patient is back to his or her normal baseline energy level. Except for prolonged lymphocytopenia, which may last up to a year after treatment, blood cell counts usually return to baseline values within several months following treatment.

Within 1 to 4 months after completion of mantle irradiation, some patients experience Lhermitte's syndrome, usually characterized by an electric shock sensation associated with neck flexion; this is transient and is not associated with late or permanent neurologic sequelae of treatment.

Patients with Hodgkin's disease have a propensity to develop herpes zoster. Although some patients have a preceding history of herpes zoster, the outbreak usually occurs within 2 years of successful treatment of Hodgkin's disease; when the outbreak occurs more than 2 years following therapy, it may be associated with recurrence of Hodgkin's disease. Usually the herpes zoster infection is confined to a single dermatomal distribution and is self-limited. The pain associated with the herpetic outbreak is often excruciating, unresponsive to anti-inflammatory or narcotic medications, and may precede the appearance of the typical vesicular lesions by a week. Acyclovir may ameliorate the course of the viral outbreak and should certainly be used if the outbreak is in a critical area or if there is any sign of dissemination.

Radiation pneumonitis occurs in less than 5 per cent of patients, usually in those who had extensive mediastinal disease, and most often within 2 to 4 months after mantle irradiation. It is characterized by a dry, hacking cough with an infiltrate confined to the radiation portals on chest roentgenogram. Symptoms may precede radiographic signs and may also include fever and shortness of breath. Although radiographic changes are usually confined to previous radiation portals, the process can extend outside the previous field and diffusely involve the lung. In patients who received combined-modality therapy, pneumocystic pneumonia must be ruled out. Rapid improvement is usually seen with the initiation of steroids (60 mg to 100 mg of prednisone daily), but some cases are not responsive. Early diagnosis and treatment are essential, as most fatalities have been associated with delay in therapy, often for histologic confirmation of the diagnosis. Prednisone may mask radiation pneumonitis, as some cases in patients receiving combined-modality therapy have been associated with steroid withdrawal. It is important to withdraw steroids slowly after treatment for radiation pneumonitis (over a period of several months), as rapid withdrawal has been associated with reactivation of the pneumonitis which may not be responsive to reinitiation of steroids.

Acute pericarditis occurs in 2 to 5 per cent of patients (usually those who had extensive mediastinal and pericardial disease) 4 to 6 months after mantle irradiation. Most patients are asymptomatic, and the diagnosis is based on plain chest roentgenograms; the condition usually resolves over a period of months without therapy. Occasionally, the patient may develop typical signs and symptoms of pericarditis including pleuritic or ischemic chest pain, shortness of breath, pericardial friction rub, paradoxic pulse, and EKG changes. Nonsteroidal anti-inflammatory medications and steroids may be effective. The patient must be observed for increasing pericardial effusion and possible tamponade, in which case emergent pericardiocentesis can be life saving.

Late Complications

Potential late complications include hypothyroidism, sterility, pulmonary fibrosis, cardiac damage, transverse myelitis, nephritis, growth abnormalities, and second malignancies.

Approximately 25 per cent of patients who receive mantle irradiation will develop hypothyroidism; periodically, thyroid functions are measured, and replacement thyroid hormone is prescribed even for asymptomatic patients who show only elevated TSH levels. With ovarian transposition to midline position at laparotomy and special testicular shields to decrease the dose of indirect radiation to the testicles from internal scatter during pelvic irradiation, sterility due to irradiation is unusual. It is important, prior to beginning pelvic irradiation in a patient who has undergone oophoropexy, to verify midline ovarian position, however, as the ovaries may detach and return to the normal anatomic position. Symptomatic pulmonary fibrosis may occur in patients in whom large mediastinal masses preclude shielding of adequate lung parenchyma; with current dose recommendations and either shrinking-field technique with radiation therapy alone or the use of chemotherapy for shrinkage of the tumor prior to definitive radiation therapy, the risk of clinically significant pulmonary damage is less than 5 per cent. Rarely, fibrotic lung that results in infectious or hemodynamic problems may be resected. The risk of radiation fibrosis is increased with the use of bleomycin. Constrictive pericarditis is an uncommon complication of mantle irradiation, usually occurring only in patients with extensive mediastinal disease with pericardial involvement in whom high doses of radiation were delivered to the whole heart. Pericardiectomy may be necessary in severe cases. Whether the risk of coronary artery disease is increased by mantle irradiation is unknown. Transverse myelitis is a rare but catastrophic complication of irradiation, usually related to poor technique in matching opposing and abutting fields; there is no known effective treatment for myelitis. Radiation nephritis occurs rarely and may be avoided with proper technique or splenectomy. If radiation nephritis results in hypertension and the contralateral kidney is functional, consideration may be given to nephrectomy.

The use of radiation therapy in children often results in hypoplastic development of the irradiated tissues and significant subsequent musculoskeletal defects, which may also contribute to psychosocial problems. The younger the child, the more significant the subsequent growth abnormalities will be. Common sequelae include a "skinny neck" and shortened interclavicular distance secondary to mantle irradiation, posterior left abdominal wall deficit from treatment of the spleen field(s), and shortened sitting height secondary to irradiation of the mantle and para-aortic fields.

Patients treated with radiation therapy alone for Hodgkin's disease do not appear to be at an increased risk over the general population for developing leukemia. There is approximately a 7 per cent risk of leukemia in patients treated with MOPP chemotherapy; patients receiving combined-modality therapy do not appear to be at a significantly increased risk over those receiving chemotherapy alone. Although there appears to be an increased risk of second solid malignancies in patients receiving radiation therapy for Hodgkin's disease compared with the general population, many of the reported malignancies are not in the previous radiation fields and are clearly related to other risk factors, such as cigarette smoking. Large numbers of patients have not been observed beyond the expected latency period for radiation-induced malignancies (5 to 30 years), and the risks due to inherent genetic deficiencies are not defined, so the relationship between second solid malignancies and the use of radiation in the treatment for Hodgkin's disease is not clear.

New Directions

As survival is in excess of 80 per cent, the emphasis in low- to intermediate-risk patients is on reduction of the late sequelae of treatment by reduction of the radiation dose and volume through shrinking-field techniques and the use of pre-irradiation chemotherapy and by the search for effective drug combinations that will be less leukemogenic and have less cardiopulmonary toxicity in combination with radiation. The emphasis in high-risk patients is improvement in survival rates through more effective combinations and sequencing of drugs and radiation. The role of ablative therapy followed by autologous bone marrow transplantation in patients with an extremely poor prognosis is also being investigated.

ACUTE LEUKEMIA IN ADULTS

method of
PHILIP L. McCARTHY, JR., M.D., and
DAVID S. ROSENTHAL, M.D.
Harvard Medical School
Boston, Massachusetts

Acute leukemia is a devastating but increasingly treatable illness. The therapeutic outcome of the acute leukemias has improved over the past ten years but the majority of patients, especially in older age groups, die of these diseases. With the advent of newer approaches, increased survival has occurred and is improving. Intensive chemotherapy and bone marrow transplantation have made cure possible.

Presentation and Diagnosis

The presenting symptoms in acute leukemia may be insidious or acute. Fatigue and malaise are common complaints often related to anemia. Gingival bleeding, epistaxis, and easy bruisability are common with thrombocytopenia. Noninfectious fever may be present, but patients with neutropenia often have an occult infection, such as a tooth abscess that has not responded to a course of antibiotics.

On physical examination, lymphadenopathy is unusual except in some cases of acute lymphoblastic leukemia (ALL). In acute myelogenous leukemia (AML), there may be minimal splenic enlargement. There are often petechiae or ecchymoses if the platelet count is low. Infiltration of the skin by leukemia and gingival hypertrophy are not uncommon. Other organ involvement is common but there are no unique physical findings.

The diagnosis is often not apparent on physical examination but is suspected on evaluation of a complete blood count. The white blood count (WBC) may be elevated, although the majority of cases present with a normal or low WBC and pancytopenia. A shift to the left with an increased number of early forms including blasts should raise the suspicion of the diagnosis.

Bone marrow aspiration and biopsy confirm the diagnosis. It is important to distinguish between AML and ALL because treatment of each leukemia is different; subtyping within the two groups is usually more for prognostic rather than therapeutic significance. Histochemical, enzymologic and immunologic marker studies for the detection of myeloid and lymphoid characteristics should be performed on bone marrow cells or on peripheral blood blast forms if an aspirate cannot be obtained. Cytogenetic analysis of leukemic cells may confirm the diagnosis and is becoming a useful adjunct in determining prognosis.

Other tests include screening chemistries with careful attention to serum potassium, calcium, phosphate, uric acid, creatinine, and blood urea nitrogen. Tumor-lysis syndrome, which is the release of intracellular ions due to rapid cell turnover or lysis, can be seen during induction chemotherapy of Burkitt's lymphoma, which is a subtype of ALL. Hyperkalemia, hyperphosphatemia and hypercalcemia can occur with the resultant medical complications. This is less common in AML. In patients with ALL, chest X-ray may disclose a mediastinal mass. Pulmonary infiltrates can be a sign of infection or leukemic infiltrates if the WBC is markedly elevated. Prothrombin time and partial thromboplastin time tests should be performed, especially if disseminated intravascular coagulation (DIC) is suspected clinically. Acute promyelocytic leukemia, a subtype of AML, is associated with DIC, and a coagulation profile should be performed and monitored with therapy. If there is focal neurologic abnormality, such as cranial neuropathy, nuchal rigidity, or severe headache, a computed tomography (CT) scan of the head should be done to look for mass lesions. If the scan is negative, a lumbar puncture should be performed to look for leukemic cells. This will necessitate early intrathecal therapy. A lumbar puncture is necessary with all cases of ALL within the first three weeks of diagnosis. A platelet transfusion is necessary for such invasive procedures if the platelet count is less than 20,000 per microliter.

Treatment

Emergency Measures

High white blood counts can be catastrophic. If the white count is over 100,000 per microliter in AML, leukostasis can result in severe respiratory distress or central nervous system (CNS) hemorrhage. The treatment is immediate leukopheresis if there is any evidence of neurologic dysfunction. In addition, 6 to 8 grams of hydroxyurea orally daily (100 mg per kg) is given for acute lowering of the white count. Platelet counts of less than 10,000 per microliter signal an increased risk of bleeding, and it is at this level that platelet transfusions are routinely given. We prefer single donor transfusions rather than platelets pooled from several donors, to reduce the exposure to multiple platelet antigens and the risk of transfusion reactions. There is evidence to suggest that increased exposure to multiple donors may make the patient refractory to future transfusions. Broad-spectrum antibiotics including a semisynthetic penicillin or third-generation cephalosporin along with an aminoglycoside are started if the patient is neutropenic (absolute neutrophil count less than 500 per microliter) and febrile. This is more of an issue during the nadir of blood counts due to chemotherapy. Severe anemia and dehydration must be corrected before chemotherapy is initiated.

Other measures include placement of an indwelling right atrial catheter for blood drawing, transfusions, and chemotherapy infusions. Vigorous hydration is performed to prevent renal insufficiency due to uric acid nephropathy. Allopurinol is given at a dose of 300 mg orally daily.

It is discontinued after 3 or 4 days as the WBC decreases, because of the high incidence of allergic skin reactions due to this medication.

The patient should be placed on the following bleeding precautions: no intramuscular injections, avoidance of subcutaneous injections, and no aspirin-containing compounds. Nonsteroidal anti-inflammatory drugs should be avoided unless clearly indicated. Neutropenic precautions include no rectal temperatures, hand washing before touching any patient, and mask-wearing if the visitor has a cold. Gloves and gowns and laminar flow rooms are usually not utilized except in a transplant setting.

Therapy of Acute Myelogenous Leukemia

Although the therapy of AML has changed over the years, some chemotherapeutic agents have become the mainstays of treatment. Treatment is usually given in two to three phases: induction and consolidation with or without maintenance. Induction therapy is designed to eliminate the leukemia, based on microscopic examination of the blood and bone marrow. Our current induction regimen consists of cytosine arabinoside (Cytosar-U) (Ara-C), 100 mg per square meter (M^2) intravenously for 7 consecutive days by continuous infusion, and daunorubicin (Cerubidine), 45 mg per M^2 intravenously by bolus daily for 3 days. On days 8, 9, and 10, Ara-C is given at a dose of 2 gm per M^{2*} intravenously over a 2-hour period every 12 hours (high-dose Ara-C), for a total of 6 doses. On day 17 after initiation of therapy, a bone marrow aspirate is performed. If the patient is in remission with a platelet count greater than 100,000 per microliter and an absolute neutrophil count greater than 1000 per microliter, the first cycle of consolidation therapy is started, consisting of Ara-C, 200 mg per M^2 by continuous infusion intravenously daily for 5 days, and daunorubicin, 60 mg per M^2 by intravenous bolus daily for 2 days. The second consolidation cycle is started as soon as possible 21 to 28 days later when the blood counts recover. This cycle consists of Ara-C, 2 grams per M^{2*} every 12 hours for 6 doses, and etoposide (VP-16), 100 mg per M^2 by slow intravenous bolus daily on days 4 and 5. The third and final cycle of consolidation chemotherapy is a repeat of Cycle 1. A bone marrow biopsy and aspirate for cytogenetics and staining is performed along with a lumbar puncture after completion of the consolidation. If the patient is in remission and does not have an HLA-identical donor or is over 50 years of age, he or she is randomized to a no-therapy arm versus autologous bone marrow transplantation

(ABMT). This randomization is to determine if ABMT will increase the percentage of long-term survivors. Those under 50 years of age and with an HLA-identical match undergo allogeneic transplantation after one cycle of consolidation.

For the ABMT, the patient's marrow is harvested after recovery from consolidation therapy and stored at $-70C$. The patient is given oral busulfan, 1 mg per kg every 6 hours for 4 days. This is followed by cyclophosphamide, 1500 mg per M^2 intravenously daily for 4 days. The patient's marrow is thawed and reinfused the day after completing the cyclophosphamide. After recovery of blood counts, the patient is observed without therapy.

If the patient does not go into remission with induction therapy, the initial therapy is repeated or high-dose Ara-C therapy is started. If these fail, other alternatives include the use of m-Amsacrine,† 200 mg per M^2 intravenously daily for a total of 5 doses; VP-16, 100 to 200 mg per M^2 intravenously daily for 5 days, with daunorubicin, 60 mg per M^2 intravenously daily for 3 days; or mitoxantrone, 12 mg per M^2 intravenously daily for a total of 3 doses, followed by VP-16, 100 mg per M^2 intravenously daily for a total of 2 doses.

All these regimens are accompanied by profound neutropenia and thrombocytopenia. If the patient becomes febrile when the neutrophil count is less than 500 per microliter, intravenous broad-spectrum antibiotics are absolutely indicated. When the platelet count is below 20,000 per microliter, single-donor platelet transfusions are given. If the patient is refractory to platelet transfusions, HLA-matched platelets or donations from blood relatives are recommended. Attention to dental care is important and the mouth should be rinsed with a dilute H_2O_2 and fluoride solution 4 times a day. A dental evaluation prior to initiation of chemotherapy is necessary and may prevent future problems during periods of neutropenia.

All patients who have an HLA-identical sibling and are under the age of 50 years are advised to undergo allogeneic transplantation. The upper limit on age has been extended to 50 years because of the utilization of anti–T cell antibodies to reduce the number of T cells in the bone marrow of the donor. This has decreased the incidence and severity of graft versus host disease, which is the major cause of morbidity and mortality with increasing age. The preparative regimen for allogeneic bone marrow transplantation includes high-dose Ara-C, VP-16, 1300 cGy

---

*Exceeds dosage recommended by the manufacturer.

†Available from the National Cancer Institute, 301-496-5223.

of total body irradiation, and high-dose cyclophosphamide.

Therapy of Acute Lymphocytic Leukemia

ALL is a disease primarily of childhood and occurs less frequently in adults. Unlike children with ALL, adults are not easily cured and relapses are common even on therapy. As with AML, a similar diagnostic workup should be performed. Cell marker studies are important because it is necessary to differentiate Burkitt's type lymphoma from typical ALL. The chemotherapy for these two entities is different and, as previously noted, tumor-lysis syndrome is more common in Burkitt's lymphoma. A lumbar puncture is usually performed within the first three weeks because of the high incidence of CNS involvement.

The treatment involves three major phases: induction, consolidation with CNS prophylaxis, and maintenance. Induction chemotherapeutic agents include doxorubicin (Adriamycin), vincristine (Oncovin), and prednisone. The induction dose of doxorubicin is 45 mg per M^2 in an intravenous bolus, with subsequent doses every 3 weeks of 30 mg per M^2 intravenously until a cumulative total of 450 mg per M^2 is reached. Vincristine is given every week at a dose of 1.5 mg per M^2 in an intravenous push (maximum 2 mg) for a 4-week induction, after which it is given every 3 weeks. Prednisone is given orally, 40 mg per M^2 daily for 21 days; consolidation consists of 120 mg per M^2 orally daily for 5 days every 3 weeks. Other agents used during consolidation include L-asparaginase, 25,000 units per M^2 intramuscularly weekly, and 6-mercaptopurine, 50 mg per M^2 orally daily for 14 days every 3-week cycle.

Because of the high incidence of CNS disease in ALL, all patients receive Ara-C, 50 mg intrathecally every week for 4 weeks and then every 18 weeks during consolidation. Cranial irradiation is given during this time at approximately 2000 to 2400 cGy, depending on the patient's eligibility for transplantation.

At week 33, maintenance chemotherapy is started with the continuation of the vincristine, prednisone, and intrathecal Ara-C. The other consolidation drugs are stopped and methotrexate, 30 mg per M^2 intramuscularly per week, and 6-mercaptopurine, 50 mg per M^2 orally daily for 14 days every 3 weeks, are started. The maintenance regimen is continued for 2 years; then all therapy is discontinued.

Because ALL in adults over the age of 20 years has a higher incidence of relapse than in children, we favor bone marrow transplantation if the patient is an adult under 50 years of age and has an HLA-identical sibling. Once the patient is in remission and is undergoing consolidation or maintenance therapy, transplantation is performed. We do not wait to complete the maintenance therapy. For patients who relapse during maintenance therapy, re-induction with doxorubicin, prednisone, and vincristine can be attempted, but the duration of second remission is short. Alternative therapy with Ara-C, 2 to 3 grams per M^{2}* intravenously every 12 hours over 2 hours for 4 to 6 days, can be used. VM-26,† 150 mg per M^2 in an intravenous bolus every 14 days for 2 doses; vincristine, 2 mg intravenously weekly for 4 doses; VP-16, 150 mg per M^2 intravenously every 14 days for two doses; and prednisone, 60 mg orally per day for 1 month, can be used as induction therapy. If remission is achieved, a consolidation/maintenance schedule of VM-26, VP-16, and Ara-C is employed. Another alternative regimen is VP-16, 100 mg per M^2 intravenously daily for 5 days, with Ara-C, 200 mg per M^2 intravenously daily for 5 days. Autologous transplantation using a monoclonal antibody to the common ALL antigen (CALLA) to purge the marrow of residual leukemia cells has had some success in children but is not yet as promising in adults.

Therapy of Patients Not in Remission

Therapy of AML and ALL patients who do not achieve remission after multiple attempts at induction should be directed toward the comfort of the patient. Similar consideration should be given to patients with multiple medical problems for whom induction chemotherapy would be intolerable. Ara-C at low doses (10 mg per M^2 subcutaneously daily for 10 to 14 days) has been tried in certain cases of AML and refractory anemias with excess blasts. It is associated with cytopenias and its side effects are not much less than continuous intravenous doses of Ara-C in the range of 100 to 200 mg per M^2. Prednisone at doses of 40 to 60 mg per day orally can alleviate the discomfort due to fever secondary to leukemia and can increase the patient's sense of well-being. Suppressive antibiotic therapy with trimethoprim-sulfamethaxazole, 1 single- or double-strength tablet per day orally, can be utilized to try to avoid hospitalization for treatment of infections. Similar regimens with a quinolone agent such as norfloxacin (Noroxin) 400 mg orally per day are alternatives. Antibiotics used for prophylaxis may decrease the time the patient has to spend in the hospital.

Major advances have been made in the treat-

---

*Exceeds dosage recommended by the manufacturer.

†Orphan drug available from the National Information Center for Orphan Drugs and Rare Diseases, 800-336-4797.

ment of acute leukemia. What was once a uniformly fatal disease is now curable with aggressive therapy. It is important that the patient and family be provided with emotional support during the initial diagnosis and subsequent chemotherapy. A team approach is utilized in assisting the patient. Social service support is often critical in helping the patient and family cope with the major disruption in their lives. Nurses who are experienced in the care of cancer patients are required to administer chemotherapy and to monitor the patient's ability to maintain the activities of daily living. Nutritional support is critical in patients who are unable to eat due to the effects of chemotherapy or to dental problems. All patients who undergo transplantation require central vein hyperalimentation and monitoring by a dietician. Twenty-four hour housestaff coverage is necessary to respond to emergencies that can lead to rapid deterioration of a patient who is at a nadir in blood counts. Psychiatric and religious liaisons can assist in the psychological maintenance of the patient and the family. A unified approach to the therapy of the patient with acute leukemia is essential.

ACUTE LEUKEMIA IN CHILDHOOD

method of
JOHN N. LUKENS, M.D.
Vanderbilt University School of Medicine
Nashville, Tennessee

As with the adult disease, acute leukemia in childhood is classified as lymphoid or myeloid in origin. Acute lymphocytic leukemia (ALL) accounts for approximately 80 per cent of the leukemias in children. The leukemias remaining are referred to collectively as the acute nonlymphocytic leukemias (ANLL). Both variants encompass a number of subtypes that differ with respect to the biology of the malignant cell and clinical patterns of disease. The ability to identify subgroups that differ with respect to prognosis has dramatically altered the treatment of these diseases. Since subgroup identification may require immunophenotyping, karyotype analysis, and electron microscopy in addition to conventional morphologic and cytochemical characterization, it is essential that the initial diagnostic evaluation be done in a pediatric cancer center. Once an appropriate therapeutic course has been charted, much of the treatment may be transferred from the pediatric oncologist to the community physician. The treatment regimens described are based on protocols developed by investigators of The Children's Cancer Study Group. While differing in details, protocols used by other pediatric oncologists are based on the same principles.

ACUTE LYMPHOCYTIC LEUKEMIA

ALL is a heterogeneous group of disorders that differ with respect to prognosis and therapeutic priorities. Most pediatric oncology centers stratify patients at diagnosis into different prognostic groups so that therapy can be tailored to anticipated needs. Definition of risk groups is based in part on the immunophenotype and cytogenetic features of the leukemic cells and in part on the clinical and hematologic features of the disease. Unfavorable features include the pre-B, B, and T cell immunophenotypes; karyotype ploidy; chromosome translocations; high white blood cell count; age less than 1 year or more than 10 years; bulky extramedullary disease in the liver, spleen, lymph nodes, or thymus; absence of anemia; French-American-British (FAB) L_2 and L_3 morphology; central nervous system (CNS) involvement; and delayed clearance of leukemic cells from the bone marrow following institution of therapy. Patients whose disease is characterized by favorable clinical and laboratory features can be expected to respond satisfactorily to standard therapy, whereas those with adverse features require newer therapeutic approaches. There is increasing evidence that novel therapeutic strategies and better supportive care will annul many adverse disease characteristics.

The goal of therapy for newly diagnosed ALL is cure. Irrespective of the risk group for which it is intended, all treatment regimens embody four major phases: remission induction, CNS prophylaxis, consolidation, and maintenance. Each contributes independently to outcome. The objectives of the induction phase are the eradication of detectable leukemia and the restoration of bone marrow function. The next phase is designed to eliminate subclinical deposits of leukemic cells in the CNS. These foci are protected from systemic chemotherapy by the blood-brain barrier. The consolidation or intensification phase, which may overlap temporally with CNS prophylaxis, is intended to reduce further residual leukemia and to prevent the emergence of drug-resistant clones. The maintenance phase utilizes less intensive chemotherapy to reduce the leukemic cell population over time while permitting the expression of host immunologic response to remaining leukemic cells. In the discussion that follows, emphasis is given to the treatment of "standard risk" leukemia, defined as patient age 1 to 21 years, white blood cell count less than 50,000 per μl, L_1 FAB morphology, absence of bulky extramedullary disease, absence of pre-B and T cell immunophenotypes, and absence of karyotype ploidy or translocations. It is inappropriate to extrapolate these guidelines to children who have clinical or laboratory features that are associated with more aggressive disease.

Treatment

Induction

The induction regimen outlined in Table 1 utilizes three drugs for the treatment of systemic disease in addition to intrathecal methotrexate for the treatment of assumed but occult CNS leukemia. A preservative-free preparation of the

TABLE 1. **Chemotherapeutic Management of Standard-Risk Childhood Acute Lymphocytic Leukemia**

Induction (28 days)
Prednisone, 40 mg/M² PO, days 0 through 28
Vincristine, 1.5 mg/M² IV, days 0, 7, 14, 21, 28 (maximum single dose 2.0 mg)
L-Asparaginase, 6000 units/M² IM, days 3, 5, 7, 10, 12, 14, 17, 19, 21 (9 doses)
Methotrexate, 6 mg (less than 1 year age); 8 mg (1 to 2 years age); 10 mg (2 to 3 years); 12 mg (3 years and over) IT, days, 0 and 14

CNS Prophylaxis/Consolidation (28 days)
Prednisone, tapered over days 0 to 14
6-Mercaptopurine, 75 mg/M² PO, days 0 to 28
Methotrexate (same dose as in induction), IT, days 0, 7, 14, 21

Maintenance (2 years)
Prednisone, 40 mg/M² PO, days 0 through 4 of each 28-day cycle
Vincristine, 1.5 mg/M² IV, day 0 of each 28-day cycle (maximum single dose 2.0 mg)
6-Mercaptopurine, 20 mg/M² PO, days 0, 7, 14, 21 of each 28-day cycle (omitted when methotrexate is given intrathecally)
Methotrexate (same dose as in induction), IT, day 0 of every third 28-day-cycle

latter drug is reconstituted with Elliott's B solution or Ringer's lactate for intrathecal use. Since the volume of the cerebrospinal fluid is a function of age rather than body surface area, the dose of intrathecal methotrexate is based on age. Patients who have adverse prognostic factors are given 4 injections of daunorubicin (Cerubidine) in a dose of 25 mg per M² at weekly intervals in addition to prednisone, vincristine (Oncovin), and L-asparaginase (Elspar). A bone marrow aspirate is taken on day 14. The persistence of intact leukemic blasts indicates a suboptimal response, requiring that therapy be escalated both for the duration of the induction phase and for the consolidation phase.

CNS Prophylaxis and Consolidation

Presymptomatic CNS treatment, begun during the induction phase, is intensified during the second month of therapy. Intrathecal methotrexate is given at weekly intervals so as to provide 6 doses within 8 weeks of diagnosis. Thereafter, intrathecal methotrexate is administered at 12-week intervals for the duration of the maintenance phase. While intrathecal chemotherapy delivered in this fashion is effective in preventing the development of symptomatic CNS disease in children with standard risk ALL, combined modality therapy is required for children with white blood cell counts in excess of 50,000 per μl as well as for those with bulky extramedullary disease ("lymphoma syndrome"). Patients in the latter groups are given cranial radiation (1800 cGy in 10 fractions) during the first 2 weeks of the consolidation phase in addition to intrathecal methotrexate. Intrathecal therapy need not be continued during the maintenance phase. Children less than 12 to 18 months of age pose a special therapeutic problem. While at high risk for CNS relapse, they are unable to tolerate cranial radiation without adverse consequences of neurologic development. High-dose methotrexate (7.2 grams per M² over 24 hours)* followed by leucovorin rescue promises to provide effective CNS prophylaxis for this group of infants. Leukemocidal concentrations of methotrexate in the cerebrospinal fluid are achieved with this dose, and leucovorin given in a delayed fashion appears to have minimal rescue effect on leukemic cells in the cerebrospinal fluid.

The systemic therapy outlined in Table 1 provides inadequate consolidation for patients with adverse prognostic features. Several more intensive regimens are currently being evaluated. Particularly promising is one developed by investigators in the Federal Republic of Germany (Berlin-Frankfurt-Münster, BFM, regimen). In addition to daily oral 6-mercaptopurine (Purinethol), this regimen utilizes intravenous cyclophosphamide (Cytoxan), 1000 mg per M² on days 0 and 14 and intravenous cytosine arabinoside (Cytosar), 75 mg per M² on days 1 to 4, 8 to 11, 15 to 18, and 22 to 25 of the consolidation phase. Following an 8-week interim maintenance phase, the BFM protocol incorporates a 7- to 8-week delayed intensification phase that utilizes dexamethasone (Decadron), L-asparaginase (Elspar), vincristine (Oncovin), doxorubicin (Adriamycin), cyclophosphamide (Cytoxan), 6-thioguanine, cytosine arabinoside (Cytosar), and intrathecal methotrexate. The BFM regimen and other protocols that utilize intensive consolidation phases, while requiring comprehensive supportive care measures, clearly improve the prospects of cure for patients in high-risk groups.

Maintenance

Administration of daily 6-mercaptopurine and weekly methotrexate is continued throughout the maintenance phase. The doses of both drugs are adjusted to maintain the absolute neutrophil count (segmented forms plus bands) between 1000 and 1300 per μl and the platelet count above 100,000 per μl. Methotrexate is given intrathecally rather than orally once every 12 weeks, and prednisone-vincristine "pulses" are given at 4-week intervals. As noted earlier, intrathecal methotrexate need not be given during

---

*This dose is higher than the manufacturer's recommended dose.

the maintenance phase if both cranial radiation and intrathecal chemotherapy are used for CNS prophylaxis in the induction and consolidation phases. The maintenance phase is continued for 2 years. Some studies suggest that a third year may be advantageous for boys. Disease-free status must be documented prior to the discontinuation of therapy. For boys at high risk for extramedullary relapse this may require bilateral wedge biopsies of the testes in addition to a bone marrow aspirate.

Relapse

Bone marrow relapse occurring during the course of therapy portends ultimately refractory disease irrespective of initial risk factors. Although a second bone marrow remission can be achieved with prednisone, vincristine, L-asparaginase, and daunorubicin in most patients, the remission characteristically is of short duration. No more than 3 per cent of such patients experience long-term disease control. Bone marrow transplantation from an HLA-identical, mixed leukocyte culture (MLC) nonreactive donor early in the second remission offers the best chance for cure (30 to 35 per cent). Chemotherapy remains the mainstay of management for children who do not have a compatible marrow donor. The selection of therapy is dictated in part by the patient's treatment prior to relapse. Since resistance to methotrexate is concentration-dependent, doses of the drug that are greater than those used in the first remission often are effective for maintaining a second remission. Methotrexate is given intravenously at 10-day intervals. The starting dose of 100 mg per M^2 is escalated by 50 mg per M^2 increments to tolerance. L-Asparaginase in a dose of 15,000 units per M^2 is given intramuscularly 24 hours after each dose of methotrexate.

Bone marrow relapses occurring more than 6 to 12 months after cessation of therapy appear to result from the regrowth of a drug-sensitive malignant clone rather than the emergence of a drug-resistant population of leukemic cells. A more intense chemotherapeutic regimen than that used with the first remission is utilized with curative intent. The regimen must include CNS prophylaxis in addition to intensive induction and consolidation phases. The type of CNS prophylaxis used is influenced by prior exposure to cranial radiation and by considerations regarding the patient's candidacy for later bone marrow transplantation. Cranial radiation should be avoided if bone marrow transplantation is an option.

Isolated CNS relapse is treated with intrathecal chemotherapy, craniospinal radiation, systemic reinduction and reconsolidation, and an additional 2 years of maintenance therapy that incorporates intrathecal methotrexate.

Boys experiencing what appears to be an isolated testicular relapse should have an imaging evaluation of the retroperitoneal nodes that drain the testes. If there is no apparent nodal involvement, radiation therapy is limited to the testes (2400 cGy in 8 fractions). As with isolated CNS relapses, patients must undergo reinduction, reconsolidation, and maintenance therapy for an additional 2 years.

ACUTE NONLYMPHOCYTIC LEUKEMIA

The French-American-British (FAB) classification defines seven variants of ANLL that differ with respect to cell line and differentiation: M-1, acute myeloblastic leukemia without differentiation; M-2, acute myeloblastic leukemia with differentiation; M-3, acute promyelocytic leukemia; M-4, acute myelomonocytic leukemia; M-5, acute monoblastic leukemia; M-6, acute erythroleukemia; and M-7, acute megakaryoblastic leukemia.

Treatment

With the exception of acute monoblastic leukemia, the acute nonlymphocytic leukemias are treated similarly. VP-16 (etoposide) and VM-26 (teniposide)* are especially active against malignant monoblasts, prompting some oncologists to incorporate one of these agents into the treatment of monoblastic disease.

What may be regarded as standard induction therapy for ANLL is summarized in Table 2. Although ostensibly simple, this therapy requires skill and the availability of intensive supportive care. Bone marrow ablation is an inevitable consequence of effective therapy in all but the promyelocytic variant, and mucositis and invasive infections are common complications. Decisions regarding the timing and intensity of second and third courses of induction therapy tax the judgment of the most experienced oncologists. The treatment of this disease should not be taken on by the uninitiated.

Cytosine arabinoside (Cytosar) is given by constant intravenous infusion for 7 days and daunorubicin (Cerubidine) by intravenous push for 3 days ("7-and-3"). For children less than 3 years of age, the doses of these drugs are based on body weight rather than on surface area. For cytosine arabinoside the dose is 3.3 mg per kg, and for daunorubicin it is 1.5 mg per kg. As for the dose of intrathecal methotrexate in ALL, the dose of intrathecal cytosine arabianoside is based on age

---

*Orphan drug available from the National Information Center for Orphan Drugs and Rare Diseases, 800-336-4797.

TABLE 2. **Chemotherapeutic Management of Acute Nonlymphocytic Leukemia**

Induction

Cycle 1

Daunorubicin, 45 mg/M^2 IV, days 0 through 2

Cytosine arabinoside, 100 mg/M^2 IV, by constant infusion, days 0 through 6

Cytosine arabinoside, 20 mg (less than 1 year age); 30 mg (1 to 2 years); 50 mg (2 to 3 years); 70 mg (3 years and over) IT, day 0

Cycle 2

Daunorubicin, 45 mg/M^2 IV, days 0 through 1 or 0 through 2

Cytosine arabinoside, 100 mg/M^2 IV, by constant infusion, days 0 through 4 or 0 through 6

Cytosine arabinoside (same dose as in Cycle 1), IT, day 0

Consolidation

Cytosine arabinoside, 3000 mg/M^2 IV over 1 hour every 12 hours for 12 doses (days 0 though 5)

Daunorubicin, 30 mg/M^2 IV, day 6

rather than on surface area or body weight. The timing and duration of the second cycle of cytosine arabinoside and daunorubicin is determined by the appearance of a day-14 bone marrow biopsy specimen. If there is persistent disease, the full 7-day cycle is repeated irrespective of marrow cellularity unless the patient is compromised by systemic infection or mucositis. If the marrow is disease-free and moderately hypocellular, the second cycle is limited to 5 days of cytosine arabinoside and 2 days of daunorubicin ("5-and-2"). If the marrow is disease-free and severely hypocellular, the "5-and-2" cycle is delayed until there is evidence of bone marrow recovery. A third cycle may be required if a bone marrow biopsy specimen is still involved by leukemia after the second cycle.

Since the prospect for cure with chemotherapy alone is less promising for children with ANLL than for those with ALL, bone marrow transplantation is recommended once remission is achieved if a compatible marrow donor is available. If transplantation is not an option, an intensive consolidation course of therapy is given following full reconstitution of blood neutrophils and platelets. The consolidation phase outlined in Table 2 utilizes high dose cytosine arabinoside at 12-hour intervals for 6 days followed by daunorubicin. For children less than 3 years of age, high-dose cytosine arabinoside is calculated as 100 mg per kg and daunorubicin as 1.0 mg per kg. Consolidation therapy is followed by 3 to 5 weeks of bone marrow aplasia. At present there is no convincing evidence that maintenance therapy following marrow recovery confers further protection from disease recurrence.

Supportive Care

The importance of comprehensive supportive care throughout all phases of treatment cannot

be overemphasized. Therapeutic approaches having curative potential mandate easy access to blood component therapy, an aggressive approach to the detection and management of infectious complications, attention to nutritional and metabolic needs, and provision of a comprehensive system of psychosocial support for the patient and family.

Venous Access

Most intensive treatment regimens require the placement of an indwelling right atrial line for venous access, especially in small children. A totally implantable system (Port-a-Cath) is well tolerated by children and is associated with fewer infectious complications than lines that exit from the chest wall (Broviac and Hickman catheters). Venous access lines are used for blood sampling as well as for the administration of drugs, blood products, and parenteral nutrition. Some severely irritating and sclerosing chemotherapeutic agents can be given only into central veins. The widespread application of venous access lines has improved the quality of life for children with cancer and has permitted the development of increasingly comprehensive treatment protocols.

Transfusion Therapy

Transfusion support is necessary for most patients during remission induction and during consolidation in the more intensive protocols. As patients who require transfusion therapy are heavily immunosuppressed, all blood products should be radiated (1500 to 5000 cGy) to prevent graft-versus-host disease. Packed red blood cells are given in increments of 10 ml per kg to maintain the hemoglobin concentration above 7 to 8 grams per dl. Platelets are given for symptomatic bleeding related to thrombocytopenia and for platelet counts less than 10,000 per μl in the absence of bleeding. The platelet count should be maintained above 30,000 per μl in patients whose white blood cell counts are in excess of 50,000 per μl and in those who require invasive procedures (such as lumbar puncture). In the unsensitized child, 1 unit of platelets per M^2 increases the platelet count by approximately 10,000 per μl.

Infectious Complications

During periods of severe neutropenia (absolute neutrophil count less than 200 to 500 per μl) patients are cautioned to avoid unnecessary exposure to crowds. Hand washing with an iodine-containing compound (Betadine, Foamaseptic) is practiced by personnel caring for the patient. The skin is prepared with povidone-iodine scrubbing before needle punctures. A stool softener (Colace,

50 to 100 mg daily) is given to prevent the development of anal fissures. The use of rectal thermometers and suppositories is avoided.

Fever occurring during periods of neutropenia is assumed to be due to bacterial disease. Broad-spectrum antibiotic coverage is instituted promptly once blood cultures have been obtained. The time-honored combination consists of cephalothin (Keflin), 170 mg per kg per day in 6 divided doses with a maximum daily dose of 12 grams; gentamicin, 6 mg per kg per day in 4 doses; and carbenicillin, 500 mg per kg per day in 6 doses with a maximum daily dose of 36 grams. Ceftazidime (Tazicef) alone in a dose of 90 mg per kg per day in 3 divided doses (maximum daily dose 6 grams) may be equally effective. Amphotericin B (Fungizone) is added if fever and neutropenia persist for more than 7 days.

Pneumocystic carinii pneumonia is more easily prevented than treated. Trimethoprim-sulfamethoxazole (Bactrim, Septra) is started following remission induction and continued for the duration of chemotherapy in a dose of 5 mg per kg of trimethoprim given in 2 divided doses 3 times weekly. For children who have not had varicella, varicella-zoster immune globulin (VZIG) is given within 72 hours of varicella exposure in a dose of 1 vial per 10 kg body weight.

Metabolic Complications

The massive destruction of leukemic cells that follows the institution of therapy may cause hyperuricemia, hyperphosphatemia, and hypocalcemia (tumor lysis syndrome). Renal failure resulting from the deposition of urate crystals in renal tubules may ensue. These potential metabolic complications must be anticipated, especially in patients with high white blood cell counts and bulky extramedullary disease. Prior to the institution of chemotherapy, a water diuresis is established with aggressive intravenous hydration (3200 ml per M^2 per day). Sodium is given as sodium bicarbonate (starting dose 40 mEq per M^2 per day) rather than sodium chloride to maintain the urine pH above 7.5. Allopurinol is given once daily in a dose of 10 mg per kg.

Psychosocial Support

The psychosocial stresses to which children and their families are exposed are enormous and are best addressed prospectively by a team that includes representatives from pediatric oncology nursing, social service, child life, and child psychiatry in addition to pediatric oncology. Patient and parent education about the disease and its treatment is of fundamental importance. Patients are encouraged to continue participation in all school and social activities to the fullest extent possible. As a corollary of this philosophy, hospitalization is avoided unless dictated by needs that cannot be provided in an outpatient setting. Community, state, and federal resources may have to be tapped to assist the family with medical expenses, transportation, and living arrangements at times when immediate access to the hospital is required.

THE CHRONIC LEUKEMIAS

method of
ARTHUR SAWITSKY, M.D., and
KANTI R. RAI, M.D.
Long Island Jewish Medical Center
New Hyde Park, New York

CHRONIC GRANULOCYTIC LEUKEMIA

Chronic granulocytic leukemia (CGL) is a hematologic and proliferative disorder involving a pluripotent stem cell common to the granulocyte, erythroid, and megakaryocytic lineages. It is characterized by a cytogenetic abnormality, the Philadelphia (Ph^1) chromosome, which represents translocation of reciprocal portions of the long arms of chromosomes 9 and 22. The Ph^1 chromosome has been found in approximately 90 to 100 per cent of dividing bone marrow cells but is not found in dividing marrow fibroblasts or in somatic cells or peripheral blood lymphocytes. The disease is considered to be a clonal neoplasm, and the clonal origin of CGL has been demonstrated not only by cytogenetic but also by enzyme glucose-6-phosphate dehydrogenase studies. CGL is predominantly a disease of young and middle-aged adults, with an equal sex distribution.

The clinical features of adult CGL include progressive splenomegaly, anemia, and a leukocytosis characterized by an increase in neutrophils, eosinophils, and basophils. A rare form of juvenile CGL differs from the adult form, is found in very young children, and is Ph^1-negative. In this form of CGL a variable degree of leukocytosis and even leukopenia may be present. An initial anemia and thrombocytopenia are usual findings. The spleen may be very large, and lymphadenopathy is noted. Treatment response is poor and overall survival short.

Approximately 3 to 5 per cent of adult patients with clinical evidence of chronic granulocytic leukemia do not show the presence of the Ph^1 chromosome; their disorder is called Ph^1-negative CGL (see section on Cytogenetics below) and has a more rapid clinical course and a poorer response to chemotherapy than Ph^1-positive CGL. At diagnosis these patients present with a lower initial leukocyte count, mild thrombocytopenia, and exceptional splenomegaly.

CGL has three phases: (1) an initial, chronic phase in which disease progression is slow and the clinical course appears to be stable, (2) an accelerated, myeloproliferative phase usually associated with the onset of anemia and/or thrombocytopenia, and (3) blast crisis, in which rapid clinical progression of disease is suggestive of acute leukemia. The hallmark of CGL at any stage is the pervasive fatigue, anorexia, and malaise present without obvious cause. Clinical findings in Ph[1]-positive patients that appear to influence the prognosis and are indicative of progressive disease include marked thrombocytosis or thrombocytopenia, progressive anemia, continuing increase in peripheral blood basophils, and marked splenomegaly or hepatomegaly, especially when these findings are not responsive to chemotherapy. The most ominous prognostic sign is an increased number of blast cells in the peripheral blood and/or bone marrow.

Cytogenetics and Molecular Aberrations

The Ph[1] chromosome is known to reflect a reciprocal translocation of small regions of chromosomes 9 and 22. These regions are closely associated with the cellular oncogenes c-abl and c-sis, and their translocation results in a shortened chromosome 22, the Ph[1] chromosome. The oncogene c-abl translocated from chromosome 9 fuses with the "breakpoint cluster region" (bcr) of chromosome 22 to form a new gene, bcr-abl. This aberrant DNA structure results in transcription of an abnormal bcr-abl mRNA that is translated into a chimeric 210-kilodalton bcr-abl protein. The tyrosine protein kinase enzymatic activity of this p210 protein differs from that of its normal homologue, a 145-kilodalton protein. This change in location of the c-abl oncogene may activate its tumor potential. It is of interest that recently it has been found that there are a small percentage of patients with Ph[1]-negative CGL leukemia who show unsuspected subchromosomal aberrations including bcr and c-abl gene rearrangements (this suggests that there may be more than one mechanism by which bcr rearrangements occur in chronic granulocytic leukemia). These latter patients appear to have a clinical course consistent with Ph[1]-positive disease, in contrast to other Ph[1]-negative patients.

Cytogenetic analysis of Ph[1]-negative CGL reveals a normal karyotype in about two thirds of these patients, and in the remainder a variety of cytogenetic anomalies, most commonly trisomy of chromosome 8.

Treatment in the Chronic Phase

We will restrict our discussion of treatment to adult Ph[1]-positive CGL. The selected treatment schedule must take into account the clinical phase of disease under treatment. Treatment strategies differ for patients in the chronic phase from those recommended for patients in the accelerated phase or in blast crisis.

During the *chronic phase* of CGL, the therapeutic objective is to reduce or maintain the total body burden of leukemic cells at as low a level as possible without producing undue toxicity. Current aggressive therapy, unless frankly ablative and requiring bone marrow transplant for support, has not shown any greater survival benefit than a more restrained approach. It can be anticipated that patients in chronic-phase CGL will be responsive to treatment by single agent chemotherapy or by radiotherapy. Many asymptomatic patients presenting in the chronic phase do not require immediate therapy. Since no survival benefit can be demonstrated by any aggressive therapeutic schedule or any special combination of chemotherapeutic agents, the choice of initial therapy frequently depends upon convenience to the patient and physician and the absence of serious toxicity.

In the past, busulfan (Myleran), an alkylating agent, has been the drug of choice for initial treatment. More recently our initial drug choice has been hydroxyurea (Hydrea). Although the exact mechanism of action of hydroxyurea is unknown, cell kill and tumor load reduction is achieved through the suppression of DNA synthesis. Therapy is begun with a drug dose of 30 to 40 mg per kg per day given orally (i.e., approximately 2.0 to 2.5 grams per day) for an average adult. The peripheral leukocyte count reduces rapidly, but with reduction of the dose of hydroxyurea or discontinuance of the drug, the peripheral leukocyte count rebounds rather quickly. Therefore, over a period of 1 to 2 weeks, doses of hydroxyurea need be adjusted so that the white blood cell count is reduced to a reasonable level, usually between 10,000 and 20,000 cells per μl. If busulfan is given, usually the initial daily dose is 0.1 to 0.15 mg per kg, with a maximum initial daily dose of 8 mg. The daily dose is gradually reduced as the peripheral white cell count declines. A rapid decrease in white blood cells or in platelet count requires prompt dose reduction.

Although hydroxyurea is no more effective than busulfan in prolonging overall survival or in stabilizing the chronic phase of CGL, we prefer hydroxyurea because its use is not attended by the severe myelosuppression or the late-appearing chronic pulmonary toxicity that may be serious complications of busulfan therapy. Regardless of which agent is used, hyperuricemia requires the simultaneous administration of allopurinol (Zyloprim), and the patient should be encouraged to have good urinary flow.

With continued initial therapy, stabilization of the chronic phase can be anticipated in the majority of patients. The stable phase is marked by a return toward normal of the abnormal pretreatment peripheral blood values as well as a reduction in the size of spleen and liver. A small minority of patients may continue to manifest a treatment-resistant large spleen during this phase. Leukocyte alkaline phosphatase values ranging from extremely low to absent at the time of diagnosis may or may not return to normal levels. The characteristic Ph^1 chromosome found in the bone marrow continues to be identified in the stable phase of CGL, although in some patients the abnormal chromosome will be found in a much lower fraction of myeloid cells. When clinical stabilization of the chronic phase has been attained, bone marrow transplant therapy should be considered.

When splenomegaly is extreme and causes significant pain or discomfort, we advise splenic radiation. Radiation therapy is frequently associated with a significant decrease in the peripheral blood leukocyte count, and we have seen severe myelosuppression and even bone marrow aplasia following its use. Although splenectomy has also been advocated, it fails to postpone or prevent blast crisis. We have not used splenectomy in any *routine* regimen.

To postpone the onset of blast crisis, unsuccessful attempts have been made to eradicate or reduce the number of malignant Ph^1 cells by aggressive multiple agent chemotherapy, including cytosine arabinoside, daunorubicin and/or cyclophasphamide.

Maintenance Therapy

We employ an intermittent treatment course schedule with hydroxyurea rather than a continuous one. We try to maintain the peripheral blood count between 10,000 and 20,000 cells per μl, as we have found this level to provide the best quality of life for the patient. When close observation of the patient is not possible during the treatment phase, busulfan may be substituted for hydroxyurea. We prefer to use as little busulfan as possible because of the relatively frequent adverse drug reactions to busulfan, including bone marrow hypoplasia, increased skin pigmentation, a wasting syndrome with features of Addison's disease, and pulmonary fibrosis. We have also seen cataracts and endocardial fibrosis. Amenorrhea may follow busulfan treatment but

the latter may also be due to the chronic leukemia seen in CGL patients.

Treatment in the Aggressive Disease Phase and Blast Crisis

The chronic phase of CGL is compatible with a good quality of life and good performance status for the patient. However, after a variable period of time—in some cases in as short a period as 10 to 12 months, but in most after approximately 2 years—a clinical change is noted. An increase in peripheral blood cells to above 50,000 per μl occurs, frequently accompanied by a decrease in hemoglobin or platelets. Peripheral basophilia, at times to levels of 20 per cent of the peripheral granulocytes, is present and a few blast cells and promyelocytes may be seen. An increasing abnormality of red cell morphology suggesting bone marrow fibrosis may be found. The development of fever without infection, increasing splenomegaly, and increasing fatigue may be initial symptoms of this phase. The previous treatment program is no longer effective and within a few weeks or months, the peripheral blast cell population becomes greater than 10 per cent and large numbers of promyelocytes are also found. Bone marrow examination at this time confirms the presence of excessive numbers of myeloblasts and promyelocytes exceeding 30 per cent of the total nucleated marrow cell count. Cytogenetic analysis may show large numbers of Ph^1-positive metaphases, and occasionally some metaphases may contain two or more Philadelphia chromosomes. In many patients, aneuploidy is also described.

When the numbers of myeloblasts and promyelocytes exceed 30 per cent either in the peripheral blood or in the bone marrow, the *blast phase* of the disease is said to be present. The prognosis is extremely grave and most patients will die within 6 months after the onset of blast phase.

Although the dominant cell in most blast crises is a myeloblast, in approximately one third of patients the blast cells have lymphoid characteristics not only in morphology but also because of the presence of the enzyme terminal deoxynucleotidyl transferase. Chemotherapy that includes vincristine and prednisone may produce an initial response in as high as 60 per cent of this latter group of patients, but the responses are brief and of no lasting benefit. Current therapy for blast crisis with myeloid expression includes varying regimens with combination chemotherapy, but none have been satisfactory. The combination of hydroxyurea, 6-mercaptopurine, and prednisone has been helpful in some patients; other combinations, including 5-azacytidine with cytosine arabinoside, and 6-thioguanine with daunomycin (with or without the addition of etoposide), have produced 20 to 30 per cent partial remission rates with only a 6- or 7-month median duration of survival. Regardless of the regimen used, marrow hypoplasia or marrow ablation is the goal of therapy. In all patients, supportive care and emotional support for patient and family becomes extremely important. Where phase 1– or phase 2–based investigational clinical trials are available, the patient should be encouraged to participate in such trials.

Alternative Approaches to Therapy

Our inability to significantly control the disease in almost all patients with CGL has given rise to many alternative approaches for therapy. None of the following treatment schedules has been proved to be materially better than current therapy, although some are still under clinical investigation and evaluation.

Radiation Therapy

Local splenic radiation has been used over the past 60 years, but no one schedule has provided results of great benefit. This modality has been reserved for the management of patients with symptomatic splenomegaly or for those patients in whom anemia or thrombocytopenia has been ascribed to hypersplenism due to the enlarged spleen. Local radiation therapy has produced good spleen size reduction; however, marrow hypoplasia has resulted in some cases, with severe adverse toxicity.

Splenectomy

Splenectomy during the chronic phase of GCL has been recommended as a rapid method of tumor load reduction as well as a means of eliminating the source of what has been thought to be the origin of a recirculating leukemic cell population. Following splenectomy, an aggressive chemotherapeutic program to eradicate the Ph[1] chromosome has been undertaken. Unfortunately, only transient benefit has resulted from this treatment plan, with no significant prolongation of survival. Early splenectomy has also been suggested to prevent the occasionally massive splenomegaly seen during the aggressive and late stages of CGL, but the results of several clinical trials evaluating early splenectomy were equivocal. Splenectomy in blast-phase CGL has, in our experience, provided little or no benefit to the great majority of patients and has frequently resulted in severe morbidity and mortality.

Interferons

Recent publications have given hope that alpha interferons may be active in CGL, and hemato-logic response has been reported in many patients. In approximately half of these, a reduction in the percentage of Ph[1]-positive cells in the bone marrow suggests a place for interferons in the treatment of patients with this disorder. Clinical trials are currently in progress, and it is yet to be demonstrated that treatment with these agents is superior to conventional therapy in terms of survival.

Bone Marrow Transplantation

A potentially curative therapy for chronic granulocytic leukemia is bone marrow transplantation (BMT). The best results have been obtained in patients brought to stable chronic phase by chemotherapy and then referred for syngeneic or allogeneic bone marrow transplantation. Present data indicate that approximately 65 per cent of patients so treated survive free of disease beyond 5 years and are "cured" of their disease. Additionally, patients treated in blast crisis have a 10 to 20 per cent chance of such disease-free survival. Unfortunately, significant morbidity and mortality still attend BMT. Because patients older than 50 years of age and patients lacking an HLA-identical donor must be excluded from BMT, only 10 to 15 per cent of patients seen in practice are eligible for this treatment. Although important strides have been made to control graft-versus-host disease utilizing cyclosporine and T-cell depleted donor marrow, further progress is required before full evaluation of this potentially curative therapy can be made.

CHRONIC LYMPHOCYTIC LEUKEMIA

During the past decade, our clinical observation suggests that following clinical and laboratory definition of the clinical stage and activity of chronic lymphocytic leukemia (CLL), treatment that induces clinical remission may be associated with prolonged survival and improvement in quality of life for the patient. There is as yet no randomized clinical trial that has properly addressed that assumption. Recent investigation of the molecular biology of the development and maturation of lymphoid disease and the sequential stages involved in B and T cell development has provided an enormous advance in our understanding of both normal and neoplastic tissues and therefore of chronic lymphocytic leukemia.

CLL is a lymphoproliferative disorder associated with the accumulation of mature-appearing lymphocytes. These cells of clonal origin are not easily stimulated in vitro and therefore are long-lived cells whose increasing tumor mass promotes progressive enlargement of the various lymphoid tissues, which if unchecked leads eventually to death of the host. The diagnosis of CLL is made by the presence of an absolute lymphocytosis in both peripheral blood and bone marrow. The diagnosis is not difficult and requires only an absolute persistent lymphocytosis equal to or greater than 5000 cells per μl, together with bone marrow infiltration of these cells equal to or greater than 30 per cent of all nucleated cells. The clonal aspect of the disease is evidenced by the predominance of a morphologically uniform mature lymphocyte population with identical surface membrane features, in which the light chain portion of the surface immunoglobulin is of a single type, either kappa or lambda. In a similar manner, idiotypic specificity of the surface immunoglobulin heavy chain type is present. Studies indicate that 95 per cent or more of all CLL patients are so characterized and therefore have B-cell CLL. Other variants of CLL, such as T-cell CLL and prolymphocytic leukemia, are unusual.

In the Western world, B-cell CLL is diagnosed in about 30 per cent of all leukemia patients and occurs in both black and white populations. In the Orient, however, CLL is much less frequently diagnosed and accounts for only 2 to 3 per cent of all leukemia. In that population, an adult T-cell form of CLL has been described. B-cell CLL is a disease of the elderly, unusual in individuals less than age 40 and rare in those less than 20 years of age, but it has been reported even in childhood. The incidence of the disease increases in each decade, with a peak in the sixth decade. New cases continue to be diagnosed even in patients in their 80's. About 90 per cent of all CLL patients are over the age of 50 at the time of diagnosis. It is likely that the incidence peak is modified not only by age but also as a function of time of onset of clinical signs and symptoms. It is well recognized that a unknown number of asymptomatic patients have undetected CLL for many years prior to diagnosis.

CLL has been observed in family members, but currently there is no evidence to prove that this disease is genetically transmitted. A related phenomenon may be the finding of abnormal alteration in immune reactivity documented in many families of patients with CLL or with other lymphoproliferative disorders.

In B-cell CLL, the major population of lymphocytes exhibits characteristics usually associated with B lymphocytes. The surface immunoglobulin is most often IgM, with frequent co-expression of IgD; infrequently, surface IgG predominates. A quantitative decrease in the surface immunoglobulin is present, and this together with the predominance of SIgM associated with SIgD, as well as a high proportion of mouse red cell rosetting

B cells, suggests that the B cell in CLL is a cell at an early stage of the B-cell differentiation pathway. Investigations utilizing monoclonal antibodies have been crucial in the attempt to interpret and define the recognized heterogeneity of the clinical presentation and response to treatment of patients whose lymphocytes are of similar morphologic appearance. These studies suggest that tumors of B-cell origin may be divided into a number of variably mature B-cell types; a pre-B-cell type as well as immature, very early, and secretory B-cell types. Most patients with B-cell CLL have a major cell population whose antigen expression would place them in the midstage of B-cell differentiation. More recently, studies have shown a commitment to the B-cell development demonstrable in the rearrangement of their immunoglobulin genes. Lymphocytes at this stage also show receptors for mouse erythrocytes, and these receptors are lost with continuing lymphocyte maturation.

Although the B cells constitute the vast majority of the cell population in the peripheral blood, it must be appreciated that there are also T cells present. In some patients, a normal helper suppressor cell ratio is maintained, but in many patients an increase in suppressor cells is noted. With progressive disease, the proportion of T cells decreases in the circulating blood, but because of the overall lymphocytosis, the absolute number of T cells may even be abnormally high. These aberrations in lymphocyte population are associated with impaired immune function that becomes progressively more evident and severe with disease progression. Numerous autoimmune phenomena may be noted, including Coombs' positive autoimmune hemolytic anemia, which is present in approximately 10 per cent of all CLL patients at some time during the course of their disease. Thrombocytopenia due to an autoimmune mechanism may be noted early in the disease, although identification of specific platelet antibodies may not be demonstrable. Increased suppressor T-cell activity may account for anemia due to red cell aplasia. The immune abnormalities produce not only B-cell–related hypogammaglobulinemia but also diminished cell-mediated immunity, which is demonstrable with clinical progression of disease.

Clinical Staging of Disease

Currently, the staging criteria for patients with CLL are those proposed by us in 1975 (the Rai staging system). The five clinical stages are outlined in Table 1. In Stages III and IV, enlargement of lymph nodes, spleen, and liver may or may not be present. The median survival time

TABLE 1. **Rai Staging System for Chronic Lymphocytic Leukemia**

Stage:
0: Lymphocytosis only of peripheral blood and bone marrow
I: Lymphocytosis plus enlarged lymph nodes
II: Lymphocytosis plus enlarged spleen and/or liver; lymph nodes may not be simultaneously enlarged
III: Lymphocytosis plus anemia (hemoglobin equal to or less than 11 grams per dl)
IV: Lymphocytosis plus thrombocytopenia (platelets less than 100×10^3 per µl)

from diagnosis was found to be 150 months for Stage 0, 101 months for Stage I, 71 months for Stage II, and 19 months for Stages III and IV. If the anemia or thrombocytopenia is of autoimmune origin (that is, due to peripheral destruction), the prognosis for that patient is better than for the patient in whom anemia and thrombocytopenia occur because of bone marrow failure. Correction of anemia and thrombocytopenia by splenectomy or by interruption of the autoimmune cell destruction process is associated with improved clinical stage and improved prognosis to that of the new clinical stage. Further study of the survival curves indicates that there may be in fact only three distinct biologic groups of patients rather than the five indicated by our staging nomenclature. Stage 0 appears to have a survival curve of its own, whereas those of Stages I and II are superimposable; similarly, the survival curves of Stages III and IV are identical. Additional prognostic factors that have been proposed include the finding of splenomegaly without lymphadenopathy, the degree of absolute peripheral blood, lymphocytosis, the lymphocyte doubling-time in the peripheral blood, and especially the pattern of lymphocyte infiltration in bone marrow biopsy. A pattern of diffuse lymphocytic infiltration of the bone marrow is associated with poor prognosis and advanced-stage CLL as compared with a nondiffuse type of bone marrow involvement.

A second staging system was proposed by Binet and his colleagues and modified the Rai staging system as follows: Patients with anemia and thrombocytopenia are grouped together in a single Stage C. All other patients are subdivided according to the number of clinically enlarged lymph node sites or regions; five regions are described that may be unilaterally or bilaterally enlarged: cervical, axillary, inguinal, spleen, and liver. In the Binet staging system, if the number of enlarged lymph node sites is equal to or greater than 3, the patient is assigned to Stage B. All other patients bearing two or fewer involved lymph node sites are placed in Stage A. When tested by a multivariant analysis, there was an excellent correlation for survival. The two systems have been integrated by an International Workshop on CLL convened in 1980 as shown in the Table 2. Both systems, however, fail to distinguish within each stage those patients whose disease remains stable or indolent from those in whom disease is active and has taken a more aggressive course. *Cytogenetic studies* may also be useful for prognosis, but more correlative data are required. Lymphocytes from patients with CLL have a very low, spontaneous mitotic index. Therefore, in the past it was not easy to define cytogenetic abnormalities. More recently, following the use of polyclonal B-cell mitogens, cytogenetic studies have shown that the presence of abnormal karyotypes such as trisomy-12 or other chromosomal abnormalities may identify patients with the poorer prognosis. The chromosomes most frequently involved in abnormalities are those associated with immune function; chromosomes 14, 2, and 22 as well as C group chromosomes 8 and 12 have been most frequently described.

Observation Phase

Before starting treatment in patients with B-cell CLL, a period of observation is necessary over a minimum period of 2 to 3 months. The exception to this general rule is the patient in obvious need of supportive or antileukemic therapy because of progressive disease. During the observation period, clinical staging and laboratory and x-ray data are obtained; when no signs or symptoms of clinical progression of disease are present, the observation period is further extended to establish a reliable baseline pattern of disease activity. The phase of observation should include an evaluation of weight loss, unexplained fever, incidence of infectious episodes, anorexia, dyspnea and/or palpitation, lymph node enlargement, and abdominal distension or discomfort.

TABLE 2. **Combined Rai and Binet Staging Systems for Chronic Lymphocytic Leukemia as Recommended by the International Workshop on CLL**

Stage	Stage Notation	Clinical Characteristics
A	A(0), A(I), A(II)	No anemia, no thrombocytopenia, and fewer than three involved lymphoid regions
B	B(I), B(II)	No anemia or thrombocytopenia and three or more involved lymphoid regions
C	C(III), C(IV)	Anemia (<10 grams/dl) and/or thrombocytopenia (<100,000 platelets/µl)

Emotional reactions to the diagnosis may vary widely and many patients will benefit from emotional support. In general, treatment is initiated if any of the following indications is present:

1. Disease-related progressive symptoms.

2. Evidence of progressive bone marrow failure—i.e., worsening anemia or thrombocytopenia.

3. Presence of autoimmune hemolytic anemia or thrombocytopenia.

4. Massive splenomegaly with or without evidence of hypersplenism.

5. Bulky lymphoid disease.

6. Progressive hyperlymphocytosis. The rate of increase of the blood lymphocyte count is a more reliable indication to start treatment than any particular threshold value. In general, in the absence of other indications it is usual practice to treat a patient whose total leukocyte count reaches 150,000 cells per μl.

7. Increased incidence of infectious episodes indicating increased susceptibility to bacterial and viral infection. Neutropenia or progressively declining neutrophilia is not a reliable criterion of need for therapy; increased numbers of infectious episodes or local infections, however, are.

Treatment Phase

Patients who have Stage 0 disease are usually asymptomatic and require no therapy. These patients should be monitored at regular intervals of 2 to 4 months. The role of chemotherapy in asymptomatic Stage I and Stage II patients is an unresolved issue. Available cell markers and other diagnostic tools do not offer any clue to differentiate these two subsets.

In a study reported by Cancer and Leukemia Group B (CALGB), asymptomatic patients with Stage I and Stage II disease were randomly assigned either to a group that received no chemotherapy or to a group treated with chlorambucil therapy. Although the patients who received chlorambucil showed evidence of some delay in progression of disease compared with those patients who were not treated, overall survival time of both patient groups was the same. Based on these data, we do not believe that cytotoxic therapy is indicated in asymptomatic patients with early-stage CLL. At present, there are no reliable guidelines for starting treatment of patients with clinical Stage I or Stage II disease. However, it is generally accepted practice to treat patients who have symptoms clearly related to their CLL.

Patients with Stage III and IV disease require therapy, and a controlled CALGB clinical trial has demonstrated that patients in these stages responding with complete or partial remission were benefited. Their median survival time increased to more than 4 years compared with nonresponding patients whose survival time remained at about 20 months.

Chemotherapy

Therapy is usually started with a single alkylator drug, and chlorambucil (Leukeran) has been the initial agent of choice. This drug is administered in an intermittent fashion at an initial dose of 0.4 mg per kg orally every 3 weeks. If reduction in lymphocytosis, lymphadenopathy, or organomegaly is deemed less than desirable, the dose schedule is adjusted to a 2-week interval. If the reduction in lymphocytosis is too great or other toxicity is noted, either dose or interval is adjusted accordingly. If no toxicity ensues, we continue the chlorambucil at the highest tolerated dose. If stable or asymptomatic disease is achieved, we continue the chlorambucil for at least 6 to 10 months thereafter.

Corticosteroids are effective in controlling autoimmune phenomena and in some patients may be used as initial therapy (i.e., for patients whose chief symptomatology is due to thrombocytopenia or hemolytic anemia). Prednisone may be used alone or, more frequently, in combination with the alkylator; when given in combination, it is given at a daily oral dose of 1 mg per kg for 10 days.

Cyclophosphamide can be used as an alternative to chlorambucil but may be accompanied by a variable degree of alopecia or cystitis. Various clinical trials using busulfan and estrogens have not been encouraging. A beneficial response in CLL must be carefully monitored and defined because although vigorous treatment will reduce the white cell count and lymph node and spleen size, it may also produce significant anemia and thrombocytopenia.

Combination chemotherapy is employed when chlorambucil or cyclophosphamide with or without prednisone becomes clinically ineffective. Unfortunately, such second-line combination chemotherapy is almost always only marginally effective in controlling advancing disease. It is also important to recognize early when first-line therapy is failing, so that bone marrow reserve is not overly compromised. The most frequent combination chemotherapy used has been cyclophosphamide (600 mg per M²), vincristine (1.5 mg), and prednisone (1 mg per kg) with or without the addition of small doses of doxorubicin. Doxorubicin has been added at a dose of about 20 to 25 mg per square meter given at 3-week intervals. More intensive programs incorporating Carmustine and L-phenylalanine mustard in combination with cyclophosphamide, vincristine, and prednisone have also been used, but this multiple drug combination has proved to be more toxic without superior benefit.

Radiation Therapy

Splenic irradiation or radiation of localized bulky lymph nodes can be very effective in the reduction of tumor when drug therapy has failed. In some patients with bulky disease who are otherwise asymptomatic, we have initiated therapy with local radiation. We do not use mediastinal irradiation because we have found that modality to be associated with unacceptable levels of toxicity and morbidity. Extracorporeal radiation produces a predictable decrease in lymphoid body burden in these patients, but unfortunately the response is very transient. Total body irradiation has been associated with significant toxicity in our experience, but has been reported by others to provide benefit in some patients.

Surgery

Splenectomy has been used in patients with serious cytopenia not responding well to corticosteroids, as well as for certain patients with a large or persistent and painful splenomegaly. Although many patients have undergone splenectomy, there has been no randomized trial that demonstrated a survival advantage for the splenectomized group. Should splenectomy become necessary, however, patients with CLL do tolerate the procedure. Supportive clinical care and good laboratory and blood bank services are essential.

Other Treatment

Therapy with biologic modifiers such as alpha interferon and monoclonal antibodies is still in the clinical investigational stage, and the results to date have not generated enthusiasm. Other studies with deoxycoformycin, fludarabinemonophosphate, and other adenosine deaminase inhibitors are currently in progress. Leukopheresis utilizing cell separation machines has proved of only temporary benefit and, if used, must be followed by adequate dosage of cytotoxic chemotherapy.

Supportive Therapy

Good supportive therapy for patients with CLL is an extremely important facet of their overall care. Transfusions are rarely required until the hemoglobin concentration is below 10 grams per dl or the patient manifests symptoms of hypoxia. In the older patient population, cardiac status must be determined during the clinical evaluation. The use of androgens to stimulate erythropoiesis has occasionally provided erythroid stimulation, and the use of danazol with prednisone has been useful to control particularly resistant Coombs-positive hemolytic anemia.

More recently we have used intravenous gammaglobulin (IVGG) to control autoimmune hemolytic anemia and autoimmune thrombocytopenia and to protect patients from bacterial sepsis. We have found that IVGG produced a favorable response and, in one patient, reversed the need for a proposed splenectomy. IVGG is given at a loading dose of 400 mg per kg daily for 3 days. The same dose is repeated at weekly intervals for 2 to 3 weeks and thereafter at 3-week intervals. Following the use of IVGG, we have been able to lower the dose of steroid to a minimal maintenance level. We have also given IVGG to patients whose serum immune globulins have fallen to hypogammaglobulinemic levels and in whom the frequency of infectious episodes has become clinically serious. In such patients we give 400 mg per kg of IVGG at 3- to 4-week intervals. This regimen has provided significant clinical benefit.

Control of infectious disease is ultimately a most troublesome and important factor for patient survival. Any fever or any evidence of secondary microbial infection requires immediate attention and laboratory workup to pinpoint the site and the identity of the causal agent. Prompt and vigorous antibacterial therapy is indicated. Herpes zoster can be especially dangerous, and at the first sign of this complication acyclovir therapy should be instituted. A fatal, generalized herpes zoster infection may occur in a patient treated casually.

NON-HODGKIN'S LYMPHOMAS

method of
PHILIP BIERMAN, M.D., and
JAMES O. ARMITAGE, M.D.
University of Nebraska Medical Center
Omaha, Nebraska

With the advent of modern combination chemotherapy it is clear that approximately 50 per cent of patients with advanced intermediate and high-grade non-Hodgkin's lymphoma can be cured of their disease. In these individuals it is of utmost importance to have accurate diagnosis and staging, since therapy with curative intent will be based on these studies. A minimal staging evaluation should include a complete history and physical examination, complete blood count and chemistry panel, chest radiograph and abdominal computerized tomography, and bilateral iliac crest bone marrow biopsies. When there is any doubt about the diagnosis, a repeat biopsy should be per-

TABLE 1. **Ann Arbor Staging Classification for Non-Hodgkin's Lymphoma**

Stage I:	Involvement of a single lymph node region (I) or of a single extralymphatic organ or site (I_E).
Stage II:	Involvement of two or more lymph node regions on the same side of the diaphragm (II) or localized involvement of an extralymphatic organ or site and of one or more lymph node regions on the same side of the diaphragm (II_E).
Stage III:	Involvement of lymph node regions on both sides of the diaphragm (III), which may also be accompanied by localized involvement of an extralymphatic organ or site (III_E) or by involvement of the spleen (III_S), or by involvement of both (III_{SE}).
Stage IV:	Diffuse or disseminated involvement of one or more extralymphatic organs or tissues with or without associated lymph node enlargement.

formed or material should be examined by pathologists experienced in the diagnosis of lymphoma who are able to perform specialized immunologic and molecular biologic techniques to arrive at a correct diagnosis.

Treatment

In general the initial treatment of non-Hodgkin's lymphoma is determined by the stage and histology. Other considerations such as patient age and co-existing medical problems often lead to individualization of treatment plans. The Ann Arbor staging classification for non-Hodgkin's lymphoma is shown in Table 1. Table 2 shows the Rappaport and corresponding Working Formulation classification for non-Hodgkin's lymphoma.

Low-Grade (Indolent) Histologies

About 15 to 20 per cent of patients have localized (stage I and "minimal" stage II) disease, and they represent a curable subset of patients with low-grade lymphoma. With 4000-cGy involved-field radiotherapy, more than 50 per cent of these patients can be expected to have disease-free survival exceeding 5 years. Patients with nodal disease appear to do better than those whose disease presents extranodally, and radiation therapy for those with stage I disease produces better results than for those with stage II disease. Since a significant fraction of patients with only minimal disease after clinical staging are found to have more extensive disease after staging laparotomy, this procedure has been advocated by some investigators, although we do not recommend this approach.

The majority of patients with low-grade lymphoma present with advanced disease. The management of these patients is controversial, and several approaches are available. These lymphomas are most often seen in the elderly and have a long natural history with a median survival of 8 to 10 years. Since these lymphomas have generally been considered incurable, a "watch and wait" approach has been advocated by many physicians. Furthermore, it has been shown that in a significant percentage of patients, lymphomas may undergo spontaneous regression, a further incentive for deferral of initial therapy.

With this approach, treatment is delayed until patients develop systemic symptoms from the lymphoma or until enlarging adenopathy causes discomfort or is cosmetically displeasing. Other reasons for treatment include mechanical problems from enlarging adenopathy, such as ureteral or bowel obstruction. Problems such as these may develop insidiously and patients should be followed extremely closely if initial therapy is deferred.

Other investigators have pointed out that the pessimism associated with treatment for low-grade lymphomas may relate to the relatively few patients who have actually been treated with aggressive chemotherapy regimens. There is evidence that some patients, particularly those with follicular mixed histology, may be cured if treated

TABLE 2. **Pathologic Classification of Non-Hodgkin's Lymphomas**

Rappaport Classification	Working Formulation Classification
Low Grade	
Diffuse lymphocytic, well differentiated	Small lymphocytic
Nodular, poorly differentiated lymphocytic	Follicular, predominantly small cleaved cell
Nodular, mixed lymphocytic-histiocytic	Follicular, mixed small cleaved and large cell
Intermediate Grade	
Nodular histiocytic	Follicular, predominantly large cell
Diffuse lymphocytic, poorly differentiated	Diffuse, small cleaved cell
Diffuse mixed lymphocytic-histiocytic	Diffuse, mixed small and large cell
Diffuse histiocytic	Diffuse, large cell
High Grade	
Diffuse histiocytic	Large cell, immunoblastic
Lymphoblastic convoluted/nonconvoluted	Lymphoblastic
Undifferentiated, Burkitt's and non-Burkitt's	Small noncleaved cell

aggressively. We think it is reasonable to attempt more aggressive treatment with regimens such as those outlined in Table 4 in young patients who present with advanced low-grade lymphomas. In other patients we would employ the "watch and wait" approach and delay treatment until signs or symptoms of disease make treatment necessary. The vast majority of patients will eventually require therapy during the course of their disease.

Treatment in this situation should be considered palliative and every attempt should be made to use the least toxic approach. Local radiation may often be used to treat "problem areas" even in the presence of more generalized disease. In this way patients can still be spared the side effects of chemotherapy.

In most trials combination chemotherapy has not been shown to be superior to single-agent therapy. For this reason we often use single-agent chemotherapy initially. Chlorambucil (Leukeran) is effective and well tolerated orally. Patients can be treated with 2 to 6 mg daily, or with 0.4 to 0.6 mg per kg every 2 to 3 weeks. Alternatively, cyclophosphamide (Cytoxan) can be used at a dose of 50 to 150 mg orally daily or 600 to 750 mg intravenously every 3 to 4 weeks.

Combination chemotherapy can be used initially or after failure of single-agent therapy. Table 3 lists several regimens that may be employed. We recommend continuing therapy for 6 to 8 weeks after complete remission or stabilization of disease. Patients are followed every 2 to 3 months for the first 2 years after treatment and then at progressively longer intervals. At relapse, disease can often be controlled with a previously used regimen, although periods of remission or disease control generally shorten progressively. Eventually patients may require treatment with more aggressive regimens such as those shown in Table 4.

It is recognized that most patients with indolent disease eventually transform into a more aggressive histology. For this reason we recommend re-biopsy of lymph nodes when relapse follows a long period of remission or if disease progresses rapidly. These patients have a poor prognosis despite aggressive therapy.

Intermediate-grade Histologies

In contrast to low-grade lymphomas, the treatment of intermediate-grade histologies is nearly always undertaken with curative intent and therefore demands a meticulous approach to diagnosis and staging.

Treatment of localized (stage I) disease is controversial. Many clinicians advocate one of the combination chemotherapy regimens detailed in

TABLE 3. **Chemotherapy Regimens for Low-Grade Lymphomas**

CVP
Cyclophosphamide, 400 mg/M^2 orally, days 1–5
Vincristine (Oncovin), 1.4 mg/M^2, day 1
Prednisone, 100 mg/M^2, days 1–5
(21-day cycles)

CHLOP
Chlorambucil, 12 mg/M^2 (maximum 20 mg), days 1–5
Vincristine (Oncovin), 1 mg/M^2, day 1
Prednisone, 100 mg, days 1–5
(21- to 28-day cycles)

ABP
Doxorubicin (Adriamycin), 75 mg/M^2, day 1
Bleomycin, 15 mg/M^2 IV, day 1, 8
Prednisone, 100 mg/M^2, days 1–5
(21-day cycles)

HOP
Doxorubicin, 80 mg/M^2, day 1
Vincristine (Oncovin), 1.4 mg/M^2, day 1
Prednisone, 100 mg, days 1–5
(21-day cycles)

C-MOPP
Cyclophosphamide, 650 mg/M^2 IV, days 1, 8
Vincristine (Oncovin), 1.4 mg/M^2, days 1, 8
Procarbazine, 100 mg/M^2, days 1–14
Prednisone, 40 mg/M^2, days 1–14
(28-day cycles)

CHOP
Cyclophosphamide, 750 mg/M^2 IV, day 1
Doxorubicin, 50 mg/M^2, day 1
Vincristine (Oncovin), 1.4 mg/M^2, day 1
Prednisone, 100 mg, days 1–5
(21- to 28-day cycles)

Table 4. Results of chemotherapy in this group are excellent, but patients are exposed to the side effects of chemotherapy. In some centers radiation therapy alone is used for localized intermediate-grade lymphomas, and 5-year disease-free survival rates exceeding 50 per cent are widely reported.

A major controversy in the treatment of clinically staged patients with stage I intermediate-grade lymphomas is whether they should receive staging laparotomies if radiotherapy alone will be used for treatment. Approximately 10 to 20 per cent of patients with clinical stage I and II disease will be found to have more extensive disease at laparotomy. Patients treated with radiation alone, following a staging laparotomy, have disease-free survival rates superior to those of clinically staged patients, and this fact has been used to support the use of staging laparotomy when radiation alone is to be used. Other investigators argue that equivalent results can be obtained if more extensive radiation fields are used or if chemotherapy is combined with radiation, and that patients can be spared the risks of laparotomy. It can also be argued that patients failing radiation therapy can be salvaged with aggressive chemotherapy regimens.

TABLE 4. **Chemotherapy Regimens for Aggressive Non-Hodgkin's Lymphomas**

First-Generation Regimens

C-MOPP*

CHOP*

BACOP
  Cyclophosphamide, 650 mg/M^2 IV, days 1, 8
  Doxorubicin (Adriamycin), 25 mg/M^2 IV, days 1, 8
  Vincristine (Oncovin), 1.4 mg/M^2 IV, days 1, 8
  Bleomycin, 5 U/M^2 IV, days 15, 22
  Prednisone, 60 mg/M^2 PO, days 15–29
  (28-day cycles)

COMLA
  Cyclophosphamide, 1.5 grams/M^2 IV, day 1
  Vincristine, 1.4 mg/M^2, days 1, 8, 15
  Methotrexate, 120 mg/M^2 IV, days 22, 29, 36, 43, 50,
    57, 64, 71; beginning 24 hr after methotrexate infu-
    sion, leucovorin, 25 mg/M^2 orally q 6 hr for 4 doses
  Cytarabine, 300 mg/M^2 IV, days 22, 29, 36, 43, 50, 57,
    64, 71
  (3 cycles with 2-week rest between cycles)

Second- and Third-Generation Regimens

COP-BLAM
  Cyclophosphamide, 400 mg/M^2 IV, day 1
  Vincristine (Oncovin), 1 mg/M^2 IV, day 1
  Doxorubicin, 40 mg/M^2 IV, day 1
  Prednisone, 40 mg/M^2 PO, days 1–10
  Procarbazine, 100 mg/M^2 PO, days 1–10
  Bleomycin, 15 mg IV, day 14
  (21-day cycles with escalation of cyclophosphamide and
    doxorubicin doses)

CAP-BOP
  Cyclophosphamide, 650 mg/M^2 IV, day 1
  Doxorubicin (Adriamycin), 50 mg/M^2 IV, day 1
  Procarbazine, 100 mg/M^2 PO, days 1–7
  Bleomycin, 10 mg/M^2 subcutaneously, day 14
  Vincristine (Oncovin), 1.4 mg/M^2 IV (maximum
    2.0 mg), day 14
  Prednisone, 100 mg PO, days 14–20
  (21- to 28-day cycles)

M-BACOD
  Bleomycin, 4.0 mg/M^2 IV, day 1
  Doxorubicin (Adriamycin), 45 mg/M^2 IV, day 1
  Cyclophosphamide, 600 mg/M^2 IV, day 1
  Vincristine (Oncovin), 1.0 mg/M^2, day 1

Dexamethasone, 6.0 mg/M^2 orally,
    days 1–5
  Methotrexate, 3.0 grams/M^2 IV, day 14; beginning 24
    hr after methotrexate is completed, leucovorin, 10
    mg/M^2 IV; then 10 mg/M^2 orally q 6 hr for 72 hr
  (21-day cycles)

ProMACE-MOPP
  Etoposide, 120 mg/M^2 IV, days 1, 8
  Cyclophosphamide, 650 mg/M^2 IV, days 1, 8
  Doxorubicin, 25 mg/M^2 IV, days 1, 8
  Methotrexate, 1.5 gm/M^2 IV, day 14; beginning 24 hr
    after methotrexate infusion is initiated, leucovorin,
    50 mg/M^2 IV, q 6 hr for 5 doses
  Prednisone 60 mg/M^2 PO, days 1–14
  (28-day cycles with cycle number determined by rate of
    tumor regression) Later MOPP given, with number
    of cycles determined by rate of tumor regression;
    additional ProMACE given for patients in remission

ProMACE-CytaBOM
  Cyclophosphamide, 650 mg/M^2 IV, day 1
  Doxorubicin (Adriamycin), 25 mg/M^2 IV, day 1
  Etoposide, 120 mg/M^2 IV, day 1
  Prednisone, 60 mg/M^2 PO, days 1–15
  Cytarabine, 300 mg/M^2 IV, day 8
  Bleomycin, 5 mg/M^2 IV, day 8
  Vincristine (Oncovin), 1.4 mg/M^2, day 8
  Methotrexate, 120 mg/M^2, day 8; beginning 24 hr after
    methotrexate infusion is initiated, leucovorin, 25 mg/
    M^2 orally, q 6 hr for 4 doses
  (21-day cycles)

MACOP-B
  Methotrexate, 400 mg/M^2 IV, weeks 2, 6, 10; beginning
    24 hr after methotrexate infusion is initiated, leuco-
    vorin, 15 mg orally q 6 hr for 6 doses
  Doxorubicin (Adriamycin), 50 mg/M^2 IV, weeks 1, 3, 5,
    7, 9, 11
  Cyclophosphamide, 350 mg/M^2 IV, weeks 1, 3, 5, 7, 9,
    11
  Vincristine (Oncovin), 1.4 mg/M^2 (maximum 2 mg) IV,
    weeks 2, 4, 6, 8, 10, 12
  Bleomycin 10 U/M^2 IV, weeks 4, 8, 12
  Prednisone, 75 mg PO daily with taper over last 2
    weeks
  (whole regimen delivered in 12 weeks)

*See Table 3 for drugs and dosage schedules.

At the University of Nebraska we do not perform staging laparotomies on clinical stage I patients. We give two cycles of CAP-BOP chemotherapy (see Table 4) followed by 4000-cGy involved field radiation therapy. To date we have seen no relapses in patients treated in this fashion.

The treatment of choice for more advanced stages of intermediate-grade non-Hodgkin's lymphoma is combination chemotherapy. With the introduction of C-MOPP chemotherapy it was recognized that patients could be cured of advanced disease. The more advanced second- and third-generation regimens employ an increasing

number of non–cross-resistant agents that are often delivered in an alternating fashion. A novel approach is exemplified by the MACOP-B regimen (see Table 4), in which the entire course of therapy is delivered over 12 weeks at a very high-dose intensity.

It is axiomatic that cure cannot be achieved without first getting the patient into a complete remission. For this reason most physicians are now using the second- and third-generation regimens that have had the highest complete response rates. With these newer regimens, the majority of patients can be expected to achieve a complete remission, and at least 50 per cent can be cured of their lymphoma. It should be emphasized that there is a lack of studies comparing the regimens in Table 4 with each other. Differences in reported results may be due in large part to variations in important prognostic variables such as patient age, histology, disease stage, and presence of bulky disease. There is no definitive evidence that any of these regimens are superior even to CHOP, although trials are under way to decide this question.

It now seems evident that patients who achieve a complete remission early in the course of their treatment have a better prognosis than those who take several cycles of chemotherapy to attain remission. It is our practice with CAP-BOP to restage patients after three cycles of chemotherapy, and after each subsequent cycle if they are not in remission. We then deliver only two additional cycles of chemotherapy after patients enter complete remission.

Patients should be restaged after treatment and followed closely thereafter. The vast majority of relapses occur in the first 2 years, and follow-up should be most frequent during this period of time. Treatment of these lymphomas requires a thorough knowledge of the chemotherapeutic agents used and their side effects, since some of these regimens have been associated with mortality rates of 10 per cent. Blood counts should be checked prior to each cycle of therapy. As a general rule we require an absolute granulocyte count of 2000 per mm^3 and a platelet count above 125,000 per mm^3 prior to initiating a cycle of therapy. Signs of bleeding require a prompt evaluation, since thrombocytopenia is often seen following treatment. Any infection or fever should be considered a medical emergency. Immediate hospitalization with empiric broad-spectrum antibiotic coverage is required for a neutropenic patient with a temperature exceeding 38.5° C.

High-Grade Histologies

Although large-cell, immunoblastic lymphomas are classified as high-grade lymphomas, they can be treated with the same regimens used for intermediate-grade lymphomas with equivalent results.

Lymphoblastic lymphomas share many clinical features with T-cell acute lymphoblastic leukemia. For this reason several regimens modeled after those used for childhood ALL have been developed. These regimens often employ cranial prophylaxis and maintainence chemotherapy lasting 2 to 3 years. The complete response rates for lymphoblastic lymphoma are very high, as in intermediate-grade histologies. However, those with high lactate dehydrogenase levels and bone marrow or central nervous system involvement make up a particularly high-risk group, and long-term disease-free survival is unusual.

We believe that patients with lymphoblastic lymphoma without these risk factors can be successfully treated with the newer regimens noted in Table 4. In those patients exhibiting high-risk features, we try to perform bone marrow transplantation once an initial remission is obtained.

The therapy for small, noncleaved cell lymphomas is similar to that for lymphoblastic lymphomas. In patients presenting with bulky abdominal Burkitt's lymphoma, an aggressive attempt at surgical debulking is indicated, since patients who are debulked have a much better prognosis. The regimens outlined in Table 4 are appropriate for treating these patients, and cure rates exceeding 50 per cent are seen in those without the high-risk factors identified for lymphoblastic lymphoma. In the high-risk patients we also recommend bone marrow transplantation after initial remission is obtained.

Salvage Therapy

Despite the success achieved in treatment of aggressive lymphomas, 30 to 60 per cent of patients will fail to achieve a remission or will relapse after attaining a remission. Without effective salvage therapy, these patients can be expected to die of their disease.

The results of salvage chemotherapy for non-Hodgkin's lymphoma have been disappointing, with few long-term disease-free survivors reported. The poor results are due in large part to poor patient tolerance from impaired marrow reserve as well as from drug resistance. A large number of conventional agents as well as investigational agents, including ifosfamide, methyl-GAG, gallium nitrate, and m-AMSA, have been used with limited success in treating refractory or relapsed patients. Mitoxantrone (Novantrone) has recently been released for general use and may show some activity in refractory lymphoma.

We have achieved the best results with the DHAP regimen consisting of dexamethasone, 40 mg intravenously or orally daily for 4 consecutive days, cisplatin (Platinol), 100 mg per square meter (M^2) via continuous infusion over 24 hours on day 1, and cytarabine (Cytosar-U), 2 grams per M^2 intravenously following the cisplatin infusion, and then repeated in 12 hours. Responses have been seen in approximately 50 per cent of patients, and about half of these responses have been complete. As with other regimens, however, very few patients achieve durable complete responses.

We believe that the best salvage treatment for non-Hodgkin's lymphoma is high-dose therapy followed by autologous bone marrow transplantation. This treatment is most effective when used early, and we believe it should be used as the initial salvage regimen for non-Hodgkin's lymphoma patients who can tolerate the considerable side effects associated with marrow transplantation. There is evidence that patients whose tumors are still sensitive to chemotherapy have better results following bone marrow transplantation than those with resistant tumors. It is our practice, when possible, to deliver 1 or 2 cycles of DHAP in an attempt to reduce tumor bulk prior to high-dose therapy and marrow transplantation.

Alternative Approaches to Salvage Treatment

Currently several biological agents are being investigated for treatment of non-Hodgkin's lymphomas, including the use of interferon in refractory lymphoma. Responses may be seen in up to 50 per cent of patients with advanced low-grade non-Hodgkin's lymphoma, but complete responses are rare and the responses obtained have generally been of short duration. There have been few responses with intermediate- and high-grade lymphomas.

Some patients with non-Hodgkin's lymphoma have been treated with anti-idiotype monoclonal antibodies, and investigational work is being carried out at some centers in which monoclonal antibodies are conjugated to radioisotopes. Other workers are investigating the role of interleukin-2 alone or with lymphokine-activated killer cells in the treatment of lymphomas. One complete response has been reported in a patient with non-Hodgkin's lymphoma, but results are quite early and there is no evidence at present that this form of therapy has curative potential in this disease.

AIDS and Non-Hodgkin's Lymphoma

The most recent criteria for the diagnosis of the acquired immunodeficiency syndrome (AIDS) includes anyone under age 60 with a primary central nervous system (CNS) lymphoma and those with small noncleaved lymphoma or large cell lymphoma and laboratory evidence of human immunodeficiency virus (HIV) infection.

The treatment of patients with AIDS-related lymphoma has been unsatisfactory, in large part because of the inability of these patients to tolerate aggressive therapy. When possible, we recommend referral of these patients to centers where they can participate in clinical trials.

The treatment of choice for primary CNS lymphoma in AIDS patients is radiotherapy, although some advocate the concurrent use of corticosteroids. Responses are seen, but most patients do not survive more than a few months.

Although 50 per cent of patients with other AIDS-related lymphomas may achieve remissions with chemotherapy, treatment is poorly tolerated owing to the development of opportunistic infections and progression in the CNS. In one series of 13 patients treated with M-BACOD, median survival was 11 months.

MYCOSIS FUNGOIDES

method of
RICHARD T. HOPPE, M.D.
Stanford University Medical Center
Stanford, California

Mycosis fungoides (MF) is a cutaneous lymphoma of T-lymphocyte origin that has a variable clinical course. Despite its generally long natural history, MF eventually becomes symptomatic in most patients, therapy is required, and death may ensue. Mycosis fungoides is an uncommon malignancy; approximately 400 new cases and 100 to 200 deaths are reported each year in the United States. This lymphoma is most common in older males. The median age of onset is about 60 and the male:female ratio is 2:1. The etiology of MF is unclear. Chemical exposure, chronic antigen stimulation, and viral causes have been proposed. A few cases of MF in association with HTLV-I infections have been reported.

Diagnosis

The diagnosis of MF is often difficult and may only be established after the disease has been present and symptomatic for many years. The typical light microscopic features of MF include a polymorphous upper dermal infiltrate that is intimate with the epidermis and has atypical mononuclear cells. These atypical mononuclear cells have hyperconvoluted ("cerebriform") nuclei, and monoclonal antibody staining reveals that they have the cell surface characteristics of helper T cells. Some of these cells must be present in the epidermis either as scattered individual cells or small clusters (Pautrier microabscesses) in order to establish a definitive diagnosis. Biopsy studies on multiple occasions are indicated when the diagnosis of MF is suspected clinically but previous biopsy results were only suggestive of that diagnosis. Since the cellular infiltrate of this disease is located in the upper dermis and epidermis, shave biopsies are generally preferable to punch biopsies in order to provide a large surface of epidermis for examination.

Clinical Appearance

The cutaneous lesions of MF are variable in appearance. Some patients present with poikilodermatous patches characterized by variable atrophy and telangiectasia. Other patients present with well demarcated erythematous scaling patches or infiltrated plaques. It is common for disease to arise initially in the bathing trunk distribution that includes the lower abdomen, upper thighs, and buttocks. The lesions of MF are generally intensely pruritic, and pruritus is often the main presenting complaint. Some patients may present with or develop frank cutaneous tumors, which may become secondarily ulcerated and infected.

Occasional patients will present with generalized erythroderma, often accompanied by marked skin atrophy. Some patients with erythroderma have abnormal cells circulating in the peripheral blood that are identical to those found in the dermal and epidermal infiltrates of the disease. These patients often have palpable lymphadenopathy and splenomegaly as well, and this constellation of findings is referred to as the Sézary syndrome. These patients usually experience severe generalized pruritus.

Staging

In staging MF, the most important considerations are the extent of skin involvement, the presence of lymph node involvement, and the presence of visceral disease. Table 1 summarizes the TNM system for staging MF. Skin involvement characterized as limited plaque implies patches or plaques involving less than 10 per cent of the total skin surface. Generalized plaque disease indicates that patches or plaques involve more than 10 per cent of the skin surface. Tumorous involvement implies frank cutaneous tumors, and erythroderma indicates total skin erythema.

Staging studies completed in these patients should include a thorough history and physical examination with careful mapping of cutaneous lesions. Examination of the skin should also include careful evaluation of the scalp, palms, soles, fingernails, and toenails. Lateral and PA chest radiographs, a complete blood count, and serum chemistry studies are indicated both to rule out extracutaneous involvement by MF and also to evaluate for the presence of other pathology. Patients with palpable lymphadenopathy should undergo lymph node biopsy. If lymph node biopsy shows involvement by MF, other staging studies should be utilized to determine the extent of extracutaneous disease. Most commonly, lymphangiography and computerized tomographic scanning of the abdomen and pelvis are helpful in this setting. If any of these studies suggest visceral involvement, biopsy documentation is warranted. Other cancers are common in patients of this age group and may account for abnormal findings on these examinations. The most common site of identifiable extracutaneous MF is in lymph nodes, and the most common visceral sites are the lungs and liver.

Treatment

Cutaneous Therapy

The potential for curative treatment of mycosis fungoides is controversial. However, most patients are symptomatic because of pruritus or are unhappy with the cosmetic deformities associated with the disease, and treatment is usually indicated. At the time of initial diagnosis, it is reasonable to use aggressive cutaneous treatment in order to clear the skin. With this approach, some patients will in fact achieve complete skin clearance, some of these will maintain clearance for variable periods of time, and occasional patients will have no evidence of return of disease activity. Furthermore, it appears that when disease on the skin can be kept at a minimal level, the likelihood that the patient will develop extracutaneous disease is exceedingly small. The topical treatment modalities utilized in this situation include topical chemotherapy with nitrogen mustard, photochemotherapy with psoralens and ultraviolet (UVA) radiation, and total skin electron beam therapy.

Topical nitrogen mustard may be utilized either in an aqueous solution or in an ointment base in a concentration of 10 to 20 mg per dl. Patients generally apply the topical nitrogen mustard to the entire cutaneous surface, sparing only the eyelids. Intertriginous areas are treated more sparingly. Cutaneous lesions are slow to respond with this therapy, and complete response, if it occurs, may require more than a year of daily treatment. It is recommended that therapy be continued during a maintenance period of 1 to 2 years following complete skin clearance.

Therapy with psoralens and ultraviolet radiation (PUVA) consists of oral 8-methoxypsoralen followed by exposure to long wave length ultraviolet light. The psoralens intercalate with DNA, which, on exposure to UVA, form cross links that inhibit DNA replication. Generally three treat-

TABLE 1. **TMN Staging System for Mycosis Fungoides**

T1—Limited plaque. Patches or plaques covering less than 10% of the total skin surface

T2—Generalized plaque. Patches or plaques covering 10% or more of the total skin surface

T3—Tumorous. One or more cutaneous tumors

T4—Erythroderma. Total skin erythema, with or without cutaneous tumors

N0—No palpable lymph nodes

N1—Palpable lymph nodes. If a biopsy is done, light microscopic appearance of specimen may be consistent with reactive changes or dermatopathic lymphadenitis, but not with actual involvement by MF

N2—Palpable lymph nodes that have been biopsied, specimen reveals MF microscopically

M0—No evidence of visceral involvement

M1—Visceral involvement present. Should be documented by biopsy

	T-Stage			
N-Stage	T1	T2	T3	T4
N0	IA	IB	IIB	IIIA
N1	IIA	IIA	IIB	IIIB
N2	IVA	IVA	IVA	IVA

Any T, N with M = 1 is Stage IVB

ments per week are given until moderate clearing has been achieved. Maintenance programs are then introduced with two treatments per week, and, subsequently, gradually tapering schedules are initiated, with treatments ultimately given as infrequently as once every 4 to 6 weeks. Generally, if treatment is discontinued completely, the disease recurs.

Total skin electron beam therapy provides the greatest likelihood of skin clearance. Electrons are a form of ionizing irradiation that penetrate to a specific depth, depending upon their energy. Electrons of appropriate energy can be used; these penetrate the skin for only several millimeters, and special techniques of treatment permit entire cutaneous therapy. Treatments are administered four days a week for about 9 weeks (total dose 30.00 to 36.00 Gy). About 80 per cent of patients will achieve complete skin clearance with this treatment. However, 50 to 75 per cent of patients who complete this therapy will have a later recurrence. Often, however, only minimal disease is present at this point, and it can be treated effectively with either topical nitrogen mustard or PUVA. The side effects of total skin electron beam therapy are more marked than those that occur with the other two topical modalities. Temporary hair loss, temporary loss of sweat gland function, and long-term skin dryness are common.

Recommendations for Cutaneous Treatment. In patients who present with the limited plaque phase of skin involvement, treatment with topical nitrogen mustard is a reasonable first line therapy. Although the time to skin clearance is quite prolonged, as many as 50 per cent of patients will achieve a complete response. Even in those who do not achieve a complete response, there is usually a significant improvement in disease with resolution of most symptoms. If the disease fails to respond to topical nitrogen mustard or progresses during therapy, institution of total skin electron beam therapy is appropriate. Patients who present with generalized plaque disease in which there is only a minimally infiltrative component and who have a long history of disease without recent progression may be treated in a similar fashion. However, in the presence of very infiltrated plaques or if there is a history of recent progression, total skin electron beam therapy is a preferable first choice of treatment. The majority of patients treated in this fashion will achieve a complete response. However, since subsequent relapse is common, it may be beneficial to institute a program of maintenance treatment with topical nitrogen mustard immediately following the completion of electron beam therapy.

Patients who present with tumorous involvement are treated initially with total skin electron beam therapy. In addition, supplemental small field irradiation with low energy x-rays to individual tumor lesions is indicated. After completion of irradiation, topical nitrogen mustard is used as a maintenance therapy.

Patients who present with erythroderma are difficult to manage inasmuch as their skin is often atrophic and very sensitive to any type of therapy. Low exposure of PUVA therapy can be successful in achieving gradual skin clearance. If either topical nitrogen mustard or electron beam therapy is utilized, the concentration or daily dose of these agents must be reduced.

Palliative Management of Skin Lesions. Frequently, despite the use of total cutaneous therapies, individual lesions develop that may be refractory and symptomatic. Local topical measures that may be helpful in this setting include topical corticosteroids, small field irradiation with either low energy x-rays or electrons, or more intensive localized treatment with higher concentrations of nitrogen mustard (i.e., 50 mg per dl).

Management of Extracutaneous Disease

The median survival of patients who develop extracutaneous disease is only one year. Systemic therapies, while occasionally achieving responses, seldom achieve complete responses, and remissions are generally brief. When extracutaneous sites are clinically localized (i.e., localized adenopathy), local field megavoltage irradiation can achieve a very good palliative and symptomatic response. Generalized systemic disease is usually treated with combination chemotherapy using agents such as cyclophosphamide, doxorubicin (Adriamycin), vincristine, and prednisone (CHOP).

TABLE 2. **5-Year Results of Treatment for Patients with Cutaneous Disease**

	Nitrogen Mustard (101 pts)		Electron Beam Therapy (170 pts)	
	Survival (%)	Freedom from Relapse (%)	Survival (%)	Freedom from Relapse (%)
Limited plaque	92	32	92	55
Generalized plaque	66	10	73	25
Tumorous	—	—	39	5

An uncommon form of systemic disease is the *Sézary syndrome*. The Sézary syndrome is incurable but usually requires treatment for relief of symptoms (i.e., pruritus). Daily treatment with chlorambucil and prednisone in addition to monitoring white blood cell counts is often successful in achieving palliative responses. When the disease becomes resistant to this approach, more intensive chemotherapy programs may be initiated, but response is unpredictable.

Prognosis

Prognosis is related to the extent of skin involvement, presence of extracutaneous disease, the type of therapy administered, and other factors such as age and intercurrent disease. The median survival of large groups of patients may be greater than 10 years, but is very dependent upon the initial extent of disease and the treatment programs utilized. Table 2 summarizes our results of treatment at Stanford, using topical nitrogen mustard or electron beam therapy in patients with disease limited to the skin.

MULTIPLE MYELOMA

method of
DANIEL E. BERGSAGEL, M.D.
Ontario Cancer Institute
Toronto, Ontario, Canada

The question of whether a patient has myeloma often starts with the discovery of an M protein (M for monoclonal) in the serum or urine. In a screening study of 10,000 Swedish subjects over the age of 25, about 1 per cent were found to have a serum M protein. The majority were asymptomatic and were classified as having monoclonal gammopathy of unknown significance (MGUS). These patients are well and require no therapy. Patients with symptomatic myeloma have a median survival of about 30 months and thus do not accumulate in the population. The prevalence of the two disorders in a population of 100,000 is about 582 for MGUS and 30 for symptomatic myeloma. Patients with symptomatic myeloma should be treated immediately; those with MGUS should be reevaluated every six months because about 2 per cent per year progress to develop plasma cell myeloma.

Patient Evaluation

The evaluation of a patient with an M protein is outlined in Table 1. For IgG M proteins and IgA peaks greater than 20 grams per liter, the serum electrophoresis strip is an accurate method of measuring the M protein, whereas radial immunodiffusion is less reliable. With IgA M proteins less than 20 grams per liter,

---

TABLE 1. Evaluation of Patient with M Protein

1. Measure the M protein by the following methods:
   Serum electrophoresis—measure M protein and albumin in grams per liter
   Urine protein—measure grams of protein excreted per 24 hours
2. Establish monoclonality of the M protein by immunoelectrophoresis
3. Hematology: hemoglobin, leukocyte and platelet counts, differential counts
4. Marrow: per cent plasma cells in marrow differential; may need to sample more than one site, since marrow plasmacytosis may be spotty
5. Biopsy of solitary lytic lesion; extramedullary plasmacytoma; skin nodules; enlarged lymph nodes
6. Evaluate renal function: serum creatinine; creatinine clearance; electrophoresis of concentrated urine to distinguish between tubular and glomerular proteinurea patterns
7. Complete skeletal survey, including skull, ribs, vertebrae, and long bones; identify lytic lesions and osteoporosis
8. Serum calcium
9. Serum β2 microglobulin (β2m)
10. Labeling index of marrow plasma cells (if available) for distinguishing progressive from indolent myeloma
11. Myelogram if there is paraspinal mass or signs and symptoms of spinal cord or nerve root compression. Send cerebrospinal fluid to lab for cytospin, cell count, and protein.
12. Special tests: serum viscosity; check for cryoglobulins; plasma volume; rectal biopsy (search for amyloid); check joint effusions for amyloid

---

the peak may be poorly defined, and the immunoglobulin is measured more accurately by nephelometry. About 60 per cent of myeloma patients excrete a light chain in the urine. The urine dipstick test for protein is designed to detect albumin and often fails to detect light chains. The electrophoresis pattern of concentrated urine should be determined. The usual lesion caused by light chain deposits in the renal tubules results in the excretion of large amounts of light chains, which migrate in the globulin region, plus some albumin. Damage to the glomerulus by deposits of amyloid or light chains results in the nonspecific leakage of all serum proteins into the urine. The glomerular urine electrophoresis pattern resembles that of serum. The bone lesions demonstrated in the skeletal survey are important in directing radiation therapy. Large lytic lesions should be irradiated before a pathologic fracture occurs. Back pain, associated with diffuse osteoporosis and vertebral collapse, usually responds better to chemotherapy than to radiation, unless a distinct lytic lesion can be identified.

Myelomatous lesions in ribs or vertebrae may extend beyond the bone and form paraspinal masses which can be visualized on vertebral radiographs. These plasma cell tumors may invade the spinal canal through an intervertebral foramen and cause spinal cord compression; paraspinal masses should be irradiated as soon as they are discovered, before neurologic complications develop. The increased bone resorption associated with plasma cell myeloma often exceeds the capacity of the kidney to excrete calcium. As a result about one third of patients present with symptoms of hypercalcemia (nausea, vomiting, constipation, polyurea, thirst, and mental confusion), and another third develop hypercalcemia during the course of the disease. Patients immobilized by bone pain are especially vulnerable to this complication. β2 microglobulin (β2m) is the light chain of the major histocompatibility complex of the cell membrane. The release of this protein into the blood is increased in active tumors with increased cell turnover. β2m is normally excreted in the urine; renal failure leads to rising serum levels. Serum β2m has proved to be a useful measurement for gauging the activity of plasma cell neoplasms; levels in the normal range (less than 3.0 mg per liter) are associated with indolent tumors (MGUS and asymptomatic, stable myeloma), whereas elevated levels indicate a more active tumor, with increased cell turnover, and possibly renal failure. The determination of the proportion of plasma cells in the DNA synthesis phase of the cell cycle (labeling index) with tritiated thymidine or bromodeoxycitidine is another useful means of distinguishing indolent from aggressive myeloma. Patients with symptomatic myeloma requiring treatment usually have plasma cell labeling indices of greater than 0.4 per cent.

Staging

Patients with symptomatic myeloma can be staged on the basis of the important prognostic factors. Those with a hemoglobin of less than 85 grams per liter, hypercalcemia, more than three lytic bone lesions, or a greatly increased M-protein (more than 70 grams per liter of IgG, more than 50 grams per liter for IgA, or more than 12 grams per 24 hours of light chain proteinuria) have a high myeloma cell mass and a poor prognosis. A simpler and more useful staging system is based on serum β2m and albumin levels. Stage 1 patients with serum β2m levels of 6.0 mg per liter, or less, and serum albumin (by electrophoresis) of 30 grams per liter, or more, have the best prognosis. Stage 2 patients have a serum β2m of more than 6.0 mg per liter, and a serum albumin of 30 grams per liter, or more. Stage 3 patients, with the worst prognosis, have both an elevated serum β2m of more than 6.0 mg per liter and albumin reduced to less than 30 grams per liter.

Treatment of Symptomatic Myeloma

General Measures

First, pain should be relieved and the patient ambulated. This requires the effective use of analgesics, and irradiation of painful lytic lesions identified by the patient and the skeletal survey. For painful rib lesions we often use a single dose of 800 cGy; for larger lytic lesions in vital areas, such as vertebrae or long bones, doses of 2000 to 3500 cGy are administered. The patient should be encouraged to get out of bed, if only to walk to the bathroom, as soon as the pain has been adequately controlled. It is important to preserve muscle strength and reduce bone resorption by

putting some stress on the skeleton. All patients should make special efforts to drink at least 3 liters of fluid a day so that the increased amount of calcium and light chains can be excreted by the kidneys. Dehydration favors the development of renal failure and hypercalcemia and the formation of tubular casts that further compromise renal function.

Initial Chemotherapy

Melphalan and prednisone are the drugs of choice as the initial form of chemotherapy. I start with a melphalan (Alkeran) dose of 9 mg per M^2 (0.25 mg per kg) before breakfast daily for 4 days every 4 to 6 weeks, along with 100 mg of prednisone in 1 dose with breakfast for 4 days. The melphalan should be administered in 1 dose at least 30 minutes before breakfast (giving melphalan with food significantly reduces the absorption of this drug). Blood counts should be repeated weekly. When an effective dose has been administered, the leukocyte and platelet count will fall to a nadir at about 3 weeks, with recovery by the fourth to sixth week.

If a significant fall in the leukocyte and/or platelet count is not observed, the next course of melphalan should be increased by 2 mg per day and, if necessary, increased by an additional 2 mg per day in subsequent courses, until a definite, transient fall in leukocytes and/or platelet counts occurs, to indicate that adequate amounts of melphalan have been absorbed. Most patients can tolerate repeat courses of melphalan and prednisone every 4 weeks, but some will have delayed marrow recovery. If the leukocyte and/or platelet counts have not begun to rise by the fourth week, the next course should be delayed by 1 or 2 weeks to prevent the development of cumulative hematologic toxicity. Some patients are distressed by the acute stimulatory effects of prednisone (hyperactivity, insomnia, dyspepsia); in these patients the prednisone can be discontinued; although prednisone does increase the response rate in myeloma, it has not been shown to improve survival.

With this therapy, 46 per cent of patients will respond with a fall in the serum and/or urine M protein to reach a stable plateau (at less than 50 per cent of the initial serum M protein concentration or at less than 10 per cent of the initial urinary M protein excreted per 24 hours), with relief of bone pain, weight gain, and improved performance status. An additional 10 per cent will become asymptomatic but will not achieve a sufficient fall in the M protein to qualify as responders, and 44 per cent will progress and require alternate forms of therapy.

Attempts to improve therapy by adding vincristine and other alkylating agents to melphalan and prednisone have failed to improve survival. There is some evidence that combining doxorubicin (Adriamycin) with alkylating agents may lead to a marginal improvement in survival.

There is no benefit in continuing therapy after a stable response has been achieved. My practice is to continue treatment with melphalan and prednisone as long as the M protein level continues to decline. After the M protein level reaches a stable plateau that persists for 4 months, I discontinue therapy but continue to see the patient at 2-month intervals to follow the course of the disease. It is impossible to monitor the management of a myeloma patient without a chronological record (flow sheet) of changes in weight, serum M protein and albumin measured by serum electrophoresis, 24-hour urine protein, serum calcium, serum creatinine, blood counts, serum β2m, and repeated skeletal surveys, along with a record of the treatment administered to the patient. Patients who achieve a stable response will remain in remission for a median of 10 to 12 months after treatment is stopped, but some will not show signs of progression for 3 years or more. Patients must be monitored carefully so that treatment can be restarted at the first sign of relapse (i.e., a progressive increase in serum and/or urinary M protein), preferably before bone pain signals progressive bony disease.

Patients treated in this way with melphalan and prednisone will survive for a median of 30 months. Those whose disease progresses despite melphalan/prednisone induction therapy have the poorest prognosis, with a median survival of 15 months; responders have a median survival of 48 months; and those who do not achieve a response but remain stable without progression also survive well, with a median of 49 months.

Second Line Therapy

The prognosis for patients whose disease is primarily resistant to melphalan and prednisone is poor, and only about 10 per cent will respond to alternate therapy. Patients whose disease responds initially to melphalan/prednisone therapy but then progresses despite reinstituted therapy have a better prognosis; about 25 to 30 per cent will respond to second line therapy.

When the disease progresses when the patient is on melphalan/prednisone therapy, I change to cyclophosphamide (Cytoxan), 500 mg (intravenously or orally) once a week, combined with prednisone, 100 mg with breakfast, on alternate days. This treatment gives the patient the advantage of high-dose prednisone, which is well-tolerated without signs of hypercorticism when administered on alternate days, and also a change in the alkylating agent to cyclophosphamide in a schedule that is well tolerated, even by patients with pancytopenia.

Patients whose disease progresses on weekly cyclophosphamide and prednisone, with clear progression of bony disease, are difficult management problems. Bone pain is best treated with irradiation, and when there are widespread lesions this may require half-body irradiation. Some patients may also respond to 4-day infusions (using venous catheter access to a large vein) of vincristine (Oncovin) and doxorubicin (Adriamycin) and 4 day courses of dexamethasone (Decadron). The treatments used at this stage of the illness require considerable clinical experience, and are best administered at centers where physicians have experience in the use of wide-field irradiation and intensive chemotherapy and have access to the required supportive care.

Management of Special Problems

Solitary Osseous Plasmacytomas

About 3 per cent of patients present with apparently solitary osteolytic lesions. These patients require a needle aspirate or biopsy from the lytic lesion to establish the diagnosis, since marrow aspirations from other sites will not show a plasmacytosis. Solitary lesions should be treated with irradiation, using a dose of about 3500 cGy. About one third of these patients will have an M protein, and this should disappear completely following irradiation. Persistence of the M protein means that myeloma cells persist, probably outside of the irradiated area. These patients must be followed carefully because in the majority the disease will eventually progress to multiple myeloma.

Extramedullary Plasmacytomas

As above, about 3 per cent of patients present with extramedullary plasmacytomas, usually in the nasopharynx or paranasal sinuses. Since the usual spread of these tumors is to the regional lymph nodes, the radiation field should include the regional nodes whenever possible. We use a radiation dose of 3500 cGy. One third of these patients will have an M protein, which should disappear following irradiation. If the M protein persists along with residual tumor, the residual tumor should be resected; the M protein will often disappear if the tumor can be resected. Extramedullary plasmacytomas can usually be controlled by local irradiation and surgical resection. Melphalan and prednisone therapy can be used for those cases that are not controlled by local measures.

Hypercalcemia

Because hypercalcemia develops frequently in myeloma patients, the serum calcium should be measured once a week in hospitalized patients and on every follow-up visit. This complication can usually be controlled in myeloma patients with a combination of hydration (using normal saline to promote the excretion of calcium, whenever possible), corticosteroids, and chemotherapy for the myeloma.

Anemia

A low hemoglobin concentration in a myeloma patient may be partially dilutional, as the plasma volume expands to accommodate the serum M protein. Red cell transfusions are not indicated and may be harmful for patients with an expanded plasma volume, especially if this is associated with hyperviscosity. The common causes of anemia, such as bleeding, should be ruled out. The usual cause is marrow failure associated with the myeloma. If anemia persists and requires transfusions in a myeloma patient whose disease is otherwise controlled by chemotherapy, I try fluoxymesterone (Halotestin), 5 mg 3 times a day with meals.* This treatment is often effective in raising the hemoglobin concentration slowly, but must be continued for 3 to 6 months before the full effect is achieved.

Renal Failure

Constant encouragement of the patient to drink 3 liters of fluid a day will do much to retard the development of renal failure. The occasional patient who presents with acute renal shut-down requires emergency treatment to clear light chains from the plasma and renal tubules. Plasmapheresis is 10 times more effective than dialysis in accomplishing this. During this emergency treatment one should also attempt to reduce the production of light chains by the myeloma cells. Melphalan should be administered with great caution, because toxicity is greatly increased when the drug cannot be excreted into the urine. In this situation I use intravenous cyclophosphamide (Cytoxan), 500 mg per week, and prednisone, 100 mg per day or every other day.

Infections

Infections occur frequently in myeloma patients and are the most common cause of death. All fevers must be monitored carefully, and antibiotics administered immediately for suspected infections. Neutropenic patients who develop a fever should be hospitalized for intravenous an-

*This use is not listed in the manufacturer's directive.

tibiotic therapy. Myeloma patients do not mount an adequate antibody response to organisms such as the pneumococcus; thus repeat infections with the same strain of pneumococcus are common. Consideration should be given to administering prophylactic penicillin to myeloma patients who have been treated for a penumococcal infection.

Experimental Therapy

Attempts to eliminate all myeloma cells with intensive chemotherapy, such as high-dose melphalan, and allogeneic or twin marrow transplantation have failed to cure patients but have succeeded in inducing prolonged remissions. Interferon has been found to reduce the self-renewal capacity of myeloma colony-forming cells, and is being tested for its capacity to prolong remissions induced by other agents.

POLYCYTHEMIA VERA AND OTHER POLYCYTHEMIC CONDITIONS

method of
HARRIET S. GILBERT, M.D.
Albert Einstein College of Medicine
Bronx, New York

Polycythemia vera (PV) is one of a group of chronic myeloproliferative disorders (MPD) involving the pluripotential hematic precursor cell. The syndromes composing MPD are low-grade hematologic malignancies characterized by monoclonal proliferation of a precursor cell that maintains its pluripotentiality and its capacity for commitment, differentiation, and maturation into the hematic populations normally derived from this cell. The result of this intrinsic growth disturbance is an expansion of the bone marrow organ throughout the medullary cavity and a reactivation of hematopoiesis in extramedullary sites that are usually active only during fetal development. The resulting panmyelosis produces increased levels of some or all circulating hematic cell progeny, as well as myeloid metaplasia of the spleen and liver. The phenotypic expression of MPD is highly variable, and nomenclature of the syndromes is based on the predominant manifestation of the proliferative process. Although they result from the same intrinsic lesion of the hematic precursor cell and share many features, the phenotypic expressions of MPD pose sufficiently different problems in diagnosis and management to justify subclassification into three variants known as polycythemia vera (PV), essential thrombocythemia (ET), and myeloid metaplasia (MyM). Erythrocythemia is the predominant manifestation of PV at the inception of the disease. With time, PV may change its phenotype, and the proliferative, erythrocythemic phase may be followed by a spent phase in which erythroid activity wanes in the absence of therapy and manifestations of myeloid metaplasia predominate. This is known as the phase of post-polycythemia myeloid metaplasia. Some patients develop progressive compromise of bone marrow function with myelofibrosis or myelodysplasia, or both. At this stage hematopoiesis becomes ineffective and bone marrow failure supervenes.

Notwithstanding the malignant nature of PV, the last four decades have seen a remarkable increase in survival from 2 years in untreated patients to a life expectancy that does not differ from that of an age-matched population without PV. This has been achieved by two strategies: reduction of the increased red cell mass by phlebotomy to reduce blood viscosity and inhibition of hematopoiesis by myelosuppressive agents. Several important observations have emerged from randomized clinical trials to evaluate these therapeutic approaches. It was found that the choice of therapy has less effect on survival than on the type of complication. Patients treated with phlebotomy show an increase in thrombotic events during the first 4 years of their course, and those managed with myelosuppression have an increased incidence of malignancy after the fourth year. Malignant transformation is both dose-related and agent-related, and administration of alkylating agents is associated with an earlier leukemic transformation than that seen with radioactive phosphorus. Extensive statistical analysis has failed to associate an elevated platelet count with a high risk of thrombotic complications. The incidence of late thrombotic events in patients treated with myelosuppression is increased so that the overall thrombosis-free cumulative survival is comparable in the phlebotomized and myelosuppressed groups.

These findings have prompted modifications in the therapy of PV in which there is a greater reliance on phlebotomy, avoidance of alkylating agents, more sparing use of radioactive phosphorus, the introduction of antiaggregating platelet therapy to prevent thrombosis, and the use of less mutagenic myelosuppressive agents, such as hydroxyurea, when myelosuppression is indicated. As survival has improved, the late complications of PV have become more of a problem. The demonstration that myelofibrosis is a reactive phenomenon rather than an intrinsic manifestation of MPD has stimulated investigations into its pathophysiology, but approaches to prevention of fibrosis and myelodysplasia have not been found, and these late, life-threatening complications of MPD still pose a difficult problem in management.

Diagnosis

A diagnosis of PV requires demonstration of an absolute increase in circulating red cells in the presence of other stigmata of panmyelosis. Adherence to rigorous diagnostic criteria serves to distinguish PV from the myriad of disorders that can produce an elevated hematocrit. Most hematocrit elevations result from a reduction in circulating plasma volume rather than an absolute increase in erythrocytes. Acute dehydration is readily appreciated clinically, but a chronic, low-grade state of dehydration may be overlooked. This may result from smoking or ingestion of caffeine or diuretics. These cause a diminution in plasma volume that is easily reversed and can be detected by hematocrit determinations before and after 72 hours of abstention. The presence of a persistently elevated hematocrit without obvious explanation necessitates direct measurement of red cell mass and plasma volume by isotope dilution to distinguish between relative and absolute polycythemia. Erythrocyte indices should be assessed prior to this determination, and if microcytosis is present, iron deficiency should be sought and corrected to elicit masked erythrocytosis. Blood volume determinations should be performed prior to phlebotomy, since the reactive changes in bone marrow proliferation induced by phlebotomy can be confused with stigmata of MPD.

Relative Polycythemia. Patients with a normal red cell mass and reduced intravascular plasma volume outnumber those with absolute erythrocytosis by a ratio of more than 5:1. The prototype is a young or middle-aged male smoker who presents with a hematocrit below 60 per cent and multiple nonspecific complaints, including headache, fatigue, dizziness, paresthesias, dyspnea, and epigastric distress. He is of stocky habitus, plethoric, and hypertensive and often has hypercholesterolemia, hypertriglyceridemia, and hyperuricemia. Patients with relative polycythemia are prone to cardiovascular disease, and their management should be directed at correction and prevention of coronary risk factors and elimination of any agents that further reduce the plasma volume, including phlebotomy.

Isolated Erythrocytosis. Documentation of an absolute increase in red cell mass to levels 25 per cent in excess of the predicted value requires further diagnostic evaluation to distinguish between isolated erythrocytosis arising from an abnormality affecting only the erythroid precursors and erythrocythemia as part of the panmyelosis of PV. One of the most significant stigmata of MPD is splenomegaly. If this organ is not readily palpable, a spleen scan is recommended to detect subclinical enlargement. An enlarged spleen combined with absolute erythrocytosis fulfills the criteria for a diagnosis of PV. Other criteria of diagnostic value are leukocytosis greater than 12,000 per cu mm, neutrophilia above 7000 per cu mm, a direct basophil count above 65 per cu mm, a platelet count above 400,000 per cu mm, increased leukocyte alkaline phosphatase activity, and an unsaturated serum vitamin B_{12} binding capacity over 2200 picograms per ml. In the absence of splenomegaly, at least two of these abnormalities should be present to fulfill the diagnostic criteria. All patients with absolute erythrocytosis should have an assessment of the adequacy of tissue oxygenation by measurement of arterial oxygen saturation and content, as well as oxygen affinity of hemoglobin. Tissue hypoxemia may be responsible for isolated erythrocytosis or may coexist with PV. Recognition of compensatory erythrocytosis is essential for proper management, since patients who have compensatory erythrocytosis require extra oxygen-carrying capacity and have different criteria for hematocrit reduction.

Causes of inappropriate erythrocytosis due to increased erythropoietin elaboration from hypoxic renal tissue or from tumors or hyperplasias of extrarenal tissues that elaborate erythropoietin inappropriately should be sought by appropriate testing, since many of these conditions are remediable. Patients with idiopathic or unclassified erythrocytosis should be observed carefully and restudied periodically for further clues to the nature of the erythrocytosis. Management should be restricted to manipulation of the circulating red cell mass with phlebotomy.

Treatment

The mainstay of therapy for PV is phlebotomy. The objective of this therapy is to maintain the hematocrit at levels of 45 per cent or less with the rationale that uncontrolled erythrocythemia with its attendant hypervolemia and hyperviscosity is the main contributory factor in the thrombotic and hemorrhagic complications of PV. These risks may be compounded further by qualitative platelet abnormalities. The presence of circulating platelet aggregates and degranulated platelets attests to in vivo hyperfunction of the platelet population. The normal stimulatory effect of phlebotomy on hematopoiesis is preserved and even exaggerated in PV. This response includes an increase in platelet count and the appearance of circulating platelets with increased hemostatic activity. The increased incidence of thrombosis during the first 4 years of a phlebotomy regimen may be attributable to this effect and suggests a role for platelet deaggregating therapy. However, this approach was rejected when a randomized study comparing high-dose aspirin (300 mg 3 times daily) combined with dipyridamole (Persantine), 75 mg 3 times daily, with radioactive phosphorus supplemented with phlebotomy not only failed to show a reduction in thrombotic complications but produced an increased incidence of gastrointestinal hemorrhage. However, in contrast to the results with high doses of deaggregating agents, patients treated with low-dose aspirin (325 mg or less per day) showed a complete absence both of thrombotic events and of significant hemorrhagic complications in two studies.

Phlebotomy and Platelet Antiaggregating Therapy

The combination of phlebotomy and low-dose aspirin is an efficacious regimen for most patients in the erythrocythemic phase of PV and is the treatment of choice at the time of diagnosis. Every patient with proved PV should have an initial series of phlebotomies to restore the hematocrit to a level between 40 and 45 per cent instead of a level that provides maximal cerebral blood flow. A phlebotomy of 500 ml should be performed every second or third day until this result is achieved. The number of phlebotomies required depends upon the degree of elevation of the red cell mass. Replacement of plasma or fluids is unnecessary, as the patient quickly reconstitutes his or her blood volume if oral hydration is maintained. Several phlebotomies may be required before a decrease in hematocrit occurs. In elderly patients or in those with cardiovascular disease, smaller phlebotomies of 350 ml are preferable to avoid abrupt changes in blood volume. Prior to or at the time of the first phlebotomy the patient should be placed on acetylsalicylic acid at a dose of 325 mg a day. A buffered form of acetylsalicylic acid or concomitant administration of antacids is recommended. In addition to its prophylactic function, this dose of aspirin produces prompt relief of symptoms attributable to small vessel stasis, such as erythromelalgia and transient ischemic attacks. Allopurinol (Zyloprim), 300 mg once a day, should be prescribed, regardless of the serum uric acid level, to reduce the excessive load of uric acid that results from increased nucleoprotein turnover. Blocking the conversion of hypoxanthine to uric acid reduces the risk of secondary gout and urate stones or nephropathy. Pruritus, related to release of histamine from basophils, may be relieved by the antihistaminic cyproheptadine (Periactin) in doses of 4 to 16 mg, as needed. The severe itching that is induced by bathing, showering, or undressing can be attenuated by administration of 4 to 8 mg of cyproheptadine one-half hour before exposure to the precipitating event.

After restoration of a normal hematocrit, the patient should be seen at 6-week intervals to assess the rate at which the hematocrit increases. Some patients display relatively indolent erythropoiesis, and the hematocrit may be kept at normal levels with four to six phlebotomies a year. Management with phlebotomy and aspirin should be employed in such patients, as well as in those with isolated erythrocytosis and in patients with polycythemia vera who are of childbearing age. Hypoferremia is an unavoidable consequence of the phlebotomy regimen but is rarely symptomatic except for producing pica manifested by a craving for crisp green vegetables (lettuce and celery) and ice. Erythrocyte indices are invariably hypochromic and microcytic. Iron replacement should not be given, since it will produce an increase in hematocrit and increase the phlebotomy requirement. A normal diet is appropriate, and no attempt to limit iron-containing foods should be made. Reactive thrombocytosis may occur following the initial series of phlebotomies. This increase in platelet count will be superimposed upon any elevation present prior to phlebotomy but is transient, and the platelet count usually returns to the prephlebotomy level within several weeks. Once the degree of erythroid and other proliferative activity and the need for phlebotomy have been assessed, visits may be reduced to every 8 to 10 weeks and phlebotomies of 500 ml performed as needed to maintain the hematocrit between 40 and 45 per cent. Aspirin should be continued at a dose of 325 mg each day unless the platelet count falls below normal or the patient has significant hemorrhagic complications. Concomitant administration of other drugs with platelet antiaggregating effects, such as nonsteroidal anti-inflammatory agents or antihistaminics, should be avoided to lessen the risk of hemorrhage. If these are indicated, aspirin should be discontinued during their administration.

Myelosuppressive Therapy

Myelosuppressive therapy should be reserved for treatment of proliferative manifestations other than erythrocythemia and used only when these become symptomatic. The most common indication is splenomegaly of sufficient degree to cause early satiety, abdominal discomfort on a mechanical basis, splenic infarction, and a hypermetabolic state manifested by weight loss, diaphoresis, and fever. These symptoms usually occur when the patient enters the phase of postpolycythemic myeloid metaplasia. Indications for myelosuppression during the polycythemic phase include a history of thrombotic events in a patient of advanced age (over 70 years) with risk factors for thrombosis; patients with extreme thrombocythemia (over 2 million per microliter) and symptoms of small vessel stasis; or inability to implement a phlebotomy regimen due to inadequate veins or adverse reactions to blood volume reduction. Myelosuppression can be achieved readily in MPD with a variety of agents, and the selection of an agent rests more on the nature of its potential toxicity than on its ability to produce the desired therapeutic effect.

Hydroxyurea (Hydrea). This agent is a nonalkylating myelosuppressive that inhibits DNA synthesis by inhibition of ribonucleoside diphosphate reductase. Prior experience with hydroxyurea has been confined to treatment of malignancies in patients with short life expectancies relative to that of PV, and in this setting mutagenesis has not been observed. The chronic nature of PV and the short-lived effect of hydroxyurea usually require continuous administration over many years. In a cohort of patients treated with hydroxyurea for a median of 5 years, there has been no increased incidence of leukemia or other malignancies, but the incidence of late onset leukemia and cancer that is characteristic of other myelosuppressive agents remains to be determined. Until this information is available, hydroxyurea is the myelosuppressive agent of choice because of the theoretical absence of mutagenesis confirmed by short-term experience and the well-established increased incidence of leukemia and cancer produced by radioactive phosphorus and alkylating agents.

An initial dose of 1 gram per day produces a response in 80 per cent of patients without untoward myelosuppression. As the spleen shrinks and the platelet count is reduced, the dose may be adjusted downward to 500 mg per day. If no effect is observed in 3 weeks, the dose may be increased to 1.5 grams per day. The blood count should be monitored frequently until an efficacious regimen is found. Since hydroxyurea induces a megaloblastic blood picture and has less effect on hematocrit levels than on platelet and leukocyte counts, supplementary phlebotomy is usually required. Toxicity is minimal at the doses employed for PV and is limited to skin rash, gastrointestinal intolerance, and fever.

Once the objective of myelosuppressive therapy has been achieved and the patient's disease activity is stabilized, it is useful to discontinue hydroxyurea administration to determine the rate at which the spleen enlarges or thrombocythemia recurs. In those patients with more indolent disease, it may be possible to interrupt chemotherapy for many months. In view of the dose-related mutagenicity of other agents, this would be preferable to continuous therapy. Unfortunately, maintenance treatment is usually required, since blood counts return to pretreatment levels within 2 weeks after therapy is discontinued.

Radioactive Phosphorus. Radioactive phosphorus (^{32}P) is a strong beta-ray emitter that irradiates the bone marrow both directly by isotope uptake and indirectly through uptake of the phosphate by surrounding bone. It is an excellent myelosuppressive agent, and it was particularly effective in controlling erythropoiesis and megakaryopoiesis in the large doses employed before its mutagenicity was appreciated. However, with the dose limitations imposed to deal with this toxicity, supplementary phlebotomies are frequently required, and splenomegaly may not respond. It has been recommended for the treatment of patients over the age of 70 because of their relatively short life expectancy, but in a physiologically young patient of 70 years with an expected survival of 13 years, disease duration will extend well beyond the 4-year period after which malignant transformation begins to occur. There may be an indication for the use of ^{32}P in elderly patients with thrombocythemia and a history of thrombosis and in patients who cannot tolerate hydroxyurea. The agent should be given intravenously in an initial dose of 2.7 mCi per square meter (up to a total dose of 5 mCi). If after 12 weeks suppression is inadequate, a second treatment at a 25 per cent dose escalation and a limit of 7 mCi may be given. A third dose may be administered at 24 weeks, if necessary, but if this is ineffective another agent should be employed. The action of ^{32}P is slow, and its full effect is seen after 3 months. Responsive patients may have remissions of 6 months to a year. Patients in whom thrombocythemia shows only a partial response can be managed with phlebotomy and platelet antiaggregating agents to minimize the amount of radiation administered.

Interferon. The antiproliferative properties of recombinant human interferon alpha may have an application in the treatment of polycythemia vera, since early experience has shown that control of thrombocythemia, leukocytosis, and the splenomegaly of myeloid metaplasia can be achieved and maintained with doses that produce minimal side effects. An induction dose of 3.5 million units per M^2 of body surface area of interferon alpha-2b given daily by subcutaneous injection for 20 weeks produced control of proliferative activity and significant reduction in spleen size, which persisted as dosage was reduced and finally discontinued. The ability to obtain cytoreduction with this biologic response modifier may avoid the problem of leukemogenicity posed by other myelosuppressive agents. Until further investigation establishes the efficacy of interferon as a first-line agent, its use in polycythemia vera is reserved for patients whose proliferative disease activity is life-threatening and cannot be controlled by conventional cytoreductive therapy.

Management of Complications

Thrombotic and hemorrhagic complications are managed in the same way as in the nonpolycythemic population. If medically indicated, anticoagulants may be employed. Platelet antiaggregating agents should be withheld in patients with hemorrhagic manifestations. Surgical morbidity and mortality are increased in PV, and elective surgery should be avoided. When surgery is indicated, the blood volume should be restored to normal with phlebotomy. Platelet deaggregating therapy should be introduced on the fourth or fifth postoperative day if there is no postoperative bleeding to prevent thrombotic complications secondary to the reactive thrombocytosis that may follow surgery.

Postpolycythemia myeloid metaplasia is often complicated by anemia. At this stage iron or folate deficiency should be sought and corrected.

Splenomegaly is accompanied by an expansion of the plasma volume, and in some patients the anemia is primarily dilutional. Measurement of the red cell mass is useful, as it may reveal normal or even increased levels of circulating red cells combined with marked hydremia. The use of diuretics may partially correct this state and relieve any symptoms of circulatory overload that are present. An absolute reduction in red cell mass may result from decreased erythropoiesis or shortened red cell survival. In the latter case, the patient may benefit from shrinkage of the spleen with hydroxyurea as described earlier.

Patients who have hypersplenism with shortened red cell survival sufficient to require transfusion therapy may benefit from corticosteroid therapy. Androgens may stimulate erythropoiesis and are worthy of a trial. Response is slow to occur, and therapy should be continued for 6 months. Splenectomy may benefit selected patients with postpolycythemic myeloid metaplasia in whom there is evidence of hypersplenism. Thrombocythemia is an absolute contraindication to splenectomy and must be corrected with myelosuppressive therapy before surgery in order to avoid a life-threatening postoperative thrombocythemia. Evidence of low grade disseminated intravascular coagulation is also a contraindication to splenectomy.

Acute leukemia develops in 1 to 2 per cent of PV patients treated with phlebotomy alone and in 10 to 20 per cent of patients treated with myelosuppressive agents. Acute nonlymphocytic leukemia is the most common type, but acute lymphoblastic or biphenotypic leukemias occur in one third of cases. Acute leukemia complicating MPD shows a poor response to conventional therapy. Thus, younger patients should be offered the opportunity to harvest and cryopreserve bone marrow during the polycythemic phase of their disease to permit aggressive chemotherapy and autologous bone marrow transplant if acute leukemia develops.

Choice of Therapy

The patient with PV presents a challenge in management, for the benefits conferred by proper treatment are dramatic in terms of improved survival and well-being. Customizing management to accommodate the factors of age, disease duration, previous and present complications, disease phenotype, and disease activity can afford the patient a long and uncomplicated course. The dilemma of myelosuppression versus phlebotomy and platelet antiaggregating therapy remains. However, equipped with the knowledge that the use of myelosuppression can be avoided or minimized in many patients and that a potentially nonmutagenic chemotherapeutic agent is now available, the physician can meet the challenge of treatment with greater optimism and expectation of even longer survival and fewer complications.

PORPHYRIA

method of
NEVILLE R. PIMSTONE, M.D.
University of California, Davis
Sacramento, California

The human porphyrias are a group of disorders that reflect bone marrow or hepatic expression of inherited and/or acquired disorders of heme biosynthesis. This is the basis for the broad classification of erythropoietic, or hepatic, porphyria (Table 1). Each syndrome results from a defect in one enzymatic step in the biosynthesis of heme; an alternate classification is by the metabolic lesion. Although uncommon, human porphyria is important not only because photocutaneous manifestations can be debilitating and disfiguring but also because individuals with most inherited hepatic porphyrias are prone to potentially lethal acute attacks associated with a rapidly progressive polyneuropathy, acute abdomen, severe psychiatric disturbance, and coma.

The wide spectrum of clinical presentation makes porphyria the domain of the gastroenterologist, hematologist, dermatologist, and neurologist. Prompt diagnosis is required not only to initiate appropriate treatment but also to provide for the institution of prophylaxis and genetic counseling for other potentially afflicted family members.

Clinical Manifestations

If the metabolic lesion is distal to the porphobilinogen (PBG) deaminase step, photosensitizing porphyrins may accumulate in the plasma and skin, resulting in photocutaneous lesions. In the hepatic porphyrias other than porphyria cutanea tarda (PCT) (Table 1), ingestion of a porphyrinogenic drug (Table 2) may result in an acute attack in which abdominal pain, polyneuropathy, or neurologic disturbances may dominate. In the erythropoietic porphyria syndromes (see Table 1) there may be hematologic abnormalities with alterations in bone marrow morphology, circulating fluorocytes (i.e., erythrocytes with increased free porphyrin), and anemia. Hepatic manifestations may occur in PCT, in which liver injury and hepatic iron may be required for expression of the metabolic lesion. In protoporphyria, hepatobiliary disorders may relate to hepatic accumulation of the excess porphyrin pigment. Thus, the main clinical expressions of the metabolic lesions in porphyria are cutaneous, hepatic, hematologic, and neurologic. These may occur singly or in combination and are summarized in Table 3.

PBG synthase deficiency porphyria, acute intermit-

TABLE 1. Classification of Human Porphyrias

I. Hepatic Porphyrias (Erythrocyte-Free Porphyrin Normal)
   Porphobilinogen (PBG) synthase deficiency
   Acute intermittent porphyria (AIP)
   Hereditary coproporphyria (HCP)
   Variegate porphyria (VP)
   Porphyria cutanea tarda (PCT)
     Sporadic PCT
     Familial PCT
     Toxic porphyria cutanea
     Renal failure
II. Erythropoietic Porphyria (Erythrocyte-Free Porphyrin Increased)
   Congenital erythropoietic porphyria (CEP)
   Protoporphyria (PP)
   Rare: Homozygous PCT (hepatoerythropoietic porphyria)

tent porphyria (AIP), hereditary coproporphyria (HCP), and variegate porphyria (VP) may be associated with acute attacks; therefore some authors classify these collectively as the acute hepatic porphyrias. This approach has not been adopted here because VP and HCP may be clinically indistinguishable from the photocutaneous PCT syndromes, and biochemically the heme precursor excretory profiles in these two disorders differ greatly in acute exacerbations of the disease when compared to the disease in remission (Table 4). In this chapter, acute hepatic porphyria and acute porphyric attack are synonymous.

Cutaneous Features. Skin lesions may result from the interaction of exciting wave bands of visible light with porphyrins and therefore occur in sun-exposed areas (i.e., the face, "V" of the neck, and extremities, particularly the hands). The lesions, which may be mild, include erosions, bullae, skin fragility, increased pigmentation, depigmented scars, and an increased downy hair growth on the face. These features are clinically indistinguishable in PCT, HCP, and VP.

Photomutilating disfigurement of the face and hands

TABLE 2. Porphyrinogenic Drugs

	Potentially Dangerous	Safe
Antimicrobials:	Dapsone	Aminoglycosides
	Griseofulvin	Cephalosporins
	Pyrazinamide	Penicillins
	Sulfonamides	Primaquine
Anticonvulsants:	Barbiturates	Bromides
	Carbamazepine	Ether
	Hydantoins	Nitrous oxide
Tranquilizers:	Glutethimide	Chloral hydrate
	Meprobamate	Lorazepam
	Methyprylon	Meclizine
Other:	Alpha methyldopa	Aspirin
	Aminopyrine	Atropine
	Dipyrone	Beta blockers
	Phenylbutazone	Codeine
	Sulfonylureas	Dicumarol
		Digitalis
		Diphenhydramine
		Insulin
		Morphine

TABLE 3. **Clinical Manifestations of Human Porphyrias**

	Cutaneous	Hepatic	Hematologic	Neurologic
PBG synthase deficiency porphyria	−	−	−	+
AIP	−	−	−	+
CEP	+ +	−	−	−
PCT	+	+	+ / −	−
HCP	+	−	−	+
VP	+	−	−	+
PP	+	+ / −	+	−

Abbreviations: PBG = porphobilinogen; AIP = acute intermittent porphyria; CEP = congenital erythropoietic porphyria; PCT = porphyria cutanea tarda; HCP = hereditary coproporphyria; VP = variegate porphyria; PP = protoporphyria.

is a function of anatomic distribution and the amount of porphyrin accumulating in the skin, and classically occurs in congenital erythropoietic porphyria (CEP). Solar urticarial syndromes and increased thickening of the skin are more characteristic of protoporphyria (PP).

Acute Porphyric Attacks. Patients with PBG synthase deficiency porphyria, AIP, HCP, and VP are prone to acute porphyric attacks. The attack may be precipitated by a variety of agents (see Table 3), many of which are slowly metabolized, lipid-soluble drugs requiring hepatic microsomal cytochrome P450 for biotransformation. This is most likely to occur when endogenous stimulation of hepatic cytochrome P450 is maximal (i.e., postpuberty and in premenstruation). Indeed, premenstrual acute porphyria may occur without antecedent ingestion of porphyrinogenic drugs. Patients also are particularly susceptible to acute attacks when on reduced calorie intake. Opinions differ regarding the hazards of pregnancy and the use of oral contraceptive pills. The risk has been reported as ranging from near zero to between 15 and 20 per cent

in pregnancy. Because of the diversity of world opinion in this regard, all female porphyric patients at risk of developing acute porphyria should be monitored closely if oral contraceptives are prescribed or if they are pregnant.

The most common clinical feature of the acute porphyric attack is vomiting, with mid-abdominal pain often radiating through the back. The abdomen usually is soft, with minimal tenderness and no rebound. Constipation and vomiting may result in a syndrome difficult to distinguish from an acute abdomen. Fever and leukocytosis may occur but are unusual. Because porphyrins in the urine result in a port wine color, the combination of abdominal pain and red urine may clinically raise the suspicion of the passage of renal stones with hematuria.

The neurologic symptoms of an acute porphyric attack are extremely variable and can be dominantly a peripheral polyneuropathy, an autonomic neuropathy, or encephalopathy. The cerebrospinal fluid is normal in acute porphyric polyneuropathy and encephalopathy. The polyneuropathy is associated with a polyax-

TABLE 4. **Heme Precursor Excretion Profiles in the Human Porphyrias**

	Urine				Stool		
Subtype	ALA (2 mg/ day)	PBG (<6 mg/day)	URO (<50 µg/day)	COPRO (<250 µg/day)	COPRO (<50 µg/gram dry wt)	PROTO (<120 µg/gram dry wt)	ISO
PBG synthase* deficiency porphyrin	+ +	N	N	N	N	N	−
PBG deaminase* (AIP)	+ +	+ +	+ +		N	N	−
UROgen III Co-synthase (CEP)	N	N	+ + +	+	N	N	−
UROD (PCT)	N	N	+ + +	+ +	+ +	N	+ +
COPROgen oxidase (HCP)							
Remission	N	N	+ −	+ +	+ +	N	−
Acute Attack	+ +	+ +	+	+ +	+ +	N	−
PROTOgen oxidase (VP)							
Remission	N	N	+	+ +	+	+ + +	−
Acute Attack	+ +	+ +	+ + +	+ +	+	+ + +	−
Ferrochelatase (PP)	N	N	N	N	N	+ +	−

*The heme precursor excretory profile in urine and stool is similar in remission to that seen in acute porphyric attacks.
Abbreviations: ALA = delta-aminolevulinic acid; PBG = porphobilinogen; URO = uroporphyrin; COPRO = coproporphyrin; PROTO = protoporphyrin; ISO = isomer; AIP = acute intermittent porphyria; CEP = congenital erythropoietic porphyria; UROD = uroporphyrinogen decarboxylase; PCT = porphyria cutanea tarda; HCP = hereditary coproporphyria; VP = Variegate porphyria; PP = protoporphyria. The normal (N) values are listed in the column headings. Abnormally elevated levels are graded from borderline (+ −) to very high (+ + +).

onal degeneration and even though the rapidity of onset and progression may lead to a total body paralysis requiring mechanical ventilation, recovery, albeit slow, usually is complete within 7 to 10 days. Autonomic neuropathy usually is manifested as hypertension and tachycardia. Encephalopathy ranges from forgetfulness, headaches, and neuroses to convulsions and deep coma. No specific neuropathologic defect has been noted, and the clinical spectrum in part may relate to inappropriate water retention, either related to the secretion of antidiuretic hormone or as a result of a direct effect of the porphyrinogen precursors on renal tubular function. The encephalopathy usually is associated with hyponatremia.

There are two prevailing theories as to the metabolic basis of the acute porphyric attack. One proposal is that the universal heme precursor delta-aminolevulinic acid (ALA), which is overproduced in all patients with acute porphyria, may have distal effects on extrahepatic cells such as neurones and renal tubules, resulting in neuropathy and/or electrolyte imbalance. The level of ALA in the urine of any patient correlates with the disease activity of that patient. This does not rule out the possibility that porphyrin precursor overproduction and excretion may be epiphenomena of the acute porphyric process.

The other prevailing theory is that when the potential for hepatic heme deficiency exists, this may be exacerbated by drugs that increase the requirement for endogenous heme synthesis by inducing microsomal cytochrome P450 synthesis. This might result in deficient synthesis of other hemoproteins such as tryptophanpyrrolase or in diminished export by the liver of heme to other organs where it may be necessary for cellular function, for example, of the neurons. Whatever the metabolic basis for acute porphyria, treatment regimens are aimed at diminishing ALA and PBG overproduction and repleting cellular heme.

Hematologic Features. In both PP and CEP, there is increased porphyrin in normoblasts and in circulating erythrocytes. These can be detected by bone marrow ultraviolet (UV) microscopy, in which the abnormal normoblasts exhibit intense red porphyrin fluorescence. The red cell smear will exhibit similar fluorescence of erythrocytes, often referred to as fluorocytes. In CEP, the bone marrow usually shows gross morphologic disturbance with dyserythropoiesis, bizarre grapelike nuclei, and evidence of intramedullary death of the porphyric normoblast population. Photohemolysis may occur in both erythropoietic porphyrias, particularly in CEP, in which the anemia may be associated with splenomegaly.

Hepatic Manifestations. Both PCT and PP are characterized by hepatic lesions. Although a specific lesion has been reported in PCT, the changes are generally nonspecific and nondiagnostic. Common in all patients with PCT is hepatic accumulation of porphyrin, which in this disease is mainly uroporphyrin and heptacarboxyl porphyrin. Thus, the best diagnostic approach is to look at the freshly procured liver biopsy core under UV light, prior to fixation, for spotty or diffuse, orange-red porphyrin fluorescence.

Histologically, 70 per cent of patients with sporadic PCT will exhibit morphologic evidence of iron overload, with stainable hemosiderin present in the liver. Iron overload usually is modest, in the order of 2 to 4 grams above normal, and in some patients may represent the heterozygote trait for idiopathic hemochromatosis. Hepatic injury may play an independent role in the expression of the metabolic lesion in PCT.

In PP, the liver disease results from accumulation of protoporphyrin in the liver. It is unknown whether this relates to endogenous hepatic protoporphyrin overproduction in this organ or to impaired hepatic clearance. Birefringent, brown protoporphyrin crystals are classic histologic features in this disease and can be detected by routine, polarization, and electron microscopy. The liver damage may vary from spotty necrosis to portal fibrosis and cirrhosis. The latter condition is rare, but when present has the propensity to rapidly deteriorate with liver failure. Gallbladder and biliary complications include the increased likelihood of gallstones which in part may be composed of protoporphyrin.

Biochemical Diagnosis

At the present moment, most laboratories do not routinely measure cell heme biosynthetic enzyme function, which would appear to be the most specific diagnostic technique. Measuring enzyme activity alone would be insufficient since there are a significant number of patients with AIP and normal PBG deaminase activity. Also sporadic PCT exhibits diminished uroporphyrinogen decarboxylase (UROD) activity in the liver tissue only; the defective enzyme thus may have normal activity but diminished substrate affinity and other kinetic abnormalities requiring tedious analyses for characterization. An immunologic approach to detect abnormal enzymes also might be difficult because even in one disease, enzyme heterogeneity exists.

A second approach that might be comprehensive and quick is to determine by chromatography the porphyrin profile on plasma and stool, which in each porphyria may be unique. This "fingerprint" approach requires analysis of every individual porphyrin either as free porphyrins or porphyrin esters. Although diagnostic, this service is not widely available. Thus, at the present time, one should rely on measurement of porphyrins and their precursors PBG and ALA in urine and stool.

Screening tests for fecal and urinary porphyrins are of little value. However, test kits for screening the urine for elevated levels of PBG are usually available in hospitals. Variants of these are known as the Watson-Schwartz and Hoesch tests (Figure 1). If negative, acute porphyria can be excluded in AIP, HCP, and VP. This is a simple test in which freshly voided urine (1 to 2 ml) is alkalinized and mixed with an equal volume of Ehrlich's reagent and shaken in a glass test tube; 0.5 to 1 ml of chloroform is added, shaken with the aqueous phase, and the chloroform allowed to settle. The immediate development of a reddish purple color complex not extractable by chloroform is highly suggestive of abnormal levels of PBG. Urobilinogen, which is the main cause of error, causes a pink color which intensifies slowly and is readily extractable with chloroform. It should be remembered that all patients with biochemically active AIP will excrete increased amounts of PBG in the urine at all times; therefore, when assessing known AIP patients, a positive screening test for PBG is of no value in evaluating acute symptoms. It also is of no value in the rare PBG synthase deficiency porphyria, in which the only elevated porphyrinogen precursor is ALA.

Quantitative measurement of porphyrins, PBG, and ALA by solvent extraction is widely available and essential in the workup of any porphyric patient. A 24-hour urine aliquot shielded from light either by aluminum foil or by a brown paper bag should be sent to the lab for quantitative estimation of porphyrin (micrograms per 24 hours) and porphyrinogen precursors (mg per dl). Also, routinely, 3 to 4 grams of stool should be sent to the same laboratory for quantitative porphyrin testing (micrograms per gram of dry-weight stool).

Referring to Tables 1 and 4, one might anticipate increased levels of urinary ALA in PBG synthase deficiency; ALA, PBG, and uroporphyrin (spontaneous formation) in AIP; urinary uroporphyrin excess in CEP; urinary uroporphyrinuria with increased coproporphyrin in the stool in PCT; urinary coproporphyrinuria with increased coproporphyrin in the stool in CEP; and coproporphyrinuria with increased protoporphyrin in the stool in VP patients in remission. Urinary uroporphyrin is the dominant pigment excreted in acute VP. In erythropoietic protoporphyria, there is no urinary excretion of porphyrins, but stool protoporphyrin levels are elevated. When CEP and PP are suspected, red cell porphyrins should be quantitated and looked for by UV microscopy.

A very simple, thin-layer chromatographic technique can detect an isomer of coproporphyrin called isocoproporphyrin in stool, which is specific marker of uroporphyrinogen decarboxylase deficiency and therefore is important in the diagnosis of PCT. Thus, in cutaneous porphyria, PCT can be differentiated from VP by a comparison of urinary uroporphyrin and fecal protoporphyrin or by measurement of the isocoproporphyrin:coproporphyrin ratio in feces. This is an important distinction, as PCT patients are *not* prone to develop acute porphyric attacks. The most widely available red cell enzyme assay is that for PBG deaminase, which, if deficient, would suggest acute intermittent porphyria.

PORPHYRIC SYNDROMES

The metabolic lesion in the heme biosynthetic pathway is usually silent, especially in the hepatic porphyrias, and biochemical/clinical expression is precipitated or modulated by endogenous or exogenous factors such as hormone activity, liver disease, drug ingestion, or hemopoietic activity.

PBG Synthase Deficiency Porphyria

This is a rare autosomal recessive disorder of hepatic heme biosynthesis, with homozygotes exhibiting a substantial decrease in a tissue PBG synthase activity. Persons with this disorder present with a history of recurrent acute attacks in childhood that resemble AIP, but with an isolated elevation of urinary ALA with normal PBG levels. As lead also inhibits heme biosynthesis at this step, lead poisoning can uncover PBG synthase deficiency, producing a toxogenetic porphyria. In tyrosinemia, because of the accumulation of succinylacetone, a potent inhibitor of PBG synthetase, a similar syndrome may occur. Treatment of the acute attack is as described below for AIP.

Acute Intermittent Porphyria (AIP)

AIP is an autosomal dominant disorder associated with a deficiency in PBG deaminase activity. It is the most common cause of acute porphyria in the United States. The first and most intensive study of this familial porphyria was undertaken in 1937 by Waldenström. Because of its high prevalence in Sweden, it was previously referred to as Swedish porphyria. The peak age of onset is in the third decade, and only a few cases have been described in children. Red cell PBG deaminase levels usually are deficient, but some patients with biochemically confirmed AIP may have normal red cell values consistent with defective enzyme action rather than an absolute deficiency of the enzyme. These patients are subject to acute attacks but will not have cutaneous porphyria.

Diagnosis

The biochemical diagnosis of AIP is confirmed by the presence of increased urinary ALA and PBG with normal stool porphyrins. This occurs both in base-line situations and during acute exacerbations. In every AIP patient, a base-line urine porphyrin and porphyrinogen precursor level should be obtained. In women, base-lines should be established both in mid-cycle and premenstrually. Once this base-line has been established, if there should be an acute clinical situation such as abdominal pain, polyneuropathy, or epilepsy, a repeat 24-hour urine quantitation of porphyrin precursors will determine if this is due to a porphyric attack. If the levels are the same as the base-line levels, one should look for another cause of the symptomatology. However, if there has been a significant change (i.e., doubling or trebling of base-line values), the patient should be aggressively treated for an acute attack.

Treatment

The cornerstone of treatment of AIP is prophylaxis. Other family members at risk should be identified by evaluation for the genetic trait by red cell PBG deaminase screening or tested for biochemical activity at regular intervals, at least until the age of 21 years. Patients at risk for acute porphyria should wear a Medic-Alert bracelet indicating the potential for developing an acute attack in response to porphyrinogenic drugs (see Table 3). Patients should be advised never to buy over-the-counter drugs. Both attending physicians and pharmacists should have a list of safe and potentially hazardous drugs.

The treatment of acute porphyria is schematically outlined as an algorithm in Figure 1. The initial approach is largely supportive, with fluid and electrolyte balance meticulously restored and maintained. Progression of paralysis to involvement of the respiratory muscles is watched for, and the patient may require artificial ventilation. If pain is prominent, it can be relieved by meperidine hydrochloride or morphine. Hypertension can be treated with beta blockers such as propanolol (Inderal), 10 to 40 mg 3 to 4 times daily. Encephalopathy with hypochloremia and hypernatremia should be treated by fluid and electrolyte correction and subsequent water restriction. When ileus is present and precludes oral administration of fluids, intravenous feeding is necessary. Salt-free solutions of dextrose may precipitate porphyric encephalopathy, and dextrose-free electrolyte solutions may aggravate the porphyric process by calorie deprivation. Therefore, saline in 10 per cent dextrose with intermittent boluses of concentrated dextrose intravenously (50 per cent W/V) is recommended to boost calorie intake in the face of fluid restriction. When the patient is able to eat, a high carbohydrate/protein diet (about 2000 calories per day) diminishes porphyrinogen overproduction and reduces porphyrinogen precursor excretion in the urine. The so-called "glucose effect" as a form of treatment is easy to achieve in any hospital setting.

More recently, intravenous hematin has been in use. Hematin, produced in 1971, has found wide acceptance and is effective in that it suppresses the rate-limiting enzyme in heme biosynthesis (i.e., ALA synthase activity) and replenishes deficient intracellular heme pools. It may also restore hepatic tryptophanpyrrolase activity. Hematin should be administered in a dose of 2 to 4 mg per kg twice daily for 3 days in association with a calorie-rich diet, particularly in the form of carbohydrate and protein calories. Hematin is generally well tolerated, but it can cause a transient coagulopathy.

Recently, heme arginate has been synthesized in Finland under the trade name Normosang (Medica, Helsinki); this may be a more stable form of heme with fewer side effects. It should be available shortly in the United States. Heme arginate is recommended at a dose of 3 mg per kg daily. The usual schedule is to dilute heme arginate in 100 ml of physiologic saline and infuse it over a 15-minute period into a peripheral vein daily for 4 consecutive days. This, combined with a high caloric intake, almost invariably results in biochemical and clinical remission. The side effects seen with hematin, such as coagulation disturbances and thrombophlebitis, have not been observed with heme arginate.

Congenital Erythropoietic Porphyria (CEP)

CEP is a rare, autosomal recessive disorder reported in less than 100 persons worldwide. It is also the most striking porphyria in terms of the severity of cutaneous photosensitivity. Synonyms are congenital porphyria, erythropoietic porphyria, and Günther's disease. The defective homozygote exhibits marked increases in porphyrins in the bone marrow, red cells, urine, and feces. Defective uroporphyrinogen III co-synthase activity results in preferential formation of isomer I rather than isomer III porphyrinogens. Isomer I porphyrinogens cannot be metabolized beyond coproporphyrinogen I and are not physiologic heme precursors.

CEP usually manifests in infancy. The first sign of the disease classically is pink-to-deep burgundy staining of the infant's diapers by urine or meconium. Severe photocutaneous lesions occur in childhood with blistering of the epidermis, bullous formation, secondary infection, and photomutilation. Hypertrichosis frequently is pres-

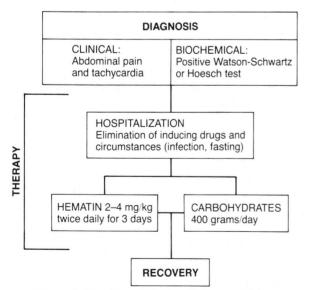

Figure 1. Algorithm of therapeutic approach to an acute porphyric attack. (Reprinted with permission of Dr. Claus Pierach.)

ent. The teeth are brown, exhibiting reddish fluorescence under UV illumination. This is due to porphyrin deposition in the dentine of the teeth (and, indeed, of the entire skeleton). Patients are usually clinically anemic with splenomegaly. The anemia is normocytic and there is usually evidence of hemolysis such as diminished serum haptoglobin and decreased red cell survival. Fluorocytes can be seen on UV microscopy of blood smears. The bone marrow morphology is grossly normal with striking dyserythropoietic changes.

Diagnosis

The diagnosis of CEP should be suspected in all cutaneous porphyric patients who become symptomatic in childhood. This can occur in CEP, PP, toxic forms of porphyria cutanea, and rare syndromes such as hepatoerythropoietic porphyria due to homozygous defects of autosomal dominantly inherited hepatic porphyria. Biochemical differentiation from rare CEP-like syndromes (e.g., hepatoerythropoietic porphyria) requires sophisticated studies of porphyrin profiles and heme biosynthetic enzyme testing. These tests are restricted to only a few research laboratories in the United States.

Biochemically, CEP is characterized by the excretion of large amounts of uroporphyrin isomer I in the urine, with relatively normal stool porphyrins. The diagnosis can be confirmed by detection of uroporphyrin in circulating erythrocytes and by the classic dyserythropoietic bone marrow on histology, with subpopulations of fluorescent normoblasts on UV microscopy.

Treatment

There is no satisfactory treatment for CEP. Sunscreen lotions are not protective, as the exciting wavebands of light extend to both the short and long wavelengths of the electromagnetic spectrum of visible light. Educating the patient to avoid sunlight by wearing protective clothing and by other measures is the only way to prevent photocutaneous skin damage.

Many studies show that hypertransfusion suppresses bone marrow activity and porphyrin production. A few reported cases have responded to a combination of weekly transfusion and splenectomy. The attendant dangers of transfusion-related iron overload and viral diseases need to be considered in determining the best clinical approach.

Activated charcoal (ActaChar) in large doses (up to 200 grams per day) has been successful in depleting plasma and skin plasma porphyrins and reversing the cutaneous lesion. This form of treatment is still in the early phase of evaluation.

Porphyria Cutanea Tarda (PCT)

PCT is recognized worldwide as the most common form of human porphyria. It is similar to CEP in that it is a purely cutaneous porphyria. However, it differs in that the photocutaneous effects appear to reflect hepatic rather than erythropoietic overproduction of porphyrins, and the pattern of porphyrin overproduction is consistent with defective hepatic uroporphyrinogen decarboxylation. A reduction of approximately 50 per cent in UROD activity has been universally reported.

In sporadic PCT, environmental factors clearly modulate clinical and biochemical expression. Red cell UROD activity is normal, which suggests that the defective UROD activity is limited to the liver. Clinical and biochemical activity is rarely spontaneous and almost invariably associated with hepatic injury, usually due to alcohol, and iron overload. Occasionally it is precipitated by the use of oral contraceptives. The cutaneous lesions are not photomutilating; they occur in sun-exposed areas, particularly affecting the hands and are clinically indistinguishable from those seen in VP and HCP. It is critical for the physician to recognize this fact because 34 per cent of VP patients may have a purely cutaneous porphyria syndrome like PCT, yet carry the potential of life-threatening acute porphyric attacks precipitated by common drugs such as barbiturates and anti-epileptics. This is not the case with PCT, which can be cured either by the depletion of hepatic iron or by eliminating the offending agent (e.g., estrogen-containing oral contraceptives).

The question of a relationship between liver carcinoma and PCT is still an open one. Two studies, made in Czechoslovakia and Spain, prior to the days of therapy, have shown increased prevalence of primary liver cancer in PCT patients. More recently, similar studies in the same countries have revealed no increased prevalence of hepatocellular carcinoma if PCT patients are treated appropriately. Rarely, a primary tumor may be the source of porphyrin overproduction and cause PCT.

Familial PCT is an autosomal dominant disorder characterized by overt, subclinical, or latent forms of the disease in which hepatic and erythrocyte UROD activity is diminished approximately 50 per cent. Although iron overload is less common, patients respond well to maneuvers to deplete iron stores.

Toxic porphyria cutanea may occur following exposure to compounds that inhibit UROD activity, such as hexachlorobenzene (HCB), which caused the first well-studied epidemic of toxic PCT in Turkey between 1956 and 1961. It also can follow exposure to other industrial toxins such as tetrachlorodibenzo-p-dioxin (TCDD). PCT and pseudo-PCT also have been observed in chronic renal failure, in which elevated plasma porphyrins may be the only abnormality.

Two rare UROD deficiency syndromes are hepatoerythropoietic porphyria (HEP), a presumed homozygous form of PCT, characterized by severe photocutaneous sensitivity exhibited from birth, liver disease, and normal bone marrow morphology; and a rare syndrome in which a dyserythropoietic anemia resembling CEP results from bone marrow expression of the gene defect for PCT.

Diagnosis

As with all porphyrias, 24-hour urine quantitative porphyrin and porphyrin precursor analysis as well as stool porphyrin assay will provide the diagnosis in 95 per cent of cases. The clear distinction from the excretory profile of VP is based on the dominance of uroporphyrin in the urine and of coproporphyrin in the stool. In contrast, in VP patients in remission, coproporphyrin is the dominant pigment in the urine and protoporphyrin is elevated in the feces. Thin-layer chromatography readily identifies isocoproporphyrin, a pigment specific for UROD deficiency states in general.

Most patients have liver function abnormalities, and liver biopsy is indicated to assess the activity and extent of the underlying liver disease. A simple, quick, and effective diagnostic maneuver is to view the fresh liver biopsy tissue core under Wood's lamp (UV light). The liver of PCT patients invariably exhibits diffuse spotty or diffuse orange-red porphyrin fluorescence. Following this test, the liver specimen passes through glass and can therefore be fixed for standard microscopy. The histopathologic features in PCT have already been described. The liver and red cell UROD activity is not routinely measured, but this can be done by special laboratories to distinguish familial from sporadic subtypes.

Treatment

General measures such as avoidance of sunlight should be adopted as much as possible, including avoidance of indirect light through glass, because visible light in the blue and red range of the electromagnetic spectrum passes through glass and can therefore cause photochemically induced skin damage. Other general measures include wearing gloves and wide-brimmed hats, avoiding hand trauma, and prompt treatment of infected bullae.

The first specific approach in PCT should be to remove the inciting agent, if this can be identi-fied. When a precipitating drug or toxin is identified, this should be discontinued. Oral contraceptive–induced PCT may disappear 3 months after withdrawal of the steroid. Removal of toxins may result in remission of toxic porphyria cutanea. However, in idiosyncratic sporadic PCT associated with alcoholic liver disease, it is unusual for alcohol withdrawal alone to result in remission.

Because iron stores are only modestly increased (1 to 2 grams) in PCT, phlebotomy with removal of 2 to 3 liters of blood usually will result in hepatic iron depletion and an associated clinical and biochemical therapeutic remission. Phlebotomy treatment should be monitored by complete blood counts, serum iron and ferritin, and 24-hour urinary porphyrin levels. If the hemoglobin falls below 11 grams per dl, or the serum iron to less than 50 micrograms per dl, treatment should be discontinued. Often it takes months for urinary uroporphyrin levels to drop and for clinical remission to occur.

Low-dose oral chloroquine at a dose of 125 mg twice weekly enhances porphyrin excretion, either by facilitating its loss from liver cells or causing a toxic necrosis of porphyrin-laden hepatocytes due to chloroquine-porphyrin interaction. This also provides an effective form of therapy. However, larger doses of chloroquine in PCT can produce an actue toxic hepatitis resembling viral hepatitis.

Newer, still experimental forms of therapy include the use of sorbents such as oral charcoal, which bind porphyrins in the gut and, by depleting the portal circulation of porphyrins, rapidly decrease porphyrins in the systemic circulation and skin. This may be useful as adjuvant therapy in rapidly achieving clinical remission while waiting for phlebotomy or chloroquine therapy to effect long-standing remission.

Hereditary Coproporphyria (HCP)

HCP is a rare, "mixed" porphyria that may present postpuberty as a purely cutaneous porphyria, an acute intermittent porphyria, or as both syndromes during the course of the disease. This autosomal dominant genetic disorder was first described in 1955; only 100 to 200 cases have been reported worldwide. Clinically, HCP resembles VP, but with a different metabolic lesion, (i.e., defective activity of the mitochondrial enzyme coproporphyrinogen oxidase). Biochemically, the disease is characterized by increased urinary and fecal excretion of coproporphyrin.

Variegate Porphyria (VP)

VP is an autosomal dominant disorder of heme biosynthesis, particularly prevalent in South Africa where more than 10,000 patients have been traced back to a marriage between a Dutch orphan girl sent to South Africa to be the wife of one of the freeburghers in 1688. The prevalence of this disease in South Africa is approximately 3 in every 1000 Caucasians. A synonym for VP is South African genetic porphyria.

The enzymatic lesion is a deficiency of the mitochondrial enzyme, protoporphyrinogen oxidase. The term *variegate* describes its variable form of presentation. VP is a postpubertal disorder that may be latent or overt. Overt cases usually present in the third decade, but the disease is biochemically apparent by the age of 20. This may reflect endogenous stimulation of hepatic heme biosynthesis by the postpubertal endogenous sex steroids in both sexes. The manner of presentation is purely cutaneous in 34 per cent of patients, and intermittent acute porphyria is the clinical presentation in 15 per cent. Cutaneous lesions occur in at least 80 per cent of patients with overt VP and are similar to those of PCT.

The acute attack is as described in the section on Clinical Manifestations. The diagnosis should always be suspected if acute abdominal pain or polyneuropathy is associated with autonomic neuropathic features (i.e., sinus tachycardia and mild hypertension). The biochemical diagnosis is summarized in Table 4. In the stool, in which protoporphyrin dominates, there is no change in the acute attack. The coproporphyrinuria of the patient changes to a uroporphyrinuria. Base-line porphyrin precursor ALA and PBG levels in the urine, which in remission are in the normal range, can increase to more than ten times normal. This underscores the importance in VP patients of always checking freshly voided urine for PBG (see the section on Biochemical Diagnosis). Unlike PBG synthase deficiency, in which ALA is the only porphyrinogen precursor in urine and unlike AIP in which ALA and PBG levels are always elevated (even when the disease is in remission), the presence of PBG by urinary screening tests in VP and HCP patients is an indicator of an acute attack. The converse also holds true; that is, in a person with a nonspecific acute clinical syndrome suspected of being acute VP, the absence of an excess of PBG in the urine excludes acute porphyria.

Treatment

Cutaneous Lesions. Treatment of cutaneous VP lesions is unsatisfactory. The skin is fragile, with easily disrupted epidermal and dermal layers. Avoiding trauma is important as a general measure. As with PCT, prompt treatment of infected bullae will help prevent scars. Avoidance of sun-

light and the use of wide-brimmed hats and gloves may be helpful. Any cholestatic episode (i.e., in reaction to drugs such as estrogens, viral hepatitis, or extrahepatic obstruction) can divert porphyrins to the plasma and cause exacerbation of cutaneous lesions. The underlying cholestatic syndromes require evaluation and treatment.

Encouraging are preliminary data suggesting that sorbents which bind porphyrins in the lumen of the gut can divert porphyrins from the portal circulation to the feces, thereby depleting systemic plasma and skin of porphyrins. This may provide more specific therapy for cutaneous VP and is still under investigation.

Acute Attack. Treatment of an established acute attack follows the same lines as for PBG synthase deficiency porphryia and AIP. The use of glucose and carbohydrates and/or hematin or heme arginate rapidly reverses biochemical and clinical activity. As with AIP, established paralysis usually resolves, although the resolution may take months to occur.

Protoporphyria (PP)

PP is regarded as an erythropoietic porphyria in which the metabolic lesion is an autosomal dominant inherited deficiency of mitochondrial ferrochelatase activity. First described in 1961 in a patient who had biliary tract disease, it is now established that PP is a disorder with childhood photosensitivity associated with the presence of porphyrin-laden circulating red cells and bone marrow normoblasts that fluoresce intensely under UV microscopy. Clinically and biochemically, the patient may exhibit erythropoietic and/or hepatic features. For this reason, the term protoporphyria may be preferable to erythropoietic protoporphyria.

In patients with PP, exposure to sunlight is followed by a tingling or burning sensation in the exposed areas, associated with intense pruritus, erythema, wheal formation, edema, and exudation. The condition has been referred to as solar urticaria or solar eczema, and the lesions rapidly subside within 24 hours. Over many years, irreversible coarsening and puckering of the skin may develop.

The hepatobiliary lesions are more subtle. Hepatic involvement in most patients with PP is absent or minimal and may only be detected by sensitive measurement of liver function, or by liver biopsy when liver function is normal. The classic histologic liver lesion is hepatic accumulation of brown pigment on routine microscopy, which fluoresces on UV microscopy and which exhibits birefringence on polarization microscopy. The pigment is crystalline in structure on electron microscopy.

Some patients exhibit a chronic active hepatitis with or without portal fibrosis, and there have been a number of reported cases of cirrhosis. In the latter condition, should jaundice supervene in the absence of a hemolytic pigment load or extrahepatic obstruction, this indicates end-stage disease and is an absolute indication for liver transplantation. At laparotomy or autopsy, the livers are black, firm, and finely granular, with evidence of portal hypertension.

The hematologic features of PP include mild anemia with slight erythrocyte hypochromia, fluorescent red cells on UV microscopy, and fluorescent normoblasts on UV microscopy of the bone marrow. Excess red cell protoporphyrin differs from that seen in lead poisoning and iron deficiency, in that in the last-named conditions protoporphyrin is present as a zinc chelate, whereas in PP the protoporphyrin is free.

Diagnosis

The 24-hour urine porphyrin and porphyrin precursor levels are normal in PP. Stool protoporphyrin levels are elevated. The hematologic features described above establish the diagnosis, especially the presence of excess red cell protoporphyrin, which on spectral analysis is free and not zinc-chelated. Liver biopsy exhibits fluorescence in many but not all cases, but the red porphyrin fluorescence is much more short-lived than in PCT. Skin porphyrin analysis will indicate a dominance of protoporphyrin.

Treatment

There is no specific treatment for PP. As with CEP, any maneuver that stimulates bone marrow activity, such as phlebotomy or blood loss, will stimulate protoporphyrin production. The disease rarely is severe enough to warrant hypertransfusion, as with CEP. Licopenes such as beta carotene (120 to 180 mg per day) can reduce or abolish skin photosensitivity. The use of sorbents such as charcoal (see page 389) has not yet been fully evaluated.

The prevention of progressive liver disease in PP is still a challenge to hepatologists. Various therapeutic maneuvers have been evaluated, such as drugs that bind porphyrins in the gut lumen (e.g., charcoal and cholestyramine), iron therapy to promote endogenous conversion of protoporphyrins to heme in the liver, and bile acids to solubilize liver porphyrin, but without uniformly good results. If photohemolysis is a feature, splenectomy may minimize bone marrow porphyrin production by increasing red cell half-life.

THERAPEUTIC USE OF BLOOD COMPONENTS
method of
PAUL D. MINTZ, M.D.
University of Virginia Medical Center
Charlottesville, Virginia

The significant risks of blood transfusion therapy compel physicians to weigh carefully the expected benefits and the hazards of blood transfusion prior to deciding to transfuse blood or blood components to a patient.

Informed Consent

The physician should document the need for transfusion in the patient's medical record. In addition, many hospitals require a process of informed consent before initiating a blood transfusion. This process should include an explanation of the recommended therapy, of the benefits and principal risks of transfusion, and of any available alternatives to transfusion therapy and their risks; a discussion of the possible consequences of not receiving a transfusion; an opportunity for the patient to ask questions; and the patient's signed consent to transfusion. The fact that the patient has provided such consent may be documented in the progress notes of the patient's chart or by a separate document placed in the chart. It is not necessary to extend this informed consent process to products that have been manufactured from blood, such as albumin or gamma globulin for intramuscular administration, which do not transmit infectious disease; however, it certainly must include coagulation concentrate preparations and should probably include gamma globulin for intravenous administration, which has been shown to transmit non-A, non-B hepatitis, although rarely. Similarly, the requirement may be waived in an emergency when a delay resulting from obtaining an informed consent would place the patient in jeopardy. However, documentation of the urgency of this situation should be included in the patient's chart.

It is reasonable to obtain informed consent only before each transfusion episode. A transfusion episode for inpatients may be defined as the total of transfusions of blood and blood components during a single hospitalization. A transfusion episode for outpatients may be defined as the total transfusions of blood and blood components required for the management of a particular disease.

Red Blood Cell Transfusion

Red blood cells are transfused to increase the oxygen-carrying capacity of the recipient's blood. There is no other indication for the transfusion of erythrocytes. In acute anemia, patients often may tolerate a reduced red blood cell mass to a hematocrit of approximately 20 per cent, so long as two conditions are met: (1) their blood volume has been maintained at a normal level and (2) their cardiac stroke volume has increased. Patients who cannot reliably increase their stroke volume begin to need to be transfused when their hematocrit falls below approximately 30 per cent. When blood loss has been monitored, such as during surgery, and the blood volume has been maintained, the hematocrit may serve as a reliable guide of the degree of loss of red cell mass. However, after trauma, the quantity of blood loss is unknown and volume has not been replaced. In such situations, extravascular fluid may take more than 72 hours to equilibrate with the depleted intravascular volume. Therefore, the hematocrit is not a reliable measurement of the loss of red cell mass.

In acute hemorrhage, the primary goal is the prompt restoration of blood volume through the use of crystalloid or colloid solutions so that tissue perfusion and oxygen delivery are sustained. Improved perfusion may restore adequate oxygen delivery despite the development of anemia. Consequently, blood components are rarely necessary as the initial choice in treating hemorrhagic shock. Because of the well-recognized risks of transfusion, such treatment is routinely best initiated by providing nonbiologic volume-expanding solutions. A healthy individual may tolerate an acute blood loss of as much as 15 per cent of his total blood volume without any signs or symptoms. Moderate hypovolemic shock develops when 20 to 40 per cent of the blood volume has been lost, and severe shock develops when volume loss is greater than 40 per cent.

In such patients, since the hematocrit is not a reliable guide to the need for transfusion, the decision to transfuse must be made on the basis of the clinical condition of the patient. Red cell transfusions are provided when volume replacement with colloid and/or crystalloid solutions has not stabilized the patient hemodynamically. Group O red blood cells may be given immediately. If more than 4 units have been transfused, we do not switch to the patient's own type (if A, B, or AB) until such cells are crossmatch compatible with the recipient's cells because of the transfused antibodies in the Group O plasma. The patient's blood group may be determined in a few minutes, and the patient may receive group-identical whole blood or red blood cells.

In chronic anemia, red cell transfusion is a strategy of final resort for the patient who cannot tolerate his or her anemia. If alternative therapies are available that can be expected to correct the anemia (e.g., iron), every effort must be made to avoid transfusion. Clearly, the decision to transfuse requires a careful assessment of the patient's symptoms and what constitutes an ap-

propriate level of activity for the patient. It is certainly preferable to permit some cardiorespiratory compensation and to tolerate a substantially reduced level of activity than to expose patients to the risks of blood transfusion. Therefore, the appropriate amount of blood to transfuse is the least amount necessary to prevent unacceptable clinical symptoms. There is a wide variability in the ability of patients to compensate for chronic anemia. Thus, there is no appropriate hemoglobin level below which patients should be transfused. Any attempt to use such an arbitrary standard will expose patients who do not need to be transfused to the substantial risks of blood products. In chronic anemia, it should never be necessary to transfuse patients whose hemoglobin level is greater than 10 grams per dl. In fact, when the hemoglobin is between 8 and 10 grams per dl, transfusion is almost always avoidable. When the hemoglobin is between 6 and 8 grams per dl, every effort should be made to try to avoid transfusions, although they may be necessary. When the hemoglobin falls below 6 grams per dl, patients frequently require transfusion, although certain patients may be able to tolerate hemoglobins of less than 6 grams per dl without requiring continuing blood transfusions. In some patients, the marrow is able to maintain a stable hemoglobin at a low level.

When patients are unable to make any red cells, their transfusion requirement will be approximately one unit per week. Of course, it is preferable to transfuse such patients 2 units every 2 weeks than to necessitate their receiving a blood transfusion each week. Patients with chronic anemia must be transfused slowly since any increase in blood volume could provoke acute pulmonary edema. This may be minimized by transfusing cells at a rate of approximately 1 ml per kg per hour. At times it may be prudent to administer a diuretic prior to or during the transfusion.

Once a patient has been transfused, every effort must be made to determine that in fact an appropriate clinical response has been obtained. It should be ascertained that the temporary relief of symptoms afforded by blood transfusions is sufficient to justify the continuing risks of further transfusions.

After transfusing patients who are making no red blood cells, it is important to realize that the red cell mass will fall at the rate of 1 unit per week. Consequently, if the patient has received 2 units of blood, the fact that the hemoglobin concentration returned to pretransfusion levels after two weeks should not be misinterpreted as an indication of decreased red cell survival.

When red blood cells are provided for neonatal

exchange transfusion, there is general agreement that the units should be less than 7 days old. Such cells provide optimum function and present less of a bilirubin load to the neonate because fewer transfused cells are destroyed in the first few hours after transfusion.

Blood products available include whole blood, which contains approximately 450 ml of donor blood collected into 63 ml of an anticoagulant preservative solution. The hematocrit of whole blood is usually between 36 and 40 per cent. Whole blood provides both oxygen-carrying capacity and blood volume. It is indicated for treating patients who are hypovolemic and have the need for increased red cell mass. For patients who need increased red cell mass but who are not hypovolemic, whole blood may result in fluid overload. Whole blood does not contain viable granulocytes or platelets; in addition, Factor V and Factor VIII levels are decreased. However, whole blood does contain albumin and normal quantities of the other coagulation factors. For patients who have required several transfusions in response to acute blood loss and who have received large quantities of red blood cells and saline, whole blood may provide sufficient quantities of coagulation factors to preclude the need for fresh frozen plasma and additional donor exposures.

Red blood cells are prepared from whole blood by removing plasma. At present, most red blood cell components are made by adding an additional amount of adenine to enhance red cell storage. Red blood cells are indicated for the treatment of reduced red cell mass in patients who are not hypovolemic. After the transfusion of 1 unit of red blood cells, the hemoglobin may be elevated by 1 to 1.5 grams per dl and the hematocrit by 3 to 4 per cent.

There is no contraindication to the provision of only 1 unit of blood. Single-unit transfusions may have been overused in the past; nonetheless, patients who require hemotherapy and for whom one transfusion will suffice should only receive 1 unit of blood. Rather than automatically transfusing 2 units, it is preferable to transfuse 1 unit, evaluate the patient, and then decide whether additional blood is required. The minimum amount of blood necessary to achieve the desired clinical response is the proper amount to transfuse.

There is no evidence that blood transfusion enhances wound healing. Red cell transfusions should not be given for this purpose.

Additional red cell products are available for selected patients. Leukocytes may be removed from red blood cells by centrifugation, filtration, or sedimentation. Such products are indicated for patients who have had repetitive nonhemolytic febrile transfusion reactions in the past. A febrile reaction is indicated by a rise of 1°C or greater in temperature attributable to a blood transfusion. Such reactions are due to recipient antibodies directed against lymphocyte, platelet, and/or granulocyte antigens in the donor. The majority of patients who have such reactions do not have repeated reactions; for those patients who have two or three reactions, the provision of leukocyte-depleted red blood cells may prevent further reactions. Leukocyte-poor products may be transfused more readily in patients on chemotherapy in whom the presence of a fever during transfusion might necessitate an extensive microbiologic investigation as well as the provision of antibiotics. In these circumstances, it is reasonable to try to avoid such reactions. In this regard, patients who have been previously transfused or who are pregnant and who are receiving transfusions may reasonably be provided leukocyte-depleted products even without a history of a febrile reaction.

Red blood cells may be washed and resuspended in saline. This process removes plasma as well as leukocytes. Washed red blood cells may be used in patients who have had repetitive allergic reactions as the result of their having been sensitized to plasma proteins or in patients who have had febrile nonhemolytic reactions. Some physicians transfuse washed cells to patients with paroxysmal nocturnal hemoglobinuria to prevent infusion of complement, but this is not a universal practice. There is no evidence that patients with autoimmune hemolytic anemia need washed cells for this purpose.

Red blood cells may be frozen for up to 10 years. Such products are valuable for patients who have antibodies directed against high-frequency red cell antigens and for whom it is difficult to find any compatible blood. The blood of such patients may be frozen for use in the future or rare blood types frozen in blood centers may be used. In addition, the blood of patients scheduled to undergo elective surgery in which large volumes of blood may be required (and for whom it would be difficult to store sufficient quantities of red cells within the 42-day liquid storage period) may be frozen so that there will be a sufficient inventory of autologous units.

There is no evidence that patients must have a hemoglobin of at least 10 grams per dl prior to surgery. It seems far more reasonable to evaluate patients individually and only expose them to the risks of transfusion when necessary.

Many patients may provide blood for themselves presurgically. It is often possible to collect 1 unit of blood per week from such patients so long as they respond to oral iron therapy. The criteria required for such donors are more lenient than for homologous blood donors. In fact, it has been shown that patients scheduled for coronary artery bypass grafting, pregnant patients, and patients older than 80 years may safely participate in autologous donation programs. Because of the significant changes that occur in blood during storage, including the dispersion of large quantities of plasticizer into the unit, and because of the always present danger of clerical error when blood is provided for transfusion, autologous blood should not be given back automatically simply because it is available. Rather, it should only be given if a need for transfusion has been established. Recent studies have shown that physicians tolerate lower preoperative nadir and discharge hematocrits in patients who have been transfused with autologous blood so as not to expose them to homologous blood. Since these patients do as well as those who receive homologous blood, it may be reasoned that patients who receive homologous blood could tolerate comparably lower hematocrit levels and could therefore receive less blood. Every effort should be made to consider every patient scheduled for elective surgery as a candidate for autologous presurgical donation. Autologous transfusion eliminates the risk of alloimmunization to red cell, white cell, platelet, and protein antigens, hemolytic transfusion reactions, and the transmission of infectious agents.

Blood should be warmed during the rapid administration of multiple transfusions (rate over 50 ml per kg per hour), during exchange transfusions in infants, for children receiving blood at a rate over 15 ml per kg per hour, for patients with clinically significant cold autoantibodies, and during rapid infusion through central venous lines. Only normal saline may be mixed with blood or blood components. All blood and blood components must be transfused through a filter. At present there is no oxygen-carrying substance available that can be used in lieu of erythrocyte transfusion.

Platelet Concentrates

Platelets are transfused to prevent or arrest hemorrhage in patients with a quantitative and/or qualitative platelet deficiency. Platelet concentrates may be prepared from whole blood donations or by selectively collecting platelets from donors on cytapheresis devices. These latter platelet concentrates, generally referred to as "single-donor platelets," contain approximately 6 to 10 times as many platelets as are found in a concentrate made from a single unit of whole blood. Single-donor concentrates reduce the number of donors to which a recipient is exposed and afford the selection of immunologically compatible donors for recipients who are alloimmunized to platelet antigens. The volume of a platelet concentrate made from whole blood is 50 to 70 ml. The volume of a single donor concentrate will vary from 200 to 500 ml.

One unit of platelet concentrate made from whole blood may be expected to increase the platelet count of a 70-kg adult by 5000 to 10,000 per microliter (μl). The usual dose is 1 unit per 10 kg body weight. Platelet transfusions are only consistently efficacious in recipients who have thrombocytopenia due to decreased production. For patients who have increased consumption of platelets (e.g., disseminated intravascular coagulation [DIC], sepsis, splenomegaly, autoimmune thrombocytopenia), transfused platelets may be consumed as readily as endogenous platelets. In thrombotic thrombocytopenic purpura, in which platelet transfusion may theoretically be harmful, platelets should not be transfused unless the patient has a life-threatening hemorrhage. Although adequate responses may be noted in consumptive processes, they occur less consistently. A reduced 1-hour post transfusion platelet count correlates well with the presence of recipient alloantibodies against HLA antigens on the transfused platelets.

The corrected count increment (CI) is calculated as follows:

$$CI = \frac{(\text{postransfusion count} - \text{pretransfusion count}) \times \text{body surface area}}{\text{platelets transfused} \times 10^{11}}$$

A patient who has a corrected CI at 1 hour of less than 10,000 per μl is likely to be alloimmunized. Recently, it has been shown that a 10-minute posttransfusion platelet count is equally useful. The transfusion of HLA-matched platelets may result in appropriate transfusion responses in such patients. Recently, platelet cross matching has also been shown to be a useful technique to ascertain if specific donors' platelets are compatible with recipients. At present, platelet cross matching and HLA typing appear to be most effective when used in combination. As with all blood products, platelet concentrates must be administered through a filter. Platelets of any ABO type may be transfused into any type recipient; routine pretransfusion red cell compatibility testing is not necessary. We screen single-donor concentrates and exclude transfusing plasma with greater than a 1:200 titer of anti-A and/or anti-B into recipients with a corresponding antigen. If a bleeding time is less than twice the upper limit of normal, it is likely that platelet dysfunction is not the cause of significant bleeding. Platelets may be transfused as fast as tolerated by the patient.

If Rh-positive platelet concentrates must be transfused to Rh-negative women who still have childbearing potential, the use of Rh immune globulin to prevent Rh immunization should be considered. Efforts should be made to provide Rh-negative platelets to such patients.

It has been suggested that the provision of single-donor concentrates in patients likely to require several platelet transfusions may reduce the incidence of alloimmunization. This is not a universal practice at present and the matter awaits further study. It has also been suggested that the provision of leukocyte-depleted concentrates may result in a reduced incidence of alloimmunization. This is not routine practice at present and this matter, too, awaits further study,.

It is necessary to have greater than 100,000 per μl normally functioning, circulating platelets to achieve normal hemostasis. However, so long as the platelet count is above approximately 50,000 per μl there are a sufficient number of platelets to control hemorrhage in patients who have no other reason to bleed. If it is necessary to achieve the most efficient hemostasis possible (e.g., during retinal or cerebral surgery), then the platelet count should be kept above 100,000 per μl at all times. Otherwise, maintaining the platelet count at greater than 50,000 per μl should suffice. Spontaneous bleeding does not arise until the platelet count falls below 20,000 per μl. The frequency of such bleeding increases markedly when the count is below 5000 per μl. There is no universal standard of practice regarding the prophylactic use of platelet transfusions in patients with counts below 20,000 per μl. A recent survey of university medical centers revealed that the majority do provide prophylactic transfusions when counts fall below 20,000 per μl, although some hospitals did not use prophylactic platelet transfusion. There is no justification for prophylactic platelet transfusion in patients undergoing open heart surgery.

Many smaller hospitals do not maintain large inventories of platelets, since they can only be stored for 5 days before outdating. Physicians who anticipate the need for platelets should notify the blood bank as soon as there is any likelihood of transfusion so that an appropriate inventory level can be obtained or maintained.

Patients with congenital platelet disorders may make antibodies to normal platelet membrane antigens and prove refractory to all allogenic platelets. Such patients may have to undergo plasmapheresis or combined plateletpheresis and plasmapheresis along with platelet infusion in order to attempt to effect hemostasis.

Patients with aplastic anemia should be transfused only if platelet counts below 5000 per μl are present for an extended period of time or if clinically significant bleeding occurs. Otherwise, platelet transfusions should be avoided because they may increase the risk of graft rejection after a subsequent bone marrow transplantation. In patients with leukemia, it is appropriate to increase the platelet count to greater than 50,000 per μl prior to an invasive procedure (e.g., lumbar puncture, catheter placement), and to maintain the count at greater than 20,000 during the healing period. Patients who have been transfused with 15 to 20 units of blood within a 24-hour period may develop a dilutional thrombocytopenia requiring platelet transfusion.

In neonatal alloimmune thrombocytopenia, consideration should always be given to utilizing the mother's platelets, which will always be compatible. Preferably, this product should be washed or volume reduced to remove plasma containing the antibody. Methods are available for depleting platelets of leukocytes to help prevent febrile transfusion reactions and for washing platelets to help prevent allergic reactions. For patients who have taken aspirin and whose bleeding time is greater than twice the upper limit of normal and for whom immediate correction of bleeding time is necessary, infusion of 2 to 4 units of random donor platelet concentrates in an adult should correct the problem, since only 20 per cent of non-acetylated platelets are necessary for adequate hemostasis in individuals who have previously ingested aspirin. Desmopressin (DDAVP) or cryoprecipitate may be preferable to platelet transfusion for the treatment of bleeding in uremia.

Granulocyte Concentrates

Granulocyte concentrates are collected from donors with a cytopheresis device. Each product contains an amount of granulocytes greater than 1×10^{10} suspended in 200 to 300 ml of plasma. The donor has usually received hydroxyethyl starch to increase the yield of granulocytes in the product. Therapeutic granulocyte transfusions should be given only to patients who have persistent neutropenia (less than 500 per μl), evidence of gram-negative sepsis that has not responded to appropriate antibiotic therapy of 48 hours' duration, and have a reasonable chance for survival. Patients who are alloimmunized to HLA antigens should receive granulocyte concentrates from HLA-compatible donors. Severely neutropenic patients with other types of bacterial infections unresponsive to antibiotics may also benefit from granulocyte transfusion. It has also been reported that therapeutic granulocyte transfusions benefitted patients with documented fungal infections. There is no basis for prophylactic granulocyte transfusions.

Granulocyte transfusions may benefit neonates with bacterial septicemia accompanied by neutropenia (less than 3000 per µl during the first week of life and less 1000 per µl thereafter). In neonates, at least 1×10^9 granulocytes per kg should be given.

All granulocyte transfusions must be cross-matched because of the quantity of red cell contamination. Because of the frequent occurrence of chills and fever during granulocyte administration, it is reasonable to infuse the product over a period of 2 to 4 hours. Granulocyte transfusions often have to be given daily to adults, although there is no general agreement regarding the duration of therapy. As with all blood products, they must be given through a filter. Granulocyte concentrates usually contain large numbers of platelets. The transfusion of a granulocyte concentrate rarely results in an increase in the patient's granulocyte count.

Plasma

Fresh frozen plasma (FFP) is plasma that has been removed and frozen from whole blood within 6 hours of collection. When plasma has not been frozen this quickly after donation, the components are called plasma and liquid plasma (hereafter collectively called plasma). FFP will have normal levels of the labile coagulation Factors V and VIII. Plasma will have equally high levels of the other procoagulants. The volume of these products is 200 to 250 ml.

A recent National Institutes of Health Consensus Conference recognized the following indications (in italics) for plasma transfusion:

1. *Replacement of isolated coagulation factor deficiencies.* Factor VIII deficiency, however, is more appropriately treated with cryoprecipitate or a specific coagulation factor concentrate. FFP is indicated for Factor V deficiency. However, plasma should have comparable levels of all the coagulation factors except for Factors V and VIII.

2. *Reversal of warfarin effect.* FFP and plasma should be equally effective in this regard. Since vitamin K will correct the prothrombin time within 6 to 12 hours, these products should only be utilized when a more rapid correction is required.

3. *Massive blood transfusion.* The coagulopathy of massive transfusion is more closely related to the duration and intensity of shock than to the number of units of blood transfused. However, it is possible to develop a dilutional coagulopathy by replacing large quantities of lost blood with red cells and saline and/or colloid. FFP may be used to replenish coagulation factors.

4. *Antithrombin III deficiency.* Either FFP or plasma may be used to replace antithrombin III.

5. *Treatment of immunodeficiencies.* The report noted that FFP is useful in infants with secondary immunodeficiency associated with protein losing enteropathy and for whom total parental nutrition has been ineffectual. Plasma should also be useful in this regard.

6. *Treatment of thrombotic thrombocytopenia purpura.* FFP is used as the replacement fluid during plasma exchange in this condition. In certain instances, infusion of FFP alone has also been associated with a beneficial response. There is no information to indicate whether plasma would also be effective. FFP is also used as the replacement fluid during plasma exchange for patients with hemolytic-uremic syndrome.

7. *Treatment of patients with other multiple coagulation factor deficiencies.* Examples are patients with liver disease who are bleeding or about to undergo invasive procedures. Although not specified in the Conference report, FFP may also replenish depleted factors in patients with DIC, although transfused procoagulants may also be consumed.

One unit of FFP should raise the coagulation factor levels of a 70-kg adult approximately 8 per cent. In addition, it should be noted that a single platelet concentrate made from a whole blood donation should raise all the coagulation factor levels except V or VIII approximately 2 per cent. Factors V and VIII may be raised approximately 1 per cent. Since it is common practice to pool 6 to 8 units of platelets, significant quantities of coagulation factors are provided during platelet transfusion as well. FFP should not be used as a volume expander or as a nutritional source.

As with all blood products, plasma must be given through a filter. Plasma is transfused only if it does not contain anti-A and/or anti-B which could react with corresponding recipient antigens. No compatibility testing is required.

Cryoprecipitate

Cryoprecipitate contains concentrated fibrinogen and Factors VIII and XIII. The volume of each bag of cryoprecipitate is approximately 15 ml, and each unit should contain approximately 250 mg of fibrinogen. Cryoprecipitate is indicated for the treatment of deficiencies of these factors. ABO-compatible cryoprecipitate should be used when possible, although, if necessary, ABO-incompatible products may be used. Each unit of cryoprecipitate may be presumed to contain 80 units of Factor VIII procoagulant activity. The transfusion of one unit of Factor VIII per kg should raise the Factor VIII level in the recipient approximately 2 per cent. Because cryoprecipitate is always administered through a filter, compatibility testing is not necessary.

At present, there is no established indication for the use of cryoprecipitate for its fibronectin content. There have been reports of successful use of cryoprecipitate to treat uremic bleeding. However, the use of DDAVP, a nonbiologic product, may be equally effective.

Coagulation Factor Concentrates

Factor VIII concentrate is used to treat patients with severe Hemophilia A. One unit of Factor VIII per kg raises the Factor VIII level approximately 2 per cent. Each lot of Factor VIII concentrate is pooled from as many as 20,000 plasma donors. Heat treatment has almost completely eliminated the risk of HIV infection but does not prevent hepatitis. However, a highly purified product has recently become available that promises to reduce the incidence of hepatitis associated with Factor VIII concentrate. Patients with moderate or mild hemophilia may be able to be treated with DDAVP.

Factor IX concentrate contains Factors II, VII, IX, and X. The product may be used to treat congenital deficiencies of these procoagulants although plasma, with its substantially lower hepatitis risk, is preferable. One unit of Factor IX per kg raises the Factor IX level approximately 1 per cent. Factor IX concentrate is heat treated to prevent transmission of HIV but carries a high risk of hepatitis. Consequently, patients with acquired deficiencies of the factors it contains are better treated with plasma. An activated Factor IX concentrate is available to treat patients with Factor VIII deficiency and high-titer Factor VIII inhibitors.

ADVERSE REACTIONS TO BLOOD TRANSFUSION

method of
YOHANNES W. YESUS, M.D.
University of Missouri
Columbia, Missouri

Despite sophisticated diagnostic methodologies, meticulous quality control procedures, and better understanding of compatibility between recipients and donors, unexpected adverse reactions are still associated with the transfusion of blood and its derivatives. Various estimates indicate that 0.5 per cent of all transfusions are accompanied by untoward side effects. These can be divided into two broad categories: immune-mediated reactions and nonimmunologic reactions.

IMMUNE-MEDIATED REACTIONS (Table 1)

Hemolytic Transfusion Reactions

Hemolytic transfusion reactions occur when antibodies in the recipient plasma interact with the corresponding antigen on the donor red cells, causing accelerated immune destruction of the transfused red cells. This may be immediate or delayed.

Immediate (Acute) Hemolytic Transfusion Reaction

A complex system of specimen and patient identification and compatibility testing has made the occurrence of this life-threatening complication a rare event. The vast majority of cases are due to clerical errors in labeling patient samples or in identifying patients to be transfused. These reactions are generally due to intravascular destruction of transfused cells by IgM antibodies, usually of the ABH antigen system. Much less frequently, anti-Le[a], anti-Jk[a], anti-Vel, and antibodies of the P system are implicated. High titered IgG antibodies that do not bind complement can also cause symptoms of acute hemolytic reaction, predominantly through extravascular sequestration and destruction of transfused cells in the reticuloendothelial organs. Antibodies against the Rhesus (Rh), Kell (K), and Duffy (Fy) blood group systems fall in this category.

The signs and symptoms of acute hemolytic transfusion reaction (outlined in Table 2) result from activation of the complement and the coagulation systems and from release of neuroendocrine mediators accompanying the antigen-antibody reaction on the red cells. The hemoglobinemia and hemoglobinuria are the result of complement activation and intravascular destruction of red cells. Generation of anaphylactic

TABLE 1. **Types of Immune-Mediated Transfusion Reactions**

Blood Component Involved	Type of Reaction
Red blood cells	Acute hemolytic reaction; delayed hemolytic reaction
White blood cells	Non-hemolytic febrile reaction; pulmonary reaction
Platelets	Post-transfusion purpura
Lymphocytes	Graft-versus-host disease
Plasma proteins	Urticarial reaction; anaphylactic reaction

TABLE 2. **Manifestations of Acute Hemolytic Transfusion Reactions**

Fever and chills
Hemoglobinemia and hemoglobinuria
Hypotension
Flushing and urticaria
Oliguria or anuria
Icterus
Pain along the veins of transfusion
Bilateral lumbar pain
Capillary or intravenous-site oozing
Anxiety
Dyspnea
Precordial discomfort

and vasoactive complement fragments such as $C3^a$ and $C5^a$ accounts for the severe hypotension. These fragments also interact with mast cells to release histamine and serotonin, which are potent vasoactive substances. Red cell membrane phospholipids and antigen antibody complexes interact with Factor XII to initiate the coagulation cascade, which may proceed to disseminated intravascular coagulation (DIC). DIC and its hemorrhagic complications, in conjunction with unexplained hypotension, may be the only prominent symptoms of acute hemolytic reaction in a comatose or anesthetized patient. The fibrin microthrombi generated during DIC may be deposited in the tubular and glomerular capillaries and contribute to renal ischemia and acute renal failure. Factor XIIa also activates the kinin system to generate bradykinin, one of the potent vasodilators responsible for severe hypotension. It is probably also responsible for the pain along the vein of the transfusion and the bilateral back pain by stimulating pain-sensitive nerve endings in the vessel walls. Catecholamines, particularly, norepinephrine, are released from the adrenal medulla in response to hypotension and precipitate anxiety, dyspnea, and precordial discomfort. In addition, norepinephrine causes the redistribution of blood flow from the splanchnic areas to vital centers such as the heart and central nevous system. This redistribution further exacerbates the ischemic renal damage. Fever is a constant feature of an acute hemolytic reaction, possibly due to the effect of the intracellular contents on the thermoregulatory center of the brain.

Successful management of an acute hemolytic transfusion reaction depends on its prompt recognition. Close monitoring during the first 15 to 30 minutes of transfusion is essential, since severe or fatal outcomes are more likely if large volumes of incompatible blood are infused. At the first sign of an adverse reaction the following steps should be taken immediately:

1. Stop the transfusion and keep the intravenous line open with isotonic saline.

2. Check the clerical information at the bedside to ensure that the patient is receiving the correct unit of blood.

3. Inform the transfusion laboratory and send them the following blood samples along with the blood bag and infusion set: (a) A clotted blood sample for serologic investigation of incompatibility; (b) An EDTA anticoagulated sample for direct antiglobulin testing and free plasma hemoglobin determination; and (c) A citrated blood specimen for base line determination of coagulation parameters.

4. Send the first voided urine specimen following the reaction for examination of free hemoglobin.

The following three preliminary tests should be performed immediately: (1) a clerical check, (2) visual examination of the post-transfusion plasma for elevated plasma hemoglobin, and (3) direct antiglobulin test (DAT) of the EDTA anticoagulated sample to detect an in vivo antigen-antibody reaction. If these tests show positive DAT and elevated free hemoglobin in plasma, therapy for hemolytic reaction should begin without further confirmatory tests.

Other confirmatory tests include retyping the patient's and donor blood and repeating the antibody screen and compatibility tests using pre- and postreaction specimens. Microbiologic checks for bacterial contamination, coagulation screening for evidence of DIC, and monitoring of renal function for evidence of renal failure will help guide therapeutic decisions. Possible laboratory abnormalities that may be seen are outlined in Table 3.

The three main objectives of therapy of acute hemolytic transfusion reaction are the prevention or treatment of shock, DIC, and acute renal failure. Since hypotension is the key factor contributing to all three conditions, aggressive treatment of hypotension with adequate crystalloid or

TABLE 3. **Laboratory Abnormalities in Acute Hemolytic Transfusion Reactions**

Elevated free plasma hemoglobin
Hemoglobinuria
Decreased plasma haptoglobin
Hyperbilirubinemia
Prolonged, aPTT, PT
Elevated fibrin split product
Decreased platelet count ($<150,000/\mu l$)
Decreased plasma fibrinogen (<150 mg/dl)
Elevated blood urea nitrogen
Elevated serum creatinine
Elevated serum LDH
Spherocytes in peripheral blood smear
Positive direct antiglobulin test

Abbreviations: aPTT = activated partial thromboplastin times; PT = normal prothrombin time; LDH = lactate dehydrogenase.

colloid solutions is mandatory. If the use of pressors is necessary, dopamine is the agent of choice, as it possesses both alpha- and beta-adrenergic effects capable of raising arterial pressure and improving cardiac output. Doses up to 1.0 mg per kg per minute also improve renal cortical blood flow, mitigating renal ischemia. Dopamine should only be used in normovolemic patients and with careful monitoring of ECG, blood pressure, and urinary output.

Diuretics should also be administered to improve renal cortical blood flow and increase urine output. The diuretics most commonly used are furosemide and mannitol. Mannitol induces osmotic diuresis when administered intravenously as a 20 per cent solution in 20-gram increments, but its value has not been established. Furosemide may be given intravenously in a dose of 20 to 40 mg and repeated, as necessary, to maintain urine output of 100 ml per hour. At the first sign of acute renal failure, a consultation must be obtained to plan for possible dialysis and for appropriate management of electrolyte and fluid balance.

Hemorrhagic manifestations may be prominent features of acute hemolytic reactions. In surgical or trauma patients, replacement of deficient plasma or cellular constituents (platelets, fibrinogen, and Factors V and VIII) with appropriate components (platelet concentrates, cryoprecipitate, fresh frozen plasma) is indicated. The therapeutic goal is to maintain platelet counts of greater than 50,000, fibrinogen of greater than 100 mg per dl, and near-normal prothrombin time (PT) and activated partial thromboplastin time (aPTT).

Although no definitive efficacy data are available, the immediate use of heparin to treat DIC has been advocated by some authors. This approach may be considered when the reaction is due to ABO incompatibility, more than 200 ml of incompatible red cells have been transfused, and no significant pre-existing bleeding is suspected. The recommended regimen is an intravenous loading dose of 5000 units followed by 600 to 1000 units per hour of continuous infusion for 12 to 24 hours. Heparin therapy should be monitored with appropriate coagulation tests to minimize bleeding complications.

Delayed Hemolytic Transfusion Reaction

When an apparently compatible blood transfusion is followed by an accelerated extravascular destruction 2 days to 3 weeks later, it is referred to as delayed hemolytic transfusion reaction. These patients have been sensitized to red cell antigens through pregnancy or previous transfusion. The initial sensitization causes low-titer antibody levels or an antibody level that decreases in time to undetectable levels. The transfusion of blood containing the sensitizing antigen acts like a booster dose, resulting in antibody levels high enough to cause red cell destruction. The majority of such patients are asymptomatic and the reactions pass undiagnosed. When the reaction is detected, the findings include an unexplained fall in hemoglobin and slight hyperbilirubinemia.

In the overwhelming majority of cases, no specific therapy is required unless large volumes of blood positive for the sensitizing antigen have been transfused and the antibodies involved are of the complement-fixing type (e.g., anti-Jk[a]); in these cases, destruction of red cells may be rapid enough to cause acute renal failure. It is therefore necessary to monitor renal function in these patients.

Nonhemolytic Febrile Reaction

The onset of fever, shaking chills, and muscle aches during or shortly after the transfusion of blood components are the commonest untoward effects of transfusion therapy. They are caused by the action of antibodies directed against granulocyte-specific or HLA antigens. These antibodies may be present in the plasma of the donor or recipient primarily as a result of multiple previous transfusions or pregnancies. The anti-leukocyte antibody and antigen reaction triggers the release of endogenous pyrogens that have properties similar to interleukin I and that are responsible for the prominent symptoms of chills and fever. The reaction is generally self-limited and resolves spontaneously. Since fever and chills are one of the more constant manifestations of hemolytic transfusion reactions, the transfusion has to be stopped until a hemolytic reaction is ruled out by the laboratory test described above.

The only treatment required is antipyretics and reassurance of the patient. Antihistamine therapy has been tried empirically and has not proved useful.

Recurrent febrile reaction to red cell transfusions can be a serious concern to patients with chronic, transfusion-dependent conditions such as sickle cell anemia or thalassemia. They can be avoided by transfusing products with reduced white blood cell constituents. In the past, red cell concentrates have been made leukocyte-poor by differential centrifugation, saline washing of units, or using frozen deglycerolized units. Convenient in-line filters are now commercially available that remove intact white cells or their membrane fragments during the transfusion of previously unmodified units.

Pulmonary Reaction

This is an uncommon but serious and life-threatening complication characterized by fever, shaking chills, respiratory distress, and bilateral pulmonary infiltrates. The antibodies are anti-HLA or granulocyte-specific agglutinins that cause trapping of agglutinated granulocytes in the pulmonary capillary bed. The classic complement pathway activation generates vasoactive substances, causing vasodilation, endothelial cell injury, and pulmonary edema.

Therapy includes intravenous dimethylprednisolone, 30 mg per kg every 6 hours for up to 48 hours; oxygen administration; intravenous diuretics; and, if necessary, positive-pressure ventilation.

Post-transfusion Purpura (PTP)

PTP is a rare, poorly understood syndrome characterized by sudden onset of thrombocytopenia, purpura, and mucosal or intracranial hemorrhage 7 to 10 days after the transfusion of blood derivatives containing platelets or platelet membrane fragments. It occurs predominantly in multiparous women or previously transfused individuals whose plasma contains anti-PlA[1] antibodies and whose platelets lack PlA[1] antigen. Although theories such as "innocent bystander" and cross-reactive antibody mechanisms have been advanced, the precise mechanism by which anti-PlA[1] antibody destroys the PlA[1]-negative platelets is not known. The disorder is usually self-limited, with the return of platelets to normal levels within 7 to 10 days. Severe thrombocytopenia, however, can be fatal during the first week.

Platelet transfusions, including PlA[1]-negative platelets, are uniformly ineffective. Variable responses have been reported to steroid therapy and therapeutic plasmapheresis. Recently, the use of high-dose (0.4 mg per kg per day for 4 days) intravenous immunoglobulin preparations has been recommended.

Anaphylactic Reactions

This rare but catastrophic reaction is characterized by hypotension, bronchospasm, and laryngeal edema. It begins within the first few minutes of transfusion in patients who are IgA-deficient and whose sera contain greater than 1:256 anti-IgA antibodies. The incidence of IgA deficiency in the general population is approximately 1 in 700 to 1000, and only 25 per cent of these individuals produce anti-IgA antibodies. There is usually no history of previous transfusion or pregnancy.

This reaction may be fatal unless promptly treated by stopping the transfusion, maintaining circulating blood volume, maintaining or establishing adequate airway, and subcutaneous administration of 0.5 ml of 1:1000 solution of epinephrine. The administration of epinephrine may be repeated every 5 minutes until symptoms resolve. Future transfusions of such patients should consist of components lacking IgA proteins, such as saline-washed units, frozen deglycerolized blood, and blood from an IgA-deficient donor.

Urticarial Reactions

This is the second most common reaction to transfusion of blood containing plasma proteins. It is characterized by hives, urticaria, wheals, and sometimes pruritus. Most often these are due to sensitization to gamma globulins. In the absence of other symptoms such as hypotension or fever, the only treatment required is to temporarily stop the transfusion, administer antihistamines, and restart the transfusion at a slower rate. No special diagnostic investigation is required.

Graft-Versus-Host Disease (GVHD)

Graft-versus-host disease is a rare complication caused by the engraftment and infiltration of the skin, gastrointestinal tract, and liver of the host by donor lymphocytes in severely immunosuppressed individuals or, very rarely, in premature infants receiving exchange transfusions. In susceptible individuals, such as those congenitally immunodeficient or those under preparation for organ transplant, blood components containing viable lymphocytes should be irradiated with 3000 rads.

NONIMMUNOLOGIC REACTIONS (Table 4)

Disease Transmission

Transmission of infectious diseases is one of the most persistent and serious complications of blood transfusion. Although any infectious organism present in the circulation of an asymptomatic blood donor may be transmitted by transfusion, in practice, the most important ones are human immunodeficiency viruses (HIV), hepatitis viruses, and cytomegalovirus.

Acquired Immunodeficiency Syndrome (AIDS)

AIDS is caused by the human immune virus (HIV), which infects and, after a variable latent period, destroys T-helper lymphocytes essential for adequate immune response. The resulting failure of the immune system may lead to the full-blown syndrome of recurrent opportunistic

TABLE 4. **Types of Nonimmunologic Transfusion Reactions**

Disease Transmission
    Acquired immunodeficiency syndrome (AIDS)
    Non-A, non-B hepatitis (NANB)
    Hepatitis B
    Delta hepatitis
    Septicemia
    Other infections

Depletion of Essential Elements
    Dilutional thrombocytopenia
    Dilution Factors V and VIIIc deficiency
    2,3-diphosphoglycerate deficiency

Accumulation of Toxic or other Unwanted Substances
    Acid load
    Hyperkalemia
    Citrate toxicity
    Microaggregates
    Hypothermia
    Fluid overload
    Iron overload

infections including *Pneumocystis carinii* and atypical malignancies such as disseminated Kaposi's sarcoma. Among the known high-risk groups are hemophiliacs and other chronic blood transfusion users, who constitute approximately 2 per cent of the reported patients with AIDS.

Steps instituted to avoid transmission include stopping donation by all those in high-risk groups and testing all units for anti-HIV antibodies. Products made from large pools of plasma, such as coagulation factor concentrates, are heat-treated or purified by monoclonal antibody affinity to inactivate or eliminate the virus. These screened blood units still pose a finite, albeit minute, risk of transmitting HIV, because some donors in the high-risk group continue to donate, and tests for HIV antibody do not detect all infected units, particularly those from recently infected persons who have not yet produced the diagnostic antibody. Current estimates are that 1 in 100,000 to 250,000 properly screened units may transmit HIV infection.

Additional measures to minimize risk include expanded use of autologous transfusion and intraoperative blood salvage procedures and strict adherence to use of transfusion only when properly indicated. In addition, 1-deamino-(8-D-arginine)-vasopressin (DDAVP) infusion, 0.3 micrograms per kg in saline over 30 minutes, may be substituted for plasma-derived products to treat mild hemophilia A and some variants of Type I von Willebrand's disease.

Hepatitis

Although public attention has been focused on AIDS, hepatitis remains one of the most common complications of transfusion therapy. Four different types of viruses—hepatitis A, hepatitis B, non-A non-B (NANB) hepatitis, and delta hepatitis agent—are responsible for the clinically similar diseases commonly called viral hepatitis.

Hepatitis A is an RNA virus responsible for epidemic outbreaks and is transmitted primarily via the fecal-oral route. Transmission by transfusion is exceedingly rare, as the viremia associated with it is of short duration and chronic asymptomatic carrier states do not occur.

Hepatitis B is caused by a DNA virus composed of a nucleic acid core surrounded by a lipoprotein coat, the hepatitis B surface antigen (HBsAg). It is transmitted parenterally during transfusion or during needle-sharing by intravenous drug users and by intimate sexual contact. The virus invades liver cells, replicates in the nucleus, and releases excess amounts of HBsAg into the circulation. Detection of HBsAg by radioimmunoassay (RIA) or enzyme-linked immunosorbent assay (ELISA) is relatively simple, but these assays are not sensitive enough to detect all infectious units. Approximately 10 per cent of post-transfusion hepatitis is caused by hepatitis B virus, despite careful testing procedures. Individuals exposed to infectious material should receive passive immunization with hepatitis B immune globulin within 24 hours of exposure. Efficient vaccines are now available from two sources (human carriers and recombinant DNA) for active immunization of health workers at increased risk.

NANB hepatitis is responsible for 80 to 90 per cent of all post-transfusion hepatitis, and it is estimated that from 5 to 10 per cent of all transfusions are responsible for this disease. Since there is no known specific virus or antigenic marker for NANB hepatitis, the diagnosis is one of exclusion of the other known hepatitis agents. Only 25 to 30 per cent of those infected show clinical symptoms. The remaining can only be detected by careful follow-up with liver enzyme alanine aminotransferase (ALT) studies. Although mild acutely, intermittent chronic elevations of ALT may be present in up to 60 per cent of these patients, with 10 to 20 per cent developing cirrhosis. Two nonspecific tests are currently used to screen blood donors: (1) the ALT and (2) antibodies to hepatitis B core antigen (anti-HBc); 3 to 5 per cent of blood donors are disqualified by these tests, and this is estimated to decrease post-transfusion NANB hepatitis by about 30 per cent.

The delta hepatitis agent is a defective RNA virus that requires co-infection with hepatitis B for replication because it shares the HBsAG of the latter; it tends to cause severe illness in chronic carriers of hepatitis B. Delta hepatitis is endemic in Mediterranean countries but rarely occurs in intravenous drug users or in individuals receiving pooled plasma products in the United States.

Cytomegalovirus

Transmission of cytomegalovirus infection through blood products containing granulocytes is well demonstrated. In healthy individuals it is of little clinical significance but results in seroconversion and latent carrier state. However, in seronegative premature neonates weighing less than 1500 grams and in patients with inherited or acquired immune deficiencies, the infection may be severe and sometimes fatal. Such patients should only be transfused with blood components from seronegative donors or with frozen deglycerolized or saline washed blood units.

Septicemia

Transfusion-induced gram-negative septicemia in its severe form is characterized by fever, chills, hypotension, shock, and death. It is caused by the transfusion of a blood product heavily contaminated with gram-negative bacteria and bacterial endotoxin. Although approximately 2 per cent of freshly drawn blood units are contaminated with small numbers of bacteria, most of these do not survive 4 or more days of refrigeration. Some strains of *Pseudomonas* species can survive cold storage, and in products that are stored at room temperature (e.g., platelet concentrates) they can grow to large numbers. This reaction is distinguished from acute hemolytic reaction by a negative DAT of the post-transfusion samples and, frequently, by the demonstration of bacteria in the transfused unit with Gram stain. The patient should immediately be started on broad-spectrum antibiotics and intravenous corticosteroids and fluids to prevent circulatory collapse.

Other Infections

On rare occasions other viral, bacterial, fungal, or parasitic infections may be transmissible by transfusion. The list includes infectious mononucleosis, brucellosis, salmonellosis, syphilis, Rocky Mountain spotted fever, malaria, trypanosomiasis, toxoplasmosis, and babesiosis.

Depletion of Essential Elements

Storage of blood causes significant functional, metabolic, and physical changes in its various components. Changes with clinical relevance during massive transfusion (greater than 1 blood volume in 3 hours) will be discussed.

Hemostatic Defects

Dilutional thrombocytopenia and abnormal bleeding may develop during massive transfu-sion, as blood stored at 4° C for a few days contains no functional platelets. Platelet counts should be monitored and hemostatic levels of at least 50,000 platelets per μl should be maintained. The labile plasma coagulation Factors V and VIII decrease to less than 50 per cent on storage; however, in the absence of DIC, dilution of these factors is unlikely to result in abnormal bleeding because Factor VIII is rapidly synthesized by the liver and only 15 to 25 per cent of Factor V activity is required for adequate hemostasis. Possible plasma coagulation factor deficiencies should, however, be evaluated with a coagulation screening test (e.g., PT, aPTT, fibrinogen and fibrinogese degradation products [FDP]), because conditions that require massive transfusion also tend to trigger DIC.

2,3-Diphosphoglycerate (DPG) Deficiency

The oxygen-releasing function of hemoglobin is facilitated by a normal intra-erythrocytic level of 2,3-DPG. Liquid storage for over 7 days significantly decreases the red cell concentration of 2,3-DPG. Massive transfusion with 2,3-DPG–depleted blood was thought to contribute to tissue hypoxia because of the inefficient oxygen delivery; however, transfused red cells regenerate their enzyme levels within 12 to 24 hours, so its real significance is not known.

Accumulation of Toxic or other Unwanted Substances

Citrate Toxicity

Citrate is the anticoagulant in the preservative for liquid storage of blood. In an individual with normal liver function and good tissue perfusion, the metabolism of citrate is rapid and complete. However, during rapid and massive transfusion (1 liter per 10 minutes or exchange transfusion in 2 hours), a marked increase in plasma citrate levels and decrease in ionized calcium may ensue. The symptoms of hypocalcemia may range from tetany and muscle twitching to ventricular fibrillation. Calcium supplementation (10 ml of 10 per cent calcium gluconate) is indicated when electrocardiography shows evidence of QT prolongation or calcium determination indicates decreased ionized calcium.

Hyperkalemia

The virtual cessation of active transport of sodium and potassium across red cell membrane during storage at 4° C results in a progressive rise in plasma potassium that approaches 30 mEq per liter after 4 weeks. Hyperkalemia is, however, an unlikely complication, unless patients are already hyperkalemic as a result of an underlying disease such as impaired renal function. Resuscitation of trauma patients with massive transfusions of stored blood usually results in hypokalemia after 24 hours, because of the influx of plasma potassium into the transfused red cells as the erythrocytes resume normal metabolism in the patient's circulation.

Acid Load

Due to the citric acid in the anticoagulant preservative and the accumulation of lactate during storage, stored blood has a base deficit of 20 to 30 mEq per liter. The transfusion of large volumes of such a fluid was thought to exacerbate the metabolic acidosis of patients already in shock. In practice, the restoration of normal intravascular volume is more pressing than the correction of the acid-base balance because, as tissue perfusion improves, citrate metabolism generates bicarbonates that will mitigate the base deficit. In patients with renal impairment and other underlying diseases, the acid load of massive transfusion may require exogenous correction.

Hypothermia

The rapid infusion (greater than 100 ml per minute) of blood stored at 4° C causes significant reduction in core body temperature. This causes the diversion of already scant metabolic energy needed for vital cellular functions to the genera-

tion of heat to maintain body temperature. Hypothermia also contributes to tissue hypoxia by increasing the oxygen affinity of hemoglobin, and to hypocalcemia and cardiac arrythmia by slowing down citrate metabolism. The use of a well-monitored blood warming device will avoid hypothermia and its potentially serious complications.

Miscellaneous Hazards

In severely anemic patients and patients with reduced cardiac reserve, rapid transfusion of blood may lead to pulmonary edema from circulatory overload. This can be prevented by monitoring central venous pressure. Patients with transfusion-dependent chronic anemia (e.g., aplastic anemia, thalassemia) will, over time, develop transfusion-induced hemosiderosis. Parenchymal deposition of iron in hepatocytes, myocardium, and other organs leads to organ failure. Although not in routine use, blood units enriched with young cells have been reported to decrease the frequency of transfusion. During storage, white cell and platelet fragments form microaggregates that can pass through a standard blood filter. Accumulation of these particles in the pulmonary microcirculation has been postulated, but its true incidence and significance is not known. Microaggregate filters may be used when rapid transfusion of large volumes of stored blood is required.

Section 6

The Digestive System

BLEEDING ESOPHAGEAL VARICES

method of
DUANE G. HUTSON, M.D.
Miami, Florida

The problem of bleeding from gastroesophageal varices can be categorized as one requiring immediate or long-term control. Achieving immediate control represents the more formidable problem, since the first episode is associated with a mortality of 30 to 80 per cent. Some plan for long-term control is mandatory, since bleeding recurs in 70 per cent of cases and is associated with a 50 per cent mortality for each recurrence. The debate regarding immediate control centers around immediate operative intervention versus nonoperative control. For long-term management, the major issue is the use of sclerotherapy versus various shunting procedures. Both of these areas remain controversial.

Management of Acute Episodes

Diagnosis

A careful history and physical examination will most often identify the presence of cirrhosis and the suspicion of portal hypertension, but the fact that 50 per cent of patients with gastroesophageal varices and hemorrhage bleed from a nonvariceal source complicates the problem. The key to the diagnosis is upper gastrointestinal endoscopy, which identifies the source of bleeding in 67 per cent of cases. Endoscopy should be done as early as possible, but if it is delayed, it should be performed during the quiescent period rather than waiting for recurrent hemorrhage, at which time the procedure may be technically impossible. If the bleeding is massive enough to preclude the use of endoscopy, treatment with lavage or vasopressin (Pitressin) should be instituted in the hope that sufficient control can be obtained to allow definitive endoscopic evaluation. If this is unsuccessful, however, visceral angiography should be considered. Angiography is not particularly effective in identifying bleeding from varices but may identify nonvariceal sources such as duodenal ulcers. If these maneuvers fail to identify the source of bleeding, operative intervention is indicated in most cases. Prolonged delays in attempting to make a diagnosis should be avoided because survival following massive transfusions with repeated episodes of hypotension is unlikely.

Resuscitation and Monitoring

Since blood loss in these patients is often massive, a large-bore catheter should be placed even though there is no evidence of bleeding at the time of examination. A setting that permits careful monitoring of vital signs is mandatory. Unstable patients with massive bleeding are best managed in an intensive care unit.

Frequent hemodynamic assessments are essential in all patients, since hematocrit changes may lag behind such parameters as pulse rate and blood pressure. Careful hemodynamic monitoring requires the placement of a Swan-Ganz catheter, which is mandatory in patients with signs of hemodynamic instability. Fluid administration is continuously adjusted as indicated by the measurements of cardiac output and wedge pressures.

The key to fluid replacement in these patients is the use of whole blood. The use of salt and fluid should be limited because of the tendency to the development of ascites. The goal should be minimal fluid and minimal salt. The use of diuretics for maintaining urinary output in most patients is condemned; however, this condition is an exception to this concept. If the patient is hemodynamically stable and the urinary output marginal, the use of small doses of diuretics is appropriate, since increasing the fluid load often leads to ascites rather than urinary output.

Hematologic Monitoring

A battery of coagulation tests, including a prothrombin time, should be ordered on admission. If the prothrombin time is low, vitamin K (phytonadione), 10 to 25 mg intramuscularly, should be given. If severe, hypoprothrombinemia may be treated with 2 to 3 units of fresh frozen plasma (FFP) given over 3 hours. Massive transfusions may lead to a deficiency in platelets and the labile factors V and VIII, which are deficient in bank blood. Thus, 1 unit of FFP and 1 to 2 units of platelet concentrate should be given for every 5 units of bank blood.

General Supportive Measures

Aspiration pneumonia is a frequent complication and can be minimized by the liberal use of an endotracheal tube. Its use is required in all patients who are massively bleeding or comatose and in those patients requiring endoscopy or balloon tamponade. Nutritional support should begin early and is best provided by a glucose solution at a concentration that allows for adequate calories (25 cal per kg) without excessive fluid volume. If a protracted course is expected, a solution with high concentration of branched chain amino acids and low concentrations of aromatic amino acids (HepatAmine) should be added. There is some evidence to suggest that prolonged coma in these patients is detrimental; therefore, the gastrointestinal tract should be cleared of blood by the use of saline enemas. Lactulose, 60 to 120 ml daily in divided doses, can be added if needed.

Control of Bleeding

Gastric Lavage

Lavage with iced saline or tap water should be the first approach, since it is simple and relatively free of complications and effectively controls bleeding in 30 per cent of cases. A standard nasogastric (NG) tube should be left in place for monitoring of further bleeding episodes and repeated irrigation. Its presence does not promote bleeding.

Vasopressin

Vasopressin produces a decrease in splanchnic blood flow and portal vascular resistance resulting in a decrease in portal pressure of 25 to 30 per cent. This reduction in portal pressure results in control of hemorrhage in 50 per cent of patients. The continuous peripheral intravenous infusion is as effective as the selective intra-arterial infusion and more effective than intermittent infusions. The side effects are rather profound and relate to generalized vasoconstriction. It produces profound coronary artery constriction and hypertension. Extravasation into the subcutaneous tissue may produce gangrene, and the antidiuretic effect may produce hyponatremia. Unusual complications such as necrosis of the tongue have been seen. Because of its cardiac effects, continuous electrocardiographic monitoring is mandatory and the presence of coronary artery disease is a contraindication to its use. The usual dose is 0.2 to 0.4 units per minute as a continuous intravenous infusion.*

---

*This use of vasopressin is not listed by the manufacturer. Also note the varying dosage listed on page 413.

High doses (0.8 units per minute) have been used with careful monitoring. Profound bradycardia and severe peripheral vasoconstriction may be seen with these doses. Despite these problems, the drug is quite safe in low doses and with adequate monitoring.

Balloon Tamponade

Balloon tamponade is the modality suggested following failure of irrigation and vasopressin. The conservative use of the device relates to a 39 per cent complication rate associated with its use. These include severe problems such as aspiration, esophageal rupture, and stenosis. The Sengstaken-Blakemore triple-lumen tube is most commonly used but requires placement of an NG tube above the inflated esophageal balloon to aspirate secretions. The Minnesota tube provides a fourth lumen for aspiration of secretions, thus eliminating the need for a second tube. We believe that all patients should be intubated prior to use of these devices.

Placement can be either oral or nasal; however, the nasal route is better tolerated. Its position in the stomach is verified by the injection of air and auscultation over the gastric area. The gastric balloon is inflated with 50 ml of air, and a chest film is taken. If in proper position, the gastric balloon is fully inflated and placed on traction. Adequate traction can be obtained by the use of a football helmet with an attached face mask. If the bleeding is not controlled by the gastric balloon, the esophageal balloon should be inflated to a pressure of 25 to 40 mm Hg. Occasionally, respiratory distress will develop with the use of this tube; should this occur, the tube should be immediately transected so as to deflate the balloons. For this purpose a pair of heavy scissors should be attached to the bed.

If bleeding is controlled over a period of 24 hours, the esophageal balloon may be deflated. The gastric balloon may be deflated if continued control is noted over the next 6 hours. Continuous tamponade should not be continued for more than 36 hours. This technique controls bleeding in 70 per cent of patients; however, bleeding recurs in approximately half of these cases.

Emergency Endoscopic Sclerotherapy

It is difficult to get a clear idea as to the usefulness of this procedure in the patient with active bleeding. There is little question that in experienced hands the procedure can be performed in the presence of active bleeding and that immediate control can be gained. This probably represents an exceptional circumstance and requires the skills of an experienced endoscopist.

Percutaneous Transhepatic Obliteration of Varices

The coronary vein represents a major direct conduit between the portal vein and the gastro-esophageal area. This arrangement permits catheterization by the percutaneous transhepatic route and successful obliteration of this vessel as well as associated collaterals in 80 per cent of cases. The materials used to produce thrombosis are gelatin foam, sodium tetradecyl sulfate, and wire coils. Despite this technical feat, the procedure is rarely used because of a 65 per cent rebleeding rate noted on long-term follow-up. In addition, portal vein thrombosis occurs in 36 per cent of patients, often producing acute hepatic failure. The procedure may be tried in a high-risk patient where other conservative measures have failed.

Emergency Nonshunting Procedure

The use of a direct operative approach to the bleeding varix is advocated in those cases where conservative measures fail. Most are disappointing. Transesophageal ligation of varices through the left chest is associated with a rebleeding rate of 33 per cent and an operation mortality of 30 per cent. The 5-year survival is a discouraging 5 per cent. If the approach is transabdominal and a devascularization is added to transection of the esophagus, the figures improve somewhat. The use of various stapling devices such as the EEA or the Russian SPTV has been advocated for esophageal transection. If the transections are combined with ligation of the coronary vein and a limited devascularization of the lower esophagus, the rebleeding rate can be reduced to 20 per cent; however, the operative mortality is 30 per cent. The Japanese have had considerable success with the Sugiura procedure (esophageal transection and gastric devascularization) for control of acute variceal hemorrhage, but this has not been duplicated in the United States. The choice of patients for these various procedures is not clear but probably depends on the interest and expertise of the surgeon involved.

Emergency Shunts

All shunting procedures effectively control variceal hemorrhage but are associated with an operative mortality of 20 per cent in Child's Class A patients and of 80 to 90 per cent in Child's Class C patients. The use of emergency shunts as the initial mode of therapy in the low-risk group is suggested by some investigators, but this approach is not widely accepted. The procedure chosen most often depends upon the interest and expertise of the surgeon involved, since there are no definitive studies indentifying the most appropriate procedure in an individual patient.

The end-to-end portacaval shunt is the procedure most commonly used, since it effectively controls bleeding and can be constructed with considerable facility. A side-to-side portacaval shunt is more appropriate, if the anatomy permits, since it tends to control ascites—which is common during this period of resuscitation—and can be reversed if the patient becomes chronically encephalopathic. The interposition mesocaval shunt is also commonly used. It is relatively easy to construct, controls bleeding, and can be easily reversed if chronic encephalopathy develops. Long-term patency of this shunt, however, is questioned by some investigators. The distal splenorenal shunt is not generally recommended in acute emergencies because of the time required for its construction and the problem of postoperative ascites. It is, however, the procedure of choice in a relatively stable patient who has maintained portal perfusion of the liver. If this procedure is considered, preoperative panhepatic angiography is essential to identify the anatomy and the status of perfusion of the liver. If perfusion through the portal vein is minimal or reversed, the procedure is not indicated. Preoperative panhepatic angiography is recommended in all cases, if readily available, since it will identify those conditions such as splenic or portal vein thrombosis that alter the surgical approach.

Long-Term Control of Bleeding

Prevention of recurrent variceal hemorrhage is dependent upon either an endoscopic or an operative procedure. Although medical control of recurrent hemorrhage is desirable, the use of propranolol (Inderal) has been ineffective and is of historic interest only. Presently, sclerotherapy is the procedure most often employed and there is considerable evidence to support its use.

Portacaval Shunt

This time-honored procedure effectively controls recurrent hemorrhage in 90 per cent of patients and is still extensively used. Dissatisfaction with the procedure developed because of the high incidence of encephalopathy reported by most investigators and the fact that survival following the operation is no different from that reported with medical management. This was thought to be related, at least in part, to the fact that the procedure produces sudden and total diversion of portal flow. This fact prompted the development of the distal splenorenal shunt (DSRS). It remains the procedure of choice, however, if portal perfusion is either reversed or minimal or if the patient has intractable ascites.

Distal Splenorenal Shunt

The DSRS procedure avoids sudden diversion of portal blood flow and is the procedure of choice when portal perfusion of the liver has been maintained. It controls recurrent hemorrhage in 90 per cent of patients and is associated with a 5 per cent incidence of chronic clinical encephalopathy. The development of collaterals over time will convert many of those selective shunts into a central shunt; however, the incidence of encephalopathy remains low at the 10-year level. This most probably relates to the slow development of this conversion. Preoperative panhepatic angiography is essential in order to demonstrate the direction of portal flow as well as patency and position of the splenic and renal veins.

Sclerotherapy

There is little question that sclerotherapy has become the procedure of choice for long-term control of hemorrhage from esophageal varices. The technique varies but consists of the injection of a sclerosing agent directly into a varix or into the adjacent tissues. The initial injection is followed by a series of injections that are continued until all varices have been obliterated. This is followed by annual endoscopic evaluation and by sclerosis of recurrent varices. This technique obliterates varices in 90 per cent of patients. Recurrent hemorrhage occurs in 20 to 30 per cent of patients, a figure that is significantly less than the 60 to 70 per cent recurrence reported in untreated patients. A randomized series comparing sclerotherapy with the DSRS suggests that survival is improved with the use of sclerotherapy as the initial form of treatment followed by a DSRS in those who rebleed. The complication rate is an acceptable 10 to 20 per cent per patient and consists of fever, ulceration, strictures, and aspiration. Despite the present enthusiasm for this procedure, adequately controlled long-term studies are presently unavailable; therefore, whether this procedure will stand the test of time is not known.

CHOLECYSTITIS AND CHOLELITHIASIS

method of
JACK PICKLEMAN, M.D.
Stritch School of Medicine,
Loyola University Medical Center
Maywood, Illinois

Although the exact incidence of gallstones is unkown in this country, it is estimated that at least 25 million

Americans harbor them. Many of these patients will never have symptoms or complications from their gallstones, but this is unpredictable in any individual patient, and gallstone-related diseases and their treatment are a major cause of morbidity and mortality. Elective operative mortality rates for patients under age 55 undergoing cholecystectomy are 0.1 to 0.2 per cent, but these figures are significantly higher in the elderly.

Symptomatic Gallstones

Treatment

Once stones become symptomatic, operative treatment will be necessary in most patients, as symptoms are likely to be repetitive and progressive. Even elderly patients with repeated episodes of biliary colic will require operation, not only to stop the persistent pain but also to prevent the development of acute cholecystitis or common bile duct stones, both of which lead to significant mortality in the elderly.

Following performance of cholecystectomy, I do not advocate routine operative cholangiography to detect occult common duct stones. If the patient has no history of jaundice or pancreatitis, has normal liver function tests, and a nondilated cystic duct and common duct at operation, the chance that he or she will have a common duct stone is less than 1 per cent. This does not justify routine operative cholangiography, with its increased operating time and cost, and the small but real risk of catheter-induced ductal injury. For the very uncommon patient who is found to have a retained common bile duct stone postoperatively, endoscopic retrograde cholangiopancreatography (ERCP) can be carried out with a papillotomy at very low risk to the patient.

Therefore, the indication for common bile duct exploration in addition to cholecystectomy is an abnormal operative cholangiogram. If the common bile duct is opened, operative choledochoscopy should be carried out before duct closure, as this technique can detect stones missed by the usual probing techniques. Although some have advocated primary common duct closure without drainage, I favor insertion of a T-tube. A T-tube cholangiogram can be carried out before hospital discharge and, if normal, the tube can be clamped off and the patient sent home. Removal of the tube can be carried out in the office a week later.

Most cholecystectomy patients can be operated on without the need for a nasogastric tube or abdominal drains. Feeding can usually be resumed on the first postoperative day, with hospital discharge on day 3 through 7, depending on the patient's overall recovery and medical status.

Asymptomatic Gallstones

Treatment

Several autopsy studies have disclosed an unexpectedly high incidence of asymptomatic gallstones, leading some to advise nonoperative treatment for all patients who do not have manifest complications of their gallstone disease. This stance is currently reinforced by the trend toward HMOs, in which a significant financial saving can be realized by not operating on patients. All authorities recognize the complications of gallstone disease—namely acute cholecystitis, common bile duct stones with cholangitis, gallstone pancreatitis, obstructive jaundice, and gallbladder carcinoma. What is not agreed upon is the incidence of these complications over the lifetime of any given patient. Although several recent studies have indicated a fairly low risk of occurrence of complications, these studies are flawed because they have looked at atypical populations or have not provided a long enough follow-up. In general, 20 to 50 per cent of patients with gallstones can expect biliary colic or one of the above complications to occur over a 10- to 15-year period after recognition of the stone disease. As the risks of cholecystectomy are clearly increased by age and perhaps increased by the development of acute cholecystitis, it is hard to imagine, given the very low operative mortality rates for elective cholecystectomy, a decreased risk over the *lifetime* of the patient by nonoperative therapy.

In the past, elective cholecystectomy for asymptomatic gallstones has been advised for only certain high-risk groups such as those patients with diabetes mellitus, large gallstones, or a calcified gallbladder. Recent studies have shown that diabetic patients do not have increased morbidity from cholecystectomy either performed electively or for acute cholecystitis. In view of these factors, I favor elective cholecystectomy for any patient below age 60 found to harbor gallstones, providing the patient has no significant medical contraindications to operation.

Acute Cholecystitis

Acute cholecystitis is generally due to impaction of a gallstone in the neck of the gallbladder or the cystic duct. This creates a cycle of edema and swelling in the gallbladder with subsequent decreased venous return, the end result of which may be gangrene and perforation of the gallbladder wall. Acalculous cholecystitis accounts for perhaps 5 per cent of cases of acute cholecystitis, and is generally associated with severe illness or sepsis, or the long-term administration of total parenteral nutrition. The disease is characterized by right upper quadrant pain and tenderness, often with a palpable mass, and by fever, leukocytosis, and, less commonly, hyperamylasemia.

Diagnosis is made by the presence of these symptoms associated with gallstones on ultrasonography. Other ultrasonographic findings include gallbladder wall thickening and pericholecystic fluid. An alternative method of diagnosis is the nuclear medicine biliary excretion (BIDA, HIDA, PIPIDA) scan. In this study, failure of isotopic visualization of the gallbladder implies cystic duct obstruction and the diagnosis of acute cholecystitis. It is important to remember that fasting patients may have a distended gallbladder and will excrete isotope normally from the liver but will have no gallbladder uptake, thus giving a false positive result indicative of cystic duct obstruction.

Treatment

The initial treatment of patients with acute cholecystitis should be intravenous fluids, nasogastric suction, volume resuscitation, and broad spectrum antibiotic administration. A second-generation cephalosporin such as cefaclor (Ceclor) will usually suffice, but in patients with evidence of bacteremia or ascending cholangitis, I prefer a combination of an aminoglycoside and clindamycin (Cleocin).

In the past, conventional management of these patients was to treat them medically until symptoms resolved, discharge them from the hospital, and then re-admit them 4 to 6 weeks later for elective cholecystectomy. The main purpose of this plan was to eliminate urgent operations, which were felt to be more technically difficult and associated with increased postoperative morbidity and mortality. This is no longer recommended for a number of reasons. (1) In up to 25 per cent of patients, the acute cholecystitis does not resolve, leading to emergency operation in a patient who has harbored sepsis for days. Mortality rates under such circumstances are considerably higher. In general, diabetic patients and those over age 60 often do not improve on medical management, but even younger, non-diabetic patients may fail to improve. (2) Many patients have recurrent acute cholecystitis during the arbitrary waiting period. (3) Often the technical problems during the subsequent operation are no less than they would have been initially. Cholecystectomy should, therefore, be carried out within 48 hours of admission when volume deficits are replaced and other medical problems have been optimized. Further delay invites considerably increased complication rates. A secondary benefit of early operation, of course, is an overall decreased length of hospital stay and cost.

An occasional patient will present with acute cholecystitis along with a grave medical contraindication for surgery, such as an acute myocardial infarction. Under these circumstances, a cholecystostomy tube can be inserted into the gallbladder under local anesthesia, and this will decompress the acutely inflamed gallbladder. Following resolution of the cholecystitis and stabilization of the medical problem, a decision regarding cholecystectomy can then be made.

Medical Treatment of Gallstones

The search continues for a nonsurgical alternative for the millions of patients in this country with gallstones. However, the current minimal operative risks for cholecystectomy and the inconsistent results of various medical treatments make most of these options unwise at the present time. Most medical treatments have many features in common. Unlike surgical removal of the gallbladder, all of these treatments are nondefinitive. In a significant percentage of patients, the gallbladder is not cleared of stones; there is significant morbidity; the cost is high; and last, gallstones will recur in almost all medically treated patients following cessation of treatment.

Chenodeoxycholic acid (CDCA), a naturally occurring bile acid, is available for oral administration. By increasing the bile salt pool, the cholesterol content of bile is decreased, and cholesterol stones may be dissolved. This drug is only effective in a patient with noncalcified or radiolucent stones in the presence of a functioning gallbladder, as determined by oral cholecystography. The National Cooperative CDCA Study disclosed that complete dissolution of stones occurred in less than 15 per cent of patients who were treated with CDCA. Other disadvantages of this drug include a significant rise in serum cholesterol and liver function tests, the long-term significance of which is unknown. Diarrhea is also a troubling complication in some patients. If gallstone dissolution is achieved, gallstones will reform in at least 50 per cent of patients within 5 years if the treatment is discontinued. Ursodeoxycholic acid (UDCA), an epimer of CDCA, is not yet approved for usage in the United States, but in several foreign trials has had roughly the same low incidence of complete gallstone dissolution but a decreased percentage of side effects.

Another recently described treatment modality is percutaneous transhepatic puncture of the gallbladder and instillation of ether compounds directly into the gallbladder. This brings about gallstone dissolution in a significant percentage of patients, but once again gallstones will reform in many of these patients unless they are placed on life-long CDCA or UDCA therapy. Most recently, various forms of laser therapy and lithotripsy are being experimented with in an effort to fragment stones to allow spontaneous passage out of the gallbladder and into the common bile duct. Some of these methods require general anesthesia. Also, the question of surrounding organ injury induced by the forces has not been answered. Most potentially disturbing is the inevitability that a certain percentage of these patients who pass their gallstones will develop gallstone pancreatitis from temporary impaction of these stones at the ampulla. This, coupled with the need for life-long gallstone dissolution agent administration postoperatively, makes recommendations for these methods premature at this time.

Because of the limitations of all of the above nonsurgical treatments, they should be reserved only for elderly or very poor-risk patients with recurrent symptomatic gallstones.

Choledocholithiasis and Ascending Cholangitis

Treatment

Common bile duct stones occur in approximately 15 per cent of patients with cholelithiasis, and in a disproportionately higher percentage of elderly patients. If common bile duct stones are noted at the time of cholecystectomy, they are easily dealt with by common bile duct exploration and stone extraction. Sometimes, however, these stones are first discovered postoperatively via a T-tube cholangiogram in patients who have recently undergone duct exploration. In this circumstance, two options are available. First, an endoscopic papillotomy can be performed and stones can be extracted at that time or they will spontaneously pass afterward. Second, the stone can be extracted under radiologic control via a basket inserted through the T-tube tract. However, it is not safe to do this initially, and 4 to 6 weeks should elapse to allow formation of a fibrous tract from the skin to the common bile duct. During this time, the patient's T-tube can be clamped.

Other patients will be discovered to harbor common duct stones long after cholecystectomy, and it is presumed that these stones have formed anew within the bile duct. In this circumstance, endoscopic papillotomy is the preferred treatment.

Some patients with common bile duct stones or other obstructing lesions of the bile duct will develop ascending cholangitis with its typical features of pain, fever, and jaundice. As this is a potentially life-threatening situation, antibiotic treatment should be initiated promptly. A combination of an aminoglycoside and clindamycin is recommended; alternatively, a newer-generation cephalosporin can be used. Ninety per cent of such patients will promptly respond to such treatment and, following radiologic definition of the biliary tract blockage, operation can be carried out. For the uncommon patients who do not promptly respond to antibiotics or for those who present with refractory sepsis and hypotension, emergency celiotomy is indicated. If the patient is very elderly or considered an unacceptably high operative risk, emergency endoscopic papillotomy can be carried out instead, and this will often bring about a resolution of the patient's symptoms. If endoscopic papillotomy is unavailable, percutaneous transhepatic cholangiography can be carried out with placement of a draining biliary tract catheter.

An occasional elderly or debilitated patient will present with cholelithiasis along with common bile duct stones and ascending cholangitis. In this circumstance, endoscopic papillotomy and stone extraction may be definitive treatment, and the patient can be left with an intact gallbladder containing stones. A subsequent decision will have to be made whether the risk of elective cholecystectomy exceeds the risk of these patients developing complications from their gallstones.

Acalculous Cholecystopathy

A small percentage of patients who present clinically with symptoms suggestive of biliary colic will be found to have a normal gallbladder ultrasound study. Such patients should undergo oral cholecystography, as this test may detect small stones previously missed. If both these tests are normal along with an upper gastrointestinal x-ray, and the patient has a *long* history of *typical* intermittent biliary colic, cholecystectomy should be considered. If the diagnosis is uncertain, a cholecystokinin (CCK) stimulated biliary excretion scan (BIDA/HIDA/PIPIDA) can be carried out, demonstrating a decreased gallbladder emptying fraction in many of these patients.

Treatment

For patients meeting all of the above criteria, cholecystectomy will relieve the pain in over 90 per cent of cases. Histologic examination of the gallbladders of these patients will generally disclose only mild chronic cholecystitis or even normal histology. However, as this is a functional gallbladder syndrome, this is no surprise, and the clinical results of cholecystectomy are excellent.

CIRRHOSIS

method of
SANJEEV ARORA, M.D., and
MARSHALL M. KAPLAN, M.D.
New England Medical Center
Boston, Massachusetts

Cirrhosis is a chronic disease of the liver characterized by widespread fibrosis of the liver and regenerating hepatic parenchymal cells, leading to nodule formation. The involvement of the liver is generalized, causing distortion of the lobular and vascular architecture. The initial insult to the liver is usually chronic destruction of hepatic parenchymal cells, which are replaced by bands of connective tissue. At the time of diagnosis there may or may not be ongoing necrosis of the liver.

The most common cause of cirrhosis in the United States and Europe is excessive consumption of alcohol. In the developing countries, chronic hepatitis B remains the most common etiology of cirrhosis of the liver. Hepatitis A virus infection does not cause cirrhosis, since it does not cause chronic hepatitis. Other, less common etiologies of cirrhosis are primary biliary cirrhosis, secondary biliary cirrhosis due to prolonged obstruction of bile flow, autoimmune chronic active hepatitis, and sclerosing cholangitis. Metabolic diseases such as Wilson's disease, hemochromatosis, tyrosinemia, glycogen storage diseases, and alpha$_1$-antitrypsin deficiency also cause cirrhosis of the liver. A more complete list of the etiologies of cirrhosis is provided in Table 1.

In 10 to 30 per cent of patients, even after a deliberate search for the etiology of cirrhosis, no definite cause can be found. The disease of this group is labeled cryptogenic or idiopathic cirrhosis.

The clinical features and complications of cirrhosis are due to two major events: the parenchymal necrosis causes hepatocellular failure and the distortion of the vascular architecture causes portal hypertension. One or both of these events are responsible for the development of jaundice, ascites, hepatic encephalopathy,

TABLE 1. **Etiology of Cirrhosis**

Alcohol	
Viral hepatitis	Chronic hepatitis B Chronic non-A, non-B hepatitis
Cholestatic liver diseases	Primary biliary cirrhosis Secondary biliary cirrhosis Sclerosing cholangitis
Metabolic liver diseases	Hemochromatosis Wilson's disease Alpha$_1$-antitrypsin deficiency Galactosemia Hereditary tyrosinemia Hereditary fructose intolerance Glycogen storage diseases
Venous outflow obstruction	Right heart failure Constrictive pericarditis Budd-Chiari syndrome
Drugs and toxins	Alpha methyldopa (Aldomet) Nitrofurantoin (Furadantin) Isoniazid (INH) Oxyphenisatin Amiodarone
Others	Autoimmune chronic active hepatitis Cystic fibrosis Small intestinal bypass Indian childhood cirrhosis Congenital syphilis Cryptogenic cirrhosis

variceal bleeding, spontaneous bacterial peritonitis, hepatorenal syndrome, and coagulopathy.

Once cirrhosis is established, it cannot be reversed. Treatment, therefore, is directed at (1) treatment of the underlying cause to arrest the progress of liver disease and (2) management of complications.

Treatment of the Underlying Cause

A careful search should be made for any treatable causes of cirrhosis of the liver. Serum ferritin levels, serum iron, and iron-binding capacity should be measured to exclude the diagnosis of *hemochromatosis*. If there is a family history of hemochromatosis or the serum ferritin is high and the transferrin is saturated greater than 50 per cent, a liver biopsy will help confirm the diagnosis of hemochromatosis. This condition is treated by weekly phlebotomies with 500 ml of blood. These are continued until iron stores are depleted, which is indicated by a fall in hemoglobin to less than 11 gram per cent or a serum ferritin below 10 ng per ml. It often takes 2 to 3 years (100 to 150 phlebotomies) to deplete iron stores. Once iron stores are depleted, maintenance phlebotomies are performed at less frequent intervals.

In patients who are anemic at the onset of treatment or develop anemia soon after initiating phlebotomies, chelation therapy with desferrioxamine may be used. Desferrioxamine is administered by subcutaneous infusion and is capable of removing 10 to 20 mg of iron per day. The prognosis is good if depletion of hepatic iron stores can be achieved, since progress of liver disease is arrested.

Wilson's disease (hepatolenticular degeneration) is another cause of cirrhosis that can be successfully treated. Patients with a family history of liver disease and all patients less than age 35 years should have a determination of serum ceruloplasmin level. If the ceruloplasmin level is low, a liver biopsy should be done to evaluate hepatic copper levels.

If the diagnosis of Wilson's disease, an autosomal recessive disorder, is established, treatment should be started with D-penicillamine, given orally in a dose of 1 to 2 grams daily given in 3 equally divided doses taken 30 minutes before each meal. The drug acts as a chelating agent and increases the urinary excretion of copper. Urinary copper should be measured to assess efficacy of the regimen. When copper depletion is achieved, a maintenance dose of 500 to 1000 mg per day of D-penicillamine is needed for life. Patients should avoid foods that are rich in copper such as mushrooms, chocolate, nuts, liver, shellfish, and dried fruits.

About 20 per cent of patients develop some side effects in the first few weeks of D-penicillamine treatment. These are often allergic in nature and consist of rash, fever, thrombocytopenia, or granulocytopenia. The drug should be stopped for 2 to 4 weeks and later started at very low doses, such as 25 mg per day, to desensitize the patients. Some patients develop more serious complications such as nephrotic syndrome, Goodpasture's syndrome, or myasthenia gravis. These patients can be treated with triethylenetetramine dihydrochloride (Trien). Treatment with oral zinc prevents absorption of dietary copper and is being evaluated as maintenance therapy once copper depletion has been achieved.

Chronic active hepatitis of the autoimmune type is a serious liver disease that can affect any age group. Young women are more often affected. If untreated, the disease has a poor prognosis with the mortality reaching 40 per cent at 6 months. There is a significant improvement in life expectancy with medical treatment, which consists of prednisone and azathioprine (Imuran). The usual dose of prednisone is 10 to 30 mg per day along with azathioprine, 1.5 mg per kg per day. The treatment improves the liver disease in approximately 80 per cent of patients. When the serum transaminases have returned to near normal levels and the serum gamma globulin level is normal, the dose of prednisone can be reduced to a maintenance dose of 10 to 15 mg per day. Steroid toxicity is a major problem. The average duration of treatment is 2 years, after which an attempt should be made to stop all treatment. In about half the patients, stopping treatment will result in relapse of the disease.

Several newer modalities of treatment for chronic liver disease are currently being investigated, some of which have been found to be beneficial. Three randomized, double-blind, placebo-controlled trials using colchicine for treatment of primary biliary cirrhosis have shown that colchicine improves the liver function tests. There is no improvement in liver histology. The usual dose is 0.6 mg twice a day. The only side effect observed was diarrhea, which improved with reduction of the dose.

One large study conducted in Mexico has recently shown the efficacy of colchicine in *alcoholic and posthepatitic cirrhosis* of the liver. The placebo-controlled, double-blind trial found that the group of patients receiving colchicine had significantly improved survival compared to patients receiving the placebo. No serious side effects were observed. Currently trials are in progress to evaluate the efficacy of antiviral therapy such as alpha-interferon for treatment of chronic hepatitis B and chronic non-A, non-B hepatitis. Any method to completely halt viral replication should arrest the progression to cirrhosis of the liver.

Patients with cholestatic liver diseases, such as primary biliary cirrhosis and sclerosing cholangitis, may have pruritus as a very distressing symptom. The drug of choice for treatment of this problem is cholestyramine, a bile salt–binding resin, given in a dose of 4 grams given 3 to 4 times daily. This often results in dramatic improvement. Patients with cholestatic liver disease may benefit from supplementation with the fat-soluble vitamins A, D, E, and K.

Management of Complications

Portal Hypertension and Variceal Bleeding

Portal hypertension is a disease state characterized by a pathologic and sustained elevation in portal venous pressure. The most common cause of portal hypertension is cirrhosis of the liver and its most common sequela is gastrointestinal bleeding from esophageal varices. Varices are dilated veins that develop as channels of communication between the portal and systemic circulation, bypassing the liver. Varices in the distal esophagus are submucosal, have little perivascular support, and protrude into the lumen, all of which make them prone to bleeding.

Bleeding from esophageal varices is a catastrophic event in the life of a patient with cirrhosis and is often the beginning of a steady downhill course. The mortality rate from a variceal bleed is as high as 50 per cent. The aims of management in a patient with cirrhosis and variceal bleeding are to stop variceal bleeding and attempt to prolong life. A patient with variceal bleeding needs intensive care. Resuscitation should be started with packed red cells, and special emphasis should be placed on correcting the coagulopathy of liver disease with fresh frozen plasma, cryoprecipitate, and/or platelets. Care should be taken to avoid excessive volume expansion, since raising the central venous pressure to unphysiologic levels exacerbates variceal bleeding; therefore, central venous pressure monitoring is often necessary.

Several controlled trials have shown that vasopressin is effective in stopping acute variceal bleeding. The drug is administered by a constant intravenous infusion, starting at a dose of 0.4 units per minute and increasing to 0.6 units per minute.* Vasopressin reduces portal pressure by causing splanchnic vasoconstriction and can therefore stop variceal bleeding. Extreme caution

---

*Also note the varying dosage listed on page 406.

has to be exercised when using vasopressin, especially in the elderly, because of its numerous side effects. It can produce bradycardia, mesenteric ischemia, coronary vasoconstriction, and even myocardial infarction. Recent studies suggest that the concomitant use of nitroglycerin may enhance the efficacy and reduce the side effects of vasopressin.

In our opinion the Sengstaken-Blakemore tube has a limited role in the management of patients with variceal bleeding because of a high risk of complications. If bleeding does not stop with intravenous vasopressin, injection sclerotherapy should be performed. This procedure involves injection of a sclerosing agent (e.g., sodium morrhuate) into or around the bleeding varix. Injection sclerotherapy can stop acute variceal bleeding in approximately 70 to 90 per cent of patients. When variceal bleeding has been stopped, the patient can then be put on a regimen of repeated endoscopic sclerotherapy with the aim of eventually obliterating the varices. Repeated sclerotherapy performed on these patients reduces the bleeding rate in patients with esophageal varices; however, it is unknown if it prolongs the survival of the patient.

Patients continuing to have recurrent variceal bleeding despite a completed course of sclerotherapy should be considered for surgical reduction of the portal hypertension. Surgery involves reduction of portal pressure by means of creating a shunt between the portal circulation and the systemic circulation. Two types of shunts are currently being performed: (1) nonselective shunts, such as the portacaval shunt, which diverts the entire portal blood flow from the systemic circulation, and (2) selective shunts, such as the distal splenorenal shunt, which decompresses a segment of the portal circulation while preserving antegrade portal vein blood flow. Shunt surgery is very effective in preventing variceal rebleeding. There is, however, a high rate of postoperative encephalopathy and hepatic failure after surgery. These complications are more frequent with the nonselective shunts than with selective shunts. The procedure of choice in patients requiring selective shunt surgery who do not have much ascites is the distal splenorenal shunt.

Studies are currently being conducted to develop medical treatment that can reduce portal pressure and therefore reduce the incidence of variceal bleeding. Some studies have shown that the use of propranolol (Inderal) in a dose sufficient to reduce the heart rate by 25 per cent may significantly reduce the frequency of variceal bleeding. Other studies, however, have failed to substantiate these findings. Propranolol therefore cannot be recommended at this time for routine treatment of portal hypertension.

Ascites

Ascites is defined as the accumulation of fluid in the peritoneal space. The patients present with increased abdominal girth and weight gain. For ascitic fluid to accumulate in the abdomen, the rate of formation of lymphatic fluid in the peritoneal space must exceed the rate of its removal by the thoracic duct. Ascitic fluid is derived both from the surface of the liver and the intestines. There is, however, a considerable amount of evidence to suggest that the vast majority of the fluid seeps out of the surface of the liver rather than that of the intestines. Cirrhosis of the liver often results in a postsinusoidal block to the outflow of blood from the liver. This results in a seven- to tenfold increase in hepatic sinusoidal pressure, leading to transudation of lymph across the sinusoidal wall and then out from the surface of the liver.

Leakage of lymph from the splanchnic capillaries occurs in response to a combination of hypoalbuminemia and increased portal pressure. However, the most important pathophysiologic mechanism for the continued formation of ascites is the avid salt and water retention by the kidneys that is seen in patients with cirrhosis of the liver. It is not known if the sodium retention by the kidney is a primary event leading to volume expansion and subsequent formation of ascites (overflow hypothesis) or if the salt and water retention by the kidney is a secondary phenomenon due to diminished effective intravascular volume secondary to primary ascitic fluid formation (underfill hypothesis).

Clinical examination is not a sensitive technique to detect small amounts of ascitic fluid in the abdomen. In contrast, an abdominal ultrasound is an extremely sensitive technique and can detect as little as 100 to 200 ml of peritoneal fluid. Most patients with new-onset ascites should have a diagnostic paracentesis performed. In a patient with chronic abdominal ascites, the development of fever, abdominal pain, encephalopathy, or unexplained deterioration in renal function should alert the physician to the possibility of infection of the ascitic fluid (spontaneous bacterial peritonitis) and a diagostic paracentesis should be performed.

The presence of ascites alone does not constitute an indication for treatment. If a patient has mild-to-moderate ascites and no other complaints, moderate sodium restriction should be used to prevent continued accumulation of ascitic fluid, and no drug therapy is necessary. Dietary restriction of sodium to 250 to 500 mg per day is very effective in preventing the accumulation of ascitic fluid. This diet, however, is often not well tolerated by patients, who may find food is unpalatable at this level of sodium intake. If the ascites limits the patient's physical activity, is accompanied by significant pedal edema, or causes respiratory embarrassment or abdominal discomfort, it should be treated with diuretics. The most important principle in treatment of ascites is the prevention of over-zealous diuresis and prerenal azotemia. Diuretic therapy reduces ascitic fluid by first diminishing intravascular volume, which in turn results in increased absorption of ascitic fluid from the peritoneal compartment. Unlike edema fluid, which can be absorbed almost immediately into the intravascular compartment, ascitic fluid can be reabsorbed only at an average rate of 400 to 500 ml per day. Therefore patients with cirrhosis who have ascites should only be diuresed to achieve a weight loss of approximately 1 pound (450 grams) per day. If there is significant pedal edema, patients can safely lose as much as 2 pounds (900 grams) per day. Large-volume diuresis in patients with ascites who do not have peripheral edema occurs at the expense of the intravascular compartment and therefore has a significant risk of hypovolemia and renal failure.

The drug of choice for treatment of ascites is spironolactone (Aldactone), which acts as an antagonist to the effect of aldosterone on the renal tubule and by actively inhibiting the release of aldosterone from the adrenal glands. The site of action is the distal tubule, where it prevents the absorption of sodium. Spironolactone should be started in a dose of 50 to 100 mg per day and the dose should be increased in a stepwise fashion until the desired effect is achieved or a dose of 400 mg per day is reached. Side effects of spironolactone are hypokalemia, gynecomastia, and metabolic acidosis. If spironolactone alone is not sufficient to achieve a desired therapeutic effect, furosemide (Lasix) should be added to the regimen. The usual dose is 20 to 40 mg per day, which can be increased gradually to a maximum of 80 to 120 mg per day. Furosemide acts by preventing salt and water reabsorption in the loop of Henle. In cirrhosis of the liver, this sodium is reabsorbed in the distal convoluted tubule, probably because of the hyperaldosteronism. Therefore, furosemide used alone is not very effective as treatment of ascites. Some patients with ascites are unresponsive to spironolactone and furosemide because of a markedly increased proximal tubular absorption of sodium, since most of the sodium is already absorbed before the fluid reaches the loop of Henle and the distal convoluted tubule. Such patients may benefit from metolazone, which can be added to a regimen of spironolactone and furosemide.

A small percentage of patients have tense ascites that is refractory to all forms of medical management and in whom ascitic fluid can be removed only at the expense of intravascular volume depletion or renal dysfunction. Such patients should be considered for peritoneal venous shunting (LeVeen or Denver shunt). This operation involves inserting a device that transports fluid from the peritoneal cavity to the central venous compartment when a pressure gradient exists between the peritoneal cavity and intrathoracic cavity. This operation is effective in relieving ascites but has many serious complications, including shunt occlusion, shunt infection, sepsis, and coagulopathy, all of which are associated with considerable morbidity and mortality.

Spontaneous Bacterial Peritonitis

Spontaneous bacterial peritonitis (SBP) (infection of the ascitic fluid) is a major life-threatening complication of ascites. The frequency of this infection in hospitalized patients with ascites has been increasing over the last 25 to 30 years. In addition to ascites, the majority of patients have other evidence of advanced liver disease such as jaundice, esophageal varices, and hepatic encephalopathy. The onset of SBP is usually characterized by fever and abdominal pain. However, as many as one third of patients with SBP have no symptoms and signs referable to the abdomen. These patients may present with worsening hepatic encephalopathy, deterioration in renal function, hypothermia, or hypotension. About three fourths of patients have leukocytosis and half have bacteremia diagnosed by positive blood cultures. The diagnosis is established by a diagnostic paracentesis.

The most reliable index of the diagnosis of SBP is a polymorphonuclear leukocyte count greater than 250 per mm^3 in the ascitic fluid. A Gram stain for the organisms is positive in only one third to one half of patients who eventually have a positive culture. Ascitic fluid protein, LDH, and glucose concentrations are not reliable indicators of the diagnosis of SBP. Some recent studies have shown that in SBP the ascitic fluid pH is reduced, and a gradient between blood pH and ascitic fluid pH greater than 0.1 may also be a reliable test for diagnosis of SBP.

Approximately 75 per cent of patients with SBP have infection with a gram-negative bacillus of enteric origin, *Escherichia coli* being the most common cause. Less commonly, other enteric organisms such as *Pseudomonas* and *Streptococcus faecalis* are found. The second most common organism detected is pneumococcus, which is found in 10 to 20 per cent of patients. Anaerobic infection is detected in only 10 per cent of cases.

The mainstay of management of patients with SBP is based on early diagnosis followed by treatment with efficacious and safe antibiotics. While awaiting the results of cultures, systemic antbiotics should be started if the polymorphonuclear count in the ascitic fluid is greater than 250 per mm^3. The conventional regimen has been a combination of ampicillin, 4 to 6 grams per day intravenously, and gentamicin intravenously to achieve appropriate blood levels. Gentamicin is administered as a loading dose of 1.5 to 2 mg per kg. Subsequent doses are adjusted for the expected creatinine clearance of the patient. We feel, however, that this regimen, although effective, is associated with considerable nephrotoxicity, to which a patient with cirrhosis may be predisposed. We recommend the use of a third-generation cephalosporin such as cefotaxime (Claforan), 1 to 2 grams intravenously every 8 hours. If the therapeutic response to intravenous antibiotics is not obvious, it is reasonable to repeat diagnostic paracentesis at 48 hours, at which time a reduction in the neutrophil count by greater than 50 per cent would indicate that the infection is being appropriately treated.

Hepatic Encephalopathy

Hepatic encephalopathy is a neuropsychiatric syndrome that encompasses all the changes in mental status occurring as a direct result of liver dysfunction. The clinical manifestations of this syndrome are diverse and can range from subtle personality changes to deep coma. The diagnosis is made by first establishing the presence of severe liver disease. The neurologic examination is suggestive of a metabolic encephalopathy. Other causes of metabolic encephalopathy such as drug overdose and renal failure should be excluded by clinical and laboratory evaluation. A deliberate search should be made to identify the factors that may have precipitated hepatic encephalopathy. The usual precipitating factors are gastrointestinal bleeding, prerenal azotemia, metabolic alkalosis, hypokalemia, systemic infection, use of sedatives, excessive dietary protein intake, and the new onset of constipation.

The first goal in the management of patients with hepatic encephalopathy is to correct or reverse any precipitating factors. If there is evidence of gastrointestinal bleeding, the blood should be evacuated from the gastrointestinal tract with a nasogastric tube and/or laxatives. Colonic blood is also effectively removed with high-colonic enemas. Hypokalemia and alkalosis can usually be corrected with intravenous potassium chloride administration. Prerenal azotemia caused by volume depletion requires the administration of crystalloids such as normal saline or colloids in the form of blood and albumin. Patients with ascites who have onset of hepatic encephalopathy should have a diagnostic paracentesis to rule out the presence of spontaneous bacterial peritonitis. In patients with advanced hepatic encephalopathy, dietary protein should be completely withheld until there is clinical improvement. Once encephalopathy is reversed, the dietary protein can be gradually increased by about 10 grams every 3 to 4 days. Patients with long-standing chronic hepatic encephalopathy may need to be maintained chronically on a low-protein diet containing approximately 30 to 40 grams of protein per day.

The next step in management is to prevent the absorption of nitrogenous breakdown products present in the digestive tract. Lactulose (1,4-galactosidofructose) is the drug of choice to achieve this goal. Lactulose is a nonabsorbable carbohydrate that reaches the colon intact, where it is broken down by the colonic bacteria to form lactic acid, formic acid, acetic acid, and carbon dioxide. The presence of these acids results in a fall in the pH of the colonic lumen to about 5.5, which in turn causes the conversion of ammonia to the ammonium ion. The low pH also results in the movement of ammonia from the intracellular compartment to the gut lumen, where it can be excreted as the ammonium ion. Lactulose also acts as a laxative and thus causes evacuation of the colonic contents. The usual dose of the drug is 15 to 30 ml administered orally 3 to 4 times a day. The desired effect is to produce 2 to 3 soft stools per day. Care must be taken to avoid diarrhea. For patients with encephalopathy who are comatose, lactulose can be administered in the form of an enema. Three hundred ml of lactulose is mixed with 700 ml of water and administered as a high-colonic enema. The major side effect of lactulose is diarrhea, which, if severe, can produce hyponatremia, hypovolemia, and azotemia.

Neomycin, a nonabosrbable antibiotic, was the drug of choice before the widespread use of lactulose. Neomycin acts by reducing the bacterial counts of urea-splitting organisms in the colon, thereby reducing the load of ammonia and other nitrogenous products absorbed into the systemic circulation. Although lactulose is the drug of choice, neomycin is a valuable adjunct to lactulose in some patients with refractory encephalopathy who have insufficient clinical effect with lactulose alone or who are not able to tolerate lactulose. The usual dose of neomycin in 500 mg to 1 gram given 4 times daily. Because 1 to 3 per cent of orally administered drug is absorbed into the systemic circulation, it has the potential for ototoxicity and nephrotoxicity, especially in patients with pre-existing renal disease.

Coagulopathy in Liver Disease

All the coagulation proteins and the inhibitors of coagulation except for the von Willebrand factor are synthesized by the liver. It is, therefore, not surprising that as many as 85 per cent of patients with liver disease exhibit some problem with hemostasis. The vast majority of these patients are asymptomatic. However, the presence of a coagulopathy becomes a significant liability in patients who have gastrointestinal bleeding from conditions such as esophageal varices and erosive gastritis. The abnormalities of coagulation in liver disease are complex and result from a combination of alterations in the level of coagulation proteins and inhibitors, platelet dysfunction, and the presence or absence of disseminated intravascular coagulation. The most common defect is a prolongation of the prothrombin time that is due to defective synthesis of the vitamin K–dependent Factors II, VII, IX, and X. Patients often have thrombocytopenia with platelet counts ranging from 50,000 to 100,000. The most common cause of thrombocytopenia is pooling of the platelets in an enlarged congested spleen. In patients with cirrhosis secondary to excessive alcohol use, bone marrow suppression may be a cause of the thrombocytopenia. In addition to thrombocytopenia, patients with cirrhosis also have defects in platelet function, and platelet adhesion to glass beads and aggregation in response to adenosine diphosphate (ADP) is impaired.

The mainstay of treatment for the coagulopathy of liver disease is fresh frozen plasma (FFP). It is useful for patients who are being prepared for elective surgery, liver biopsy, angiography, or other invasive procedures. Patients with cirrhosis who are actively bleeding and have a prolonged prothrombin time should also receive FFP. FFP contains all the coagulation factors in their inactive forms; in addition, it contains components of the fibrinolytic and inhibitor systems. Patients with thrombocytopenia may need platelet transfusions. Infusions of cryoprecipitates have also been found to be useful in some patients who are not responding adequately to FFP alone. Two new forms of treatment which are currently being investigated are antithrombin III and desmopressin (DDAVP). Antithrombin III concentrates have been found to be useful in patients with disseminated intravascular coagulation, fulminant hepatitis, and fatty liver of pregnancy. Desmopressin is an analogue of vasopressin that produces an increase in the plasma concentration of Factor VIII and von Willebrand's factor. It may also decrease the prothrombin time and raise the level of Factors VII, IX, and XII.

DYSPHAGIA AND ESOPHAGEAL OBSTRUCTION

method of
NEIL J. SEVY, M.D., and
WILLIAM J. SNAPE, JR., M.D.
Harbor-UCLA Medical Center
Torrance, California

Dysphagia, or difficulty swallowing, may be caused by a disturbance in the transport of food from the oropharynx to the esophagus (oropharyngeal dysphagia) or by an abnormality in the passage of food down the esophagus. In either category, impairment of transport may be due to mechanical obstruction from an intrinsic or extrinsic lesion or abnormalities in the coordinated movement of muscles. The history and physical examination will often suggest the proper diagnosis. All patients, however, should undergo an air-contrast barium swallow as their first diagnostic test. Video- or cineradiography should be performed as part of this examination, especially if one suspects an oropharyngeal disorder. Pharyngoscopy and esophagoscopy may be necessary if these tests do not identify the cause of symptoms or if a biopsy is necessary. If an esophageal motility disorder is suspected, an esophageal motility study should be done. Various provocative agents may be used during the study to precipitate symptoms or motility abnormalities, or both.

OROPHARYNGEAL DYSPHAGIA

Patients with pharyngeal symptoms or dysphagia localized to the neck may have esophageal abnormalities or combined disorders of the oropharynx and esophagus. Coughing or choking during swallowing strongly suggests an abnormality in the oropharynx. Dentition, size and contour of the tongue, and neurologic function of the oropharynx must be assessed.

Neuromuscular disorders account for at least 75 per cent of oropharyngeal dysphagia by causing either weakness of the tongue, pharynx, or cricopharyngeus muscle or a decrease in coordinative movements between these structures. A cine- or videoesophagram is the best way to make a diagnosis. An isolated abnormality of the cricopharyngeus, the cause of "cricopharyngeal spasm," is often cured by cricopharyngeal myotomy. Oropharyngeal dysphagia can be caused by primary muscular disorders such as polymyositis, dermatomyositis, and oculopharyngeal muscular dystrophy; secondary muscular disorders

associated with thyroid disease, amyloidosis, and chronic steroid administration; central nervous system disorders such as tumor, stroke, Parkinson's disease, multiple sclerosis, amyotrophic lateral sclerosis, poliomyelitis, Huntington's disease, and syringomyelia; and disease of the motor end plate in myasthenia gravis.

Mechanical obstruction is a less common cause of oropharyngeal dysphagia. Tumors, infections such as severe pharyngitis or tonsillitis, inflammation secondary to irradiation or caustic burns of the oropharynx, and trauma causing hematoma formation can mechanically obstruct the esophagus. A Zenker's diverticulum or false diverticulum of the hypopharynx may cause dysphagia by an extrinsic compression due to enlargement or by an abnormality of the cricopharyngeus that often accompanies the diverticulum. Poor dentition, ill-fitting dentures, and structural abnormalities of the mandible, maxilla, tongue, and palates will occasionally cause dysphagia.

Treatment leading to improvement or resolution of dysphagia is available for a number of disorders of the oropharynx and includes L-dopa and related compounds for Parkinson's disease, phenothiazines and haloperidol (Haldol) for Huntington's disease, cholinesterase inhibitors for myasthenia gravis, steroids for poly- and dermatomyositis, appropriate treatment of hypo- and hyperthyroidism, withdrawal of causative agents (e.g., steroids), cricopharyngeal myotomy, diverticulectomy or diverticulopexy for Zenker's diverticulum, and surgical reconstruction of anatomic defects of the oropharynx. Diet modification, strengthening of weakened muscle groups, and changes in swallowing techniques can help patients with chronic neurologic disorders.

ESOPHAGEAL DYSPHAGIA

Motility Disorders

Achalasia

Achalasia is an esophageal motility disorder due to an abnormality in the myenteric plexus of unknown etiology, which presents with progressive dysphagia for solids and liquids in 90 per cent of patients. Regurgitation, and aspiration with secondary pneumonia, may also be present. Significant weight loss suggests secondary achalasia associated with a carcinoma. Approximately 25 per cent of patients also complain of chest pain that is usually retrosternal and may radiate to the back, shoulders, jaw, or arms, often mimicking angina. Chest pain is more common in a variant form of achalasia called *vigorous achalasia*. In patients with chronic symptoms, a barium swallow may show a dilated esophagus with a smoothly tapered distal esophagus often referred to as a "bird's beak." Peristalsis is absent and an air-fluid level demonstrates retained food in the esophagus. Manometric findings include low-amplitude, nonperistaltic contractions in the lower two thirds of the esophagus (smooth muscle portion) and incomplete relaxation of the lower esophageal sphincter (LES). Resting LES pressure is usually elevated. The subgroup of patients with vigorous achalasia will have nonperistaltic body contractions with high amplitude (>50 mm Hg) in addition to the abnormalities in the lower esophageal sphincter. Endoscopy must always be done to rule out tumor at the gastroesophageal junction, which can cause a motility abnormality identical to achalasia (secondary achalasia). Achalasia may also rarely be caused by Chagas' disease resulting from infection with *Trypanosoma cruzi,* which is endemic in South America. The incidence of carcinoma of the esophagus is thought to be increased in patients with primary achalasia and some physicians recommend yearly screening endoscopy with cytology and biopsy.

Treatment is usually directed at reducing LES pressure. Dilation with mercury or equivalent bougies will give only transient relief of symptoms. Pneumatic dilation of the LES is the treatment procedure of choice. The patient should be on a liquid diet for approximately 24 hours and fasted overnight. The patient should be sedated adequately with a benzodiazepine and meperidine (Demerol), and a local anesthetic is sprayed into the oropharynx. A nasogastric tube is placed into the esophagus to remove retained material. The balloon dilator is introduced orally and passed down the esophagus to the LES. Under fluoroscopic guidance the balloon is positioned so that the tight LES can be seen to compress the balloon at its midportion. If a very tortuous esophagus has been noted on prior endoscopic examination, a guide wire may be passed via the endoscope and the balloon catheter may then be passed over the wire under fluoroscopic guidance. The balloon is then filled with air to a pressure of 200 mm Hg for approximately 30 seconds. During this time the patient will complain of pain and one should see the waist of the balloon expand. The balloon is usually then deflated and removed. The balloon will often be blood-tinged due to the traumatic rupture of muscle bundles in the LES. The incidence of perforation is 2 to 8 per cent. After the procedure, a water-soluble contrast agent is used to examine the esophagus radiographically to rule out perforation. A widely patent LES may not be noted at this time due to early post-dilation edema. The patient is then fasted for an additional 6 hours and if asymptomatic may then leave the hospital. Some physicians may elect to keep the patient hospitalized overnight for observation, with discharge in the morning. Pre- and post-dilation radionuclide scans may be used to document improvement with treatment.

Perforation may require emergency thoracotomy if the patient does not stabilize with intravenous antibiotics. Therefore, a patient who is unable to tolerate a thoracotomy should not have pneumatic dilation. We recommend a repeat dilation 2 weeks later if the first one results in a suboptimal response. Pneumatic dilation is associated with a successful response approximately 70 per cent of the time, with an average resultant resting LES pressure of approximately 15 mm Hg. If a patient fails two to five dilation attempts, surgery may be the best way to treat the obstruction.

There are various modifications of the Heller myotomy, which consists of incision of the circular muscle fibers at the gastroesophageal junction. This usually results in a decrease of LES pressure to about 10 mm Hg, giving relief to approximately 90 per cent of patients. In the past, up to 30 per cent of patients have developed significant postsurgical gastroesophageal reflux, with many of these ultimately requiring surgery for intractable reflux. Therefore many surgeons perform a concomitant loose fundoplication with the myotomy. For those patients who refuse surgery, who are not surgical candidates, or who have had partial responses to dilation or myotomy, several drugs are available that may offer some relief of symptoms. Nifedipine (Procardia), a calcium channel blocker, can decrease resting LES pressure significantly as well as reduce peak contraction amplitude in the esophagus; thus, this drug is suitable for use in achalasia, especially vigorous achalasia. It can be used in doses of 10 to 30 mg 30 minutes to 1 hour before meals and at bedtime. Anticholinergic agents such as propantheline bromide (Pro-Banthine), 15 to 30 mg, and dicyclomine hydrochloride (Bentyl), 20 to 40 mg, may also be used either at bedtime, because of the additional action of decreasing secretions, or before meals. Nitrates and beta-adrenoceptor agonists may also provide some relief of symptoms. Frequent bouginage may be attempted as a last resort in those patients who are not candidates for any of the above therapies.

Diffuse Esophageal Spasm

Diffuse esophageal spasm (DES) is a primary disorder of esophageal motility that usually presents with intermittent chest pain (present in 80 to 90 per cent of patients) that may mimic angina. Chest pain may or may not be precipitated by eating. Dysphagia also occurs in about 70 per cent of these patients. Barium swallow may show distortion of the esophagus with tertiary contractions. Manometric findings may include a 30 to 80 per cent frequency of nonperistaltic swallows with a higher than normal amplitude. LES pressure and relaxation are usually normal. A patient with chest pain, a normal cardiac evaluation, and a normal manometry should have a repeat manometry using the provocative agent edrophonium (Tensilon). Cholinergic stimulation with edrophonium may lead to a positive diagnosis of DES in a patient with an otherwise normal baseline tracing if the patient has pain after administration of the drug.

When there is acute chest pain, treatment should include either nitroglycerin, 0.4 mg sublingually, or nifedipine (Procardia), 10 to 30 mg sublingually. If chest pain occurs frequently, treatment may be instituted with either nifedipine (Procardia), 10 to 30 mg, or an anticholinergic agent such as dicyclomine hydrochloride (Bentyl), 10 to 40 mg; propantheline bromide (Pro-Banthine), 15 to 30 mg; or isosorbide dinitrate (Isordil), 10 to 20 mg, 30 minutes to 1 hour before meals and at bedtime. Since nifedipine is more effective at decreasing LES pressure, it should be used in those patients with elevated LES pressure. Since the anticholinergics also inhibit acid secretion they might preferentially be used in patients with concomitant reflux disease so long as side effects are tolerated.

Most patients respond to medical therapy. In those that continue to have dysphagia with elevated LES pressures or incomplete LES relaxation, bouginage may be helpful. Pneumatic dilation may be indicated for patients with elevated LES pressures and incomplete LES relaxation. Rarely chest pain is refractory to the above therapy, and in these cases one may consider a long esophagomyotomy with extension to the LES if it is abnormal. If the LES is also incised, most surgeons will do an antireflux procedure as well.

Nutcracker Esophagus

Nutcracker esophagus is characterized by very high-amplitude peristaltic contractions seen on manometry. Almost all patients have chest pain and some have dysphagia. Some contractions may be prolonged, and approximately 40 per cent of patients will have a hypertensive LES. Approximately 40 per cent of patients will also have evidence of esophageal reflux. Some feel that this entity may be a harbinger of DES, and indeed progression to DES has been documented in a few patients.

Treatment in patients with a normal LES may be accomplished with an anticholinergic agent (see dosages in preceding section) since these are more efficacious than nifedipine in decreasing the amplitude of esophageal body contractions. Anticholinergics are also preferable in patients with reflux because of their effect on acid secretion. Nifedipine (Procardia) (see dosages in preceding section) will be most appropriate for patients with concomitant LES pressure elevation. (Anticholinergics and nifedipine may be used in conjunction.) Refractory dysphagia may improve after bouginage in patients with LES hypertension. Pneumatic dilation may rarely be indicated for refractory dysphagia in this subgroup. Esophagomyotomy should be a last resort, given the preservation of peristalsis in this disorder; however, chest pain and dysphagia refractory to medical therapy may necessitate surgery with or without extension to the LES and an antireflux procedure.

Hypertensive Lower Esophageal Sphincter

Hypertensive lower esophageal sphincter occasionally will present as an isolated abnormality on manometry. Patients may present with intermittent dysphagia and/or chest pain. Generally this condition is of clinical significance only if incomplete LES relaxation is present.

Treatment is usually successful with nifedipine (Procardia) or anticholinergic agents in the previously mentioned doses. Refractory cases may be managed with bouginage, pneumatic dilation, and in extreme cases LES myotomy.

Scleroderma

Scleroderma is often associated with esophageal abnormalities. Manometry characteristically reveals low-amplitude waves that may be peristaltic in the early stages, but aperistaltic during later stages of the disease. LES resting pressure is very low. The combination of an incompetent LES and poor peristalsis predisposes the patient to frequent and significant reflux with poor clearing of refluxed material from the esophageal body, resulting in significant esophagitis. The incidence of erosive esophagitis and stricture formation is significant. These findings may also be present in other collagen vascular diseases such as mixed connective tissue disease.

Treatment is directed at control of reflux (see Reflux Esophagitis section below). Metoclopramide (Reglan), 5 to 10 mg 30 minutes before meals and at bedtime, has recently been shown to be effective in this disorder. Since strictures are common, periodic bouginage with tapered mercury-filled (Maloney) dilators or hollow plastic (Savary) dilators is often necessary. If surgery is deemed necessary to control intractable esophagitis, care must be taken not to make the fundoplication too "tight," since the poor peristalsis may precipitate postsurgical dysphagia.

Gastroesophageal Reflux

Gastroesophageal reflux is occasionally associated with motility disorders. A small number of patients, most often with stricture or Barrett's esophagus, will have an abnormal number of nonperistaltic low-amplitude contractions. A significant number of patients with nutcracker esophagus will have concomitant reflux with a positive Bernstein test (pain with instillation of 0.1 N HCl) on manometry. A small number of patients with reflux will have squeezing, retrosternal chest pain that can may be demonstrated with a Bernstein test. Therapy consists of those measures described in the section on Reflux Esophagitis.

Miscellaneous Disorders

Amyloidosis, diabetes mellitus, and chronic alcohol abuse may lead to nonspecific motility disorders. Patients with neuropathic intestinal pseudo-obstruction may also have abnormal peristalsis on esophageal manometry. These disorders are usually asymptomatic and require no treatment. Other primary motility abnormalities seen on manometry include esophageal contractions of prolonged duration and localized segmental spasm or a small localized area of esophagus with changes similar to those seen in DES. Treatment with nifedipine or anticholinergic agents in symptomatic patients may be of benefit.

ESOPHAGITIS

Reflux Esophagitis

Reflux esophagitis is caused by the reflux of acid-containing material from the stomach into the esophagus, usually because of an incompetent lower esophageal sphincter. Diagnosis is most often made by endoscopy with or without biopsy and by a positive Bernstein test or 24-hour pH monitoring.

Treatment consists of (1) avoiding smoking and foods and drugs that decrease LES pressure and (2) administration of drugs that increase sphincter pressure, decrease gastric acidity, or help injured tissue to "recover."

Elevating the head of the bed on 6-inch blocks allows gravity to better reduce both the frequency and duration of reflux, and weight loss may decrease intra-abdominal pressure. Coffee, tea, chocolate, alcohol, smoking, dietary fat, theophylline, anticholinergics, and the progesterone in birth control pills may decrease lower esophageal sphincter pressure and should be avoided. Patients should eat small meals, taking care not to eat for 3 hours before reclining at night. Bending at the waist, heavy lifting, and wearing tight-fitting corsets should be avoided.

Histamine$_2$ (H$_2$) receptor antagonists, cimetidine, ranitidine, and famotidine may be used in doses that maximally suppress gastric acid secretion. Antacids may be used liberally throughout the day for symptoms. Metoclopramide (Reglan), 5 to 10 mg 30 minutes before meals and at bedtime, will increase LES pressure and gastric emptying. A significant number of patients with esophageal reflux also have delayed gastric emptying. Bethanechol (Urecholine), 10 to 50 mg in a similar dosing schedule, may also increase LES pressure. Sucralfate (Carafate), 1 gram dissolved in 30 ml of water, may be taken 3 times daily and at bedtime. This may both "coat" and protect injured mucosa. These drugs may be used in a stepwise manner if changes in habits and the use of antacids do not provide relief. H$_2$ antagonists are usually tried first, followed by metoclopramide and bethanechol. Sucralfate may be used to treat acute inflammation and then also may be used in a nightly dose for maintenance. If a patient has documented reflux disease and clearly is refractory to maximal medical management, a surgical fundoplication may be recommended. However, the patient should be advised that a fundoplication with time may "unravel," necessitating an additional surgical procedure. Surgery is usually reserved for those patients with refractory, erosive esophagitis, stricture formation, or Barrett's esophagus with refractory esophagitis. Those patients who develop Barrett's esophagus, a complication of chronic reflux disease, should have esophagoscopy with biopsy on a yearly basis to screen for development of adenocarcinoma of the esophagus, which occurs in 2 to 10 per cent of cases.

Infectious Esophagitis

Both the *Candida* organism and the herpes simplex virus may cause esophagitis in immunocompromised patients and, rarely, in otherwise normal patients. *Candida* infection also may be seen in patients with poorly controlled diabetes and in patients with significant stasis secondary to severe motility disorders. Diagnosis is made via endoscopy with biopsy, brush cytology, and cultures. Cytomegalovirus (CMV) has been isolated from the esophagus in patients with immunosuppression, especially those with the acquired immune deficiency syndrome (AIDS), and may be a significant cause of esophagitis in these patients. Other unusual causes of esophagitis usually found in immunocompromised patients include various bacteria, *Blastomyces, Torulopsis,* tuberculosis, and sarcoidosis.

Treatment of mild candidal esophagitis in non-immunocompromised patients includes oral nystatin (Mycostatin), 200,000 to 600,000 units 4 times daily, or clotrimazole (Mycelex) troches given every 2 hours. If the infection is severe, if the above therapy has failed, or if the patient is significantly immunocompromised, ketoconazole (Nizoral), 200 to 400 mg per day, is the drug of choice. Patients with clearly documented candidal esophagitis who do not respond to the above regimen will require therapy with intravenous amphotericin B. A test dose of 1 mg dissolved in 100 ml of D5W is infused over 1 to 2 hours while the patient is carefully monitored. If the patient tolerates this dose, he or she may be given 0.25 mg per kg dissolved in 500 ml of a 5 per cent dextrose solution over 6 hours on the following day. Daily therapeutic doses range from 0.25 to 1 mg per kg per day, depending on the response of the patient. Patients are usually given diphenhydramine (Benadryl), 50 mg, and acetaminophen (Tylenol), 650 to 1000 mg, as well as an antiemetic prior to the first few doses, to minimize a possible febrile reaction and the nausea and vomiting that may occur. Hydrocortisone, 50 mg, is also infused with the amphotericin B. Toxicity includes hypotension, bronchoconstriction, hypokalemia, anemia, thrombophlebitis, hepatocellular damage, and both early and late renal failure. A complete blood count, electrolytes, and hepatic chemistries must be drawn at least weekly, and a serum creatine drawn twice weekly. Significant toxicity or abnormalities in these tests will necessitate a decrease in dosage and perhaps cessation of the drug.

Herpes esophagitis is usually self limited in the otherwise normal patient; it can be treated in immunocompromised patients with acyclovir (Zovirax), 5 mg per kg intravenously every 8 hours for 1 week, if renal function is normal. There is no acceptable treatment for presumed CMV esophagitis. *Blastomyces* infection can be treated with amphotericin B. Esophagitis secondary to bacterial infection, sarcoidosis, or tuberculosis is treated as one would treat the systemic disease and is based on appropriate cultures of esophageal tissue and blood.

Caustic Esophagitis

Ingestion of caustic substances either accidentally, as usually occurs in children, or in a suicide attempt, as usually occurs in adults, can cause significant damage to the esophagus. Anteroposterior and lateral chest radiographs that demonstrate mediastinal air suggest perforation. Antiemetics are contraindicated and lavage is controversial, some physicians recommending very gentle lavage so as not to cause reflux or emesis of caustic material from the stomach into the esophagus. Careful dilution with water in the immediate post-ingestion period is reasonable. Careful endoscopy with a small-caliber endoscope within 24 hours, if there are no signs of perforation, is recommended to evaluate the degree of esophageal injury. One must proceed with extreme caution, especially when significant oropharyngeal damage is evident. If there are any symptoms or signs of perforation, a water-soluble contrast swallow should be performed for evaluation.

Treatment of these patients is controversial. Most agree that patients with mild injury need no specific treatment unless symptoms develop. If esophageal injury is moderate to severe, a small-caliber nasogastric tube may be placed to maintain luminal patency for likely future dilations. Antibiotics, usually a penicillin and either an aminoglycoside or a third-generation cephalosporin, may be used as a prophylactic measure while the patient is being observed in the hospital. Some physicians recommend the use of steroids acutely in doses equivalent to 60 to 80 mg per day of prednisone, with a quick taper. There are no well-controlled clinical trials that support the use of antibiotics or steroids. Prophylactic bouginage may be started at the end of the first week unless injury is severe, in which case it may have to be delayed. Others recommend bouginage when symptoms occur. Most agree that early surgery is indicated in the setting of perforation. Periodic endoscopy is required in those patients that have swallowed alkaline substances, especially lye, because of the increased incidence of esophageal squamous cell carcinoma in this population.

Injury to the esophagus may also result from ingestion of certain types of pills that may lodge in the esophagus, causing localized esophagitis with or without erosions or ulcerations. Doxycycline, tetracycline, quinidine compounds, iron, and potassium chloride have commonly been described in this setting; aspirin and non-steroidal anti-inflammatory drugs have been infrequently involved. We treat these patients with sucralfate (Carafate), 1 gram dissolved in 30 ml of water 4 times daily, or with frequent antacids until symptoms have resolved for approximately 1 week. Prophylaxis includes swallowing pills with adequate amounts of water in a non-recumbent position. Liquid preparations and crushing larger tablets will also be of benefit.

Esophageal sclerotherapy commonly results in erosions or ulcerations at the site of injection.

Treatment during sclerotherapy may be instituted with sucralfate in the above-mentioned doses.

Radiation therapy and certain types of chemotherapy may cause esophagitis. Treatment includes sucralfate, antacids, or H_2 blockers. All of the caustic agents described above may lead to esophageal strictures, the treatment of which is discussed below.

MECHANICAL OBSTRUCTION

Foreign Bodies

After obtaining a history of ingestion of a foreign body, anteroposterior and lateral radiographs of the neck as well as a supine and upright radiograph of the abdomen should be done to better localize the foreign body and rule out perforation. If a patient has swallowed a radiolucent object, a barium swallow with dilute barium may locate the object. Coins can usually be removed from the esophagus endoscopically with alligator forceps, taking care not to drop the coin as it is being pulled past the larynx. Coins already in the stomach may be allowed to pass, followed radiographically on an outpatient basis. Sharp objects may be removed from the esophagus as long as the sharp edge trails. Otherwise they may be pushed into the stomach and removed with an overtube placed over the endoscope and the object, thus protecting the mucosa. Meat that has impacted in the esophagus may pass, with sedation and 1 mg of glucagon given intravenously. If this fails, it can sometimes be pulled out with a grasping device placed through the endoscope. If this fails, one can attempt to carefully push the meat into the stomach, especially if one can see no obstruction distal to the meat, using a small pediatric endoscope. Meat tenderizer (papain) should be avoided because there have been numerous reports of complications. Disc batteries should be removed immediately because of their potential to cause significant burns and secondary perforation. Foreign bodies seen at the level of the pharynx and cricopharyngeus are best removed with a surgical grasper (e.g., Kelly clamp) while directly viewing the object with a rigid laryngoscope. If the removal procedure has been traumatic or if there are any signs or symptoms of post-procedure perforation, a water-contrast swallow (e.g., Gastrografin) should be done. Perforation requires immediate intravenous antibiotics and surgery. After a foreign body has been removed from the esophagus, a full diagnostic workup must be done to rule out stricture, tumor, or motility disorder as the precipitating cause of the obstruction.

Tumors

Most tumors of the esophagus are squamous. Tumors associated with Barrett's epithelium and those that are at the gastroesophageal junction are usually adenocarcinomas. Only 5 to 10 per cent of patients survive at 5 years despite treatment with radiotherapy, surgery, or chemotherapy alone. Most patients present with dysphagia and weight loss. Definitive diagnosis is usually made at endoscopy with tissue biopsy. Limited data suggest a significant decrease in mortality in those patients that undergo both preoperative radiation therapy and chemotherapy and who on resection have no evidence of malignant disease. The mortality data from series comparing surgery alone and surgery with preoperative radiation are mixed. If after a computed tomography (CT) scan of the chest and abdomen an esophageal cancer is thought to be resectable, we recommend inclusion of the patient in a randomized controlled study for treatment if one is available. If not available, we recommend preoperative radiation and resection. If metastatic or local extension of disease on CT scan suggests tumor unresectability, we recommend either palliative radiation or laser therapy. The CT scan may be repeated after radiation to see if tumor regression has occurred to a point where resection is possible. Frequent dilations with tapered mercury-filled (Maloney) dilators, or tapered dilators placed over a guide wire (Savary dilators) if the esophagus is tortuous, may provide some temporary relief of dysphagia and obstruction. This also may be attained through laser therapy or placement of an esophageal stent (especially in the presence of a tracheoesophageal fistula) via the endoscope.

Strictures

Strictures may occur as a result of tissue injury secondary to reflux, with or without Barrett's epithelium, caustic ingestions, prolonged nasogastric intubation, radiation, chemotherapy, esophageal variceal sclerotherapy, prior surgery (especially when an esophageal anastomosis is present), and malignancy. All strictures should be closely examined at endoscopy and biopsies taken, when appropriate, to rule out malignancy.

Treatment of benign strictures involves withdrawal of offending agents, medical treatment of esophagitis, and, if dysphagia develops, peroral bouginage of the stricture. Dilation is most easily accomplished with the patient in the sitting or standing position but may also be adequately accomplished with the patient in the left lateral decubitus position. The patient should fast for 6 to 8 hours prior to the procedure. Tetracaine, 2 per cent, is topically applied to the pharynx and hypopharynx. Occasionally premedication with meperidine (Demerol), 25 to 100 mg intravenously or intramuscularly, is required, especially if the stricture is tight. We use tapered mercury-filled (Maloney) or Savary dilators. The size of the first dilator is chosen depending upon endoscopic and radiographic findings. The top of the dilator is guided into the hypopharynx with the index finger and the patient is asked to swallow, allowing the dilator to enter the esophagus. The combination of the weight of the dilator and gentle pressure from the examiner allows the dilator to pass down the esophagus. Some resistance may be felt. Too much pressure applied to pass the stricture increases the risk of perforation. In general, three or four dilators of progressively larger diameters are used in a single setting. The procedure may be repeated every 2 or 3 days until a No. 48 to 50 French (Fr) dilator (approximately 16 to 17 millimeters in diameter) passes through the stricture. Repeat dilations may then be done as patients become symptomatic. If the esophagus is very tortuous, Savary dilators may be used. These are hollow, radiopaque dilators composed of a polyvinyl material, which are passed over a guide wire passed either via fluoroscopy or directly through the endoscope. In addition, radial balloon dilators are available that can be passed through the endoscope and then inflated with direct endoscopic guidance and observation. Surgery is occasionally required for a stricture that cannot be adequately dilated.

Miscellaneous Abnormalities

Schatzki's ring consists of a constriction at the gastroesophageal junction, usually composed of mucosa and submucosa. It may cause intermittent dysphagia for solid foods. Treatment consists of endoscopy, which itself may tear the ring, followed by dilation with a No. 50 Fr mercury dilator.

Muscular rings may occur just above the gastroesophageal junction and are often associated with motility disorders. Treatment of dysphagia consists of adequate therapy of the motor disorder.

Upper esophageal webs, if symptomatic, usually are torn with the endoscope and further dilated with a No. 50 Fr dilator if necessary. They should be carefully examined at endoscopy for evidence of cancer, which has an increased incidence in this disorder.

Vascular compression of the esophagus by an aberrant artery (dysphagia lusoria) can rarely be a cause of dysphagia. A double aortic arch or aberrant right subclavian artery is usually the culprit. Surgery depends on the extent and type of associated anomalies.

Congenital esophageal stenosis is caused by one or more strictures that may contain bronchial remnants. Treatment consists of surgical resection.

Esophageal atresia is often associated with a tracheoesophageal fistula. Treatment includes prevention of aspiration and surgical reconstruction.

DIVERTICULA OF THE ALIMENTARY TRACT

method of
GARY W. FALK, M.D.
The Cleveland Clinic Foundation
Cleveland, Ohio

While diverticula of the gastrointestinal tract are most commonly located in the colon, they can also be found in the esophagus, stomach, and small bowel. The pathogenesis of alimentary tract diverticula is poorly understood, and their clinical significance ranges from that of an intellectual curiosity to a surgical emergency.

ESOPHAGEAL DIVERTICULA

Esophageal diverticula are an outpouching of one or more layers of the esophageal wall. They may occur just above the upper esophageal sphincter (Zenker's diverticulum), in the midesophagus, or just proximal to the lower esophageal sphincter.

Pharyngoesophageal Diverticula

A pharyngoesophageal (Zenker's) diverticulum is an acquired herniation of pharyngeal mucosa through a defect in the posterior hypopharyngeal wall just above the cricopharyngeus. Although the cause of Zenker's diverticula is unclear, motor incoordination of the cricopharyngeal muscle has been implicated in the pathogenesis of these diverticula. Symptoms include transient dysphagia, regurgitation of food, halitosis, and gurgling. Pulmonary complications such as aspiration, coughing, and hoarseness may also develop. Diagnosis is confirmed by barium studies or by endoscopic evaluation under direct vision.

Treatment

Surgery is the primary method of therapy once a pharyngoesophageal diverticulum becomes symptomatic. If the diverticulum is small, cricopharyngeal myotomy alone may be sufficient. For moderate- to large-sized sacs, one-stage diverticulectomy or inversion of the diverticulum may be performed. It is unclear at present whether or not a cricopharyngeal myotomy should accompany this technique. Recurrences may be seen after surgery, but are uncommon. Complications of surgery are uncommon, but may include cervical esophageal stenosis, esophageal-cutaneous fistula, vocal cord paralysis, and wound infection.

Mid-esophageal Diverticula

Mid-esophageal diverticula are typically asymptomatic. Symptoms such as episodic dysphagia, chest pain, regurgitation, or obstruction by a bolus of food may occasionally occur. However, it may be difficult to determine whether these symptoms are caused by the diverticulum or by motor abnormalities of the esophagus that have been associated with these diverticula. If symptoms occur, esophageal manometric studies may allow for diagnosis of any such motility disorder.

Treatment

Treatment is not necessary in the asymptomatic individual or if the diverticulum is small. If an associated motor abnormality is present, it should be treated by appropriate medical therapy. Should symptoms continue, an esophageal myotomy may be necessary.

Epiphrenic Diverticula

Epiphrenic diverticula are rare outpouchings of the distal esophagus occurring just above the lower esophageal sphincter. They also have been shown to be associated with a variety of motor disturbances of the esophagus such as achalasia and diffuse esophageal spasm. Symptoms such as dysphagia, regurgitation, or chest pain are usually caused by the underlying motility disturbance and not by the diverticulum. In patients symptomatic from an epiphrenic diverticulum, esophageal manometric studies will help define any underlying motor dysfunction, and endoscopy may be helpful in delineating any structural abnormality.

Treatment

Treatment is necessary only for symptomatic individuals. Calcium channel blockers such as diltiazem (Cardizem), 30 to 60 mg four times daily, or nitrates should be initial therapy for spasm, achalasia or nutcracker esophagus. Achalasia may require pneumatic balloon dilation. A minority of patients will have intractable symptoms for which surgical intervention is required. When surgical therapy is indicated, the diverticulum should be excised and the underlying motor disturbance corrected with an esophageal myotomy.

GASTRIC DIVERTICULA

Gastric diverticula are rare clinical entities typically discovered as incidental radiologic or endoscopic findings. Over 75 per cent are found on the posterior wall of the stomach in close proximity to the lesser curvature and just distal to the esophagogastric junction. Approximately 15 per cent are located in the antral region, often in the setting of previous peptic ulcer disease, surgery, or tumor. Pouches in this location may be difficult to distinguish from a neoplastic process, thereby necessitating endoscopic confirmation and biopsy. The least common location of gastric diverticula is in the body of the stomach. Gastric diverticula are generally asymptomatic. When present, symptoms are nonspecific and are often related to concomitant gastrointestinal disease. Symptoms attributed to gastric diverticula include intermittent postprandial upper abdominal pain (which may be relieved by assuming a supine position), nonspecific dyspepsia, early satiety, nausea, and vomiting.

Treatment

Since the majority of gastric diverticula are asymptomatic, no treatment is necessary except for reassurance. When symptoms are present, they may well be related to associated gastrointestinal disorders, which should then be treated accordingly. The efficacy of nonspecific measures such as antacids, postural drainage, or dietary changes is difficult to evaluate. In the minority of patients with severe refractory symptoms, surgical excision may become necessary. Surgical therapy is clearly indicated for the rare complications of bleeding, perforation, or inflammation.

SMALL INTESTINAL DIVERTICULA

Diverticula of the Duodenum

The duodenum is the second most common site for diverticula in the alimentary tract after the colon. Most duodenal diverticula are solitary lesions that arise in the second part of the duodenum in close proximity to the ampulla of Vater. The majority are asymptomatic and are discovered incidentally during barium studies. Symptoms are nonspecific and include postprandial upper abdominal pain, nausea, vomiting, anorexia, and weight loss. As such, symptomatic duodenal diverticula may be difficult to differentiate from other disorders such as peptic ulcer, biliary tract diseases, or pancreatic diseases. However, complications of duodenal diverticula can occur and include diverticulitis, ulceration, hemorrhage, perforation, fistula formation, duodenal obstruction, chronic and acute pancreatitis, and common bile duct obstruction with ascending cholangitis.

Treatment

No therapy is required for asymptomatic duodenal diverticula. The occurrence of symptoms in the absence of complications that can clearly be related to duodenal diverticula is unusual. Elective surgery for persistent discomfort is rarely indicated, and symptoms are best managed in a conservative fashion.

Surgical therapy is warranted for complications of duodenal diverticula such as perforation, hemorrhage, common bile duct obstruction, recurrent episodes of pancreatitis, and diverticulitis. Significant morbidity and mortality have been associated with surgery of duodenal diverticula because of their retroperitoneal location and close association with the pancreatic duct, common bile duct, and major blood vessels. Currently, there is no agreement on the ideal operation for these diverticula. Some physicians advocate excision of the diverticulum after carefully defining the relationship between it and the ampulla of Vater. This approach is especially useful in cases of perforation or obstruction. Others recommend a Roux-en-Y duodenojejunostomy as therapy, especially in the setting of recurrent pancreatico-biliary disease. The value of endoscopic sphincterotomy and surgical sphincteroplasty is currently speculative.

Diverticula of the Jejunum and Ileum

Diverticula of the jejunum and ileum are uncommon, with an incidence of less than 1 per cent in postmortem examinations. These diverticula are acquired outpouching of mucosa, submucosa, and serosa projecting through the mesenteric border. They typically are more common after age 40, decrease in frequency as one moves distally, and may be solitary or multiple.

Though usually asymptomatic, jejunoileal diverticula have been associated with a variety of nonspecific clinical manifestations. When present, symptoms such as intermittent pain, distention, and nausea and vomiting are often suggestive of low-grade obstruction. It has been observed that chronic intestinal pseudo-obstruction may be the cause of symptoms in some of these patients. The diverticula may be associated with local stagnation and subsequent bacterial overgrowth. The consequences of this may include weight loss, megaloblastic anemia from vitamin B_{12} deficiency, and steatorrhea secondary to bile acid deconjugation. In addition to these chronic symptoms, acute complications associated with jejunoileal diverticula include hemorrhage, perforation, diverticulitis, volvulus, obstruction, and abscess formation.

Treatment

Therapy is indicated for symptomatic individuals or for those with acute complications. Bacterial overgrowth may be treated with a 7- to 10-day course of tetracycline at a dose of 250 to 500 mg 4 times daily or metronidazole (Flagyl) at a dose of 500 mg 3 times daily. In many patients, a single course of therapy will result in a resolution of symptoms; in others, symptoms may recur rapidly. In relapsing patients, intermittent antibiotic therapy for 1 out of every 6 weeks may be an alternate therapeutic modality. For patients with underlying intestinal pseudo-obstruction, the new prokinetic agent cisapride is currently undergoing evaluation in clinical trials and may provide long-term symptomatic relief without the need for antibiotics. The only currently available prokinetic agent, metoclopramide (Reglan), at a dose of 10 to 20 mg before meals, is on occasion effective if there is underlying pseudo-obstruction.

Nutritional therapy is necessary if megaloblastic anemia, steatorrhea, or other nutrient deficits are present. Vitamin B_{12} is administered in monthly intramuscular injections of 100 micrograms. Acquired lactose deficiency may develop and can be treated by a lactose-free diet. Dietary fat requirements may be met by using medium-chain triglycerides.

Surgery is indicated for acute complications, such as obstruction, volvulus, hemorrhage, diverticulitis, or perforation. Treatment consists of resection of the involved segment with primary anastomosis. Surgical intervention may also be considered if symptoms secondary to bacterial overgrowth are refractory to medical therapy.

Meckel's Diverticulum

Meckel's diverticulum is the most common congenital abnormality of the gastrointestinal tract. Located on the antimesenteric border of the terminal ileum, it arises from incomplete obliteration of the vitelline duct and may be connected to the umbilicus by a fibrous band. It is a wide-mouthed diverticulum containing all layers of the intestinal wall. The sac may be lined with normal ileal mucosa or heterotopic gastric, pancreatic, duodenal, or colonic mucosa. Symptoms are uncommon after childhood years, and, when present, they are usually due to complications. Bleeding is the most common complication, resulting from ulceration of ileal mucosa adjacent to ectopic gastric mucosa. It is usually painless and typically presents as iron deficiency anemia secondary to chronic blood loss, although melena and hematochezia may also be seen. Obstructive symptoms may develop from intussusception, volvulus around a persistent fibrous remnant of the vitelline duct, or stricture formation. Diverticulitis may be clinically indistinguishable from acute appendicitis. Diagnosis, even when suspected, can be difficult, and may best be achieved by the small bowel enema (enteroclysis) technique.

Treatment

Treatment consists of excision of the diverticulum only if symptoms develop. Resection of the ileal segment containing the sac may be necessary if ulceration or inflammation is present. Resection of asymptomatic Meckel's diverticula encountered at laparotomy or discovered by small bowel x-rays cannot be justified at the present time.

DIVERTICULAR DISEASE OF THE COLON

Diverticular disease of the colon is an increasingly common problem in Western societies. While the true prevalence of this disorder is unknown, it is rarely seen before the age of 40 and increases with age thereafter. Autopsy studies have demonstrated an incidence of 50 per cent by age 80. While rarely reversible, the condition is asymptomatic in the overwhelming majority of cases.

Uncomplicated Diverticular Disease

Colonic diverticula are acquired deformities in which the basic abnormality is a pseudodiverticulum of mucosa and submucosa through the circular muscle of the colon. The most common location for this is in the sigmoid colon, although more proximal involvement may also be seen. Development of diverticula is thought to be preceded by thickening of the circular smooth muscle layer. It has been hypothesized that contraction of this thickened smooth muscle of the sigmoid narrows the bowel lumen, divides it into discontinuous segments, and allows for the development of high-pressure zones. The resulting transmural pressure gradient then permits the herniation of colonic mucosa through a zone of diminished resistance corresponding to the cleft in smooth muscle through which penetrating arteries reach the submucosa. This sequence of events has been thought to be precipitated by a deficiency in dietary fiber intake. While conclusive proof for this theory has not yet been demonstrated, proponents of it cite the striking rarity of the condition in Africa and other developing nations where intake of dietary fiber is far greater than in the Western world.

Uncomplicated diverticular disease is asymptomatic in the majority of patients and is often diagnosed incidentally by endoscopy or barium enema. Patients who do have symptoms classically complain of left lower quadrant aching or pain, often with some component of colic. This discomfort, which may be variable in intensity, may persist for hours or days and is often exacerbated by meals and relieved by defecation. Accompanying complaints may include abdominal distention, flatulence, and nausea. As such, uncomplicated symptomatic diverticular disease has many of the same clinical characteristics as irritable bowel syndrome. Physical examination is usually unremarkable except for variable lower quadrant tenderness. Basic laboratory data, most notably leukocyte count, should be normal. Diagnosis requires structural studies, such as barium enema and flexible sigmoidoscopy, or colonoscopy to rule out more significant structural abnormalities such as colon carcinoma. If diarrhea with flatulence is a presenting complaint, consideration should be given to lactose intolerance or infection with *Giardia*. One caveat, however, is that demonstration of diverticula does not prove that symptoms are related to them.

Treatment

Therapy of uncomplicated diverticular disease is based on relieving symptoms. There is no proof that therapy prevents the development of complications. It is thought that the abnormalities in colonic function that contribute to the pathogenesis and symptoms of diverticular disease may be related to the low-fiber diet prevalent in Western societies. The addition of indigestible fiber to the diet increases fecal bulk and is thought to decrease intraluminal pressure in the colon. Dietary fiber represents the undigested components of fruits and vegetables such as cellulose, lignin, gums, and pectins. It increases stool bulk by mechanisms such as the water-holding capacity of undigested fiber and by production of osmotically active metabolic breakdown products by the intestinal microflora. Limited studies have demonstrated a trend toward decreasing symptoms by increasing the consumption of dietary fiber. Given the low risk and cost, dietary fiber supplementation has become the primary therapy of uncomplicated diverticular disease.

Several strategies of dietary fiber supplementation may be followed. The best results have been obtained with whole wheat bran at a dose of 10 to 25 grams per day with meals. Five slices of whole wheat bread daily provide a similar amount of fiber. Other good sources of fiber include breakfast cereals such as Shredded Wheat and bran; fruits such as bananas, apples, and pears; and vegetables such as broccoli, tomatoes, carrots, and peas. Fiber supplementation may initially cause symptoms such as bloating and flatulence, which generally subside after several weeks. This can be avoided by gradually increasing dietary fiber. There are no good data to support dietary restriction of vegetables or fruits containing seeds.

An alternative strategy to dietary fiber supplementation is the use of nonprescription fiber formulations. Hydrophilic colloids, such as psyllium or methylcellulose, may be better tolerated than dietary manipulation. Products such as Metamucil or Perdiem Plain may be added to cereal, juices, or water in gradually increasing doses beginning with 1 or 2 teaspoons and increasing to several tablespoons per day. Products that contain stimulant laxatives should be meticulously avoided. If the above measures do not allow for easy defecation or relief of pain, the nonabsorbable sugar lactulose may be added to the therapeutic program. Initial dosage is 1 to 2 tablespoons daily, but this may be titrated to achieve the desired results.

While there is no proven role for anticholinergics or antispasmodics in the therapy of painful diverticular disease, a short clinical trial with such an agent may be warranted in patients with continued symptoms. Tincture of belladonna, 10 drops in a glass of water, or dicyclomine (Bentyl), 10 to 20 mg prior to meals, may be prescribed. Use of analgesics in painful diverticular disease should be discouraged. Similarly, other remedies advocated in the past, such as stool softeners, antibiotics, sedatives, and tranquilizers, have no rational role in the therapy of uncomplicated diverticular disease.

Diverticular Bleeding

It is now apparent that the incidence of lower gastrointestinal tract bleeding secondary to diverticular disease has been overestimated. This is because most estimates of the frequency of diverticular bleeding were based on diagnostic techniques that did not demonstrate a bleeding site. Therefore, in approaching an individual with lower gastrointestinal bleeding, other diagnostic possibilities, such as angiodysplasia, carcinoma, polyps, inflammatory bowel disease, and upper tract etiologies, warrant adequate consideration. Typically, the bleeding is painless and occurs in an individual with previously uncomplicated disease. Bleeding may be continuous or intermittent, and spontaneous cessation of bleeding is the most common course.

Treatment

Management of patients with presumed diverticular bleeding depends on the patient's hemodynamic status and the pace of bleeding. If the patient is orthostatic or actively bleeding, volume resuscitation with crystalloid solutions should be started immediately. Blood transfusion with packed red cells should be aimed at maintaining the hemoglobin at 10 grams per dl. In addition to the hemoglobin and hematocrit, coagulation parameters should be determined.

Once the patient has been stabilized, a nasogastric tube should be passed to aspirate gastric contents. If the aspirate is negative for blood, an upper tract lesion is less likely but is by no means excluded. A flexible sigmoidoscopic examination should then be performed to help assess the amount of bleeding as well as the status of the rectosigmoid region.

In patients who have stopped bleeding, or if bleeding is not massive, the diagnostic test of choice is colonoscopy after a rapid oral purge with 4 or more liters of an electrolyte solution such as GoLYTELY. Colonoscopy can be performed safely and effectively in this setting. It is a technique that permits accurate diagnosis of a bleeding site, and now permits therapeutic intervention with the heater probe or bipolar electrocoagulation in certain bleeding lesions.

If the patient is stable and colonoscopy is unrevealing, upper endoscopy to evaluate upper tract disease should be the next diagnostic step. If this too is negative, serious consideration should be given to [99m]technetium-labeled red blood cell scanning, which allows for detection of intermittent bleeding at a rate of 0.1 ml per minute or greater for 24 hours after administration of the tracer. Should this be negative, a dedicated small bowel barium study to evaluate the small bowel and angiography to identify vascular abnormalities would complete the evaluation.

Management differs in the hemodynamically unstable patient with massive rectal bleeding. Angiography should be the first diagnostic study, although some advocate antecedent radionuclide imaging to help localize the angiographic area of interest. Angiography generally requires the bleeding rate to be 0.5 ml per minute or greater and is positive if there is demonstration of injected radiopaque material in the colonic lumen. Although the data are limited and uncontrolled, angiographic therapy with selective infusion of vasopressin at a dose of 0.2 to 0.4 units per minute may control bleeding effectively. Duration of infusion is uncertain, but a minimum of 12 to 24 hours should be considered. Arterial embolization with absorbable gelatin sponge (Gelfoam) or oxidized cellulose (Oxycel) has been reported, but its role is not yet established.

Should angiographic therapy fail, or if bleeding recurs while the patient is in the hospital, surgical therapy is indicated. Prior to surgery every effort should be made as outlined above to define the bleeding site. This allows for a more limited segmental resection of the involved colon. Subtotal or blind hemicolectomy, as advocated in the past, is to be discouraged. The role of elective surgery in a patient in whom bleeding has been controlled needs to be critically evaluated, because previous recommendations were based on studies in which bleeding sites were infrequently identified.

Diverticulitis

The most common complication of colonic diverticulosis is diverticulitis. It begins with inflammation at the apex of a diverticulum that then extends to peridiverticular tissue with necrosis, microperforation or macroperforation, and serosal and mesenteric inflammation. The process, however, is usually localized by the surrounding tissues. Clinical manifestations of peridiverticulitis classically consist of an acute onset of left lower quadrant pain accompanied by fever and leukocytosis. Pain may on occasion be suprapubic or right lower quadrant in location. Anorexia, nausea, vomiting, and change in bowel habits may occur as well.

Flexible sigmoidoscopy is useful in excluding other structural abnormalities of the distal large bowel. While barium enema findings of extraluminal barium, pericolic mass, fistula, or a narrowed segment of bowel with normal mucosal pattern may suggest the diagnosis, controversy exists as to the proper timing of such a study. Computed tomography (CT) scans can demonstrate extramural extent of disease in a noninvasive manner. Colonoscopy may be necessary to adequately exclude colon carcinoma, ischemic bowel disease, ulcerative colitis, or Crohn's disease.

Treatment

Precise information concerning the efficacy of medical therapy for diverticulitis is unavailable. The majority of patients are managed successfully with rare recurrence of symptoms. The goals of therapy are bowel rest and resolution of infection. The patient should be given nothing by mouth, and a nasogastric tube is placed only if nausea and vomiting are present. Intravenous fluids should be administered to maintain intravascular volume. Parenteral antibiotics should be administered and provide coverage against *Escherichia coli*, enterococci, and anaerobes. If inflammation is clinically mild, ampicillin alone, 500 mg every 6 hours, may be sufficient therapy. However, for severe infection, coverage should be broadened to include clindamycin, 600 mg every 6 hours, or metronidazole, 500 mg every 6 hours, and gentamicin or tobramycin, 1 to 1.7 mg per kg every 8 hours adjusted for renal function. Alternatively, single-agent therapy with cefoxitin, 2 grams every 6 to 8 hours, or imipenem, 1 gram every 6 to 8 hours, may be used. Therapy should generally be continued for 7 to 10 days. In most uncomplicated cases symptoms resolve in 3 to 4 days. A liquid diet can then be started and advanced as tolerated. With resolution of symptoms, deferred diagnostic studies should be performed. Upon hospital discharge, treatment with a regimen similar to that employed for uncomplicated diverticular disease is appropriate.

Surgical therapy for acute diverticulitis should be reserved for patients who fail to respond to medical therapy or for those in whom complications develop. Indications for prophylactic surgery after acute diverticulitis are controversial and can probably be justified only in cases of recurrent disabling attacks (see Table 1).

Other Complications of Diverticulitis

When the process of peridiverticulitis is not contained locally or fails to respond appropriately to medical therapy, a number of complications may ensue.

Abscess. Persistent temperature elevation, leukocytosis, and abdominal pain may be clinical features of abscesses, which can develop anywhere in the abdominal cavity. Computed tomog-

TABLE 1. **Indications for Surgery in Diverticulitis**

1. Failure to improve with medical therapy
2. Hemorrhage
3. Intra-abdominal abscess
4. Fistula
   Colovesical
   Colovaginal
   Coloenteric
5. Large bowel obstruction
6. Generalized peritonitis
7. Inability to rule out carcinoma

raphy (CT) is the best means to confirm the diagnosis. Preliminary work indicates that CT-guided percutaneous drainage of an abscess prior to surgical resection simplifies the surgical approach and allows for single-stage resection with primary reanastomosis.

Fistula. Extension of the inflammatory process into surrounding structures can result in fistula formation. Common locations include colovesical, colovaginal, coloenteric, and colocutaneous fistulas. Treatment involves elective surgical resection, which, whenever possible, can be performed as a one-stage procedure.

Obstruction. Single or multiple episodes of diverticulitis may result in complete or partial large bowel obstruction. Furthermore, acute small bowel ileus may be a feature of acute diverticulitis. Progressive luminal narrowing is often indistinguishable from colon carcinoma. Resection of the involved segment is the surgical objective.

Generalized Peritonitis. Acute perforation presents with typical findings of an acute abdomen with severe abdominal pain, rigidity, and hemodynamic instability. Emergency surgery is indicated in these individuals after initial resuscitative efforts with fluids and antibiotics. Increasingly, the procedure of choice is resection of the involved segment accompanied by proximal colostomy and mucous fistula, or closure of the distal bowel as a Hartmann's pouch. Primary resection has been shown to decrease morbidity and mortality of the procedure. The timing of a second procedure to restore bowel continuity is uncertain. In general, several months should pass prior to attempting reanastomosis.

ULCERATIVE COLITIS

method of
KIRON M. DAS, M.D.
*University of Medicine and Dentistry
of New Jersey
Robert Wood Johnson Medical School
New Brunswick, New Jersey*

Ulcerative colitis is a chronic inflammatory disease of unknown etiology, affecting the mucosa of the rectum and variable length of colon. It is characterized by rectal bleeding and diarrhea during exacerbation, which usually undergoes remission with treatment. The pathogenesis of the disease is considered to be an autoimmune process where specific auto-antibodies develop to colonic epithelial cell components. The common age of onset is during the second and third decades of life, although it can become manifest as early as the neonatal period or after 60 years of age. There is no difference in sex distribution. There is a significantly higher incidence among the family members, particularly first degree blood relatives. The diagnosis is usually made on the basis of clinical symptoms and the demonstration of an uniformly involved mucosal inflammation by sigmoidoscopy. The diagnosis is supported by chronicity; negative stool examinations for bacteria, viruses, and parasites capable of causing colitis, and the characteristic findings on proctoscopy, colonoscopy, mucosal biopsy, and barium enema.

There is no medical cure for ulcerative colitis. Medical therapy, however, does offer comfort to at least 80 per cent of these patients and improves their lives. Surgery can provide a cure but requires the very high price of total colectomy and ileostomy. Newer surgical procedures creating either a continent ileostomy or one of several types of ileoanal anastomoses may be more appealing cosmetically. These techniques, however, are still evolving, and their results are not always completely satisfactory. The aims of medical therapy are to maintain nutritional status, provide symptomatic relief, and hopefully to reverse the bowel inflammation itself.

Supportive Treatment

There is no specific diet for ulcerative colitis. Patients should be encouraged to eat well and maintain an adequate caloric intake with whatever food they prefer and can tolerate. They need to avoid only those foods that clearly provoke symptoms. Some patients may be consistently lactose intolerant; others may find that alcohol provokes diarrhea or that spices aggravate their symptoms. During an acute exacerbation, excess dietary roughage, although not contraindicated, may precipitate bleeding from a friable colonic mucosa or may increase the number of bowel movements. Roughage, however, is helpful in patients with constipated colitis usually due to left-sided or distal colon involvement.

Patients with ulcerative colitis often find that their overall food intake is limited because of diarrhea, anorexia, or abdominal pain, and thus they may suffer a variety of nutritional deficiencies, compounded by gastrointestinal protein, fluid, and blood loss. Anemia, electrolyte and fluid deficiencies, and evidence of malnutrition must be corrected during the initial phases of the medical treatment, particularly in patients with moderately severe disease who have hypoalbuminemia and anemia. The most aggressive efforts to reverse nutritional disturbances have focused on various regimens of parenteral hyperalimentation. While this approach may certainly reverse specific deficiencies and maintain body protein, it has no role as primary therapy for acute exacerbations of disease. Oral preparations, if tolerated, may have a similar supportive role. Parenteral nutrition or oral supplements are useful in acute episodes of illness by maintaining hydration and potassium supplement and nutritional intake until the disease undergoes remission.

Psychotherapy

General emotional and psychologic support is very helpful. No specific emotional disorder is prominent in the ulcerative colitis group; however, individual psychotherapy and group and family therapy can be beneficial, particularly in children and adolescents.

Sulfasalazine Therapy

The most commonly prescribed medication for ulcerative colitis is sulfasalazine (Azulfidine; S.A.S.-500), a drug that was developed by linking a sulfonamide and a salicylate by an azo (N=N) bond. This drug has been used for over 40 years, and its effectiveness in treating mild ulcerative colitis and in preventing relapse has been amply confirmed in randomized controlled trials. Unfortunately it is of little or no benefit in 20 to 30 per cent of patients with ulcerative colitis.

Pharmacokinetics

Studies have shown the pattern of absorption, metabolism, and excretion of sulfasalazine in patients with ulcerative colitis and Crohn's disease are the same as in healthy subjects.

Absorption and Metabolism. The metabolic pathway of sulfasalazine is depicted in Figure 1. Only 20 to 30 per cent of an oral dose of sulfasalazine is absorbed from the upper gastrointestinal tract. When the bulk of an orally administered dose of sulfasalazine arrives in the colon, bacterial action causes cleavage to its active metabolites sulfapyridine (SP) and 5-aminosalicylic acid (5-ASA). Azo reduction by intestinal flora has been shown to be the major metabolic route for a number of other azo compounds and can be accomplished by most strains of bacteria. Therefore, concomitant administration of antibiotics may influence the metabolism of sulfasalazine. In addition, sulfasalazine breakdown may be reduced if transit time of the drug is shortened, a condition that can occur in diarrheal states caused by large-bowel disease such as ulcerative colitis or colonic Crohn's disease or following ileal resection.

The foregoing observations on the role of bacteria in sulfasalazine metabolism, combined with clinical evidence, led to the prediction that sulfasalazine would be a useful agent in ulcerative colitis or colonic Crohn's disease, but not in disease limited to the ileum. The clinical relevance of this point is discussed later.

Excretion. Most of the sulfasalazine absorbed from the small intestine is excreted into the bile

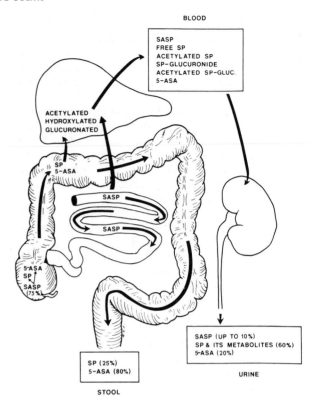

Figure 1. Metabolic pathway of sulfasalazine. Numbers in parentheses indicate percentage of administered dose normally absorbed, metabolized, or excreted. SASP, sulfasalazine; SP, sulfapyridine; 5-ASA, 5-aminosalicylic acid. (From Das KM, Sternlieb I: Salicylazosulfapyridine in inflammatory bowel disease. Am. J. Dig. Dis. 20:971–976, 1975.

without being metabolized in the liver. About 1 to 10 per cent of the ingested sulfasalazine is excreted unchanged in the urine. Most of SP and only a negligible amount of the 5-ASA that is liberated by bacterial action is absorbed from the colon. Absorbed SP is metabolized in the liver and excreted by the kidney as SP and its metabolites. Individuals vary genetically in their rate of SP metabolism in the liver, which may affect steady-state serum concentrations. The capacity to acetylate SP is dependent on individuals being slow or fast acetylators. The latter group acetylate the drug fast and excrete quickly. The combination of slow acetylation and slow hydroxylation causes the serum SP to rise to twice the normal level and these patients are prone to side effects as discussed below.

Drug Interactions. Sulfasalazine, but not SP or 5-ASA, inhibits absorption of folic acid by competitive inhibition of the jejunal brush border enzyme folate conjugase, which hydrolyzes folate polyglutamate to the monoglutamate form essential for intestinal absorption. Administration of folic acid is therefore helpful, especially when a large dose (more than 3 grams per day) of sulfasalazine is given. Cholestyramine and ferrous sulfate combine with sulfasalazine and prevent its absorption from the small intestine. Concurrent administration of sulfasalazine and digoxin may reduce the bioavailability of digoxin by about 25 per cent.

Clinical Use and Dosage

Several randomized controlled trials have established the effectiveness of sulfasalazine therapy in mild to moderate cases of symptomatic ulcerative colitis at a dosage of 3 to 4 grams per day. While about one third of placebo-treated patients show improvement, about three fourths of patients with ulcerative colitis are expected to improve with sulfasalazine. Although studies have shown sulfasalazine to be effective in mild to moderate cases of ulcerative colitis, it appears that concomitant steroid therapy is superior for rapid improvement of an acute attack. However, the effectiveness of sulfasalazine (not of steroids) for maintenance of remission in ulcerative colitis has been shown in several studies. One showed that 86 per cent of patients with quiescent ulcerative colitis who were given 2 grams per day of sulfasalazine remained symptom-free, compared to less than 20 per cent of patients on placebo. The usual initial dose is 3 to 4 grams per day. A few patients will respond better to doses up to 6 grams per day but at the cost of possible side effects, unless they are fast acetylators. The drug can be continued indefinitely at a dose of 1.5 to 2 grams per day as prophylaxis in patients with ulcerative colitis who have gone into remission.

Side Effects

The incidence of the side effects related to sulfasalazine in different series ranges from a low of 5 per cent to as high as 55 per cent. Side effects are frequent during the initial 6 to 8 weeks of treatment, but in patients on long-term therapy, the incidence is 12 per cent. Some side effects such as drug rash, fever, and hepatitis, are due to hypersensitivity reaction. Most of the others seem to be dose related and reflect total serum SP concentration and slow acetylator phenotype. Side effects are more frequent with a daily dose of 4 grams or more. Total SP concentrations usually in excess of 50 µg per ml serum may manifest itself through one or another adverse reaction. Commonly observed toxic reactions include nausea, vomiting, anorexia, headache, fever, rash, arthralgia, anemia with reticulocytosis due to increased RBC fragility or folic acid deficiency, leukopenia, thrombocytopenia, asthmatic bronchitis, and decreased sperm motility with infertility in young men. Recently, sulfasalazine was found to induce exacerbation of ulcerative colitis after oral or rectal administration probably related to 5-ASA moiety.

Desensitization

Although numerous reports have documented the side effects of sulfasalazine, few have considered desensitization to the medication, which can be accomplished easily and effectively. This is clinically important because of the established value of sulfasalazine in preventing relapses. In one study, 26 of 28 patients with inflammatory bowel disease who suffered toxic effects from sulfasalazine were successfully desensitized. After temporarily stopping the drug for 1 to 2 weeks, side effects usually subside, allowing its readministration in gradually increasing doses, starting with 0.25 or 0.5 gram daily and then gradually increasing the dose by half a tablet (250 mg) every week until the final dose of 2 to 3 grams is achieved. A history of agranulocytosis or frank hemolysis and hepatitis during sulfasalazine treatment contraindicate desensitization. Other reports confirm successful desensitization of patients to sulfasalazine starting with an even smaller dose.

Mode of Action

The mechanism of beneficial effects of sulfasalazine in ulcerative colitis is still not clear. For a long time it was unknown whether the clinical efficacy of sulfasalazine resided in the unsplit sulfasalazine or in its metabolites. Recent studies in patients with distal colitis using sulfasalazine, SP, and 5-ASA demonstrate that both sulfasalazine and 5-ASA are clinically effective, but not SP. It is thought that sulfasalazine serves as a vehicle for the delivery of active metabolites, especially 5-ASA, to the colon in higher concentrations than can be achieved by oral administration of 5-ASA alone.

5-ASA may be topically active through an anti-inflammatory effect or by inhibiting prostaglandin production. The improved transportation of sodium and water in the colon by sulfasalazine is independent of mucosal prostaglandin production. Improvement may be related to an antidiarrheal effect observed in patients treated with sulfasalazine. Abnormal immunologic functions observed in patients with inflammatory bowel disease revert to normal following treatment with sulfasalazine alone. During treatment with sulfasalazine, 5-ASA, or steroids, there is decreased release of prostaglandin E2 and F2, thromboxane A2, and prostacyclin metabolites from the rectal mucosa. Sulfasalazine and 5-ASA block the synthesis of several products of the lipoxygenase pathway related to inflammatory cellular response. The beneficial action of sulfasalazine and its metabolites may be related to one or more of these effects.

Pregnancy and Nursing. Sulfasalazine crosses the placenta. Mean concentrations in cord serum are approximately one half those in maternal serum. Despite the exposure of the fetus to sulfasalazine and its metabolites there is no evidence of fetal harm. The concentration of sulfasalazine in milk may be as high as 30 per cent of that found in the maternal serum. The concentration of free sulfapyridine is as much as 50 per cent of that in maternal serum, while 5-ASA concentration is negligible. There appears to be no harm to the fetus or evidence of kernicterus related to this exposure. The evidence suggests that sulfasalazine can be used to treat ulcerative colitis during pregnancy. There is no evidence suggesting that therapy must be stopped near the time of delivery or that use by a nursing mother will harm the infant. However, reduction of dose to 1.5 grams per day seems appropriate.

5-ASA (Mesalamine) Therapy

Pharmacokinetic studies suggest that 5-ASA is probably the important therapeutic moiety of sulfasalazine and that SP is related to most of the side effects. 5-ASA, like aspirin, when given orally, is exclusively absorbed from the upper small intestine, and only a small amount reaches the site of inflammation in the colon. This short-coming has been corrected by the development of a timed-release capsule containing 5-ASA, which avoids small bowel absorption and is capable of reaching the terminal ileum/colon, thus avoiding side effects related to the sulfonamide component. 5-ASA enema preparations (2 to 4 grams per enema) have been developed for patients with distal colitis and proctitis. Suppositories containing 5-ASA will also soon be available.

Enema Treatment

A study of 5-ASA enemas confirmed that 5-ASA is poorly absorbed from the colon. The retrograde spread of an enema is volume-dependent. A comparison of 4-ASA (4-aminosalicylic acid [para-amino salicylate; PAS]) (2 g) and 5-ASA (2 g) enemas in mild to moderately severe distal colitis showed that about 80 per cent of the patients in both groups improved clinically and sigmoidoscopically after 2 weeks. Another controlled study showed that 4-ASA enemas (1 to 2 g) were superior to placebo. However, early reports suggest that more than half of the patients experience flare-up following stoppage of treatment with these salicylate enemas, and therefore the treatment may need to be continued for an indefinite period.

Rowasa (Reid-Rowell) is the first 5-ASA enema preparation approved by the FDA. Each enema contains 4 grams of mesalamine in 60 ml suspension. The enema can be given as a retention enema once or twice a day for patients with proctitis and proctosigmoiditis.

Oral Treatment

To overcome the rapid absorption of 5-ASA, several slow- or delayed-release preparations have been manufactured. Other azo compounds have also been synthesized using a carrier other than SP. At present several mesalamine preparations are close to being approved. They all have different formulations.

Asacol (Tillot) is a tablet of mesalamine covered with an acrylic polymer that is soluble at pH 7 and above. 5-ASA is released in the lower ileum and in the colon. Pentasa (Marion) is a preparation of mesalamine in 1-mm granules individually coated with an ethylcellulose membrane with amphionic properties. The microgranules are available in the small intestine, and up to 53 per cent of the dose is excreted in the urine. Thus this preparation appears well suited for treatment of small bowel disease and possibly colonic disease.

The most extensively studied new azo compound is azodisal sodium (olsalazine or Dipentum) in which two 5-ASA molecules are linked together by an azobond. Like sulfasalazine, only a small amount of intact olsalazine is absorbed from the small intestine, and of this a considerable amount enters the enterohepatic circulation without being split. The half life is considerably longer than for sulfasalazine. Sulfasalazine and olsalazine are distributed somewhat differently in the body. The concentrations of 5-ASA in the feces are doubled when sulfasalazine is replaced by the same equivalent dosage of olsalazine.

Clinical Use, Tolerance, and Toxicity

Asacol and olsalazine have been given to large numbers of patients; Pentasa is being clinically evaluated in the United States. About 75 per cent of patients with mild to moderately severe ulcerative colitis improved, with partial to complete remission, when treated over a 6-week period with either Asacol (4.8 grams per day) or olsalazine (up to 4 grams per day). However, when Asacol and olsalazine were given to sulfasalazine-intolerant patients, it was necessary to stop treatment because of side effects, in 24 per cent and 14 per cent of patients, respectively.

The commonest side effect of olsalazine is watery diarrhea which appears to be dose dependent and occurs in one third of patients taking a 4 gram dose. Common side effects of asacol are muscle aches, headache, and dizziness in about one third of the patients. Bloody diarrhea with fever, nausea, and abdominal cramps have been described with both 5-ASA preparations.

Corticosteroid Therapy

Clinical Use

Corticosteroids given orally, parenterally, or by enema are beneficial in the treatment of either limited or extensive ulcerative colitis that is unresponsive to sulfasalazine alone or disease that initially is more severe. Local rectal instillations are useful for distal ulcerative colitis. When there is more extensive involvement, systemic administration is necessary.

For distal ulcerative colitis, hydrocortisone enemas (Cort-enema) may be given once or twice daily until significant clinical improvement is achieved, which may require 3 to 6 weeks or longer. Treatment is then tapered to one enema at bedtime, then to one every other night, and then discontinued. The foam (Cortifoam) is easier to tolerate but is only effective for localized proctitis. The enemas contain 100 mg of hydrocortisone; the foam, 80 mg. Advances are being made in the development of topical corticosteroid therapy, which results in minimal systemic corticoid side effects. Tixocortol pivalate and beclomethasone dipropionate enemas have been extensively studied but are not yet approved for distal ulcerative colitis therapy.

Oral therapy is usually initiated with 30 to 60 mg of prednisone daily. This dose is continued for approximately 10 to 14 days and then decreased by 5 mg every 7 to 10 days. The dose can be given as a single morning dose or in 2 divided doses; reducing the evening dose helps minimize side effects. If there is a relapse, the prednisone dose will need to be increased again. Once disease control is achieved, the tapering process is resumed. Corticosteroids do not have a prophylactic role in ulcerative colitis and should be discontinued in patients with quiescent disease.

In patients with severe symptoms, parenteral hydrocortisone therapy can be beneficial. Hydrocortisone (300 mg daily) is preferred for patients who have received corticosteroids prior to hospitalization. It can be given as a continuous intravenous infusion or every 6 to 8 hours for 5 to 7 days. Once maximal benefit is achieved, oral prednisone is substituted.

Pharmacology and Adverse Effects

Oral corticosteroid absorption in severe colitis may be delayed, but total absorption is normal. Intravenous therapy results in higher and more prolonged plasma levels than the oral route. The mechanism by which corticosteroids exert their clinical usefulness is also unknown. The toxicity of corticosteroid therapy at the doses used to suppress active ulcerative colitis is appreciable. Adverse effects include facial mooning, acne, ecchymoses, petechial bleeding, striae, hirsutism, infection, hypertension, peptic ulcer, bone abnormalities, emotional disturbances, and many others. These complications generally resolve with the withdrawal or reduction of the dose and with specific therapy for the complications.

Pregnancy. Corticosteroids are well known to cause fetal abnormalities in animals. Studies in humans, however, have failed to demonstrate significant harmful effects. Fetal complications are more common when the mother's disease is active and untreated than when she is treated with corticosteroids during pregnancy.

Antibiotic Therapy

Antibiotics do not have a role as primary therapy for ulcerative colitis. On the contrary, they may affect intestinal bacteria, disturbing the metabolism of sulfasalazine, and may cause *Clostridium difficile*–associated colitis. The toxin of this organism may induce or aggravate the underlying ulcerative colitis.

Immunosuppressive Therapy

Azathioprine (Imuran)* or 6-mercaptopurine (Purinethol)* may be helpful in a rare case, but they have little role in the usual patients with ulcerative colitis. Their toxic side effects, which include infection, pancreatitis, and the potential development of malignancy, generally outweigh their benefits. Cyclosporin A has not been especially successful in the few patients in whom it has been used.

Approach to the Patient

The first step in choosing therapy is to make a global assessment of the disease activity and to exclude any specific pathogen(s) by appropriate stool cultures. There is no uniform measurement of disease activity available. A simple activity index one can follow is to ascertain the disease to be *in remission* when the patient has 2 to 3 bowel movements per day without any mucus and blood; *mild* when there are 4 to 6 stools daily, including minimal rectal bleeding and mucus; *moderate* when there are 7 to 9 stools daily with rectal bleeding, mucus, anorexia, or nausea and some weakness; *severe* when there are 10 or more stools daily with mucus and blood and one or more of the following signs of colitis are present; abdominal tenderness,

---

*This use is not listed in the manufacturer's directives.

pulse rate greater than 100 per minute, and a body temperature above 37.5°C. The disease is *fulminant* when the patient has 10 or more bowel movements daily with significant bleeding plus a body temperature higher than 38°C, anemia, hypoalbuminemia or colonic dilatation on plain abdominal x-rays (greater than 6 cm in diameter).

The appearance of the rectal mucosa at proctoscopy adds important objective information for the assessment of disease activity. Mild to moderate colitis activity is indicated by a red mucosa that is finely granular and easily friable and has a vascular pattern obliterated by edema. Spontaneous bleeding, prominent ulcerations, or mucosal sloughing indicates more severe activity. The proctoscopic appearance may be more severe than the clinical colitis activity and may help predict a flare-up of disease in the near future indicating the need for prompt therapy. In addition, improvement of the rectal mucosa may lag behind clinical recovery during therapy. This should mandate slower reduction of drug doses to prevent disease recurrence. Occasionally, in a patient with chronic ulcerative colitis, especially after receiving topical steroids, the rectal mucosa may appear relatively spared and may not accurately reflect the total colitis activity.

Mild to Moderate Disease Activity

Ambulatory patients with mild to moderate ulcerative colitis activity should be given sulfasalazine initially at a dose of 1.5 grams per day, slowly increasing to 3 to 4 grams per day, if tolerated. Since most patients will achieve a good response within 2 to 3 weeks, this time period seems reasonable before drawing conclusions regarding effectiveness. Patients who cannot tolerate sulfasalazine may benefit from one of the newer preparations without SP such as Asacol,* olsalazine, or Pentasa.*

Those who fail therapy with sulfasalazine or who are very uncomfortable will generally require the addition of steroids. Topical therapy may be used for distal colitis; hydrocortisone enemas for disease distal to the splenic flexure; or foam when disease is confined to the rectum (proctitis). Topical therapy is given once or twice daily for 2 to 4 weeks, at which time a clinical response should be observed. Therapy is then continued once before bedtime until remission is achieved, usually over the subsequent 3 to 6 weeks, and then may be reduced to alternate nights for several weeks. Assuming the patient remains well, topical agents can then be discontinued, with sulfasalazine continued as a maintenance dose of 1 to 2 grams per day. Patients with proctosigmoiditis refractory to topical steroid therapy may benefit from topical salicylate enemas as described previously. If the response to topical therapy is inadequate or there is more

---

*Investigational drugs, not yet approved.

extensive colonic disease, prednisone, 30 to 60 mg per day orally, will be required. This dose is continued for 7 to 14 days and then tapered over approximately 2 months as the symptoms improve. The continuation of high doses of prednisone for prolonged periods is not recommended. Intramuscular ACTH-gel occasionally can be used (40 to 80 units daily) to supplement sulfasalazine in patients with milder disease activity when a long course of oral prednisone is unnecessary.

A variety of preparations, including antidiarrheals, anticholinergics, tranquilizers, and analgesics, may be of symptomatic benefit. However, these agents should be avoided as much as possible because of side effects and possible toxic dilatation of the colon with high doses.

A trial of avoidance of lactose and raw vegetables may also be worthwhile during a flare-up. Proper nutritional balance, supplemental vitamins and iron, and adequate rest are important, but strict bed rest is not necessary.

Severe to Fulminant Disease Activity

The patient with severe activity will generally require corticosteroids and often hospitalization. Oral feedings should be encouraged if they are tolerated, but very ill patients will require bowel rest or even nasogastric suction. Intravenous fluids and electrolytes will be required to insure adequate hydration. If a full diet will not be reinstituted within 10 to 14 days, total parenteral nutrition should be considered. If there is any suspicion of a suppurative complication, antibiotics are given after all appropriate cultures are collected. Sulfasalazine alone is generally not helpful. Its onset of action is slow, and it may be poorly tolerated owing to the side effects of gastric intolerance. If tolerated, I prefer oral suspension (rather than tablets) of sulfasalazine (about 3 grams per day). Oral prednisone can be used as previously described. If this has failed to induce improvement by 10 to 14 days or if oral intake is not tolerated, parenteral therapy will be necessary. ACTH (120 units daily) or hydrocortisone (300 mg daily) is given as a continuous intravenous infusion or 100 mg three times daily. Intravenous ACTH is preferred for the patient not already on steroid therapy. After 7 to 10 days of intravenous infusions, therapy is continued with 30 to 60 mg of oral prednisone. Once prednisone is tapered, sulfasalazine is added to the medical regimen if it has not already been started. Hydrocortisone enemas may also be useful, especially when the patient is on a lower prednisone dose (10 to 20 mg daily). This may allow continued reduction of the prednisone and reduced overall corticosteroid side effects. Patients who do not improve with vigorous medical therapy should be considered for surgery. This is especially true for patients with complications such as profuse bleeding or toxic megacolon and is mandatory when there is a free colonic perforation.

In the ill hospitalized patient, twice-daily physical examinations and frequent abdominal radiographic observations are necessary. Toxic megacolon or perforation may develop quickly and without obvious clinical signs in these very ill patients on high doses of steroids. Toxic megacolon may be induced by diagnostic procedures such as a barium enema or colonoscopy or by hypokalemia, hypomagnesemia, or anticholinergic, antidiarrheal, or analgesic therapy. Avoiding these procedures, correcting the deficiencies, and eliminating the offending drugs are essential. Failure to improve after 48 to 72 hours of intensive therapy or deterioration is an indication for early surgery; prolonging the medical therapy significantly increases the overall mortality and morbidity.

Remission

Once disease activity has subsided, withdrawal of steroids must be attempted; sulfasalazine is continued indefinitely. Unfortunately, some patients are not able to be withdrawn from steroids without a flare-up of their disease. A continued requirement of more than 15 mg daily of prednisone for more than 1 year is a relative indication for surgery.

Cancer Surveillance

The risk of colon cancer in ulcerative colitis begins to increase after 8 years among those with extensive disease. The cumulative risk of cancer by 20 years is about 12 per cent or 32 times the risk of cancer in a normal population. The risk is also higher among those with disease confined to the left colon, but its onset appears delayed about 10 years.

Patients with continuous symptoms are at risk for cancer and have a poor quality of life, and their general health is at risk. They should be encouraged to undergo total colectomy. The cancer issue is but one more indication for surgery.

Patients who are relatively well but at risk for cancer should be in a continued surveillance program. These patients require annual colonoscopy, including multiple colonic biopsies. Surgery may be indicated if definite high-grade dysplasia is noted, especially if associated with a mass lesion. These patients are at very high risk or may already have cancer. Lower grades of dysplasia require close observation, with repeat colonoscopy and biopsy at 6-month intervals.

CROHN'S DISEASE

method of
WILLIAM J. TREMAINE, M.D.
Mayo Clinic
Rochester, Minnesota

Crohn's disease is a chronic inflammatory disorder of unknown cause that can involve any portion of the digestive tract from the mouth to the anus. Most commonly, the disease affects the colon or the terminal ileum, or both areas. Histologically, lesions develop as areas of focal inflammation adjacent to epithelial crypts which progress to transmural inflammation, fissures, and ulcers. In addition to the direct involvement of the digestive tract, there may be coexistent inflammation in the joints, skin, eyes, and liver. The clinical course of the disease is unpredictable, with varying durations of exacerbations and remissions, and this makes it difficult to determine the efficacy of different therapies.

Management

Nutrition

Diet. Food intolerances occur four times as often in patients with Crohn's disease as in healthy individuals, particularly for vegetables, cereals, and dairy products. Patients should be encouraged to eat a balanced diet and to avoid only those foods that clearly cause symptoms. Careful attention should be paid to maintaining nutrition, particularly in children, as growth failure in children with Crohn's disease is due mainly to malnutrition. Lactose intolerance is particularly common and should be looked for, either by a trial of a lactose-free diet and assessment for improvement in symptoms, or by a lactose breath hydrogen test. There is no need to avoid milk products unless there is evidence of intolerance. For patients who have steatorrhea, due to either previous resections of portions of the terminal ileum or extensive disease, dietary fat should be restricted to 40 to 60 grams per day. In the presence of steatorrhea, hyperoxaluria may occur because of decreased intraluminal binding of oxalate to calcium and increased absorption. Patients who have hyperoxaluria should avoid foods that are high in oxalate such as rhubarb, grapefruit, tea, and colas. High-fiber foods should be avoided if there are strictures of the bowel with partial obstruction.

Vitamin and Mineral Supplements. A water-soluble multiple vitamin should be taken daily by patients who are on restricted diets. Vitamin B_{12} should be given monthly, 100 micrograms intramuscularly, to patients who have had 60 centimeters or more of the terminal ileum resected or who have active disease involving this amount or more of the ileum. The patient can be instructed in self-administration. Calcium carbonate or calcium gluconate, in a dose of 1.5 grams per day or more, and vitamin D, in a dose of 50,000 units per week or more, should be given to prevent osteoporosis and osteomalacia in patients with steatorrhea who have laboratory evidence of calcium or vitamin D malabsorption. Subsequently, more precise doses should be determined by urinary calcium and serum vitamin D levels. Folic acid should be given orally as a tablet, 1 mg per day, to patients who have low serum folate levels. Patients who have extensive small intestinal disease or who have undergone major small intestinal resections are at risk for vitamin E deficiency, which can cause progressive neuromuscular disease; serum vitamin E levels should be monitored in these patients and low levels should be treated with oral supplements of 200 mg twice a day or more. Deficiencies of vitamins A and K are rare except in patients with short bowel syndrome; serum levels should be monitored or prophylactic treatment should be given to these patients.

Supportive Therapy

Education and Emotional Support. Patients and their families may not have heard of Crohn's disease until the diagnosis has been made. A knowledgeable physician can explain the disease to them, and excellent patient literature can be obtained from the National Foundation for Ileitis and Colitis (NFIC).* Patients benefit from the ongoing care of a physician during times of active disease and during remission. Also, there are local chapters of the NFIC where patients can share experiences with other patients and gain support. Psychiatric illness is a result, not a cause, of Crohn's disease, and patients more commonly have psychiatric problems, particularly depression, than other patients with medical illness. Anti-anxiety and anti-depressant medications may be indicated in some patients, but in most the best solution is to bring the underlying disease under control.

Control of Diarrhea. The most common symptom of Crohn's disease, diarrhea, usually improves with treatment of the inflammatory disease (see below). Mild symptoms may be controlled with only a bulk agent such as psyllium (Metamucil; Hydrocil; Perdiem Fiber), 1 to 2 teaspoons, once or twice daily, or methylcellulose (Citrucel), 1 tablespoon 1 to 3 times a day. Diphenoxylate 2.5 mg with atropine sulfate 0.025 mg (Lomotil), one or two doses as tablets or liquid 1 to 4 times

daily, or loperamide (Imodium), 1 to 8 tablets per day, can be used for the temporary relief of mild symptoms. For more troublesome diarrhea, a deodorized tincture of opium, 6 to 10 drops 2 to 6 times a day, can be used. These anti-diarrheal agents should not be used in patients who have severe diarrhea due to colonic disease, because of the risk of precipitating toxic megacolon.

Patients who have undergone one or more resections of the terminal ileum (usually less than 100 cm, total) may have bile acid (cholerrheic) diarrhea due to the inadequate resorption of bile from the terminal ileum with the direct stimulation of fluid secretion from the colonic mucosa by the bile acids. These patients usually have postprandial watery diarrhea, which can be controlled with cholestyramine (Questran) 2 to 4 grams 2 to 4 times daily, or colestipol (Colestid), 5 grams 1 to 4 times daily. Because these anion exchange resins also bind fat-soluble vitamins and a number of other medications, the lowest effective dose should be used. Cholestyramine and colestipol should not be used in patients who have steatorrhea; instead, a low-fat diet is the recommended treatment.

Treatment of Active Disease

Anti-inflammatory Therapy

A number of different medications are used, alone or in combination, for the treatment of inflammation.

Sulfasalazine. Sulfasalazine (Azulfidine)* is the first line of treatment for mild or moderately active Crohn's disease when there is involvement of the colon, with or without ileal involvement. Sulfasalazine requires bacterial action for breakdown to its components sulfapyridine (SP) and 5-aminosalicylic acid (5-ASA). It is not effective for the treatment of small bowel disease alone, probably because of the lack of breakdown of the drug there. Sulfasalazine should be started in a dose of 1 gram per day (500 mg twice daily) and gradually increased over a week to a final dose of 3 to 4 grams per day in divided doses, although some patients may be able to tolerate 5 to 6 grams per day. The complete blood count should be checked after 1 week to look for drug-induced hematologic problems (hemolysis, leukopenia, thrombocytopenia, or pancytopenia). Folic acid can be given prophylactically in a dose of 1 mg per day as a tablet, or the serum folate levels can be monitored periodically to look for drug-induced folate deficiency. Up to 45 per cent of patients develop dose-related toxicities such as nausea, vomiting, or headaches on high-dose therapy, and

---

*444 Park Avenue South, New York, NY 10016-7374.

*This use is not listed in the manufacturer's directive.

these usually resolve with reduction of the dose. After 6 weeks of treatment, about 45 per cent of patients show improvement.

5-Aminosalicylic Acid. 5-ASA (mesalamine) accounts for most of the anti-inflammatory action of sulfasalazine. It has few side effects when administered as an enema or orally. Mesalamine enemas (Rowasa) have recently been released in a 4-gram dose for the treatment of distal ulcerative colitis; they may also be useful for the treatment of distal Crohn's colitis, although they have not been approved for this indication. Several forms of oral Mesalamine are available in Europe and in Canada for treatment of inflammatory bowel disease; however, none of these oral preparations have been approved for use in the United States.

Corticosteroids. Corticosteroids are the first line of treatment for Crohn's disease in patients with severe symptoms and in those with only ileal involvement; they are also used as adjunctive treatment for patients with mild or moderate symptoms. Adrencorticotropic hormone (ACTH) is no more effective than oral or intravenous steroids. Alternate-day therapy with steroids does not usually give satisfactory results when the disease is symptomatic but is sometimes effective when the symptoms subside and the dose of steroids is being tapered. Patients who have severe symptoms with abdominal pain, diarrhea, and fever should be kept NPO and on intravenous fluids and treated with prednisolone, 30 to 60 mg intravenously, or with hydrocortisone (Solu-Cortef), 200 to 400 mg per day in divided doses, until symptoms improve. Prednisone, 30 to 60 mg per day in divided doses, can be used when the patient with severe symptoms has improved and is no longer NPO and on intravenous fluids, and doses of 20 to 40 mg per day can be started in patients with less severe symptoms. The response to prednisone should be seen in 3 to 7 weeks; with improvement, the dose should be gradually tapered over the subsequent 2 to 3 months to the lowest dose that controls the symptoms, and eventually the prednisone should be discontinued, if possible. To minimize problems with insomnia, prednisone usually can be given as a single morning dose in patients who are on 30 mg or less. Hydrocortisone enemas as a solution (Cortenema) or as a foam (Cortifoam) can be used in patients with distal colonic disease, with one enema taken at bedtime if the patient has good anal continence.

Metronidazole. For patients with mild to moderately active colitis or ileocolitis who are intolerant to sulfasalazine or in whom sulfasalazine has not been effective, metronidazole (Flagyl),*

in an initial dose of 20 mg per kg (250 to 500 mg 3 to 4 times a day) may be helpful. This drug has been particularly useful when perianal involvement is present. Metronidazole may be used in combination with prednisone to achieve a steroid-sparing effect, although there are no studies to support this strategy. Metronidazole should be tapered gradually to the lowest dose that controls symptoms. The most worrisome side effect of metronidazole is peripheral neuropathy, manifested by burning paresthesias in the toes and feet and sometimes in the hands. These paresthesias usually resolve with discontinuing treatment, although it may take months for full resolution.

6-Mercaptopurine and Azathioprine. These drugs are usually reserved for the patient with chronic severe disease that cannot be controlled with other forms of treatment or for patients who cannot be tapered from high doses of steroids because of a resulting flare-up in symptoms. 6-Mercaptopurine (Purinethol)* and its derivative azathioprine (Imuran)* have similar biological effects; either drug may be used in a dose of 50 mg to 100 mg per day in adults or 25 mg per day in children. Neither should be used as a single initial agent for treatment of Crohn's disease as it may take up to 4 months before there is a response to treatment. The major drawbacks with these drugs are the serious side effects (bone marrow suppression, fever, and pancreatitis), which occur in 10 per cent of patients, and the small risk of inducing malignancy, either carcinoma or lymphoma. The hemoglobin, white cell count, and platelet count should be monitored weekly while the patient is receiving one of these drugs.

Nutritional Therapy

Enteral Nutrition. Two randomized studies have shown an elemental diet (Vivonex) to be as effective as prednisone in inducing a remission in Crohn's disease, although the remissions may not last as long. A trial of elemental feeding for 3 to 4 weeks as the sole source of calories, along with prednisone, can be considered in patients who have not previously responded to sulfasalazine, prednisone, or metronidazole. The volume should be calculated for the patient's ideal body weight and with one kcal per ml, usually 1500 to 2500 ml per day of the preparations are needed. The expense (from $700 to $950 for 3 weeks) and taste fatigue are major drawbacks.

Central Parenteral Nutrition. Two randomized studies showed no added benefit of bowel rest in the induction of remission in Crohn's disease.

---

*This use is not listed by the manufacturer.

*This use is not listed by manufacturer.

However, central hyperalimentation is helpful prior to surgical resection in the stabilization of the malnourished patient with obstructive symptoms; 3 weeks of therapy are usually needed to achieve improvement in protein stores.

Medical Treatment During Remission

No medication has been shown to be effective in maintaining remission in patients with Crohn's disease. Likewise, no medication has been shown to reduce the rate of recurrence in patients who have undergone surgical resection of all evidence of disease.

Surgery

More than 60 per cent of patients with Crohn's disease will require one resection and over half will need a second operation. It is important not to err in sending the patient for surgery before a reasonable trial of medical options; on the other hand, surgery should not be delayed when the disease is refractory to treatment. The indications for surgery are (1) chronic obstruction due to stricture, (2) uncontrollable diarrhea due to enteroenteric fistulae, (3) free perforation and intraabdominal abscess, (4) massive bleeding, (5) toxic megacolon, and (6) intractable symptoms due to a limited area of involvement. Stricturoplasty, in which a stricture is opened horizontally and closed vertically without resecting bowel, has recently been shown to be effective in patients with obstructive symptoms due to multiple skip areas of involvement.

Treatment During Pregnancy

Neither sulfasalazine nor corticosteroids have caused significant problems when used in pregnant women with Crohn's disease, and either drug may be used to control active disease. As neither drug prevents relapses of inactive disease, prednisone and sulfasalazine should be discontinued in the asymptomatic patient. Both may be used in the nursing mother, if indicated. Azathioprine, 6-mercaptopurine, and metronidazole should be avoided during pregnancy. Nutritional treatment in pregnant patients with Crohn's disease should be prompt and aggressive and may be administered as enteral or parenteral hyperalimentation.

Extraintestinal Complications

Joint, skin, mouth and eye symptoms are much more common with colonic involvement than when the disease is confined to the small intestine.

Arthritis. Peripheral arthritis is the most common extraintestinal problem and occurs in about one fourth of patients. The joint symptoms usually parallel the activity of the bowel disease, and the most effective therapy is to control the bowel inflammation. In addition to reducing intestinal inflammation, sulfasalazine probably acts directly to reduce joint inflammation. Also, a nonsteroidal anti-inflammatory drug such as naproxen (Naprosyn), 250 to 500 mg twice a day, is helpful.

Spondylitis. Ankylosing spondylitis and sacroileitis occur in HLA-B27–positive patients and do not follow the course of the bowel disease. Therapy is directed at the joint disease and includes the use of sulfasalazine and nonsteroidal anti-inflammatory drugs and physical therapy.

Skin and Oral Manifestations. Erythema nodosum occurs in about 10 per cent of patients who have colonic involvement and in 4 per cent of patients with only small bowel disease. It occurs synchronously with the activity of the bowel disease and resolves with treatment of the bowel inflammation. Pyoderma gangrenosum occurs in less than 2 per cent of patients and is treated with high-dose systemic steroids and usually improves as the bowel symptoms resolve, although in some cases it persists despite remission or resection of the involved bowel. Aphthous stomatitis occurs in about 10 per cent of patients, usually with other extraintestinal symptoms, and resolves with control of the bowel disease.

Eye Manifestations. Eye disorders due to conjunctivitis, recurrent episcleritis, or uveitis occur in more than 10 per cent of patients with colonic disease and are rare with only ileal involvement. Topical steroid drops can be used for therapy, under the direction of an ophthalmologist. The symptoms are usually synchronous with the bowel disease activity.

Hepatobiliary Abnormalities. Cholesterol gallstones are common in patients who have extensive terminal ileal disease or who have undergone terminal ileal resections because of the diminished bile acid pool. Cholecystectomy is the treatment of choice for symptomatic gallstones. Primary sclerosing cholangitis occurs rarely in association with Crohn's disease, and treatment of the Crohn's disease has no effect on the liver disease; so far, no medical therapy has proved to be effective.

Urinary Tract Abnormalities. Nephrolithiasis occurs in 5 to 10 per cent of patients because of dehydration due to chronic diarrhea and also because of increased colonic oxalate absorption. Prophylactic therapy for the calcium oxalate stones was discussed earlier. Right ureteral obstruction with hydronephrosis occurs because of contiguous inflammation in the overlying terminal ileum and colon and may require temporary stenting of the ureter.

IRRITABLE BOWEL SYNDROME

method of
FRED M. SUTTON, M.D.
Baylor College of Medicine
Houston, Texas

Most of us at one time or another suffer an alteration in bowel habits in conjunction with stressful situations. In fact, 14 to 30 per cent of the general population at some point will have some bowel dysfunction. Patients who have regular recurring symptoms of abdominal pain, constipation, and/or diarrhea and no organic cause identified are designated as having the irritable bowel syndrome. In addition to the symptoms of diarrhea, constipation, and abdominal pain, patients may also complain of nausea, vomiting, headaches, or belching, or they may exhibit evidence of neurotic traits. Although the spectrum of illness presentation is wide, most of the patients will fit into three major symptom groups (Table 1). Many patients will complain of their symptoms on a regular basis but will relate that the symptoms are exacerbated by conditions that they find stressful.

Diagnosis

The diagnosis of irritable bowel syndrome can be made on a prospective basis. That is, following a history and physical examination, the physician can usually decide that irritable bowel syndrome is the most likely diagnosis and only a few tests would be required in order to exclude other reasonable diagnostic possibilities. One can feel reasonably confident about the diagnosis. The patient often presents with a long history of symptoms compatible with irritable bowel syndrome without evidence of organic disease. Symptoms of weight loss, fever, bloody stool, nocturnal pain, or nocturnal diarrhea should provoke physicians to consider the possibility of other problems complicating the irritable bowel syndrome.

One of the first questions that must be addressed is: Why did the patient come to the doctor? (What was the iatrotropic stimulus?) For example, many patients relate that their symptoms began after a recent traumatic event such as a family death, accident, or the identification of a carcinoma in a friend or relative. Probing of such a patient's history usually reveals that the symptoms were present long before that stressful event and were only exacerbated with the current stress.

TABLE 1. **Patterns of Irritable Bowel Syndrome**

Spastic colitis
Left lower quadrant abdominal pain
Constipation
Abdominal distention
Dyspepsia
Mucous colitis
Predominantly diarrhea
Spastic/mucous colitis
Mainly alternating diarrhea and
constipation

Differential Diagnosis

In most patients, the long history and the obvious good health of the patient make other diagnoses very unlikely. Patients who present with diarrhea may have underlying carbohydrate malabsorption, such as lactose intolerance, and it is often worth considering a trial of lactose elimination. Other patients may have diarrhea that is due to excess sorbitol in the diet. Sorbitol is being consumed in the form of sugar-free gum, dietetic ice cream, or other dietetic foods. A careful history should identify such patients. In patients with a recent change in bowel habits and in those older than 45 years, it is useful to perform a sigmoidoscopic examination to exclude rectal pathology and to look for the presence of melanosis coli. A rectal biopsy should be performed in those patients presenting with diarrhea to search for the presence of colitis. Finally, a basic laboratory evaluation, including a complete blood count, urinalysis, and biochemistry profile such as a sequential multiple analyzer (SMA), is useful to screen for the presence of other diseases.

Treatment

General Management

Patient education and a good doctor-patient relationship are the heart of the management of the patient with irritable bowel syndrome. The patient should understand that total resolution of the symptoms may not be practical.

Diet

Patients should be instructed to avoid foods that are known to exacerbate their symptoms. As mentioned earlier, lactose malabsorption or the excess ingestion of poorly absorbable carbohydrates such as sorbitol should be considered. Patients should be instructed to attempt to attain some regularity in their lives, which includes eating three balanced meals per day and obtaining adequate exercise. Many of the patients are sedentary, and a program of walking or other simple exercise often has been quite beneficial in terms of bowel habits.

Fiber

One of the mainstays of therapy has been to increase the amount of fiber in the diet. The increase in dietary fiber content has been associated with an increase in the fecal weight and an improvement in intestinal transit time (decreased transit time in those with constipation and increased transit time in those with diarrhea). The simplest methods of adding fiber to the diet are to suggest that the patient consume one third to one half cup of a bran cereal each day or, alternatively, to use one of the psyllium-containing products such as Metamucil. Patients may complain of abdominal bloating when initially increasing the amount of fiber in the diet. They should be cautioned that this might happen and that they should add the increasing amounts of fiber over a period of several weeks.

Laxatives

A small group of patients with refractory constipation may require the use of chemical laxatives. Many patients with constipation are habitual laxative users, and attempts should be made to wean them from laxatives and switch them to a high-fiber diet. An occasional use of magnesium hydroxide such as Milk of Magnesia or bisacodyl (Dulcolax) may be required.

Antidiarrheals

In most instances, diarrhea is adequately controlled by the addition of one of the psyllium-containing products. In some cases, small doses of loperamide (Imodium) may be required. Loperamide is preferred over diphenoxylate (Lomotil), as there is no risk for substance abuse with Imodium.

Anticholinergics

In the past, anticholinergics were prescribed for the abdominal cramping but they seem to benefit only a minority of the patients. A number of such products are available. Typically, the dose should be titrated to achieve a desired clinical effect and yet avoid the common anticholinergic side effects, including blurred vision, dizziness, and urinary hesitancy.

Antidepressants

Many of the patients presenting to a physician with symptoms of irritable bowel syndrome suffer from depression or identifiable neuropsychiatric disturbances. The fact that depression is present should be identified in the history and questions should always be asked about sexual function and sleep disturbances. The treatment of the depression with imipramine (Tofranil) or amitriptyline (Elavil) may be beneficial. These drugs are typically begun at bedtime, and their anticholinergic side effects may preclude their prolonged administration. Anxiolytic drugs such as diazepam (Valium) or chlordiazepoxide (Librium) are rarely indicated in the treatment of irritable bowel syndrome.

Psychotherapy

Formal psychiatric consultation is rarely required. A caring physician can usually provide adequate psychotherapy in the form of frequent visits, reassurance, and establishment of a good doctor-patient relationship.

Prognosis

Patients with irritable bowel syndrome have a normal life expectancy. Several studies have shown that the majority of patients continue to have symptoms. Therefore, irritable bowel syndrome is considered a chronic condition for which treatment is primarily symptomatic. This emphasizes that support and reassurance are needed to manage these patients.

HEMORRHOIDS, ANAL FISSURE, AND ANORECTAL ABSCESS AND FISTULA

method of
JOHN J. MURRAY, M.D.
Lahey Clinic Medical Center
Burlington, Massachusetts

HEMORRHOIDS

Hemorrhoids are a normal part of human anatomy and may contribute to anal continence. They consist of a network of arterioles and dilated veins in a supporting matrix of smooth muscle and connective tissue that serves to anchor the hemorrhoid to the internal anal sphincter. Organized as discrete submucosal cushions in the proximal anal canal, hemorrhoids typically occupy the left lateral, right anterior, and right posterior segments of the anal circumference. Although the pathogenesis of symptomatic internal hemorrhoids is unclear, it is presumably related to downward displacement of these vascular cushions as a result of repeated straining at defecation. With disruption of the supporting connective tissue framework of the hemorrhoidal cushion, vascular engorgement develops.

Prolapse and bleeding are the primary features of symptomatic internal hemorrhoids. The blood shed is bright red, and bleeding may be quite brisk because of the presence of arteriovenous communications within the hemorrhoid. Anal seepage and mucous drainage associated with prolapsing hemorrhoids produce perianal dermatitis. With progressive displacement of the internal hemorrhoids, a second series of veins distal to the dentate line becomes engorged. These veins have a tendency to thrombose and constitute the external hemorrhoid network. In the absence of thrombosis, pain is usually not a feature of symptomatic hemorrhoids. Patients complaining of pain should be evaluated for the presence of anal fissure, abscess, or neoplasm.

Examination of patients with symptomatic hemorrhoids should include sigmoidoscopy and anoscopy. Evaluation of the proximal colon with flexible sigmoidoscopy or air-contrast barium enema study should be undertaken in those patients whose symptoms are atypical or whose age or medical history places them at risk for colorectal carcinoma.

Classification of internal hemorrhoids by degree of prolapse aids in selecting appropriate therapeutic options. First-degree hemorrhoids bleed but do not prolapse. Prolapse associated with second-degree hemorrhoids reduces spontaneously, and prolapse associated with third-degree internal hemorrhoids requires manual reduction. Fourth-degree internal hemorrhoids are chronically prolapsed and cannot be reduced.

Treatment

Because hemorrhoids are a feature of normal anatomy, treatment of patients with hemorrhoids should be undertaken only to alleviate symptoms. First-degree hemorrhoids that are infrequently or minimally symptomatic may respond to a high-fiber diet possibly supplemented with any of the commercially available psyllium seed bulk agents. Such a regimen will alleviate symptoms by reducing the need for excessive straining at defecation. Perianal dermatitis associated with symptomatic hemorrhoids should be treated with topical ointments containing hydrocortisone. The value of such agents in treating other symptoms of hemorrhoids is unproved.

Office Procedures

Office procedures available for treatment of patients with symptomatic first-degree, second-degree, and small third-degree internal hemorrhoids include sclerotherapy, rubber band ligation, and infrared photocoagulation. The goal of each of these procedures is the creation of focal areas of inflammation and subsequent fibrosis at the apex of the hemorrhoid, which restores fixation to the internal sphincter and reduces vascular engorgement. These procedures can be performed without anesthesia because the apex of the hemorrhoid is normally devoid of sensory innervation. Injection sclerotherapy is more cumbersome technically than the other options and has been shown to produce poorer long-term results in comparative trials with rubber band ligation. Rubber band ligation uses a special applicator to encompass a tuft of mucosa and submucosa within a rubber band at the apex of the hemorrhoid. The involved tissue subsequently necroses and sloughs. One or more hemorrhoids may be treated at a single time. Mild

discomfort lasting 24 to 72 hours and responding to mild analgesics and sitz baths is experienced by 5 to 40 per cent of patients. Serious complications include delayed active bleeding (1 per cent) and thrombosis of external hemorrhoids (2 to 3 per cent). Rare cases of potentially life-threatening perineal infections after rubber band ligation have been reported. The scarcity of these reports has made it impossible to identify precipitating factors. Long-term follow-up in patients treated with rubber band ligation reveals appreciable improvement in 80 to 90 per cent of patients. Infrared photocoagulation uses infrared radiation to produce a focal area of protein coagulation at the apex of the hemorrhoid. The procedure is associated with minimal discomfort. Comparative trials with rubber band ligation have demonstrated equivalent results in treating patients with first-degree and small second-degree internal hemorrhoids.

Operative Measures

Operative measures for treatment of patients with symptomatic hemorrhoids include cryotherapy, anal dilatation, and hemorrhoidectomy. Cryotherapy is classified as an operative procedure because it requires local anesthesia if not general anesthesia. As many as two thirds of patients treated will require inpatient hospital care, and the postoperative course is characterized by moderate to severe pain and a profuse, malodorous discharge that may persist for weeks. For these reasons, cryotherapy has few advocates.

Anal manometric studies in patients with symptomatic hemorrhoids have identified a group with elevated resting and squeeze pressures. These patients tend to be young men with first-degree internal hemorrhoids. On the premise that this abnormality reflects a constricted anal outlet predisposing to excessive straining at defecation, disruption of the internal sphincter by anal dilatation or internal sphincterotomy has been advocated as primary treatment for internal hemorrhoids. Although comparative trials have demonstrated results equivalent to those obtained with rubber band ligation, the necessity for anesthesia and the possibility of temporary difficulties with continence make this a poorer therapeutic option.

Hemorrhoidectomy is the preferred treatment for most patients with third-degree and for all patients with fourth-degree internal hemorrhoids. Depending on patient and physician preference, the procedure can be performed on an inpatient or outpatient basis under local, regional, or general anesthesia. Hemorrhage (1 per cent), acute urinary retention (10 per cent), and anal stenosis (1 per cent) are common short-term and long-term complications associated with the procedure. Long-term follow-up reveals a high degree of patient satisfaction, with only 5 to 8 per cent suffering recurrent symptoms.

Laser Therapy

Enthusiasm for the use of lasers in medicine has extended to their application in the treatment of patients with hemorrhoids. Lasers have been used in a variety of ways to excise internal hemorrhoids or to restore fixation to the internal sphincter. The benefit of such measures over currently available techniques has not been demonstrated convincingly.

Treatment of External Hemorrhoids

Patients with external hemorrhoids require specific treatment only when the hemorrhoids are complicated by acute thrombosis. Patients presenting with severe discomfort are best treated with excision of the thrombosed hemorrhoid under local anesthesia. Simple incision and evacuation is prone to early recurrence and is not advised. Patients seen several days after onset of symptoms, when the discomfort is beginning to subside, are best treated with sitz baths and bulk laxatives. Complete resolution will occur in six to eight weeks but may be associated with a residual skin tag.

ANAL FISSURE

Anal fissure is the most common cause of chronic perianal pain. It is characterized by a linear tear extending distally from the dentate line to the anal verge. In its chronic stage, anal fissure becomes a fibrotic ulcer. Edema at the lower pole resulting from chronic infection produces the characteristic sentinel pile. The initiating event in development of an acute anal fissure is traumatic injury to the anal canal, most commonly from passage of a large, hard fecal bolus. Fissures tend to occur in young and middle-aged adults. Primary or idiopathic anal fissures are confined to the anterior or posterior midline of the anal canal. Although posterior fissures predominate, anterior anal fissures are found more commonly in women than in men.

The factors responsible for progression of an acute anal fissure to its chronic stage are uncertain. Anal manometry has demonstrated a tendency for spasmodic contraction of the internal sphincter in patients with chronic anal fissures. Whether this abnormality represents a primary or secondary phenomenon is unproved. Anal fissure may also represent a secondary manifestation of other diseases. Anal fissures in an aberrant location should suggest the possibility of associated Crohn's disease, ulcerative colitis, anal tuberculosis, syphilis, or leukemia.

Patients with anal fissure usually complain of pain on defecation, which may become continuous and disabling. Bleeding tends to be minimal but is often the symptom that brings the patient to the physician. Anal seepage, pruritus, dysuria, and dyspareunia may be related complaints. An anal fissure can usually be demonstrated by gently separating the buttocks to expose the anal margin. Although evaluation of patients with symptoms of anal fissure requires sigmoidoscopy and anoscopy, this may not be possible in patients who are acutely symptomatic. Examination under anesthesia is occasionally required for those patients too uncomfortable to examine without anesthesia or in whom other pathologic conditions cannot be excluded.

Treatment

Treatment of patients with acute anal fissure should focus on interrupting the cycle of constipated bowel movements producing pain, sphincter spasm, further injury, and suppression of the urge to defecate. Such a program should include use of bulk agents to alter stool consistency and sitz baths to alleviate muscle spasm and pain. Regimens employing topical ointments and suppositories, local anesthetics, and anal dilators are without lasting benefit or effectiveness.

Those individuals who fail to respond or who present with a fissure that is chronic in appearance or duration of symptoms will require operation. Although proposed surgical options are many, they all result in the increased potential diameter of the anal canal and the interruption of internal sphincter spasm. Excision of the fissure as part of these procedures has no impact on successful outcome.

Lateral subcutaneous internal sphincterotomy accomplishes the goals of operation in a simple fashion. This procedure involves division of the distal portion of the internal sphincter through a puncture wound at the anal margin. The procedure provides rapid resolution of symptoms, permits early return to work, and results in healing of the fissure in 95 per cent of patients. Although it can be performed under local or general anesthesia, comparative trials have demonstrated a higher incidence of fissure recurrence when sphincterotomy is performed under local anesthesia. Potential complications include bleeding (1 per cent), abscess or fistula (2 per cent), and minor, temporary difficulties with continence (3 per cent). Postoperative care involves use of bulk agents and sitz baths. Healing of the fissure is usually complete in three to four weeks.

Anal dilatation under general anesthesia to disrupt bluntly the internal sphincter has been reported to produce results comparable to those obtained with internal sphincterotomy. Extensive perianal hematoma formation and a higher incidence of treatment failure have also been reported, making anal dilatation a less attractive alternative.

ANORECTAL ABSCESS AND FISTULA

Anorectal abscess and fistula represent acute and chronic phases of the same disease process. Acute abscess develops after obstruction of one of the anal glands as it discharges into one of the anal crypts at the dentate line. These glands are situated primarily in the anterior and posterior quadrants of the anal canal. They ramify in the submucosa and extend through the internal sphincter to end in the intersphincteric plane. A mixed pyogenic infection occurs as a consequence of obstruction and develops into a localized abscess in the intersphincteric plane. The process may then extend cephalad, caudad, or laterally through the external sphincter to present clinically as an intermuscular, perianal, or ischiorectal abscess. The acute process resolves with spontaneous drainage or as a result of intentional incision and drainage and leads to a focus of chronic infection that persists as a fistula in ano. Although this process accounts for the majority of anorectal abscesses and fistulas, other potential sources include infected sebaceous cysts, pilonidal disease, furunculosis, inflammatory bowel disease, foreign bodies, bartholinian abscess, and hidradenitis suppurativa.

In the acute phase, patients present after several days of progressive, throbbing perianal pain and swelling. With intersphincteric or postanal space abscesses, no external signs may be present to suggest an underlying infection. Digital rectal examination will usually demonstrate a focal area of induration and tenderness. In the chronic stage, patients will usually complain of variable amounts of feculent or purulent perianal drainage with associated pruritus. The physician should be alert for symptoms of underlying inflammatory bowel disease, as this condition will influence management of the perianal problem. Physical examination at this stage reveals an external sinus with associated induration. Sigmoidoscopic examination is performed at some point during the course of the illness to exclude underlying neoplasm or inflammatory bowel disease as the source for the abscess or fistula.

Treatment

Use of antibiotics as primary or temporizing treatment for anorectal abscess is to be condemned. Effective treatment requires incision and drainage under local, regional, or general anesthesia. Adjunctive antibiotic therapy may be employed in individuals with associated cellulitis or compromising systemic disorders, such as diabetes. Although treatment of carefully selected patients with perianal or small ischiorectal abscesses under local anesthesia in the office is often possible, the morbidity and mortality that can attend the management of anorectal abscess are frequently related to inadequate initial drainage.

Treatment of patients with fistula requires that the origin in the offending anal crypt and the distal tract be completely unroofed and allowed to heal by secondary intention. This process usually involves division of at least a portion of the internal sphincter and a segment of the external sphincter as well, which usually can be accomplished with minimal disturbance of continence as long as the puborectal muscle remains intact. Treatment of patients with more complicated fistulas may involve use of a seton, a piece of heavy suture material, or a rubber band, which is passed along the course of the fistula. With repeated traction on the suture or gradual tightening of the rubber band, the seton will slowly divide the encompassed sphincter muscle. With high transsphincteric fistulas, suprasphincteric fistulas, or any anterior fistula in a woman, this approach minimizes the consequences to continence by providing more gradual division of the involved muscle and preventing wide separation.

Recent experience with the successful use of endoanal advancement flaps to obliterate the origin of the fistula while preserving sphincter muscle represents an alternative option for treating patients with complicated fistulas. Primary fistulotomy at time of initial treatment for anorectal abscess is warranted with small abscesses or with postanal space abscesses if the anatomy can be easily defined. In general, however, delayed fistulotomy will spare unnecessary destruction of sphincter muscle and is associated with less morbidity.

Extrasphincteric fistulas are completely outside the ring of sphincter muscles, arising from traumatic, neoplastic, or inflammatory processes in the rectum or from acute inflammatory processes in the pelvis that necessitate an approach through the perineum. Patients with extrasphincteric fistulas originating in the rectum usually require temporary colostomy as part of a staged therapeutic approach. Patients with extrasphincteric fistulas arising from intra-abdominal pathologic conditions require laparotomy for definitive treatment. No local anorectal procedure is necessary.

GASTRITIS

method of
WILLIAM S. HAUBRICH, M.D.
University of California, San Diego, School of Medicine
La Jolla, California

Gastritis can be broadly defined as inflammation of the stomach, but the term, used in a casual way, surely would be near the top of any list of overused diagnostic terms. For most patients who are merely dyspeptic, "upset stomach" would be more apt. A bona fide diagnosis of gastritis requires endoscopy and, in some cases, biopsy; inflammation in the gastric mucosa is not reliably evident in radiographic contrast films. Unfortunately, it is often difficult to satisfactorily reconcile even endoscopic and biopsy findings with a given patient's symptoms. Nonetheless, gastric mucosa is liable to inflammatory reaction and, bearing in mind these disclaimers, there are several forms of gastritis for which therapy can be considered.

Patchy Erythema of the Gastric Mucosa

This probably is the single most frequently reported finding at gastroscopy. But often gastroscopic observation is liable to exaggerated interpretation. A few patches of redder than usual mucosa, especially in the prepyloric antrum, are seldom significant. No therapy is required. The prudent clinician looks elsewhere for a cause of the patient's dyspepsia.

Erosive Gastritis

This is the most commonly encountered form of gastric mucosal injury, and the usual cause is exposure to a noxious chemical agent, either a drug or alcohol. Notoriously injurious to the gastric mucosa in susceptible persons are aspirin and other nonsteroidal anti-inflammatory drugs (NSAIDs). The reaction can be as mild as mere erythema or as severe as extensive ulceration. Fortunately, gastric mucosa is capable of healing rapidly, once the noxious agent is removed. Treatment, first and foremost, is withdrawal of the imputed offender.

However, often the patient cannot manage well without aspirin or NSAIDs. In most cases, if a satisfactory substitute cannot be found, palliative therapy, using one or another of the measures described below, will suffice to allay the patient's dyspepsia, even when the NSAID therapy is cautiously continued.

True *corrosive* gastritis is seldom encountered. Concentrated acids or alkalis, when deliberately or inadvertently swallowed, wreak havoc mainly in the esophagus.

Reflux Gastritis

Bile and pancreatic juice, normally abundant in the duodenum, are potentially injurious to gastric mucosa when it is exposed by reflux. Reflux of duodenal content occurs normally but is abated by the barrier of the intact pylorus and by prompt clearing from the stomach. Endoscopic evidence of bile-stained fluid entering the stomach from the duodenum is *not* to be construed as evidence of reflux gastritis. Of more concern is the circumstance wherein the pylorus has become distorted (as after pyloroplasty) or ablated (as after antrectomy) or when gastric emptying is impaired. Even in these instances, a degree of mucosal reaction is to be expected and should not precipitate a hasty decision for further surgical intervention. Palliative treatment, with watchful waiting, should be the rule. Cholestyramine (Questran), once suggested as a remedy for bile-reflux gastritis, has been found ineffective and is no longer recommended.

Hemorrhagic Gastritis (Stress Ulceration)

The pathogenesis here, insofar as it is understood, is principally hemodynamic. Any inflammatory component is probably secondary to the vascular lesion. The condition is observed usually in patients subject to the stress of hypovolemia. The typical locale is the intensive care unit. Bleeding is common and covers a broad spectrum of severity, from little more than a few flecks of blood issuing from an indwelling nasogastric tube to exsanguinating hemorrhage.

The risk of hemodynamic injury to gastric mucosa in any stressed patient is sufficient to warrant consideration of preventive measures. Needless to say, the most effective preventive or therapeutic measures are those undertaken to relieve the injurious stress. These include correction of hypovolemia, restoration of circulatory perfusion, and control of sepsis.

The injured mucosa suffers from back-diffusion of hydrogen ions, so it makes sense to inhibit or counteract gastric acid secretion. Thus, the use of H_2 receptor antagonists or antacids, as described below, is well advised. Another approach is to bolster mucosal resistance. Sucralfate (Carafate) seems to be helpful in this way. Experimental evidence suggests that prostaglandins, especially those of the PGE type, when they become available for clinical use, will be beneficial. Therapy, when the lesion becomes evident, is a stepped-up version of these preventive measures.

Hemorrhage consequent to stress ulceration can be life-threatening. Such circumstance calls for more vigorous measures. Endoscopically guided cautery by heater probe, electrocoagulation, or laser therapy can be tried, but often the lesions are so numerous and widespread that cautery is futile. In extreme instances, emergency total gastrectomy may be necessary.

Infectious Gastritis

The stomach is notably resistant to bacterial infection, and this is rarely a problem, with one important exception. Recent investigation has shown that gastric mucosa, particularly in older patients, can harbor the organism *Campylobacter pylori* (a species distinct from *C. jejuni* that is well known to cause enteritis). The relation between *C. pylori* infection and gastritis or mucosal ulceration is not yet clear, but if mucosal inflammation is associated with infection by curved bacilli, as evident in silver-stained biopsy sections, then more specific therapy can be considered. Interestingly, *C. pylori* is eradicated more efficiently by bismuth (readily available as the subsalicylate in the form of Pepto Bismol, 30 ml or 2 tablets—about 500 mg 3 times daily for 5 to 7 days), than by more conventional antibiotic agents. When prescribing bismuth, remember to tell the patient to expect to see black stools. Evidence is yet insufficient to promote bismuth as rational therapy in all cases of gastritis, but its easy availability, apparent safety, and low cost are commendable features.

An exceedingly rare form of infection in the stomach is phlegmonous gastritis, a suppuration involving the entire stomach wall. This occurs in a setting of sepsis, typically streptococcal, and requires intensive, parenteral penicillin therapy.

Gastric Mucosal Atrophy

This is mentioned here because often it is referred to as "atrophic gastritis." The lesion, however, is primarily a disintegration of gastric epithelium, caused by a yet incompletely understood immune reaction. Any inflammatory component is secondary. Gastric mucosal atrophy is significant when it is attended by deficiency of intrinsic factor and impaired absorption of vitamin B_{12}. The treatment is that for vitamin B_{12} deficiency (see p. 308).

General Methods of Treatment

With the possible exception of *C. pylori* infection, as noted above, there is no specific therapy for the various types of gastritis. Hence, the following are offered as generally applicable measures. Just as reaction in gastric mucosa ranges widely from mild to severe, so the intensity of treatment should be modulated accordingly.

Diet

Most patients with symptomatic gastritis will have blunted appetite and some nausea; therefore, they are amenable to prescription of a light, soft diet. When nausea is severe and attended by vomiting, food should be withheld, and parenteral fluid and electrolyte supplements will be required.

Antacids

These agents constitute first-line therapy and often are the only medication required. Antacids combine with H^+ in the lumen of the stomach, thus preventing the potentially injurious back-diffusion of acid. Antacids should be given in liquid form (diluted if necessary to facilitate delivery through a nasogastric tube) and in ample volume (one can hardly give too much or too frequently). An average antacid dose (e.g., Mylanta II) would be 15 ml every 1 or 2 hours. The only drawbacks to the use of antacids are the necessity for frequent dosage and lack of compliance by the patient. A minor side effect of magnesium-containing antacids is diarrhea. This is easily corrected by substituting aluminum hydroxide (e.g., Alternagel).

H_2 Receptor Antagonists

Gastric acid secretion can be effectively inhibited by cimetidine (Tagamet), ranitidine (Zantac), and famotidine (Pepcid), and by this means back-diffusion of H^+ is reduced. Moreover, for severely ill patients these agents can be given intravenously. Continuous intravenous infusion, rather than repeated boluses, is recommended for both efficacy and reduced cost.

If cimetidine is chosen, the usual schedule calls for an initial intravenous "priming" dose of 300 mg and then a steady infusion of 37.5 mg to 75 mg per hour, dissolved in the running fluid. If the patient has an indwelling nasogastric tube, the stomach contents can be aspirated from time to time and checked for pH. The aim is to keep the pH above 4; the running dose of cimetidine can be regulated accordingly.

Patients less acutely ill can be given medication orally: cimetidine, 300 mg every 6 hours; ranitidine, 150 mg every 12 hours; or famotidine, 20 mg every 12 hours. If medication is being used prophylactically, the frequency of doses can be halved.

Antacids and H_2 receptor antagonists are compatible, although—as in the case of the fellow who wears both belt and suspenders—the combination may amount to more caution than is necessary.

If antacids or H$_2$ receptor antagonists are administered in such a way as to totally eliminate gastric acid secretion in the stomach of an acutely ill patient, there is a risk of complication by nosocomial infection, that is, pneumonitis resulting from aspiration of bacterially contaminated gastric juice. This does not happen often, but because of the possibility, care should be taken to avoid unduly vigorous therapy.

Other Measures

Another approach is to use measures for bolstering mucosal defense. This involves agents that are said to confer "cytoprotection."

Sucralfate (Carafate) can be given orally, 1 gram (1 tablet) every 4 to 6 hours on an empty stomach, both for prevention of mucosal injury and as therapy. While efficacy is not always certain, safety is assured. Following is a simple and useful technique for administering sucralfate to a patient with an indwelling nasogastric tube. Place a tablet of sucralfate (1 gram) in the empty barrel of a 60-ml syringe. Replace the plunger and draw up 20 ml of water. Let the syringe stand with its tip up for about 5 minutes, gently shaking the syringe occasionally. The tablet will disintegrate, forming a sucralfate suspension that can be injected through the nasogastric tube. This can be repeated every 3 or 4 hours.

Prostaglandins of the PGE type can be administered orally. Experimental trials suggest a dose of 37.5 micrograms twice daily. While showing promise of efficacy and safety, this class of agents has yet to be released for clinical use. Prostaglandins doubtless will eventually be approved and will then be a useful addition to the armamentarium of agents available for the prevention and treatment of gastritis.

ACUTE AND CHRONIC VIRAL HEPATITIS

method of
RICHARD B. SEWELL, M.D.
Austin Hospital, University of Melbourne
Melbourne, Australia

ACUTE VIRAL HEPATITIS

Acute viral hepatitis refers by convention to cases of acute hepatic cell necrosis caused by the hepatitis A, hepatitis B, delta hepatitis, and non-A, non-B hepatitis agents. Other viral infections, including infectious mononucleosis and cytomegalovirus, may produce hepatitis and should be considered in the appropriate clinical setting. If serologic evidence of viral infection is absent, consideration should be given to causes such as alcohol, drug-induced hepatitis, and extrahepatic cholestasis. The majority of cases of acute viral hepatitis are subclinical, especially in children, and are only recognized by coincidentally measured elevations of serum transaminases. Hepatitis A virus (HAV) causes type A hepatitis and is usually acquired by the fecal-oral route and has an incubation period of 20 to 50 days. Hepatitis B virus (HBV) causes type B hepatitis and is acquired by percutaneous introduction or by close personal contact; it has an incubation period of 28 to 150 days. Delta hepatitis virus (HDV) causes type D hepatitis and is a small, defective RNA virus dependent on HBV for its replication. Non-A, non-B hepatitis (NANB) is caused by three or more viruses that have not been unequivocally identified. It can be spread by both percutaneous introduction, with either a short or long incubation period, or by personal contact in the "sporadic" form. Hepatitis A is usually uncomplicated and never runs a chronic course. Hepatitis B is self limited and uncomplicated in 90 per cent of cases. Delta hepatitis is more often associated with a severe and sometimes fulminant outcome. Hepatitis NANB tends to produce a mild disease; when acquired following blood transfusion, there is a significant (10 to 40 per cent) incidence of indolent chronic liver disease or cirrhosis. Clinical severity tends to increase with age.

Treatment

Standard treatment is conservative and has little effect on the course of acute viral hepatitis. The patient should be observed and monitored for potential acute complications and to ensure that chronic disease does not develop. Initial blood should be taken for biochemistry, including standard liver function tests, and serology, including tests for hepatitis B surface antigen (HBsAg) and IgM anti-HAV. The main purposes are confirming the diagnosis, planning protection of contacts, and predicting fulminant hepatitis.

Hospitalization. The patient can usually be managed at home. Hospitalization is reserved for patients at risk of developing complications, particularly fulminant hepatic failure, those requiring special diagnostic procedures, and those who cannot be adequately isolated and cared for at home. Dehydration, altered consciousness, prolonged prothrombin time, and bruising or development of ascites warrant hospitalization.

Bed Rest. Although bed rest has not been proved to alter the course of the illness, it is usually advised while the patient is symptomatic. Patients should not work while jaundiced and during the postictal malaise (usually 1 to 4 weeks). Activity should be increased in parallel with clinical improvement.

Diet. The choice of diet is at the discretion of the patient. Fluid input should be maintained. A low-fat, high-carbohydrate diet is usually acceptable. Abstinence from alcohol is advisable for 3 to 4 months. If parenteral fluids or nutrition are necessary, the patient should be hospitalized.

Drugs. There is generally no place for drugs in most cases of hepatitis. If medication is given, allowance should be made for altered, and usually impaired, drug metabolism. Special care is required for drugs that may precipitate encephalopathy, including sedatives and analgesics. Corticosteroids are not indicated and in HBV may predispose to chronicity.

Isolation. Patients with hepatitis A are most infective prior to the development of jaundice but can shed the virus for up to 2 weeks from its onset; they should be isolated while potentially infectious and special care should be taken to prevent fecal-oral contamination. Patients with hepatitis B or NANB do not require isolation. These patients should be advised about routes of hepatitis spread; those with hepatitis are potentially infectious until serum antibodies appear. Blood and body fluids are potentially infectious. Toothbrushes, razors, and so forth should not be shared. Sexual intercourse need not be disallowed, but a condom is advised, and the partner should be vaccinated. For the patient hospitalized with HBV, NANB, or HDV hepatitis, the institutional guidelines for handling the patient's blood and secretions should be carefully followed.

Patient Contacts. Those in close contact with a patient who develops acute hepatitis A should generally receive normal immunoglobulin; if the contact already has anti-HAV antibodies, immunoglobin is not indicated. Immunoglobulin is not officially recommended for contacts of patients with NANB hepatitis. Close contacts of a patient with HBV (e.g., spouse, sexual partner, children under 5 years) should be vaccinated if they are HGsAg-negative and antibody-negative.

Convalescence and Recovery. In the typical patient, improvement is evident by the end of the second or third week of illness. The period of convalescence should be approximately twice the symptomatic period. Follow-up biochemical studies (bilirubin and transaminase) should be performed initially at weekly and then at monthly intervals until recovery is complete. Prior to return to work and usual routines, the patient should be free of symptoms, with normal serum bilirubin and transaminase.

A gradual return to full activity should be planned. If HBsAg remains positive for 3 months or if transaminase abnormalities persist, follow-up studies must be continued to check for possible progression to chronic hepatitis.

Relapses. Relapses occur in 5 to 10 per cent of patients. They may be mildly symptomatic or there may be only an increase in serum transaminases or bilirubin. Treatment is as for the initial episode. Subsequent recovery is usually complete.

Complications

Prolonged Cholestasis. Occasionally prolonged cholestasis may complicate the convalescent phase despite symptomatic improvement. Jaundice may persist for up to 6 months. Treatment is usually unnecessary, although cholestyramine may be used. If the diagnosis is in doubt, cholangiography or needle biopsy of the liver should be performed. Laparotomy is to be avoided.

Fulminant Hepatitis. Fulminant hepatic failure is a rare complication of acute viral hepatitis, more common with hepatitis B and NANB hepatitis than with hepatitis A. There is a high mortality rate (70 to 90 per cent); however, if recovery occurs, liver function and architecture return to normal. Management is best undertaken in a specialized intensive care unit, with careful observation and monitoring of vital functions. The major causes of death are related to the development of hepatic encephalopathy, gastrointestinal bleeding, and renal failure.

The goal of therapy is to provide support while hepatic regeneration occurs. Careful monitoring of cardiovascular, renal, respiratory, hematological, hepatic, and neurological function is mandatory. Impending hepatic encephalopathy is treated with neomycin and lactulose. Hypoglycemia may impair consciousness and is treated with 10 per cent dextrose infusion. Mannitol may be required if signs of cerebral edema develop. Protein intake should be stopped and nutrition maintained enterally or parenterally. Coagulation studies determine the need for replacement therapy with fresh frozen plasma, clotting factor concentrates, or platelets. Heparin is ineffective. Prophylactic histamine$_2$ (H$_2$) antagonists decrease the incidence of complicating gastrointestinal bleeding. Corticosteroid therapy is not recommended.

A number of temporary hepatic support systems have been tried. These include exchange blood transfusions, plasmapheresis, cross-circulation, extracorporeal pig liver perfusion, hemodialysis, and charcoal column hemoperfusion. There is no clear-cut evidence that any of these measures are of value in improving survival.

Where there is access to a center performing liver transplantation, early consultation during stage I or II of hepatic precoma is recommended.

Hepatitis During Pregnancy. In women with poor socioeconomic backgrounds, the clinical course may be more severe. Therapeutic abortion may add risk to the mother and does not alter the course of the illness. There is no evidence that hepatitis produces congenital malformations; however, there is evidence of transmission of HBV and NANB to the infant when infection occurs in the third trimester.

Aplastic Anemia. Bone marrow hypoplasia is a rare complication of acute viral hepatitis.

CHRONIC VIRAL HEPATITIS

Chronic Hepatitis B

Persistent infection with HBV for more than 6 months occurs in up to 10 per cent of patients following hepatitis B, regardless of the initial severity. Liver biopsy shows that approximately one third of patients have chronic active hepatitis and two thirds have chronic persistent hepatitis. In other cases, chronic viral hepatitis is not preceded by a clearly recognizable acute attack. Cirrhosis may be present, and hepatocellular carcinoma represents a late event. Patients with chronic hepatitis B often have serum markers of viral replication, such as serum HBV DNA, Dane particles, hepatitis B e antigen (HBeAg) and DNA polymerase. These patients convert from HbeAg-positive to anti-HBe at the rate of about 10 per cent per year. In addition to losing markers of viral replication, HBeAg seroconversion is usually accompanied by normalization of transaminases. HBsAg seroconversion, on the other hand, occurs rarely. Care should be taken in giving HBV-positive patients blood or blood products since a minute inoculum of HDV may induce severe disease.

Delta Agent. The delta agent (HDV) is a small incomplete RNA hepatitis virus that is dependent on coexisting hepatitis B infection for its replication. It is highly virulent and parenteral transmission may occur simultaneously with exposure to HBV or as a superinfection in a hepatitis B carrier. Both fulminant hepatitis and progressive liver disease occur with HDV infection. No specific therapy is available. Serologic evidence of delta agent should be sought in relapse of chronic hepatitis B.

Clinical Relapse. This can occur during spontaneous conversion from HBeAg-positive to negative and is marked by increasing fatigue and raised serum transaminase values. It may occur due to added HDV infection. Rarely, spontaneous reactivation from HBeAg-negative to positive has been described. Clinical deterioration may mark development of hepatocellular carcinoma.

Treatment

The patient must be counseled about personal infectivity, and close family and sexual contacts should be considered for hepatitis B vaccination. Alcohol excess should be avoided since this may potentiate the HBV damage. Antiviral therapy should be considered particularly in a patient likely to disseminate the disease.

Corticosteroid Therapy. Although immunosuppressive therapy is of proven benefit in *autoimmune* chronic active hepatitis, corticosteroid therapy may have deleterious effects in chronic hepatitis B. Viral replication is increased by steroid therapy. Prednisolone should be considered only in HBeAg-negative chronic hepatitis B when the patients are symptomatic and the biopsy shows severe chronic active hepatitis. In these cases the drug should be given for 3 to 6 months and withdrawn if there is no improvement. Small trials have shown that immunostimulant substances are not successful in therapy.

Antiviral Therapy. Results have been encouraging in trials using the antiviral agents adenine arabinoside (ara-A) and soluble adenine arabinoside monophosphate (ara-AMP), which inhibit viral DNA polymerase. Viral replication ceases while the patients are on therapy; in some, the effect is sustained, and seroconversion from HBeAg to anti-HBe occurs. Similar improvement has been noted in some patients treated with various interferons. Studies with these and other antiviral agents are continuing, but as yet they are not available for routine clinical use.

Chronic Non-A, Non-B Hepatitis

Chronic hepatitis occurs in more than 50 per cent of patients with NANB hepatitis following blood transfusion and less commonly after sporadic infection. Liver biopsy will disclose chronic persistent hepatitis in 30 per cent, chronic active hepatitis in 60 per cent, and cirrhosis in 20 per cent of these cases. The course of NANB is characterized by relapses and remissions, especially in transaminases. Regular supervision is necessary, and in the absence of controlled studies, prednisolone cannot be recommended.

Complications

Hepatic encephalopathy, variceal hemorrhage, ascites, renal failure, and bacterial infections may complicate chronic hepatitis and cirrhosis following both hepatitis B and NANB hepatitis. Hepatocellular carcinoma may develop in both cirrhotic and noncirrhotic carriers of hepatitis B and possibly NANB hepatitis. Resection is possible in less than 1 per cent, and chemotherapy with doxorubicin (Adriamycin) induces remissions in around 20 per cent of cases.

PREVENTION

Hepatitis A. Personal hygiene and proper sanitation are mandatory. Separate toilet facilities are desirable. Bedding and clothing should be autoclaved or separately laundered. General handling of food or water by patient or contacts should be prevented. The use of disposable crockery and cutlery is encouraged. Because virus shedding in stools begins at least 2 weeks before the illness, quarantine is unlikely to influence the spread of disease in the community.

Hepatitis B. High-risk groups include certain hospital and dental staff (e.g., oncology, hemodialysis-transplantation, gastroenterology, intensive care units, diagnostic laboratories, surgical units), staff in institutions for the mentally handicapped, patients receiving blood and blood products, drug addicts, male homosexuals, and the families of chronic carriers (Table 1). For high-risk hospital personnel, a program of continuing education concerning hepatitis transmission, monitoring of clinical practices, and regular serologic surveillance for hepatitis B is recommended.

Disposable material and equipment must be used whenever possible; nondisposable equipment should be sterilized by autoclaving for 15 minutes, boiling for 20 minutes, or exposing to dry heat for 1 hour. Equipment that cannot be heat-sterilized should be disinfected with sodium hypochlorite (60 grams per 9 liters of water) or 2 per cent glutaraldehyde. The wearing of gloves and protective clothing by medical and dental staff is advised when they are working in a field contaminated with blood or other body fluids. All blood donors must be screened for HBsAg. Blood products should be used sparingly and only for specific indication.

Transmission of HBV from mother to neonate is the commonest route of infection. The risk to the infant of an HBeAg-positive carrier mother of becoming a chronic HBsAg carrier is about 90 per cent. Carrier risk to infants of HBV carriers who have anti-HBe antibodies is low (5 to 10 per cent), but acute hepatitis may occur. HBsAg screening of mothers whose likely prevalence of HBV carriage is relatively high is probably cost effective. Infants of all HBV carriers should receive combined active/passive vaccination as soon as possible after birth.

Non-A, Non-B Hepatitis. Most transfusion-re-

TABLE 1. **Prevalence of HBV Exposure and Annual Hepatitis B Attack Rates in Different Groups**

Group	Prevalence of HBV Markers (%)	Annual Attack Rate (%)
Health-Care Workers		
Dialysis staff	34–39	3–11
Oral surgeons	30	5
Staff of custodial institutions	22–33	13–20
Surgeons	23–28	5
Nurses in high-risk units	7–47	1–11
Blood-bank workers	6–26	1–2
Laboratory technicians	11–26	1–3
Physicians (general)	12–19	2
Dentists (general)	14–15	2
Surgical house officers	10–17	4–10
Nurse (general)	5–21	1
High-Risk Patients		
Dialysis patients	42–59	3–14
Hemophiliacs	76–96	13–20
Institutionalized Persons		
Mentally retarded	50–90	1–10
Prisoners	42	5–10
Other Groups		
Homosexual men	60–68	12–19
Intravenous drug users	50–71	4–33
Household contacts of HBsAg carriers	26–61	2–5
Promiscuous heterosexuals	15–31	2–5
Military	7–20	0.5–12
General U.S. Population	5–10	0.1

From Mulley AG, Silverstein MD, Dienstag JL: N Engl J Med *307*:651, 1982.

lated hepatitis is NANB hepatitis. Exclusion of paid donors and those with a past history of hepatitis will reduce the risk. Exclusion of blood from volunteer donors who have serum glutamic pyruvic transaminase (SGPT) levels greater than 2.25 times the standard deviation (SD) above the mean will reduce the incidence of NANB hepatitis about one third while excluding less than 2 per cent of blood donors. Prevention of posttransfusion NANB hepatitis awaits identification of the viruses involved and development of reliable screening tests.

Immune Globulin

Hepatitis A. Immune serum globulin (ISG) is effective in preventing or modifying hepatitis A. The dose recommended by the United States Public Health Service Advisory Committee on Immunization Practices is 0.06 ml per kg administered once, as soon as possible after exposure, to people in close contact with patients with acute type A hepatitis, especially in households, institutions for the mentally retarded, and prisons. It is not recommended in the postexposure situation for casual contacts in schools, hospitals, offices, and factories, unless an overt epidemic develops.

ISG may be effective prophylactically in individuals traveling to tropical and developing countries. The recommended dose is 0.06 ml per kg at 4- to 6-month intervals, unless the period of exposure is less than 3 months, in which case it can be given in a dose of 0.02 ml per kg immediately before the visit.

Hepatitis B. Hepatitis B immune globulin (HBIG) is prepared from persons who have high titers of antibody to HBsAg. The United States Public Health Service Advisory Committee recommends that HBIG, 0.06 ml per kg, be administered within 24 hours of parenteral (needle-stick) exposure to HBsAg-positive blood and again 1 month later. Active vaccination should be commenced immediately as well.

All infants born to HBsAg-positive mothers (especially those positive for HBeAg) should be given HBIG (total dose 0.5 ml) within 24 hours of birth, followed by vaccination. It is not currently recommended that HBIG be given to sexual contacts of acute type B hepatitis patients.

Although there is a theoretical risk of immune complex disease if HBIG is given to an HBsAg-positive individual, this has not been reported and it is not necessary to test the recipient prior to treatment.

Non-A, Non-B Hepatitis. Although one study indicated that ISG in standard doses appears to offer significant protection against non-A, non-B hepatitis, other studies failed to confirm this and firm recommendations can not be given.

Vaccination

Hepatitis A. Vaccines against this virus are under development but are not yet available.

Hepatitis B. A successful immunization trial against acute hepatitis B using inactivated HBsAg prepared from the plasma of asymptomatic carriers (Heptavax B, Merck) led to licensing for its clinical use in the United States in 1982. Most side effects recognized to date have been mild. Although the vaccine is made from human serum, purification includes steps to inactivate all known pathogens, including the slow viruses, and three separate studies have excluded any association between the vaccine and the acquired immune deficiency syndrome (AIDS). A similar vaccine has been prepared and used in France (Pasteur, Hevac B).

The high cost and limited availability of these first-generation vaccines require that priorities for immunization be ascertained. Strategies will differ between countries. In countries with a high incidence of HBsAg carriage and vertical transmission, an immunization program should be directed at infants and young children. Hepatitis B vaccine and HBIG can be given simultaneously without diminishing the efficacy of either, and infants born to HBsAg-positive mothers should receive both at birth.

In developed countries, immunization should be offered to high-risk groups. It is believed that protection will last for at least 5 years. Injection should be given into the deltoid. Seroconversion is lower with increasing age and in the immunocompromised; a check for HBs antibody is recommended in these groups, if not in all subjects. The most cost-effective way of immunizing a high-risk, high–previous exposure group is to perform serologic testing for hepatitis B markers and to immunize only those who are not immune. In contrast, a high-risk, low–previous exposure group will be most effectively protected by immunization without prior testing.

Alternative vaccines using recombinant DNA technology are now available, and synthetic vaccines have shown encouraging results with the added benefit of superior safety. The lower cost of these second- and third-generation vaccines should eventually allow an immunization program world-wide.

THE MALABSORPTION SYNDROMES

method of
T. RAYMOND FOLEY, M.D., and
FREDERICK A. WILSON, M.D.
Pennsylvania State University
Hershey, Pennsylvania

Malabsorption, which is failure to assimilate one or more ingested foodstuffs normally, can result from a large, diverse group of disorders. Classically, the impaired absorption is classified according to the disturbance in fat absorption (Table 1). The sequential steps in fat absorption are the lipolytic, micellar, mucosal, and delivery phases. Although fat, protein and carbohydrate malabsorption often occur together, protein and carbohydrate malabsorption can occur in the absence of fat malabsorption in protein-losing gastroenteropathies and disaccharidase deficiencies, respectively.

The presence of malabsorption is suspected in patients with progressive symptoms of weight loss, fatigue, bulky stools, diarrhea, abdominal distention, tetany, or bone pain (calcium and vitamin D deficiency). Physical examination and routine blood work can reveal abnormalities that indicate multiple nutritional deficiencies, such as easy bruisability (vitamin K), anemia (iron, vitamin B_{12}, folate) and edema (hypoproteinemia). Once malabsorption is suspected, however, more specialized tests of absorption are required

TABLE 1. **Classification of Malabsorption**

Insufficient Intraluminal Activity
  Pancreatic insufficiency
  Bile acid deficiency

Mucosal Disease
  Celiac disease
  Lactase deficiency
  Whipple's disease
  Tropical sprue
  Eosinophilic gastroenteritis

Impaired Lymphatic Delivery
  Lymphangiectasia

Multiple Defects
  Bacterial overgrowth
  Postgastrectomy
  Short bowel syndrome
  Gastrinoma (Zollinger-Ellison Syndrome)

Unknown Causes
  Parasitic infections
  Systemic mastocytosis (urticaria pigmentosa)
  AIDS

to identify the specific absorptive defect prior to initiating therapy.

Fat absorption is best assessed by a 72-hour stool collection while the patient is ingesting 60 to 100 gram of fat daily. A Sudan III stain for fat in the stool may be a useful screening test for steatorrhea. The D-xylose test measures the functional integrity of the proximal small bowel mucosa, whereas the Schilling test for vitamin B_{12} absorption assesses the absorptive capacity of the distal small bowel. Renal failure, ascites, and intestinal bacterial overgrowth can cause artifactually low measurements of xylose absorption. In addition to ileal disease, vitamin B_{12} absorption may be abnormal in patients with bacterial overgrowth and pancreatic insufficiency. These two entities may be distinguished from ileal disease by the return of vitamin B_{12} absorption to or toward normal following a course of pancreatic enzymes or broad-spectrum antibiotics. When an abnormal D-xylose test suggests a mucosal defect, an endoscopic or suction capsule biopsy of the small intestine should be performed for a histologic diagnosis. If available, radiolabeled or hydrogen breath tests can be useful in the diagnosis of bacterial overgrowth (^{14}C bile acid and ^{14}C D-xylose), fat malabsorption (^{14}C triolein), disaccharidase insufficiency (^{14}C lactose hydrogen), or pancreatic insufficiency (newly described cholesteryl-[1-^{14}C]octanoate). The bentiromide test, pancreolauryl test, and secretin stimulation tests assess pancreatic exocrine function. The intestinal clearance of alpha-1-antitrypsin is a useful test for protein-losing enteropathy. A suggested algorithm for the diagnostic approach to malabsorption is shown in Figure 1.

INSUFFICIENT INTRALUMINAL ACTIVITY

Lipolytic Defects

Disorders characterized by lipolytic defects include chronic pancreatitis, pancreatic carcinoma, pancreatic resection, cystic fibrosis, and Schwachman's syndrome.

The diseases listed above can result in insufficient intraluminal pancreatic enzyme activity. Although impairment of protein and carbohydrate digestion occurs, the defect in lipolysis is the major contributor to malabsorption. As much as 90 to 95 per cent of pancreatic exocrine function must be lost for steatorrhea to occur. Because of the intensity of fat loss through the stool (fecal fat can exceed 50 grams per day), bulky stools and weight loss are typical features.

Treatment

Once a baseline measurement of fecal fat excretion is obtained, treatment with pancreatic enzyme replacement therapy is begun. A wide variety of commercial enzyme preparations is available. They are essentially purified hog pancreas and contain all essential digestive enzymes including lipase, protease, and amylase. Because protease and amylase are relatively acid-resistant, most enzyme preparations will correct protein and carbohydrate malabsorption. Correcting fat malabsorption is more difficult because lipase is actively destroyed at a pH <4 and because of the marked variability in lipase content in different preparations. The actual and stated enzyme contents can be quite disparate. It has been reported that Ilozyme is the most potent preparation, containing approximately 3600 units of lipase per pill. Pancrease, Ku-Zyme HP, Festal, Cotazym, and Cotazym-S each contain from 2000 to 3000 units of lipase per pill; Viokase has from 1000 to 2000 units per pill. In general, 10,000 lipase units given with a meal will result in at least a 50 per cent reduction in steatorrhea. Tablet and capsule preparations appear equally effective; however, enteric-coated tablets (Festal) may not be bioavailable. In contrast, enteric-coated microspheres (Pancrease, Cotazym-S) have predictable enzyme activity.

If significant steatorrhea persists, more lipase can be made available to the duodenum in three ways. The first is to increase the dosage. This is often limited by patient acceptance and expense. The second is to protect the enzyme, (i.e., the more expensive, enteric-coated microsphere formulations may be more useful in some patients). The third is to decrease gastric acidity. Four sodium bicarbonate tablets (1.3 grams) with meals or 30 ml of aluminum hydroxide before and after meals can result in a significant reduction in steatorrhea. Calcium carbonate and magnesium-aluminum hydroxide are not recommended, as they can increase steatorrhea. If symptoms persist, one may try an H_2 blocker such as cimetidine (Tagamet), 300 mg 4 times daily before meals.

Dietary therapy is usually not required. A high-protein, high-carbohydrate diet with 30 to 50 grams of fat may relieve symptoms in the

Suggestive clinical history of malabsorption

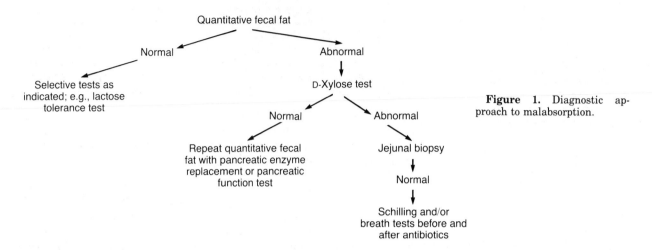

Figure 1. Diagnostic approach to malabsorption.

challenging patient with persistent steatorrhea and diarrhea. Medium-chain triglycerides, which do not require pancreatic enzyme for absorption, will provide added calories if needed. Vitamin deficiencies should be corrected, but long-term vitamin supplementation is usually not required. If symptoms persist despite the above measures, other causes of malabsorption should be considered (e.g., Zollinger-Ellison syndrome, celiac disease, bacterial overgrowth). A suggested treatment plan for pancreatic insufficiency is shown in Figure 2.

Micellar Defects

Any disease or process that interrupts the enterohepatic circulation of bile acids (e.g., extrahepatic

biliary obstruction, intrahepatic disease, or ileal disease, bypass, or resection) may result in defective micellar solubilization of fatty acids and beta-monoglycerides. Isolated steatorrhea with no malabsorption of other major dietary constituents and normal tests of proximal small bowel mucosal integrity are present. The steatorrhea is usually mild (<20 grams stool fat per 24 hours).

Treatment

Treatment may be directed to the condition that is interrupting the enterohepatic circulation, such as extrahepatic biliary obstruction. Exogenous treament with bile or bile acid may be tried but is usually of limited success and expensive and may worsen the diarrhea if ileal disease or resection is present. General nutritional support,

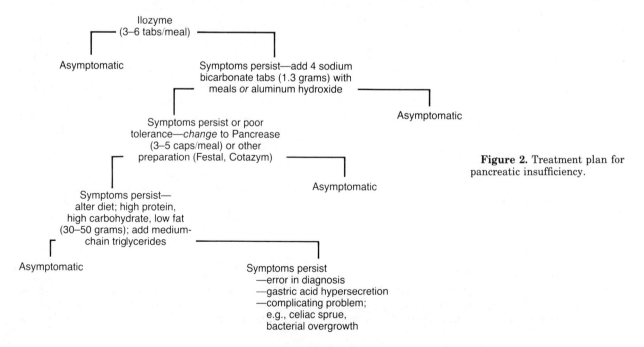

Figure 2. Treatment plan for pancreatic insufficiency.

such as medium-chain triglycerides, fat-soluble vitamins and defined formula diet supplementation, is helpful in most instances.

MUCOSAL DISEASE

Celiac Disease

Celiac disease (gluten-sensitive enteropathy; celiac sprue) is a condition in which the small intestinal mucosa of susceptible persons is damaged after eating gluten-containing foods. The damaged intestinal mucosa affects the absorption of usually more than one dietary constituent. An abnormal D-xylose test suggests mucosal disease, but a small bowel biopsy is necessary to establish the diagnosis. The characteristic small bowel biopsy consists of villous flattening, cuboidal epithelial cells, crypt hypertrophy, and infiltration of the lamina propria with lymphocytes and plasma cells.

Treatment

The mainstay of therapy is a gluten-free diet. Improvement in well-being is often noted within 2 to 3 days, but complete remission may take weeks, months, or even years. Gluten is ubiquitous, and a gluten-free diet is very difficult for most patients to achieve and maintain. Gluten is contained in wheat, barley, rye, and probably oats. Obvious sources of gluten (e.g., breakfast cereals, bread, pasta, baked goods) are easy to identify and avoid; however, it is much more difficult to avoid wheat flour, which is used in many processed foods including some ice creams, salad dressings, canned soups and vegetables, and alcoholic beverages (i.e., beer, scotch, bourbon, vodka, rye, gin). Ketchup, mustard, most meat sauces, and many candy bars also contain gluten.

Extensive counseling of the patient by physician and dietician is very important. Patients must be encouraged to examine food labels carefully and suspiciously. Young patients must be educated as to the importance of a gluten-free diet in ensuring full physical and intellectual development. Membership in the Celiac Sprue Society* can be educational and supportive. This society will provide a list of gluten-free products as well as products that appear safe but contain gluten. Other sources for gluten-free product lists are provided in Table 2.

It is not clear whether oats are toxic to all patients with celiac disease. Some patients who are very sensitive to small amounts of wheat flour can tolerate oats without ill effects; others develop symptoms a few hours after eating oat-containing foods. Initially, oats should be completely eliminated from the diet. Once remission

*45 Gifford Avenue, Jersey City, NJ 07304

TABLE 2. Sources of Gluten-Free Product Lists

CPC International Avenue
Best Foods Search Center
Union, NJ 07083

Ener-G Foods, Inc.
PO Box 24723
Seattle, WA 98134

Featherweight
Chicago Dietetic Supply Inc.
Dept 25, PO Box 529
La Grange, IL 60525

General Foods Kitchens
250 North Street
White Plains, NY 10625

Henkel Corporation
Dietary Specialties
4620 West 77th
Minneapolis, MN 55435

Med-Diet Laboratories Inc.
695 Hopkins Crossroad
Minnetonka, MN 55343

Metabolic Research Dietician
Clinical Research Center Rc-14
University Hospital
University of Washington
Seattle, WA 98105

has been achieved, oats can be carefully reintroduced.

Patients with severe disease should receive appropriate replacement therapy for vitamin and mineral deficiencies. Anemia usually results from iron or folate deficiency; vitamin B_{12} deficiency is unusual. Pyridoxine may be tried in daily doses of 200 to 400 mg orally in patients whose anemia has not responded to other treatment. A prolonged prothrombin time can be corrected with parenteral vitamin K. To correct deficiencies and prevent mobilization of skeletal calcium, calcium carbonate (500 mg twice daily) and vitamin D_2 (calciferol, 1.25 mg or 50,000 units daily) should be given until malabsorption has been corrected and osteomalacia is controlled. Hypokalemia and hypomagnesemia should be corrected. Zinc deficiency is relatively common in celiac disease and can result in loss of appetite and taste. This can be readily treated with oral zinc sulfate, 220 mg 3 times daily.

About 80 per cent of celiac patients should respond within 3 weeks of initiating a gluten-free diet. In patients who fail to respond to the above manipulations, a poor adherence to diet, either consciously or unconsciously, is the most common culprit. A genetic or acquired lactase deficiency may require restriction of dietary dairy products. Short-term steroid therapy (prednisone, 0.5 mg per kg per day) may be useful in the patient who is unable to maintain health despite a strict milk-free, gluten-free diet, in the patient who refuses or is unable to tolerate a gluten-free diet, or in the presence of complicating disorders such as ulcerative jejunitis. Finally, in patients who fail to respond or who relapse despite apparent adherence to diet, the development of lymphoma (up to 7 per cent of patients) or collagenous sprue should be considered.

Lactase Deficiency

With the exception of people of Northern European extraction, certain African tribes and the natives of certain areas of India, most of the world's adults have a relative lactase deficiency. This is transmitted in an autosomal dominant fashion but can also be acquired if the small intestine is affected by other mucosal disease. Acute infectious enteritis can result in low lactase activity for several weeks following the acute event, as can prolonged parenteral hyperalimentation in a patient who is taking nothing by mouth. Chronic intestinal diseases such as celiac disease, tropical sprue, giardiasis, and inflammatory bowel disease also can produce lactase deficiency.

Lactase, a small intestinal brush border enzyme, cleaves lactose into glucose and galactose. Failure to do so increases the osmotic load delivered to the small intestine. When lactose is metabolized by intestinal bacteria, the osmotic load increases further, and gas also is produced. Clinically, this is manifested after milk intake by cramping and abdominal distension, which may be quickly relieved by diarrheal stools and flatus. Because the disorder is benign, a symptomatic response to treatment is usually sufficient for diagnosis. The lactose tolerance test or breath hydrogen test can be employed if the diagnosis needs to be confirmed.

Treatment

The treatment of lactase deficiency consists of avoiding dietary lactose, which is found principally in dairy products. Many patients discover this relationship themselves and therefore consume a low-calcium diet. Low-lactose milk, cheese, ice cream, and lactose-free yogurt preparations can be substituted for unmodified dairy products. Commercially prepared semipurified yeast lactase (Lactrase, LactAid) is available. This can be taken at mealtime with dairy products (1 to 3 capsules or tablets) or added to milk (5 to 15 drops LactAid per quart of milk); in the latter circumstance, within 24 hours most lactose will be converted to glucose and galactose. A continued source of calcium, vitamin D, and protein is particularly important in children and adolescents with high nutritional requirements, as well as for middle-aged, postmenopausal women, who have a high predilection for osteoporosis. If dietary milk intake is restricted in this last group, supplemental calcium carbonate, 500 mg 2 to 3 times per day, and vitamin D should be provided.

Whipple's Disease

Whipple's disease is an uncommon cause of malabsorption that usually affects middle-aged men. The disease should be suspected in individuals with weight loss, diarrhea, arthralgias, and abdominal pain, particularly if the arthralgias precede other symptoms by months to years. Central nervous system and cardiac involvement has been described. More than 90 per cent of untreated patients will have steatorrhea. The proximal small bowel undergoes the most severe histologic changes, and a small bowel biopsy is the diagnostic procedure of choice. The intestinal mucosa characteristically shows infiltration of the lamina propria with PAS-positive macrophages. The bacilli implicated as the causative agent may be seen within macrophages by electron microscopy or specially prepared light microscopy.

Treatment

Treatment of Whipple's disease consists of appropriate use of antibiotics. The choice of antibiotic and the duration of therapy are somewhat empiric, but the risk of relapse (especially central nervous system involvement) suggests that treatment should be continued for at least a year. Suggested daily regimens include intramuscular procaine penicillin G (1.2 million U) with intramuscular streptomycin (1 gram) or with parenteral chloramphenicol (4 grams in divided doses). Two weeks of either regimen is followed by 1 year of therapy with trimethoprim-sulfamethoxazole (Bactrim, Septra), 1 double-strength tablet twice daily. This regimen can be complicated by folic acid deficiency, and supplemental folate may be required. Supplemental iron, calcium, or magnesium also may be needed. Repeat small bowel biopsy showing absence of bacilli should be performed to confirm adequacy of treatment.

Tropical Sprue

Tropical sprue is a chronic diarrheal illness acquired in endemic tropical areas including Puerto Rico and Cuba. It is characterized by progressive small bowel dysfunction resulting in the development of nutritional deficiencies. Although it usually occurs after many months or years in an endemic area, visitors to these areas may develop tropical sprue within weeks. Lassitude, weight loss, and gastrointestinal complaints (diarrhea, flatulence, abdominal distension and cramping) dominate the clinical picture. The anemia that develops in all untreated patients is usually megaloblastic secondary to folate and/or vitamin B_{12} deficiency. The anemia may be dimorphic, reflecting a concomitant iron deficiency. A small bowel biopsy reveals villous atrophy and marked lymphocytic and plasma cell infiltration of the lamina propria. Present evidence suggests a bacterial origin for this disease.

Treatment

While supportive therapy may be necessary for individuals with electrolyte depletion, protein deficiency, or dehydration, most persons respond remarkably well to folate and antibiotic therapy. Treatment with pharmacologic doses of folate (5 mg daily by mouth) leads to striking chemical and hematologic improvement. Correction of anemia, disappearance of glossitis, and return of appetite with resulting weight gain usually precede the abatement of gastrointestinal symptoms. Patients with "megaloblastic madness" who receive parenteral folate become rational within 48 to 72 hours. Oral folate therapy (5 mg daily) should be continued for 1 year.

Antibiotic therapy should be combined with folate therapy for optimal results, particularly in patients with long-standing symptoms (greater than 4 months). Tetracycline, 500 mg by mouth 4 times daily for 1 month and then twice daily for an additional 5 to 11 months, or trimethoprim-sulfamethoxazole (Bactrim, Septra), 1 double-strength tablet twice daily for 6 to 12 months, is recommended. Patients who contract this disease in the tropics and then return to temperate climates may only need treatment for several weeks. Long-standing tropical sprue tends to recur even after long-term antibiotic treatment.

Parenteral vitamin B_{12} therapy should be administered to patients with long-standing symptoms or patients with documented B_{12} deficiency. A daily dose of 100 micrograms of vitamin B_{12} is administered parenterally for 1 week; thereafter, 100 micrograms of vitamin B_{12} is given monthly.

Dietary modification is usually not necessary. Alcohol can exacerbate symptoms and should be avoided. An acquired lactase deficiency may be present. Failure to respond to treatment with antibiotics and folate should prompt an investigation into other causes of diarrhea, particularly parasitic infections.

Eosinophilic Gastroenteritis

Eosinophils can infiltrate any of three layers of the intestinal wall (mucosa, muscularis, serosa). Malabsorption is usually seen with mucosal disease. Patients note varied and frequently intermittent gastrointestinal complaints that may be precipitated by certain foods. A peripheral eosinophilia is usually seen, and small bowel biopsy confirms the diagnosis.

Treatment

If certain foods obviously cause symptoms, they should be avoided. Otherwise, elimination diets can be tried but produce variable responses. A short course of steroids (prednisone, 20 to 30 mg per day for 7 to 10 days) usually produces a dramatic response, and some patients will remain asymptomatic for years. Other patients may require low-dose steroid (prednisone 5 to 10 mg) alternate-day therapy for control of symptoms.

Oral disodium cromoglycate,* 800 to 1200 mg daily in 4 doses, has been reported to be useful for this condition. If effective, cromoglycate may prevent the need for long-term steroid therapy.

IMPAIRED LYMPHATIC DELIVERY

Lymphangiectasia

Interference with the flow of lymph from the small intestine can result from either congenital lymphatic malformation or from an acquired obstruction to lymph flow (e.g., lymphoma, other neoplasms, severe constrictive pericarditis). Ruptured lacteals with a resultant enteric loss of plasma proteins, chylomicrons, and lymphocytes results in hypoproteinemia, fat malabsorption, and lymphocytopenia. Enteric loss may be documented by an elevated intestinal clearance of alpha-1-antitrypsin. Small bowel biopsy revealing dilated lacteals can confirm the diagnosis of lymphangiectasia.

Treatment

In patients with congenital lymphangiectasia, enteric protein loss usually decreases during treatment with a low-fat diet. Long-chain triglycerides stimulate intestinal lymph flow. Medium-chain triglycerides do not require intestinal lymphatic transport and can supply additional calories. This can be given as an oil (MCT oil, Mead Johnson), or, more palatably, as Portagen. Peripheral lymphedema should be treated with external elastic support. Diuretics are of limited value. Fat-soluble vitamins can be supplied in oral form.

Treatment of an acquired lymphangiectasia consists of identifying the underlying abnormality and then instituting appropriate therapy. Chemotherapy and/or radiation therapy may improve lymphangiectasia secondary to lymphoma. Surgical repair of severe constrictive pericarditis may ameliorate the secondary lymphangiectasia.

MULTIPLE DEFECTS

Bacterial Overgrowth

The predisposing conditions associated with small intestine bacterial overgrowth are legion (Table 3). The absence of gastric acid, delay in intestinal transit, internal fistulization of the intestine and resection of the ileocecal valve predispose to bacterial overgrowth. Overgrowth of aerobic and anaerobic bacteria results in malabsorption secondary to (1) intraluminal bacterial assimilation or metabolism of intestinal contents (vitamin B_{12} malabsorption), (2) intraluminal bacterial deconjugation of bile salts (fat malabsorption), and (3) mucosal injury (carbohydrate malabsorption). ^{14}C D-xylose and hydrogen breath tests can confirm the

---

*Oral form not available in the United States.

TABLE 3. **Causes of Bacterial Overgrowth**

Blind loop after surgery
Crohn's disease
Diabetes
Gastric achlorhydria
Intestinal fistula
Intestinal pseudo-obstruction
Radiation enteritis
Resection of ileocecal valve
Scleroderma
Short bowel syndrome
Small bowel diverticulum

diagnosis, but empiric antibiotic trials are often used in the proper clinical setting.

The first step in the treatment of bacterial overgrowth is identifying and correcting any surgically correctable cause (e.g., long afferent loop after Billroth II gastrojejunostomy, isolated small bowel diverticulum, intestinal fistula). Most causes of bacterial overgrowth are not amenable to surgical correction. If malabsorption and/or malnutrition are present, broad-spectrum antibiotic therapy should be instituted. Tetracycline, 250 mg to 500 mg 4 times daily, or metronidazole (Flagyl), 250 mg 3 times daily, can be given alone or together for 7 to 10 days. Most patients will respond to this regimen and will not need retreatment for months. Less frequently, patients will require intermittent treatment (e.g., 1 week out of every 6) or a prolonged initial course of treatment. For those individuals who fail to respond, chloramphenicol, 50 mg per kg per day in 4 divided doses; clindamycin (Cleocin), 75 to 150 mg 4 times daily; or a combination of metronidazole or clindamycin with an oral first-generation cephalosporin are useful alternatives.

Continued malabsorption despite optimal antibiotic therapy may require restricting long-chain triglycerides and substituting medium-chain triglycerides. A concomitant lactase deficiency may be present, and restricting dairy products may be useful. Deficiencies of vitamin B_{12}, fat-soluble vitamins, and calcium should be corrected.

Postgastrectomy

Although diarrhea is not infrequent following a vagotomy and pyloroplasty, steatorrhea is unusual. Steatorrhea is seen more frequently after a subtotal gastrectomy and is more common with a Billroth II than with a Billroth I anastomosis. Usually the fat loss is minimal, ranging from 7 to 10 grams daily. Following a subtotal gastrectomy and gastrojejunostomy (Billroth II) or a total gastrectomy, steatorrhea and malabsorption are usually due to (1) loss of reservoir function, with rapid emptying and dispersion of food through the small intestine, thereby diluting the normal output of pancreatic enzymes; or (2) stasis with

bacterial overgrowth of an afferent loop. Because the duodenum is the primary site for the absorption of calcim and iron, a Billroth II anastomosis predisposes to calcium and iron deficiencies. Vitamin B_{12} deficiency can be seen after a subtotal gastrectomy and is inevitable after a total gastrectomy because of the loss of intrinsic factor.

Treatment

Many remedies have been proposed in this setting. Because of a functional pancreatic insufficiency, pancreatic extracts (see Chronic Pancreatitis) have been tried with inconsistent results. When combined with broad-spectrum antibiotics (ampicillin or tetracycline, 1 gram daily in divided doses), fat absorption may improve. Deficiencies of iron, calcium, vitamin B_{12} and fat-soluble vitamins should be sought for and corrected.

Dietary measures consist of six small feedings daily, with carbohydrate being restricted in favor of protein. Liquids should be taken between, rather than with, meals. Lactase deficiency may complicate the treatment of postgastrectomy malabsorption. The use of commercially prepared semipurified yeast lactase (LactAid, Lactrase) can be useful and is preferable to avoidance of dairy products by these patients, who are already prone to calcium deficiency.

Short Bowel Syndrome

Crohn's disease, mesenteric thrombosis, abdominal trauma, small bowel obstruction with infarction, and severe radiation injury are the most common conditions resulting in extensive small bowel resection. Improvement in perioperative management have resulted in increasing numbers of persons who survive with a short bowel. Maldigestion and malabsorption can pose formidable management problems, and the underlying etiologic mechanisms are complex. Contributory factors include a reduction in small intestinal absorptive surface; decrease in small bowel transit time; diminution of the bile salt pool after ileal resection; loss of the stimulatory effects of cholecystokinin (CCK) and secretin; removal of the ileocecal valve with resultant bacterial overgrowth, gastric hypersecretion, and disaccharidase deficiency, which prolongs the malabsorptive state. If large bowel is also resected, fluid and electrolyte problems are compounded. The functional integrity of the remaining small and large bowel is very important in the long-term management of these patients.

Treatment

Proper treatment of these individuals begins in the immediate postoperative period with the institution of total parenteral nutrition. Variations in the extent of resection and functional integrity of the remaining bowel dictates individual variations in the introduction of enteral feedings. In those patients whose bowel sounds return and are passing flatus, an enteral feeding regimen can be begun within a week of surgery. It is important to remember that enteral nutrients are necessary for intestinal adaptation to occur. Patients with massive bowel loss should be started on elemental formula diets containing medium-chain triglycerides (Vital, Vivonex). Because of their unpalatable character, they are best administered through a soft, small-bore feeding tube. These solutions are hyperosmolar and should be diluted to one fourth to one third strength initially. A continuous 24-hour infusion beginning at 25 ml per hour is recommended, and incremental increases in the strength of the solution are made as tolerated. Diarrhea can be treated with antimotility agents (diphenoxylate and atropine [Lomotil], up to 2 tablets 4 times daily; loperamide [Imodium], 4 mg initially and then 2 mg after each unformed stool, up to 16 mg daily; codeine, 30 to 60 mg 4 times daily; or deodorized tincture of opium, 10 drops 2 or 3 times daily. Parenteral nutrition should be continued as enteral feedings are introduced and advanced. Soy protein/casein-based preparations (Isocal, HCN Osmolite) contain medium chain triglycerides and no lactose and are very useful. Patients with short bowel syndrome may have a lactase deficiency and lactose-containing formulas (e.g., Carnation Instant Breakfast) should be avoided.

Recent evidence suggests that persons with an intact colon and at least 75 cm of small bowel or patients who have had a colon resection but have at least 150 cm of small bowel, will be able to satisfy their nutritional needs with oral intake and will not require home hyperalimentation. As the diet is advanced, conventional philosophy has been to introduce a low fat (less than 40 grams daily), low lactose diet with frequent small feedings (5 to 6 meals daily). Medium chain triglycerides can be added in the diet of all patients for their caloric value as well as their ability to aid the absorption of fat soluble vitamins. 15 ml of MCT oil (Mead-Johnson) given 4 time daily provides 370 calories per day. Patients can also substitute MCT oil for vegetable oil when cooking and in salad dressing. It has recently been shown that a high fat diet does not have detrimental effects in these patients and that long-term fat restriction is not necessary.

High-oxalate foods (spinach, chocolate, rhubarb) are avoided to minimize the tendency to form calcium oxalate kidney stones. Patients with short bowel syndrome usually require supplementation of fat-soluble vitamins (A, D, and K) and mineral supplementation (calcium, magnesium, iron, and zinc). Magnesium replacement should be given parenterally (magnesium sulfate) because oral magnesium preparations can aggravate diarrhea. Although vitamin B_{12} deficiency may not become evident for years, patients with ileal resection greater than 6 to 8 feet usually require intramuscular vitamin B_{12} therapy (100 micrograms monthly).

Serum gastrin levels should be measured because many of these patients have gastric hypersecretion. If elevated, an H_2 blocker (cimetidine [Tagamet], 800 mg daily; ranitidine [Zantac], 300 mg daily; or famotidine [Pepcid], 40 mg daily) may help alleviate diarrhea. Patients with ileal resections of less than 100 cm may show improvement in bile acid–induced diarrhea after treatment with cholestyramine (Questran), 8 to 12 grams daily in divided doses. Pancreatic supplements high in lipase may reduce steatorrhea. Broad-spectrum antibiotics are used when bacterial overgrowth is present. If malabsorption and malnutrition persist despite these measures, home hyperalimentation can be employed.

Gastrinoma (Zollinger-Ellison Syndrome)

Diarrhea including steatorrhea occurs in one third to one half of patients with gastrinoma and may be the initial manifestation in up to 35 per cent of patients. The diagnosis of gastrinoma is usually made by demonstrating elevated serum gastrin levels (fasting levels greater than 1000 picograms per ml) or gastric acid hypersecretion (basal output greater than 15 mmol per hour) in a patient with ulcer disease, unexplained diarrhea, or symptoms of hypercalcemia. A secretin stimulation test with measurement of serum gastrin levels can confirm the diagnosis.

Treatment

Large doses of histamine H_2-receptor antagonists form the mainstay of treatment. In recent studies, the median daily doses of cimetidine (Tagamet), ranitidine (Zantac), and famotidine (Pepcid) were 3.6 grams (range, 1.2 to 12.6 grams) 1.2 grams (0.45 to 6 grams) and 0.25 gram (0.05 to 0.8 gram), respectively. Dosage requirements tend to increase with time. Symptom relief does not reflect effectiveness of therapy. A reduction in gastric acid secretion to less than 10 mmol in the hour preceding the next dose of medication reliably reflects adequacy of treatment.

In patients with multiple endocrine neoplasia, type 1 (MEN-1) syndrome, correction of hypercalcemia facilitates control of gastric hypersecretion. Although many patients are maintained adequately with medical treatment, most patients should be evaluated for the possibility of tumor resection. Although it is not presently available, it seems likely that the H^+-K^+-ATPase inhibitor omeprazole (investigational) will become the drug of choice for gastrinoma.

UNKNOWN CAUSES

The etiologic role of viruses, atypical mycobacteria, or other unrecognized enteric pathogens in malabsorption is unclear. The role of malnutrition, including zinc deficiency, is speculative. It has been reported that in patients with *Pneumocystis carinii* pneumonia and diarrhea, treatment with trimethoprim/sulfamethoxazole resulted in a resolution of the diarrhea as the pneumonia resolved. In the absence of a specific etiologic agent, generalized nutritional support with medium-chain triglycerides, fat-soluble vitamins, and defined formula diet supplementation should be employed.

Parasitic Infections

Most parasitic intestinal infections do not produce malabsorption. Giardiasis, coccidiosis, and strongyloidiasis can produce malabsorption in the immunocompetent and the immunocompromised individual, although the specific cause(s) for the malabsorption is unknown. The diagnosis of giardiasis is made by recovering the trophozoite by proximal small bowel biopsy and/or aspiration or by stool examination for *Giardia* cysts. Marked clinical improvement follows treatment with metronidazole (Flagyl), 250 mg orally 3 times daily for 10 days. If symptoms recur, patients are retreated for 3 to 4 weeks. If the patient has an underlying IgA deficiency, initial therapy should be continued for 6 weeks.

Chronic enteric infections with species of coccidia (*Cryptosporidium* sp. and *Isospora belli*) can produce secretory diarrhea and malabsorption. For the treatment of *I. belli* infections, trimethoprim-sulfamethoxazole (Septra, Bactrim), 1 double-strength tablet 4 times daily for 10 days and then twice daily for 3 weeks, has been recommended and can provide rapid relief. Recurrences have been described in patients with AIDS.

In the immunocompetent host, cryptosporidiosis is usually self-limited. In immunocompromised patients, *Cryptosporidium* infection can be severe and persistent. Effective therapy remains to be established. Spiramycin, 1 gram orally 3 or 4 times daily, has alleviated symptoms in some, but not in all, patients. This drug is not commercially available, but can be obtained through the FDA's Division of Anti-infective Drug Products.

Although more common in tropical climates, *Strongyloides stercoralis* has a worldwide distribution. Treatment with thiabendazole (Mintezol) is highly effective. Twenty-five mg per kg of body weight is given after meals twice daily for 2 days. In immunocompromised individuals or those exhibiting disseminated strongyloidiasis, treatment is continued for at least 5 days. After treatment, monthly stool exams should be performed for 2 to 3 months.

Systemic Mastocytosis (Urticaria Pigmentosa)

A disorder characterized by recurrent episodes of flushing, headache, pruritus, and tachycardia, systemic mastocytosis is an unusual cause of diarrhea and malabsorption. Cimetidine (Tagamet), 300 mg 4 times daily, and oral disodium cromoglycate*, 100 mg 4 times daily, can relieve diarrhea and abdominal cramping, but treatment of malabsorption has not been successful.

AIDS

Diarrhea has been reported to be a problem in 50 to 60 per cent of patients with the acquired immune deficiency syndrome (AIDS). This may be due to gastrointestinal tract infestation with a unique group of opportunistic pathogens or to a malignancy involving the gastrointestinal tract (Kaposi's sarcoma or non-Hodgkin's lymphoma). In 40 to 75 per cent of AIDS patients with diarrhea, weight loss, and malnutrition, an identifiable cause cannot be found. This has been termed AIDS enteropathy. D-Xylose and ^{14}C-glycerol tripalmitate absorption tests are frequently abnormal. Small bowel biopsy specimens reveal partial villous atrophy, crypt hyperplasia, and lymphocytic infiltration of the lamina propria. Treatment of opportunistic pathogens and general nutritional support are the goals of therapy.

ACUTE PANCREATITIS
method of
MARION C. ANDERSON, M.D.
Medical University of South Carolina
Charleston, South Carolina

In the United States the most common cause of acute pancreatitis is chronic alcohol abuse (60 to 70 per cent), followed by biliary tract disease (20 to 25 per cent). A variety of less common causes, including abdominal trauma, make up the remaining group.

Clinical symptoms include severe, steady upper abdominal pain that develops suddenly, often following a heavy intake of food and drink. The pain frequently radiates directly posteriorly into the lower dorsal area of the back and usually is accompanied by nausea and vomiting. Associated ileus may result in abdominal distention.

The initial hemoglobin and hematocrit may be increased, reflecting hypovolemia secondary to fluid losses into the interstitium of the gland and into the peripancreatic area, retroperitoneum, peritoneal cavity, and bowel lumen. Severe, acute pancreatitis can produce a reduction of plasma volume in the range of

---

*Oral form not available in the United States.

30 to 40 per cent. This in turn results in tachycardia and hypotension with associated vasoconstriction of splanchnic, renal, and peripheral arterial beds. Urine volume is reduced and the blood urea nitrogen and creatinine may be increased. Leukocytosis is usually present with a left shift in the differential count. Serum amylase is increased in two thirds of cases, but high levels do not correlate with the severity of an attack. There may be substantial losses of electrolytes including sodium and potassium. Hypocalcemia is common and persistently low levels are associated with severe disease.

Plain films of the abdomen are helpful in excluding obvious free air and may show areas of segmental ileus. Usually there is little to suggest a diagnosis of acute pancreatitis. Patients with advanced chronic pancreatitis may have calcification which is associated with the ductal obstructive changes characteristic of this form of the disease, which is nearly always secondary to chronic alcohol abuse. Ultrasonography is helpful in assessing the biliary tract for stones and demonstrating pancreatic and peripancreatic fluid collections. Computed tomography (CT) scans also provide considerable detail regarding the magnitude of pancreatic enlargement and the presence of pancreatic fluid collections. Ranson's correlations of CT scan findings with previously defined clinical prognostic signs are shown in Table 1. The more severe CT changes were found to be predictive of serious complications such as pancreatic abscess (Table 2).

Acute pancreatitis ranges from a mild edema to an overwhelming hemorrhagic necrosis. Fortunately, the latter comprises only 5 to 10 per cent of cases in any given series. Most of the remainder are self-limiting and respond to simple therapeutic measures. In contrast, the severe form is associated with a high morbidity and mortality in spite of all types of treatment currently available. Utilization of predictive criteria such as those shown in Table 1 are helpful in the identification of patients with the severe form of the disease.

Treatment

Patients with acute pancreatitis should be hospitalized and placed at bed rest.

TABLE 1. **Ranson's Prognostic Signs**

On Admission
Age >55 years
WBC >16,000
Blood glucose >200 mg/dl
LDH >350 IU/liter
SGOT >250 units/dl
Markedly elevated amylase

During Initial 48 Hours
Hct ↓ of >10%
BUN ↑ of >5 mg/dl
Serum Ca^{++} <8 mg/dl
Arterial Po_2 <60 mm Hg
Base deficit >4 mcg/liter
Fluid sequestration >6 liters

Fluid and Electrolyte Replacement

As indicated above, hypovolemia secondary to fluid losses from the pancreatic microcirculation is a hallmark of the disease. Fluid replacement should be initiated promptly with 5.2 D/S solution containing 40 mEq of potassium per liter. A urethral catheter should be placed, and with rare exceptions the volume of fluid replacement can be determined by maintaining an hourly urinary output in the range of 30 to 50 ml per hour. Milder forms of acute pancreatitis respond to relatively small replacement volumes. Fluid loss increases with severity of disease and these patients often benefit from central venous pressure measurements to guide fluid replacement more precisely. Unstable patients should be monitored with a Swan-Ganz catheter. The most serious error is to underestimate the magnitude of fluid loss in the patient with severe pancreatitis. The resulting hypovolemia triggers splanchnic vasoconstriction, which in turn may intensify local vascular and tissue injury associated with the disease. Volumes in the range of 10 to 15 liters may be required in the initial 24 hours to maintain an adequate urinary output in this small group of seriously ill patients.

Pain Control

Even in the mild forms of the disease, pain can be severe and usually can be controlled with adequate doses of meperidine (Demerol). Morphine produces spasm in the ampullary sphincter and duodenum and is therefore contraindicated. Epidural blocks or continuous epidural infusions have been employed; however, I have not found it necessary to employ these techniques.

Antibiotic Therapy

Simple acute pancreatitis is not a product of bacterial action, and therefore antibiotic therapy is rarely necessary. One exception to this rule is acute biliary pancreatitis that results from migration of small stones through the biliary tract. The stones produce obstruction as they pass through the ampullary area and thereby initiate the attack. There is a high incidence of associated bactobilia which most studies show should be treated with broad-spectrum antibiotics. Severe forms of acute pancreatitis may produce areas of pancreatic necrosis that are at high risk for bacterial infection and ultimately progression to abscess formation. For this reason patients with severe pancreatic inflammation should be aggressively treated with broad-spectrum antibiotics, such as the third-generation cephalosporin imipenem (Primaxin).

TABLE 2. **Identification* of Patients at High Risk for Pancreatic Abscess**

CT Grade**	Positive Prognostic Signs†								
	0	1	2	3	4	5	6	7	8
A	0000	00000	00		0				
B	0000 000	0000	00	000	0	0 +			
C	0000 000 P	000	000	0 a	a				
D	00 a	000	00	0	00	A			
E		a	0000 aaaaa	00 aa		00 aA	0 AA		aA

*Based on the occurrence of local pancreatic complications related to the initial CT findings and the number of positive prognostic signs listed in Table 1.

**A = normal; B = pancreatic enlargement only; C = peripancreatic inflammation; D = one fluid collection; E = more than one collection.

†0 = no complication; a = abscess with survival; A = death from abscess; P = persistent pseudocyst; + = death without abscess.

From Ranson, J. H. C., et al. Annals of Surgery 201:656, 1985.

Gastrointestinal and Pancreatic Rest

Gastrointestinal ileus is a common feature of acute pancreatitis, probably related to the inflammatory involvement of autonomic plexuses located adjacent to the celiac axis and superior mesenteric artery. Gastric distention with associated nausea and vomiting is common and benefits from the placement of a nasogastric tube, which also reduces the chance of aspiration. In the past, nasogastric suction and more recently the use of H_2 blockers and antacids were employed to decrease gastric acid and in turn diminish secretin release and the resulting increase of pancreatic secretion. Several well-controlled studies have failed to demonstrate any beneficial effect on the inflammatory process from either removal or reduction of gastric acid. The latter, however, may be useful in preventing upper gastrointestinal erosion and bleeding during the course of the disease.

Ventilatory Support

In the milder forms of acute pancreatitis severe respiratory failure rarely is a problem. In severe forms of the disease respiratory insufficiency may be insidious and its presence can be detected early with serial blood gas determinations. These patients benefit from increased oxygen delivered through nasal prongs or by mask. More severe respiratory failure requires intubation and assisted mechanical ventilation employing positive pressure ventilation and PEEP (positive end-expiratory pressure) to maintain adequate oxygenation.

Peritoneal Lavage

This treatment has been recommended in the approximately 10 per cent of patients who fail to respond promptly to conventional therapy. A peritoneal dialysis catheter is inserted under direct vision through a small mid-line incision inferior to the umbilicus. Dialysis is carried out with an isotonic electrolyte solution containing 15 grams of dextrose per liter. Heparin and ampicillin may be added to the solution. Two liters are infused, allowed to remain in the peritoneal cavity for 30 minutes, and then drained by gravity. This cycle is repeated hourly for 24 to 72 hours. The technique permits the removal of the inflammatory exudate which accumulates in the peritoneal cavity. Some patients show clinical improvement, including a reduction of serum amylase levels and leukocyte count and stabilization of vital signs; however, it is unclear whether this treatment modifies the ultimate outcome in cases of severe pancreatitis.

Experimental Forms of Treatment

A number of experimental studies have suggested that a variety of agents may be beneficial in the management of acute pancreatitis. Atropine decreases pancreatic secretions and relaxes the ampullary sphincter; glucagon is a potent inhibitor of pancreatic secretion; similar properties are ascribed to 5-fluorouracil and somatostatin; aprotinin (Trasylol) is a protease inhibitor. Most clinical studies involving the use of these agents have failed to clearly demonstrate a beneficial effect. A recent review of these therapeutic approaches points out that highly variable animal models employed for the study of pancreatitis and inadequate numbers of patients in clinical trials may have contributed to a less than optimal evaluation of these agents.

Role of Surgery

In the 1920s Lord Moynihan recommended surgical intervention in all patients with acute pancreatitis. By the 1940s surgical exploration was considered detrimental except in the management of pancreatic abscess. In the 1960s several authors again advocated early exploration, particularly in cases where the diagnosis was in doubt and to exclude potentially remediable problems such as intestinal strangulation, which can be difficult to differentiate from severe acute pancreatitis. The advent of new diagnostic modalities such as the CT scan has reduced the need for diagnostic laparotomy. However, surgical intervention continues to be used in the management of pancreatic abscess.

As indicated above, a high percentage of patients with acute pancreatitis have a self-limiting disease which abates with the aforementioned therapeutic measures. As the patient improves, gastrointestinal function returns with the passage of flatus and stool and loss of abdominal distention. Oral intake should be initiated with clear liquids followed by low-fat foods. Every effort should be made to identify the cause of the attack. Patients with proven biliary tract disease should have this corrected prior to discharge from the hospital to eliminate the possibility of recurrent episodes.

Complications

Hypocalcemia

Hypocalcemia may occur, especially in the severe forms of the disease (see Table 1). When present, this metabolic abnormality often indicates the presence of tissue necrosis and hence the possibility of a poor prognosis. Ionized calcium can be replaced intravenously, utilizing calcium chloride or calcium gluconate; however, therapy should be reserved for those patients manifesting clinical evidence of hypocalcemia such as a positive Chvostek's or Trousseau's sign.

Abscess

Sepsis secondary to tissue necrosis and subsequent bacterial invasion is the most common cause of morbidity and mortality in patients with severe pancreatitis. The development of abscess occurs later in the course of an attack, usually during the second or third week. CT provides the most detailed information in cases of pancreatic abscess (see Table 2). Often, small mottled collections of air can be demonstrated in one or more collections of pancreatic fluid. Fluid collections also may occur in the peripancreatic areas. Definitive diagnosis can be achieved with percutaneous skinny needle aspiration of fluid to determine the presence or absence of bacteria.

When a single infected collection is present, percutaneous drainage with a stent can be successful. In our own experience, 12 of 17 patients (71 per cent) with infected collections were successfully managed with this technique.

When multiple infected collections are present,

early operative management consisting of wide débridement is indicated. It is important to mobilize the pancreatic head and explore the lateral gutters posterior to the right and left colon, which often are involved by extension through the retroperitoneum. The area should be extensively drained with soft sump and Penrose drains. Recently, several studies have recommended that the area be left open with extensive packing, which requires repeated removal, further débridement, and repacking under general anesthesia every 48 hours in the early stages. Later repacking can be accomplished in a treatment room without need for anesthesia. Ultimately, the abdominal wound is closed, leaving drains in the residual cavity to prevent recurrent abscess formation. Early results with this method have been encouraging.

Respiratory Failure

Respiratory failure also is associated with a substantial morbidity and mortality. Although the precise mechanism for the pulmonary injury is not entirely clear, the release of lecithinase from the inflamed pancreas is thought to result in loss of pulmonary surfactant and possibly the liberation of free fatty acids, which in turn produce pulmonary capillary injury. Respiratory failure develops as a consequence of increased capillary permeability with an increase in pulmonary extravascular water and alveolar collapse. Replacement of extracellular fluid losses must be accomplished with great care to avoid further accumulation of extravasated pulmonary fluid. This is most likely to occur after 24 to 48 hours when extracellular fluid losses associated with the disease have been replaced.

Early in the course of respiratory failure an increase in inspired oxygen may be adequate treatment. The patient must be carefully followed with serial blood gases and, when indicated, endotracheal intubation and maintenance on a ventilator should be employed, often with the addition of PEEP. The use of diuretics may be helpful in mobilizing pulmonary extravascular water. Adult respiratory distress syndrome (ARDS) secondary to severe acute pancreatitis is associated with a high mortality.

Pseudocyst Formation

Peripancreatic fluid collections are quite common in the early stages of acute pancreatitis. In approximately 20 per cent of cases the fluid collection is merely an acute inflammatory exudate which can be expected to resorb spontaneously as the patient recovers (acute cysts). True pseudocysts develop as a consequence of ductal disruption associated with the pancreatic inflammatory process. The fluid, which has a high enzyme concentration, is contained by surrounding structures including the upper gastrointestinal tract, transverse mesocolon, and colon. Ultimately a dense

fibrous wall evolves to confine the collection. A high
percentage of pseudocysts that persist develop secondary to attacks of alcohol-induced pancreatitis which
is associated with ductal strictures; therefore exocrine
obstruction contributes to the persistence of the fluid
collection.

As indicated above, early in the course some fluid
collections disappear spontaneously and the incidence
of serious complication is low during the initial six
weeks. Thereafter, the chance of spontaneous resolution is minimal and there is an increase in major
complications such as spontaneous cyst rupture, cys-
tenteric fistula, and major vascular erosion. Also, during the initial six weeks, the pseudocyst wall undergoes
maturation to a dense fibrous layer capable of holding
sutures when operative correction is required.

Based on the above evidence, most surgeons
prefer to observe patients with pseudocyst for
approximately six weeks before recommending
surgical correction. Occasionally a pseudocyst
may become infected early in the course and
require external drainage either percutaneously
with a stent or by the operative route. Also, some
patients present with a pseudocyst of unknown
duration. A CT scan can be helpful in assessing
the thickness and density of the cyst wall in such
cases.

Over the years, operative internal drainage
utilizing direct cystogastrostomy and cystoduo-
denostomy or cystojejunostomy (Roux-en-Y) has
been the standard approach. Smaller cysts may
be incorporated into a lateral pancreaticojejunos-
tomy which is used to correct an underlying
ductal obstruction, a hallmark of pancreatitis
secondary to alcohol abuse. It is important to re-
emphasize that most pseudocysts occur in this
group of patients, and simple internal drainage
of the cyst does not correct the associated ductal
obstructive problem. Accordingly, the incidence
of recurrent attacks of pancreatitis and recurrent
pseudocyst formation can be expected to be high.

Hemorrhage

Severe pancreatitis may result in intrapancreatic
and peripancreatic hemorrhage. This often is associated with a drop in the hematocrit, requiring blood
replacement. In most cases the bleeding is contained
in the surrounding retroperitoneum and rarely requires operative intervention to achieve control. As
indicated above, pseudocysts may erode adjacent vascular structures such as the splenic artery and gastro-
duodenal artery; less frequently the common hepatic
artery, celiac axis, superior mesenteric artery, and
even the aorta may be involved. This complication
represents the most formidable surgical problem associated with pancreatitis. Whenever possible, the location of the vascular erosion should be identified with
splanchnic angiography. This may demonstrate a pseudoaneurysm in the wall of the pseudocyst or filling of
the cyst with contrast media.

In some cases it is possible to embolize the
affected vessel. Since the most commonly involved vessel is the splenic artery, it may be
possible in some cases to obtain proximal control
prior to operation with a balloon catheter placed
into the splenic artery. When the pseudocyst is
located in the proximal body or tail of the gland,
operative control of the proximal splenic artery
can be achieved, followed by resection of the cyst
and involved proximal gland. In other cases it is
necessary to open the cyst and attempt direct
suture ligation of the bleeding vessel followed by
external drainage of the cyst. This latter method
may not provide permanent control. The mortality rate in this group of patients remains in the
range of 50 per cent.

CHRONIC PANCREATITIS
method of
GEORGE L. JORDAN, JR., M.D.
Baylor College of Medicine
Houston, Texas

Following an attack of acute pancreatitis from which
the patient recovers, the future course of any specific
patient is unknown. Some patients have only one
attack and then remain well for the rest of their lives.
Others have recurrent mild attacks of acute pancreatitis that are not severely disabling; some have recurrent severe attacks of pancreatitis, but with intervening periods in which the patient is clinically normal.
Other patients develop deficiency syndromes and/or
chronic pain. A variety of terms have been applied to
these different clinical syndromes, including recurrent
pancreatitis, recurring pancreatitis, acute relapsing
pancreatitis, chronic relapsing pancreatitis, and, at
times, simply chronic pancreatitis. This last term is
often limited to patients who have a persistent and
continuing problem with the pancreas, secondary to
inflammatory disease. There is destruction of a significant portion of the normal cellular population of the
gland and replacement with fibrous tissue. The most
common symptom is chronic pain, whereas other manifestations of chronic disease include exocrine insufficiency and/or diabetes due to destruction of the islets
of Langerhans. In the United States the development
of calcification of the pancreas, which can be seen
radiographically, is most commonly due to chronic
pancreatitis; in other countries nutritional deficiencies
may result in this pathologic change.

Etiology

Chronic pancreatitis has been reported in patients
with all types of pancreatitis but is relatively rare in
patients with gallstone disease. Approximately 50 per
cent of patients with gallstone pancreatitis will have
recurrent attacks of acute pancreatitis if not treated

surgically. In these individuals, however, the gross and microscopic appearance of the pancreas usually returns to normal after each attack, and the function of the gland remains normal. The development of chronic pain and exocrine or endocrine deficiency is uncommon, occurring in no more than 2 to 3 per cent of patients with gallstone pancreatitis. Even some of this small percentage of patients with gallstone pancreatitis who develop chronic pancreatitis also indulge excessively in alcohol ingestion. The primary etiologic factor leading to typical chronic pancreatitis is alcohol. Chronic pancreatitis also develops in a significant percentage of patients with congenital pancreatitis, but congenital pancreatitis is uncommon and thus accounts for very few cases. The other major type of pancreatitis that may progress to chronic form is idiopathic pancreatitis. It may also occur in patients having strictures of the pancreatic duct (for example, following trauma) and is due to failure of emptying of the distal ductal system.

The exact pathogenesis of chronic alcoholic pancreatitis is not fully understood. In the past, it was presumed that it resulted from secretion of pancreatic juice under pressure against a sphincter in spasm, both factors resulting from the ingestion of alcohol. In more recent years proteinaceous plugs have been observed in the small ducts of the pancreas of patients with alcoholic pancreatitis secondary to metabolic alterations due to the alcohol ingestion. These plugs are believed to produce obstruction.

Diagnosis

In the majority of patients who develop chronic pancreatitis, the onset of their disease is an acute episode, followed by multiple acute episodes before the manifestations of chronicity are apparent. Although some patients present because of exocrine or endocrine insufficiency, or because of the presence of pancreatic calcifications, in the majority pain is the presenting symptom. In many of these patients, the pancreas is hard, firm, and somewhat shrunken but not sufficiently changed in size or contour that the pathology is easily demonstrable by ultrasound or computed tomography (CT) scan examination. In some patients, however, particularly those with severe cystic changes in the head of the pancreas, the image presented by these techniques can suggest carcinoma, and occasionally this differential diagnosis may be difficult. Changes also may be seen on barium studies of the upper gastrointestinal tract that may mimic those seen in carcinoma. In the majority of patients, however, the clinical course leaves little question concerning the diagnosis.

The most important test is endoscopic retrograde cholangiopancreatography (ERCP), with studies of both the pancreatic and common bile ducts. In the typical case there are multiple strictures of the pancreatic duct with intervening areas of ductal dilatation—the so-called "chain-of-lakes" appearance. Not all patients with alcoholic pancreatitis develop this pattern, however, and it cannot always be determined how much of the pain is due to the secretion of pancreatic juice against the partially obstructed duct, how much is due to the inflamed pancreas itself, or how much is due to inflammation of the peripancreatic tissue. Narrowing of the pancreatic duct, or even complete obstruction in some cases, is also observed in carcinoma, but the roentgenographic appearance of these two types of pancreatic ductal obstruction are sufficiently different that the diagnostic accuracy is very high.

Patients who complain of diarrhea should have an evaluation of exocrine function. At least 85 to 90 per cent of pancreatic function must be lost before there is clinical evidence of pancreatic insufficiency. Patients with chronic pancreatitis are at risk for the development of diabetes, and thus their carbohydrate metabolism should be evaluated. Periodic determinations of urine and/or blood sugar should be performed in order to recognize and treat this problem if it occurs.

There are a number of complications of chronic pancreatitis other than those that arise from destruction of the gland itself. The most common of these are obstructive jaundice due to constriction of the common bile duct as it passes through the head of the inflamed gland; pseudocyst formation; and obstruction of the duodenum due to cicatricial stenosis. When common duct obstruction is suspected, hepatic function tests and other appropriate tests should be performed. Pseudocyst is best diagnosed by CT scan or ultrasound studies; the latter is less expensive and probably more specific concerning cyst formation. Stricture of the duodenum with obstruction is fortunately much less common than with carcinoma of the pancreas, but symptoms of duodenal obstruction may occur, and this diagnosis is best made on the basis of barium meal radiography of the upper gastrointestinal tract. Other, relatively rare extrapancreatic complications include colon obstruction, which usually involves the transverse colon but may involve either the splenic or hepatic flexures, and vascular complications. There can be erosion of either the arterial or venous system with hemorrhage, as well as thrombosis of the portal or splenic vein, with portal hypertension. In rare instances, the patient with chronic pancreatitis will present with massively bleeding esophageal varices secondary to this complication. Appropriate radiographic studies will delineate colonic or vascular abnormalities, but unless the diagnosis of chronic pancreatitis has been made in the past, the findings at surgery will come as a surprise.

Management

Nonoperative Therapy

There is some evidence that reduction of serum lipids in patients with hyperlipidemia, representing an uncommon type of pancreatitis, may be of value in preventing recurrent attacks. It is recommended that patients with alcoholic pancreatitis totally abstain from alcohol ingestion, although it is not certain that cessation of alcohol ingestion will interrupt the course of the disease after the pancreatitis has reached the chronic stage. However, management of the problem of alcoholism is important in these patients, whether or not it changes the course of pancreatitis, because it is well documented that alcoholic patients have a greatly reduced life expectancy compared to the general population.

Other than these two specific recommendations, it is difficult to demonstrate that any medical treatment influences the course of the disease. There is, on the other hand, much that can be done to aid specific problems which these patients encounter. A low-fat diet to reduce pancreatic stimulation may be tolerated better than a high-fat diet. Patients who have developed diabetes should have proper management of their carbohydrate metabolism. Administration of oral pancreatic enzyme supplements are of value in patients with exocrine insufficiency.

The symptom that causes the greatest distress for patients with chronic pancreatitis is pain. The pain is often severe, intractable, and disabling. Many alcoholic patients continue to drink in an attempt to relieve the pain; when the pain is not relieved, many then take more potent narcotics and reach the point of addiction. A small percentage of patients do not have severe pain, and their main problems relate to their endocrine and exocrine deficiency syndromes. Those patients are appropriately treated nonoperatively, as there is no good evidence that any surgical procedure improves either exocrine or endocrine deficiency in such patients.

Patients with chronic pancreatitis should be followed not only for the control of the inflammatory disease but also because of the risk of carcinoma, with the diagnosis made difficult by the already existing disease. Reports have suggested that patients with chronic pancreatitis are at a higher risk for carcinoma than the population at large. General experience does not support this conclusion, but it is also true that chronic pancreatitis does not protect the pancreas from the development of carcinoma.

Although many patients with chronic pancreatitis may be shown to have some increased loss of fat in the stool on the basis of specific testing, there is no indication for treatment in the absence of diarrhea and/or weight loss due to malabsorption. When such treatment *is* necessary, the use of oral pancreatic enzymes is indicated. Viokase and Cotazym have been the most efficacious preparations in my experience. A high carbohydrate diet is also recommended, as the sugar is well absorbed, as is adequate protein to maintain good nutrition. The amount of fat in the diet can be regulated to provide as much as can be tolerated without the production of diarrhea. Predigested, so-called elemental diets are advocated by some as dietary supplements, and in the occasional patient they may be helpful. However, they are not necessary in most patients and are very poorly tolerated by others. The diabetes that develops in patients with chronic pancreatitis is an insulin-deficient diabetes due to direct damage of the islet cells. The damage may also impair the secretion of glucagon, and most patients do not require more than 20 to 40 units of insulin daily. Furthermore, some patients may have episodes of hypoglycemia, similar to that which occurs following pancreatectomy.

Surgical Therapy

Patients with severe pain are best treated surgically; such procedures can be performed safely and many patients have good long-term pain relief.

The single test that should unequivocally be performed before operative intervention is *retrograde pancreatography* to determine the status of the pancreatic duct, which may be normal, may have one area of stricture with dilatation of the duct distal to that point, or may have multiple strictures with intervening areas of dilatation of the duct ("chain-of-lakes" appearance).

When there is ductal obstruction at or near the ampulla, with dilatation of the entire ductal system beyond, or when there are multiple strictures, the treatment of choice is a *lateral pancreatojejunostomy*. This consists of opening the duct throughout the entire tail, body, and neck of the pancreas, and carrying the incision to the region of the pancreatoduodenal artery where it crosses the anterior surface of the pancreas (Puestow procedure). There are several techniques for anastomosis of the pancreas to a Roux-en-Y loop of jejunum, with no unequivocal evidence that one is definitely superior to the others; all strictures should be divided and drainage of the entire pancreas should be accomplished. Simple amputation of the tail with anastomosis to the duct at this point has not proved to be as efficacious.

Pain relief in the early postoperative period has been gratifying, with relief reported in 60 to 85 per cent of patients. Some studies report a recurrence of pain within a few years in some patients, but lasting pain relief may be achieved in over 50 per cent of patients. It has not been shown that lateral pancreatojejunostomy significantly improves the flow of digestive juice into the bowel to improve fat absorption significantly. Nevertheless, many patients gain weight following this procedure because the relief of pain, particularly following ingestion of food, allows them to increase their dietary intake significantly. This procedure also does not prevent the subsequent development of diabetes; thus, these patients need to be followed over a period of many years to monitor pancreatic function. If pain recurs, a repeat retrograde pancreatogram is indicated to rule out or demonstrate stenosis of the anastomosis. Such patients should have a second operation to re-establish the pancreatojejunostomy, as the potential for relief of recurrent pain is good.

The second surgical procedure of value is *pancreatic resection*. Whereas in most cases of chronic pancreatitis there is involvement of the entire gland, in some patients the disease is limited to either the head or the tail of the gland, and resection of the involved portion can be anticipated to give excellent results. There is not full agreement concerning the removal of the distal portion of the pancreas versus pancreatoduodenectomy in patients with diffuse disease; either procedure may be successful. When the head of the pancreas is severely diseased, pancreatoduodenectomy is likely to be the best procedure, particularly if there are multiple retention cysts. When treating pancreatitis, there is not a great deal of difference between the mortality rate with the Whipple operation and with distal pancreatectomy, in contrast to reported data concerning treatment of cancer of the pancreas. The mortality rate using the Whipple operation for pancreatitis should be below 5 per cent, and some studies have shown much lower mortality rates. In fact, there is now an increasing number of reports of low mortality rates following pancreatoduodenectomy for carcinoma of the pancreas as well.

Total pancreatectomy might seem to be the treatment of choice when this operation can be performed with an acceptable mortality rate. Good results have been reported after total pancreatectomy, but they are not significantly better than after a pancreatoduodenectomy, leaving the body and tail of the pancreas intact; thus, this more extensive operation is justified only in selected patients. One of the major problems of total pancreatectomy is the resulting diabetes. Attempts have been made to prevent this by autotransplantation of the islet cells in the resected pancreas; and by total division of all nerve supply to the body and tail of the pancreas following the Whipple operation, leaving the denervated pancreas in situ; by in situ autotransplantation; and by transplantation of the body and tail of the pancreas into the groin. Each of these procedures has been successful in preventing diabetes in some patients, but uniform success was not achieved.

The last operation that should be mentioned is *splanchnicectomy* for relief of pain. This operation can be performed safely and provides some pain relief in many patients. Although splanchicectomy is indicated for selected patients, the results are significantly inferior to those previously described; although initial results may be good, recurrence of pain is frequent.

In addition to procedures to relieve the pain of pancreatitis, surgical procedures may be specifically indicated in the treatment of other complications. Chronic pancreatitis is the most common etiology in pseudocyst production. The treatment of choice is internal drainage, which can be performed safely. Although various data suggest that one procedure may be better than another, there is no uniform consensus. The type of internal drainage should be dictated more by the location and pathology of the cyst than considerations of mortality and of long-term results. In special circumstances, resection of a pseudocyst may be the treatment of choice when it can be performed without sacrificing any organ except a portion of the pancreas, and in some patients external drainage is still employed. In most instances internal drainage not only will be safe but will be efficacious. Many patients with chronic pancreatitis who have drainage of a pseudocyst not only will have correction of the cyst but will have good relief of pain by this procedure alone. Obstruction of the common bile duct may require choledochojejunostomy; obstruction of the duodenum will require gastrojejunostomy. Stenosis of the colon and segmental portal hypertension, at times with bleeding esophageal varices, may also require surgical intervention.

Other procedures that have been utilized in the management of chronic pancreatitis include sphincterotomy, occlusion of the pancreatic duct with ligatures, and obstruction of the pancreatic ductal system by injection of nonabsorbable materials. In my opinion, for the patient with chronic pancreatitis none of these procedures is as valuable as those described in detail above. Opinion varies about the value of sphincterotomy of the minor papilla in patients with pancreas divisum; those patients reported to have good results have had relatively mild recurring pancreatitis, and even in this group, selection of patients for surgery may be difficult. There have not been good results in patients whose pancreas is chronically inflamed and fibrotic.

My experience with chronic pancreatitis indicates that these patients, as a group, do not have a normal life expectancy. Individual patients may do well and live out their lives without further difficulty, dying of other causes. Those patients who develop diabetes are at risk for the complications of this disease; those with severe exocrine insufficiency may have chronic nutritional problems; and other patients develop complications of alcoholism involving organs other than the pancreas.

Despite the fact that surgical treatment of

chronic pancreatitis is not always successful, the success rate is sufficiently high and the surgical mortality rate is sufficiently low that an aggressive surgical approach to this disease is warranted. Procedures to interrupt the course of the disease by preventing recurrent attacks or to relieve pain should be instituted prior to the time that the patient is hopelessly addicted to narcotics or has developed life-endangering complications.

PEPTIC ULCER

method of
JAMES H. LEWIS, M.D.
Georgetown University Medical Center
Washington, D.C.

The pathogenesis of peptic ulcer disease (PUD) is multifactorial, and it is important that any therapeutic approach to ulcer healing address all factors that may be associated with an increased risk of PUD. These factors include smoking, the use of aspirin and other nonsteroidal anti-inflammatory drugs (NSAIDs), certain underlying diseases (e.g., chronic lung disease, chronic renal failure, hyperparathyroidism) and environmental and emotional stress, among others. Diet therapy has never been shown to significantly alter the course of duodenal ulcer (DU) disease and has been relegated to a position of minor importance. The Inglefinger diet (three regular meals daily with avoidance of a bedtime snack or any foods or beverages that cause symptoms) seems the most sensible.

The natural history of PUD is one of recurrent exacerbations and remissions. Although the overall incidence of DU appears to be declining, the complication rate from ulcer disease has remained relatively constant, despite the introduction of the H_2 blockers and other new ulcer agents. Whether or not PUD ever eventually "burns itself out" after one or more decades (as has been suggested) is not known with any certainty. As a result, ulcer disease should be regarded as a chronic disorder and treated accordingly.

The role played by *Campylobacter pylori* in the pathogenesis of ulcer disease and its inherent tendency to relapse remains controversial. *C. pylori* is currently regarded as an important cause of nonerosive gastritis, which is found in most (but not all) patients with PUD, and which has been associated with many instances of ulcer relapse. However, since *C. pylori* is also seen in approximately 20 per cent of asymptomatic individuals (nearly all of whom harbor unsuspected nonerosive gastritis), the relationship between the organism and dyspeptic symptoms has not been fully defined. Nor has the issue of whether to look for and/or treat *C. pylori* infection been settled, as will be discussed below.

TREATMENT

Duodenal Ulcer

Short-Term Therapy

Several dozen pharmacologic agents have been developed for the treatment of duodenal ulcer.

These drugs fall into four general categories: (1) acid-neutralizing agents, (2) antisecretory drugs, (3) cytoprotective compounds, and (4) compounds with both antisecretory and cytoprotective properties (Table 1). No clinically important differences exist in the ability of any of these agents to heal ulcers acutely or to relieve ulcer symptoms. Between 60 and 80 per cent of DUs heal endoscopically at 4 weeks. Continuing therapy for an additional 2 or 4 weeks will increase healing to 90 per cent or more. In general, the antisecretory potency of a drug does not appear to correlate with its ability to heal an ulcer. Even ulcers treated with placebos heal 25 to 60 per cent of the time depending on geographic location.

Since healing and symptom relief are similar regardless of which agent is prescribed, the remaining factors that govern the rational choice of ulcer therapy must center on the issues of drug safety (adverse effects and drug interactions) and patient acceptability (compliance and cost) as discussed below.

Antacids. Antacids are a time-honored therapy for peptic ulcer disease but are inconvenient because of a dosing schedule that generally calls for 30 to 60 ml of a liquid suspension to be taken 1 and 3 hours after meals and at bedtime. Even the use of lower acid neutralizing capacity products or tablet antacid regimens requires dosing at least four times daily. Bowel dysfunction is common, with diarrhea resulting from magnesium-containing preparations and constipation from aluminum-containing products. Mineral and electrolyte disturbances, variable sodium content, the ability to interfere with the absorp-

TABLE 1. **Ulcer-Healing Drugs**

Class	Examples
Acid neutralizing	Antacids
Antisecretory	
H_2 receptor antagonists	Cimetidine, ranitidine, famotidine
Muscarinic receptor antagonists	
Nonselective	Anticholinergics, atropine
Selective	Pirenzepine*
Gastrin antagonists	Proglumide*
Tricyclic antidepressants	Trimipramine*
Cell activation inhibitors	
Calcium entry blockers	Verapamil,* nifedipine*
Proton pump inhibitors	Omeprazole*
Cytoprotective	
Sulfated disaccharides	Sucralfate
Colloidal bismuth	De-Nol,* TDB*
Licorice derivatives	Carbenoxolone,* Caved-S*
Antisecretory-Cytoprotective	
Prostaglandins E_1, E_2	Misoprostol,* Enprostil*

*Not approved by the U.S. Food and Drug Administration for ulcer treatment.

tion of numerous drugs (including cimetidine, ranitidine, digoxin, tetracycline, and isoniazid) and the fact that the cost of therapeutic amounts of many antacids is considerably more expensive than other classes of agents are several additional reasons why antacids are currently unattractive to many patients as well as physicians.

H_2 Blockers

These agents reduce acid secretion through competitive inhibition of the histamine-2 receptor on the parietal cell. Tens of millions of patients have been treated with cimetidine (Tagamet) and ranitidine (Zantac), and the safety and compliance profiles that have emerged for each drug are excellent. Short-term healing rates and symptom reduction are virtually identical for the two medications. The compounds are, however, structurally dissimilar, cimetidine having an imidazole ring and ranitidine a furan ring. This chemical difference probably accounts for some, if not all, of the important clinical differences that have become apparent between the two drugs. Famotidine (Pepcid) and nizatidine (Axid) are the two newest agents in this class. Both possess a thiazole ring structure. However, clinical experience has been limited in comparison with cimetidine and ranitidine, and the complete safety profiles of famotidine and nizatidine remain to be defined. Neither agent appears to offer any advantages in terms of clinical efficacy, safety, or compliance as compared with ranitidine. Perhaps the most important distinction to be made among the H_2 blockers is the inhibitory effect of cimetidine on the hepatic cytochrome P450 mixed-function oxidase (MFO) system. The result of this MFO inhibition is a reduction in hepatic clearance, leading to an increased serum concentration of many drugs, including warfarin, theophylline, phenytoin, benzodiazepines, lidocaine, and propranolol. In some patients these increased blood levels may result in clinically evident toxicity: e.g., bleeding from warfarin; arrhythmias, diarrhea, and convulsions from theophylline; nystagmus, ataxia, and confusion from phenytoin, and so on. Ranitidine, famotidine, and nizatidine have only one-tenth the affinity of cimetidine to inhibit the P450 MFO system, and suspected instances of pharmacologic drug interactions are very rare.

The antiandrogenic effects seen with cimetidine (impotence, gynecomastia, and breast tenderness) generally do not occur unless the drug is taken in large doses for long periods of time (e.g., in Zollinger-Ellison syndrome). Ranitidine is not antiandrogenic and has been used successfully in patients with these cimetidine-induced antiandrogenic effects. Both famotidine and nizatidine appear to be devoid of antiandrogenic side effects. Headaches are probably the most commonly reported side effect seen with ranitidine and famotidine. Mental confusion has been reported with all four drugs, but would appear to be more common in cimetidine recipients, especially those with multiple organ failure in an intensive care unit (ICU) setting.

None of the currently available H_2 blockers is intrinsically hepatotoxic, although mild hepatic dysfunction and rare instances of overt hepatitis have been reported for all four agents. The incidence and clinical severity of hepatitis appears similar for cimetidine and ranitidine. Instances of hepatitis were identified during clinical trials of both famotidine and nizatidine, and the true incidence of hepatic injury remains to be defined for these two newer H_2 blockers. There are no reports of hepatitis from the intravenous use of these drugs. The potential use of cimetidine in the prevention of hepatic injury from acute acetaminophen overdose remains theoretical and investigational. No instances of acetaminophen-induced liver injury have been reported in volunteers or patients receiving ranitidine.

Each H_2 blocker is effective when used twice daily, and all have been approved for use as a single bedtime dose to control nocturnal acid and improve patient compliance. The move to bedtime dosing (800 mg cimetidine; 300 mg ranitidine; 40 mg famotidine; and 300 mg nizatidine) is based in part on the pioneering work on vagotomy conducted more than 40 years ago by the American surgeon Lester Dragstedt. His studies suggested it is nocturnal acid secretion that is most important in terms of ulcer pathogenesis. Recent studies indicate that taking the H_2 blocker just after the evening meal may be an even more effective means of controlling acid and healing ulcers.

Other Antisecretory Drugs. *Anticholinergics* are not suited for primary therapy of peptic ulcer disease because of inferior healing rates and unwanted side effects. Their role is presently confined to that of adjunctive therapy in certain patients with the Zollinger-Ellison syndrome and other hypersecretory states that are poorly controlled with H_2 blockers. But even here, newer agents (e.g., omeprazole) may soon make this role obsolete.

Tricyclic antidepressants are not officially approved for use in peptic ulcer disease, but they have been successfully employed in ulcer patients requiring psychotropic drug therapy. Whether or not their effects are additive to those of H_2 blockers or other agents remains speculative. *Pirenzepine* is a drug with selective antimuscarinic and tricyclic antidepressant properties that is in use outside of the United States. Clinical experience has not demonstrated any advantages over H₂ blockers. *Omeprazole* (investigational drug), a substituted benzimidazole, is a potent inhibitor of the H^+/K^+ ATPase (proton) pump of the parietal cell. Although it was temporarily suspended from clinical investigation in 1985 owing to reports of gastric enterochromaffin-like (carcinoid) tumors in rats, it is presently being used in Zollinger-Ellison syndrome patients without apparent toxicity, and clinical trials have resumed in DU patients. This agent appears to be particularly effective in patients with refractory DU and reflux esophagitis because of its extremely potent antisecretory effects.

Cytoprotective Drugs. Agents that heal ulcers through mechanisms other than inhibition or neutralization of gastric acid are termed "cytoprotective." *Sucralfate* (Carafate) has been in use for more than 15 years and has proved to be an excellent alternative agent for short-term therapy of peptic ulcer disease. Although some patients have complained of slower initial pain relief compared with H₂ blockers, overall healing efficacy and symptom reduction at the end of 4- to 8-week trials are not significantly different from other agents.

Constipation is the most commonly reported side effect with sucralfate, the result of the high aluminum content of the compound. Since sucralfate is very poorly absorbed, no systemic side effects are expected. However, it may interfere with the absorption of other agents, such as tetracycline and phenytoin. Accordingly, it should not be given concomitantly with other drugs and should be taken at least 30 minutes prior to meals to avoid being bound to food. Although initially designed to be given as 1 gram four times daily, twice daily regimens may be equally effective but are not currently approved by the FDA.

Prostaglandin analogs of the E1 and E2 classes are presently in use for DU outside of the United States. While healing efficacy is similar to that of the H₂ blockers, no advantages over these or other agents have emerged and concerns about safety (e.g., diarrhea and potentially abortifacient effects) continue to delay FDA approval.

Combination Ulcer Therapy

Antacids are widely prescribed with H₂ blockers and other agents to help control ulcer symptoms, although they are usually unnecessary for this purpose. Only a few studies have examined the usefulness of two or more therapeutically active agents taken together to promote ulcer healing. In one well-controlled trial, no advantage was found for the combination of cimetidine

plus sucralfate (both given four times a day) compared with either agent used alone. It is doubtful that any other combination would be of additional benefit. Combination therapy for bleeding ulcers or refractory ulcers has not been well studied.

Follow-Up

In contrast to gastric ulcers, it is generally not necessary to document healing of a DU following short-term therapy. If ulcer symptoms remain well controlled throughout the course of treatment, most physicians do not repeat the endoscopy or upper GI series, even though it is well known that there is a poor correlation between symptoms and the presence or absence of the ulcer after therapy with H₂ blockers. On the other hand, if the symptomatic response at the end of therapy is not satisfactory, it may be useful to document healing (or nonhealing) and the presence or absence of *C. pylori* to help determine the direction that future therapy or additional diagnostic evaluation should take.

Prevention

Up to 80 per cent of healed ulcers will relapse endoscopically within 1 year after therapy is withdrawn. This relapse rate is virtually the same, regardless of whether healing is accomplished with antacids, H₂ blockers, or other antisecretory agents and no matter how long the acute therapy is extended prior to being discontinued. The one exception appears to be bismuth compounds, which are associated with significantly lower relapse rates after acute healing than occur after treatment with H₂ blockers. This has been attributed to the eradication of *C. pylori* infection and resolution of the accompanying gastric (and possibly duodenal) inflammation.

Since most DUs remain in remission only during the time that active therapy is being administered, a number of long-term treatment approaches have been developed. The most commonly employed method utilizes a low dose of an H₂ blocker (usually half of the nocturnal dose used for short-term healing, e.g., cimetidine, 400 mg; ranitidine, 150 mg; famotidine, 20 mg; or nizatidine, 150 mg) given daily at bedtime. One-year DU relapse rates can be reduced from 80 per cent to 20 or 30 per cent using these agents, with the relapse rate for patients on ranitidine thought to be somewhat lower than that for cimetidine. Much less information and clinical experience is available for other agents. Maintenance therapy with sucralfate, 1 gram twice daily, is effective but is currently awaiting

FDA approval for this indication. Antacids given several times throughout the day have been shown to be as effective as other agents. They are not effective when given only at bedtime and are not recommended by this author for patients with a severe underlying ulcer diathesis.

A small number of patients will experience a "breakthrough" relapse while on maintenance therapy. These relapses tend to be clinically mild, relatively easy to re-heal, and less likely to be associated with ulcer complications compared with relapses that develop in individuals not receiving preventative therapy.

To date, the longest controlled maintenance trials conducted with H_2 blockers have lasted only 5 to 6 years. However, cumulative relapse rates suggest that an ulcer that remains healed during the first year of maintenance therapy will continue to do so during subsequent years. Just how long such preventative therapy can or should be continued is unclear at this time. Few adverse side effects from long-term continuous administration of the H_2 blockers in maintenance doses have been observed or are expected. While some individuals have expressed concern that gastric cancer might develop from prolonged exposure to these agents, this complication remains more theoretical than practical, as it has not been borne out in experimental or clinical studies. Nevertheless, in an effort to avoid continuous long-term therapy in selected patients, an "intermittent" treatment approach has been devised. Initiated by the physician for a documented or suspected ulcer relapse, full-dose medication (generally an H_2 blocker) is restarted and continued for at least 2 weeks after symptoms abate. The average DU patient will require treatment for only 5 to 6 weeks per year using this alternative approach. For individuals with frequent symptomatic relapses (especially smokers, chronic NSAID users, patients with a long history of DU disease) and those with a history of hemorrhage or other ulcer-related complications, the use of continuous (daily) low-dose maintenance therapy, or ulcer surgery, is recommended over the use of "intermittent" therapy.

For patients in whom chronic (perhaps several years and even possibly life-long) maintenance therapy is recommended but is not acceptable for any number of reasons, consideration should be given to a surgical means of ulcer prevention. The favored operation in some centers is a parietal cell vagotomy. Although it has a lower perioperative and postoperative morbidity and mortality rate compared with more conventional operations, it also has a higher recurrence rate and has fallen out of favor with some surgeons. Nevertheless, its recurrence rate of 2 to 3 per cent per year compares quite favorably with an annual relapse rate of 20 to 30 per cent for medical therapy.

Gastric Ulcer

Short-Term Therapy

The same drugs used in DU therapy are used to treat gastric ulcers (GU), but the healing rates are generally 10 to 25 per cent lower than those observed for DU, reflecting, in part, differences in the pathophysiology of the two conditions.

Prepyloric and pyloric channel ulcers are anatomically in the stomach but behave clinically in fashion similar to that of DU and should be treated similarly. A careful history concerning the ingestion of aspirin and other NSAIDs should always be taken. Discontinuing the offending agent is sometimes all that is necessary, but the addition of sucralfate (for its cytoprotective properties) or an H_2 blocker for a few weeks is sometimes recommended. It is probably unnecessary to perform a biopsy of a benign-appearing channel ulcer or a prepyloric ulcer that has been confidently ascribed to an NSAID or other agent. In contrast, the risk of a non–drug-related GU being malignant (approximately 1 to 3 per cent) mandates that most if not all GUs be followed endoscopically or radiographically until they heal completely. A combination of endoscopically directed biopsies and brushings for cytologic findings can accurately exclude malignancy in over 99 per cent of cases and should be obtained early in all patients in whom the endoscopic or radiographic findings are equivocal or suspicious for gastric cancer.

Drug-induced and prepyloric (peptic-type) gastric ulcers can be expected to heal after 6 to 8 weeks of therapy with sucralfate or an H_2 blocker. For other types of GU, up to 15 weeks may be required for healing, depending on their size. It should be remembered that even a malignant GU can partially heal on therapy. Therefore, any GU that does not heal completely on an intensive medical regimen after an appropriate length of time (e.g., 8 to 12 weeks for ulcer diameter < 2.5 cm and 12 to 15 weeks for an ulcer > 2.5 cm) should be seriously considered for surgery.

Refractory Ulcers

Approximately 10 to 25 per cent of DUs remain unhealed after 4 to 8 weeks, regardless of the agent employed. Noncompliance with the prescribed treatment regimen, cigarette smoking, the continued use of NSAIDs, and gastric acid hypersecretion are the most common reasons why ulcers fail to heal. Several reports of "cimetidine-resistant" DUs that were subsequently responsive to ranitidine have appeared. However, in most instances the initial treatment period was only 4 to 6 weeks. This may have been too short a time to label an ulcer as truly "resistant," and it is equally as likely that continued treatment with cimetidine for an additional 2 to 4 weeks would have resulted in the same rate of healing as was accomplished by switching to ranitidine. Actual "resistance" to an active agent due to genetic or other factors is thought to be exceedingly rare.

If, however, an ulcer is judged to be refractory to a standard course of H$_2$ blocker therapy, treatment options include (1) continuing the same drug at the same or a higher dose, (2) trying a different H$_2$ blocker, or (3) switching to a completely different class of agent, e.g., sucralfate or omeprazole. In our unit many patients with refractory ulcers have been found to have idiopathic hypersecretion of acid. We have had good success treating these patients with increased doses of H$_2$ blockers to keep the basal acid output (BAO) below 10 mEq per hour.

Special Circumstances

Ulcer Disease in Pregnancy. Pregnancy is normally associated with a lower incidence of DU relapse and ulcer complications than is the nonpregnant state, although some patients may require treatment during gestation. While none of the generally prescribed ulcer healing drugs is approved for use during pregnancy, antacids and sucralfate are probably safe, especially after the first trimester. H$_2$ blockers are excreted in breast milk and are not recommended for nursing mothers.

Ulcer Disease in Children. The same drugs used in adults may be used to heal PUD in children, recognizing that there is far less experience with these agents in the younger age groups.

Treatment of *Campylobacter pylori* Infection

The in vitro sensitivity of *C. pylori* to many agents correlates poorly with their actual in vivo effects. The treatment combination of a bismuth compound for the first 7 days (e.g., Pepto Bismol two tablets or 30 ml four times daily on an empty stomach) plus the addition of a concomitant antibiotic (e.g., amoxicillin, 500 mg four times daily; erythromycin, 500 mg four times daily; or metronidazole, 50 mg three times daily) for the next 10 to 14 days produces an eradication rate of only 50 to 60 per cent. Relapse rates of *C. pylori* infection are high, and follow-up biopsy, culture, or urea breath testing is recommended following treatment to assess the clearance of *C. pylori* infection.

Side effects of bismuth generally are only cosmetic (e.g., black stools and darkening of the tongue), but encephalopathy is reported with prolonged use. Antibiotics in this setting have been associated with the usual hypersensitivity reactions and *Clostridium difficile*–related colitis (even among those receiving metronidazole). Thus, the decision to treat *C. pylori* with these agents must take such risks into account. Since ulcers have been shown to heal quite well with H$_2$ blockers, despite the presence or persistence of *C. pylori* infection, treatment of *C. pylori* is not necessary if the therapeutic response to conventional ulcer therapy is satisfactory. However, if dyspeptic symptoms persist after treatment with H$_2$ blockers or if ulcer relapses are frequent when therapy is discontinued, the knowledge that *C. pylori* is present may provide for a reasonable treatment alternative.

TUMORS OF THE STOMACH

method of
CHARLES W. CHAPPUIS, M.D., and
ISIDORE COHN, JR., M.D.
Louisiana State University School of Medicine
New Orleans, Louisiana

The majority of primary gastric tumors are malignant, and, of these, adenocarcinoma is the most common histologic type. Benign tumors of the stomach are rare and can be classified as either submucosal (intramural) or mucosal (polyps). The most common presenting symptoms of both benign and malignant tumors are pain, weight loss, nausea and vomiting, and bleeding. Although still a useful diagnostic tool, the upper gastrointestinal series has all but been replaced by fiberoptic endoscopy as the diagnostic procedure of choice. The reported accuracy rate for combined endoscopy with biopsy is 98.8 per cent. Computed tomography has been useful in evaluating patients for extragastric spread of disease. Information regarding gastric wall thickness, extension into adjacent organs, nodal enlargement, liver metastasis, and ascites may be useful in treatment planning.

BENIGN TUMORS

Submucosal Lesions

Benign submucosal lesions are usually single and include leiomyomas, ectopic pancreas, fibromas, vascular tumors, lipomas, and neurogenic tumors. Leiomyoma is the most common benign submucosal tumor. The majority of these lesions are discovered incidentally during endoscopic or roentgenographic examination or incidentally at operation. Attempts at endoscopic biopsy are frequently unrewarding because of the submucosal location of these tumors. If there are no significant contraindications, these lesions should be surgically excised. Attempts at enucleation should be avoided because of the difficulty in distinguishing between benign and malignant varients. Tumors on the greater curvature can often be removed with a wedge excision. Large lesions and those situated on the lesser curvature may require formal gastrectomy for extirpation.

Mucosal Lesions (Polyps)

Gastric polyps can be defined as either adenomatous or hyperplastic. Approximately 75 per cent of gastric polyps are hyperplastic or inflammatory and rarely undergo malignant change. They are frequently multiple and are usually distributed evenly over the antrum and fundus. The histology should be determined by endoscopic biopsy. Unless they are symptomatic they do not require any specific therapy.

Adenomatous polyps tend to be located in the antrum and are more often single. The likelihood of malignancy is related both to size and histologic type. Polyps greater than 2 cm in diameter have a 25 to 50 per cent chance of malignancy. Adenomatous polyps may be categorized into three histologic types: tubular, tubulovillous, and villous adenoma. The incidence of carcinoma in a tubular adenoma is 5 per cent, whereas the incidence in villous adenoma has been reported to be as high as 50 to 70 per cent.

Treatment of gastric polyps depends on the size, number, and location. All polyps should be biopsied endoscopically to determine the histologic type and whether malignancy is present. Hyperplastic polyps usually do not require removal unless they are symptomatic or malignancy cannot be excluded. Pedunculated adenomatous polyps can usually be removed by endoscopic polypectomy, and a thorough histologic evaluation for malignancy should be carried out. Sessile and large pedunculated polyps often require operative removal.

MALIGNANT TUMORS

Adenocarcinoma is the most common malignancy involving the stomach (95 per cent). Gastric lymphoma constitutes about 4 per cent of gastric malignancy and the remaining 1 per cent includes leiomyosarcoma, squamous cell carcinoma, angiosarcoma, and carcinoid. The incidence of gastric carcinoma is decreasing in the United States. Stomach cancer deaths have rap-

idly declined from a rate of 30 per 100,000 in 1930 to 8 per 100,000 today. Conditions associated with gastric malignancy include pernicious anemia, chronic atrophic gastritis, previous subtotal gastrectomy, immunodeficiency disorders, adenomatous polyps, and hypertrophic gastropathy. Several studies have shown a relationship between certain dietary factors and gastric cancer. Food items that have been implicated include starch, pickled vegetables, salted fish, and meat. Foods containing nitrosamines or polycyclic hydrocarbons such as benzpyrene have also been implicated in the development of gastric cancer.

The majority of gastric cancers are located in the distal stomach with at least half originating in the antrum, particularly along the lesser curvature. Tumors can be classified into one of three categories based on gross morphology and are as follows: (1) the infiltrating type, which in the latter stages is referred to as linitis plastica; (2) the ulcerating type, commonly found in the antrum along the lesser curvature; and (3) the polypoid type of tumor, more commonly found in the body and fundus of the stomach. Early gastric cancer as described by the Japanese is limited to the mucosa and submucosa regardless of lymph node status.

Surgical Resection

The two major factors that influence survival in resectable lesions include the depth of invasion through the gastric wall and the status of regional lymph node involvement. Carcinoma of the stomach can only be cured by surgical resection. Treatment depends on the ability to resect the primary lesion. Radical subtotal gastrectomy yields the highest survival statistics for those lesions resected for cure. Proximal third lesions often require total gastrectomy; however, this procedure should not be done for palliation. Approximately 50 per cent of patients operated on for gastric cancer undergo what is thought to be a curative resection. Resection of the primary lesion is the best form of palliation and is indicated even when cure is not possible.

The overall 5-year survival rate for patients with gastric cancer is 7.5 per cent, and approximately 25 per cent for patients with curative resection. The absence of lymph node involvement improves the 5-year survival rate by two- to fourfold. Tumors classified as early gastric cancers have the most favorable 5-year survival rates, in the range of 95 per cent.

Chemotherapy

Although often used in patients with advanced disease, the results with chemotherapy as a primary mode of therapy are generally poor. Chemotherapy as an adjuvant to surgical treatment has been reported to prolong survival and delay recurrence in treated patients. Combination drug therapy using FAM (fluorouracil [5-FU], doxorubicin [Adriamycin], and mitomycin C [Mutamycin]) has been used as an adjuvant to curative resection with positive response rates reported to approach 40 to 50 per cent.

Radiation Therapy

The use of radiation therapy alone to treat gastric cancer does not prolong survival. Combined radiotherapy and chemotherapy has been evaluated but does not seem to offer any benefit. Good results have been reported in palliation of obstructing cancers of the gastroesophageal junction and distal stomach. The results of radiation therapy in gastric lymphoma as an adjunctive measure as well as for palliation have been much better than for adenocarcinoma.

TUMORS OF THE COLON AND RECTUM

method of
LASALLE D. LEFFALL, JR., M.D.
Howard University College of Medicine
Washington, D.C.

COLORECTAL CANCER

Colorectal cancer is the second most common cancer (excluding skin cancer) in the United States, exceeded in incidence and mortality only by lung cancer. In 1988 there were an estimated 147,000 new cases (105,000 colon and 42,000 rectal) with approximately 61,500 deaths. The disease occurs with almost equal frequency in both sexes, although colon cancer is somewhat more frequent in females and rectal cancer is slightly more frequent in males. Approximately one in 20 American adults will have cancer of the colon and rectum during their lives. Three tests are important in the early detection of colorectal cancer: (1) digital rectal examination, (2) stool blood test, and (3) proctosigmoidoscopic examination (rigid or flexible).

To aid in the proper use of these procedures, the American Cancer Society has issued the following guidelines for the cancer-related checkup for colorectal cancer: (1) men and women over age 50 years should have a stool blood test every year, (2) men and women over age 50 should have

annual sigmoidoscopic examinations until two consecutive examinations are normal and thereafter every 3 to 5 years, and (3) men and women over age 40 should have a digital rectal examination every year.

Persons who are at a high risk for colorectal cancer should receive more frequent and intensive examinations beginning at an earlier age. This includes persons with familial polyposis, Gardner's syndrome, ulcerative colitis, a personal history of colorectal polyps or cancer, and a family history of colorectal polyps or cancer and endometrial cancer.

Epidemiology and Etiology

Almost all colorectal cancers progress through a polyp (adenoma) phase before they become malignant. These adenomas range in diameter from several millimeters to several centimeters. That the great majority of colorectal cancer patients are over 40 years of age evidently reflects the unusually long induction time for a cancer to become clinically apparent—perhaps 5 to 10 years or longer. Since it takes so long for an adenoma to develop and then transform into a carcinoma, it is understandable that the incidence of colorectal cancer increases with age. Only a small proportion of adenomas develop into cancer, but the presence of an adenoma puts a patient at increased risk for colorectal cancer. The removal of adenomas detected by sigmoidoscopy sharply reduces the incidence of rectosigmoid cancer in the examined bowel.

The cause of colorectal cancer is unknown, but three predisposing factors are genetics, environmental toxins, and diet. Most of the current evidence, however, suggests that colorectal cancer may be attributable to a dietary imbalance, specifically to a high-fat, low-fiber diet. As with the environmental toxins, the evidence is primarily correlational and therefore does not establish a cause-and-effect relationship.

Since almost all colorectal cancers arise from adenomas, the primary high-risk factor for colorectal cancer is the presence of an adenoma or adenomas. Histologically, there are three types of colorectal adenomas: (1) tubular adenomas (most common), (2) villous adenomas, and (3) tubulovillous adenomas. The vast majority (95 per cent) of colorectal adenomas never become malignant; only about 5 per cent actually progress to cancer. Tubular adenomas have a low malignant potential, whereas adenomas with a villous component have the greatest potential for malignancy. The probability of adenomas becoming malignant is related directly to their number, size, degree of villous transformation, and presence or absence of dysplasia.

Inflammatory bowel disease constitutes about the only nongenetic predisposition to colorectal cancer, although the disease itself may be an inherited condition. Regardless of age, a patient with long-standing ulcerative colitis is five to ten times more likely to become affected by colorectal cancer than is the general population—about 35 to 50 per cent of such patients develop cancer. Crohn's disease (granulomatous enterocolitis) is considered to be premalignant, especially when the age of onset is before age 21 years. The magnitude of the risk for colorectal cancer, however, is much less than that associated with ulcerative colitis. There is low incidence of small bowel adenocarcinoma associated with both Crohn's disease and Gardner's syndrome.

Clinical Manifestations

Although detection of asymptomatic colorectal cancer is the ideal, in reality clinical manifestations most often alert the clinician to the possibility of cancer. The signs and symptoms of colorectal cancer differ, depending on the location, size, and stage of the disease, but sometimes include abdominal pain or discomfort, blood in or on the stool, and change in bowel habits.

Rectal bleeding is the most common symptom of colorectal cancer. In right colon cancer, blood is usually dark or mahogany red and mixed in the stool, while in lesions of the left colon and rectum, it is a brighter red and coats the surface of the stool. The passage of bloody mucus usually indicates cancer, polyps, or, less commonly, ulcerative colitis.

Abdominal pain is another significant symptom of colon cancer. In right colon cancer, the pain is vague, dull, and annoying and may be confused with gallbladder disease or peptic ulcer. The characteristic feature of the pain is that it is uncharacteristic. In left colon cancer, pain is usually secondary to obstruction of the colon and produces what the patient often refers to as "gas" or "cramps." Pain is a late manifestation in patients with rectal cancer.

Other clinical manifestations of right colon cancer include anemia (secondary to bleeding) and a palpable mass in the right lower quadrant of the abdomen. In left colon cancer, pain and bleeding are accompanied by a decrease in the caliber of stools, change in bowel habits, and increased use of laxatives. A common complication of left colon cancer in the adult is acute large bowel obstruction, usually in the region of the sigmoid or rectosigmoid, although other sites may be involved. These patients present with increasing abdominal distention, abdominal pain, vomiting, and constipation progressing to obstipation. Cancer of the cecum or ileocecal valve must always be considered in older patients with symptoms of appendicitis or low small bowel obstruction. Emergency barium enema examination is indicated in these cases.

Signs and symptoms of rectal cancer, other than bright red bleeding, include a sense of incomplete evacuation and tenesmus. Cancer of the anus also produces bright red bleeding and local discomfort and may be confused with hemorrhoids. Rectal bleeding in adults should never be ascribed to hemorrhoids (even in those patients with a history of hemorrhoids) without first searching for additional lesions by proctosigmoidoscopy, barium enema study, and/or colonoscopy. Enlarged inguinal nodes, secondary to metastases, may be found in patients with anal cancer.

Patients with suspicious findings of colorectal cancer must be thoroughly examined for signs of metastatic cancer. These include supraclavicular adenopathy (Virchow's nodes); an enlarged nodular liver; ascites; Blumer's rectal shelf; palpably enlarged, firm ovaries (Krukenberg's tumors), and nodules in the region of the umbilicus.

In addition to routine physical examination and history taking, four diagnostic procedures should be performed on most patients suspected of having colorectal cancer: (1) digital rectal examination, (2) proctosigmoidoscopy (flexible or rigid), (3) barium enema study, and (4) colonoscopy.

Digital rectal examination was once sufficient to detect 30 per cent of all colorectal lesions, but with a proximal redistribution of neoplasia occurring over the past 20 years, it now can detect only about 10 per cent of all such lesions Similarly, the estimated yield with the standard proctosigmoidoscopic examination has decreased from 75 per cent to about 50 per cent.

Barium enema study and colonoscopy are complementary and thus aid in determining the presence or absence of synchronous lesions. The use of colonoscopy in patients with colorectal cancer begins preoperatively. Two to 5 per cent of such patients will have a synchronous carcinoma elsewhere in the colon and 40 to 50 per cent will concurrently have one or more adenomas. Patients in whom obstructive tumor, clinical condition, or incomplete bowel preparation precludes preoperative total colonoscopy should undergo this procedure within 3 to 5 months after operation. The high risk of subsequent metachronous carcinoma (3 to 5 per cent) and adenoma (10 to 30 per cent) in these patients has led many clinicians to adopt annual total colonoscopy as the primary means of intraluminal surveillance. However, the adequately performed barium enema study with air contrast in a well-prepared colon remains of value in diagnosis and follow-up and may be used to complement colonoscopy, with colonoscopy and barium enema alternating on an annual or biannual basis. If either is unsatisfactory, the other should be performed.

Screening and Survival

Preliminary results of screening for colorectal cancer seem promising. However, there are insufficient data now available to know whether the use of the stool blood test can decrease mortality from colorectal cancer. Clinical trials are now under way, and their early results are expected in 4 to 5 years. Because of the limitations of the test and the intermittent nature of bleeding from colorectal cancer or adenomas, all persons over 50 years of age should be regularly followed in the health care system regardless of the outcome of the stool blood test. The following screening tests are important in the early detection of colorectal cancer: (1) the digital rectal examination, (2) the stool guaiac slide test, and (3) the proctosigmoidoscopic examination (rigid or flexible).

The fecal occult blood test will detect 90 per cent of all patients who actually have colorectal lesions that bleed. It is a relatively sensitive and specific test with acceptable false-negative and false-positive rates when used appropriately.

The use of commercially available guaiac-impregnated slides is a valuable, simple, inexpensive, and esthetically acceptable method of testing the feces for blood. Several studies have conclusively shown that the test can detect cancer in asymptomatic persons, when the disease tends to be in an early stage. This is especially important, as recent data indicate that about half of all colorectal cancers lie beyond the reach of the rigid sigmoidoscope. The test can also detect a large proportion of polyps (adenomas). The American Cancer Society recommends an annual stool guaiac slide test for all persons aged 50 years and over.

Whenever possible, the stool guaiac slides should be mailed to patients prior to a checkup. Patients are asked to prepare two separate stool samples at home on each of three consecutive stool specimens and to bring the slides at the time of the checkup as soon as the six samples have been collected. To increase the accuracy and discriminating ability of the stool analysis, a meat-free, vitamin C–free, high-fiber diet should be implemented at least 48 hours before the first slide is prepared. Iron and aspirin should be avoided because they may cause gastric irritation, yielding false-positive results, whereas vitamin C can interfere with the peroxidase reaction, causing false-negative results.

Specimens should be stored for no more than 4 days before testing. All test results should be recorded as positive or negative. Testing is done without hydration to decrease the incidence of false-positive reactions. Doubtful readings should be recorded as negative and trace readings as positive. A single positive slide should be handled as if all slides are positive. All positive tests should be followed up by complete radiologic and/or endoscopic examination.

Early enthusiasm for carcinoembryonic antigen (CEA) determinations as a screening test for colorectal cancer has waned following evidence that the test is positive in both cancerous and noncancerous lesions. Its greatest potential value will probably be to help to determine the effectiveness of therapy and indicate prognosis. Further immunologic studies of CEA are being conducted.

Treatment

For those patients in whom a diagnosis of colorectal cancer is established, surgical resection is the treatment of choice. The preoperative evaluation includes a general medical workup, blood tests including carcinoembryonic antigen (CEA), chest radiography, intravenous pyelography, and liver scan, if indicated.

An adequate cancer operation involves removal of the primary tumor and wide excision of the mesentery with its contained regional lymph nodes and lymphovascular pathways.

Cancer of the right colon is treated by right hemicolectomy with an end-to-end ileotransverse colostomy. An extended right hemicolectomy is preferred for lesions of the hepatic flexure or proximal transverse colon. Cancer of the left colon is treated by left hemicolectomy, whereas lesions in the region of the splenic flexure are managed best by extended left hemicolectomy. Lesions of the mid-transverse colon may be treated adequately by transverse colectomy. For lesions in the mid-portion of the sigmoid colon, sigmoid resection with anastomosis may be performed; however, for lesions in the distal sigmoid or the upper rectum (above 12 cm from the anal verge), anterior resection is preferred. For lesions in the mid-rectum (8 to 12 cm from the anal verge), low anterior resection or abdominotranssacral resection is performed in an attempt to have a 2.0 to 5.0 cm margin of normal rectum distal to the cancer. The absolute minimum is 2.0 cm if local recurrence is to be decreased.

Lesions of the low rectum are treated by the Miles abdominoperineal resection. Usually this operation is required for lesions located from 0 to 8 cm from the anal verge.

Solitary metastases in the liver, if readily accessible, should be removed. If metastatic disease is confined to the lateral segment of the left lobe of the liver, this segment may be removed. However, right hepatic lobectomy is generally not advocated for metastatic colon cancer, although it may be performed in selected cases. An arteriogram is performed before a proposed hepatic resection. Furthermore, there is increased use of hepatic artery infusion of chemotherapeutic agents for metastatic liver disease. The value of this modality is still being evaluated. Even in the presence of multiple hepatic or peritoneal metastases, palliative resection of the colon is generally indicated, if the patient's condition will permit, in order to decrease the possibility of perforation, hemorrhage, or obstruction. The roles of radiation therapy and chemotherapy are still being evaluated in the treatment of rectal cancer. Preliminary data suggest that these modalities improve survival in Dukes B and C lesions. Further study is needed.

COLORECTAL POLYPS

Patients with polyps typically present with rectal bleeding, prolapse through the anus, and, rarely, intussusception. The most common polypoid lesion is the adenomatous polyp (tubular adenoma), occurring almost eight times more frequently than the villous adenoma. Juvenile polyps are found principally in children under 12 years of age but occasionally may develop in adults. Multiple polypoid lesions are usually noted in patients with familial polyposis or Gardner's syndrome. Patients with these hereditary disorders will usually have colorectal cancer by the age of 40 to 50 years unless total colectomy is performed. Thus, families with a history of these conditions must be followed very carefully.

Colonoscopy and barium enema examination with air contrast are essential in the differential diagnosis of cancer. The larger the polyp, the greater the risk of cancer; lesions larger than 1.5 cm to 2.0 cm are more likely to be malignant than those smaller than 1 cm.

INTESTINAL PARASITES
method of
CHAU NGUYEN, M.D., and
RALPH E. WARREN, M.D.
University of Toronto
Toronto, Ontario, Canada

The importance of intestinal parasites has steadily increased throughout the 1980s as a direct outcome of the epidemic of acquired immunodeficiency syndrome (AIDS) and recognition of the "gay bowel syndrome." A wider spectrum of physicians is, therefore, continuing to encounter and treat patients with intestinal parasites more frequently. Treatment is often challenging and sometimes unsuccessful when the immune system is persistently suppressed. Travelers are increasingly adventurous and are visiting more exotic and less restricted places, sometimes with greater health risks. Immigration from developing countries continues to be encouraged.

History

The most important question is: "Where have you been?" Epidemics and endemics vary in different parts of the world. The history obtained from the patient should go back over a considerable period of time, as certain parasites such as *Strongyloides stercoralis* and *Entamoeba histolytica* can survive in humans for several years without causing symptoms. Exposure to tropical bodies of fresh water should create a suspicion of schistosomiasis. Contact with pets or farm animals is associated with some nontyphoidal *Salmonella* infections, hydatid cyst disease, toxocariasis, and several other parasitic and bacterial infections.

Children in day-care centers have a high incidence of *Giardia* and *Cryptosporidium* infections. A significant proportion of immigrants from Southeast Asia have hookworm, *Clonorchis,* and *Strongyloides* infections. Patients infected with the human immunodeficiency virus (HIV) may be harboring the parasites *Giardia, Cryptosporidium,* and *Isospora.* Other organisms such as *Candida,* cytomegalovirus, and atypical mycobacteria may coexist and complicate the clinical findings.

Symptoms

The spectrum of signs and symptoms is broad, ranging from absence of symptoms in a carrier to an acute abdominal crisis. Parasites can infect organs other than the abdomen, creating difficulties in diagnosis. The asymptomatic patient may be passing *Entamoeba histolytica* cysts or *Schistosoma mansoni* ova. Acute travelers' diarrhea is usually self limited, but the presence of blood in the stool or high fever indicates invasive disease caused by *Shigella, Campylobacter, Salmonella,* or *Entamoeba histolytica.* Patients recently treated with antibiotics should have stool specimens evaluated for the toxin assay and culture of *Clostridium difficile.*

Schistosomiasis may present with bleeding gastroesophageal varices secondary to portal hypertension. Cysticercosis often presents with a seizure because of cerebral cysts. A cough or transient pneumonitis may be seen during the migratory stage of hookworm, *Ascaris,* or *Strongyloides* infestation. The fish tapeworm *Diphyllobothrium* may cause vitamin B_{12} deficiency. Amebic abscess may be found in the liver, lung, or brain.

Chronic travelers' diarrhea has not been widely investigated. It can be caused by *Giardia, Entamoeba histolytica, Aeromonas,* tropical sprue or, by exclusion, the postinfectious irritable bowel syndrome. Nonparasitic conditions such as adult celiac disease, ulcerative colitis, and Crohn's disease may become unmasked by an episode of travelers' diarrhea.

Parasites infecting the small bowel, such as *Giardia* and *Strongyloides,* may cause upper gastrointestinal symptoms, such as bloating, flatulence, and cramps in giardiasis and peptic ulcer–like symptoms in strongyloidiasis. Lower abdominal symptoms are seen with parasitic infection of the large bowel (e.g., *Entamoeba histolytica*) or in heavy infections of *Trichuris trichiura.*

Patients may pass adult worms by mouth or per rectum. Large adult worms may be seen with *Ascaris,* smaller ones with *Anisakis, Trichuris,* and occasionally *Enterobius.* Worm fragments are most commonly passed per rectum with *Taenia.*

Treatment

Intestinal Parasites

Drug therapy for intestinal protozoa and helminths are summarized in Tables 1 and 2.

Amebiasis. Infection with amebae is discussed in a separate article in Section 2 of this text.

Ascaris. The adult worm usually lives less than a year in the human small bowel. Drugs of choice are mebendazole and pyrantel pamoate, and both are well tolerated. If a patient requires more than one drug for multiple parasitic infections, ascariasis should be treated first because some drugs will induce migration of ascarids into the biliary-pancreatic tree. Mebendazole (Vermox) can occasionally cause abdominal pain, diarrhea, and rarely leukopenia. Pyrantel pamoate (Antiminth) may cause gastrointestinal disturbance, headache, rash, dizziness, and fever.

If an ascarid is lodged in the common bile duct or pancreatic duct, constant nasogastric suction and parenteral fluids should be tried first for several days to encourage the worm to return to the duodenum. Endoscopic retrograde cholangiopancreatography (ERCP) with or without papillotomy may be required to remove the worm. Rarely is surgery required.

Balantidium coli. This ciliated protozoan rarely infects man. The majority of patients have had prior contact with pigs or pig excrement. Symptoms are similar to amebiasis, including fulminating dysentery. Treatment using tetracycline, iodoquinol (Yodoxin), or metronidazole is effective.

Blastocystis hominis. This protozoan may cause diarrhea when present in large numbers. Treatment often decreases symptoms and the parasitic burden, but recurrences are common. Iodoquinol (Yodoxin) is the best treatment. Its major toxic reaction is subacute myelo-optic neuropathy (SMON) after prolonged use. In doses recommended for treating intestinal protozoa, iodoquinol does not cause optic atrophy. However, it

may cause thyroid enlargement and interfere with thyroid function tests for several months. It is contraindicated in patients with iodine intolerance or hepatic damage. Asymptomatic *Blastocystis* carriers should probably not be treated unless they are food handlers or otherwise at risk of contaminating others.

Cryptosporidium. This is a coccidian protozoan recently recognized as a cause of severe, protracted diarrhea in immunocompromised patients and of significant, although self-limited, enteritis in the immunocompetent host. It is a common cause of diarrhea worldwide, infecting as many as 7 per cent of children in the developing world. Prevalence in day-care centers in the United States ranges from 6 to 54 per cent.

Most AIDS patients infected with *Cryptosporidium* have severe diarrhea (up to 25 times per day), with voluminous watery bowel movements (up to 20 liters per day), associated with severe dehydration, wasting, and cachexia. Cryptosporidial cholecystitis and cholangitis have been described in immunocompromised hosts. In immunocompetent hosts, diarrhea usually lasts an average of 10 to 14 days without treatment. Clinically, the infection closely resembles giardiasis and isosporiasis.

There is currently no known effective therapy for cryptosporidial infection. Successful management has only occurred when the immune defect could be reversed by discontinuation of immunosuppressive therapy. Spiramycin has a modest efficacy, with a lack of toxicity, and is used extensively. Permission to use spiramycin is obtained through the Division of Anti-Infective Drug Products, United States Food and Drug Administration; telephone (301) 443–4310. The drug itself must be obtained from Rhone-Poulenc Pharmaceuticals in Montreal, Canada; telephone (514) 384–8220.

Alpha-difluoromethylornithine (DFMO) (investigational) for treatment of cryptosporidial infection was recently studied in several trials with mixed success. Unfortunately, severe toxicity (bone marrow suppression and gastrointestinal irritation) has limited its use.

Dientamoeba fragilis. This protozoan, a flagellate, is seen frequently in association with pinworm infection. It may cause diarrhea and abdominal pain. Treatment consists of iodoquinol (Yodoxin), tetracycline, paromomycin (Humatin), or diphetarsone (Bémarsal).

Enterobius vermicularis (Pinworm). Although pinworm infection is not of special importance in travelers or immigrants, pinworm eggs are occasionally found when stools of such patients are examined. Whole families are often affected, so that the entire family and close contacts should

TABLE 1. **Drug Therapy for Intestinal Protozoan Parasites**[1]

Parasite	Drug	Adult Dose[2]	Pediatric Dose[2]	Availability
Balantidium coli	Tetracycline[3] or	As per *D. fragilis*	As per *D. fragilis*	
	Iodoquinol[3] or	As per *D. fragilis*	As per *D. fragilis*	
	Metronidazole	750 mg tid × 5 days	35–50 mg per kg per day in 3 divided doses × 5 days	Flagyl (Searle)
Blastocystis hominis	Iodoquinol or	As per *D. fragilis*	As per *D. fragilis*	
	Metronidazole	750 mg tid × 10 days	35–50 mg per kg per day in 3 divided doses × 10 days	Flagyl (Searle)
Cryptosporidium	Spiramycin[4]	3 grams/day in divided doses for 2–4 weeks	As per *E. histolytica* for 5 days	Rovamycin (Rhone-Poulenc/Montreal) (tablets)
Dientamoeba fragilis	Iodoquinol or	650 mg tid × 20 days	40 mg per kg per day in 3 divided doses × 20 days (max, 2 grams per day)	Yodoxin (Glenwood, Inc.) (tablets)
	Tetracycline or	500 mg qid × 10 days	10 mg per kg qid × 10 days (max, 2 grams per day [use only for children over 7 years of age])	
	Paromomycin or	25–30 mg/kg/d in 3 doses × 7 days	25–30 mg/kg/d in 3 doses × 7 days	Humatin (Parke-Davis) (tablets)
	Diphetarsone[5]	500 mg tid × 10 days	<1 yr: 50 mg/kg 1–3 yr: 250 mg bid 3–5 yr: 250 mg tid 5–10 yr: 500 mg bid >10 yr: Adult dose[5]	Bémarsal (Rhone-Poulenc) (tablets)
Entamoeba histolytica	See separate article on amebiasis			
Giardia lamblia	Quinacrine HCl or	100 mg p.c. tid × 5 days	2 mg per kg p.c. tid × 5 days (max. 300 mg/day)	Atabrine (Winthrop-Breon) (tablets)
	Metronidazole[3]	250 mg tid × 5 days	5 mg per kg tid × 5 days or <25 kg: 35 mg/kg	Flagyl (Searle) (tablets)
	or	2 grams once daily × 3 days	25–40 kg: 50 mg/kg >40 kg: Adult dose (once daily × 3 days)	
	Furazolidone	100 mg (tablet) qid × 7–10 days	1.25 mg per kg qid × 7–10 days (suspension)	Furoxone (Norwich-Eaton) (tablets and suspension)
Isopora belli	Trimethoprim/ sulfamethoxazole[3] (TMP/SMX) or	160 mg TMP and 800 mg SMX qid × 10 days, then bid × 3 weeks; chronic suppression with 1 tablet daily may be necessary		Bactrim (Roche) Septra (Burroughs Wellcome) (tablets)
	Pyrimethamine	50–75 mg daily for sulfonamide-sensitive patients		Daraprim (Burroughs Wellcome) (tablets)

[1]Adapted from previous editions of this text and The Medical Letter.
[2]All recommended drugs given by mouth.
[3]Considered investigational for this indication by the FDA.
[4]Not approved in the United States. Permission to use this drug must be obtained from the FDA, telephone (301) 443-4310. *Cryptosporidium* is self-limiting in immunocompetent patients (see text).
[5]Not available in the United States; permission must be obtained from the Bureau of Drugs, Health Protection Branch, Ottawa, Canada.

TABLE 2. **Drug Therapy for Intestinal Helminths**[1]

Parasite	Drug	Adult Dose[2]	Pediatric Dose[2]	Availability
Ascaris lumbricoides	Mebendazole or	100 mg bid × 3 days	Same as adult dose (for children over 2 years)	Vermox (Janssen) (tablets)
	Pyrantel pamoate or	11 mg per kg single dose (max. 1 gram)	Same as adult dose (max, 1 gram)	Antiminth (Pfipharmecs) (suspension)
	Piperazine citrate	75 mg per kg per day × 2 days (max, 3.5 grams per day)	Same as adult dose (max, 3.5 grams per day)	Antepar (Burroughs Wellcome) (syrup)
Enterobius vermicularis (pinworm)	Pyrantel pamoate or	11 mg per kg single dose; (max, 1 gram; repeat after 2 weeks)	Same as adult dose (max, 1 gram)	
	Mebendazole	100 mg single dose; repeat after 2 weeks	Same as adult dose (for children over 2 years)	
Hookworm: *Necator americanus*	Mebendazole or	As per *Ascaris*	As per *Ascaris*	
Ancylostoma duodenale	Pyrantel pamoate[3]	As per *Ascaris* daily for 3 days	As per *Ascaris* daily for 3 days	
Intestinal flukes: *Fasciolopsis buski*	Praziquantel[3] or	25 mg per kg tid for 1 day	Same as adult dose	Biltricide (Miles) (tablets)
	Niclosamide	As per *T. saginata*	As per *T. saginata*	Niclocide, Yomesan (Miles) (tablets)
Heterophyes heterophyes	Praziquantel	As per *F. buski*	As per *F. buski*	
Metagonimus yokogawai	Praziquantel	As per *F. buski*	As per *F. buski*	

Liver flukes:
  Clonorchis sinensis
  Opisthorchis viverrini
	Praziquantel[3]	25 mg per kg tid for 2 days	Same as adult dose	

Fasciola hepatica	Bithionol[3]	30 to 50 mg per kg on alternate days × 10 to 15 doses	Same as adult dose	Bitin (Parasitic Disease Service, Centers for Disease Control, Atlanta, GA) (tablets)
Schistosomiasis: *Schistosoma mansoni*	Praziquantel or	20 mg per kg tid for 1 day	Same as adult dose	Biltricide (Miles) (tablets)
	Oxamniquine	Caribbean & South American strains: 15 mg per kg single dose	10 mg per kg bid	Vansil (Pfipharmecs) (tablets)
		African strains: 15 mg per kg bid × 1 day East Africa; × 2 days Egypt and South Africa	Same as adult dose	
Schistosoma japonicum	Praziquantel	As per *S. mansoni*	As per *S. mansoni*	
Schistosoma mekongi	Praziquantel	As per *S. mansoni*	As per *S. mansoni*	
Schistosoma haematobium	Praziquantel	As per *S. mansoni*	As per *S. mansoni*	
Strongyloides stercoralis	Thiabendazole	25 mg per kg bid × 2 days (max, 3 grams per day)[4]	Same as adult dose	Mintezol (Merck, Sharp and Dohme) (tablets)

Tapeworms:
  Taenia saginata
  Taenia solium
  Diphyllobothrium latum and
  pacificum
	Niclosamide
	or
		Single dose of 4 tablets (2 grams) chewed thoroughly	11–34 kg: single dose of 2 tablets (1 gram), >34 kg: single dose of 3 tablets (1.5 grams)	Niclocide, Yomesan (Miles) (tablets)

Dipylidium caninum	Praziquantel[3]	10 to 20 mg per kg once	Same as adult dose	Biltricide (Miles) (tablets)
Hymenolepis nana	Praziquantel[3] or	25 mg per kg once	Same as adult dose	
	Niclosamide	Single 2-gram dose (4 tablets) followed by 1 gram (2 tablets) daily × 6 days	11–34 kg single dose of 2 tablets (1 gram) × 1 day then 1 tablet (0.5 gram) daily × 6 days, >34 kg: a single dose of 3 tablets (1.5 grams) × 1 day, then 2 tablets (1 gram) daily × 6 days	
Trichostrongylus sp.	Thiabendazole[3] or	As per *Strongyloides*	As per *Strongyloides*	
	Pyrantel pamoate[3]	As per *Ascaris*	As per *Ascaris*	
Trichuris trichiura	Mebendazole or	As per *Ascaris*	As per *Ascaris*	
	Diphetarsone[5]	As per *Dientamoeba fragilis*, Table 1	As per *D. fragilis*, Table 1	

[1]Adapted from previous editions of this text and The Medical Letter.
[2]All recommended drugs given by mouth.
[3]Considered investigational for this indication by the FDA.
[4]For disseminated strongyloidiasis, thiabendazole should be continued for at least 5 days.
[5]Not available in the United States; permission must be obtained from Bureau of Drugs, Health Protection Branch, Ottawa, Canada.

be treated simultaneously, with either a single dose of pyrantel pamoate or mebendazole. Treatment should be repeated in 2 weeks.

Close attention to personal hygiene (i.e., handwashing before meals and after use of the toilet, grooming of nails, thorough laundering of all bedclothes, sheets, and towels, etc.) should be encouraged.

Flukes. Praziquantel (Biltricide) is effective against all liver, lung, and intestinal flukes. It may cause sedation, gastrointestinal discomfort, fever, and eosinophilia. There are limited data on the effectiveness of praziquantel in *Fasciola hepatica* infection. Bithionol (Bitin), an investigational alternative drug for *Fasciola* infection, often causes vomiting, abdominal pain, diarrhea, urticaria, and photosensitivity.

Giardia lamblia. Infection with this parasite is worldwide in distribution. It is the most common pathogenic parasite detected in stool samples in public health laboratories. It is often seen in campers and hikers as well as travelers returning from many regions, including the Soviet Union. Outbreaks in day-care centers are common, and several water-borne outbreaks have occurred in the western and northeastern United States. Male homosexuals appear to be at great risk of infection.

Patients suspected of harboring *Giardia,* but with negative stool examinations, may require duodenal aspiration or small bowel biopsy for verification of giardiasis. Quinacrine (Atabrine) is the drug of choice and is very effective. Side effects include dizziness, headache, vomiting, and diarrhea. Yellow staining of skin, nightmares, rash, and blood dyscrasias also are occasionally seen. Toxic psychosis is a rare side effect; therefore, a prior history of neuropsychiatric disorders is a contraindication for the use of this drug. It is also poorly tolerated in children. Like metronidazole, it can cause a disulfiramlike reaction with alcohol intake, and like chloroquine, it exacerbates psoriasis and porphyria.

Metronidazole (Flagyl), although somewhat less effective, is better tolerated than quinacrine. Equally effective and more convenient is a short course of metronidazole, 2 grams in a single dose for 3 consecutive days, taken before breakfast or at bedtime. Side effects are nausea, diarrhea, cramps, metallic aftertaste, and a disulfiram-like reaction with any alcohol intake. Metronidazole is both mutagenic and carcinogenic in experimental animals but has been used extensively for over 30 years in pregnant women without apparent deleterious effects. However, its use should be avoided in pregnancy, especially in the first trimester, unless the severity of the illness warrants the risk.

Furazolidone (Furoxone), a second alternative for treatment of giardiasis, is better tolerated in children than quinacrine. It may cause headache, nausea, vomiting, allergic reactions, a disulfiramlike reaction to alcohol, and hemolysis in the presence of glucose-6-phosphate dehydrogenase (G6PD) deficiency.

In patients with chronic giardiasis, combination use of metronidazole (750 mg 3 times daily) and quinacrine (100 mg 3 times daily) for 14 days has been found to be quite effective. Chronic giardiasis has been frequently diagnosed in cases of primary hypogammaglobulinemia.

Hookworms. Although severe anemia is less frequently seen with hookworm infection than in the past, this infection is still important in recent immigrants, especially children. Mebendazole and pyrantel pamoate are effective. Iron therapy may also be required. It is not necessary to retreat until the stools no longer contain eggs unless there are major persistent symptoms.

Isospora belli. The coccidial parasites *Isospora belli* and *Cryptosporidium*, both cause chronic watery diarrhea and weight loss in AIDS patients. Trimethoprim-sulfamethoxazole (Bactrim, Septra) has been used successfully for isosporiasis. Long-term treatment may be required in some immunocompromised patients because the rate of recurrence is high. In sulfonamide-sensitive patients, pyrimethamine, 50 to 75 mg daily, has been effective.

Schistosomiasis. Praziquantel (Biltricide) is the drug of choice for all forms of schistosomiasis. Any patients shedding ova in their stools should be treated. Praziquantel is well tolerated. Because of an increased abortion rate in experimental animals, pregnancy is a relative contraindication for its use. Sclerotherapy of gastroesophageal varices may be useful to minimize the risk of further hemorrhage after variceal rupture in the hepatosplenic form of schistosomiasis.

Strongyloides stercoralis. This worm is unusual in several respects: in light infections, it is difficult to detect and may cause no symptoms; its cycle of auto-infection allows it to remain active for prolonged periods (over 20 years); and it may become a systemically invasive opportunistic infection, with fatal consequences, when malignancy or AIDS develops or when immunosuppressive therapy is prescribed (e.g., corticosteroids). It frequently causes persistent mild eosinophilia. If this occurs and stool specimens are negative for *Strongyloides* larvae, duodenal drainage and small bowel biopsies should be performed for further searches, especially in immigrants, even if they arrived several decades previously. A course of thiabendazole is justified in patients with unexplained eosinophilia who are to receive immunosuppressive therapy, who have resided in the tropics, and in whom thorough investigations for *Strongyloides* have produced negative results.

Thiabendazole (Mintezol) is usually effective in uncomplicated infections, using a 2-day course. In disseminated strongyloidiasis, treatment should be continued for at least 5 days and immunosuppressive therapy should be discontinued. When immunosuppression cannot be reversed and the worms cannot be irradicated, monthly 2-day courses of thiabendazole may be administered to prevent hyperinfection. Thiabendazole is often poorly tolerated because of nausea, vomiting, and vertigo. Alternative drug choices are albendazole (Zental) and ivermectin (Mectizan).

Tapeworms. Uncomplicated intestinal tapeworm infections with *Taenia saginata* (beef tapeworm), *Taenia solium* (pork tapeworm), *Diphyllobothrium latum* and *pacificum* (fish tapeworms), and *Dipylidium caninum* (dog tapeworm) are best treated with a single dose of niclosamide (Niclocide) or praziquantel (Biltricide). In the case of *Hymenolepis nana,* praziquantel is the drug of choice.

Caution should be used in treating *Taenia solium.* Therapy with niclosamide or praziquantel results in the release of the eggs of *Taenia solium* from the proglottids, which are then passed as free eggs per rectum. In the absence of strict enteric precautions, these eggs can inadvertently be transmitted to the patient's mouth (external auto-infection) or that of others, and ingestion can result in cysticercosis. In the past, an oral purge of magnesium sulfate (15 to 30 grams) has been recommended. This may decrease the risk of internal auto-infection causing cysticercosis; however, if marked diarrhea ensues, careful personal hygiene may be more difficult to practice, increasing the risk of external auto-infection and subsequent cysticercosis.

Trichuris trichiura (Whipworm). *Trichuris trichiura* is the second most commonly detected parasite on mass survey in the United States and is frequently seen in association with other parasite infections. Patients are usually asymptomatic unless the colon contains a heavy worm load. One course of mebendazole removes most of the worms, and it is not necessary to re-treat until the stools no longer contain eggs.

Nonpathogenic Protozoa

Several nonpathogenic amebae and flagellates are commonly detected on stool examination. These nonpathogens include *Entamoeba hartmanni, Entamoeba coli, Endolimax nana, Iodamoeba butschlii, Chilomastix mesnili, Trichomonas hominis, Retortamonas intestinalis,* and *Enteromonas hominis.* Their presence indicates that the host has ingested fecally contaminated food or water, but their presence does not usually cause symptoms. Therefore, treatment is not necessary, even in food handlers. Occasionally, technicians may misinterpret some of these protozoa for pathogenic ones such as *Entamoeba histolytica.*

Section 7

Metabolic Disorders

BERIBERI
(Thiamine [Vitamin B$_1$] Deficiency)

method of
AKIHIRO IGATA, M.D.
University of Kagoshima
Kagoshima, Japan

Classic beriberi, once prevalent in Asian rice-eating countries, is widespread in alcoholics in the United States and Europe. The prevalence has decreased, perhaps as a result of economic improvement and the spread of medical knowledge about thiamine deficiency and its prevention.

Thiamine deficiency can occur with manifestations of beriberi. Beriberi can occur in persons who have inadequate nutritional intake, malabsorption, malignancy, anorexia nervosa, or other wasting diseases; possibly, it occurs during dialysis in those with renal insufficiency. It can be easily prevented by the administration of thiamine. Infantile beriberi that is due to inadequate intake of thiamine by the mother is also preventable.

Even in improved nutritional conditions, latent thiamine deficiency can occur as a result of poor selection or unbalanced food intake. This is exemplified by the resurgence of beriberi in Japan from 1973 to 1979. We found that this was partly due to the high intake of sugar contained in soft drinks, since artificial sweeteners, such as saccharine, were banned because of the danger of carcinogenicity.

The thiamine requirement in adults is approximately 0.5 mg per 1000 calories (kcal), or 1.5 mg or more per day (although requirements may vary in each country), depending on body weight. Ideal balance of food energy requires that carbohydrate should be lower than 60 per cent of total energy with sufficient thiamine. The requirement increases if there is fever, infection, heavy physical exercise, hyperthyroidism, or pregnancy. Growing children should be assured of having adequate thiamine. The prevention of beriberi is quite easy if we eat a well-balanced diet. Beriberi should be prevented by adequate food intake and not by the administration of thiamine as a drug. These problems should be settled by social education regarding the importance of balanced nutrition and customs of daily diet. We should always be aware of foods that are rich or deficient in thiamine content.

In malnutrition, beriberi appears along with deficiencies of other nutrients like niacin and vitamin B$_{12}$, so that pure beriberi is rare. It is also said that beriberi can sometimes combine with pellagra. Thus, the diagnosis of multivitamin deficiency can be more applicable in many cases. Sometimes, in malnutrition of total energy insufficiency, the requirement of thiamine becomes rather low if the intake of carbohydrates is low. Thiamine is present in legumes, fresh vegetables and fruits, sweet potatoes, nuts, and meats, especially pork. In Japan, dietary change involving less rice and focusing more on other foods has been the major cause of disappearance of beriberi.

Polished rice with poor other foods, which is still popular in Japan, should be avoided. Although thiamine-rich rice, fortified with synthetic thiamine, is now being sold in Japan, this has not been widely accepted.

Some foods contain thiaminase, which inactivates thiamine. These include some kinds of Chinese tea, Japanese ferns, and other items. However, the occurrence of beriberi due to such foods is quite rare and easily avoidable.

Diagnostic Considerations

Even now, latent deficiency of thiamine is prevalent in rice-eating countries. The symptoms include general malaise and anorexia. Thiamine deficiency can be confirmed by nutritional study of inadequate thiamine intake; biochemical analysis, such as low thiamine and high pyruvate levels in blood; low excretion of thiamine in urine with rapid and transient increase after thiamine administration; and low transketolase activity in blood cells and its increase by thiamine pyrophosphate (TPP).

The symptoms of beriberi center on neurologic as well as cardiovascular manifestations. Numbness and sensory impairment of extremities of the glove-and-stocking type, sometimes combined with perioral numbness, are common neurologic complaints. Diminished or absent deep tendon reflexes are also a cardinal sign. Muscle tenderness, especially in the calves, is a characteristic sign of beriberi. In severe cases, there is weakness, especially in the lower extremities. If symptoms are left untreated, persistent paresis with muscle atrophy leading to a bedridden state can occur. Muscle cramps are also fairly common. Cranial nerve signs are usually absent, although aphonia and deafness have been rarely noted.

Bilateral pedal edema is the most common sign along with other cardiovascular manifestations. In severe cases, ascites, pleural effusion, facial edema, and sometimes anasarca can be seen. Such cases are termed wet beriberi. Cardiomegaly is the most prominent symptom. Tachycardia with palpitations, breathlessness with low diastolic pressure, and a wide pulse pressure can be found in almost all cases. The high cardiac output can be improved by administration of thiamine.

All these manifestations can be diagnosed as beri-beri, especially if supplemented by the aforementioned biochemical and nutritional studies. Patients with severe, untreated cases are susceptible to infection and sudden death. These symptoms are similar to beriberi in chronic alcoholics as a result of dietary restriction and heavy daily alcohol drinking. High incidence of Wernicke's encephalitis is reported among alcoholics.

Infantile beriberi is also very rare. Its characteristics include onset within the first year of life, dominant cardiac involvement (fulminant form), vomiting, restlessness, dyspnea, edema, tachycardia, anorexia, and insomnia. Sometimes these are complicated with convulsions.

Treatment

The prevention and early diagnosis of latent thiamine deficiency are the most important steps for its treatment. Oral administration of thiamine is satisfactory for the treatment of beriberi except for acute and emergent cases. Usually, 25 to 50 mg per day of thiamine is given, although 75 to 150 mg is also given in severe and acute cases. Intramuscular or intravenous administration is recommended in emergent cases. Drug administration need not be continued beyond the acute stage if suitable thiamine-containing foods are provided. The effectiveness of thiamine administration can be noted by the disappearance of symptoms, especially of edema, palpitations, and cardiomegaly, and later by recovery of polyneuropathy. The reappearance of deep tendon reflexes within several weeks can be confirmed after all other symptoms disappear.

Needless to say, the most important treatment of beriberi is diet therapy. Attention should also be paid to the coexisting deficiency of other nutritional constituents. A parenteral route should be employed in malabsorption syndrome or in cases with vomiting. Infantile beriberi sometimes presents as an emergency, but children respond promptly to thiamine administration by any route.

Beriberi is now regarded as a disease of the past, and its importance can sometimes be forgotten to the extent of a misdiagnosis. Aggravating factors, like infection or high fever, hyperthyroidism, or severe physical exercise, should be avoided in patients with latent deficiency. The more important step should be adequate health to prevent thiamine deficiency. Concerning the treatment of Wernicke's encephalitis, immediate and large doses of thiamine are necessary as in emergent cases of beriberi.

DIABETES MELLITUS IN ADULTS

method of
N. V. EMANUELE, M.D.,
M. A. EMANUELE, M.D., and
A. M. LAWRENCE, M.D., Ph.D.
Loyola University of Chicago Stritch School of Medicine
Maywood, Illinois

Over 10 million Americans have diabetes mellitus, which is one of the world's most common and important diseases. Most adults with diabetes have the Type II disease and are not prone to ketosis. Almost a decade ago the National Diabetes Data Group formulated new diagnostic criteria for diabetes mellitus, applicable to the diagnosis of both Type I and Type II disease, and applicable to all age groups (Table 1).

Treatment

As in any chronic disease, perhaps the most important management strategy that can be undertaken is patient education. The four major areas of therapeutic intervention continue to be diet, exercise, sulfonylureas, and insulin.

Diet

Diet has been, and continues to be, the mainstay of treatment for the majority of adults with diabetes mellitus. Nutritional recommendations for the individual patient with diabetes are similar to those of the American Heart Association, the American Cancer Society, and the 1986 U.S. Dietary Guidelines. A registered dietitian with expertise in diabetes management should be closely and frequently involved in the meal plan and its implementation.

TABLE 1. **Diagnostic Criteria: Diabetes Mellitus in Nonpregnant Adults***

A. Fasting plasma glucose $\geq$ 140 mg/dl on more than one occasion. If this criterion is met, oral glucose tolerance test (OGTT) is not required.

Or

B. If fasting plasma glucose is less than in A, diagnosis can be made by OGTT, showing sustained elevation of glucose concentration on more than one occasion defined as follows:

Both the 2-hour plasma glucose sample and some other sample taken between administration of the 75-gram glucose dose and 2 hours later must be $\geq$ 200 mg/dl.

Or

C. Presence of the classic symptoms of diabetes, such as polyuria, polydipsia, ketonuria and rapid weight loss, together with gross and unequivocal elevation of plasma glucose.[†]

*Criteria are different for children and pregnant adults (see Diabetes 28:1039–1057, 1979).

[†]The National Diabetes Data Group did not define "gross and unequivocal elevation of plasma glucose."

The number of calories prescribed should be tailored to achieve and maintain a desirable body weight. In general, caloric allotment should be distributed consistently throughout the day with three regular meals, a bedtime snack, and one or more between-meal snacks. The distribution of the calories should be divided into the following: carbohydrate, protein, and fat allowances:

1. The carbohydrate content can be liberal, with 55 to 60 per cent of the total calories given as carbohydrate. Close individualized attention to the impact on blood glucose and lipid levels in the patient is mandatory. Unrefined carbohydrates with fiber should be substituted for highly refined carbohydrates, which tend to be lower in fiber content. Although modest amounts of sucrose and other refined sugars appear to be acceptable, careful attention must be paid to the patient's metabolic profile and body weight.

2. The recommended dietary allowance for protein is 0.8 gram per kg of body weight for adults, with the qualification that elderly subjects may require more than this. If renal insufficiency is a concomitant problem for the patient, protein restriction would need to be advocated.

3. Total cholesterol and fat intake should be restricted, with total fat composing less than 30 per cent of the total calories and cholesterol less than 300 mg per day. Saturated fat should be replaced with unsaturated fat as often as possible, since this may slow the progression of atherosclerosis. While it is felt that monounsaturated fats and eicosapentanoic acid (fish oil) are acceptable in the diabetic diet, more research is necessary to define their value.

In addition to the distribution of total calories into carbohydrate, protein, and fat, the sodium intake should not be more than 1000 mg per 1000 kilocalories and not to exceed 3000 mg per day. Caution must be exercised regarding salt restriction in patients with poorly controlled diabetes, postural hypotension, or fluid imbalance. Vitamins and minerals may be necessary in certain selective instances, but there is no evidence to support supplementation of the diabetic patient with vitamins and minerals in general. Similarly, calcium supplements may be necessary only under special circumstances but are not a strict recommendation for an individual with diabetes. Fiber supplementation is beneficial only if given with a diet comprising at least 50 per cent of the calories as carbohydrate. An intake of up to 40 grams of fiber per day or 25 grams per 1000 kilocalories of food appears to be advantageous. The use of nutritive and nonnutritive sweeteners is acceptable, but to offset the possible disadvantages that may result from excessive consumption of a single agent, the use of several nonnutritive sweeteners is encouraged.

A meal plan appropriate for the individual's lifestyle and based on the patient's diet history should be determined prior to the initiation of the diabetic diet. It is essential that the meal plan, education, and counseling program be tailored for the patient. The meal plan must be realistic and provide as much flexibility as possible, allowing integration of therapeutic measures into the daily routine. For the obese patient dietary intervention directed at weight reduction appears to have a great impact on morbidity and mortality. The metabolic improvements achieved with weight reduction in obese patients include not only diminution in hyperglycemia, hyperlipidemia, and hypertension, but also proteinuria, improved pulmonary function and operative risk, and reduction in musculoskeletal difficulties. With weight reduction the need for oral hypoglycemic agents or insulin may be reduced or eliminated. Thus, the benefits of weight loss relative to the progression of diabetes may be critical to the long-term prognosis of the patient and must be emphasized.

Exercise

The second aspect of the management of the patient with diabetes mellitus is exercise. It is necessary to distinguish clearly between the acute effects on carbohydrate metabolism of a single period of exercise and the long-lasting, chronic effects of regular repeated exercise over months and years (training effect).

Acute Effects of Exercise in the Diabetic. The acute effects of exercise on glucose metabolism apply primarily to Type I diabetics or Type II patients receiving insulin. In nondiabetics increased uptake of glucose by muscle during exercise is matched by increased hepatic output of glucose, so that circulating plasma glucose concentrations are generally kept within the normal range. This beautiful example of precise metabolic engineering is accomplished, at least in part, by a fall early in the exercise period of plasma insulin coupled with a rise in glucagon and epinephrine during prolonged exercise. Although the increased uptake of circulating glucose by exercising muscle is largely, if not completely, insulin-independent, the enhanced hepatic provision of glucose by accelerated glycogenolysis and gluconeogenesis is critically dependent on the fall in insulin. Patients taking insulin are therefore vulnerable to hypoglycemia, since the circulating insulin levels (largely derived from exogenous insulin administration) may not fall and, thus, may not allow for unleashing of hepatic glucose output to match the increased muscle demands for fuel. This danger of exercise-induced hypoglycemia is compounded by the exercise-induced increase in absorption of insulin from injection sites and, if patients exercise regularly, increased sensitivity to the effects of insulin. Besides hypoglycemia during or immediately after exercise, hypoglycemia may be delayed, occurring as late as 6 to 15 hours *after* unusually strenuous exercise is completed.

In contrast to hypoglycemia, exercise may sometimes actually worsen hyperglycemia. This is liable to happen if a patient starts exercising when in poor metabolic control (i.e., a plasma glucose level greater than 300 mg per dl). Presumably, these patients are underinsulinized and exercise leads to increases in circulating glucagon and epinephrine; in the face of inadequate insulin action this leads to exuberant hepatic glucose output with worsening of the plasma glucose and, in some cases, unmasking of ketosis. This underscores the point that other aspects of diabetic therapy cannot be neglected when the patient is exercising.

Limitations imposed by the complications of diabetes and other medical conditions need to be taken into account in tailoring the program for the diabetic. Some general guidelines are:

1. Patients should exercise regularly—daily, if possible.

2. The program must include forms of exercise that the patient enjoys; our patients usually start with walking.

3. Patients should not exercise if the blood glucose is high (> 300 mg per dl), since exercise may worsen glucose levels in this situation.

4. Because of the potential for exercise-induced hypoglycemia, on exercise days patients should decrease insulin dosage by 15 to 20 per cent and should increase carbohydrate intake prior to exercising. The actual insulin dose decrement and calorie increase should be adjusted, based on the effects of this initial regimen on plasma glucose, as determined by home blood glucose monitoring.

5. Limitations imposed by cardiac, peripheral vascular, or neurologic status, as well as by other concurrent disease processes, have to be taken into account. Analysis of cardiac reserve capacity may be indicated in selected patients. Some investigators have cautioned that diabetics with proliferative retinopathy should avoid strenuous exercise because of concern that exercise-associated rises in blood pressure, transmitted to the fragile retinal vasculature, may result in vitreous hemorrhage. In addition, since exercise leads to proteinuria and since some believe that proteinuria itself worsens diabetic nephropathy, the presence of proteinuria is theoretically a *relative* contraindication to intense exercise.

Chronic Effects of Exercise in the Diabetic. While it is clear that exercise has acute effects on blood glucose level (with acute defined as up to 15 hours after the exercise period), whether regular exercise can lead to reduced blood sugars beyond 15 hours after exercise (training effect) is doubtful. That long-term exercise enhances insulin sensitivity is supported by the observation that nondiabetic trained athletes have excellent glucose tolerance, despite much-reduced insulin secretory responsiveness. It seems clear that in Type I and Type II diabetics, as in nondiabetics, insulin sensitivity is enhanced by exercise but, interestingly, this has *not* consistently been translated into lower blood glucose levels between exercise periods. There are some reports showing that regular physical training can improve blood glucose levels between bouts of exercise in Type II diabetics, but this has not been the universal experience. We are aware of only one report showing such a training effect on blood glucose levels in Type I diabetics among many other communications that did not demonstrate lower blood glucoses *between* exercise periods in active versus nonactive persons. This may be explained by increased food intake on exercise days offsetting the effects of increased insulin sensitivity. The main impetus for exercising should be the expectation of a decrease in certain risk factors for atherosclerotic vascular disease, of increased work capacity, and of an increased general sense of well-being.

Oral Hypoglycemic Agents

Historically, the use of sulfonylureas as part of the therapeutic regimen for Type II diabetes is rooted in the serendipitous observations of the French physician Marcell Janbon during World War II, who noted that patients treated for typhoid fever with government-supplied sulfonylurea, 2255-RP, had symptoms of hypoglycemia.

Acutely sulfonylureas seem to lower blood glucose by promoting both basal and secretagogue-stimulated insulin release (Table 2). For the most part, this stimulation wanes and, after weeks to months of sulfonylurea therapy, even with blood glucose reductions maintained, serum insulin levels are no higher and may actually be lower than pretreatment levels. A major mechanism of action of chronic sulfonylurea therapy is to decrease insulin resistance in all major insulin target tissues—muscle, liver, and adipocytes. Although early studies suggested that this decreased insulin resistance was primarily accomplished by increasing insulin receptors, it has subsequently been shown that improved insulin action can be accomplished without increased insulin receptor binding, consistent with the current view that insulin resistance in patients with

TABLE 2. **The Sulfonylureas**

	Site of Metabolism	Activity of Metabolite(s)	Route of Excretion	Duration of Activity (hr)	Dose Range (mg)
First-Generation					
Tolbutamide (Oramide, Orinase)	Liver	Inactive	Kidney	6–8	500–3000
Chlorpropamide (Diabinese)	Liver	Conflicting data	Kidney	Up to 60+	100–500
Acetohexamide (Dymelor)	Liver	Highly active	Kidney	12–18	250–1500
Tolazamide (Tolinase)	Liver	Weakly active	Kidney	12–18	100–1000
Second-Generation					
Glyburide (DiaBeta, Micronase)	Liver	Weakly active	Kidney Bile	16–24	1.25–20
Glipizide (Glucotrol)	Liver	Inactive	Kidney Bile	12–18	2.5–40

Type II diabetes mellitus is located distal to the binding site of insulin with its receptor. It should be noted that one of the second-generation agents, glipizide, has been reported to cause continued improvement in insulin secretion for 2 years or more after initiation of therapy.

We start sulfonylureas if several months of dietary therapy has failed to reduce blood sugar to levels reasonable for that particular patient. Analysis of thousands of patients indicates that those most likely to respond to sulfonylureas are patients with normal or excess body weight, age of onset of diabetes at 40 years or older, duration of diabetes of less than 5 years at the time oral therapy is initiated, and a previous history of insulin treatment of less than 20 units per day or no history of insulin treatment. None of these are hard and fast rules.

Sulfonylureas either are contraindicated or should be used with greatest of caution in those patients who would be most vulnerable to prolonged, unrecognized hypoglycemia, in particular elderly patients who live alone or are otherwise poorly monitored, the malnourished with little metabolic reserve to rebound from hypoglycemia, those with hepatic and/or renal insufficiency and consequent impaired ability to degrade and excrete sulfonylureas, and patients taking other medications that might enhance the hypoglycemic activity of the sulfonylureas (see below). Other contraindications to sulfonylurea use are most cases of Type I diabetes, pregnancy, lactation, and known allergy to sulfa drugs. Although still considered experimental, combined use of insulin and a sulfonylurea is being studied.

The introduction of the second generation of sulfonylureas (Table 2) has increased the physician's therapeutic options. These newer drugs differ from the first-generation agents in that the side groups attached to the basic sulfonylurea structure are large and relatively nonpolar.

These structural changes confer greater intrinsic hypoglycemic activity to the second-generation sulfonylureas as compared with the first-generation agents. However, on a weight basis, both first- and second-generation agents lower blood sugar levels to about the same degree when used at maximum recommended doses. Thus, in terms of therapeutic efficacy, the second-generation agents are not clearly superior to the first generation of sulfonylureas.

Do the second-generation agents confer any advantage, in terms of reduced side effects? The major side effects of sulfonylureas are hypoglycemia, hyponatremia, and the disulfiram (Antabuse) syndrome (attacks of facial flushing that occur when a patient receiving an oral hypoglycemic agent drinks alcohol). Severe hypoglycemia has been reported to occur with all of sulfonylureas, but about half the reported cases have been associated with chlorpropamide (Diabinese). However, glyburide (DiaBeta, Micronase) may cause severe hypoglycemia as well. It is important to appreciate that sulfonylurea-induced hypoglycemia may be extremely refractory to therapy, sometimes requiring continuous 10 per cent glucose infusion for days and occasionally up to 2 weeks.

Hyponatremia caused by sulfonylurea potentiation of the action of antidiuretic hormone (ADH) and perhaps by stimulation of ADH secretion is also seen, mainly with chlorpropamide (Diabinese). This would occur rarely—if ever— with the second-generation agents or with other first-generation sulfonylureas, most of which have a slight diuretic rather than antidiuretic effect. The disulfiram reaction has classically been associated with chlorpropamide (Diabinese) but can also be seen with the second-generation agents.

First-generation sulfonylureas are bound to circulating albumin by ionic forces, whereas second-generation agents having a nonpolar side chain are not as highly charged and are attached to albumin by nonionic forces. First-generation sulfonylureas may be displaced from albumin by ionically charged medicines (e.g., salicylates, chloramphenicol, phenylbutazone, and coumadins), and this displacement results in increased hypoglycemic potency. In theory, since the second-generation agents are not ionically bound to albumin, this should not occur, a contention supported by some in vitro evidence. Whether this will prove to be a clinically significant advantage of second-generation agents will require time to determine. On the other hand, drugs that impair glucose tolerance will antagonize the hypoglycemic actions of insulin as well as the first- or second-generation sulfonylureas. These drugs include pharmacologic doses of thiazide diuretics, corticosteroids, estrogens, phenytoin, calcium channel blockers, nicotinic acid, and excessive doses of thyroid.

Finally, the metabolism of the second-generation sulfonylureas is different in that they are metabolized by the liver and excreted in the bile and urine (Table 2). It has been speculated that this may be advantageous to the patient with reduced renal function.

Thus, although the second-generation agents do not have any clear therapeutic superiority over the first-generation agents, they may be advantageous in causing fewer significant side effects and have less interaction with other drugs.

Some general guidelines on the use of first- or second-generation sulfonylureas are:

1. Start with the lowest possible dose and give it 30 minutes before meals. As we have tried to indicate, the second-generation agents are not a panacea for certain problems encountered with first-generation drugs. Choosing one over the other rests on a consideration of duration of hypoglycemic activity (prolonged hypoglycemic activity may be convenient in some patients and contraindicated in others, such as the elderly and frail), other medications the patient is taking, and the presence of hepatic or renal disease, which would interfere with metabolism or excretion.

2. Increase doses at 5- to 7-day intervals until the desired blood sugar level has been achieved or until the maximum dose of the particular agent is reached.

3. If the first agent does not work, try another. When a patient is switched to a second-generation agent, the first-generation agents should be discontinued for several days (for chlorpropamide, approximately 1 week). Remember also that causes for primary or secondary failure may sometimes (but not always) be transient and

reversible; such causes include dietary inadherence or intercurrent illness, especially infection.

4. If the second sulfonylurea tried does not work, the patient is probably a candidate for insulin.

Insulin Therapy

The decision to initiate insulin therapy is a function of a number of variables, including the degree of hyperglycemia, the amount of remaining endogenous insulin secretion, and the size of the patient, including the degree of obesity. A safe initial dose for most adults is 0.2 to 0.5 unit per kg of intermediate-acting insulin (NPH or Lente) in the morning. Subsequent dosage adjustments can be made according to the plasma glucose values obtained by home glucose monitoring. When insulin is initiated, we ask patients to check their blood sugar four times a day. Recommended times are 7:00 a.m., 11:00 a.m., 4:00 p.m., and 8:00 p.m., and as necessary in between if symptoms of hypoglycemia develop. If the afternoon blood sugar has normalized but the fasting blood sugar the following day remains elevated, a split dose of insulin should be instituted with two thirds of the total dose given in the morning and one third in the early evening, prior to dinner. An occasional patient may demonstrate persistence of fasting hyperglycemia, and in this instance the second dose of insulin may be given at bedtime rather than dinner. Recent evidence has suggested that if the hyperglycemia resulting from the "dawn phenomenon" (early morning hyperglycemia, related to a surge of growth hormone between 5:00 and 6:00 a.m.) can be controlled, the patient has a better chance of remaining euglycemic throughout the day. If a patient is started on a second dose of insulin prior to dinner or bedtime, an evening snack should always be ingested. Once the fasting and afternoon blood sugars have been normalized, fine tuning of the patient's diabetes can be achieved by reviewing the 11:00 a.m. and 8:00 p.m. (postprandial) blood sugar values. If hyperglycemia is present at these times, regular insulin should be added to the morning and afternoon dosages of NPH or Lente. A reasonable proportion of regular insulin is to give one third of the total morning or evening dose as regular and two thirds as NPH or Lente. This is the most popular insulin regimen and is commonly referred to as a "mixed-split" regimen. Other alternative insulin schedules include a morning dose of Ultralente in combination with Semilente, with an additional dose of Semilente at each meal. This regimen, while quite effective, involves 3 or 4 injections of insulin per day and may be inconvenient for many patients. Alternatively, Ultralente and Semilente can be given in the morning, Semilente at the noon meal, and a second dose of Ultralente with Semilente before supper.

If hypoglycemia develops, it is reasonable to decrease the total dose by 2 to 4 units of intermediate or regular insulin, depending on when the hypoglycemic episode has occurred. Also, a possible change in the patient's dietary intake or physical activity should be considered. All insulin schedules assume that the patient is receiving an optimum diabetic diet and that reliable plasma glucose data are available based on home glucose monitoring.

The complications of insulin therapy include lipodystrophies (atrophic lipodystrophy or lipoatrophy and hypertrophy) and antibody formation leading to insulin resistance and allergy, in addition to hypoglycemia and insulin edema. The major complications of insulin have been linked to impurities in the insulin preparation, and most of these have been substantially reduced with the markedly purified preparations available today.

Human insulin is now readily available and is produced by one of three methodologies: the enzymatic conversion of pork insulin; recombinant DNA, in which genetically altered bacteria make human insulin; and total chemical synthesis. Because of the extraordinary complexity of the manufacturing process, chemically synthesized insulin is available in only limited quantities. Both human insulin and purified pork insulin provide a source of highly purified product for those diabetics who desire or need it. There are no data at the present time to indicate whether human insulin is clearly superior to purified pork insulin in the treatment of patients with complications of insulin therapy, although recombinant DNA human insulin is absorbed more quickly than animal-source insulin and has a shorter duration of action. This tends to improve postprandial metabolic control but might allow for elevation in the next day's fasting blood sugar. The clear indications for switching a patient from a mixed beef-pork preparation to a more purified form of insulin include short-term insulin requirements, including gestational diabetes; problems with insulin allergy; insulin resistance; or insulin lipoatrophy. It is the authors' belief that all hospital pharmacies should carry only human insulin, so that when a patient enters the hospital he or she will automatically be put on this preparation. This will alleviate all potential problems with insulin allergy in the patient inadvertently placed on a beef-pork preparation who had been maintained on either human or pure pork insulin. In time, human insulin may be the only insulin available and all newly diagnosed patients will be started on this insulin preparation.

Intranasal insulin administration is attractive, as it is injection-free, but drawbacks include cost, since large amounts of intranasal insulin are needed to achieve levels comparable to those of injection, and the problem of variable absorption. Although insulin pumps have enjoyed popularity in the past, patients appear to be discouraged by the continual need for frequent blood glucose monitoring and insulin dose adjustments. If a patient elects to begin using an insulin pump, caution must be exercised since precipitous ketoacidosis in the face of near-normal or minimally elevated blood glucose values may occur. Also, the patient must be able to trouble-shoot for mechanical problems, such as blocked tubing and "runaway pump" leading to hypoglycemia. The recent release of an insulin preparation specific for insulin pumps (Humulin BR, Eli Lilly and Co.) has helped diminish problems with insulin binding to the tubing. Before a patient invests in a pump, it is imperative that he or she research several different types and decide on one that best fits his or her particular lifestyle.

Different insulin injecting devices have been marketed to assist patients with needle phobias and to improve the discomfort of the injection process. Again, it is recommended that a patient examine and experiment with several competing brands prior to investing in a particular injecting device.

Assessing Metabolic Control. Crucial to the proper use of various management strategies is careful assessment of metabolic control. No method of monitoring is perfect, and each must be used with a clear understanding of its limitations.

Blood glucose determinations give information about only a single moment in time. In Type I diabetics there may be enormous (tenfold or more) variations in blood glucose within a single day. In both Type I and Type II patients there may be substantial fluctuations in plasma glucose levels measured at the same time on different days. Although fasting or postprandial levels of glucose in Type II diabetics are not as labile as those in patients with Type I, readings obtained in clinic visits might not reflect the prevailing metabolic milieu if the patient has been unusually careful to stay within the limits of therapy just prior to the clinic appointment. This is highlighted in one study of sulfonylurea-treated patients in which blood glucose levels measured at surprise home visits were almost twice as high as levels obtained at visits to physicians' offices.

The finest measure of "moment-to-moment" metabolic control available to the outpatient is self-monitoring of capillary blood glucose with strips read visually or with a readout photometer.

This is a remarkable educational tool, allowing patient involvement to a degree never before possible since the patient can almost immediately see the effects of dietary adherence or indiscretion, of exercise or inactivity, and of changes in insulin or sulfonylurea regimens. Furthermore, it is a therapeutic tool since it affords physician and patient the ability to adapt therapy based on blood glucose measurements. The optimum frequency for capillary blood glucose monitoring should be established. Common sense dictates that patients should monitor themselves frequently (1) just after the time of diagnosis of diabetes, during which period the specific therapeutic regimen is being established; (2) at the times of metabolic instability occasioned by intercurrent illness or other factors; and (3) during pregnancy. At other times, when control is stable, monitoring can be less frequent. The issue, of course, is what constitutes "frequent" monitoring. There is no clear answer, but some would use a regimen of four measurements per day—measurement of glucose before each meal and at bedtime with occasional (once or twice per week) 90-minute postprandial assessments. Others would say that a frequent regimen of monitoring is seven times per day—before each meal, 90 minutes after each meal, and at bedtime, arguing that this seven-point assessment correlates significantly with sampling done in research studies 22 times per day. Finally, it is worthwhile to note that measuring fasting and 90-minute post-breakfast blood glucose has been shown to correlate with mean glycemia determined from 24-hour continuous monitoring of blood glucose. Thus, the frequency of monitoring to be recommended to a patient depends on the physician's assessment of metabolic stability or instability and the patient's willingness and capability to cooperate.

Hemoglobin A_{1c} (Hb A_{1c}) or glycosylated hemoglobin has proved a useful tool to assess integrated metabolic control over longer time intervals. Hb A_{1c} is formed by nonenzymatic binding of glucose to the N-terminal valine of the beta chain of adult hemoglobin. In all persons, Hb A_{1c} makes up a certain percentage of total Hb A. Since the formation of Hb A_{1c} occurs continuously throughout the life span of red blood cells and is largely (though not completely) irreversible, diabetics by virtue of their higher ambient glucose level can be expected to have a higher level of Hb A_{1c} than nondiabetics. Indeed, Hb A_{1c} levels have correlated well with a variety of parameters of metabolic control. Thus, Hb A_{1c} readings provide a good measure of average, but not moment-to-moment, metabolic control over the previous 1 to 2 months. As such, it needs to be used in conjunction with home blood glucose monitoring, which reflects glycemia over shorter periods of time.

Several observations warrant caution in the interpretation of hemoglobin A_{1c} levels. First, the stable form of Hb A_{1c} can increase after as little as 1 to 4 weeks of persistent hyperglycemia, whereas Hb A_{1c} levels become normalized only 4 to 6 weeks *after* normoglycemia has been achieved, since red blood cells having high Hb A_{1c} levels have been eliminated. Put another way, relatively *short* periods of poor metabolic control can lead to Hb A_{1c} levels that are elevated for a *long* time. Thus, clinicians should realize that a single elevated Hb A_{1c} determination may not accurately reflect overall metabolic control. The second important interpretative consideration regarding Hb A_{1c} is that, depending on the method used for its determination in the particular laboratory, factors other than ambient glucose can raise or lower Hb A_{1c} levels; for example, uremia can raise the Hb A_{1c} level, whereas hemolysis or blood loss can lower it. With these caveats in mind, the following guidelines may prove useful in interpreting Hb A_{1c} levels:

1. When conditions that artificially lower Hb A_{1c} levels can be ruled out, one normal Hb A_{1c} level almost always indicates good average metabolic control over the previous 1 to 2 months.

2. If a condition that artificially raises glycosylated hemoglobin can be ruled out, repeatedly elevated levels are an indication of poor metabolic control. As noted previously, a single elevated measurement cannot be used with confidence to identify consistently poor metabolic control.

In the near future, measurement of glycosylated albumin and/or fructosamine may supplant or join Hb A_{1c} measurements as indices of integrated metabolic control, as they measure integrated diabetic control over a shorter period of time.

The usefulness of spot-checking urine glucose levels is severely limited by a number of factors. A given urine glucose value can reflect a rather wide range of blood glucose concentrations. Renal thresholds for urinary glucose spillage vary from person to person and may vary over time in the same person. Retention of urine in the bladder for hours is another problem. Furthermore, several studies have shown that when well-informed diabetics were given urine aliquots with known amounts of glucose added, 50 to 80 per cent of the patients determined these levels incorrectly. Determinations were most likely to be correct when either no glucose or large amounts of glucose were added to the urine. Even with these limitations in mind, information obtained from spot urine checks is not totally worthless. For example, a patient who generally does not spill glucose and who starts to do so consistently should realize that something is wrong, and the patient and/or physician should attempt to identify the problem and correct it as soon as possible. As noted above, spot-checking urine is also useful for the recognition of acetonuria. But urine glucose estimations should almost never be used, in our opinion, to "fine tune" insulin dosages.

Twenty-four-hour testing for urine glucose, either total 24-hour samples or quantitative fractional samples, is cumbersome to patients; and assessment of integrated control is better provided by Hb A_{1c} determinations.

Parenthetically, all Type I patients must be instructed to monitor urinary ketones with Keto-Diastix whenever they experience illness, nausea, or poor diabetic control and to report ketosis to their physician immediately.

Complications

Diabetic Neuropathy

Probably the most common complication of diabetes mellitus is neuropathy, and the most common and troublesome of the neuropathic syndromes of diabetes mellitus is clinically significant peripheral neuropathy with its pain and/or any of a variety of other unpleasant symptoms. The story, still in evolution, of the unraveling of the multifaceted pathophysiologic basis of this problem has been an exciting one. Although promise for therapeutic advances lies with such studies, information gains so far have not yet been translated into significantly improved management of this particular complication.

Proof of therapeutic efficacy for symptomatic neuropathic problems really requires double-blind, placebo-controlled trials of drugs currently being evaluated. The attainment of good metabolic control has been shown to improve or normalize diminished nerve conduction velocity in neurologically asymptomatic diabetic humans and animals. Further, it is of interest that hyperglycemia dereases pain threshold, but it is not clear that the symptoms of neuropathy are helped by attainment of good metabolic control. Analgesics, from mild to potent, may be required for some patients. About 10 per cent of Type I diabetics have associated pernicious anemia, which can present as symptomatic peripheral neuropathy amenable to vitamin B_{12} therapy. Vitamin B_{12} levels should be checked in neurologically symptomatic Type I diabetics. Symptomatic diabetics may not have diabetic peripheral neuropathy, and other causes, sometimes correctable,

such as herniated disc disease or alcoholic neuropathy, should be considered.

With regard to symptomatic neuropathy, we are aware of three properly controlled studies, indicating that amitriptyline (Elavil) (generally up to 150 mg at bedtime) is useful in the treatment of symptomatic neuropathy; there is no proof that the addition of fluphenazine (Prolixin) does anything more than amitriptyline alone. Two controlled studies indicate that imipramine (Tofranil) (up to 100 mg at bedtime) may also be useful. It would appear that these two antidepressants act by mechanisms other than by treatment of depression, although relief of depression might be useful in some severely symptomatic patients. Remember that when efficacy is established in these sorts of trials it does not mean that every patient responds favorably, nor does it necessarily mean that responding patients experience full symptomatic relief.

Other hopes for the future management of distressful neuropathic symptoms include the use of aldose reductase inhibitors (mixed results in clinical trials so far), intravenous lidocaine, and mexilentine, a close structural analogue of lidocaine that can be taken orally. Pentoxifylline and other drugs that increase erythrocyte flexibility and improve blood flow in the microvasculature are currently being evaluated as to efficacy.

Diabetic Nephropathy

Diabetic nephropathy continues to be the major cause of death in patients with Type I diabetes mellitus and accounts for approximately 25 per cent of all patients beginning dialysis in the United States.

Recent evidence suggests that the earliest marker for diabetic nephropathy is microalbuminuria, which appears to be a predictor for overt diabetic nephropathy in both Type I and Type II diabetes. Microalbuminuria is defined as an increased urinary albumin excretion as measured by radioimmunoassay. Persistent microalbuminuria is indicated by the finding of 20 to 200 micrograms per minute or 30 to 300 mg per 24 hours in at least two of three urine samples collected within 6 months. When a patient is categorized as having microalbuminuria, other transient or reversible causes must be excluded. These include urinary tract infections, physical exercise, essential hypertension, cardiac insufficiency, and water loading. These patients may have no proteinuria on standard screening tests.

Pathophysiologically, increased albumin excretion is associated with a decrease in the synthesis of heparan sulfate. Depletion of heparan sulfate compromises the anionic barrier to albumin, leading to increased excretion of this protein. Increased albumin excretion results in increased mesangial deposition and basement membrane thickening, and thus the morphologic picture of diabetic nephropathy.

Glycemic control as assessed by glycosylated hemoglobin and home glucose monitoring closely correlates with the albumin excretion rate in early diabetic renal disease, but the impact on the progression of established diabetic nephropathy has yet to be proved by the NIH Control and Complications Trial.

Treatment of albuminuria begins with establishing good metabolic control. An underlying urinary tract infection must always be excluded and treated if present. Aggressive antihypertensive therapy has also been proved to have a clear beneficial effect on slowing the progressive rate of nephropathy. The angiotensin enzyme inhibitors are of particular value in the antihypertensive regimen in the diabetic patient with proteinuria, although careful monitoring of renal function and serum potassium levels must be done. Dietary intervention with a low-protein diet also slows the progressive decline of renal function and prolongs life in patients with moderate to severe renal disease. Although aldose reductase inhibitors reduce proteinuria in the rat model, to date no human studies have been reported on the effect of this class of agents on either overt proteinuria or the microalbuminuria of early diabetic nephropathy.

Careful monitoring of the patient's initial renal status should be performed, including determination of baseline 24-hour urine creatinine clearance and microalbumin excretion rates in addition to serum creatinine and blood urea nitrogen measurements. These studies should be repeated on an annual basis and early referral should be made to a nephrologist, if indicated.

DIABETES MELLITUS IN CHILDREN AND ADOLESCENTS

method of
DAVID E. GOLDSTEIN, M.D., and
MELBA R. HOEPER, R.N.
*University of Missouri-Columbia
Columbia, Missouri*

Diabetes mellitus is one of the most common serious chronic diseases of children and adolescents, with an annual incidence of nearly 15 per 100,000; by age 18 years, approximately 1 in 500 individuals in the United States have been diagnosed as having diabetes mellitus. In children almost all cases are insulin-dependent (Type I diabetes or IDDM), which is associated with destruction of pancreatic beta cells and life-long dependence on exogenous insulin for survival. Following diagnosis, patients may show a rapid decline in insulin requirements, the so-called "honeymoon," which can persist for months to years. However, pancreatic beta cell destruction is usually complete within 1 to 2 years of diagnosis.

Diagnosis

It is not necessary to perform an oral glucose tolerance test to diagnose diabetes in children. The diagnosis can be made if either a random plasma glucose value is greater than 200 mg per dl with a typical history (polyuria, polydipsia, weight loss) or if the fasting plasma glucose is greater than 140 mg per dl.

Although diabetic children usually present with polyuria, polydipsia, polyphagia, and weight loss, the disease may present with life-threatening coma or be suspected because of fatigue, enuresis, or candidal vaginitis. Infants and young children may show only nonspecific symptoms such as irritability or poor feeding. The immediate precipitating event is often an acute viral illness.

DIABETIC KETOACIDOSIS

Diabetic ketoacidosis (DKA) may be part of the initial presentation of IDDM or may occur in a child previously diagnosed. DKA should be considered a medical emergency; delay in treatment of even a few hours can be fatal. The condition is caused by severe insulin deficiency, which leads to profound alterations in carbohydrate, lipid, and protein metabolism. Key features include *dehydration* due to massive urinary loss of fluid secondary to hyperglycemia and glycosuria, *ketosis* leading to progressive acidosis, and *urinary loss of amino acids and electrolytes,* including sodium, potassium, chloride, and phosphorus. As the metabolic deterioration progresses, patients begin vomiting and dehydration becomes severe; vascular volume and glomerular filtration decrease; and serum osmolality increases, leading to shock, coma, and death.

Diagnosis

The diagnosis of DKA should offer no difficulties in a child with or without a previous diagnosis of diabetes who presents with a history of polyuria, polydipsia, weight loss, vomiting, and changes in sensorium. Patients typically show characteristic Kussmaul respirations, which are deep and rapid. The breath has a peculiar fruity odor caused by the excessive ketones. Some patients present with abdominal pain suggesting a primary intra-abdominal disorder such as appendicitis. The condition can be both triggered and masked by a wide variety of precipitating factors, such as trauma or infection. Laboratory findings include the following: positive urinary glucose and ketones; hyperglycemia, with blood glucose values generally greater than 250 mg per dl; positive serum ketones; and serum CO_2 less than 17 mEq per liter. Kidney function studies generally show evidence of dehydration with elevated blood urea nitrogen and creatinine. Serum sodium may be falsely low because of the hyperglycemia, while the serum potassium may be low, normal, or elevated. Hematologic studies reveal elevated hematocrit and leukocytosis.

Treatment

Treatment of DKA is aimed at correcting the acidosis and the fluid and electrolyte losses, and treating any precipitating disease if present. Treatment is usually initiated in an intensive care setting and can be facilitated by construction of a flowsheet for charting the patient's progress and laboratory data. An intravenous line should be placed and blood obtained for "stat" measurements of glucose, BUN, creatinine, electrolytes, pH, CO_2 (or bicarbonate), calcium, and phosphorus. A 12-lead EKG should be obtained with a long lead II rhythm strip. Other studies may be indicated depending on possible precipitating causes.

A number of serious complications can develop during treatment and should be considered at the outset. These include the following:

1. Hypoglycemia occurs secondary to excessive insulin treatment.

2. Hypokalemia results from a rapid shift of potassium ion from the extracellular space into cells during correction of the acidosis.

3. Vascular thrombosis is due to dehydration. A contributing factor is a further fall in intravascular volume when hypotonic fluids are used for initial fluid treatment.

4. Cerebral edema can occur during the first 18 hours of therapy. The cause of this edema is unknown, but the complication may result in brain herniation and death.

Fluid and Electrolyte Replacement

Deficits should be estimated. On average, patients are 10 per cent dehydrated (e.g., a 30 kg child has a fluid deficit of 3 liters). Sodium, potassium, and chloride deficits are 3 to 4 mEq per kg. Except for potassium deficits, which require several days to replace, fluid and electrolyte deficits should be fully replaced within 12 to 24 hours. Fluid replacement should begin as soon as a tentative diagnosis is made. Normal saline (0.9 per cent sodium chloride) or Ringer's lactate should be given at 20 ml per kg over the first

hour. Then normal saline is given at a rate of 10 to 15 ml per kg per hour; the rate is adjusted based on calculated deficits, maintenance, and ongoing losses. After 3 to 4 hours of therapy, a switch should be made to a slightly hypotonic solution (one-half normal saline). After approximately 8 to 12 hours of therapy, fluids can be switched to one-quarter normal saline at a maintenance rate. Dextrose should be added to intravenous fluids when the blood glucose level reaches 250 to 300 mg per dl. We attempt to maintain plasma glucose concentrations between 150 and 300 mg per dl during the first 12 hours of therapy.

Potassium. All patients with DKA are severely potassium-depleted even if the serum potassium level is normal or elevated. Replacement is begun if the serum potassium level is not elevated, and if the patient is producing urine; with correction of the systemic acidosis, the serum potassium will fall precipitously if potassium is not administered at a rate of 30 to 40 mEq per liter. Frequent serum potassium determinations are mandatory. As an aid to monitoring serum potassium levels, T waves can be followed on lead II EKG rhythm strips obtained every 1 to 2 hours. Progressive loss of T waves or formation of U waves suggests hypokalemia and should prompt "stat" measurement of serum potassium. There is debate concerning the use of potassium phosphate instead of potassium chloride. Serum phosphate levels fall during treatment, and there are some theoretical advantages of replenishing the phosphate, which is important for synthesis of red blood cell 2,3-diphosphoglycerate, an important factor in hemoglobin-oxygen dissociation. However, clinical trials have shown no benefit from phosphate administration. We use only potassium chloride for replacement therapy, although some experts use 50 per cent potassium chloride and 50 per cent potassium phosphate. One risk of phosphate therapy is hypocalcemic tetany; if phosphate is administered, serum calcium levels should be monitored.

Bicarbonate. The use of bicarbonate is controversial. We do not use bicarbonate routinely unless the pH is less than 7.0 or there is hypotension or other evidence of impaired myocardial function. Administration of bicarbonate may decrease sensorium due to a paradoxical decrease in cerebrospinal fluid pH for several hours after bicarbonate administration. In addition, bicarbonate administration can contribute to a rapid fall in serum potassium. If bicarbonate is administered, the amount should be calculated to correct the serum bicarbonate level to only 15 mEq per liter, and it should be given over 4 to 6 hours, not as a bolus. The usual total dosage is approximately 4 to 6 mEq per kg.

Insulin Therapy

Continuous intravenous administration of regular insulin is recommended for most cases. First, regular insulin, 0.1 unit per kg, is given as an intravenous bolus. Then, regular insulin is administered intravenously, 0.1 unit per kg per hour. Regular insulin can be mixed in normal saline and infused piggyback to the rehydration intravenous fluids. For convenience, 50 units of regular insulin can be added to 500 ml of saline and infused at 1 ml per kg per hour, which is equivalent to 0.1 unit of insulin per kg per hour. If insulin administration is adequate, serum CO_2 and pH will rise steadily. Initial improvement in hyperglycemia is more often attributable to adequate fluid replacement than to insulin administration. If after 2 hours of intravenous insulin therapy the serum CO_2 has not increased by at least 5 mEq per liter, the infusion line should be checked for any obstruction; if the line is clear, the insulin infusion rate should be doubled.

Insulin should be infused until the blood glucose level has stabilized in the 200 to 300 mg per dl range and the serum CO_2 is greater than 15 mEq per liter. Generally this requires 6 to 12 hours. Then subcutaneous regular insulin injections, every 6 hours at an initial dosage of 0.25 unit per kg, are begun. The insulin infusion is discontinued 30 minutes after the first subcutaneous insulin injection. The subcutaneous insulin dose is adjusted every 6 hours based on blood glucose, urine glucose, and ketone testing results just prior to the next dose. Most patients require 1 to 2 units per kg per 24 hours for the first 24 to 48 hours.

Occasionally, patients present with very mild DKA and with only minimal acidosis and dehydration. In this situation, we sometimes administer regular insulin every 6 hours by the subcutaneous route, beginning with 0.25 unit per kg. However, with even minimal dehydration we administer fluids by the intravenous route as described above.

LONG-TERM MANAGEMENT

Diabetes mellitus is a chronic disease with potentially serious complications. Management is difficult and requires proper patient and family education from the start. Specific goals include (1) elimination of symptoms due to hyperglycemia, which include polydipsia, polyuria, and polyphagia; (2) prevention of DKA; (3) prevention of serious hypoglycemia; (4) maintenance of normal growth and development; (5) promotion of emotional well-being; and (6) prevention of chronic complications of diabetes.

Although the evidence relating hyperglycemia to complications is not yet conclusive, most experts believe that families should strive for the best possible glycemic control with a clear understanding that risks of hypoglycemia limit attempts to normalize blood glucose levels.

Diabetes Education

The term "diabetes education" refers to the sum total of all diabetes teaching performed by the health care team. This includes teaching about diet, insulin therapy, monitoring, and so forth. For children and adolescents, it is critical that the health providers have an organized approach to the educational process and that the proper resources be available for this teaching. In our institution, we use a diabetes "team" approach to education and ongoing care. The team includes a pediatrician, dietitian, nurse educator, and social worker. Team members are all experienced in management of children and adolescents with diabetes. We generally hospitalize children for 1 to 2 weeks at onset of their diabetes. The inpatient setting is optimal for teaching the patient and family the many new routines that will be necessary to obtain optimal control of the diabetes. Our institution contains a public school and child life specialists who can provide many structured activities for the children so the hospital stay can be a pleasant experience.

Our goal is for families to achieve relative independence in diabetes management after hospital discharge, and for school-age children to return immediately to school. Routine follow-up visits in the outpatient clinic are scheduled three times per year, but care team members are available 24 hours a day if problems develop.

The education must be individualized and adapted to the particular family situation and to the patient's age and stage of psychologic development. The burden of responsibility for the diabetes care of infants and young children is on the parents, and the main goal is to have the infant accept the routine care procedures that must be performed, such as finger sticks or injections. Infants and young children generally make an excellent adjustment to blood testing and injections if the parents are relaxed and matter-of-fact about the need to perform these procedures.

As children reach the age of 3 to 5 years, they can be gently encouraged to participate in their care. Whatever they do in helping with their care should be praised. For example, 3- or 4-year-olds can be taught to indicate where their injection site will be, to wipe off their finger with alcohol before a finger prick, or to help read the blood glucose number on the reflectance meter.

In the age range of 5 to 10 years, progressively more responsibility can be given to children, but continued supervision by the parents is critical. We do not encourage children to give their own injections on a regular basis, but if they show interest, we recommend that they be allowed to do some. During this developmental stage, many children learn what is expected of them in respect to blood and urine test results, and if they are allowed to perform the procedures without supervision, they may not provide accurate results. Also, parents should be warned that children may be embarrassed about their diabetes and skip necessary snacks at school for fear of calling attention to their diabetes.

During the adolescent years, patients can be given increased responsibility for their diabetes care and increasingly complex information about their diabetes. This can, however, be a very difficult age in managing diabetes. The adolescent process is largely concerned with establishing independence from parents. The adolescent does not want parental supervision, yet he is not able to accept full responsibility for management of his diabetes. The adolescent may use the diabetes as a weapon in dealing with parents. We try to avoid "taking sides" and negotiate separately with the parents and with the adolescent as to who will be responsible for what aspects of the diabetes, and what the expectations are. We strive to make clinic visits pleasant and try not to make unrealistic demands.

Insulin Therapy

We initially treat all patients with two daily injections of a mixture of NPH and regular human insulins, proportioned as 2 parts NPH to 1 part regular insulin. The insulin is premixed by the pharmacy, for example, 3 ml regular insulin and 6 ml NPH in a 10-ml sterile bottle, to avoid syringe-mixing of insulins, which increases risks of dosing errors. Two thirds of the total daily dose is given in the morning one half hour before breakfast, and the remaining one third is given one half hour before supper. The initial dosage is determined by the previous 24 hours' total dosage of regular insulin given subcutaneously every 6 hours. For example, if the patient presented with DKA and was treated with intravenous insulin and then switched to subcutaneous insulin every 6 hours for 36 hours, and if the previous 24 hours' insulin requirements were 60 units, we would start the patient with 40 units of the 2:1 NPH:regular mixture before breakfast and give the remaining 20 units before supper. The total

daily insulin dosage is increased or decreased by "steps" (one "step" equals 2 units of the 2:1 mixture in the morning dose and 1 unit in the dose given before supper) based on urine and blood testing results (urine tests for glucose and ketones before breakfast, lunch, supper, and bedtime, and capillary blood glucose testing before breakfast, lunch, supper, and bedtime, and at 3 a.m. to monitor for nocturnal hypoglycemia). Table 1 shows an example of a step chart for insulin dose changes. Initially, our goals are to maintain the urine glucose-free and to prevent hypoglycemia. If the previous day's urine tests were completely negative for glucose, or if the patient had a hypoglycemic reaction, the insulin dosage is decreased by one "step" the next day. If the patient shows positive urine glucose tests and no hypoglycemia, the insulin dosage is increased by one "step" each day. Generally, by one week of therapy, insulin dosage requirements are on a steady decline; urine is almost always glucose-free, and blood glucose values are generally less than 150 mg per dl. We continue to decrease the insulin dosage by "steps" based on monitoring results until the total daily insulin dosage reaches 0.25 unit per kg. We maintain the insulin dosage at this level even if the urine and blood glucose tests are near normal. This "honeymoon" phase can last for months or even years before insulin requirements gradually increase again to an average of 0.8 to 1 unit per kg per 24 hours in patients with no endogenous insulin secretion.

Approximately 50 per cent of our newly diagnosed children with IDDM reach the minimal insulin dose level; in others, particularly children under age 2 years, the dose does not fall appreciably.

Parents are taught how to make insulin adjustments at home based on urine and blood testing results. Particularly during the first few months after diagnosis, we recommend that urine test results (rather than blood) be used primarily for adjusting the insulin dosage. Rules for home insulin dose changes are as follows: If the urine tests for glucose are negative 2 days in a row, the day's insulin dosage is decreased one "step," but not below the level 0.25 unit per kg; if the urine is positive for glucose 2 days in a row, the insulin dosage is increased one "step."

Families should use blood testing results to "fine tune" the insulin dosage. Target blood glu-

TABLE 1. **A 2:1 NPH: Regular Insulin "Step Chart"**

Total units for 24 hours	48	45	42	39	36	33	30
Breakfast dose	32	30	28	26	24	22	20
Supper dose	16	15	14	13	12	11	10

cose levels are shown in Table 2. If urine test results are consistently negative for glucose, but if blood testing shows many values greater than 150 mg per dl, the insulin dosage should be increased one "step" with frequent (at least once per week) blood monitoring at 3 a.m. for hypoglycemia. If the patient shows frequent daytime or nocturnal hypoglycemia, it is necessary to decrease the insulin dosage even if some urine samples are positive for glucose or some blood glucose levels are high during the day. For the patient who has either high or low blood glucose levels at only one particular time during the day, a minor change in the meal plan can usually improve the situation.

For very young patients, for whom the insulin dosage is very small, we use diluted insulin. Insulin manufacturers will supply buffering solutions free of charge that can be used to dilute the insulin to whatever strength is necessary. Insulin can be diluted to one-half strength (50 units per ml), one-quarter strength (25 units per ml), and one-tenth strength (10 units per ml), still maintaining the 2:1 NPH:regular proportions. Thus, an infant whose insulin dosage is 2 units before breakfast and 1 unit before supper of a 2:1 mixture can be given this as U-10 (9 parts diluting fluid and 1 part insulin) with 0.2 ml insulin "mix" in the morning dose (this shows as 20 units on the syringe) and 0.1 ml in the evening dose. We use diluted insulin if the dosage is less than 10 units (0.1 ml). Although any pharmacist can obtain the diluting fluid and mix the insulins, most families can be easily taught to mix and dilute insulins correctly. Recently, at least one pharmaceutical company has marketed a 70:30 NPH:regular mixture.

Occasionally, the insulin regimen presented above does not control the diabetes well throughout the day. Regular insulin can be added to the morning or evening injections of "mix" or administered as a supplemental injection before lunch or at bedtime. If the fasting blood glucose level is above goals yet the patient experiences nocturnal hypoglycemia, some physicians recommend splitting the evening dosage as 1:1 NPH:regular with the regular component given before supper and the NPH at bedtime.

On average, children require about 0.8 to 1 unit insulin per kg after 12 to 18 months of diabetes. During adolescence, the insulin dosage frequently rises by 15 to 20 per cent (total daily

TABLE 2. **Target Blood Glucose Levels**

Fasting	60–120 mg/dl
Preprandial	60–120 mg/dl
2 hours postprandial	70–150 mg/dl
3 a.m.	≥65 mg/dl

dosage 1 to 1.5 units per kg). In any patient, a total daily dose greater than 2 units per kg should suggest insulin resistance or nonadherence to the treatment regimen.

Intensified Therapies

With the development of home glucose monitoring, intensified insulin therapies have been developed to more closely simulate normal plasma insulin profiles and blood sugar patterns during the day. Most commonly, the treatments use either multiple daily injections of insulin (MDI) or continuous subcutaneous insulin infusion using a portable pump (CSII). With all intensified regimens, the goal is to achieve normal blood glucose patterns by providing a continuous "basal" dosage of insulin throughout the day and night and "boluses" of insulin before meals. One relatively simple MDI regimen provides NPH insulin before breakfast and supper in equal amounts (or Ultralente insulin once daily) as the basal component (about one-half the total daily dosage) and boluses of regular insulin, syringe-mixed with the NPH before breakfast, before lunch, and syringe-mixed with the NPH before supper. A fourth daily injection of regular insulin is given at bedtime if blood glucose values are above goals. The basal insulin dosage is adjusted based on 3 a.m. and fasting blood glucose levels. The bolus injections are adjusted individually based on blood glucose levels preprandially and 1½ to 2 hours postprandially.

CSII has been used with success in adults at many centers; its use in children is controversial. The pump is a very small battery-powered infusion apparatus that is worn externally. The pump is programmed to deliver a basal rate of insulin between meals and during the night and boluses of insulin before meals. The pump uses a syringe filled with insulin and an infusion set with a needle that is placed in the subcutaneous tissue, usually in the abdomen and secured with tape. The needle must be changed daily.

We do not often recommend the use of CSII in children, and do not recommend any form of intensified therapy for patients of any age who are having difficulty in achieving well-controlled diabetes on more conventional forms of treatment. The CSII and MDI regimens are most useful in mature patients who are very committed to their diabetes care and who have a specific reason for choosing this treatment approach, such as an unusual work schedule or a desire to have more control over their diabetes treatment. Intensified therapies require major time commitments from patients and health professionals. Intensive forms of treatment, particularly CSII, should not be used unless the diabetes care team is highly skilled in the use of these treatments and can supervise the patient's care. All forms of intensified therapy carry with them increased risks of hypoglycemia. In addition, the use of an insulin infusion pump entails much-increased cost compared with more conventional treatments. These factors must be carefully weighed in making a decision to use an intensified therapy.

Monitoring Control

Monitoring allows the physician and patient to determine if the diabetes treatment is "on track." Patients should monitor both blood and urine glucose at home on a regular basis. Urine glucose testing is simple and inexpensive, but it has limitations. Patients do not have glycosuria unless the blood glucose level has been above the kidney threshold for glucose, which is approximately 180 mg per dl. In patients who have either high or low thresholds, results will not accurately reflect blood glucose levels. Also, urine that is negative for glucose does not provide any specific information concerning hypoglycemia. Nonetheless, home urine testing is useful and well accepted by children. We recommend one of the newer urine strip methods, such as Chemstrips UgK, that measures both glucose and ketones. The glucose results are given in a range of 0 to 5 per cent.

For patients treated with conventional (two daily injections of a 2:1 NPH:regular mixture) insulin therapy, urine glucose should be tested at least three times daily for determining routine insulin dose changes.

Blood Glucose Testing

Self blood glucose monitoring (SBGM) represents a very important advance in diabetes management. We recommend that all patients use this method of monitoring on a regular basis. SBGM is particularly useful in monitoring for hypoglycemia. The procedure should be taught by a diabetes educator experienced in the use of SBGM, and the patient's and family's accuracy in performing the procedure should be tested against laboratory glucose determinations. Capillary samples can be obtained using a spring-loaded lancet device. If performed properly, the test is nearly painless, and even young children can be taught to do SBGM. In summary, the lancet device pricks a finger at the side, near the nail bed. The finger is squeezed to obtain a large drop of blood, which can then be placed on a reagent strip pad. The exact timing and wiping technique for the specific strip used must be followed precisely. With most strips, the result can be read visually by comparison with a color chart, or the strip can be placed in a reflectance meter. Testing results should be recorded in a log book so that the results can be reviewed by the patient, family, and health care team. An important part of the diabetes education process is education in the use of SBGM. The parents and child should be taught what normal blood glucose values are, what treatment target values are, and what to do if values are above or below target levels.

Monitoring schedules depend on the patient's or family's preferences, but, in general, patients should monitor blood glucose at home not less than twice daily. For those who do not wish to monitor urine glucose routinely, we recommend a minimum of three blood tests daily with fasting (prebreakfast) and presupper blood samples, and either prelunch, bedtime, or 3 a.m. blood testing. Patients should vary the times during the day when they test. For most patients treated with conventional insulin regimens, we recommend a combination of blood and urine glucose testing. On average, our patients test two to three urine samples and two blood samples per day. For patients who have chosen an intensified insulin therapy, frequent SBGM is mandatory, with at least three tests daily and one 3 a.m. test per week. For all patients, urinary ketones should be checked during illness, if blood glucose values are consistently greater than 200 mg per dl, or if urinary glucose values are 3 per cent or greater.

Glycosylated Hemoglobin. A major advance in monitoring is the development of the glycosylated hemoglobin (GHb) test. The term glycosylated hemoglobin (also called glycated hemoglobin, hemoglobin A1, hemoglobin A_{1c}) refers to a series of linkages between hemoglobin and sugars that are formed inside the red blood cell through a nonenzymatic reaction. The rate of the reaction depends only on the glucose concentration to which the red blood cells are exposed. Red blood cells live approximately 120 days; thus, determination of GHb serves as an index of the average blood glucose during the preceding weeks to months. The test is now widely used for routine management of diabetes, and should be performed at each clinic visit in children and adolescents with diabetes. The test can provide patients and their families with an overview of the patient's blood glucose control and complements nicely the home blood and urine testing, which provides day-to-day information. The test, though widely available, has not yet been standardized, so that numbers obtained in different laboratories cannot be easily related to one another. Table 3 shows the relationship between GHb measured in our laboratory and average blood glucose. For

TABLE 3. **Relationship Between Glycosylated Hemoglobin (Hb A$_{1c}$) and Average Blood Glucose**

Hb A$_{1c}$ (%)	Average Blood Glucose (mg/dl)
4–6*	60–120
6–8	120–180
8–10	180–240
>10	>240

*Nondiabetic. Values in this range are rarely observed in children with IDDM except during the "honeymoon" period. The average in our clinic is about 7.5 per cent.

most children and adolescents with diabetes, we aim for GHb levels as close to the normal range as possible without frequent episodes of hypoglycemia. Few patients are able to safely achieve and maintain levels in the normal range except during the honeymoon period. In our clinic, the average level in children and adolescents with IDDM is approximately 7.5 per cent (nondiabetic range, 4 to 6 per cent). Values greater than 3 per cent above the upper limit of normal reflect very poor diabetes control.

As with any other laboratory test, a major discrepancy between test result and clinical impression should be investigated. For example, hemoglobinopathies such as hemoglobin S and C can falsely lower results with some assay methods, while hemoglobinopathies such as fetal hemoglobin can falsely elevate results with some assay methods.

Diet

Another cornerstone of diabetes management is diet. The three nutritional goals of diabetes management are to achieve appropriate blood glucose and fat levels, to achieve and maintain reasonable body weight, and to provide good and satisfying nutrition. Strict adherence to the meal plan is essential for optimal control of the diabetes. For most patients and families adherence to the meal plan represents by far the most difficult aspect of diabetes care. We use the American Diabetes Association guidelines in developing meal plans based on exchange lists. A nutritionist who is knowledgeable about diabetes, and in particular about the special needs of infants, children, and adolescents with diabetes, is an essential member of the care team.

We recommend three meals and three snacks with sufficient calories to promote normal growth. The snacks are very useful in moderating the caloric load at any one meal and in preventing hypoglycemia. Some children will resist taking the midmorning and midafternoon snacks at school, but this can usually be worked out satisfactorily by the parents and school personnel.

Patients and families are taught that the exchange system allows great flexibility in food choices while allowing the patient to achieve excellent blood glucose control. We tend to recommend many more within-day and between-day adjustments in the meal plan than in the insulin regimen to compensate for differences in activity. We emphasize the importance of adjusting the total caloric level to the patient's appetite rather than adjusting the total calories to improve glycemic control.

For patients who are overweight and who wish to lose weight, caloric restriction is recommended, but this is also carried out using a structured meal plan. We recommend that 50 to 60 per cent of the total calories be derived from carbohydrate, most of which is complex carbohydrates, 30 to 35 per cent of calories be derived from fat, and 15 to 20 per cent of total calories be derived from protein. We do not recommend special dietetic foods, nor do we encourage frequent use of artificial sweeteners. Although we recommend that patients use the exchange system and start out weighing portion sizes, with experience patients can "guesstimate" portion sizes quite accurately. For convenience in dining out, particularly for "fast foods," patients can count calories rather than exchanges.

Given sufficient training and encouragement, most patients and families become quite expert with the meal plan, and most patients will follow the meal plan acceptably well. Proper nutritional instruction takes a minimum of 5 to 10 hours at the outset with frequent reinforcement over time. With very young children, achieving adherence to the meal plan can be difficult because of fluctuations in appetite. It is useful initially to provide slightly fewer calories than the patient will require for normal growth. This approach quickly gets the "picky eater" to eat the meals and snacks in a consistent manner. Thereafter, the calories can be gradually increased provided the child continues to eat satisfactorily. Parents should not show anxiety or anger, nor should they try to bribe children to eat. Otherwise, behavior patterns will develop that can be very difficult to correct. Children and adolescents should be encouraged to communicate openly with their parents and health care providers about their meal plan; if they are not provided with sufficient food to satisfy them, most children will "cheat," leading to maladaptive behavior, guilt, and poor glycemic control.

Exercise

All persons with diabetes, including children and adolescents, should be encouraged to exercise on a regular basis. Exercise can improve glycemic control, help prevent excessive weight gain, improve cardiovascular disease risk factors, and give patients a sense of well-being. Particularly for adolescents who are not active, it may be helpful for the physician to "contract" with the patient for some regular exercise. Patients and their families should be alerted to the dangers of exercise if the diabetes is poorly controlled; in this situation, exercise can further increase hyperglycemia and ketone production. Patients should be taught to eat extra food with exercise to prevent hypoglycemia.

Hypoglycemia

Hypoglycemia is a serious risk of insulin in all patients, but particularly in children who may not easily recognize or communicate their symptoms. The risks of hypoglycemia are increased as treatment goals become more stringent. All patients should be taught the dangers of hypoglycemia and how to recognize the signs and symptoms, which include tremulousness, sweating, dizziness, hunger, headache, pallor, lethargy, and confusion. In children, recurrent nightmares may be the result of nocturnal hypoglycemia. Monitoring blood glucose levels at home decreases considerably the risks of serious hypoglycemia by detecting asymptomatic hypoglycemia, which should prompt consideration of changes in insulin dosage or the meal plan.

All episodes of hypoglycemia must be considered as potentially serious and should be treated promptly. Mild to moderate reactions can be treated with 10 to 15 grams of carbohydrate, which can be given as 2 to 3 teaspoons of table sugar, about 4 oz (120 ml) of orange juice, or two glucose tablets. We do not recommend the routine use of candy bars or other sweets to treat reactions. Milk (4 oz or 120 ml) is generally quite effective in raising the blood glucose level. For mild reactions just prior to a scheduled meal, the patient can just begin the meal early. For reactions that are treated with simple sugars, this should always be followed by some complex carbohydrate and protein, such as milk. Otherwise the hypoglycemia may recur in a relatively short period of time.

For more severe reactions in which the patient is conscious but cannot self-administer food, honey, syrup, or cake frosting can be placed in the person's mouth. But the most effective means of raising the blood glucose in this situation or when the patient is unconscious is to inject 0.5 to 1 mg of glucagon subcutaneously. All patients and their families should be taught how to use glucagon and to keep the medication readily available for emergencies. Glucagon is supplied in a vial containing 1 mg of lyophilized glucagon and 1 ml of diluent. The medication should not be reconstituted except immediately before administration. Glucagon will reliably raise the blood glucose level, but it may also induce severe vomiting.

Following severe reactions many patients have intense headaches and even confusion for many hours. Thus, any reaction with loss of consciousness may require medical observation until the patient demonstrates normal behavior and ability to take food by mouth without vomiting. With any severe reaction it is very important to determine the cause, if possible, and to institute measures to prevent recurrence. The risks of hypoglycemia are particularly great in small infants, whose initial symptoms may be very nonspecific, such as crying or fussing, and in any patients who do not show typical adrenergic symptoms.

Sick Day Rules

An important part of diabetes education is to teach patients and families how to manage the diabetes during intercurrent illnesses. Children and adolescents with well-controlled diabetes are not at increased risk for infections compared to nondiabetics. However, with infections, insulin requirements usually increase dramatically. With illness we recommend that patients check urine glucose and ketones and blood glucose every 4 to 6 hours. For patients taking two daily injections of NPH/regular insulin mixture, the prebreakfast and presupper insulin doses can be increased up to 4 "steps," depending on the blood and urine glucose and urine findings. (For example, for blood glucose greater than 200 mg per dl, urine sugar 3 to 5 per cent, and positive urinary ketones, the prebreakfast insulin can be increased from 40 units to 48 units and the presupper insulin from 20 units to 24 units.) If the urine is positive for ketones and glucose, and the blood glucose is greater than 200 mg per dl before lunchtime and bedtime, supplemental regular insulin should be given at a dose of 0.1 to 0.3 unit per kg. It is very important that patients maintain adequate hydration. For vomiting, patients can be given frequent small sips of sugar-containing solutions such as soda, soup, popsicles, and Jell-O. If vomiting persists more than 6 hours with positive urinary ketones, the physician should be contacted. For patients being treated with intensive therapies, supplementation should be given with only regular insulin every 6 hours at a dose of 0.1 to 0.3 unit per kg, again based on blood and urine test results.

Occasionally, patients have gastrointestinal

symptoms such as nausea, vomiting, and diarrhea, or cannot maintain their usual caloric intake for some other reason, but do not show significant hyperglycemia and glycosuria (blood sugar less than 150 mg per dl and urine glucose less than 1 per cent). In this situation, we recommend giving two thirds of the usual insulin dosage to prevent possible hypoglycemia.

Surgery

For children and adolescents with diabetes undergoing any surgical procedure that necessitates general anesthesia or requires cessation of oral intake for several hours, certain precautions are recommended. Elective procedures should be scheduled early in the day if possible. Prior to the morning insulin injection, an intravenous infusion should be started with 5 per cent dextrose in saline to run at maintenance (e.g., about 80 ml per hour for a 60-kg person). Two thirds of the usual morning insulin injection should be administered, and the blood glucose level should be monitored every 1 to 2 hours with a goal of 100 to 200 mg per dl. When the patient is able to tolerate oral fluids well, the intravenous infusion can be discontinued. For more extensive surgery, it may be useful to administer regular insulin subcutaneously every 4 to 6 hours, or intravenously as discussed in the section on treatment of DKA.

Routine Follow-Up Visits

We schedule routine clinic visits every 3 to 4 months. At each clinic visit, the patient and family meet with the physician and other diabetes care team members. The home blood and urine testing results are reviewed, and the patient's overall success in adhering to the prescribed care plan is assessed. Psychosocial factors that might influence diabetes care, such as school performance or extracurricular activities, are discussed. A complete physical examination is performed at each clinic visit to include measurements of height and weight and examination of insulin injection sites, looking for any lipoatrophy or hypertrophy; thyroid gland (20 per cent of children and adolescents with IDDM have chronic lymphocytic thyroiditis); eyes, including undilated funduscopic examination; and feet. At each clinic visit, blood is obtained for measurement of GHb. At diagnosis and every other year thereafter, blood is obtained for measurements of serum thyroxine, thyroid-stimulating hormone, and thyroid antimicrosomal antibodies. We recommend yearly ophthalmologic evaluations beginning at about age 10 years.

The Future

Diabetes mellitus is a chronic disease with potentially devastating complications. Proper treatment requires commitment by the patient, family, and health care providers. Management issues much more often revolve around psychosocial issues than strictly medical ones. No current treatment approaches can be considered optimal; consistently normal blood glucose patterns are not achievable, and attempts to reach such goals can precipitate serious hypoglycemia. Regardless, most patients with diabetes are capable of safely achieving much better control of their diabetes than they do achieve at present. Poorly controlled diabetes generally reflects inadequate diabetes education or failure of the patient and family to follow the care prescription.

Research is under way to develop more effective means of treatment using pancreatic transplantation, implantable insulin infusion pumps, and other innovative approaches, but these are highly experimental at present. Other research studies are under way to determine if near-normal blood glucose levels long-term can truly improve the outcome for persons with diabetes. One such study, called the Diabetes Control and Complications Trial (DCCT), is being sponsored by the National Institutes of Health and is a long-term clinical trial involving 27 clinical centers in the United States and Canada and 1400 volunteers with IDDM, ages 13 to 39 years.

HYPERURICEMIA AND GOUT

method of
W. NEAL ROBERTS, M.D.
The Medical College of Virginia
Richmond, Virginia

Gout is a heterogeneous group of diseases. In more than 90 per cent of patients, renal tubular defects prevent normal excretion of uric acid. Enzyme defects leading to overproduction of uric acid play a prominent role in other patients. Gout has long been a model of physiologically based medicine, and a number of historically interesting methods have been used in its treatment.

Gout has an increased prevalence of about 3 per cent in the older age groups. Drug toxicities from medication used to treat gout are also more common in the older age group, and the potential for these toxicities creates most of the difficult management choices. Uncertainties of gout management revolve around three problematic areas: (1) the use of allopurinol and alternatives to it; (2) treatment when renal insufficiency coincides with gout and hyperuricemia; (3) the roles for diagnostic maneuvers, including polarized light microscopy of joint fluid for crystals, radiographs, 24-hour urine determination of uric acid, and colchicine trials. Less often, exacerbating factors such as diet, alcohol and aspirin consumption, and the interactions of allopurinol with cytotoxic drugs such as azathioprine and cyclophosphamide complicate management.

Treatment

Treatment is designed to avoid harmful outcomes in the natural history of gout, including uric acid nephrolithiasis, urate nephropathy, tophi, erosive disease of the joint, and, most commonly, acute painful gout attacks. However, urate nephropathy and the variable presentation of gouty arthritis constitute two aspects of the natural history that potentially add to the complexity of management. Urate nephropathy is rare and has no apparent impact on renal function or survival in epidemiologic studies. The main significance of urate nephropathy is that it is sometimes invoked as a reason for treating moderate (7 to 10 mg per dl) asymptomatic hyperuricemia with allopurinol—a clinical decision that is usually incorrect. Almost all cases of urate nephropathy have been reported in patients with overt gouty arthritis instead of asymptomatic hyperuricemia. Finally, there are several clinical presentations of acute crystal deposition in and around joints. The joint affected by a typical gout attack resembles a septic joint, but some attacks appear clinically more like cellulitis over a joint. The classic picture is one of very painful podagra, but joints in the hand, multiple joints, or joints exhibiting only moderate pain may represent gout.

Management of Asymptomatic Hyperuricemia

The conventional classification of gout into four phases—asymptomatic hyperuricemia, acute arthritis, intercritical gout between attacks, and chronic tophaceous gout—does not necessarily imply progression between phases. Most patients with hyperuricemia never have gout, and most patients with gout never develop tophi. In addition, one third of acute attacks occur in people with normal serum uric acid levels. Despite the epidemiologic association between the two, a serum urate value is a poor predictor of a clinical event in the individual patient.

Of the four stages of gout outlined in the conventional scheme, asymptomatic hyperuricemia is the most common, occurring in as many as 5 per cent of the male population. Most allopurinol is incorrectly prescribed for this indication. Several times more allopurinol is sold in the United States than would be used by every symptomatic gout patient taking 300 mg daily.

These figures imply that most of the rare deaths from the hepatotoxicity or exfoliative dermatitis due to allopurinol occur among patients who did not need hypouricemic therapy. The rationale that lowering serum uric acid will protect the kidneys from urate nephropathy is usually ill-founded, since in most patients any decrease in renal function can be attributed to an accompanying disorder such as hypertension, atherosclerosis, or diabetes. These disorders are associated with hyperuricemia but are not affected by treatment of it. Correction of hyperuricemia in non-gouty subjects did not favorably affect renal function in a 2-year randomized, placebo-controlled trial.

Consequently, for most patients who have not experienced their first acute gout attack or episode of nephrolithiasis, the prescription of life-long medication to lower the serum uric acid is unnecessary. Initial therapy is indicated for a few patients who meet criteria for a greater than 50 per cent risk of nephrolithiasis and acute gout: greater than 1100 mg of uric acid in a 24-hour urine collection; greater than 13 mg per dl serum urate on repeated measurements in men; greater than 10 mg per dl in women; anticipated lysis of cells due to cytotoxic chemotherapy or radiation of lymphoma or leukemia. For the more usual patient in an office setting, the risk of side effects from allopurinol and the inconvenience and expense of lifelong therapy make treatment of asymptomatic hyperuricemia impractical and, on balance, harmful. Thiazide diuretics cause many cases of asymptomatic hyperuricemia in office practice. These cases will resolve completely with the choice of an alternative antihypertensive regimen. Weight loss will decrease uric acid in others.

Management of Acute Gout

Acute gout can be treated with nonsteroidal anti-inflammatory drugs (NSAIDs), corticosteroid injection, oral corticosteroids, oral colchicine, intravenous colchicine, and combinations of these agents. One of the most successful regimens for acute gout is a double dose of indomethacin (Indocin) (50 mg three to four times daily) for 2 days followed by a 2-day transition to a usual dose of 25 mg three times a day. Such a regimen permits the patient to avoid both prolonged high-dose NSAID treatment, with its increased risk of gastrointestinal bleeding, and high doses of oral colchicine, which often lead to diarrhea just at the dose that is effective in controlling the gout. Four days of treatment is often sufficient; the earlier treatment begins, the less prolonged it must be.

Alternative treatment employing oral colchicine alone calls for up to 6 mg in the first 24 hours and a dose limit of 8 mg during the first 3 days. An important difference between the NSAID protocol and the colchicine protocol is that the former relies upon a rigid schedule, whereas colchicine is titrated against the pain within strict limits upon total dose. Both oral and intravenous colchicine should be reduced from their maximum dosage in proportion to renal function. This caution particularly applies to intravenous colchicine given as 1 to 3 mg diluted in 30 ml of normal saline over 30 minutes. A scalp vein needle ("butterfly") should not be used as the intravenous access, because extravasation of the colchicine leads to painful local inflammation. Intravenous colchicine has the advantage of being the most rapidly effective of all drugs used against acute gouty arthritis. This feature makes it particularly useful in the emergency room. Intravenous colchicine carries the disadvantage of having the smallest therapeutic index of any drug used in acute gout. A dosage error with NSAIDs may result in vomiting, and the same is true with oral colchicine. In contrast, intravenous colchicine usually bypasses gastrointestinal side effects, but a two- or threefold dosage error by this route may occasionally lead to neutropenia, sepsis, and death without preceding nausea. Intravenous colchicine should be reduced according to the percentage of renal function remaining by using the assumption that a young person with normal renal function will get a maximum of 4 mg total dose with no repeat course within 2 weeks. For the elderly, 3 weeks should elapse between courses of intravenous colchicine. For older people the upper limit calculated in proportion to renal function is often about 2 mg of intravenous colchicine per attack.

Oral or intra-articular corticosteroids for treatment of acute gout are often overlooked. Their disadvantage is that occasionally gout symptoms rebound on the third or fourth day after treatment. As with NSAID therapy, initial corticosteroid treatment can be supplemented by maintenance oral colchicine (0.6 mg orally twice per day) as prophylaxis against recurrent gout after the initial 72 hours.

For acute gout, then, NSAIDs are the most frequently used agents. Indomethacin (Indocin) is the most common individual agent, but any nonsteroidal will work. Intravenous colchicine is the single most effective agent but also the most dangerous if a dosage error should occur.

Management of Intercritical Gout

The decision to treat intercritical gout is usually made either to prevent subsequent kidney stones in a patient who has already experienced one or to prevent subsequent acute attacks of gouty arthritis in a patient who is experiencing attacks at a rate of four or more per year. Fewer attacks can justify lowering the serum uric acid if they are debilitating and prolonged. There are two approaches to preventing attacks of arthritis. Prophylaxis against attacks of arthritis can be achieved conveniently with 0.6 mg oral colchicine twice daily, or with relatively low doses of NSAIDs such as 25 mg Indocin twice daily if colchicine is inappropriate. The second approach is to lower the serum uric acid using allopurinol or probenecid. Indications for choosing the uricosuric approach (probenecid) or xanthine oxidase inhibition (allopurinol) are listed in Table 1. If the patient does not meet the criteria for hypouricemic therapy described in Table 1 and the acute attacks of gouty arthritis are not disabling, a more convenient and less expensive approach is to allow the patient to treat attacks at home at

TABLE 1. **Indications for Hypouricemic Treatment of Gout**

Indication	Explanation
Frequent (2–4/year) and disabling attacks of gouty arthritis	How frequent and how disabling varies according to patient's inclination to comply with a daily medication schedule
Tophaceous deposits in soft tissues	These imply high total body stores and more potential for joint and renal damage
Destructive gouty joint disease	Erosions on radiograph, crystal-proven gout
Recurrent urolithiasis; most recent stone within last 2 years	One stone and severe hyperuricemia or urinary uric acid >800 mg/day is sufficient if patient can be convinced to take daily medication
Severe hyperuricemia (>13 mg/dl in men; >10 mg/dl in women; >15 mg/dl in renal failure)	Risk of arthritis and stones very high; theoretical risk of urate nephropathy unquantified
Severe uric acid overproduction (urinary uric acid excretion >1100 mg/day)	High risk of nephrolithiasis
Prevention of acute uric acid precipitation in renal tubules in patients with leukemia/lymphoma about to receive cytotoxic treatment	
Gout with renal damage	Never proved in practice; most patients considered for this criterion qualify because of severe hyperuricemia. Control of any associated hypertension is more critical than control of serum uric acid

the earliest perception of pain using a standby supply of an NSAID or colchicine. If the patient is properly educated regarding early initiation of therapy, this approach is often successful. As with asymptomatic hyperuricemia, there is a tendency to overtreat intercritical gout. Gout manifested as only two or three manageable attacks per year may not justify a lifelong commitment to daily medication. A poorly understood feature of treatment with hypouricemic agents is the propensity of the patient to develop more frequent acute gout attacks during the first 6 months of hypouricemic treatment. To counteract this propensity, prophylaxis with daily oral colchicine is indicated while the serum urate is declining toward a plateau in the patient on hypouricemic therapy. Once the serum value stabilizes, prophylaxis can be discontinued.

The dose range for allopurinol is 100 to 600 mg daily in a single dose. The usual dose is 300 mg per day. An effective policy is to use the minimum dose that keeps the serum uric acid to a level of about 7 mg per dl. The dose is adjusted every 2 weeks, in order to find the correct level for the individual patient. With both allopurinol and probenecid, beginning at the lowest dose and working up avoids wide swings in serum urate, which tend to bring on attacks. Allopurinol can exacerbate an acute attack and should be added only during an intercritical period.

Probenecid (Benemid) inhibits renal tubular uric acid reabsorption and can be used to reduce serum uric acid. The side effects of probenecid include skin rash and gastrointestinal upset. Gastric intolerance is less common at lower doses. Sulfinpyrazone (Anturane) has a similar mechanism but carries greater risk of bone marrow suppression. The starting dose of probenecid is 250 mg twice daily, increasing to 1 gram per day over 2 weeks. Up to 3 grams per day are sometimes tolerated, but gastrointestinal side effects can limit the total dose and leave the patient with an overall decrement in uric acid of only 2 mg per dl. Because the mechanism of probenecid is to increase renal excretion of uric acid, the drug is contraindicated in patients with nephrolithiasis or greater than 800 mg per day of uric acid excretion in urine. Forced fluids up to 3 liters a day initially, alkalinization of urine to pH 6.5 with Shohl's solution, and prophylactic oral colchicine are necessary adjuncts to use of uricosuric treatment in tophaceous gout to prevent nephrolithiasis and acute attacks.

Management of Tophaceous Gout

Tophaceous gout is one of the stronger indications for hypouricemic treatment (Table 1). Tophi are crystallized deposits of urate and imply risk of joint and renal damage; joint erosions on radiographs also represent crystalline deposits and are equally strong indications for allopurinol or probenecid. Every effort should be made to reduce the serum uric acid to 7 mg per dl in order to mobilize urate in tophaceous gout. Because practical use of probenecid often results in only a 2 mg per dl decrement in serum uric acid, probenecid is often insufficient for patients with tophaceous gout. Specific indications for choosing allopurinol over probenecid include creatinine clearance less than 80 mg per minute, stones, or 24-hour urinary uric acid greater than 800 mg. Rarely a patient with a strong indication for lowering of the serum uric acid will exhibit hypersensitivity to allopurinol. The active metabolite of allopurinol, oxypurinol, which can cross react, is available. Desensitization to allopurinol is possible.

Management of Gout in Renal Insufficiency

Renal disease is the most dangerous special situation in the treatment of gout, complicating therapy of both intercritical and acute gout. Doses of every drug used for gout, except corticosteroids, are affected by renal function. Allopurinol dosage needs to be drastically reduced in the presence of diminished renal function. For an anephric patient the dose can go as low as 100 mg every third day. A creatinine clearance of 10 ml per minute implies an allopurinol dose of 100 mg every other day; 20 ml, 100 mg daily; and 40 ml, 200 mg daily. In patients with renal insufficiency, 0.6 mg of colchicine by mouth twice daily occasionally leads to a myopathy with elevated creatine kinase or to a peripheral neuropathy. These cases are diagnostic problems mimicking polymyositis and uremic neuropathy. Patients with creatine clearances less than 50 ml per minute should probably try gout prophylaxis with 0.6 mg only once per day. Probenecid is not able to increase uric acid excretion substantially in patients with renal insufficiency; it should not be used. Sulindac probably has the least effect upon intrarenal prostaglandin production and glomerular filtration pressure. However, every nonsteroidal can result in this reversible decrease in glomerular filtration. Dehydrated patients who already exhibit some decrement in creatine clearance are the most vulnerable to NSAID-induced acute renal failure. Prominent in this latter group are older patients exhibiting serum creatinines within normal limits but who have small muscle masses and actual creatinine clearances of 30 to 40 ml per minute.

Sometimes the least problematic regimen for acute gout in renal insufficiency is one that begins with oral or injectable corticosteroid (10 or

15 mg of prednisone orally for 3 days is often adequate), accompanied by an optional reduced regimen of oral colchicine (0.6 mg daily) to prevent the rebound sometimes seen after corticosteroid treatment of gout. Moderate doses of prednisone produce surprisingly little perturbation in glucose control in most diabetic patients. Rebound after steroid treatment may not occur, especially if injectable steroids have been used, and in any case rebound can be avoided with reduced doses of nonsteroidals or oral colchicine that would, by themselves, be inadequate to control the acute attack. The feared complications of corticosteroids rarely if ever occur, owing to the short courses of treatment needed for gout.

Emergency Room Setting

In the emergency room when a quick resolution of gout symptoms is important, narcotic analgesia may play a role. Narcotics are particularly helpful when angina or myocardial infarction occurs with acute gout. A 2 mg infusion of intravenous colchicine can produce a very rapid analgesia (usually within 3 hours) through its specific anti-inflammatory effect. Rapid response to intravenous colchicine serves a diagnostic function as well. Safe use of intravenous colchicine in the emergency room requires that the drug not be given in doses beyond 1 or 2 mg until renal function has been assessed. An initial trial of 1 mg intravenously is appropriate for older patients.

Diagnostic Problems Affecting Therapy

Several diagnostic questions frequently affect treatment choices in acute and intercurrent gout. These questions include the following: (1) when to omit arthrocentesis with crystal diagnosis and substitute another method such as radiographs, colchicine trial, or assessment of general clinical picture; (2) when to obtain a radiograph; (3) when to obtain a 24-hour urine collection for uric acid measurement; (4) when to revise the diagnosis and consider entirely different monoarticular diseases such as peripheral arthritis of ankylosing spondylitis, psoriatic arthritis, or Reiter's syndrome.

There is seldom urgency to make a specific diagnosis of gout. However, when such a diagnosis is needed there is no substitute for arthrocentesis and examination for crystals under polarized light. Owing to the similarity between the appearance of septic joints and gouty joints, certain situations absolutely prohibit omission of the arthrocentesis. In particular, patients who have fever and uncertain follow-up, uncertain compliance, or diabetes and an inflamed joint in the foot all need arthrocentesis. Patients whose attacks elude crystal-proved diagnosis and respond to treatment slowly may have another type of monoarthritis. A radiograph is rarely helpful in the first few years of the course. If there have been multiple attempts at crystal diagnosis via arthrocenteses and multiple attacks over several years, then it is reasonable to order a radiograph to look for the characteristic erosion with an overhanging edge. In contrast, when there have been only one or two attacks a radiograph ordered in the emergency room is of little value. In particular, an acute septic joint cannot be ruled out by radiograph. A 24-hour urinary uric acid measurement is most useful in resolving indecision about starting uricosuric therapy or xanthine oxidase inhibition, especially if renal function is abnormal. For a patient whose overall clinical situation (including stone history and frequency and severity of attacks of arthritis) is almost sufficient to justify a lifelong prescription, hyperexcretion (a 24-hour urine collection with uric acid above 800 mg) will sway the decision in favor of starting allopurinol. All patients who are about to receive probenecid should have a 24-hour urine collection to determine that they do in fact have uric acid excretions less than 800 mg per day. This policy precludes the possibility of giving a uricosuric agent to someone who is already predisposed to form uric acid kidney stones.

Cautions Regarding Individual Agents

Nonsteroidal anti-inflammatory drugs can cause perforations in patients with peptic ulcer disease or inflammatory bowel disease. Serious allopurinol toxicity characterized by eosinophilia, exfoliative dermatitis, fever, hepatocellular damage, acute renal failure, and vasculitis occurs more often in patients taking thiazide diuretics and patients with renal insufficiency. Ten to 20

TABLE 2. **Errors in Gout Management**

Prescription of allopurinol for asymptomatic hyperuricemia, or for hyperuricemia due to diuretics

Failure either to adjust doses of colchicine or allopurinol for renal insufficiency or to substitute corticosteroids

Prescription of allopurinol and an interacting drug such as azathioprine, cyclophosphamide, or warfarin without reduction in dosage

Daily intravenous colchicine for patient unable to take medication by mouth

Failure to recognize gouty erosions on radiograph as equivalent to tophi as indications for hypouricemic treatment

Failure to reconsider the diagnosis when treatment fails and gout is not crystal-proven (alternative diagnoses include Reiter's syndrome, psoriatic arthropathy, peripheral joint involvement in spondyloarthropathy)

Arthrotomy for presumed septic joint, especially in the hand, in a setting compatible with gout, prior to arthrocentesis and examination for crystals per cent of these rare idiosyncratic reactions are fatal. Allopurinol is the agent for gout that exhibits the most interaction with other drugs. Warfarin (Coumadin), azathioprine (which is metabolized by xanthine oxidase), and cyclophosphamide are all potentiated by allopurinol. When azathioprine is prescribed with allopurinol, the azathioprine should be reduced to a one-third dosage. Allopurinol and ampicillin prescribed together frequently cause a rash. The major limitations of probenecid are that in practical use it seldom produces more than a 2 mg per dl decrease in serum uric acid and that because of the risk of nephrolithiasis it cannot be used in patients with hyperexcretion.

With one exception, deaths from colchicine have been described only in patients who received at least some of the drug intravenously and in whom a dosage error was made. Sources of dosage errors are: (1) the assumption that patients who can take nothing by mouth can have their oral colchicine replaced mg for mg with intravenous colchicine over a period of days; (2) failure to follow the total dosage guidelines; (3) the impression that a 4-mg course of intravenous colchicine can be repeated for the same attack if unsuccessful the first time; (4) overestimation of an elderly patient's creatinine clearance; and (5) the prescription of intravenous colchicine in unusual situations that exacerbate colchicine's toxicity or interfere with its metabolism. These latter situations include inflammatory bowel disease, combined liver and renal disease, and a pre-existing regimen of a drug such as cyclophosphamide, which suppresses bone marrow and potentiates the capacity of an overdose of colchicine to produce neutropenia and sepsis.

Pitfalls in the treatment of gout are outlined in Table 2. From the public health standpoint, the greatest impact comes from the excessive use of allopurinol for asymptomatic hyperuricemia. Adjustments of colchicine and allopurinol dosages for renal insufficiency are also important for a small number of patients.

HYPERLIPOPROTEINEMIA

method of
NEIL J. STONE, M.D.
Northwestern University School of Medicine
Chicago, Illinois

Cholesterol and triglycerides can be viewed as independent entities in the detection and evaluation of hyperlipidemia. Cholesterol is ubiquitous among animals because of its key role in cell membranes, adrenal hormones, and the various forms of vitamin D. It is not found in vegetable products. Triglycerides are sources of storage fat. Fatty acid chains are attached to the glycerol backbone of triglycerides. These fatty acid chains determine whether the fat will be in the form of saturated fats, which raise cholesterol levels, or monounsaturated or polyunsaturated fats, which, if substituted for saturated fat in the diet, lower cholesterol levels.

Cholesterol and triglycerides, however, are insoluble and must be packaged into large macromolecular complexes called lipoproteins. Treatment then requires that the problem of hyperlipidemia be restated in terms of lipoprotein excess or deficiency. The four major lipoprotein classes include (1) the triglyceride-rich lipoproteins called *chylomicrons,* which carry dietary glyceride, (2) the *very-low-density lipoproteins* (VLDL), which are produced in the liver, (3) the *cholesterol-rich* lipoproteins called the *low-density lipoproteins* (LDL), which are either produced from intravascular conversion from VLDL or secreted from the liver, and (4) the *high-density lipoproteins* (HDL), which are secreted as cholesterol-poor precursors from liver and intestine.

The LDL usually carry about 70 per cent of the plasma cholesterol. These are small particles that depend for clearance on cell-surface receptors (LDL receptors). These receptors function to provide the cells with an adequate supply of cholesterol. Subunits of LDL called apoproteins (apo) help the LDL receptor recognize LDL. The liver, which is the major site for LDL removal, has LDL receptors that recognize at least two kinds of these surface components of LDL, known as apo B100 and apo E. Diet influences the liver's cholesterol production through remnants of chylomicron metabolism, which also interact with the LDL receptor. Normally, a lesser amount of LDL is cleared by macrophages through a non–LDL-receptor-mediated process.

Excess cholesterol and saturated fat in the diet elevate blood cholesterol through the LDL receptor mechanism. The liver cells deal with the increased cholesterol from LDL by reducing intracellular production of cholesterol. This is accomplished by inhibition of the enzyme that controls the rate-limiting step in cholesterol synthesis, HMG CoA reductase. As a consequence, fewer LDL receptors are produced to prevent dietary cholesterol from overloading the cell. When an inherited defect causes less than the usual number of functioning LDL receptors, plasma LDL cholesterol (LDL-C) concentrations rise and there is a proportionate increase in CHD.

HDL is an even smaller lipoprotein than LDL. HDL carry about 20 to 25 per cent of the plasma cholesterol. This protein-rich class of lipoproteins functions to remove cholesterol from tissues and transport it to the liver. HDL also provide cholesterol to lipoproteins and serve as a reservoir of apoproteins for triglyceride-rich lipoproteins to aid in their efficient metabolism. Commonly when triglyceride levels are high owing to impaired catabolism, HDL cholesterol (HDL-C) levels are low. Families with elevated HDL-C have a low rate of CHD. Moreover, since the initial observation that men with myocardial infarction (MI) had low levels of HDL-C, numerous epidemiologic and angio-

TABLE 1. **Six-Year Coronary Heart Disease Death Rates per 1000 as a Function of Quintiles of Blood Cholesterol, Smoking Status, and Diastolic Blood Pressure (DBP) in MRFIT Trial**

Blood Cholesterol (mg/dl)	DBP < 90 mm Hg		DBP > 90 mm Hg	
	Nonsmokers	*Smokers*	*Nonsmokers*	*Smokers*
≤181	1.6	5.2	3.7	6.3
182–202	2.5	5.5	4.0	10.0
203–220	2.7	7.3	5.6	15.5
221–244	3.8	10.2	5.6	16.6
245 or more	6.4	13.3	10.7	21.4

graphic studies have confirmed that low HDL-C is a powerful, independent predictor of an increased risk of CHD. The Framingham Study noted that the ratios of cholesterol/HDL-C or LDL-C/HDL-C in persons over age 50 were useful summary predictors of coronary events. Values for the cholesterol/HDL-C exceeding 6 and the LDL-C/HDL-C exceeding 4 were shown to signify a high risk of CHD. Clinicians are cautioned, however, that a single ratio is not always as informative as the individual fractions that make up the estimate.

Detection and Assessment of Hypercholesterolemia

The large data set of more than 350,000 persons screened in the Multiple Risk Factor Intervention Trial showed that with increasing cholesterol levels, the risk of CHD was exponential, with strikingly higher rates at levels above 240 mg per dl. Below 200 mg per dl the risk seemed lower, but there did not appear to be a threshold above which risk commenced. Although atherosclerosis is seen in persons with values from 150 to 220 mg per dl, clinical CHD is less likely and occurs later in life at any level of risk factors in this group.

Clearly, the presence of CHD or risk factors for CHD increase the risk of CHD at any given cholesterol value. In the MRFIT trial, the risk of CHD for hypertensive smokers with the lowest cholesterol values was similar to the risk of CHD for normotensive nonsmokers with the highest cholesterol values (Table 1).

Thus, further evaluation is required when an individual has elevated blood cholesterol (more than 240 mg per dl) or has a cholesterol level between 200 and 239 mg per dl and either definite CHD or two or more of risk factors for CHD (Table 2). If elevated blood

TABLE 2. **Risk Factors for Coronary Heart Disease**

Male sex
Hypertension
Cigarette smoking (currently smokes more than 10 cigarettes per day)
Diabetes
Low HDL cholesterol (less than 35 mg/dl as measured at least twice)
Family history of CHD (parent or sibling affected before age 55)
Marked obesity (greater than 30%)
Presence of definite cerebrovascular or occlusive peripheral vascular disease

cholesterol is determined in a mass screening program, it is important to confirm this value with a repeat test in a standardized laboratory. If two values differ by more than 30 mg per dl, then a third test should be performed. The action required once blood cholesterol and risk factor status for CHD is determined is outlined in Table 3.

Those at higher risk for coronary events require specific therapy. Lipoprotein analysis (to determine LDL-C and HDL-C) is needed to guide total risk assessment and therapy. Fortunately, total cholesterol, triglycerides, and HDL-C can be measured on a single fasting blood sample. The following formula is used to calculate the LDL-C value:

$$LDL\text{-}C = \text{Total cholesterol} - (HDL\text{-}C) - (\text{triglyceride}/5)$$

(This assumes a specimen obtained after a 12- to 16-hour fast, a triglyceride level less than 400 mg per dl, and the absence of the rare dysbetalipoproteinemia [Type III] disorder.)

The LDL-C determination should be repeated within 1 to 6 weeks to provide an average value that is a more reliable baseline measurement. If values vary by more than 30 mg per dl, a third determination should be done.

Table 4 shows how to proceed after LDL-C values are determined. When there is a primary elevation of LDL (i.e., no secondary cause such as hypothyroidism, obstructive liver disease, or nephrosis), a goal LDL-C can be set. The recommended goals are set to be minimal goals. In many cases, lower levels can be encouraged and easily achieved, resulting in even further reduction of CHD risk. Also, family members should be screened for high blood cholesterol.

Table 5 illustrates that once there is evidence of response to dietary therapy, total cholesterol can act as a surrogate for LDL-C in monitoring progress over the long term. This is especially true if HDL-C values are within the normal range. Nonetheless, it is prudent to measure LDL-C values periodically and assess the relationship between total cholesterol and LDL-C in the individual patient.

Hypertriglyceridemia

Borderline hypertriglyceridemia is defined as triglyceride values from 250 to 499 mg per dl. Definite hypertriglyceridemia is defined as values of 500 mg per dl and above. Although elevated triglyceride values have not been proved to be independent risk factors

TABLE 3. **Cholesterol Screening Guidelines**

Blood Cholesterol Value (mg/dl)	CHD or Two Risk Factors	Recommendations
<200	Absent	Repeat again in 5 yrs Provide general dietary and risk factor education
<200	Present	Same as above, but some physicians may wish to check HDL*
200–239	Absent	Re-evaluate annually Provide Step One diet
200–239	Present	Measure lipoproteins: HDL-C and LDL-C Further assessment
≥240	Absent or present	Measure lipoproteins: HDL-C and LDL-C Further assessment

*To see if familial hypoalphalipoproteinemia is present as a risk factor for CHD.

for CHD, high triglyceride levels are commonly seen in CHD. Hypertriglyceridemia due to overproduction of VLDL particles by the liver is associated with CHD. This should be suspected when elevated triglyceride levels are associated with either a personal or family history of abnormal lipids or lipoproteins (elevated LDL-C and/or low HDL-C), when there is elevated apo B, or when there is a personal or family history of CHD. Look for metabolic influences (e.g., pregnancy), dietary factors (e.g., alcohol excess), medications (e.g., estrogens and steroids), or diseases (e.g., insulinopenic diabetes) that can exacerbate existing hypertriglyceridemia such that triglyceride levels exceed 1500 mg per dl (creamy plasma is seen) and acute pancreatitis occurs. This requires prompt diet and drug therapy.

Dietary Treatment

Effect of Diet on CHD

The link between diet and CHD is inferred from data gathered from regression experiments in Rhesus monkeys and epidemiologic studies in humans. The most convincing of the latter was a landmark observational study involving groups of men in seven countries showing strong correlations between dietary saturated fat intake and serum cholesterol levels. Moreover, detailed die-

tary data showed striking correlations between saturated fat intake and CHD. Data from two prospective studies with detailed dietary records and lipid assessments at baseline showed that 20-year rates of CHD were highly correlated with dietary cholesterol intake despite small effects on blood cholesterol values. These studies also showed that regular consumption of fish in the diet was associated with lower rates of CHD. This suggests that diets rich in dietary cholesterol can have adverse effects on atherosclerosis even in those with mild blood cholesterol elevations. Although it is tempting to recommend fish oil capsules to patients because of various studies showing beneficial effects of oils rich in eicosapentanoic acid, there are no long-term data showing efficacy or toxicity of current preparations in Western populations. This contrasts with the excellent data supporting the recommendation of frequent consumption of fish.

Finally, two intervention trials give compelling evidence that a diet lower in saturated fat and dietary cholesterol can lower lipid and lipoprotein values and also reduce risk of CHD. The Oslo study examined hard endpoints for CHD in middle-aged men with severe hypercholesterolemia who were randomly assigned to receive either

TABLE 4. **Use of LDL-C to Determine Dietary or Drug Therapy***

LDL-C Value (mg/dl)	CHD or Two or More Major Risk Factors	Action
1. <130 (desirable LDL-C)	Absent or present	Repeat cholesterol measurements in 5 years General dietary, risk factor education
2. 130–159 (borderline high risk LDL-C)	Absent	Reevaluate status annually Provide information on the Step One diet
3. 130–159 (borderline high risk LDL-C)	Present	Clinical evaluation† Goal LDL-C < 130
4. 160 or more (high risk LDL-C)	Absent	Clinical evaluation† Goal LDL-C < 160
5. 160 or more (high risk LDL-C)	Present	Clinical evaluation† Goal LDL-C < 130 mg/dl

*LDL-C determined by formula; average of two or three measurements.
†Rule out secondary factors and familial causes with history, exam, and laboratory tests. Consider influence of age and sex.

TABLE 5. **Values for Goal LDL-C and Total Cholesterol**

Clinical Status	Goal LDL-C (mg/dl)	Surrogate Goal Blood Cholesterol (mg/dl)
No CHD and less than two risk factors for CHD	<160	<240
Definite CHD or two or more risk factors for CHD	<130	<200

diet and smoking advice or no intervention. The intervention group showed a 13 per cent fall in blood cholesterol and a decline in smoking, with a 47 per cent less incidence of sudden death and MI than the control group. Another study of the effects of vegetarian diet in moderately hypercholesterolemic men with angina who underwent coronary angiography before diet and 2 years later showed disease progression to be significant in patients whose total/HDL cholesterol ratios were greater than 6.9. Yet no growth in coronary lesions was seen in patients who had values less than 6.9 or whose higher values were significantly lowered by diet.

The Step One and Step Two Diets

The Step One diet is recommended as the initial dietary intervention to achieve the total cholesterol and LDL-C goals. This diet restricts total fat to 30 per cent of calories, saturated fat to less than 10 per cent of calories, and dietary cholesterol to 300 mg per day. If lipid measurements at 4 to 6 weeks and again at 3 months do not show that the cholesterol and LDL-C goals are achieved and adherence seems satisfactory, then the Step Two diet is recommended. This dietary pattern restricts saturated fat to no more than 7 per cent of total calories and limits dietary cholesterol to 200 mg per day or less. This dietary pattern will require the assistance of a dietitian for optimal adherence. Table 6 compares these diets with a typical American diet. For those with hypertriglyceridemia, it is important to stress

weight reduction toward ideal weight and regular exercise as an initial step. Also, excess calories from alcohol must be curtailed.

Meat fat, dairy fat, commercial baked goods, egg fat, and fat used in preparation and processing of foods represent the major contributors of saturated fat and cholesterol in the diet. Physicians should be aware of dietary alterations in these five areas that can improve adherence to a lower-fat diet. Table 7 gives some practical suggestions. Lists such as this can be photocopied and given to patients. Having patients walk through the grocery store reading labels so they can get a better idea of the range of products made with saturated fats like coconut oil, palm oil, palm kernel oil, and cocoa butter is as instructive as it is enlightening. For those with mild elevations of cholesterol, maintenance of desirable weight and regular exercise may be all that is required to lower blood cholesterol. Weight loss and exercise both also have the advantage of raising levels of HDL-C. Alcohol raises HDL-C as well as the triglyceride level. Alcohol's beneficial effect on CHD incidence does not appear to be mediated through its effects on lipoproteins. The HDL-3 fraction, not the protective HDL-2 fraction, is raised with chronic alcohol usage. Prescribing alcohol to raise HDL-C is not recommended.

Adherence to and success of the diet will vary greatly with patients. For those with mild hypercholesterolemia (up to 240 mg per dl), physician endorsement, prescription, and encouragement of the Step One diet may be the only stimulus needed. For these individuals, successful lipid reduction can be expected to occur within 3 to 6 months. Studies suggest that a switch from a high-fat, typical American diet to the Step One diet could reduce blood cholesterol levels by at least 30 mg per dl. For those with higher cholesterol values, diet alone may be insufficient to achieve the minimal goal levels. In these cases, more frequent contact with the registered dietitian can best accomplish dietary change. Periodic monitoring with blood or LDL-C values gives the

TABLE 6. **The Step One and Step Two Diets versus a Typical American Diet**

Constituents of Diet	Typical American	Step One	Step Two
Dietary cholesterol (mg per day)	500	<300	<200
Total calories		Achieve and maintain ideal weight	
		Below Given as Percentage of Total Calories	
Total fat	40	<30	<30
Saturated fat	17	<10	<7
Polyunsaturated fat	6	Up to 10	Up to 10
Monounsaturated fat	17	10–15	10–15
Carbohydrates	40	50–60	50–60
Protein	20	10–20	10–20

TABLE 7. **Diet Modifications to Achieve a Lower Fat Diet**

Category	Ask Regarding:	Advise
Meal frequency	How many meals per day? How many are out?	Regular, balanced meals Lower fat selections
Meat ingestion	Beef, pork, lamb, veal? Portion size? Organ meats like liver? Eating fowl with skin? Hot dogs, sausages eaten?	Leaner cuts of meat 4 ounces or less Avoidance Eating without the skin Eating more sparingly
Egg yolks	How many per week?	Egg white omelettes or recipes with fewer yolks; egg substitutes
Dairy products	Whole milk? Whole milk products? Cheeses? Ice cream?	Skim milk (or 1%); low-fat cheeses; low-fat ice cream or yogurt
Invisible fats	Baked goods: doughnuts, cakes, cookies, pies?	Products whose labels show no coconut, palm, or palm kernel oils Watch calories
Cooking and table fats	Cook with lard, butter, shortening? Creamy salad dressings?	Soft margarine or unsaturated oils Clear dressings using mono- or polyunsaturated oils
Snacks	Ice cream, cake, candy bars, cookies, or chips?	Products without saturated fats or snacks of fruit or whole-grain products
Spirits	How many drinks per week? (Drink is 1 oz of liquor, one can of beer, one glass of wine)	Moderation (restrict intake if high triglycerides)

needed feedback for continued progress toward goal values. It is helpful to warn patients who may prefer drug therapy without a reasonable dietary trial that medication is not curative and that the convenience of a pill must be balanced against the cost not only in dollars spent, but in the potential for side effects.

Drug Therapy

The cutpoints for initiating drug therapy were set high so as to discourage drug usage. Drug therapy should be considered for those with LDL-C above 190 mg per ml despite rigorous diet for at least a 6-month period or those with LDL-C above 160 mg per ml and a high risk status. Those needing drugs often have familial lipoprotein disorders.

Familial Disorders

Those with inherited defects in cholesterol metabolism, such as the patient with *familial hypercholesterolemia* (FH) whose cholesterol values run 2 to 3 times normal, require lipid-lowering medication as well as diet. Clinically, heterozygotes for FH are recognized by having cholesterol values 325 to 450 mg per dl despite diet, tendon xanthomas involving most commonly the Achilles tendons and the extensor tendons over the metacarpals, and premature CHD with more than 50 per cent of close relatives experiencing CHD before age 60. In these families, the defi-

ciency of functioning LDL receptors is seen in successive generations, as it is inherited as an autosomal dominant trait. Family screening is productive, as there is a 50 per cent chance that each close relative (even children) will be affected.

Other inherited disorders also affect lipid levels. *Familial combined hyperlipidemia* is the commonest genetic lipid disorder among survivors of MI. In affected families, multiple family members are found to have abnormal levels of either cholesterol or triglyceride or both. Elevated levels of apo B may be a useful marker to detect affected family members. Xanthomas are not seen, and children are usually not affected. In *polygenic hypercholesterolemia* multiple family members have cholesterol values elevated above the population norm. Also, rare cases of *familial dysbetalipoproteinemia* (also referred to as Type III hyperlipoproteinemia) are recognized by markedly elevated cholesterol and triglyceride levels along with palmar and tuberous xanthomas. In families with this disorder, a high prevalence of early peripheral vascular disease as well as CHD is seen.

Drug Evaluation

The ideal cholesterol-lowering drug would effectively lower LDL-C and raise HDL-C. It would be proved to reduce both total mortality and hard endpoint for CHD. It would have no long-term toxicity. It would be an inexpensive, easily taken medication and relatively free of side effects. Currently, drugs of first choice include the bile acid resins such as cholestyramine (Questran), colestipol (Colestid), and niacin; also highly considered after these is gemfibrozil (Lopid). They are chosen owing to their proven efficacy in lowering LDL-C and/or raising HDL-C and their relatively safe, long-term profiles. Newer drugs should be considered when first-line drugs cannot be tolerated or when the severity of the problem mandates a more aggressive approach. Lovastatin's ability to treat severely elevated cholesterol effectively makes this drug increasingly attractive. While the exact role for probucol has not been determined, its antiatherosclerotic effects must be considered for certain patients (Table 8).

The maintenance dosages suggested will be those likely to be used in patients with FH. Patients with nonfamilial, milder forms of hypercholesterolemia will often reach their goals for LDL-C with lower dosages.

Bile Acid–Sequestering Resins. These agents are considered front-line therapy because they are not absorbed systemically. The two agents available are cholestyramine (Questran) and colestipol (Colestid). By exchanging chloride ions for bile acids in the gut, they prevent the enterohepatic circulation of bile acids and promote their fecal excretion. This causes increased cholesterol conversion to bile acids in the liver cells with an increase in LDL receptors. This increase is only partial, as there is a compensatory rise in cholesterol synthesis. Both resins are packaged in cannisters and packets. Most patients tolerate the resins best by starting off with just one packet or scoop (4 grams of cholestyramine or 5 grams of colestipol) and increasing the dosage gradually. Those with nonfamilial hypercholesterolemia often respond well to 2 to 3 scoops or packets daily, while those with FH will need 4 to 6 scoops or packets of resin daily to approach goal LDL-C values.

EFFICACY. In patients with severe hypercholesterolemia likely to have FH, declines in cholesterol and LDL-C of 20 per cent and 27 per cent are seen with doses of 4 scoops or packets taken daily. HDL-C is also raised. For those with mild hypercholesterolemia, low doses are likely to be effective. With time, there can be a waning of these effects. Resins have been shown to decrease hard events of CHD in men without overt CHD. The magnitude of the effect appears to depend on the amount of LDL lowering, with each 1 per cent decline in LDL-C linked to a 2 per cent decline in CHD events.

TOXICITY. The drug is nonsystemic. Gastrointestinal side effects predominate. Constipation, aggravation of hemorrhoids, bloating, distention, and cramping can be seen. Use of a high-fiber diet and/or psyllium derivatives seems to help. Some tolerate the drugs well even at high doses of 20 to 24 grams per day, while others are intolerant at low dosage. If triglycerides are elevated (above 250 mg per dl), resins should not be used alone, as they will elevate triglycerides further.

EASE OF USE. The resins are gritty powders that are mixed with liquids like fruit juice or milk and taken twice daily. The cost is moderate, with convenient packets usually more expensive than dosing from large cannisters with a prepackaged scoop. Resins interfere with other medications such as digoxin, antibiotics, thiazides, warfarin, and thyroxine. One study showed that digoxin capsules were less likely than tablets to be affected by cholestyramine. Resins need to be taken 1 hour after other medications or at least 4 hours before. Since resins are best given on a twice-daily regimen, many physicians find it convenient to give medications like digoxin and vitamins at noon, with resin doses given in the morning and at night.

Niacin. Niacin is vitamin B_3. It should be contrasted with niacinamide, which has useful vita-

TABLE 8. **Guide for Selecting Lipid-Lowering Therapy**

Category	Drugs
First-line drugs	Resins (cholestyramine, colestipol)
	Niacin
	Gemfibrozil
Most powerful LDL-C–lowering drug	Lovastatin (may be first-line in future; no long-term trial data at present)
Safest long-term	Resins (nonabsorbable)
Cheapest	Unmodified niacin
Easiest to use	Lovastatin, gemfibrozil, probucol
Raises HDL-C	Niacin, gemfibrozil, lovastatin; mildly so, resins
Lowers triglycerides	Niacin, gemfibrozil, lovastatin
Raises triglycerides	Resins
Combinations to try in familial hypercholesterolemia	Resins and niacin; resins and lovastatin; resins and probucol; in some, triple therapy
Combinations to avoid	Lovastatin and gemfibrozil; clofibrate and probucol

min effects but is not effective in lowering lipid levels. Niacin inhibits fatty acid release from adipose tissue and decreases secretion of VLDL from the liver by decreasing the turnover of apo B. Niacin also causes a decrease in the fractional catabolic rate of HDL, leading to higher serum levels of HDL-C, through an increase in the HDL-2 subfraction. Niacin is available in tablet form or in a sustained-release preparation. The initial dosage is either 100 or 250 mg of drug taken two or three times daily with food. FH patients often require 2 to 4 grams per day for good effect, and some patients who tolerate the drug well can be treated with more.

EFFICACY. Niacin lowers cholesterol, LDL-C, and triglycerides and raises HDL-C. It is effective in a dose-dependent manner in mild to severe hypercholesterolemia. It is particularly useful when triglycerides are elevated as well. It was used at a dosage of 3 grams per day in the Coronary Drug Project study, in which it lowered nonfatal MI rates and on follow-up 14 years later was shown to reduce mortality by 11 per cent as compared with placebo.

TOXICITY. Niacin can cause abnormal liver function tests, ulcers, hyperglycemia, and gout. Dry skin or acanthosis nigricans can occasionally be seen. Since niacin irritates the stomach, its use is contraindicated in active peptic ulcer disease. Time-release preparations appear to cause a greater number of gastrointestinal side effects and fatigue and significantly greater increases in alkaline phosphatase.

EASE OF USE. USP niacin comes in 100 mg and 500 mg tablets. Use of the drug would be more widespread were it not for the invariable facial and truncal flushing and itching that accompanies its use. This is due to prostaglandin-mediated vasodilation. It can be inhibited, but not completely prevented, by taking an aspirin tablet one half hour before its use. The reaction is mild in some and more severe in others. In those with severe reactions, the timed-release form may be of benefit. Most patients can tolerate the unmodified form if warned about this flushing, learn to always take niacin with food, and avoid concurrent hot liquids or alcohol. Starting at a low dosage and building up the dosage gradually helps patients acclimate to the effects of niacin as well. In most, tolerance will gradually develop.

Gemfibrozil. Gemfibrozil is a fibric acid derivative with potent effects on triglycerides and HDL-C. It appears to act by decreasing production of VLDL and increasing its clearance. It comes in 300-mg tablets that are taken twice daily. The usual maintenance dosage is 600 mg twice daily.

EFFICACY. Initially, gemfibrozil was approved only for triglyceride values above 750 mg per dl

to prevent pancreatitis. The Helsinki trial showed that in men with moderately severe hypercholesterolemia (cholesterol 270 mg per dl) at baseline, gemfibrozil lowered cholesterol by 11 per cent and LDL-C by 10 per cent, and increased HDL by more than 10 per cent. In agreement with previous studies, LDL-C reductions were largest in those with the highest baseline LDL-C, and in those with LDL-C 160 mg per dl or less, LDL-C actually rose. There was a reduction of 34 per cent in hard cardiac endpoints in this study, and the effect became evident in the second year of the study.

TOXICITY. Although gemfibrozil increases biliary cholesterol saturation in healthy persons, significant increases in cholecystectomies were not seen in the Helsinki trial. This is unlike clofibrate, which clearly increases gallstone incidence.

EASE OF USE. There is a mild increase in upper gastrointestinal symptoms with gemfibrozil.

Lovastatin. Lovastatin (Mevacor) is the newest lipid-lowering agent to be approved. It is a competitive inhibitor of HMG CoA reductase, the rate-limiting enzyme of intracellular cholesterol synthesis. The resultant increase in LDL receptors causes marked lowering of LDL-C. The current dosage form is a 20-mg pill, which produces a better blood level when it is taken concurrently with the evening meal. Maximal dosage is 40 mg twice daily.

EFFICACY. Cholesterol and LDL cholesterol are lowered dramatically even in familial forms of hypercholesterolemia. In a multicenter trial of severe hypercholesterolemia, lovastatin 40 mg twice daily lowered total cholesterol 34 per cent and LDL-C 42 per cent, which was roughly twice the lowering seen with 24 grams per day of cholestyramine. There are no large-scale clinical trial data available.

TOXICITY. There is a 1.9 per cent incidence of hepatic side effects, and liver enzymes should be monitored frequently during therapy. This effect is usually seen after 3 months. Myositis is seen rarely; an increased incidence including rhabdomyolysis is seen in patients on cyclosporine for immunosuppression or on concomitant gemfibrozil. Lovastatin should not be used with these medications. Moreover, any muscle tenderness, fever, or dark urine should be cause for stopping the drug, measuring creatine phosphokinase levels, and observing for rhabdomyolysis.

Finally, although there has been much concern regarding lens opacities, no evidence for drug-induced lens opacities has been noted.

EASE OF USE. There is a low incidence of gastrointestinal side effects.

Probucol. Probucol (Lorelco) lowers both LDL-C

and HDL-C by affecting LDL structure rather than by stimulating LDL receptor activity. This non–receptor-mediated mechanism is thought to be the basis for the tissue cholesterol mobilization seen in hypercholesterolemic rabbits and homozygous cases of FH. Probucol comes as 250-mg tablets. The dosage is 500 mg given twice daily.

EFFICACY. Probucol appears to lower cholesterol by 15 to 20 per cent, and LDL-C by a lesser amount on average, since HDL-C also is reduced. Probucol has no effect on triglycerides. One randomized but nonblinded multifactorial intervention trial with small numbers of patients who used probucol and clofibrate did not show a decreased incidence of CHD after 5 years. Probucol and clofibrate together lowered HDL-C severely.

TOXICITY. Probucol prolongs the QT interval. No arrhythmogenic effect in man has been noted. The side effects are gastrointestinal. Probucol is stored in adipose tissue and slowly excreted in the bile.

EASE OF USE. Mild diarrhea is seen in some patients.

Combination Drug Therapy. Combination therapy is indicated for the patient who cannot reach the goal LDL-C value because of either the severity of the hypercholesterolemia (e.g., FH heterozygous and homozygous cases) or the toxicity and side effects that occur when large dosages of any single agent are used. This strategy can allow resins to be used in a lower, better-tolerated dosage. In a study of men with previous coronary bypass surgery, colestipol and niacin lowered LDL-C below 100 mg per dl on average and caused a marked reduction in progression of CHD seen on follow-up coronary angiography. Resins and lovastatin or resins and probucol are examples of combinations reported to be useful. Triple therapy with resins, niacin, and lovastatin should be considered in severe cases.

OBESITY

method of
GEORGE A. BRAY, M.D.
University of Southern California
Los Angeles County/USC Medical Center
Los Angeles, California

Treating individuals with weight problems has many similarities to treatment of other chronic illnesses. Although hypertension can be effectively treated by current medications, the side effects of treatment and the need to treat individuals who may have no symptoms from their hypertension lead to high levels of therapeutic failure, including unwillingness of the hypertensive individuals to seek medical help, unwilling-

ness to maintain treatment once prescribed, and termination of treatment because of some of the side effects of medications. Treatments for overweight, like those for hypertension and many other chronic illnesses, are palliative, not curative. By cure is meant a treatment that when terminated produces a permanent remission, with no further treatment required. A simple example is appendectomy, in which the patient is cured by surgical removal of the diseased appendix. Comparable results with treatment for overweight are rare. One example would be effective treatment for Cushing's disease in which the primary presenting problem was obesity. For most cases, however, we are seeking palliation and alleviation of symptoms associated with obesity, not a cure.

Recidivism, or regaining of lost weight, is another reality of treatment for obesity. Of those who lose weight on any treatment program, a significant percentage will fail to maintain this weight loss. Identification of those individuals who will lose weight successfully as opposed to those who will be less successful is at best imprecise. Some suggestive indicators include the initial 1-week weight loss, frequency and regularity of attendance at a weight loss program, and the patient's belief that one can control one's own destiny. However, additional insight is needed before it will be possible to distinguish at the beginning of the treatment successful individuals from those who will be unsuccessful.

Risk Associated with Obesity

Since all treatments entail some risk, the first essential for deciding whether treatment for obesity is appropriate and what that treatment should be is the assessment of the risk associated with the degree and distribution of excess weight. Two independent varia-

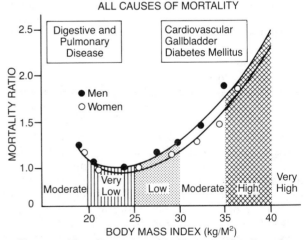

Figure 1. Mortality ratio and body mass index. Data from the American Cancer Society study have been plotted for men and women to show relationship of body mass index to overall mortality. At a body mass index below 20 kg/M² and above 25 kg/M² there is an increase in relative mortality. The major causes for this increased mortality are listed, along with a division of body mass index groupings into various levels of risk.

TABLE 1. **Body Weights in Pounds According to Height and Body Mass Index**

Height (in)	Body Mass Index (kg/M²)													
	19.0	20.0	21.0	22.0	23.0	24.0	25.0	26.0	27.0	28.0	29.0	30.0	35.0	40.0
	Body Weight (lb)													
58.0	90.7	95.5	100.3	105.0	109.8	114.6	119.4	124.1	128.9	133.7	138.5	143.2	167.1	191.0
59.0	93.9	98.8	103.8	108.7	113.6	118.6	123.5	128.5	133.4	138.3	143.3	148.2	172.9	197.6
60.0	97.1	102.2	107.3	112.4	117.5	122.6	127.7	132.9	138.0	143.1	148.2	153.3	178.8	204.4
61.0	100.3	105.6	110.9	116.2	121.5	126.8	132.0	137.3	142.6	147.9	153.2	158.4	184.8	211.3
62.0	103.7	109.1	114.6	120.0	125.5	130.9	136.4	141.9	147.3	152.8	158.2	163.7	191.0	218.2
63.0	107.0	112.7	118.3	123.9	129.6	135.2	140.8	146.5	152.1	157.7	163.4	169.0	197.2	225.3
64.0	110.5	116.3	122.1	127.9	133.7	139.5	145.3	151.2	157.0	162.8	168.6	174.4	203.5	232.5
65.0	113.9	119.9	125.9	131.9	137.9	143.9	149.9	155.9	161.9	167.9	173.9	179.9	209.9	239.9
66.0	117.5	123.7	129.8	136.0	142.2	148.4	154.6	160.8	166.9	173.1	179.3	185.5	216.4	247.3
67.0	121.1	127.4	133.8	140.2	146.5	152.9	159.3	165.7	172.0	178.4	184.8	191.1	223.0	254.9
68.0	124.7	131.3	137.8	144.4	151.0	157.5	164.1	170.6	177.2	183.8	190.3	196.9	229.7	262.5
69.0	128.4	135.2	141.9	148.7	155.4	162.2	168.9	175.7	182.5	189.2	196.0	202.7	236.5	270.3
70.0	132.1	139.1	146.1	153.0	160.0	166.9	173.9	180.8	187.8	194.7	201.7	208.6	243.4	278.2
71.0	135.9	143.1	150.3	157.4	164.6	171.7	178.9	186.0	193.2	200.3	207.5	214.6	250.4	286.2
72.0	139.8	147.2	154.5	161.9	169.2	176.6	183.9	191.3	198.7	206.0	213.4	220.7	257.5	294.3
73.0	143.7	151.3	158.8	166.4	174.0	181.5	189.1	196.7	204.2	211.8	219.3	226.9	264.7	302.5
74.0	147.7	155.4	163.2	171.0	178.8	186.5	194.3	202.1	209.9	217.6	225.4	233.2	272.0	310.9
75.0	151.7	159.7	167.7	175.6	183.6	191.6	199.6	207.6	215.6	223.5	231.5	239.5	279.4	319.4
76.0	155.8	164.0	172.2	180.4	188.6	196.8	205.0	213.2	221.4	229.5	237.7	245.9	286.9	327.9

TABLE 2. **Body Weights in Kilograms According to Height and Body Mass Index**

Height (cm)	Body Mass Index (kg/M²)													
	19.0	20.0	21.0	22.0	23.0	24.0	25.0	26.0	27.0	28.0	29.0	30.0	35.0	40.0
	Body Weight (kg)													
140.0	37.2	39.2	41.2	43.1	45.1	47.0	49.0	51.0	52.9	54.9	56.8	58.8	68.6	78.4
142.0	38.3	40.3	42.3	44.4	46.4	48.4	50.4	52.4	54.4	56.5	58.5	60.5	70.6	80.7
144.0	39.4	41.5	43.5	45.6	47.7	49.8	51.8	53.9	56.0	58.1	60.1	62.2	72.6	82.9
146.0	40.5	42.6	44.8	46.9	49.0	51.2	53.3	55.4	57.6	59.7	61.8	63.9	74.6	85.3
148.0	41.6	43.8	46.0	48.2	50.4	52.6	54.8	57.0	59.1	61.3	63.5	65.7	76.7	87.6
150.0	42.8	45.0	47.3	49.5	51.8	54.0	56.3	58.5	60.8	63.0	65.3	67.5	78.8	90.0
152.0	43.9	46.2	48.5	50.8	53.1	55.4	57.8	60.1	62.4	64.7	67.0	69.3	80.9	92.4
154.0	45.1	47.4	49.8	52.2	54.5	56.9	59.3	61.7	64.0	66.4	68.8	71.1	83.0	94.9
156.0	46.2	48.7	51.1	53.5	56.0	58.4	60.8	63.3	65.7	68.1	70.6	73.0	85.2	97.3
158.0	47.4	49.9	52.4	54.9	57.4	59.9	62.4	64.9	67.4	69.9	72.4	74.9	87.4	99.9
160.0	48.6	51.2	53.8	56.3	58.9	61.4	64.0	66.6	69.1	71.7	74.2	76.8	89.6	102.4
162.0	49.9	52.5	55.1	57.7	60.4	63.0	65.6	68.2	70.9	73.5	76.1	78.7	91.9	105.0
164.0	51.1	53.8	56.5	59.2	61.9	64.6	67.2	69.9	72.6	75.3	78.0	80.7	94.1	107.6
166.0	52.4	55.1	57.9	60.6	63.4	66.1	68.9	71.6	74.4	77.2	79.9	82.7	96.4	110.2
168.0	53.6	56.4	59.3	62.1	64.9	67.7	70.6	73.4	76.2	79.0	81.8	84.7	98.8	112.9
170.0	54.9	57.8	60.7	63.6	66.5	69.4	72.3	75.1	78.0	80.9	83.8	86.7	101.2	115.6
172.0	56.2	59.2	62.1	65.1	68.0	71.0	74.0	76.9	79.9	82.8	85.8	88.8	103.5	118.3
174.0	57.5	60.6	63.6	66.6	69.6	72.7	75.7	78.7	81.7	84.8	87.8	90.8	106.0	121.1
176.0	58.9	62.0	65.0	68.1	71.2	74.3	77.4	80.5	83.6	86.7	89.8	92.9	108.4	123.9
178.0	60.2	63.4	66.5	69.7	72.9	76.0	79.2	82.4	85.5	88.7	91.9	95.1	110.9	126.7
180.0	61.6	64.8	68.0	71.3	74.5	77.8	81.0	84.2	87.5	90.7	94.0	97.2	113.4	129.6
182.0	62.9	66.2	69.6	72.9	76.2	79.5	82.8	86.1	89.4	92.7	96.1	99.4	115.9	132.5
184.0	64.3	67.7	71.1	74.5	77.9	81.3	84.6	88.0	91.4	94.8	98.2	101.6	118.5	135.4
186.0	65.7	69.2	72.7	76.1	79.6	83.0	86.5	89.9	93.4	96.9	100.3	103.8	121.1	138.4
188.0	67.2	70.7	74.2	77.8	81.3	84.8	88.4	91.9	95.4	99.0	102.5	106.0	123.7	141.4
190.0	68.6	72.2	75.8	79.4	83.0	86.6	90.3	93.9	97.5	101.1	104.7	108.3	126.4	144.4
192.0	70.0	73.7	77.4	81.1	84.8	88.5	92.2	95.8	99.5	103.2	106.9	110.6	129.0	147.5
194.0	71.5	75.3	79.0	82.8	86.6	90.3	94.1	97.9	101.6	105.4	109.1	112.9	131.7	150.5
196.0	73.0	76.8	80.7	84.5	88.4	92.2	96.0	99.9	103.7	107.6	111.4	115.2	134.5	153.7
198.0	74.5	78.4	82.3	86.2	90.2	94.1	98.0	101.9	105.9	109.8	113.7	117.6	137.2	156.8
200.0	76.0	80.0	84.0	88.0	92.0	96.0	100.0	104.0	108.0	112.0	116.0	120.0	140.0	160.0

TABLE 3. **Desirable Body Mass Index Range in Relation to Age**

Age Group (Years)	Body Mass Index (kg/M^2)
19–24	19–24
25–34	20–25
35–44	21–26
45–54	22–27
55–64	23–28
65+	24–29

bles are involved in the risk related to obesity. The first is the risk associated with total body fatness. Underweight individuals have increased risk for respiratory disease, tuberculosis, digestive disease, and some cancers. For overweight individuals, on the other hand, cardiovascular disease, gallbladder disease, high blood pressure, and diabetes are the primary risks. From a clinical point of view, these relationships of overweight, expressed as body mass index (BMI), to mortality are depicted schematically in Figure 1. The body weights associated with a BMI of 20 to 25 kg per M^2 show little or no increased risk. When the BMI is below 20 kg per M^2 or above 25 kg per M^2, risk increases in a curvilinear fashion. Individuals with a BMI of 25 to 30 kg per M^2 have low risk, those with a BMI between 30 and 35 kg per M^2 have moderate risk, those with a BMI of 35 to 40 kg per M^2 have high risk, and those with a BMI above 40 kg per M^2 are at very high risk from their obesity. Tables 1 and 2 present body mass index for different heights and weights. Table 3 is a guide to recommended ranges of body mass index for different ages.

A second component of risk related to body fat is the distribution of that fat. In a quantitative sense, the higher the proportion of body fat in the abdominal or truncal region, the greater is the risk. The ratio of the circumference of the abdomen to that at the hips or gluteal region is defined as the abdominal gluteal ratio (AGR). Figure 2 is a nomogram for estimating abdominal-gluteal (waist-hips) ratio. At any given level of body mass index the risk to health is increased with greater AGR. A value above 0.85 for women and 0.90 for men carries increased risk. Other factors included in Figure 1 that increase risk from obesity include the presence of medical problems such as diabetes mellitus, hypertension or hyperlipidemia, age less than 40, and male sex. Table 4 provides a way of including both total body fat, as estimated from the BMI, and a distribution of body fat in making decisions about relative treatment groupings.

Evaluation

To guide the physician in evaluating the overweight patient, we have developed the algorithm shown in Table 5. It summarizes a series of measurements and their interpretation that are appropriate for all obese individuals. In this algorithm, the patient is evaluated for hypertension and its possible causes, for hypothyroidism, for glucose intolerance, for hypertriglyceride-

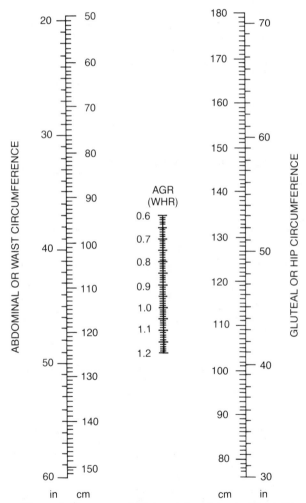

Figure 2. Nomogram for determining abdominal (waist) to gluteal (hips) ratio. Place a straight edge between the column for waist circumference and the column for hip circumference and read the ratio from the point where this straight edge crosses the AGR or WHR line. The waist or abdominal circumference is the smallest circumference below the rib cage and above the umbilicus, and the hip or gluteal circumference is taken as the largest circumference at the posterior extension of the buttocks. (Copyright 1987, George A. Bray).

TABLE 4. **Risk Classification for Obesity**

Body Mass Index	Complicating Factors*	
	No	Yes
<25	Very low risk	Low risk
25–30	Low risk	Moderate risk
30–35	Moderate risk	Moderate risk
35–40	Moderate risk	High risk
>40	High risk	High risk

*Complicating factors include elevated abdominal-gluteal ratio, diabetes mellitus, hypertension, hyperlipidemia, male sex, and age less than 40 years.

TABLE 5. **Algorithm for Evaluating the Overweight Patient**

The criteria for abnormality are shown elsewhere. This reference includes tables for evaluating desirable body weight and body mass index as well as establishing appropriate glucose and blood pressure levels.

1. Overweight is defined as:
   Body weight: From upper limit of "acceptable" to 20% above that limit.
   Body mass index: 25 to 30 kg/M²

2. Obesity is defined as:

	Men	Women
Triceps plus subscapular skinfold (mm)	>43	>58
Body mass index (kg/M²)	>30	>30
Body fat (% body weight)	>25	>30

3. Blood pressure readings (mm Hg) taken with a large cuff that encircles 75 per cent of the arm:

	Systolic	Diastolic
Normal	120–140	<90
Mild	140–160	90–104
Moderate	160–190	105–114
Severe	>190	>115

4. Cortisol suppression: less than 3 µg/dl at 8 a.m., 9 hr after 1 mg of dexamethasone orally.

5. Thyroid function:

	Serum Thyroxine (Corrected) (µg/dl)	Serum Thyrotropin (TSH) (µU/ml)
High	>12	<7
Normal	5.5–12.0	<7
Borderline low	4.0–5.5	7–10
Low	<4.0	>10

In the presence of severe illness, a low serum thyroxine must be interpreted cautiously; it may be a bad prognostic sign but is not indicative of hypothyroidism unless TSH is elevated.

6. The diagnosis of diabetes in nonpregnant adults is based on the following:
   a. Unequivocal hyperglycemia and classic symptoms of diabetes mellitus
   b. Fasting venous plasma glucose above 140 mg/dl on more than one occasion
   c. Fasting venous plasma glucose below 140 mg/dl, but with values of venous plasma glucose of above 200 mg/dl at some point between 0 and 2 hr, and at 2 hr after an oral glucose tolerance test with 75 gram glucose (for children 1.75 grams/kg of ideal body weight, not to exceed 75 grams).

7. Suggested upper limits* of serum lipids for normal adults:

Females

Age	Cholesterol (mg/dl) Total	LDL	HDL	Triacylglycerol (mg/dl)
0–19	200	—	—	—
5–19	—	140	35	—
10–19	—	—	—	130
15–19	—	—	—	—
20–24	230	160	35	170
25–29	235	160	35	170
30–34	245	170	35	170
35–39	255	175	35	195
40–44	270	185	35	210
45–69	285	200	35	230
70	295	215	35	240

Males

Age	Cholesterol (mg/dl) Total	LDL	HDL	Triacylglycerol (mg/dl)
0–19	200	—	—	—
5–19	—	130	—	—
10–19	—	—	—	—
15–19	—	—	30	150
20–24	220	145	30	200
25–29	245	165	30	250
30–34	255	185	30	265
35–39	270	190	30	320
40–44	270	185	25	320
45–69	275	205	30	290
70	270	185	30	260

8. Testosterone >300 ng/dl in females. One should be very suspicious with a value of 100 to 300 ng/dl.

*95th percentile for total cholesterol, LDL cholesterol, and triglycerides; 5th percentile for HDL cholesterol.

mia, for potential pulmonary problems, for headaches, and for reproductive abnormalities. Once the risks, if any, associated with obesity have been identified, treatment can be selected.

Treatment

Risk-Benefit Assessment of Treatment

Treatments for obesity can be grouped according to their relative risk as shown in Table 6. They can be further divided by whether they influence the energy intake or energy loss. In a quantitative sense, treatments that reduce energy intake have a greater potential for acute weight loss than those directed at increasing energy expenditure by exercise. Since all of our energy comes from food, we can reduce nutrient intake to zero (starvation). Energy expenditure, on the other hand, has a minimum level associated with the energy required to maintain body temperature and to repair tissues and maintain function of the heart and other organs. Thus, simply staying in bed and spending no time in physical activity reduces energy expenditure to approximately 0.8 kcal per minute (1150 kcal per day). High levels of physical activity can increase this by not much more than three to four fold over 24 hours. Thus, for initial weight loss, decreasing food intake has the most to recommend it, while changes in energy expenditure through physical activity appear to have a particular attractiveness in efforts at long-term maintenance of changed body weight and composition.

Diet

Any diet must reduce caloric intake below daily caloric expenditure for an individual to sustain a net loss of body fat. To determine the appropriate level of caloric restriction requires an assessment of caloric needs. This can be done in two ways. The first way to estimate caloric expenditure is to multiply desirable body weight in kg by 30 to 35 kcal for men (14 to 16 kcal per lb), and for women by 25 to 30 kcal per kg (12 to 14 kcal per lb). Alternatively, actual body weight can be multiplied by 22 kcal per kg (10 kcal per lb) for

TABLE 6. Risks Associated with Various Treatments for Obesity

Caloric Intake	Caloric Loss
Low Risk	
1. Behavior modification	1. Behavior modification
2. Diets	2. Exercise
3. Appetite suppressants	3. Thermogenic drugs
4. Jaw wiring	4. Inhibit absorption
5. Gastric surgery	5. Jejunoileal bypass
High Risk	

TABLE 7. Estimating Energy Needs

Resting metabolic rate (RMR)
  Men   = 900 + 10 × (wt in kg)
  Women = 800 + 7 × (wt in kg)
Daily energy requirement
  RMR × Activity factor

Activity Level	Activity Factor
Low (sedentary)	1.2
Moderate	1.4
High (regular exercise or manual labor)	1.6

women or 26 kcal per kg (12 kcal per lb) for men. The second method multiplies estimated resting metabolic rate (RMR) by an activity factor. Resting metabolic rate for men and women can be reasonably approximated with the formulas shown in Table 7.

After caloric requirements are assessed, a reasonable average caloric deficit can be selected. If the average daily intake is 500 kcal below estimated needs, approximately 3500 kcal per week will be withdrawn from stored energy, producing a loss of approximately 0.45 kg (1 lb) of fat tissue each week.

Table 8 gives a list of diets divided according to the levels of energy. These range from fasting or the zero-calorie diet to diets with conventional levels of reduced calorie intake (above 800 to 1000 kcal per day). With all diets there are two phases to the weight loss. The first phase is more rapid and reflects the loss of significant amounts of water associated with catabolism of glycogen and protein. After 24 to 72 hours, glycogen stores are reduced or depleted and the associated water has been excreted. Gluconeogenesis from protein is at a maximum at this time. After the first several days the rate of weight loss begins to fall, reflecting the reduced losses of body protein and the associated water and electrolytes. The second phase begins after 7 to 10 days, when catabolism of fat becomes the principal mechanism for weight loss. Weight loss on any diet is slower after the excess fluids and readily mobilized body tissues have been depleted. Frustration with

TABLE 8. Classification of Diets

I.   Starvation (less than 200 kcal/day)
II. Very-low-calorie (200 to 800 kcal/day)
III. Low-calorie (800 to 1200 kcal/day, provided that the intake is less than the patient's needs for maintenance of body weight)

  A. Balanced
     1. Natural food
     2. Formula

  B. Unbalanced
     1. Low carbohydrate
     2. Low fat
     3. Fad (emphasizing a single food)

slower weight loss is compounded by the decrease in caloric expenditure that occurs with most if not all diets containing less than 800 kcal per day. The metabolic rate can decline by as much as 15 to 20 per cent.

Starvation. During therapeutic starvation, the initial rate of weight loss may be high, often reaching 1 to 1.5 kg per day. After 2 to 3 weeks, however, it slows to 0.5 kg per day. Loss of nitrogen declines to levels of about 5 grams per day, while the loss of potassium in the urine levels off at 30 to 40 mEq per day. Several deaths have been reported in patients who were fasting, and this has been associated with cardiac arrhythmias. Total fasting should be done only in the hospital, where fluid losses, blood pressure, and electrocardiogram can be monitored. The rise in ketones with fasting inhibits uric acid excretion and may precipitate urate renal stones if the patient is not appropriately treated.

Very-Low-Calorie Diets. Very-low-calorie diets (below 400 kcal per day) will reduce the net loss of nitrogen to less than 1 gram per day, down from levels of 4 to 6 grams per day found during starvation. However, there is little evidence that the net loss of protein is completely stopped with any of these diets. Protein from egg, casein, or soy composes between 33 per cent and 100 per cent of the energy in most of these diets. However, it is desirable for these diets to contain at least 25 per cent of their calories as carbohydrate. Supplements of electrolytes, including potassium, magnesium, and other inorganic salts, as well as vitamins, including folate, pyridoxine, and thiamine, should be given. Very-low-calorie diets composed of digested collagen have been associated with a number of deaths. Fatalities occurred in 16 young and middle-aged women and one man who had stayed on such a diet for more than 8 weeks and lost more than 23 kg (50 lb). Autop-

TABLE 9. **The Basic Four Food Groups**

Food Group	Recommended Servings Daily	Examples	Serving Size	Kilocalories per Serving	Major Contribution to Health
Vegetables and Fruits	4	Cooked or canned vegetables	½ cup	25–100	Vitamins Minerals Fiber
		Cooked or canned fruits (water packed)	½ cup	30–100	
		Raw orange, apple, or banana	1 medium	70–95	
		Grapefruit	½ medium	40	
		Cantaloupe	¼ medium	30	
		Raw salad greens	1 cup	20	
Bread and Cereal	4	Bread	1 slice	60	B vitamins Fiber
		Bun (hamburger or hot dog)	½ bun	56	
		English muffin	½ muffin	70	
		Dinner roll	1 roll	60–120	
		Pancake	1 (4 inch)	70–105	
		Cooked cereals, rice, or noodles	½ cup	65–100	
Milk and cheese	2 (adult) 3 (children)	Whole milk	1 cup (8 ounces)	160	Calcium Protein
		Low fat (2%) milk	1 cup	140	
		Skim milk	1 cup	90	
		Ice milk	⅔ cup	135–140	
		Yogurt (plain, without fruit)	1 cup	120–150	
		Cheese	1–1⅓ ounces	80–120	
		Cottage cheese, creamed	2 ounces	60	
		Ice cream	1⅓ cups	340–500	
Meat, poultry, fish, and beans	2	Cooked lean meat, poultry, or fish	2 ounces	50–125	Protein
		Hot dogs	2 ounces	250	
		Lunch meats	2 ounces	120–190	
		Tuna fish (oil packed)	2 ounces	120	
		(water packed)	2 ounces	75	
		Eggs	2	160	
		Dried beans or peas	1 cup (cooked)	160–230	
		Nuts	½ cup	400–600	
		Peanut butter	4 tablespoons	345	

sies showed abnormalities of the myocardium with premorbid evidence of a cardiac arrhythmia called "les pointes de Torsades." It would therefore be desirable for low-calorie diets to use high-quality protein, to have some carbohydrate and essential fatty acids, to be supplemented with vitamins and minerals, and to be used only under medical supervision.

Conventional Diets and Nutritional Education

TYPES OF DIETS. Conventional diets, with more than 800 kcal per day, can be divided into two categories: balanced diets and unbalanced diets. In a balanced diet, calories have been restricted, but no single food or food group predominates. In unbalanced diets, on the other hand, one type of food predominates. In this latter group are the very-low-carbohydrate diets (less than 25 grams per day) and many other diets identified by special names, such as the grapefruit diet, the banana diet, the ice cream diet, and the candy diet. The unbalanced diet has one major advantage: it is monotonous. For this reason it is usually not continued for prolonged periods. While eating fewer than 1000 calories each day it is difficult, if not impossible, to achieve an adequate intake of all needed nutrients, and supplemental vitamins and minerals should usually be given.

ENERGY VALUE OF FOOD. There are at least two ways for patients to determine energy intake. The first is to "count calories." Patients can weigh or measure the foods they eat and determine the caloric values from various tables. A second way is to use the information published on the nutrition labels of many packaged foods. A typical nutrition label shows the serving size, the number of servings per container, and the calories, the protein, carbohydrate, and fat and the percentage of the recommended daily intake of eight selected nutrients in each serving. This is followed by the ingredients listed in order of weight from highest to lowest.

FOOD GROUPS. Use of the Four Basic Food Group system provides a useful guide to nutrition. Table 9 lists the recommended daily servings for each food group and examples of foods that can provide these servings along with the major nutrient(s) associated with each food group. There is a wide variation in the number of calories provided by equivalent nutritional servings within each food group. For example, skim milk has 90 calories per serving, while an equivalent nutritional serving of ice cream (1⅓ cups) has 380. Peanut butter provides 400 calories in a serving, whereas water-packed tuna has only 75.

TABLE 10. **Appetite-Suppressant Drugs**

Generic and Proprietary Names	Suppliers	Dosage (mg)	Administration (mg)	Peak Blood Concentration (hr after oral dose)	Half-Life in Blood (hr)	Per Cent Excreted Unchanged in Acidic Urine
*Schedule II**						
Amphetamine						
Benzedrine and others		5, 10, 15	5 to 10 before meals (tid)	1–2	5	55
Methamphetamine						
Desoxyn	Abbot	5, 10, 15	2.5 or 5 before meals (tid) 10 or 15 in morning	1–2	13	45
Phenmetrazine						
Preludin	Boehringer	25, 50, 75	25 (bid or tid)	—	—	19
*Schedule III**						
Phendimetrazine						
Plegine and others	Ayerst	35	35 before meals	—	4	—
Benzphetamine						
Didrex	Upjohn	25, 50	25–50 before meals	1–2	—	—
*Schedule IV**						
Diethylpropion						
Tenuate	Merrell	25, 75	25 before meals (tid)	1–2	8–13	24
Tepanil	Riker		75 in morning			
Fenfluramine						
Pondimin	Robins	20	20–40 before meals	1	20	20
Mazindol						
Sanorex	Sandoz	1, 2	1 before meals	2	13	22
Mazanor	Wyeth		2 in morning			
Phentermine						
Fastin and others	Beecham	15, 30	15 tid	—	Free 7–8	75
Ionamin (resin)	Pennwalt		30 in morning	1	20–24	

*The Federal Controlled Substances Act of 1970 places the prescription anorexiants into five Schedule categories.
—: Data not available.

Changing Behavioral Patterns of Eating

The basic principles of behavioral approaches to obesity can be summarized under "the ABCs of eating." The "A" stands for antecedent. Eating is often a response to events in the environment. These antecedent events may then serve to trigger eating. The "B" stands for the behavior of eating itself. This includes, among other things, the place, rate, and frequency with which an individual eats. Limiting the act of eating to one area with a single small plate and place setting may help to provide control over eating. Finally, the "C" in these ABCs is the consequence of the eating. The feelings an individual has about eating can be altered, and rewards for changing eating patterns can be instituted. Behavioral programs for treatment of obesity provide the elements for long-term changes that can increase success rates.

Exercise and Physical Activity

The only part of energy expenditure that is amenable to significant manipulation is physical activity. The lowest level of energy expenditure occurs during sleep and is approximately 0.6 to 0.8 kcal per minute. Thus, if an individual sleeps for an entire 24 hours, between 850 and 1150 kcal will be expended. Upon waking, the value rises to 0.8 to 0.9 kcal per minute. Reclining increases this level to approximately 1.0 kcal per minute. Very light activity (the level at which most people spend much of their time) consumes between 1.1 and 3.0 kcal per minute, while moderate activity consumes 3.5 to 7.0 kcal per minute and heavy activity 7.0 to 12 kcal per minute. Obese and diabetic patients should be encouraged to increase their physical activity for two reasons. First, it consumes calories. Second, and more important, exercise increases glucose utilization and may improve insulin sensitivity.

Appetite Suppressant Drugs

Although most appetite-suppressant drugs can increase locomotor activity and stimulate the central nervous system, their relative potency differs considerably. Some features of these drugs are summarized in Table 10. Amphetamine and methamphetamine are the most potent stimulants of the central nervous system and have no place in the treatment of obesity. Fenfluramine (Pondimin) is the least potent, and although it may be a depressant, it has almost no effect on locomotor activity. Cardiovascular effects are frequently observed in patients treated with appetite-suppressant drugs. Heart rate and blood pressure may increase, particularly with the drugs in Schedule II and some of those in Schedule III, but the effects are less for drugs in Schedule IV.

TABLE 11. **Comparison of Bypass Operations for Obesity**

	Jejunoileal	Gastric
Mortality (early)	0–11.5%	1–4
Vomiting	Rare	Common
Diarrhea	Common	Rare
Electrolyte depletion	Common	Rare
Peptic ulceration	Rare	1–2%
Liver failure	5%*	0
Urinary calculi	1–32%*	1%
Osteomalacia	17–48%*	?
Revision (inadequate weight loss)	5–20%	10–40%
Reversal (complications)	1–23%	1%
Follow-up	26 years	11 years

*Late complications.

The effectiveness of these drugs has been reviewed by the Food and Drug Administration based on evidence provided in 105 new drug applications submitted to the agency. The applications included reports on more than 200 controlled trials, about 160 of which compared placebo and active drugs. Overall, the patients treated with drugs lost an average of 0.25 kg per week more than did those in the placebo-treated group. Since this review by the FDA, there have been several other long-term trials with appetite-suppressant drugs. In one of these trials, 186 patients were treated for 12 months and then observed for an additional 12 months without treatment. Weight loss plateaued at an average of 10 kg (22 lb) below the starting point and remained at this level for 12 months. When treatment was discontinued, the patients regained an average of 9 kg. The data on the few studies of 20 weeks or longer suggest that some patients might maintain their ability to reset the internal control systems that regulate body fat at a lower level for a prolonged period of time if they continued to ingest the appetite-suppressant drugs.

The safety of appetite-suppressant drugs has been the subject of considerable discussion. Amphetamine, methamphetamine, and phenmetrazine reportedly have been more frequently abused than have other drugs in this group. The two most common side effects of these drugs are insomnia and dry mouth. With fenfluramine, depression and diarrhea, rather than dry mouth and constipation, are the most frequently observed side effects. If appetite suppressants are to be used, they should be adjuncts in the treatment of obesity. Several rules for the use of these drugs should be borne in mind. First, they should be used only in persons whose body mass index is greater than 30 kg per M^2 (those with Class III obesity). Second, because of the potential for drug abuse, the compounds in Schedule IV should be the agents of choice. Such drugs should not be used for the treatment of pregnant women, or in obese children who are still growing. My first choice of drugs is phenylpropanolamine, with phentermine (Fastin), fenfluramine (Pondimin), diethylpropion (Tenuate), and mazindol (Sanorex) in second place. For patients with a history of depression or mental illness, mazindol and diethylpropion merit first choice, and fenfluramine should probably not be used. For diabetic patients, fenfluramine is usually my preference. For hypertensive patients, I generally think of mazindol or diethylpropion. The potential of intermittent or interrupted courses of therapy should also be kept in mind. Three- or 6-week courses of therapy, discontinued for a period half the length of the original treatment time, have been advocated and may be desirable.

Surgery

Diets, exercise, behavioral change, and anorectic drugs have generally been less successful for massively obese patients (those in Class V) with a body mass index above 40. The increased risk to the life of such patients from obesity has led to surgical procedures for obesity, including gastric and intestinal bypass operations.

Gastric Bypass. The gastric bypass was pioneered by Mason and colleagues, who had become discouraged with some of the untoward results seen with small bowel bypass. They tried several different procedures, including gastric exclusion, partial gastric exclusion, and total gastric transection. Problems with hemorrhoids, rectal discomfort, and diarrhea, which were frequently observed in patients with jejunoileal bypass, were not seen in patients with gastric bypass. Similarly, fatigue, lethargy, and bloating were not observed in the gastric bypass group. Of more interest was the fact that the late complications of liver disease, renal stones, and polyarthritis, which represent a major group of difficulties for patients undergoing jejunoileal bypass, were uncommon in the individuals with a gastric bypass. Long-term results with this procedure are somewhat disappointing in that patients may regain weight as the gastrointestinal tract adapts.

Intestinal Bypass. Two types of intestinal bypass have been used most widely. The end-to-side operation attaches a segment of jejunum, measuring approximately 35 cm (14 in), from the ligament of Treitz to the side of the ileum 10 cm (4 in) from the ileocecal valve. The end-to-end operation attaches the same length of jejunum to the end of the ileum and anastomoses the separated ileal end to the colon. Weight loss with these operations ranges from 4 to 68 kg (10 to 150 lb) in the first year, depending on the length of bowel left in continuity. A comparison of complications between gastric and intestinal operations is shown in Table 11. The mortality from this procedure runs up to 10 per cent, but averages overall about 4 per cent. In addition, there are many short- and long-term complications, including liver failure, fluid and electrolyte imbalance, protein malnutrition, renal stones, blind loop syndrome, and metabolic bone disease. For these reasons, the intestinal bypass operations are now done infrequently.

PELLAGRA

method of
JOSÉ ERNESTO DOS SANTOS, M.D.
Universidade De São Paulo
São Paulo, Brazil

Pellagra is a disease caused by nutritional deficiencies, frequently multiple, in which niacin and tryptophan inadequacies predominate. There is evidence for the participation of other vitamin and mineral deficiencies in the etiology of the disease. It is diagnosed mainly in alcoholic patients and less frequently in food faddists, elderly people, and persons with malabsorption syndromes or other illnesses that cause an increased requirement for niacin and its precursor, such as the malignant carcinoid syndrome. In this syndrome, 60 per cent of the dietary tryptophan is converted to serotonin (in contrast to only 1 per cent in a normal situation), with a consequent decrease in niacin coenzyme synthesis. Pellagra-like skin lesions have been reported in 7 per cent of patients with carcinoid syndrome. Another disease associated with pellagra is Hartnup disease, a familial abnormality in monoaminomonocarboxylic amino acid absorption by the intestine and reabsorption by renal tubules.

Primary pellagra, in which diet is the only etiologic factor, is observed in underdeveloped countries where corn, millet, and jowar *(Sorghum vulgare)*, cereals with low niacin and tryptophan contents, are staple foods. The disease is rare in countries where corn is treated with alkali before human consumption, probably as a consequence of the liberation of niacin bound to peptides or carbohydrates by the alkali treatment. The effect of excess leucine (as in jowar) as an inhibitor of niacin coenzyme synthesis is also considered a possible explanation.

The clinical picture of pellagra is characterized by diarrhea, symmetric scaling and sometimes ulcerating dermatitis on sun-exposed skin surfaces, irritability, anxiety, depression, and ultimately psychosis. Other frequent clinical signs are scarlet glossitis and fatigue. As a multiple deficiency state, it is frequently associated with anemia, peripheral neuropathy, and other signs related to deficiency of other nutrients.

Prevention

The most important preventive method is the provision of a diet with sufficient amounts of energy, protein, vitamins, and minerals. Such a diet includes vegetables, cereals, meat, dairy products, and fruits. A daily intake of 2400 to 2800 kcal, 45 to 55 grams of protein of high biologic value, and 20 niacin equivalents (NE) (1 NE is equal to 1 mg of niacin or 60 mg of dietary tryptophan) will prevent pellagra in healthy adults. For patients who cannot or should not eat, a multivitamin supplementation given orally, by tube, or parenterally must be added to the prescription. The Food and Nutrition Board of the National Academy of Sciences in the United States (1980) recommends 6 to 9 NE for healthy infants, and 11 to 19 NE for older children and adults. For lactating or pregnant women, it is advisable to supplement the normal diet with 5 or 2 NE, respectively.

Treatment

The acute manifestations should be treated with 150 to 300 mg of niacinamide orally. For children, the dose must be reduced to 60 to 150 mg a day. Usually this amount is prescribed for a period of 15 days. When diarrhea and anorexia are also present, the utilization of tube feeding or parenteral nutrition is indicated. In this case, commercial products should contain the recommended amounts of vitamins. With appropriate treatment, the skin signs and other symptoms disappear in 10 to 20 days.

RICKETS AND OSTEOMALACIA

method of
MICHAEL D. FALLON, M.D.
University of Pennsylvania
Philadelphia, Pennsylvania

Osteomalacia is a metabolic bone disease resulting from defective mineralization of the osteoid matrix of the cortical and trabecular bone, whereas rickets results from defective mineralization of the cartilage matrix at the epiphyseal growth plate. Children will exhibit a combination of rickets and osteomalacia as long as the growth plate cartilage remains open. In contrast, adults will manifest only osteoid (bone) changes following epiphyseal closure.

Clinically, affected patients may present with bone pain, weakness, bone deformities, and skeletal fragility, despite the fact that the apparent bone mass (density) will be increased (osteosclerosis), normal, or decreased (osteopenic). These definitions are not meant to connote a specific disease state but rather a syndrome, or group of clinical disorders, that shares in common an abnormality of skeletal matrix mineralization.

REGULATION OF MINERAL HOMEOSTASIS

Calcium and phosphorus levels are maintained by the action of parathyroid hormone (PTH) and vitamin D.

Parathyroid Hormone

When serum calcium concentration falls, PTH secretion elevates the calcium level by (1) increasing osteoclastic bone resorption, (2) augmenting renal tubular calcium reabsorption, and (3) indirectly, via stimulation of intestinal calcium absorption, through the regulation of vitamin D metabolism. In addition, PTH reduces serum phosphate by promoting phosphaturia. PTH also stimulates osteoblasts and the osteogenic mesenchyme, resulting in increased production and secretion of alkaline phosphatase.

Vitamin D

Vitamin D_3 (cholecalciferol) is photosynthesized from the action of ultraviolet light on epidermal 7-dehydrocholesterol. Vitamin D_2 (ergocalciferol) is an irradiated plant sterol widely used to fortify foods and multivitamins. Once ergocalciferol is ingested, metabolism appears to be similar to that of cholecalciferol. Both sterols are stored in body fat and are equipotent in their calcium tropic effects, but subsequently undergo a series of bioactivation steps.

Vitamin D is converted initially in the liver to 25-hydroxycholecalciferol, or 25(OH)D, which is then converted to the most potent metabolite, 1,25-dihydroxycholecalciferol, or $1,25(OH)_2D$, in the kidney. The renal 1-hydroxylase activity is stimulated by PTH and inhibited by phosphate; $1,25(OH)_2D$, in turn, stimulates intestinal absorption of calcium and phosphorus and at higher concentrations stimulates bone resorption. Because parent vitamin D is fat-soluble, intestinal absorption of vitamin D requires normal fat absorption, with intact biliary and pancreatic function, and intestinal mucosal integrity.

REGULATION OF MINERALIZATION

Mineralization is promoted by optimum ambient calcium and phosphorus concentrations, the levels of which are maintained by the aforementioned hormones. It is unclear whether vitamin D metabolites play a direct role in osteoid synthesis, maturation, and mineralization or whether they promote mineralization seondarily by maintaining serum calcium and phosphorus levels. Mineralization is facilitated by the osteoblast chondrocyte enzyme alkaline phosphatase, which may function to remove endogenous crystallization inhibitors, such as pyrophosphates. Other exogenous agents, such as metal ions, fluoride, and synthetic diphosphonates, may act as crystal poisons and may inhibit mineralization.

GENERAL GUIDELINES FOR THERAPY

The principles for therapy are outlined in Table 1. The diagnosis of rickets and osteomalacia can generally be made on the basis of the clinical history, physical findings, and radiographic and biochemical findings. Defective mineralization is confirmed, with confidence, by examining nondecalcified tetracycline-labeled bone biopsy tissue, obtained by needle biopsy of the iliac crest under local anesthesia. Defective mineralization is characterized by increased quantities of unmineralized matrix (i.e., osteoid excess) in conjunction with abnormal tetracycline deposition at mineralization fronts.

The pathogenic mechanisms responsible for the clinical conditions associated with rickets and osteomalacia are numerous (Table 2). Ideally, treatment should be directed at correcting the underlying primary process. For example, a gluten-free diet may improve intestinal absorption, and surgical reversal of intestinal bypass operations may prevent malabsorption. Usually, these maneuvers are not practical or are impossible, and pharmacologic doses of vitamin D will be required along with mineral supplementation.

Establishing the correct diagnosis is also important to prevent any toxicity that may be attended by significant clinical sequelae: nephrocalcinosis and renal failure. If the underlying pathogenetic process is understood, the abnormality in mineral metabolism may be circumvented. The selection of the appropriate dose and rate of administration of vitamin D, or its metabolite, will be determined by the existing abnormality in vitamin D metabolism and the status of vitamin D body stores. For example, simple nutritional vitamin D deficiency may be treated with oral parent

---

TABLE 1. **Therapy Outline for Rickets and Osteomalacia**

I. Confirm Diagnosis of a Mineralization Defect and Establish the Pathogenesis
 1. History
 2. Physical examination
 3. Biochemical studies
 4. Radiologic examination
 5. Bone biopsy

II. Correct Any Underlying Conditions
 1. Gluten-free diet
 2. Surgical reversal of intestinal bypass
 3. Pancreatic enzyme supplement
 4. Renal transplantation
 5. Advice on nutrition and habits
 6. Discontinuance of phosphate-binding antacids

III. Vitamin D Therapy
 A. Select metabolite and route of administration appropriate for the site of altered sterol metabolism
   1. Dietary vitamin D deficiency—ergocalciferol
   2. Malabsorption of vitamin D—ergocalciferol, parenteral
   3. Altered hepatic bioactivation—calcifidiol
   4. Abnormal renal bioactivation—calcitriol
 B. Select dose of metabolite
   1. Replacement dose
   2. Maintenance therapy

IV. Mineral Supplements
 A. Calcium therapy
   1. Yes: Complex pathogenesis; alteration of sterol and mineral metabolism
   2. No: Simple vitamin D deficiency
 B. Phosphorus therapy
   1. Yes: Phosphate depletion states
   2. No: Simple hypophosphatemia due to secondary hyperparathyroidism

V. Follow up—Monitor Treatment
 A. Initially monitor replacement therapy
   1. Successful response—disease remission
   2. Parameters
     a. Alkaline-phosphatase
     b. Urine calcium
     c. 25(OH)D level
     d. Radiologic improvement
     e. Biopsy-proven changes
 B. Subsequently monitor maintenance therapy
   1. Prevent relapse; prevent toxicity
   2. Parameters
     a. 25(OH)D
     b. 24-hour urine calcium excretion—hypercalciuria
     c. Serum calcium—hypercalcemia
 C. Plan
   1. Adjust dosages with changes in diet or concurrent use of interfering drugs (phenytoin, thiazides)
   2. Adjust dosages with progression or remission of disease

---

TABLE 2. **Pathogenic Mechanisms of Rickets and Osteomalacia**

 1. *Vitamin D deficiency*
   Dietary deprivation and lack of sunlight exposure
 2. *Vitamin D malabsorption*
   a. Postgastrectomy states
   b. Small bowel disease, surgical resection, or bypass operations
   c. Pancreatic insufficiency
   d. Biliary obstruction
 3. *Impaired 25-hydroxylation of vitamin D*
   a. Premature infants
   b. Neonatal hepatitis
 4. *Increased catabolism or excretion of vitamin D*
   Enzyme induction, anticonvulsant drugs
 5. *Impaired 1-hydroxylation of 25(OH)D*
   a. Vitamin D–dependent rickets, Type I
   b. Hypoparathyroidism and pseudohypoparathyroidism
   c. Chronic renal failure
   d. X-linked hypophosphatemia
   e. Oncogenic osteomalacia
 6. *Impaired target-organ response to $1,25(OH)_2D$*
   a. Vitamin D–dependent rickets, Type II
   b. Anticonvulsant drugs
 7. *Hypophosphatemia*
   a. X-linked hypophosphatemia
   b. Sporadic hypophosphatemia
   c. Oncogenic osteomalacia
   d. Antacid-induced osteomalacia
 8. *Metabolic acidosis*
 9. *Inhibitors of mineralization*
   a. Aluminum
   b. Fluoride
   c. Disodium etidronate
 10. *Miscellaneous*
   a. Hypophosphatasia
   b. Fibrogenesis imperfecta ossium
   c. Calcium deficiency in children
   d. Parenteral nutrition

TABLE 3. **Treatment of Osteomalacia and Rickets with Pharmaceutical Preparations of Vitamin D Sterols**

	Ergocalciferol	Dihydrotachysterol	Calciferol	Calcitriol
Abbreviation	D_2	DHT	25(OH)D	1,25(OH)$_2$D
Trade name	Calciferol, Drisdol	DHT, Hytackerol	Calderol	Rocaltrol
Dosage form	Capsules: 1250 µg (50,000 IU) Liquid: 200 µg/ml Injection: 12.5 mg/ml	Tablets: 125, 100, and 400 µg Liquid: 250 µg/ml	Capsules: 20 and 50 µg	Capsules: 0.25 and 0.5 µg
Daily dosage in vitamin D deficiency	5–75 µg	20–100 µg	1–6 µg	0.25–1.0 µg
Normal serum levels	0.5–18 ng/ml	—	11–47 ng/ml	27–70 pg/ml
Estimated daily dosage range in resistant cases	1–10 mg	0.1–1 mg	50–200 µg	1–5 µg
Time to reach maximum effects	4–10 weeks	2–4 weeks	4–20 weeks	½–1 week
Persistence of biologic effect after cessation	6–30 weeks	2–8 weeks	4–12 weeks	½–1 week

vitamin D, whereas severe malabsorption and secondary vitamin D deficiency may require parenteral administration of vitamin D. If hepatic or renal disease impairs vitamin D bioactivation, specific metabolite replacement with 25(OH)D or 1,25(OH)$_2$D, respectively, is potentially available.

Pharmaceutical Preparations

Four forms of vitamin D are available in the United States (Table 3). The Food and Drug Administration (FDA) has approved 25(OH)$_2$D$_3$ (calciferol [Calderol]) and 1,25(OH)$_2$D$_3$ (calcitriol [Rocaltrol]) for use in the treatment of renal osteodystrophy. Dihydrotachysterol (Hytakerol), a synthetic analogue of 1,25(OH)$_2$D, as well as Rocaltrol is approved for treatment of the hypocalcemia of hypoparathyroidism.

These vitamin D metabolites have potential advantages in selectively circumventing abnormalities in vitamin D bioactivation. In addition, each metabolite has a more rapid onset of action and a shorter biologic half-life than the parent sterol. Preparations for minerals are shown in Tables 4 and 5.

Complications

Therapy with vitamin D poses the risk of vitamin D intoxication. Characteristically, a rising urinary cal-

cium level, falling serum alkaline phosphatase levels, and 25(OH)D levels exceeding 200 ng per ml herald the onset of vitamin D intoxication with hypercalciuria, with attendant hypercalcemia.

Monitoring Therapy

Biochemical parameters are the most useful means of following treatment. The initial response to treatment is an increase in alkaline phosphatase, or "flare," and a small rise in the urine and serum calcium. Parathyroid hormone levels may fall as secondary hyperparathyroidism is ameliorated.

Improved skeletal mineralization may be noted within a few weeks by sensitive, noninvasive quantitative bone density determinations, i.e., single or dual photon absorptiometry or quantitative computed tomography (CT). Radiographic improvement with normalization of endochondrial ossification may take months. The determination of serum 25(OH)D is the best indication of total body stores of vitamin D and may be used to confirm sterol repleteness.

PRIMARY VITAMIN D DEFICIENCY

Risk Factors

In healthy individuals, the minimum daily requirement of vitamin D necessary to prevent this

TABLE 4. **Treatment of Osteomalacia and Rickets with Calcium Supplements**

Preparation	Trade Name	Per Cent Elemental Calcium	Dosage Form	Amount Containing One Gram of Elemental Calcium	Comments
Calcium carbonate	Titrilac	40	Suspension Tablets: 420 mg, 650 mg	12.5 ml 6 tablets 4 tablets	May cause constipation, flatulence
Calcium lactate		13	Tablets: 325 mg, 650 mg	24 tablets 12 tablets	May be poorly absorbed by some people
Calcium gluconate		9	Tablets: 650 mg, 1000 mg	17 tablets 11 tablets	Fewer gastrointestinal complaints
Calcium glubionate	Neo-Calglucon	7	Syrup	43.5 ml	Fewer gastrointestinal complaints

TABLE 5. **Treatment of Osteomalacia and Rickets with Phosphate Supplements**

Preparation (Trade Name)	Amount Containing One Gram of Phosphorus	Comment
Neutra-Phos	4 capsules*	
Neutra-Phos-K	4 capsules*	
K-Phos Neutral	4 tablets	
K-Phos Original	9 tablets	
Fleet Phospho-Soda	6.7 ml	More diarrhea than with other preparations

*Each capsule is reconstituted with 75 ml of water, fruit juice, or cola. A powder concentrate is also available.

deficiency is just 10 micrograms (400 IU) for children and 2.5 micrograms (100 IU) for adults. Primary deficiency of vitamin D is generally found in individuals who, because of economic, social, or cultural factors, do not receive sufficient exposure to sunlight (5 to 20 minutes several times weekly) for adequate cutaneous synthesis of vitamin D_3 and whose diets do not contain sufficient foodstuffs fortified with vitamin D. Institutionalized patients, the poor, the elderly, food faddists, and some religious groups (because of diet and dress) are most likely to be affected. Infants who are breast-fed generally receive sufficient antirachitic sterol; however, babies who are bottle-fed with nonfortified milk are likely to become vitamin D–deficient.

Diagnosis

Measurement of circulating 25(OH)D is useful when a diagnosis of vitamin D deficiency is not readily achieved by routine medical history, physical examination, or biochemical and radiographic studies. Blood levels less than about 6 ng per ml (normal: 10 to 50) are considered diagnostic of vitamin D deficiency.

Treatment

Children with nutritional rickets respond to ergocalciferol in doses of 25 to 50 micrograms daily combined with 1 gram per day of a calcium supplement (Table 6). For children who are too young to swallow even small capsules, a liquid preparation of vitamin D_2 is available. The child should receive 4000 IU of vitamin D_2 (100 micrograms) daily for several months. With successful therapy, detectable biochemical and radiographic improvement can often be documented as early as 7 to 10 days after treatment is instituted. However, a follow-up visit for radiographic and biochemical studies after 2 months of therapy is appropriate. Once there has been healing, as demonstrated by radiographic and biochemical studies, patients can then receive the recommended daily allowance (RDA) of 400 IU per day in their food, either by consuming adequate amounts of fortified foods (dairy products) or by supplementation with pediatric multivitamin preparations that contain the RDA for vitamin D. For children who can take capsules, one 50,000

TABLE 6. **Summary of Therapeutic Modalities**

| | Nutritional Vitamin D Deficiency | | Vitamin D Malabsorption | Impaired 25-Hydroxylation | | Vitamin D–Dependent Rickets | | Chronic Renal Failure | X-Linked Hypophosphatemia |
	Children	Adults		Premature Infants	Anticonvulsant-Associated	Type I	Type II		
Ergocalciferol	25–50 µg up to 100 µg per day for infants Liquid—200 µg/ml Older children—1250 µg capsules/week	5–75 µg per day	1250–5000 µg per day or injection: 1–2.5 mg IM monthly	—	1250 µg 1 to 3 times a week	1250–5000 µg per day	May be 10 mg or more per day	2.5 mg or more per day	No longer recommended
Calcifediol	—	—	20–200 µg per day	—	Usually not required	50–100 µg per day	200 µg or more per day	50–100 µg per day	—
Cacitriol	—	—	1–2 µg per day	0.05 µg/kg per day	0.25–0.5 µg twice a day	1–3 µg a day	5–20 µg a day up to 40 µg/day	1–2 µg per day	0.25 µg twice a day, up to 3–4 µg/day
Elemental calcium	1–2 gram per day	800–1000 mg per day	1–2 gram per day	100–120 mg per kg/day	800–1000 mg per day	—	—	1000 mg per day	—
Phosphate	—	—	—	60–70 mg per kg/day	—	—	—	May need to restrict	1–4 gram per day in 4 to 6 divided doses
Elemental magnesium	—	—	350–750 mg per day	May be required	—	—	—	—	—

IU capsule (1.25 mg) of vitamin D_2 orally once weekly for three or four doses is an inexpensive, simple, and effective replacement regimen prior to RDA maintenance doses.

Adults have been successfully treated with 5 to 75 micrograms per day of ergocalciferol. Such small doses of vitamin D may result in supranormal levels of serum $1,25(OH)_2D$ within 72 hours, whereas $25(OH)D$ levels show only modest increases. The supranormal concentrations of serum $1,25(OH)_2D$ are probably a result of the accompanying secondary hyperparathyroidism inducing rapid 1-hydroxylation. In several patients, histologic resolution of vitamin D deficiency has been achieved with 0.5 microgram of calcitriol twice daily.

SECONDARY VITAMIN D DEFICIENCY

Risk Factors

Despite adequate sunlight exposure and a diet fortified with vitamin D, in some instances a deficiency of vitamin D may develop as a result of a variety of gastrointestinal, pancreatic, or hepatobiliary disorders. The mechanisms responsible for the vitamin D deficiency and deranged mineral metabolism are often complex.

Vitamin D and its principal metabolite—$25(OH)D$—are fat-soluble sterols that undergo enterohepatic circulation. Bile salts are necessary for their absorption; hence, hepatobiliary disease or short bowel syndrome may result in steatorrhea and both malabsorption of dietary vitamin D and depletion of endogenous vitamin D_2 and D_3 stores. Malabsorption of vitamin D and calcium may, however, be selective and not be reflected by the degree of steatorrhea, amount of small bowel disease, severity of pancreatic insufficiency, or duration of gastrointestinal disease. Also, in addition to having poor absorption, some patients with gastrointestinal disease may also have reduced exposure to sunlight, may have a poor intake of dietary vitamin D, and may consume drugs, like cholestyramine, that alter intestinal absorption of vitamin D.

Diagnosis

Assay of circulating $25(OH)D$ levels is performed to document vitamin D deficiency and, subsequently, to monitor replacement therapy. In some instances, however, symptomatic osteomalacia in patients with gastrointestinal disease may occur with a paucity of clues. Furthermore, in as many as two thirds of these patients, there may be a reduction in bone volume, i.e., osteoporosis, rather than an increase in osteoid, i.e., osteomalacia. In these cases, an examination of a tetracycline-labeled iliac crest undecalcified bone biopsy specimen may be useful to confirm the presence of a mineralization or defect.

Treatment

Although the pathogenesis of this type of rickets or osteomalacia is often complex and involves malabsorption of antirachitic sterols as well as minerals, therapy is generally straightforward and should often lead to gratifying results. Since patients with rickets or osteomalacia secondary to these disorders are a heterogeneous group, adequate therapy will require an individualized approach and careful follow-up. Pharmacologic doses of ergocalciferol (vitamin D_2) given orally often prove effective and are relatively inexpensive. Vitamin D_2 is readily converted to $25(OH)D_2$ even when there is parenchymal liver disease.

Patients with biopsy-proven osteomalacia should be treated with calcium supplements (calcium carbonate, 1200 to 1600 mg per day) and vitamin D. If ergocalciferol is used, doses range from 1250 to 5000 micrograms per day. With calcifediol, doses are 20 to 200 micrograms per day. Serum $25(OH)D$ levels are valuable in monitoring vitamin D therapy in malabsorption, and the goal is to achieve normal mean concentrations. In patients with intestinal disease or resection, calcitriol may be utilized at 1 to 2 micrograms per day. With metabolite therapy, the onset of biologic effects is faster, individual dosage requirements are more easily established, and toxicity is more quickly reversed.

Healing of osteomalacia with vitamin D therapy will be delayed if hypomagnesemia is present, and many patients with gastrointestinal disease (especially after intestinal bypass surgery for obesity) will require a magnesium supplement. Magnesium oxide tablets contain 60 per cent magnesium oxide. A daily dose of 350 to 750 mg of elemental magnesium may be needed. Serum magnesium levels should be monitored to avoid hypermagnesemia in patients with a decreased creatinine clearance. Although oral supplementation with vitamin D_2 is usually successful for this group of clinical disorders, intramuscular injection of vitamin D_2 should be considered if the patient's vitamin D status is not corrected. Vitamin D_2 is dissolved in sesame oil in this parenteral preparation. This pharmaceutical, therefore, will have delayed bioavailability. Vitamin D_2 release will persist for several months after one dose. Increased circulating $25(OH)D$ levels will be observed for several weeks. A single intramuscular injection of about 500,000 IU (1 ml) every few months should provide effective and continuous vitamin D_2 supplementation.

It must be emphasized that therapy for any

disorder with pharmacologic doses of vitamin D_2 requires periodic follow-up. Patients may need changes in their therapeutic regimen as rickets or osteomalacia heals and as underlying gastrointestinal or hepatobiliary disease evolves or responds to therapy. Assay of circulating 25(OH)D levels about 1 month after beginning therapy (and continuing about every 6 months thereafter) can be used to confirm successful oral absorption of vitamin D. Assays of calcium and creatinine excretion in 24-hour urine collections before, and periodically during, therapy (1) should reveal correction of hypocalciuria, (2) should suggest improvement in skeletal mineralization, and (3) should help to guard against vitamin D_2 toxicity (which will often present as hypercalciuria).

IMPAIRED 25-HYDROXYLATION

Anticonvulsant Drug Associated

Rickets and osteomalacia have been reported in institutionalized subjects with seizure disorders who are receiving anticonvulsant medication. This observation led to extensive studies of the effects of anticonvulsant drugs on mineral homeostasis. It was subsequently found that defective bone mineralization could be attributed to primary deficiency of vitamin D caused by poor diets and limited solar exposure.

Double tetracycline-labeled bone biopsies in ambulatory patients with epilepsy who are on chronic anticonvulsant therapy often fail to document osteomalacia and reveal normal mineralization rates and evidence of secondary hyperparathyroidism. The unique direct effects of anticonvulsant drugs in decreasing target-organ responsiveness to calcium-regulating hormones result in drug-induced hypocalcemia.

Treatment

Patients who receive significant doses of phenytoin or phenobarbital should also receive 50,000 IU of vitamin D_2 orally once weekly, with periodic assay of levels of circulating 25(OH)D and urinary calcium and creatinine in 24-hour collections if initial values are low. Treatment with vitamin D can correct the hypocalcemia, may reduce the degree of secondary hyperparathyroidism, and may decrease the number of seizures. Calcitriol, 0.25 to 0.5 microgram twice daily, has been successful in early trials.

Hepatic Disease

Severe hepatic disease is not usually associated with osteomalacia. Low levels of 25(OH)D in affected patients are probably due to nutritional vitamin D deficiency, limited sunlight exposure, and interruption of the enterohepatic circulation of vitamin D metabolites. Patients with primary biliary cirrhosis or alcoholic cirrhosis usually exhibit normal 25-hydroxylation capacity if supplied with adequate amounts of vitamin D substrate. Osteomalacia, if found in a patient with biliary cirrhosis, may be treated in a fashion similar to that for patients with malabsorption syndromes.

Premature infants and those with neonatal hepatitis may have impaired hepatic 25-hydroxylation. For rickets in the premature infant, liberal calcium and phosphorus supplementation may be required to supply the rapidly growing skeleton. Fetal calcium and phosphorus requirements in the last trimester are 100 to 120 and 60 to 75 mg per kg per day, respectively. Magnesium salts may also be necessary. Rapid radiologic improvement in these patients has been noted with calcitriol in doses of 0.05 microgram per kg per day.

VITAMIN D RESISTANCE

Vitamin D–Dependent Rickets, Type I

This autosomal recessive syndrome is an inborn error of vitamin D biosynthesis, with defective conversion of 25(OH)D to $1,25(OH)_2D$.

This defect, at the level of renal 25(OH)D, 1-alpha-hydroxylase, can be overcome by pharmacologic doses of vitamin D_2 (20,000 to 60,000 IU per day), which increase circulating 25(OH)D levels. Since there is no defect in the liver's ability to convert vitamin D_2 to $25(OH)D_2$, administration of vitamin D_2—rather than metabolite—is less expensive yet appropriate therapy. Pharmacologic doses of 25(OH)D or physiologic amounts of $1,25(OH)D_2D_3$ (0.25 to 2.0 micrograms per day) are also effective but are more expensive than vitamin D_2 supplementation.

Although these metabolites are an expensive approach to therapy, they offer an advantage: the circulating and physiologic half-lives of these metabolites are much shorter than those of vitamin D_2, such that excessive dosing will respond rapidly to modification.

Hypoparathyroidism

Hypoparathyroidism and pseudohypoparathyroidism are characterized by reduced serum $1,25(OH)_2D$ concentrations as a result of impaired stimulation of 1-hydroxylation by parathyroid hormone. Although a mineralization defect may accompany hypoparathyroidism, the primary clinical problem is that of hypocalcemia. Therapy consists of 1 gram per day of supplemental calcium and calcitriol (0.5 to 1.5 micrograms per day in two or three divided doses).

Impaired Target-Organ Response to 1,25(OH)$_2$D

In vitamin D–dependent rickets, Type II, a defect in target organ sensitivity to 1,25(OH)$_2$D has been recognized. Sometimes associated with alopecia, this disorder may have autosomal recessive inheritance or may be sporadic. Therapy with calcitriol must surpass the endogenous serum 1,25(OH)$_2$D levels, which may be as high as 140 to 745 pg per ml. Remission has occurred with 5 to 20 micrograms per day of calcitriol, resulting in serum levels of 200 to 4000 pg per ml. Extraordinarily high doses of other vitamin D preparations have sometimes proved successful but also increase the risk of prolonged vitamin D intoxication.

HYPOPHOSPHATEMIC STATES

X-Linked Hypophosphatemia

X-linked hypophosphatemia (XLH) is the most common form of hereditary rickets and osteomalacia. Also known as vitamin D–resistant rickets, familial hypophosphatemia, and phosphate diabetes, XLH is characterized by a primary defect in the renal transport of phosphorus, resulting in hypophosphatemia and inappropriately low 1,25(OH)$_2$D concentrations. Phosphorus supplementation alone improves calcification in the cartilage but may barely modify the osteomalacic process at the trabecular bone surface.

Treatment

Multidose therapy is required, and 1 to 4 grams per day of phosphorus should be given in four to six divided doses. In the past, concurrent ergocalciferol therapy was utilized to increase the efficiency of phosphorus and calcium absorption in order to minimize the required dose of oral phosphorus and to minimize the increased secretion of parathyroid hormone induced by long-term phosphorus administration. Calcitriol currently allows better control and is the agent of choice. Short-lived episodes of hypercalcemia have been rapidly controlled by lowering the dosage of calcitriol. Serum ionized calcium levels and the urinary calcium:creatinine ratio should be monitored bimonthly, since hypercalciuria usually develops before hypercalcemia.

Treatment should be started with 0.25 microgram of calcitriol twice daily and may require up to 3 to 4 micrograms per day to normalize mineralization. Unfortunately, only 0.25 and 0.50 microgram capsules of 1,25(OH)$_2$D$_3$ (Rocaltrol) are commercially available at this time, and there is no liquid preparation. For young children these small capsules may be dissolved in applesauce. A therapeutic (pharmacologic) dose of approximately 50 ng (0.050 microgram) per kg of body weight once daily should be achieved, after a 2- to 3-month period, by gradually increasing the dose. Serum phosphorus levels should be maintained at greater than 3 mg per dl and are best sampled about 45 minutes after an oral dose. With effective therapy, the serum alkaline phosphatase activity returns to levels normal for the age of the patient and serum parathyroid hormone levels should not be increased.

Lifelong treatment appears to be necessary. A small decrement in the daily calcitriol dose may be necessary during prolonged bed rest (e.g., after corrective orthopedic surgery), but usually calcitriol and phosphorus therapy can be maintained without immobilization hypercalcemia. Osteotomies are best postponed until growth has ceased or at least until medical management achieves persistently adequate phosphorus levels as well as a reduction in the serum alkaline phosphatase activity.

Sporadic Hypophosphatemia

Renal phosphorus wasting may also occur without a family history and is managed in a manner similar to that of XLH. The development of adult-onset hypophosphatemic osteomalacia, however, must be diagnosed with caution, and the presence of potentially curable oncogenic osteomalacia must be excluded.

Fanconi's Syndrome

Renal phosphorus wasting is a frequent complication of proximal renal tubular dysfunction in Fanconi's syndrome. Therapy with 1,25(OH)$_2$D$_3$ and phosphorus is appropriate in Fanconi's syndrome associated with rickets or osteomalacia. However, urinary calcium levels must be monitored carefully, since hypercalciuria is more likely to occur in Fanconi's syndrome than in XLH.

Oncogenic Osteomalacia

Rickets or osteomalacia that remits after resection of a coexisting tumor is apparently caused by the secretion of a tumor factor that inhibits renal tubular reabsorption of phosphorus and the 1-hydroxylation of 25(OH)D. Hypophosphatemic osteomalacia has been described with a wide variety of tumors. When resection of a tumor is not possible, inorganic phosphate supplementation and $1,25(OH)_2D_3$ therapy, often with pharmacologic doses of $1,25(OH)_2D_3$, will be necessary.

Antacid-Induced Osteomalacia

Chronic consumption of excess phosphorus-binding antacids can cause hypophosphatemic osteomalacia. Bone pain and weakness may be incapacitating, but the excessive use of antacids may be overlooked by the physician. Antacid-induced phosphorus depletion is characterized by hypophosphatemia with hypophosphaturia, hypercalciuria, and nephrolithiasis; by increased gastrointestinal absorption of calcium; by a tendency to borderline high serum calcium concentrations; and by elevated serum alkaline phosphatase activity levels. Patients with a history of abdominal pain, peptic ulcer disease, or esophagitis and renal transplant recipients given antacids should be monitored for antacid-induced hypophosphatemia. Discontinuation of antacid use and the institution of phosphorus supplements (2 to 4 grams per day) are required for healing of the bone disease.

METABOLIC ACIDOSIS

Rickets and osteomalacia occur in patients with chronic hyperchloremic acidosis from renal tubular disorders or following surgical procedures that place a segment of bowel in continuity with the urinary tract. The pathogenetic mechanisms are complex, but the skeletal disease responds well to vitamin D_2 supplementation and alkali therapy (divided doses of 10 to 15 grams of sodium bicarbonate daily). Alkali therapy to correct the acidosis is important and should be continued after pharmacologic doses of vitamin D_2 help to correct the mineralization defect. Vitamin D_2, about 1.25 mg (50,000 IU) three times a week, is indicated until healing occurs. However, urinary calcium and creatinine must be monitored frequently, since acidosis per se will promote hypercalciuria. Finally, calcium and potassium supplementation may be necessary at the onset of alkali therapy to guard against tetany and hypokalemia.

CHRONIC RENAL FAILURE

Renal osteodystrophy encompasses the array of vitamin D mineral and skeletal derangements that attend chronic renal failure. Virtually all patients with end-stage renal disease can be shown to have some uremic bone disease. Skeletal disease results from secondary hyperparathyroidism (in which bone remodeling is rapid) and from concomitant osteomalacia, the pathogenesis of which is complex. Hyperphosphatemia must be controlled before calcium and vitamin D supplementation is started. Phosphorus accumulation can be prevented by dietary phosphorus restriction to about 600 mg per day. Aluminum-containing antacids may be required to bind dietary and gastrointestinal endogenous phosphorus. Serum phosphorus levels should be maintained at 4 to 5 mg per dl. The addition of 1200 mg per day of calcium (1 teaspoon of calcium carbonate suspension three times daily) may help raise the serum calcium level. Although dihydrotachysterol and calcifediol have been used successfully in renal osteodystrophy, calcitriol has a biologic advantage, since it specifically replaces the hormone missing in uremia. Initial doses of 0.25 microgram twice daily should be increased every 2 to 3 weeks until the serum calcium begins to rise. The increased phosphorus absorption that occurs with calcitriol therapy may require the use of additional phosphorus-binding antacids. Calcitriol can improve muscle strength, decrease bone pain, and help prevent and treat secondary uremic hyperparathyroidism. Mild hypercalcemia is common after 10 to 15 months of therapy and is predicted by a decrease toward normal of the serum alkaline phosphatase activity. The syndrome of osteomalacic dialysis osteodystrophy is characterized by a sporadic occurrence, debilitating bone pain and myopathy, skeletal fragility, hypercalcemia with sensitivity to calcitriol, and, in some cases, dialysis dementia. Contributing factors may be phosphorus depletion, prior parathyroid surgery, and intoxication with trace metals. Aluminum in contaminated dialysate and from antacid therapy has been proposed as one cause of this syndrome. Therapy generally consists of altering the antacid regimen. In some cases, deferoxamine (Desferal) has been reported to be a useful chelating agent for aluminum, reversing the mineralization defect.

RICKETS AND OSTEOMALACIA CAUSED BY INHIBITORS OF BONE

Mineralization

Rickets or osteomalacia can occur from excessive ingestion of inhibitors of bone mineralization:

1. *Aluminum.* Rare case reports suggest that defective bone mineralization can occur in otherwise healthy individuals when high concentrations of aluminum are leached into food from cookware. More frequently, patients with uremia who ingest excessive quantities of aluminum-containing antacids may be affected, with subsequent aluminum deposition in bone.

2. *Fluoride.* Pharmacologic doses of sodium fluoride (60 to 80 mg or more per day), given for prolonged periods of time (9 to 12 months or more) in an attempt to treat osteoporosis, may result in osteomalacia by complexing in the bone mineral and preventing further crystal formation. Defective bone mineralization will respond to discontinuation of the fluoride therapy.

3. *Disodium Etidronate.* This diphosphonate compound is used to treat patients with Paget's bone disease and to prevent heterotopic calcification in individuals who undergo hip replacement surgery. Excessive doses (greater than 10 to 15 mg per kg) or prolonged drug therapy will lead to rickets or osteomalacia.

CALCIUM-DEFICIENT RICKETS

Dietary calcium deprivation in children may cause rachitic changes, and bone biopsies in children receiving less than 200 mg of calcium per day have revealed increased osteoid and a delay in mineralization. Hypocalcemia, hypocalciuria, and elevated serum alkaline phosphatase activity levels may be present, and secondary hyperparathyroidism may be severe. Calcium supplementation (1 gram per day) heals the bone disease.

MISCELLANEOUS DISORDERS

A variety of rare inherited or sporadic conditions present with rickets or osteomalacia even though circulating concentrations of calcium and phosphorus are normal or even increased. There is no specific medical therapy for these disorders. A correct diagnosis at the onset is important because therapeutic "trials" of vitamin D (or its metabolites) or calcium supplementation may lead to hypercalcemia and hypercalciuria.

Hypophosphatasia is an inherited inborn error of metabolism characterized biochemically by subnormal circulating alkaline phosphatase activity. Defective skeletal mineralization appears to be a direct result of deficient alkaline phosphatase activity in osseous tissue.

Fibrogenesis imperfecta ossium, a disorder reported in a few sporadic cases, appears to be due to defective skeletal mineralization stemming from a primary defect in the organic matrix of bone.

SCURVY AND VITAMIN C DEFICIENCY

method of
WILLIAM B. BEAN, M.D.
Iowa City, Iowa

Although clinical scurvy is considered a rare disease, it may occur and is likely to be overlooked because of its alleged rarity. The street people, the homeless, alcoholics, the elderly, persons who live alone, and those depressed from loss of a mate should be thought of as potential victims—the desolate, bewildered, and sometimes lost as derelicts in modern metropolitan areas. Lind's classic controlled studies in the British navy demonstrated that lemon juice was a specific cure and indeed preventive well over 200 years ago. It took the British Admiralty nearly 80 years to come around to using what one of their naval surgeons had discovered. The British tar used to be called a "limey" because at that time lemons were called limes. In days of overseas expansion from Europe the Portuguese and British developed spectacular overseas empires because they understood the role of lemons better than others. On very long voyages their ships carried enough to last for the voyage to the Orient. The Portuguese stopped and replenished their larder with lemons in South Africa.

In experimental scurvy produced by removing vitamin C from the diet, blood levels decline rapidly, well before any symptoms occur. The plasma is the first to lose vitamin C, then the nucleated cells, which hold on to it pretty well, particularly the platelets. Ultimately it disappears. As with other vitamin deficiencies, a stage of chemical depletion exists for a time without clinical manifestations. Signs and symptoms (Table 1) come unpredictably and sometimes with explosive violence. Vascular lesions in experimental scurvy may occur in the conjunctivae, and peripheral neuropathy also may appear. Rarely the sicca syndrome may occur.

Prevention

Citrus fruits and tomatoes provide the best natural source of vitamin C, but the vitamin is present in many foods in sufficient amounts to provide ample safety (Table 2). Ripe fruits and vegetables contain much more vitamin C un-

TABLE 1. **Clinical Features of Scurvy**

Skin
  Perifollicular hemorrhage
  Hyperpigmentation
  Bleeding gums
    Note: If the person has no teeth, the gums do not show
    the characteristic hemorrhage
  Poor healing of wounds
Blood Vessels
  Easy bruising
  Hemorrhage, which often is extensive and occasionally
    occurs in sheets along fascial planes
Bones and Joints
  Subperiosteal hemorrhages
  Scorbutic rosary in children
  Fractures
  Bone tenderness
  Hemorrhage into joints
Central Nervous System
  Lassitude
  Irritability
  Emotional changes
  Motor deterioration

TABLE 2. **Approximate Vitamin C Content in Single Portions of Common Foods**

Broccoli	140 mg	Cauliflower	69 mg
Brussels sprouts	135 mg	Spinach	50 mg
Orange juice	124 mg	Boiled potato	36 mg
Orange	113 mg	Lima beans	29 mg
Cantaloupe	90 mg	Asparagus	25 mg
Strawberries	88 mg	French fried potato	16 mg

cooked than they do in the cooked state. Losses also may occur from storage. Green vegetables supply additional amounts. Broccoli, kale, Brussels sprouts, and turnip greens are good sources. Even vegetables not very high in ascorbic acid if eaten in large quantities provide the necessary amount. These include white potatoes, green beans, peas, apples, bananas, onions, cauliflower, turnips, and parsnips. Times of high metabolic requirement such as rapid growth, pregnancy, lactation, and certain illnesses, especially severe chronic ones, increase the requirement. The recommended daily allowance of ascorbic acid ranges from 35 mg a day for infants to 60 mg a day for adults. Women have slightly lower requirements than men except during pregnancy and lactation. Recommended allowances usually include a surplus, because there is considerable variation from person to person in what is necessary.

Treatment

In an adult subject with clear-cut scurvy, which indicates profound deficiency, it is wise to give approximately 2 grams of ascorbic acid a day early in treatment. Though it can be given intravenously either in isotonic salt solution or in 5 per cent glucose solution, usually oral medication is satisfactory. Infusion should be given slowly. The level of vitamin C in the fluid should not be higher than 2 per cent. In edentulous patients or those whose gums are not seriously involved, oral therapy is satisfactory. In infants and children the vitamin may be given either way. Approximately 0.5 gram daily for the first few days restores the depletion and saturates the tissues. A larger amount than the usual daily allowance should be given during the first few weeks of convalescence. An older notion that vitamin C improved wound healing has not been confirmed, although severe vitamin C depletion will delay or prevent wound healing. It is doubtful that vitamin C is helpful in patients with leukemia, and it has not been demonstrated to have any role in the treatment of poisoning, stress, shock, or hyperthyroidism. In theory prolonged diarrhea, diuresis, or excessive sweating might lower the stores of vitamin C, but from a practical point

of view this has not proved important. The anemia of scurvy does not respond to iron, folic acid, or vitamin B_{12} but is relieved by vitamin C. Vitamin C is relatively nontoxic, and when it is given in very large doses the surplus is rapidly excreted in the urine. It is best to have the person with acute scurvy or long-standing scurvy remain in bed during the early phase of treatment. Treatment in addition to vitamin C is mainly supportive.

VITAMIN K DEFICIENCY

method of
JAMES J. CORRIGAN, JR., M.D.
University of Arizona Health Sciences Center
Tucson, Arizona

Vitamin K comprises a group of fat-soluble 1,4-naphthoquinones that are required for normal hemostasis. The vitamin is involved in the biosynthesis of four procoagulants (Factors II, VII, IX, and X) and two natural inhibitors (protein C and protein S). Vitamin K is found in a wide variety of foods. The highest concentrations (as phylloquinone, K_1) are in green leafy vegetables; the next greatest amounts (as menaquinones) are in meat and dairy products. As with other fat-soluble vitamins, bile salts and normal fat absorption are required for efficient oral intake of vitamin K.

The minimal daily requirement of vitamin K, estimated at less than 100 micrograms, is provided mainly by diet. In addition, vitamin K is synthesized by certain microorganisms in the colon, although this source may not be important under normal circumstances. Since body stores of vitamin K are limited, a deficiency can occur within days to several weeks in circumstances of reduced intake or absorption.

Causes

The major cause of vitamin K deficiency is decreased intake by persons who are anorectic or in whom oral alimentation is restricted, such as the normal newborn infant, patients exclusively on parenteral hyperalimentation, and those recovering from major gastrointestinal surgery. Moreover, vitamin K deficiency may result from diminished absorption owing either to diffuse intestinal mucosal disease or to diminished flow of bile. Accordingly, obstructive jaundice of any cause may result in bleeding secondary to vitamin K deficiency. Another factor contributing to vitamin K deficiency is administration of broad-spectrum antibiotics, which may eradicate vitamin K–producing intestinal bacteria and/or inhibit vitamin K metabolism. Hemorrhage due to deficient vitamin K action at the cellular level may result from the presence of a vitamin K antagonist, such as the warfarin or indanedione anticoagulant. A coagulopathy due to a reduction in the vitamin K–dependent coagulation factors has been described in patients with gram-negative septicemia; this disorder is unrelated to antibiotic use or disseminated intravascular coagulation. The cause and significance of this observation is poorly understood.

Vitamin K deficiency occurs in most newborn infants because stores are nonexistent, bacterial colonization is absent, and oral intake is minimal, particularly during the first several days of life. It may occur especially in neonates who are breast fed, since human breast milk contains little vitamin K. Prophylactic vitamin K shortly after birth, recommended by the American Academy of Pediatrics in the early 1960s, has been extremely effective in reducing the frequency of hemorrhagic disease of the newborn.

Clinical Manifestations

The only clinical manifestation of vitamin K deficiency is excessive hemorrhage, usually following local trauma but occurring spontaneously in severe cases. Signs and symptoms of bleeding include easy bruising, mucosal bleeding (epistaxis, gastrointestinal hemorrhage, menometrorrhagia, and hematuria), and oozing from puncture sites, cutdowns, and surgical incisions. Intracranial bleeding or bleeding into the retroperitoneal space may cause severe morbidity.

The laboratory manifestations of vitamin K deficiency are prolonged prothrombin time (PT) and prolonged partial thromboplastin time (PTT). The platelet count and plasma fibrinogen level are normal. If needed, specific assays for Factors II, VII, IX, and X or laboratory tests for detecting the noncarboxylated protein precursors of the vitamin K–dependent procoagulants can be performed.

Treatment

Patients with striking laboratory abnormalities or clinical bleeding manifestations are best treated with parenteral vitamin K. This is most usually the natural derivative vitamin K_1 (AquaMEPHYTON). The dose varies with the size of the patient; 0.5 to 1 mg is adequate for premature and term infants, 2 to 3 mg for children, and 5 to 10 mg for older children and adults. Slow intravenous infusion is only rarely associated with hypotension and anaphylaxis. The vitamin can also be given subcutaneously. The intramuscular route should be avoided, since it can be associated with hematomas. The advantage of intravenous administration is prompter delivery of the vitamin to the hepatocytes, resulting in the rapid onset of carboxylation of precursor proteins. The carboxylated proteins may even then take as long as 24 hours to reach plasma levels sufficient to alter coagulation tests. Prevention of vitamin K deficiency in the highly susceptible patient often can be managed by oral administration of a water-soluble synthetic vitamin K analogue, 5 mg twice to three times weekly.

In most instances, vitamin K therapy is followed over the next 12 to 24 hours by cessation of hemorrhage and normalization of the PT and PTT. The usual practice is to repeat these studies 24 hours after parenteral vitamin K therapy. If a decrease in bleeding and partial improvement in laboratory studies have not occurred by this time, the diagnosis is incorrect or the patient has other associated coagulation disturbances.

Following initial replacement therapy, subsequent doses of vitamin K should be given twice to three times weekly if the underlying problem (malabsorption, broad-spectrum antibiotics, long-term parenteral alimentation) persists. For the patient who is hemorrhaging, vitamin K may not be immediately effective, even if a large dose (20 to 50 mg) is utilized. In this setting, fresh frozen plasma or rarely a prothrombin complex concentrate (Proplex or Konyne) may be indicated in instances of severe bleeding. Prothrombin complex concentrates should be avoided if at all possible; they are associated with a high risk of hepatitis and can cause thrombosis, especially in patients with associated liver disease. In other circumstances of vitamin K deficiency, plasma replacement therapy is rarely required. As in the treatment of other acquired hemorrhagic disorders, aggressive management of the underlying disease is mandatory.

OSTEOPOROSIS

method of
ROBERT LINDSAY, M.B., CH.B., PH.D.
Columbia University
New York, New York

Osteoporosis is a group of conditions characterized by low bone mass, which leads to increased risk of fracture. It is only after fractures have occurred that osteoporosis becomes clinically important. However, prevention of bone loss is so significantly more successful than treatment of the condition after fracture that identification of the asymptomatic patient at greatest risk has assumed major importance. The disorder affects postmenopausal women, particularly of Caucasian and Oriental origins, more frequently than it does men. Therefore, such groups constitute those at maximum risk. Many other factors that might change risk have been described, but the contribution of any of these is often difficult to evaluate for an individual patient. The most frequently cited risk factors include early menopause, oophorectomy, family history of osteoporotic fractures, slight body build, low calcium intake, and prolonged physical inactivity. Other factors that may increase risk are excessive consumption of alcohol, cigarette smoking, excess glucocorticoids (given therapeutically, or endogenous as in Cushing's syndrome), liver disease, gastrectomy, loop diuretics, excessive thyroid hormone replacement, and perhaps thyrotoxicosis. Indeed, any chronic disorder associated with long-term disability and disuse may potentially increase the likelihood of osteoporosis.

All of these are superimposed on the basic pattern of skeletal changes that occur throughout life. Thus, they may interfere with the attainment of peak bone mass during growth or during the period of skeletal consolidation that follows cessation of linear growth, or may accelerate the age-dependent loss of bone mass that occurs in all adults in all populations studied thus far, accompanying the reduction in muscle mass that occurs with increasing age. Loss of ovarian function, for example, either at menopause or even in the pre-menopausal years (e.g., amenorrhea of the competitive athlete, or in anorexia nervosa, or hyperprolactinemia) will superimpose an accelerated phase of bone loss on the normal age-related decline in bone mass. The greater incidence and prevalence of fractures in the female population is a reflection of their lower peak bone mass and the acceleration of bone loss consequent to estrogen deficiency. Vertebral crush fractures are the most common presentation of osteoporosis in the postmenopausal population, occurring at least ten times more commonly than in the male population. Hip fracture, the most serious of the osteoporotic fractures, affects women only twice as commonly as it affects men, suggesting that there may be different controlling mechanisms for bone loss at the hip super-imposed, in women, on the bone loss of ovarian deficiency. Classification of the disorder by fracture expression has been suggested as a result of these findings, but with our current state of knowledge about therapy this is scarcely of benefit to the clinician.

Despite the recognition of the many factors that can increase risk of bone loss, their presence or absence in any individual cannot be used to assess or predict skeletal mass. Therefore, for proper identification of the person most at risk of developing fractures as a result of low bone mass, a measurement of the skeleton using one of the noninvasive techniques for bone mass quantification must be obtained. The presence of low bone mass in any individual, even if asymptomatic, increases the urgency for aggressive intervention.

Prevention

For any asymptomatic individual for whom intervention is considered necessary, the initial approach is one of behavior modification to elim-inate all potential factors that might exaggerate risk. Many of these are sufficiently detrimental to general health and well-being that they should be discouraged for reasons other than their po-tential to aggravate osteoporosis. Reduction of alcohol intake and cigarette consumption and improvement in the ongoing level of physical activity are logical initial steps. At the same time, most would recommend increasing calcium intake to at least adequate levels. Prevention of the postmenopausal acceleration of bone loss re-quires estrogen therapy, while calcitonin may be an alternative for those who do not wish to take estrogens.

Calcium

The rationale for increasing calcium intake is based on the assumption that an inadequate intake will require utilization of skeletal calcium to maintain adequate levels of serum calcium. It is impossible to define an adequate intake for each individual patient, since that would require measurement of both usual intake and absorption efficiency, and therefore "average" intake levels are recommended for segments of the population, based on the elegant balance studies of Heaney. For estrogen-replete women a total daily intake of about 1000 mg is probably adequate, but for the estrogen-deficient woman the estimated cal-cium requirement increases to 1500 mg per day. These intake levels, which include calcium from all sources, whether dietary or supplements, are probably sufficient to ensure that calcium defi-ciency does not exacerbate bone loss. It seems likely, however, that these levels of intake will not maintain calcium balance at all times or in all women, given the other stresses that are placed on the organism. Thus a high calcium intake, by itself, will not prevent bone loss due to estrogen deficiency or glucocorticoid excess.

Although an adequate intake can be obtained from dietary sources, in practice this is difficult to achieve. The major source of bioavailable cal-cium is dairy products (1 quart of milk contains approximately 1200 mg of calcium), but many individuals will avoid milk because of true lac-tase deficiency, vague discomfort after consump-tion, or the calorie and fat content, or simply because of dislike.

Where an adequate calcium intake cannot be obtained from dietary sources, calcium supple-ments are required. Calcium carbonate is the usual recommended calcium salt, since this salt has the highest percentage of calcium (40 per cent) of any of the available preparations. The carbonate requires acid conditions for solubility, and absorption efficiency has been reported to be low in patients with achlorhydria. The relevance of this in calcium supplementation of the elderly, in whom lower production rates of gastric HCl are likely to prevail, is not clear. However, we recommend that the supplement be taken with meals, and in divided doses, to circumvent any absorption difficulty and to reduce side effects. Generally doses of no more than 200 to 500 mg of calcium should be taken at any one time.

Recently it has been recognized that some calcium carbonate products may not meet FDA guidelines for solubility, and presumably may be less bioavailable. We suggest that patients obtain name-brand products, since these seem to be more reliable, and that they check the solubility by leaving a tablet in 8 oz of vinegar for 45 minutes. If the tablet has not dissolved, the product should be exchanged. Calcium citrate may provide an alternative that bypasses the solubility problem with carbonate, and other salts are also available, although with lower concentrations of calcium. However, supplements prepared from clay or bone meal should be avoided, since they may be contaminated with lead or other heavy metals.

Side effects of calcium supplementation if practiced in this conservative fashion are minimal and consist of constipation, usual fairly minor, eructation, especially if carbonate is used, and a potential risk of renal stones. Except for those who have a history of active renal stone disease, this latter complication appears more theoretical than real. If concern exists, the citrate salt is to be preferred. In addition to being taken with food, supplements should be temporally separated from other medication by at least 1 hour; this is especially true for iron, phenothiazines, L-dopa, and tetracyclines.

Estrogens

The period of rapid bone loss that follows cessation of ovarian function is preferentially prevented with replacement of ovarian hormones. Considerable data, obtained in carefully controlled trials, have demonstrated that estrogens reduce skeletal turnover, and thus bone loss, when provided to estrogen-deficient women. These changes in bone are accompanied by improved efficiency in utilization of dietary calcium. The effects appear to last as long as the hormones are given (at least 10 years), and retrospective and case control data indicate that skeletal preservation can be translated into prevention of fracture. Our prospective data suggest that vertebral fracture incidence can be reduced by as much as 90 per cent, while other data suggest a 50 per cent reduction in hip fracture incidence. Since the consequence of estrogen treatment is reduction of loss of skeletal tissue, treatment is most effective if begun close to menopause, and when continued for as long as possible. However, estrogens can be shown to reduce bone turnover in any estrogen-deficient woman. Menopausal acceleration of bone loss therefore becomes the single most preventable event in the pathogenesis of osteoporosis, since its onset (roughly speaking) is marked by cessation of menses, and therapy is clearly effective.

While other reasons may exist for intervention with estrogen at this time point, the introduction of estrogen for prevention of osteoporosis is confounded by the difficulty in determining the exact degree of risk to which any individual is exposed. In general, we suggest that the presence of major risk factors be considered as guidelines for therapy, recognizing that bone mass at menopause is independent of the presence or absence of these factors. Thus, estrogen might be considered for the small, thin white or Oriental woman who has an earlier than expected menopause (or oophorectomy) and who has a family history of osteoporotic fractures. If nutrition and lifestyle also contribute to risk, the argument for aggressive intervention is even stronger. However, it appears that the major determinant of subsequent risk of osteoporosis (defined as low bone mass increasing fracture risk) is low peak bone mass, or low bone mass at time of menopause. Since mass can be determined only by measurement, we recommend that the physician obtain a bone mass measurement when considering estrogen therapy specifically for prevention of osteoporosis. Noninvasive techniques of bone mass measurement are becoming more commonly available. While a measurement of the spine is probably the most useful, the physician should become familiar with and obtain whichever measurement is available.

The majority of the data obtained about prevention of osteoporosis have been about use of oral estrogen therapy. The minimum effective dose appears to be 0.625 mg of conjugated equine estrogen per day, or its equivalent. Many regimens for estrogen administration have been described. Currently we are prescribing estrogen daily (continuously) for all patients, adding a progestogen for the first 14 days of each calendar month for all patients with an intact uterus. Preliminary data suggest that the route of administration is not critical, and percutaneous, subcutaneous, or transdermal routes may be equally effective, provided the dose is adequate. However, confirmatory data are required on this issue.

The side effects of estrogen therapy are probably also dependent on the dose, route, and accompanying medication. The use of long-term high-dose oral estrogen has been demonstrated to increase the risk of endometrial carcinoma perhaps as much as eight to ten times. Other side effects include an increase in the risk of gallstones and a potentially increased risk of thromboembolic phenomena; the latter requires confirmation and seems likely to be associated only with the use of contraceptive agents, under certain specific circumstances, rather than the use of estrogens after menopause. Although the issue has been studied many times, it is still not clear whether there is any alteration in the risk of breast malignancy with the use of estrogens. It seems reasonable that if this is a risk of estrogen treatment, it must be very small. In some patients there may be an idiosyncratic increase in blood pressure, although in general blood pressure changes are small, and downward changes may also occur. Some of these effects may be minimized by introducing progestogens, or using other routes of administration of estrogens. However, the return of menstrual bleeding as a result of progestogen withdrawal is problematic for some individuals. Progestogens in currently prescribed doses may negate the proposed beneficial effects of estrogen on cardiovascular disease, which are thought to occur through changes in lipid metabolism.

Calcitonin

The hormone calcitonin has been shown to reduce bone loss in several well-designed studies in patients with established osteoporosis. Thus, calcitonin is an alternative to estrogen for those patients who cannot or will not take estrogens. The usual dose is 50 to 200 units daily given by subcutaneous or intramuscular injection. The major attraction of calcitonin is its safety. Side effects are nausea and vomiting after the injection in occasional patients, and flushing involving the blush area. These problems can be controlled by giving the dose at night and adding an antiemetic about 30 minutes before the injection, if necessary. The main problems with calcitonin at present are its route of administration and its cost. Recently intranasal delivery of calcitonin has been described, and although the bioavailability is low, this is an attractive alternate delivery system that may supersede parenteral administration. Detailed clinical testing has yet to be done, however, using this route.

Treatment

Although the therapeutic agents available for treatment of patients who present with fracture syndromes are identical to those above, there are certain general strategies that can be proposed for this group of patients. In all circumstances, secondary causes of osteoporosis should be excluded and other diagnoses (such as myeloma) eliminated. For those with fractures of the hip, the initial approach is almost always surgical. For those with vertebral fractures, when back pain is an acute problem, specific measures to relieve the symptoms may be required. Bed rest may be required at this stage, but should be for as short a period as possible, and the patient should usually be mobilized within 72 hours.

When pain is persistent, a spinal support may be useful to accelerate mobilization, but the patient should be weaned off the support as early as possible. Adequate analgesia is appropriate, but should be accompanied by alternative means of relieving the pain, including hot packs, transcutaneous nerve stimulation, and hydrotherapy. Acetaminophen and codeine usually suffice, but occasionally stronger narcotic analgesics are required. Muscle relaxants may be required for the severe muscle spasms that occasionally accompany the acute episode.

More commonly patients will present with chronic low back pain that is probably muscular in origin, secondary to the muscular disadvantage created by kyphosis. The pain can usually be controlled with nonsteroidal anti-inflammatory agents or acetaminophen, in combination with heat, transcutaneous nerve stimulation, and hydrotherapy. Stronger analgesics should be avoided if possible. Each patient should be instructed in an exercise program designed to strengthen the back extensors, while flexion of the spine should be avoided. Swimming is an excellent exercise for these individuals.

Pharmacologic Therapy

In the established disorder the principles of therapy are similar to those for the younger population. The appropriate treatment for secondary causes of osteoporosis is elimination of the problem directly responsible. Cushing's syndrome, thyrotoxicosis, and hyperparathyroidism are examples of disorders that require treatment before the introduction of antiresorptive therapy. If the patient is on steroid therapy, re-evaluation of the need for steroids must be a priority, since there is, as yet, no effective treatment for this form of osteoporosis. Pharmacologic approaches therefore follow the general guidelines to prevention outlined in this article. An adequate intake of calcium is recommended for all patients, either from dietary sources or using supplements following the guidelines described above. Prevention of further bone loss can be achieved using estrogens or calcitonin. Calcitonin may be advantageous in the acute phase of the disorder, since it has a dramatic analgesic effect in some patients. Except for use in patients over 70 years of age, there is no place for vitamin D in the treatment of osteoporosis. For the elderly routine supplementation with vitamin D should be provided, using physiologic doses (<1000 units per day). At present no other therapeutic agents are approved for treatment of osteoporosis. However, a number are in development or clinical trials.

New Therapeutic Approaches

While ongoing research tries to find alternative antiresorptive agents, such as diphosphonates that will be safer for use among the elderly population, the goal of many developments in this field is to find an effective, safe therapeutic agent or regimen that will increase bone mass significantly. While preliminary data are encouraging, none is sufficiently well documented to be used in the routine management of fracture patients. Sodium fluoride is hardly a new preparation, but is now undergoing controlled investigation for the first time. About 60 per cent of patients given fluoride in doses of approximately 1 mg per kg will exhibit increases in spinal mineral of about 30 per cent. Since the crystal size is changed by the addition of the fluoride atom, the strength of the newly formed bone has been questioned. No changes in bone in the peripheral skeleton have been found (including the hip). Since there is a high incidence of side effects, including gastric irritation and periarticular pain in the weight-bearing joints, general use of fluoride must await the outcome of the formal clinical trials. Anabolic agents may be useful in patients with severe fracture syndromes, acting mostly as antiresorptive agents. However, their use is limited because of side effects, including their negative effects on serum lipids. One uncontrolled study suggests that parathyroid hormone may be anabolic to the skeleton when given by injection, perhaps in combination with 1,25-$(OH)_2$-D_3 (calcitriol) to improve calcium absorption. There does not appear to be a significant role for the active metabolite of vitamin D except in this restricted and defined mode. Other approaches to therapy include a variety of regimens designed to stimulate bone turnover while inhibiting the resorption phase of the bone remodeling cycle, using an antiresorbing agent such as calcitonin, estrogen, or a diphosphonate. This remains at this time a theoretical approach, and considerably more documentation will be required before it becomes generally available.

PAGET'S DISEASE OF BONE

method of
ROY D. ALTMAN, M.D.
University of Miami School of Medicine
Miami, Florida

Paget's disease of bone can be defined as a remodeling of isolated areas of the skeleton whereby bone initially undergoes increased resorption. This results in subsequent deposition of bone that is disorganized, often enlarged, interspersed with areas of fibrosis, and, although often heavily calcified, structurally weak.

The diagnosis of Paget's disease can occasionally be made on clinical examination by the findings listed in Table 1. Most often the diagnosis is made in the pursuit of an elevated serum alkaline phosphatase or on the typical appearance on a radiograph. The bone scan can verify the extent of bony involvement. Bone biopsy is rarely needed unless sarcoma or metastatic disease is suspected.

It is estimated that 80 per cent of patients with Paget's disease are elderly and without clinical findings or complications. Table 1 lists the complications of Paget's disease that may require therapy. Since the newer medications have some risk and cost, there should be a definite objective in therapy. One should construct a therapeutic program for individual patients with consideration of complications of the disease. It should be remembered, however, that most often the disease is localized and asymptomatic and does not require therapy.

Treatment

General Measures

The patient should be advised that Paget's disease is rarely a serious illness. Most often symptoms are mild and readily suppressed by a therapeutic program. In patients with sympto-

TABLE 1. **Complications of Paget's Disease of Bone**

Symptom or Finding	Pathologic Anatomy
Bone pain	Cause unknown, periostitis, "bone angina," osteomalacia
Deformity	Softened bone
Fracture	Advancing osteolytic wedge, structurally weak bone, stress fracture of bowed extremity, compression fracture vertebra
Secondary osteoarthritis	Juxta-articular Paget's disease, change in joint congruity, altered gait dynamics
High-output cardiac state	Extensive skeletal involvement; i.e., over one third of the skeleton, serum alkaline phosphatase > 4 × upper normal
Malignancy	Sarcomatous degeneration of involved bone, metastatic malignant disease to pagetic bone
Dizziness/headache	Cause unknown, massive skull involvement platybasia (with occipital headache)
Hearing loss	Eighth nerve compression, otosclerosis, invasion of cochlea by pagetic bone
Change in mental status	Platybasia with compression of fourth ventricle
Paraparesis/paraplegia	Cord compression, "spinal artery steal syndrome"
Back pain	Altered gait dynamics, secondary osteoarthritis, active spinal Paget's disease, spinal stenosis, lateral recess syndrome
Hypercalcemia	Hyperparathyroidism, immobilization
Visual loss	Rupture of angioid streak of fundus, optic nerve entrapment

matic disease, an array of physical, medicinal, and surgical measures are often effective in controlling the disease. Death from Paget's disease is almost limited to the less than 1 per cent of patients who develop sarcomatous changes of the pagetic lesion.

Mechanical devices such as orthotics often correct symptoms related to bowed lower extremities or pelvic deformity. Often a heel lift, or occasionally a medial wedge, will suffice. Orthopedic procedures indicated for Paget's disease include osteotomy for tibial or femoral deformity, open or closed reduction for fracture, joint arthroplasty for secondary osteoarthritis, and spinal decompression for cord compression. Fractures or osteotomies may require intramedullary rods for stabilization. Since the fractured bone is often soft and tends to bow, the intramedullary rod is often left in place indefinitely for continued stabilization. Although fractures most often heal without event, occasional nonunions do occur. The fracture callus is often pagetic. During orthopedic surgery, pagetic bone may be hard and difficult to cut or may be soft and bleed excessively. Medicinal therapy prior to orthopedic surgery may reduce the excessive bleeding.

Anti-inflammatory Drugs

High-dose salicylates have been used for their analgesic and anti-inflammatory properties. In addition, they have been shown to retard collagen production and reduce hydroxyproline excretion in pagetic patients. Suppression of prostaglandin levels by indomethacin and other anti-inflammatory agents is felt to decrease skeletal vascularity and bone resorption. In many patients with Paget's disease, pain is related to secondary osteoarthritis. Symptoms related to osteoarthritis may be partly controlled by the use of anti-inflammatory agents.

Guidelines for Suppressive Therapy

Patients who require treatment have symptoms related to Paget's disease, demonstrate active disease by elevated serum alkaline phosphatase, and show radiographic evidence of Paget's disease at the symptomatic site.

There are no uniformly accepted guidelines for the treatment of Paget's disease. The author's indications for therapy are outlined in Table 2. Most would agree that pain related to Paget's disease and not due to another phenomenon such as secondary osteoarthritis is an indication for suppressive therapy.

One should be cautious in the therapy for lumbar spine involvement with Paget's disease. Although back pain is a common complaint in patients with Paget's disease, it is an uncommon

TABLE 2. Indications for Medicinal Therapy of Paget's Disease

	Calcitonin	Diphosphonates
Bone pain due to Paget's disease	+	+
Spinal Paget's disease with paraparesis/paraplegia	+	+
Preoperative orthopedic surgery	+	+
Immobilization hypercalcemia	+	−
Nonunion pagetic fracture	−	+
Osteolytic wedge of long bone on x-ray	+	?
Skull symptoms—headache, dizziness (not platybasia)	+	+
High-output cardiac failure	+	+
Prevent progression of disease (i.e., not correction of existing defect)	+	+
Hearing loss (Paget's disease of the petrous ridge)	+	+
Osteoarthritis (juxtaarticular Paget's disease)	+	+
Deformity (Paget's disease of long bones)	+	+
Asymptomatic increase in serum alkaline phosphatase without complications listed above	−	−

Key: + = useful; − = not indicated.

cause of symptoms. More often symptoms are due to an arthritic process resulting from the Paget's disease.

Paraparesis or paraplegia related to Paget's disease has often been reversed, at least in part, by medicinal therapy in poor surgical candidates for decompression. It is believed that this dramatic improvement is due to reversal of a "spinal artery steal" syndrome rather than alteration of bone from the spinal canal.

Pagetic bone has been described by orthopedic surgeons as structurally soft and highly vascular. Pretreatment with one of the suppressive agents appears to decrease the vascularity of the pagetic bone and may limit blood loss during orthopedic surgery. The treated bone is likely to heal more normally. Immobilization-induced hypercalcemia should be treated specifically with calcitonin.

Our experience with nonunion fractures has been favorable using diphosphonates. Nonunion pagetic fractures often heal shortly following high-dose diphosphonate therapy, although the reasons are not yet understood.

The long-bone osteolytic phase of Paget's disease may require high-quality x-rays for diagnosis. This complication is not common, occurring in about 10 per cent of x-rays in our series. Calcitonin consistently induces radiographic "healing" during therapy. However, withdrawal of calcitonin often is followed by rapid progression of disease, implying that therapy should not be discontinued. Disodium etidronate inconsistently will induce radiographic "healing" and is sometimes associated with progression.

A possible set of indications for suppressive therapy for Paget's disease are dependent upon the hypothesis that suppressive therapy will prevent additional complications of the pagetic process. It can be argued that suppressive therapy inhibits disease activity and that progressive abnormalities may at least in part be retarded or prevented. However, none of these therapies are expected to correct existing hearing loss, deformity, or osteoarthritis. Activity of disease should be followed by periodic testing of Paget's disease of bone, namely the serum alkaline phosphatase and, if possible, 24-hour urine total peptide hydroxyproline excretion.

Calcitonin Therapy. The first approved agent demonstrating dramatic effectiveness in the therapy for Paget's disease was the recently discovered hormone calcitonin. Calcitonin is a 32–amino acid hormone of the thyroid C cells. It has been demonstrated to lower plasma inorganic calcium concentration by action on bone and kidney. It inhibits osteoclastic bone resorption with loss of the ruffled resorption surface of osteoclasts within 1 hour, having some effect within 15 minutes. This effect is probably mediated by cyclic adenosine monophosphate (cAMP) accumulation and results in reduction in the number of osteoclasts. Even though there is no deficiency of calcitonin in Paget's disease, calcitonin has been demonstrated to suppress clinical and chemical disease. Antibodies to synthetic salmon calcitonin (Calcimar) have been demonstrated in patients receiving this agent. It is uncertain if resistance to synthetic salmon calcitonin is related to high titers of neutralizing antibodies. Reduction of symptoms with synthetic salmon or synthetic human calcitonin may occur by the end of the first month of therapy, sometimes occurring dramatically in the first few weeks. Calcitonins induce a more normal bony histologic picture, with more lamellar than woven bone.

Although considerable variation occurs, synthetic salmon calcitonin suppresses the chemical expressions of Paget's disease to about 50 per cent of pretreatment levels, with a slight loss of effect after 3 to 6 months. After 18 to 24 months chemical exacerbation often occurs. If calcitonin is discontinued, most patients will have chemical exacerbation within 6 months. Antibodies can occur without clinical resistance and are not present in all patients with resistance to salmon calcitonin. Synthetic human calcitonin (Cibacalcin) does not lose its suppressive chemical effect in most patients as long as the drug is being administered; however, the net chemical suppression of chemistries is usually somewhat less than might be expected with salmon calcitonin. Chemical relapse and clinical relapse do not necessarily coincide; indeed, most patients have a considerable delay in exacerbation of symptoms after withdrawal of calcitonin.

The usual dose of synthetic salmon calcitonin is 100 IU, 0.5 ml subcutaneously or intramuscularly daily, for the first month. The dose can be decreased or the interval between doses later increased depending on the severity of disease and response to therapy. Even though there is no histologic confirmation of benefit, the chemistries can be controlled on as little as 50 IU 3 times weekly in many patients. Salmon calcitonin should be kept cool. It is supplied as 400 IU per 2-ml vial.

Synthetic human calcitonin is supplied as 5 doses of 0.5 mg per box. Each dose is supplied with desiccated calcitonin and the diluent separated in a syringe. The patient breaks the seal between the diluent and the powder, mixes, reaspirates the solution, and injects. Similar to synthetic salmon calcitonin, the initial dose of synthetic human calcitonin is a single dose daily for the first month, with increases of the interval between doses depending on the clinical and chemical response.

The most important adverse reactions to the calcitonins are gastrointestinal symptoms (nausea, vomiting, diarrhea, abdominal pain, cramps), vascular symptoms (flushing of face, tingling of hands and feet), pain at the injection site, urinary frequency, rash, and occasional angioedema. Most symptoms occur within several minutes of injection and last about 1 hour. Hyperparathyroidism, believed to be secondary to calcitonin therapy, has been reported. Adverse reactions are most common during the initial period of therapy and tend to decrease or disappear with continued administration. Combined plicamycin and calcitonin have been proposed for severely afflicted patients. In the patient with uncomplicated Paget's disease, calcitonin therapy may be discontinued after 2 years. In the presence of a Paget's disease–induced lytic bony lesion, calcitonin probably should be continued indefinitely.

If resistance to salmon calcitonin is suspected, one can test for a calcitonin effect on serum calcium. Serum calcium is determined after an overnight fast. Serum calcium is determined 3 to 6 hours after synthetic salmon calcitonin (100 IU) is injected intramuscularly. Breakfast is allowed. If the calcitonin is effective, a decrease of 0.5 mg per dl or more in serum calcium is seen. A decrease of 0.3 mg per dl or less of serum calcium is evidence of calcitonin resistance.

Another calcitonin (eel calcitonin) is under investigation, as well as alternate methods of administration (synthetic salmon calcitonin by nasal spray).

Diphosphonates. Diphosphonates, or bisphosphonates, the newer approved suppressive agents for Paget's disease, are pyrophosphate analogues that replace the central oxygen of pyrophosphate with a carbon; they are resistant to pyrophosphatase activity. Serum alkaline phosphatase contains pyrophosphatase activity. Diphosphonates inhibit the precipitation of calcium phosphate, block the transformation of amorphous calcium phosphate to hydroxyapatite, and inhibit aggregation of calcium apatite crystals into clusters. In addition, they retard dissolution of calcium crystals, disaggregate apatite crystal clusters, peptidize crystals (transform crystals into a colloidal state), and form polynuclear complexes in the presence of calcium. Diphosphonates can inhibit both soft and hard tissue calcification and inhibit bone resorption.

At very high doses in animals, disodium etidronate (Didronel) was shown to inhibit vitamin D absorption from the gastrointestinal tract—a phenomenon not yet demonstrated in man. Diphosphonates have a direct effect on macrophage function. Osteoclasts appear to be macrophage-like cells with the same stem cell origin. Pagetic osteoclasts appear particularly sensitive to the diphosphonates.

Short- and long-term clinical and chemical suppression of Paget's disease was demonstrated in several studies utilizing disodium etidronate at doses of 5 mg per kg per day for periods of 6 months. Continuation of therapy beyond 6 months does not provide increased clinical or chemical effectiveness. Higher doses can be used for shorter periods of time but are not usually necessary in the initial course of therapy. Clinical improvement may occur after the first month of therapy but is often not apparent until 3 to 6 months, and occasionally not until after therapy has been discontinued. Between 15 and 40 per cent of patients receive prolonged clinical and chemical remission from disodium etidronate therapy. The duration of response may be related to the initial dose of medication but more likely correlates with the pretreatment level of hydroxyproline excretion and serum alkaline phosphatase. Generally the number of retreatments needed can be predicted by the height of the initial chemical values (i.e., the higher the initial chemical value, the more likely retreatment will

be needed). Retreatment, when used at a frequency of less than once yearly, is usually effective. Approximately 15 per cent of patients treated with disodium etidronate become refractory to the drug. Patients refractory to 5 mg per kg per day may respond to higher doses. If treatment with disodium etidronate is administered at high dosage or for prolonged periods of time, or if a course of therapy is required more than once a year, the patient is at risk to become refractory to the drug or to develop adverse reactions.

In the United States, there appear to be regional differences in the frequency of adverse reactions, such as bone pain. It is tempting to attribute these differences to climate (sun exposure—vitamin D) or hereditary factors.

The usual dose of disodium etidronate for Paget's disease is 5 mg per kg per day or 400 mg daily for a 45-kg (100-pound) to 80-kg (176-pound) patient. The drug is supplied as 200 mg and 400 mg tablets. The entire disodium etidronate dose should be administered at one time, midway between breakfast and lunch (or at bedtime) with either fruit juice or water. Disodium etidronate adheres to food and milk or dairy products, preventing absorption.

Adverse reactions to disodium etidronate include abdominal cramps and diarrhea, hyperphosphatemia, increasing bone pain, and a possible increase in fractures. Abdominal symptoms often subside by altering the dose or time of drug administration. Hyperphosphatemia appears to be due to a direct renal effect of disodium etidronate in humans that does not occur in animals. Hyperphosphatemia in humans is not related to changes in parathyroid, vitamin D, calcitonin, or calcium homeostasis.

Under investigation is intravenous administration of disodium etidronate* as well as other diphosphonates such as dichloromethylene diphosphonate ($MDCl_2$) and aminohydroxypropylidene diphosphonate (APD). Diphosphonates have been combined with calcitonin; this program seems of particular value in severely afflicted patients. There is clinical and laboratory evidence that, when used sequentially, disodium etidronate should be followed, rather than preceded, by calcitonin.

Plicamycin. The first agent that seemed to attack effectively the progression of Paget's disease was plicamycin (Mithracin). (This drug is not approved by the Food and Drug Administration for use in Paget's disease.) Plicamycin is a yellow

---

*The intravenous form of disodium etidronate, Didronel IV, manufactured by Norwich Eaton, has been approved by the FDA for use in hypercalcemia of malignancy.

crystalline antibiotic derived from the microorganism *Streptomyces plicatus*. It is an inhibitor of deoxyribonucleic acid (DNA)–directed ribonucleic acid (RNA) synthesis, probably by binding, but not DNA-altering. Intravenous administration of 25 micrograms per kg daily for 10 days results in clinical and chemical benefit in most patients. Smaller doses (10 to 15 micrograms per kg daily for 10 days) may give similar results. Prolonged remissions of disease may occur. Clinical response to plicamycin is often dramatic. In resistant patients, combination with other agents may be effective. Widespread use of plicamycin should be limited. Adverse reactions to this agent include hepatotoxicity, nephrotoxicity, hematotoxicity, and dermatologic reactions. It is often associated with hypocalcemia, nausea, and vomiting during administration. Many physicians reserve plicamycin for the most seriously afflicted patients, especially those who do not respond or become resistant to alternative therapies.

PARENTERAL NUTRITION IN ADULTS

method of
STEVEN B. HEYMSFIELD, M.D.,
ROBERT FERRARO, M.D., and
NICHOLAS H. E. MEZITIS, M.D.
*Columbia University College of Physicians and
    Surgeons*
New York, New York

Nutritional Assessment

Malnutrition is a nonspecific term that encompasses over 25 nutrient deficiency syndromes. The most common of these syndromes in hospitalized patients is protein-energy malnutrition (PEM). PEM is multicausal, involving reduced energy-protein intake, increased energy-nitrogen losses, or a combination of the two.

The core evaluation of patients suspected of or at risk of developing PEM includes a food intake and weight history and measurement of body weight and height (Table 1). A simple battery of directed questions can elucidate if and why food intake is inadequate. A more quantitative approach is to secure the services of a dietitian, who can perform a recall food history. The best method of estimating actual food intake is to request the dietitian to assist in a 48- to 72-hour in-hospital calorie count. The adequacy of intake can be established relative to Recommended Daily Allowance tables. In simple terms negative energy and nitrogen (N) balance ensues when caloric and N intake in the nonstressed patient falls below 30 to 35 kcal per kg and 0.5 to 1.0 gram per kg, respectively.

Body weight is expressed as a percentage change from pre-illness weight, as a percentage of desirable

TABLE 1. **Core Components of
Nutritional Assessment**

History
Appetite and recent food intake
Eating preferences and food aversions
Alterations in taste or smell
Physical disabilities that limit food ingestion
Food allergies and nutrient intolerance
Gastrointestinal disturbances
Potential drug-nutrient interactions

Physical Examination
Appearance
Weight (check for edema)
Height
Calculate: Percentage weight change
              Percentage desirable weight
              Body mass index

Ancillary Studies
Anthropometric measurements
Serum proteins
Selected mineral and vitamin levels

weight, and as body mass index (weight in kg divided by body surface area in M^2). A significant weight loss is considered a reduction in weight from the pre-illness value of 10 per cent. Desirable weight can be calculated from available tables adjusted for height or estimated at the bedside as: $100 + [5 \times (\text{height} - 60)]$ for females, and $106 + [6 \times (\text{height} - 60)]$ for males, where weight is in pounds and height is in inches. Weight less than 90 per cent of the desirable weight is considered subnormal. The body mass index in healthy lean adults ranges between 19 and 26 kg per M^2.

While inadequate food intake, weight loss, and underweight are the hallmarks of present or impending PEM, other ancillary studies should be considered. These include anthropometric measurements and serum proteins. The readily available serum albumin level, a classic marker of PEM, is correlated with outcome. Low levels (<2.5 grams per dl) generally signify a poor prognosis. Serum levels of transferrin, prealbumin, and retinol-binding protein, if available, can serve as markers of repletional adequacy; caution is warranted in their application owing to nonnutritional confounding factors. Anthropometric measurements, often performed by members of the nutrition support team, are useful in evaluating and monitoring patients receiving long-term nutritional therapy. Selected tests of mineral or vitamin nutriture are indicated when suspicions of a specific deficiency are aroused during the initial evaluation.

The patient's diet history, weight record, clinical examination, and ancillary tests are then used to establish if and to what extent PEM or other deficiencies will develop.

Indications for Parenteral Nutrition

Protein-energy malnutrition that is present or impending in the viable patient requires nutritional therapy. Parenteral feeding is reserved for patients whose food ingestion is inadequate for a maximum of 5 to 7 days and who will not tolerate gastrointestinal tube feeding at a rate sufficient to meet their requirements. Also included are patients for whom the enteral route is proscribed owing to surgical or other conditions. Parenteral nutrition support is administered via a peripheral vein in patients who require short-term (<10 to 14 days) maintenance feeding. Peripheral intravenous feeding can be combined with partial food or formula ingestion.

Access Routes

The hypertonic central formulas have an osmolality of 1800 mosm per liter and therefore require an inflow site that provides prompt mixing and distribution. In addition, the selected location should provide maximum convenience for the patient and easy access for dressing change. The venous access of choice is the superior vena cava, entered via either the subclavian or the internal jugular vein. These two sites, particularly the subclavian location, are comfortable, convenient, and associated with a low risk of infection and thrombosis. The cannulation should be performed using aseptic technique by a physician who regularly does this procedure. Catheter placement should be confirmed radiographically.

A variety of catheters are available for cannulating central veins. Single-lumen catheters are dedicated to the infusion of the nutrient formula and can remain in place for long periods. Multi-lumen catheters provide additional portals for the delivery of medications and blood component transfusions. The frequent manipulations associated with their use mandate a change of the catheter over a guidewire every 4 days and a change in access site after two replacements in an effort to prevent catheter-related infection. Catheters inserted through a subcutaneous tunnel (Hickman, Broviac) are less likely to be associated with infection and are thus suited for long-term outpatient parenteral support.

Infection, phlebitis, venous thrombosis, pneumothorax, chylothorax, and hemothorax are all complications of central vein catheterization. Infection is usually heralded by shaking chills, spiking temperatures, and glucose intolerance. Cultures of the formula, the catheter tip, and blood are indicated.

Peripheral veins will tolerate osmolalities of up to 900 mosm per liter. Large veins with good flow should be selected, and it is advisable to inspect and rotate the site at frequent intervals.

Delivery Systems

A stock glucose–amino acid mixture can be prepared in the pharmacy and stored for up to 2 weeks. The final mixture, including vitamins and trace elements, should be infused within 24 hours. The solution should be kept refrigerated prior to use. The maximum safe time for hanging the unrefrigerated mixture during use is 24 hours, and the formula should be discarded if the bottle is cracked, seals are broken, or cloudiness appears. A pump and filter system are recommended.

Lipids, which are not filtered, can be infused parallel to the dextrose—amino acid solution. Admixture systems are now available that allow the formulation of lipids, carbohydrate, protein, and other nutrients in a single container. While this approach is simple and convenient, the risks of infection, "oiling-out" (disruption of emulsion), and wastage are increased.

Peripheral infusions can be supplied with either a pump or a drip chamber.

Formulas

Although the central intravenous formula is theoretically complex to prescribe, most hospital pharmacies now offer several standard options that will satisfy the needs of most patients. The key decisions that must be made when ordering the parenteral formula include amount and distribution of calories, fluid volume, and electrolyte content.

Energy

The goal in most patients is maintenance of energy balance, although some severely malnourished individuals will require repletion. Maintenance of body weight and energy stores in the stable patient requires 25 to 35 kcal per kg. An improved estimate of requirements can be obtained by use of the Harris-Benedict equations to calculate resting metabolic rate for men,

$$66.0 + 13.7 \, \text{Wt} + 5 \, \text{Ht} - 6.8 \, \text{Age},$$

and for women

$$655 + 9.6 \, \text{Wt} + 1.7 \, \text{Ht} - 4.7 \, \text{Age},$$

where age, height, and weight are in years, centimeters, and kilograms, respectively. With injury, sepsis, and extensive burns, the resting requirements for energy are increased by approximately 30 per cent, 60 per cent, and 100 per cent, respectively. Some hospitals now have the facilities for measuring resting energy expenditure using indirect calorimetery.

The resting metabolic rate should be adjusted upward to account for energy expended in physical activities. The usual approach is to add 25 to 30 per cent extra calories above the resting level established for nonstressed, afebrile patients. The physical activity adjustment is not needed in paralyzed or ventilator-dependent patients.

Weight gain requires a formula infusion rate exceeding that for the calculated or measured maintenance requirement. An infusion set at 1.3 to 1.5 times the maintenance requirement will result in a reasonable and safe rate of weight gain.

The available energy sources include fat (9 kcal per gram), glucose monohydrate (3.4 kcal per gram), and amino acids (4 kcal per gram). Most dextrose–amino acid mixtures provide about 1.0 kcal per ml; and 10 per cent and 20 per cent lipid preparations are 1.1 and 2.0 kcal per ml, respectively. Recall that the amino acids in protein have a dual role, to supply energy to selected organs and tissues, and to preserve or replenish the body's functional protein mass.

Carbohydrate. The primary available carbohydrate is glucose monohydrate, which comes in concentrations that range between 5 and 70 per cent. Glucose is protein-sparing, which in healthy adults requires a minimum infusion rate of 1 mg per kg per minute. With increasing infusion rates glucose is progressively oxidized, supplying in the process high-energy intermediates and releasing carbon dioxide. Unoxidized glucose is stored as either glycogen or triglyceride. The synthesis of triglyceride from glucose, a process referred to as lipogenesis, results in a further release of carbon dioxide. The optimal glucose infusion rate is between 2 and 4 mg per kg per minute.

In the stressed state endogenous glucose production is increased, insulin responsiveness is lowered, and glucose clearance is reduced. The glucose infusion rate that maximally spares protein is higher in the stressed patient than in the stable hospitalized individual.

Three important complications and/or side effects of central venous infusions are in part attributable to glucose. First, there are reports of fatty liver appearing during large glucose infusions. Second, the relatively large release of carbon dioxide in the process of lipogenesis can have an adverse impact on respiratory status in susceptible patients. Both fatty liver and glucose-related hypercapnia are minimized by adjusting formula infusion rate so as to avoid positive energy balance and by reducing glucose by use of fat.

The third complication related to glucose infusion is glucose intolerance, manifested as hyperosmotic nonketotic coma or hyperglycemia. In addition to reducing formula infusion rate and glucose content, crystalline (regular) insulin can be added directly to the intravenous formula. The

amount to be added remains a clinical decision. It should be noted that roughly half the added quantity is made unavailable through adsorption to the container and the tubing, while the remainder remains stable for 24 hours at room temperature. The half-life of intravenous insulin is 40 minutes, and good glucose control is possible in most patients.

The amount of glucose that can be provided for parenteral nutrition ranges between 35 and 80 per cent of total calories, assuming a formula protein content of 10 to 15 per cent of calories. The precise amount provided depends upon the lipid prescription, which is discussed in the following section.

Glycerol (4.3 kcal per gram), which forms a stable solution when combined with amino acids and electrolytes, is used as the energy source in a commercially available peripheral formula.

Lipid. Intravenous fat sources are available that consist of 10 and 20 per cent soybean and/or safflower oil emulsions. The isotonicity and good endothelial tolerance of these preparations, combined with their high caloric density (1.1 and 2.0 kcal per ml) make them well suited for the central or peripheral intravenous feeding program.

Healthy adults require a minimum of 1 to 2 per cent of energy intake as the two essential fatty acids (EFA), linoleic and alpha-linolenic. EFA needs can be satisfied in the stable patient by infusing 500 ml of 10 per cent lipid emulsion two times per week. EFA deficiency, manifested by reduced growth, scaly skin, fatty liver, and coagulation abnormalities, requires treatment dosages above the normal requirement. The needs for EFA are also increased in the stressed or hypercatabolic patient.

Following an overnight fast, the normal adult can clear intravenous fat at a daily rate of 2.5 grams per kg. Prolonged fasting and the stress of injury increase the maximal clearance rate of lipid. The patient's lipid tolerance is checked by first confirming acceptable blood triglyceride levels (less than 400 to 500 mg per dl). The formula is next infused at a rate of 1 ml per minute for 15 to 30 minutes in order to identify an early adverse reaction. The lipid preparation is then infused at a rate of 50 ml per hour over 10 hours and the triglyceride level is measured again 4 to 6 hours after infusion; levels in the acceptable range indicate adequate intravenous fat clearance. The infusion should then be started at a rate of 500 ml per day as a 10 per cent solution and increased over 72 hours to a maximal daily rate of 2.5 gram per kg.

A consensus does not exist on how much lipid to provide the individual patient. Daily allowances may range from 2 mg per kg to 2 grams per kg, delivered either continuously or over an 8- to 10-hour period. The expense relative to dextrose and the potential complications should be balanced against the benefits: provision of a large isotonic caloric load in minimum volume, low carbon dioxide production, and reduction in insulin requirements. A conservative approach favors lipid infusion at a rate providing 30 per cent of total daily calories, in accordance with current dietary guidelines.

Protein

The crystalline L-amino acids provided in the intravenous solution are the building blocks of tissue protein. Of the 26 amino acids, 8 to 10 are essential or semi-essential, while the remainder are nonessential. The stable adult can balance nitrogen (N) losses in stool, skin, and urine by ingesting a minimum of 0.5 to 0.6 gram per kg of a high-biologic-value protein (e.g., egg albumin) in which essential amino acids are 18 to 20 per cent of total amino acids and energy is ingested in the ratio 250 to 300 kcal per gram N. Growing infants, recovering malnourished patients, and injured or stressed individuals require a relative increase in essential amino acids and a decrease in kcal per gram N.

Available solutions typically supply 40 to 48 per cent of amino acids in the essential form. The recommended ratio of kcal per gram N is 300:1 for stable patients and 100:1 to 150:1 for catabolic stressed and injured patients. The standard guidelines for protein requirements (grams N × 6.25) are 1 gram per kg (15 per cent of total kcal) and 1.2 to 1.5 grams per kg (20 per cent total of kcal) for stable and stressed patients, respectively.

Protein homeostasis is established at the simplest level by following body weight and monitoring serum albumin levels; if available, measurements of the shorter half-life serum proteins (e.g., retinol-binding protein, prealbumin) are useful but nonspecific. Finally, clinical N balance studies are used when uncertainty persists and the patient can provide an accurate urine collection.

Nitrogen balance (in grams per day) is estimated as formula N − (urinary urea N + 3.5). The coefficient 3.5 is an approximation of fecal, dermal, and nonurinary urea N losses. This N balance method assumes no major pathologic fecal or dermal N losses and no significant rise in total body urea N during the collection period. Results of −2 to +2 grams per day indicate approximate N equilibrium. More negative or positive values represent protein depletion or accretion, respectively.

Minerals and Trace Elements

The recommended daily parenteral requirements for sodium, potassium, magnesium, calcium, and phosphorus in patients with normal renal function are presented in Table 2. Appropriate adjustments of these values should be made in cases of renal and cardiac insufficiency as well as in conditions of increased loss. The need for rapid weight gain may necessitate supplementation of these elements beyond the level indicated in Table 2.

Commercial additives that contain zinc, copper, chromium, and manganese in amounts conforming to AMA and FDA guidelines are now available (Table 3). Although trace elements are usually not required during brief periods of nutritional support, it is now accepted practice to add them to the parenteral formulation on a daily basis. A dosage adjustment is usually required in patients with renal failure or biliary obstruction. Requirements for some elements may also be increased for patients in the catabolic state or those with large gastrointestinal fluid losses or diarrhea.

Iron deficiency can be corrected by adding iron dextran or citrate to the nutritional formula for infusion.

Selenium supplements should be considered in the catabolic or malabsorptive state. Deficiency in this element has been associated with cardiomyopathy.

Iodide and molybdenum supplements are not usually provided in patients receiving parenteral nutritional support.

Vitamins

The AMA-FDA recommendations for parenteral vitamin formulations are presented in Table

TABLE 2. **Proposed Intravenous Macromineral Requirements for Adults**

Ion	Requirement
Sodium	60 mEq or more
Potassium	60 mEq or more
Magnesium	12–20 mEq or more
Calcium	10–25 mEq
Phosphorous	450 mg or more

TABLE 3. **Suggested Intravenous Trace Element Requirements for Adults**

Element	Requirement
Zinc	2.5–4.0 mg
Copper	0.5–1.5 mg
Chromium	10–15 mg
Manganese	0.2–0.8 mg
Iron	0.5–2.0 mg
Selenium	120 μg
Iodine	50–120 μg

*See text for further comments.

TABLE 4. **Proposed AMA-FDA Intravenous Vitamin Requirements for Adults**

Vitamin	Requirement
Vitamin A	0.99 mg (3300 IU)
Vitamin C	400 mg
Vitamin D_2	5.0 μg (200 IU)
Vitamin E	10.0 mg (10 IU)
Vitamin K_1	0 mg
Thiamine (hydrochloride)	3.0 mg
Riboflavin (phosphate)	3.6 mg
Niacin (phosphate)	40.0 mg
Pyridoxine (hydrochloride)	4.0 mg
Pantothenate (dexpanthenol)	15.0 mg
Biotin	60.0 μg
Folic acid	400.0 μg
Cyanocobalamin (vitamin B_{12})	5.0 μg
Ascorbic acid	100.0 mg

4. Most commercial preparations meet these minimum daily requirements. One unit dose of the multivitamin preparation is added to the nutrient formula each day. Vitamin K (5 mg) should be added to the solution once each week or administered intramuscularly.

Special Considerations

Congestive Heart Failure

Fluid must be kept to a minimum. Sodium intake is limited to 50 mEq per day or less. Potassium is provided as needed based on serum concentration.

Hepatic Failure

Protein is restricted to 40 grams per day and conventional management (neomycin, lactulose) is initiated. Sodium and fluid are limited to 25 to 50 mEq per day and 1000 to 1500 ml, respectively. In encephalopathy refractory to the above measures, use of a nutrient formulation with a high branched-chain to aromatic amino acid ratio may be considered.

Respiratory Failure

The calorie allowance is limited to maintenance or less during nonmechanical ventilating periods, and lipid is infused in preference to dextrose.

Renal Failure

Protein is restricted to 0.5 to 0.6 gram per kg. Even less may be given if an essential amino acid–enriched formula is available. The protein allowance is increased to 1 gram per kg for patients on dialysis. Maintenance energy requirements are met, preferably with glucose. The electrolyte concentration and fluid volume are adjusted according to clinical and laboratory studies.

Monitoring

Vital signs, urine fractional concentrations, and fluid balance measurements are recorded every 6 to 8 hours. Body weight may be a more reliable indicator of fluid balance, and should be recorded daily. Serum levels of glucose, blood urea nitrogen, creatinine, electrolytes, albumin, and liver enzymes must be measured at least twice weekly.

Home Parenteral Nutrition

Technologic advances now permit managing the patient on chronic parenteral nutrition in the home setting. Nutrient solutions are prepared by commercial vendors and delivered to the patient's residence every 2 weeks on the average, where they are stored in a special refrigerator until used.

Vitamins and insulin are added to the individual formulation by the patient or a designated assistant on the day of use. Solutions are infused over a 12-hour period ("cycling"), usually at night, using an infusion pump and filter system similar to that employed in the hospital. Supplies are provided to maintain aseptic technique in connecting and disconnecting the nutrient solution. The patient and other persons responsible for providing parenteral fluids should master the necessary techniques in the hospital prior to discharge.

A physician experienced in parenteral nutrition should maintain a supervisory role and modify the formula as changes in laboratory studies and the clinical situation dictate. Home monitoring is usually performed by visiting nurses, who also ensure that samples for required laboratory studies are obtained and processed according to schedule.

The major complication in this setting is infection, and strict guidelines must be adhered to when symptoms even remotely related to infection are reported. Under proper care, patients may live a productive, gratifying life while being sustained with parenteral nutrition.

PARENTERAL FLUID THERAPY FOR INFANTS AND CHILDREN

method of
STANLEY HELLERSTEIN, M.D.
University of Missouri–Kansas City School of Medicine
Kansas City, Missouri

Fluid therapy may be approached by dividing water and electrolyte requirements into those needed for maintenance, for repair of the deficit, and for the replacement therapy of abnormal losses. Calculations of expenditures in each of these categories are based on the physiologic and pathologic processes involved, on clinical evaluation of the patient, and on estimation or measurement of losses (e.g., in nasogastric suction or stool losses). It should be recognized that these divisions are artificial. A patient's kidneys, skin, and respiratory tract do not differentiate molecules of maintenance water from those provided for replacement of abnormal losses or those given for deficit therapy. There is, however, a sound reason for using these divisions, since different bases of reference are needed for estimation of fluid requirements in each of the categories.

Maintenance fluid expenditures are a function of *metabolic rate*.

Deficit fluid requirements reflect losses *per kilogram of body weight*.

Replacement therapy is based on *measurement* or *estimation* of *continuing abnormal losses*.

These concepts serve as the basis for provision of fluids whether by the oral or the parenteral route.

Maintenance Water

Maintenance therapy, or "usual maintenance therapy," consists of the provision of water and electrolytes equivalent to that expended in the course of normal physiologic activities such as breathing, excreting wastes, and regulation of body temperature. These are continuous losses which must be met during sickness as well as health. Maintenance requirements are defined in terms of metabolic rate, since both insensible water loss, which amounts to about 45 ml per 100 kcal per 24 hours, and the renal water allowance, which is about 50 ml per 100 kcal per 24 hours, can be related to caloric expenditure. Table 1 shows data relating normal expenditures of water to the number of calories metabolized per 24 hours. If kidney function is not significantly impaired and the homeostatic mechanisms for

conservation and excretion of water are intact (no adrenal insufficiency, diabetes insipidus, or inappropriate secretion of ADH), the usual expenditures of water may be safely met with 100 to 150 ml of water for each 100 kcal metabolized.

The problem of providing a patient with appropriate quantities of maintenance water actually resolves itself into that of estimating metabolic rate under clinical conditions. The various "systems of fluid therapy" are essentially different ways of estimating metabolism. Water is given so that 100 to 150 ml is available for each 100 kcal metabolized (Table 1). Using the method developed by Holliday and Segar (Table 2), the number of calories metabolized per 24 hours may be estimated from body weight.

Modification of Maintenance Water Expenditures

It is frequently necessary to modify the quantity of fluid provided for maintenance water because of alterations in the "usual" rate of these expenditures. Maintenance fluid expenditures are based on estimates of water lost from the skin, from the lungs, and in stool and that needed for excretion of renal solute. Significant alterations in the rate of loss of water from the skin, from the lungs, or in stool necessitate modification in the maintenance water allowance. When kidney function is impaired or the homeostatic mechanisms for conservation and excretion of water are not intact, maintenance water requirements must be based on urine volume and other measurable expenditures and weight changes.

Insensible water loss results from the diffusion of water from the lungs and skin. The rate of loss depends upon the vapor tension in the environmental air, air movement, and respiratory rate and depth. Dry air, active air currents, and hyperventilation increase the rate of insensible water loss. High humidity decreases this expenditure.

Sweat, or the loss of visible water from the skin, seems to be present in some degree even in neutral environmental conditions. Metabolic studies and clinical experience have indicated that an allowance of 5 to 20 ml per 100 kcal is satisfactory in most instances. Sweat losses as

TABLE 1. **Usual Expenditure of Water Per 100 Kilocalories Metabolized**

		Water Expended (ml per 100 kcal)
Insensible		45
Lungs	15	
Skin	30	
Sensible (sweat)		5–20
Stool		5–10
Urine		30–80
	Total	100–150

Modified from Darrow DC, Pratt EL: JAMA *143*:365, 432, 1950.

TABLE 2. **Estimation of Maintenance Water Requirement**

Weight Range	Water Requirement
2.5–10 kg	100 ml/kg
10–20 kg	1000 ml + 50 ml/kg over 10 kg
≥20 kg	1500 ml + 20 ml/kg over 20 kg

Modified from Holliday MA, Segar WE: Pediatrics *19*:823, 1957.

100 ml of water provided for each 100 kcal metabolized.

TABLE 3. **Modifications of Usual Maintenance Water Estimates**

Clinical Situation	Effect on Metabolic Rate	Water Expenditure per 100 kcal			
		Insensible Water Loss		Sweat	Maintenance Water per 100 ml*
		Lungs	Skin		
No modifying features	None	15	30	10	100 ml
Neonate:					
1st day	50 kcal/kg	15	30	(?) 10	50 ml
2nd–6th day	75 kcal/kg	15	30	(?) 10	75 ml
7th day and after	100 kcal/kg	15	30	(?) 10	100 ml
Coma (↓ body temperature and activity)	↓ 10% per °C below 37° (R)	15	30	10	↓ 10 ml per °C below 37° (R)
Persistently ↑ temperature	↑ 10% per °C above 38° (R)	↑	↑	↑	↑ 10 ml per °C below 38° (R)
High humidity	None	(↓ 50%)	(↓ 20%)		(Expect ↑ volume of dilute urine)
(ambient temperature normal)		7	25	10	100 ml
Hyperventilation (afebrile)	Some ↑ due to exertion of breathing	↑ 25–40 or more	30	10	110–120 ml or more

*Estimated using method of Holliday MA, Segar WE: Pediatrics *19*:823, 1957.
(R) = rectal temperature.

large as 100 ml per kg per 24 hours have been recorded in infants in a warm, dry environment.

Stool losses tend to be small in the absence of diarrhea. Breast fed infants will usually lose about 10 ml of water per 100 kcal, while infants on cow's milk and older persons on an ordinary diet expend about 5 ml per 100 kcal. Stool losses of 40 to 60 ml per kg per 24 hours are not unusual in infants and children with commonly encountered viral or bacterial diarrhea. Stool losses may reach 100 ml or more per kg per day in secretory diarrheas such as those due to cholera or infections with enterotoxigenic *Escherichia coli*. Stool water losses are relatively easy to measure in infants and young children if disposable diapers are used for stool collection. The plastic outer surface of the diaper prevents loss of water, so the change in weight of the soiled diaper is a close measure of the water content of a diarrheal stool.

Renal excretion of water is the physiologic effector mechanism for regulation of the concentration of solute in body fluids. The volume of water needed to handle the renal solute load depends upon the size of the solute load and the concentration of solute in the urine:

$$\text{urine volume} = \frac{\text{renal solute load}}{\text{concentration}}$$

When water is provided with sufficient carbohydrate to minimize tissue breakdown, the endogenous solute load is 10 to 15 mOsm per 100 kcal metabolized. Maintenance electrolytes added to the glucose and water contribute about 10 mOsm per 100 kcal, bringing the solute load in the maintenance solution to 20 to 25 mOsm per 100 kcal. A solute load of 20 mOsm per 100 kcal could be excreted in 80 ml of water at a concentration of about 250 mOsm per liter or in 30 ml at a concentration of 666 mOsm per liter. The usual infant is able to vary the urinary solute concentration from 100 to about 700 mOsm per liter by the fifth day of life and after the first few months can excrete urinary solute at concentrations from about 75 to 1000 mOsm per liter. Assuming normal homeostatic regulatory mechanisms and intact renal function, the 20 to 25 mOsm of renal solute for each 100 kcal metabolized may be excreted in as little as 20 to 30 ml or urine or in 80 ml or more. By regulating the solute concentration of urine, renal mechanisms can compensate for usual variations in water intake and extrarenal water expenditures.

Table 3 shows some approximations that are useful for modification of maintenance water allowance in a clinical setting. Adjustments of fluid allowances should be made at appropriate time intervals (often 8 to 12 hours in the infant) based on careful monitoring of weight, clinical condition, and urine volume and concentration.

Maintenance Electrolytes

Maintenance electrolyte requirements are not as well defined as those for water. The aim is to supply slightly more than the minimal need, but cause no excess burden on the renal excretory mechanisms. The electrolyte concentration of usual fluid expenditures are shown in Table 4.

Maintenance water and electrolyte requirements may be met if solutions containing 20 to 30 mEq per liter of sodium, chloride, and potassium in 5 to 10 per cent carbohydrate are infused at a rate that provides maintenance water.

Parenteral Fluid Therapy

Pediatric patients requiring parenteral fluids usually have some degree of dehydration with or without a disturbance in body solute (sodium) concentration. The deficits in body water and solute must be replaced to permit restoration of normal body composition and function.

Volume of the Deficit

Clinical estimates of the severity of dehydration are at best crude. This is due, in part at least, to the fact that the clinical features of "dehydration" are really signs of extracellular volume depletion. The child with hyponatremic dehydration has a loss of sodium and chloride out of proportion to water. Since osmotic equilibrium is maintained in body fluids, there is a transfer of extracellular water into the cells. With a given decrease in total body water, the extracellular volume loss is more marked in a patient with hyponatremic dehydration than in one with isonatremic dehydration. Quite the opposite situation occurs with hypernatremic dehydration. The major water deficit is intracellular, so the extracellular volume tends to be supported and clinical signs of dehydration are minimal in spite of large losses of body water. The volume of the deficit may be taken as 100 ml per kg or greater in the pediatric patient with a serum sodium concentration over 150 mEq per liter even though physical examination does not suggest severe dehydration. (Hypernatremia occasionally indicates salt excess rather than water deficit. In these instances un-

usual fluid losses have not occurred and there is a history of ingestion of excess salt.)

Table 5 shows a clinically useful system for estimation of the size of the water deficit in patients with isonatremic dehydration. The clinician's skill in estimation of degrees of dehydration may be sharpened by following the changes in body weight during rehydration. In the absence of a surgical procedure, loss or gain in body weight in excess of about 0.5 per cent per day probably reflects changes in body water.

Composition of the Deficit

An estimate should be made of the extracellular and intracellular electrolyte losses (sodium, chloride, and potassium) to permit rational restoration of fluid and electrolytes. The composition of the replacement fluid should reflect the losses in major body electrolytes. Table 6, which is derived from recovery balance studies on dehydrated infants, shows that the tonicity of body fluids, as reflected by serum sodium concentration, may serve as an index of the magnitude of the electrolyte deficits in dehydrated pediatric patients.

Management of Dehydrated Patients

Management of patients who are significantly dehydrated usually consists of two phases, *initial hydration* and *deficit plus maintenance therapy*. Initial hydration is necessary for the patient with a significant reduction in extracellular volume. The mildly to moderately dehydrated patient with a satisfactory blood pressure, good tissue perfusion, and adequate urine output does not require rapid expansion of the extracellular volume. Therapy for the latter patient consists of deficit plus maintenance fluids mixed together and infused over a 24-hour period.

Initial Hydration

There should be minimal delay in starting an intravenous infusion in a severely dehydrated patient. Frequently it is necessary to select the solution for initial expansion of the extracellular volume without knowing the results of the initial laboratory studies. The key information needed

TABLE 4. **Electrolyte Concentrations in Usual Fluid Expenditures**

Fluid	Electrolytes (mEq/L)			Water per 100 kcal (ml)
	Na	*K*	*Cl*	
Insensible				45
Skin	0	0	0	
Lungs	0	0	0	
Sweat (variable)	10–30	5–15	10–30	5–20
Urine (variable)	0–much	5–much	0–much	30–80
Stool	20–25	50–60	15–30	5

Usual expenditures are met using 2–3 mEq of Na, Cl, and K per 100 ml of maintenance water.

TABLE 5. **Estimation of Size of Fluid Deficit**

Severity of Dehydration	Percentage of Body Weight Lost	Volume of Deficit (ml/kg)
Mild	3–5	30–50
Moderate	5–9	50–90
Severe	10 or more	100 or more

These estimates refer to patients with isonatremic dehydration.

TABLE 6. **Probable Deficits of Water and Electrolytes in Severe Dehydration**

Condition*	Water (ml/kg)	Na⁺	K⁺	Cl⁻
			(mEq/kg)	
Diarrheal dehydration				
Hyponatremic				
[Na] <130 mEq/L	20–100(?)	10–15	8–15	10–12
Isonatremic				
[Na] 130–150 mEq/L	100–120	8–10	8–10	8–10
Hypernatremic				
[Na] >150 mEq/L	100–120	2–4	0–6	0–3
Hypertrophic pyloric stenosis	100–120	8–10	10–12	10–12

*[Na] refers to the serum or plasma Na⁺ concentration.

in selecting an initial hydrating solution relates to the tonicity of the patient's body fluids, since rapid infusion of a moderately hypotonic solution (Na <75 mEq per liter) in the patient with hyponatremic body fluids may induce water intoxication. Unfortunately, neither history nor physical examination is a reliable indicator of the tonicity of body fluids, so the initial hydrating solution selected should be satisfactory for rapid expansion of the extracellular volume regardless of the initial tonicity of the patient's body fluids. Table 7 shows solutions that we have found satisfactory for initial hydration of dehydrated pediatric patients.

An infusion rate of 30 to 40 ml per kg per hour is suitable for most infants weighing up to about 15 kg. An infusion rate of 500 to 600 ml per hour may be used for initial hydration of patients weighing 15 to 25 kg, and a rate of 20 to 25 ml per kg per hour for those weighing more than 25 kg. Slower rates of infusion should be employed

TABLE 7. **Initial Hydrating Solutions**

	Na⁺	K⁺	Cl⁻	HCO₃⁻	Glucose (grams)
		mEq			
Dehydration with acidosis (nondiabetic)					
1000 ml ½ isotonic NaCl in 5% glucose	77	0	77	0	50
25 ml 1M NaHCO₃	25	0	0	25	0
Approximate concentration per liter	100	0	75	25	50
Dehydration with alkalosis					
1000 ml ½ isotonic NaCl in 5% glucose	77	0	77	0	50
25 ml in 1M NaCl	25	0	25	0	0
Approximate concentration per liter	100	0	100	0	50
Diabetic ketoacidosis					
1000 ml ½ isotonic NaCl in H₂O	77	0	77	0	0
25 ml 1M NaHCO₃	25	0	0	25	0
Approximate concentration per liter	100	0	75	25	0

for dehydrated children with impaired cardiac function, those with elevated blood pressure or diseases commonly complicated by elevated blood pressure (e.g., acute glomerulonephritis), and patients who may have or may be at risk for increased intracranial pressure (e.g., those with meningitis or encephalitis).

Deficit Therapy

Deficit therapy consists in provision of both deficit and maintenance fluids, and is instituted initially in the patient who does not require volume expansion and in the more severely dehydrated patient once he or she is out of shock and excreting reasonable volumes of urine. The fluids administered should provide water and electrolytes to correct the existing deficits, to meet the usual maintenance requirements, and to cover continuing abnormal losses. The solution for maintenance plus deficit therapy is arrived at by adding together the fluids needed to meet maintenance expenditures plus those to repair the deficit. Table 8 shows maintenance plus deficit solutions suitable for pediatric patients with hyponatremic, isonatremic, and hypernatremic dehydration.

As a general rule, the volume of fluid for replacement of a deficit should not exceed 10 per cent of body weight, or 100 ml per kg, in a single 24-hour period. Children with hypernatremic dehydration are a special problem. The volume of the deficit may be taken as 100 ml per kg or greater in the pediatric patient with a serum sodium concentration over 150 mEq per liter even though physical examination does not suggest severe dehydration. The major water deficit is intracellular, so the extracellular volume tends to be supported and clinical signs of dehydration are minimal in spite of large losses of body water. These children are at risk for seizures with rapid reduction of body fluid tonicity, so the rule is to limit the fluid for deficit repair to 50 ml per kg per 24 hours.

The volume of the solution infused during the period of repair of the deficit is derived by adding

TABLE 8. **Solutions Providing Maintenance Plus Deficit Fluid**

Type of Dehydration	H_2O (ml)	Na$^+$	K$^+$	Cl$^-$	Ac	PO$_4$ (mM)	Glucose (grams)
				mEq			
Hyponatremic: [Na] <130 mEq/L							
900 ml 5% glucose in H_2O	900						45
80 mM NaCl	80	80		80			
20 mM KAc	10		38		20	12	
4 mM K phosphate*	4						
10 ml Ca gluconate (10%)	10						
Approximate concentration per liter		80	38	80	20	12	45
Isonatremic: [Na] 130–150 mEq/L							
900 ml 5% glucose in H_2O	900						45
55 mM NaCl	55	55		55			
20 mM KAc	10		38		20	12	
4 mM K phosphate	4						
10 ml Ca gluconate (10%)	10						
Approximate concentration per liter		55	38	55	20	12	45
Hypernatremic: [Na] >150 mEq/L							
950 ml 5% glucose in H_2O	950						45
25 mM NaCl	25	25		25			
20 mM KAc	10		38		20	12	
4 mM K phosphate	4						
10 ml Ca gluconate (10%)	10						
Approximate concentration per liter		25	38	25	20	12	45

*Potassium phosphate: contains a mixture of KH_2PO_4 and K_2HPO_4: K = 4.4 mEq/ml and PO_4 = 3 mM/ml.

the maintenance fluid (Table 2) plus the deficit fluid (Table 8) and infusing this volume over a 24-hour period. For example, an 8-kg infant with severe isonatremic dehydration is re-evaluated following initial rehydration. Circulation has improved and 12 ml of urine has been passed. The patient is appraised as severely dehydrated, but not in shock.

Maintenance fluid: 100 ml per kg =   800 ml
Deficit fluid: 100 ml per kg =   800 ml
      Total 24-hour requirement = 1600 ml

Using the solution providing maintenance plus deficit fluid for a patient with isonatremic dehydration, the rate of infusion would be 67 ml per hour (1600/24 = 67).

A 4-kg infant with severe hypernatremic dehydration is irritable, but has good circulation and a wet diaper. Initial hydration is not needed. Although a fluid deficit of at least 100 ml per kg is present, only 50 ml per kg of deficit will be replaced in a single 24-hour period.

Maintenance fluid: 400 ml per kg
Deficit fluid: 200 ml per kg
Total 24-hour requirement = 600 ml

Using the solution providing maintenance plus

deficit fluid for a patient with hypernatremic dehydration, the rate of infusion would be 25 ml per hour (600/24 = 25).

A 16-kg child with mild to moderate hyponatremic dehydration is unable to tolerate oral fluids. The deficit is estimated as 50 ml per kg.

Maintenance fluid: 1300 ml
Deficit fluid: 800 ml
Total 24-hour requirement = 2100 ml

Using the solution providing maintenance plus deficit fluid for hyponatremic dehydration, the

TABLE 9. **Composition of Fluids for Replacement of Abnormal Losses**

Type of Fluid Loss	Na$^+$	K$^+$	Cl$^-$	*HCO$_3^-$
		mEq		
Sweating				
Normal person	60–75	20–30	50–75	20–25
Cystic fibrosis	100–130	20–30	75–100	20–25
Gastric	75–100	30–40	100–140	0
Small intestinal	100–140	20–30	75–110	20–40
Diarrheal	40–60	30–40	40–60	30–40

*Actual bicarbonate or its metabolic equivalent such as lactate or acetate.

Note that these fluids for replacement of an ongoing abnormal expenditure are not identical in composition with the fluid actually lost. Gastric juice, for example, approaches an isotonic solution of HCl in composition at high rates of secretion.

rate of infusion would be 88 ml per hour (2100/24 = 88).

Replacement Therapy

The replacement of ongoing abnormal losses should be done on a volume-for-volume basis using a fluid similar in composition to that being lost (Table 9). The rate at which an abnormal loss is replaced depends on the rate at which fluid is being lost and the size of the patient. In the small infant even modest abnormal losses should be replaced each 2 to 4 hours. In the larger patient abnormal fluid expenditures may be replaced each 4 to 8 hours, but in all instances large ongoing fluid losses should be replaced promptly enough to avoid the pathophysiologic effects of depletions.

Close monitoring of the patient's clinical status, urine output, and weight is essential for good management. Measurements of serum electrolyte, urea nitrogen, and creatinine concentrations, and at times pH and P_{CO_2}, may be needed for adequate assessment. It is not uncommon to reintroduce oral feedings in pediatric patients with diarrheal dehydration after 24 hours of parenteral rehydration. Regardless of the indication for continued parenteral fluid therapy, if nutritional requirements are not being met after 24 to 48 hours, total or partial parenteral nutrition should be part of the regimen.

Section 8

The Endocrine System

ACROMEGALY

method of
JOHN A. LINFOOT, M.D.
Providence Hospital
Oakland, California

Acromegaly is an uncommon endocrinopathy resulting from the hypersecretion of growth hormone (GH). The prevalence of acromegaly is estimated at five to six cases per 100,000 population, with an estimated yearly incidence of three to four cases per year. It is the second most common cause of pituitary hyperfunction. Excessive growth hormone secretion originates (1) usually from an adenoma of somatotropic cells of the anterior lobe of the pituitary; (2) occasionally from hyperplasia of pituitary somatotropic cells from stimulation by growth hormone–releasing hormone (GHRH) by nonpituitary tumors; and (3) rarely from ectopic nonpituitary tumors producing growth hormone. Excessive growth hormone secretion, occurring prior to puberty when linear growth can occur, results in gigantism. The term acromegaly describes the bony and soft tissue overgrowth of the acral segments such as hands, feet, nose, chin, and forehead. Acral changes tend to be less conspicuous in children suffering from gigantism. The clinical manifestations result from several major causes: (1) excessive growth hormone secretion, (2) deficiencies of other pituitary tropic hormones, and (3) local invasion of parasellar, neural, vascular, and bony structures.

Evaluation

Growth hormone has multiple effects on most tissues. Some of the actions of growth hormone are direct and other indirect through the generation of somatomedin (SM). Somatomedins are proinsulin-like peptides that are synthesized and released by a variety of tissues in response to growth hormone and act either as local growth factors (paracrine) and/or as systemic growth factors (endocrine) in concert with growth hormone. Insulin-like growth factor I (IGF-I) or somatomedin C (SM-C) is the major somatomedin in man. Elevated levels of GH hormone and SM-C can be used to diagnose and to monitor the treatment of patients with acromegaly and gigantism.

An understanding of the pathophysiology of growth hormone secretion is important in the selection and implementation of treatment of this disease. The regulation of GH level at the pituitary level is by dual control of growth hormone–releasing hormone (GHRH), which is the stimulatory factor, and somatostatin (SRIH), which is the inhibitory factor. The neurophysiologic pathways for stimulation and inhibition of GH are important to understand, since a variety of tests (e.g., the paradoxical rise of GH following thyroid-releasing hormone [TRH]) and medical treatments (e.g., dopamine agonists) are based on this new data. In addition, a number of pathophysiologic states have elevated GH levels without acromegaly or gigantism.

The classification of pituitary adenomas based on tinctorial staining affinities of cell cytoplasm has no value because it does not take into consideration hormone production or cytogenesis and fails to correlate structural features and the endocrine activity. It has been shown conclusively that the substantial majority of the chromophobic adenomas produce one or more hormones, such as growth hormone prolactin, adrenocorticotropic hormone (ACTH), thyroid-stimulating hormone (TSH), follicle-stimulating hormone (FSH), luteinizing hormone (LH), and/or the alpha subunit of these glycoproteins. Acidophilic adenomas have been linked to acromegaly and gigantism; however, using modern morphomimetric classifications there are at least six different cell types that are associated with growth hormone hypersecretion. Thus acidophilic adenomas may discharge hormones other than growth hormones, may synthesize prolactin or TSH, and may be hormonally nonfunctioning tumors.

The role of the hypothalamus in the pathogenesis of acromegaly remains controversial. The majority of patients with pituitary adenomas are successfully treated by tumor removal, and the incidence of relapse has been less than expected if persistent hypothalamic stimulation were the cause of tumor development. Twenty to 40 per cent of acromegalic patients secrete both GH and prolactin (PRL), and in most acromegalic patients there is a parallel release of GH and PRL in response to GRH regardless of whether there was basal hyperprolactinemia. A stimulation of both growth hormone and prolactin by GHRH may explain the development of bihormonal tumors. An explanation for the abnormal responses to hypothalamic and other physiologic stimuli in patients with acromegaly may be that somatotropic tumors, like many other endocrine tumors, remain partially responsive to normal stimuli and may show aberrant responses to a variety of secretagogues, such as TRH, GHRH, dopamine, and glucose.

Acromegaly and gigantism in families is rare, although other endocrine neoplasms occur in acromegaly. Hyperparathyroidism is the most common associated endocrinopathy. Hyperthyroidism (TSH-mediated) and galactorrhea-amenorrhea syndrome also occur. These endocrinopathic associations should be distinguished from multiple endocrine neoplasia (MEN) syndromes. MEN type I is a syndrome characterized by multiple endocrine tumors involving the parathyroid, pituitary, pancreatic islets, and adrenal cortex. MEN type I is an uncommon syndrome in my series of over 400 patients with acromegaly. MEN type II, or Sipple's syndrome (medullary thyroid carcinoma, hyperparathyroidism, pheochromocytoma), is not associated with acromegaly or gigantism.

Acromegaly and gigantism are associated with a variety of complications. Important systemic manifestations include swelling and disfigurement of the extremities, face, and skull; glucose intolerance; diabetes; hypertension; nerve entrapment; severe arthropathy; and cardiac disease. Because of the delay in diagnosis (averaging approximately 10 years in our series) these tumors tend to be larger and more invasive than other pituitary tumors. Invasiveness may result in extraocular motor nerve palsies, parasellar vascular displacement or invasion, bony erosion, and hypopituitarism. The morbidity of the disease is substantial and the mortality increased. It has been emphasized in one series that 50 per cent of 100 patients died before the age of 50 years and that 89 per cent died before the age of 69. The leading cause of death is cardiovascular disease.

Surgical Management

The transsphenoidal approach to pituitary tumors was resurrected in the 1960s primarily because of Gerard Guiot, a French neurosurgeon who had trained with Norman Dott of Edinburgh. Dott had continued to use Harvey Cushing's transsphenoidal approach and taught it to Guiot, who in turn taught the technique to Jules Hardy of Montreal while he was studying in France. Hardy introduced the operating microscope, intraoperative fluoroscopy, and the concept of selective pituitary adenectomy. Since this time, many surgeons have performed these techniques, capitalizing on the advances in endocrinology and neuroradiology that complement the management of these patients. The reduced morbidity and low mortality rates existing with this procedure make this a treatment of choice. Tumor tissue can be exposed and surgically separated from the normal pituitary gland. Pressure on adjacent tissues is promptly relieved, and within

TABLE 1. **Therapeutic Goals in the Treatment of Acromegaly**

1. Permanent control of tumor growth
2. Permanent normalization of hormone hypersecretion
3. Minimal tropic hormonal side effects
4. Minimal CNS side effects
5. Minimal surgical and/or anesthetic morbidity and mortality

TABLE 2. **Treatment of Acromegaly**

A. Surgical treatment
  1. Transfrontal craniotomy
  2. Transsphenoidal microsurgery
B. Radiotherapy
  1. Photon radiation or "conventional radiation," high voltage x-ray, 60 CO, and linear accelerator
  2. Heavy particle (Cyclotron), alpha particle (Berkeley) proton beam, Bragg peak (Boston)
  3. Stereotaxic radiosurgery (Stockholm)
C. Pharmacologic treatment
  1. Bromocriptine
  2. Sandostatin
D. Combined therapy
  1. Radiation and pharmacologic treatment
  2. Multiple surgeries
  3. Surgery plus irradiation
    a. Heavy particle
    b. Photon
  4. Surgery and pharmacologic treatment

minutes blood levels of growth hormone drop to normal range. However, total effectiveness of the operation is limited by the tumor size and any extension into the surrounding intrasellar and parasellar structures. Use of an anatomic classification suggested by Hardy and modified by others is essential in predicting the outcome of treatment. Microadenomas measuring 10 ml or less in diameter (Grade I tumors) and larger enclosed noninvasive (Grade II tumors) without parasellar or suprasellar extension can be treated with high degrees of success by an experienced neurosurgeon. The incidence of hypopituitarism is generally low. Larger invasive tumors (Grade III and IV) are associated with lesser degrees of success and, in terms of complete resection, correction of biochemical abnormalities and complications. Cure or remission rates range from 78 to 97 per cent for microadenomas, less than 10 ml in diameter and from 33 to 90 per cent for larger tumors or macroadenomas. Surgical success rates, thus, will vary depending upon the size, location, type of extension, invasiveness, and resectability of tumors as well as the skill and experience of the neurosurgeon.

Basal GH levels of less than 10 ng per ml and more recently 5 ng per ml have been traditionally regarded as evidence of therapeutic success. However, neither is evidence of a cure. The cutoff value of normalcy of GH has decreased over the years and differs among reported series, thus making comparisons difficult. The majority of treated patients fail to exhibit normal growth hormone regulation when basal GH levels are above 2 ng per ml. Thus, it would appear that the majority of patients are controlled rather than cured. Follow-up examinations of evidence for regression of acromegaly and the development of hypopituitarism is indicated in all patients.

Normalization of SM-C levels usually does not occur unless the GH levels are well below 2 ng per ml. In my experience, the SM-C levels may be misleading unless they are performed in extremely experienced research or reference laboratories.

Complications of surgery include hypopituitarism (in 5 to 15 per cent), cerebrospinal rhinorrhea (in 1 to 5 per cent), meningitis (in 0.5 to 2.5 per cent), and permanent diabetes insipidus (0.5 to 1 per cent). About half of the patients will develop transient diabetes insipidus postoperatively. Other complications from a transsphenoidal approach are uncommon. The mortality rate is low (less than 1 per cent). Serious complications include (1) hemorrhage or damage to the hypothalamus or other intracranial structures; (2) carotid arterial laceration, thrombosis, or spasm with resulting hemorrhage, embolism, or stroke; (3) optic nerve injury resulting in blindness, and (4) cranial nerve injury in the cavernous sinus resulting in diplopia. Cerebrospinal rhinorrhea with or without meningitis may require reoperation for repair. Nasal injury (perforation, deformity, or infection), dental disturbance, and/or numbness of the upper lip may occur but usually represent minor complications.

Transcranial pituitary surgery is now limited to large tumors with extensive suprasellar or parasellar extension. The advantage of the craniotomy approach is that it affords the surgeon a complete view of the large pituitary tumor. The optic nerves and optic chiasm can be directly visualized and any extension of the pituitary tumor into the anterior or middle flossa behind the anterior clinoids along the clivus can be visualized. Extensions into the third ventricle producing obstructive hydrocephalus can also be managed by this route. Lesions that mimic pituitary tumors, such as craniopharyngioma and meningiomas and aneurysm, will also require the craniotomy approach for effective surgical management.

Other indications for the surgical management of patients with acromegaly include pituitary apoplexy, evidence of progressive mass effect, either optic chiasmal or extraocular palsies, and finally failure of prior therapy in patients treated with radiation or medical treatment or a previous surgical procedure.

Patients treated for either transsphenoidal or transcranial surgery require an adrenal steroid coverage preoperatively, operatively, and postoperatively, even in the event of normal preoperative endocrine evaluation. High-dose steroid support is best given until the patient is up and about and has normal urinary output; at that point it can be rapidly tapered over a 3- to 4-week period (see management of adrenal insufficiency). Vasopressin can be used in the same fashion (see management of diabetes insipidus). In pituitary-deficient patients, protective doses of steroids are given until the patient has recovered from the immediate stress of surgery, and then standard pituitary replacement cortisol and thyroid is instituted as indicated. Postoperatively, patients should be evaluated with base-line pituitary hormone functional assessment, which would include testosterone or estradiol measurements, and an evaluation with fourth generation computed tomographic (CT) or magnetic resonance imaging (MRI) scans (using 1 to 3 mm per slice) should be performed after surgery to confirm the presence of any unsuspected hormone deficiencies or residual tumor.

TABLE 3. **Complications of Treatment for Acromegaly**

A. Surgery
  1. Anesthesia and surgical events
  2. Hemorrhage
  3. CSF leak
  4. Meningitis
  5. Diabetes insipidus
  6. Hypopituitarism
  7. Cranial nerve damage
  8. Empty sella syndrome
B. Radiotherapy
  1. Epilation (photon therapy only)
  2. Postirradiation necrosis
    a. Extraocular motor nerve impairment
    b. Optic chiasm
    c. Temporal lobe impairment
    d. Empty sella syndrome
    e. Hypopituitarism
C. Pharmacologic treatment
  1. Variable and often incomplete human growth hormone suppression
  2. Failure to have a consistent and clear-cut effect on tumor growth
  3. Rapid rise of human growth hormone to pretreatment levels after discontinuation of medication
  4. Drug reaction

Radiotherapy

Pituitary irradiation can be achieved by external or teletherapy delivery or by implantation of radioactive sources. The latter has been employed successfully at a few centers in the United Kingdom and in Europe but has never been popular in this country because it combines the complications of both surgery and irradiation. External irradiation can be given as either conventional photon (x-ray or gamma ray) therapy or as heavy particle (alpha particles or protons). Particle therapy was originally developed in California at Berkeley Cyclotron in the late 1950s, and later

TABLE 4. **Desired End Points of Treatment of Acromegaly**

A. Physical findings
  1. Cessation of acral growth
  2. Cessation of hyperhidrosis and skin tag (fibroma) formation
  3. Soft tissue regression
  4. Improvement in fatigue and lethargy
  5. Stable visual fields and neuroophthalmologic examination
B. Radiographic findings
  1. Lack of recurrence as documented by CT or MRI scans
  2. Remineralization of sella
  3. Remineralization of metacarpal medullary space
  4. Stabilization or variable regression of heel pad and other soft tissue thickening
C. Metabolic
  1. Improvement in diabetic state and/or glucose tolerance
  2. Loss of insulin resistance
  3. Fall in elevated serum phosphorus levels
D. Growth hormone
  1. Fasting human growth hormone levels less than 5 ng per ml, preferably less than 2 ng per ml
  2. Absent paradoxic rise to thyroid-releasing hormone and other pharmacologic stimulation
  3. Partial return of suppressibility to glucose stimulation
  4. Normal serum somatomedin levels

proton beam therapy was introduced at the Massachusetts General Hospital.

Prior to the 1960s, radiation therapy alone, often without biopsy, was frequently used for the management of pituitary tumors. In our early studies with the GH radioimmunoassay, we found that many patients who were treated years previously with photon therapy had elevated growth hormone levels. In studying our own patients who had received alpha-particle pituitary radiation, we found elevated levels in recently treated patients and discovered that several years were required before the normal levels were achieved. Later, we observed that the response to treatment was more rapid in the smaller tumors or microadenomas than in the larger tumors. Similar results have been observed with photon therapy and with proton beam therapy. Currently, photon therapy is largely used as an adjunctive therapy to surgery and is reserved for patients who have had incomplete tumor removal or persistent elevated growth hormone postoperatively. Occasionally, it is used as the sole therapy in patients who are not surgical candidates. Currently, photon therapy appears to control tumors with reasonable effectiveness in many cases of acromegaly. Only a little more than one third of patients will have growth hormone levels lower than 10 ng per ml by 2 years, but by 5 years three fourths of the patients will have growth hormone levels less than 10 ng per dl. Patients who have had prior transsphenoidal or transcranial surgical procedures will have slower responses to treatment but will ultimately achieve growth hormone levels less than 10 ng per dl. The coexistence of pleural hormone secretion does not clearly influence the effect of control in acromegaly, although some investigators have reported a better response in patients with both elevated GH and PRL. My own experience cannot confirm this. In patients treated with alpha-particle therapy, the complications of radiotherapy were infrequent. The response to treatment is more rapid, and the incidence of hypopituitarism is less than with conventional irradiation. The alpha-particle pituitary irradiation program at Berkeley was discontinued in 1981; proton-beam therapy is available in Boston.

Parasellar radionecrosis is determined by the type and size of the radiation field, total days of therapy, and dose delivered per fraction. During the mid 1960s and early 1970s there was a trend toward increasing the total dose and the rate per fraction with the idea that therapy could be improved. With doses of 50 to 60 gray (Gy) (1 Gy = 100 rad), the effect on tumor growth and hypersecretion was apparently improved; however, there was a slight but significant increase in complications from radiation. Minor complications of photon therapy include epilation of the scalp and occasionally mild headache; acute tumor swelling due to infarction and hemorrhage into a tumor rarely occurs. Epilation is much less common with the new linear accelerators.

In the past few years there has been a trend to reduce the total radiation dose as well as the dose per fraction, and as a result complications have been infrequent. Delayed complications of radiation therapy include a postponed or incomplete fall in GH, hypopituitarism, optic nerve and brain necrosis, and carcinogenesis. The incidence of optic nerve damage seems to be higher in patients with acromegaly than in other types of pituitary tumors. This may be related to the invasiveness of the lesions or the associated vascular disease. Radionecrosis described with alpha-particle and proton beam tends to be more localized because of the focal and precise localization of these beams.

Medical Management

There are only two pharmacologic treatments that have been used with any degree of success, namely bromocriptine (Parlodel) and somatostatin. Typically, the ergot derivatives produce an increase in GH secretion; however, patients with acromegaly demonstrate a paradoxical response, and GH levels fall when most ergot drugs are administered. Currently, the only approved ergot derivative for acromegaly is bromocriptine, a long-acting dopamine agonist. Since the effect of a single dose lasts 6 to 8 hours, daily treatment with 2 to 4 divided doses is usually required. Treatment is best initiated with 1.25 mg, with a gradual increase over several weeks. The total dose normally ranges between 7.5 and a maximum of 30 mg per day. Responses to bromocriptine can be predicted if a 55 per cent or higher fall in a basal GH level occurs after a single 2.5 mg oral dose. While such a trial test is not always essential, the administration of the initial dose under observation avoids annoying side effects, which often accompany the first dose of medication. Bromocriptine rarely normalizes growth hormone, but at least a 50 per cent lowering of growth hormone is seen in the majority of patients. Interestingly the symptoms of acromegaly have improved without complete normalization of GH levels. A similar finding is observed following irradiation therapy. Side effects include postural hypotension, blanching of the fingers, and mild constipation. Intolerance to bromocriptine and rapid return to pretreatment levels occur upon discontinuation of the medication.

Bromocriptine has been demonstrated to reduce GH effectively in acromegalic patients undergoing radiation therapy when GH levels are gradually declining but have not returned to normal. The response to GH bromocriptine should be contrasted to that observed in patients with hyperprolactinemia, in which complete suppression of prolactin can be achieved in the majority of patients. The limited secretory effect is associated with a limited cytogenic inhibition of somatotropic cells. The prominent effect of bromocriptine on shrinking macroprolactinomas is infrequent in tumors secreting GH and is apparently independent of coexisting hyperprolactinemia.

Bromocriptine is seldom used as an initial treatment of acromegaly. Currently, it should be restricted to elderly, symptomatic patients who are not suitable candidates for surgery, or it should be used as an adjunctive therapy in patients who have undergone unsuccessful surgical hyposectomy or radiation therapy. Its most important role is probably as a temporary adjustive treatment in patients who have received radiation therapy and are awaiting the full effects of treatment. Bromocriptine should always be administered during or after meals, since the most common side effect is nausea, which can be substantially curtailed by not giving the medication on an empty stomach.

Somatostatin infusions promptly lower growth hormone, but the effects are fleeting. An analogue, sandostatin, has a more prolonged effect. Recent reports indicate that cytogenesis is not affected and tumor size is not influenced by somatostatin. The disadvantage of this treatment is that three injections per day are required to give optimal treatment. Sandostatin has not been released for treatment and remains an investigative drug. Other dopamine agonists have not demonstrated any significant advantage over bromocriptine. Other drugs, such as glucocorticoids, medroxyprogesterone, chlorpromazine, and estrogens, that have been proposed as treatment have been abandoned owing to lack of therapeutic efficiency and side effects.

ADRENOCORTICAL INSUFFICIENCY

method of
I. IRONY, M.D., and
E. G. BIGLIERI, M.D.
University of California, San Francisco
San Francisco, California

The clinical presentation of subacute or acute adrenal insufficiency has not changed, but the causes of adrenal destruction or impairment have increased in number. This is in part a result of new infections (human immunodeficiency virus, HIV) and newer drugs that impair adrenocortical steroid production. At least 90 per cent destruction of the adrenal gland must occur to produce the clinical and laboratory findings that are due to a deficiency of glucocorticoid, mineralocorticoid, and androgenic hormones. However, zonal destruction and/or impairment can result in selective mineralocorticoid (zona glomerulosa) or glucocorticoid deficiencies. Steroid deficiency may range from the loss of a single or multiple steroids, resulting in a variable spectrum of deficiencies. As a consequence, the clinical manifestations may vary.

PRIMARY ADRENOCORTICAL INSUFFICIENCY (ADDISON'S DISEASE)

Etiology

Addison's disease occurs in 1 per 15,000 population and is twice as common in females between the third and fourth decades of life. In 80 per cent of cases the major cause of adrenocortical insufficiency is still idiopathic (Table 1), probably autoimmune in nature, and often associated with other autoimmune endocrine failures (thyroid, parathyroid, gonads, pancreas). The HLA-DW3 phenotype is found in most patients. About 20 per cent of the cases are due to tuberculous or fungal adrenal infections such as coccidiomycosis. However, in the acquired immunodeficiency syndrome (AIDS), adrenal insufficiency will eventually occur in 5 per cent of patients. Rare causes include adrenal hemorrhage during sepsis or co-

TABLE 1. **Adrenocortical Failure**

Primary
1. Autoimmune: adrenalitis (idiopathic)
2. Infections: tuberculosis, fungal, sepsis
3. Infiltrative: metastatic, lymphomas, amyloidosis
4. Vascular: hemorrhage, infarction
5. Congenital: hypoplasia, familial glucocorticoid deficiency
6. Iatrogenic: surgical ablation, radiotherapy, op'DDD, anti-coagulants
7. Enzymatic deficiencies:
   Congenital: 21-, 11-, and 17-hydroxylase, CMO types I and II
   Iatrogenic: metyrapone, ketoconazole, aminoglu-thethimide

Secondary
1. ACTH deficiency: pituitary tumors, necrosis, surgery, chronic glucocorticoid therapy
2. Renin deficiency: hyporeninemic hypoaldosteronism, chronic renal failure, iatrogenic (indomethacin, converting enzyme inhibitors)

agulation disorders, metastatic replacement, hemochromatosis, radiotherapy, enzymatic inhibitors (e.g., metyrapone and ketoconazole), and cytotoxic agents (e.g., mitotane). Specific deficiencies are present in some congenital disorders: glucocorticoid deficiency in the 21-hydroxylase deficiency syndrome (with androgen excess), familial glucocorticoid deficiency, and congenital adrenal hypoplasia; mineralocorticoid deficiency in the salt-losing congenital enzymatic disorders (21-hydroxylase deficiency syndrome and corticosterone methyloxidase type II deficiency syndrome); gonadal deficiency in the 17-hydroxylase deficiency syndrome (with mineralocorticoid excess).

Acute adrenocortical insufficiency may occur in partially deficient steroid patients undergoing surgery, infection, or trauma or in those in whom rapid destruction is observed, such as after hemorrhage, septicemia, or embolus formation. It is the initial presentation in approximately 25 per cent of patients with Addison's disease.

Clinical Features

Subacute Presentation

Progressive adrenal insufficiency may take place over a period of years before an acute crisis occurs. Manifestations such as asthenia, weakness, nausea, vomiting, amenorrhea, loss of libido, scant pubic and axillary hair, low blood pressure, weight loss, hyperpigmentation, and salt hunger as well as symptoms related to hypoglycemia are present. Orthostatic hypotension, hyperkalemia, and hyponatremia are usually late findings and represent the destruction of the zona glomerulosa, with subsequent aldosterone deficiency.

Acute Adrenocortical Insufficiency

This is a medical emergency, and when clinically suspected, vigorous replacement with fluids and steroids is required. Confirmation of the diagnosis can be made after stabilization. A plasma cortisol level less than 5 micrograms per dl at that initial presentation would be diagnostic. Shock, fever, profound weakness, and dehydration are hallmarks of the crisis. Volume contraction due to lack of mineralocorticoid leads to hypotension; increased hematocrit, creatinine, and blood urea nitrogen; hyponatremia; and hyperkalemia. Cortisol deficiency impairs gluconeogenesis, and hypoglycemia is present. If the inciting cause (e.g., infection or specific trauma) can be determined, it must be vigorously treated at the same time.

Treatment of Chronic Adrenocortical Insufficiency

The ideal glucocorticoid for therapy is hydrocortisone, 20 to 30 mg per day, in divided doses (two thirds in the morning and one third in the afternoon). Children can be treated with a dose of 15 mg per M^2 of body surface area. Hydrocortisone is preferred over other synthetic steroids because of its shorter half-life and some intrinsic mineralocorticoid activity. Prednisone, 7.5 mg per day, or dexamethasone, 0.5 to 1.0 mg per day, can also be used. The mineralocorticoid routinely used in maintenance replacement therapy is fludrocortisone acetate in oral doses between 0.05 and 0.2 mg per day. Fludrocortisone may increase blood pressure and deplete body potassium with doses higher than 0.2 mg per day. When infection with fever is present, or during the pre-, intra-, and postoperative periods, cortisol should be increased to 200 mg parenterally per day, given as either hydrocortisone phosphate or hydrocortisone hemisuccinate, with particular attention given to blood pressure and electrolyte concentrations.

The patient should carry a medical alert bracelet indicating diagnosis, replacement medication, and acute management.

Treatment of Acute Adrenocortical Insufficiency

A suspicion of the diagnosis is an adequate indication to initiate therapy. A blood sample should be drawn for electrolyte, glucose, blood urea nitrogen, creatinine, and steroid concentrations followed by intravenous administration of 100 mg of hydrocortisone hemisuccinate or hydrocortisone phosphate followed by rapid intravenous infusion of 5 per cent dextrose in normal saline, as the overall clinical status permits. The intravenous hydrocortisone should be continued every 6 to 8 hours until hydration is achieved and electrolyte concentration is normalized. Persistent shock that is refractory to this emergency treatment will require vasopressor agents such as norepinephrine or pharmacologic doses of methylprednisolone (0.5 to 2.0 grams) intravenously for the initial dose and then intramuscularly (every 6 hours), or even oral hydrocortisone may be administered. Mineralocorticoids are not necessary during the acute phase, since hydrocortisone at high doses (greater than 100 mg per day) has mineralocorticoid properties and abundant sodium chloride is being given.

When the patient is stable, the dose can be reduced to 50 mg every 6 hours and tapered to the maintenance dose in a period of 5 days. At this point, we recommend adding a mineralocorticoid, such as fludrocortisone, as part of the treatment. Proper antibiotic and supportive therapy is required for precipitating infections.

Diagnosis of Adrenocortical Insufficiency

When considering global failure of adrenocortical steroids, the plasma cortisol concentration gives the most information and can be readily determined. A level of less than 5 micrograms per dl at 8 a.m. is highly suggestive of adrenal insufficiency. It is important to remember that these levels can be seen in the early morning as part of the circadian rhythm of the hypothalamic-pituitary-adrenal axis. Cosyntropin (adrenocorticotropic hormone [ACTH]) given as an intravenous bolus of 0.25 mg with plasma samples at 0 and 60 minutes is an effective screen for adrenocortical insufficiency. Values greater than 22 micrograms per dl at 60 minutes imply normal adrenocortical function. Increases of cortisol by 100 per cent or more but below 22 micrograms per dl although indicative of adrenal responsiveness are not necessarily equated with adrenal reserve. An accurate diagnosis must be made because replacement is for life. The best way to establish the diagnosis of adrenal insufficiency is to replace maintenance cortisol with 1 mg of dexamethasone (which does not interfere with cortisol measurements) and administer 20 IU of ACTH gel intramuscularly every 8 hours for 3 to 5 days; cortisol levels increase to at least 35 micrograms per dl. This maneuver also helps to identify those patients with partial adrenal insufficiency, namely individuals who have normal but fixed cortisol levels, high ACTH concentrations, and no response to prolonged ACTH treatment. High ACTH levels are part of the diagnosis of adrenal insufficiency due to intrinsic adrenal disease. Reduced ACTH levels are crucial to the diagnosis of glucocorticoid deficiency secondary to pituitary destruction. Prolonged ACTH treatment as described above will show a gradual increase of cortisol.

Primary Aldosterone Deficiency

There are rare causes of primary aldosterone deficiency in which treatment consists of fludrocortisone in doses of 0.05 to 0.2 mg per day. Corticosterone methyloxidase deficiency type II (18 dehydrogenase deficiency) is an aldosterone deficiency state with renal salt wasting, hyperkalemia, and normal cortisol production. The defect is the inability to dehydrogenate 18 hydroxycorticosterone, the immediate precursor of aldosterone, to form aldosterone.

SECONDARY ADRENAL INSUFFICIENCY

ACTH Deficiency

ACTH is the main regulator for glucocorticoids. The most common cause of ACTH deficiency is prolonged glucocorticoid therapy. ACTH suppression results in adrenocortical atrophy. Sudden withdrawal of glucocorticoids may lead to secondary adrenal insufficiency. Adrenocortical tumors secreting cortisol (Cushing's syndrome) suppress ACTH secretion, with contralateral adrenal atrophy. Removal of the tumor may cause secondary cortisol deficiency because of ACTH and adrenal suppression. Replacement hydrocortisone may be required for 6 to 12 months before recovery occurs. Other causes for ACTH deficiency are pituitary tumors, hemorrhage and necrosis, irradiation, and infections. Since the primary regulator for aldosterone is renin and not ACTH, there is no mineralocorticoid depletion in ACTH deficiency; however, as cortisol is responsible for free-water excretion, its secondary deficiency alone may result in water retention and hyponatremia. The diagnosis is made by measurement of plasma ACTH, which is low or inappropriately normal in face of *low* cortisol, and by a metyrapone or insulin tolerance test, which reveals subnormal ACTH release.

In this disorder only glucocorticoid replacement is usually necessary. Synthetic glucocorticoids such as prednisone or dexamethasone can be used in doses equivalent to 20 to 30 mg of hydrocortisone. In panhypopituitarism, replacement of glucocorticoids should be done prior to the administration of thyroid hormones, since the latter accelerate cortisol metabolism and aggravate glucocorticoid insufficiency.

Secondary Aldosterone Deficiency (Hyporeninism)

Renin is the major stimulus for aldosterone secretion. Deficiency of renin results in only mineralocorticoid deficiency. Renin is chronically suppressed by aldosterone-producing tumors. When these tumors are removed, transient hypoaldosteronism secondary to renin deficiency occurs, with hyperkalemia transiently observed. The same pathogenesis can be applied to the early phase of treatment of 11β- and 17α-hydroxylase deficiencies with glucocorticoids, when renin and aldosterone are suppressed by high deoxycorticosterone levels. Renin secretion is also impaired in diabetic nephropathy, tubulointerstitial nephritis, obstructive uropathy, renal transplantation, and administration of prostaglandin synthesis inhibitors. The diagnosis is established by the presence of hyperkalemic hyperchloremic metabolic acidosis and by renin levels that do not respond to stimulatory maneuvers such as postural stimulation and diuretic administration. The patients are treated only with fludrocortisone at a dose of 0.05 to 2.0 mg orally per day.

CUSHING'S SYNDROME

method of
DAVID E. SCHTEINGART, M.D.
University of Michigan Medical School
Ann Arbor, Michigan

Cushing's syndrome results from prolonged exposure to high levels of glucocorticoid hormones. The cause can be exogenous, due to the administration of glucocorticoids or adrenocorticotropic hormone (ACTH), or endogenous, due to a primary increased secretion of cortisol or ACTH.

ACTH-dependent Cushing's syndrome accounts for 70 per cent of all cases. ACTH is secreted in excessive amounts by the pituitary gland or is secreted ectopically by an extrapituitary neoplasm. In pituitary ACTH-dependent Cushing's syndrome, the feedback relationship between the pituitary and the adrenal cortex is preserved but is abnormal. In contrast, in ectopic ACTH syndrome, pituitary ACTH release is suppressed by the excessive production of cortisol, which is in turn stimulated by an unsuppressible overproduction of ACTH from the ectopic source. In patients with ACTH-independent types of Cushing's syndrome, pituitary ACTH secretion is suppressed by excessive cortisol production originating either in autonomous nodular hyperplastic glands or in adrenocortical adenomas or carcinomas. Single adrenocortical tumors account for 20 per cent of patients with Cushing's syndrome.

The clinical manifestations of Cushing's syndrome involve many organ systems and biochemical processes. While some of these manifestations (hypertension, diabetes, androgen-type hirsutism, and acne) are commonly seen among patients without primary glucocorticoid excess, the following findings increase the suspicion of Cushing's syndrome: (1) symptoms and signs of protein catabolism, (2) truncal obesity, (3) lanugal hirsutism, (4) tinea versicolor, (5) wide purple striae, and (6) hyperpigmentation. In addition to cortisol excess, the presence of high levels of ACTH, prolactin, androgens and mineralocorticoids will account for the clinical picture that emerges. Biochemical manifestations of Cushing's syndrome are the loss of normal circadian rhythm of ACTH and cortisol secretion and of the negative feedback regulation of ACTH release. While relative suppressibility of ACTH release by corticosteroids is maintained in the majority of these patients, up to 40 per cent exhibit resistance to suppression and resemble patients with ectopic ACTH syndrome. Unusual abnormal patterns of release of ACTH and cortisol have been described, in which episodes of hypersecretion occur for hours or weeks and are interrupted by periods of normal secretion. Periodic hormonogenesis can occur with or without ACTH-secreting pituitary adenomas.

Diagnostic Evaluation

Biochemical evaluation of Cushing's syndrome is necessary for confirmation of the clinical diagnosis and for determination of the presence of Cushing's syndrome in patients with an equivocal clinical presentation. Preliminary testing includes measurement of urinary-free cortisol and of the ability to suppress with a low dose of dexamethasone. In patients with Cushing's syndrome, urinary-free cortisol usually exceeds 150 micrograms per day. Serum cortisol obtained 9 hours after the oral administration of 1 mg of dexamethasone at 11 p.m. fails to decrease to less than 5.0 micrograms per dl, and plasma ACTH levels fail to decrease to less than 40 pg per ml. Once the preliminary diagnosis has been determined, final confirmation is carried out according to a more extensive protocol. This protocol includes measurement of serum cortisol and plasma ACTH levels at various times of the day in order to determine the absence of circadian rhythm and the pituitary response to metyrapone and dexamethasone in order to ascertain the presence of abnormal feedback regulation of ACTH and cortisol secretion. Metyrapone (Metopirone), an 11β-hydroxylase inhibitor, is given in doses of 750 mg orally every 4 hours for six doses, while dexamethasone is given in doses of 0.5 mg every 6 hours for eight doses followed by 2 mg every 6 hours for eight doses. Patients with Cushing's syndrome, regardless of etiology or type, exhibit high baseline urinary 17-hydroxycorticoids, and free-cortisol and cortisol levels lack a normal circadian rhythm. Occasionally, the early morning cortisol levels may be indistinguishable from normal, but levels obtained between 10 p.m. and midnight are clearly higher than those in normal people. The response of plasma ACTH levels to metyrapone and dexamethasone depends on the type of Cushing's syndrome. Baseline levels are high (70 to 100 pg per ml) in ACTH-dependent types and low (less than 50 pg per ml) in ACTH-independent types. While ACTH levels are frequently in the upper limits of normal in patients with a pituitary etiology, they may range from 200 to 1000 pg per ml in patients with the ectopic type. A positive response to metyrapone is present in patients with pituitary ACTH-dependent syndrome. Lack of normal suppression of cortisol with low doses of dexamethasone is found in all types of Cushing's syndrome, but in the majority of patients with pituitary ACTH-dependent Cushing's syndrome, suppression occurs with high doses of dexamethasone to values below 50 per cent of the baseline levels. Less than 10 per cent of patients with ectopic ACTH syndrome respond in this manner. In patients with ACTH-dependent Cushing's syndrome, high ACTH levels and lack of response to either metyrapone or dexamethasone should strongly suggest the possibility of ectopic ACTH syndrome. Additional information regarding the source of ACTH can be obtained through corticotropin-releasing hormone (CRH) administration. Ovine CRH given as an intravenous bolus injection (1 microgram per kg) stimulates plasma ACTH and cortisol in 85 to 90 per cent of patients with Cushing's disease. Patients with ectopic ACTH syndrome rarely respond to this maneuver.

Anatomic Localization

Detection of Pituitary Lesions. Once the diagnosis of Cushing's syndrome has been established on clinical and biochemical grounds, the presence of a pituitary lesion should be further determined by computed tomographic (CT) scan of the sella turcica. Large adenomas secreting ACTH are extremely rare at the time the initial diagnosis of Cushing's syndrome is made. Large-size tumors are frequently associated with the development of Nelson's syndrome when the pituitary tumor enlarges following a bilateral total adrenalectomy. Small (less than 10 mm in diameter) pituitary microadenomas can be detected by CT scanning of the pituitary gland using coronal cuts in approximately 30 per cent of patients with pituitary ACTH-dependent Cushing's syndrome. The lesion usually appears as a hypodense or enhancing abnormality within the pituitary gland. The isodense lesions may be missed, and many patients with Cushing's syndrome fail to show a distinct intrapituitary abnormality. Magnetic resonance imaging (MRI) also allows for detection of these microadenomas, although the yield is not higher than that which is obtained with CT scans. Petrosal sinus sampling with or without CRH stimulation is also used for localization of pituitary lesions. Blood is drawn simultaneously from both inferior petrosal sinuses and peripheral veins. A plasma ACTH concentration gradient (petrosal sinus/peripheral vein ACTH greater than or equal to 1.6) verifies the pituitary source of ACTH. A right-to-left discrepancy in levels may also help to lateralize ACTH secretion and aids in the preoperative localization of the lesion.

Detection of Adrenal Lesions. Techniques for the anatomic localization of adrenal lesions include abdominal CT scan and adrenal scintigraphy with 6-beta-(^{131}I)-iodomethyl-19-norcholesterol. These techniques are noninvasive and provide good definition of structure and function of the adrenal glands. Adrenocortical masses can be easily detected by CT scanning. Scintigraphy with iodocholesterol provides not only an image reflective of the structure of the adrenal gland but also information about its function. Patients with bilateral adrenocortical hyperplasia demonstrate bilaterally increased adrenal uptake of iodocholesterol. Patients with cortisol-secreting adrenocortical adenomas that suppress pituitary ACTH secretion and the function of the contralateral gland demonstrate unilateral concentration of the tracer. Patients with Cushing's syndrome secondary to an adrenocortical carcinoma fail to show uptake of the tracer in either side, since the relatively low functional activity of carcinomas decreases their ability to concentrate iodocholesterol. Patients with primary macronodular hyperplasia may show asymmetrical uptake, with greater activity on the side of the predominant nodules. This finding is important in determining the presence of bilateral adrenocortical disease, since a CT scan of the adrenal glands may show a mass on one side, but surgical resection of that mass may not result in remission if the contralateral gland is also abnormal.

Localization of ectopic sources of ACTH involves a variety of procedures, including CT scans of the chest and abdomen, thyroid scan, and selected venous catheterization and blood sampling in search of ACTH concentration gradients. Approximately 50 per cent of these tumors are within the thorax (oat cell carcinomas, bronchial carcinoids, thymomas), and thoracic CT scans will usually localize the lesion. Other ACTH-secreting tumors are found in the pancreas (islet cell tumors), the thyroid (medullary carcinoma), and the adrenal medulla (pheochromocytoma). Ectopic ACTH-secreting bronchial carcinoids may be small and slow growing, and up to 12 years may elapse before they become radiographically apparent. Bronchoscopy and repeat CT scans of the chest may help in the detection of these lesions. Tumors secreting ectopic CRH or CRH and ACTH have also been described. These tumors have been bronchial carcinoids, oat cell carcinoma of the lung, intrasellar gangliocytoma, and metastatic medullary carcinoma of the thyroid. In patients with ectopic ACTH production, pituitary ACTH concentration is low, and only Crooke's changes have been observed in pituitary corticotropes. In contrast, patients with ectopic CRH secretion demonstrate corticotropic hyperplasia. In addition, biochemical studies of these tumors show that while patients with ectopic ACTH syndrome fail to respond to metyrapone or suppress with dexamethasone, those secreting CRH may respond to feedback maneuvers. The presence of an ectopic ACTH-secreting tumor should be suspected in patients who behave biochemically like those with pituitary ACTH-dependent disease but who have a rather rapid clinical course and high plasma ACTH levels.

The differential diagnosis between mild Cushing's disease and the hypercortisolism of depression can be a problem. A consistent constellation of neuropsychiatric disturbances is found in patients with Cushing's disease, including impairment in affect (depressed mood and crying), cognitive functions (decreased concentration and memory), and vegetative functions (decreased libido and insomnia). In about 50 per cent of these patients, the psychiatric manifestations can be severe. There is a statistically significant relationship between overall neuropsychiatric disability and cortisol and ACTH levels. Patients with high cortisol and ACTH levels usually exhibit more severe depression. There are several features that distinguish the depression of Cushing's disease from that which occurs in patients with primary endogenous major depressive illness. Each depressive episode is usually of limited duration (1 to 3 days) and is not associated with unrelenting, unremitting inability to experience pleasure, which is characteristic of patients with primary depression. Also, patients with primary depressive illness have milder abnormalities of cortisol secretion and do not exhibit the clinical stigmata of Cushing's syndrome. The biochemical abnormalities of cortisol secretion observed in depression are usually reversed by treatment of the depressive illness. In contrast, the depression of Cushing's disease is ameliorated by medical or surgical correction of the hypercortisolemia.

When the results of the evaluation of Cushing's syndrome are inconclusive, periodic hypersecretion of cortisol should be suspected. Long-term, repeated monitoring with weekly urine collections for free cortisol will help uncover this periodic pattern.

Rarely, factitious Cushing's syndrome is encountered. If the patients have been taking synthetic glucocorticoids, their endogenous adrenocortical function will be suppressed. There will be a paradoxical finding of clinical manifestations of Cushing's syndrome with suppressed ACTH and cortisol levels.

Treatment

Pituitary pathology is found in 95 per cent of patients with typical preoperative endocrine testing for pituitary ACTH-dependent disease and in 55 per cent of those with atypical testing results. Four approaches are presently used in the management of pituitary ACTH-dependent Cushing's syndrome: pituitary surgery, pituitary irradiation, drug therapy, and adrenal surgery. The treatment of choice is the microsurgical removal of microadenomas or macroadenomas. When the presence of a pituitary adenoma or microadenoma can be demonstrated by radiographic techniques, resection through a transsphenoidal approach to the pituitary gland should be the preferred treatment. When a tumor is not detected by imaging techniques, a transsphenoidal exploration of the pituitary gland is still in order, since a tumor can still be found in approximately 90 per cent of patients. Even with considerable suprasellar extension, the tumor can be resected transsphenoidally. If the tumor is invasive into the dura, total resection may be impossible, but good remission rates of 45 to 75 per cent have been described. The microsurgical transsphenoidal selective resection of ACTH-secreting pituitary microadenomas is currently the most common treat-

ment of Cushing's syndrome and comes closest to the ideal form of treatment for this condition. If a microadenoma can be identified and totally resected, the remaining pituitary tissue will continue to function, and patients can enjoy remission without loss of endocrine function. It is common, however, after selective adenoma resection for patients to experience transient (6 months to 2 years) adrenal insufficiency requiring maintenance hydrocortisone replacement. If the cortisol levels do not return to the normal range, a recurrence is more likely. If a specific adenoma cannot be identified during surgery, then a decision must be made whether to perform a partial or total hypophysectomy. If preoperative inferior petrosal sinus sampling has been carried out and is clearly lateralizing, an appropriate hemiresection of the hypophesis should be performed. If the endocrine studies strongly indicate a pituitary origin but the petrosal sinus sampling is not lateralizing and the patient does not wish to have children, then a total hypophysectomy should be considered but only after a lengthy preoperative discussion with the patient regarding this possibility. If the patient wishes to have children, alternative forms of therapy, including medical treatment or a total adrenalectomy, must be considered. With transsphenoidal surgery, permanent anterior or posterior pituitary hormone deficiencies are rare. Transient diabetes insipidus may occur during the early weeks following surgery. Permanent diabetes insipidus and cerebrospinal fluid rhinorrhea are uncommon complications with an initial procedure but may occur more commonly with repeated transsphenoidal surgery. Treatment failures are most common in patients with pituitary macroadenomas or in those in whom a distinct microadenoma has not been found.

When transsphenoidal surgery has failed or alternative forms of treatment are desired, pituitary irradiation is an option. The most widely used type of pituitary irradiation is high voltage irradiation provided by ^{60}Co. The total dose recommended is 4000 to 5000 rad and favorable results can be effected in about 50 per cent of patients. The best responders are patients with the juvenile form of the disease or in adults under 40 years of age. When successful, ^{60}Co irradiation has several advantages. Remission occurs with preservation of pituitary and adrenal function, panhypopituitarism seldom develops, normal reproductive function is restored when the patient is in remission, steroid replacement therapy is not needed, recurrence is rare, and normal cortisol secretion may be restored (circadian rhythm and normal suppressibility on dexamethasone). The major disadvantage is the slow therapeutic response to pituitary irradiation: Six to 18 months may elapse before clinical and biochemical remission is achieved. Clearly, ^{60}Co irradiation alone is not adequate in patients who have severe Cushing's syndrome. Symptoms may progress if one waits for a remission, and severe, perhaps irreversible complications may result. Heavy particle beam irradiation and Bragg peak proton irradiation therapy, with a rate of improvement or remission as high as 80 per cent, appear to be more effective than ^{60}Co irradiation in the treatment of Cushing's syndrome; however, the prevalence of postirradiation panhypopituitarism is high.

In patients with advanced Cushing's syndrome in whom transsphenoidal surgery has failed, bilateral total adrenalectomy is the preferred treatment. The major disadvantage of adrenalectomy is that it fails to attack the cause underlying the hypersecretion of ACTH. In addition, complications may occur months or years later owing to Nelson's syndrome, with hyperpigmentation and an ACTH-secreting pituitary macroadenoma becoming clinically apparent after adrenalectomy. These ACTH-secreting tumors may become locally invasive and difficult to control by surgery or radiation therapy.

Various drugs have been used in the treatment of Cushing's syndrome. Some of these drugs act on neurotransmitters and decrease the secretion of ACTH. Cyproheptadine, a serotonin antagonist, and bromocriptine, a dopamine receptor agonist, can suppress ACTH secretion and cause remission of Cushing's syndrome. However, the effect of these drugs is temporary, lasting while the drug is being administered. Recurrence of the disease occurs after interruption of therapy. Undesirable weight gain has been reported as a consistent side effect of cyproheptadine therapy. Various inhibitors of adrenal function—aminoglutethimide, metyrapone, and ketoconazole—have been used to suppress cortisol secretion in patients with Cushing's syndrome. These drugs, however, have only temporary effects, while the drug is being administered. Aminoglutethimide (Cytadren) is given in doses of 1 to 2 grams daily in four divided doses. It decreases cortisol secretion by inhibiting cholesterol desmolase. Aminoglutethimide has gastrointestinal (anorexia, nausea, vomiting) and neurologic (lethargy, sedation, blurred vision) side effects and can cause hypothyroidism in 5 per cent of patients. A skin rash is frequently observed during the first 10 days of treatment which usually subsides despite continuation of treatment. Metyrapone (Metopirone) is an 11-beta-hydroxylase inhibitor and is given in doses of 2 grams daily in divided doses. It may cause hypertension and hyperkalemic alkalosis

as a result of the accumulation of 11-deoxycorticosterone. Ketoconazole (Nizoral) can be given in doses of 800 to 1200 mg a day in divided doses. Another drug, mitotane (Lysodren), is the only one that both inhibits biosynthesis of corticosteroids and destroys adrenocortical cells secreting cortisol without interfering with aldosterone production. A combination of ^{60}Co irradiation of the pituitary gland with selective suppression of cortisol secretion with mitotane has been employed in the treatment of patients with Cushing's disease. Eighty per cent of these patients treated with mitotane and pituitary irradiation underwent clinical and biochemical remission of Cushing's syndrome. In addition to suppressing cortisol secretion, mitotane appears to have a partial suppressive effect on ACTH. After suppression of cortisol secretion, there is a minimal feedback increase in ACTH production, and in 70 per cent of patients treated with this drug, an actual decrease in ACTH levels is observed. This is in contrast to the increase in ACTH levels in patients treated by adrenalectomy or other adrenal inhibitors, such as metyrapone. Mitotane is a selective inhibitor of the reticularis and fasciculata zones of the adrenal cortex. Aldosterone secretion is usually spared, and patients treated with mitotane do not require mineralocorticoid replacement when they develop adrenal insufficiency. Side effects with mitotane therapy include anorexia, nausea, diarrhea, somnolence, pruritus, hyperlipoproteinemia, and hypouricemia. Elevated alkaline phosphatase levels can also occur as the result of hepatotoxic effects of mitotane. The combined treatment with pituitary irradiation and mitotane chemotherapy can be given as a primary medical treatment of Cushing's syndrome when surgery is contraindicated or as the next modality of therapy when transsphenoidal pituitary surgery fails to bring about remission of the disease. The dose of mitotane employed for the treatment of Cushing's syndrome is 2 to 4 grams daily. Treatment may be initiated with a dose of 500 mg twice daily and increased to 1 gram four times daily as needed to achieve adrenal suppressive effects. Response occurs either early, within 4 months of therapy, or late, gradually over a period of 1 year. The urinary-free cortisol excretion should be monitored, and the dose of mitotane should be titrated to maintain urinary-free cortisol excretion in the low normal range. If adrenal insufficiency is suspected, hydrocortisone should be given orally. Since mitotane induces liver monooxygenases (P-450 enzymes) that metabolize steroids and other drugs, an adequate dose of fludrocortisone or hydrocortisone may be higher than expected. As the effect of radiation therapy becomes apparent with suppression of ACTH secretion, the treatment with mitotane can be gradually discontinued.

Treatment of ectopic ACTH syndrome involves the surgical resection of the primary tumor followed by radiation therapy or chemotherapy, depending on the type of neoplasm producing ectopic ACTH production. In patients whose neoplasm cannot be resected, the use of adrenal inhibitors may ameliorate clinical manifestations of Cushing's syndrome. Patients may become severely pigmented when ACTH levels are very high. Bilateral adrenalectomy is an alternative approach but frequently not a practical one for patients with progressive metastatic disease. RU-486, a glucocorticoid antagonist, has been shown effectively to antagonize hypercortisolism causing Cushing's syndrome. It is well tolerated and nontoxic at doses ranging from 10 to 20 mg per kg per day. RU-486 is still an investigational drug, and its use is limited to investigational protocols.

Adrenocortical adenomas should be surgically removed with cure of the Cushing's syndrome. Because of suppression of the hypothalamic-pituitary-adrenal axis in these patients, replacement therapy with physiologic doses of cortisol is usually required until recovery has taken place. This may take 6 to 16 months.

Adrenal carcinomas causing Cushing's syndrome are highly malignant neoplasms that result in a shortened life expectancy. Their treatment has not been well standardized, and the prognosis has been poor regardless of therapy. Several approaches to therapy have been used. One method is surgical excision of the primary tumor and of large neoplastic abdominal masses. While temporary remission of the disease frequently occurs with this approach, recurrence and eventual death from metastatic disease is the rule. Another approach is radiation therapy and nonspecific chemotherapy; these have been generally effective only for palliation of local disease. Agents that block steroid hormone production by the tumor have also been used. While effective in reversing the metabolic consequences of these tumors, these drugs do not alter the progression and eventual fatal outcome of the disease. Since its clinical introduction, mitotane has been the only drug that has proved effective in patients with metastatic adrenocortical carcinoma. Most of the experience with mitotane comes from its use in patients with obvious metastatic disease. Its effectiveness under those conditions has been disputed in the literature. Decreases in elevated urinary steroid levels, measurable disease response, and overall clinical response have been described. However, mean survival when the drug is used after the appearance of metastatic disease is short (8.4 months). Isolated case reports have described impressive remissions and even cures of adrenocortical carcinoma following mitotane therapy. In general, survival appears to depend on the size of the primary lesion and the degree of local and distal extension of the neoplasm at the time of initial surgery. Criteria for staging adrenal cancer have been suggested. Patients with primary tumors less than 5 cm in diameter and without local or distal extension appear to have a relatively good prognosis and long survival. It has been generally concluded that if mitotane therapy is to be effective, it should be instituted early following resection of the primary tumor and before local extension or distal metastases occur. Adverse effects of mitotane therapy are found to be dose dependent and prohibitive when doses higher than 6 grams per day are administered. Thus, early chemotherapy of adrenal carcinoma with low doses of mitotane following resection of the primary tumor or debulking resection of recurrent tumor appears to be associated with prolonged survival.

Postoperative Steroid Replacement

Since a successful transsphenoidal operation in Cushing's syndrome and removal of an autonomous adrenal adenoma lead to a period of adrenal insufficiency, glucocorticoids must be replaced. Insufficiency of the hypothalamic-pituitary-adrenal axis can last as long as 1 year. Intraoperatively and during the first 2 postoperative days, patients should be given doses of 150 to 200 mg of hydrocortisone or its equivalent. After tapering the dose of hydrocortisone to physiologic replacement and once the patient has recovered from the surgical procedure, patients are maintained on doses of hydrocortisone of 20 to 30 mg daily. The replacement dose of hydrocortisone should be tapered if there is evidence of recovery of hypothalamic-pituitary-adrenal function. This can be ascertained periodically by measuring the serum cortisol level at 8 hours prior to the patient's receiving the first dose of hydrocortisone for the day. If levels have been increasing into the low normal range, the replacement dose can be further decreased. At that time, the patient can also be tested with a short ACTH stimulation test (cosyntropin 250 micrograms given intravenously and cortisol measured at 60 and 90 minutes). If the response to this test is normal (plasma cortisol above 20 micrograms per dl), replacement hydrocortisone therapy can be discontinued. If the test is not normal, therapy may be continued for another 2 to 3 months and the test repeated. The majority of patients can discontinue glucocorticoid replacement within 1 year postoperatively. During this interval, the patient should be given extra glucocorticoid replacement during stress. All patients should wear medical badges indicating that they are receiving glucocorticoid replacement therapy.

DIABETES INSIPIDUS

method of
ARTHUR GREENBERG, M.D., and
JOSEPH G. VERBALIS, M.D.
University of Pittsburgh School of Medicine
Pittsburgh, Pennsylvania

In diabetes insipidus, diminished antidiuretic hormone (ADH) levels or effect leads to abnormal urinary losses of solute-free water with resultant polyuria, polydipsia, hypertonicity, and hypernatremia. Central diabetes insipidus is characterized by an impairment in the hypothalamic-pituitary response to hypertonicity. Release of ADH is subnormal in the partial form of central diabetes insipidus and absent in the complete form. In nephrogenic diabetes insipidus, ADH release is normal, but renal sensitivity to its hydro-osmotic effect is impaired or absent.

Central diabetes insipidus is caused by any of a variety of acquired or congenital anatomic lesions that disrupt the hypothalamic-posterior pituitary axis, including pituitary surgery, tumor, trauma, hemorrhage, thrombosis, infarction, or granulomatous disease. Severe nephrogenic diabetes insipidus is most commonly hereditary and congenital, but relief of chronic urinary obstruction or therapy with lithium or other drugs may cause an acquired form severe enough to warrant specific treatment. Short-lived nephrogenic diabetes insipidus from hypokalemia or hypercalcemia responds to correction of the underlying disorder and, like the mild concentrating defect associated with chronic renal failure that does not by itself cause sufficient water loss to lead to hypertonicity, will not be considered further. Other causes of polyuria include primary polydipsia and solute diuresis from glycosuria, mannitol, or diuretic therapy or resolving acute renal failure. Solute diuresis can be excluded by demonstrating that the urine osmolality is below 150 mosm per kg or that the specific gravity is below 1.005. A formal water deprivation test is dangerous and unnecessary when severe hypertonicity is already present but may be essential for the diagnosis of partial diabetes insipidus or in cases in which treatment has already been initiated. The urinary response to exogenous ADH distinguishes central from nephrogenic diabetes insipidus in most cases. ADH levels are confirmatory and helpful in equivocal cases but not available on an emergent basis.

Treatment

The general goals of treatment are (1) a correction of any pre-existing water deficits and (2) a reduction in the ongoing excessive urinary water losses. The specific therapy required varies with the clinical situation. Awake ambulatory patients with normal thirst have little water deficit but benefit greatly from relief of the polyuria and polydipsia that disrupt normal activity. Comatose patients with acute diabetes insipidus after head trauma are unable to drink in response to thirst; in them, hypertonicity may be life-threatening.

Correction of Water Deficit

The established deficit may be estimated using the following formula:

$$\text{Water deficit} = 0.6 \times \text{premorbid weight} \times \left(1 - \frac{140}{[\text{Na}]}\right)$$

where [Na] is the serum sodium concentration. This formula is dependent on three assumptions: (1) total body water is 60 per cent of weight, (2) no solute was lost as hypertonicity developed, and (3) the premorbid [Na] was 140 mEq per liter.

To reduce the risk of central nervous system damage from protracted exposure to severe hypertonicity, the serum tonicity should be rapidly lowered to 330 mosm per kg. Tonicity may be estimated most easily as twice the [Na] if there is no hyperglycemia, and measured osmolality may be substituted if there is no azotemia. The brain increases intracellular osmolality by generating "idiogenic osmoles" as a protection against shrinkage during hypertonicity. Because these idiogenic osmoles cannot be immediately dissipated, further correction should be spread over 24 to 48 hours to avoid cerebral edema during treatment.

The above formula does not take into account ongoing water losses and is, at best, a crude estimate. Frequent serum and urine electrolyte determinations should be made, and the administration rate of oral water or 5 per cent dextrose in water should be adjusted accordingly. Note, for example, that the estimated deficit of a 70 kg patient whose [Na] is 160 mEq per liter is 5.25 liters of water. In such an individual, administration of water at a rate greater than 200 ml/hour would be required simply to correct the established deficit over 24 hours. Additional fluid would be needed to keep up with ongoing losses until a response to definitive treatment has occurred.

Useful Pharmacologic Agents

The various agents and dosages currently recommended for treatment of diabetes insipidus are listed in the table.

Arginine Vasopressin (Pitressin). This is a synthetic form of naturally occurring human vasopressin (ADH). Because of the drug's short half-life and propensity to cause hypertension when given intravenously, this route should be avoided. The aqueous solution contains 20 units per ml. This agent is mainly used for acute situations such as postoperative diabetes insipidus. Repeated dosing is required and should be titrated to achieve the desired reduction in urine output. Arginine vasopressin is not useful in nephrogenic diabetes insipidus.

Desmopressin Acetate (DDAVP). One of a number of synthetic congeners of vasopressin, desmopressin (1-desamino-8-D-arginine vasopressin) was developed for drug use because it has a longer half-life than the native form and is devoid of the latter's pressor activity. The drug of choice for chronic administration, the intranasal form is provided as an aqueous solution containing 100 micrograms per ml in a bottle with a calibrated tube applicator. To use the applicator, the tube is filled to the appropriate graduation line and bent in a U shape. Taking care to retain the fluid within the catheter, one end of the tube is placed in the mouth and the other approximately 1 cm into the anterior nares. The drug is then puffed into the midportion of the nose deep enough to avoid runoff out the nose but not so far back as to propel the hormone into the throat. Patients require training in how to use the applicator to deliver the prescribed dose reliably.

The parenteral form is supplied as a solution containing 4 micrograms per ml and may be given by intravenous, intramuscular, or subcutaneous route. Although the parenteral form is said to be 5 to 10 times more potent than the intranasal preparation, the recommended dosage is somewhat less. Desmopressin is not useful in nephrogenic diabetes insipidus.

Chlorpropamide (Diabinese). Primarily used as an oral hypoglycemic agent, this sulfonylurea also potentiates the hydro-osmotic effect of ADH in the kidney. It is of no value in nephrogenic diabetes insipidus or in most patients with complete diabetes insipidus, but it can be a useful adjunct in partial central diabetes insipidus. Caution regarding development of hypoglycemia, particularly in patients with anterior pituitary insufficiency, is necessary. Several days' treatment is required before maximal effect is seen.

Thiazide Diuretics—Chlorthalidone (Hygroton) and Others. The natriuretic effect of the thiazide class of diuretics is conferred by their ability to block sodium absorption in the cortical diluting site. When combined with dietary sodium restriction, the drugs cause modest hypovolemia. This stimulates isotonic proximal tubular solute reabsorp-

tion and diminishes solute delivery to the more distal diluting site, whose concentrating activity has already been partially poisoned. Together, these effects markedly diminish renal diluting ability and free-water clearance independent of any action of ADH. Thus, agents of this class are the mainstay of therapy for nephrogenic diabetes insipidus. Although they can also be useful adjuncts in central diabetes insipidus, the more direct antidiuretic therapies available for these patients are generally preferred. Monitoring for hypokalemia is recommended; supplementation is occasionally required. The dosage of a long-acting thiazide, chlorthalidone, is given in Table 1, but the thiazides are interchangeable. Any drug of the thiazide class may be used with equal potential for benefit, and the physician is advised to use the one with which he is most familiar from use in other conditions.

Nonsteroidal Anti-inflammatory Agents—Indomethacin (Indocin) and Others. Prostaglandins increase renal medullary blood flow and diminish medullary solute reabsorption, effects that modestly decrease the interstitial gradient for water reabsorption. By blocking renal prostaglandin synthesis, drugs of this class can increase non–ADH-mediated water reabsorption and minimal urine osmolality, thereby reducing free-water clearance and urine output. Although these agents may also be effective in central diabetes insipidus, their main usefulness is in nephrogenic diabetes insipidus, in which direct antidiuretic therapies are more limited. Indomethacin* (Indocin), tolmetin* (Tolectin), and ibuprofen* (Motrin, Rufen) have been used beneficially. Although ibuprofen may be less effective, indomethacin may not be tolerated chronically because of gastrointestinal side effects. The drugs should be given in three divided doses.

Other Agents. Arginine vasopressin tannate in oil has a 24- to 72-hour duration of action. Because of variable bioability, it has been supplanted by desmopressin. Clofibrate (Atromid-S) and carbamazepine (Tegretol) augment release of vasopressin in partial diabetes insipidus, but significant side effects preclude recommending their routine use. Other sulfonylureas share chlorpropamide's effect but are less potent.

Specific Situations

Acute Postsurgical or Posttraumatic Central Diabetes Insipidus. A frequent complication of pituitary surgery or severe head trauma, this diagnosis is obvious from the clinical situation. Hypernatremia may develop rapidly, is apt to be

---

*This use of these agents is not listed in the manufacturers' directives.

TABLE 1. **Drugs Useful in Treatment of Diabetes Insipidus**

Drug	Dose	Onset of Action (Hours)	Duration of Action (Hours)	Comments
Aqueous vasopressin (Pitressin)	5 to 10 units subcutaneously	1 to 2	4 to 8	Avoid intravenous use owing to risk of hypertension
Desmopressin (DDAVP)	50 to 200 microliters intra-nasally	1 to 2	6 to 24	Drug of choice for chronic use
	2 to 4 micrograms intrave-nously or subcutaneously	1 to 2	6 to 24	
Chlorpropamide* (Diabinese)	100 to 500 mg daily	delayed	24 to 48	Potentiates renal effect of ADH
Chlorthalidone* (Hygroton)	50 to 100 mg daily	2 to 4	24 to 48	Reduces renal water clearance Useful in nephrogenic diabetes insipidus Comparable doses of other thiazides equally effective
Idomethacin* (Indocin)	100 to 150 mg daily	2 to 4	6 to 8	Decreases renal water clearance Useful in nephrogenic diabetes insipidus

*Not approved for this use.

severe, and warrants specific therapy with intravenous 5 per cent dextrose in water at a rate estimated from the deficit calculation described previously. Parenteral aqueous vasopressin in a dosage of 5 U subcutaneously or desmopressin in a dosage of 1 to 2 micrograms intramuscularly or subcutaneously should be started to reduce urine flow rate and simplify fluid management. Frequent monitoring of urine output and serum electrolytes is required. After the acute phase, partial or complete resolution of diabetes insipidus often occurs. In some patients, the initial phase of diabetes insipidus is followed by axonal necrosis with uncontrolled ADH release potentially leading to water retention and hyponatremia and then by axonal death with cessation of ADH production and recurrent diabetes insipidus; this is the so-called triphasic pattern. ADH requirements may thus vary. To ensure detection of recovery or a period of inappropriate antidiuresis, the dosage interval for parenteral desmopressin or aqueous vasopressin should be empirically tailored to allow a brief recurrence of polyuria. Postsurgical patients who do not recover will need chronic outpatient therapy.

Chronic Central Diabetes Insipidus. Patients with complete central diabetes insipidus should be treated with intranasal desmopressin. Unless the hypothalamic thirst center is also affected by the primary lesion, patients will develop thirst when hypertonic. Severe hypertonicity is therefore not a risk in the patient who is alert, ambulatory, and able to drink. Polyuria and polydipsia are thus inconvenient and disruptive but not life-threatening. Hypotonicity is largely asymptomatic and may be progressive if water intake continues during a period of continuous antidi-

uresis. Therefore, treatment must be designed to minimize polyuria and polydipsia without an undue risk of hyponatremia from overtreatment. It is best to permit brief intermittent polyuric episodes, ideally on a daily basis, but alternatively at least weekly, at the patient's convenience. Treatment must be individualized, usually with an inhospital trial to determine optimal dosage and interval. This also permits careful education of patients on how to administer the drug intranasally and how to ensure a polyuric phase. Starting at 50 microliters, the dose that results in 12 to 24 hours of control should be determined. Most patients require twice daily dosing, but in some once daily dosing suffices. Even so, multiple small doses may be preferred because of the high cost of desmopressin. Chlorpropamide may lower the required desmopressin dose and produce an additional economy. Patients with partial central diabetes insipidus can be readily managed with desmopressin, but chlorpropamide alone may be sufficient and simpler in some cases.

Nephrogenic Diabetes Insipidus. By definition, patients with nephrogenic diabetes insipidus are resistant to ADH. Useful treatment measures include sodium restriction and thiazides to reduce renal diluting capacity combined with a prostaglandin synthesis inhibitor. Indomethacin,* tolmetin,* and ibuprofen* have been used in this setting, although the last may be less effective than the others. The combination of thiazides and a nonsteroidal anti-inflammatory agent will not increase urinary osmolality above that of plasma, but the lessening of polyuria is nonetheless beneficial to patients.

---

*This use of these agents is not listed in the manufacturers' directives.

SIMPLE GOITER

method of
MARY KORYTKOWSKI, M.D., and
DAVID S. COOPER, M.D.
Johns Hopkins University School of Medicine
Baltimore, Maryland

The term goiter refers to any visible or palpable enlargement of the thyroid gland. The enlargement may be diffuse or nodular (i.e., containing one or more nodules) and generally results from hyperplasia of thyroid follicular cells. Simple goiters are those goiters that have no clear etiology and are therefore justifiably also called idiopathic or sporadic goiters. Thyroid function in individuals with simple goiters is usually normal, although hyperthyroidism is occasionally seen (toxic nodular goiter or Plummer's disease).

The etiology of simple goiter (i.e., goiter occurring in a nonendemic goiter region) is far from clear. In the United States, iodine deficiency as a cause of goiter was eliminated with the introduction of iodized salt in the 1920s; however, the prevalence of goiter still varies from 0.4 to 7.2 per cent. Disorders of thyroid hormone biosynthesis account for only a very small percentage of goiters; such patients are usually identified in childhood and are often hypothyroid. As with other disorders of the thyroid gland, women are affected more frequently than men.

Numerous factors have been postulated in the etiology of simple goiter. These include genetic predisposition, an increased sensitivity of the thyroid gland to the growth-stimulating effects of thyroid-stimulating hormone (TSH), or cyclic periods of clinically undetectable thyroid hypofunction, with subsequent increases in TSH. Recently, thyroid growth-stimulating immunoglobulins have been identified in the sera from a large proportion of patients with simple goiters, suggesting that autoimmunity may be important. In some geographic areas, environmental pollutants may contribute to goiter development. Certain drugs, especially iodine-containing medications (e.g., amiodarone) and lithium, have been associated with goiter, particularly in individuals with underlying subclinical autoimmune thyroid disease. Not uncommonly, patients with a past history of head and neck irradiation will also develop the disease with a small diffuse or nodular goiter.

Diagnosis

Any patient presenting with either a nodular or diffuse goiter should have thyroid function tests performed, including serum thyroxine (T_4) level determination, T_3 resin uptake (T_3RU), thyrotropin (TSH) level determination, and antithyroid antibodies; serum triiodothyronine (T_3) levels should be obtained if hyperthyroidism is suspected clinically. Radioisotope scanning is indicated to rule out the presence of a dominant hypofunctioning region, particularly if a nodule is enlarging or if there is a history of head and neck irradiation. Thyroid ultrasonography is not particularly useful in the evaluation of goiter.

The presence of antithyroid antibodies and/or an elevated serum TSH is evidence for autoimmune (Hashimoto's) thyroiditis. If a dominant cold area is noted on radioisotope scan, needle biopsy is indicated, especially if there is a history of rapid growth, compressive symptoms, or radiation exposure. While nodular goiters are not premalignant, malignancy can arise in a pre-existing goiter, making detection more difficult.

Therapy

In treating the patient with a simple goiter, several factors need to be considered, including the age of the patient, the length of time the goiter has been present, the consistency of the goiter (diffuse or nodular), the patient's thyroid function, and whether there has been a recent increase in the size of the goiter.

Patients with a small diffuse goiter and normal thyroid function do not necessarily require treatment unless they find the presence of a goiter cosmetically unacceptable. If suppressive treatment with thyroid hormone is not initiated, patients are followed up initially at 6 months and then at yearly intervals to monitor the size of the thyroid gland and the potential development of nodules.

Long-term therapy with L-thyroxine (Synthroid, Levothroid) is the cornerstone of therapy for patients with simple goiters. The goal of treatment is to suppress the patient's endogenous TSH secretion and therefore to remove a potent stimulus for thyroid gland growth. In general, an L-thyroxine dose of 2 micrograms per kg is required to render circulating TSH undetectable; smaller doses should be used in the elderly. Regression of the size of the goiter occurs in about 60 percent of patients. Some goiters, however, function independently of TSH and may continue to grow even though TSH secretion is completely inhibited. Regression in the size of the gland is dependent on (1) the size of the goiter at the initiation of treatment, with large goiters showing less response, and (2) the duration of treatment, with greater regression occurring with longer treatment. A lack of response is usually due to the presence of cysts, fibrosis, and calcifications within long-standing goiters as well as the presence of foci of autonomous function. Continued growth despite suppressive therapy is an indication for biopsy or surgery because of the concern about malignancy.

In patients with one or more autonomously functioning thyroid nodules, L-thyroxine therapy may cause iatrogenic thyrotoxicosis due to continued function of the nonsuppressible nodular tissue. Because of the possibility of autonomous function within a goiter, caution must be used in starting patients on L-thyroxine, especially individuals older than 60 years of age or those with a history of cardiovascular disease. Iatrogenic thyrotoxicosis can be minimized by seeing the patient 4 weeks after the initiation of treatment for repeat thyroid function studies and by starting elderly and cardiac patients on low doses of L-thyroxine. Thyroid scanning *while the patient is taking L-thyroxine* is the best way to document the presence of autonomously functioning nodules (suppression scanning). Patients with autonomous nodules can also develop hyperthyroidism when exposed to iodide-containing medications and contrast media (jodbasedow phenomenon). These compounds should be avoided in individuals with nodular goiters.

Surgical management of simple goiter becomes necessary when the goiter is unresponsive to thyroid hormone therapy and/or becomes large enough to cause local pressure symptoms, such as shortness of breath, wheezing, dysphagia, or hoarseness, or if there is concern about malignancy. Some patients with large asymptomatic goiters may choose surgical management as the initial therapy for cosmetic reasons. Postoperative thyroid hormone is then prescribed to prevent recurrence of the goiter.

HYPERPARATHYROIDISM AND HYPOPARATHYROIDISM

method of
W. ROBERT GRAHAM, M.D., and
LEONARD J. DEFTOS, M.D.
University of California
San Diego, California

HYPERPARATHYROIDISM

The parathyroid glands act in concert with other endocrine glands to regulate skeletal and mineral metabolism. They synthesize and secrete parathyroid hormone (PTH), which mediates the mobilization of calcium from bones and enhances renal calcium reabsorption. In addition to these direct effects, PTH also stimulates the production of 1,25-dihydroxycholecalciferol (1,25-DHCC) in the kidney. The net effect of PTH is to raise the serum calcium concentration. Hyperparathyroidism results from increased serum PTH activity, and hypoparathyroidism results from decreased serum PTH activity. Both conditions are characterized by abnormalities in serum calcium concentration, and therapeutic interventions are directed at restoring this concentration to normal. However, therapeutic strategies must also take into account the underlying causes of abnormal PTH activity and the presence of coexisting diseases.

Diagnostic Considerations

Hyperparathyroidism may be divided into primary and secondary forms. *Primary hyperparathyroidism* is due to the hypersecretion of PTH by an adenomatous or hyperplastic parathyroid gland, or occasionally by a carcinoma. Primary hyperparathyroidism is thus a disease of the parathyroid glands. An elevated serum calcium level is the sine qua non of primary hyperparathyroidism. Patients may be asymptomatic or have manifestations such as renal stones, peptic ulcer disease, hypertension, pancreatitis, and skeletal demineralization. Central nervous system (CNS) manifestations may range from lethargy to coma.

Secondary hyperparathyroidism occurs when there is increased PTH secretion in response to a hypocalcemic stimulus, such as occurs in renal disease and in abnormalities of vitamin D physiology and metabolism. The increased PTH secretion may maintain the serum calcium concentration near normal by enhancing calcium mobilization from bone.

Primary and secondary hyperparathyroidism are well-defined pathophysiologic states. Less well defined is "tertiary hyperparathyroidism." This term is used to identify the consequences of a protracted and severe hypocalcemic stimulus to the parathyroid glands. The parathyroid glands become hyperplastic and "escape" from the regulatory control of serum calcium. Their excessive PTH secretion overcompensates for the hypocalcemia and produces hypercalcemia. The symptoms of hypercalcemia then become superimposed on the underlying disease initially responsible for the hypocalcemia. Tertiary hyperparathyroidism is described most commonly in patients with years of renal failure and poorly controlled secondary hyperparathyroidism, including those who undergo renal transplantation.

Therapy

Primary Hyperparathyroidism

The mainstay of therapy for primary hyperparathyroidism is surgical resection of the abnormal parathyroid tissue. In the large majority of cases, this represents removal of a single adenoma. Hyperplasia of the parathyroid glands occurs much less commonly and the occurrence of multiple adenomas is debated. Carcinoma is very rare. Once the diagnosis of primary hyperparathyroidism is established, the physician may proceed directly to surgical exploration. Alternatively, noninvasive procedures may be used in an attempt to localize the abnormal parathyroid tissue, so that the surgery can be limited to the involved side of the neck. These procedures include computed tomography (CT) scanning, ultrasonography, [^{72}Se]selenomethionine scanning, thermography, cine-esophagography, and nuclear magnetic resonance imaging (MRI). Whether these techniques will be sufficiently reliable to guide surgical resection depends on the resources and experiences of a particular institution. In many centers, preoperative localization procedures are not considered to be adequate substitutes for a skilled and experienced surgeon. In most cases, surgical removal of a single parathyroid adenoma is curative. Evaluation of the ipsilateral gland by inspection or biopsy can rule out hyperplasia. If hyperplasia is present, it will involve all glands and a subtotal parathyroidectomy is performed in which all but a small amount (50 to 100 mg) of tissue is removed. Additionally, the surgeon should identify all glands and consider the possibility that parathyroid tissue may exist in aberrant locations.

Medical therapy for symptomatic primary hyperparathyroidism has met with some success, but, in general, it is reserved for those patients who are unable or unwilling to undergo surgery. Estrogens, particularly ethinyl estradiol at a dose of 30 micrograms daily, have been used to effectively lower calcium concentrations and reduce bone resorption in postmenopausal women with primary hyperparathyroidism. Oral phosphorus can lower serum calcium levels, but increased PTH secretion may result. In addition, it may result in ectopic calcification, which makes its use potentially hazardous, although this is a more common complication of parenteral phosphorus administration.

The diphosphonates available in the United States are not useful in primary hyperparathyroidism. Some of the newer analogues are potent inhibitors of bone resorption and effectively lower calcium levels in patients with primary hyperparathyroidism as well as with malignancy. However, these drugs are still investigational, and their toxicity has not been fully evaluated. Calcitonin can lower serum calcium levels acutely, but its long-term efficacy has not been established, and its usefulness is limited by the need for parenteral administration. Cimetidine and beta-adrenergic agents have been reported to lower blood calcium in primary hyperparathyroidism, but they are not generally effective. Recently, a parathyroid hormone antagonist, [Ty-34]bPTH-(7-34)amide, was reported to inhibit the effects of PTH in experimental animals. Such antagonists hold promise for future therapy.

There is no consensus on the approach to patients with primary hyperparathyroidism who are asymptomatic. For many, their course is benign, and our ability to identify those who will become symptomatic is limited. However, the high rate of success of surgery when compared with its low rate of significant complications warrants its serious consideration for most patients with primary hyperparathyroidism. A high serum calcium concentration (set by some at greater than 11 mg per dl), excessive hypercalciuria, increased bone resorption, compromised renal function, a young age, and the female gender are each an additional impetus to surgery.

Secondary and Tertiary Hyperparathyroidism

The initial goal of therapy for secondary hyperparathyroidism is to maintain a normal serum calcium concentration. In renal failure this is accomplished by adequate dietary calcium, phosphate restriction, and the judicious use of vitamin D preparations such as 1,25-DHCC. In diseases due to decreased calcium absorption, 1,25-DHCC is the mainstay of therapy. Patients with chronic renal failure who have evidence of secondary hyperparathyroidism typically require a daily calcium intake of approximately 1.5 grams. Although doses of vitamin D in the range of 50,000 to 200,000 IU per day are recommended in some texts, great caution must be used in treating any patient with high doses of long-acting vitamin D metabolites. It is preferable to give shorter-acting metabolites whose effects can be frequently monitored. (See the discussion of hypoparathyroidism for more details of vitamin D and calcium therapy.)

If medical measures fail to control the increased PTH secretion and consequences of secondary hyperparathyroidism develop, such as severe bone pain, fractures, intractable pruritus, and cutaneous gangrene, parathyroid resection should be considered. Subtotal parathyroidectomy should also be considered in patients with symptomatic tertiary hyperparathyroidism, particularly in cases in which the hypercalcemia threatens the integrity of a transplanted kidney. Transplanting parathyroid tissue to an accessible site can be considered for some patients with secondary or tertiary hyperparathyroidism but not for primary hyperparathyroidism.

Hypercalcemia of Malignancy

Many tumors are known to cause hypercalcemia. This may be due to direct invasion and resorption of bone by the tumor. More often, however, the neoplastic cells release humoral factors that stimulate the resorption of bone, often by stimulating osteoclasts. In malignancy, the rise in serum calcium may be abrupt and severe. Initial therapy is directed at rapidly lowering the serum calcium concentration. This is first accomplished by infusing solutions such as isotonic saline, which expand the intravascular volume and increase glomerular filtration. Barring any relative contraindications, such as cardiopulmonary or renal dysfunction, 1 to 2 liters of isotonic saline may be infused over the first several hours. Once the intravascular volume has been adequately expanded, intravenous furosemide (Lasix) is given in small doses (in the range of 20 mg) to increase urinary excretion of calcium. Further Lasix and isotonic saline may be titrated to produce an adequate diuresis and lowering of the serum calcium level: roughly, 200 to 300 ml of isotonic saline per hour and doses of Lasix that cause the urinary output to run only slightly behind input. In this setting, the patient's volume status will need to be monitored closely. Careful bedside evaluation, weighing when feasible, and monitoring of the fluid balance are usually sufficient, but the use of a central venous pressure monitor may be required in difficult cases. Frequent measurements of serum electrolytes, particularly K^+ and Mg^{++}, should be performed. Once the serum calcium concentration has been lowered, the problem becomes one of maintaining it within a reasonable range.

The nature of the underlying malignancy influences the choice of therapy. In patients with multiple myeloma and certain other hematologic malignancies, prednisone, 40 to 60 mg per day, may be effective. Prednisone is not effective in solid tumors except in some patients with carcinoma of the breast. Indomethacin (Indocin), 50 mg four times daily, has been disappointing in the treatment of the hypercalcemia of malignancy. Oral phosphorus, 500 to 1500 mg per day, has been used with some success in lowering blood calcium, but it is inconvenient to administer, commonly causes gastrointestinal distress, and poses the risk of ectopic calcification. Parenteral phosphate therapy can be very effective, but it carries a considerable risk of ectopic calcification. Salmon calcitonin (Calcimar), administered as 100 to 200 units subcutaneously every 12 hours, is often initially successful in lowering the blood calcium level. However, its use is limited by the rapid development of resistance to its hypocalcemic action. The concomitant use of glucocorticosteroids may enhance the action of calcitonin. Plicamycin (mithramycin), 25 micrograms per kg given as an intravenous infusion, can be very effective in lowering the serum calcium concentration for several days to a week following its administration. However, the need for an intravenous infusion and hematologic and hepatorenal complications make its long-term use difficult. Dichloromethylene diphosphonate, 5 mg per kg per day, or aminohydroxypropylidine diphosphonate, 30 mg per day, effectively lowers serum calcium concentrations when given as an intravenous infusion. These and other new diphosphonate analogues hold promise for treating hypercalcemia, but none has been approved for general use in the United States.

HYPOPARATHYROIDISM

Hypoparathyroidism is characterized by decreased serum PTH activity resulting in hypocalcemia and hyperphosphatemia. Several pathogenic mechanisms explain this low PTH activity: reduced secretion of PTH by the parathyroid glands, resistance of the target organs to the actions of PTH, and production of a nonfunctional hormone. When reduced secretion is encountered, it may result from surgical or, more rarely, radiational ablation of the parathyroid glands; from idiopathic destruction of the glands (which may be associated with autoimmune destruction of other glands); or from factors that interfere with PTH release such as a magnesium deficiency. Production of a nonfunctional hormone is a rare entity; it may occur in some patients with pseudohypoparathyroidism in whom a PTH inhibitor has been postulated. However, pseudohypoparathyroidism classically refers to hypoparathyroidism that is caused by an inability of the target organs to respond to PTH. In some cases, this target organ resistance is due to abnormal guanine nucleotide binding protein (G or N protein) activity. The G protein activity is responsible for coupling the PTH-generated extracellular signal to the intracellular cyclic adenosine monophosphate (cAMP) response. In one form of pseudohypoparathyroidism, known as Albright's hereditary osteodystrophy, the patient has typical phenotypic features: short stature, round face, short thick neck, obesity, low intelligence, subcutaneous calcification, and bony abnormalities (shortening of the metacarpals and metatarsals). The cells from patients with Albright's hereditary osteodystrophy exhibit abnormal G protein activity. Laboratory evaluation is required to distinguish the various forms of hypoparathyroidism. A low or undetectable PTH level in the face of hypocalcemia indicates PTH deficiency, whereas an elevated or normal PTH level suggests target organ resistance. The diagnosis of PTH deficiency may be confirmed by demonstrating an adequate rise in urinary cAMP following administration of PTH.

The signs and symptoms of hypoparathyroidism are primarily attributable to the hypocalcemia. Neuromuscular irritability is one of the earliest signs of hypocalcemia. At the bedside, this irritability may be elicited by demonstrating Chvostek's sign or Trousseau's sign. Patients may have cataracts; dry, flaky skin; coarse hair; and sparse eyebrows. Severe hypocalcemia may produce an altered mental status or seizures.

Therapy

Restoration of the serum calcium concentration is the main goal of therapy in patients with hypoparathyroidism. A secondary goal, which may aid the first one, is to decrease a high phosphorus concentration when it is present. Blood calcium should be maintained close to the normal range. However, it should be kept in mind that the patient with decreased PTH activity is at increased risk for hypercalciuria; therefore, the physician should attempt to maintain the patient's calcium level near the lower limit of the normal range. Dietary supplementation with elemental calcium may be all that is required to achieve eucalcemia. Calcium gluconate and calcium carbonate are the most commonly used oral preparations; 1 to 2 grams should be given daily in four divided doses. Although milk products contain abundant calcium, their use is limited by their lactose content and their high phosphorus content. If the patient remains hypocalcemic in spite of a reasonable intake of oral calcium, a vitamin D preparation should be added. Ergocalciferol (vitamin D_2) and cholecalciferol (vitamin D_3) are commonly used vitamin D preparations. They are inexpensive but must be given cautiously because their prolonged half-life may dispose the patient to hypercalcemia and hypercalciuria. Effective doses of vitamin D can be variable, and frequent monitoring of both blood and urinary calcium should be performed, especially during the early phases of therapy. Doses may range from 25,000 units of vitamin D twice a week to 100,000 units per day. The need for high doses should signal the possibility of resistance to the action of the hormone. 1,25-DHCC, the biologically active metabolite of vitamin D_3, and dihydrotachysterol (DHT), a monohydroxylated analogue of vitamin D, are therapeutically advantageous because of their relatively short half-lives, but are more expensive when compared with the long-acting preparations. Also known as calcitriol, 1,25-DHCC is given in doses ranging from 0.25 to 5 micrograms per day, and DHT is given in doses ranging from 0.2 to 1 mg per day. The use of phosphate-binding gels should be considered in the hyperphosphatemic patient.

Thiazide diuretics to conserve renal calcium have a disadvantageous benefit to risk ratio.

For treating acute and severe hypocalcemia, calcium must be given intravenously. For emergencies, as may occur following parathyroid surgery, approximately 200 mg of elemental calcium diluted in 50 to 100 ml of D5W should be infused over 10 minutes. Intravenous preparations of elemental calcium include calcium chloride (a 10-ml ampule contains 272 mg elemental calcium), calcium gluceptate (a 5-ml ampule contains 90 mg elemental calcium), and calcium gluconate (a 10-ml ampule contains 90 mg elemental calcium). Intravenous calcium must be given cautiously in digitalized patients or those with underlying cardiovascular disease. If necessary, intravenous calcium can be continued at an approximate rate of 500 mg per 24 hours in order to maintain the serum calcium close to normal. Every attempt should be made to wean the patient from calcium in order not to suppress parathyroid gland function. For similar reasons, vitamin D therapy should be reserved for only the most persistent hypocalcemia.

Magnesium deficiency can produce hypocalcemia by decreasing PTH secretion or interfering with its biological effects. Replenishing the magnesium deficit restores parathyroid activity. Magnesium deficiency is primarily seen in the hospitalized alcoholic, and measurements of the serum magnesium concentration should be performed in these patients. However, because magnesium is primarily an intracellular cation, significant magnesium deficiency may exist in the presence of a normal serum magnesium level. If hypocalcemia is encountered in a patient who is likely to have a deficiency of magnesium, cautious replacement may be initiated in spite of a normal serum level. Elemental magnesium is generally given as magnesium sulfate by intramuscular or intravenous administration. There are intramuscular preparations of $MgSO_4$ that can be given at doses of 8 to 16 mEq every 4 to 6 hours. However, because these patients are often volume depleted and require isotonic saline, it is convenient to begin initial therapy by adding one or two ampules of magnesium sulfate (one ampule is 2 ml, which contains 8.1 mEq of elemental magnesium) to the first liter of isotonic saline and infuse it over 4 to 6 hours for several days. Up to 100 mEq per day may be given. The extent of magnesium replacement, however, should be guided by the response of the serum calcium and magnesium. It must be emphasized that magnesium should be given cautiously in patients with renal compromise.

HYPOPITUITARISM

method of
ANDREW G. FRANTZ, M.D.
*Columbia University College of Physicians
and Surgeons
New York, New York*

Hypopituitarism is defined as a deficiency of one or more anterior pituitary hormones. It is important to remember that pituitary disease of any kind can result in deficiencies that are single or multiple and that virtually any combination of deficiencies may coexist. With some hormone-secreting tumors (e.g., with prolactinomas or with adenomas causing acromegaly), excess production of one hormone may be accompanied by deficiencies of others. In practice, gonadotropin deficiency is among the most commonly encountered. Growth hormone deficiency may also be shown by stimulation tests in many patients with pituitary disease, although its diagnosis is not clinically important in the adult because no replacement therapy is currently given to adults. Somewhat less frequently encountered are clinical deficiencies of adrenocorticotropic hormone (ACTH) and thyroid-stimulating hormone (TSH), although with these disorders, the diagnosis is of clinical importance because of the necessity of instituting therapy. Prolactin deficiency occurs very rarely, and replacement therapy is not given for this condition.

Pituitary tumors are among the commonest causes of hypopituitarism in adults. Treatment of the mass lesion itself by surgery, radiotherapy, or tumor-shrinking drugs (e.g., bromocriptine for prolactinomas) may infrequently correct a deficiency of a tropic hormone that was caused by compression of the gland itself or the stalk. Prolactin reduction may also correct a functional defect in gonadotropin secretion caused by hyperprolactinemia. The decision to treat hypopituitarism is made by careful assessment of each of the individual hormones. It must also be remembered that with mass lesions, hypopituitarism not present initially may develop gradually over the course of months or years either as a result of progression of the lesion itself or as a late result of treatment, especially after radiotherapy.

GONADOTROPIN DEFICIENCY

Hypogonadotropic hypogonadism could in theory be treated by giving either gonadotropins or gonadal steroids. In practice, except when fertility is desired, gonadal steroids are always chosen for reasons of convenience and expense.

Males

Testosterone administered orally is ineffective because of rapid degradation and inactivation by the liver. Derivatives have been synthesized that resist degradation; all of these oral preparations carry a small risk of causing cholestatic jaundice, which is reversible on discontinuation of the drug. The oral replacement dose for an adult male with 17α-methyltestosterone (Oreton Methyl, Metandren, Neo-Hombreol-M) is 20 to 50 mg per day (e.g., 10 to 25 mg twice daily). A buccal tablet, to be dissolved slowly in the cheek pouch and not swallowed, is said to be about twice as effective as the oral preparation and should therefore be given in half the above dose; some individuals find this route of administration annoying. Fluoxymesterone (Halotestin, Ultandren, Ora-Testryl) is another androgen about as effective as methyltestosterone and should be given orally in total doses of 10 to 20 mg per day, preferably twice daily.

In my experience the oral androgens are frequently not as effective as one could wish, and I prefer the administration of a long-acting testosterone ester intramuscularly. Testosterone enanthate (Delatestryl) and testosterone cypionate (Depo-Testosterone) are available in sesame oil preparation of 200 and 100 mg per ml. Maximal effects are produced by administering 400 mg intramuscularly every 2 weeks, and it is probably never necessary to exceed this dose for replacement therapy. Administration of 200 mg every 2 weeks or 300 mg every 3 weeks provides an adequate replacement dose for most men.

Side effects of androgen therapy include variable degrees of fluid retention, sometimes seen as worsening of pre-existing congestive heart failure; gynecomastia, which may regress with continued therapy; and male pattern baldness in individuals genetically predisposed. With oral preparations, in addition to cholestatic jaundice, peliosis hepatis (blood-filled cysts of the liver) and hepatoma have rarely been noted.

In treating previously virilized males who have become hypogonadal, I generally start out with full doses of parenteral steroids. Therapy may then be tapered somewhat to what seems a satisfactory dose, depending on degree of libido and sexual performance. For reasons of convenience, one may experiment at this point with oral androgens if the patient so desires, but he should be advised that they may be less effective. In inducing virilization for the first time in a patient who has failed to go through a normal puberty, it is generally desirable to proceed at a slower rate because of profound and potentially unsettling psychic changes that may accompany too rapid virilization. In young men with concomitant growth hormone deficiency whose epiphyses are unfused and who are short, one may also wish to use low doses or to defer therapy pending the use of growth hormone. The object in this case is to achieve as much statural growth as possible before epiphyseal closure occurs.

Not all male hypogonadism requires treatment. Patients often make what are to them satisfactory long-term adjustments to reduced or absent libido. Disturbance of a long-established pattern by the induction of desires that the patient is ill equipped to fulfill may do him a real disservice. Such therapy should be undertaken only after careful consideration and discussion with the patient. Finally, it should be mentioned that impotence due to hypogonadism of long duration, particularly that associated with pituitary tumors, may be quite resistant to androgenic replacement therapy; sometimes there is no therapy that is entirely satisfactory for these patients.

Fertility is rarely restored in hypogonadotropic males by treatment with androgens alone, but prior use of androgens does not impair the subsequent effectiveness of gonadotropin therapy. The usual approach is therefore to use androgens until the point at which fertility is actively sought. At this time treatment is changed to parenteral hCG (human chorionic gonadotropin, a lutenizing hormone–like preparation of placental origin derived from pregnancy urine), which is given three times weekly for many weeks to months. In some cases this is adequate to initiate spermatogenesis, but additional parenteral therapy with a preparation having follicle-stimulating hormone (FSH) activity (Pergonal, derived from the urine of postmenopausal women) is usually also required. Treatment may be necessary for as long as 6 to 12 months, is expensive, and on the whole is less successful than corresponding treatment to induce fertility in women.

In both men and women with hypogonadotropism due to hypothalamic deficiency (who constitute the majority of those with "idiopathic" hypogonadotropism), considerable success has recently been achieved in inducing fertility by means of luteinizing hormone–releasing hormone (LHRH) delivered subcutaneously in pulsatile fashion by means of a special pump.

Females

Young women in the premenopausal age range who are clearly hypogonadal should usually be treated, with the object of preventing premature osteoporosis, maintaining normal secondary sex characteristics and skin texture, and possibly reducing susceptibility to coronary artery disease. Low cyclic doses of estrogen should be used, as well as a progestational agent to ensure normal withdrawal bleeding. A satisfactory regimen is either 10 to 20 µg of ethinyl estradiol (Estinyl) or 0.625 to 1.25 mg of conjugated estrogens (Premarin) once a day for the first 25 days of each month. An oral progestin such as medroxy-progesterone acetate (Provera), 10 mg, is then given once a day for days 16 through 25 inclusive.

Side effects of estrogens that have been reported when they are used for birth control purposes include edema, a somewhat increased risk of thromboembolic disease as well as of endometrial cancer, hypertension, hepatic adenoma, and hepatocellular carcinoma. These risks are small, and it is unclear whether they even exist to a significant degree when estrogen is used in low doses as suggested for replacement in hypogonadotropic hypogonadism. Recently, a transdermal form of estrogen (Estraderm) has become available to be applied to the skin as a patch twice weekly. It may decrease some of these risks still further, as a result of bypassing the liver after absorption, but whether it has advantages over oral estrogen for the treatment of hypopituitarism is uncertain.

Libido may be depressed in women with hypopituitarism, and if so, it is usually not restored with estrogens alone. In women who complain of diminished libido, a trial of low-dose androgen therapy, e.g., 25 mg of testosterone enanthate (Delatestryl) or testosterone cypionate (Depo-Testosterone) intramuscularly every 4 to 6 weeks, may be worthwhile. There is danger, however, in the use of androgens because women who respond favorably may want to continue them indefinitely; prolonged use even at these low dose levels may lead to irreversible deepening of the voice as well as hirsutism, clitoromegaly, and acne. The physician should be alert to these changes and should discuss the possibility of them in advance with the patient.

Fertility in women with hypopituitarism, if desired, is usually brought about with the use of exogenous gonadotropins. The length of treatment required is shorter, and the success rate is considerably higher than when these agents are used for men, as mentioned previously. Because of the risks involved, which include the ovarian hyperstimulation syndrome and multiple births, such treatment should be undertaken only by physicians familiar with this form of therapy.

ACTH DEFICIENCY

Hypoadrenocorticism, when present in patients with hypopituitarism, is seldom as severe as that seen in patients with Addison's disease or after bilateral adrenalectomy. Glucocorticoid production, although impaired, usually persists to some degree. Furthermore, since aldosterone production is not primarily under ACTH control, replacement mineralocorticoid is rarely required.

Hydrocortisone production rate in the normal adult is of the order of 15 to 20 mg per day, and this defines the usual replacement dose. I prefer to give either hydrocortisone, 10 mg twice daily, or cortisone acetate, 12.5 mg (one-half tablet) twice daily. A higher dosage than this is rarely necessary in hypopituitarism. Some argument could be made for giving more of the total dose in the morning and less in the late afternoon, to mimic more closely the normal secretory pattern, but the above regimens are usually satisfactory. Prednisone, 2.5 mg twice daily, may also be given. Occasionally, a patient with hypopituitarism may appear to be borderline with respect to the need for steroid replacement. On such occasions I sometimes give hydrocortisone, 5 mg twice a day, or 10 mg in the morning and 5 mg in the afternoon. Hypothyroidism, if present in the patient with hypopituitarism, may diminish the need for steroid replacement by slowing the degradation of circulating steroids. Under these circumstances, treatment of the hypothyroidism may necessitate the simultaneous institution of glucocorticoid therapy. In all cases, patients should be advised to increase their steroids to double or triple the usual daily dose in the event of unusual stress or minor febrile illnesses. They should be in touch with their physician at once in case of severe illness, and if any delay in securing medical help is anticipated, particularly in the event of severe vomiting, they or a family member should be provided with an injectable form of steroid such as dexamethasone sodium phosphate (Decadron), available as 4 mg in 1.0 ml in a disposable syringe, to be taken intramuscularly. This may be repeated after 6 to 8 hours if a doctor is not available. Patients with hypoadrenocorticism should also wear a medical information bracelet or necklace with information about their condition. Such devices are obtainable from the Medic-Alert Foundation International, P.O. Box 1009, Turlock, CA 95381-1009 (telephone 1-800-344-3226). In the event of severe or life-threatening infections or stress, including major surgery, hospitalized patients with hypopituitarism should be treated like addisonian patients, with large total daily steroid doses of the order of 300 mg per day of hydrocortisone equivalents given intravenously or intramuscularly in divided doses. Therapy is frequently initiated with a bolus dose such as 4 mg of dexamethasone phosphate intravenously (or sometimes intramuscularly, in preparation for operation) followed by 100 mg of hydrocortisone sodium succinate (Solu-Cortef) every 6 to 8 hours by slow intravenous drip.

TSH DEFICIENCY

Sodium L-thyroxine is the drug of choice for treating hypothyroidism. The daily replacement is 50 to 200 micrograms, given as a single oral dose, with 150 micrograms being appropriate for the majority of both older children and younger adults. In these individuals, therapy may be started directly with this dose. In older patients, and particularly in those with coronary artery disease, a lower starting dose should be used, generally not more than 50 micrograms per day and sometimes as low as 25 micrograms or even 12.5 micrograms if angina is present and severe. This can be increased in 25- to 50-microgram increments every 3 to 4 weeks, depending on the clinical response and the serum thyroxine (T_4) measurements. With optimum therapy the serum T_4 will generally be at the upper end of the normal range and may even slightly exceed it in some cases. Serum triiodothyronine (T_3) will be normal, however, unless the patient is being overtreated. It has been shown that when L-thyroxine therapy is substituted for desiccated thyroid in a dose that is therapeutically equivalent, serum T_4 will rise by approximately 3 micrograms per dl, and serum T_3 (which may have been elevated on desiccated thyroid therapy) will fall. For practical purposes, serum T_3 measurements are usually unnecessary, particularly if the patient feels well and serum T_4 is not elevated.

As noted previously, consideration should be given to the possible need for instituting, or increasing the dose of, glucocorticoid therapy when L-thyroxine therapy is begun in hypopituitary patients, who may have defects of ACTH secretion as well as of TSH.

GROWTH HORMONE DEFICIENCY

Growth hormone deficiency in hypopituitarism is not treated unless the patient is of short stature and the long bone epiphyses are unfused. If these conditions exist, however, growth rates approximating those of a normal child may be achieved with parenteral growth hormone therapy. Growth hormone obtained from cadaver pituitaries is no longer available in the United States because of the development of Creutzfeldt-Jakob disease in a small number of patients after long-term treatment with this preparation. Two human growth hormone preparations made biosynthetically by recombinant DNA techniques (Protropin and Humatrope) are currently available. The usual dose is in the range of 0.1 to 0.2 IU per kg, given intramuscularly three times a week. Therapy is expensive and must be continued for many months to years. It is desirable to withhold sex hormone therapy and to treat concomitant ACTH deficiency, if the latter is present, with the minimum necessary dose of glucocorticoid, in order to prevent steroid antagonism of growth hormone action.

HYPERPROLACTINEMIA

method of
CHARLES FOUAD ABBOUD, M.B., B.Ch.
Mayo Medical School
Rochester, Minnesota

Prolactin is a polypeptide hormone produced by the anterior pituitary lactotroph. Its secretion is under dominant hypothalamic inhibitory regulation, primarily by dopamine.

Hyperprolactinemia expresses itself clinically by galactogenic effect on the breasts, suppressive effect on the hypothalamic-pituitary-gonadal axis, and stimulatory effect on androgen production by the adrenal cortex. The clinical manifestations of hyperprolactinemia are outlined in Table 1.

Hyperprolactinemia can be either physiologic or pathologic in origin. *Physiologic hyperprolactinemia* is seen in pregnancy, postpartum state, stress, and in response to acute medical or surgical illness. *Pathologic hyperprolactinemia* is almost always caused by excessive prolactin secretion by the pituitary lactotroph. This is usually due to primary pituitary disease (pituitary tumors, empty sella, hypophysitis), or it may be secondary to hypothalamic stalk disease with consequent loss of dopaminergic inhibition. Very rarely, hyperprolactinemia can result from ectopic prolactin production by hypernephroma or bronchogenic carcinoma.

Prolactinomas, prolactin-producing pituitary tumors, comprise 60 to 70 per cent of all pituitary tumors and are the most common organic cause of hyperprolactinemia. They are variable in size and in extent: Tumors less than 1 cm in diameter are called microadenomas, and those more than 1 cm in diameter are called macroadenomas. Macroprolactinomas may be confined to the sella or may have extrasellar extension. Prolactinomas are preponderantly benign. The natural history of microprolactinoma is unknown, but it is believed that at least a few will increase in size and become macroprolactinomas. The sex distribution of prolactinomas is approximately equal, although microprolactinomas are found much more commonly in young females, presumably because of earlier recognition of the endocrine consequences of hyperprolactinemia.

Hyperprolactinemia may occur with other pituitary tumors. Functioning pituitary tumors may produce more than one pituitary hormone, and hyperprolactinemia has been noted in some patients with acromegaly or Cushing's syndrome. Alternatively, a nonfunctioning tumor may be associated with hyperprolactinemia if it has a suprasellar extension impinging on the pituitary stalk or hypothalamus and interfering with hypothalamic inhibition of prolactin secretion.

Hypothalamic hyperprolactinemia may be functional (related to use of drugs, chest wall and spinal disorders, renal/hepatic failure, and primary hypothyroidism) or organic (related to structural diverse pathologic states such as traumatic, inflammatory/infiltrative, vascular, and neoplastic disorders).

The clinical steps in the diagnostic approach to hyperprolactinemia include (1) serum prolactin levels, (2) a careful drug history and general medical evaluation to exclude functional causes (drugs, chest wall lesion, primary hypothyroidism, chronic renal/hepatic failure), (3) serum thyroxin and thyroid-stimulating hormone (TSH) levels to exclude primary hypothyroidism, (4) computed tomographic/magnetic resonance imaging scans of the pituitary region, visual fields, and pituitary function tests to delineate organic hypothalamic pituitary disease. The two most common diagnostic entities are prolactinomas and idiopathic hyperprolactinemia.

Idiopathic hyperprolactinemia refers to those patients in whom no discernible cause for the hyperprolactinemia is found after a thorough evaluation. Follow-up is critical in these patients, since some of them may harbor microprolactinomas or other hypothalamic pituitary space-occupying lesions that are too small to be detected by our present radiologic techniques.

TREATMENT

The primary objective of management is to identify and to treat the underlying cause. If the cause is not identifiable or cannot be effectively removed or reversed, then management is directed at the treatment of the hyperprolactinemia itself.

Resolution of hyperprolactinemia due to an identifiable disorder can be achieved, for example, by discontinuation of an offending drug, thyroid hormone replacement therapy in a patient with primary hypothyroidism, renal transplantation in a patient with chronic severe irreversible renal failure, or surgical/radiotherapeutic ablation of tumors in or around the pituitary area.

The objectives of treatment of hyperprolactin-

TABLE 1. **Clinical Manifestations of Hyperprolactinemia**

Female
Galactorrhea
Ovulatory and menstrual dysfunction
Short luteal phase
Anovulation, infertility
Oligo/amenorrhea, hypoestrogenism
Hyperandrogenicity
Hirsutism
Acne
Decreased libido
Male
Libido and potency impairment
Oligospermia, infertility
Galactorrhea, gynecomastia (rare)
Both sexes
Delayed puberty

emia include (1) the achievement of fertility in a patient who has hyperprolactinemia-related infertility; (2) reversal of hypogonadism and recovery of sexual and gonadal functions (in the long run this prevents the development of osteoporosis and premature coronary heart disease); (3) correction of galactorrhea, which may be copious or continuous and interfering with the patient's quality of life; and (4) compliance with the desire for reassurance by the informed patient who is apprehensive about potential growth of an underlying tumor or the long-term effects of hyperprolactinemia.

Prolactinomas

The goals of therapy of prolactinomas are (1) to treat the tumor and to correct or to prevent its anatomic complications, (2) to normalize prolactin secretion and to reverse or to prevent its clinical effects, (3) to maintain or to restore normal pituitary functions, (4) to prevent tumor recurrence, and (5) to achieve all of these objectives with no mortality or morbidity.

The current options for therapy of prolactinomas include bromocriptine, surgery, and radiation therapy. Although no single mode of therapy presently available can achieve all the therapeutic objectives, in most patients these therapeutic modalities singly or in combination can control the disease adequately and safely.

Bromocriptine (Parlodel), the only dopamine agonist presently approved for clinical use in the United States, is a semisynthetic ergot derivative. It is administered orally, and its duration of action is 8 to 12 hours. It has a direct effect on the lactotrophs, binding to their dopamine receptors and resulting in suppression of prolactin secretion and synthesis.

Bromocriptine suppresses prolactin secretion in 80 to 90 per cent of patients wih hyperprolactinemia regardless of the etiology. This suppression leads to reversal of the manifestations of hyperprolactinemia, and the beneficial effects include increased libido, resolution of galactorrhea, and normalization of gonadal function. In addition, in patients with prolactinomas, it has an antineoplastic effect that results in tumor shrinkage in 60 to 75 per cent of treated patients. The size of reduction in the tumor averages 50 to 70 per cent and is caused by a decrease in both nuclear and cytoplasmic size.

The main side effects encountered with bromocriptine therapy include anorexia, nausea, and vomiting in about 50 per cent of patients; postural hypotension, headaches, and nasal stuffiness in about 20 per cent of patients; and depression and peripheral vasospasm in 10 to 15 per cent of patients. Most of these symptoms are transient and disappear within a few days of the onset of treatment; in a few patients, however, they persist and preclude continued use of the drug. Rarely, in less than 1 to 2 per cent of patients, psychotic reactions occur that are schizophrenic-like; these do occur in patients with and without prior psychiatric history.

To minimize these side effects, bromocriptine therapy is started with a low dose, which is increased gradually to reach the lowest effective dose. The drug is always administered with food. I usually start therapy with 1.25 mg of bromocriptine given at bedtime with food and increase the dose by 1.25 mg at weekly intervals to reach a dose of 2.5 mg twice a day. At that time I check serum prolactin levels, and if hyperprolactinemia persists, I increase the dose of bromocriptine further and gradually until the serum prolactin is normalized or until side effects become the limiting factor. The usual effective dose is 5 to 7.5 mg per day, although doses as low as 1.25 mg and as high as 20 mg per day* may be needed in some patients. Drug interactions are few: Antidopaminergic drugs may interfere with the effect of bromocriptine on the lactotroph, and estrogen can increase prolactin production by a direct effect on the lactotroph.

It is important to remember that the therapeutic effects of bromocriptine are limited to the period of drug use. Discontinuation of the drug is followed, in most patients, by resumption of hyperprolactinemia, and in those patients with prolactinoma, by regrowth of the pituitary tumor. Therefore, in the management of prolactinomas, use of bromocriptine in most patients has to be on a long-term, indefinite basis. Bromocriptine has been available worldwide for approximately 15 years and in the United States for approximately 8 years; its long-term effects, therefore, are unknown.

Surgery. Craniotomy via the transfrontal approach is employed only for tumors with considerable parasellar and suprasellar extension. Otherwise, the preferred surgical approach is transsphenoidal selective adenomectomy. Neurosurgical expertise, modern fluoroscopic and microsurgical technique, and perioperative endocrine support have made such a surgical approach safe and effective. Mortality is less than 1 per cent and is seen only with large invasive tumors and with management by inexperienced physicians. Morbidity, which varies between 1 and 5 per cent and also depends on the expertise of the neurosurgeon, includes cerebral spinal fluid (CSF) rhinorrhea, bacterial or aseptic meningitis,

---

*This dose exceeds the manufacturer's recommended dose.

hemorrhage, permanent diabetes insipidus, sinusitis, central nervous system (CNS) damage, and the development of secondary empty sella.

Radiotherapy. Radiotherapy has received less attention and favor because of the effectiveness of the alternatives of bromocriptine and transsphenoidal microsurgery and because of the concern for possible postradiation damage to anterior pituitary function, especially the gonadal axis in patients of reproductive age. Radiotherapy can be used as primary therapy or as an adjunct to surgery in patients who refuse, cannot tolerate, or fail bromocriptine therapy, or it can be used in those patients with postoperative persistent disease.

Radiotherapy is administered most commonly via conventional (supervoltage) radiation, whereby 4000 to 5000 rad are delivered in 4 to 5 weeks or via heavy particle (proton beam and alpha particle) radiation (currently available in only a few centers with the cyclotron), in which the radiation dose is delivered in 1 day. Stereotactic implantation of ^{90}Y pellets, although an effective alternative, has been abandoned because of the frequency of complications, including improper placement of the pellets and CSF rhinorrhea.

Radiotherapy leads to a slow and progressive fall in serum prolactin. Arrest of tumor growth is seen in the majority of patients. The disadvantages of radiotherapy are (1) long latent period; (2) frequent occurrence of hypopituitarism, estimated between 20 and 50 per cent in 10 years; (3) very infrequently damage to the surrounding structures; (4) rarely increased risk of acute swelling of the tumor during the administration of the therapy; (5) occasional occurrence of pituitary apoplexy following therapy; (6) occasional development of secondary empty sella and prolapse of the optic chiasm into the sella and development of chiasmal syndrome; and (7) very rarely the occurrence of sarcoma or brain necrosis. Radiotherapy is contraindicated in patients with more than minimal suprasellar extension for fear of damage to the optic pathways and other brain structures.

Microprolactinomas

Accumulating evidence over the past decade indicates that in most women microprolactinomas will show stability in endocrine and growth potential, at least over a 10- to 15-year period of observation. Only 4 to 5 per cent of patients with microprolactinomas will show increase in the size of the tumor over this period of follow-up. At present, however, it is not possible to identify which patients will show progression to a macroprolactinoma. If the patient has a microprolacti-

noma and no significant endocrine effects from the hyperprolactinemia, observation without active treatment is an option. If that option is chosen, the patient is monitored closely, with serum prolactin levels evaluated every 6 to 12 months and with a radiologic study of the sella (CT or MRI scanning) every 1 to 2 years.

The need for active treatment of a patient with a microprolactinoma is based on the need for management of hyperprolactinemia and the desirability of preventing possible effects of tumor expansion.

Selective transsphenoidal microadenomectomy is widely available. In experienced anesthetic and neurosurgical hands it carries an overall mortality of 0.03 per cent and morbidity of 0 to 2 per cent. Microadenomectomy gives an initial cure rate of 70 to 85 per cent; patients with smaller tumors and with prolactin levels less than 200 ng per ml have the most favorable results. The reported incidence of recurrence of hyperprolactinemia varies between 0 and 50 per cent, with most authorities reporting a 15 to 20 per cent incidence. The true recurrence of identifiable tumor is very low (less than 3 per cent) over the first 10 to 15 years of follow-up. The options of therapy for patients who have persistent or recurrent hyperprolactinemia following transsphenoidal microadenomectomy are bromocriptine or postoperative pituitary irradiation and interim bromocriptine therapy.

Pharmacologic Therapy. The advantages of bromocriptine in the management of microprolactinomas are suppression of hyperprolactinemia and reversal of its manifestations in 80 to 90 per cent of patients and shrinkage of the tumor mass. But bromocriptine has the following disadvantages:

1. If bromocriptine is discontinued, prolactin returns to pretreatment levels in 2 to 4 months in almost all patients, and the tumor resumes its potential for growth. This lack of permanent effect necessitates continual administration of the drug; there is at present no information available about the potential adverse effects of chronic lifelong therapy.

2. Most patients will need 5 to 7.5 mg of bromocriptine per day for achievement of the therapeutic goals; this translates into a cost of $50 to $75 per month.

3. Escape from the side effects of bromocriptine occurs but is rare; all bromocriptine-treated patients should have serum prolactin levels checked every year and a radiologic study (CT or MRI scanning) done every 2 years or earlier should it be deemed necessary by the development of symptoms and signs suggestive of tumor growth.

4. If fertility is restored and the patient wishes to conceive, certain considerations apply as discussed later in this article.

Spontaneous infarction of the pituitary tumor leads to resolution of the tumor and associated hyperprolactinemia. This is estimated to occur in less than 5 per cent of patients with microprolactinoma; therefore, bromocriptine needs to be stopped every 1 to 2 years. If hyperprolactinemia recurs, therapy is reinstituted.

In patients who choose bromocriptine as their primary treatment, transsphenoidal microadenomectomy may become necessary if the patient becomes drug intolerant because of significant side effects or becomes drug resistant (i.e., no change in prolactin levels or in the size of the tumor during therapy), if the desired goals of therapy are not achieved, and if the patient refuses to take the drug for a long time because of cost or fear of ill health.

Radiotherapy. Radiotherapy is effective in 30 to 50 per cent of patients and leads to a slow and progressive fall in the level of the serum prolactin. It may take 2 to 10 years or more for serum prolactin levels to reach normal. Bromocriptine can be used as interim therapy in the interval while awaiting the beneficial effects of radiotherapy; it is stopped periodically to determine whether resolution of hyperprolactinemia and its many manifestations have occurred.

The decision as to which therapeutic option will be used in a particular patient with microprolactinoma will depend upon a frank, thorough discussion with the patient of each therapeutic option and its implications. The patient should make an informed decision.

Macroprolactinoma

The presence of a macroprolactinoma dictates active treatment. Therapeutic objectives include the treatment of the tumor mass, restoration of gonadal function, and the restoration or maintenance of normal pituitary function. Observation is not a management option for patients with macroprolactinomas.

Bromocriptine can correct the hyperprolactinemia (80 to 90 per cent), reduce tumor size (60 per cent), reverse neurophthalmologic impairment (90 per cent), and, in some patients, restore anterior pituitary endocrine function (10 to 20 per cent). Significant reduction in tumor size may occur rapidly in 1 to 3 weeks or may be slow, taking 6 months or even up to 12 months before maximum effect is achieved. It is not possible to predict which patient will respond to medical therapy. Careful and repeated neurophthalmologic evaluation during bromocriptine therapy is essential. Deterioration of visual function is a call for aborting the pharmacologic trial and for prompt neurosurgical decompression. There is no correlation between size reduction and prolactin levels before and during drug therapy. Decreases in serum prolactin levels always precede reduction in the size of the tumor. However, tumor involution does not always correlate with the degree of fall in serum prolactin.

Because of these very satisfactory results, many authorities regard long-term bromocriptine therapy as the treatment of choice for macroprolactinomas. If such an option is chosen as definitive therapy, bromocriptine is continued indefinitely. Alternatively, surgery or radiotherapy can be pursued later.

When bromocriptine therapy is stopped, hyperprolactinemia recurs in a few weeks to a few months, often to levels substantially less than pretreatment values, and the tumor resumes its anatomic growth, usually but not always returning to its original size. This tumor reexpansion may occur rapidly, and extreme caution needs to be exercised during bromocriptine withdrawal.

Surgery. Transsphenoidal surgery is the usual surgical approach; transfrontal surgery is employed only for tumors with massive suprasellar or parasellar extension. In comparison with surgical management of microprolactinomas, the surgical results in patients with macroprolactinomas are poor (25 to 40 per cent), the recurrence rates are high (20 to 80 per cent), and the morbidity and mortality rates are higher (about 10 per cent and 1 per cent, respectively). It is clear that surgical management of macroprolactinomas is not for cure but for debulking of the tumor to decrease the size and reverse its extrasellar effects.

Most authorities recommend preoperative bromocriptine for a period of a few weeks to a few months in an attempt to reduce tumor size preoperatively and to improve the surgical result. For patients with persistent postoperative disease, bromocriptine therapy or radiotherapy and interim bromocriptine is recommended. Radiotherapy is indicated if a large volume of the tumor remains, if the tumor is nonresponsive to bromocriptine, or if the tumor is invasive or aggressive in its behavior.

Radiotherapy. Radiotherapy can be used as primary or as adjunctive therapy. Reduction of hyperprolactinemia, which occurs in almost all patients, is gradual and slow and may take years to achieve. Normoprolactinemia is restored in about 30 per cent of patients.

It is important to remember that if the patient has a sellar mass with suprasellar extension and a serum prolactin level that is mild to modestly elevated, the mass is definitely not a prolactinoma. It could be a nonfunctioning pituitary tumor or another mass lesion (e.g., craniopharyngioma or meningioma). The treatment options are surgery or radiotherapy. Bromocriptine may suppress the hyperprolactinemia but does not have any antineoplastic effect on these tumors.

Bromocriptine Therapy and Pregnancy

Restoration of normal gonadal function by bromocriptine in hyperprolactinemic women implies restoration of fertility potential. If the patient does not desire fertility, mechanical contraception should be used. If the patient desires fertility, several important points need to be emphasized:

1. Usage of the drug to achieve ovulation and pregnancy has not been associated with increased incidence of fetal loss or congenital anomalies.

2. The drug should be discontinued as soon as possible after the diagnosis of pregnancy is made; to ensure early diagnosis of pregnancy after institution of bromocriptine, the patient should use a mechanical contraceptive until the regular menstrual cycle is established for at least 3 months before attempting pregnancy. At the first missed period, bromocriptine should be stopped and a pregnancy test performed.

3. In patients with underlying pituitary tumor, pregnancy can lead to increased rate of growth of the tumor, which may result in headaches, visual impairment, and diabetes insipidus; the incidence of such a development in patients with microprolactinomas is less than 5 per cent, and in those with macroprolactinomas it is 25 to 35 per cent.

Based on these considerations the following recommendations are made:

1. Patients who harbor macroadenomas and desire fertility should be actively treated with either surgery or radiotherapy prior to the use of bromocriptine for restoration of fertility.

2. Careful follow-up during pregnancy is indicated in all bromocriptine-treated patients who harbor a prolactinoma. In patients with microprolactinomas the visual field is checked every 3 months and in those with macroadenomas every month or as dictated by development of symptoms and signs of tumor expansion.

3. If the complication of increased pituitary tumor growth arises during pregnancy, the options of therapy include resumption of bromocriptine or surgical excision/decompression of the pituitary tumor.

Idiopathic Hyperprolactinemia

Two issues necessitate management of this disorder. First, a minority of these patients during follow-up will manifest findings of a prolactinoma or other identifiable disorder causing hyperprolactinemia. Close long-term follow-up is therefore mandatory. Second, consideration must be taken in a given patient of the usual indications for treatment of hyperprolactinemia. If such indications are present, bromocriptine is the therapeutic option of choice. In the absence of these indications for treatment, close observation is instituted. The patient is informed of the symptoms that suggest clinical progression and is advised to return promptly for reevaluation should these occur. Otherwise, serum prolactin levels are checked annually, and CT or MRI scanning of the hypothalamic-pituitary area is performed biannually.

Other Dopaminergic Agonists

Pergolide and lisuride (Cuvalit) achieve results similar to those of bromocriptine but offer little advantage over bromocriptine. They are not presently approved for use by the Food and Drug Administration in the United States.

HYPERTHYROIDISM

method of
JAMES C. SHEININ, M.D., and
ARTHUR B. SCHNEIDER, M.D., PH.D.
Michael Reese Hospital and Medical Center
Chicago, Illinois

The presence of hyperthyroidism (thyrotoxicosis) and its underlying cause can be readily detected with current diagnostic techniques. Although available therapeutic modalities satisfactorily result in the reversal and eventual correction of the metabolic abnormalities, their major shortcoming is that they are usually directed at the result (e.g., the overactive thyroid or the excess thyroid hormone) rather than the pathogenesis (e.g., thyroid-stimulating immunoglobulins in Graves' disease) of the condition. Before discussing the options for treating hyperthyroidism, it is helpful to understand how the newer "high sensitivity" thyroid-stimulating hormone (TSH) assays facilitate diagnosis. It is also important to highlight some steps in the differential diagnosis, so that the appropriate therapeutic choices can be considered.

Measurement of total thyroxine (T_4) and free thyroxine index (FTI) remains the first step in evaluating thyroid function. TSH assays that allow for the clear distinction between normal and low TSH levels are now widely available. Hyperthyroidism is associated with immeasurably low TSH levels (the very rare TSH-producing pituitary tumors are an exception). It appears that these TSH assays obviate the need for TRH stimulation testing. A normal TSH level, as measured by one of the new assays, virtually eliminates the possibility of hyperthyroidism. This can be especially helpful in patients with changes in levels of or with abnormalities of thyroxine-binding proteins. Occasionally, an undetectable TSH level may be found in patients with autonomous functioning nodules or Graves' disease who are euthyroid. Such patients require no treatment but close follow-up for evidence of hyperthyroidism.

The physical examination often establishes the cause of hyperthyroidism. Finding infiltrative ophthalmopathy (exophthalmos and/or extraocular muscle weakness) establishes Graves' disease, a nodular goiter suggests toxic multinodular goiter, and characteristic pain establishes subacute thyroiditis. In other cases the cause can be determined without further tests. Thyrotoxic states can be divided into those with elevated or normal uptake and those with low uptake. Of the former, Graves' disease can be treated with antithyroid drugs or ablative therapy with radioactive iodine (^{131}I) or surgery. Toxic multinodular goiter or toxic adenomas are best treated with ablative therapy. Therapy must be directed at the rare tumors that produce TSH or human chorionic gonadotropin (hCG). Causes associated with low uptake (subacute thyroiditis, painless thyroiditis, thyrotoxicosis factitia, and other rare causes) are often self-limited and require no treatment or palliative treatment. Other tests may be helpful. Low serum thyroglobulin is characteristic of thyrotoxicosis factitia. High triiodothyronine (T_3) levels may establish hyperthyroidism when T_4 levels are normal or borderline high, while normal T_3 levels when T_4 levels are elevated may help identify states of abnormal T_4-binding proteins in the blood.

GRAVES' DISEASE

Graves' hyperthyroidism is an organ-specific autoimmune disorder in which thyroid-stimulating immunoglobulins (TSIs) cause overactivity of the thyroid gland independent of normal hypothalamic-pituitary control. Hence, the thyroid in Graves' disease can be thought of as the victim and not the culprit. It is a lifetime disease that is characterized by spontaneous exacerbations and remissions. In time, up to 20 per cent of patients may spontaneously develop overt or subclinical hypothyroidism. The ophthalmopathy and dermopathy of Graves' disease appear to be separate but related organ-specific autoimmune disorders that do not occur in all patients with Graves' disease. They may occur before or after the onset of hyperthyroidism and may occur in euthyroid or hypothyroid patients with Hashimoto's thyroiditis.

Unfortunately, no treatment of Graves' hyperthyroidism now available will regularly bring about permanent cure of the disorder without causing untoward effects. Current treatments limit the response of the thyroid to the thyroid-stimulating immunoglobulins and thereby control the production of thyroid hormones. Unlike other forms of hyperthyroidism, Graves' hyperthyroidism may go into remission, so all three therapeutic alternatives may be considered. These are inhibition of thyroid hormone synthesis with thioureylene drugs, ablation of thyroid tissue with ^{131}I, and ablation with surgery. Recent surveys in the United States and in Europe show that there is no consensus among endocrinologists in the approach to Graves' hyperthyroidism. Most favor a trial of thioureylene therapy as the initial management of young adult women, a view that we share. In older patients we most frequently recommend ^{131}I therapy. A recent report suggests that children and adolescents with Graves' hyperthyroidism are less likely to go into a thioureylene-related remission than adults. For them we prefer long-term thioureylene therapy and consider subtotal thyroidectomy if a remission is not achieved. The theoretic possibility of unforeseen problems with ^{131}I therapy is greatest for young patients. However, we have no lower age limit for its use and make recommendations on a case by case basis. Clearly, no single treatment is optimal for all patients. When, as in many patients with Graves' hyperthyroidism, two or all three therapeutic alternatives would be appropriate, the patient should be an enlightened participant in the decision-making process.

Thioureylene Drugs

Since the thioureylene drugs cause no permanent damage to the thyroid gland, permanent hypothyroidism does not occur as a consequence of their use. Most recent data suggest that there is about a 50 per cent likelihood of a remission following treatment with thioureylene drugs for 2 years. It has been suggested that the likelihood of remission following thioureylene therapy is inversely related to dietary iodine intake and that more frequent remissions are being seen now because of decreased dietary iodine.

Thioureylene drugs inhibit thyroid hormone biosynthesis by inhibiting incorporation of iodide into the tyrosine residues in thyroglobulin. In addition, one of the thioureylene drugs, propylthiouracil (PTU), inhibits 5'-deiodinase activity and thereby inhibits peripheral conversion of T_4 to the more active hormone T_3. Thioureylene drugs do not block the release of preformed, stored thyroid hormone into the circulation. Consequently, thyroid hormone levels may not fall, and peripheral manifestations of hyperthyroidism may not abate until stored hormone is depleted. This may take 2 to 3 weeks after initiation of treatment. Therapeutic measures that block release of stored hormone and control peripheral manifestations of circulating hormones will be discussed subsequently.

Increasing evidence indicates that thioureylene drugs may have a direct or indirect immunosuppressive effect on the autoimmune disorder underlying Graves' disease. Clearly, however, the putative immunosuppressive effect does not assure that a sustained remission will occur in all patients treated with thioureylene drugs. Characteristics of patients that tend to be associated with sustained remission are short duration of disease, mild disease, and small goiter. Conversely, long duration of disease, large goiter, ophthalmopathy, other autoimmune disorders, and family history of autoimmune thyroid disorders are associated with a greater chance of relapse.

There is controversy involving several fundamental aspects of thioureylene therapy, including selection of drug, size and timing of dosage, and duration of therapy. The therapeutic efficacy and side effects of PTU and methimazole (Tapazole) are quite similar. The potency of methimazole is about tenfold that of PTU. The serum half-lives of methimazole and PTU are about 5 and 1 hours, respectively. In most clinical settings either drug would be appropriate. There are some situations in which the longer half-life of methimazole or the inhibition of 5'-deiodinase activity by PTU makes one or the other the preferred drug. Our preponderant experience has been with PTU, and we have found it to be remarkably effective and safe. We begin therapy with 100 to 200 mg of PTU or 10 to 20 mg of methimazole every 8 hours. To maximize compliance, we recommend taking the medication upon arising, in midafternoon, and at bedtime. We see patients every 3 weeks for the first 6 weeks until the patient is euthyroid. Because of the postulated immunosuppressive effect of thioureylene drugs and because of recent data suggesting that higher dosages of thioureylene drugs may be associated with a higher incidence of remission, it is uncertain whether the dosage of thioureylene drugs should be decreased or be kept at a relatively high level with thyroid hormone added to maintain a euthyroid state. A recent survey of European endocrinologists found that 55 per cent favored the former, and 45 per cent favored the latter. Until recently, we favored the former approach, but reassessment now seems warranted, except in pregnancy. Parenthetically, thyroid enlargement in a patient on thioureylene therapy may be an important clue to development of hypothyroidism resulting from stimulation of the thyroid by TSH.

Another unresolved aspect of treatment is the frequency of administration of thioureylene drugs. Although there have been advocates of giving either drug as a single daily dose, methimazole clearly appears more appropriate for such a regimen because of its longer half-life. If we felt that single daily dose therapy would enhance patient compliance, we would select methimazole but initiate therapy every 8 hours and switch to a single daily dose when the patient became euthyroid. Once a euthyroid state and a stable medical regimen are established, we monitor our patients every 3 months, reverting to 3- to 6-week intervals should the clinical state or medical regimen change.

Yet another area of uncertainty involves the optimal duration of thioureylene therapy. Reports of duration of therapy range from as little as 3 months to 4 years or more. Although remissions may occur in as little as 3 months, sustained remissions apparently are more likely to occur after 1 to 2 years of therapy and may be even more likely to occur after more prolonged therapy. Although thioureylene therapy has been given for many years without untoward effects, the bulk of thioureylene-related sustained remissions appear to occur within 2 years of initiation of therapy.

Unfortunately, none of the currently available clinical or laboratory parameters assessed before or during thioureylene therapy are reliable predictors of thioureylene-related sustained remission. Therefore, after 1 to 2 years, we withdraw patients from thioureylene therapy as a clinical trial. Such patients should be seen every 4 to 6 weeks for the first 3 months and at 3-month intervals for the remainder of the first year off therapy, since this is the period of time during which hyperthyroidism is most likely to recur. However, as patients are followed for prolonged periods, more will relapse, and some will develop overt or subclinical hypothyroidism. Hence, we recommend that patients be seen at least once a year for their lifetime.

Untoward effects of thioureylene drugs occur in 1 to 5 per cent of patients, with fever, rash, urticaria, and arthralgia or arthritis most commonly seen. More significant but less frequent reactions include a lupuslike syndrome, toxic hepatitis (with PTU), and cholestatic jaundice (with methimazole). All patients treated with thioureylene drugs must be told about the small risk of acute agranulocytosis and should be instructed to stop the drug and to contact their physician immediately if they develop fever or sore throat. Agranulocytosis occurs in less than one half of 1 per cent of patients treated, nearly always within 3 months of starting therapy. It should be noted that although neutropenia is common in untreated Graves' hyperthyroidism and that a dose-related neutropenia is associated with thioureylene therapy, agranulocytosis is acute, idiosyncratic, and not dose-related and cannot be predicted from previous blood counts.

Ablative Therapy

Radioactive Iodine

Optimally, ablative therapy with ^{131}I or surgery would be sufficient to damage or to remove sufficient thyroid tissue to control the hyperthyroidism but not enough to cause lifetime hypothyroidism. Unfortunately, neither form of ablative therapy reliably fulfills this expectation.

Various approaches to ^{131}I therapy have been used in Graves' hyperthyroidism. These include doses calculated to attempt to achieve the above optimal goal, smaller doses that attempt to minimize the incidence of post–[131]I hypothyroidism, and larger doses that attempt to ablate the gland totally, accepting hypothyroidism and treating it with thyroid hormone replacement. The size of the ^{131}I dose is directly related to the incidence of hypothyroidism within the first year of therapy and is inversely related to the failure of the dose to restore a euthyroid state. However, the increasing incidence of hypothyroidism with time is independent of size of the ^{131}I dose given. It should be noted that up to 28 per cent of patients may develop transient hypothyroidism soon after ^{131}I therapy and subsequently may become either euthyroid or hyperthyroid again.

We calculate the ^{131}I dose to be given using the following formula:

$$\text{Dose (mCi)} = \frac{\text{base dose (}\mu\text{Ci per gram)} \times \text{estimated thyroid weight (grams)}}{\text{fractional 24-hour }^{131}\text{I uptake} \times 1000}$$

In an uncomplicated case of Graves' hyperthyroidism we use a base dose of 80 μCi per gram. With this dose, we find that about 90 per cent of patients are rendered euthyroid within 6 months, that there is an incidence of hypothyroidism of about 10 to 20 per cent in the first year after therapy, and that there is a continuing incidence of hypothyroidism of about 2 to 5 per cent per year thereafter. Consideration is given to using thioureylene drugs, iodides, or beta blockers after ^{131}I therapy if more prompt restoration to a euthyroid state or if blocking peripheral manifestations of hyperthyroidism is desired. After ^{131}I therapy, we follow our patients at 6-week intervals for the first 3 months, at 3-month intervals for the remainder of the first year, and once a year for their lifetime.

Complications of ^{131}I therapy are rare. Radiation-induced thyroiditis or sialitis and mild exacerbations of hyperthyroidism may occur. Radiation-induced thyroid storm, which tends to occur in elderly patients, patients with complicating diseases, patients with long-standing hyperthyroidism, and patients with large glands, can be prevented by thioureylene drug treatment to restore a euthyroid state and deplete the gland of stored thyroid hormone prior to ^{131}I administration. To date, there is no evidence for increased incidence of any long-term genetic or neoplastic complications of ^{131}I therapy.

Surgery

Subtotal thyroidectomy carries with it not only the benefits and risks of ^{131}I therapy but the additional risks of a surgical procedure. It does result in prompt resolution of the hyperthyroid state. We favor the standard preparation for surgery, consisting of thioureylene drugs for 6 weeks to restore a euthyroid state and deplete the gland of stored thyroid hormone and potassium iodide as Lugol's iodine, 5 to 15 drops three times a day, or a saturated solution of potassium iodide (SSKI), 1 to 3 drops three times a day, for the 10 days just prior to surgery to decrease the vascularity of the gland. We feel that preparation for thyroid surgery using beta blockers and potassium iodide is less effective because it leaves the gland with a large amount of stored thyroid hormone and therefore should be limited to situations in which surgery cannot be delayed. Even in the hands of experienced thyroid surgeons and anesthesiologists, in addition to the minimal risk of intraoperative mortality, the risks of recurrent laryngeal nerve damage and permanent hypoparathyroidism are reported to be about 3 per cent. There may also be a minimal risk of thyroid storm, even after preoperative preparation. The risks of persistent or recurrent hyperthyroidism and of short- and long-term permanent hypothyroidism are correlated with the amount of residual thyroid tissue, which is not unlike the situation with ^{131}I therapy. Studies have demonstrated a 6 to 12 per cent incidence of persistent or recurrent hyperthyroidism—unacceptably high in our perspective—and up to about a 50 per cent incidence of hypothyroidism, depending on the amount of residual thyroid tissue and duration of follow-up. As with ^{131}I therapy, transient hypothyroidism may occur in up to 20 per cent of patients in the first postoperative year.

Adjunctive Therapy and Thyroid Storm

Beta-adrenergic blocking agents have proved to be valuable adjuncts because they ameliorate the peripheral sympathomimetic effects of hyperthyroidism. Propranolol (Inderal) has the additional advantage of inhibiting peripheral conversion of T_4 to T_3. Beta blockers are particularly useful in patients with supraventricular arrhythmias. Although they have been used as the sole therapy for Graves' hyperthyroidism and as preparation for surgery, we feel that such treatment is suboptimal. They are an essential part of the treatment of thyroid storm. Representative doses of propranolol in hyperthyroidism as adjunctive therapy are 40 to 160 mg daily, and in thyroid storm they are 160 to 480 mg daily or 1 to 10 mg intravenously.

Iodides are used to block release of stored thyroid hormone in thyroid storm and in other settings in which prompt lowering of thyroid hormone levels is desirable; they are also used to decrease the vascularity of the thyroid gland preoperatively. In thyroid storm, SSKI is given as 8 drops every 6 hours and 1 to 3 drops three times a day in other settings. Because iodides are incorporated into thyroid hormone, they should not be given until hormone biosynthesis is blocked by an initial dose of thioureylene drugs. Recently, iodinated contrast agents such as ipodate* (Oragrafin) and iopanoic acid* (Telepaque) have been used in thyroid storm. They are extremely effective in blocking the conversion of T_4 to T_3, but their exact role remains to be determined.

High dosages of glucocorticoids have been used empirically to treat thyroid storm due to "relative adrenal insufficiency," but it has been shown that such dosages inhibit peripheral conversion of T_4 to T_3 and may inhibit thyroid hormone secretion. In thyroid storm, 100 mg of hydrocortisone every 8 hours is recommended.

Since thyroid storm often occurs in association with a precipitating illness, the latter should be searched for and treated vigorously. Also, the systemic manifestations of thyroid storm, including fever, fluid loss, and cardiac complications, should be treated aggressively.

Complicating Illnesses

There are certain clinical settings that favor one therapeutic modality or contraindicate another. There are patients for whom hyperthyroidism is a more significant risk, e.g., the elderly patient, patients with antecedent or hyperthyroidism-related cardiovascular disease, or patients with related autoimmune endocrine disorders such as adrenal insufficiency or insulin-dependent diabetes mellitus. Such patients require therapy that will promptly block the peripheral effects of hyperthyroidism, will rapidly restore a euthyroid state, will prevent release of stored thyroid hormone that may adversely affect their condition or may provoke thyroid storm, and will ensure no recurrence of hyperthyroid-

*This use of these agents is not listed in the manufacturers' directives.

ism. We initiate treatment of such patients with higher doses of PTU, 200 mg every 8 hours, and with propranolol, 40 to 240 mg daily in single long-acting or divided doses, for 6 weeks to render the patient euthyroid and to deplete the gland of stored hormone. Propranolol is continued, PTU is stopped for 3 to 5 days, and ^{131}I therapy is administered using the formula given above with 120 μCi per gram of thyroid used as the base dose.

Pregnancy

Accurate assessment of thyroid status in pregnancy, in which thyroxine-binding globulin is elevated, requires estimation or measurement of the concentration of free T_4. Free T_4 is unchanged in normal pregnancy. It is estimated by the FTI (calculated from the T_3 resin uptake, which is low or low normal, and the total T_4, which is high in normal pregnancy) or measured by equilibrium dialysis. Graves' disease tends to abate or to remit in the second and third trimesters of pregnancy, possibly owing to immunologic alterations during pregnancy, and to exacerbate post partum. Because of the risk of thioureylene-induced fetal goiter and hypothyroidism, the dose of thioureylene drugs should be minimized and the mother should be kept at a high normal or minimally elevated free T_4 level. Thyroid hormones do not effectively cross the placenta, so that giving thyroid hormone medication to the mother will not prevent fetal goiter. PTU clearly is preferred to methimazole in pregnancy and lactation because it crosses the placental barrier about one fourth as much as methimazole and is concentrated in milk about one tenth as well. The suggestion that methimazole may be associated with congenital skin defects recently has been challenged. No teratogenic effects have been attributed to PTU.

Clearly, ablative therapy with ^{131}I is contraindicated during pregnancy. Should thioureylene therapy not be tolerated or should high doses be required, subtotal thyroidectomy in the midtrimester of pregnancy following the usual preoperative preparation is an appropriate and safe alternative. The safety of beta blockers in pregnancy has not yet been established. Because of the natural history of the disease during and after pregnancy and because of the desirability of minimizing PTU dosage, we follow our pregnant patients with Graves' hyperthyroidism at 4- to 6-week intervals during and for 3 to 6 months after pregnancy.

Recurrent Graves' Disease

Finally, the question arises of how to treat patients with persistent or recurrent Graves' hyperthyroidism following thioureylene therapy, subtotal thyroidectomy, and ^{131}I therapy. A patient who has not become euthyroid within 6 months after ^{131}I should be given a second dose, calculated with 120 to 150 µCi per gram of thyroid as the base dose. Second operations carry with them significantly greater risks of hypoparathyroidism and laryngeal nerve injury, so patients with recurrent hypothyroidism following subtotal thyroidectomy should be given [131]I. The surveys previously alluded to demonstrate a clear lack of consensus on the approach to patients with persistent or recurrent hyperthyroidism following thioureylene therapy. Since most thioureylene-related remissions will occur within the first 2 years of therapy, hyperthyroidism will be controlled, but remission will occur infrequently after additional thioureylene therapy. Although long-term thioureylene has been well tolerated, we and most others would recommend ablative therapy, and we prefer ^{131}I therapy in all but the youngest patients. Should there be an exacerbation of hyperthyroidism after a sustained remission of years, we would favor another course of thioureylene therapy.

OTHER FORMS OF HYPERTHYROIDISM

Toxic Multinodular Goiter

The considerations for treatment of this form of hyperthyroidism are very similar to those for Graves' disease. Since toxic multinodular goiters do not go into spontaneous remission, thioureylene drugs are only indicated as a preparatory measure for ablative treatment with ^{131}I or surgery. Such preparatory treatment to deplete the gland of stored hormone is often indicated because toxic multinodular goiters occur most frequently in older patients. Preparatory treatment with PTU, 100 to 200 mg every 8 hours, should be continued until thyroid hormone levels fall into the normal range. These goiters tend to be more difficult to treat with [131]I. It is likely that this resistance occurs because different parts of the gland have different levels of function and autonomy. Therefore, larger doses of ^{131}I are usually given using the formula noted previously, with 150 µCi per gram of thyroid as the base dose, and repeated treatments are sometimes required. Adjunctive therapy with beta blockers, as described previously, should be used as necessary.

Solitary Toxic Adenoma

Hyperthyroidism caused by a single overactive thyroid nodule is effectively treated with [131]I. The "hot" nodule concentrates ^{131}I, while the remainder of the thyroid has reduced uptake, resulting from suppression of pituitary TSH secretion, and is protected. It should be remembered that a "warm" nodule does not cause hyperthyroidism. The continued function of the remaining thyroid tissue indicates that pituitary TSH secretion has not been suppressed. Further, while all "hot" nodules are functioning autonomously, not all of them cause hyperthyroidism. Surgery is an acceptable, but usually unnecessary, alternative to ^{131}I therapy. The surgical procedure is limited to removal of the nodule and therefore is relatively safe.

Thyroiditis

Two forms of thyroiditis may present as hyperthyroidism. One form (subacute, de Quervain's or giant cell thyroiditis) is associated with a painful thyroid gland. The other form (silent, painless, or lymphocytic thyroiditis) is not associated with pain and often occurs in the postpartum period. In both instances, hyperthyroidism is caused by a process that destroys the thyroid gland, resulting in leakage of hormone into the circulation. Therefore, neither thioureylene drugs nor ablative therapy has a role in treatment. Both forms of thyroiditis resolve spontaneously, although lymphocytic thyroiditis may recur after subsequent pregnancies. In the acute phase, treatment is directed at controlling the peripheral manifestations of hyperthyroidism and controlling discomfort. The former may be treated with beta blockers and the latter with aspirin (up to twelve 325-mg tablets per day in divided doses) or other nonsteroidal anti-inflammatory agents. In unusually resistant cases, prednisone may be used, starting with 40 mg per day and rapidly tapering the dose. The hyperthyroid phase of the disease may be followed by transient and rarely permanent hypothyroidism.

HYPOTHYROIDISM

method of
INDER J. CHOPRA, M.D.
University of California School of Medicine
Los Angeles, California

Hypothyroidism is a clinical syndrome resulting from a deficiency of thyroid hormones causing a slowing of several metabolic processes. The term *myxedema* refers to a characteristic manifestation of chronic hypothyroidism, which consists of mucinous edema resulting from a collection of hydrophilic mucopolysaccharides (predominantly hyaluronic acid) and water in interstitial tissues. A deficiency of thyroid hormones may be the result of a primary thyroidal disease (primary hypothyroidism) or it may be secondary to decreased production of thyroid-stimulating hormone (TSH) by the anterior pituitary (secondary hypothyroidism). Pituitary secretion of TSH may be decreased not just in pituitary disorders but also in hypothalamic disorders associated with decreased production of thyrotropin-releasing hormone (TRH). Hypothyroidism associated with hypothalamic disorders has been referred to as tertiary hypothyroidism. Serum TSH is characteristically elevated in primary hypothyroidsm, whereas it is low or normal in secondary (or tertiary) hypothyroidism. Secondary and tertiary hypothyroidism usually manifest as one component of multiple deficits in the endocrine function of the pituitary gland. Rarely, hypothyroidism is a result of resistance to tissue effects of thyroid hormones. Patients with this disorder, which may be familial, manifest hypothyroidism even when serum concentrations of thyroid hormones are entirely normal and may actually be elevated. Serum TSH may be normal or high in instances of peripheral resistance to thyroid hormones.

Table 1 lists the various causes of hypothyroidism. Primary thyroid failure is a very common disorder. Its prevalence has been estimated to approximate 0.8 per cent. In patients over 50 years of age, 3 to 10 per cent may demonstrate elevated serum TSH levels. Chronic (Hashimoto's or lymphocytic or autoimmune) thyroiditis and spontaneous (idiopathic) thyroid atrophy are the most common causes of hypothyroidism, explaining almost 50 per cent of cases. Iatrogenic hypothyroidism following treatment with radioactive iodine (e.g., for treatment of hyperthyroidism) or surgery (subtotal or total thyroidectomy for hyperthyroidism, thyroid nod-

TABLE 1. Causes of Hypothyroidism*

A. Thyroidal disorders:
 1. Atrophy: spontaneous (idiopathic), possibly autoimmune.
 2. Destruction: chronic autoimmune thyroiditis, radioiodine therapy, surgical thyroidectomy, external radiation, cancer, infiltrating disease (e.g., sarcoidosis).
 3. Inflammation: postpartum thyroiditis, subacute thyroiditis.
 4. TSH receptor blocking antibodies in autoimmune thyroid disease.
 5. Developmental aberration: thyroid dysgenesis.
 6. Abnormalities in hormone production: inborn errors in hormonal synthesis, goitrogens, antithyroid drugs, iodide excess, iodine deficiency.
B. Hypophyseal disorder (e.g., postpartum infarction, tumors, granulomatous disease such as sarcoidosis, and therapeutic irradiation) presenting as panhypopituitarism or isolated TSH deficiency.
C. Hypothalamic disorder (e.g., hypothalamic tumors, therapeutic irradiation, or hypothalamic disorder occurring transiently during a serious systemic illness) leading to decreased production of TRH.
D. Peripheral tissue disorder: resistance to intracellular action of thyroid hormone.

*Primary thyroid dysfunction (A above) is much more common as a cause of hypothyroidism than pituitary, hypothalamic, and peripheral tissue disorders (B, C, and D above).

ules, or carcinoma) is the next most common cause of hypothyroidism, explaining about 30 to 40 per cent of cases. Drugs (antithyroid agents such as propylthiouracil, methimazole, lithium carbonate, and iodide or iodine-containing agents like amiodarone) are also important causes of hypothyroidism. Antibodies directed against the TSH receptor may block thyroidal growth and stimulation by TSH; they have been recently implicated in the pathogenesis of hypothyroidism in autoimmune thyroid disease. This form of hypothyroidism may remit or may even be followed by hyperthyroidism when there is concurrence of an excess of thyroid-stimulating antibodies with TSH receptor–blocking antibodies.

Hypothyroidism may be transient, lasting a few weeks to months, and may follow a phase of hyperthyroidism in subacute thyroiditis and postpartum thyroiditis. Hypothyroidism associated with postpartum thyroiditis may recur following subsequent pregnancies. Antithyroid antibodies are usually present in high titers in patients with postpartum thyroiditis but not in those with subacute thyroiditis. Other thyroid causes of hypothyroidism listed in Table 1 are much less frequent than those mentioned previously. Additionally, secondary (or tertiary) causes and peripheral resistance to the action of thyroid hormones are infrequent and explain hypothyroidism only in 1 to 2 per cent of cases.

Clinical Manifestations

The clinical presentation of hypothyroidism varies with age of onset and severity. Recent studies with screening of newborns with serum TSH and/or thyroxine (T_4) measurements have revealed that hypothyroidism occurs in 1 in 5000 newborns. Many of these newborns show little or no clinical signs of hypothyroidism, and diagnosis requires a routine neonatal screening and/or a high index of suspicion. When present, clinical features of congenital hypothyroidism include respiratory difficulties, cyanosis, persistent jaundice, poor feeding, hoarse cry, umbilical hernia, and bone retardation. It is extremely important for optimal brain development that the diagnosis be made as soon as possible and that treatment be started; permanent mental deficiency occurs if treatment is delayed. There is evidence that reduction in intelligence quotient (IQ) is minimal if treatment is instituted before 3 months of age.

Thyroid hormone deficiency beginning early in infancy and in early childhood is characteristically associated with growth retardation (short stature and delayed bone maturation), mental deficiency, and delayed dentition. Growth retardation is treatable, but mental retardation can persist despite treatment with thyroid hormones. Adolescents with primary hypothyroidism may manifest, in addition to growth retardation, an enlarged sella turcica and rarely precocious puberty.

Clinical features of hypothyroidism in adult patients include lethargy, easy fatigability, diminished energy, dry skin, excessive loss of hair, muscle weakness, sleepiness, impaired memory, weight gain, increased pallor, diminished hearing acuity, paresthesia, and/or menometrorrhagia. Additionally, myxedema may result in coarse features, periorbital edema, enlarged tongue, hoarseness, carpal tunnel syndrome, and pleuropericardial effusions. Heart failure may result from myocardial dysfunction and/or pleural and pericardial effusions. Mental impairment and myxedema madness are usually observed in older individuals, and they manifest as emotional instability, delusions, hallucinations, and/or frank psychosis. Myxedema coma is a true emergency and the mortality rate can be very high (greater than 50 per cent) despite treatment. Usual precipitating factors include some form of severe stress, including infection, trauma, and exposure to cold. Clinical presentation may include hypothermia temperature as low as 24° C [75° F], shock, hypoventilation and CO_2 narcosis, severe hyponatremia, and other features suggestive of inappropriate antidiuretic hormone (ADH) syndrome.

Typical physical findings include absence of palpable thyroid tissue or a firmer than normal, diffusely enlarged thyroid (of chronic thyroiditis), bradycardia, pallor and characteristic deep tendon reflexes with delayed relaxation (hung-up reflexes).

Laboratory Findings

Hypothyroidism is characteristically associated with decreased serum T_4 concentration (T_4 radioimmunoassay) and decreased free T_4 concentration or free T_4 index. It is important to measure free T_4 concentration or free T_4 index, since serum T_4 may be low in the absence of hypothyroidism when the serum binding of T_4 is reduced, as in patients with systemic nonthyroidal illness and those in whom serum concentration of thyroxine-binding globulin (TBG) is reduced as a result of either an inherited disorder, ingestion of some drugs (e.g., androgens), high dose corticosteroid and asparginase administration, or loss in urine (e.g., nephrotic syndrome). Serum concentration of free T_4 is essentially normal in these instances. Free T_4 index is also normal in these situations, except in systemic nonthyroidal illnesses, in which it may be low in apparently euthyroid individuals. Serum T_3 concentration as measured by radioimmunoassay (RIA) and free T_3 are decreased in the majority of hypothyroid patients but are within the normal range in about 15 to 20 per cent of cases. Furthermore, serum T_3 (RIA) and free T_3 are subnormal in a variety of systemic illnesses, including hepatic and renal diseases. Therefore, low serum T_3 (RIA) and/or free T_3 concentrations are not very helpful in the diagnosis of hypothyroidism.

Serum TSH is characteristically elevated in primary hypothyroidism. Ultrasensitive immunoradiometric (or immunoassay) methods of TSH measurement are now available that can easily detect 0.05 μU per ml TSH and differentiate among low, normal, and high values. Normal range of serum TSH in assays approximates 0.5 to 4.5 μU per ml. A serum TSH value of greater than 20 μU per ml and a low T_4 and free T_4 are diagnostic of primary hypothyroidism. However, a mildly elevated serum TSH of up to 15 to 20 μU per ml is at times seen in euthyroid patients with systemic illnesses, especially during their recovery phase and in some acute psychiatric disorders. I prefer to wait about 2 to 3 weeks in these cases of mild TSH elevation and repeat T_4 and TSH measurements before considering treatment with thyroid hormones. Serum TSH is low normal or low in patients with secondary (or tertiary) hypothyroidism. Serum TSH response to TRH is exaggerated in primary hypothyroidism, decreased (often absent) in secondary (pituitary) hypothyroidism, and normal with a delay in the peak response in tertiary (hypothalamic) hypothyroidism.

Some patients demonstrate normal serum T_4 (and free T_4) and elevated serum TSH. This combination of laboratory findings has been considered to signify diminished thyroid hormone reserve or compensated hypothyroidism. It may be seen in patients with chronic thyroiditis and in those with a history of subtotal thyroidectomy or of treatment with radioiodine or antithyroid drugs. A high serum TSH in these patients signifies that the patient can maintain an euthyroid state only on the basis of increased stimulation of the thyroid. If baseline serum TSH is clearly elevated (i.e., greater than 20 μU per ml) and/or serum TSH response to TRH is exaggerated, I prefer to initiate treatment with thyroid hormone replacement. Such treatment ensures euthyroidism and prevents further enlargement of the thyroid.

Treatment

Choice of Agents

The daily production rate of T_4 in normal man approximates 100 micrograms, while that of T_3 approximates 30 micrograms. The majority (greater than 75 per cent) of T_3 produced daily derives from extrathyroidal conversion of T_4 to T_3. Normal human thyroid contains little T_3 relative to T_4. T_4 to T_3 ratio (T_4/T_3) in the normal thyroid approximates 15 to 20 to 1 (15 to 20/1). Serum T_4 and T_3 levels in man show little change in a day. Serum half-life of T_4 approximates 6 to 7 days, while that of T_3 approximates 1 day.

The treatment that most closely mimics the physiologic situation is administration of synthetic T_4 (levothyroxine, or L-thyroxine [Synthroid, Levothroid]). Once-daily ingestion of replacement doses of T_4 is associated with normal serum levels of both T_4 and T_3, and there is little if any fluctuation in their levels throughout the day. Absorption of T_4 from the gastrointestinal tract has been observed to approximate 70 to 90 per cent. The gastrointestinal absorption of T_4 remains essentially normal in systemic illnesses except in patients with severe diarrhea and hypermotility of gastrointestinal tract and in those following a major gut resection. These various considerations suggest that treatment with synthetic T_4 is the treatment of choice for hypothyroidism. The usual daily replacement dose of T_4 in adults is about 0.1 to 0.2 mg, approximating 1.7 micrograms per kg per day. The mean replacement dose of T_4 in an adult man is 0.125 mg per day. The requirement for thyroxine changes with age. It is higher in newborns, infants, and children than in adults, and it decreases with age: It may decrease as much as 50 per cent at 80 years of age compared with the requirement at 20 years of age. The dose of T_4 in infants has been suggested to be 100 micrograms per square meter per day. Alternatively, one may treat term neonates with a daily T_4 dose of 25 micrograms, and the dose may be increased gradually to 50 micrograms by 1 year of age. Doses up to 7 micrograms per kg body weight have been used to achieve clinical euthyroidism in infants. The daily T_4 replacement dose in children is 100 micrograms per square meter or 3 micrograms per kg body weight. A word of caution appears appropriate, however, when one uses generic preparations of L-thyroxine. Several studies have suggested that the L-thyroxine content of generic preparations can vary considerably, sometimes to as much as 34 to 127 per cent of the stated content.

Adequacy of treatment with T_4 is assessed by clinical examination, coupled with normalization of serum T_4, T_3, and TSH levels. When equilibrium has been reached during replacement T_4 therapy, the serum TSH concentration is normal or low, the serum T_4 concentration is high normal or slightly elevated, and the serum T_3 concentration approximates mean normal value. Although the elevated serum TSH of primary hypothyroidism falls steadily soon after T_4 treatment is initiated, it may not normalize for several weeks, sometimes as long as 8 to 12 weeks. Therefore, in the first several weeks of treatment I prefer to gauge the adequacy of T_4 treatment on the basis of serum thyroid hormone levels. It is, of course, necessary to determine the adequacy of treatment of seconday hypothyroidism on the basis of serum thyroid hormone levels; as mentioned already, serum TSH is low or normal to begin with in these patients. It is not necessary to continue follow-up of serum T_3 levels during treatment with T_4. Follow-up should be based on serum TSH and serum T_4 and free T_4 index; the latter measurements are less expensive than serum T_3 concentration measurements in most institutions. Serum TSH levels may not fall to normal despite treatment with adequate doses of T_4 in infants. This is presumably a result of immaturity of the CNS-hypothalamic-thyrotropic axis. Therefore, adequacy of treatment with T_4 in the first 1 to 2 years of life should be based mainly on clinical examination and on rendering serum T_4 (and T_3) concentrations to levels that are appropriate for the age of the child.

Thyroid Hormone Preparations Other Than Oral Thyroxine

Besides treatment with T_4, hypothyroidism may be treated with synthetic T_3 (liothyronine, Cytomel). Over 90 per cent of T_3 is absorbed after oral ingestion. However, T_3 is more expensive than T_4 and results in unphysiologic levels of serum T_4 and T_3. Thus, serum T_4 is subnormal, while serum T_3 varies markedly during a day. Serum T_3 during treatment with a replacement dose of T_3 (approximately 50 μg per day) is two to four times the upper limit of normal at 2 to 4 hours after ingestion, while it is high normal at 24 hours after ingestion. A similar problem of peaking T_3 levels occurs after ingestion of preparations that contain mixtures of synthetic T_4 and T_3 (usually in a ratio of 4:1) (e.g., Liotrix, Thyrolar, Euthroid) or preparations from animal thyroids (e.g., desiccated thyroid U.S.P. and Thyrar from pork and beef thyroids, respectively, and Proloid from pork thyroglobulin). Desiccated thyroid U.S.P. is easily available and is the least expensive form of thyroid hormone treatment available for oral ingestion. However, one hears of batches of variable potency and occasional batches of inactive preparations. Overall, I rank desiccated thyroid after synthetic T_4 as a treatment of choice for hypothyroidism. The usual replacement dose of desiccated thyroid approximates 65 to 130 mg (1 to 2 grains) per day. The biologic activity of 100 micrograms of synthetic T_4 approximates that of 25 micrograms of Cytomel; 65 mg (1 grain) of desiccated thyroid U.S.P., Thyrar, or Proloid; or 1 tablet of a mixture of 50 micrograms synthetic T_4 plus 12.5 micrograms synthetic T_3 (Thyrolar I or Euthroid I). Among the various thyroid preparations, only synthetic T_4 is available at this time for parenteral use. It should be used in patients with hypothyroid emergencies; for example, those in myxedema coma or those not able to swallow or to absorb oral preparations of thyroid hormones. The replacement dose for intravenous T_4 is about 70 to 80 per cent that of an oral preparation.

I do not recommend treatment of hypothyroidism with T_3 (Cytomel) except for a short period (about 4 weeks) in patients with thyroid cancer who have already undergone thyroidectomy and are being prepared for thyroid and total body radioiodine scanning. In my experience, symptoms of hyperthyroidism and cardiac aberrations (e.g., worsening of angina, tachyarrhythmias, and congestive heart failure) are more frequent during treatment with T_3 than with T_4.

Initiation and Assessment of Treatment

In a young patient with mild hypothyroidism and in the absence of cardiac disease, treatment may be started with nearly a replacement dose of about 100 micrograms per day. In older patients and in those with known cardiac disease, institution of rapid treatment with a full replacement dose of desiccated thyroid may be associated with angina pectoris, tachyarrhythmias, myocardial infarction, and/or congestive heart failure. I am not yet aware of a similar experience during treatment with synthetic T_4. However, it is prudent to start therapy with a low (usually 50 micrograms per day and sometimes as low as 25 micrograms per day) initial dose of T_4, and if no adverse effects appear, the dose may be increased gradually in 25-microgram-per-day increments at about 4-week intervals until a full replacement dose of about 0.125 mg per day has been achieved and the adequacy of replacement treatment has been verified by normal serum thyroid hormone and TSH levels. In children, however, appropriate progression of growth (height, weight, and skeletal maturation) should also be monitored periodically. Treatment of hypothyroidism is lifelong in most instances, except in transient hypothyroidism, as noted previously.

Other Considerations

1. Associated conditions. Patients with hypothyroidism and myxedema may demonstrate adrenal insufficiency, which is typically permanent in patients with multiple endocrine deficiency syndrome and in secondary hypothyroidism but is temporary in patients who are suffering adrenal effects of severe hypothyroidism. Adrenal cortical reserve may be tested using the cosyntropin test, and if it is compromised, the patient should be treated with replacement doses of glucocorticoids and mineralocorticoids. Hydrocortisone (10 to 20 mg in the morning and 10 mg in the evening) is a reasonable treatment.

Patients with multiple endocrine deficiency syndrome may manifest, besides hypothyroidism and adrenal insufficiency, hypoparathyroidism, diabetes mellitus, ovarian failure, pernicious anemia, and vitiligo. Hypoparathyroidism is also a concern in patients with postsurgical hypothyroidism. Physician attention to these possible syndromes may add to the well-being of the patient.

2. Pregnancy. Serum T_4 concentration increases in pregnancy mainly because the serum concentration of thyroxine-binding globulin (TBG) is increased. Serum concentration of free T_4 and free T_4 index is normal in pregnancy. Replacement doses of T_4 are not changed in pregnancy. Adequacy of treatment with T_4 should be judged by clinical examination, normal free T_4 index, normal free T_3 index, and normal or suppressed serum TSH levels. Alternatively, sufficient T_4 is given to raise serum total T_4 concentration to a value appropriate for pregnancy (12 to 16 micrograms per dl, normal range 5 to 12). Increases in serum concentrations of TBG and in thyroid hormones in patients taking estrogen (e.g., oral contraceptives) are similar to those in pregnancy.

3. Toxic effects of thyroid preparations. The issues of possible cardiac catastrophes in older patients with arteriosclerosis and coronary artery disease have been mentioned. Allergic reactions to synthetic T_4 tablets have rarely been reported. Studies have suggested that the reported symptoms of pruritus and skin rash were most likely a result of an allergic reaction to a dye in the T_4 tablet (e.g., tartrazine or another excipient) rather than to T_4 per se. Another important concern is that of hyperthyroidism due to an overdosage of exogenous thyroid hormones (i.e., thyrotoxicosis factitia). Symptoms of hyperthyroidism in these patients will be associated with low thyroid radioiodine uptake, low serum thyroglobulin, and absence of goiter.

4. Drug interactions. Serum concentrations of thyroid hormones may remain low in patients taking adequate replacement T_4 therapy when the patients are simultaneously treated with agents such as phenytoin (Dilantin), which occupies T_4-binding sites on TBG, or agents such as androgen and asparginase, which lower serum TBG concentration. Serum concentration of free T_4 or free T_4 index changes little when TBG decreases and should be helpful in appropriate evaluation of the patient. Some drugs (e.g., cholestyramine [Questran]) and the soybean contained in some infant formulas may bind T_4 in the gut and prevent its absorption. Serum TSH will remain high and serum T_4 (and T_3) low despite T_4 replacement in patients ingesting these agents. Higher than usual oral replacement doses of exogenous T_4 will be needed in these instances to normalize serum TSH and T_4 (and free T_4 index). A similar situation exists in cases in which the absorption of a T_4 dose is reduced because of severe diarrhea or following a major gut resection. Parenteral administration of T_4 is rarely necessary in these patients. High doses of thyroid hormones may aggravate glucose intolerance and hence prompt the need for increased doses of hypoglycemic agents. On the other hand, thyroid preparations may potentiate the effects of several drugs, including sympathomimetic agents (e.g., epinephrine), anticoagulants (e.g., warfarin), and tricyclic antidepressants (e.g., imipramine).

5. Surgery in hypothyroidism. It has been generally held, and I fully agree, that hypothyroidism should be corrected prior to an elective surgical procedure. Recent studies suggest, however, that complications of anesthesia or surgery are no more frequent or severe in mild hypothyroidism than in normal (euthyroid) subjects. More severely hypothyroid patients may, however, be

subject to shock, cardiac arrhythmias, congestive heart failure, or gastrointestinal and psychiatric difficulties with a greater frequency than euthyroid subjects. There is also a concern about occurrence of myxedema coma during and after surgery in patients with severe hypothyroidism. If emergency surgery is necessary for a life-threatening situation in a severely hypothyroid patient, perhaps hypothyroidism should be treated aggressively, as for myxedema coma. A careful study is needed, however, to examine this issue closely.

6. Treatment of myxedema coma. Myxedema coma is a serious emergency with a high mortality. It clearly requires aggressive treatment. I usually recommend (1) parenteral (intravenous) T_4: 400 to 500 micrograms to replace the extrathyroidal pool of T_4 followed by 100 micrograms daily intravenously for several days when the patient is comatose followed by 0.1 to 0.15 mg daily orally when the patient is awake; (2) treatment of precipitating disorders, if known (e.g., antibiotics for an infection such as pneumonia), and attention to trauma; and (3) supportive treatment consisting of blankets to reduce heat loss (active warming is not helpful and may lead to peripheral vasodilation), intravenous fluids and blood transfusion for shock (use of pressor agents requires careful monitoring for cardiac arrhythmias), ventilatory assistance with intubation or tracheostomy for CO_2 retention, fluid restriction and/or hypertonic saline if serum sodium is less than 120 mEq per liter, hydrocortisone approximately 150 mg per day intravenously on the first day (it is to be tapered gradually over 5 to 7 days as the patient improves), attention to plasma glucose levels (which may be low in some cases), and cautious use of diuretics and digoxin for congestive heart failure.

THYROID CANCER

method of
COLIN G. THOMAS, Jr., M.D.
University of North Carolina
Chapel Hill, North Carolina

Cancer of the thyroid has an annual incidence of 10,600, with approximately 1100 deaths annually. Of these cancers, 7700 are in women, with 700 deaths, and 2900 are in men, with 400 deaths. Although an uncommon cause of death, cancer of the thyroid has received emphasis because of the frequency of nodular thyroid disease (4 to 7 per cent of adults, 20 to 30 per cent of radiation-exposed patients), from which it needs to be differentiated.

Cancers of the thyroid should be classified according to histopathologic characteristics that have predictive value to the surgeon in determining the type and extent of surgical treatment (Table 1). Other factors playing a major role in the prognosis of thyroid neoplasms are stage of the disease and age and sex of the patient. Less well understood are (1) hormonal sensitivity, (2) functional activity of the cancer, (3) presence of initiating and promoting factors, and (4) immunologic and endocrine status of the patient. Cognizance of the spectrum of thyroid neoplasms and the effect that these various factors have on the clinical course of the disease are necessary in attempting to select the most effective management.

Treatment

Selection of Patients for Surgical Treatment

Most patients with nodular/neoplastic thyroid disease are euthyroid. Confirmation of their metabolic status can be made by determining the free thyroxine index. When laboratory studies are not consistent with the clinical impression, the serum thyroid-stimulating hormone (TSH) and radioimmunoassay (RIA) of triiodothyroxine (T_3) may identify the patient with associated hypothyroidism or the rare patient with T_3 thyrotoxicosis.

Selection of patients for surgical treatment is based on identifying the common causes of thyromegaly and those individuals in whom a dominant mass is most likely to represent a tumor. The physical characteristics of a mass in the thyroid are best determined by a bidigital examination, thereby gaining a three-dimensional concept of the size, consistency, and topography of the thyroid gland. The functional state of the thyroid can be portrayed by a thyroid scan following the administration of short-lived radionuclides (^{99m}Tc, ^{123}I). Scanning permits definition of the size and configuration of the thyroid as well as determination of the function of macroscopic areas within the gland. Areas of abnormal function must be carefully correlated with the clinical findings. A "nodule" is a clinical, not a

TABLE 1. **Classification of Cancers of the Thyroid**

I. Well-differentiated (from follicular epithelium)
  A. Papillary or papillary-follicular
    1. Minimal thyroid cancer (<1.5 cm or occult sclerosing)
    2. Invasive
  B. Follicular
    1. Low-grade encapsulated
    2. High-grade, angioinvasive
    3. Hürthle cell
II. Medullary with amyloid (from parafollicular cells)
III. Undifferentiated (anaplastic, spindle, giant-cell, small-cell)
IV. Lymphoma
V. Others (epidermoid, sarcoma, teratoma, metastatic)

radiologic, finding. Thyroid adenomas, malignant tumors, and cysts are usually nonfunctioning, or "cold." Adenomatous nodules characteristically demonstrate hypofunction; however, degenerative changes, hemorrhage, fibrosis, and cyst formation may cause them to be nonfunctional.

Ultrasonography using the B mode is of value in determining the cellularity of tissue and defines hypofunctioning or nonfunctioning thyroid nodules as solid, cystic, or mixed with solid components. Solid lesions are most likely to be adenomas, carcinomas, or adenomatoid nodules. Ultrasonography is of chief value in measuring change in size of a specific lesion and in identifying lesions that are impalpable.

Since neither thyroid imaging nor ultrasonography will differentiate benign from malignant lesions, the cytologic/histopathologic characteristics of a nodule should be appraised prior to rendering judgment as to the need for surgical excision. The cytologic characteristics are studied by aspiration of cells through a fine needle (No. 22, No. 19) with staining by Papanicolaou techniques. The overall diagnostic accuracy of needle aspiration (aspiration biopsy cytology) is estimated to be greater than 90 per cent by experienced cytopathologists. The test is most helpful when smears are read as malignant, indeterminate, or benign. The first usually represents papillary carcinoma or, less frequently, medullary or anaplastic carcinoma or lymphoma. Indeterminate smears will be encountered with cellular follicular adenomas and follicular adenocarcinomas. Benign findings are usually associated with a cyst, adenomatous nodule, or thyroiditis. An inadequate specimen is procured in approximately 10 per cent of patients and requires reaspiration. An alternative technique is to remove a core of tissue using a cutting needle (Vim-Silverman or Tru-Cut) biopsy technique for routine microscopy.

Utilizing the clinical history, physical findings, and appropriate laboratory studies, patients with a hyperfunctioning nodule, thyroid cyst, chronic thyroiditis, and TSH-dependent nodular goiter can usually be identified. Surgical intervention is indicated in those patients with an established diagnosis of cancer and in patients in whom the histocytologic/pathologic findings are indeterminate because of the inability to distinguish between follicular adenoma and follicular adenocarcinoma.

Operative Management

The primary method of treatment of thyroid malignancies is surgical excision. Argument exists as to the desirability of carrying out a "total" thyroidectomy in all patients. Such arguments relate to removal of both lobes because of multifocal disease, a lower incidence of recurrent disease, the facilitation of radioiodine therapy, the perceived better survivorship, and the ability to accomplish total thyroidectomy with an acceptably low morbidity. The most cogent argument against routine total thyroidectomy is that the prognosis is not significantly improved over that of more conservative surgery (e.g., lobectomy with isthmusthectomy or lobectomy with partial excision of the remaining lobe) and that morbidity in terms of hypoparathyroidism and recurrent nerve damage is significantly increased. A more selective approach in keeping with the biology of a particular tumor is recommended (i.e., histopathologic characteristics, age and sex of the patient, extent of disease, as well as the experience of the surgeon).

In the removal of a solitary mass in which a cytologic/histopathologic diagnosis has not been established, incisional biopsy or enucleation of the nodule is to be condemned because of the danger of tumor dissemination as well as the possibility of providing the pathologist with an inadequate specimen. Complete lobectomy with removal of capsular lymph nodes and preservation of the recurrent laryngeal nerve and parathyroid glands is the most desirable procedure. A frozen section examination will identify most thyroid cancers but may not be able to differentiate follicular adenoma from follicular adenocarcinoma. Should permanent sections confirm the initial impression of benignancy (e.g., adenomatous goiter or adenoma), no further surgery need be carried out; only a decision is required as to the need for supplemental thyroid hormone in order to reduce the incidence of recurrence of the disorder in the opposite lobe. This is particularly true in nodular goiter because the goitrogenic stimulus not only still exists but also may have been aggravated by the partial thyroidectomy.

A diagnosis of "cancer" of the thyroid should be regarded as unacceptable. The surgeon and pathologist should make every effort to further categorize the lesion in order to plan the most appropriate treatment.

Well-Differentiated Adenocarcinoma of the Thyroid

PAPILLARY OR PAPILLARY-FOLLICULAR CARCINOMA. Tumors less than 1.5 cm in diameter in the absence of lymph node metastases or gross multifocal disease and without a history of low-dose irradiation are well managed by lobectomy with isthmusthectomy. Tumors greater than 1.5 cm in diameter and particularly those with capsular invasion, nodal metastasis, or gross involvement of the opposite lobe and in patients with a poor prognosis (men over 40 years of age and women over 50 years of age) require more aggressive treatment. A lobectomy on the side of the primary lesion with a near-total thyroidectomy on the contralateral side is recommended. Preservation of an adequate blood supply to the parathyroid glands is facilitated by preserving the posterior capsule of the contralateral lobe. This will usually ensure against the development of postoperative hypoparathyroidism.

Total thyroidectomy is indicated (1) in order to excise all gross disease; (2) in the case of more aggressive neoplasms, as determined by size, local infiltration, regional metastases, and age and sex of the patient; and (3) in the presence of distant metastases (pulmonary, bone), anticipating the need for therapy with radioiodine. The need to remove all thyroid tissue by performing total thyroidectomy to facilitate subsequent radioiodine therapy has been overemphasized. The potential benefit from the prophylactic use of radioiodine therapy in well-differentiated thyroid cancer has not been demonstrated.

The integrity of recurrent nerves and the parathyroid glands should be maintained at essentially "all costs." Despite its seeming adherence to the overlying neoplasm, in most circumstances the recurrent nerve can be dissected free. Excision of one recurrent laryngeal nerve is justified only if this is the limiting factor in the surgeon's ability to excise all gross neoplasm completely.

The indication for removal of cervical lymph nodes is the presence of metastatic cancer. The extent of the dissection will depend on the magnitude of node involvement as well as the location of the primary lesion. In neoplasms arising from the inferior pole of the thyroid without capsular invasion and with two or three lymph node metastases along the recurrent laryngeal nerve and no evidence of enlarged lymph nodes along the course of the midjugular or inferior jugular chain, excision of pretracheal areolar tissue as well as the lymphatic tissue along the recurrent nerve is indicated. More extensive involvement of lymph nodes along the internal jugular vein requires a modified type of neck dissection with removal of lymphatic drainage peculiar to the thyroid. The sternocleidomastoid muscle and internal jugular vein can usually be preserved along with the eleventh nerve.

FOLLICULAR CARCINOMA. Encapsulated follicular carcinoma of the thyroid is considered a low-grade malignancy but with a significant potential for distant metastasis in patients over 60 years of age and in lesions greater than 3.5 cm in diameter. Complete excision of the tumor with a margin of normal thyroid parenchyma is best accomplished by a lobectomy with inclusion of the isthmus or medial portion of the opposite lobe—depending upon the location of the tumor.

Although lymph nodes are rarely involved, if enlarged or firm, they should be excised and examined by frozen section for evidence of metastatic disease. Because of the increased incidence of distant metastasis and local recurrence in patients over age 60 and with lesions greater than 3.5 cm and the possibility of the need for radioactive iodine therapy, a total/near-total lobectomy should be carried out on the contralateral side, according to the gross findings and the ability of the surgeon to preserve the integrity of the recurrent nerve and parathyroid gland.

Infiltrating follicular carcinoma is usually a more aggressive tumor and more likely to require postoperative therapy with radioactive iodine. This lesion is best treated by a complete lobectomy on the side of the lesion and total/near-total lobectomy on the contralateral side.

Medullary Carcinoma. Medullary carcinoma represents approximately 5 to 7 per cent of all cancers of the thyroid. It may be a component of Sipple's syndrome (concomitant hyperparathyroidism, pheochromocytoma, and mucosal neuromas). The measurement of calcitonin in the peripheral blood by radioimmunoassay following a provocative test with pentagastrin has provided a sensitive and specific test for identification of this neoplasm. The multiple sites of origin and propensity for bilateral lymph node metastasis associated with a biologic aggressiveness midway between well-differentiated and undifferentiated cancer of the thyroid justify the recommendation for "total" thyroidectomy and removal of involved lymph nodes by a modified neck dissection.

Undifferentiated Carcinoma of the Thyroid. Undifferentiated thyroid carcinoma is frequently sufficiently extensive that surgical treatment other than biopsy is unwarranted. When, however, the disease seems confined to its primary site of origin and/or regional nodes, the results of an aggressive surgical attack, although poor, warrant thyroidectomy and a radical neck dissection. In view of the propensity for tracheal invasion and compression, every effort should be made to remove this tumor from about the trachea at the initial operation. In general, these tumors are best treated with external irradiation and, in selected patients, chemotherapy.

Lymphoma. The problem is primarily that of diagnosis, since these tumors are highly radiosensitive and radiation is the treatment of choice. The diagnosis of lymphoma is difficult to establish by fine needle aspiration and requires, at a minimum, a cutting (core) needle biopsy. An open biopsy is the best method to provide the pathologist with an adequate specimen to classify the disease. For the rare localized intralobular tumor, lobectomy establishes the diagnosis. Staging of the disease should then be carried out to determine whether mantle irradiation is adequate or whether multimodal chemotherapy is necessary.

Postoperative Management

All patients with thyroid cancer should be placed upon thyroid hormone therapy for life. The rationale for TSH suppression is based on the documented dependency of some thyroid cancers on TSH, the role of TSH as a promoting factor in experimental thyroid cancer, and the presence of TSH receptor sites in most well-differentiated thyroid cancers. Clinical findings also suggest that recurrence rates are lower and survivorship is better in patients on thyroid hormone. Finally, thyroid hormone is essential to maintain euthyroidism. T_4 in a dosage of 0.15 mg to 0.20 mg will cause adequate suppression of TSH in most patients. Hyperthyroidism should be avoided. Ultrasensitive serum TSH levels should be measured to evaluate the dosage and to monitor compliance.

Radioiodine. Evaluation with radioiodine scintiscan in the immediate postoperative period will identify any remnant of thyroid, whether in the region of the posterior capsule, pyramidal lobe, or superior pole, and will serve as a baseline for future evaluation in the event of recurrent disease.

Radioactive iodine has been used both prophylactically and therapeutically in the management of well-differentiated cancers. Its value prophylactically is not well documented. Its prophylactic use would seem justified in older patients with well-differentiated carcinomas who are likely to have more aggressive disease. Radioiodine is clearly indicated therapeutically in patients with residual or recurrent cervical neoplasms not amenable to surgical excision and in patients with distant metastases, primarily lung and bone. Treatment is repeated at yearly intervals until there is no longer uptake by the neoplasm, avoiding pulmonary fibrosis and bone marrow damage. Serum thyroglobulin serves as a useful marker of well-differentiated thyroid cancer, and in the absence of any normal thyroid tissue it can be used as an index of persistent or recurrent disease demonstrating the need for further radioiodine therapy. Radioiodine therapy has no place in the management of medullary or poorly differentiated carcinomas.

External Irradiation. External beam therapy given by megavoltage x-rays, cobalt (^{60}Co) gamma rays, or high-energy electrons is indicated primarily for lymphomas, undifferentiated carcinomas, and those well-differentiated tumors not amenable to surgical excision, thyrotropin suppression, or radioiodine therapy.

Chemotherapy. There has been very limited success in the management of undifferentiated carcinomas with chemotherapy, which has been used primarily as an adjunct to radiation therapy. Somewhat encouraging results have followed the use of doxorubicin. Chemotherapy has no role in the treatment of well-differentiated neoplasms.

PHEOCHROMOCYTOMA

method of
SHELDON G. SHEPS, M.D.
Mayo Clinic and Mayo Medical School
Rochester, Minnesota

Just over a century ago (1886), Fränkel described a young woman with symptoms of pheochromocytoma in whom, at autopsy, bilateral adrenal tumors were found. In 1922, Labbé reported a case and was the first to attribute the symptoms to the adrenal tumors. The next year, Professor Villard of Lyon operated on a patient who died in shock. In 1926, C. H. Mayo, at the Mayo Clinic, and G. Roux, in Switzerland, successfully removed adrenal tumors and dramatically reversed hypertensive episodes.

Epinephrine was isolated in crystalline form and the chemical structure was elucidated in 1897. The hormone was synthesized in 1904 and later was shown to be present in increased amounts in pheochromocytomas. Some years later, identification of norepinephrine, dopamine, other precursors, and metabolites led to rapid advances in the biochemical diagnosis of pheochromocytoma. Precision in the measurement of these compounds was further refined by high-pressure liquid chromatography and radioisotopic labeling techniques, which have greatly contributed to the preoperative diagnosis and follow-up in patients with catecholamine-producing tumors.

Incidence

Pheochromocytoma is a rare tumor that occurs at any age, but the peak incidence is in the fourth through the sixth decades. Among the general population in Olmsted County, Minnesota, pheochromocytoma occurs in one or two adults per 100,000 per year, whereas in Sweden, occurrence is one fourth that rate. Among hypertensive persons, the incidence of pheochromocytoma has decreased because essential hypertension has been diagnosed in an increased number of persons in recent years. From 1973 to 1975, the annual incidence of pheochromocytoma at the Mayo Clinic was estimated to be 0.4 per 1000 hypertensive persons with diastolic pressures of 95 mmHg or more.

Pheochromocytoma may be part of a polyglandular endocrine derangement or may be associated with other neuroectodermal disorders. There is an increased incidence in families, particularly those of children with pheochromocytoma and especially when pheochromocytoma is present in both adrenal glands. Autosomal dominant inheritance is seen in multiple endocrine neoplasia, Type II (MEN Type II), in association with pancreatic islet cell tumors, and in neuroectodermal disorders (neurofibromatosis and von Hippel-Lindau disease). Families with multiple adrenal and extra-adrenal pheochromocytomas unassociated with other tumors or syndromes also have been reported.

Pathologic Features

Pheochromocytoma is a tumor of chromaffin cells located in the adrenal medulla. The cells are derived from the cells of the neural crest, which also contribute to the central nervous system and sympathetic ganglia. Neuroblastomas, ganglioneuromas, and pheochromocytomas may arise from these tissues. Mixtures of these cell types may be present in the tumors. These cells are part of the amine precursor uptake and decarboxylation (APUD) cell system and retain the biochemical mechanisms to synthesize, store, and secrete many biogenic amines and peptides. This development explains some of the isolated and familial polyglandular tumor relationships and the many potential secretory products.

Ninety per cent of pheochromocytomas arise in the adrenal medulla. Solitary lesions are more common on the right. About 5 per cent of occurrences are bilateral, and about 10 per cent of tumors are extra-adrenal and solitary. The location of extra-adrenal chromaffin tissue may be anywhere from the base of the brain to the testicle, including the interatrial cardiac septum. Extra-adrenal tumors account for up to 19 per cent of catecholamine-producing tumors. Most are within the abdomen, but a few are within the chest and neck. About 10 per cent of tumors recur.

Malignancy is a difficult problem because of the potential for multicentric origin of pheochromocytoma and because of the lack of specific histologic, biochemical, and electron microscopic criteria of malignancy. For malignancy to be diagnosed, tumor cells must be found in sites where chromaffin tissue does not normally occur (for example, lymph nodes, liver, bone, muscle, and lung). The incidence of malignant disease may range from 3 to 14 per cent. Hosaka and associates performed nuclear DNA studies on ploidy by flow cytometry in 75 patients with pheochromocytomas who had a follow-up of 10 years. All patients with a normal DNA histogram had a benign course, whereas 30 to 40 per cent of those with aneuploid or tetraploid-polyploid DNA had evidence of malignant disease. The importance of these observations in the diagnosis and follow-up of patients operated on remains to be clarified.

Clinical Features

Nearly all tumors produce symptoms or signs related to the excessive production and release of catecholamines; even manipulation of a "nonfunctioning" tumor at surgery can release catecholamines. Symptoms are not related to the size, location, or histologic appearance of the tumor. Symptoms, entirely or in part, are episodic in most patients. The episodes usually are uniform in composition, although they tend to vary in duration and increase in severity and frequency with time. The onset of each episode is characteristically sudden, and peak severity is reached within a few minutes. The duration is less than 15 minutes in half the patients and shorter than an hour in most. The paroxysms either are spontaneous or are elicited by exercise, bending over, urination, defecation, pressure on the abdomen, induction of anesthesia, or injection of histamine, guanethidine, glucagon, droperidol, tyramine, metoclopramide, cytotoxic drugs, saralasin, tricyclic antidepressants, or phenothiazines.

The clinical clues to pheochromocytoma are symptomatic paroxysms, including headache, pallor, perspiration, and palpitations; unusual lability of blood pressure; accelerated hypertension; a pressor response to induction of anesthesia or to any antihypertensive drugs; and a suprarenal or midline abdominal mass. Hypertension may appear only with a paroxysm or may be more persistent. Rarely, hypotension is a presenting feature; when it is, the patient usually has a tumor that secretes predominantly epinephrine, dopa, or dopamine.

Multiple endocrine neoplasia, Type II (MEN Type II) consists of medullary carcinoma of the thyroid gland, pheochromocytomas, and parathyroid disease. A variant of this syndrome, MEN Type IIB, is manifested as an abnormal phenotype and rarely includes parathyroid disease. Pheochromocytomas in MEN Type II are asymptomatic in about half the patients and are diagnosed by biochemical testing, indicated by detection of abnormalities in the thyroid and parathyroid glands or by a positive family history (autosomal dominant inheritance). In this syndrome, the thyroid tumor and pheochromocytomas are preceded by hyperplasia of the appropriate cell type, and the tumors are multiple, bilateral, and potentially malignant with metastasis.

Catecholamine Metabolism

Norepinephrine is synthesized from tyrosine by way of dopa and dopamine in the brain, chromaffin tissue, and sympathetic nerve endings (Fig. 1). In mammals, epinephrine is formed from norepinephrine almost entirely in the adrenal medulla. Small amounts of epinephrine and norepinephrine are excreted unchanged or conjugated, but the rest is excreted primarily as the respective catechol O-methyl derivatives (metanephrine and normetanephrine) and, after additional oxidation of the amine group, as vanillylmandelic acid (VMA).

Diagnosis

Diagnostic studies generally include measuring the urinary excretion of norepinephrine, epinephrine, dopamine, total metanephrines, and VMA and the plasma concentrations of norepinephrine and epinephrine. The urinary determinations may be done on specimens collected during 24 hours or less, and the results may be expressed as either 24-hour rates, hourly rates, or per milligram of creatinine. The determination of total metanephrines has given the fewest false-negative results, from 1 to 2 per cent, and has

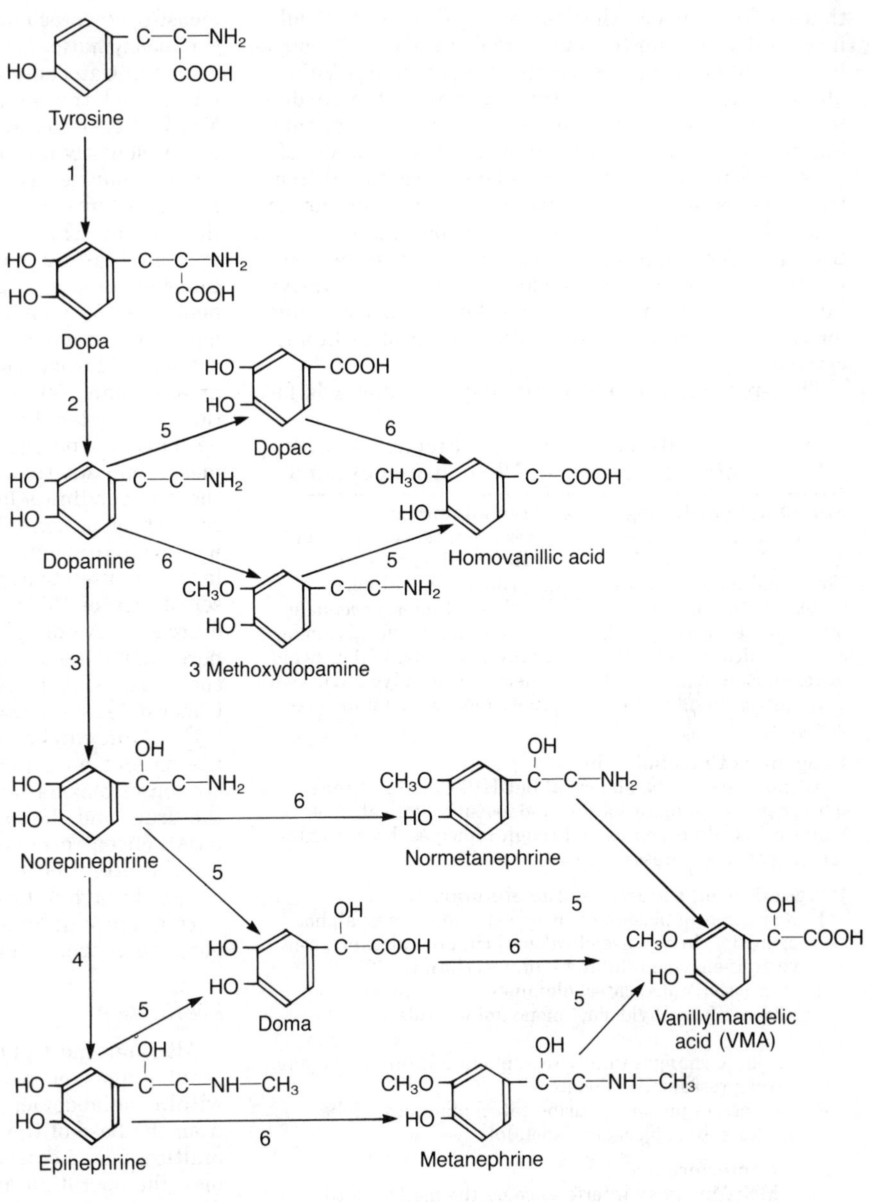

Figure 1. Pathways and enzymes of catecholamine metabolism: 1, tyrosine hydroxylase; 2, aromatic amino acid decarboxylase; 3, phenylamine beta-hydroxylase; 4, phenylethanolamine N-methyltransferase; 5, monoamine oxidase plus aldehyde dehydrogenase; and 6, catechol O-methyltransferase. (From Sheps, S. G.: Pheochromocytoma. *In* Spittell JA Jr (ed): Clinical Medicine. Vol. 7. Philadelphia, Harper & Row, Publishers, 1984, pp 1–26. Used by permission.)

been our choice for a screening test because of its accuracy and the ease of processing many specimens every day. Methylglucamine, a component of many iodinated contrast media used in radiology, may cause metanephrine values to be falsely normal for as long as 72 hours after its use. Determinations of VMA are positive in about 90 per cent of patients with pheochromocytoma.

Methods that use high-pressure liquid chromatography (HPLC) for the determination of fractionated catecholamines (norepinephrine, less than 80 micrograms in 24 hours; epinephrine, less than 20 micrograms in 24 hours; and dopamine, less than 400 micrograms in 24 hours) in urine are highly sensitive: More than 95 per cent of tumor patients have had positive results (norepinephrine and epinephrine, greater than 100 micrograms in 24 hours). At these diagnostic decision levels, the clinical specificity of the test is relatively low. Higher decision levels (norepinephrine of greater than 170 micrograms in 24 hours or epinephrine of greater than 35 micrograms in 24 hours) provide good clinical specificity (greater than 95 per cent), even in patients receiving antihypertensive medications, while maintaining the same level of sensitivity for tumor detection. Examining both the norepinephrine and the epinephrine values and considering an increase of either catecholamine to be positive are important. From 50 to 70 per cent of patients have increased values of epinephrine, and 75 to 80 per cent have increased values of norepinephrine. When norepinephrine and epinephrine are considered together, more than 95 per cent of patients have increased concentrations of either. Dopamine adds little diagnostic information except in relatively rare situations when extraordinary amounts are secreted.

One must be aware of clinical situations and drugs

that could influence the test result (Table 1). Mildly increased values for total metanephrines may be noted in 10 to 20 per cent of patients without tumor. Values above the normal range in these patients often are due to interference by drugs or unusual urine pigments. Special precautions that we have described enable these interfering substances to be differentiated from true increases in metanephrines. The combination of determination of urinary metanephrines as a screening test and confirmation by determination of urinary fractionated catecholamine excretion is a noninvasive laboratory regimen that has excellent predictive value for the identification of the patient with pheochromocytoma.

The application of much more specific methods for

TABLE 1. Situations and Drugs Interfering with Biochemical Diagnosis of Pheochromocytoma

Stimulation of Endogenous Catecholamines

Plasma and urine catecholamines are most sensitive, but metanephrines and VMA can be abnormal as well: emotional and physical stress, surgery, acute central nervous system disturbance (stroke, hemorrhage, tumor, encephalopathy), acute coronary ischemia, angiography, hypoglycemia, caffeine, nicotine, diazoxide, theophylline, drug withdrawal (alcohol, clonidine), vasodilator therapy (nitroglycerine, sodium nitroprusside, calcium channel blockers administered acutely).

Exogenous Catecholamines

All the tests can be abnormal but HPLC and radioenzymatic assays are more specific and sensitive for catecholamines: nose drops, sinus and cough remedies, bronchodilators, appetite suppressants.

Drugs Altering Catecholamine Metabolism

1. Reduction in plasma or urine catecholamines: alpha$_2$ agonists, chronic use of calcium channel blockers, converting-enzyme inhibitors, bromocriptine.
2. Decreased VMA; catecholamines and metanephrines increased: methyldopa,* monoamine oxidase inhibitors.†
3. Variable changes in any test: phenothiazines,† tricyclic antidepressants,† L-dopa.†
4. Increase in plasma or urine catecholamines: alpha$_1$ blockers, beta blockers, labetalol.

Specific Interference

1. ↓ MN: MN assay interference by the methylglucamine‡ in radiographic contrast medium.
2. ↓ Urinary catecholamines: mandelamine destroys catecholamines in bladder urine.
3. VMA ↓: clofibrate.
   VMA ↑: nalidixic acid, anileridine.
4. Labetalol: metabolite(s) interfering with all tests.

*HPLC assays can accurately determine catecholamines and metanephrines in presence of methyldopa.

†Drugs with prolonged half-lives may need to be discontinued for 2 to 3 weeks before accurate determinations can be made.

‡Methylglucamine destroys a reagent in the Pisano metanephrines assay; this is most pronounced in urine collected the same day as the contrast medium is administered but may last up to 72 hours.

HPLC, high-pressure liquid chromatography; MN, metanephrines; and VMA, vanillylmandelic acid.

From Sheps, S. G., Jiang, N.-S., and Klee, G. G.: Diagnostic evaluation of pheochromocytoma. Clin Endocrinol Metab *17*:397, 1988.

measuring catecholamine concentrations in plasma (radioenzymatic, HPLC) also has added to diagnostic acumen. Catecholamines in plasma are chemically labile, and the samples must be handled carefully. Many alterations in physiologic and pathologic states can profoundly affect the concentration of plasma-free norepinephrine. To enhance accuracy, one must pay careful attention to blood drawing and preparation of the patient. The variability associated with age, sex, and renal failure is uncertain. Even when samples are collected properly, plasma measurements of norepinephrine and epinephrine are not as sensitive as urinary measurements for the detection of pheochromocytoma. Plasma norepinephrine concentrations of greater than 750 pg per ml or epinephrine concentrations of greater than 110 pg per ml are found in 90 to 95 per cent of patients with tumors, but as with urinary measurements, the specificity of the measurements at these upper limits for normal subjects is not good for separating patients with tumors from other patients with similar symptoms. When high diagnostic decision levels are used to overcome the specificity problem, the sensitivity of the measurements for tumor detection decreases. At decision levels of 2000 pg per ml for norepinephrine or 200 pg per ml for epinephrine, the specificity is about 95 per cent, but the sensitivity for tumor detection drops to about 85 per cent.

Clonidine can be given orally to distinguish between the patient with pheochromocytoma, whose hypersecretion of plasma norepinephrine does not respond to the drug, and the patient without tumor, whose high basal concentration is decreased to normal by the drug. Careful attention to the procedure of this test is necessary to avoid false-positive results, for example, during concomitant administration of propranolol. Provocative pharmacologic tests are rarely necessary.

Localization

Although most pheochromocytomas arise in the adrenal glands or nearby and almost all are located within the abdomen, the tumors may exist anywhere from the base of the brain to the scrotum and may be multicentric. Localization methods help the surgeon plan the operation and reduce the chance of negative findings at laparotomy if the tumor happens to be outside the abdomen. However, the surgeon still must determine whether there are multiple and bilateral tumors. At present, computed tomography (CT) is the most reliable method for preoperative localization: Well over 90 per cent of the tumors are visible if included in the area of examination. CT is accurate, noninvasive, and reproducible; magnetic resonance imaging (MRI) and CT are the only imaging techniques that can visualize normal adrenal glands when the diagnosis is equivocal. MRI may emerge as a desirable procedure for extra-adrenal locations and in pregnant patients. In adrenal MRI, relaxation times of pheochromocytomas are often dramatically greater than those of normal adrenal tissue. More experience is needed to evaluate this observation. CT-guided percutaneous adrenal biopsy in unsuspected pheochromocytoma has been associated with cardiovascular crises.

Scintigraphy with ^{131}I,meta-iodobenzylguanidine

(MIBG) is an exciting new method for localizing pheochromocytomas. MIBG concentrates in adrenergic vesicles, and where these vesicles are sufficiently numerous, an image can be produced. Catecholamine-producing tumors and metastatic lesions have been demonstrated throughout the body; the normal adrenal medulla in humans generally is not imaged. About 10 per cent of tumors are not demonstrated; false-positives are rare (1 to 2 per cent). Positive studies can be used to direct CT scanning efforts to provide precise anatomic localization of the tumor or tumors. MIBG may also image other APUD tumors. At present, CT, because of general availability, should be used for initial localization attempts, first to scan the adrenals and, if results are negative, next to study the entire abdomen and pelvis. MIBG scintigraphy should be used if results of this study are negative or if metastasis or familial disease is considered likely. MRI can be directed at any extra-abdominal site for further anatomic localization.

Treatment

Surgical excision is the definitive therapy. Proper preparation for surgery has greatly reduced the previously high surgical morbidity. Most institutions now prepare their patients with alpha-adrenergic blocking agents (phenoxybenzamine [Dibenzyline], prazosin [Minipress], terazosin [Hytrin], phentolamine [Regitine]) until they have been normotensive and free of spells for about a week. Preoperative volume expansion is seldom necessary with this approach. Beta-adrenergic blocking drugs are added for several days before the operation, particularly if the patient has had arrhythmia. Caution should be taken with the addition of beta-adrenergic blocking agents if cardiomegaly or evidence of cardiomyopathy exists. Labetalol or other alpha- and beta-adrenergic blocking agents can be very effective, but the proportion of the alpha and beta blockades in the drug may not be applicable to all patients with pheochromocytoma. If the blocking drugs are not well tolerated, metyrosine (Demser) may be used preoperatively. Additional drugs that have been useful in some cases are calcium channel blocking agents and converting-enzyme inhibitors. Preoperative preparation with glucocorticoid should be done in patients likely to have bilateral adrenalectomy, such as those with MEN Type II. Attempts to preserve the adrenal cortex have occasionally been successful.

A transabdominal approach is generally necessary to allow thorough exploration of all chromaffin tissue in the abdomen, and associated intra-abdominal disease, particularly cholelithiasis (occurring in almost 30 per cent of patients with pheochromocytoma), can be corrected at the same time. The posterior approach, although safe, usually entails excessive manipulations of the tumor. During surgery, careful attention to anesthesia, cardiovascular hemodynamics, and blood volumes contributes to greatly reduced surgical mortality. The present consensus is that enflurane is the anesthetic agent of choice because it does not sensitize the myocardium to exogenously administered catecholamines or stimulate the release of catecholamines from the tumor or sympathetic system. During the operation, the electrocardiogram, central venous pressure, and mean arterial pressure are monitored continuously. A Swan-Ganz catheter is used almost routinely to measure the filling pressures of the left ventricle. Intraoperative blood pressure crises are handled with infusions of sodium nitroprusside or nitroglycerin; phentolamine (Regitine) and labetalol (Normodyne, Trandate) can also be used. Arrhythmias can be treated by parenterally administered beta-adrenergic blocking drugs and lidocaine.

The operative mortality at the Mayo Clinic from 1980 to 1986 was 1 in 77 patients (1.3 per cent). In our previous experience, the 5-year survival rate was 96 per cent for patients with benign tumors and 44 per cent for those with malignant tumors.

After curative surgery, 10 per cent of patients have recurrence; thus, catecholamine and metabolite levels should be measured annually for at least 5 years and perhaps longer—and certainly promptly if symptoms appear or hypertension recurs. The recent findings of flow cytometry suggest that patients with abnormal DNA patterns should have closer and longer follow-up to detect malignant disease earlier.

For inoperable or metastatic tumors, consideration has been given to surgical intervention and therapeutic embolization to reduce tumor load and catecholamine production. Repeated therapeutic doses of MIBG have not produced a substantial long-lasting benefit. Radiation therapy is generally successful if doses of 40 Gy or more can be administered to the area because the tumors are relatively radioresistant. Chemotherapy trials have not had a persistent benefit on catecholamine production or tumor growth, although striking transient decreases have been reported with cyclic administration of cyclophosphamide, vincristine, and dacarbazine. The effects of excess circulating catecholamines can be controlled by the use of alpha- and beta-adrenergic blocking agents, alone or in combination with the previously mentioned drugs.

THYROIDITIS

method of
NADIR R. FARID, M.B., B.S.
Memorial University of Newfoundland
St. John's, Newfoundland, Canada

Traditionally, thyroiditis has been classified temporally as acute, subacute, and chronic, with these descriptions often superimposed upon other relevant characteristics, e.g., acute suppurative or chronic goitrous. The recent recognition of the clinical entity of painless thyroiditis (associated or unassociated with pregnancy) has further complicated this classification. Silent thyroiditis unassociated with pregnancy is subacute in duration, whereas postpartum thyroiditis may fall in the categories of subacute to chronic. In the latter event, it would be important to differentiate postpartum from chronic autoimmune thyroiditis, as the management is different. A viable alternative to the traditional classification of thyroiditis has, however, not emerged.

ACUTE (SUPPURATIVE) THYROIDITIS

Acute thyroiditis is now rarely seen in adults except in immunocompromised patients. It is usually associated with infection with Gram-positive organisms. It presents as an acute inflammatory process with exquisite localized swelling and tenderness, lymphadenopathy, fever, and leukocytosis. In the event of recurrent attacks or in the involvement of the left lobe, pyriform sinus fistula should be suspected. Appropriate parenteral antibiotics should be instituted immediately while awaiting the results of bacteriologic culture. Aspirates of the affected area should be cultured both aerobically and anaerobically, and antibiotic therapy should be altered accordingly. Surgical intervention may be necessary if an abscess is formed.

Although they do not present acutely, tuberculosis and (even more unusually), syphilis, and fungal infections can result in suppurative thyroiditis.

SUBACUTE (DE QUERVAIN'S) THYROIDITIS

Pain is generally a cardinal feature of subacute thyroiditis; unusual patients presenting with protracted malaise have been described. Subacute thyroiditis is probably due to viral and rickettsial infections of the thyroid triggering cell-mediated injury. This form of thyroiditis predominantly occurs in the summer and early fall, particularly around the Great Lakes. The pain over the thyroid area may be flitting in nature and may be transmitted. The thyroid gland is tender to touch and presents a localized or generalized "woody"

texture. More severe cases are associated with marked systemic symptoms, including fever, malaise, and hyperthyroidism. The diagnosis is made on clinical grounds, corroborated by mild to moderate hyperthyroxinemia in the presence of thyroidal radioiodine uptakes greater than 5 per cent and high erythrocyte sedimentation rates; thyroid autoantibody titers are usually negative to low.

Reassurance of the patient and anti-inflammatory agents usually suffice in the case of mild attacks. Coated aspirin, 600 mg every 6 to 8 hours, for a week to 10 days is prescribed with gradual reduction of the dose thereafter. Steroids should be used in severe attacks as well as for recurrent mild bouts. Dexamethasone (Decadron) is started at a dose of 8 mg per day and is rapidly halved by 7 to 10 days and then reduced slowly thereafter, with the view to discontinuing therapy by the end of a month. In the event of recurrence of symptoms on reducing or discontinuing the drug, the lowest dose compatible with symptom control should be reinstituted. Symptoms of hyperthyroidism should be controlled with propranolol (Inderal) 20 to 40 mg every 8 hours.

With severe attacks or after several recurrences, patients may experience symptomatic hypothyroidism; this is usually short lived and does not require replacement therapy. Permanent hypothyroidism is not a usual sequela of subacute thyroiditis.

PAINLESS THYROIDITIS

Painless thyroiditis is immunogenetically and immunologically allied to autoimmune thyroiditis. The reason these conditions are usually self-limiting, whereas chronic autoimmune thyroiditis is not, is unknown. They generally run a subacute course associated with variable degrees of thyroid dysfunction. The condition is characterized by lymphocytic infiltration of the thyroid associated with no to moderate goiter formation, and variable degrees of hyperthyroxinemia followed by no to fairly severe thyroid insufficiency; during the acute phase the 24-hour radioactive iodine uptake ≤ 5 per cent. This condition tends to occur preferentially postpartum, and then it is more likely to be associated with goiter, a symptomatic acute hyperthyroid phase, and severe prolonged hypothyroidism. In some areas postpartum hypothyroidism is not usually preceded by a thyrotoxic phase; the extent to which variation in diagnostic criteria, dietary iodide intake, and disease severity contribute to this phenomenon is unclear. Mothers with elevated titers of antimicrosomal antibodies in the second/third trimester of pregnancy are at approximately 50 times the risk for postpartum thyroiditis than are antibody-negative women. The prevalence of postpartum thyroiditis is 6 per cent in these women, and they stand a 25 to 30 per cent chance of recurrence in future pregnancies. Thyroid autoantibody titers are lower in painless thyroiditis not related to pregnancy.

Painless thyroiditis unrelated to pregnancy at most requires symptomatic control of the hyperthyroid phase with beta-adrenergic blockers; rarely do these patients become symptomatically hypothyroid. The hyperthyroid phase of postpartum thyroiditis usually requires symptomatic management. Thyroid replacement therapy is necessary in about 30 per cent of patients with postpartum thyroiditis. While hormone replacement may be necessary for several months to a year, we have seen patients who required treatment, albeit at a reducing dosage for up to 4 years after a single episode of postpartum thyroiditis. The need for continued thyroid replacement therapy should be reviewed on a 6-month basis after discontinuing the drug for 4 to 5 weeks. Circulating thyroid hormones, basal, and if necessary thyroid-releasing hormone (TRH)–stimulated thyroid-stimulating hormone (TSH) should be measured. When in doubt as to whether postpartum hypothyroidism is related to chronic or postpartum thyroiditis, I elect to manage the patient in the same fashion as I would a patient with postpartum thyroiditis. Recovery from painless thyroiditis is often associated with a decline and even a disappearance of thyroid autoantibodies.

CHRONIC AUTOIMMUNE THYROIDITIS

Chronic autoimmune thyroiditis may or may not be associated with diffuse (goitrous) goiter (Hashimoto's thyroiditis) and atrophic (idiopathic myxedema) thyroiditis, respectively. The underlying pathologic processes, lymphocytic infiltration, thyroid cell death, and attempts at regeneration and fibrosis, are common to both conditions; in goitrous thyroiditis, thyroid growth predominates over destruction. The manifold increase in the prevalence of goitrous thyroiditis over the last 3 decades has been attributed to the increase in iodide intake. Atrophic thyroiditis affects an older group more readily than does the goitrous variety. In Hashimoto's thyroiditis, goiter is diffuse and may reach large proportions even in iodide-sufficient areas. The vast majority of patients with autoimmune thyroiditis remain euthyroid and asymptomatic, although it remains the most important cause of noniatrogenic thyroid failure.

The diagnosis of goitrous autoimmune thyroiditis is confirmed by high titers of antimicrosomial antibodies; although a patchy pattern on thyroid scintiscan provides further confirmation, it is not necessary to establish a diagnosis. Serum (preferably serum-free) thyroxine and basal TSH should be measured; slight elevations of serum TSH are an indication for TRH stimulation tests. On the basis of this battery of tests, different degrees of thyroid failure may be established: from minimal, with normal serum thyroid hormone concentrations and increased pituitary TSH reserve, to severe, associated with marked symptoms, very high basal TSH, and low serum thyroxine concentrations. Atrophic thyroiditis is uncovered in epidemiologic or hospital surveys or in patients found to be hypothyroid in the absence of goiter.

The purpose of thyroxine treatment should be to correct symptomatic hypothyroidism and limit or suppress goiter growth. Epidemiologic data suggest that symptomatic individuals who are positive for thyroid autoantibodies and having a slight elevation of serum TSH may drift in and out of a euthyroid state. Unless they have an expanding goiter, these patients do not require therapy but should be maintained under close surveillance. Symptoms of mild thyroid failure may be subtle, and therapeutic trials may sometimes be justified. No control studies are available to date to separate the placebo effect from a physiologic effect of such a policy.

The goal of therapy of thyroid failure is to correct symptoms and to normalize serum TSH. The advent of high-sensitivity TSH assay has made it unnecessary for most patients to undergo the TRH stimulation test to ascertain suppression of pituitary TSH. Despite claims to the contrary, most of these TSH assays cannot confidently separate "undetectable" from normal serum TSH, and concomitant free-serum thyroxine measurement may be necessary. Overreplacement is particularly relevant in the older patient, as even mild hyperthyroxinemia may induce insomnia, weight loss, or cardiac symptoms. In younger patients with goiter in whom the goal is complete suppression of pituitary TSH secretion, mild hyperthyroxinemia may be well tolerated. Older recommendations concerning optimal replacement doses of L-thyroxine ($L-T_4$) were recently revised as the amounts of the bioavailable hormone in older formulation (before 1985) were apparently overestimated. This phenomenon was reflected by the need to reduce the L-thyroxine dose of patients on stable chronic doses. Patients with symptomatic hypothyroidism should be advised not to expect improvement for 3 to 5 weeks after onset of therapy. Younger patients with moderate to severe hypothyroidism may be started on 0.075 to 0.1 mg of thyroxine and followed up some 6 weeks later for clinical assessment and measurement of serum-free thyroxine and high-sensitivity TSH, with dosage adjusted accordingly. Patients above the age of 55, particularly if they have symptoms or ECG evidence of ischemic heart disease, are started on 0.025 mg per day, with a stepwise increase by 0.025 mg per day every 4 to 6 weeks, and thyroid function is reassessed when a dose of 0.075 mg per day is attained. The dose of L-thyroxine may then be adjusted to bring serum TSH within the normal range. In patients with moderate to severe symptoms of ischemic heart disease, a smaller dose of thyroid and/or prior institution of beta-adrenergic blockers may be necessary. Clearly, the thyroid replacement dose should be individualized on the basis of thyroid function tests. Because in some patients the autoimmune injury is progressive, the dose of L-thyroxine may have to be adjusted depending on symptoms, goiter progression, and thyroid function tests after many months of apparent stable activity. There is no place for the use of thyroid extracts of L-triiodothyronine (L-T_3) for the correction of hypothyroidism or suppression of goiter growth. The physician should stress to the patient the importance of compliance with chronic thyroid replacement.

It is good practice to monitor shrinkage of goiter in patients with goitrous thyroiditis. Unequal reduction of goiter may be due to a coincidental nodule or thyroid lymphoma and warrant further investigations. Infrequently, the goiter may continue to grow despite suppression of serum TSH, and surgery is indicated if evidence of pressure on underlying or retrosternal structure is suspected.

RIEDEL'S THYROIDITIS

Riedel's thyroiditis is a rare condition in which the thyroid and surrounding structures are involved in a progressive fibrotic process. Patients with retroperitoneal fibrosis and biliary cirrhosis are particularly prone to this disorder. The thyroid is stony hard. Surgery may be required to relieve pressure symptoms, and thyroid hormones may be necessary if hypothyroidism supervenes.

The Urogenital Tract

BACTERIAL INFECTIONS OF THE URINARY TRACT IN MALES

method of
PHILIP M. HANNO, M.D.
Hospital of the University of Pennsylvania
Philadelphia, Pennsylvania

Asymptomatic infections of the urinary tract are rare, present in less than 0.6 per cent of men under 60 years, 1.5 per cent of men 60 to 69 years, and 3.6 per cent of men over 70 years. The incidence of symptomatic infection is 10 per cent that of women, and infections in adult males mandate urologic investigation. Cystitis is normally secondary to a primary infection of the prostate or kidney or to recent instrumentation or urologic surgery. In the absence of lower urinary tract obstruction, urinary stasis, a foreign body (e.g., catheter), or calculus disease, recurrent urinary infections will usually be traced to bacterial persistence in prostatic fluid. A prostatic antibacterial factor has been isolated from prostate fluid. It is a zinc salt that along with the protective length of the male urethra may be an important extrinsic defense mechanism against infection in men. Intrinsic bladder defense mechanisms include hydrokinetic clearance of bacteria through voiding (compromised in patients with outlet obstruction and residual urine), bacterial antiadherence activity of luminal mucopolysaccharides of the bladder mucosa, and possibly some bacterial growth-inhibitory characteristics of urine.

Diagnosis and Localization of Urinary Tract Infection

Segmented bacteriologic localization cultures will differentiate cystitis from urethritis and allow determination of whether the prostate is the source of infection. Following cleansing of the glans, the patient initiates urination, and the physician collects 5 to 10 ml of urine first voided in a sterile container (VB 1). A sterile midstream urine is next obtained (VB 2). The patient is asked to stop voiding and prostatic massage is conducted, following which the expressed prostatic secretion is collected from the meatus (EPS). Finally, the patient completes voiding, and the fourth specimen is collected (VB 3). Quantitative culture and sensitivity data are collected from each of the above specimens.

If VB 1 is positive and greater than VB 3, the diagnosis is urethritis. If EPS or VB 3 is greater than VB 1, a prostatic infection is primary. If VB 2 indicates greater than 10^4 organisms of pure culture, the patient has cystitis and needs to be treated for 5 days with an appropriate antimicrobial (Table 1) that does not diffuse into the prostate (e.g., nitrofurantoin macrocrystals), following which cultures are repeated to determine the source of the infection.

Bacterial Cystitis

This presents with some combination of urinary frequency, urgency, dysuria, nocturia, suprapubic discomfort, low back pain, and hematuria. Systemic symptoms of fever, chills, and rigors are generally absent unless acute bacterial prostatitis or pyelonephritis is concomitant. Urine culture confirms the diagnosis, showing at least 10^5 colonies of pathogen. *Escherichia coli* is found in 80 per cent of infections. *Klebsiella, Enterobacter, Proteus, Pseudomonas,* and *Serratia* organisms are also found. Other pathogens include *Streptococcus faecalis* and *Staphylococcus.* Treatment requires 10 to 14 days of oral antibiotics, the choice determined by culture and sensitivity data. Urologic investigation to rule out complicating anatomic or functional pathology in the urinary tract is carried out during or after completion of therapy.

Acute and Chronic Bacterial Prostatitis

Acute bacterial prostatitis is manifested by the sudden onset of chills, fever, pain in the lower back and perineum, and difficulty in urination. The urine sediment is positive for white cells and bacteria. On rectal examination the prostate is exquisitely tender. Excessive prostatic palpation

TABLE 1. **Oral Antibiotics Commonly Given for Urinary Tract Infection in Adult Males**

Antibiotic	Recommended Dose
Nitrofurantoin macrocrystals (Macrodantin)	50 mg four times daily
Trimethoprim-sulfamethoxazole (Septra, Bactrim)	Two tablets (160 mg trimethoprim, 800 mg sulfamethoxazole) twice daily
Carbenicillin indanyl sodium (Geocillin)	One to two tablets four times daily
Cephradine (Velosef)	250 to 500 mg four times daily
Norfloxacin (Noroxin)	400 mg twice daily

can induce septicemia. This condition is usually treated on an inpatient basis with 5 to 10 days of parenteral antibiotics, chosen according to bacterial sensitivities. Empiric therapy with a penicillin or cephalosporin in conjunction with an aminoglycoside is recommended prior to tailoring therapy after sensitivity data become available. Following parenteral treatment, outpatient treatment for another 2 weeks is the rule with oral antibiotics. As opposed to chronic bacterial prostatitis, there is good penetration of antibiotic into the acutely inflamed gland, and the choice of drug is not as critical.

Chronic bacterial prostatitis, in contrast, is insidious in onset. In most cases, the patient has no history of acute prostatitis, and there is no fever. Patients usually present with a history of recurrent bacterial cystitis but may be surprisingly asymptomatic in the intervals. They may have perineal pain and a tender, "boggy" prostate on examination. Diagnosis is made on the basis of the localization studies already described. Treatment is prolonged, as diffusion of antibiotics into the non–acutely inflamed prostate is poor, and 6 to 8 weeks of oral antibiotic therapy is not uncommon. Trimethoprim-sulfamethoxazole (Septra, Bacterim), carbenicillin indanyl sodium (Geocillin), and norfloxacin (Noroxin) reportedly give adequate prostatic levels of antibiotic in many cases. One should not confuse true bacterial prostatitis with nonbacterial prostatitis and prostatodynia, much more common conditions for which antibiotics are *not* indicated.

Special Circumstances

Patients with chronic indwelling catheters and asymptomatic bacterial colonization should not be treated, as sterilization of the urine is virtually impossible, and resistant organisms are likely to establish residence in the presence of long-term antibiotic supression. Treatment should only be instituted for symptoms of acute infection. Asymptomatic bacteriuria in elderly patients, although associated with an increased mortality rate, has not been found to be the cause of the mortality. This condition is difficult to cure and probably should not be treated.

BACTERIAL INFECTIONS OF THE URINARY TRACT IN FEMALES

method of
JOHN A. MATA, M.D.
Louisiana State University Medical Center
Shreveport, Louisiana

Urinary tract infection (UTI) in adult women is a common and often frustrating problem. Up to 50 per cent of adult women experience at least one episode of dysuria, half of which have a culture-proven bacterial UTI. The prevalence rate of bacteriuria (2 to 10 per cent) increases with age, so that it is not uncommon that patients with symptoms of a UTI make up 10 per cent of a general practice. Luckily, the vast majority of UTIs in females are uncomplicated and respond promptly to treatment or resolve spontaneously. However, there is a small cohort of patients who have complicating factors (Table 1), such as diabetes, pregnancy, or stone disease, that may create a life-threatening infection or who have recurrent or persistent UTI.

Etiology/Diagnosis

Although there are inherent vaginal and bladder defense mechanisms, the most common cause of UTI is bacterial ascent from periurethral colonization by organisms that normally constitute the fecal flora. The most common include *Escherichia coli, Staphylococcus* species, and strains of *Proteus, Klebsiella,* and *Enterobacter.* The majority of infections occur in the lower tract (cystitis, urethritis), not in the upper tract (pyelonephritis), and in over 90 per cent of the cases the infections are uncomplicated but prone to recurrence. The signs and symptoms of UTI in adult females are characteristic but not specific in that the bladder and urethra respond similarly to a variety of irritative factors. Dysuria, frequency, and urgency are commonly present; however, fever, flank pain, or costovertebral angle tenderness may herald an upper tract infection in 50 per cent of cases.

For accurate diagnosis I rely on a bacterial culture and sensitivity of a clean-catch, midstream, or catheterized urine specimen. A preliminary office urinalysis (UA) may be suggestive of a UTI, but pyuria or bacteriuria alone is not pathognomonic. Although 100,000 bacteria per ml of urine is the statistical sine qua non of a UTI, counts of 10,000 colonies per ml of an appropriately collected urine sample can be considered significant.

MANAGEMENT

Antibiotic Selection

The majority of commonly used antimicrobials in UTI therapy are effective and safe. Since uncomplicated UTIs respond rapidly to treatment, short-term to single dose regimens have become popular and cost effective. Table 2 lists

TABLE 1. **Complicating Factors in Female Urinary Tract Infection**

Diabetes	Pregnancy
Carcinoma-in-situ	Vaginitis
Neurogenic bladder	Urethral diverticulum
Urethral syndrome	Urethral stenosis
Vesicoureteral reflux	Congenital anomalies
Tuberculosis	Interstitial cystitis
Stone disease	Immunosuppression
Chronic catheter	Foreign body

TABLE 2. **Antibiotic Therapy for Female Urinary Tract Infection**

Antimicrobial	Single-Dose Regimen	3 to 7 Day Oral Regimen
Amoxicillin	3 grams	250 mg twice daily
Nitrofurantoin (Macrodantin)	100 mg	50 to 100 mg four times daily
Trimethoprim-sulfamethoxazole (TMX) (Bactrim/Septra)	160 mg/800 mg	1 double-strength tablet twice daily
Sulfisoxazole (Gantrisin)	2 grams	1 gram four times daily
Ciprofloxacin (Cipro)	750 mg	250 mg twice daily
Cephalexin* (Keflex)		250 to 500 mg four times daily

*There are several other oral cephalosporins available now.

the commonly used oral antibiotics and their dosages and schedules in UTI treatment. A brief review of the drugs and their common side effects follows.

Penicillins. The aminopenicillins such as ampicillin and amoxicillin are commonly prescribed bactericidal agents in nonallergic patients; however, up to 25 per cent of organisms may be resistant. The more expensive beta-lactamase inhibitor amoxicillin plus clavulanic acid (Augmentin) is effective against the majority of isolates resistant to the aminopenicillins. Adverse reactions common to the penicillin family include nausea, diarrhea, rashes, and a propensity for vaginitis due to *Candida* species (10 to 15 per cent).

Sulfonamides. These are bacteriostatic agents effective in over three-quarters of the urinary pathogens. Common agents include sulfisoxazole (Gantrisin) and sulfamethoxazole (Gantanol). They are inexpensive, and side effects include rashes, nausea, and headaches.

TRIMETHOPRIM. This bacteriostatic agent is available as a single agent (Trimpex, Proloprim), 100 mg twice daily or 200 mg daily, and is effective in over 90 per cent of UTI isolates. It is suitable for prophylaxis. Side effects include rash and nausea.

TRIMETHOPRIM/SULFAMETHOXAZOLE (TMX). This synergistic combination available as Bactrim/Septra or in a generic preparation is quite popular because of its effectiveness, low cost, and twice daily dosage. Side effects reflect the component drugs but also include leukopenia and falsely elevated creatinine levels. It is not recommended in the frail, elderly population or in patients with significant renal insufficiency or autoimmune disorders.

NITROFURANTOIN. A urinary specific drug, nitrofurantoin (Macrodantin) is active against gram-negative and gram-positive organisms. Its side effects include nausea, vomiting, and rash. Prolonged therapy may be associated with pulmonary fibrosis. This drug is contraindicated in patients with a glomerular filtration rate (GFR) less than 40 ml per minute.

CEPHALOSPORINS. These are safe, effective antimicrobials with few adverse side effects. There are many preparations now available since the original cephalexin (Keflex), 250–500 mg orally four times daily, became available. These include cefaclor (Ceclor), cefuroxime (Zinacef), and cephradine (Anspor, Velosef). Vaginitis due to *Candida* species occurs in up to 15 per cent of women treated with these agents.

FLUOROQUINOLONES. Norfloxacin (Noroxin), 400 mg orally twice daily and ciprofloxacin (Cipro), 250 mg orally twice daily, are recent antimicrobial additions offering oral antipseudomonal coverage. They are more potent than the older quinolone nalidixic acid (NegGram), offering a broader gram-negative and gram-positive spectrum. These are generally not first line drugs for UTI but are welcome additions for those women with resistant or complicated UTIs. They are contraindicated in children and in pregnancy at this time. Potential side effects include nausea, vomiting, diarrhea, headache, and vaginitis due to *Candida* species.

Uncomplicated Simple Infections

The majority of women with UTI have a simple infection that may or may not be recurrent. These infections respond rapidly to appropriate treatment, although occasionally some women may benefit from urinary analgesics or antispasmodics such as phenazopyridine (Pyridium), 100 mg orally three times a day, or flavoxate (Urispas), 100 mg orally twice daily. Rarely in the woman without UTI risk factors do I need to call back the patient for a resistant culture report in order to change antibiotics. I have the patient return for a routine symptom check and to repeat the urine culture (now off treatment) to document a sterile specimen.

The greatest risk factors in patients with simple infections include sexual activity (by far the greatest), recent use of a diaphragm contraceptive, and a past history of a simple UTI. Plenty of fluids, frequent bladder emptying (especially after intercourse), and occasionally a pericoital antibiotic in patients with recurrent "honeymoon cystitis" are helpful in reducing risk.

Recurrent Urinary Tract Infections

UTIs in women are prone to recurrence. Recurrence means reinfection with a new organism, although it may still be *E. coli* but of a different serotype. Unfortunately, the majority (80 per cent) of women will have another symptomatic UTI within a 2-year period. Again, assuming there is no reason to suspect a complicated UTI, treatment is routine. Prophylactic therapy is indicated in this group of patients, if these recurrences are at frequent, closely spaced intervals, such as two or more infections in a 6-month period or less. I tend to use a bedtime dose of nitrofurantoin, 50 mg, trimethoprim, 50 mg, or TMX single strength over a 3- to 6-month period. This can be a frustrating problem for the patient and physician. If these episodes break through despite prophylaxis or continue, I evaluate the problem initially with a voiding cystourethrogram (VCUG) and a renal/bladder ultrasonogram. Occasionally, cystourethroscopy is indicated, but this is generally reserved for patients with abacterial cystitis, such as interstitial cystitis or urethral syndrome (these patients by definition do not have recurrent UTI).

Acute Pyelonephritis

Pyelonephritis is the term denoting infection in the renal pelvis and parenchyma. Physicians are alert to this diagnosis in patients with a UTI accompanied by fever and flank pain. I treat these patients with a 2-week course of therapy with TMX, amoxicillin, or a cephalosporin and order an intravenous pyelogram (IVP) or a kidney, ureter, and bladder (KUB) plain film and renal ultrasonogram early on. Sensitive tests for true bacterial localization exist, but they require invasive procedures (although antibody-coated urine has been called a reliable marker for renal infection). Ill patients, of course, benefit from hospital admission, intravenous fluids, and parenteral antibiotics as well as early radiographic or sonographic imaging. Failure to respond promptly to therapy may indicate a complicated UTI, i.e., lobar nephronia, obstruction, stones, or perinephric abscess. Follow-up urine cultures are then obtained after the patient's treatment.

TABLE 3. **Diagnosis in Complicated Urinary Tract Infections**

Upper Tract
Emphysematous pyelonephritis
Xanthogranulomatous pyelonephritis
Acute bacterial nephritis (lobar nephronia)
Renal cortical abscess
Perinephric abscess
Pyonephrosis
Lower Tract
Cystitis cystica/glandularis
Eosinophilic cystitis
Malakoplakia
Interstitial cystitis
Cystitis emphysematosa
Vesicointestinal fistula

Urinary Infections in Pregnancy

Symptomatic or asymptomatic bacteriuria in pregnant females should be treated. Safe drugs include the penicillins and cephalosporins and nitrofurantoin. A 3- to 5-day course suffices for most lower tract infections followed by a repeat urine culture 2 to 3 days after treatment. Acute pyelonephritis unresponsive to antibiotics mandates that one rule out obstruction. Early on, a KUB and renal ultrasonogram may be diagnostic but because of the hydronephrosis of pregnancy, often a two- to three-shot IVP is required.

Complicated Urinary Tract Infections

A small cohort of female patients may have persistent or unresolved bacteriuria secondary to a complicated UTI. These patients generally have complicating factors (see Table 1) causing these difficult infections (Table 3). Their management may require intravenous antibiotics and radiographic and urologic evaluation, and often endourologic or surgical therapy is necessary. A high index of suspicion is mandatory in these patients.

Geriatric or neurogenic patients with chronic Foley catheter insertion may present special problems with recurrent UTIs secondary to stones or candidal overgrowth. Asymptomatic or colonized bacteriuria is not treated unless associated with systemic symptoms or if stone-forming pathogens such as *Proteus* species are cultured.

Candiduria may be treated with a three-way indwelling urethral catheter using a 5 mg per dl suspension of amphotericin B (50 mg in 1 liter sterile water) at 40 ml per hour or 1 liter per day over 5 to 7 days. Often, simply discontinuing chronic antibiotics and removing foreign bodies (catheters), if possible, will clear up a noninvasive fungal infection of the urinary bladder.

URINARY TRACT INFECTIONS IN FEMALE CHILDREN

method of
BRUCE BROECKER, M.D.
Emory University School of Medicine
Atlanta, Georgia

Urinary tract infections (UTIs) are a common cause of morbidity and an occasional cause of mortality in children. Five to six per cent of girls will have at least one bacterial urinary tract infection during childhood, and many will have multiple recurrences. Pediatric UTIs occur predominantly in girls (female to male ratio of 30:1) except during the first 30 days of life, when males predominate by a ratio of 10:1. During the past 30 years, the treatment of UTIs has become highly successful as a result of the many effective antibacterials that concentrate in the urine, but the pathophysiology of individual susceptibility and the natural history continue to be less well understood despite intense research efforts.

Urinary tract infections may be classified in ways that are useful in selecting therapy and further diagnostic evaluation. One such classification divides UTIs into (1) neonatal, (2) uncomplicated cystitis, (3) recurrent cystitis, and (4) acute pyelonephritis. It should be recognized that this classification is clinical and that by parameters such as bacterial localization there may be significant overlap. It should also be recognized that the symptoms in each of these categories may be caused by nonbacterial infections (from *Chlamydia, Candida,* and *Adenovirus* species) as well as by noninfectious conditions.

Methods of anatomically localizing bacteria have been exhaustively studied in an effort to tailor therapy more objectively. As yet, those methods that are noninvasive (antibody-coated bacteria, c-reactive protein capsular antigen, lactate dehydrogenase (LDH) isoenzyme) are unreliable. The most reliable techniques (bladder washout and ureteral catheterization) are invasive, requiring general anesthesia and, therefore, are not generally employed.

The most common organism responsible for bacterial UTIs continues to be *Escherichia coli,* followed by *Enterococci, Pseudomonas, Klebsiella,* and *Proteus* species.

Treatment and Evaluation

Neonatal

Neonatal UTIs occur predominantly in males, with an incidence of approximately 1.5 per cent (male) and 0.15 per cent (female), respectively. Neonatal UTIs are distinguished from UTIs in older children by clinical symptoms and laboratory findings that suggest a hematogenous rather than an ascending route of infection. The most common organism is *E. coli,* accounting for 80 per cent of the infections. These are serious infections and must be treated promptly and aggressively. Recommended treatment is with ampicillin and an aminoglycoside (gentamicin, tobramycin, amikacin) (Table 1) until an organism is identified and sensitivity tests are available. Peak and trough aminoglycoside levels should be obtained regularly to monitor and adjust dosage. Treatment should be continued for 10 to 14 days, at which time a urinalysis should be acellular. A urine culture should be repeated 5 to 7 days after completion of therapy. The incidence of anatomic abnormalities in these children is significant (30 to 50 per cent), with vesicoureteral reflux being the most common. All infected neonates should be evaluated radio-

TABLE 1. Treatment of Urinary Tract Infections in Female Children

Type of Therapy	Dose/Kg/Day	Daily Doses
Parenteral		
Ampicillin	100 mg	4
Amoxicillin	50 mg	3
Cefazolin (Ancef)	50 mg	4
Cefamandole (Mandol)	100 mg	4
Gentamicin (Garamycin)	5 to 7 mg	3
Tobramycin (Nebcin)	5 mg	3
Amikacin (Amikin)	15 mg	3
Oral		
Ampicillin	100 mg	4
Amoxicillin	40 mg	3
Cefradine (Velosef)	25 mg	4
Erythromycin	30 mg	4
Nitrofurantoin (Furadantin)	5 to 7 mg	4
TMP/SMX* (Bactrim, Septra)	0.5 to 1 ml	2
Prophylactic		
Nitrofurantoin	3 mg	1
TMP/SMX	0.5 ml	1

*TMP/SMX = 8 mg of trimethoprim and 40 mg of sulfamethoxazole per ml.

graphically (Table 2). A renal ultrasonogram should be done early in the course of a neonatal infection to rule out obstruction. The timing of delayed evaluation is not critical, but generally it is carried out between 2 and 4 weeks after the completion of treatment. It is desirable, however, for the child to take oral antibiotics until the evaluation is completed.

Radiographic evaluation should include a voiding cystourethrogram (VCUG) and a renal nuclear scan or an intravenous urogram (if the VCUG demonstrates vesicoureteral reflux). The urogram or nuclear scan is preferred in infants with demonstrable reflux because of its better delineation of subtle degrees of reflux nephropathy. It has been recommended that the neonate with a febrile UTI and normal radiographic studies should have a follow-up ultrasonogram at age 2 years, since the evolution of renal scarring may take this long to appear on imaging studies.

TABLE 2. Evaluation of Female Child with UTI

Neonate
1. During therapy (early): renal/bladder ultrasonogram*
2. After resolution of UTI (delayed): VCUG*

Uncomplicated Cystitis
1. Greater than 5 years of age: renal/bladder ultrasonogram
2. Less than 5 years of age: VCUG, renal ultrasound (IVP)

Recurrent Cystitis
VCUG, renal ultrasonogram (IVP)

Acute Pyelonephritis
As per neonatal UTI

*Further studies (intravenous pyelogram [IV], renal scan, CT scan) may be indicated by abnormalities discovered on the above studies.

Uncomplicated Cystitis

Uncomplicated cystitis denotes a bacterial infection of the bladder occurring for the first time in an anatomically normal urinary tract. This infection occurs overwhelmingly in females, generally with irritative voiding symptoms and without fever. Radiographic evaluation is indicated in all children who present with clinical symptoms of uncomplicated cystitis and have a culture-proven bacterial infection. The particular imaging studies may, however, be tailored to the patient's age. It is my practice to evaluate older children (over 5 years) with a first afebrile infection with ultrasonography alone. If that study is normal, no further imaging studies are done. A child with an abnormal study is evaluated with additional studies as dictated by the abnormal findings. In younger children (less than 5 years) or in any child with febrile or recurrent infections, a VCUG is done in addition to the ultrasonographic examination. The ultrasonographic examination of a child with a UTI should include views of both the kidneys and bladder.

Treatment of uncomplicated cystitis is extremely effective. The following antibiotics are all useful: sulfisoxazole (Gantrisin), ampicillin, amoxicillin, erythromycin, cefradine (Velosef), trimethoprim-sulfamethoxazole (TMP/SMX) (Bactrim, Septra), trimethoprim, and nitrofurantoin (Furadantin) (see Table 1). The appropriate length of treatment has been the subject of a number of articles over recent years. The standard treatment course of 10 to 14 days has been challenged by courses lasting 7, 5, 3, and 1 day(s). Advocates of the shortest regimen point to advantages of decreased cost, decreased toxicity, greater compliance, and comparable success rates, while those advocates of the longer courses argue that there is a greater recurrence rate with abbreviated treatment. For uncomplicated cystitis this author favors a 3- to 5-day course of one of the above antibiotics, most commonly TMP/SMX or nitrofurantoin.

Recurrent Cystitis

Recurrent cystitis denotes a repetitive UTI and is a particularly prevalent feature of UTIs in children. Up to 75 per cent of children with a UTI will develop one or more recurrent infections. A recurrent infection is defined as a second new infection and is to be distinguished from bacterial persistence, which means failure of eradication of the original organism. This differentiation is usually readily done with the urine culture and sensitivity test. Even when infections are closely spaced, recurrent infection is the rule. Bacterial persistence generally occurs only with bacterial resistance (wrong antibiotics), treatment non-

compliance, or anatomic abnormalities. Nitrofurantoin and TMP/SMX are the most useful antibiotics in this category, with a dosage modification for prophylactic use (see Table 1). In those children in whom the recurrent infections are closely spaced (several days to a week), it is my feeling that the infection has altered the normal bladder defensive mechanisms, rendering the child susceptible to an early recurrence. I have found a prophylactic dose of TMP/SMX or nitrofurantoin for 4 to 6 weeks immediately following the therapeutic course useful in interrupting this process. In the child whose recurrences are more widely spaced (weeks to months), I use the parameter of three infections in 6 months or four infections in 1 year as indication for prophylactic therapy lasting 3 to 6 months. Infections occurring at less frequent intervals are treated individually with a 3- to 5-day therapeutic course of one of the standard antibiotics mentioned earlier.

Acute Pyelonephritis

This category consists of those children with an acute febrile urinary tract infection associated with leukocytosis and flank pain. It is a serious upper urinary tract infection that needs prompt and effective treatment to prevent renal damage. These children should have an ultrasonogram of the kidneys and bladder early during treatment to rule out obstructive anomalies of the urinary tract. Further imaging studies are postponed until after resolution of the infection. Parenteral antibiotics with ampicillin and an aminoglycoside are indicated as initial therapy until culture and sensitivity studies are available. Parenteral therapy should continue until the patient has been afebrile for 24 hours and the urinalysis is without pyuria or bacteriuria. Oral antibiotics are continued for a total of 14 days.

CHILDHOOD ENURESIS

method of
H. GIL RUSHTON, M.D.
Children's Hospital National Medical Center
Washington, D.C.

Enuresis is the involuntary voiding of urine beyond the age by which normal control is expected. Nocturnal enuresis refers to persistent wetting during sleep past the age of 5. Primary enuresis is defined as bed wetting in patients who have never been dry for extended periods of time. In contrast, secondary enuresis is the onset of wetting following a continuous dry period greater than 6 months.

Nocturnal enuresis is prevalent in as many as 15 to 20 per cent of 5-year-old children. Approximately 15 per cent of bed wetters will achieve nocturnal control each year, so that by age 15 only 1 to 2 per cent of adolescents remain enuretic. Approximately 15 per cent of bed wetters also have diurnal enuresis (wetting while awake).

Treatment

Although many etiologic theories for enuresis have been proposed, the bulk of data supports a biologic basis in most patients. Cystometrogram evaluation in up to 85 per cent of enuretic children reveals a persistent pattern of infantile-type detrusor instability, with uninhibited bladder contractions and a small capacity. Enuresis is considered by most to represent a "maturational lag" of normal inhibitory control by the central nervous system. Genetic factors clearly appear to contribute to enuresis. In one survey, when both parents had a history of enuresis, 77 per cent of the children were enuretic. When only one parent had a history of enuresis, 44 per cent of the children were enuretic. When neither parent had a history of enuresis, only 15 per cent of the children were enuretic. Sleep and/or arousal disorders have also been implicated in some enuretics. This relationship is poorly understood, and supporting data are both equivocal and conflicting. Although most enuretics do not suffer from underlying psychopathology, emotional stress can at times manifest as secondary or "onset" enuresis. In a recent retrospective study of 1265 children, the factors most predictive of the age of attainment of bladder control were a family history of enuresis, the child's developmental level at 1 and 3 years of age, and the child's early sleeping patterns.

Evaluation and treatment is contingent upon the pattern of enuresis, physical examination, and urinalysis and culture. Physical examination should include abdominal and genital examination, observation of the child while voiding, and neurologic evaluation. Neurologic evaluation should include checking peripheral reflexes, evaluation of perineal sensation and anal sphincter tone, and inspection of the lower back for evidence of sacral dimpling or cutaneous anomalies suggestive of spina bifida occulta.

Uncomplicated Enuresis

The incidence of organic uropathology in children with nocturnal enuresis, normal physical examination, and negative urine culture does not appear to be significantly higher than in the normal population. Frequently, these children will have associated mild daytime frequency or enuresis with a normal urinary stream, a positive family history of enuresis, and perhaps slightly delayed developmental milestones. No further urologic evaluation is indicated in most of these patients.

Numerous therapeutic programs for uncomplicated nocturnal enuresis have been recommended. These include psychotherapy, hypnotherapy, diet therapy, motivational therapy, drug therapy, and behavioral modification (conditioning) therapy. Although no single therapeutic plan is ideal for all patients, the last two approaches are the most effective and practical. There is no objective evidence that withholding fluids in the evening, random awakening of the child to void, or punitive measures result in significant cessation of enuresis.

Drug Therapy. A number of pharmacologic agents have been used to treat enuresis. Tricyclic antidepressants, particularly imipramine (Tofranil), have been used with the best results. The exact pharmacologic mechanism of action on the bladder is not well understood. However, it does appear to result in a measurable increase in functional bladder capacity when it is effective. Imipramine should not be used to treat enuresis in children under age 6 to 7 years and should be kept out of the reach of small children, owing to its extreme toxicity in excessive doses. Success rates are best in older children, with complete cessation of enuresis reported in up to 40 per cent and improvement in 10 to 20 per cent. However, the relapse rate following discontinuation is high, particularly when the drug is stopped abruptly or prematurely, and many children escape control, requiring an increasingly higher dosage for effectiveness. The dose of imipramine is 25 mg taken 1 to 2 hours prior to bedtime for patients 6 to 8 years old and 50 to 75 mg in older children and adolescents (not to exceed 1.5 mg per kg day). A new sustained-release form (Tofranil PM) may be most effective. Therapy should be continued for at least 2 weeks prior to assessing efficacy and possibly adjusting the dosage. The optimal duration of therapy in patients who respond favorably is uncertain. Generally, I recommend treatment for 3 to 6 months, at which time the patient is "weaned" by gradually reducing the dose and/or frequency, i.e., every other night over 3 to 4 weeks. Should relapse occur, a repeat course of treatment can be started. Often, imipramine will work on a "prn" basis, and use may be reserved for times when staying dry is particularly important to the child (sleepovers, camp).

Side effects from treatment with imipramine are uncommon but include anxiety, insomnia, and adverse personality changes. Overdoses have been reported secondary to excessive ingestion and can cause potentially fatal toxicity with cardiac arrhythmias and conduction blocks, hypotension, and convulsions. Physostigmine therapy is used to manage life-threatening imipramine toxicity.

Anticholinergic drugs, specifically oxybutynin* (Ditropan), reduce or abolish uninhibited bladder contractions and may be particularly beneficial in patients who also have daytime frequency or enuresis. The dose in children over 6 years old is usually 5 mg two to three times daily. Common side effects include dryness of the mouth and facial flushing. Excessive dosage may result in blurring of vision.

Behavioral Modification (Conditioning) Therapy. Behavioral modification therapy revolves around use of a signal alarm device that is electrolytically triggered when the child voids, awakening the patient. Initially, the child wakens after or during voiding. A conditioned response is gradually evoked by the association of awakening and inhibition of micturition. Long-term success rates of 75 per cent have been reported following 4 to 6 months of treatment. Essential to the success of such a program are strong patient compliance and motivation.

Numerous systems are available at reasonable cost. Occasional complications have been reported with pad and buzzer systems such as "buzzer ulcers" of the skin or alarm failure if the child is not positioned properly on the pad. A modification of the alarm system, known as the "Wet-Stop" (Palco Labs, Santa Cruz, CA), uses a small sensor that is placed into a cotton pocket in the child's underwear and an alarm that is attached to the child's pajama collar. These units are compact, safe, and effective and avoid many of the problems associated with a pad and buzzer.

As success depends on a cooperative and motivated child, behavioral modification therapy is generally used in patients over 7 years old. In some children who fail to awaken to the alarm or who awaken in a confused state, a low dose of imipramine in conjunction with the alarm system may be beneficial. Adjunctive measures that will increase the effectiveness of the alarm system include positive reinforcement programs in which the child receives a "reward" following a predetermined number of successive dry nights. The child is encouraged to keep a record of progress, such as using a calendar with stars for each dry night. Parental support, empathy, and patience are key elements in successful management of the child with enuresis. Likewise, reassurance, periodic feedback, and encouragement of the parents and child by the physician are necessary for optimal results.

---

*Safety and efficacy of this drug in children under 5 years of age have not been established.

Complicated Enuresis

Patients with a positive urine culture or history of urinary tract infection, abnormal neurologic examination, or a history of significant voiding dysfunction characterized by either infrequent voiding or severe frequency associated with incontinence, poor urinary stream, and/or encopresis have complicated enuresis. These patients should be further evaluated with a renal/bladder sonogram and voiding cystogram (with spine films) to exclude vesicoureteral reflux and/or hydroureteronephrosis associated with a thickened, unstable bladder. The latter findings indicate the need for further urologic and/or urodynamic evaluation. Neurosurgical evaluation may also be indicated in some of these patients to exclude spina bifida occulta or a tethered cord.

In those patients with secondary onset enuresis associated with severe voiding dysfunction, including infrequent voiding and encopresis, a careful family and social history may reveal underlying psychosocial stresses. Treatment of these children is initially directed toward emotional support. Those patients with bladder or upper tract damage secondary to severe voiding dysfunction who do not have an organic obstructive or neurologic lesion may also benefit from timed voidings, anticholinergic therapy, and/or biofeedback therapy. Occasionally, renal damage may be so severe as to necessitate a program of intermittent catheterization if bladder emptying cannot be achieved by other means. In some cases psychotherapy or professional counseling may also be warranted.

URINARY INCONTINENCE

method of
EDWARD J. McGUIRE, M.D.
University of Michigan
Ann Arbor, Michigan

Incontinence may be due to abnormalities of urethral or bladder function. Bladder abnormalities include poor reservoir function manifested by decreased compliance or an increase in pressure with increasing volume. These abnormalities are relatively subtle and often poorly diagnosed and poorly managed. Abnormalities of the control of bladder reflex activity are probably the most common reason for incontinence, although the etiology of this kind of abnormality is multiple. In addition, "paradoxic" or overflow incontinence results from lack of reflex bladder contractility.

Treatment

Bladder-Related Incontinence

Disorders of Compliance. An abnormal increase in intravesical pressure with filling, indicating loss of bladder reservoir function, occurs after radical pelvic surgery, in cases of peripheral neuropathy, in patients with myelodysplasia, and in those with sacral cord or sacral root injuries or disease. These disorders are frequently associated with lack of reflex bladder contractility, but the major abnormality is a loss of low pressure volume accommodation. The increased pressure volume relationship has a direct hydraulic effect on ureteral delivery of urine to the bladder and induces leakage across a fixed continence mechanism at low to moderate vesical volumes. The intent of treatment is to empty the bladder periodically and to preserve and to protect low pressure storage of urine. This can usually be accomplished by intermittent catheterization and anticholinergic drugs. If vesical pressures cannot be kept below 35 cm of H_2O at the volumes obtained at the time of intermittent catheterization, some method to improve reservoir function is essential to preserve upper tract function. This can be by augmentation cystoplasty using bowel tissue or by reducing the outlet resistance and lowering the pressure at which leakage occurs (with the acceptance of more incontinence). Increasing urethral resistance to improve continence is directly prejudical to upper tract function if vesical compliance (volume tolerance at pressures under 35 cm of H_2O) is indicated.

Disorders of Control of Reflex Vesical Activity. These disorders may be associated wtih spinal cord injury or disease and multiple sclerosis, in which case control of reflex bladder activity is poor or absent and both the storage and voiding phases of bladder activity are disordered. Approximately 70 per cent of the patients can be managed by anticholinergic medication and intermittent catheterization. Because the major effect of such lesions in men is related to upper tract changes related to high bladder pressure, sphincter obviation procedures and condom catheter drainage are frequently used—these sacrifice continence. In women, bladder pressures are lower, and continence is of major importance. Interruption of reflex pathways at the trigone, sacral root, or cord levels or partial cystectomy and augmentation cytoplasty can be used to achieve good vesical storage function, with intermittent catheterization used for periodic bladder emptying. Quadriplegic women are a special problem; provision for a continent stoma to allow self-catheterization permits avoidance of treatment by Foley catheter drainage or ileal loop diversion; both methods have a dismal long-term outlook. Treatment of male spinal-injured patients by ileal loop diversion, cutaneous ureterostomy, suprapubic tube, or Foley catheter drainage is associated with equally dismal long-term complications.

"Idiopathic" Detrusor Contractile Incontinence. Poor control of reflex vesical activity without high pressure bladder dysfunction is a fairly common problem that is frequently encountered in the elderly, those with cerebrovascular disease or lesions of the basal ganglia, adult men and women without neurologic disease, and children. The urodynamic finding is basically a sudden bladder contraction that occurs unwillingly.

Warning of detrusor events is poor, and reflex contractility is provoked by volume. Treatment is directed at delay of the reflex bladder response with anticholinergic agents such as oxybutynin chloride (Ditropan), 5 mg three times daily; propantheline bromide (Pro-Banthine), 15 to 30 mg three times daily; dicyclomine (Bentyl), 20 mg four times daily; or imipramine (Tofranil), 10 to 25 mg three times daily or 50 mg at bedtime. These should be coupled with a regular program of timed voiding, which tends to short-circuit the uninhibited response of the bladder to filling. Urodynamically, no qualitative differences distinguish hyperactive bladder activity in one group from that in another. Poor response to one agent often can be circumvented by using two agents that act differently—e.g., imipramine, 10 mg three times daily, and oxybutynin, 5 mg three times daily.

Obstructive Uropathy. Poor control of reflex vesical activity is also associated with obstructive uropathy, most commonly, benign prostatic hyperplasia. Residual urine or symptoms suggesting obstruction, e.g., hesitancy or a slow stream, should prompt investigation and initially contraindicate anticholinergic therapy.

Stress Incontinence

Stress incontinence related to poor urethral support in women, associated with visible urethral hypermobility, responds most predictably to surgical repair. Alternative methods include tampon use to achieve urethral support, and temporary treatment with drugs with alpha-stimulating properties (e.g., phenylpropanolamine, 25 mg three times daily, or imipramine, 25 mg three times daily). These agents have not been approved by the Food and Drug Administration for this usage and have somewhat limited value.

Weakness of urethral sphincter function in elderly women, not associated with urethral hypermobility with an increase in intra-abdominal pressure, responds reasonably well to intravaginal Premarin (one third of an applicator at night) and imipramine (10 mg three times daily). Men with very mild postprostatectomy incontinence *may* respond to alpha-stimulating agents, but this does not happen often.

When internal sphincter function is absent in

patients with myelodysplasia and following radical prostatectomy, and occasionally following radical surgery for uterine or rectal malignant disease, medication is of no benefit, and usually complicated surgical procedures are required for relief.

EPIDIDYMITIS

method of
JOHN R. RICHARDSON, JR., M.D.
Dartmouth-Hitchcock Medical Center
Hanover, New Hampshire

Epididymitis is a painful swelling due to an inflammatory process involving the epididymis on one or both sides. It is thought to occur most often secondary to reflux of infective material down the vas deferens. The process can be seen in children and older men, but most cases occur in young, sexually active males. The infecting agent is usually whatever is the most common uropathogen in the afflicted age group. In children and older men it is *Escherichia coli,* whereas in young adults it is usually *Gonococcus, Chlamydia,* or a nonspecific agent. Rarely, epididymitis can be seen in such systemic diseases as tuberculosis, brucellosis, or cryptococcosis. Noninfective causes of epididymitis are trauma and the antiarrhythmic agent amiodarone. In the latter instance, only the head of the epididymis tends to be involved, and the process responds to withdrawal of the drug.

This disease occurs in an acute or, less often, in a chronic form. Acute epididymitis usually involves the lower pole, or globus major, of the epididymis, since this is the location of the attachment to the offending vas deferens. The epididymis is red, hot, tender, painful, and swollen. Likewise, the vas deferens tends to be swollen and tender. Analysis of the urine often demonstrates white blood cells and bacteria. A urine culture may be positive.

Chronic epididymitis usually presents with an aching, tender, lumpy epididymis. The vas deferens is usually palpably normal, and the urine analysis is often normal.

For obvious reasons, epididymitis must be differentiated from two other serious pathologic processes, namely, torsion of the spermatic cord, and testicular tumor. In cases of torsion of the cord, the urine is usually normal, and a radionuclide testicular scan demonstrates absent blood flow. In cases of testicular tumor, an ultrasonographic examination identifies a hypoechoic mass beneath the tunica albuginea. If either of these conditions cannot be ruled out, surgical exploration is indicated—immediately in the former case, urgently in the latter.

Vigorous palpation of the prostate is to be avoided in cases of epididymitis prior to the institution of antibiotics. This may cause increased reflux of infected material down the affected vas deferens, or it may convert a unilateral process to a bilateral one. There is also danger of provoking urosepsis.

Treatment

Treatment of all cases of epididymitis involves rest, heat, and elevation. Rest means that the patient should spend most of his time lying down, preferably in bed. Heat means that he should sit in a hot bathtub three to four times a day for 20 minutes at a time. This regimen promotes comfort and increases local blood flow. If a tub is not available, a hot wet washcloth may be used instead. Elevation means that when lying down, the patient should have a crushed bath towel placed between his thighs to elevate his scrotum. When upright, he should wear an athletic supporter.

In addition, infective epididymitis is treated with a broad-spectrum antibiotic pending the results of the urine culture. A good choice is oxytetracycline (Terramycin) 250 mg four times daily for 10 days.

In acutely painful cases, 10 ml of 2 per cent lidocaine (Xylocaine) with epinephrine can be instilled into the spermatic cord. The cord may be located one fingerbreadth above and one fingerbreadth medial to the pubic tubercle at a depth of 2 to 4 cm beneath the skin. In some cases, an oral analgesic such as codeine 30 mg may be given every 3 to 4 hours for the first 24 to 48 hours. If the inflammatory reaction is severe, there may be a role for a nonsteroidal antiinflammatory agent such as ibuprofen (Motrin). Usually, aspirin works as well.

Epididymitis is often slow to resolve. Definite improvement should be noted after 48 to 72 hours of therapy. Reasonably complete resolution may not occur for 1 to 2 weeks or perhaps longer.

Complications include abscess formation, infertility, and chronic pain, although most cases eventually resolve completely.

GLOMERULAR DISORDERS

method of
MARC J. SADOVNIC, M.D., and
W. KLINE BOLTON, M.D.
University of Virginia School of Medicine
Charlottesville, Virginia

Patients with glomerular disorders may present with complaints such as edema, oliguria, and macroscopic hematuria, or they may be asymptomatic with abnormalities in urinary protein excretion, urinary sediment, or elevated serum creatinine levels detected on routine screening. Occasionally, a renal biopsy is not necessary, as in the child with nephrotic syndrome, or when history, physical findings, and laboratory data support the diagnoses of poststreptococcal glomerulonephritis or Schönlein-Henoch purpura. In the majority of cases, however, the diagnosis cannot be made on clinical grounds, and information from renal biopsy with specimens processed for light, electron, and immunofluorescent microscopy is required to determine therapy and prognosis. It has also become evident that examination of biopsy material alone cannot always distinguish between the primary (idiopathic) and various secondary causes of certain glomerular disorders. When a secondary cause exists, as with infection-associated glomerulonephritis, therapy is often best directed at the cause rather than the glomerulopathy itself.

The term acute glomerulonephritis is used to denote the syndrome of decreased glomerular filtration rate (GFR), edema, hypertension, and hematuria usually with red cell casts. Nephrotic syndrome denotes the finding of proteinuria of 3.0 grams or more per 24 hours. Hypoalbuminemia, edema, and hyperlipidemia are frequently but not always present.

Hypertension, either predating or secondary to glomerular disorders, should be treated aggressively, since if uncontrolled, it may contribute substantially to deterioration in renal function and nonrenal morbidity. Nutrition is also an important consideration both in the nephrotic patient with massive urinary protein loss and in the patient with progressive deterioration in renal function.

POSTSTREPTOCOCCAL GLOMERULONEPHRITIS (PSGN)

PSGN follows a minority of infections caused by certain nephritogenic strains of Group A beta-hemolytic streptococcus, typically pharyngitis or impetigo. There is a latent period that varies from 7 to 15 days with pharyngitis; this period is longer with impetigo. The majority of affected individuals have subclinical disease with microscopic hematuria. Red cells are characteristically fragmented and bizarrely dysmorphic, unlike cells of nonglomerular origin. Acute nephritis, the classic presentation in symptomatic individuals, is seen in roughly 40 per cent of these patients. Hematuria is universal and macroscopic in approximately one third. Proteinuria is seen in over three quarters of cases but is rarely of nephrotic proportions. Hypertension is equally common and often mild but rarely may precipitate encephalopathy. About one half of the patients will give a history of decreased urine output. Rarely, oliguria and hypertension will precipitate pulmonary edema. A majority of patients will have some azotemia, and some will have BUN greater than 80 mg per dl. Diagnosis is based on clinical and serologic findings. Approximately 90 per cent of patients will have decreased levels of complement C_3. The combination of antistreptolysin O (ASO), antihyaluronidase (Altase), and streptozyme tests, if obtained

later than 2 weeks into the course, will detect recent streptococcal infection in the majority of patients. Organisms can be recovered from the pharynx or skin in only a minority of cases. Treatment of infection will not prevent the nephritis but will prevent spread in epidemic outbreaks. It will also lower ASO titers.

The nephrotic syndrome usually begins to resolve in less than 1 week. Microscopic hematuria and mild proteinuria may persist for over a year and do not affect prognosis. The majority of patients, especially children, do well with supportive therapy, which includes fluid and sodium restriction, diuretics, and antihypertensives. Only a small proportion of patients will require dialysis. Adults have a somewhat greater tendency to develop chronic disease with progressive deterioration in renal function or superimposed rapidly progressive glomerulonephritis (see discussion under Rapidly Progressive Glomerulonephritis). If C_3 remains depressed for a period longer than 8 weeks (see discussion under Membranoproliferative Glomerulonephritis), or oligoanuria and deteriorating renal function suggest rapidly progressive glomerulonephritis (RPGN), we obtain a renal biopsy.

Treatment

Supportive therapy directed at control of hypertension, fluid overload, and azotemia (see discussion under Supportive Therapy) is often required and may include dialysis. Patients with uncontrolled hypertension, evidence of encephalopathy (altered mental status, ophthalmologic changes, vomiting), severe anemia, evidence of pulmonary vascular congestion including pulmonary edema, or BUN greater than 50 mg per dl should be hospitalized. Bedrest without hospitalization during the acute phase is indicated in those with less severe but significant involvement. Patients and family members should have throat cultures and cultures of suspicious skin lesions. We recommend treating all patients and only those family members with cultures positive for Group A beta-hemolytic streptococcus with a 10-day course of penicillin or, for those with allergy to penicillin, erythromycin. Adults with a clinical presentation of RPGN, 3 to 4 days of oligoanuria, and/or greater than 20 per cent cellular crescents on renal biopsy should be treated for RPGN. Dialysis may be necessary. Children usually recover full renal function despite anuria and extensive crescent formation and are usually not treated for RPGN if the diagnosis of PSGN is secure.

OTHER INFECTION-ASSOCIATED GLOMERULONEPHRITIS

Glomerulonephritis has been described in association with a variety of infections of bacterial, fungal, viral, protozoal, and helminthic origin, the common denominator being long-standing antigenemia with immune complex formation. More common examples include bacterial endocarditis, visceral abdominal abscess, and ventriculojugular, -atrial, and -peritoneal shunt infection. In the United States, syphilis, typhoid fever, histoplasmosis, infectious mononucleosis, quartan and falciparum malaria, and trichinosis are less commonly encountered causes of glomerulonephritis. Whenever possible, treatment should be supportive and directed at eliminating the infection. Often, recovery of renal function will then be complete. Plasmapheresis, high dose corticosteroids, and immunosuppressants such as cyclophosphamide or azathioprine generally should not be considered while infection is still active. Our view is that it is better to risk permanent loss of renal function provided the patient can be maintained on dialysis than to risk therapy-related morbidity and mortality due to sepsis. Circumstances will vary, however, and there may be a role for immunosuppressants in diseases of viral or other origin when the threat to patients posed by their immune response outweighs the cytopathic effects of the infectious agent.

Subacute and chronic bacterial endocarditis are usually associated with only mild azotemia and urinary abnormalities of which the patient is unaware, such as non-nephrotic proteinuria and microscopic hematuria. These are usually overshadowed by the other consequences of valvular cardiac involvement. Serum complement is typically depressed. Renal biopsy is often unnecessary but typically shows a proliferative or necrotizing glomerulonephritis. Biopsy is of value in distinguishing glomerulonephritis fom iatrogenically induced renal dysfunction, such as drug-associated interstitial nephritis or acute tubular necrosis (ATN), ATN resulting from hypotension secondary to valvular incompetence and cardiac decompensation, or renal damage from bland or septic emboli. After proper therapy, renal function often returns to premorbid levels.

Ventriculojugular, -atrial, and -peritoneal cerebral spinal fluid shunts inserted to relieve hydrocephalus may become infected and result in persistent fevers. Blood cultures may be negative, while culture of shunt fluid is diagnostic. Although the clinical picture may resemble that of endocarditis, there is less of a tendency toward hypocomplementemia, anemia, and hepatosplenomegally. Proteinuria may be severe, and nephrotic syndrome is seen in roughly one quarter

of cases. Nephritis has also been reported with an infected Le Veen shunt. Membranoproliferative glomerulonephritis (MPGN, see following discussion) is the most common renal biopsy finding, although other forms of proliferative glomerulonephritis are seen. With eradication of the infection, renal function often improves but reverts to premorbid levels less frequently than with endocarditis. Although there are reports of clearing of infection through the use of a combination of synergistic antibiotics, especially when given through an indwelling ventricular reservoir, usually the shunt must be removed, with placement of a new device after the infection has been eradicated.

Treatment

Specific treatment aimed at glomerulonephritis is justified only after infection has been eradicated and the clinical picture and renal biopsy support a diagnosis of RPGN.

IMMUNOGLOBULIN A (IgA) NEPHROPATHY (BERGER'S DISEASE)

Patients with Berger's disease typically have episodes of gross hematuria often within a few days of an upper respiratory tract infection. There is no prolonged latent period as with PSGN. Hematuria and proteinuria are universal findings with active disease, and nephritic or nephrotic presentations may be seen. There is also a tendency to recurrence and reversible increases in the serum creatinine. Although glomerular crescents are common in renal biopsies showing the mesangial IgA deposits characteristic of Berger's disease, a course consistent with RPGN is not common.

With the accumulation of data on patients with recurrent disease followed over a period of decades, the prognosis of patients with this disorder, once thought to be uniformly excellent, has been modified. Roughly one quarter of such patients go on to develop end-stage renal disease over a period of 20 years. Microscopic hematuria with proteinuria above 2 grams per 24 hours at presentation is associated with a worse prognosis than macroscopic hematuria, as is male sex, advanced age, Oriental versus Caucasian race, hypertension, and biopsy findings of extensive crescent formation or chronic changes of interstitial fibrosis and glomerulosclerosis.

Treatment

There are few data to support any specific therapy. Phenytoin lowers serum IgA levels and tetracycline lowers urinary red cell count, but neither drug appears to affect the course of disease. Corticosteroids, cyclophosphamide, anticoagulants, and plasmapheresis have enjoyed anecdotal success. We use aspirin, 325 mg, and dipyridamole (Persantine), 75 mg three times daily, in patients with progressive disease. We treat patients with nephrotic syndrome with the regimen of oral prednisone used for membranous nephropathy (see discussion later on). Those with the clinical course of RPGN and a renal biopsy showing greater than 20 per cent crescent formation, we treat as we would RPGN (see discussion later on).

While IgA nephropathy may recur in allografts, disease progresses slowly, so that there is no contraindication against renal transplantation.

SCHÖNLEIN-HENOCH PURPURA

Schönlein-Henoch purpura is a leukocytoclastic vasculitis involving skin, gut, kidneys, and joints. Renal biopsy is unnecessary when there is classic presentation. Characteristic signs and symptoms are nonthrombocytopenic purpura of the buttocks and lower extremities, abdominal pain, glomerulonephritis indistinguishable clinically or pathologically from Berger's disease, and nondeforming arthritis. Biopsy of unaffected skin may show IgA deposition on immunofluorescent microscopy, and serum IgA levels are often elevated. While Schönlein-Henoch purpura is predominantly a disease of children under 5 years of age, it may be seen in adults.

Treatment

For the most part, this disease is a self-limiting disorder. The abdominal pain often responds to low dose corticosteroids, while rash, glomerulonephritis, and arthritis typically do not. When the course suggests RPGN, we confirm this with renal biopsy and treat accordingly. Schönlein-Henoch purpura, like Berger's disease, may recur in renal transplants but rarely leads to graft loss.

MEMBRANOPROLIFERATIVE GLOMERULONEPHRITIS (MPGN)

MPGN may occur as a primary disorder or as secondary to a variety of nonrenal processes such as chronic active hepatitis or visceral abscess. A majority of patients present with nephrotic syndrome or asymptomatic proteinuria often in association with microscopic or recurrent macroscopic hematuria. Acute nephritis is seen in roughly one quarter of cases. A history of preced-

ing upper respiratory tract infection, the finding of an elevated ASO titer, or depressed C_3 is not uncommon. Unlike PSGN, complement remains depressed for longer than 8 weeks. Findings on renal biopsy have been categorized into three types, with Type I the most common. Immune deposits are subendothelial in Type I disease, intramembranous in Type II (dense-deposit disease), and subepithelial in Type III.

Spontaneous remissions of MPGN are rare but have been reported. The tendency is toward deterioration in renal function, with 50 per cent of patients progressing to end-stage disease at 10 years. Persistent nephrotic syndrome, hypertension, decreased glomerular filtration rate at presentation, and Type II disease are poor prognostic signs. The course of Type III disease is variable, with prognostic factors similar to those of Type I.

Treatment

Corticosteroids, cyclophosphamide, aspirin, dipyridamole, and warfarin have been used in therapy. Patients with Type II or III disease have been too few in number in controlled trials for specific recommendations to be made, and they are treated as patients with the more common Type I disease. No controlled trial has shown a favorable effect of treatment on proteinuria. We treat nephrotic syndrome with the same regimen of oral prednisone used for RPGN. With remission of proteinuria and maintenance of GFR for a period of 1 month, we move to the next step in the prednisone regimen. Approximately half of these patients have shown a decrease in proteinuria, and three fourths have improvement or stabilization of serum creatinine. We add aspirin, 325 mg, and dipyridamole (Persantine), 75 mg, three times a day indefinitely, if tolerated. Patients with the clinical course of RPGN, irrespective of percentage crescents, are treated with pulse methylprednisolone with a high rate of improvement and discontinuance of dialysis support. MPGN may recur or arise de novo in renal transplants and may lead to loss of graft function but is not a contraindication to transplantation. Recurrence is more common with Type II MPGN than with Type I, but the course is usually more severe with the latter, so that the incidence of graft loss due to recurrence is approximately 10 per cent with each type. Graft loss may occur within the first year after transplantation.

LUPUS NEPHRITIS

Although renal involvement may be found in almost all patients with systemic lupus erythematosus if renal biopsy is obtained, a minority of patients will require biopsy or specific therapy for renal involvement. Persistent heavy proteinuria with or without nephrotic syndrome or reduced GFR is the principal reason for pursuing tissue diagnosis. Hematuria and hypocomplementemia are common findings. Clinically significant renal involvement, if it will occur, usually presents early in the course of the disease. Biopsy findings are diverse and include normal glomeruli, mesangial proliferative glomerulonephritis, focal and diffuse proliferative glomerulonephritis, membranous lupus glomerulopathy, interstitial nephritis, and advanced sclerosing glomerulonephritis. Superimposed crescents may be seen as well, and the course may be that of RPGN.

The prognosis for lupus glomerulonephritis is variable even among the different subtypes, and survival figures have not been firmly established. Membranous lupus glomerulonephritis, in general, has a more indolent course than either focal or diffuse proliferative lupus glomerulonephritis. Of the three, the latter has the worst prognosis but with treatment may have a 5 year survival rate of over 60 per cent.

Treatment

It is difficult to justify the treatment of those with advanced chronic lesions or minimal disease. Of the glomerular disorders, we recommend treatment for focal and diffuse proliferative and membranous lesions as well as for RPGN. The latter two are treated as their primary counterparts (see the following). With focal or diffuse proliferative glomerulonephritis, we treat with prednisone, 1 mg per kg daily, for 4 to 8 weeks, then taper the dosage over the next 4 weeks to maintenance levels required to control nonrenal symptoms. If there is no response or abnormalities in urinary sediment persist, we add cytotoxic agents. We favor the use of a combination of oral azathioprine* (Imuran) and cyclophosphamide* (Cytoxan), each up to 1 mg per kg per day, or intravenous cyclophosphamide given every 3 months at doses of 0.5 to 1.0 g per M^2 of body surface area. Intravenous cyclophosphamide is given over 1 hour and is accompanied by vigorous hydration over the following 24 hours to produce a dilute urine. Frequent voiding is encouraged, and dosage is reduced for creatinine clearance below 30 ml per minute or is reduced to maintain a total leukocyte nadir above 2000 per mm^3. Cytotoxics are then continued up to 4 years with

---

*This use of these agents is not listed in the manufacturer's directives.

alternate day low dose prednisone. If remission is achieved and maintained, we believe that conversion to azathioprine (Imuran), 2 to 3 mg per kg per day, is justified to reduce the risk of hematologic malignancy.

MINIMAL CHANGE DISEASE (MCD)

Minimal change disease is the most common cause of nephrotic syndrome in children, especially in those between the ages of 1 and 6 years, and accounts for up to 20 per cent of cases of idiopathic nephrotic syndrome in adults. Heavy proteinuria is the rule. Gross hematuria is uncommon but does occur, while microscopic hematuria is seen in about 20 per cent of patients. Occasionally, mild azotemia is evident. Renal biopsy is often unnecessary in children with typical presentation who respond to a therapeutic trial of corticosteroids but is usually obtained in adults. As this is essentially a diagnosis of exclusion, it is particularly important that a biopsy specimen be processed for all three forms of microscopy. Malignancies are occasional secondary causes of minimal change disease, with Hodgkin's disease being most common, although other lymphomas and even carcinomas have been associated with minimal change disease. Nephrosis has resolved with successful treatment of the malignancy and reappeared with recurrence.

Treatment

With or without treatment, minimal change disease is characterized by remission and recurrences, and it is unusual for the disease to progress to renal failure. Treatment frequently produces remission in proteinuria, likely does not affect renal prognosis, and is associated with its own morbidity and mortality, which must be balanced against those of prolonged nephrotic syndrome.

For the initial treatment of nephrotic syndrome in children, we recommend oral prednisone, 60 mg per M^2 of body surface area per day, up to a total of not more than 80 mg per day once daily until remission (under 200 mg of urinary protein per 24 hours) or up to a maximum of 4 weeks. The dose is then doubled but given on alternate days and gradually tapered over the next 8 to 10 weeks. With adults we have found high dose alternate day oral corticosteroids to be well tolerated and favor treatment with alternate day prednisone as described for MPGN. We have found that this regimen helps stabilize or improve renal function in over 90 per cent of patients with minimal change disease and decreases proteinuria to a non-nephrotic range, with a greater than 50 per cent decrease from baseline in over 80 per cent. With relapse during the period of the taper, we resume higher alternate day dosages and taper more slowly.

While more than 90 per cent of patients remit with therapy, relapses occur in the majority of such patients. A full course may be repeated, but we recommend limiting these in children to no more than three times per year. Those who relapse may benefit from the addition of daily doses of either cyclophosphamide* (Cytoxan), 2 mg per kg, or chlorambucil* (Leukeran), 0.15 mg per kg, to prednisone therapy for a period of 8 weeks in an attempt to induce a sustained remission. Cyclophosphamide may be extended for an additional 4 weeks if nephrotic syndrome is disabling. Hematocrit, leukocyte, and platelet counts should be followed weekly while the patient is on alkylating agents, and dosage should be reduced or discontinued with evidence of hematologic toxicity. Malignancy, gonadal toxicity, alopecia, hematologic toxicity, and cystitis have been reported with either chlorambucil or cyclophosphamide but are unusual with this regimen. Patients with well-tolerated proteinuria are best treated with supportive measures rather than frequent courses of corticosteroid or alkylating agents.

FOCAL GLOMERULAR SCLEROSIS

Focal glomerular sclerosis is found in approximately 10 per cent of patients with idiopathic nephrotic syndrome and is the primary cause of steroid unresponsive nephrotic syndrome in children. Associated secondary causes include intravenous heroin abuse and reflux nephropathy. Proteinuria is universal and usually heavy at presentation. These patients have a greater tendency to present with hematuria, more commonly microscopic than gross, and hypertension, especially with progression, than is seen in those with minimal change disease or membranous nephropathy.

While the course is quite variable, most patients with focal glomerular sclerosis will have unremittant heavy proteinuria, develop persistent hypertension, and have progressive deterioration in GFR, requiring dialysis over a period ranging from 3 to 10 years. Previous renal biopsy showing minimal change disease, response to corticosteroids, and persistent non-nephrotic proteinuria indicate a more favorable prognosis.

*This use of these agents is not listed in the manufacturer's directives.

Treatment

In addition to supportive therapy, we recommend a trial of corticosteroids for nephrotic proteinuria if there are no contraindications and serum creatinine is under 2 mg per dl. We treat with the same regimen described for MPGN and have found that this helps to stabilize or to improve renal function in 50 per cent of patients with focal glomerular sclerosis and decreases proteinuria to a non-nephrotic range, with a greater than 50 per cent decrease from baseline in 30 per cent. In patients who are not steroid responsive, or if therapy with corticosteroids is not undertaken, we treat with aspirin, 325 mg, and dipyridamole (Persantine), 75 mg three times a day, indefinitely in an effort to preserve renal function.

If the patient proves steroid responsive but relapses after an interval of 6 or more months, we recommend another course of alternate day prednisone. In steroid-dependent cases we attempt to produce a prolonged remission of proteinuria by adding cyclophosphamide* (Cytoxan), 2 mg per kg per day, or chlorambucil* (Leukeran), 0.15 mg per kg per day, for 8 to 10 weeks to another course of alternate day prednisone. If there is further relapse, we treat with aspirin and dipyridamole as described above.

MEMBRANOUS NEPHROPATHY

Membranous nephropathy is, in most series, the most common cause of nephrotic syndrome in adults, although it is rarely found in children. Asymptomatic proteinuria is found in less than one fifth of patients at presentation, and while microscopic hematuria is common, gross hematuria is rare. Secondary causes of membranous nephropathy should be pursued, and these include systemic lupus erythematosis, hepatitis B, drugs such as captopril, organic gold, D-penicillamine, and neoplasms, especially carcinoma of lung, breast, and gastrointestinal tract. Perhaps 10 to 15 per cent of those over 55 years of age with membranous nephropathy will have or develop malignancy. In patients over age 50 we recommend a thorough physical examination, which includes evaluation of liver, breasts, lymph nodes, pelvic and rectal examination, chest radiograph, complete blood count, measurement of liver enzymes, and evaluation of three stool specimens for occult blood. If there are any abnormalities, or if history so suggests, more specialized tests such as colonoscopy or mammography are indicated. Also, patients with membranous nephropathy seem more predisposed to renal vein and other deep venous thromboses than other patients with nephrotic syndrome. Findings that suggest thromboembolic phenomena, including pulmonary embolism, should be pursued and anticoagulation begun if these are documented.

Secondary membranous nephropathy often remits if the inciting cause can be eliminated. The prognosis in primary membranous nephropathy is variable. In general, children do well, with over a 90 per cent 10 year survival rate. Approximately 25 per cent of adults will have complete remission or significant reduction in proteinuria without deterioration in GFR without treatment, while another 25 per cent have stable GFR with continued proteinuria. In the remaining 50 per cent, there will be a progressive decrease in GFR with or without remission in proteinuria, with end-stage renal disease or patient death at about 15 years' duration. Adult age, male sex, persistent nephrotic proteinuria, associated factors such as deep venous thrombosis, hypertension, and reduced GFR at presentation are poor prognostic signs, whereas GFR is often preserved in those patients with remission to non-nephrotic proteinuria.

Treatment

The slow course and partially remitting nature of membranous nephropathy make treatment controversial. The potential benefit to those with progressive disease must be balanced against the potential harm to those who would remit without treatment. We treat with high dose alternate day oral prednisone as described in treatment for MPGN. We have found that this regimen helps to stabilize or to improve renal function in over 80 per cent of patients with membranous nephropathy and decreases proteinuria to a non-nephrotic range, with a greater than 50 per cent decrease from baseline in over 70 per cent of patients. In patients with deteriorating renal function, more aggressive therapy should be considered using methylprednisolone, 1 gram given intravenously for 3 consecutive days, followed by 6 months of alternating cycles each of 1 month's duration, beginning with prednisone, 0.5 mg per kg daily, followed by chlorambucil* (Leukeran), 0.2 mg per kg daily. Chlorambucil dosage must be lowered if the leukocyte count falls below 5000 per mm³.

CRYOGLOBULINEMIA AND LIGHT CHAIN NEPHROPATHY

The cryoglobulinemias are a heterogeneous group of disorders. Cryoglobulins are circulating

---

*These uses of these agents are not listed in the manufacturers' directives.

cold-precipitable immunoglobulins that may be associated with a variety of acute and chronic infectious disorders, systemic vasculitis, collagen vascular disease, lymphoproliferative disorders, or idiopathic (essential) disorders. In Type I the cryoglobulin is monoclonal, as in certain instances with Waldenström's macroglobulinemia or multiple myeloma. In Type II there is a monoclonal as well as a polyclonal component, while in Type III there are polyclonal but no monoclonal cryoglobulins. Types II and III are called mixed. Glomerular involvement is variable, as are clinical findings, which in essential mixed cryoglobulinemia include urticaria, purpuric skin lesions, Raynaud's phenomenon, arthralgias, and hepatosplenomegally. Exposure to cold may lead to signs and symptoms resulting from intravascular cryoglobulin precipitation.

Glomerular damage may also result from the deposition of circulating monoclonal immunoglobulin light chains. These are most often of the kappa type. The findings on renal biopsy resemble the nodular glomerulosclerosis of diabetes mellitus, with which it may be confused.

Treatment

With cryoglobulinemia or light chain nephropathy, therapy should first be directed at the primary cause, i.e., infection or lymphoproliferative disorder. Cold should be avoided if it aggravates symptoms. With fulminant extrarenal or renal involvement, we recommend plasmapheresis using 4-liter exchanges three times per week in conjunction with oral prednisone, 60 mg per day, and oral cyclophosphamide* (Cytoxan), 2 to 3 mg per kg, while monitoring cryoglobulin or light chain levels. As symptoms improve and levels fall, plasmapheresis is tapered, then discontinued. Prednisone is then tapered while maintaining the dosage of cyclophosphamide. The latter may then be discontinued after prolonged remission.

We have had very good success in treating light chain nephropathy isolated to the kidney with melphalan* (Alkeran), 0.25 mg per kg per day for 4 days up to a maximum dose of 16 mg, plus prednisone, 2.0 mg per kg per day for 4 days. This is repeated at 6-week intervals for six courses, checking the leukocyte count at 2 weeks after melphalan is completed.

SYSTEMIC VASCULITIS

RPGN or less fulminant forms of glomerulonephritis may be seen with the vasculitides, which include polyarteritis nodosa, its microscopic variant, Wegener's granulomatosis, and hypersensitivity vasculitis. Hematuria, either gross or microscopic, proteinuria, and rising serum creatinine levels indicate renal involvement. Many patients will have circulating antibodies to neutrophil cytoplasmic antigens. Renal biopsy supports the diagnosis but rarely distinguishes among the subtypes, and nonrenal tissue should be sought to obtain a definitive diagnosis. An open renal biopsy to obtain a wedge that includes medullary tissue is often helpful when other biopsies, including percutaneous renal biopsy, have been unsuccessful. We routinely obtain open renal biopsy with both wedge and needle specimens when there is difficulty in making the diagnosis of vasculitis.

Prognosis for patient survival and preservation of renal function is variable. Supportive measures, including aggressive control of hypertension, have a significant impact on reducing morbidity.

Treatment

For polyarteritis nodosa and hypersensitivity vasculitis uncomplicated by RPGN, we recommend an initial trial of oral prednisone or intravenous prednisolone of 1 mg per kg per day for 4 weeks. This is given in three or four divided doses over the first 1 to 2 weeks, then is consolidated to a single daily dose over a period of several days to complete a month's course. Over the next 2 months, prednisone, 2 mg per kg, is given on alternate days. Subsequently, alternate day prednisone is slowly tapered over a period of 3 to 6 months. If the initial course is fulminant, or response is minimal over the first week or two of therapy, we add oral cyclophosphamide* (Cytoxan), 2 mg per kg per day, and continue this, reducing dosage as necessary to maintain adequate leukocyte, neutrophil, and platelet counts for a period of 1 year following a complete remission. Cyclophosphamide is then tapered by increments of 25 mg every 2 months.

With Wegener's granulomatosis, cyclophosphamide is the mainstay of therapy. We start with a dose of 2 to 3 mg per kg per day supplemented with prednisone, 1 mg per kg per day, given initially in divided doses as with polyarteritis nodosa. After 4 weeks, cyclophosphamide is reduced to 1 to 2 mg per kg per day, and prednisone is tapered and discontinued over the next 8 weeks. Cyclophosphamide may be tapered after 1 year.

Cyclophosphamide is held, or dosage is reduced so as to maintain total leukocyte count above

---

*These uses of cyclophosphamide are not listed in the manufacturer's directive.

3500 per mm^3, neutrophil count above 1500 per mm^3, or platelet count above 100,000 per mm^3. Dosage is halved for creatinine clearance under 10 ml per minute.

When any form of vasculitis is associated with RPGN, we use high dose pulse methylprednisolone and a longer course of prednisone (see discussion under RPGN) in addition to cyclophosphamide.

GOODPASTURE'S SYNDROME

Goodpasture's syndrome is characterized by pulmonary hemorrhage and antiglomerular basement (anti-GBM) antibody-associated glomerulonephritis. Pulmonary manifestations may include life-threatening hemoptysis or the incidental finding of pulmonary hemosiderosis. Renal involvement may be minimal, with only microscopic or gross hematuria, mild proteinuria, and relatively normal GFR but may progress to irreversible anuria over a period of hours.

Diagnosis is made, in the proper clinical setting, by the demonstration of circulating anti-GBM antibody or the characteristic linear indirect immunofluorescent pattern of anti-GBM antibody in either lung or kidney. Anti-GBM antibodies may also be demonstrated without the full syndrome in idiopathic RPGN (see below) and systemic vasculitis. A necrotizing vasculitis is also seen occasionally with Goodpasture's syndrome. Prognosis is variable and depends on the severity of pulmonary and renal involvement as well as their response to therapy. Patients with oligoanuria who are on dialysis, those with greater than 50 per cent crescents on renal biopsy, or those with serum creatinine levels above 6 mg per dl have a very poor prognosis. We have never seen improvement in GFR after oligoanuria arises, despite therapy.

Treatment

With well-preserved renal function, no evidence of vasculitis, and primarily pulmonary involvement, we treat with pulse methylprednisolone and prednisone using the same dosage and schedule as that for RPGN (see the following discussion). If renal involvement is severe, renal function deteriorates acutely, or pulmonary hemorrhage does not respond to corticosteroids, we add plasmapheresis, initially on a daily basis, using 4-liter exchanges with 5 per cent normal serum albumin replacement and supplemental fresh frozen plasma if there is bleeding. Cyclophosphamide* is added when plasmapheresis is necessary or when there is evidence of vasculitis. We use 2 to 3 mg per kg ideal body weight for a period of 3 months. Anti-GBM antibody titers are followed, and plasmapheresis is switched to alternate days then tapered further as these fall. With intractable pulmonary hemorrhage of life-threatening proportion, bilateral nephrectomy is advocated as a heroic measure. Recurrent Goodpasture's syndrome has been noted in native and transplanted kidneys but is unusual. Transplantation should not be attempted during active disease or with high antibody titers.

RAPIDLY PROGRESSIVE GLOMERULONEPHRITIS (RPGN)

RPGN is a clinical syndrome characterized by deterioration of GFR by greater than 50 per cent within a period of 3 months with a biopsy documenting glomerulonephritis. While usually associated with crescents, RPGN can occur without them. RPGN may arise de novo or may be associated with other forms of glomerulonephritis. The onset of disease may be insidious, with the patient presenting with a history of generalized complaints and symptoms of well-advanced renal failure, or less commonly it may present abruptly, with the development of acute nephritis. Hematuria, often macroscopic, and proteinuria are universal findings unless the patient is anuric. Oliguria and mild to moderate normocytic, normochromic anemia are common, while hypertension is not. RPGN may arise infrequently in the course of vasculitis.

With idiopathic RPGN, three renal biopsy patterns are recognized on immunofluorescent microscopy: linear immunoglobulin deposits (anti-GBM) indistinguishable from those of Goodpasture's syndrome, granular deposits, and no deposits. The anti-GBM type is associated with a worse prognosis than the other varieties. With conventional therapy, a worse prognosis is portended for all types with oliguria, advanced renal insufficiency (serum creatinine levels above 6 mg per dl), extensive crescent formation (greater than 50 per cent of glomeruli), extensive glomerular tuft necrosis, and interstitial fibrosis. This poor prognosis is altered by pulse methylprednisolone therapy and plasma exchange.

Treatment

There have been few randomized studies of the various proposed treatment modalities in this dramatic but infrequently encountered syndrome. We have had success with the following protocol: Pulse methylprednisolone, 30 mg per kg up to a total of 3 grams, is administered intravenously over exactly 20 minutes every other day for three doses in the volume replete patient. We then add oral alternate day prednisone on a mg per kg basis (or ideal body weight for the very obese patient) beginning with 2.0 for 0.5 months, then 1.75 for 1 month, 1.5 for 3 months, 1.25 for 6 months, 1.0 for 6 months, 0.75 for 6 months, 0.5 for 6 months, 0.25 for 6 months, 0.125 for 12 months, concluding with 0.0625 mg per kg for 12 months. Patients over 60 years of age receive full pulse therapy but have their oral prednisone dose reduced by 25 per cent. With remission of proteinuria and normalization of GFR for a period of 1 month, we move to the next step in the prednisone regimen. Otherwise, the regimen is followed as described. With this regimen, the 75 per cent failure rate for conventional therapy is reversed, and about 75 per cent of patients will improve, including those with oligoanuria, those on dialysis, and those with greater than 60 per cent glomerular crescents. It is critical to obtain the biopsy and to start treatment early in these diseases. A 4-week delay in starting therapy is associated with a slight decrease in the immediate response rate and a significant decrease in the long-term response rate.

When RPGN is associated with Goodpasture's syndrome or is idiopathic with anti-GBM antibody, we add plasmapheresis and cyclophosphamide (see discussion of Goodpasture's syndrome) if there is inadequate response to corticosteroids. Cyclophosphamide is also used in RPGN associated with systemic vasculitis (see preceding).

SUPPORTIVE THERAPY

Supportive therapy, besides providing for relief of symptoms, may significantly reduce morbidity and mortality associated with glomerular disorders. It is the only available therapy for glomerular disorders such as diabetic nephropathy or most forms of amyloidosis. Hypertension should be treated as in nonglomerular disorders, although special attention to dosage is required with drugs that may adversely affect GFR or accumulate in renal insufficiency. Calcium channel blockers, angiotensin-converting enzyme inhibitors, and peripheral vasodilators such as prazosin and hydralazine are effective antihypertensives. Edema is initially best treated with salt restriction. Daily intake should be kept under 80 mEq of sodium, and this should be verified with 24-hour urine collections. In more severe cases, diuretics are required. These are usually well tolerated in states of fluid overload but may cause difficulty when effective circulating plasma volume is depleted because of severe hypoalbuminemia. We use hydrochlorothiazide, 25 to 50 mg daily or twice a day if GFR is above 50 ml per minute. With more severe renal insufficiency, we use a loop diuretic such as furosemide. Diuresis with these is not as prolonged as with the thiazides, so that shorter dosing intervals may be required. The dose of the loop diuretic should be sufficient to produce a diuresis. There is no beneficial cumulative effect from smaller dosages. For refractory edema, we add hydrochlorothiazide or metolazone to a loop diuretic. Worsening of renal function with any of these agents is most often a result of prerenal azotemia, but the possibility of acute interstitial nephritis should be recognized. Therapy rarely abolishes edema but may substantially reduce the risk for skin breakdown or infection.

Proper nutritional therapy in nephrotic syndrome is not well established. We recommend that all patients with glomerular disorders follow a diet containing sufficient protein of high biologic value to maintain positive nitrogen balance. Excessive protein intake leading to glomerular hyperfiltration may lead to progressive deterioration in renal function and should be avoided. In the absence of heavy proteinuria we recommend a diet containing 0.6 to 0.7 gram per kg of ideal body weight of protein. Nutritional status may be followed with nitrogen balance studies and serum albumin and transferrin levels. With severe nephrosis, replacement of urinary losses of vitamin D, zinc, iron, and copper may be necessary as well as infusion of intravenous human immune globulin if hypoglobulinemia leads to frequent infection. Rarely, with intractable nephrotic syndrome, we have used nonsteroidal anti-inflammatory drugs such as indomethacin or meclofenamate or renal ablation to reduce or abolish GFR and thus decrease proteinuria.

SIDE EFFECTS OF SPECIFIC THERAPY

The complications attributed to long-term therapy with corticosteroids are well known and include cushingoid facies, cataracts, osteoporosis, psychosis, infections, skin lesions, glaucoma, hirsutism, edema, hypertension, glucose intolerance, hyperlipidemia, hypokalemia, negative nitrogen balance, venous thrombosis, cerebrovascular accident, and possibly peptic ulcer. Immediate side effects attributed to pulse methylprednisolone therapy include metallic taste, nausea, psychotropic effects, myalgias, arthralgias, hypotension, and cardiac arrhythmias. Pulse therapy is administered only to patients who are volume repleted. Diuretics should be withheld 3 hours before and 24 hours after the drug dose, which is given over a period of no more than 20 minutes. Contraindications further include active gastric ulcer, major surgery in the preceding 5 days, severe debi-

litation, psychosis, or inadequately treated systemic bacterial or fungal infection.

Adverse reactions with cyclophosphamide include bone marrow suppression, alopecia, gastrointestinal disturbances, pulmonary fibrosis, myocarditis with congestive heart failure with large doses, gonadal dysfunction, sterile hemorrhagic cystitis, bladder fibrosis or carcinoma, and other neoplasms. Patients should be kept well hydrated and encouraged to void frequently to help protect against bladder injury from active metabolites. Permanent gonadal toxicity is uncommon when the total dose is kept below 200 mg per kg. Chlorambucil has a similar spectrum of toxicity. Hemorrhagic cystitis is not seen, and gonadal toxicity is more prominent than that with cyclophosphamide. Reactions to azathioprine include drug fever, gastrointestinal disturbances, bone marrow suppression, hepatocellular necrosis, and cholestasis. Dosage must be reduced in patients concurrently taking allopurinol. All of these cytotoxic agents should be avoided during pregnancy.

Adverse reactions to aspirin are well known and will not be reviewed here. Dipyridamole has been associated with headaches, dizziness, gastrointestinal disturbance, and rash.

Plasmapheresis may produce thrombocytopenia, coagulation abnormalities, and hypogammaglobulinemia. We recommend replacement with intravenous immune globulin when plasma IgG levels fall below 500 mg per dl.

PYELONEPHRITIS

method of
ROBIN BENNETT, M.D.
Alexandria, Louisiana

ACUTE PYELONEPHRITIS

Acute pyelonephritis represents acute interstitial inflammation and tubular necrosis due to bacterial invasion of the kidney and pelvis. The most common organism causing this disorder in both inpatients and outpatients is *Escherichia coli*, although the proportion of other gram-negative organisms and enterococci increases in both inpatients and patients who have had their urinary tracts instrumented recently. Fungi, such as *Candida* and *Mycobacterium* species, may also infect the urinary tract and cause pyelonephritis, although this situation is decidedly less common. The most common route of infection of the kidneys is ascension of the pathogen from the bladder or prostate. Hematogenous spread occurs in less than 3 per cent of patients and is common only in children less than 2 years of age.

On a clinical basis, it is often difficult to separate patients who have true pyelonephritis from those who have a lower urinary tract infection. In general, individuals with recurrent rigors and fever of 101° F or higher, back and loin pain (particularly costovertebral angle tenderness), abdominal pain with nausea and vomiting, and dysuria with frequency and nocturia should be considered to have pyelonephritis. Pyuria is usually present with greater than 7 white cells per high-power field, with the presence of white blood cell casts being most consistent with pyelonephritis. In an unspun urine specimen, the presence of bacteria in each high-power field correlates well with a colony count of greater than 100,000. The localization tests for pyelonephritis, such as antibody-coated bacteria, bladder washout, or renal biopsy, are of little clinical usefulness at present.

Pyelonephritis can cause acute renal failure with oliguria. Acute pyelonephritis may cause overt sepsis, especially with an underlying problem such as obstruction or abscess formation. This is particularly important in diabetics, who may develop papillary necrosis with subsequent obstruction.

Treatment

In individuals with mild symptoms, the use of a single oral dose of antibiotic can differentiate lower tract from upper tract infection. In young women this is an effective means of treating cystitis. Drugs that have been used for single-dose therapy include amoxicillin, 3 grams; trimethoprim-sulfa-methoxazole (Bactrim, Septra), two double-strength tablets; sulfisoxazole (Gantrisin), 2 grams; and trimethoprim, 400 mg. At the time of this writing, the new antibiotic agents ciprofloxacin and norfloxacin have not yet been tried as a single-dose agent. Patients with overt pyelonephritis who appear toxic or have a temperature of 101° F or higher should be admitted for fluid management and parenteral antibiotics. With pyelonephritis, there is often a defect in salt and water conservation and in acidification. These patients should be treated with adequate volume repletion with generation of good urine flows to help remove bacteria. The antibiotics given should be based on Gram stain and urine culture. Individuals who have normal renal function should be given ampicillin, 1 gram intravenously every 6 hours, and an aminoglycoside such as gentamicin (Garamycin), 1.5 mg per kg loading dose followed by 1 mg per kg every 8 hours intravenously for at least the first 48 hours. In individuals with renal insufficiency, a third gen-

eration cephalosporin, imipenem (Primaxin), aztreonam (Azactam), or ticarcillin/clavulanate (Timentin) should also be considered as initial therapy. Most patients will improve dramatically within the first 24 hours. After initial culture results are obtained and as the clinical situation warrants, the patient may be changed to oral antibiotics, which should be continued in most cases for 4 to 6 weeks. The relapse rate is approximately 50 per cent in individuals treated for only 2 weeks. The urinalysis and urine CNS should be repeated at the end of the 4 to 6 week period and again after 3 to 6 months.

An anatomic evaluation is warranted (1) in individuals who have infections that do not respond within 48 to 72 hours to evaluate for possible abscess; (2) in children, especially those less than 5 years old (after the infection subsides); (3) in men; and (4) in women with recurrent upper tract infections after at least 6 weeks of therapy or who have broken through suppressive therapy.

CHRONIC PYELONEPHRITIS

Chronic pyelonephritis is more difficult to define and presently is restricted to cases that have unequivocal evidence of pelvocaliceal inflammation, fibrosis, and deformity. In the majority of patients with chronic pyelonephritis, the bacterial infection is actually superimposed on an anatomic urinary tract anomaly, an obstruction, or vesicoureteral reflux (especially in children). Radiographs show pelvocaliceal scarring. These individuals manifest physiologic derangements that are usually more striking than their infectious symptoms and include hypertension, salt wasting, a decreased ability to concentrate or to acidify their urine, and hyperkalemia, all of which are out of proportion to the degree of renal failure. The presence of increasing proteinuria indicates a poor prognosis for renal survival. Children with chronic bacteriuria and vesicoureteral reflux should be treated with suppressive therapy to avert renal failure. Suppressive therapy should also be considered in any adult who manifests chronic scarring on anatomic evaluation and persistent bacteriuria.

TRAUMA TO THE GENITOURINARY TRACT

method of
PHILIP M. HANNO, M.D., and
ALAN J. WEIN, M.D.
Hospital of the University of Pennsylvania
Philadelphia, Pennsylvania

Genitourinary injuries account for up to 10 per cent of traumatic injuries seen in the emergency department. Often, in the patient with severe multiple trauma, injuries to the genitourinary tract assume secondary importance, and their definitive management may take place months later.

The major protection of the urogenital tract against traumatic injury lies in its ability to move and thus cushion itself from severe impact. Mobility prolongs the period of deceleration, thereby limiting the shock to affected organs. The chief exception to this concept is the membranous urethra, which is immobilized by the urogenital diaphragm and is subject to shearing injuries in pelvic fractures.

UPPER URINARY TRACT TRAUMA

Blunt Renal Trauma

The kidney is the most commonly injured organ in the urogenital system. The kidneys are mobile organs, surrounded by fat and fixed only by their attachments to the aorta, vena cava, and ureter. The renal capsule is a strong membrane that resists rupture. When it is torn, there usually has been significant parenchymal damage. Gerota's fascia surrounds the kidney and tends to stop renal hemorrhage via a tamponade effect. If it is not intact, bleeding can be massive, as the retroperitoneal space has a tremendous potential capacity.

Renal injury should be suspected in patients who have (1) sudden deceleration injury, (2) injury to flank soft tissue, (3) microhematuria or gross hematuria following trauma, (4) flank or abdominal mass, (5) shock following blunt trauma, and (6) fractures of lower ribs or upper lumbar vertebrae. Blunt renal injury is usually associated with sudden deceleration of the human body. Motor vehicle injuries account for more than half of all renal injuries. Contact sports also are responsible for many. Although well protected by the psoas and quadratus lumborum muscles posteriorly and the viscera anteriorly, the kidney moves one to three vertebral levels on the pedicle and is thrust against the ribs, resulting in renal contusion. Rib fractures occurring at the time of renal displacement may result in renal laceration. Fracture of the transverse process of one of the upper lumbar vertebrae is often associated with renal contusion or laceration. Sudden deceleration injuries may also result in renal arterial intimal tear, with subsequent arterial thrombosis and/or disruption of the ureteropelvic junction, the latter most commonly appearing in children.

Indications for Consultation. Hematuria following trauma is the major indication of renal injury. One must keep in mind, however, that from 10 to 40 per cent of patients with significant renal injury from blunt trauma may not have hematuria and that the degree of correlation between the amount of hematuria and the severity of renal injury is poor. Any of the situations described above, even without the presence of hematuria, is sufficient to proceed with urologic evaluation.

Diagnostic Procedures. Following urinalysis, radiographic studies are indicated. Abdominal and chest radiographs are helpful in searching for bony fractures. Ground-glass density or obliteration of the psoas shadow suggests a retroperitoneal hematoma or urinary extravasation. Despite all of the newer diagnostic modalities available, the cornerstone for the evaluation and initial management of blunt renal trauma remains the intravenous urogram with nephrotomography. The results of the urogram are used to categorize the type of renal injury.

The four large classifications of renal injury include (1) renal contusions—subcapsular hematomas or bruises associated with an intact renal capsule and collecting system, (2) minor lacerations—superficial cortical disruptions not involving the medulla or collecting system, (3) major lacerations—parenchymal disruptions involving the medulla and/or collecting system and also "fractured kidneys," and (4) pedicle injuries—occlusions or tears of the renal artery and/or vein.

When the results of the intravenous urogram are abnormal or indeterminate (poor visualization), computed tomography (CT) is now being used extensively on an emergent basis to help determine the extent of injury and to identify associated injuries in other organ systems. It is available in most trauma centers on a 24-hour basis. Arteriography has generally been supplanted by CT in the evaluation of renal trauma except in the situation of complete nonvisualization of the kidney on urography. Renal pedicle injury must be considered in this instance, and arteriography gives more precise data on the arterial or venous injuries, which may be critical to their proper management. Risks of arteriography in children may make digital subtraction angiography, CT, or nuclear studies better choices for evaluation of nonfunction on urography.

While patient instability may call for immediate operative intervention, at least a one-film urogram should be obtained in the trauma suite, with contrast injected directly into the intravenous lines used for resuscitation in order to indicate the presence of kidneys and the general extent of renal injury. Retrograde pyelography is rarely indicated unless avulsion of the ureter is suspected.

Management. Patients with microhematuria and a normal urogram can be discharged. They should limit activities and continue outpatient follow-up until the hematuria resolves.

If gross hematuria is present and the urogram is consistent with a contusion or minor cortical laceration, with or without urinary extravasation, the patient is admitted and treated with bed rest. Vital signs and serial physical examinations are important to assess the patient for signs of expanding hematoma or urinoma. Complete blood counts are recorded, and the patient's urine samples are taped to the bedside for quick determination of any change in the degree of hematuria. The vast majority of these patients are successfully managed conservatively. Repeat CT is ordered if the clinical condition deteriorates, and a repeat urogram is routinely obtained later in the recovery period to verify the status of the upper tracts.

Patients with multiple severe lacerations or shattered kidneys—manifested by unstable vital signs, the need for multiple transfusions, or an expanding flank mass—require prompt surgical exploration. Preoperative CT or arteriography is helpful. Patients with renal nonfunction on urography and evidence of a pedicle injury on arteriography require prompt exploration if hope for renal salvage is entertained. If the only possible operation is nephrectomy and the patient is clinically stable, the patient need not undergo operation on an emergent basis and can be followed until nephrectomy is necessary on an elective basis.

Patients operated on in the acute setting should be explored through a midline incision. The peritoneal cavity is explored, the renal pedicle is isolated through a dorsal parietal peritoneal incision over the aorta just medial to the inferior mesenteric vein, and vascular control is obtained. The colon is then reflected medially, and Gerota's fascia is opened.

Approximately 85 per cent of patients have minor injuries and can be managed expectantly. Five per cent of patients have severe injuries and unstable or unstabilizable vital signs and require immediate exploration. Management of the remaining 10 per cent of patients with severe renal injury and evidence of renal function (making pedicle injury unlikely) is controversial. One school believes that exploration is mandatory if maximum salvage of renal function is to be obtained. Others believe that more renal tissue is salvaged by nonoperative management, transfusion as necessary, close clinical monitoring, and absolute bed rest. Complications are managed if they occur, and nephrectomy is carried out in an elective setting if necessary. Logistics probably demand the former approach on a busy trauma service.

Penetrating Renal Trauma

Eighty per cent of penetrating renal injuries have associated intra-abdominal wounds. After penetrating trauma, Gerota's fascia cannot be relied upon to tamponade renal bleeding. For both of these reasons, penetrating renal injuries should have operative exploration.

Evaluation of the patient consists of intravenous urography and eventual laparotomy. If a bullet wound shows both entry and exit points on the body, missile velocity can be assumed to have been great, and extensive blast injury can be suspected. Small caliber, low velocity wounds, as from .22-caliber bullets, rarely produce major injury unless damage to a significant vessel or the collecting system has occurred. Drainage and tamponade of the bullet hole with fat suffices to treat parenchymal injury. High velocity bullet wounds are associated with more significant injury from the blast effect. Arteriography can help to estimate the extent of devascularization, but time often does not permit it.

Anterior stab wounds should probably be explored. However, if the general surgeon feels comfortable, on the basis of a minilaparotomy or peritoneal lavage, that no major intra-abdominal injury has resulted, the renal injury can be managed expectantly as outlined under the section on Blunt Renal Trauma. Flank and posterior stab wounds need not be explored unless extravasation or obvious signs of injury are noted by intravenous urography or CT studies or gross hematuria is present.

All patients with significant renal trauma should have at least one follow-up visit, with a urogram performed, 9 to 12 months after injury, as calcification, segmental nonfunction, and hypertension may occasionally result.

Ureteral Trauma

As the ureter is well protected anatomically, traumatic injuries are relatively uncommon, and the majority of injuries are iatrogenic, related to gynecologic or urologic surgery. The blood supply to the ureters comes in medially from above and laterally in its lower third. Ureteral trauma should be suspected in the following situations: (1) penetrating injury in the vicinity of the ureter; (2) presence of gross or microscopic hematuria; (3) deceleration injury with hyperextension of the spine, especially in children; and (4) presence of a flank mass.

Indications for Consultation. Hematuria is usually associated with ureteral injury, but urinalysis may be normal at the time of presentation.

If injury is secondary to a penetrating wound, the course of the knife or missile should lead to suspicion of possible ureteral injury. Sudden deceleration injuries in children associated with hyperextension of the spine can cause ureteropelvic junction disruption, as the ureter tenses like a bowstring and snaps against the psoas or vertebral column. Without a high index of suspicion, these injuries may go undiagnosed for days or weeks until a painful flank mass appears.

Diagnostic Procedures. When a ureteral injury is suspected, and time permits, an intravenous urogram should be performed prior to exploration. A normal urogram does not rule out ureteral injury, and a retrograde ureterogram may be necessary. A high index of suspicion is necessary to make the diagnosis of ureteral injury. Immediate recognition is important if sequelae of fistula and stricture (and potentially nephrectomy) are to be avoided. If ureteral injury is first suspected during surgical exploration, intravenous injection of indigo carmine is helpful in detecting urinary extravasation. In the area of injury, the ureter must be completely dissected, with care taken to avoid injury to the adventitia, through which the ureteral blood supply courses.

Management. Injuries to the ureter below the iliac vessels are often managed by reimplanting the ureter into the bladder. Injury to the upper ureter can be managed by one of several pyeloplasty techniques. Uncomplicated injuries to the middle third of the ureter can be treated with ureteroureterostomy. In debriding the ureter after bullet wounds, one must be careful to debride back to viable tissue, taking into account damage from the blast effect of the missile. Repairs may require stenting and nephrostomy placement to ensure adequate healing. In a patient with numerous life-threatening injuries, a cutaneous ureterostomy or insertion of a diverting stent into the renal pelvis from a point below the injury site and brought out to the skin may be an adequate temporizing measure.

LOWER URINARY TRACT TRAUMA

Urethral Trauma

The portions of the urethra most susceptible to injury are those that are least mobile—the bulbous urethra and the membranous urethra. The former is commonly injured via a straddle injury and the latter is injured subsequent to pelvic fracture.

Anterior Urethral Injury

Indications for Consultation. There is often a history of a fall and, in some cases, a history of instrumentation. Bleeding from the urethra, difficulty in voiding, perineal pain, and perineal or penile hematoma may be present. Tenderness and a palpable mass may be noted in the penis in the event of a pendulous urethral injury, or these signs may be noted in the perineum if the injury is in the bulbous urethra.

Diagnostic Procedures. The patient is instructed not to void, so as to prevent urinary extravasation. A retrograde urethrogram should demonstrate the site of injury. With urethral contusion alone, no extravasation will be noted. Catheterization prior to radiologic visualization of the urethra is to be avoided, so as to prevent inadvertent further injury to the urethra.

Emergency Management. Contusion can be treated with catheter drainage or observation alone if the patient can void and the urine is clear. A partial rupture can either be treated with indwelling catheter drainage for 7 to 10 days or suprapubic urinary drainage. Penetrating injuries should be debrided and cleansed and may be managed with either immediate reconstruction or cystostomy drainage. Urethral injuries are rare in women. Bleeding may be significant and can often be controlled endoscopically.

Posterior Urethral Injury

Indications for Consultation. Five per cent of patients with pelvic fracture will have partial or complete rupture of the posterior (prostatomembranous) urethra. The classic triad leading to suspicion of such an injury is blood at the urethral meatus, urinary retention, and a distended bladder. Findings of a pelvic fracture and an upwardly displaced, boggy prostate on rectal examination mandate radiologic evaluation.

Diagnostic Procedures. As with anterior urethral injuries, the "diagnostic catheter" is to be condemned. A retrograde urethrogram is the study of choice. Loss of urethral continuity implies rupture. If there is extravasation, but some contrast material leaks into the bladder, a partial tear is diagnosed. No extravasation of contrast material is an indication to insert a catheter so that cystography can be performed.

Emergency Management. Controversy exists regarding the ideal approach to posterior urethral injury. One technique involves manipulating the urethra through the bladder and penis after a suprapubic cystostomy is performed. Interlocking sounds establish urethral continuity, and an indwelling urethral retention catheter is placed on traction to approximate the severed ends of the urethra. Others advocate placement of perineal traction sutures through the prostatic capsule rather than balloon catheter traction for urethral approximation.

A second method involves immediate dissection of the severed urethral ends at initial surgery, with primary anastomosis and placement of a urethral catheter as a stent.

Perhaps the most commonly used approach currently is simple placement of a suprapubic tube with delayed urethral reconstruction in 3 to 6 months following appropriate radiologic study of the status of the injury at that time. Advantages of this approach include reduced blood loss, no need for a urologic specialist, speed, the possibility of spontaneous urethral closure if the laceration was only partial, and possibly a decreased likelihood of erectile impotence. All patients with posterior urethral injury should be warned of the potential complications of stricture and impotence regardless of the approach used in the initial treatment.

Bladder Trauma

Mechanisms of injury to the bladder include direct injury from a bone fracture, the explosive hydraulic injury resulting from blunt trauma to a filled bladder, and penetrating trauma.

Indications for Consultation. Five to ten per cent of patients with a fractured pelvis will have an associated bladder rupture. When both pubic rami are fractured, the incidence climbs to 20 per cent. From 50 to 80 per cent of bladder ruptures secondary to pelvic fracture are extraperitoneal. Blunt trauma to a distended bladder generally results in rupture of the dome into the peritoneal cavity. Aside from pelvic fracture, bladder injury should be suspected in patients with a history of trauma who have lower abdominal pain, hematuria, or an inability to void. If diagnosis is delayed, the presentation may be that of an acute abdomen. Any penetrating lower abdominal or pelvic wound should also be investigated for bladder injury.

Diagnostic Procedures. Abdominal plain films may demonstrate pelvic fracture. Intravenous urography will ensure upper tract integrity, deliniate bladder configuration, and diagnose 15 per cent of bladder ruptures. A carefully performed three-phase cystogram is essential to rule out bladder injury. Fifty ml of contrast material is instilled to demonstrate a massive rupture. If no extravasation is seen, an additional 250 ml are instilled to distend the bladder fully. Finally, a postevacuation film is reviewed. A diagnosis of contusion, intraperitoneal rupture, or extraperitoneal rupture can be made based on the cystogram.

Emergency Management. Penetrating injuries must be explored both to repair the bladder and to treat any associated injuries. Patients with blunt vesical injuries with evidence of intra-abdominal trauma (positive peritoneal lavage) and those with intraperitoneal bladder rupture are managed in a similar fashion. A large suprapubic tube is used for vesical drainage in males, while in females a urethral catheter is generally used to perform drainage. The bladder is repaired, and the prevesical space is drained.

Patients with extraperitoneal rupture can be explored or can be treated nonoperatively with urethral catheter drainage provided that (1) there is no reason to expect complicating injuries requiring exploration, (2) diagnosis is made within 12 hours, and (3) the urine is sterile.

INJURIES TO THE GENITALIA

The relative mobility of the genitalia tends to protect them from serious injury in civilian life. Genital injuries can be classified as avulsion, penetrating, crush, or burns. The penis itself may be subject to amputation, fracture, or strangulation injury.

Nonpenetrating wounds of the penis and scrotum may be associated with marked edema of the tissues because of the elastic nature of the skin and fascial layers. Cold packs, rest, elevation, and occasionally pressure dressings are indicated when damage to the testes and corpora is *not* suspected. Persistent hemorrhage will require open surgical hemostasis and drainage. Ultrasonography may be helpful in diagnosing rupture of the corporal bodies or testes if physical examination alone is equivocal. Rupture of the testes or corporal rupture (penile fracture, usually during sexual activity) requires surgical exploration and repair.

Penetrating trauma of the genitalia is treated similarly to penetrating trauma elsewhere on the body. Retrograde urethrography may be important to document urethral integrity. Lavage, debridement, removal of foreign bodies, hemostasis, repair of underlying structures, and primary wound closure (unless there is gross contamination) are the mainstays of therapy.

Avulsion of the penile and scrotal skin is usually secondary to machinery accidents. Skin separation occurs along relatively bloodless planes superficial to Buck's fascia in the penile shaft and just beneath the dartos fascia of the scrotum. Immediate treatment consists of analgesics; application of sterile, moist saline packs; broad-spectrum antibiotics; tetanus and gas gangrene antitoxin; and emergency surgical repair within hours of the injury. Split-thickness skin grafts are used to cover the denuded penile shaft. Skin distal to the avulsion should be debrided to the area of the corona (leaving a small cuff on which to anchor the graft) to prevent marked lymphedema. An indwelling urethral catheter and pressure dressing complete the procedure.

Contrary to the management of avulsion injuries of the penis, in scrotal trauma all viable scrotal skin should be salvaged so the testicles may be covered primarily with scrotal skin whenever possible, as scrotal tissue will return to normal size and consistency in a matter of months. If skin is insufficient to provide testicular housing, the testes may be implanted immediately beneath the skin of the thigh.

BENIGN PROSTATIC HYPERPLASIA

method of
MICHAEL E. MAYO, M.B.B.S.
University of Washington
Seattle, Washington

In benign prostatic hyperplasia (BPH) there is an enlargement of a small volume (5 per cent) of tissue surrounding the central third of the urethra. The urethra is usually elongated and both lateral and middle lobes may enlarge and distort the neck and trigone of the bladder. This prevents the normal funneling of the bladder neck, obstructing voiding. BPH is an age-related condition rarely found before age 40 but is present in 80 per cent of men over 80 years of age. Today, there is a 29 per cent probability that a 40-year-old man will have a prostatectomy during his lifetime.

The history of prostatism typically encompasses two sets of symptoms: obstructive and irritative. Hesitancy, poor stream, intermittency, terminal dribbling, double voiding, and incomplete emptying are the commonest obstructive symptoms. Men with BPH rarely strain to void unless chronic retention has developed. The irritative symptoms of frequency and urgency are present in most patients, and these are often more troublesome than the obstructive ones, especially when sleep is disturbed by nocturia. Incontinence (urge and overflow), retention (acute and chronic with azotemia), infection (producing pain on urination), and hematuria are all less common forms of presentation. Physical examination should include an assessment of the size and consistency of the prostate. Although size does not always correlate with the degree of obstruction, a very large gland may need a different surgical approach and any suspicion of malignancy will usually require a tissue diagnosis before treatment can be planned. Physical signs of retention of urine or neuropathy should also be sought.

Initial investigations should be noninvasive, and a flow rate determination is the most useful screening test. Urinalysis, and culture if indicated, a hemogram, and blood chemistry are standard investigations in all cases. Although upper tract imaging is not essential, except when there is a history of stones or hematuria, an ultrasonogram and/or excretory urogram will allow for an estimate of trabeculation and residual urine without the necessity for urethral instrumentation. Cystoscopy will be indicated if a decision on the management of prostatism cannot be made or if there is any suspicion of other bladder pathology, especially a tumor. A simple cystometrogram (CMG) may demonstrate detrusor muscle instability, which is present in 60 to 70 per cent of men with prostatism but is rarely helpful in deciding on treatment. The CMG may document a large capacity bladder with reduced sensation in men with chronic retention; however, to determine the contractility of the detrusor muscle, a complex multichannel urodynamic study with voiding pressure is required. Any man with a neuropathy and possible obstruction should also have a urodynamic evaluation to determine the significance of each component. The commonest indications for intervention in BPH are the symptoms of prostatism. Men with moderate symptoms (nocturia of twice or less) have a good chance of remaining the same or improving over time, and, indeed, a large placebo effect has been found in controlled trials of drug treatment for BPH. Therefore, in men with mild to moderate symptoms a period of observation is advisable. Retention (acute or chronic with azotemia), recurrent infection and persistent hematuria are much less common but more urgent reasons for intervention.

Treatment

Nonsurgical

Surgical removal of the obstructing tissue is still the most effective treatment but there are nonsurgical therapies that should be discussed with the patient and recommended if there is a high surgical risk.

Alpha-Adrenergic Antagonists. The prostate and bladder neck contain a large number of alpha-adrenergic receptors, and inhibition of these has been shown to improve both the obstructive and irritative symptoms in many well-controlled trials. The drug most often used is phenoxybenzamine* (Dibenzyline), 10 mg per day orally, increasing as tolerated over a period of 1 week to 30 mg per day. Prazosin* (Minipress), 1 mg orally, increasing as tolerated to 4 mg per day, is also effective and may be associated with fewer side effects (dizziness, lack of concentration, stuffy nose). A reduction in circulating testosterone by using estrogens or performing orchiectomy will often allow atrophy of a benign gland but is not generally acceptable in men without disseminated cancer of the prostate. However, the intracellular conversion of testosterone to dihydrotestosterone can be blocked by inhibiting the enzyme 5 α-reductase, which is responsible for this conversion; therapeutic trials of a 5 α-reductase

---

*This use of these agents is not listed in the manufacturers' directives.

inhibitor are now in progress. Balloon dilation of the prostatic urethra is also under therapeutic trial.

Surgical

Transurethral Surgery. Transurethral resection of the prostate (TURP) has become the surgical treatment of choice in most cases. Resection of relatively small glands (less than 20 grams) seems to be associated with a higher incidence of bladder neck contracture, and the early results of incising the bladder neck and prostate (transurethral incision of the prostate [TUIP]) are excellent. It remains to be seen if a TURP will be required more often in the TUIP patients at a later date.

Open Surgery. Only 10 per cent of prostatectomies are performed by open procedure, the indications being very large glands, inadequate urethral size for the resectoscope, and the presence of certain bladder pathologies. In a *suprapubic* prostatectomy the gland is approached through the bladder, and in the *retropubic* prostatectomy the anterior prostate capsule is incised directly just below the bladder neck. In the *perineal* prostatectomy the posterior prostatic capsule is incised in the perineum, but the latter procedure is rarely indicated because of significant impotence and incontinence problems that ensue.

In all resection procedures the objective is to remove the adenoma, leaving the surgical capsule. Clearly, the open procedure is more complete but is usually associated with a higher morbidity.

Anesthesia. Spinal or epidural anesthesia is excellent for a transurethral approach and may be adequate for open surgery if high enough to give adequate relaxation of the abdominal muscles. General anesthetic is required if there are contraindications to spinal or epidural anesthesia. It is also possible to do the procedure under local anesthetic, infiltrating the prostate from both the perineal and urethral aspects.

Antibiotics. Appropriate antibiotic therapy should be started parenterally at least 12 hours prior to surgery and continued for 5 days after catheter removal in patients with bacteriuria and in those with indwelling urethral catheters. Even if the urine from the Foley catheter is sterile, there is an increase in urethral colonization around it. Prophylactic antibiotics given to patients with sterile urine and no preoperative catheters appear to reduce postoperative bacteriuria but do not show any benefit in reducing the rare but serious complications of septicemia. Also, in the majority of patients, this postoperative bacteriuria is asymptomatic and transient. Prophylactic antibiotics should, however, be given to high-risk patients with diabetes, neurogenic bladder, and immunosupression and to those with cardiac and other prostheses.

Blood Transfusion. It is rare to need blood transfusion in transurethral surgery, and cross-matching is not performed routinely unless the preoperative hematocrit is borderline. In open prostatectomy blood is more often required and should be cross-matched beforehand.

Postoperative Care. Bleeding with obstruction of the drainage catheters is probably the most troublesome problem. It is not important which type of catheter and method of irrigation are used as long as the nursing staff caring for the patient is thoroughly familiar with their management. There is a real advantage to having all postoperative prostatectomy patients on a designated urology nursing unit. The catheter is removed usually in 1 to 3 days after a TURP when the urine has cleared to a light pink or brown if there are no other factors such as fever, a large perforation, or other active medical problem that would compromise a voiding trial. The patient should be warned to expect some increased frequency, urgency, and even urge incontinence. Unless the voided volumes are very small, the stream should be noticeably better than before operation. Bleeding should be monitored by saving the three most recent urine samples. The postvoid residual should be determined if there is any clinical suspicion of incomplete emptying.

Complications

Early Complications

Mortality. Traditionally, the operative mortality (death within 30 days of surgery) for open prostatectomy and TURP was thought to be less than 2 per cent and less than 1 per cent, respectively. However, recent figures based on health-care claims data have revealed the mortality (occurring in or out of hospital within 91 days of prostatectomy) is 3.1 per cent for open prostatectomy, and 2.8 per cent for TURP in teaching hospitals. This compares with a high figure of 6.1 per cent and 9.0 per cent for TURP for small nonteaching hospitals (less than 150 beds). Within 1 year of TURP 9 per cent of men age 55 to 69 years of age die as compared with a predicted rate of 3.5 per cent in age-matched men not undergoing surgery. If these figures are confirmed, it is clear that in high-risk patients, with poor life expectancy, alternative management of prostatic enlargement should be carefully considered.

TURP Syndrome. An average of 1 liter of irrigation fluid is absorbed in a TURP and this causes little clinical or biochemical disturbance. However, if large venous sinuses are opened or if large perforations in the prostate capsule or bladder neck are made and large amounts of irrigating fluid are extravasated, considerable amounts of fluid may enter the patient's circulation. The irrigating fluid used is usually a slightly hypotonic solution of glycine or sorbitol, which causes a dilutional hyponatremia that is responsible for most of the chemical manifestations (nausea, vomiting, confusion, coma, bradycardia, hypertension, and muscle paralysis). Many patients will correct the clinical and metabolic problem of the TURP syndrome with diuresis, which may, if necessary, be induced by diuretics. Attempting to correct the hyponatremia with hypertonic saline may be indicated in patients with coma, but cardiac failure is likely to be precipitated.

Hemorrhage. Venous bleeding at the end of the procedure can usually be controlled with gentle catheter traction and tamponade of the bladder neck and prostatic fossa for a few hours. Heavy arterial bleeding restarting after the procedure will usually require a recystoscopy under anesthetic with evacuation of clots and coagulation of the bleeding point.

Secondary venous hemorrhage is often brought on by straining, and readmission to hospital with cystoscopy is occasionally required. Patients should be advised not to be too active and to try to avoid straining for defecation, and they should not allow the bladder to become overdistended.

Urinary Tract Infection. The use of preoperative antibiotics, whether for treatment or prophylaxis, has been discussed. If antibiotics are not used, it is advisable to check a urine culture before discharge and at 3 to 4 weeks, as asymptomatic bacteriuria that does not clear may be associated with delayed healing of the prostatic fossa and increased scarring. Urinalysis will usually reveal pyuria and microhematuria for 6 weeks until the prostatic fossa has reepithelized, and urine culture is needed to confirm bacteriuria and to check sensitivities. Epididymitis occurs in 2 per cent of patients after TURP, and vasectomy does not appear to prevent it.

Wound Infection. The incidence of wound infection may be as high as 20 per cent even in patients with uninfected urine. The source of these organisms is probably the distal urethra, and prophylactic antibiotics are advisable in open procedures and will usually halve the risk. The condition of osteitis pubis is rarely seen now that most urinary tract infections can be adequately treated prior to surgery.

Incontinence. Detrusor muscle instability present in 60 to 70 per cent of men prior to surgery may cause urgency incontinence for several months after operation; however, 60 per cent of these patients will lose their instability within 6 months. Sphincter weakness incontinence is seen in less than 1 per cent of patients in the long run, although it may be present for a few days after removal of the catheter. Sphincter incontinence after prostatectomy is usually due to damage to the passive component of the distal sphincter. The patient may be able to prevent leakage by active pelvic floor contraction, but when this voluntary muscle fatigues, a slow drip will occur when the patient is upright. Improvement in sphincter function will occur over time and with pelvic floor exercises. Surgical correction with an artificial sphincter is not usually considered for 6 to 12 months, which will allow spontaneous improvement to occur.

Impotence and Retrograde Ejaculation. Potency may decrease in a number of men after suprapubic and retropubic prostatectomy, TURP, or TUIP but rarely can an organic cause be found for this. Sexual activity often decreases at this time of life, and the prostatectomy, with the associated local discomfort, adds a further psychologic factor. Ejaculation is nearly always partly or largely retrograde after surgery except in patients who have had a TUIP. Preoperative counseling should include a generally positive outlook with regard to change in potency but should contain a warning about the problem of retrograde ejaculation, especially if the patient is relatively young and may want to father more children.

Inadequate Emptying. This may be due to persistent adenoma or hypocontractility of the detrusor muscle. It is important to determine which of these is present before undertaking further surgery, and this evaluation may require at least a CMG, or preferably multichannel urodynamics to determine detrusor contractility during attempted voiding. If obstructing tissue is still present, further resection is generally indicated. Hypocontractility should be treated with a further period of catheter drainage, preferably by a self-intermittent catheterization program, or if this cannot be performed, a Foley catheter may be inserted for a few weeks. The patient may have to learn to void by straining or Credé's method. The addition of parasympathetic agents (bethanechol [Urecholine] orally 25 mg three times per day) may be tried but is usually ineffective unless much larger doses are taken, in which case unacceptable side effects will occur.

Late Complications

Urethral Strictures. These occur in approximately 6 per cent of patients after TURP and are commonest in the submeatal area. Attempting to use instruments and catheters that are too large for the urethra may predispose to stricture, and the meatal and submeatal areas may be damaged by allowing dried blood and secretions to build up on the catheter. Treatment consists of dilation and occasionally internal urethrotomy, but if the stricture is in the membranous urethra, gentle and repeated dilations only should be performed, otherwise the passive sphincter may be damaged.

Bladder Neck Contracture. This is a scarring of the bladder neck that constricts in ringlike fashion and prevents adequate funneling. It seems to be commoner after small TURPS or if the bladder neck is resected too deeply. The condition presents with obstructive and irritative symptoms, often with infection. Endoscopic incision rather than resection is the treatment of choice, and this may have to be done more than once. Occasionally, an open Y-V plasty is necessary to resolve the problem.

Regrowth of Prostatic Tissue. Health-care claims data have revealed a much higher incidence of repeat prostatectomy than the 10 per cent quoted from traditional retrospective studies. For patients surviving 8 years, the cumulative probability for a second operation is 20 per cent for TURP and 10 per cent for open operation.

PROSTATITIS

method of
RICHARD K. LO, M.D.
Stanford University School of Medicine
Stanford, California

The term prostatitis has been used by most physicians to describe a constellation of symptoms, including perineal pain, ejaculatory and voiding dysfunction, and nonspecific complaints of pain or discomfort in the groin, pelvic, and perineal regions. Confusion over the etiology of the painful syndromes in these patients has further compounded the poor understanding of the treatment strategies and the lack of systematic studies of the disease. Prostatitis can be classified into three main categories: bacterial prostatitis, nonbacterial prostatitis, and prostatodynia. Careful analysis of segmentally voided urine specimens and microscopic examination of the prostate fluid will allow proper identification and stratification of the patient into these categories, with treatment tailored accordingly.

Segmental collection and culture of the urine samples should be performed by the examiner to ascertain the adequacy of the specimens and the technique of the collections. The bladder urine should be sterile at the time of localization; otherwise, the localization should be deferred and the patient given an appropriate antibiotic that does not penetrate the prostate, such as nitrofurantoin or ampicillin. Culture of the first 5 to 10 ml of voided urine (voided bladder 1, VB1)

shows urethral organisms. Voided bladder 2 (VB2), the classic midstream collection, demonstrates organisms resident in the bladder. The prostate is then massaged vigorously to obtain prostate fluid, which is called expressed prostatic secretions (EPS), which will reflect prostatic organisms. The first 5 to 10 ml of urine voided after prostatic massage (VB3) are then obtained to show prostatic and urethral organisms. Bacterial infection is localized to the prostate if the colony count in the EPS or VB3 specimen is at least 10-fold higher than that found in the VB1 specimen. Those with documented bacterial infections will therefore be classified under bacterial prostatitis.

The EPS should also be examined microscopically to detect the presence of inflammatory cells. Under a high dry field examination the presence of more than 12 leukocytes is indicative of prostatic inflammation, a true definition of prostatitis. It is not uncommon to see clumps of white blood cells even in those patients whose prostatitis is clinically quiescent. Oval fat bodies are macrophages laden with cholesterol and appear brown under the low power field in prostatitis, especially in bacterial prostatitis. Interpretation of microscopic findings in the EPS is meaningless without simultaneously examining the VB1 sediments to exclude urethral inflammation. The same is true for an isolated culture of the EPS, without information on the other specimens. Patients with a normal EPS and no demonstrated bacterial infection are classified under prostatodynia.

BACTERIAL PROSTATITIS

Gram-negative bacteria, such as *Escherichia coli, Proteus, Enterobacter, Klebsiella, Serratia,* and *Pseudomonas* species, are the most common organisms associated with bacterial prostatitis. In the male, recurrent bacterial urinary infections with *Enterococcus* species probably represent colonization of the prostate by this organism. Other gram-positive organisms are commensal organisms in the male urethra, which are at times recovered from the EPS and VB1; the role of these organisms in bacterial prostatitis is uncertain.

Acute Bacterial Prostatitis

Patients with acute bacterial prostatitis usually present with high fevers; chills; perineal and low back pain; symptoms of bladder outlet obstruction, including hesistancy, intermittency, retention; and irritable symptoms of dysuria, urgency, and frequency. Rectal examination shows an exquisitely tender and swollen prostate gland, which is at times nodular. The physician should, however, refrain from performing a prostatic massage to avoid the risk of disseminating bacteria into the bloodstream and causing sepsis. Invariably, bacteria can be recovered from the urine to confirm the diagnosis.

Most of these patients are acutely ill, some with urinary retention, and require hospitalization. With the severe inflammatory changes associated with acute bacterial prostatitis, the usual barrier of the prostate gland to diffusion of antimicrobials from the serum is broken down. Intravenous aminoglycoside and ampicillin should be used empirically (gentamicin [Garamycin] or tobramycin [Nebcin], 3 to 5 mg per kg per 24 hours in three divided doses; ampicillin at 2 grams every 6 hours) for approximately 3 to 4 days. The patient can then be started on sulfamethoxazole-trimethoprim (Bactrim, Septra), 800 mg TMP/160 mg SMX twice daily, for a total of 4 weeks, unless the culture and sensitivity indicate otherwise or are contraindicated by the patient's allergy to the sulfas. Acute bacterial prostatitis is a rare indication in which long-term, full dose antimicrobials should be used to treat a urinary tract infection, since there is a good chance of curing the infection using this regimen and of avoiding a relapse. Urethral instrumentations should be avoided; if the patient is in retention, a percutaneous suprapubic catheter should be inserted instead of an indwelling urethral catheter. General supportive measures, such as bed rest, antipyretics, analgesics, and stool softeners, should be instituted. Rarely, prostatic abscesses form, despite the use of antibiotics. Transrectal drainage or transurethral resection to unroof the abscess may be indicated.

Chronic Bacterial Prostatitis

The diagnosis of chronic bacterial prostatitis is made by recognizing the pattern of chronic relapsing bacterial cystitis that is caused by the same organism. The presentation of these patients during an infectious episode is less dramatic than that of an acute bacterial prostatitis. They usually complain of dysuria, frequency, nocturia, chronic perineal ache, and at times hemospermia. In older males, the bacteriuria may be silent and is recognized only incidentally. There may or may not be a history of an antecedent episode of acute bacterial prostatitis, even though failure to eradicate all bacteria in acute bacterial prostatitis is often the etiology of the recurring chronic bacterial prostatitis. Palpation of the prostate is often unremarkable, showing maybe only benign enlargement of the gland. The diagnosis is confirmed by lower tract localization utilizing segmental cultures and examination of the EPS, as described previously.

Attempts to eradicate bacteria totally from the prostate are often a frustrating exercise. Bacterial infections of the prostate may involve the ducts and acini, calculi, and even the stroma and interstitium. The high alkalinity of the prostatic fluid in men with chronic bacterial prostatitis prevents diffusion of most antimicrobials into the prostate in bactericidal levels. Two exceptions may be carbenicillin indanyl sodium (Geocillin), 764 mg orally four times daily, and sulfamethoxazole-trimethoprim, 800 mg TMP/160 mg SMX twice daily. Patients are given a full dose of these agents for 8 to 12 weeks, and the lower tract localization is repeated at the conclusion of treatment. Unfortunately, less than 50 per cent of these patients are cured.

When full dose antibiotics fail to eradicate the chronic bacterial prostatitis, the patient is given antibiotic prophylaxis. Sulfamethoxazole-trimethoprim, 200 mg TMP/40 mg SMX, or half of a single strength tablet once daily, or nitrofurantoin (Macrodantin), 50 to 100 mg daily, is preferred, since each of these drugs is almost completely absorbed at the small bowel level and will not affect the fecal flora. The harbored bacteria are not exposed to the antimicrobial, and the sensitivity therefore remains unchanged. The duration of treatment is at least 6 months; most of the patients, however, will relapse and will require a lifelong treatment with this low dose regimen. Despite the chronicity and inconvenience of a lifelong treatment, good control of the irritable bladder symptoms from bacteriuria can be achieved. Radical transurethral resection of the prostate and total prostatectomy are rarely indicated. The former is often unsuccessful because transurethral resection does not remove the peripheral zone of the prostate where the infection and infected calculi are most often located. Impotence and incontinence are the main drawbacks in recommending total prostatectomy.

NONBACTERIAL PROSTATITIS

Patients with nonbacterial prostatitis suffer from the same perineal pain and voiding and ejaculatory dysfunction as those with acute or chronic bacterial prostatitis. On evaluation, the prostate may appear boggy and tender, and the microscopic examination of the EPS may show a specimen loaded with many leukocytes and oval fat macrophages. These patients, however, do not have a history of bacteriuria, and the culture of the EPS will fail to demonstrate bacterial infections. The inflammation appears to be secondary to an unidentified bacteria or perhaps even to a nonbacterial agent: *Mycoplasma, Trichomonas,* or *Chlamydia* species or even viruses. Since the etiology is poorly understood, rational treatment is empirical at best. This syndrome accounts for about three quarters of the men with an inflamed prostate as indicated by the EPS findings.

A clinical trial of doxycycline, 100 mg twice daily, tetracycline, 500 mg four times a day, or erythromycin, 500 mg four times a day, can be given for 3 to 4 weeks. Most often there is no relief of the symptoms. These patients are then started on an oral anti-inflammatory agent: ibuprofen, 600 mg four times daily, indomethacin, 25 mg four times daily, aspirin, 325 mg four times daily, or oxyphenbutazone, 100 mg three times daily. Since these medications have significant gastrointestinal side effects, their use in patients with a previous history of peptic ulcer disease should be monitored closely. The results in some patients can be dramatic, even after years of suffering from nonbacterial prostatitis. The patient is given instructions to start the medication at full dosage, and after he obtains relief and is stabilized for 2 to 3 weeks, the dose is tapered slowly and eventually to a maintenance dose of one pill daily or every other day. When there is an exacerbation in symptoms, he will immediately return to the full dose schedule and repeat the tapering process when the symptoms subside.

PROSTATODYNIA

Prostatodynia literally means prostate pain. Patients who have identical symptoms as those with chronic bacterial prostatitis and acute bacterial prostatitis but who have no evidence of inflammation on examination of the EPS are categorized under this syndrome. The etiology of prostatodynia is unknown, although pelvic floor spasms, adrenergic overactivity, stress, and psychologic disturbances of neurosis have been implicated. Often these patients are younger than ones from the other groups. During an interview, they may admit to or volunteer information regarding stresses at work or at home or the relationship of ingestion of alcohol, coffee, or spices to periods of exacerbation. Treatment is difficult and is tailored to the individual. Empiric use of an alpha-blocking agent such as prazosin (Minipress), 1 to 3 mg one to three times daily, slowly increasing the dose to minimize orthostatic hypotension, or phenoxybenzamine (Dibenzyline), 10 mg three times daily with the same precautions, can sometimes be helpful. In addition, muscle-relaxants and antispasmodics, diazepam (Valium), 5 mg four times daily, or baclofen (Lioresal), 10 mg three times daily, have been successful in a subgroup of these patients, although identification of these patients a priori is not possible. Avoidance of inciting agents (alcohol, caffeine) may be appropiate in isolated situations. General supportive measures such as sitz baths, scrotal elevation, and prostatic massage are sometimes utilized, although the value of the latter is questioned. The clinician should avoid dismissing voiding and ejaculatory complaints of patients with prostatodynia refractory to treatment. Cystoscopy with biopsies should be performed to exclude the presence of interstitial cystitis, bladder tumor, carcinoma in situ of the bladder, or ductal carcinoma of prostatic ducts in these patients. When these are absent, the physician should reassure the patient that there is no life-threatening situation but instead a nuisance he will probably have to learn to accept and live with.

ACUTE RENAL FAILURE
method of
MICHAEL I. SORKIN, M.D.
University of Pittsburgh and Veterans Administration Medical Center
Pittsburgh, Pennsylvania

Any decrease in renal function characterized by a short and relatively severe course is called acute renal failure. The decrease in renal function is detected by an increasing BUN and creatinine, which is usually (but not always) coupled with decreasing urine output. The major diagnostic problem is to differentiate disease affecting the kidney (renal failure) from factors affecting the blood flow to the kidney (prerenal) and from factors obstructing the urinary tract (postrenal). Both prerenal and postrenal factors may produce renal failure if not corrected, so an accurate diagnosis and rapid correction of these factors are essential to preserving renal function.

Prerenal Factors

The ischemic kidney preserves renal blood flow by preventing loss of fluid. It invokes mechanisms to cause maximum reabsorption of sodium and water, thereby producing "concentrated urine" with high osmolality, low sodium concentration, a high specific gravity, and a relatively large concentration gradient between urine and blood of solutes that are not affected by active tubular reabsorption (creatinine and urea are the most useful clinically). This concentrated urine can be produced only as long as tubules are healthy. Glomerular filtration is normal until parenchymal damage occurs. Since urea is reabsorbed passively but creatinine is not reabsorbed at all, when renal blood flow decreases, the ratio of BUN to creatinine rises from 10 past the normal upper limit of 20.

These prerenal manifestations appear any time renal perfusion is reduced, regardless of the etiology. Hemorrhage, heart failure, and dehydration are all the same to the kidney.

Postrenal Factors

Postrenal factors encompass urinary tract obstruction, which interferes with urine output. Bladder outlet obstruction caused by a large prostate is the most common postrenal factor. One should be alert to the unilateral ureteral obstruction in the patient with only one kidney. A history of periods of anuria interspersed with polyuria is the classic presentation of obstruction. Although renal failure caused by obstruction has several phases, for practical purposes it has all the laboratory features of renal failure. High intratubular pressure damages the tubular epithelium and results in urine osmolality that is nearly the same as plasma osmolality and high urine sodium concentration.

Renal Failure

Any insult to any component of the nephron can result in enough damage to cause acute renal failure. The usual mechanisms are ischemia and nephrotoxins, but immunologically mediated injury also occurs.

Damage to tubules interferes with the capacity to concentrate urine by blocking the ability to reabsorb filtered sodium and water, resulting in rising urine sodium concentration and falling osmolality. Damaged tubular cells may slough off the tubular basement membrane and appear either free in the urine, as renal tubular cell casts, or, as the cells deteriorate, the dirty brown granular casts characteristic of that variety of renal failure known as acute tubular necrosis (ATN).

Damage to glomeruli is characterized by falling glomerular filtration rate and increasing plasma creatinine. Early in the course of acute glomerular disease (e.g., acute poststreptococcal glomerulonephritis), swelling of glomerular components may reduce blood flow and produce the classic signs of prerenal factors. Damage to the glomerulus, especially by inflammation, causes hematuria and red blood cell casts.

Damage to the interstitium causes white blood cell casts, and allergic damage to interstitium causes eosinophiluria and eosinophilia (e.g., acute interstitial nephritis from methicillin).

Acute on Chronic Renal Failure

Patients with some degree of renal failure may also develop pre- or postrenal factors that influence renal function. These patients are lacking the critical adaptive mechanisms that allow them to "autoregulate" renal blood flow and to produce concentrated urine. Therefore, prerenal factors will produce laboratory findings indistinguishable from those of true acute renal failure. One should be suspicious of an element of chronic renal failure in patients who have diseases that may be associated with renal failure, especially diabetes mellitus or hypertension. A serum creatinine at the upper limits of normal or a creatinine within the normal range but higher than expected for apparent muscle mass indicates renal failure. In this case, prerenal factors must be excluded by determining that they are not present or by correcting them. A prompt improvement in renal function with correction of prerenal factors indicates that they played a role in producing the laboratory findings suggestive of renal failure.

History

The cause of renal failure is frequently obvious, as when it follows major trauma, surgery, or burns. Sometimes the specific cause cannot be determined because many potential causes are present, as is encountered in the intensive care unit setting. Nevertheless, a careful history will reveal helpful information. The complaint of thirst is an important clue to dehydration. Nocturia is caused by the loss of the normal concentrating mechanism early in chronic renal failure. Unexpected exposure to drugs and poisons will come to light only if all drugs are considered potential causes of renal failure. Underlying systemic diseases may cause acute renal failure or predispose to renal failure if other factors appear (e.g., dehydration, radiocontrast agents, chemotherapy). Dehydration potentiates the effects of renal ischemia and nephrotoxins to produce acute renal failure. Table 1 lists most of the common causes of acute renal failure.

Physical Examination

Accurate evaluation of volume status is the single most important part of the physical examination. The presence of any detectable edema means the patient has at least 3 kg of extra fluid and is not likely to be volume depleted. Central venous pressure (CVP) is estimated by the height of the column of blood in a neck vein (or any vein) using the level of the right atrium as reference. Volume depletion is unlikely if the CVP is above 5. Orthostatic hypotension occurs with inadequate blood volume, but it also occurs with autonomic neuropathy and prolonged bed rest. Heart failure, a common cause of reduced renal blood flow, may be difficult to detect. Other more subtle signs may be helpful (e.g., absence of sweat, poor skin turgor, dry mucous membranes).

The skin may indicate systemic diseases that cause renal failure. The presence of scleroderma, purpura (Henoch-Schöenlein's), petechiae or necrotic areas (atheromatous or cholesterol emboli), the butterfly rash of systemic lupus erythematosus, and spider angioma of cirrhosis are only a few examples.

Diagnostic Studies

First, bladder outlet obstruction should be eliminated. If a catheter inserted into the bladder after an attempt at voiding drains a large volume, the diagnosis of obstruction is confirmed and also treated. Any postvoiding residual urine over 50 ml suggests that some component of obstruction is present.

Urinalysis, including dipstick and microscopic examinations, is of critical importance. Table 2 gives a quick reference to the diagnostic features of the urinalysis. Cultures should be performed if more than a few white cells per high power field are present, but infection is a very rare cause of acute renal failure even if it is present.

Prerenal factors may not be obvious. The laboratory studies in Table 3 should help in this decision. More sophisticated tests and calculations have been devised, but they are more complex that those listed and add little information in most cases.

TABLE 1. **Causes of Acute Renal Failure**

Glomerular
  Postinfectious acute glomerulonephritis
  Goodpasture's syndrome
  Wegener's granulomatosis
Tubular/Interstitial
  Acute tubular necrosis
  Acute interstitial nephritis
  Hepatorenal syndrome
  Myeloma
  Leptospirosis
Obstruction
  Prostatic hyperplasia
  Stones
  Retroperitoneal fibrosis
Vascular
  Acute renal artery occlusion
  Cholesterol emboli
  Aneurysm
  Vasculitis
  Malignant hypertension
Drugs
  Acetaminophen (overdose)
  Allopurinol
  Aminoglycosides
  Amphotericin B
  Angiotensin-converting enzyme inhibitors
  Antineoplastic agents
    Cisplatin
    Nitrosoureas
    CCNU/Methyl-CCNU
    Methotrexate
    Mithramycin
    Radiation
  Cimetidine
  Gold salts
  Methicillin (and penicillin, ampicillin, oxacillin,
    carbenicillin, nafcillin, amoxicillin)
  Nifedipine
  Nonsteroidal anti-inflammatory drugs
  Phenytoin
  Radiographic contrast agents
  Tetracyclines
  Thiazides
Poisons
  Carbon monoxide
  Carbon tetrachloride
  Ethylene glycol
  Lead
  Mercury
Rhabdomyolysis
  Alcohol
  Heat stroke
  Trauma
Hemolysis
  Malaria
Transfusion reaction

TABLE 2. **The Urinalysis in Acute Renal Failure**

Finding	Disease
RBC casts	Glomerulonephritis
WBC casts	Interstitial nephritis
Eosinophils	Allergic interstitial nephritis
Pigmented granular casts	Acute tubular necrosis
Dipstick positive for blood but few RBCs	
With pink tinged serum	Hemolysis with hemoglobinuria
With normal serum	Rhabdomyolysis with myoglobinuria
Foamy urine	Nephrotic syndrome
Foamy urine with little protein on dipstick	Myeloma
Foamy yellow urine	Hepatobiliary disease

failure, especially in patients who have chronic renal failure, who are elderly, or who have diabetes or myeloma. The IVP frequently gives no more information than the scout film because failing kidneys do not concentrate the contrast agent. A retrograde pyelogram is not nephrotoxic but does carry the risks of instrumentation. It has been implicated in the production of ureteral obstruction by causing local edema. Therefore, it should be performed on only one ureter and should be reserved for situations in which there is still a question of ureteral obstruction in spite of the ultrasonogram.

Radionuclide studies show renal blood flow and cortical function as well as obstruction. The procedure carries little risk. Usually, it adds little information to the sonogram but may be helpful when ultrasonography cannot determine renal blood flow.

Renal biopsy is useful if renal failure is suspected to be associated with a systemic disease or if no reasonable etiology can be found. If potentially dangerous drugs are planned, a specific diagnosis should be available to guide treatment.

Other studies may be helpful in special circumstances but only after the preceding have been considered.

Treatment

The single most important therapeutic maneuver must be to optimize the patient's volume status. Diuretics should not be used until the patient is clearly at least euvolemic. Normal saline should be used to correct hypotension rapidly (or salt-poor albumin if edema is present)

Ultrasonography is usually the next step. The sonogram has no known adverse effects and can usually be performed at the bedside if necessary. It reveals information about obstruction, the number of kidneys, kidney size, and renal blood flow. Echoes from the renal cortex may help diagnose acute tubular necrosis and acute interstitial nephritis.

Radiographic studies have limited usefulness. A scout film may show renal outlines or stones. The intravenous pyelogram (IVP) may produce acute renal

TABLE 3. **Laboratory Diagnosis of Prerenal Factors**

	Prerenal	Renal	Postrenal
BUN/creatinine	> 20	10	10
Urine sodium	< 20	> 40	> 40
Urine osmolality	> 500	serum	serum
Ucr/Scr	> 40	< 20	< 20
Specific gravity	> 1.020	1.010	1.010

Ucr = urine creatinine in mg per dl; Scr = serum creatinine in mg per dl and to raise CVP into the upper range of normal. If this fails to improve urine output, an intravenous bolus of furosemide (Lasix), 120 mg, may restore function or convert oliguric to nonoliguric renal failure. If there is no response within an hour, an additional dose of 240 mg may be tried. If there is no response within an hour, conservative measures must be started immediately. Restrict fluid to insensible loss (roughly 500 ml per day) plus other fluid losses (including urine). Half normal saline is a good choice for starting maintenance fluids since many of the fluids lost (including urine) will be equivalent to half normal saline. Maintenance fluids should be adjusted according to measurements of sodium lost in output and the serum concentration of sodium, potassium, and bicarbonate. Daily blood tests are adequate unless there is reason to expect sudden changes (e.g., surgery, respiratory failure).

Hyperkalemia is a potentially lethal complication, especially in oliguric renal failure. It is not usually a problem if urine output is greater than 1 liter per day. A few patients will present with weakness, but most of the time hyperkalemia is found on routine electrolyte monitoring or during review of the ECG. Mild elevation of serum potassium (up to 6.5) with only peaked T waves on the ECG can be treated by restricting potassium intake and correcting acidosis as long as urine output is in the range of 500 to 1000 ml per day. More severe situations require, in addition, calcium gluconate, 1 gram intravenously, to correct cardiac effects (with no effect on serum potassium), and at the same time (but in a different line to avoid calcium carbonate precipitation) sodium bicarbonate, 50 to 100 mEq (even if there is no acidosis), and glucose, 25 grams followed by 10 per cent dextrose in water infusion (to lower serum potassium by moving it into cells). Insulin is not required in patients who do not have diabetes. If in doubt, 10 units of regular insulin for each 100 grams of glucose should be added to the glucose infusion. Potassium should then be removed by increasing urine output. If urine output is low and cannot be increased, the potassium must be removed by giving the ion exchange resin sodium polystyrene sulfonate (Kayexalate), 25 to 50 grams, in sorbitol 20 per cent, 100 to 200 ml either orally or as a retention enema. Hemodialysis is more effective if available. Peritoneal dialysis is much less effective than either hemodialysis or Kayexalate administration and should be started early if it is the only choice possible.

Expect a weight loss of 0.25 to 0.5 kg per day and confirm the appropriateness of the fluid replacement rate by following daily weights, blood pressure, and examination for edema or rising CVP. Glucose, 100 grams daily, will minimize protein catabolism, but early use of hyperalimentation should be considered if the patient is unable to eat.

A major effort must be made to prevent additional damage to the kidney and the patient. Avoid nephrotoxic agents (be especially careful of antibiotics) when possible and modify dosage when potentially nephrotoxic agents must be used. Do not use magnesium or phosphate-containing compounds unless serum magnesium or phosphate is low. Remove indwelling catheters as soon as possible. With low daily urine volumes, I prefer to catheterize the patient daily if he is unable to void, since indwelling catheters are a source of infection.

Conservative management is all that is required for ATN, since most will recover renal function within 1 to 2 weeks. More aggressive treatment may be required for the other diseases, and other sources should be consulted for specific details.

Indications for emergency (immediate) dialysis are pulmonary edema, life-threatening hyperkalemia, and uremia with malignant hypertension or seizures. Hypervolemia and uremia require dialysis soon (within several days depending on severity) but are not emergencies. Uremia (the clinical syndrome consisting of anorexia, nausea, vomiting, pericarditis, bleeding disorder) must be distinguished from azotemia (elevation of BUN and creatinine), since azotemia by itself is not an indication for urgent dialysis.

CHRONIC RENAL FAILURE

method of
SUHAIL AHMAD, M.D.
University of Washington
Seattle, Washington

Chronic renal failure (CRF) has not been well defined; however, the term suggests chronic and generally irreversible failure of renal function. Each year 50 to 150 persons per million population either require dialysis or renal transplant or die of renal failure. Thus, at any time a large number of patients are in chronic renal failure. Various therapeutic methods can be used to maintain these patients in a state of well-being and to slow the rate of progression of renal failure. Serum creatinine and creatinine clearance are clinically useful methods to assess and follow renal function. Creatinine clearance is generally equivalent to glomerular filtration rate (GFR). If lean body mass does not change, then creatinine generation and excretion remain constant, and serum creatinine reflects creatinine clearance. Recently, the reciprocal of serum creatinine (1/creatinine) has been utilized to reflect renal function. Blood urea nitrogen (BUN) concentration depends on factors other than GFR and is not a reliable indicator of renal function.

CLINICAL MANIFESTATIONS

Among different patients and sometimes in the same patient at different times, signs and symptoms of renal failure are extremely variable. Table 1 shows a broad outline of manifestations of renal failure at various stages of progression of the disease. Generally, symptoms of renal failure are not evident until GFR (as measured by creatinine clearance) declines below 20 to 30 ml per minute. Dialysis is usually not required until the GFR is less than 5 to 10 ml per minute.

Common signs and symptoms include general malaise, lack of energy, easy fatigability, unexplained normochromic normocytic anemia, fluid excess, hypertension, and nocturia. Itching, nausea, vomiting, and disturbance of the senses of smell and taste appear late in the course of the disease. With careful management and early institution of dialysis, complications such as severe acidosis, uremic frost, pericarditis, uremic lungs, and various neurologic manifestations, formerly typical in the uremic patient, are rare.

The exact pathogenesis of uremic manifestations is not known, but they are probably caused by retained metabolic products. Deficiency of erythropoietin contributes to anemia, and deficiency of active vitamin D to renal osteodystrophy. Hyperparathyroidism is quite common and has been suggested to play a pathogenic role in certain uremic manifestations.

TREATMENT

Specific management of CRF depends on symptoms and the degree of physiologic derangement that the patient displays at various stages in the course of the disease (see Table 1). However, certain general principles of management can be applied to all patients with CRF.

General Considerations

Reversible Factors

In chronically diseased kidneys, renal function can be further compromised by several potentially reversible factors. Thus it is imperative, as the first step, to identify these factors.

Hypoperfusion. Kidneys may be underperfused as a result of extracellular fluid (ECF) depletion secondary to overzealous use of diuretics or because of heart failure. Hypoperfusion causes a decline in GFR and increased tubular reabsorption of glomerular filtrate along with urea. Thus, renal function deteriorates suddenly with a disproportionate increase in BUN relative to increase in serum creatinine. Presence of orthostatic changes in blood pressure (BP) and heart rate, signs of congestive failure, an increased ratio of BUN to creatinine ($>3:1$), and decreased urinary sodium (fractional excretion of sodium <1 per cent) are helpful in identifying hypoperfusion. For ECF depletion, the discontinuation of diuretic alone may be sufficient to improve renal perfusion. In severe cases, however, liberalization of salt intake or even careful intravenous infusion of half normal saline may be required. Treatment of congestive cardiac failure, if present, also may improve renal function.

Urinary Tract Obstruction. Obstruction of any type at any site along the urinary tract may further aggravate renal failure. Sonography is a good noninvasive technique to rule out significant obstructions, although this may not be helpful in the occasional case of partial obstruction. If possible, contrast studies should be avoided because of the nephrotoxicity of contrast medium.

Nephrotoxins. The three most common nephrotoxins associated with worsening of renal function are nonsteroidal anti-inflammatory drugs (NSAIDs), aminoglycosides, and contrast media. Deterioration of renal function with these agents is usually reversible if recognized early. Nephrotoxicity associated with NSAID is more often encountered if other risk factors are present. These factors include already impaired renal function, nephrotic syndrome, advanced age of the patient, and severe heart disease. Some NSAIDs, such as clinoril (Sulindac), are reported to be less nephrotoxic than others; however, cau-

TABLE 1. **Manifestations and Plan for Management of Renal Failure**

Creatinine Clearance (ml/min)	Serum Creatinine (mg/dl)	Manifestations	Management
>50	1.5–2.4	Manifestations of primary renal disease	Work-up and treat primary disease; control HTN*; ?Diet
30–50	1.5–3.0	Anemia, HTN, tiredness	Work-up and treat anemia; control HTN, reversible causes; drug precautions; ?Diet
10–29	3.0–10.0	HTN, $\uparrow PO_4$, $\downarrow Ca$, acidosis, uremia	Control HTN; PO_4 Binders, Ca, vitamin D; Diet, consultation
<10	>8	Uremia (pericarditis, neuropathy, bleeding, diathesis, seizures)	Dialysis and/or transplant

*HTN = Hypertension.

tion should be used in high-risk patients with all medications of this class.

Worsening of renal function has been reported following excretory urography, angiography, cholecystography, and computed tomography. Contrast media are particularly risky in patients with Bence-Jones nephropathy or diabetic nephropathy. If contrast medium has to be used in patients with CRF, then use of the minimal dose possible, of volume expansion, and of mannitol (12.5 to 25 grams) before and after the procedure will maintain good urine flow and reduce the risk of nephrotoxicity.

Certain drugs, such as diuretics, sulfa, and allopurinol, cause interstitial nephritis, and this possibility should be considered. High-risk drugs should be avoided; if use cannot be avoided, the dosage should always be adjusted for the reduced renal function.

Infection. Uncomplicated urinary tract infection (UTI) usually does not cause significant reduction in renal function. However, complicated UTI may cause severe renal damage and worsening of renal function. Recognition of UTI, correction of the underlying cause, and aggressive yet judicious treatment of UTI is important for the preservation of renal function. Until the infecting organism is recognized, a broad-spectrum penicillin or cephalosporin can be used.

Other Reversible Factors. Hypercalcemia (serum calcium >12 mg per dl) may worsen renal function. Sudden deterioration of renal function in a nephrotic patient, particularly in the presence of thromboembolic phenomena, may be caused by renal vein thrombosis. If diagnosis is confirmed by radiologic studies, anticoagulation is indicated. Pregnancy in patients with CRF may result in further deterioration of renal function. Patients with already compromised renal function should be warned about this possibility. If pregnancy occurs, renal function should be carefully monitored and blood pressure controlled to prevent worsening of renal function.

Control of Hypertension

More than 80 per cent of patients with a GFR below 30 ml per minute have elevated blood pressure. Control of hypertension is the most important factor influencing the rate of progression of renal failure. Good control of blood pressure reduces the rate at which renal function deteriorates. This effect is well documented in patients with diabetic nephropathy. Initially, good control of blood pressure may be associated with a transient decline in renal function. Despite the possibility of transient worsening of renal function, blood pressure should always be controlled, since the hazards of uncontrolled hypertension exceed those of worsening of renal function. Apart from influencing the rate of progression of renal failure, uncontrolled hypertension also has been shown to be the single most important factor causing accelerated atherosclerosis, thus influencing survival of these patients both before and after starting dialysis. Control of hypertension, therefore, should receive major emphasis in the patient's overall treatment regimen.

Most hypertensive patients with CRF have ECF excess; consequently, control of salt intake and the use of diuretics are usually the first step in the treatment of hypertension. If GFR is <30 ml per minute, milder diuretics such as the thiazides are generally not effective, and loop diuretics such as furosemide (Lasix) must be used. Potassium-sparing diuretics and potassium supplements are usually contraindicated because of the risk of hyperkalemia. If diuretics alone are not effective, then any of the following can be added: vasodilators such as hydralazine (Apresoline), calcium channel blockers such as nifedipine (Procardia), or beta-blockers such as metoprolol (Lopressor). Drugs that are metabolized by the kidney, such as atenolol (Tenormin), and pindolol (Visken), may accumulate in renal failure and should be used with caution and the dose should be adjusted accordingly.

Recently, the angiotensin-converting enzyme (ACE) inhibitors such as enalapril (Vasotec) have been proposed to slow the rate of progression of renal failure, particularly in patients with diabetic nephropathy. These drugs are supposed to reduce the intraglomerular pressure, thereby slowing the progression of glomerulosclerosis. More work is needed to further define the role of these drugs in CRF. If they are used, renal function, proteinuria, and bone marrow function should be carefully monitored to detect drug toxicity.

Diet

Protein. In the past, protein restriction had been shown to ameliorate uremic symptoms. In recent years, with the wide use of dialysis and due to the potential of protein malnutrition, severe protein restriction became controversial. This controversy has recently taken a new form. In animal work and a few human studies, moderate protein restriction has been shown to slow the progression of renal failure (as judged by 1/creatinine values). In chronic renal disease individual glomeruli are thought to be hyperfiltering; persistent hyperfiltration is associated with progressive sclerosis of the glomeruli. A low-protein diet is thought to reduce glomerular hyperfiltration, thereby slowing the progression of glomerulosclerosis. Additional studies are needed to validate this hypothesis and also to determine whether the protein restriction is safe and does not cause malnutrition or tissue loss and whether patients are compliant with the restricted diet. Studies addressing these issues are presently being conducted.

Supporters of protein restriction argue that if the proper protocol is carefully followed, negative nitrogen balance does not occur. The protocol suggests 0.6 gram per kilogram of protein, of which 75 per cent should be of high biologic value, with daily caloric intake of 30 to 35 kilocalories per kg. If protein is restricted, these patients should be carefully followed with anthropometric measurements, creatinine and urea generation rates, total plasma protein, and transferrin and C_3 levels to detect protein malnutrition.

Additional Dietary Modifications. With advancing renal failure (GFR <20), more stringent dietary restrictions may have to be applied. If ECF excess is present, sodium should be restricted to about 60 mEq per day; if the serum potassium rises, then the daily allowance should not exceed 60 mEq. Hyperphosphatemia is usually treated by restricting dairy product intake and using phosphate (PO_4) binders. Most patients maintain good water balance with a daily allowance of total water limited to between 1000 and 2000 ml.

Calcium Phosphate Metabolism and Renal Osteodystrophy

As shown in Figure 1, there are four major defects in bone metabolism: (1) renal retention of phosphorus and hyperphosphatemia, which causes a reduction in serum calcium and also reduces the synthesis of 1,25-dihydroxy-D_3 (1,25[OH]$_2$-D_3) in the kidney; (2) loss of renal parenchyma, where vitamin D is converted to 1,25(OH)$_2$-D_3, the most active form. With loss of renal parenchyma, the synthesis of 1,25(OH)$_2$-D_3 is reduced. Dihydroxy-vitamin D_3 has several effects: it enhances gut absorption of calcium and bone mineral resorption and inhibits parathyroid hormone. These effects are impaired when renal failure occurs. (3) As patients become anorectic, reduced calcium intake may result in more profound hypocalcemia. (4) Because of hypocalcemia the parathyroid hormone (PTH) is stimulated and hyperparathyroidism occurs. However, in uremia bones are relatively resistant to PTH and serum calcium does not increase proportionally. Thus, in CRF there is hyperphosphatemia, relative hypocalcemia, and hyperparathyroidism (elevated alkaline phosphatase and n terminal PTH activity).

As the GFR declines to less than 30, serum PO_4 increases, and serum calcium may decline. If calcium and PO_4 product are higher than 55,

there is risk of soft tissue calcification. Therefore, PO_4 concentration should first be lowered (below 6 mg per dl) before calcium supplements are used. Hyperphosphatemia is controlled by restricting intake of dairy products and aluminum hydroxide (Al[OH]$_3$) administration, which binds PO_4 in the gut and prevents its absorption. In severe cases dialysis may be needed to reduce PO_4 concentration. With use of Al(OH)$_3$ over several years, there is some indication that aluminum absorption may lead to aluminum intoxication. Unfortunately, ingestion of magnesium-containing antacids may result in magnesium accumulation; thus, their use has been limited. Recently $CaCO_3$ has been used as a PO_4 binder in dialysis patients, but its value and possible risk factors need to be more clearly established. About 1 to 2 grams of $CaCO_3$ daily in divided doses with each meal can be used. Serum Ca and PO_4 should be closely monitored. If PO_4 is uncontrolled or if Ca starts increasing, then Al(OH)$_3$ should be used. Chronic use of Al(OH)$_3$ requires monitoring of aluminum levels.

Metabolic Acidosis

With severe renal failure, the usual daily excretion of 60 to 80 mEq of H^+ is impaired. This results in positive H^+ balance and metabolic acidosis. Associated with this is the kidney's inability to excrete unmeasured anions such as HPO_4, resulting in accumulation of these anions and increase in the anion gap. The second type of metabolic acidosis, seen with even milder renal failure, is a tubular defect contributing to acidosis; hence it is called renal tubular acidosis (RTA). RTA is associated with normal anion gap.

Usually, acidosis is well tolerated unless the serum bicarbonate (HCO_3) drops below 15 mEq per liter. Although chronic acidosis would be expected to worsen osteodystrophy by the consumption of bone buffers, there is little evidence to support this. If it is decided to treat the acidosis, however, 20 to 40 mEq of $NaHCO_3$ or sodium citrate (Shohl's solution) a day is needed to combat acidosis. In the presence of hypertension or ECF excess these sodium salts should be used with caution. With the use of citrate solution two points should be considered: (1) To avoid hyperkalemia, only Na citrate (not Na-K citrate) should be used; (2) there is some evidence that if citrate is used with Al(OH)$_3$, it results in excessive absorption of aluminum and risk of aluminum intoxication. Consequently, citrate and aluminum should not be administered together.

Anemia, Hyperkalemia, and Hyperuricemia

Anemia is quite common with advanced renal failure and usually is multifactorial in origin.

CHRONIC RENAL FAILURE

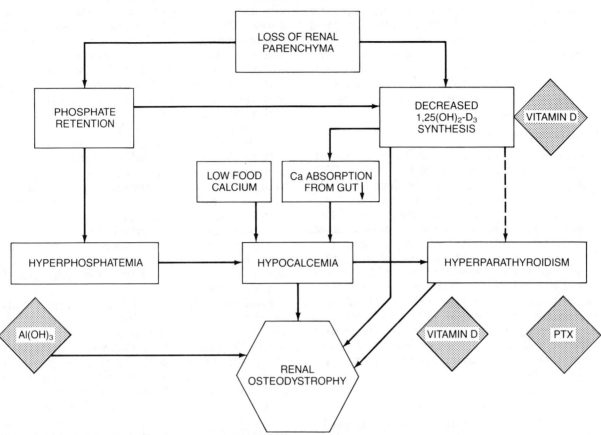

Figure 1. Calcium and phosphate metabolism and renal osteodystrophy in patients with chronic renal failure. Shaded squares indicate treatment; PTX = parathyroidectomy. Vitamin D = Calcitriol (Rocaltrol), 0.25 micrograms per day.

Reduced synthesis of erythropoietin by the diseased kidney is probably the most important contributing factor. However, other treatable causes of anemia, such as nutritional deficiency and excessive blood loss, should be ruled out. Although no specific therapy is currently available, recombinant human erythropoietin has been recently tried successfully in dialysis patients and may soon be available for clinical use.

Tubules have remarkable capacity to secrete potassium; thus, hyperkalemia is uncommon until the terminal stage of renal failure. An exception are patients with type IV RTA who have an impaired capacity to handle potassium and can easily develop life-threatening hyperkalemia. Dietary potassium restriction and avoiding potassium-sparing diuretics, potassium salts, and drugs usually reduces the risk of hyperkalemia. Hyperuricemia is common in CRF; however, uric acid values under 11 mg per dl generally do not cause any problems. Allopurinol (Zyloprim) is used for patients with gout or a uric acid level of >11 mg per dl, with the dose being adjusted according to the severity of renal failure.

Drug Dosage

Four general principles should be remembered whenever patients with CRF are prescribed medicine: (1) *Metabolism:* If a drug and its active metabolites are eliminated by the kidney, the dose should be adjusted. (2) *Nephrotoxicity:* Certain drugs such as NSAIDs (see earlier section) have the potential to produce further renal damage and should either be avoided or used with caution. (3) *Hyperkalemia:* Drugs such as potassium-sparing diuretics and salt substitutes can cause life-threatening hyperkalemia. (4) *Side effects:* Certain side effects of drugs may be more common in the presence of renal failure and should be monitored (e.g., peripheral neuropathy from nitrofurantoins, digoxin toxicity, and toxicity of aminoglycosides).

Vascular Access

Preservation of arm veins for the later creation of vascular access for hemodialysis is one of the most important considerations in the management of CRF patients. Unfortunately, this is often ignored and causes tremendous problems later on. Forearm veins in these patients should not be used for infusions, transfusions, and diagnostic venipunctures. If possible, veins in the wrist and leg or central veins should be used. Two to four months before dialysis is to start, an arteriovenous fistula should be created. This gives sufficient time for the fistula vein to develop. Only a surgeon with extensive experience in angioaccess should do the surgery.

Psychosocial Aspects

Very few diseases cause as drastic an adjustment in almost all aspects of life as does CRF. The patient, spouse, and family should be given details of the various aspects of the disease and its management in simple and clear terms. These discussions should be carried out in a relaxed, sympathetic, and nonthreatening fashion. It is best to see the patient and family frequently, with continued discussions in a frank and friendly atmosphere. Younger patients take longer to adjust to necessary changes in lifestyle and need more support and time to comprehend. At an appropriate time, exposure to other well-adjusted and well-informed patients is often very helpful. Group therapy and counseling may also be beneficial.

Specific Therapy

Generally, when definitive therapy is needed for uremic symptoms, fluid overload, hyperkalemia, or severe acidosis, the BUN is above 100 and creatinine is more than 6 to 8 mg per dl. In patients with diabetic nephropathy, dialysis is usually required earlier. Once a patient has reached the terminal renal failure stage, three choices are available. These are (1) dialysis, (2) transplantation, or (3) protein restriction and palliative treatment. It is important to have an ongoing discussion about these alternatives, including various considerations involved with the dialysis and transplant options, well before the end-stage is reached. The third choice of limiting therapy to diet restrictions is the most difficult for family and physician to accept, since it means accepting the eventual death of the patient. However, if the patient is terminally ill with other incurable conditions and makes a well-informed decision not to receive dialysis, such a decision should be honored.

Dialysis

In broad terms, two types of dialysis therapy are available: hemodialysis and peritoneal dialysis.

Hemodialysis. During hemodialysis, blood is passed through a cartridge (dialyzer) where it is separated from a rinsing fluid (dialysate) by a semipermeable membrane. The procedure usually lasts about 4 hours and is repeated 3 times a week. Predialysis BUN and creatinine concentrations generally are in the range of 80 to 100 and 8 to 14 mg per dl, respectively. ECF is controlled by ultrafiltration of plasma across the dialyzer membrane. Patients can either dialyze at outpatient dialysis units or can be trained to dialyze at home. Home dialysis is less expensive and allows a more normal lifestyle for the patient, and these patients are generally healthier.

With dialysis, control of hypertension is easier, and uremic symptoms (such as vomiting and neuropathy) improve. However, other problems such as osteodystrophy, anemia, cardiovascular disease, and sexual problems persist and require continued attention. Survival of dialysis patients has improved over the last decade. The leading cause of death is cardiovascular disease. Control of hypertension and cessation of smoking greatly improve survival.

Peritoneal Dialysis. Intermittent cycling of dialysate into and out of the peritoneal cavity through an implanted catheter is called peritoneal dialysis. The procedure commonly involves infusion of 2 liters of sterile dialysate into the peritoneal cavity from a plastic bag, and draining it out after about 6 hours. The cycle is repeated 4 times throughout a 24-hour period, and the procedure is called continuous ambulatory peritoneal dialysis (CAPD). CAPD has to be performed around the clock every day. An alternative is the use of an automated system ("cycler") to cycle 2 liters of fluid every 2 to 3 hours at night while the patient is sleeping. Sometimes, with this technique, 2 liters of fluid are left in the peritoneal cavity during the day; this process is called continuous cycling peritoneal dialysis (CCPD). Peritonitis is a major problem with both CAPD and CCPD. Peritoneal dialysis provides less overall clearance of solutes than does hemodialysis. Thus, for patients with a large dialysis requirement (e.g., a large man with zero GFR) it may be inadequate to maintain well-being. Overall dropout rate of patients on CAPD or CCPD is much higher than for patients on hemodialysis.

Transplantation

A successful transplant provides a better quality of life than is seen with either peritoneal dialysis or hemodialysis. However, the limited availability of cadaveric kidneys and the surgical risk, side effects of immunosuppression, bone disease, and rejection of transplanted kidneys are major problems with this alternative to dialysis. Transplants from a living related donor and cadaveric transplants have both been carried out successfully. Rejection episodes and immunosuppression-related problems are less common with a matched, related-donor transplant than with cadaveric transplants. With new immunosuppressive agents (e.g., cyclosporine) the future of renal transplantation may be better than in the last 20 years.

Summary

The three modes of specific therapies should be viewed by the practitioner as mutually complementary measures to be used according to patient preference and needs. It is common for the patient to start on dialysis therapy and then receive a transplant when circumstances are right. If rejection of the renal graft occurs, peritoneal dialysis or hemodialysis is again employed. Because of the developments over the last two decades, physicians can now offer several alternatives to death for patients with CRF.

GENITOURINARY TUBERCULOSIS

method of
ARNOLD C. CINMAN, M.D.
University of California School of Medicine
Los Angeles, California

The introduction of effective chemotherapeutic agents has dramatically reduced the incidence of pulmonary tuberculosis. However, the occurrence of genitourinary (GU) tuberculosis has not paralleled this decline. This may be due to the long latent period preceding the appearance of tuberculosis in extrapulmonary sites; moreover, in Western Europe and the United States it may be due to the massive influx of people from developing countries where the incidence of tuberculosis is higher.

Treatment

The primary therapy for genitourinary tuberculosis is medical. Surgical intervention is reserved for the treatment of complications or for the correction of postchemotherapeutic sequelae. The principles of chemotherapy include the simultaneous use of multiple antituberculous drugs, prolonged therapy, regular follow-up, and diligent monitoring to ensure adequate disease control, drug compliance, and early return to a normal lifestyle. Ideally, the drugs should be bactericidal, taken orally, free of serious side effects, and reasonably inexpensive. Except for preventive treatment of persons in contact with patients recently diagnosed as having tuberculosis and with recent tuberculin skin converters, the use of single-drug treatment is condemned, since it rapidly causes the development of resistant organisms. Adult converters should be closely monitored, and chest radiographs should be obtained every 3 to 6 months. Child converters should be treated with isoniazid (INH), 10 to 15 mg per kg body weight, in two divided daily doses for 1 year.

Commitment to a sanitarium or isolation is unnecessary for renal tuberculosis. However, proper precautions should be taken when disposing of urine. Ideally, a male patient with positive urine cultures should use his own toilet and avoid any urinary spillage. Men are instructed to void in the sitting position. A nourishing diet, adequate rest and minimal, nonfatiguing activity represent integral parts of the general management of patients with urinary tuberculosis.

Chemotherapy

Treatment is not commenced until the diagnosis is firmly established. Although short-term therapy of 6 to 9 months is recommended in treating pulmonary tuberculosis, it has been customary to treat patients with genitourinary tuberculosis for 2 years. For the first 8 to 12 weeks triple-drug therapy, namely isoniazid (INH), rifampin (RMP), and ethambutol (ETB), is used. A double-drug regimen is then instituted for the remaining treatment period based on the results of sensitivity testing. The recommended regimen consists of isoniazid, 300 mg; rifampin, 600 mg; and ethambutol, 15 mg per kg body weight in a single daily oral dose. The most effective double-drug therapy to be continued for 2 years is isoniazid, 300 mg, and rifampin, 600 mg, in single daily doses. Substitution of ethambutol for rifampin, 1000 to 1200 mg in a single daily dose, in conjunction with isoniazid is effective but is not as desirable because ethambutol is bacteriostatic and has a higher incidence of side effects. To prevent isoniazid-induced polyneuritis, 100 mg of pyridoxine (vitamin B_6) is given as a daily supplement.

In children the recommended regimen is isoniazid, 10 mg per kg (up to 300 mg), and rifampin, 10 to 20 mg per kg, not to exceed 600 mg per day in single or divided doses. Ethambutol is not recommended for children younger than 13 years of age.

No incidence of relapse has been observed with the above treatment regimens. In most instances urine cultures become negative within 1 month after initiation of treatment, which is a positive indication of the effectiveness of therapy. Patients are followed with urine cultures at 1 month, 3 months, and every 6 months thereafter for the first 2 years. If the culture taken at 1 month is negative, the 3-month study is not performed. A final culture is obtained 1 year after cessation of treatment. An intravenous pyelogram or nuclear renogram is obtained twice a year for the first 3 years. Periodic follow-up once a year and radiographic studies once every 2 to 3 years are necessary to ascertain the long-term arrest of the disease.

More recent data suggest that double-drug therapy using two bactericidal drugs, namely isoniazid and rifampin, for 6 to 9 months is as effective as the previously recommended regimen (Table 1). The rationale for using a triple-drug regimen for the first 8 to 12 weeks is that ethambutol is a bacteriostatic drug (affects both intra- and extracellular organisms) and therefore, at least on theoretical grounds, inhibits development of resistant mutants.

Other antituberculous agents are available, although they are used to a lesser extent and are defined as second- and third-line drugs.

First-Line Drugs

ISONIAZID. Isoniazid (INH) is the least toxic of currently used antituberculous drugs and is bactericidal to both intra- and extracellular organisms. Peripheral neuropathy occurs more often in malnourished patients and is largely prevented by the administration of 100 mg of pyridoxine daily. Hypersensitivity reactions such as fever, skin eruptions, lymphadenopathy, vasculitis, and occasionally fatal hepatitis are rarely encountered. Central nervous system reactions, including seizures, toxic encephalopathy, and psychosis, have been reported. Caffeine and amphetamine derivatives, both CNS stimulants, must be avoided while taking isoniazid. The usual oral dosage is 5 mg per kg per day for adults (up to 300 mg) and 10 to 15 mg per kg per day for infants and children (up to 300 mg per day).

RIFAMPIN. Rifampin (RMP; Rifadin, Rimactane) inhibits DNA-dependent RNA polymerase activity and is a bactericidal drug. Because it occasionally causes liver dysfunction, concomitant administration of hepatotoxic agents must be avoided. It crosses the placental barrier, and therefore neonates of rifampin-treated mothers should be carefully observed. While undergoing treatment with RMP, patients should be given liver function tests every 4 to 6 months. Renal impairment is not a contraindication, since the drug is excreted by the liver. It causes orange-colored urine. The usual dosage is 600 mg per day for adults and 10 to 20 mg per kg per day for children, not to exceed 600 mg per day.

ETHAMBUTOL. Ethambutol (ETB; Myambutol) is a bacteriostatic drug affecting intra- as well as extracellular organisms. It induces reversible optic neuritis, although this is rarely encountered with doses of 15 mg per kg daily. Patients should therefore be tested for visual acuity and red-green color discrimination prior to commencing therapy and every 3 months thereafter, unless visual acuity diminishes in the interim. If this happens, an ophthalmologic examination should be carried out immediately, and the drug should be temporarily discontinued. Skin rashes may also occur. The usual daily dose is 15 to 25 mg per kg. In patients with reduced renal function, the dosage should be smaller because the drug is excreted mainly by the kidneys.

Second-Line Drugs

These drugs are always used in combination with first-line drugs and are only used when treatment failure occurs with primary drugs or when retreatment is required. Although these drugs are effective, their side effects are greater than those encountered with first-line drugs.

STREPTOMYCIN. Streptomycin is bacteriostatic to extracellular organisms but causes eighth nerve toxicity, with auditory and vestibular impairment. It should be used cautiously in older patients or in those with renal impairment be-

TABLE 1. **First-Line Drugs in Short-Course Chemotherapy of Tuberculosis**

Drug	Dosage		Activity
	Daily	*Twice Weekly*	
Bactericidal Drugs			
Isoniazid	5–10 mg/kg, usually 300 mg orally	15 mg/kg, usually 900 mg	Active in both extracellular and intracellular bacilli
Rifampin	10 mg/kg, usually 450–600 mg orally	10 mg/kg, usually 450–600 mg	As above, particularly on closed lesion "persistors"
Streptomycin	15–25 mg/kg, 5 days/week intramuscularly	25–30 mg/kg	Active in neutral or slightly alkaline pH against extracellular bacilli in cavities
Pyrazinamide*	30–35 mg/kg, usually 1.5–2 grams orally	50–60 mg/kg, usually 1.5–2 grams	Active in acid pH medium on intracellular bacilli
Capreomycin*	0.75–1 gram, 5 days/week intramuscularly	1.5 gram	Same as streptomycin
Bacteriostatic Drug			
Ethambutol†	15–25 mg/kg, usually 1200–1600 mg orally	50 mg/kg	Acts both on intracellular and extracellular bacilli to inhibit development of resistant mutants

*Safety and efficacy of these drugs in children have not been established.
†Not recommended for children under 13 years of age.

cause of its nephrotoxicity. Vestibular function studies and audiograms in conjunction with BUN and serum creatinine should be obtained prior to treatment. Patients should be carefully monitored during treatment. The peak serum concentration should not exceed 20 to 25 micrograms per ml in persons with decreased renal function. During initial treatment, streptomycin is given intramuscularly in doses of 15 to 25 mg per kg (up to 1 gram) on a daily basis. After 6 to 8 weeks, a twice-weekly regimen is instituted using doses of 25 to 30 mg per kg.

PYRAZINAMIDE. Pyrazinamide is the synthetic analogue of nicotinamide and is bacteriostatic to intracellular organisms. Hepatotoxicity is the most common serious side effect. It may induce hyperuricemia because it inhibits excretion of urate, and acute episodes of gout have been described in patients taking the drug. Elevation of plasma glutamic-oxaloacetic acid as well as glutamic pyruvic transaminase is the earliest abnormality induced by the drug. Close monitoring of serum glutamic-oxaloacetic transaminase (SGOT), serum glutamic-pyruvic transaminase (SGPT), and serum uric acid is mandatory during its administration. The usual dosage is 15 to 30 mg per kg, up to 2 grams, given orally in three to four divided doses. When administered on a twice-weekly basis, the dosage is 50 to 70 mg per kg.

CYCLOSERINE. Cycloserine* (Seromycin) is a broad-spectrum antibiotic that is bacteriostatic to both intra- and extracellular organisms. Its untoward effects commonly involve the central nervous system; psychotic states, paranoid reactions, personality changes, and convulsions have been described. Alcohol use during the administration of the drug aggravates the psychiatric problems. The usual dosage is 10 to 20 mg per kg or 250 mg orally twice a day. At this dosage the risk of adverse reactions is small. In order to minimize toxicity, plasma levels should not exceed 30 micrograms per ml. Side effects may be prevented with 100 mg of pyridoxine given daily.

Third-Line Drugs. These drugs are less commonly used and include the following.

CAPREOMYCIN. Capreomycin† (Capastat) is bactericidal to extracellular organisms in cavities. It is nephrotoxic and causes eighth nerve damage. Vestibular function studies, audiograms, and BUN and serum creatinine should be obtained at frequent intervals during drug administration. The usual daily dose is 15 to 30 mg per kg intramuscularly up to 1 gram. The drug should be used cautiously in older patients, and its use should be avoided in those with decreased renal function.

KANAMYCIN. Kanamycin (Kantrex) is bactericidal to extracellular organisms. Side effects and dosage are the same as those for capreomycin.

ETHIONAMIDE. Ethionamide (Trecator-SC) is bacteriostatic to both intracellular and extracellular organisms. It induces gastrointestinal disturbances and is hepatotoxic, thus requiring close monitoring of SGOT and SGPT. It has a metallic taste. Divided doses may minimize gastrointestinal side effects. Use of the drug should be avoided during pregnancy. The usual dosage is 15 to 30 mg per kg up to 1 gram daily.

PARA-AMINOSALICYLIC ACID. Para-aminosalicylic acid (PAS) is bacteriostatic to extracellular organisms only. The importance of this drug in the management of tuberculosis has decreased markedly since more active agents have been developed. It induces irritation of the gastrointestinal tract and, at times, severe diarrhea. Patients with peptic ulcers tolerate the drug poorly. Hypersensitivity reactions are common. Because it may cause hepatic damage of varying degrees, SGOT and SGPT levels should be monitored. This drug may induce acidosis, especially in children, because it is a relatively strong organic acid. When the sodium salt is used, excessive sodium loading may result. The usual dose is 150 mg per kg up to 12 grams daily in three or four divided doses.

Several general principles should be followed in the chemotherapeutic management of genitourinary tuberculosis: (1) selection of drug regimen should be based on susceptibility testing, (2) the regimen should contain two bactericidal drugs, and (3) the concomitant use of drugs with the same type of side effects should be avoided whenever possible.

Hypoadrenalism (Addison's syndrome) caused by tuberculosis is rare today but should be looked for and treated appropriately.

Surgical Therapy

Whereas surgical management of GU tuberculosis was widely used in the 1950s and 1960s, today operative therapy has become the exception rather than the rule. The indications for surgical intervention in genitourinary tuberculosis are (1) obstruction, (2) destruction, and (3) reconstruction. Occasionally, diagnostic surgery may be indicated to confirm the presence of tuberculosis prior to instituting chemotherapy. Tuberculotic patients should be on antitubercular chemotherapy for at least 3 weeks prior to undergoing surgery.

---

*Safety and dosage of this drug have not been established for pediatric use.

†Safety and efficacy of this drug in children have not been established.

Obstruction. The most common sites of urinary tract obstruction in tuberculosis occur in areas of anatomic narrowing. The process may be silent, causing unrecognized loss of a kidney, and may be accelerated during the healing phase, while the patient is on chemotherapy. Partial nephrectomy or cavernotomy may be necessary to treat intrarenal obstruction, whereas strictures at the ureteropelvic junction are amenable to standard pyeloplasty techniques. Ureteric strictures have been successfully treated with transcystoscopic dilations, with or without steroids. Transluminal balloon dilation of ureteric strictures has been reported and can be performed via a percutaneous nephrostomy if difficulty is encountered with ureteric instrumentation. Internal double-J stents are of great value in keeping ureteric strictures patent. Surgical resection followed by ureteroureterostomy, ureteroneocystostomy, or ileal interposition is reserved for the management of cases that cannot be managed with the preceding more simple treatments.

Destruction. A unilateral nonfunctioning kidney, especially associated with calcification, pain, hematuria or hypertension, should be removed after adequate antituberculotic coverage. The poorly vascularized kidney may be a reservoir for viable mycobacteria, which may reactivate the disease when the patient's immunity is weakened as the result of old age or debilitating diseases. Epididymectomy is performed only rarely in patients with enlarged, fistulizing lesions or for diagnostic purposes in the differential diagnosis of an intrascrotal mass lesion.

Reconstruction. Augmentation enterocystoplasty or ileocecocystoplasty is advised for managing the contracted bladder of "burnt-out" tuberculosis. The bowel-to-bladder anastomosis should be made as wide as possible to prevent the development of stenosis. Vasovasostomies or vasoepididymostomies may be the only method of restoring fertility to males with tuberculotic vasal strictures.

MALIGNANT TUMORS OF THE UROGENITAL TRACT

method of
JOSEPH A. SMITH, JR., M.D.
University of Utah School of Medicine
Salt Lake City, Utah

PROSTATE CARCINOMA

Adenocarcinoma of the prostate is the most common cancer in men in the United States and the second leading cause of death from cancer. The disease is uncommon in men under age 50 and increases in incidence with advancing age. Autopsy studies show that the pathologic incidence of the disease greatly exceeds the rate of clinical recognition. Thus, the disease remains clinically occult in the majority of patients while developing into a cause of considerable morbidity or death in others. The inability to predict this course with accuracy in an individual patient contributes to the controversy and dilemma regarding treatment of prostatic cancer.

Detection and Diagnosis

Early stage prostatic cancer is asymptomatic. Bladder outlet obstruction, hematuria, perineal pain, or ureteral obstruction appear with locally advanced disease. Metastatic carcinoma of the prostate usually presents as bone pain, although weakness, weight loss, and anorexia may also be observed.

Digital palpation of the prostate is the most common method for detection of prostatic cancer. Induration, nodularity, or asymmetry of the prostate should be considered with a high index of suspicion for carcinoma. Although digital rectal examination is a relatively insensitive method for detection of prostatic cancer, it remains the most accepted method for screening and detection of early stage disease.

Transrectal ultrasonography for screening and early detection of prostatic cancer has received a great deal of attention and has been the subject of much discussion. Well-designed studies testing the ability of ultrasonography to detect early prostatic cancer have not been conducted. Currently, it seems likely that transrectal ultrasonography alone will not have a sensitivity or specificity that makes it useful as a screening method for prostatic cancer. The procedure does appear to be of some value for staging local extent of disease, although its superiority over rectal examination has not been demonstrated definitively.

A core needle biopsy of the prostate remains the most common method for obtaining tissue for histologic documentation of disease. Increasingly, transrectal aspiration biopsies of the prostate are being performed. In experienced hands, this technique has a sensitivity at least equal to that of core needle biopsy but with reduced morbidity.

A radioisotope bone scan should be obtained in all patients with prostatic cancer to rule out metastatic disease to bone. An elevation in serum prostatic acid phosphatase usually indicates systemic disease. Prostate-specific antigen has proved to be more sensitive than prostatic acid phosphatase and is a more reliable indicator of disease response or progression. Prostate-specific antigen is elevated in over 95 per cent of men with prostatic cancer metastatic to bone, while prostatic acid phosphatase is elevated in 75 to 80 per cent.

Treatment

The appropriate treatment of patients with carcinoma of the prostate, especially in early stages, remains a subject of great controversy. In part, this is due to the variable natural history of the disease and the inability to predict reliably the prognosis for an individual patient. The treatment options relate directly to the stage of disease at the time of diagnosis.

Stage A

The category of stage A includes patients found to have histologic evidence of adenocarcinoma in prostate tissue removed for symptoms of presumed benign prostatic hyperplasia (BPH). Accordingly, the disease by definition occurs in men in whom there is no palpable abnormality of the prostate. Approximately 10 per cent of men undergoing prostatectomy for presumed BPH are found to have carcinoma in the specimen. Stage A carcinoma has been subdivided into A1 and A2 disease. The disease is considered A1 when less than 5 per cent of the specimen contains carcinoma or, alternatively, when fewer than 5 foci of disease are identified. Additionally, all high-grade carcinomas are considered to be stage A2.

Most often, a diagnosis of stage A1 prostatic cancer implies that the patient is unlikely to develop clinically significant disease, and no treatment is indicated. With long-term follow-up, some 15 per cent of patients with stage A1 disease may develop progression of carcinoma. Treatment may be indicated in a small subset of young patients who will be at risk for disease recurrence for a prolonged time.

Nearly one third of patients with stage A2 carcinoma of the prostate have metastatic disease to the pelvic lymph nodes at the time of diagnosis. For patients with negative nodes, treatment by radical prostatectomy or external irradiation is indicated if the patient otherwise has a life expectancy of more than 10 years.

Stage B

Stage B prostatic cancer consists of a nodule or an area of induration that is palpably confined within the capsule of the prostate. Approximately 30 per cent of patients with prostatic cancer are found to have stage B disease at the time of diagnosis.

Radical prostatectomy is the most commonly performed treatment for stage B prostatic cancer in most centers. In patients with histologically negative lymph nodes and disease confined to the prostate, 10-year survival rates after radical prostatectomy approximate those for a healthy age-matched population. Urinary incontinence occurs in less than 5 per cent of patients after radical prostatectomy. Modifications in technique allow the surgeon to preserve the neurovascular bundle, which is responsible for potency. In the hands of most surgeons, approximately 50 per cent of patients retain erectile potency after radical prostatectomy.

Excellent long-term survival rates have also been achieved with external irradiation for stage B prostatic cancer. A high incidence of positive biopsies after external irradiation has been documented but the impact of this upon ultimate survival is uncertain.

Stage C

Stage C disease occurs when there is palpable extracapsular extension of tumor. These patients generally are not considered candidates for radical prostatectomy. Over 50 per cent of patients with stage C disease are found to have histologic lymph node metastasis. For patients with negative pelvic lymph nodes, external irradiation is the treatment of choice. There is an apparent favorable impact of treatment by external irradiation in these patients, although most patients eventually experience disease progression.

Stage D

After the pelvic lymph nodes, the most common site of metastatic prostate cancer is bone. Over one third of patients with prostatic cancer are found to have metastatic disease at the time of diagnosis. Hormonal therapy remains the most effective initial treatment for patients with metastatic carcinoma of the prostate. Approximately 80 per cent of patients experience disease remission with a median duration of 18 months. There is no evidence that any method of treatment that adequately deprives the cancer cell of testicular sources of androgen is superior to others. Furthermore, although the concept of total androgen suppression of both testicular and adrenal sources of androgens has received a great deal of attention in the lay press, large randomized studies have shown no clinical benefit with this form of therapy over treatment methods that suppress testicular testosterone alone.

Orchiectomy is a simple and safe surgical procedure that can be performed under local anesthesia. Circulating levels of serum testosterone are suppressed to the castrate range (less than

50 ng per dl) within 12 hours. Oral diethylstilbestrol (DES) is an effective alternative to orchiectomy. However, DES at dose levels that reliably suppress testosterone (3 mg per day) has been associated with major cardiovascular or thromboembolic morbidity in up to 20 per cent of patients. There is apparent decreased cardiovascular toxicity with 1 mg daily of DES, but serum testosterone may be incompletely suppressed. After a short period of stimulation, luteinizing hormone–releasing hormone (LHRH) analogues suppress testosterone to the castrate range and are an effective alternative therapy for patients with prostatic metastatic cancer. The only LHRH analogue approved by the Food and Drug Administration is leuprolide (Lupron), which should be administered subcutaneously in doses of 1 mg per day. Vasomotor hot flashes occur in approximately 60 per cent of patients on LHRH analogues. A transient elevation in serum testosterone occurs but usually is of no clinical significance. However, LHRH analogues probably should not be used as initial treatment in patients with impending neurologic compromise or in those with immediate life-threatening disease. Various antiandrogens are undergoing testing, but none is currently approved for use in the United States.

UROTHELIAL TUMORS—TRANSITIONAL CELL CARCINOMA

Transitional cells line the urothelium from the renal calices to the prostatic urethra. Transitional cell carcinoma may occur at any of these points and is often a "field change" tumor that affects different areas simultaneously or in sequence.

Detection and Diagnosis

The most common presenting sign or symptom in patients with transitional cell carcinoma is gross painless hematuria. Flank pain may occur in patients with upper tract tumors associated with the passage of blood clots. Irritative voiding symptoms such as urinary frequency and urgency are seen sometimes in patients with bladder involvement.

Since malignant cells are sloughed readily, cytopathologic examination of the urine is often capable of detecting malignant cells. Flow cytometry analyses of DNA are increasingly being used to predict tumor behavior. The diagnosis is confirmed by endoscopic visualization of tumors in the bladder and by transurethral resection or biopsy. For upper tract tumors, the diagnosis is usually made based on a typical appearance of a filling defect on intravenous pyelography.

CARCINOMA OF THE RENAL PELVIS

Transitional cell carcinoma may occur in the renal pelvis or the caliceal system. Except in situations in which there is a solitary kidney or compromised renal function in the opposite kidney, nephroureterectomy is the preferred treatment. In patients with solitary kidneys, a conservative approach is warranted. If feasible, partial nephrectomy is performed. Alternatively, neodymium:YAG laser treatment or electrocautery fulguration can be performed. For low-stage, low-grade tumors, the prognosis after treatment is excellent. High-grade tumors are associated with a poor prognosis. After nephroureterectomy for a renal pelvic transitional cell carcinoma, there is approximately a 5 per cent incidence of an asynchronous tumor in the opposite kidney.

URETERAL CARCINOMA

Transitional cell carcinoma of the ureter most often involves the distal one third. Nephroureterectomy traditionally has been the form of treatment for these lesions. Increasingly, more conservative approaches are used when the tumor is in the distal ureter. Distal ureterectomy with reimplantation of the ureter into the bladder using either a psoas hitch or Boari's flap allows preservation of the ipsilateral kidney. Endoscopic management through ureteroscopes sometimes is feasible. When more conservative approaches are used for proximal ureteral tumors, tumor recurrence in the ureter distal to the lesion is frequent. Consistent with a theory of "field change" as well as with tumor cell implantation, there is a high incidence of subsequent tumor within the bladder, especially near the ipsilateral trigone, in patients with a history of carcinoma of the ureter.

BLADDER CARCINOMA

There are approximately 36,000 new cases of bladder cancer diagnosed annually in the United States and 12,000 deaths from this disease. There is a male-to-female ratio of approximately 3 to 1. Certain chemical carcinogens have been definitely associated with bladder cancer, especially beta naphthalene and certain dyes. Chronic bladder irritation from indwelling Foley catheters or infection with schistosomiasis is associated with squamous cell carcinoma of the bladder. Finally, there is a definite and strong association with cigarette smoking.

Approximately 80 per cent of bladder cancers occur in a superficial, low grade, low stage form. Patients with superficial bladder cancer are treated by transurethral electrocautery resection or neodymium:YAG laser photocoagulation.

Laser therapy offers some practical advantages for patients, but both treatments are equally effective in eliminating visible tumors. After either electrocautery resection or laser treatment, there is a greater than 50 per cent recurrence rate. Because of the high recurrence rate, patients must undergo close surveillance after treatment of tumors. In general, cystoscopy and cytologic examination of the urine are performed every 3 months for a period of 1 year, then every 6 months for another year, and then yearly unless tumor recurs. Most recurrences are superficial. However, there is a 15 per cent incidence of progression in grade or stage in patients who initially present with superficial tumors.

Intravesical chemotherapy or immunotherapy is capable of decreasing the recurrence rate of superficial bladder cancer. Treatment should be given to any patient with recurrent tumors, multiple tumors at the time of diagnosis, tumors larger than 4 cm in size, or dysplasia or carcinoma in situ in adjacent areas of the bladder. Thiotepa is the most frequently used chemotherapeutic agent and is given intravesically in doses of 30 mg weekly for 6 weeks. A white blood cell count should be monitored, since intravascular absorption and myelosuppression may occur in as many as 10 per cent of patients. Mitomycin C (40 mg intravesically weekly for 6 weeks) is also active against superficial bladder cancer but is quite expensive. Bacillus Calmette-Guérin (BCG), an attenuated strain of *Mycobacterium tuberculosis,* is probably the most effective intravesical agent for prophylactic treatment of superficial bladder cancer. Although the drug is not approved by the Food and Drug Association for this purpose, it is one of the most commonly used treatments in this country. Various strains of the organism exist, but none is known to be therapeutically superior to others. The exact mechanism of action is uncertain but local immunologic response within the bladder is likely. Tuberculosis skin tests (intermediate PPD) may convert to positive in patients after intravesical BCG therapy, and bladder biopsies often show granuloma formation in the bladder wall. Therapy is usually well tolerated, although irritative voiding symptoms are common and fever and malaise may be seen on the day of drug administration. Systemic infections with BCG develop in a few per cent of patients and are manifested as granulomatous hepatitis, pulmonary disease, or prostatitis. Systemic antituberculous therapy is indicated in this situation. When used in a prophylactic manner after removal of existing bladder tumors, approximately 80 per cent of patients have had no evidence of recurrence after intravesical BCG therapy. In addition, the drug is the most effective intravesical treatment for carcinoma in situ of the bladder.

Transitional cell carcinoma that invades the detrusor muscle is usually high grade and not manageable by transurethral resection. Neodymium:YAG laser treatment can offer reasonable survival rates in patients with only superficial muscle invasion but is ineffective for tumors that invade the deep muscle of the bladder wall or extend into the perivesical fat. Partial cystectomy with removal of only the involved segment of the bladder is indicated in the unusual situation in which the remainder of the bladder is normal and the tumor is located in a mobile portion of the bladder wall. Most often, the tumor involves the bladder trigone or there is an antecedent history of tumors in other portions of the bladder. Radical cystectomy is the most proven form of therapy for muscle invasive transitional cell carcinoma of the bladder. In men, this includes removal of the prostate and seminal vesicles, while in women the uterus, fallopian tubes, ovaries, and anterior portion of the vagina are removed along with the bladder. Pelvic lymph node dissection should be performed in all patients. Approximately one fourth of patients with invasive bladder cancer have histologic nodal metastasis, and a distinct minority of these are cured by surgery alone. The value of pelvic irradiation prior to cystectomy has been debated for many years. However, recent randomized studies have shown no benefit for patients receiving pelvic irradiation, and this is usually eliminated except in patients undergoing segmental cystectomy, in which the risk of tumor cell implantation in the wound is increased. An ileal conduit remains the most common form of urinary reconstruction after bladder removal, but there are alternatives that can be used depending upon patient preference. Using a detubularized right colon segment and a tapered and reinforced distal ileum and iliocecal valve, a continent form of supravesical urinary diversion can be performed without excessive increased morbidity. The patient catheterizes the reservoir through the skin stoma every 4 hours but is not required to wear a collecting device otherwise. Methods of internal reconstruction, with voiding through the urethra, can also be successful in men. Patients selected for this procedure should not have diffuse carcinoma in situ or tumor invasion of the prostatic urethra, since total urethrectomy is indicated in these patients. Various bowel segments can be used to form a low pressure reservoir which can be anastomosed to the urethra. One of the simplest is to use a detubularized segment of the sigmoid colon. Continence rates during the day are usually good, although there may be some urinary leakage at night.

As an alternative to cystectomy, radiation therapy can be curative in some patients. Methods of bladder preservation using radiation plus chemotherapy are being explored. In general, though, radiation is reserved for patients who refuse or who are not candidates for radical surgery, since the cure rates are less than with bladder removal and radiation does not prevent the formation of new tumors.

METASTATIC DISEASE

Approximately 10,000 people annually die in the United States from metastatic transitional cell carcinoma, usually with the bladder as the primary site. Lung, liver, and bone are the primary sites of distant metastatic disease, but local pelvic recurrence or involvement of retroperitoneal lymph nodes is not uncommon. Cisplatinum and methotrexate are the most active single cytotoxic agents for metastatic transitional cell carcinoma. The best reported response rates have occurred using a combination of methotrexate, vincristine, doxorubicin (Adriamycin), and cisplatinum, the so-called M-VAC regimen. Objective response has been documented in as many as 70 per cent of patients, with approximately one third having a complete response. The complete responses have been of sufficient duration that a survival advantage for treated patients can be anticipated. The regimen is toxic and requires adequate renal function. The role of adjuvant chemotherapy either before or after radical surgery is being explored.

TESTICULAR CARCINOMA

Germ cell tumors of the testis are the most common malignancy in men between the ages of 25 and 39 years. Less commonly, juvenile embryonal cell carcinoma is seen in young children, and there is a somewhat increased incidence of seminoma in men in the sixth decade of life. Testicular tumors are quite uncommon in blacks. A history of cryptorchidism introduces an increased risk for development of testicular cancer.

The presentation is most often as a hard, sometimes irregular mass intrinsic to the testis. The tumors typically are asymptomatic and nontender, but pain may occur when there is hemorrhage within the tumor or associated epididymitis. Scrotal ultrasonography can sometimes help distinguish testicular tumors from other common scrotal masses such as epididymitis, but in general, inguinal exploration of the testis should be performed whenever physical examination raises suspicions of tumor. Inguinal orchiectomy with removal of the entire spermatic cord to the level of the internal inguinal ring should be performed.

Local recurrence is unusual unless there has been violation of the scrotal sac. The first echelon of metastatic disease is to the retroperitoneal lymph nodes near the origin of the spermatic vessels. Computed tomographic (CT) scanning is the best single staging procedure for detection of retroperitoneal nodal disease. A chest radiograph is obtained in all patients, and lungs are the most common site of disease beyond the retroperitoneum. Serum levels of alpha$_1$-fetoprotein and/or beta-human charionic gonadotropin (HCG) are elevated in nearly 70 per cent of patients with metastatic nonseminomatous testis tumors and can be followed as markers of tumor response or recurrence. Beta-HCG is sometimes modestly elevated in patients with seminoma, but elevated levels of alpha$_1$-fetoprotein are diagnostic of nonseminomatous elements.

Seminoma

Seminoma is the most common single histologic variety of testis tumors. In addition, its natural history and response to treatment are different from nonseminomatous tumors. Most patients have clinical stage I disease at the time of presentation with no evidence of residual tumor after orchiectomy. Although the substantial majority of these patients could be anticipated to have no recurrence without treatment, retroperitoneal irradiation provides a cure rate of over 95 per cent with low morbidity. Treatment is delivered to the retroperitoneal nodes and ipsilateral pelvic nodes. Supradiaphragmatic irradiation is not indicated in this group. Excellent cure rates are also achieved with radiation in patients with small-volume retroperitoneal disease. When retroperitoneal nodes exceed 5 cm in size or when there is evidence of disease outside the retroperitoneum, chemotherapy should be used. Various cisplatin-based regimens of chemotherapy have been shown to be active against seminoma. Often, the same combinations that are used against nonseminomatous tumors are employed for seminoma, with response rates that equal or exceed those for nonseminomatous lesions.

Nonseminomatous Tumors

Although this term incorporates a variety of histologic types, it is a valid grouping since evaluation, treatment, and follow-up are generally identical for embryonal cell carcinoma and teratocarcinoma as well as for tumors with mixed elements. Pure choriocarcinoma accounts for less than 1 per cent of testis tumors, is associated with a poor prognosis, and should be treated with aggressive combination chemotherapy. Treatment for other nonseminomatous testis tumors depends on stage at the time of diagnosis. Because of the inaccuracies of clinical staging, retroperitoneal lymph node dissection has been the recommended form of therapy for patients with stage I disease. If the retroperitoneal lymph nodes histologically are normal, no treatment is needed and recurrence rates are under 10 per cent. In patients with microscopic involvement of the retroperitoneal lymph nodes, two courses of cisplatinum-based chemotherapy are given, with a cure rate of over 95 per cent with this approach. Using a technique that preserves the sympathetic nerves responsible for ejaculation, only a minority of patients are rendered infertile because of retroperitoneal lymphadenectomy. However, there is an overall increased incidence of infertility in men with testis tumors because of abnormalities in the semen pattern seen in these patients. Some patients with stage I tumors can be observed carefully without lymphadenectomy. Although no randomized studies are available, cure rates approach those obtained in patients treated with lymphadenectomy. However, this approach applies only to a minority of patients with testis tumors. To be considered for such a protocol, a patient should have a primary tumor that does not invade the epididymis or spermatic cord, an unequivocally normal CT scan and lymphangiogram of the retroperitoneum, a normal chest radiograph, and normal serum levels of alpha$_1$-fetoprotein and beta-HCG. Furthermore, the patient must be both willing and able to comply with a stringent follow-up regimen. Physical examination, chest radiograph, and blood studies should be obtained monthly for two years and a CT scan at least every 3 months. Approximately 25 per cent of the tumors can be expected to recur and require chemotherapy.

Chemotherapy should be used initially in patients with metastatic disease beyond the retroperitoneum or in those with retroperitoneal lymph nodes that are greater than 5 cm in size. In the past, the most frequently used regimen of chemotherapy was the combination of cisplatinum, vinblastin, and bleomycin. Excellent response rates are observed, and over 70 per cent of patients with metastatic disease can be cured. A recent study has shown that VP-16-213 (etoposide) can be used to replace bleomycin while maintaining the same response rate but decreasing morbidity from pulmonary fibrosis and mucositis. In patients who have not undergone lymphadenectomy, a residual retroperitoneal mass often is evident. Fibrosis is found after surgical removal in approximately 40 per cent of patients, while another 20 per cent have residual malignant elements. In the other 40 per cent of patients, mature teratoma is identified. Teratoma

must be resected completely because subsequent enlargement may compromise adjacent organs, or malignant degeneration may occur. No further treatment is indicated if a mature teratoma is resected completely, but additional chemotherapy should be used if malignant elements are present. Treatment with ifosfamide can induce a response in some patients not responding to other chemotherapy.

TUMORS OF THE KIDNEY

Over 90 per cent of tumors that arise from the renal parenchyma are malignant. Sarcomas or metastatic tumors to the kidney are seen occasionally. However, the substantial majority of kidney tumors are renal cell carcinomas in adults and Wilm's tumors in children.

Renal Cell Carcinoma

Renal cell carcinomas arise from the proximal tubular epithelium and are adenocarcinomas. These tumors are commonly referred to as hypernephromas. The classic triad of symptoms associated with hypernephroma—flank pain, a palpable mass, and hematuria—is seen rarely. Increasingly, renal cell carcinomas are being detected incidentally on abdominal imaging studies performed for evaluation of other organs. Because they may produce no symptoms and the kidney is not readily palpable on physical examination, renal cell carcinomas may attain great size before they are detected. Lung, bone, and brain are the most common sites of metastatic disease, but renal cell carcinomas are notorious for having unusual patterns of metastasis. Tumor-associated findings such as anemia, erythrocytosis, liver function abnormalities, and hypercalcemia are not uncommon. The diagnosis of renal cell carcinoma most often is made based on a characteristic appearance on CT scan. Occasionally, a benign angiomyolipoma of the kidney is mistaken for a renal cell carcinoma, but a CT scan showing fat within the tumor is diagnostic of an angiomyolipoma. Oncocytomas are not distinguishable from renal cell carcinoma on CT scan and are considered to be probably benign tumors. Arteriography was used frequently in the past but is rarely indicated now for either diagnosis or staging of renal cell cancers. Percutaneous needle biopsy of renal masses is not usually rewarding. A diagnosis based on radiographic findings provides sufficient clinical accuracy, and a biopsy showing only benign elements does not exclude the presence of a renal cell carcinoma.

Radical nephrectomy is the treatment of choice for renal cell carcinomas when there is a normal contralateral kidney. Gerota's fascia and its contents are removed en bloc, including the kidney, the perirenal fat, and the ipsilateral adrenal gland. Lymphadenectomy provides prognostic information but probably little therapeutic value. Prognosis for tumors confined within the renal capsule is fairly good, with a 70 per cent 5-year survival. If the tumor penetrates into the perirenal fat, 5-year survival after radical nephrectomy is around 50 per cent. Radical surgery is rarely curative in patients with positive regional lymph nodes. In solitary kidneys or in situations in which there is compromised function of the contralateral kidney, parenchymal sparing procedures are indicated. For polar lesions, partial nephrectomy with a margin of normal kidney is indicated. Sometimes, tumor size or location makes enucleation of the tumor or resection with precarious margins necessary. Under these circumstances, a neodymium:YAG laser can be used to extend the treatment margin another 5 to 10 mm.

Some 10 to 15 per cent of renal cell cancers invade the renal vein or inferior vena cava. In the absence of distant metastatic disease, surgical removal can provide surprisingly good cure rates if regional lymph nodes are not simultaneously involved. Cardiac bypass and complete circulatory arrest have been used for some tumors that extend into the right atrium. Most often, the caval thrombus does not actually invade the wall of the inferior vena cava and can be extracted through a vena cavotomy.

Metastatic renal cell carcinoma has been one of the most resistant tumors to chemotherapy. No cytotoxic agent has been identified that produces satisfactory response rates or that has been shown to improve survival. Hormonal therapy, often medroxyprogesterone acetate (Depo-Provera) 10 mg intramuscularly once a week, is sometimes used but probably is ineffective. Removal of the primary tumor in patients with known metastatic disease usually is not indicated unless there is pain or recurrent bleeding. Although spontaneous regression of metastatic disease after removal of the primary lesion has been documented, it occurs in fewer than 1 per cent of patients. Interferons generally have provided around a 15 per cent response rate without any evidence that survival is improved. An objective response rate of nearly 50 per cent has been reported for a combination of leukocyte-activated killer cells (LAK) and interleukin-2. Most responses are partial, but durable complete responses have been observed. Response is improved if the primary tumor is removed. Treatment is extremely expensive and toxic, but the response rates are the most promising report for metastatic renal cell cancer.

Wilms' Tumor

Wilms' tumors are composed histologically of renal blastema epithelial and stromal components. They are rare beyond childhood and are detected most often before age 6. The National Wilms' Tumor Study Group has conducted numerous studies that have established current treatment recommendations. A palpable abdominal mass is the most frequent sign. Bilateral tumors are observed in 5 per cent of patients. Therefore, surgical removal should be accomplished through a transperitoneal incision so that the opposite kidney can be examined. Nephrectomy on the most involved side, with partial nephrectomy for the kidney with the smaller tumor, should be performed if feasible. If surgical removal is not possible or hazardous, chemotherapy should be given prior to an attempt at surgical removal. Adjuvant chemotherapy is used for 15 months after surgical resection. Radiation therapy is not used unless there has been surgical violation of the tumor capsule or extension of the tumor to soft tissue. Unfavorable histologic stage in the primary tumor (sarcomatous changes) is associated with a relatively poor prognosis. With favorable histologic stage, surgical removal, and chemotherapy, cure rates exceed 80 per cent.

TUMORS OF THE PENIS

Squamous cell carcinoma of the penis is the most common cancer seen in some countries but accounts for less than 1 per cent of tumors in men in the United States. Squamous cell carcinoma of the penis is exceedingly rare in men who underwent neonatal circumcision. The disease is most often seen in the sixth or seventh decade of life but may occur earlier. The primary lesion usually involves the glans penis or prepuce. Typically, the tumors are painless, and patients may not present until the lesion has attained a large size. Secondary infection with purulence and drainage is common. A biopsy is used to establish the diagnosis. The first site of metastatic disease is the inguinal lymph nodes. Palpable lymph nodes at the time of presentation may be reactive, but fine needle aspiration can help distinguish this tumor from metastatic disease. In the presence of abnormal lymph nodes, inguinal lymphadenectomy should be performed. When the nodes palpably are normal, a limited dissection and sentinal node biopsy are performed if the primary tumor is high grade and infiltrative. While a negative sentinal node biopsy does not ensure negative lymph nodes elsewhere, this approach seems preferable to observation alone. The primary morbidity of inguinal lymphadenectomy, skin flap necrosis and lower extremity edema, can be prevented by avoiding excessive thinning of the skin flap and dissection of the lymphatic channels lateral to and behind the femoral vessels. Lymphadenectomy can be curative in almost half of patients who have metastasis limited to the inguinal lymph nodes. Pelvic node involvement or distant disease is associated with a very poor prognosis. Cisplatinum, methotrexate, and bleomycin are the most frequently used cytotoxic drugs, but none has been shown to increase survival.

Extensive primary tumors with involvement of the proximal corpora cavernosa may require total penectomy and perineal urethrotomy. Usually, the primary lesion can be excised with an adequate margin if partial penectomy is performed approximately 2 cm proximal to the glans penis. For minimally infiltrative tumors, a neodymium:YAG laser has provided excellent local control rates with functional and cosmetic results that are superior to those obtained with partial penectomy.

ADRENAL TUMORS

Adrenal cortical carcinomas are tumors that arise from the adrenal cortex. The majority of these tumors are hormonally functional and may produce Cushing's syndrome from excessive glucocorticoids or virilization from excessive androgen production. When the tumors do not retain endocrine function, they may remain asymptomatic until they attain great size.

Aggressive surgical resection should be performed for adrenal carcinomas. This may require ipsilateral nephrectomy but the prognosis for unresectable or metastatic adrenal carcinoma is dismal. Mitotane (*o,p′*DDD) (Lysodren) is an insecticide that has shown some activity against metastatic adrenal carcinoma. However, the drug has severe side effects and has not been shown to improve survival. In patients with steroid-producing cancers, periodic steroid excretion tests can be used to monitor patients postoperatively, since recurrent tumors may be detected by a rising steroid excretion.

Pheochromocytomas may arise anywhere along the sympathetic chain in the retroperitoneum or the mediastinum. However, the most common intra-abdominal location is the adrenal medulla. Only 10 per cent of pheochromocytomas are malignant, and histologic features of the primary tumor are unreliable in determining whether the lesions are malignant. Most often the diagnosis of malignancy is based upon the presence of nodal metastasis or metastatic disease. Aggressive surgical resection is indicated, but the prognosis for malignant pheochromocytomas is poor.

URETHRAL STRICTURE

method of
ROY WITHERINGTON, M.D.
Medical College of Georgia
Augusta, Georgia

Postinfective strictures are common, involve the anterior urethra, can be treated in many ways, and frequently recur. Posttraumatic strictures involve either the prostatomembranous or bulbous urethra and respond well to excision and reanastomosis. A tentative diagnosis can be made when a small latex catheter will not pass into the bladder, and diagnosis can be confirmed by urethrography. When associated with inflammation or trauma, preliminary suprapubic cystostomy is indicated to allow for reaction to subside and for scar to mature. A properly planned approach to management requires a knowledge of location, cause, extent, and severity of the lesion.

Management

General Methods

Urethral Dilation. Urethral dilation is still the gold standard, and most patients can be managed on a long-term basis by simple dilation. To be successful, it is imperative that progressive dilation rather than forceful tearing be accomplished. Tears heal by scarring, and stricture can be worsened by overzealous treatment. Tight strictures are best managed using filiforms and Phillips followers (either catheters or bougies). After passage of a small follower (8 F), progressively larger followers are passed until resistance is met. The instrument is removed and voiding is usually much improved. Repeat dilation is accomplished at 7- to 10-day intervals, and each time the urethra can usually be dilated to a larger diameter. LeFort sounds can be substituted for Phillips followers after the first or second session. Once dilated to 22 to 24 F, Van Buren sounds can be used instead of filiforms and followers or LeFort sounds. When the urethral diameter reaches 26 to 28 F, dilations are required less frequently. Patients in urinary retention with particularly dense strictures that cannot be dilated beyond 8 to 10 F initially can be managed by leaving a catheter-type follower indwelling. It is held in place by two silk ties, which are placed around it just distal to the meatus and carefully taped to the penis. After 2 to 3 days, progressive dilation can be accomplished with ease. Once the lumen of the urethra is enlarged to 16 to 18 F, placement of a Foley catheter can accomplish soft dilation. The catheter can be changed to a larger size every 2 to 3 days until the desired caliber is reached. Successful long-term management depends on careful atraumatic dilation every 3 to 6 months.

Internal Urethrotomy. Incision of urethral strictures can be accomplished by either a blind or visual technique. Blind urethrotomy is done using an Otis urethrotome. The device is 16 F in diameter and therefore cannot be used initially to treat tight strictures. The shaft of the instrument is made larger by turning a proximally positioned wheel, and changes in size can be read from a calibrated dial on the instrument. A dull knife blade is inserted on the top of the shaft and when properly introduced is hidden at the distal end. Once the instrument has been inserted and enlarged to the point where it is snug within the urethra, the knife is quickly drawn through the stricture to produce a clean dorsal cut. The urethra can be enlarged to any desired diameter, usually 28 to 30 F, by repeated cuts. Proper use requires that overzealous stretching not occur prior to making any cuts. A Teflon-coated latex catheter that must be 2 F smaller than the incised urethra is left indwelling for 3 weeks to allow epithelium to grow across the incised area and to enlarge the urethral lumen. Visual urethrotomy necessitates a distal urethral lumen of fairly large caliber to permit introduction of the urethrotome. The stricture is visualized and a small ureteral catheter passed through it to maintain access and orientation. The blade is extended and clean cuts made through the stricture in one or more locations to enlarge the diameter to 26 to 30 F. This method of management is best for clean iris diaphragm–type strictures, and extensive tight strictures often cannot be successfully treated in this way. If the stricture is small and not very fibrotic, posttreatment catheterization may not be necessary. When extensive incisions are made, a short period of catheterization for both hemostasis and diversion or urine is wise. Following urethrotomy, residual stricture is usually present and can be managed by either periodic dilations or repeat internal urethrotomy.

Open Surgical Techniques

Patch Graft Urethroplasty. Strictures in the distal bulb and pendulous urethra can be managed by patch graft urethroplasty. A ventral incision is made through the stricture, and it is extended at least 1 to 1.5 cm proximally and distally into normal urethra. A free full-thickness graft of distal dorsal prepuce is harvested, tailored to fit, and sewn into the defect over a stenting catheter. All subdermal tissue is excised, and epidermis is placed toward the lumen. With particularly severe segmental strictures, it may be necessary to excise the strictured area and to interpose a tubularized graft. The stenting catheter is left indwelling for 10 to 14 days. Pedicle island grafts of penile or scrotal skin can be substituted for free patch grafts in many instances. Long-term results from both free and pedicle graft urethroplasties appear good.

Excision of Stricture with Urethrourethrostomy. Short posttraumatic bulbous and prostatomembranous urethral strictures can easily be managed by excision and accurate spatulated urethrourethrostomy over a stenting catheter. The stent is left indwelling for 10 to 14 days.

Multistaged Procedures. These techniques initially externalize the strictured area when adjacent penile or scrotal skin is sewn directly to the incised urethra (first stage). The externalized area is allowed to become soft and pliable prior to urethral reconstruction (second stage). The strip of epithelium used for urethral reconstruction must be wide enough to produce a tube of adequate caliber, and a small fenestrated catheter is left in the urethra to act as an internal drain. The multistage techniques can be applied to strictures located anywhere from the prostatomembranous junction to the distal penis. They are most often used for proximal bulbous strictures.

Suprapubic cystostomy at the time of urethroplasty or urethral reconstruction by any technique is wise, so that proximal urinary diversion can be accomplished should there be extravasation from the repair site following removal of the urethral stent.

Treatment of Stricture by Location

Meatal Strictures. Simple postinfective meatal strictures can be managed by doral or ventral meatotomy. Dorsal meatotomy using the Otis urethrotome results in a good cosmetic result and in an absence of splayed stream. Following dorsal meatotomy, a catheter must be left indwelling for a few days to allow for hemostasis to occur. Then, self-dilation to maintain the caliber of meatus is necessary until healing is complete. Ventral meatotomy is accomplished by incision of the ventral meatal area and suture approximation of skin to urethral epithelium. With ventral meatotomy, the cosmetic result is not good and splaying of the urinary stream often occurs. Meatal stricture secondary to balanitis xerotica obliterans is best managed by meatoplasty. Here, the strictured area is incised ventrally until normal urethra is encountered. A U-shaped skin flap is created on the ventral surface of the penis near the frenulum which is sewn into the urethral meatus to enlarge its caliber. The cosmetic result is not pleasing but the functional result is usually quite acceptable.

Pendulous Urethral Strictures. These may be managed by periodic dilations, internal urethrotomy, either patch graft or pedicle graft urethroplasty, and multistaged urethroplasty. The multistaged technique is particularly applicable to dense panurethral postinfective strictures.

Bulbous Urethral Strictures. Posttraumatic bulbous urethral stricture is best treated by excision and accurate spatulated urethrourethrostomy. Distal bulbous postinfective strictures can be managed by periodic dilations and by either patch graft or pedicle island graft urethroplasty. The very proximal bulbous postinfective stricture can be managed by periodic dilations but should not be managed by patch graft urethroplasty because the lesion is adjacent to the active part of the urethra (sphincter). This stricture is best managed by a two-stage procedure. A popular technique is to use a perineally based skin flap in which the tip extends onto the scrotum, as advocated by Blandy. The urethra is incised proximally and distally at least 1 to 1.5 cm from the stricture, and the flap is sewn in place. The externalized area is carefully observed over the next 6 months, and if either granulation tissue or synechiae appear, they are destroyed. The externalized urethra is allowed to become soft and pliable. Adequate caliber of stomas (28 to 30 F) must be assured before second stage urethroplasty is accomplished.

Prostatomembranous Urethral Strictures. These nearly always follow trauma and are best handled by excision and accurate spatulated urethrourethrostomy. With short strictures, a transperineal approach gives excellent results. Long or complex strictures with associated fistulas, sinuses, diverticula, and bone spicules within the urethra are best managed by a combined retropubic and perineal approach. The combined approach allows appropriate treatment of associated lesions, accurate urethral anastomosis, and placement of a pedicle graft of omentum around the repair site, which lends blood supply, fills dead space, and prevents excessive postoperative fibrosis. Short prostatomembranous strictures can sometimes be managed satisfactorily by transurethral incision and periodic dilations.

RENAL CALCULI

method of
ROBERT I. KAHN, M.D., and
FELIX O. KOLB, M.D.
Pacific-Presbyterian Medical Center
San Francisco, California

Renal stones are common, affecting 0.1 to 0.3 per cent of the population annually and 5 to 10 per cent of people sometime in their lifetime. There are about 300,000 admissions to hospitals for renal stone disease per year, and since only about one third of patients are admitted to a hospital, the true incidence may exceed 1 million per year. There has been an increased incidence of renal stones throughout the world in the past 20 years. Males predominate over females by a ratio of 3 to 4:1, and individuals between the ages of 20 and 60 pass 80 per cent of stones. After passing one stone, there is a 20 per cent recurrence rate within 5 years. After more than one stone has been passed, 80 per cent further recurrences are likely in 2 years. The overall recurrence rate in untreated patients is roughly 7 per cent per year. This has a major economic impact. Calcareous stones account for 80 to 95 per cent of stones and are primarily composed of calcium oxalate and calcium phosphate, usually occurring in mixtures. The remaining stones are composed of struvite, uric acid, and cystine.

A specific cause can be identified in roughly two thirds of patients with renal stones, but rapid progress in the understanding of the pathophysiology of stone formation and diagnostic differentiation has led to effective treatment in the vast majority of patients with recurrent renal calculi. Removal of stones has been greatly facilitated by newer techniques, such as lithotripsy.

Clinical Presentation

Renal calculi can present with a wide variety of symptoms. These depend on the size and location of the stones and also whether infection is present. Renal calculi that migrate into the ureteropelvic junction or further into the ureter present with classical renal colic. Milder flank pain may be indicative of a larger stone within the renal pelvis. Small calyceal calculi are often asymptomatic; however, some calculi within calyces do cause mild pain.

Virtually all calculi are associated with microscopic or gross hematuria. The bleeding is seldom significant enough to cause alterations in the blood count.

Pyelonephritis or cystitis may result from infection secondary to a stone. Infection can also compound the presentation of an obstructing ureteral calculus by infecting the renal unit above the obstruction. If severe enough, these infections can precipitate septic shock.

Obstruction from stones may be unilateral or bilateral. In the latter situation, the patient may present with anuria. In the former situation, unless the patient has a solitary kidney, the contralateral kidney will maintain sufficient renal function.

Diagnosis

The clinical presentation often suggests the diagnosis of an upper urinary tract calculus. Urinalysis will reveal microscopic or gross hematuria. It is also important to measure the pH, although an isolated measurement is not diagnostic of any particular stone composition. A pH diary may be kept by the patient and will suggest, for example, a tendency toward acid or alkaline urine. More than 80 per cent of urinary calculi are visible on a plain abdominal radiograph of the kidney, ureter, and bladder (KUB). An intravenous pyelogram (IVP) will give some functional information with regard to the involved kidney and the state of the uninvolved contralateral kidney. Most importantly, the IVP shows the size, shape, and position of the offending stone. Some nonopaque calculi can be appreciated by IVP, but often a retrograde pyelogram is necessary to further delineate them. A CT scan of the kidneys without contrast material will reveal nonopaque or poorly opaque calculi that are otherwise not visible on the KUB radiograph. Diagnostic ultrasonography can also reveal whether hydronephrosis is present and is excellent in detecting calculi.

Metabolic Diagnosis

The key to the proper diagnosis is an accurate stone analysis, preferably by polarizing microscopy that identifies the nucleus and surrounding crystalline structure of the stone. Crystals in the urine occur frequently but by themselves are not diagnostic, except for cystine crystals. The urinary pH is important. A consistently acid concentrated urine predisposes to uric acid stones, and struvite stones are found in highly alkaline-infected urines. A relatively fixed urinary pH of 5.5 suggests renal tubular acidosis.

Calcium stones are most common, and in the majority of cases they are due to hypercalciuria. Roughly 5 per cent of patients harbor parathyroid tumors, which must be removed surgically. Several fasting serum calcium levels, with a proper parathormone assay, will usually ascertain the diagnosis.

The other causes of calcium stones include hypercalciuria due to either excessive renal losses (renal hypercalciuria) or hyperabsorption (absorptive hypercalciuria), hyperuricosuria, hyperoxaluria, hypocitraturia, and hypomagnesiuria. The diagnosis rests on properly collected 24-hour urine specimens for calcium, phosphorus, creatinine, oxalate, uric acid, citrate, and magnesium with the patient maintaining his usual diet. A calcium load test with 1000 to 1500 mg of oral calcium for 3 days will reveal patients who are hyperabsorbers. Excess oxalate is due either to diet, excessive intestinal absorption (e.g., ileitis), or, rarely, congenital factors. Hypocitraturia is a consequence of metabolic acidosis (e.g., diarrheal states) or thiazide-induced hypokalemia or is due to unknown causes. Excessive excretion of uric acid can predispose to calcium oxalate stone formation. Hypomagnesiuria is probably dietary in origin and often coexists with hypocitraturia.

Noncalcareous stones are less common (8 per cent of all stones). Uric acid stones frequently occur in association with gout, but the majority of uric acid stones occur in a highly acid, concentrated urine in patients on high protein diets.

Cystine stones account for about 3 per cent of stones in patients with congenital hypercystinuria. The hexagonal urinary crystals, especially in an acidified specimen, are diagnostic.

Struvite stones (magnesium ammonium phosphate stones) develop only in highly alkaline urine, usually secondary to urinary tract infection with urea-splitting organisms.

Rare stones include triamterine, silicone dioxide, renografin, or hypaque. Artifacts may be passed as "renal stones" by emotionally disturbed patients, who are often previous stone formers.

The evaluation of patients with a single stone episode need not be extensive, but should include blood screen (calcium, phosphate, electrolytes, creatinine, uric acid), urine culture, crystal count in sediment, and the 24-hour urine measurements outlined above.

In recurrent stone formers, more extensive work-up, including parathyroid hormone assay, 1-25 dihydroxyvitamin D assays, and calcium load or restriction tests, is required. At times, the response to treatment (e.g., thiazide unmasking hyperparathyroidism) helps to establish the diagnosis.

Expectant Therapy

A patient who presents with an obstruction from a ureteral calculus most commonly can be managed without any interventions. This, of course, depends on the size of the stone, the severity of symptoms, the degree of renal functional impairment, whether infection is present, and the social situation.

The principal factor determining whether a ureteral calculus will pass spontaneously is its size. Calculi with sizes from several millimeters up to 8 mm in diameter may be expected to pass spontaneously with an inverse relationship of size to probability of passage. The degree of impaction, which is partially determined by the length of time a stone remains in one position, will also determine the likelihood of spontaneous passage. Radiographic evaluation can reveal the degree of obstruction and impaction.

A stone may be allowed to pass spontaneously if symptoms are not too severe and if the social situation of the patient permits the time that may be necessary for this to occur. Patients with urinary tract infections have a more complicated situation, which may require intervention. However, mild infections may be treated with oral or intravenous antibiotics, with spontaneous passage the eventual outcome. With more severe infections, the stone should either be removed directly after loading with intravenous antibiotics, or a temporary diversion (a ureteral catheter or percutaneous nephrostomy) may permit rapid resolution of the septic condition. Later, elective stone removal may be undertaken.

Medical Treatment

All patients should be managed with a high fluid intake sufficient to produce a urine output of at least 2 liters per day and by avoidance of dietary excesses. More aggressive and specific treatment regimens with drugs are indicated for active stone disease, and their effectiveness should be determined with serial blood and urine chemical tests.

Therapy of Calcium Stones

A diet reasonably restricted in calcium and vitamin D is generally desirable in absorptive hypercalciuria. It is not indicated in renal hypercalciuria, since over prolonged periods it may lead to depletion of the bone mineral stores. Thiazide therapy is highly effective in renal hypercalciuria, and to a lesser extent in absorptive hypercalciuria. Cellulose phosphate, which is effective in absorptive hypercalciuria, is expensive, not readily available, and may lead to hyperabsorption of oxalate and to magnesium depletion. Neutral phosphate therapy, such as K-Phos Neutral, 2 tablets (0.5 grams phosphate) three to four times per day is highly effective and can be combined with thiazides. It is also helpful in patients who have renal phosphate leaks. Since thiazides lead to potassium depletion, which causes hypocitraturia, the addition of amiloride is advisable. Triamterene should be avoided, since it can cause stone formation. Many patients tolerate amiloride HCl-hydrochlorothiazide (Moduretic), ½ to 1 pill daily, or chlorthalidone (Hygroton), 25 to 50 mg with added potassium, preferably as citrate. Patients who do not tolerate thiazides can be managed with potassium citrate in a long-acting form (Urocit-K), 20 to 60 mEq per day in divided doses. Restriction of oxalates and ascorbic acid in the diet is moderately successful in hyperoxaluric states, with the addition of pyridoxine, 50 to 150 mg, and also magnesium oxide, 400 to 800 mg per day.

Patients with enteric hyperoxaluria, in addition to dietary restriction of oxalate, added pyridoxine, and magnesium, may need reduction of dietary fats, large doses of calcium carbonate or calcium citrate (up to 3 to 4 grams or more per day), and rarely the addition of crystalline vitamin D (Calderol).

In hyperuricosuric calcium oxalate stone formers, the addition of a low purine diet and allopurinol (Zyloprim), 200 to 600 mg per day, is effective in addition to thiazides. Patients who have idiopathic hypocitraturia are readily managed with long-acting citrate.

Struvite stones require attempts at urinary acidifications, e.g., ascorbic acid, 1 to 4 grams per day, antibiotics to eliminate urea-splitting infection, and, rarely, acetohydroxamic acid, a urease inhibitor. Once stones have formed, however, surgical removal is usually required to remove the bacteria embedded within the stones.

Uric acid stones are effectively treated with low purine diets, alkalinization of the urine with citrus fruit or potassium citrate, and allopurinol in doses of 200 to 600 mg per day if serum and urine uric acid remain elevated.

Cystine stones are treated by forcing large volumes of fluid, especially at night, alkalinization, which must be aggressive to raise the pH above 7.0, and cautious use of penicillamine, 250 mg two to eight capsules per day. The latter has significant side effects and often has to be stopped. A low methionine diet and sodium restriction can reduce urinary cystine excretion further to keep the urine crystal free.

Once an effective medical treatment has been prescribed, periodic follow-up is needed to ensure the effectiveness of the program, to detect potential side effects, and to make adjustments in drug dosages.

Interventional Treatment

Calculi that should be removed include the following: (1) stones that are symptomatic and that are too large for spontaneous passage; (2) stones associated with bacteriuria or symptomatic infection; (3) stones that are causing severe, acute renal functional impairment or chronic severe renal functional impairment; (4) stones that despite adequate conservative management are producing severe and persistent symptoms such as pain, nausea, ileus; (5) stones that for whatever reason warrant removal because of an individual's social situation, e.g., travel to a remote area without the possibility of medical attention; and (6) stones that cannot be dissolved.

Depending upon the size, location, and associated signs or symptoms, a calculus can be removed by a variety of endoscopic, surgical, and extracorporeal methods. With recent technological advances, the need for open surgical removal is rare.

Endoscopic Methods

Traditionally, small calculi in the distal ureter were commonly removed with a cystoscope and stone basket that was passed up the ureter either "blindly" or under fluoroscopic guidance. The stones would become trapped in the basket and would be removed. This technique is highly successful in the hands of a skilled operator. However, complications, including avulsion and failure to grasp the stone in the basket occur more commonly than with the methods described below.

Ureteroscopic stone removal is an endoscopic method in which a small caliber rigid or flexible instrument is passed up the ureter to the stone. The stone is then either trapped in a basket and removed in one piece, or various forms of mechanical lithotripsy (ultrasound, electrohydraulics, laser, microexplosives) are used to fracture the stone and remove it. This method is highly successful in the distal ureter but is also safe and effective in the mid- and proximal ureter, with the latter being less successful.

A third method of endoscopic stone removal is percutaneous nephrostolithotomy. A nephrostomy tract is established through the parenchyma of the kidney and on into the collecting system so that a rigid or flexible nephroscope can be introduced directly into the upper urinary tract. Stones may be removed intact if they are small enough to fit through the 1 cm tract. Otherwise, lithotripsy performed with ultrasound, electrohydraulics, laser, or microexplosives may be performed to reduce the size of the larger stones. The various nephroscopes may view the entire renal collecting system along with the upper two thirds of the ureter. This method is particularly suitable for large renal stones, stones associated with congenital anomalies such as ureteropelvic junction obstruction or calyceal diverticulum, and impacted ureteral stones that have failed treatment by other methods. The results are highly successful, and the complications are minimal, although the patient does require insertion of a nephrostomy tube for several days.

Extracorporeal Shock Wave Lithotripsy (ESWL)

Extracorporeal shock wave lithotripsy (ESWL) is a method by which shock waves are generated by an energy source external to the body, and these waves are focused onto the target stone. The shock waves travel through a water medium and enter the soft tissues of the flank. The stone is positioned by means of x-ray or ultrasound localization, so that it lies directly at the focus of the shock waves. A series of these waves then pulverize the stone so that the resultant fragments are small enough for easy, spontaneous passage. A variety of machines are available for this procedure. Some require anesthesia, while others require none. Some localize the stone with ultrasound and others with fluoroscopy or plain radiographs. The energy source producing the shock waves may be an electric spark, electromagnetic energy, or ultrasound.

The limitations of ESWL are principally stone size (less than 2.5 cm), stone hardness (calcium oxalate monohydrate and cystine are difficult to fracture), and obstruction distal to the path of the stone. Ureteral stones often have to be manipulated back into the kidney prior to ESWL because of the relatively poor results for treatment of stones in situ in the ureter. Overall, 80 to 90 per cent of all calculi that require removal can be treated by this method. The success rate is directly correlated with the adherence of the preceding limiting criteria for patient selection.

Surgery

Until recently, open surgical removal of calculi was considered to be the standard of practice. However, with the previously described new procedures, it is probably responsible today for removal of only 1 per cent of all calculi. Although highly successful for most calculi, the resultant morbidity from a surgical incision and the required rehabilitation and healing time offer significant disadvantages compared with the newer procedures. Surgery along with endoscopic methods is most useful for treatment of complications of the newer procedures, treatment of very large complex calculi, or treatment of some stones associated with congenital anomalies that cannot be treated by percutaneous nephrostolithotomy.

Other Interventional Methods

Other procedures that may be ancillary to the preceding are important in the treatment of renal calculi. An obstructing ureteral stone may be manipulated back into the kidney without removal in planning for ESWL treatment. With obstructing pyelonephritis, a stone may either be bypassed by a ureteral catheter or stent, or a percutaneous nephrostomy drainage tube may be introduced to permit quick resolution of the infection so that elective removal can be performed later. Also, many of the above procedures may be used in combination as a planned multistage stone removal procedure or with the secondary procedure being utilized to treat a complication of the original procedure. For example, after ESWL a condition known as "steinstrasse" may develop from obstruction secondary to numerous small fragments occluding the ureter. Ureteroscopic stone manipulation may be necessary to resolve this condition. Some large staghorn calculi may be treated percutaneously, and if all the stone is not removed at the first session, either a repeat percutaneous session or extracorporeal shock wave lithotripsy may be necessary.

Sexually Transmitted Diseases

CHANCROID

method of
ALLAN R. RONALD, M.D.
University of Manitoba
Winnipeg, Manitoba

Chancroid has reemerged in the United States and other Western countries as an important sexually transmitted disease. Epidemics of this disease are occurring throughout the United States and Canada. Nonvesicular genital ulcers must be investigated by darkfield examination and serologic test to exclude syphilis and must be cultured for herpes to exclude herpetic ulceration. A clinical diagnosis, to ascribe etiology to any agent, is not good practice and does not permit adequate treatment or control of sexually transmitted ulcers. The etiologic agent for chancroid is *Haemophilus ducreyi.* This organism is difficult to grow in vitro, and many laboratories still are unable to culture it. However, a swab of ulcer pus cultured promptly on vitamin-supplemented gonococcal agar with added vancomycin and incubated at 100 per cent humidity in a candle jar for 72 hours at a temperature of 33° C will yield *H. ducreyi* in about 70 per cent of men with chancroid. This procedure should be available in most urban communities.

Genital ulcers due to *H. ducreyi* often are associated with tender lymphadenitis. This may progress to suppurative buboes. If these are not aspirated, inguinal abscesses may develop.

In about 5 per cent of patients with chancroid, a second sexually transmitted pathogen, *Treponema pallidum* or *Herpes simplex,* may be present concomitantly.

Genital ulcer disease facilitates the transmission of human immunodeficiency virus (HIV). Early treatment of epidemiologic contacts is a strategic priority for the control of HIV transmission.

Treatment

Sulfonamides have been the optimal treatment for chancroid, but during the past decade, widespread resistance to sulfonamides, ampicillin, tetracyclines, and kanamycin has developed. All resistance is mediated by plasmids.

Untreated, genital ulcers persist for weeks and even months. Buboes frequently develop. In women particularly, sexual activity may continue with ongoing spread of ulcers to sexual partners. Treatment with an effective agent leads to rapid resolution of symptoms and gradual healing of the ulcer over 7 to 10 days.

Chancroid should be treated immediately once syphilis and herpetic infection have been excluded by appropriate laboratory tests regardless of proof of *H. ducreyi* infection based on results of culture. Five treatment regimens have been shown by two or more investigators to be effective.

Trimethoprim-sulfamethoxazole (Bactrim, Septra), prescribed in a dose of one double-strength capsule orally, twice daily for 7 days, is an effective regimen. In Kenya, a single-dose regimen of four double-strength tablets of trimethoprim combined with a sulfonamide cured over 90 per cent of patients with chancroid. The recent emergence of trimethoprim-resistant strains of *H. ducreyi* in Thailand is of some threat to the ongoing efficacy of this regimen. The dose of amoxicillin combined with clavulanic acid (Augmentin) prescribed as 375 mg three times daily for 3 days cured over 95 per cent of men with chancroid. Clavulanic acid blocks the beta-lactamase enzyme and permits amoxicillin to inhibit the growth of *H. ducreyi.* Erythromycin, 500 mg orally four times a day for 7 days, is very effective. A single dose therapy with ceftriaxone (Rocephin), 250 mg intramuscularly, is equally effective. Ciprofloxacin prescribed as a single oral dose of 1 gram also has been shown to cure all patients treated. Both these two single-dose regimens need not be repeated. Ulcers and buboes resolve once *H. ducreyi* has been eradicated from the lesion. Relapse of infection at the site of the original ulcer without sexual reexposure occurs in 2 to 5 per cent of patients and responds to a second course of treatment. Patients with coexisting HIV infection have an increased propensity to relapse.

Some patients will require needle aspiration of buboes. This usually can be done on one or two occasions without complications. Bubo pus is almost always sterile.

Sexual partners should be examined for ulcers and treated with the identical regimen that has been shown to be effective for the index patient. Most sexual partners have ulcers, which in females are often asymptomatic and found only with careful observation.

GONORRHEA

method of
WILLIAM O. HARRISON, M.D.
Balboa Naval Hospital
San Diego, California

Because of major changes in the antibiotic sensitivity of *Neisseria gonorrhoeae* in many areas of the world during the past decade, recommendations for treatment of gonorrhea have undergone significant revision. Unless otherwise noted, all therapy applies equally to men and women.

Treatment

Uncomplicated Gonorrhea (Urethritis, Cervicitis, Symptomatic and Asymptomatic Proctitis)

Drugs of choice in areas where antibiotic resistance is not a problem are listed alphabetically as follows:
1. *Parenteral*
   a. Aqueous procaine penicillin G, 4.8 million units intramuscularly, accompanied by 1 gram of probenicid orally.
   b. Ceftriaxone (Rocephin), 250 mg intramuscularly.
   c. Spectinomycin hydrochloride (Trobicin), 2 grams intramuscularly.
2. *Oral*
   a. Amoxicillin, 3.0 grams orally, accompanied by 1 gram of probenecid.
   b. Ampicillin, 3.5 grams orally accompanied by 1 gram of probenicid.

In addition, tetracycline hydrochloride, 500 mg orally four times daily for 7 days, or doxycycline (Vibramycin), 100 mg orally twice daily for 7 days, should be included.

All of these regimens are essentially equal in efficacy for the above conditions. Since they are single-dose regimens, problems with compliance are minimized. Tetracycline analogues are no more effective than tetracycline hydrochloride but may have better acceptance.

Tetracycline is included with all antigonococcal regimens because of the high incidence of coexisting chlamydial infections. Gonococcal isolates in many parts of the world, including the United States, may be more resistant to tetracycline; thus tetracycline alone is no longer recommended.

Patients who have concomitant incubating syphilis but who have no physical signs and have negative serology will generally have such an infection aborted by the penicillin regimen. Because data do not exist for other regimens, all patients treated for gonococcal infections should have a serologic test for syphilis done at the time of such treatment, with a follow-up serologic test 6 to 10 weeks afterwards.

Uncomplicated gonococcal infections can be treated in the outpatient setting.

Penicillinase-Producing Neisseria gonorrhoeae (PPNG)

Despite excellent early control measures in North America and Western Europe, this strain of gonococcus has become the predominate one in many parts of the world. It has also established itself in significant numbers in circumscribed areas of the United States and Europe. Because of the increasing antibiotic resistance of gonococcus to both penicillin and other drugs, it is recommended that patients who have been treated with penicillin and who have failed such treatment have repeat cultures prior to retreatment. These isolates must also be tested for the presence of penicillinase (beta-lactamase). Such testing is available through many laboratories and state health departments as well as through the Centers for Disease Control, Atlanta, Georgia. Patients with a history of sexual exposure in geographic areas known to have a high incidence of resistant strains should be initially treated primarily with either spectinomycin or a third-generation cephalosporin.

Treatment of documented or suspected PPNG should be with spectinomycin hydrochloride (Trobicin), 2 grams intramuscularly. Unfortunately, isolates of gonococcus completely resistant to both penicillin and spectinomycin are occurring with increasing frequency. Thus, a PPNG infection that fails to respond to 2 grams of spectinomycin may be retreated with any of the following regimens:

1. Ceftriaxone (Rocephin), 250 mg intramuscularly.
2. Cefoxitin (Mefoxin), intramuscularly, either 1 or 2 grams in a single dose (either regimen is equally effective), accompanied by 1 gram of oral probenecid.
3. Cefotaxime (Claforan), 1 gram intramuscularly.

4. Norfloxacin (Noroxin), 600 mg twice daily for 1 day.*

Chromosomally mediated resistant *N. gonorrhoeae* (CMRNG) and tetracycline-resistant gonococci may also be treated with the above regimens.

Complicated Gonococcal Disease

Salpingitis (Pelvic Inflammatory Disease [PID]). Women with suspected salpingitis who do not appear to be seriously ill may be treated as outpatients. The agent(s) causing the infection may be gonococci, aerobic or anaerobic vaginal or enteric flora, chlamydia, or any combination of these. If the gonococcus is not identified by endocervical culture, therapy may need to be modified, but antigonococcal therapy should be started as soon as cultures are obtained.

Outpatient regimens include any of the following:

1. Amoxicillin, 3 grams orally.
2. Ampicillin, 3.5 grams orally.
3. Procaine penicillin G, 4.8 million units intramuscularly, or cefoxitin (Mefoxin), 2 grams intramuscularly, each accompanied by 1 gram of oral probenecid.
4. Ceftriaxone (Rocephin), 250 mg intramuscularly.

All of these regimens should be followed by one of the following:

1. Tetracycline, 500 mg orally four times daily for 10 days.
2. Doxycycline (Vibramycin), 100 mg orally for 10 days.

Pregnant women should receive erythromycin, 500 mg twice daily for 10 days, instead of tetracycline.

Hospitalization is recommended for patients who may have pelvic abscess or other surgical complications, signs or symptoms of sepsis, or apparent failure of outpatient treatment. Patients who are pregnant or who cannot tolerate outpatient treatment should also be hospitalized. Some authorities recommend that *all* women with PID be hospitalized.

Effective inpatient therapy consists of one of the following:

1. Intravenous aqueous crystalline penicillin G, 20 million units daily in four to six divided doses, plus doxycycline, 100 mg intravenously twice daily.
2. Cefoxitin (Mefoxin), 2.0 grams intravenously four times daily, plus doxycycline as above.
3. Clindamycin (Cleocin), 600 mg intrave-

nously four times daily, plus gentamicin (Garamycin), 1.5 mg/kg three times daily.

If the patient improves rapidly, a change to oral therapy can be accomplished using the regimens noted previously to complete a 10-day course of combined treatment. Tetracycline should not be used in pregnancy and may need dose adjustment in patients with renal failure, as may gentamicin.

Epididymitis. The cause of epididymitis may be either gonococcal or nongonococcal. Older men tend to have nongonococcal infection, whereas younger men usually have gonococcal epididymitis. Outpatient treatment with scrotal suspension, sitz baths, and analgesics in addition to antibiotics is usually satisfactory. Occasionally, patients require bed rest.

The antibiotic of choice is procaine penicillin G, 4.8 million units intramuscularly, accompanied by 1 gram of probenecid orally and followed by 500 mg of ampicillin orally four times daily for 10 days. If gonococci cannot be demonstrated by Gram's stain or culture of urethral secretions, the regimen of choice is tetracycline hydrochloride, 500 mg orally four times daily for 10 days. Epididymitis caused by PPNG may be effectively treated with intravenous cefoxitin or intramuscular ceftriaxone in the doses listed previously.

Pharyngitis (Symptomatic). Symptoms are treated with warm saline solution gargles and analgesics in addition to antibiotics. It should be noted, however, that gonococcal pharyngitis does not respond well to most of the regimens listed for uncomplicated gonorrhea.

The treatment of choice is procaine penicillin G, 4.8 million units intramuscularly accompanied by 1 gram of probenecid orally. A sucessful alternative regimen is ceftriaxone, 250 mg intramuscularly, or sulfamethoxazole-trimethoprim* (Bactrim, Septra), 9 tablets in a single dose daily for 5 days. These latter two regimens have been shown to be very effective against pharyngitis associated with PPNG.

There is some debate as to whether asymptomatic pharyngeal infection requires treatment. It often resolves spontaneously and may not be readily communicable, although there are several recent reports of pharynx-to-genital infection.

Conjunctivitis. Gonococcal conjunctivitis in adults is being seen with increasing frequency. It may be successfully treated using ceftriaxone (Rocephin), 250 mg intramuscularly daily for 3 to 5 days. There is limited data on the use of tetracycline for treating conjunctivitis, and its use for this purpose should probably be avoided.

---

*Exceeds the maximum daily dose of 800 mg listed in the manufacturer's official directives.

*This use of sulfamethoxazole-trimethoprim is not listed in the manufacturer's official directives.

Disseminated Gonococcal Infection (DGI, Dermatitis/Arthritis Syndrome). The milder forms of this syndrome may be managed on an outpatient basis. Patients who manifest severe or purulent arthritis, high fever, and heart murmur or who might not comply with an outpatient regimen should be hospitalized.

Several outpatient regimens are effective. Amoxicillin, 3 grams; or ampicillin, 3.5 grams orally; or procaine penicillin G, 4.8 million units intramuscularly, each accompanied by 1 gram of probenecid orally initially, should be followed by 500 mg of either amoxicillin or ampicillin four times daily for 7 days. For penicillin-allergic patients, tetracycline, 500 mg four times daily for 7 days, or erythromycin, 500 mg four times daily for 7 days, is adequate therapy.

Hospitalized patients should receive intravenous aqueous crystalline penicillin G, 10 million units daily in four or six divided doses for 7 days. If the patient improves rapidly, therapy can be changed to ampicillin or amoxicillin, 500 mg four times daily, to complete the 7-day course. Ancillary measures for treatment of arthritis, such as bed rest, joint aspiration, or immobilization, should be used as necessary. Irrigation of infected joints with antibiotic solutions is contraindicated. Open drainage of infected joints other than the hip is not necessary.

Disseminated gonococcal infection with PPNG has been reported in small numbers but with increasing frequency. The preferred treatment is cefoxitin (Mefoxin), 1 or 2 grams intravenously every 6 hours for 7 days, or spectinomycin hydrochloride (Trobicin), 2 grams intramuscularly every 12 hours for 7 days, or ceftriaxone (Rocephin), 1.0 gram intravenously daily for 7 days.

Gonorrhea in Pregnancy

Any of the penicillin/ampicillin/amoxicillin regimens is adequate for treating gonococcal infection in a pregnant woman. For therapy in a pregnant woman who is allergic to penicillin, cefoxitin, or ceftriaxone, spectinomycin hydrochloride is an effective alternative. The safety of these drugs in pregnancy has not been thoroughly proved. Erythromycin is useful only in combination with a parenteral therapy.

Gonococcal Infections in Children

Children weighing 45 kg or more should receive adult doses of antibiotics and may be treated as outpatients if not seriously ill. Others should be hospitalized and treated with aqueous crystalline penicillin G, 75,000 to 250,000 units per day in two to four doses for 7 to 10 days. Children allergic to penicillin should be given

spectinomycin hydrochloride* (Trobicin), 40 mg per kg per day intramuscularly (maximum dose, 2 grams) or cefotaxime (Claforan), 200 mg per kg per day intravenously in four divided doses. There have been no reported cases of complicated gonococcal infections caused by PPNG in children.

Epidemiologic Treatment

Patients, particularly women, who have been exposed to known gonococcal infections should be treated as soon as cultures have been obtained, without waiting for culture results, and regardless of whether symptoms are present.

Test-of-Cure Cultures

All patients treated for gonorrhea should have test-of-cure cultures obtained at 3 to 7 days following therapy from each site that was infected prior to treatment. Additionally, women with endocervical gonorrhea should have anal canal cultures obtained at the follow-up visit.

Inadequate Regimens

Antibiotics that are not recommended include benzathine penicillin G, oral penicillin V, bacitracin ophthalmic ointment, penicillin ophthalmic drops, and tetracycline or its analogues in *single-dose* therapy.

NONGONOCOCCAL URETHRITIS

method of
MARC S. COHEN, M.D.
*The University of Texas Medical Branch
Galveston, Texas*

Nongonococcal urethritis (NGU) is largely a diagnosis of exclusion in that it is made when *Neisseria gonorrhoeae* cannot be detected by urethral culture or Gram's stain in a patient with urethritis. Although a number of organisms may be responsible for a nongonococcal urethritis (*Corynebacterium, Staphlococcus, Gardnerella, Herpes simplex, Trichomonas,* yeast), the most commonly implicated organisms are either *Chlamydia trachomatous,* which is recovered from 25 to 60 per cent of new onset cases of urethritis (and less than 5 per cent of recurrent or persistent cases), or *Ureaplasma urealyticum,* which is found in 30 to 40 per cent of acute cases, 40 to 50 per cent of persistent cases, and 10 to 20 per cent of recurrent cases. Nongonococcal urethritis represents more than one half of patients seen for a urethral discharge.

The urethritis associated with nongonococcal organ-

---

*The safety of spectinomycin in children has not been established.

isms usually occurs after an incubation period of 1 to 5 weeks and is generally less symptomatic than that seen with gonorrhea (resulting in longer delays before presentation for medical treatment). Symptoms frequently include dysuria and pruritus. In patients with minimal symptoms, clinical findings may be most evident in the morning, prior to voiding. A urethral discharge need not be present, but when one is encountered, it is usually less profuse and purulent than that seen with gonorrhea. Other clinical findings, such as lymphadenopathy, hematuria, or testicular or perineal pain, suggest concurrent or other causes for the urethritis. The findings of concomitant arthritis, conjunctivitis, and dermatitis may suggest Reiter's syndrome. As part of the physical examination, a thorough inspection of the genitalia for cutaneous lesions and adenopathy should be undertaken. The urethral length is palpated for induration, abscess, or foreign bodies. If a urethral discharge is evident on examination, a collection is made on a glass slide and is examined with methylene blue or preferably Gram's stain. The appearance of more than four polymorphonuclear leukocytes under oil immersion (1000 ×) is consistent with urethritis. The presence of intracellular diplococci (gram-negative) is thought to be highly sensitive (90 to 95 per cent) and specific (95 to 100 per cent) in men with symptomatic gonococcal urethritis. The absence of these organisms is taken as presumptive evidence for nongonococcal urethritis. In this manner, most men with nongonococcal urethritis can be distinguished from those with gonococcal urethritis, and specific therapy can thus be initiated. In equivocal or recurrent cases or in those nonresponsive to therapy, urethral cultures for *N. gonorrhoeae* should be obtained. In such cases, the use of cultures and/or rapid detection systems (fluorescent smear, enzyme immunoassay) for *Chlamydia* species and cultures for *Ureaplasma* species and *Herpes simplex* are available and may be helpful in distinguishing these more complex cases.

Treatment

Once suspected, nongonococcal urethritis is usually treated empirically with tetracycline hydrochloride, 500 mg every 6 hours for 7 days. In individuals in whom a Gram's stain is equivocal or not obtained, the physician may find some reassurance in the fact that this therapy is effective in most cases of gonococcal urethritis as well as nongonococcal urethritis. Minocycline (Minocin) or Doxycycline (Vibramycin), 100 mg twice a day for 7 days, is equally effective for NGU, and patients may be more compliant with the daily dosage regimen but may have to assume increased medication cost. For patients in whom tetracyclines are contraindicated, erythromycin base, 500 mg every 6 hours for 7 days, is usually an effective alternative. Other drugs recognized as being effective against *Chlamydia* species but whose efficacy in treating NGU is not well documented include sulfisoxazole, 500 mg every 6

hours for 10 days, sulfamethoxazole (160 mg)-trimethoprim (800 mg) (Bactrim, Septra), twice a day for 10 days, or rifampin (Rifadin, Rimactane), 600 mg every day for 6 days.

As previously mentioned, recurrent or persistent NGU requires redocumentation and reevaluation. Because *U. urealyticum* is frequently encountered in this situation, a course of erythromycin base, 500 mg every 6 hours for 10 days, in patients refractory to tetracycline or in whom *U. urealyticum* has been isolated may be effective. In the evaluation of patients with persistent or recurrent NGU, it is recommended that wet mounts of the urethral discharge or a urethral smear be examined for motile *Trichomonas vaginalis* and that the exudate be mixed with 10 per cent potassium hydroxide to check for fungal hyphae. In patients with urethritis and negative evaluations for an infectious etiology, a proximal inflammatory source such as urethral stricture disease, urethral neoplasm, prostatitis, or cystitis should be considered.

Nongonococcal urethritis patients with infections should be counseled regarding the transmission of the disease and the necessity for treatment of their sexual partners. Sexual abstinence for the period of treatment and until resolution of symptoms is recommended.

GRANULOMA INGUINALE
(Donovanosis)

method of
THOMAS A. CHAPEL, M.D.
Wayne State University
Detroit, Michigan

Granuloma inguinale is a slowly progressive, ulcerative, anogenital infection caused by an intracellular gram-negative bacillus, *Calymmatobacterium granulomatis*. *Calymmatobacterium granulomatis* is demonstrated by Wright or Giemsa stain of biopsy or crush preparations of granulation tissue taken from the periphery of a lesion. This condition is traditionally classified as a venereal disease, although its sexual transmission is controversial.

Treatment

The treatment of choice is tetracycline, 2 grams daily for 10 to 21 days or until the lesions have healed. Healing is usually apparent within 3 weeks. If tetracycline fails, streptomycin should be used, 0.5 to 1.0 gram intramuscularly twice daily for 10 to 15 days. Alternative therapies, given for 10 to 21 days, include chloramphenicol,

500 mg every 8 hours orally; gentamicin (Gara-mycin), 40 mg twice daily intramuscularly; and co-trimoxazole (trimethoprim 160 mg, sulfameth-oxazole 800 mg) twice daily. In pregnant women, erythromycin, 500 mg every 6 hours, may be effective.

LYMPHOGRANULOMA VENEREUM

method of
THOMAS A. CHAPEL, M.D.
Wayne State University
Detroit, Michigan

Lymphogranuloma venereum (LGV) is a systemic, sexually transmitted disease caused by *Chlamydia trachomatis* strains of the L_1, L_2, or L_3 serovars. The disease is characterized by a small, transient initial lesion usually located on the genitalia or perineum. This is followed by regional lymphadenitis and/or chronic inflammation in the adjacent connective tissue of the infected areas.

Treatment

The recommended treatment regimen is tetracycline hydrochloride, 500 mg four times daily for 3 weeks. Success of therapy can usually be monitored by resolution of clinical signs. If lymphadenopathy fails to respond within 10 to 14 days or if a relapse occurs, an alternative antimicrobial should be used. Alternative regimens include 2- to 6-week courses of either sulfamethoxazole, 1.0 gram orally twice daily, or erythromycin, 500 mg orally four times daily. The latter is preferred in women who are pregnant.

Fluctuant lymph nodes should be aspirated with a large bore needle and a syringe. Rectal stricture sometimes seen with LGV should be managed by dilation at 2-week intervals, and refractory cases may require surgery.

SYPHILIS

method of
EDWARD W. HOOK III, M.D.
The Johns Hopkins Hospital
Baltimore, Maryland

The treatment of syphilis varies with the clinical stage of disease. For therapeutic purposes, clinical staging of syphilis is divided into incubating, early (primary, secondary, or early latent), and late (late latent or tertiary) syphilis based on historical factors, physical examination, and laboratory test results.

Lumbar puncture is recommended as part of the evaluation of patients with late syphilis to determine the presence or absence of neurologic involvement, which would modify the approach to therapy and follow-up.

Currently, penicillin in varying forms, dosages, and durations is the mainstay of syphilotherapy. In general, the long division time (33 hours to 5 days) of *Treponema pallidum,* the causative agent of syphilis, dictates a need for relatively long durations of therapy. Fortunately, however, there is little evidence that *T. pallidum* has developed significant resistance to penicillin or other antibiotics. As a result, parenterally administered benzathine penicillin G, a long-acting preparation that provides low serum levels of penicillin for periods of up to 3 weeks following a single 2.4 million unit injection, may be used to treat most syphilis not involving the central nervous system. Other penicillin formulations, including high-dose penicillin G for neurosyphilis, multiple injections of procaine penicillin, or courses of oral ampicillin or amoxicillin, appear equally useful for syphilis treatment; however, there is far less experience with these regimens than with benzathine penicillin. Nonpenicillin alternatives for syphilis therapy are relatively few and are far less well characterized. Tetracycline hydrochloride in doses of 500 mg four times daily for 15 days may be shown to be nearly as effective as benzathine penicillin G for patients with early syphilis. Other agents for the treatment of early syphilis are cephalexin, an oral cephalosporin, and cephaloridine or ceftriaxone, two parenterally administered cephalosporin antibiotics. Erythromycin is no longer recommended as a result of increased appreciation of unacceptable failure rates. Although many other antibiotics have activity against *T. pallidum* in experimental animals and thus may be effective for syphilis, the body of experience with penicillin therapy relative to all other antibiotics is so great that every effort should be made to treat patients with penicillin. Therapy utilizing benzathine penicillin G has the added advantage of overcoming potential compliance problems, since a single injection provides the prolonged serum levels required for therapy.

INCUBATING SYPHILIS

Patients sexually exposed to partners with early syphilis in the 90 days preceding evaluation are referred to as having incubating syphilis. Patients in this category have no clinical findings suggestive of syphilis and have nonreactive serologic tests for syphilis. Thus, these patients are actually being treated prophylactically rather than for proven infection. If untreated, the probability of developing active syphilis following exposure to a patient with untreated early syphilis is 30 to 50 per cent. The 90-day cutoff for defining incubating syphilis was chosen based on observations that the average time between exposure and development of syphilis is 21 days, although in occasional patients this may be prolonged. It is exceedingly rare for syphilis to develop after more than 90 days following exposure. Patients sexually exposed to partners with syphilis more than 90 days prior to evaluation who have no clinical findings and nonreactive serologic tests need simply to be followed with serologic tests for syphilis rather than be treated prophylactically.

The recommended treatment for patients with incubating syphilis is 2.4 million units of benzathine penicillin G intramuscularly. A not uncommon clinical problem, however, is how to deal with patients treated for gonorrhea who are subsequently discovered to have been exposed to syphilis at the same time. Fortunately, most patients treated for gonorrhea using aqueous procaine penicillin G are probably adequately protected against syphilis exposure and thus may be followed with serial serologic tests rather than having to be treated a second time with benzathine penicillin G. The ampicillin (or amoxicillin)/probenecid or ceftriaxone regimens currently recommended for gonorrhea may also be active against incubating syphilis; however, the utility of these regimens for aborting incubating syphilis is poorly studied, if at all. Spectinomycin has no activity against *T. pallidum,* thus exposed patients treated for gonorrhea with spectinomycin should be retreated for incubating syphilis with agents effective against *T. pallidum.* Tetracycline hydrochloride for a period of 7 days may also be effective for treatment of incubating syphilis. All patients with incubating syphilis should have monthly follow-up serologic tests for a 3-month period following treatment for incubating syphilis.

EARLY SYPHILIS

For therapeutic purposes patients with primary, secondary, or early latent syphilis are collectively considered under the category of early syphilis. Primary syphilis is diagnosed based on the presence of an ulcerative lesion at a site of sexual exposure (a chancre), demonstration of *T. pallidum* using darkfield or immunofluorescence microscopy, and/or a newly reactive serologic test for syphilis. Approximately 20 to 30 per cent of patients with untreated primary syphilis, particularly those who have only had their lesions for a brief (less than 4 to 5 days) period of time, will have nonreactive serologic tests for syphilis. Secondary syphilis is diagnosed based on physical findings, which may include a skin rash (classically located on the palms and soles, but which may also be diffuse and located anywhere else on the body), the presence of mucosal lesions such as condylomata lata or mucous patches, alopecia, generalized lymphadenopathy,

or generalized flulike illness. Some patients with secondary syphilis may still have a resolving chancre present. For practical purposes, nearly all patients with secondary syphilis have reactive serologic tests for syphilis. Patients with early latent syphilis have no clinical findings suggestive of syphilis, but a reactive serologic test for syphilis is present, and it can be *documented* that the patient had a nonreactive serologic test for syphilis at some point in the preceding 12 months. Patients for whom there is no documentation of a recent nonreactive serologic test for syphilis cannot be considered to have early latent syphilis. Their disease is termed syphilis of *unknown duration* and should be treated with regimens effective for late rather than early syphilis.

The therapy of choice for early syphilis is a single intramuscular injection of 2.4 million units of benzathine penicillin G. For patients with documented penicillin allergy, tetracycline hydrochloride, 500 mg four times daily for 15 days, is nearly as effective as benzathine penicillin G. However, this multiple dose, prolonged course of therapy may be compromised by difficulties in patient compliance. Few other well-tested alternatives to the penicillins or tetracyclines are available at the present time, and should a patient be encountered who is unable to be treated using penicillin or tetracyclines, consultation with an expert is advised.

Following treatment, approximately 50 to 60 per cent of patients experience a Jarisch-Herxheimer reaction, which may present with intensification of the rash (if present), feverish feeling, sweats, myalgias, arthralgias, and a generalized flulike illness. The cause of the Jarisch-Herxheimer reaction is unknown; however, conservative treatment with oral fluids and aspirin is generally helpful, and the reaction subsides spontaneously within 24 hours of onset.

Because all early syphilis is felt to be highly infectious, any patient having sexual contact with these individuals within 90 days of diagnosis should be referred for evaluation, including serologic tests for syphilis and careful physical examination. The contacts can then be characterized as either established syphilis (and therefore either a "spread" or "source" case) or as incubating syphilis. In either instance, however, if still untreated at the time of evaluation, these patients should be expeditiously treated.

LATE SYPHILIS

Patients with syphilis of more than 1 year's duration are considered to have late syphilis. Most patients with late syphilis have late latent syphilis with a reactive serologic test for syphilis and no clinical findings. Also included among patients with late syphilis are those with tertiary syphilis, manifested as neurosyphilis, cardiovascular syphilis, or gummatous syphilis. Currently, all forms of tertiary syphilis are relatively rare. Most patients with late latent syphilis will have acquired their disease at some time in the past and are discovered on serologic testing done for screening purposes. Patients in whom there are no clinical findings and no history of prior serologic test for syphilis (syphilis of unknown duration), irrespective of age, should be treated and evaluated as though they had late syphilis. For patients with late syphilis, lumbar puncture is recommended to detect that subset of individuals who have neurosyphilis, which is most often asymptomatic. Although the need for lumbar puncture in patients with latent syphilis is a subject of considerable debate, this conservative approach continues to be the recommendation of the Centers for Disease Control. Recommended therapy for patients with late latent syphilis, syphilis of unknown duration, and tertiary syphilis other than neurosyphilis is benzathine penicillin G, 2.4 million units intramuscularly weekly for 3 consecutive weeks. For patients with penicillin allergy, alternative therapy is tetracycline, 500 mg orally four times daily for 30 days. Patients with neurosyphilis require more intensive therapy.

All recent sex partners of patients with late syphilis should undergo serologic testing for syphilis. Patients with reactive serologic tests should be staged in the same manner as other patients with syphilis. Treatment of seronegative sexual partners of patients with late syphilis is generally not required because the late stages of syphilis are considerably less infectious than the early stages. For sexual contacts of patients with syphilis of unknown duration, however, the safest approach, because of the possibility that the index patient may have early rather than late syphilis, is to treat these individuals using benzathine penicillin G.

NEUROSYPHILIS

Neurologic involvement in syphilis may be present at all stages of disease. Thus, patients with primary, secondary, or early latent as well as late syphilis may present with neurologic abnormalities attributable to central nervous system involvement. Neurosyphilis is generally subdivided into asymptomatic neurosyphilis; meningeal syphilis, which may present as a subacute or chronic meningitis; meningovascular syphilis, in which blood vessel involvement may result in a strokelike presentation; or parenchy-

mal neurosyphilis, which may manifest as either tabes dorsalis or general paresis. Gummatous neurosyphilis is rarely seen. In patients with neurologic involvement, the most common categorizations are asymptomatic, meningeal, and meningovascular syphilis. Of patients with neurosyphilis, the other organs most often involved are the eyes (iritis, retinitis, or oculomotor abnormalities) and the eighth cranial nerves. Lumbar puncture is of diagnostic importance in patients with suspected neurosyphilis, and the presence of any cerebral spinal fluid (CSF) abnormality, whether cells, protein, or a reactive CSF-VDRL, is evidence supporting the diagnosis of neurosyphilis. Due to low central nervous system penicillin levels in patients treated with benzathine penicillin G, neurosyphilis should be treated using higher doses of antibiotics than recommended for syphilis not involving the central nervous system. For patients with neurosyphilis, recommended therapy consists of either aqueous penicillin G, 10 to 20 million units intravenously per day in divided doses or alternatively, for patients who wish to remain outpatients, aqueous procaine pencillin G, 2.4 million units intramuscularly daily for 10 to 14 days given concomitantly with probenecid, 500 mg orally four times a day. Following completion of 10 to 14 days of high-dose therapy, continued therapy using 2.4 million units of benzathine penicillin G weekly for 3 weeks is recommended by the Centers for Disease Control although many experts feel that this additional therapy is not necessary. Although still listed by the Centers for Disease Control as an alternative therapy for neurosyphilis, treatment using 2.4 million units of benzathine penicillin G weekly for 3 weeks is not recommended by the author on the basis of multiple studies showing that this regimen fails to reliably provide measurable cerebrospinal fluid penicillin levels. Patients with neurosyphilis should have follow-up serologic tests for syphilis performed at monthly intervals for the first 3 months, then at 3-month intervals for at least 2 years. In addition, follow-up lumbar punctures are recommended at 6-month intervals to document resolution of CSF abnormalities.

SYPHILIS IN PREGNANCY

Pregnant women with syphilis are likely to give birth to children with congenital syphilis, a disease that has increased in recent years. Screening serologic tests for syphilis are recommended for all pregnant women in the first trimester of pregnancy, and for high-risk patients a second serologic test should be obtained during the third trimester. Treatment for pregnant women with syphilis should utilize the same regimens as recommended for nonpregnant patients. There is no documented need for more intensive therapy of pregnant patients. Children born to mothers with syphilis during pregnancy, however, should be carefully evaluated both clinically and serologically following birth for the possibility of congenital syphilis; cases of congenital syphilis have been reported in children born to mothers treated for syphilis during pregnancy. These mothers, as well as their children, need retreatment.

Pregnant women who have received appropriate treatment for syphilis in the past need not be retreated unless there is clinical, serologic, or epidemiologic evidence of relapse or reinfection. This evidence includes lesions found to be positive on darkfield examination, a fourfold rise in titer of a serologic test for syphilis, or history of recent exposure to a partner with early syphilis. Since tetracycline is not recommended during pregnancy, treatment with erythromycin was formerly suggested for patients with penicillin allergy; however, because of increasing numbers of treatment failures, this is no longer recommended. Presently, it is suggested that penicillin-allergic pregnant women be hospitalized, carefully desensitized to penicillin, and treated using penicillin. If this is impossible, treatment with erythromycin is a poor compromise, and very close follow-up of both the patient and the child are essential.

SYPHILIS IN PATIENTS WITH HUMAN IMMUNODEFICIENCY VIRUS (HIV) INFECTION

Recent reports suggest that the natural history and response to treatment of syphilis may be modified by concurrent HIV infection. Genital ulcerations irrespective of cause are emerging as contributors to enhanced risk for acquisition of HIV, perhaps by facilitating virus transmission through disrupted epithelial surfaces. Case reports describing delayed serologic response to infection, possibly accelerated courses of disease, and failures of recommended therapy in HIV-infected patients should be considered numerator figures. The impact of HIV infection on syphilis and the response to currently recommended therapy are unknown. In the interim, patients with syphilis and concurrent HIV infection should be carefully followed for treatment failure or possible relapse. Should documented treatment failure occur, retreatment using doses of penicillin recommend for neurosyphilis should be considered.

RESPONSE TO TREATMENT

In patients with early syphilis, resolution of cutaneous manifestations of infection may take 2 to 3 weeks. Serologic follow-up is recommended at 3, 6, and 12 months following treatment. In early syphilis patients, quantitative serologic tests for syphilis (VDRL or RPR tests) will generally decline to nonreactive or low (1:1 or 1:2) titers within 1 year following treatment with penicillin. Serologic tests may decline more slowly if patients have had syphilis in the past or if they are treated with alternative antimicrobial agents. In patients with late syphilis, serologic response to therapy tends to be somewhat slower than in patients with early syphilis, thus serologic follow-up should include quantitative serologic tests for syphilis at 3, 6, 12, 18, and 24 months. Retreatment of patients treated for syphilis should be considered if clinical signs or symptoms of syphilis persist or recur, if there is a fourfold increase in quantitative serologic tests for syphilis, or if an initial high titer nontreponemal test for syphilis fails to show a fourfold decrease in titer within 1 year following treatment. Patients who require retreatment should be treated as recommended for late syphilis. In patients in whom treatment fails, strong consideration should also be given to cerebrospinal fluid examination.

SIMULTANEOUS INFECTIONS

Patients at risk for syphilis are often at risk for other sexually transmissible infections as well. Until recently, syphilis was more common among homosexual or bisexual men than among heterosexuals. This trend seems to have changed recently. In addition, however, it has also been noted that genital ulcerations may act as cofactors for acquisition of infection with the human immunodeficiency virus (HIV). Thus, patients with syphilis should be carefully screened for other potential infections: not only infection with HIV but also the possibility of gonorrhea, chlamydia, genital warts, or other sexually transmitted diseases. In addition, other transmissible agents that are common in patients with syphilis may well include hepatitis A and B, Epstein-Barr virus, and cytomegalovirus infections. Patients with concurrent infections should be treated and counseled appropriately for those diseases in addition to receiving appropriate therapy for syphilis.

Diseases of Allergy

ANAPHYLAXIS, ANAPHYLACTOID REACTIONS, AND SERUM SICKNESS

method of
D. BETTY LEW, M.D., and
HENRY G. HERROD, M.D.
University of Tennessee
Memphis, Tennessee

ANAPHYLAXIS AND ANAPHYLACTOID REACTIONS

Anaphylaxis is a potentially life-threatening systemic reaction that is mediated by antigen-induced IgE or possibly IgG_4. The clinical reaction usually has its onset within a short period, often minutes, after exposure to antigen in previously sensitized individuals. Symptoms and signs of anaphylaxis are most often diaphoresis, flushing of skin, pruritus, urticaria, angioedema, stridor, wheeze, cough, shortness of breath, chest tightness, hypotension, shock, arrhythmias, dysphonia, dysphagia, abdominal pain, vomiting, diarrhea, and/or incontinence. Anaphylactoid reactions are nonimmunologically mediated reactions resulting in similar end-organ responses. The most frequent causative agents are listed in Table 1.

Precautions/Prevention

1. Avoidance
   a. A structurally unrelated drug should be used as a substitute for any drug to which the patient has had reactions.
   b. Whenever possible, drugs should be administered orally rather than by a parenteral route.
   c. Patients should be educated concerning cross-reacting allergens to a known allergen or anaphylactoid agent.
   d. Individuals sensitive to hymenoptera should be appropriately instructed to minimize the likelihood of insect stings.
2. A patient receiving a drug or injection in an office setting should remain in the office for 30 minutes after medication for observation.

3. Predisposed patients should carry an anaphylactic kit consisting of a preloaded epinephrine injector (EpiPen) at all times.
4. Patients with documented anaphylaxis to hymenoptera venom should receive appropriate venom immunotherapy. Desensitization to some drugs, insulin, and animal antisera has been successful.
5. If a radiographic contrast study is essential in an individual with a history of a previous reaction, pretreat with:
   a. Diphenhydramine (Benadryl), 50 mg intramuscularly 1 hour before the study.
   b. Prednisone, 50 mg orally every 6 hours beginning 19 hours before the study (the third dose is given 1 hour before the study).
   c. Cimetidine, 300 mg orally, may be added 1 hour before the study.
   d. For emergency procedures when adequate time for pretreatment with oral prednisone and antihistamine is not available, hydrocortisone 200 mg or methylprednisolone 40 mg IV should be administered before

TABLE 1. **Common Causative Agents of Anaphylaxis or Anaphylactoid Reactions**

Anaphylaxis (IgE-Mediated)	Anaphylactoid (Non–IgE-Mediated)
Antibiotics—penicillin, cephalosporin, tetracycline, etc.	Radiographic contrast media
Heterologous antisera	Opiates
Adrenocorticotropic hormone (ACTH)	Highly charged antibiotics
Insulin	Muscle relaxant
Chymopapain (meat tenderizer, soft contact lens cleaning agents, etc.)	Dextrans
Stinging insect venom	Captopril
Foods—milk, egg white, shellfish, nuts, wheat, etc.	Aspirin
Allergen extracts	Food or drug additives—tartrazine, benzoate, and sulfite
Local anesthetics (may be either IgE-mediated or non–IgE-mediated)	Recurrent idiopathic reactions
Sulfite (may be either IgE-mediated or non–IgE-mediated)	
Exercise (commonly associated with ingestion of shellfish or celery prior to exercise)	

the procedure and at 4-hour intervals until the procedure is completed. Diphenhydramine, 50 mg intramuscularly, should also be given before the procedure.

6. Para-aminophenyl–free local anesthetics are preferable for those with a history of a reaction to a local anesthetic. These include lidocaine, mepivacaine, and dibucaine. The drug should be administered in a carefully monitored serial dilution fashion over a period of 2 hours.

7. Predisposed individuals should avoid propranolol or other beta-blocking agents, as these drugs interfere with the action of epinephrine, which is used to control anaphylactic reactions.

8. Exercise-induced anaphylaxis is being more commonly reported. Individuals should be educated to avoid ingestion of suspected foods (e.g., alcohol, shellfish, or celery) prior to exercise. Wearing a tight garment should be discouraged. The individual should stop exercising at the first warning symptoms and signs of exercise-induced anaphylaxis. A desensitization program consisting of a gradual increase in exercise level may be useful. For scheduled activities, albuterol (Proventil, Ventolin) inhaler 2 puffs 5 minutes before exercise and/or cromolyn (Intal) 20 mg by Spinhaler 30 minutes before exercise is recommended.

9. All predisposed individuals should wear Medic-Alert bracelets or necklaces.

Treatment

1. Administration of subcutaneous or intramuscular epinephrine at the first sign of anaphylaxis can prevent more serious manifestations from occurring. The dose is 0.01 ml per kg up to 0.5 ml of a 1:1000 concentration. If the reaction is secondary to an insect sting or follows an injection, a dose of 0.1 ml into the site of injection may be useful. Injections may be repeated every 15 minutes until an effect is achieved or until arrhythmias, tachycardia, or other untoward side effects supervene. For severe cardiovascular shock or loss of consciousness, intravenous administration of 0.01 ml per kg up to 0.3 ml in children and 0.5 ml in adults of a 1:10,000 solution should be given cautiously over a period of approximately 5 minutes.

2. When anaphylaxis follows an injection or insect sting, a tourniquet should be placed proximal to the site of the injection or sting. This tourniquet should be removed for a 2- to 3-minute period every 10 to 15 minutes.

3. Nasal oxygen should be started.

4. The patient should be placed in the recumbent position with the feet elevated. The head of the patient should be turned to the side to prevent aspiration of vomitus.

5. Adequate intravenous access should be established.

6. Vital signs should be monitored every 10 to 15 minutes for the duration of the attack.

7. The airway should be checked immediately and at frequent intervals after the attack.

8. An antihistamine, such as diphenhydramine (Benadryl) at a dose of 10 to 25 mg for infants and younger children and 25 to 50 mg for older children and adults, should be administered intravenously.

9. The development of airway obstruction requires the establishment of an artificial airway. Tracheostomy may be performed if intubation cannot be done. When severe bronchospasm is part of the clinical picture, administration of intravenous aminophylline may be of benefit. The dose of the initial bolus is 4 to 7 mg per kg given at a rate of 10 mg per minute, followed by a continuous intravenous aminophylline drip, 0.5 to 1.0 mg per kg per hour.

10. In the treatment of shock, fluids and plasma expanders are mandatory. Intravenous administration of a colloid material, preferably albumin, is indicated. However, rapid infusion of isotonic saline, 20 ml per kg in children and 500 ml in adults, can be used initially. This is followed by slow infusion adjusted according to clinical responses. A vasopressor agent such as metaraminol (Aramine), 0.4 mg per kg, mixed in 500 ml of 5 per cent dextrose water or saline injection solution and given slowly, may be used in patients with severe hypotension.

11. A large dose of intravenous glucocorticosteroid in the form of methylprednisone, 2 mg per kg up to 120 mg, or an equivalent dose of hydrocortisone (Solu-Cortef) should be administered initially and every 4 hours as needed.

12. The patient who responds poorly to the above procedures should have therapy continued in an intensive care unit with appropriate careful monitoring of cardiovascular status and blood gases.

SERUM SICKNESS

Acute serum sickness results when antigen-antibody complexes formed in the circulation disseminate, localize in tissue, and produce inflammation. Historically, serum sickness was first described by von Pirquet and Schick in 1905 when they postulated that the clinical symptoms of rash, fever, lymphadenopathy, joint involvement, and rarely glomerulonephritis and neuritis in patients who had received therapeutic horse serum administration were initiated by the interaction of the foreign protein and host antibody.

Today serum sickness–like reactions are most likely to occur following administration of nonprotein drugs such as penicillin. The most common manifestations are urticaria, angioedema, fever, arthralgias, and lymphadenopathy. Rarely neurologic complications such as Guillain-Barré syndrome, glomerular disease, and myocardial damage may occur. The syndrome develops 7 to 10 days following primary exposure to the antigens and persists for 4 to 14 days. The diagnosis is based on an exposure history and clinical symptoms.

Treatment

Human immune serum to various agents such as tetanus toxoid can now be used in place of horse serum. Whenever possible serum from human sources should be utilized rather than serum from animal sources. Most cases of serum sickness resolve spontaneously within 2 weeks of onset. Aspirin at 30 to 60 mg per kg per day in children and 600 mg every 4 to 6 hours in adults generally relieves joint symptoms. Antihistamines such as diphenhydramine at a dose of 25 mg four times per day may be given for pruritus; this treatment may even be effective as a prophylaxis in patients who must receive heterologous serum.

In more severe cases, corticosteroids, 1 to 2 mg per kg up to 60 mg per day in adults, may be necessary. The drug can frequently be tapered rapidly, but in severe cases therapy of up to 10 to 14 days may be indicated because of the frequency of relapse during corticosteroid withdrawal.

ASTHMA IN THE ADOLESCENT AND THE ADULT

method of
MARTA M. LITTLE, M.D., and
THOMAS B. CASALE, M.D.
University of Iowa College of Medicine
Iowa City, Iowa

Asthma symptoms most frequently develop during childhood and often diminish or resolve completely dur-

ing adolescence. Nevertheless, symptomatic asthma frequently recurs or develops de novo in adults. Among adults, asthma remains a relatively common disease and is estimated to affect approximately 5 per cent of the general population.

Diagnosis

Currently there is no universally accepted definition of asthma. Nevertheless, *airway hyperresponsiveness* to various stimuli and *reversible airway obstruction* are clinical features that have become the cornerstones for diagnosis of asthma. While the exact mechanisms underlying airway hyperresponsiveness in asthma are not known, factors that potentially contribute include abnormalities in airway geometry, airway epithelium, airway smooth muscle, and autonomic nervous system regulation of airway tone. Potential imbalances in autonomic neural control of airway tone, specifically beta-adrenergic hyporesponsiveness and cholinergic hyperresponsiveness, have particular clinical relevance, since current diagnostic and therapeutic maneuvers commonly involve the use of agonists and antagonists of these nervous systems.

The degree of airway hyperresponsiveness, the frequency and severity of airway obstruction, and the large variety of stimuli that may trigger acute episodes make asthma a very heterogeneous disease clinically. Asthma has traditionally been classified as *extrinsic* when allergic sensitivity is involved in triggering asthmatic episodes, and *intrinsic* when no allergic cause is readily apparent. It may also be classified in terms of severity and chronicity as *intermittent* asthma when acute obstructive episodes are separated in time by relatively long symptom-free periods without airway obstruction, and as *chronic* asthma when obstruction is more frequent and prolonged without complete resolution between episodes. Classification of asthma by both its triggers and its chronicity bears important therapeutic implications for individual patients.

While many patients with asthma present with a very charactertistic clinical history of episodic wheezing and dyspnea, it is important to remember that not all patients with asthma present in this way. Patients may instead complain of vague tightness in the chest or of recurrent cough without overt wheezing. Also, it is important to remember the old adage, "not all that wheezes is asthma," since a number of disease processes may similarly present with wheezing. Thorough consideration of alternative diagnoses is particularly important in the adult patient at risk for cardiovascular disease or chronic lung disease related to smoking. In addition to a thorough history and physical examination, a plain chest roentgenograph, pulmonary function testing, and sputum analysis may be particularly helpful in assessing the diagnostic possibilities. In uncomplicated asthma, the chest roentgenograph may show hyperinflation but is otherwise normal. During an asymptomatic period, spirometric (forced vital capacity [FVC] and forced expiratory volume in 1 second [FEV_1]) and peak flow measurements may be totally normal, but residual volume (RV) and total lung capacity (TLC) are frequently increased owing to air trapping. Diffusion capacity is normal to increased.

During a period of acute asthma, there is a significant reduction in FEV_1, peak expiratory flow rate, and FEV_1/FVC ratio. Sputum from asthmatics is remarkable for the presence of eosinophils. Characteristic Charcot-Leyden crystals and Curschmann's spirals may also be noted.

To establish a definitive diagnosis of asthma, it is essential to demonstrate reversible airway obstruction or airway hyperreactivity, which are the hallmarks of this disease. Airway reversibility and hyperreactivity can often be easily demonstrated by monitoring changes in pulmonary functions before and after inhalation of therapeutic or provocative agents. When initial spirometric measurements are abnormal, administration of an inhaled $beta_2$ agonist followed by repeat spirometry 15 minutes later is useful in assessing reversibility. Traditionally, an increase in FEV_1 or flow rates by 15 to 20 per cent or greater has been considered diagnostic. A few patients with chronic airway obstruction will not respond to inhaled beta agonist medication, but will have significant reversal of airway obstruction following a trial of oral prednisone, 40 to 60 mg daily for 1 to 2 weeks. Such a corticosteroid trial may be critical in distinguishing asthma from nonreversible chronic obstructive lung disease. When initial spirometric measurements are normal, hyperreactivity of the airways can be confirmed by bronchoprovocation challenges with methacholine (cholinergic agonist), histamine, or exercise testing. In a patient with a suggestive clinical history, a decline in FEV_1 or flow rates by 20 per cent or greater during the provocative test is strongly supportive of a diagnosis of asthma, especially if the decline occurs in response to low concentrations of the provocative agent or during minimal exercise.

Treatment

Chronic Maintenance Therapy

The goal of maintenance therapy should be to provide long-term, symptom-free existence with minimal side effects from the medications used. Greatest success is achieved when the therapeutic approach includes both avoidance of provoking stimuli and a carefully individualized therapeutic regimen. The first step is a comprehensive history and physical examination, particularly aimed at identifying triggers of acute attacks and at gauging the intensity of therapy required. A history of the degree of symptom control achieved with previous therapeutic regimens is also useful. To identify triggers that may precipitate asthma in an individual patient, it is particularly important to note the following:

1. Exposures to potential provocative agents found in the home and workplace (e.g., pets, dust, mold, irritants, and industrial chemicals such as isocyanates).

2. Smoking (active or passive exposure).

3. Seasonal pattern to symptoms suggesting sensitivity to aeroallergens.

4. Relationship of asthma symptoms to exercise.

5. Relationship of asthma symptoms to ingestion of foods, preservatives, and medications, especially metabisulfites, aspirin, and beta blockers.

6. Relationship of asthma symptoms to upper and lower respiratory infections.

Skin testing for allergic sensitivity to inhalant allergens is a useful adjunct to a thorough history in identifying triggers of asthma. Once identified, these provocative agents should be removed or avoided as much as is practically possible. Avoidance measures may involve counseling the patient in ways to minimize exposure to dust, molds, or animal danders in the home environment or to irritants and sensitizing chemicals in the workplace. It may involve instructions to stop smoking or to discontinue use of prescription and nonprescription drugs felt to be exacerbating factors.

Pharmacologic therapy of asthma begins with an aerosolized $beta_2$ agonist as the first-line medication. Every adult asthmatic should have ready access to and know how to use an aerosolized $beta_2$ agonist. Whether or not this and other medications will be required on a regular basis for maintenance therapy can largely be predicted from the chronicity of symptoms (intermittent versus chronic) and previous medication needs. Thus, a previously untreated patient who experiences only mild intermittent asthma may require a $beta_2$ agonist inhaler only for acute symptoms. A patient with chronic asthma, however, would benefit from regular use of an aerosolized $beta_2$ agonist every 4 to 6 hours plus stepwise addition of additional agents as needed. The aim of therapy is to provide long-term symptom-free periods. In severe asthma, however, this may mean weighing residual asthmatic symptoms against the side effects caused by further increases in therapy, especially therapy with corticosteroids.

Beta$_2$-Adrenergic Agonists. Most of the beta-adrenergic agonist medications currently used in asthma are beta$_2$ selective. However, this selectivity is relative and varies with the dosage and route of administration. Thus, while the predominant action of these medications is to stimulate lung beta$_2$ receptors, other beta receptors may also be stimulated, resulting in side effects of palpitations and tremor. These medications are thought to be therapeutic in asthma by increasing cAMP levels in airway smooth muscle and in mast cells, causing bronchodilation and inhibiting mast cell mediator release, respectively. Beta-adrenergic agonists are available in 3 forms: (1) aerosol formulations including metered dose inhalers (MDIs) and solutions for delivery by a compressor-driven jet nebulizer, (2) oral tablets, and (3) preparations for parenteral (subcutaneous) administration. Parenteral therapy is most appropriate for emergency room management and will be discussed under therapy for the acute attack. Table 1 shows the aerosol and oral beta$_2$ agonist medications currently available and their recommended dosages. In general, the beta$_2$ agonist aerosols are preferred over the oral tablets, since the oral preparations may not be as effective as aerosols and cause more side effects. The aerosol medications are administered directly to the airway by inhalation and result in more rapid onset of bronchodilation at relatively small doses.

Maximal deposition of aerosolized drug in the airways and maximal therapeutic effect are achieved only when proper inhalation technique is followed. For optimal use of an MDI, the patient should hold the inhaler 2 inches in front of his or her open mouth, inhale slowly from end tidal volume to total lung capacity, trigger the inhaler to deliver medication at the beginning of the inhalation, and hold his or her breath for 10 seconds before exhaling. Patients should be thoroughly instructed and made to demonstrate proper MDI use during future clinic visits. Patients who find it difficult to precisely coordinate inhalation and actuation of the inhaler may benefit from use of a volume reservoir or spacer. When attached to the MDI, the spacer acts as a holding chamber from which the aerosolized medication can be inhaled without the need for coordination of activation and inhalation. Administration of aerosolized beta$_2$ agonists via a powered nebulizer unit also obviates the need for coordinated ventilatory maneuvers, but this is typically reserved for treatment of acute asthma attacks. Nebulizers are less suited for chronic maintenance therapy, as they are not portable and much more expensive.

When administered as aerosols in recommended dosage, the selective beta$_2$ agonists listed in Table 1 (albuterol, bitolterol, metaproterenol, terbutaline and pirbuterol) differ from each other only slightly in potency and length of action. For many patients, these medications are equally effective, and individual patient preference and cost may be the best determinants for selecting one for chronic use.

Theophylline. Theophylline has been used in the treatment of asthma for more than 50 years and has a proven record of effectiveness. Despite this long history of use, precisely how theophylline mediates its therapeutic effect remains unclear. Today, theophylline's most important role is as oral maintenance therapy in the management of patients with chronic asthma. Intravenous administration of theophylline for acute attacks of asthma is discussed later.

An important guide to optimal therapy with theophylline is measurement of the serum theophylline level. Theophylline is most effective when serum levels are in the range of 10 to 20 micrograms per ml, although some patients are benefited at lower levels. Serum theophylline levels above 20 micrograms per ml should be avoided because of frequent side effects and potentially serious toxicity. While these serum levels are reliable therapeutic standards, the theophylline dosage regimen that maintains these serum levels varies considerably among patients and among different formulations of theophylline. A typical maintenance dosage of oral theophylline for a generally healthy, nonsmoking adult is 10 to 12 mg per kg per day, usually administered in divided doses. Multiple factors may, however, alter the pharmacokinetics of the drug. Factors that decrease theophylline metabolism and result in a lower dosage requirement include advanced age, liver disease, congestive heart failure, and concurrent use of macrolide antibiotics (erythromycin) or cimetidine. Factors that increase theophylline metabolism and result in higher dosage requirements include younger age, smoking, and concurrent use of certain other medications such as phenytoin.

TABLE 1. **Beta$_2$-Adrenergic Agonists**

| Drug | Dosage per Treatment (mg) | | | Duration of Action (hr) |
	Metered Dose Inhaler	*Nebulizer*	*Oral*	
Albuterol (Proventil, Ventolin)	0.18 (2 puffs)	2.5	2–4	4–6
Bitolterol (Tornalate)	0.74–1.11 (2–3 puffs)			4–6
Metaproterenol (Alupent, Metaprel)	1.3–1.95 (2–3 puffs)	10–15	10–20	3–4
Terbutaline (Brethaire, Brethine)	0.40 (2 puffs)		2.5–5	4–6
Pirbuterol (Maxair)	0.2–0.4 (1–2 puffs)			4–6

Theophylline is available in rapidly absorbed, short-acting formulations and in slow-release, sustained-action formulations. The slow-release compounds are preferred for maintenance therapy because of longer dosing intervals (resulting in better patient compliance) and less variation in serum concentrations. A large number of slow-release theophylline (either bead-filled capsules or tablets) are currently available (Table 2). The manufacturers recommend 12-hour dosing intervals for most of these slow-release theophyllines. However, some patients with very rapid elimination of the drug may require 8-hour dosing intervals. In addition to the 8- to 12-hour slow-release theophyllines, two 24-hour ultra-slow-release theophyllines are now on the market in the United States. These once-a-day preparations have been associated with variable absorption and greater fluctuation in serum concentrations. They may not be optimal for use in patients who require tight maintenance of therapeutic serum theophylline concentrations to avoid breakthrough asthma, but may be used to treat selected patients with milder disease. Maintenance theophylline therapy should be initiated gradually by incremental increases in dosage over 1 to 2 weeks. This avoids many of the minor adverse side effects (nervousness, tremor, gastrointestinal symptoms) associated with rapid initiation of therapy. After the anticipated maintenance dosage has been reached, serum theophylline measurements should be used to make any final dose adjustments.

Cromolyn Sodium. Cromolyn is a prophylactic agent for asthma that may, in part, act by stabilizing mast cell membranes. Cromolyn has no bronchodilator action of its own and is thus of no benefit in acute asthma. In fact, because of its irritating effects on the airway, it should be avoided during acute attacks. Cromolyn is poten-tially useful as a substitute for theophylline in chronic maintenance therapy, especially in children, for whom it has been shown to be most effective. While cromolyn has generally been disappointing in the management of asthma in adults, there are a few situations in which it may be the drug of choice. In particular, if the patient can identify a certain event or exposure that precipitates asthma attacks, then the prophylactic use of cromolyn can be highly effective. For example, cromolyn can be effectively used just prior to exercise or prior to anticipated exposure to a pet or laboratory animal known to trigger asthmatic symptoms.

Cromolyn is poorly absorbed when given orally and must be given by inhalation. Cromolyn is available as a powdered capsule for use in a Spinhaler, but this has largely been superseded by the introduction of a cromolyn MDI (Intal). The dose for the MDI is 2 puffs four times daily, and a 6-week trial is necessary before efficacy can be adequately assessed.

Corticosteroids. Rational use of corticosteroids in asthma takes into account two variables: Corticosteroids are the most potent agents in the asthma pharmacopeia, but their use for long periods is associated with severe side effects such as weight gain, cataracts, osteoporosis, glucose intolerance, hypertension, poor wound healing, and immunosuppression. Fortunately, short (1- to 2-week) courses of high-dose corticosteroids (such as oral prednisone, 40 to 60 mg per day) followed by a rapid taper are both well-tolerated and extremely effective in managing exacerbations of asthma. In patients with frequent exacerbations of asthma who require frequent short courses of prednisone, chronic maintenance therapy with steroid inhalation should be tried. Inhaled steroid therapy can be administered chronically without the severe side effects associated with chronic systemic corticosteroid use. The major side effects of inhaled steroids are dysphonia and oral candidiasis. The risks of these side effects can be minimized by using a spacer and by rinsing the mouth after inhaler use.

The steroid inhalers currently available in the United States and their recommended dosages are shown in Table 3. The recommended dosage

TABLE 2. Slow-Release Theophylline Compounds

| Brand Name | Available Doses (mg) | |
	Capsules	Tablets
Elixophyllin SR	125, 250	
Slo-bid Gyrocaps	50, 100, 200, 300	
Slo-Phyllin Gyrocaps	60, 125, 250	
Somophyllin-CRT	100, 200, 250, 300	
Theobid Duracaps	130, 260	
Theo-Dur Sprinkle	50, 75, 125, 200	
Theovent LA	125, 250	
Theo-24*	100, 200, 300	
Theo-Dur		100, 200, 300
Theolair-SR		200, 250, 300, 500
Uniphyl*		200, 400

*Once-a-day preparations.

TABLE 3. Corticosteroid Inhalers

Drug	Recommended Dosage
Beclomethasone dipropionate (Vanceril, Beclovent)	2 puffs (84 μg) 3 or 4 times daily
Flunisolide (AeroBid)	2 puffs (500 μg) twice daily
Triamcinolone acetonide (Azmacort)	2 puffs (200 μg) 3 or 4 times daily

can be doubled if necessary to suppress activity of the disease, but side effects of systemic steroid treatment may become evident with chronic administration of higher doses. The patient who is well maintained on inhaled steroids may occasionally need a short burst and taper of oral prednisone for exacerbations of asthma. It should be noted that inhaled steroids, although useful in maintenance therapy, are not as useful in treatment of acute exacerbations of asthma. We generally recommend that inhaled steroids be preceded by inhaled beta agonists.

For a minority of steroid-dependent patients, inhaled steroids are not sufficient, and chronic oral prednisone is necessary for adequate control of symptoms. If possible, such patients should be maintained on alternate-day prednisone therapy to decrease adrenal suppression and side effects. Patients with the most severe steroid-dependent asthma may, however, notice significant diminution of lung function on the alternate days off steroids. These patients often require daily prednisone, usually 10 to 15 mg per day, for maintenance therapy. Overall, the goal should be to determine the minimum dose of prednisone necessary to control asthma adequately while being very careful not to withhold steroids when they are needed. Indeed, inappropriate withholding of corticosteroids and too rapid withdrawal of corticosteroids have been repeatedly implicated as contributing factors in cases of fatal asthma.

Anticholinergic Agents. Since the cholinergic nervous system is the most important regulator of airway tone, and asthmatics have cholinergic hyperresponsiveness, anticholinergic agents should theoretically be effective in treatment of asthma. Anticholinergic agents in the form of datura leaves and stramonium were among the earliest bronchodilators used. Nevertheless, administration of atropine and related tertiary ammonium compounds is associated with troublesome side effects that limit their usefulness in asthma. The recent introduction of ipratropium bromide, a quaternary ammonium compound that is poorly absorbed and is associated with negligible systemic side effects, has allowed further analysis of the efficacy of anticholinergic agents in asthma. The amount of bronchodilation produced by ipratropium inhalation varies from subject to subject. In general, older asthmatics and those with intrinsic asthma seem to have the most favorable response. For most patients, anticholinergic agents are less potent than $beta_2$-adrenergic agents, but the combination may have an additive bronchodilatory effect. A particular situation in which anticholinergic agents may be significantly more effective than $beta_2$-adrenergic agents is in bronchospasm resulting from, or occurring in a patient on, beta blockers.

In general, inclusion of ipratropium in maintenance therapy should be considered for patients who have not had full bronchodilatory response to $beta_2$ agonists and theophylline. It is important, however, to evaluate its efficacy in the individual patient before commitment to long-term therapy. Efficacy can be estimated by measuring the bronchodilatory response 30 to 60 minutes (the time to peak effect) after inhalation of ipratropium. The recommended dose for ipratropium administered via an MDI (Atrovent) is 2 puffs (36 micrograms) four times daily.

Other Agents. Desensitization to allergens, which has been shown to be effective in the treatment of allergic rhinitis, may also benefit selected patients whose asthma is exacerbated by common aeroallergens. Other therapeutic considerations that should not be overlooked are the importance of physical conditioning and attention to recommended vaccination schedules. With proper instruction to avoid cold air and in using a $beta_2$ agonist or cromolyn inhaler prior to exercise, even patients with chronic asthma can tolerate some form of regular exercise, particularly swimming. This type of regular exercise program is rewarded by improved functional capacity. Patients with chronic asthma and other chronic pulmonary diseases should receive the polyvalent pneumococcal vaccine and annual influenza vaccinations. New therapies being investigated for potential efficacy in chronic management of asthma, including calcium channel blockers, antiallergic agents (azelastine, ketotifen), and methotrexate, may prove to be significantly useful in steroid-dependent asthmatics.

Emergency Room and Hospital Management of Acute Asthma

Initial rapid assessment of the patient with acute asthma should include a pertinent history and physical examination aimed at ruling out other causes of wheezing and dyspnea (pneumonia, pulmonary embolism, congestive heart failure) and at assessing the severity of the asthma attack. Historical details that are helpful in assessing severity and in predicting how well the asthmatic obstruction will respond to bronchodilator therapy include the duration of symptoms, precipitating factors, current medications, and severity of previous attacks. For example, an asthmatic patient who presents to an emergency room with a several-day history of a viral upper respiratory infection and asthmatic symptoms that have worsened despite frequent use of a beta agonist inhaler at home is unlikely to have immediate and full response to bronchodilator therapy in the emergency room. The maximum bronchodilation possible from relaxation of bronchial smooth muscle may already have been achieved. The remaining obstruction is predominantly the result of inflammation, mucosal edema, and mucus plugging, and successful management will require use of corticosteroids.

Of the findings on physical examinations, the most ominous is a disturbance of consciousness, as this suggests respiratory failure and need for immediate aggressive therapy, possibly including mechanical ventilation. Other physical findings and observations that are indicative of relatively severe obstruction include tachycardia (above 120 beats per minute), use of accessory muscles of respiration, diaphoresis, inability to lie flat, and severe breathlessness during speech. Generalized wheezing is typically present, and the absence of wheezing may be an ominous sign indicative of very severe obstruction.

The clinical findings noted above are very useful guides, but they are not by themselves completely reliable. Severe physiologic impairment can be present in the absence of many of the clinical findings suggesting severity. Objective measurement of lung function with spirometry is therefore imperative. FEV_1 measurements no higher than 30 per cent of predicted value and peak expiratory flow rates (PEFR) of 130 liters per minute or less are evidence of severe asthma requiring immediate intensive therapy. Arterial blood gases (ABG) to assess gas exchange are essential in patients with severe obstruction (including those too ill to perform spirometric maneuvers) but are of limited value in patients with mild to moderate attacks. In severe asthma, the ABG provides an important clue to impending respiratory failure (rising Pco_2 in a tiring patient) and a means to check for adequacy of supplemental oxygen therapy.

Many of these clinical parameters have been used to develop an index or formula for determining which patients presenting to the emergency room will need to be hospitalized. Nevertheless, the decision to hospitalize a patient for acute asthma is ultimately made when, in the physician's clinical judgment, outpatient management is unlikely to be successful or when an initial attempt at outpatient management has already failed.

As in chronic maintenance therapy, the first-line medications in emergency treatment of asthma are sympathomimetics, including beta-adrenergic agonists. Patients may be treated with epinephrine (1:1000), 0.3 ml, or with terbutaline (1 mg per ml), 0.25 ml subcutaneously at 20-minute intervals for a maximum of 3 doses. Alternatively, 0.5 ml of 0.5 per cent isoproterenol or 0.3 ml of metaproterenol or albuterol (Table 1) can be administered via a wet nebulizer every

TABLE 4. **Adult Dosages of Intravenous Aminophylline and Theophylline**

	Aminophylline	Theophylline (in 5% dextrose)
Loading dose (mg/kg)	5–7	4–6
Maintenance dose (mg/kg/hr)		
Nonsmoker	0.5–0.7	0.4–0.6
Smoker	0.9	0.6
Elderly	0.4	0.3
Heart failure or liver dysfunction	0.2–0.3	0.2

20 minutes for 3 doses. The patient should be re-evaluated clinically and by spirometry after each treatment. In a patient not previously taking theophylline, additional bronchodilation may be achieved by theophylline loading in the emergency room. Theophylline loading may be accomplished with an oral loading dose of a rapid-release preparation or, more rapidly, by intravenous administration of aminophylline, 5 to 7 mg per kg, or theophylline, 4 to 6 mg per kg (Table 4). A loading dose should not be given to a patient already taking theophylline unless a serum theophylline concentration is used as a guide to appropriately adjust the loading dose. In some patients with limited response to sympathomimetics and theophylline, anticholinergic medication such as atropine, 0.025 to 0.035 mg per kg, via a nebulizer may be of benefit.

If there has been a good response to bronchodilators, the patient may continue management as an outpatient after release from the emergency room on an intensified maintenance program and with close medical follow-up. In most cases the medications upon release from the emergency room will include a burst and taper of prednisone. If response has been poor, with either little clinical improvement or failure of FEV_1 to improve to above 40 to 50 per cent of normal, the patient should be hospitalized for further intensive bronchodilator therapy plus intravenous corticosteroids. In the hospital setting, maintenance theophylline or aminophylline may be given by continuous intravenous infusion. Guidelines to adult dosage of aminophylline and theophylline, including suggested alterations in special clinical situations, are shown in Table 4. Because of considerable variability in theophylline metabolism between patients, therapy must be monitored with serum theophylline levels and adjusted to maintain equilibrium levels between 10 and 20 micrograms per ml. The physician should be cognizant of the signs of theophylline toxicity, including nausea, vomiting, restlessness, arrhythmias, and convulsions, and know how to treat these toxic effects. The response to corticosteroids may take several hours, and steroid therapy should be instituted without undue delay. Intravenous corticosteroid doses are empirical, but hydrocortisone, 100 to 200 mg every 4 hours, and methylprednisolone, 40 to 60 mg every 6 hours, have both been effective. Response to this intensive therapy can be followed by spirometry and arterial blood gases. Once steady improvement is demonstrated, the therapy can be gradually converted to a regimen of inhaled and oral medications that can be continued on an outpatient basis with close follow-up after discharge.

ASTHMA IN CHILDREN

method of
KARL M. ALTENBURGER, M.D.
Seventeenth Street Medical Center
Ocala, Florida

It has been estimated that between 7.5 and 10 per cent of children have asthma. There is some suspicion of late that this incidence is increasing. Because it is so common, it underlies a large proportion of doctor visits and, when taken together with associated allergic illness, it probably represents the single most common reason for ill children to visit the doctor. Over the past 15 years our understanding of this disorder has improved greatly. We view this now as a spectrum of disease ranging from the very severe, even life-threatening, to the very mild. Some asthmatic diseases have a major allergic component, whereas others have no significant allergic triggering factors. For some patients, the onset is in early infancy, for others in early childhood, and still others manifest their disease only during adolescence. The course may be severe and unremitting or it may improve and become quiescent. If there is anything that can be said about the child with asthma, it is that each child is unique both in the presentation of disease and in the response to treatment. In spite of our advances and the greater availability of trained personnel, the rate of hospitalization for asthma and the mortality rate for asthma appear to be increasing. Asthma is now the leading diagnosis for children admitted to the hospital. Many problems, therefore, remain. It is hoped that by focusing more attention on the pathophysiology of this disorder and on its impact on the child and family, these figures can be reversed.

There are goals in caring for the asthmatic child, and these goals should be reviewed and shared with the child and family. The first goal is to keep the child out of the hospital. The second goal is to keep the child out of the physician's office, walk-in clinic, or emergency room. The third goal is to keep the child in school. The final goal is to keep the child socially and physically active so that a normal interaction with his or her peer group is possible. Accomplishing these goals usually, but not always, requires focusing our efforts on normalizing a child's pulmonary functions.

Experience in performing and interpreting basic spirometry is essential if adequate care is to be delivered. If management of asthma is successful, the child and the family are placed in control of the patient's asthma. It is an all too common tragedy to see this disease process unnecessarily control the patient and family.

Diagnosis

Before a rational treatment plan can be developed a precise diagnosis needs to be established. Usually this diagnosis is quite easy, especially when the asthma is more severe. The diagnosis is much more difficult when the asthma is very mild or when it presents in a fashion that is not familiar to the clinician. It is all too common to see a child visit a physician's office six to eight times each winter for "bronchitis" or "pneumonia." It should be noted that this is distinctly unusual unless that child has an immunodeficiency disorder or an underlying chest problem. The former is distinctly rare, and the latter problem is usually asthma. The diagnosis of asthma can be made by demonstrating reversibility by simple spirometry. This is easily performed on children as young as 6 years of age. However, in older children whose baseline lung functions are normal, a methacholine challenge is useful. Several standard protocols are available (see Chest 82:15, 1982). Methacholine challenges can even be performed on very young children in whom the diagnosis is often more difficult because a simple test for quantitating air flow obstruction is not widely available.

TREATMENT

There are four basic approaches to the outpatient management of the child with asthma: (1) manipulating the environment as a way of controlling the patient's exposure to allergens and irritants, (2) controlling bronchospasm and the inflammatory component with medication; (3) altering the patient's immune response to environmental allergens (immunotherapy, hyposensitization); and (4) educating the patient and family to improve their ability to adequately manage this chronic illness.

Environmental Control

Controlling the asthmatic patient's environment is a critical aspect of care. The single most important substance for the asthmatic child to avoid is tobacco smoke. It is impossible to overestimate the harmful effects of this potent irritant on the lung. Passive cigarette smoking harms even the nonasthmatic lung, and its effects have been shown to increase the frequency and severity of acute asthmatic episodes. This has been especially correlated with maternal cigarette smoking; however, both parents need to be encouraged to stop smoking completely. In addition, no one else should smoke in the house or car at any time. This irritant continues to pose a problem for the asthmatic child in public facilities. However, we are inexorably moving toward a smoke-free society, and in the future this will be less of a problem. There are a number of resources and aids to assist a child's parents in discontinuing this harmful habit, and the physician needs to be supportive of them in this regard. In addition, asthmatic teenagers, even those who had very mild disease in infancy and who are now asymptomatic, should be strongly discouraged from smoking. The risks of developing chronic lung disease in this group appear to be very high.

Attention also should be paid to other sources of irritants, especially wood-burning stoves, fireplaces, assorted oil-based heaters, and various chemicals (formaldehyde, cleaning products, etc.) that are products of our modern lives. Many asthmatic children have significant IgE-mediated triggering factors. Dust mite allergy is especially common, and house dust must be avoided to the best of the family's ability. This cannot be accomplished completely, and most suggestions for providing a dust-free environment are rather complex and expensive. Table 1 provides a basic sample. Special attention needs to be paid to the

TABLE 1. **House Dust Avoidance: General Guidelines**

1. All pillows, mattresses, and boxsprings should be *encased* in plastic covers. These should be wiped weekly. Mattress pads, washed weekly, are permitted. Many department stores carry zippered plastic covers, or, alternatively, they can be ordered from a number of allergy supply companies (e.g., Allergy Products Directory, P.O. Box 640, Menlo Park, California 94026).
2. Limit furniture and wall hangings. Toys, books, and so forth should be kept to a minimum. Shades should be vacuumed weekly. Curtains or drapes are permitted, but should be washed weekly.
3. Bare floors are preferred. These should be damp mopped weekly. Cotton throw rugs may be used if washed frequently. Carpeting should be vacuumed several times a week and shampooed yearly.
4. All room air vents should be closed or covered with five to six layers of cheesecloth. Wash and replace this monthly. The central fiberglass furnace filters should be changed at least every 3 to 6 weeks.
5. Closets should contain only the current season's clothes. The doors to the closet should be kept closed at all times.
6. Preferably, no animals should be kept in the house, and certainly, no animals should be allowed in the bedroom at any time. If an animal is kept in the house, doors to the bedroom should be kept closed.
7. The bedroom should be dusted daily. Be sure to clean underneath beds as well. The child should not be in the immediate area when the room is being cleaned. The room should be aired thoroughly after cleaning. If the person doing the cleaning has allergies, a pollen and dust mask may be worn. These are available at most drug stores.

child's bedroom, because young children spend fully half of their lives in this one room. Animal allergens are potent triggering factors and, where identified, these should be removed completely from the home. Even after an animal has been removed, a significant amount of allergen remains and is circulated through central air conditioning systems. Allergy to airborne fungi is an especially difficult problem. Avoidance is practically impossible, although a number of suggestions have been made in an attempt to decrease exposure inside the home. To this end, the use of a dehumidifier in an attempt to keep the general area as dry as possible should be considered. Avoidance of allergenic pollens is, to all intents and purposes, impossible.

Air purification systems may be especially useful. Room units can be purchased for the bedroom (see Consumer Reports, January, 1985). These should be run 24 hours per day, and the filter should be changed frequently; the child should not perform this task. Central air purification systems can be purchased, and the combination of these two air purifiers is most effective. Unfortunately, the installation of central air cleaner systems is often quite expensive (approximately $500 to $1000) and beyond the reach of most families. A humidistat (Honeywell) can be easily installed in homes with central air conditioning and heating systems as an aid in controlling humidity inside the home.

The major pathogens implicated in triggering asthma in children include *Mycoplasma*, parainfluenza virus, rhinovirus, respiratory syncytial virus, adenovirus, and influenza virus. These are very troublesome for most asthmatics because there is little that can be done to prevent exposure. Except for the use of erythromycin for *Mycoplasma* infections, and possibly ribavirin (Virazole), for respiratory syncytial virus (RSV), no effective treatment is available once an infection begins. Consideration can be given to removing young children from day-care settings. Hand washing should be emphasized for all those caring for these children, including their parents. The use of influenza vaccine should be encouraged.

Although environmental control is an important aspect of the asthmatic child's care, its success is often limited by parental resistance to changes in their immediate environment and life style. In addition, many children find that their asthma is triggered by stimuli that simply cannot be affected using any method currently available. It is for this reason that the pharmacologic management of asthma remains the cornerstone of the patient's care.

Pharmacotherapy

Our understanding of the drug treatment of asthma has improved greatly over the past 15 years. We have a much firmer rational basis for the use of many older medications, and a number of newer medications have been added to our armamentarium. It must be kept in mind that the use of any of these medications needs to be individualized and, while guidelines are provided, every child responds to and tolerates these drugs differently. Side effects occur and, while most parents will forgive you if you are unable to make their child better, very few will be as forgiving if you make the condition worse. Specific drug therapy is always preferred. There is no indication for the use of various fixed drug combinations (Marax, Tedral).

Theophylline

Theophylline remains the most commonly prescribed drug for asthma in this country, although its precise mode of action is unclear. It had been erroneously assumed in the past that theophylline acted as a phosphodiesterase inhibitor, but it now appears that other mechanisms are responsible for theophylline's effect. This drug is especially useful for maintenance therapy. The improvement in lung functions with theophylline is dose dependent and follows a linear relationship. It is well absorbed from the oral route, and the pharmacokinetics of many preparations have now been well defined. The major benefit of theophylline is that it has been used in the treatment of asthma for over 50 years. There appear to be no long-term side effects with the use of this medication. This makes it especially useful for the treatment of children. The symptoms of theophylline toxicity have been well described. Gastrointestinal upset (nausea, reflux, vomiting) occurs at serum levels over 20 micrograms per ml. Headache generally does not occur until the level reaches 30 micrograms per ml. Serious signs of theophylline toxcity (seizures) generally do not occur until the level reaches 40 micrograms per ml, although, rarely, these have been reported at lower levels.

Many children have difficulty tolerating any dose of theophylline, and at times the signs of intolerance can be quite subtle. Irritability, restlessness, nightmares, decreased attention span, sleep walking, misbehavior, enuresis, and poor school performance are not uncommon complaints. Teachers can easily identify these children, and their observations should be noted. These adverse affects may be observed even at doses of theophylline that produce serum levels in the therapeutic range or below.

When theophylline is first introduced to the child, it should be introduced slowly. In the outpatient management of chronic asthma there is rarely a need to reach an optimal level rapidly. Attempts should also be made to simplify the administration of theophylline as much as possible. For young children, theophylline capsules should be used (Slo-bid, Slo-Phyllin, Theo-Dur Sprinkles). Capsules can be opened and the contents placed in any food; they should be administered at least three times per day. At times, beginning the administration once a day, and then after a few days increasing to twice a day, and finally to three times a day is appropriate, especially when a history of theophylline intolerance is suspected. Even young children can be taught to swallow (using M & M's, for example), and this makes life much easier for their parents. For children who can swallow theophylline, tablets or capsules can be prescribed, although some children have more trouble swallowing tablets. Tablets may begin to dissolve in the esophagus, causing epigastric discomfort, unless they are taken with a full glass of water. Alternatively, they can be taken before or during meals.

Theophylline levels should be measured and will guide adjustments in therapy. It is not uncommon to find children who are using several different oral theophylline preparations at the same time and who are on such a complicated regimen that it is difficult for the physician to figure out exactly what the child is taking. There is rarely a need to divide capsules. Furthermore, there is rarely a need to administer this medication every 8 hours on a strict schedule. An attempt should be made to balance the practical with the ideal, and this is usually possible. If good compliance is to be obtained, the parents should be able to administer these medications without a major disruption in their lives.

There is rarely a need for oral liquid theophylline preparations. On occasion, especially during episodes of gastroenteritis, rectal theophylline solutions (Somophyllin Rectal Solution) are helpful in maintaining a therapeutic level. These *solutions* are rapidly and reliably absorbed and are rarely required for longer than 12- to 24-hour periods. In contrast, rectal suppositories should never be used because of their erratic absorption.

When adjusting the theophylline level it is important to note that very small increases in the oral theophylline dose can, especially as one approaches the therapeutic range, produce very large increases in the child's serum theophylline level.

Most of our patients and their parents do not like the idea of the child's having to take medication, especially on a chronic basis. Recognizing this fact and verbalizing it to the child and his or her parents is an important part of developing and sustaining rapport. The fact is that many children with asthma benefit by using various medications on a chronic basis, and for some such use is life-saving. I often tell the family that having asthma is very similar to the need for glasses. A person who wears glasses has a problem with his or her eyes. We cannot remove the eyes and give a person new ones, so he or she must wear glasses to correct the problem. Nobody likes wearing glasses, but it is better than not being able to read or otherwise see properly. Similarly, asthma involves a problem with the lungs. We cannot remove the lungs and give the child new lungs, so medications are often required to keep the problem under control. For the patient with poor eyes, when glasses are removed the eye problem persists. Similarly, for the child with chronic asthma, asthma remains after medications are discontinued. Reassurance concerning the safety of many of the medications used in the treatment of asthma is important, and this issue needs to be addressed frequently.

Beta-Adrenergic Agonists

These drugs have been known and used for at least five thousand years. First used by the Chinese as *ma huang,* the active ingredient was later identified as ephedrine (1924). Both ephedrine and epinephrine were being used for the treatment of asthma in the early part of this century. With the identification of beta$_1$ and beta$_2$ receptors, more specific beta$_2$ agonists have been developed and are now in wide use. These drugs are available as either oral preparations (liquids or tablets) or inhaled preparations (metered dose inhalers or nebulizer solutions). All of these preparations are useful for the treatment of asthma. Many children who are intolerant of theophylline benefit greatly by the use of oral or inhaled beta$_2$ agonists. In addition, they can be used concomitantly with theophylline to achieve additional effects. The drugs are generally well tolerated, although an increased heart rate, tremor, and irritability can be problems. These side effects tend to decrease with time, but this is not always the case. The major drugs currently available include metaproterenol (Alupent, Metaprel), terbutaline (Brethine, Bricanyl), bitolterol (Tornalate), albuterol (Ventolin, Proventil), and pirbuterol (Maxair).

Oral medications are useful for the treatment of both acute and chronic asthma. When used for treatment of the acute form, liquid preparations and tablets are rapidly absorbed from the gastrointestinal tract. They often produce hyperactivity and, occasionally, tremor, although most patients, especially during acute episodes, will tolerate this. This is more troublesome when these drugs need to be used routinely. These drugs can be used interchangeably, although some patients, for no apparent reason, seem to tolerate one form better than another. Terbutaline is the preferred inhaled and oral drug for the treatment of the occasional child with asthma who is pregnant. The inhaled forms of these medications are particularly useful because of their rapid onset of action. Their use is limited only by the patient's ability to coordinate activation of the metered inhaler and inhalation. While this sounds simple, it is very difficult or even impossible for many patients. The technique for administration (Table 2) must be reviewed with the patient at the beginning of therapy and at frequent intervals thereafter. In children who are unable to utilize metered dose inhalers properly, reservoir spacer devices (Inhal-Aid, Inspirease) can be used. Although they are a bit more complicated for the family, these devices clearly improve the delivery of the aerosol into the lungs. Pausing (at least 3 minutes) between inhalations significantly improves the effect of these medications. This should be encouraged during acute asthmatic episodes but is not necessary when these inhalers are used routinely. When asthma is especially troublesome, especially when frequent acute episodes occur, the use of nebulized beta-adrenergic drugs can be especially helpful. These are delivered using a compressor (Pulmo-Aide, DeVilbiss, Somerset, Pennsylvania 15501). Many types are available. More important than the make and model that the patient purchases is the service available to the patient after the purchase. Of special concern is the availability of a replacement compressor should the unit malfunction at any time. The physician should also inquire about the costs of these units, because they vary widely even in the same community. Compressors are suitable for very young children. For these children, the medication may be delivered by mask. Because the amount entering the oropharynx, and then the lungs, is much less concentrated than when the medication is inhaled with a mouthpiece, the concentration of the medication used in the nebulizer needs to be increased. For example, one may wish to use metaproterenol nebulizer solution 0.2 ml plus 2 to 3 ml of normal saline for a child who is able to use a mouthpiece, but for a child who requires a mask one may wish to increase the amount of drug to 0.3 ml. The use of passive nebulization treatments in the home can significantly reduce the severity of acute asthmatic episodes and the need for frequent emergency room visits or hospitalizations. Of course, the use of all beta-adre-

TABLE 2. Sample Instruction Sheet for Patients Describing the Use of Metered Dose Inhalers

Asthma is best controlled when the bronchial tubes are maintained open and normal. "Asthma inhalers" are especially useful in this regard. Some inhalers such as albuterol (Proventil, Ventolin), bitolterol (Tornalate), metaproterenol (Alupent, Metaprel), terbutaline (Brethaire), and pirbuterol (Maxair) also provide rapid relief from sudden attacks of airway narrowing (asthma). Others such as beclomethasone (Beclovent, Vanceril), cromolyn (Intal), flunisolide (AeroBid), and triamcinolone (Azmacort) are used to control inflammation in the bronchial tubes and are generally not used during severe attacks.

These inhalers must be used CORRECTLY if the desired beneficial effects are to be achieved. Instructions for their safe and effective use will be found below. Read them carefully. Remember, it is important that you use the inhaler(s) *only as often as directed by your doctor*. If you are having trouble using these, please contact us.

Step 1 *Shake* the inhalers well before each inhalation. Remove the dust cap to expose the mouthpiece.
Step 2 *Tilt* your head back to straighten out your airway. This is a very important step. If your head and neck are bent, more of each spray will impact on the back of the throat. With the head tilted back, more medication will reach the lungs.
Step 3 *Breathe* out fully (but not *forcefully*), expelling as much air from your lungs as possible. Hold the inhaler between your index finger and thumb (using both hands provides greater stability).
Step 4 *Place* the mouthpiece just outside your wide-opened mouth and direct it toward the back of your throat.
Step 5 *Inhale* (through the mouth only *slowly and evenly* and, at the same time, firmly *press* down the top of the canister. Continue to inhale fully and *slowly*.
Step 6 *Hold* your breath for as long as possible (5 to 10 seconds). This will allow the finer particles to deposit where they can do the most good. Now exhale.
Step 7 *Wait* and then repeat Steps 1 through 6 for each subsequent inhalation. *Shake* the inhaler well before each inhalation.
Step 8 At the end of each day remove the metal canister and rinse the plastic case in warm water. After drying, place the canister in the case and replace the dust cap.

Call if you have any questions.

nergic drugs must be carefully supervised, but under appropriate conditions their safety has been established.

Cromolyn (Intal)

The precise mechanism of action of cromolyn has not been firmly established. It had been thought to be a mast cell stabilizer, although other mechanisms are no doubt involved. Cromolyn appears to prevent bronchospasm and to have anti-inflammatory effects as well. Therefore, there are many good reasons why this drug should be considered as a first line drug in the treatment of asthma. It has practically no side effects, and it should be considered for use especially in children who cannot tolerate theophylline or beta-adrenergic agents. It must be used prophylactically, and most children require its administration at least three times a day. However, once adequate control has been obtained, and after routine use, many children can be adequately maintained on lower doses.

Cromolyn is available for administration in three forms. The oldest form available is as a capsule containing 20 mg of cromolyn in a lactose carrier. The capsule is opened using a Spinhaler, and the medication and substrate are actively inhaled into the lungs with a normal inspiration. Because no coordination is required, it is especially suitable for young children. Demonstrating the correct technique for administration is important, and it is often useful to develop a standardized instruction sheet that the patient can refer to frequently. Lactose is present inside the capsule and can be swallowed and, in the lactose intolerant patient, this can cause gastrointestinal symptoms. Intal is also available as a metered dose inhaler, and because this is less complicated and easier to use than the capsule and Spinhaler, it is a better choice for many older children and adolescents. Again, repeated demonstration of the correct technique for inhalation is important. This medication is best used after a beta-adrenergic inhaler. This ensures better penetration into the lungs. It may be utilized alone, but it takes longer for the patient to feel the beneficial effects. In addition, these medications are not suitable for the treatment of acute episodes, and the patient will need to have something for this in any event. After a month or two, if appropriate, the beta-adrenergic inhaler can then be withdrawn and used only as needed to treat acute episodes. Finally, Intal is made as a nebulizer solution. It is produced as a 10 mg per ml solution and comes in 2-ml ampules. The directions for opening these glass ampules must be carefully followed to avoid breaking the glass and cutting the fingers. The solution is then poured into a nebulizer chamber, and usually a beta-adrenergic nebulizer solution is added. It is not necessary to use a nebulized adrenergic agent and then a second nebulizer treatment with Intal.

Corticosteroids

Corticosteroids are very effective drugs in the treatment of acute and chronic asthma. They clearly enhance the response of bronchial smooth muscle to beta-adrenergic drugs. They are the only medication that effectively treats the inflammatory component present in most asthmatic disease. They accomplish this by decreasing mucus secretion and vascular permeability, improving mucosal edema, and inhibiting the late-phase reaction and the release of leukotrienes C_4 and D_4 (formally known as slow reacting substance of anaphylaxis). They interfere with eosinophilic chemotactic activity, reducing the cytotoxic effects of the mediators released from eosinophils. While their effects can be life-saving, the side effects of long-term oral corticosteroid therapy limit its usefulness.

Various topical preparations manufactured for use by inhalation have been introduced (beclomethasone [Beclovent, Vanceril], flunisolide [AeroBid], triamcinolone [Azmacort]). These drugs are well absorbed into the systemic circulation, but are metabolized so rapidly that systemic effects rarely occur. For asthmatic patients who are not maintained adequately on bronchodilator therapy alone, the addition of these anti-inflammatory agents often results in dramatic clinical improvement. Improvement in lung functions is usually noted as well. The key to initiating such therapy is to achieve adequate control of the airways. This usually requires a short course of an oral corticosteroid. Usually 20 mg of prednisone twice a day for 5 to 7 days and then once a day for an additional 5 to 7 days is sufficient. Once the patient reaches once-a-day dosage, I would prescribe the use of an inhaled corticosteroid routinely after an inhaled beta-adrenergic drug. This allows better penetration of the anti-inflammatory agent into the lungs. All patients should be encouraged to rinse their mouths out after using these agents (easily accomplished by drinking a glass of water or using the medications before meals). This avoids nonspecific throat irritation which is occasionally noted with these agents, and the development of oral candidiasis. The latter complication can usually be prevented by using spacer devices between the metered dose inhaler and the mouth. Once clinical improvement has been noted, the smallest dose of these medications that provides the desired clinical effect should be continued. While most of the inhaled preparations are not recommended for children under 6 years of age, many of these children often benefit significantly by their use. They can be easily administered using either spacer tubes or various aerochambers. Their use often prevents the frequent use of oral corticosteroids. In children who continue to experience difficulty even using optimal doses of inhaled bronchodilators and inhaled anti-inflammatory agents and who require large doses of oral corticosteroids frequently to treat acute episodes, consideration should be given to alternate-day corticosteroid therapy. The use of alternate-day corticosteroids will often provide optimal control of the child's asthma and may in the long run result in lower total doses of corticosteroids

being administered. Again, control of the airway should be achieved using larger doses of prednisone as suggested earlier and then tapering to 20 to 40 mg every other day. If the child remains well on this dose after 6 to 8 weeks, the dose should be slowly tapered to the lowest tolerable dose.

Prednisone tablets are readily available and inexpensive. For a child who cannot swallow, these tablets may be crushed and added to any food (e.g., jelly, honey), although their bitter taste is very difficult to hide. Palatable liquid preparations of prednisolone have been introduced (Prelone, 15 mg per 5 ml; Pediapred, 5 mg per 5 ml). Prelone is more concentrated and less expensive; however, it is mixed in 5 per cent alcohol. Pediapred is alcohol-free. Prednisone must be metabolized to its active form in the liver, whereas prednisolone and methylprednisolone (Medrol) are already active. Therefore, the latter drugs may be necessary for patients who have significant liver dysfunction. Dexamethasone is not suitable for the therapy of childhood asthma because its longer half-life increases the risk of adrenal suppression.

Atropine and Ipratropium Bromide (Atrovent)

Atropine is a well known anticholinergic agent that in most, but not all, asthmatic children has significant bronchodilator properties. It has been widely used in the treatment of asthma in the West for almost two centuries. Currently it is utilized only rarely in children. There are occasional children who benefit by receiving nebulized atropine sulfate. This can be readily made by the pharmacist, using atropine 0.6 mg tablets. These tablets are easily dissolved in normal saline (without preservatives) to a concentration of 1 mg per ml and sterile filtered; 1 to 2 ml of this nebulizer solution is placed in the nebulizer chamber and may be mixed with a beta-adrenergic bronchodilator or cromolyn or both. This drug is well absorbed into the systemic circulation, and, therefore, anticholinergic side effects (typically dried mouth, blurred vision, and altered heart rate) can occur.

Ipratropium bromide is a quaternary isopropyl derivative of atropine and, because it is poorly absorbed, it has few systemic effects. It has been available in Europe for over 10 years, and a number of studies have already appeared in the pediatric literature attesting to the efficacy and safety of this product in children. It is available in the United States as Atrovent, and has been approved by the Food and Drug Administration only for use in adults. There are a number of children, however, who may benefit by its use. It is marketed as a metered dose inhaler that delivers 18 micrograms to the patient per actuation. The recommended effective dose in children is approximately 40 micrograms (2 inhalations), although more may be needed. Improvement in lung functions (FEV_1) is noted 15 minutes after administration and peaks at 45 to 60 minutes. Administration three to four times a day will probably be required. Of particular interest is that ipratropium bromide seems to produce significant bronchodilation *after* maximal effects have been achieved from beta-adrenergic drugs. This has implications in the emergency treatment of asthma, and a nebulizer solution, although not yet available, will soon be introduced.

Other Medications

Antihistamines, usually in combination with decongestants, often carry a notice warning of their use in asthma. However, a number of studies have shown that they can be safely used even in patients with severe asthma, and they may, in fact, have bronchodilator effects. Certainly many asthmatic patients have nasal congestion either from inhalant allergy or upper respiratory tract infections, and the benefit of these drugs should not be denied to them.

Antibiotics are over-used in the treatment of asthma, and their routine use cannot be justified. However, sinusitis should be rigorously treated as it is an important, often subtle, triggering factor in many children (see the article on sinusitis). Erythromycin in milder cases of asthma is often necessary to treat *Mycoplasma* infections. Erythromycin and triacetyloleandomycin (Tao) seem to have corticosteroid-sparing effects. Because these drugs decrease the clearance of theophylline, the theophylline dose needs to be adjusted (decreased at least 25 to 33 per cent) when initiating therapy.

Expectorants (guaifenesin, iodides) have not been demonstrated to benefit the child with asthma. Therefore, their use cannot be recommended. Medications for anxiety and sedation are contraindicated.

Approaches to Treatment

Mild Asthma. Mild asthma occurs in the child troubled only infrequently by his or her asthma and who, between acute exacerbations, is essentially asymptomatic. Older children should have normal or near normal pulmonary functions when they are well. This group includes those with exercise-induced bronchospasm, those who present only with a cough, and those who have fewer than two or three mild, non–life-threatening, acute asthmatic episodes per year. These children generally require only the intermittent

use of medications and rarely require corticosteroids.

Children with exercise-induced bronchospasm only should be managed with an inhaled beta-adrenergic bronchodilator (2 sprays of a metered dose inhaler). Albuterol (Proventil, Ventolin) has a longer duration of effect and is the drug of choice, especially for children who are unable to determine the time of their exercise or who are frequently active. Cromolyn sodium (Intal), 2 sprays of a metered dose inhaler or 1 capsule by Spinhaler, is a good alternative. These should be taken 15 to 20 minutes before exercise. An adequate warm-up period will also improve these children's responses to exercise. Some children, especially the very physically active, will benefit by using the beta-adrenergic inhaler followed 5 to 10 minutes later by cromolyn. This combination seems to work better than either drug alone.

Acute exacerbations in the child with mild asthma can generally be treated with inhaled beta-adrenegic agents. In small children these can be delivered using various aerochambers at a dose of 2 sprays every 4 to 6 hours. It may be necessary to administer an oral agent as well. Oral agents are usually helpful in children who are unable to use the inhaled agents. The oral beta-adrenergic agents work faster than theophylline and, if tolerated, are the drugs of choice for this group. Doses for albuterol and metaproterenol (Table 3) are provided as guidelines only. Treatment is begun with the smaller dose, increasing, if needed and tolerated, to the larger dose. Therapy with these agents should be continued for 5 to 7 days after the child is well. This allows adequate clearing of the inflammatory component from the lung. Some children benefit by continuing these medications for longer periods of time.

Moderate to Severe Asthma (Chronic Asthma). Children with chronic asthma have frequent acute exacerbations that have significantly affected their ability to function normally at their age level. Such children include those who have abnormal lung functions even when "well" and those who require frequent emergency room or

TABLE 3. **Dosing Guidelines for Beta-Adrenergic Agents**

Age (years)	Albuterol (2 mg/5 ml) or Metaproterenol (10 mg/5 mg)
<2	¼–½ tsp. tid or qid
2–6	¼–¾ tsp. tid or qid
6–12	½–1½ tsp. tid or qid
>12	½–2 tsp. tid or qid

office visits. These children generally require the continuous use of medication. Theophylline is an excellent medication for this purpose. Various dosing schemes have been developed to minimize adverse reactions and decrease the number of theophylline levels required (J. Pediatr. 109:351–354, 1986). I would start at 10 to 15 mg per kg per day and deliver the dose three times a day for children under the age of 12 and twice a day for children over the age of 12. There are a number of children over the age of 12 who are hypermetabolizers of theophylline, and they may need to take this medication three times a day. However, compliance is more of a problem in this age group and efforts to simplify the regimen are worthwhile. The dose should be rounded slightly higher or lower to accommodate the theophylline preparation selected. For example, a 20-kg, 5-year-old child would start at approximately 200 to 300 mg per day. To begin, try Slo-bid Gyrocaps, 100 mg, three times a day. If the child is doing well, no further adjustments are necessary. If the child requires more, and most children will at this level, increase the evening dose of Slo-bid Gyrocaps or switch to a 125-mg capsule. Most pharmaceutical companies will freely provide samples to physicians, and these are of great benefit to these families as you proceed through this process. Most of these children should be shown how to use a metered dose inhaler. Even if this is not required for routine use, it is very helpful in the treatment of acute attacks. If the asthma is not sufficiently controlled, the next step would be to add an anti-inflammatory agent such as cromolyn or inhaled corticosteroids. These should be given initially three to four times a day, and, after a response is noted, the dose can be tapered to the lowest tolerable dose. On occasion, the routine administration of oral or inhaled beta agonists or both is also needed for adequate control. Once the goals of treatment have been accomplished, the regimen should be reviewed to ensure that all medications are tolerated (physiologically and socially) and that compliance is not only possible but probable.

Severe Acute Asthma (Status Asthmaticus). The treatment of acute asthma requires an understanding of the child's past history, the duration and tempo of the present episode, and the child's treatment prior to his presentation. This can be accomplished in a few minutes while other preparations for his care are undertaken. Once treatment has begun, the remainder of the child's history can be obtained. Ideally, this should be accomplished in a quiet and unhurried environment, and the child should be attended by similarly disposed personnel. This problem is common enough in most emergency rooms or busy clinics to justify separate treatment areas.

Nebulized terbutaline (1 to 2 ml plus 1 to 2 ml of normal saline) is administered with oxygen unless the child has been receiving terbutaline at home. In that case another nebulizer solution (e.g., Alupent unit dose 2.5 ml, which is sulfite free; albuterol) should be given. A pharmacologic dose of Solu-Medrol should be administered intravenously (approximately 4 mg per kg). This can be administered with a butterfly inserted in a peripheral vein (hand) for this purpose only. If the acute episode is very mild, oral prednisolone may be sufficient. Intravenous fluid administration is rarely needed unless the patient is dehydrated. In this case, losses should be replaced but care should be taken not to overhydrate the patient. Nebulizer treatments are repeated every 20 minutes as long as the heart rate remains acceptable (less than 80 per cent of predicted maximum). If there is no satisfactory response after two or three treatments, and certainly sooner if the patient's condition deteriorates, hospitalization for prolonged treatment and observation is probably necessary. Short-stay areas, if available, are ideal for many patients.

The patient rarely requires injections of epinephrine, unless the asthmatic episode is part of a systemic anaphylactic reaction. In this case, they are the treatment of choice. Limiting or preferably eliminating injections helps to decrease the child's anxiety, and this improves the chances of achieving a satisfactory response. Intravenous theophylline does not appear to add significantly to the bronchodilator effects of beta-adrenergic agents. It does, however, contribute significantly to side effects observed as a consequence of treatment. Oxygen should be administered during most acute asthmatic episodes but, with improvement of the patient's condition, should be discontinued. In young children its benefit needs to be carefully weighed against the anxiety produced by holding a mask in place. For older children nasal cannulas are ideal.

With few exceptions, there is no clear benefit to the patient in performing various laboratory tests or radiologic examinations. Complete blood counts are frequently ordered; however, because of the effects of various medications, they seldom, if ever, provide useful information. Electrolyte evaluations are useful if dehydration is suspected. Chest x-ray examinations are rarely necessary unless the presence of pneumothorax or pneumonia is considered likely. Arterial blood gas determinations should always be obtained if there is any question as to how the child is responding and certainly if the development of ventilatory failure is suspected. A theophylline level may be useful especially to assess compliance or to rule out toxicity.

Once a satisfactory response has been achieved, it is essential that a treatment plan for the next 10 to 14 days be carefully considered and reviewed with the patient and parents. Oral corticosteroids should be administered in all patients who are already using oral or inhaled corticosteroid preparations or cromolyn (e.g., children under 6 years of age or those who cannot swallow can take Prelone, ½ to 1 tsp. twice a day for 5 days, then ½ to 1 tsp. once a day for 5 days; children over 6 years of age who can swallow tablets can take prednisone 20 mg twice a day for 5 days then once a day for 5 days). Although less certain, corticosteroids appear to be beneficial in all other asthmatics as well, hastening resolution of the acute episode and preventing relapses that otherwise occur all too frequently (approximately 25 per cent of the time). Adequate follow-up with the primary care physician should be arranged so that a long-term treatment plan

that makes the treatment of acute asthma unnecessary can be developed.

Immunotherapy

It is clear that asthma can be triggered by the inhalation of many different allergens. Small particles (dust mite, mold spores, animal danders, and so forth) are especially troublesome because they penetrate easily into the lower airways. However, larger particles (pollens) can also cause difficulties because these are present in the air as small fragments, and the antigens themselves can be leached into small water droplets (pollen vapor), which are then inhaled into the lung. Allergic reactions in the lung also increase nonspecific bronchial reactivity (e.g, to exercise, cold air, irritants).

A great deal of attention has recently been focused on the late-phase reaction mediated by specific IgE. Immunotherapy appears to achieve its effects at least in part by blunting this response. Immunotherapy is indicated only for children who, by appropriate testing, have been demonstrated to have significant allergic triggering factors. Immunotherapy will not cure asthma and is not a substitute for appropriate environmental modification or pharmacotherapy. Immunotherapy is administered only against those allergens that cannot be avoided. Although a number of studies have demonstrated the efficacy of immunotherapy in this population, not all children respond satisfactorily and, in some, the condition can be made worse. Systemic reactions to allergenic extract are not uncommon, and these should not be administered cavalierly. The child should be observed carefully for 20 to 30 minutes after each injection, and injections should be administered only when and where a physician is available to treat adverse reactions. Certainly, there is no place for immunotherapy using bacterial vaccines or against tobacco, histamine, or food allergens. The characterization and standardization of allergenic extract remains a formidable challenge for the future, and controlled studies are needed to answer many remaining questions. Until this is accomplished, the precise role of immunotherapy in asthmatic children cannot be determined.

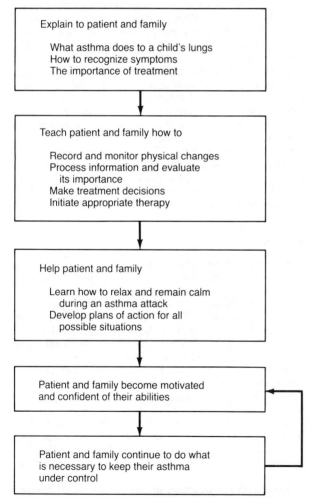

Figure 1. The essentials of successful asthma management. (Adapted from Creer, TL. Is your asthma patient his own worst enemy? J Respir Dis 7(10):27–32, 1986.

Education

To many patients and families asthma remains a mystery. They are angry about having the problem, confused about what triggers it, and frustrated in their attempts to deal with it. The goal of any educational program then is to acknowledge these issues and convince the family that they are able, with help and support, to control this problem. The physician's attitude in this regard is critical. There is no substitute for spending enough time if one seeks to change the outlook of the entire family (even involving three generations). This cannot be accomplished in one or two brief office visits. But as the journey of a thousand miles begins with one step, it is important to direct the family on a course toward the goal of asthma management (Figure 1). The family must understand the pathophysiology of this disorder. Their ability to receive and process this information should not be underestimated. Many informative booklets and pamphlets have been developed to assist both physician and patient. Excellent materials can be obtained from the Asthma and Allergy Foundation of America (1717 Massachusetts Ave. N.W., Suite 305, Washington, D.C., 20036, (202) 265–0265) and the American Lung Association (1740 Broadway, N.Y., N.Y., 10019, (212) 315–8700). A number of self-management programs (Airpower, Openairways, Airwise, Living With Asthma) have been developed and are frequently sponsored by the local chapters of these organizations. The facts learned in these programs must be reinforced by the family's physician. Patients are taught how to recognize the early onset of problems and the options that are available for treatment.

It must be acknowledged that no one, not even physicians, likes to have a child take medication. The physician must be supportive of this concern. Explaining side effects and being open to making changes if these occur is crucial. The family must be provided with a protocol to help them manage illnesses and acute asthmatic episodes. Certainly they will learn a great deal by trial and error, but mistakes can be minimized by providing timely and compassionate feedback. Armed with this knowledge, the patient and family can more easily deal with the stress that accompanies an acute episode, making relaxation possible. In time, the family will develop a more positive attitude. The stability brought to their lives by adequate control of their child's asthma will allow them to more confidently perform the tasks required. Compliance then becomes a certainty and continued control a reality.

ALLERGIC RHINITIS DUE TO INHALANT ALLERGENS

method of
ELI O. MELTZER, M.D.
University of California, San Diego
San Diego, California

Rhinitis, a general term for disorders of the nasal mucosa, chronically affects over 40 million Americans.

Of all mechanisms involved in chronic rhinitis, allergy is the most common, affecting approximately 10 per cent of the population. A national survey in 1975 estimated that, as a result of allergic rhinitis, in 1 year Americans were restricted in activity 28 million days, were bedridden 6 million days, and lost 2 million school days. Furthermore, this illness cost Americans 500 million dollars for physician services and medications. Thus, substantial morbidity is caused by allergic rhinitis.

Pathogenesis

The allergic mechanism involves genetically predisposed atopic individuals who mount, within the lymphoid tissue of the respiratory tract, a high and prolonged IgE antibody response on exposure to inhaled allergens. Within minutes of re-exposure to the specific inhaled allergen, reactions are initiated by the cross-linking of specific IgE molecules bound to basophilic cells found within the nasal lumen or on intraepithelial surfaces of the nasal mucosa. This process releases mediators such as histamine, leukotrienes, kinins, and prostaglandins and also releases chemotactic factors that lead to an influx to the nose of eosinophils, neutrophils, and basophils. These events provoke the nasal symptoms of obstruction, mucus secretion, itching, and sneezing.

Investigators have discovered that the nasal mucosa may be hypersensitive to a rechallenge after an initial challenge. This may be due to the inflammatory damage of the mucosal barrier allowing more irritant or antigen to penetrate to the target cells or because of the migration of additional target cells, such as basophils, into the mucosa. This empowers subsequent lower amounts of a specific allergen or a second allergen to cause significant symptoms. Disturbance of the usually well-balanced autonomic nervous control of nasal function further magnifies the rhinitis.

Evaluation

Many patients who have allergic rhinitis can identify siblings, children, parents, or even grandparents who have similar symptoms. For most people, rhinitis begins in childhood, when it is often mistaken for recurring colds. However, the onset may occur at any age and present in differing degrees indefinitely. The symptoms may vary in frequency from intermittent to seasonal to unremitting and in severity from mild to annoying to distressing. Perennial inhalant precipitants may include dust mites, animal danders, and mold spores, while seasonal inhalant allergens are usually pollens. An increase in wind conditions tends to aggravate pollen exposure, humidity increases dust mite exposure, and the presence of increased wind and humidity increases the effect of ambient mold spores. Airborne irritants complicate upper airway inflammation.

The nasal examination of the patient with allergic rhinitis is variable. The mucosal color can be a normal lip color pink or more often is slightly or moderately pale. Either the inferior or middle turbinates or both are typically swollen to partially or significantly compromise the airways. The nasal secretions are often increased and usually thin and colorless.

The physical examination for individuals with complaints of allergic rhinitis must include, besides the nose, the eyes, ears, sinuses, and mouth. A similar IgE-mediated pathogenetic mechanism leads to the ocular signs of puffy eyelids, conjunctival injection, and tearing as well as ocular and palatal pruritus. Nasal obstruction can also lead to venous pooling in the suborbital area, referred to as allergy shiners. Allergic rhinitis appears to be a risk factor for otitis media with effusion by contributing to the obstruction of the eustachian tubes. Sinusitis also appears to be more common among allergic patients than in the nonallergic population. The most common symptoms and signs are chronic rhinorrhea, cough, sore throat, and bad breath. Some investigators have reported that as many as 70 per cent of allergic children presenting with chronic rhinitis have abnormalities found when their sinuses are x-rayed. Another frequent consequence of allergic rhinitis is the necessity for mouth breathing. This reduces the important nasal physiologic functions of olfaction, air filtration, and air conditioning, and results in both a duller facial appearance and the development of lengthened facial features including a narrowed maxillary arch and greater palatal and anterior facial height.

Nasal cytologic analysis is a critical tool in differentiating among allergic, nonallergic, and infectious forms of rhinitis. In allergic rhinitis, eosinophils predominate; basophils and goblet cells are also common. A blood total eosinophil count, however, is usually of no major help in the evaluation of rhinitis.

The value of the total serum IgE as a screening test is also limited. Patients with low levels (less than 50 IU per ml) can still have significantly positive test reactions that correlate with their histories. Specific IgE tests can be performed on the nasal mucosa, the skin, or the serum. The nasal tests are the most specific but are cumbersome for routine clinical application. The serum tests (RAST, FAST, MAST) are the least sensitive because there is relatively less IgE in the serum than is fixed to dermal cells. Thus, skin testing is the generally preferred technique because of its good sensitivity, rapid turnaround time, and lower cost per tested antigen.

Treatment

Optimal management of allergic rhinitis depends on an understanding of the various available therapeutic modalities. A patient's assurance of the physician's concern for his or her long-term health is the first important factor. Patients should be thoroughly educated in the symptoms, causes, and course of allergic rhinitis and the aim and specific types of treatment. A high level of compliance is most likely if a patient feels informed, involved, and self-reliant.

Control of Allergen Exposure

Avoidance of rhinitis triggers is the second principle of management. Environmental controls to decrease exposure to such allergens as animal danders, dust mites, mold spores, and pollens are important. Effective measures include keeping fur-bearing pets outside the home, using polyester pillows, enclosing the bedroom mattresses and box springs in zippered, heavy vinyl, airtight encasements, covering the bedroom windows with washable curtains or blinds, removing the bedroom carpeting, keeping the windows closed to reduce the influx of outdoor mold and pollen, and simplifying the bedroom, allowing only limited numbers of knickknacks, books, and toys. Additional steps may be required or helpful in the home and workplace and involve the elimination of chores associated with allergen exposure, maintaining the ambient relative humidity at about 50 per cent, and the purchase of air conditioning and filtering systems. Temperature changes, bright lights, alcohol ingestion, infections, and irritants such as perfumes, automobile exhaust, and tobacco smoke further aggravate the hyperirritable airway. Insofar as possible, avoidance of these precipitant factors should also be attempted.

Antihistamines

The third measure required in the management of allergic rhinitis is the use of specific pharmacologic agents to control symptoms. The most commonly used are the antihistamines (Table 1), which are chemically different groups of compounds with the similar pharmacologic property of competitively antagonizing histamine at its H_1 receptor site on goblet cells, submucous glands, and postcapillary venules in the nasal mucosa. In general, better therapeutic results in allergic rhinitis are achieved when antihistamines are taken routinely rather than sporadically, since receptor sites can be blocked before histamine is released. Certain antihistamines may also inhibit mediator release, and many antihistamines possess anticholinergic effects, which may be of further benefit. Antihistamines effectively prevent mucus secretion, itching, and sneezing but are less valuable against the problem of nasal congestion. These agents are pharmacodynamically diverse and differ in potency, duration of action, side effects, and also cost. Sedation, the most common troublesome effect of this class of drugs, can be lessened by dosing at bedtime only with some of the usual antihistamines such as chlorpheniramine and hydroxyzine (Atarax, Vistaril), or by prescribing one of the newer, less sedating compounds such as terfenadine (Seldane), loratadine, or astemizole (Hismanal).

Oral decongestants are sympathomimetic amines that reduce mucosal edema and the symp-

TABLE 1. **Classes of Antihistamines**

Chemical Class	Generic Name	Trade Name	Comments
Ethanolamine	Carbinoxamine Clemastine Diphenhydramine Doxylamine	Clistin Tavist Benadryl	This group of antihistamines has substantial anticholinergic activity. They also commonly cause CNS depression; with usual doses, drowsiness occurs in 50% of patients. Incidence of adverse GI effects is low.
Ethylenediamine	Methapyriline Pyrilamine Tripelennamine	 In combinations PBZ	Relatively weak CNS effects; however, drowsiness in some patients. Adverse GI effects are common.
Alkylamine	Brompheniramine Chlorpheniramine Dexchlorpheniramine Triprolidine	Dimetane Chlortrimeton Polaramine Actidil	Cause less drowsiness and more CNS stimulation than others and are thus suitable for daytime use.
Piperazine	Hydroxyzine HCl Hydroxyzine Pamoate	Atarax Vistaril	Hydroxyzine is used as a tranquilizer, sedative, antipruritic. Anticholinergic effects and drowsiness common.
Phenothiazine	Methdilazine Promethazine Trimeprazine	Tacaryl Phenergan Temaril	Used as antipruritic and antiemetic.
Piperidine	Azatadine Cyproheptadine	Optimine Periactin	Cyproheptadine causes weight gain and pronounced sedation.
Miscellaneous	Acrivastine* Astemizole* Azelastine* Cetirizine* Ketotifen* Loratadine* Mequitazine* Terfenadine	 Hismanal Zaditen Primalan Seldane	Most of this group causes significantly less sedation than other classes.

*Investigational drugs.

tom of nasal congestion by vasoconstriction due to alpha-adrenergic activity. Nervousness and elevated blood pressure are the most common side effects. These drugs are available as single entity agents (such as pseudoephedrine and phenylpropanolamine) or combined with antihistamines. Studies have demonstrated that the efficacy of these combination drugs in the management of allergic rhinitis is superior to the efficacy of either component alone. Topically applied sympathomimetics may be catecholamines (such as phenylephrine) or imidazole derivatives (such as oxymetazoline [Afrin]). Both types of drugs cause marked nasal vasoconstriction and decreased edema without any systemic effects. However, unlike the oral decongestants, if used in a prolonged manner, these agents can cause rebound congestion and result in rhinitis medicamentosa. Topical decongestants are most useful in the treatment of allergic rhinitis prior to the initiation of intranasal cromolyn (Nasalcrom), or intranasal corticosteroids to improve the penetration of those medications.

Cromolyn

Intranasal cromolyn acts by stabilizing the membranes of mast cells to inhibit the immunologic release of chemical mediators of nasal inflammation which produce the early- and late-phase reactions that result in allergic rhinitis. Cromolyn can be used prophylactically prior to allergen exposure and therapeutically in chronic allergic rhinitis to reduce the symptoms of sneezing, itch, and rhinorrhea. It has been found to be less effective in preventing nasal congestion. Efficacy is dose-related and is probably due to both the medication and the frequent rinsing of the membrane by the spray. Application of a saline mist to the nasal mucosa similarly soothes irritated tissue, liquefies tenacious mucus, and flushes particulates and allergens. Cromolyn is available in a 4 per cent solution delivering approximately 5 mg per spray. A usual starting dose is one spray in each nostril four or five times a day. Compliance with multiple dosing may be poor, so the frequency recommendation should be adjusted downward as symptoms abate. Except for some mild local irritation, the safety record of cromolyn is excellent.

Corticosteroids

The last major family of medications prescribed for allergic rhinitis are the corticosteroids. Treatment with this group of agents leads to decreased vasodilation and edema in the inflamed tissue, decreased sensitivity of irritant or sneeze receptors, decreased glandular response to cholinergic stimulation, and decreased neutrophilic, eosinophilic, basophilic, and goblet cell inflammation of the epithelium. Newer, highly potent, topically active, and rapidly metabolized corticosteroid sprays such as beclomethasone dipropionate (Beconase, Vancenase), flunisolide (Nasalide), triamcinolone acetonide (Azmacort), budesonide (investigational), and fluocortin butyl (investigational) are extremely effective in decreasing itching, sneezing, rhinorrhea, and congestion without suppression of the hypothalamic-pituitary-adrenal axis; twice daily is the usual dosing regimen. Recently released pump spray delivery systems are less locally irritating; some of the older available pump and aerosol sprays are frequently reported to sting or cause discomfort from the force of their impact. Care should be taken not to direct the spray toward the septum, as perforations from the trauma and vasoconstriction have occurred. At times, a course of oral corticosteroids may be necessary to relieve symptoms and to reduce the nasal inflammation and obstruction adequately to permit effective use of topical corticosteroids. A tapered course beginning with 30 to 40 mg over 7 days is usually satisfactory for allergic rhinitis. Once improvement is evident, every attempt should be made to control the disorder without systemic corticosteroids. Although intranasal turbinate injections of corticosteroid have been reported as effective and safe in the management of allergic rhinitis, no prospective study has ever documented this, and in addition, both cortisol suppression and loss of vision have been adverse consequences. Considering this information, intranasal corticosteroids sprays would appear to be a much better choice than intranasal injections in the initial management of corticosteroid-responsive allergic rhinitis.

Immunotherapy

Immunotherapy, sometimes referred to as desensitization, is a fourth management measure and is indicated for seasonal or perennial allergic rhinitis that is not adequately controlled by environmental avoidance and tolerated medications. It has been shown to generate antigen-specific IgG-blocking antibody, reduce specific IgE antibody, decrease basophilic cell sensitivity, and increase antigen-specific suppressor T cells. Consultation with an allergist trained and experienced with this treatment modality and familiar with the patient is most likely to produce a safe and effective regimen. In general, about 80 per cent of appropriately selected patients will report amelioration of symptoms, usually observed after a year of immunotherapy. Assuming this improvement, a course of at least 3 years is recommended so that the recurrence of symptoms can be minimized. Current research is directed toward better and more standardized antigen extracts that will result in decreased frequency of required treatments, less likelihood of adverse local or systemic reactions, and improvement of the allergy-induced symptoms.

ADVERSE REACTIONS TO DRUGS

method of
GEORGE R. GREEN, M.D.
Abington Memorial Hospital
Abington, Pennsylvania

Classification of adverse drug reactions can be based upon many factors, such as type of reaction, organ involvement, or causal mechanisms (Table 1).

Nonimmunologic Adverse Drug Reactions

Side effects are predictable but often unwanted actions that are likely to occur even when a drug is used properly and in normal dosage. Side effects, such as the sedation that occurs with antihistamines, tranquilizers, and antidepressants or the dryness of mouth seen with anticholinergics, are common and must be considered in the selection of specific treatment. Often these side effects are variable in incidence and degree, such as the impotence associated with methyldopa (Aldomet) or the risk of bleeding with aspirin, but patients should be alerted to these likely possibilities. Occasionally, side effects may be useful, as in the platelet effect of aspirin, which, although it may induce bleeding, may also prevent stroke and myocardial infarction.

Individual *intolerance* to the usual dosage of medication relates to predictable side effects that occur at unusually small doses. Common examples are nausea and vomiting with quinidine or theophyllines, sleeplessness with ephedrine-containing cold remedies, or excessive bradycardia with beta blockers. These tend to be reproducible with any given patient and carry through to other drugs of the same class, thus limiting the therapeutic alternatives for that patient. Drugs of

TABLE 1. **Classification of Adverse Drug Reactions**

Nonimmunologic
Side effects
Intolerance
Idiosyncratic
Toxic
Secondary effects
Special circumstances
Immunologic

a different class but with a similar mode of action may be tolerated, as in the case of patients who develop excessive tinnitus as a reaction to aspirin but who tolerate nonsalicylate anti-inflammatory drugs such as ibuprofen (Motrin) without difficulty.

Idiosyncratic reactions are pharmacologically unexpected reactions to drugs that occur in relatively few patients, but usually are characteristic of a given drug or class. Examples would be dystonic reactions with prochlorperazine (Compazine), which is usually easily reversed with diphenhydramine (Benadryl), or psychosis from atropine.

Some idiosyncratic reactions are now known to be genetically controlled. For example, hemolytic anemia may occur after treatment with oxidant drugs (such as the antimalarials, phenacetin, or dapsone) in patients with G6PD deficiency, a sex-linked recessive disorder most common among persons of Mediterranean ancestry. Another example is the prolonged paralysis sometimes seen with succinylcholine chloride used for muscle relaxation during surgery in patients with a cholinesterase deficiency.

Many idiosyncratic reactions are "pseudoallergic" or "anaphylactoid," and may be caused by dosage-related release or activation of vasoactive inflammatory mediators such as histamine or leukotrienes. A common example is the reaction that occurs following use of iodinated contrast dyes in radiology. Another group of these idiosyncratic reactions are related to the pharmacologic effect of the drug on an unrelated abnormal system or organ. Bronchospasm occurring with beta-blocking agents in asthmatics or similar reactions occurring with aspirin or the nonsalicylate anti-inflammatory drugs in some patients with nasal polyps and asthma are examples. Even simple chemicals may cause such reactions; for example, sulfites added as preservatives to foods may exacerbate asthma in some instances.

Toxic effects of drugs can be expected with an excessive dose of practically any drug. This most commonly occurs with drugs that have a very narrow therapeutic-toxic index, such as warfarin (Coumadin), which requires very frequent laboratory monitoring to achieve the desired anticoagulant effect without inducing hemorrhage. Many commonly used and important drugs have fairly narrow therapeutic-toxic ratios and must be monitored regularly for the patient to receive optimal benefit without toxicity.

Drug toxicity may be markedly enhanced by impaired metabolism or delayed elimination of the drug and its metabolites. Any patient with known or suspected liver, circulatory, or renal impairment must be managed with great care, with dosage modified and/or drug levels monitored much more frequently than usual. These patients may also respond adversely to many over-the-counter medications and should be educated to the increased risk associated with all medications.

A third area of drug toxicity refers to *drug-drug interactions*. Many patients take two or more drugs to treat their condition or are treating several conditions (often under the care of two or more physicians) simultaneously. This has become such a common problem that many pharmacists have drug interaction programs built into their computer systems. Patients, however, often circumvent even these clever devices by purchasing their medications at two or more pharmacies. These drug interactions often occur because of competition for binding sites for metabolism or excretion, such as between warfarin and phenylbutazone (Butazolidin) or theophyllines and barbiturates. Another compounding difficulty with such interactions is the fact that these may occur with over-the-counter medications that patients often do not consider medications (aspirin and tolbutamide [Orinase] or even with foods (monoamine oxidase inhibitors and cheese).

A final consideration of toxic effects is that of *withdrawal*. This is inherent with the use of many drugs, and the most common examples are alcohol and nicotine. The potential for withdrawal from narcotics, amphetamines, and barbiturates is well known, but it is necessary to be aware that this is a common phenomenon with many chronically used medications, especially when tachyphylaxis or tolerance has required the dosage to become unusually high; for example, the use of decongesting nasal sprays and drops. A related problem is the risk of prolonged shock when steroids have been discontinued after chronic usage.

Finally, certain patients must be labeled as being sensitive to multiple drugs, often with unknown or varied mechanisms, and should be very cautious regarding all medication usage.

Immunologic Adverse Drug Reactions

The classic distinguishing feature of immunologic reactions is the need for prior exposure (sensitization) and the fact that minute dosages can cause violent reactions. Ideally, immunologic sensitivity should be confirmed by the finding of specific antidrug antibodies or sensitized lymphocytes, but, unfortunately, reliable tests are frequently unavailable. This problem is compounded by the fact that the reaction may be to a metabolite rather than to the drug itself.

Penicillin has been the most well studied drug in regard to immunologic reactions. The reactions due to IgE-mediated sensitivity have been found to be most commonly related to the development of IgE antibodies to the penicilloyl hapten, which rapidly develops when penicillin is administered. This hapten binds strongly to serum proteins and is highly immunogenic. Persons who develop IgE antibodies to this penicilloyl protein complex may have an allergic reaction if penicillin or other beta-lactam antibiotics are administered subsequently. Additionally, some patients develop IgE antibodies to penicillin itself, or possibly to other breakdown products such as the benzylpenicilloate hapten (minor determinant). Fortunately, most of the patients sensitized to penicillin can be evaluated with skin testing to penicilloyl-polylysine (Pre-Pen) and penicillin G. In the future there may be a preparation available containing benzylpenicilloate and possibly other degradation products. However, studies with the currently available agents have shown that the reaction rate to penicillin or other beta-lactam antibiotics is only 3 per cent or less in patients who have a history of penicillin allergy and negative skin tests to penicilloyl-polylysine (Pre-Pen) and penicillin G. This reaction rate is similar to that occurring in most populations without a history of penicillin allergy. Other drugs cause IgE-mediated Type I allergic reactions, but skin testing is reliable for only a very few proteins or polypeptides such as horse serum, insulin, streptokinase, and chymopapain.

Management of other drugs suspected of causing allergic reactions involves avoidance or, very rarely, if the drug is essential, readministration of a small test dose under carefully controlled circumstances. Drugs and chemicals that cause contact dermatitis can be identified using a patch test. This causes a limited reproduction of the original reaction and may define a single component of a complex mixture to which the patient is sensitive.

Drugs may occasionally cause reactions by other immunologic mechanisms. High doses of penicillin cause a sufficiently large quantity of the penicilloyl hapten to be bound to red cells that if a patient has enough IgG antibody to penicilloyl, it will cause agglutination of the red cells and hemolysis. Similar immune mechanisms may also be responsible for other cases of anemia as well as for leukopenia and thrombocytopenia.

Approach to the Patient with Adverse Drug Reaction

The problem of an adverse drug reaction is most often raised by a cutaneous rash. Certain drugs are much more commonly associated with cutaneous reactions, for example, penicillin and other beta-lactam antibiotics, sulfonamides, blood and serum products, iodinated contrast media, and possibly erythromycin and barbiturates. However, many commonly used drugs, such as digoxin, antacids, phenothiazines, nitrates, theophyllines, beta blockers, steroids, acetaminophen, antihistamines, and iron, are rarely associated with cutaneous reactions. A more difficult problem is unexplained fever in the patient who is receiving multiple drugs. Here the possibilities tend to parallel to some extent drugs that cause cutaneous reactions. Some drugs are much more commonly associated with drug fever, such as the beta-lactam antibiotics, sulfonamides, and methyldopa (Aldomet). In either case, it is usually more likely that a recently introduced drug will be the cause of the reaction than one that has been tolerated for a prolonged time.

Hematologic reactions such as anemia, granulocytopenia, thrombocytopenia, and agranulocytosis are more often associated with specific drug groups. The risk with chloramphenicol is well known, but other groups such as the anticonvulsants, antimalarials, gold salts, and coal tar derivatives have also been implicated. Damage to specific organs also calls for a careful review of drug history. Hepatic damage has been associated with a wide range of drugs. Similarly, renal toxicity is a potential side effect of many agents, but this is a more common problem with the aminoglycoside antibiotics and nonsalicylate anti-inflammatory drugs.

Prevention of Adverse Drug Reactions

A history of prior adverse reactions should be a routine part of the medical record. If such a history is obtainable, more specific information related to the type of reaction, the variety of agents the patient was taking at the reputed time of the reaction, the type of illness being treated, the interval between the beginning of the course of medication and the onset of the prior reaction, as well as the time interval since that reaction can be helpful in assessment of the real risk of a recurrent reaction. Certain patients have been identified as having multiple drug sensitivities and should be considered at increased risk of future reactions from any drug.

When all of the above factors have been evaluated, a more rational clinical decision can be made, with the likelihood of an adverse drug reaction being weighed against the clinical disease to be treated, with consideration of the alternate treatments that are available. Cross-reactivity among groups of drugs, such as penicillin and cephalosporins, or sulfa-oral hypoglycemics and thiazides, may also be a factor in this evaluation. The chance of an adverse drug reaction will be reduced if the drugs are used only for essential indications. However, occasionally there is a strong indication for the use of an agent despite a clear history of a prior adverse reaction. Local anesthetics are an example of a group of agents for which a history of sensitivity is fairly common but true severe allergic reactions are very uncommon. Consultation and evaluation may be preferable to subjecting the patient to the repetitive risk of general anesthetics, since many of these patients are found to be able to tolerate drugs despite a history of adverse reactions.

Iodinated contrast dyes are also a common cause of adverse reactions. Nevertheless, many patients with such a history have strong indications for a repeat study. This problem can be handled by a series of risk reduction procedures such as re-evaluating the need for the radiographic study or using nonionic contrast media and premedication of the patient with a combination of high-dose steroids, antihistamines, ephedrines, and H_2 antagonists. In addition, the physician must be prepared to deal with a reaction, should it occur, by having an intravenous line in place and emergency equipment at hand.

A history of allergy to penicillin or other beta-lactam antibiotics is important; denying these drugs to the large group of patients with such histories would certainly affect the outcome of treatment of serious infectious diseases. Evaluation should first involve assessing the risk of using substitutes for the beta-lactam antibiotics. If this risk is significant, skin testing to penicillin and penicilloyl-polylysine (Pre-Pen) can give very useful information regarding the true risk of an immediate allergic reaction. If the skin tests are negative and indications are strong, careful use of the appropriate antibiotics could be warranted. The relatively few patients who have a positive skin test are at considerable risk of an immediate allergic reaction, but occasionally the life-threatening nature of the infection may still require their use. One would use the least related antibiotic, for example, a second- or third-generation cephalosporin, and administer the antibiotic using a desensitization technique under very carefully controlled circumstances in a hospital setting. Recent information suggests that aztreonam (Azactam) may not be cross-reactive with beta-lactam antibiotics, but further studies are still in progress.

Treatment of an Adverse Drug Reaction

Immediate discontinuation of the suspect medication is usually all that is required to manage most adverse drug reactions. Cutaneous reactions may require other symptomatic measures including antihistamines for itching, such as hydroxyzine (Atarax or Vistaril), 25 to 100 mg every 6 to 8 hours, or diphenhydramine (Benadryl), 25 mg every 6 hours. Topical steroids may be used for contact dermatitis, but systemic steroids are usually not needed unless there is exfoliative dermatitis or extensive mucous membrane involvement.

Reactions occurring immediately after the initiation of the drug or those that progress rapidly, even if only urticarial, must raise concern of anaphylaxis. The patient should be placed supine and vital signs monitored. Epinephrine 1:1000 in a 0.3 ml dose should be given immediately, and a rapid-acting antihistamine such as diphenhydramine (Benadryl), 25 mg, may be added. If the reaction persists, an intravenous line should be placed and emergency treatment continued with repeated doses of epinephrine, antihistamines, and intravenous steroids while the patient is transported to a hospital emergency room.

ALLERGIC REACTIONS TO INSECT STINGS

method of
MACY I. LEVINE, M.D.
Pittsburgh, Pennsylvania

In the past 10 years immunotherapy with Hymenoptera venoms has become recognized as an effective means of preventing serious reactions to stings in patients allergic to Hymenoptera insects. Allergic reactions to insect stings are very common and are responsible for about 40 deaths each year in the United States. Therefore, proper diagnosis and management is of crucial importance in minimizing the seriousness of reactions to these stings. It should be noted that insects of the order Hymenoptera, which includes bees, hornets, wasps, yellowjackets, and fire ants, are responsible for the vast majority of allergic reactions to insect stings in the United States.

Local Reactions

The insect sting may produce no visible reaction or it may produce a welt up to 1 cm in diameter with itching. The patient may require no treatment, a local cold compress, or an oral antihistamine, such as diphenhydramine (Benadryl), 25 to 50 mg every 4 hours. If there is a stinger from a bee present, it must be scraped or flicked away so as not to introduce more venom into the skin. It should not be pulled out.

A large local swelling at the site of the sting and in the contiguous area may occur, frequently causing apprehension or even panic, especially when the face, eyelids, and mouth are affected. As long as the airway is not compromised, these large local reactions are not serious or dangerous. They are due not to any allergic mechanism, but to an inflammatory reaction to the venom constituents. Furthermore, they do not appear to be forerunners of more serious allergic reactions. Treatment is symptomatic with local cold compresses, oral antihistamines and analgesics, explanation, and reassurance. Subcutaneous injection of epinephrine (1:1000), 0.2 to 0.3 ml at the sting site, if on the trunk or an extremity, may help reduce the swelling. The patient must be observed closely if the swelling involves the airway so that additional therapeutic measures may be instituted if necessary. Patients with large local reactions do not require allergy testing or immunotherapy.

At times the sting site becomes infected and requires treatment similar to that for other local infections.

Systemic Reactions

A systemic reaction may develop within minutes or up to 1 hour following an insect sting. Generally, any reaction beginning after that time is not likely to be serious. Symptoms include urticaria, angioedema, shortness of breath, coughing, wheezing, abdominal cramps, or diarrhea. Symptoms may be very mild or very severe, with anaphylactic shock being the most severe reaction. Anaphylaxis usually develops within minutes of the sting and includes the above symptoms in addition to a fall in blood pressure, sweating, pallor, weakness, tachycardia, nausea, and vomiting.

Systemic reactions represent allergic reactions to some constituent of the insect venom, mediated by an IgE antibody.

Systemic reactions demand immediate attention beginning with the administration of epinephrine hydrochloride (1:1000), 0.2 to 0.5 ml subcutaneously, and followed by an antihistamine, such as diphenhydramine or chlorpheniramine, either by mouth or by intramuscular administration, depending on the severity of the reaction. A small dose of epinephrine may be repeated in 15 to 20 minutes if there has been no satisfactory response. A tourniquet should be applied proximal to the sting site when the sting is on an extremity. Aminophylline, 250 to 500 mg, should be administered intravenously over a period of 30 minutes for bronchospasm. Oxygen and vasopressor agents may be given if necessary. Antihistamines and ephedrine, 25 mg, may be given every 4 hours by mouth if the symptoms continue. If the patient does not respond within 15 or 20 minutes, arrangements for hospitalization and further therapy must be made as quickly as possible. Whether corticosteroid agents should be administered remains a matter of opinion, since there have been no controlled studies of the use of these drugs in serious allergic reactions or anaphylaxis. On theoretical grounds, corticosteroids should not be helpful for acute allergic reactions or anaphylaxis and, therefore, are not recommended by many experts.

On rare occasion the patient may have the serum sickness type of reaction to the insect sting, with urticaria, angioedema, fever, and arthralgia. Other rare reactions include neuritis, nephrosis, vasculitis, or encephalopathy. The mechanism for these reactions is not understood. The treatment is symptomatic.

Immunotherapy

Immunization with specific Hymenoptera venoms has been well documented as a preventive of serious reactions to stings in persons known to have reacted previously. Children appear to be at much less risk from repeated stings than adults and require immunization only if they have had a life-threatening reaction, such as severe urticaria, severe angioedema, or anaphylaxis.

Children who have had severe allergic reactions and adults who have had any type of allergic reaction should be tested with the Hymenoptera venoms as the initial diagnostic procedure. The purpose of this testing is to identify the presence of IgE antibodies to the insect venoms, which signify that the patient has some degree of risk from another insect sting. Testing begins with scratch or prick tests and proceeds to intradermal testing using venoms containing up to 1.0 microgram of venom per milliliter. A two-plus or greater reaction to any venom test is considered a positive test and indicates that the patient is a candidate for immunization therapy. Patients with negative tests do not require immunization therapy.

If the insect causing the sting and reaction has been positively identified, the patient may be immunized only with the venom of that insect. If the insect has not been identified, the patient should be immunized with each venom that produces a significant positive reaction.

In some situations it may be preferable to obtain RAST tests to measure sensitivity to the insect venoms. For example, when the patient has had a life-threatening or anaphylactic reaction and there is some concern about the safety of skin testing, a RAST test with the specific sting venom or venoms could be obtained. Again, a significant positive RAST test indicates that the patient is at risk and requires immunotherapy.

Immunotherapy is given with a specific insect venom or venoms by means of deep subcutaneous injections at weekly intervals beginning with a strength of venom containing 0.001 to 0.1 microgram of venom per milliliter. Injections are given at weekly intervals as a rule following a schedule that comes with the commercial extract or appears in most textbooks of allergy. The dose should be increased up to a maintenance dose of 100 micrograms of the venom. The interval between injections is gradually extended to 4 weeks for the first year of therapy, then to 6 weeks. Some experts increase the interval to 8 weeks. Other schedules have been used, depending largely on physician's preferences and patients' requirements.

Until recently it was recommended that immunization therapy be continued indefinitely. Studies are now in progress to determine the criteria for discontinuation of therapy. At the present time it appears that if the skin test reactions or RAST results become negative, immunotherapy may be discontinued. Some experts have suggested that treatment be stopped after 5 years. However, the long-term reaction rate from repeated stings has not been established, so that at this time there are no firm guidelines for discontinuation of therapy. It is recommended that treatment be continued until specific recommendations can be made.

Fire Ant Allergy

In ten southern states along the Gulf Coast, the fire ant is an important cause of insect sting allergy. Fire ant venom is not commercially available, so that whole-body extracts have been used for testing and for immunization. The principles of diagnosis and therapy are the same for fire ant allergy as for other Hymenoptera allergy. Studies are being conducted with fire ant venom to determine its effectiveness and usefulness so that it may be determined whether this should become commercially available.

General Directions for Patients

Patients who have had reactions to insect stings should be advised to follow certain precautions in order to avoid further stings. These directions include avoidance of the insects that have produced reactions, avoiding situations where stings are likely to occur, wearing long-sleeve shirts, stockings, and shoes when outdoors, avoiding perfumes and other cosmetics that may attract insects, and avoiding foods and beverages that attract insects.

Those who are at risk from another insect sting should carry some antihistamine, such as diphenhydramine (Benadryl), 25 mg, or chlorpheniramine (Chlor-Trimeton), 4 mg, to be used in case of any sting. In addition, the patient who has had an allergic reaction should have available a kit containing epinephrine, a tourniquet, and an antihistamine in case of any reaction. An insect sting kit such as the AnaKit is commercially available. Epinephrine in the form of the EpiPen (Center Laboratories) is available for immediate injection.

Diseases of the Skin

ACNE VULGARIS AND ROSACEA

method of
DAN K. CHALKER, M.D.
Medical College of Georgia
Augusta, Georgia

ACNE VULGARIS

The onset of acne vulgaris coincides with puberty and peaks in the mid-teens. Even so, a large number of adults present with acne vulgaris for the first time. The lesions consist of papules and pustules with open and closed comedones (blackheads and whiteheads). The face, back, and chest are more commonly involved. Acne is a product of the sebaceous follicle. The initial event may be a hyperkeratosis of the follicular orifice. This narrowing of the follicular opening allows retention of sebaceous gland secretions and proliferation of *Propionibacterium acnes (P. acnes)*. This resident bacterium is an anaerobic diphtheroid. The overgrowth of this organism and subsequent production of chemotactic substances attracts neutrophils into the follicle. The ingestion of *P. acnes* by the neutrophils results in the release of hydrolytic enzymes, rupture of the follicle wall, and extrusion of follicular contents into the dermis. Inflammation results and presents as a papule or pustule to the clinician. The mechanism for formation of the comedonal lesions (blackheads and whiteheads) is less clear.

Treatment

The patient should be made aware that treatment is long term and response slow. A history of medications the patient is taking can be helpful. Certain medications, notably corticosteroids, ACTH, testosterone, Dilantin, isoniazid, and lithium may aggravate or produce acne eruptions. Certain medications, food, antacids, and diet supplements may interfere with absorption of oral antibiotics. It is important to tell the patient how to take or apply the medication. A topical medication should be applied over the entire affected area, not just on individual lesions. The goal of therapy is prevention of new lesions. Some patients have the idea that acne is related to dirt or uncleanliness and attempt to scrub lesions away. It should be emphasized that topical treatment is to be done gently and medication applied in a thin layer. Excessive irritation is not a goal. In some patients, simply stopping the scrubbing with soaps and abrasives (especially if a brush or other such appliance is used) results in improvement.

Topical Therapy

Many cases of acne can be handled by topical means alone. Initially a combination of topical and systemic therapy may be used and, as response is obtained, topical therapy alone may suffice.

Tretinoin. Tretinoin (Retin-A) is widely used in the treatment of acne. It decreases the cohesiveness of epidermal cells and stimulates cell turnover. A frequent problem is skin irritation. Most patients are unable to apply medication twice daily initially. I initiate therapy with applications 3 times a week for 4 to 6 weeks and then increase applications to every other day, and then to daily use as tolerated. If necessary, applications may be increased to twice daily. If significant irritation occurs, the patient should discontinue medication. A flare-up may occur sometime around the sixth week of therapy. In most cases this is temporary; however, in some it may persist and medication may have to be discontinued. Patients may find a moisturizer beneficial. Retin-A is available in a liquid, cream, and gel. Concentrations vary from .01 per cent to 0.1 per cent. I use the .01 per cent gel or the .05 per cent cream when initiating therapy. The strength may be increased, according to tolerance and response.

Benzoyl Peroxide. Benzoyl peroxide is probably the most widely used agent in the treatment of acne. It is available over-the-counter and by prescription. Benzoyl peroxide works by its antibacterial and keratolytic effect. A recent study suggested an anti-inflammatory ability. Benzoyl peroxide is available in creams, lotions, washes, gels, and soaps. It is available in strengths of 2.5, 5, and 10 per cent. There is no evidence that the 10 per cent concentration is more efficacious than the lower concentrations. I prefer the 5 per cent benzoyl peroxide gels. I have the patient apply this once daily for the first 3 to 4 weeks and, with tolerance, increase to twice-daily applications. Although allergic sensitization is possible, I have found this very uncommon, if not rare. It should be cautioned that benzoyl peroxide can bleach colored garments or hair. Benzoyl peroxide may be combined with either tretinoin (Retin-A) or one of the topical antibiotics, with the patient applying one in the morning and the other in the evening.

Topical Antibiotics. A number of topical antibiotics have been introduced for the treatment of acne vulgaris. These include tetracycline, erythromycin, clindamycin and meclocycline sulfosalicylate. They are available in liquids, gels, saturated pads, creams, and ointments. The topical antibiotics work through antibacterial and anti-inflammatory mechanisms. In cases of mild to moderate inflammatory acne, these can be used alone. The usual application is twice daily. A combination therapy using either Retin-A or benzoyl peroxide in the morning and the antibiotic at night or vice versa may be employed. This has the advantage of two mechanisms of action. If antibiotic and benzoyl peroxide are applied at the same time, the benzoyl peroxide neutralizes the antibiotic. When using tretinoin (Retin-A) or benzoyl peroxide, the patient may experience dryness, and use of an antibiotic cream or ointment may be desirable. Meclocycline sulfosalicylate (Meclan) cream and erythromycin ointment (Akne-mycin) are available. In cold dry climates or in certain patients with sensitive skin, a cream or ointment may be preferred. A tinted topical erythromycin solution (Ery-Sol) is available. Some patients prefer this tinted solution, especially under make-up.

A combination of 5 per cent benzoyl peroxide and 3 per cent erythromycin (Benzamycin gel) is available. It is mixed when dispensed and requires 3 ml of alcohol mixed with a powder to form a gel (I note on the prescription that the medication should be mixed with grain alcohol). It is applied once or twice daily. Benzamycin has been shown to be effective in the treatment of inflammatory as well as comedonal acne.

The numerous over-the-counter (OTC) acne products include astringents, lotions, soaps, and so forth. Most of these contain sulfur, resorcinol, alcohol, and salicylic acid. Salicylic acid is mildly keratolytic and comedolytic. The mechanism and efficacy of sulfur and resorcinol is not well established. These products can be useful in mild cases of acne.

Oral Antibiotic Therapy

The most commonly used antibiotic in the treatment of acne vulgaris is tetracycline. Tetracycline is administered in a dose of 500 to 2000 mg orally per day. I usually start with 500 mg twice daily. This is useful in inflammatory acne when there is a significant number of papules and pustules. In almost all cases I use a topical agent in conjunction with the oral antibiotic. The goal is to continue the therapy for several months, decrease the oral medication, and maintain on topical therapy alone.

Problems in administration of tetracycline consist primarily of gastrointestinal upset and vaginal yeast infection. Tetracycline will bind with divalent cations in the intestine. The patient should be asked about consumption of milk and of medications or vitamins containing iron and antacids. The medication is best given on an empty stomach. Phototoxic eruptions may occur with tetracycline, and its effect on bones and teeth must also be kept in mind.

Doxycycline (Vibramycin) and minocycline (Minocin) are also useful in acne therapy. They are absorbed better than tetracycline and are not as easily chelated to cations in the bowel. The dosage for Vibramycin is 50 to 100 mg orally per day. Minocin is given as 50 mg once or twice daily. If given in higher dosages it may result in vertigo. Minocin may cause a bluish discoloration of the skin. This is an infrequent and reversible complication.

Erythromycin in a dosage of 500 to 2000 mg per day orally is commonly employed therapy for acne. The usual dosage is 500 mg twice daily by mouth. Chelation and decreased absorption is not as much a problem as with tetracycline. Gastrointestinal disturbance with erythromycin may prohibit its use.

Trimethoprim-Sulfamethoxazole (Bactrim, Septra) may be beneficial in patients not responding to other antibiotic therapy. I use it in selected cases.

Clindamycin (Cleocin) has also been used in treating acne vulgaris and is very effective. However, the possible development of pseudomembranous colitis and its complications has all but precluded its use.

Hormone Therapy

The dosage of estrogen required to suppress the sebaceous gland is such that I rarely, if ever, use this therapy in ordinary acne vulgaris. Spironolactone in a dosage of 150 to 200 mg orally per day is anti-androgenic. This drug is restricted to use in female patients due to its feminizing effects. I have used it in selected cases; however, I do not recommend it in the treatment of the ordinary case of acne vulgaris.

Accutane Therapy

Isotretinoin (Accutane) is now available and is indicated for cases of severe acne resistant to conventional therapy. These are usually severe cases of cystic acne. Accutane is effective through its anti-keratinizing effect and inhibition of the sebaceous gland.

The possible complications of Accutane therapy will be considered here before discussing the dosage. A primary concern is the teratogenicity of Accutane (the drug is teratogenic but not mutagenic), which should be discussed with the patient. The drug should be used with extreme caution in women of childbearing potential. These patients should be checked for pregnancy prior to therapy and should practice an effective method of birth control during and for at least one month following treatment.

A generalized dryness on the skin and mucous membranes is expected. Cheilitis is experienced by most patients. Skin fragility and pruritus are common. Other side effects include peeling of the palms and soles, thinning of hair, conjunctivitis, dry eyes, dry nose, epistaxis, increased sensitivity to sunlight, formation of granulation tissue, increased tendency to form keloids, nasal colonization by staphylococci, hyperostosis, musculoskeletal discomfort, decreased night vision, and headache. Elevated triglyceride, cholesterol, creatinine phosphokinase, uric acid, and liver function studies have been reported and should be monitored. The hyperostosis may or may not return to pre-treatment condition, but other problems usually resolve after Accutane is discontinued. Patients should not take vitamin A while on Accutane therapy.

The dosage of Accutane is 0.5 to 2.0 mg per kg daily. The usual dose is 1 mg per kg per day. The medication is administered for a period of 4 to 5 months. The response may be slow and a flareup of the acne may occur (usually around the second month of therapy). Although there may be little improvement over the 4- to 5-month period, the medication should be stopped at that point, and a response may still occur.

Corticosteroid Therapy

Systemic corticosteroids are uncommonly used in the therapy of acne vulgaris, due to the prolonged course of acne and the side effects of systemic corticosteroid therapy. In a few instances, such therapy may be indicated for a brief period—for example, for a patient with an acute flare-up of acne while on Accutane therapy or a patient that has an acute limited flare-up. Prednisone in a dose of 40 to 60 mg per day on a decreasing dose schedule over 10 to 14 days is usually effective.

Corticosteroid therapy in a topical form may initially improve acne; however, it is contraindicated due to its acneogenic potential. One can create acne in the facial area by application of potent topical corticosteroid preparations. Intralesional corticosteroid therapy may be used in patients with cystic or large inflamed lesions. The dosage is 2.5, 5, or 10 mg per ml of Kenalog. This is injected directly into the lesions. There may be a slight depression in some lesions after injection; however, this is usually reversible.

Miscellaneous Therapy

Cosmetics. The use of oil-free cosmetics is advised in the acne patient. Abstention from cosmetics is ideal; however, this advice is not practical with most patients. Eye shadow, lipstick, and a dry blush are preferred, but if patients persist in using make-up, I advise cleansing the skin thoroughly when removing make-up and applying Velmasque (an OTC acne treatment mask), allowing it to dry for 10 to 15 minutes, and gently rinsing it off. This should be followed by a warm compress for 10 to 15 minutes.

Diet. Dietary manipulation and restrictions have been used in acne therapy. There is no objective evidence of effectiveness and I do not use dietary restrictions.

Ultraviolet Light. Sunlight and obtaining suntans have been advocated as acne therapy in the past. The only purpose it serves is to mask the disorder.

Acne Surgery. A direct approach to removal of the lesions, particularly comedones, is with a comedone extractor. This is best done after the patient has been on topical therapy for at least a month. Opening of whiteheads with a small needle prior to using the extractor is recommended. The use of the comedone extractor usually leaves areas of erythema that are highly visible for the next day or so. It is wise to ask patients if they have a social function to attend within the next 48 to 72 hours prior to instituting this therapy.

Face Peels. I use a mild peel, trichloroacetic acid (TCA), on selected patients. The concentration is 25 to 35 per cent. It is most useful for comedonal acne in fair-skinned individuals. An active herpes simplex lesion must not be present. Although an easy technique, instruction in the procedure is necessary.

ROSACEA

Rosacea is an acneiform eruption that usually occurs in people in their thirties and beyond. It is seen primarily on the face; however, lesions may be scattered over the trunk. Rosacea differs from acne vulgaris in that the lesions include papules, pustules, erythema, and telangiectasias. Comedones are not a feature of rosacea. Previously it was felt that alcohol ingestion played a significant role in this disorder; however, recent studies have shown that this is not true.

The nose may develop swollen areas secondary to sebaceous gland enlargement, a condition called rhinophyma. The eyes may be involved with a blepharitis, conjunctivitis, keratitis, and less commonly iritis.

Treatment

The treatment of rosacea is primarily systemic antibiotic therapy. Most effective is tetracycline orally in a dosage of 500 to 2000 mg per day. Most cases will show improvement over a period of 6 to 8 weeks. Long-term antibiotic therapy is necessary; however, a reduction in dosage can often be made after 3 to 4 months and dosage maintained at the lowest possible dose (usually 250 to 500 mg orally per day). The improvement is seen primarily in the papules and pustules. The ocular problems, if present, usually improve. Other antibiotics, notably erythromycin in the same dosage, may be used to treat rosacea. Other forms of tetracycline such as minocycline (Minocin) and doxycycline (Vibramycin) may be used. The dosage of these is the same as for acne vulgaris.

Topical therapy is not as effective as in acne vulgaris. I have used topical tetracycline (Topicycline) in patients with mild to moderate rosacea. Topical erythromycin does not appear to be as efficacious. Sodium sulfacetamide (Sebazon lotion) may be beneficial. I have not found benzoyl peroxide to be as helpful, and it may irritate the patient's skin.

Rhinophyma may be treated by excision of the offending nodules on the nose. This may be done with cold steel, dermabrasion, laser, or other surgical techniques.

The most difficult problems to treat in the rosacea patient are the erythema and telangiectasia. Telangiectasias may be treated with fulguration by an experienced operator; erythema is more difficult to treat. Patients with rosacea have been advised to avoid hot foods, both in temperature and spice content. They have also been advised to abstain from alcohol. As stated earlier, alcohol is not an etiologic agent in rosacea, although it may make the lesions more apparent once they are present. I have advised patients to decrease their intake of hot foods, spicy foods, and alcohol and to avoid exposure to extreme hot or cold. I have found this to be of limited value.

HAIR DISORDERS
method of
WILMA F. BERGFELD, M.D.
The Cleveland Clinic Foundation
Cleveland, Ohio

To understand hair disorders (Table 1), it is essential to be aware of normal hair growth patterns. Scalp hair grows in an asynchronous pattern with 85 to 95 per cent of hair in an anagen growth phase (active) and 10 to 15 per cent in a telogen phase (resting). Any alteration of hair growth will present clinically as increased shedding of scalp hair, a telogen or dystrophic anagen shed. In addition, variations of hair growth are normally observed with age, sex, and season.

Office techniques that aid in the diagnosis of hair disorders include visual examination of the scalp, skin, body hair, and nails. Specific diagnostic techniques include hair pulls, hair plucks, light microscopy examination of hair fibers and scalp scales, and scalp biopsies (Tables 2 and 3).

Alterations of Hair Growth Cycles. The complaint from a patient that his or her hair is coming out by the roots represents an alteration in the cyclic growth pattern of scalp hair, which may present as either a telogen or an anagen shed. The mechanism of action appears to reside in the degree of insult to the growing germinal center of the anagen hair follicle. A minimal insult will initiate the formation of early telogen or resting hair follicles; a maximal insult will partially or totally interrupt the active metabolism of the anagen germinal center and cause an anagen arrest or cessation of growth of this hair follicle. This results in abrupt shedding of the deformed or dystrophic hair fiber. A slower insult will result in the shedding of an abnormal telogen hair (Table 4).

ANDROGENIC ALOPECIA

Androgenic alopecia is the most common form of baldness observed in genetically predisposed

TABLE 1. **Classification of Hair Disorders**

Nonscarring
  Alterations in hair growth cycles
  Telogen shed
    Androgenic alopecia
  Anagen shed (effluvium)
  Alterations of hair shaft (trichodystrophies—fragile hair)
    Congenital hair shaft abnormalities
    Acquired trichodystrophies
      Trichotillomania
      Physical and chemical damage
    Tinea capitis

Scarring
  Lupus erythematosus, chronic
  Lichen planopilaris
  Pseudopelade
  Scleroderma
  Sequela of suppurative skin inflammation
    Tinea capitis
  Physical and chemical damage

TABLE 2. **Normal Scalp Hair Growth Patterns**

Average total number of scalp hairs is 100,000.
Fastest growth is between 15 and 30 years of age.
Slow growth occurs in the elderly.
Average rate of growth is 0.35 mm/day.
Faster growth occurs in summer than in winter.
Active growth period is 2 to 5 years prior to replacement.
Average daily loss is 25 to 100 hairs/day.
Female hair grows faster than male hair.
Fiber diameters and shapes vary in different races and nationalities.

TABLE 4. **Causes of Hair Loss**

Telogen Shed
Childbirth (postpartum)
Androgenic alopecia
Febrile illness (postfebrile)
Surgical shock
Drugs
Alopecia areata
Endocrinopathies
Nutritional and metabolic deficiencies
Chronic infection
Collagen vascular disease

Anagen Shed
Anticoagulants
Antimetabolites
Cytotoxic agents
Alkylating agents
Alopecia areata

individuals whose hair follicles are highly sensitive to androgen hormones as compared with those of normal, nonalopecic individuals. Essentially in the predisposed individual, there is a gradual reduction of scalp hair density. In males, there is also a gradual transformation of terminal (large) anagen hair to fine vellus hair in a pattern distribution. In females, there is a slowly progressive, diffuse reduction of scalp hair density without vellus hair formation. Rarely, the male presents with a female pattern, and vice versa. Androgenic alopecia most commonly presents as a telogen shed or effluvium and is considered an autosomal dominant disorder observed in both sexes. It may occur in the early teens or late adult life. Clinically, the earlier the presentation, the greater the loss of scalp hair and, ultimately, the worse the condition.

Female androgenic alopecia appears in women with strong family histories of baldness and a personal history of normal or abnormal menses with or without associated androgen excess signs. In women, androgenic alopecia may occur in youth and in paramenopausal and postmenopausal states. The younger women have an increased incidence of acquired adrenal hyperplasia, polycystic ovaries, or both. The older female has relative estrogen depletion with relative testosterone excess and only occasionally the same

TABLE 3. **Diagnosis of Hair Disorders**

Local Examination
Pattern of hair loss
Length and diameter of hair fiber
Hair pull, pluck (trichodystrophy)
Light microscopy examination of hair
Scalp skin condition
Fungal culture
Scalp biopsy

Laboratory Examination—Screen
CBC, differential, SMA-12
Serologic tests
Serum iron
Thyroid screen (T4, TSH, microsomal antibodies)
Special studies as indicated by history and physical examination; androgen excess screen, testosterone, dehydroepiandrosterone, androstenedione, urinary adrenal profile

findings as the young female. These women are best evaluated by androgen screening tests, which would include serum testosterone, free testosterone, dehydroepiandrosterone, and androstenedione. Urinary adrenal steroids can be done to further elucidate the androgen excess.

Treatment

The treatment of androgenic alopecia is less than desirable. In men, the treatment consists of creative hair styles, hair pieces, hair transplantation, and scalp reduction. Most recently, the topical use of 2 per cent minoxidil twice a day has been advocated. In women, similar treatment modalities are available; in addition, antiandrogens and estrogens are employed. These agents* include estrogen-dominant products such as norethynodrel with mestranol (Enovid-E) and ethynodiol with mestranol (Ovulen) or topical progesterones in solution. Oral spironolactone (Aldactone) in doses of 50 to 200 mg daily has also been used successfully. When there is a need for adrenal suppression, dexamethasone in doses of 0.125 to 0.25 mg daily is used for 4 or more months. Contraindications to antiandrogen therapy include a strong family history of carcinoma, especially breast carcinoma and colon cancer, thrombophlebitis, and severe vascular headaches.

ANAGEN SHED

Anagen shed (effluvium) is the result of an extreme alteration or cessation of growth of the growing anagen matrix. This results in dystrophic or deformed hair fibers that are weak and easily shed from the scalp and other hairy areas. These sheds are observed 1 to 2 weeks after the

---

*The use of these agents is not specifically mentioned in the manufacturers' official directives.

insult to the growing hair. As a result of the altered growth, multiple trichodystrophies or abnormal hair fibers are observed on examination. The use of chemotherapeutic drugs such as antimetabolites, alkylating agents, and cytotoxic agents is the insult that usually causes cessation of growth. Alopecia areata has also presented as an anagen dystrophic shed.

ALOPECIA AREATA

Alopecia areata classically presents as an anagen dystrophic shed and is thought to be an autoimmune disease associated with other autoimmune diseases such as Hashimoto's thyroiditis and vitiligo. While the chronic presentation of the insidious, patchy discoid lesions commonly is as a mixed telogen and an anagen dystrophic shed, the most common history is an abrupt onset of discoid alopecic lesions that have a 1 per cent incidence of further progression within weeks or months to alopecia totalis or universalis.

The clinical presentation of patchy, discoid alopecia areata is often difficult to differentiate from trichotillomania or tinea capitis. Diagnostic techniques to differentiate the three disorders include a scalp biopsy and fungal culture. A scalp biopsy specimen of alopecia areata demonstrates characteristic lymphocytic cuffing around germinal centers of the anagen hair and negative fungal cultures.

Treatment

The treatment varies from topical irritant, hypersensitivity therapy to topical corticosteroids and oral corticosteroids. Duration of treatment varies from weeks to years. For children, it is advisable to use topical medications rather than oral corticosteroids. Multiple vitamins and minerals have been used successfully in children.

PHYSICAL AND CHEMICAL DAMAGE

Physical and chemical damage to hair is infrequently secondary to sunlight and harmful hair care techniques. These techniques injure the hair shaft and produce fragile hair that is easily broken with normal handling. These hair disorders may be corrected by discontinuing the inducing agent or practice for at least 12 months with gradual cutting off of the damaged hair. Shampoos and hair conditioners are helpful, but until the hair regrows and replaces itself, the damage remains. Chronic repetitive physical and chemical damage may result in a permanent scarring alopecia.

TRACTION ALOPECIA

Hair loss secondary to traction, pulling, or tugging on the scalp hair will also produce alterations in the growth cycle and abnormalities of the hair shaft. If traction on the hair is repetitive and chronic, it may induce irreversible scarring alopecia. Such hair care techniques that commonly induce alopecias include braiding, ponytails, elastic hair bands, hair rollers, and extreme and repetitive teasing of the scalp hair.

TRICHOTILLOMANIA

Trichotillomania is a traction alopecia that is produced by a patient who pulls, tugs, plucks, or cuts the hair in a bizarre pattern. This condition is commonly associated with psychological disorders and is frequently seen in children and elderly females. Clinically, the patient is observed to have incomplete hair loss with a short stubble of hair on the scalp, eyebrows, or other hairy areas. If the eyelashes and eyebrows are involved, hair restoration will take at least 3 months after manipulation has ceased. Diagnosis is confirmed by light microscopy of the clipped hair, which demonstrates fracture of the terminal, pigmented ends. A scalp biopsy is helpful in identifying increased numbers of resting, telogen hair follicles, follicular cysts with evidence of trichomalacia (pigmented, broken hair fibers), and perifollicular hemorrhage and scarring. Therapy is psychological counseling and treatment.

TRICHORRHEXIS NODOSA

Trichorrhexis nodosa is a common trichodystrophy that can be a congenital or acquired defect of hair keratinization. The acquired defects are a result of various physical and chemical processes that induce a structural defect of the intracellular cement of the cuticle that cause defective keratinization of the external root sheath. On rare occasions, trichorrhexis nodosa may be associated with an inborn error of metabolism, aminoaciduria.

The acquired form of trichorrhexis nodosa clinically may be of two varieties: a proximal nodal lesion and a distal nodal lesion. The proximal nodal lesions represent a distinct disorder of the black population, whereas the distal nodal lesions are more commonly observed in whites. The usual complaint is that the hair is short and of good density but fails to grow. The history reveals indulgence in a variety of hair care techniques such as hair straightening, hot combing, reverse permanent waves, and coloring. Characteristically, the hair breaks off suddenly and becomes strikingly short in the affected areas, which may be patchy or diffuse. The treatment of choice is discontinuation of all hair care products except for normal shampooing and the use of hair conditioners. This condition may last for 2 to 6 years or indefinitely.

TINEA CAPITIS

Tinea capitis presents as an inflammatory or noninflammatory scalp condition. A noninflammatory type presents as a papulosquamous patch or scaling with decreased hair, whereas the inflammatory type is an indurated suppurative plaque with prominent folliculitis. The papulosquamous form is most frequently caused by *Microsporum canis* or *M. audouinii* and *Trichophyton tonsurans*. The suppurative form, kerion, is caused by *T. mentagrophytes, M. gypseum, T. ferrugineum,* and *T. schoenleini.* Wood's light examination of the involved scalp may demonstrate green fluorescence when the causative agent is *M. canis.* A potassium hydroxide (KOH) examination of plucked hair or scales for spores or hyphae is diagnostic. Fungal cultures of hair and scales are frequently necessary to confirm the diagnosis.

Treatment

Treatment of choice for both disorders includes local cleansing and débridement, topical antifungal agents (imidazoles), and oral griseofulvin. When a kerion is present, adjunctive use of antibiotics may be necessary.

INFLAMMATORY SCARRING ALOPECIA

Inflammatory scarring alopecias of the scalp are most commonly diagnosed as chronic lupus erythematosus, lichen planopilaris, pseudopelade, and morphea scleroderma.

Lupus erythematosus, of the discoid or chronic type, may present with or without systemic disease. It is characterized by alopecic, indurated papulosquamous plaques on the scalp or sun-exposed areas of the skin. A biopsy of the active lesion demonstrates intense inflammatory reaction around hair follicles with ultimate destruction. Biopsy of older lesions demonstrates fibrosis and obliteration of all the dermal appendages, including the hair follicles. Diagnosis of lupus erythematosus can be made by clinical presentation, skin biopsy, and direct immunofluorescence. Serologic testing for collagen vascular disease may be negative. Therapy consists of topical and oral corticosteroids and antimalarial drugs.

Lichen planopilaris is a rare, patchy, scarring alopecia of the scalp that presents as a papulosquamous patch with follicular prominence. It occurs primarily in adults and is difficult to differentiate from lupus erythematosus. The presence of skin lesions of lichen planopilaris associated with the scarring alopecia may be helpful in arriving at the diagnosis. The use of direct immunofluorescence techniques and biopsy specimens may differentiate the two disorders. Discoid lupus erythematosus demonstrates a band fluorescence at the dermal-epidermal junction and the follicular junction of IgG and C3. Lichen planopilaris demonstrates a globular deposition of IgG, IgA, and fibrinogen adjacent to the superficial epithelium and follicular epithelium, but not involving the dermal-epidermal junction. The treatment of lichen planopilaris is similar to that of discoid lupus erythematosus. The use of systemic and topical corticosteroids and antimalarial agents has been helpful in limiting the progression of the disorder. Regrowth of hair in the scarred alopecic areas will not occur. When there are scarred areas, the preferred treatment is hair transplantation, scalp reduction, or both.

Pseudopelade is an uncommon, slowly progressive, patchy alopecic condition of unknown etiology that affects males and females in their mature years. Clinically it resembles end-stage discoid lupus erythematosus and lichen planopilaris. A scalp biopsy reveals two types: noninflammatory and inflammatory, with an end-stage of scarring and permanent alopecia. Treatment is unrewarding; however, treatments reported include corticosteroids, high-dose tetracycline, antimalarial agents, Fulvicin, and isotretinoin, alone and in combination.

Localized scleroderma is a rare cutaneous disorder that may present as a mild inflammatory scarring alopecia. The clinical and histologic presentation is classic and demonstrates the scarring alopecia with prominent dermal sclerosis and patchy mononuclear perivascular infiltrate. Active localized scleroderma has responded to parenteral antimalarial drugs. The disease is generally self-limited, and the quiescent lesions can be cosmetically treated with hair transplantation, scalp reduction, or both.

TUMORS OF THE SCALP

Benign and malignant neoplastic tumors of the scalp will interrupt or destroy the hair follicles. Clinically, the patients will have an alopecic patch or a palpable tumor. Skin biopsy of the localized involved area is generally diagnostic. The most common neoplasms of the skin include pilar cysts, nevocytic nevi, organoid nevi, basal cell carcinomas, warts, sarcoidosis, and metastatic lesions from the breast, lung, and gastrointestinal tract.

CANCER OF THE SKIN
method of
MICHAEL J. ALBOM, M.D.
New York, New York

Several modalities are suitable for the treatment of epithelial cancers of the skin. To arrive at a proper treatment for a particular case, one must assess (1) the gross and microscopic type of neoplasm; (2) whether it is primary or recurrent; (3) the size and depth of penetration; (4) the anatomic location; (5) the general history of the patient, judged from a detailed history of pertinent disease (e.g., hypertension, and whether a pacemaker is being worn), medications currently being taken, allergies, bleeding tendencies, and problems with wound healing (e.g., keloids); and (6) cosmetic considerations.

Biopsy

The type of neoplasm can usually be diagnosed by clinical examination. Nevertheless, a biopsy of the lesion should be done and histologic confirmation or correction of the clinical diagnosis should be sought before definitive treatment is planned. Skill in clinical dermatology and histopathology is a prerequisite to intelligent choices of proper methods of biopsy. For example, if one were to plan to treat a basal cell carcinoma with curettage and electrodesiccation, a biopsy should be done by shave with a scalpel or sharp curet. The reason is that in order to extirpate a basal cell carcinoma by curettage and electrodesiccation, the dermal base under the lesion must be intact so that the soft material of the cancerous tissue can be distinguished from the firmness of normal uninvolved dermis, which resists removal by curettage. If a biopsy by punch is unwisely chosen, penetration into superficial subcutaneous fat is likely, and such removal of full-thickness of dermis instantly cancels the use of curettage and electrodesiccation as a proper procedure. If a lesion is suspected of being a malignant melanoma, it is necessary if at all feasible to perform a biopsy of the gross lesion in toto in order to furnish the pathologist an adequate specimen to judge its characteristics, especially thickness. If a lesion suspected of being malignant melanoma is too large or so situated that biopsy in toto is not feasible, then biopsy in part may be done and planned to include a portion of the lesion that is likely to reveal the true thickness of the neoplasm. Definitive surgical treatment of a malignant melanoma and the prognosis depend upon proper histologic evaluation.

NON-MELANOMA SKIN CANCERS
Treatment

It makes a vast difference whether a cutaneous cancer is a primary or recurrent lesion. Most primary basal cell carcinomas under 1 cm in diameter ordinarily do not extend more than 4 mm beyond their apparent margins. However, recurrent lesions may spread several centimeters beyond their clinically evident borders, assuming that clinical borders are evident, which is not always the case. The depth of the penetration of a cutaneous cancer never can be accurately assessed by gross inspection or palpation. For recurrent malignancies especially, complete extirpation can be done with confidence only by microscopically controlled surgery (Mohs' micrographic surgery).

With respect to gross size of the cutaneous cancer, lesions over 2 cm in diameter, except for superficial basal cell carcinomas, squamous cell carcinomas in situ (Bowen's disease), and those palpable into subcutaneous tissue, should be ablated by surgical excision. The excised specimen should then be submitted for microscopic study of its margins to determine completeness of removal. Basal cell and squamous cell carcinomas that have invaded most of the reticular dermis are difficult to evaluate in true depth by means of clinical inspection. A shave biopsy would not reveal the maximum depth of invasion. In such a case, the operator must be prepared to choose another method of extirpation if, for example, curettage and electrodesiccation had been started and then the curet was found to fall into subcutaneous fat. The operator should then resort to surgical excision of the entire site of the malignancy.

Anatomic sites are important factors in planning methods of treatment. The nasolabial groove is an embryonal fusion plane. Surgical excision is best in this site when coupled with histologic analysis of the margins to ensure completeness of the excision. Recurrence in this site is hazardous and has potential for extensive spread in planes difficult of access. Lesions around the inner canthi are best managed by serial excisions with microscopic control. Recurrences in these sites may jeopardize eyes and at worst necessitate exenterations. For a cutaneous malignancy in skin over the superficial temporal artery, surgical excision and ligation of that vessel would be best utilized for ablation of the tumor, and postoperative bleeding would thus be avoided. For a lesion situated over the midsternum, the patient should be forewarned that no matter which method of treatment is practiced, a keloid may occur postoperatively.

The general health of the patient may dictate choice of treatment. A severely debilitated individual could tolerate noninvasive superficial x-ray therapy, but not surgery of any complexity. For a patient who has an implanted cardiac pacemaker, the use of electrocoagulation devices is hazardous during surgery, because their action may adversely affect the function of the pacemaker.

Although eradication of a malignancy is the primary goal in the management of a cutaneous malignancy, the cosmetic result merits thought in the plan of operation. The patient must understand that cure takes precedence over cosmesis. In the worst cases, a conscientious surgeon who has assuredly cured a complicated malignancy may subsequently undertake revision of unsightly scars, but cosmetic considerations must never be permitted to compromise cure.

Curettage and Electrodesiccation

This method is suitable for small (that is, approximately 1 cm in diameter) primary basal cell and squamous cell carcinomas. The technique is feasibly practiced in an outpatient facility and is convenient for the patient because treatment time is short and the procedure can be completed in one visit. It is not suitable for treatment of morphea basal cell carcinomas, recurrent malignancies, or basal cell carcinomas on the nose, in the nasolabial groove, in the periorbital area, on the scalp, or in the postauricular sulcus.

The method of curettage and electrodesiccation is as follows:

1. Local anesthesia is induced in a field block fashion around the periphery of the lesion and in depth. In the case of squamous cell carcinomas, care should be taken not to invade the actual lesion during the process of injection. Although it is uncommon, the malignancy may be spread along the needle tracks used to obtain local anesthesia.

2. The lesion is then repeatedly "scraped" with a curet of a size commensurate with the size of the lesion. The cancerous tissue is highly cellular and therefore soft and easily removed. When normal tissue has been attained below and around the lesion, it will be found that nothing more can be curetted. Some operators finish the procedure by using curets of smaller sizes to explore for and dislodge small extensions of malignant tissue that may have escaped a large curet.

3. The entire base and sides of the wound are then electrodesiccated lightly or heavily, depending upon bleeding and surety of extirpation.

4. The process of curettage and electrodesiccation is repeated at least once more. For larger lesions, as many as three or more passes of the curet followed by electrodesiccation may be advisable. By the end of the procedure, the curettage and electrodesiccation should encompass a surrounding border of normal-appearing skin up to 3 to 5 mm. This will ensure that no microscopic foci of malignancy in the epidermis has been left.

5. Postoperative care of wounds of curettage and electrodesiccation on exposed surfaces (e.g., the face and hands) consists of washing the wound once daily with hydrogen peroxide, followed by the application of a topical antibiotic ointment and a dressing as simple as a Band-Aid. For covered areas such as the trunk, the wound should be swabbed several times a day with isopropyl alcohol to induce drying. Unsutured wounds on the trunk often ooze and become macerated if covered continuously.

The time for complete healing varies with the size and location of the wound. Follow-up visits are planned appropriately to observe the healing progress.

Cryosurgery

This method is suitable for most small primary basal and squamous cell carcinomas anywhere except near the inner canthi, on the scalp, along the external canals of the ears, or in the nasolabial groove. It is not suitable for morphea basal cell carcinomas and recurrent basal cell and squamous cell carcinomas.

Liquid nitrogen has an operative temperature of $-196°C$ and is the most commonly used cryogen to treat cutaneous cancers. Although it has been found that a temperature range of -25 to $-30°C$ is lethal to malignant tissue in vivo, the highest kill rate of malignant cells in suspensions occurs at $-50°C$, which is the temperature at which all cellular electrolytes crystallize. Cryosurgery is done by a double freeze-thaw cycle whereby the lesion is first frozen (usually with a spray apparatus) and then allowed to thaw, with this sequence immediately repeated a second time.

Radiation Therapy

Radiotherapy is particularly useful for elderly and debilitated patients who cannot tolerate surgical procedures. It is suitable for the treatment of basal cell and squamous cell carcinomas on the nasal alae, lips, eyelids, and pinnae of the ears. It is not suitable for recurrent lesions. In cases of very extensive malignancies that are inoperable, radiation therapy may reasonably provide palliation. The following factors must be considered in the treatment plan: (1) radiosensitivity of the neoplasm, (2) skin tolerance, (3) quality of radiation, (4) field size, and (5) fractionation of total dosage.

In the treatment of skin cancer, radiation therapy is such a specialized modality that it must be performed or supervised by a highly trained and experienced physician who can properly integrate all the variables involved in assessing appropriate treatment plans.

5-Fluorouracil Therapy

As a topical preparation in concentrations of 1 to 5 per cent, 5-fluorouracil is an effective drug in the treatment of superficial basal cell carcinomas and squamous cell carcinomas in situ (Bowen's disease and erythroplasia of Queyrat). Patient compliance is often difficult to obtain, because the drug must be applied daily for at least 2 months and attainment of a satisfactory therapeutic response may entail considerable discomfort.

Surgical Excision

Conventional surgery is suitable for most primary basal cell and squamous cell carcinomas, small or large. Whenever possible, the excised specimen should be checked immediately by frozen sections for completeness of ablation. Surgical operations range from simple excisions and primary closures to complex procedures requiring grafts or flaps. In any event, they require careful planning. With the exception of small excisions, which can easily be closed in a side-to-side fashion, if complete ablation cannot be obtained with certainty, larger excisions may have to be left unrepaired until results of permanent histopathologic margin analysis are returned to the operator. Since permanent sections may take 4 or more days to be processed, wound healing would begin by second intention until postoperative surgical repair could be safely performed. Flaps should not be done without complete margin analysis, since tissue planes are altered during flap procedures and possible residual tumor could be inadvertently buried.

If tumor persists after adequate microscopic examination, then further excision or Mohs' micrographic surgery should be done until complete extirpation of disease is accomplished. It is incumbent upon the surgeon to know the method of margin analysis utilized by the pathologist. Often the margins of the tissue specimen are "sampled" rather than thoroughly studied. The importance of critical margin analysis is obvious. If the margins are incompletely processed, and the pathologist indicates that the margins are free of tumor (in the face of an inadequate examination), the surgeon will proceed with false confidence in his repair of the surgical defect. If the disease persists subclinically, as it often does, it may be months to years before it is once again detected. By that point, it may have caused severe problems for the patient.

Following are general principles of the practice of conventional surgery for cutaneous malignancies.

Method. The skin is cleansed with alcohol, followed by wash of a solution with povidone-iodine or chlorhexidine gluconate. At the surgical site, projected lines of excision and surrounding lines of skin tension are drawn with a sterile solution of a dye such as gentian violet. These lines are drawn prior to infiltration by local anesthetic, because the process of injecting local anesthetic solution may distort tissue planes and lines of skin tension. Local anesthesia is achieved in a field-block fashion of injections of a solution of 1 per cent lidocaine with epinephrine. A wait of 5 to 10 minutes following the injections will maximize the effects of the epinephrine and minimize bleeding during surgery.

The lesion is first curetted so that the surgeon can get an idea of both the depth and peripheral spread of the process. If the peripheral extent of the neoplasm is greater than anticipated, new lines of incision may have to be drawn. Next, the operating assistant presses on the skin at the surgical site, in order to minimize tissue movement as the operator incises the cutaneous surface with a scalpel (usually a #15 blade). The blade should be carried to the superficial subcutaneous tissue at the first stroke. Once incisions are complete, the mass of skin to be excised is raised with forceps and cut from its underlying bed with a scissors. The depth of separation is at the dermosubcutaneous junction or beyond, depending on the type of lesion that has to be excised. Bleeding vessels clamped with a jeweler's forceps are spot-coagulated using a biterminal electrocoagulator. Skin edges are undermined sufficiently (usually at the dermosubcutaneous junction) to facilitate side-to-side closure. On the scalp and areas of the back, excisions may extend to deep subcutaneous fascia, and undermining, under these circumstances, is carried out in the deeper layers of tissue. As needed, two-layered closures are done with deep dermal sutures (absorbable polyglycolic acid derivatives) followed by simple interrupted sutures on the surface of the skin with monofilament nylon material.

The wound site is washed with hydrogen peroxide and dried, and a thin coat of antibiotic is applied along the suture line. A layered dressing composed of a Telfa pad cut to the wound size, cotton balls, and either plastic or paper tape is firmly applied. The dressing is removed in 48 hours. Thereafter, a daily change of dressing consisting of hydrogen peroxide wash and application of ointment, Telfa pad, and paper tape is made until the time of removal of sutures. The sutures are removed as early as 5 days after operation when possible; on the extremities, it may be necessary to leave them in place for up to 2 weeks in order to prevent dehiscence of the wound. Prior to the surgical procedure, the patient should be warned of possible postoperative complications such as hematoma formation, infection, and spread of scar.

Mohs' Micrographic Surgery

In the early 1930s, Dr. Frederic Mohs, Professor of Surgery at the University of Wisconsin, conceived a form of treatment for skin cancer that he described as "chemosurgery." Initially, a chemical fixative (a paste of zinc chloride) was applied to the surface of the skin cancer, after which the surgeon removed the chemically treated tissue for microscopic analysis. The surgically removed tissues were painted with special color-coded dyes, and at the time of surgery, orientation of these tissues was provided by a precise map (or diagram) of the surgical site, which was drawn and color-coded identical to the color-coding of the tissues.

Next, the tissues were microscopically analyzed by the surgeon in a laboratory located on-premises within the surgical facility. If persistent tumor was discovered in the tissues, the surgeon drew on the map the exact location of these tumor cells. The map became the Mohs surgeon's guide to perform additional surgery in order to ultimately eradicate the entire skin cancer.

The process of chemical application, surgery, color-coding of tissues, construction of maps, and microscopic analysis was repeated as many times as necessary until the cancer was fully eradicated. This was a very complex and time-consuming procedure that often required several days to complete. Remember, *the Mohs surgeon was functioning in the capacity as both surgeon and pathologist in this technique.* It was such a rigorous and difficult method that very few physicians were willing to devote the time and effort to learn it.

In 1953, Mohs reported that he had eliminated the use of zinc-chloride paste fixative in certain cases, and thus was able to reduce the treatment time from several days to several hours. Other than the elimination of the paste, the essential elements of the treatment remained the same. In the 1960s, others corroborated his findings. In 1986, the American College of Chemosurgery replaced the name "chemosurgery" with the up-to-date term, Mohs' micrographic surgery (MMS). In 1987, to maintain consistency with the change in terms, the College changed its name to the American College of Mohs Micrographic Surgery and Cutaneous Oncology. It is important to reiterate that except for the deletion of the chemical fixative and minor technical refinements in the procedure, the essential principles are the same for both the modernized Mohs' micrographic surgery and previous Mohs' chemosurgery.

The procedure has several indications. This method is excellent for small primary basal cell and squamous cell carcinomas in important anatomic sites such as the inner canthi of the eyes, dorsum of the nose, nasal alae, nasolabial grooves, pinnae of the ears, digits, and genitalia. The method is particularly useful for longstanding, large primary (i.e., previously untreated) neoplasms, morphea basal cell carcinomas, and especially recurrent malignancies.

The procedure must be performed by individuals who have acquired the necessary skills in a formal training program. The American College of Mohs Micrographic Surgery and Cutaneous Oncology has approved several one-year fellowships for training in MMS. The graduates of these one-year fellowship programs receive extensive training in all the intricate components of the MMS procedure.

In brief, the basic techniques of MMS are as follows:

1. A local anesthetic is injected into the surgical site.

2. The bulk of the tumor mass is reduced with a curet.

3. A tissue specimen encompassing the gross tumor and a small amount of clinically normal-appearing tissue is removed by a scalpel. The tissue is placed on a tray in which its orientation is maintained identical to that of its original position on the patient.

4. A map is drawn corresponding to both the tissue that was removed and the surgical site.

5. The excised specimen of tissue is divided into segments, the edges of which are color-coded for identification during microscopic processing.

6. The segments of tissue and their respective colored edges are drawn to scale on the map.

7. The tissue is taken into the surgeon's on-premises laboratory where frozen sections are obtained from the undersurfaces of the segments of tissue.

8. If residual malignancy is seen during microscopic examination of the frozen sections, the surgeon codes this on a map that correlates the precise location and exact position of remaining tumor within the patient.

9. The surgeon excises additional tissue from the area containing residual tumor.

10. Mapping, surgical excisions, and microscopic analysis are repeated as necessary, until complete removal of malignant tissues has been achieved.

The wound may heal by second intention, or reconstructive surgery can be done.

MMS is a method for precise and complete removal of skin cancer whereby the surgeon can precisely extirpate the tumor with the maximal preservation of normal, healthy tissue. Because of its precision, MMS offers the highest cure rates of any form of treatment for the removal of skin cancers.

MALIGNANT MELANOMA

Malignant melanoma is the most serious of cutaneous malignancies because it has the capability to metastasize and cause death. A full review of treatment of malignant melanomas is beyond the scope of this discussion. Certain important factors, however, will be discussed briefly here.

Biopsy

Whenever possible, biopsy in toto is preferable to biopsy in part. If a biopsy in part must be done, it should be taken at the deepest penetration. Histologic thickness of a lesion is a guide to the choice of definitive therapy and to prognosis (Breslow's classification). Some newer evidence suggests that tumor volume, determined by a computer analysis of microscopic step-sections, may be a better indicator as to the best choice of therapy and prognosis.

Treatment

Surgical excision, based upon microscopic invasion of the deepest portion of the malignant melanoma, is the treatment of choice in Stage 1 disease. There has been considerable controversy in recent years concerning the amount of normal-appearing tissue to be excised adjacent to the lesion of malignant melanoma. Within the last 5 years, the trend has been to reduce the amount of skin that is excised surrounding the lesion. In recently published literature, there are still variable guidelines for determining surgical margins based upon microscopic thickness of tumor. Here are some examples:

1. For tumors less than 0.85 mm in microscopic thickness, 1.5-cm surgical margins are chosen.
2. For tumors less than 1.0 mm in microscopic thickness, 2.0-cm surgical margins are chosen.
3. For tumors greater than 0.85 mm in microscopic thickness, 3.0-cm surgical margins are chosen.
4. For tumors greater than 1.0 mm in microscopic thickness, no less than 3-cm margins are chosen.
5. For facial lesions, irrespective of microscopic depth, the requirements for surgical margins are altered if the process of excision would compromise or sacrifice a major anatomic structure such as an eye.

Entire books have been written to account for the many factors, variables, and subtleties involved in the evaluation and treatment of malignant melanoma. The controversy in determining surgical margins is only one of many ongoing complex issues that require resolution.

Concurrent or subsequent lymph node dissection is determined principally by thickness of tumor, location of disease, and evidence of metastatic disease. When the thickness of the malignant melanoma is such that metastatic disease is possible or likely, the patient should be referred to a physician who specializes in the care of such patients.

If properly treated in its earliest stages, malignant melanoma has a good prognosis.

PAPULOSQUAMOUS ERUPTIONS

method of
WALTER H. C. BURGDORF, M.D.
University of New Mexico School of Medicine
Albuquerque, New Mexico

Papulosquamous eruptions are as much a diagnostic as a therapeutic problem. In addition to the conditions covered in this section, drug eruptions and secondary syphilis frequently enter into the list of possible diagnoses.

SEBORRHEIC DERMATITIS

Seborrheic dermatitis is a common rash affecting everyone at some stage of their life. The eruption is erythematous and scaly and may often acquire a waxy crust if severe or untreated. Common areas of involvement include the scalp (e.g., cradle cap in infants and dandruff in adults) and face (e.g., scaling and redness of the eyelids, nasolabial folds, and retroauricular areas and along the hair line). The disease may be widespread, and typically the sternal and intertriginous regions are involved; this type of seborrheic dermatitis is a possible precursor of erythroderma in the elderly.

Except in rare cases with unusual distribution, secondary infection, or inappropriate prior therapy, the diagnosis is usually obvious on inspection.

Management

The mainstay of management of seborrheic dermatitis is frequent shampooing. The daily use is more important than the type or brand of shampoo; however, there are at least four major shampoo types with the following different active ingredients:

1. Zinc pyrithione (Head and Shoulders, DHS Zinc, Sebulon, Zincon)
2. Selenium sulfide (Selsun, Exsel)
3. Salicyclic acid (Ionil, Sebulex, Vanseb)
4. Tar. The tar shampoos range from old-fashioned, smelly but effective products (Polytar, Zetar, Ionil, Sebutone) to newer, more cosmetically elegant preparations (T Gel, Ionil T Plus, DHS Tar Gel). In addition to enjoying better patient acceptance, products in the latter group are less likely to stain blond or grey hair.

Patients should be instructed to wash their hair, rinse, reapply the shampoo, wait 2 to 3 minutes, and rinse again. It is perfectly appropriate to use rinse and/or conditioner; some are made especially for such patients (Ionil rinse, DHS conditioner). A minimum interval is shampooing every other day; for most patients daily shampoos are necessary. Patients with hair styles that do not allow such frequent shampooing may have to choose between their style and their scalp disease. In addition, many patients find that they do better if they alternate different types of shampoos.

Recalcitrant scalp disease, especially that with thick crusts, may require pre-soaking. Generations of young mothers have discovered the application of baby oil to the scalp for an hour or overnight, followed by shampooing and use of a scrub brush will loosen most scales. Baker P&S Liquid is a more sophisticated solution for the same purpose.

Finally, topical corticosteroids may be needed, with particular attention to vehicle and strength. On the scalp itself, a relatively mid- to high-potency steroid in either a spray (Kenalog Spray), gel (Lidex or Topicort Gel), lotion (Maxivate Lotion), or solution (Synlar or Halog) should be applied once a day to thickened or itchy areas. The patient should be cautioned not to use the expensive corticosteroid as a hair-dressing alternative, but to apply it sparingly to "bad" areas.

A milder corticosteroid in a less drying vehicle must be used on the hairline, face, and other areas. Seborrheic dermatitis does not respond well to high-potency steroids. Have the patient start with 1 per cent hydrocorticosone cream (Hytone), applying it 2 or 3 times daily. If this does not work, usually the explanation is noncompliance or failure to shampoo. However, slightly more potent steroids such as desonide cream 0.05 per cent (Desowen, Tridesilon) or 0.025 per cent triamcinolone cream (Kenalog, Artistocort) may be tried.

PSORIASIS

Psoriasis is a common skin disease; 1 to 3 per cent of the population are estimated to suffer from the "heartbreak" disease. The diagnosis may be made on physical examination. Lesions are usually erythematous with a thick, silvery scale; they are most commonly seen over the knees, elbows, and scalp. On the scalp, severe seborrheic dermatitis and psoriasis merge imperceptibly; the old term sebopsoriasis is useful. There may be other clues: nail changes (pitting, oil spots, subungual debris) and gluteal cleft redness are helpful. Treated lesions notoriously lose the above features and become harder to diagnose.

A type of psoriasis rarely identified by patients or nondermatologists is the guttate variant. Usually seen in children and young adults and often triggered by a streptococcal infection, guttate psoriasis is characterized by many small erythematous papules that appear suddenly, primarily on the trunk, without other stigmata.

Patients with psoriasis show a wide spectrum of disease. Those with localized disease are easily managed by any physician. As they develop more widespread disease, simple topical therapy becomes less helpful and affordable, and other approaches must be developed. In a small subset, the disease becomes so widespread as to involve the entire body (erythroderma), may have an acute pustular component with widespread sterile pustules, or may be associated with arthritis.

Management

Most psoriatics need a friendly doctor. Taking the time to explain their disease to them and promising to work with them to control but not cure the disorder are more important contributions than any prescription. Possible triggering factors occasionally can be eliminated; these include drugs (lithium and the beta blockers are notorious for causing psoriasis to flare up) and trauma (psoriasis tends to appear in areas of trauma, such as on the hands of manual laborers).

The mainstays of management of localized psoriasis, adaptable to almost any practice setting, are topical corticosteroids, tar, and anathralin (Table 1). Topical corticosteroids are cosmetically elegant and preferred by patients. One can start with the most cost-effective product, 0.025 per cent triamcinolone cream (Kenalog, Aristocort); however, stronger, far more expensive products are usually needed. In any event, one can then move up through the therapeutic range; I usually employ Lidex because it is quite potent and available in many forms (cream, emollient cream, ointment, gel, lotion). Many patients will want

TABLE 1. **Management of Psoriasis**

	Localized Plaque-type Psoriasis (<30% body surface)	Widespread Plaque-type Psoriasis, Eruptive Guttate-type	Generalized Pustular Psoriasis	Erythrodermic Psoriasis
Treatment (in order of preference)	Tar plus topical corticosteroids *or* Anthralin plus topical corticosteroids	(1) Anthralin plus ultraviolet light *or* Goeckerman Regimen (2) PUVA	Methotrexate *or* Oral retinoids	Methotrexate *or* Oral retinoids
Ideal setting of treatment	Outpatient	Day-care center or inpatient unit	Inpatient unit	Inpatient unit

Courtesy of Chung-Hong Hu, M.D.

to use a cream or emollient cream in the morning, but prefer a messier but less drying ointment at night. Patients should be encouraged to apply their medication twice daily or at most 3 times daily.

Several tricks are available to increase the potent effect of topical corticosteroids. Cheapest to use is Saran Wrap occlusion; some areas of the body are more amenable to this than others. Intralesional triamcinolone, 2.2 to 5.0 mg per ml (Kenalog or Aristocort) can be used for localized plaques, injected with either a needle and Luerlok syringe or a air-powered injection device (Derma-jet, Mada-jet). Finally, a number of extremely potent topical corticosteroids are now available in the United States for short-term pulse treatment, often on a once-daily basis. They include 0.05 per cent clobetasol propionate (Temovate cream or ointment), 0.05 per cent diflorasone diacetate (Psorcon ointment), and 0.05 per cent betamethasone dipropionate (Diprolene AF cream). None should be used for more than 2 weeks without special indications, because in addition to the well-known topical side effects such as atrophy, telangiectasia, striae, and infections, these new agents increase the possibility of adverse systemic reactions.

Two clinically relevant phenomena have been described with topical corticosteroid therapy. First, tachyphylaxis occurs (that is, patients or their disease become tolerant to a given compound with time); thus, it is appropriate to alternate products. Second, when high-potency corticosteroid therapy is stopped, often there is a rebound flare-up of psoriasis. For these reasons most physicians employ either tars or anthralin as adjunctive therapy, even in localized disease. While both products were messy and difficult to use in the not too distant past, major advances in their formulations have been made, and patient compliance is now much higher because of the more cosmetically elegant forms.

Tars are now available in alcoholic bases (psoriGel, Estar gel) and creams (Fotocar cream).

Thus, it is rarely necessary to struggle to find a pharmacist who can mix one of the old crude coal tar "recipes." Tars can be applied directly to the patches of psoriasis; I typically have a patient use a topical steroid in the morning and then in the evening apply tar, let it dry, and then cover with the steroid. The choice between gel and cream is dependent on patient tolerance. Tar can also be used for simple home phototherapy. Before exposing their lesions to sunlight, patients can either bathe in a tar bath (3 capfuls Balnetar in a half-filled tub) or apply a tar product to the lesions.

Anthralin is also available in varying percentages as creams (0.1, 0.2, 0.4, 1.0 per cent Lasan Cream; 0.1, 0.25, 0.5, 1.0 per cent Drithocream or ointments; 0.1 0.25, 0.5, 1.0 per cent AnthraDerm ointment). It can be applied, as described above for the tar products, in the evening. The patient should start with the lowest concentration and work up to 0.5 per cent. Alternatively, short contact use of 1.0 per cent anthralin can be made; the patient applies the product to the psoriatic lesions, waits 30 to 60 minutes, and removes it with a bath or mineral oil. Both anthralin and tar stain bedclothes and sheets.

Psoriasis presents unique problems in certain areas:

1. Scalp: Manage just as seborrheic dermatitis.

2. Flexural areas: Inverse psoriasis, involving the axillae and groin, is also similar to seborrheic dermatitis and does better with low-potency corticosteroids. Tar and anthralin should be avoided in these areas.

3. Palmar and plantar lesions: Treatment with topical corticosteroids, tars, and short-contact anthralin therapy should be tried.

Management of More Extensive Cases

Cases which fail to respond to the above measures generally require more complicated therapy; it may be troublesome because of expense, need for special equipment, or use of dangerous medications. Such approaches should probably be left to physicians with a special interest in psoriasis who have both the experience to choose between competing regimens and the facilities to provide most cost-effective care. Several approaches are possible (see Table 1).

Goeckerman Regimen. Patients receive tar and ultraviolet light, either in a day-care of inpatient setting. This represents the safest, most time-tested approach to severe psoriasis, but has the least patient acceptance because it requires so much of the patient's time.

Antimetabolites. Because psoriasis is a hyperproliferative disorder, it is not surprising that a variety of antimetabolites will help control the disease. Methotrexate has been best studied; a single daily weekly dose of 10 to 30 mg has proved very effective. The success of the relatively lower dosages in rheumatoid and psoriatic arthritis has encouraged me to use a weekly regimen of 7.5 to 15 mg. I currently have no patients on the larger doses. The role of liver biopsies in methotrexate patients remains controversial; if greater than 15 mg per week is used, there is a general consensus that a pretreatment biopsy and biopsies every 2 years are appropriate while the patient is on therapy. With lower dosages, the recommendations vary but one should keep a log of total methotrexate dosage and at least get a biopsy after ingestion of total dosage of 1.0 to 1.5 grams. Patients cannot be allowed to conceive or father a child while on methotrexate therapy; the safe washout period is felt to be 2 to 3 months. Other antimetabolites such as 5-fluorouracil and hydroxyurea may also be employed but are much less widely used than methotrexate.

PUVA Photochemotherapy. Patients take the photosensitizing drug psoralen *(P)* and are exposed to high-intensity ultraviolet A *(UVA)* light in a special light box. PUVA is very effective but causes skin aging and cataracts and increases the risk of skin cancers.

Retinoids. Oral retinoids are now available in this country in the form of etretinate (Tegison), which is approved for psoriatic erythroderma and pustular psoriasis as well as for severe psoriasis not responsive to standard measures. It may also be used as adjunctive therapy with PUVA to reduce the UVA dose and speed the response. Etretinate has a very long half-life and is a potent teratogen. I am reluctant to treat female patients with it. The lengthy package insert should be followed in detail should this drug be required for its potential life-saving role in erythroderma or a pustular flare-up.

PITYRIASIS ROSEA

Pityriasis rosea is an idiopathic acute papulosquamous eruption, which is diagnosed on clini-

cal examination. Patients typically describe a single initial scaly patch, often misdiagnosed as tinea corporis. Multiple oval-shaped macules then develop, often in a Christmas-tree pattern following skin lines on the trunk. In Caucasians, the arms, legs, and head are usually spared, although in blacks these areas may be involved (inverse variant). Since secondary syphilis can exactly mimic pityriasis rosea, a Venereal Disease Research Laboratory (VDRL) test should be considered.

Management

If the patient with pityriasis rosea is not itching, management consists of lubrication and reassurance. Generally, a mild soap (e.g., Dove) and post-bathing or showering lubrication (e.g., Alpha-Keri bath oil, Cetaphil) suffice. When pruritus occurs, antihistamines and distractors can be used. I typically prescribe hydroxyzine, 25 mg twice daily and 50 mg at bedtime, but other regimens and drugs are acceptable. I mix 0.025 per cent menthol with Cetaphil as an effective, inexpensive distractor; Sarna may also be used. Topical steroids can also be employed but are disappointing; they are an expensive way to lubricate and a poor way to control itch. When extreme pruritus occurs or in blacks with facial involvement or pigmentary changes, a short burst of systemic corticosteroids may be needed. I employ prednisone, 60 mg daily for 3 days, 40 mg daily for 3 days, and 20 mg daily for 3 days, taken all at once in the morning; any comparable regimen will do.

PITYRIASIS LICHENOIDES ET VARIOLIFORMIS ACUTA (PLEVA)

This tongue-twister is actually an identifiable papulosquamous eruption of teenagers and young adults. It looks like "bad chronic chickenpox" with necrotic (varioliform) papules and macules with scale; the patient looks terrible but feels fine. The main differential considerations are guttate psoriasis and pityriasis rosea. Since PLEVA is characterized by lymphocytic vasculitis and hemorrhage, it can usually be identified by skin biopsy.

Management

PLEVA is generally a self-limited disease and requires no therapy. However, most patients desire something for such a severe-looking disease. Topical lubricants and distractors can be employed, as for pityriasis rosea. In addition, oral antibiotics may be helpful. Either tetracycline,

1.0 gram daily, or minocycline (Minocin), 100 mg daily, may be tried. Extremely low-dose methotrexate* (5.0 to 10 mg week) is amazingly effective; unfortunately, PLEVA occurs in an age group where a teratogen such as methotrexate can rarely be justified for a benign disease.

LICHEN PLANUS

Lichen planus is another acute idiopathic dermatosis, characterized by violaceous, polygonal, flat-topped papules. Typical areas of involvement are the wrists, ankles, and genitalia. The oral mucosa may also be involved, either with lacy white streaks or with ulcerations. Similarly, the palms and soles may either be hyperkeratotic or ulcerated. In addition, atrophic and bullous lesions can occur. Because of the widespread and varied clinical appearance, a biopsy is often necessary; the typical band-like infiltrate of lymphocytes at the epidermal-dermal junction usually resolves the diagnostic dilemma. The disease usually persists for 3 to 6 months; almost all cases resolve by 12 months except for oral, genital, and plantar variants, which are more chronic.

Management

Treatment of the pruritus is the goal of therapy. Topically, for limited disease, high-potency topical corticosteroids such as 0.05 per cent fluocinonide cream (Lidex) may be useful for limited areas; on the genitalia, a milder form such as 0.05 per cent desonide cream (Tridesilon, DesOwen) should be used. Application is 2 to 3 times daily. In addition, distractors such as 0.025 per cent menthol in Cetaphil can be used.

Antihistamines are used as for any other pruritus. Hydroxyzine has traditionally been favored, in a dosage of 25 mg 2 to 3 times daily and 50 mg at night, but newer nonsoporific agents such as terfenadine (Seldane), 60 mg, or combination blockers such as doxepin (Sinequan, Adapin), 50 to 75 mg at night and 25 mg in the morning, may be useful.

Finally, systemic corticosteroids are often needed for relief from itching. I usually prescribe 60 mg per day of prednisone in the morning tapered over a 3-week period, with consideration of alternate-day steroids if this regimen helps but the disease recurs. Griseofulvin, 500 mg twice a day, may also be tried, especially in the presence of a dermatophyte infection, but also in patients with no other indications. For the oral disease, either topical Kenalog in Orabase or 0.025 per cent isotretinoin gel (Retin-A) may be used.

---

*This use of methotrexate is not listed in the manufacturer's directive.

CONNECTIVE TISSUE DISORDERS: LUPUS ERYTHEMATOSUS, DERMATOMYOSITIS, AND SCLERODERMA

method of
JOSEPH L. JORIZZO, M.D.
*Bowman Gray School of Medicine
of Wake Forest University
Winston-Salem, North Carolina*

LUPUS ERYTHEMATOSUS

Proper treatment of the patient with lupus erythematosus (LE) is dependent on the following therapeutic classification:
I. Vessel-based lesions in patients with acute systemic lupus erythematosus (ASLE)
II. Lesions characterized by a lymphocytic infiltrate at the dermal-epidermal (DE) junction
   A. Discoid lesions—Patient may have chronic cutaneous lupus erythematosus (CCLE) or ASLE
   B. Subacute cutaneous lupus erythematosus (SCLE)
   C. Poikiloderma—A feature of ASLE
III. Special lesions
   A. Lupus panniculitis
   B. Vesiculobullous lesions

Vessel-Based Lesions in Patients with ASLE

A number of different vascular reactions occur in patients with ASLE including small vessel necrotizing vasculitis (including urticarial vasculitis), large vessel necrotizing vasculitis, miscellaneous serum sickness–like reactions, erythemas, erythema multiforme–like reactions, and other vascular reactions. Vasculitic lesions are particularly important to identify in patients with ASLE as they may be the first sign of a major flare of systemic disease.

Lesions Characterized by Lymphocytic Infiltrate at the DE Junction

Therapeutic classification within this group of lesions is crucial. Patients with lesions having this histologic pattern may be at the benign cutaneous end of the LE spectrum (CCLE), may be at an intermediate point (SCLE), or may have potentially life-threatening disease (ASLE). The patient with discoid lesions must be evaluated by a complete history, physical examination, and laboratory screening, evaluation including antinuclear antibody profile (ANA), urinalysis, complete blood count, and chemistry profile, to look for American Rheumatologic Association criteria for systemic disease (i.e., to diagnose CCLE by excluding ASLE). Patients with cutaneous lesions of SCLE require a similar evaluation. The ANA test may be negative in SCLE if traditional rat tissue substrates are used; therefore, tests for Sjögren's syndrome antibodies (i.e., SSA [Ro] and SSB [La]) should be ordered if SCLE is suspected. The finding of poikiloderma (i.e., the presence of epidermal atrophy, telangiectasia, and hyper- and hypopigmentation) in a patient with LE indicates ASLE. Poikiloderma is a more technically correct and specific term than "malar rash."

Treatment

General Measures

Sunscreens with a high solar protection factor (SPF) (e.g., SPF 29) must be used faithfully. Patients are often more compliant if these agents can be applied every morning "like after-shave" or "like moisturizer." Re-application should precede significant sun exposure and should follow if the skin becomes wet. Daily outdoor activities should be concentrated in the hours of reduced ultraviolet B (UVB) intensity, such as before 9 to 10 AM and after 5 to 6 PM. A patient who works under high-intensity fluorescent light bulbs may have significant ultraviolet A (UVA) exposure. Mylar filters may be placed over the fluorescent bulbs.

Patients should be made aware of the existence of local, state and national lupus societies. These groups provide useful support and patient education.

Physicians should be aware of drug-induced ASLE and of drug effects on patients and should question the patient about the use of medications such as procainamide, hydralazine, and oral contraceptives that affect ASLE. Pregnancy is an important issue for patients with ASLE, as the disease may flare up during pregnancy or during the postpartum period and also because of the potential effects on the developing fetus of the medications used to treat ASLE.

Topical Therapy

Topical corticosteroids are the mainstay of topical therapy for lesions of lupus erythematosus. As a general rule, mild corticosteroids, such as 1 per cent hydrocortisone, are used for atrophic lesions (e.g., poikiloderma of ASLE), middle strength corticosteroids, such as 0.1 per cent triamcinolone, are used for lesions of SCLE and possibly for initial therapy of discoid lesions in CCLE or ASLE. The most potent topical corticosteroids or intralesional corticosteroids (triamcinolone 2.5 to 5.0 mg per ml, or 0.1 ml per cm using a 30-gauge needle) may be cautiously used for the thickest discoid lesions. Cutaneous atrophy and steroid acne of the face are complications of excessive topical corticosteroid therapy.

Antimalarial Therapy

Antimalarial therapy is a mainstay of therapy for photodistributed, lymphocyte-predominant lesions in CCLE, SCLE, and ASLE. In my opinion, this therapy is not useful in the treatment of vessel-based lesions. Three different antimalarials are used: chloroquine diphosphate (Aralen), hydroxychloroquine sulfate (Plaquenil), and quinacrine (Atabrine).* Oral hydroxychloroquine in a dose of 200 to 400 mg per day is the most commonly used treatment. The ceiling of 400 mg per day should not be exceeded, because of the significant increase in retinal toxicity at higher doses. Ophthalmologic evaluation should occur at baseline and at 3- to 6-month intervals during treatment. Quinacrine, 100 mg in daily oral dose, can be added to a maximal dose of hydroxychloroquine if more therapeutic efficacy is needed. Quinacrine causes the skin to turn a yellowish color, which limits its acceptability to patients as monotherapy, in which higher doses would be needed. Other side effects that can occur with any of the antimalarials include gastrointestinal upset; myopathy; pigmentary changes of skin, hair, and nails; cutaneous eruptions and pruritus; leukopenia and anemia (aplastic anemia has been reported); and in addition to the irreversible retinopathy, ocular keratopathy and cycloplegia, which are more frequently seen and are reversible.

Other Therapies

Cutaneous lymphocyte-mediated lesions alone of CCLE, SCLE, and ASLE are, with rare exception, not an indication for systemic corticosteroid therapy. When this treatment is used to treat other conditions there is tremendous potential for rebound of cutaneous and systemic lesions if systemic corticosteroids are tapered too rapidly.

Experimental or less well-substantiated oral therapies include dapsone, sulfapyridine, thalidomide (no longer available for this use), and isotretinoin (Accutane).† Isotretinoin is used for 16 weeks in a dose of 1 to 2 mg per kg to regain control of flaring lesions: however, long-term therapy with isotretinoin is not possible, due to unacceptable side effects. Familiarity by the prescribing physician with side effects of this treatment, especially teratogenicity, is mandatory.

---

*This treatment indication is not listed by the manufacturer for chloroquine or quinacrine.

†This use is not listed by the manufacturer.

Therapy for Special Lesions

Antimalarial therapy and possibly intralesional corticosteroid therapy are particularly useful in treating lupus panniculitis (i.e., lupus profundus). Oral dapsone,* 50 to 200 mg per day, is useful in the treatment of vesiculo bullous lesions of ASLE. Careful hematologic monitoring and baseline glucose-6-phosphate dehydrogenase (G6PD) levels are required before therapy. Experience with the use of this potentially toxic agent is important.

DERMATOMYOSITIS

Dermatomyositis is an idiopathic inflammatory disorder that primarily affects the skin and muscle. The cutaneous eruption may precede all other disease manifestations by months to even years. Poikiloderma occurs in dermatomyositis; however, in contrast to ASLE, the color in dermatomyositis is violaceous. The name given to the violaceous poikiloderma of dermatomyositis occurring with periorbital edema is the "heliotrope sign"; when it occurs over the knuckles it is called Gottron's sign. Periungual telangiectasia and cuticular dystrophy are other typical features.

Dermatomyositis occurs in a biphasic age distribution. The childhood form is more likely to be associated with vasculitis; the adult form may occur in association with occult malignancy. Current practice suggests a directed malignancy evaluation (i.e., pursue leads from history, physical examination and screening laboratory studies) rather than a routine "million dollar workup" for affected adults.

The following diagnostic criteria are used for dermatomyositis:

1. Clinical signs and symptoms of proximal muscle weakness
2. Elevation of muscle enzymes (e.g., aldolase, creatine phosphokinase [CPK])
3. Electromyographic changes of myositis
4. Typical histologic changes of myositis from muscle biopsy
5. Typical cutaneous eruption

Treatment

General Treatment Measures

Initial hospitalization allows for the diagnosis to be confirmed and for the necessary bed rest. A program of gradually increasing activity from full bed rest to passive range-of-motion exercises and then to increasing exercise is best coordinated by physical and occupational therapy con-

---

*This use is not listed by the manufacturer.

sultants. A high-protein diet may also be beneficial during the acute stage of the disorder.

Topical Therapy

Dermatomyositis, like lupus erythematosus, is characterized by a cutaneous eruption with a photosensitivity component. Sunscreens should be used as described for lupus erythematosus.

The poikilodermatous eruption, by definition, is characterized by epidermal atrophy. Potent topical corticosteroid therapy should be avoided due to the potential to exacerbate this atrophy. Emollients and mild topical corticosteroids (1% hydrocortisone) may be of benefit in alleviating pruritus.

Cosmetics such as Covermark, which are compounded to the patient's specific skin color, may be beneficial. The cutaneous eruption does not follow the course of the muscle disease. Many patients have cutaneous morbidity that persists long after they are asymptomatic from their muscle disease. These patients no longer perceive themselves as being acutely ill; however, physician support and understanding must continue through this period.

Systemic Therapy

Corticosteroids. Systemic corticosteroid therapy is the treatment of choice for the myositis of dermatomyositis. The usual precautions should be taken both prior to initiating therapy and during the course of long-term systemic corticosteroid therapy. Physicians should be familiar with the significant and varied complications of therapy with this agent.

Therapy is initiated with prednisone, approximately 1 mg per kg per day in a single morning dose. Extensor muscle strength and laboratory assessment of muscle enzymes should be monitored carefully. Aggressive therapy should be maintained at least until a steady plateau of improvement is reached. Response is variable; some patients improve dramatically within 2 weeks and others show very little change after 3 to 6 months. Divided daily-dose prednisone therapy, or single dose therapy of up to 100 mg per day, in some cases with the addition of immunosuppressive agents, can be used for patients with refractory disease. Pulse therapy, with massive doses of 1 gram equivalent of prednisone per day for 3 to 5 days, has also been described as treatment for dermatomyositis, with subsequent requirement of lower maintenance doses of prednisone. Hospital monitoring is usually required for this still experimental therapy.

As improvement occurs, the prednisone dose can be reduced slowly; with careful monitoring of muscle strength and serum enzymes on each clinic visit. An initial dosage reduction of 10 to 25 per cent can be used, followed by a 5-mg reduction every 2 to 4 weeks. If relapse occurs, a prompt substantial increase in dosage is required with a slower subsequent taper. Dermatomyositis responds well to a single-dose, every-other-day regimen. This can often be accomplished after 6 months of daily-dose therapy when prednisone dosage is in the range of 20 to 30 mg per day. Since 60 mg of prednisone on alternate days represents a significant taper from 30 mg per day, several weeks of intermediate therapy are often helpful—for example, 50 mg alternating with 10 mg; other published guidelines are available for changing to alternate-day therapy.

Maintenance prednisone therapy is usually required for a minimum of 2 years. Most patients can eventually stop therapy, but as many as 25 per cent may require therapy for more than 5 years.

Methotrexate. Methotrexate* can be added to the regimen of prednisone and supportive care if control of disease activity is not achieved with prednisone alone after 2 to 4 months or if prednisone-sparing effects are required. The dosage regimen popularized by dermatologists in the treatment of psoriasis is appropriate, and 10 to 25 mg can be given in a single weekly oral dose. Full benefit may not be derived for 3 to 4 months. Pre-existing liver disease and chronic alcohol use are contraindications to therapy, as are pregnancy, severe renal disease, and blood dyscrasias. With decreased disease activity, methotrexate can be tapered by lowering the weekly dose. The usual precautions with methotrexate therapy should be followed.

Azathioprine. Azathioprine (Imuran)* can be used instead of methotrexate. A dosage of 2 to 3 mg per kg per day in divided doses is usual. Again, several months of therapy may be required to assess full benefit. Hematologic toxicity, in particular, requires close monitoring. The rare but potential risk of development of malignancy exists with therapy with any immunosuppressive agent.

Antimalarials. As the cutaneous eruption does not always respond to the aforementioned therapies, adjunctive therapy for the poikiloderma may be required. Therapy for patients with refractory cutaneous lesions of dermatomyositis is initiated as described for patients with lupus erythematosus.

Other Drugs. Cyclophosphamide, chlorambucil, and 6-mercaptopurine have been used in the management of dermatomyositis, but are not standard therapies.

*This use of these agents is not listed in the manufacturers' official directives.

Plasmapheresis. Plasmapheresis may have a role in the treatment of resistant cases of dermatomyositis. Maintenance corticosteroid therapy is still necessary.

SCLERODERMA

Scleroderma is a chronic disease with the potential for significant cutaneous as well as systemic morbidity. The pathogenesis remains unknown, and therapies that are as dramatically effective as systemic corticosteroid therapy for lupus erythematosus or dermatomyositis are unavailable for scleroderma. The disease is characterized by dermal sclerosis, fibrosis of other organs, inflammation and autoantibody formation, and obliterative, proliferative, and vasospastic vascular abnormalities.

Scleroderma has a localized, primarily cutaneous subset called morphea. Plaque, guttate, generalized, and linear (includes the "en coup de sabre" variant on the face) forms of morphea occur. The linear form, especially in children, may be associated with autoantibody formation and mild systemic rheumatologic features; however, in general the primary effect of these localized variants is to produce dermal sclerosis. The linear variants are the least likely to resolve spontaneously and are more likely to involve deep underlying structures, producing hemiatrophy on the face or joint contractures on the extremities.

Eosinophilic fasciitis is a variant of scleroderma characterized by dramatic proximal extremity or truncal cutaneous induration without the acral changes of scleroderma which will be discussed. Lesions often occur after localized trauma. Histologically inflammation and thickening of the fascia with eosinophilia are seen. Systemic features do occur but are generally mild. These patients usually respond well to systemic corticosteroid therapy.

Systemic scleroderma occurs in two general forms: the CREST form (Calcinosis, Raynaud's phenomenon, Esophageal dysmotility, Sclerodactyly, and Telangiectasia) (often used synonymously with acrosclerosis) and diffuse, or progressive systemic sclerosis. Although patients with both forms can suffer from severe vasospasm, gastrointestinal involvement, hypertension, scleroderma kidney, cardiac conduction abnormalities, and pulmonary hypertension and fibrosis, patients with the CREST form generally do not have significant shortening of their lives (patients are often elderly women), whereas patients with diffuse systemic sclerosis (younger men and women) may have a five-year survival rate of only 50 per cent.

Although systemic therapies are sometimes

used for the treatment of the subset morphea (described above) general therapy (e.g., emollients, physical therapy for linear variants) and intralesional corticosteroid therapy are the most frequently used approaches.

Overlap syndromes of scleroderma with lupus erythematosus, dermatomyositis, and rheumatoid arthritis exist. One overlap syndrome, mixed connective tissue disease, is characterized by autoantibody to ribonucleoprotein (RNP). Although these overlap syndromes are described as corticosteroid responsive, long-term follow-up has shown that many of these patients are have pulmonary fibrosis and hypertension as seen in scleroderma. The following discussion relates to therapy of the patient with systemic scleroderma.

Treatment

General

Patients with scleroderma are often frustrated by the lack of a single dramatically effective therapy for this disease; therefore, emotional support is critical. Patients may benefit greatly from membership in the United Scleroderma Foundation, Inc. Emollients are important in making the "hidebound" skin more tolerable for the patient. Avoidance of smoking is crucial, as the local digital vasospasm associated with smoking may be synergistic with the vasospasm of Raynaud's phenomenon and result in digital necrosis. Not only cold exposure of the hands but also generalized cooling should be minimized by protective clothing and by other appropriate measures.

Areas of cutaneous calcinosis or acral erosions are particularly predisposed to secondary infection. Topical clindamycin or erythromycin or Silvadene cream can be useful in preventing recurrent infection after treatment of acute tissue infection with the appropriate systemic antibiotic.

Physical therapists can be vitally important in helping the patient maintain range of motion and in preventing contractures. Occupational therapists work with the patient's hands to maintain maximum function. Both these health professionals are invaluable partners in the total management of the scleroderma patient.

The typical "crow's beak" esophagus of scleroderma results in large part from esophageal reflux which follows esophageal dysmotility. Scleroderma patients should be treated with an antireflux program which might include: elevation of the head of the bed, antacid and H_2-antihistamine therapy.

Systemic Therapy—Vasoactive Agents

Vasoactive agents have been used primarily to treat Raynaud's phenomenon and its sequelae. It is believed that some of these therapies may also modify basic disease mechanisms.

Topical Nitroglycerin. These vasodilating agents were originally developed to treat Raynaud's phenomenon, but their use diminished because of the rebound cardiac vessel spasm that followed the use of excessive amounts. If dosage is carefully restricted, these agents can improve signs and symptoms of Raynaud's phenomenon and promote healing of digital ulcers.

Arteriolar Dilators. Methyldopa (Aldomet), and more recently prazosin (Minipress), has been beneficial, as described with the topical nitroglycerins.

Alpha Blockers. Phenoxybenzamine (Dibenzyline) and tolazoline (Priscoline) have been used.

Beta-Agonists. Terbutaline (Brethine) has been used to treat Raynaud's phenomenon.

Angiotensin-Converting Enzyme Inhibitor. Captopril (Capoten) has been used for the hypertensive crisis associated with scleroderma, but with increasing frequency it is being reported to benefit Raynaud's phenomenon and its sequelae. Some investigators believe that cutaneous sclerosis is also ameliorated.

Calcium Channel Blockers. Nifedipine (Procardia) and verapamil (Calan) have also been successfully used to treat Raynaud's phenomenon and digital ulceration.

Other Vasoactive Agents. Ketanserin, a selective type-II serotonin antagonist, has been used with success. Intra-arterial therapy with reserpine and methyldopa, and more recently with prostacycline infusions, is of benefit and may be used when oral systemic therapies are no longer beneficial and when digital gangrene is imminent.

Hematologic Therapy

Therapy with stanozolol (Winstrol), a fibrinolytic agent, corrects laboratory fibrinolytic abnormalities and may be associated with clinical improvement in digital ulceration. Antiplatelet therapy with dipyridamide (Persantin) and aspirin may also be beneficial. Pentoxifylline (Trental), an agent that affects blood viscosity, has also been claimed to benefit digital ulceration.

Lathyrogens

D-Penicillamine alters aldehyde cross-links of Type-I collagen. In addition to effects on collagen, D-penicillamine also has immunomodulating effects. Therapy with this agent (250 to 750 mg per day) may be associated with reduced dermal sclerosis and possibly with improvement in organ involvement and with increased survival. Significant side effects of D-penicillamine therapy include leukopenia, thrombocytopenia, induction of autoimmune disorders such as lupus erythematosus, pemphigus and myasthenia gravis, renal toxicity such as the nephrotic syndrome, and cutaneous eruptions.

Immunosuppressive Therapy

Azathioprine, cyclophosphamide, and chlorambucil have been used alone in dosages like those described above (see ASLE) or in combination with plasmapheresis for the treatment of life-threatening or potentially crippling scleroderma. Results have been equivocal, but many patients may have had significant improvement in visceral organ function. Meticulous monitoring of the patient for acute and chronic toxicity is mandatory. Experience by the prescribing physician with the use of these therapies is important.

Other Therapies

Lymphapheresis is currently an investigational therapy. Phenytoin (Dilantin) has been claimed to benefit dermal sclerosis. Therapy with antimalarials, potassium aminobenzoate, colchicine, and dimethyl sulfoxide each have their advocates, although experimental evidence of benefit in patients with dermal sclerosis and other manifestations of scleroderma is lacking.

CUTANEOUS VASCULITIS

method of
EDUARDO TSCHEN, M.D., and
ALICIA B. MONROE, D.O.
The University of New Mexico
Albuquerque, New Mexico

Vasculitis is a reaction characterized by inflammation and damage to blood vessels in response to a variety of internal and external stimuli. Cutaneous vasculitis results when the process affects those vessels of the skin from postcapillary venules to the larger vessels located in the deep dermis or subcutaneous fat. It may be the sole manifestation of an ongoing immunologic event or a marker of severe underlying systemic involvement. No single classification scheme exists to satisfy all clinicians. However, the important factors to be considered that may influence eventual outcome include clinical and cutaneous manifestations, histopathological pattern, degree of systemic involvement, size and type of blood vessel affected, and response to therapy.

This discussion will focus on leukocytoclastic vasculitis in adults and Henoch-Schönlein purpura in children as the prototypes of cutaneous vasculitis. Other vasculitides that are important to consider because they may potentially result in significant morbidity and mortality include Wegener's granulomatosis, polyarteritis nodosa, allergic granulomatosis, giant cell arteritis, Behçet's disease, Kawasaki's disease, and thromboangiitis obliterans. These are characterized by extracutaneous involvement, and the type of blood vessels affected are larger than in the primarily cutaneous variant.

Classical cutaneous vasculitis presents as "palpable purpura," exhibiting nonblanching purpuric papules and plaques most often on dependent areas. Variants can be seen ranging from livedo reticularis, vesicles, pustules, and ulcerations to nodules. Small vessel vasculitis as seen in leukocytoclastic vasculitis can occur at any age and in both sexes, manifested by purpuric papules that may occur in waves, each one lasting 7 to 28 days. Lesions can vary in size from 1 mm to greater than several centimeters and vary in number from several to over several hundred. Recurrences are common and new crops may continue to occur for weeks to months. They most often appear on the lower legs and dorsum of the feet, although the thighs, buttocks, and lower abdomen can be affected. The upper extremities are rarely involved. The lesions may itch, sting, or burn, or they may be slightly painful and heal with some degree of postinflammatory hypo- or hyperpigmentation, leaving a yellow or brown macule. General malaise, swelling of the legs, and arthralgias may accompany the cutaneous signs. Systemic involvement can be found in up to 50 per cent of patients, most often reflected in the kidney as glomerulonephritis and by the appearance of microscopic hematuria and proteinuria. This process can be triggered by many factors, including infection, drugs, chemicals, underlying connective tissue diseases, endogenous antigens such as tumor antigens and others, as shown in Table 1.

The Henoch-Schönlein variant of leukocytoclastic vasculitis is seen most commonly in children between the ages of 3 and 10. In addition to skin and renal lesions, gastrointestinal vasculitis may occur, manifested by anorexia, nausea, vomiting, melena, abdominal pain, and possible perforation. Lung involvement can also be seen. This variant often appears following an upper respiratory infection caused by beta hemolytic streptococcus or viral organisms. Edema of the face and distal extremities is more commonly seen than in the adult variety, as is a pronounced arthritic component.

Evaluation

The aim of the evaluation is to identify a possible antigen producing the syndrome and determine the extent of cutaneous and or systemic involvement. Most of this information is obtained with a complete physical examination and a good history. The skin examination as well as evaluation of other systems is likely to give details about whether the problem is purely cutaneous or co-exists with systemic involvement. A minimum of laboratory studies is necessary, such as cell blood count, erythrocyte sedimentation rate, liver function tests, and urinalysis. Other tests that may be helpful are complement studies, skin biopsies, chest x-ray studies, antinuclear antibodies, rheumatoid factor, cry-

TABLE 1. Causes of Leukocytoclastic Vasculitis

Infectious Agents
    Streptococcus
    Mycobacteria
    Hepatitis B virus
    Influenza virus
    Mononucleosis
    Histoplasmosis
    Candida
    Schistosomiasis

Drugs and Other Agents
    Aspirin
    Penicillin
    Sulfonamides
    Serum proteins—vaccines, hyposensitization antigens
    Chemicals—herbicides, insecticides, petroleum products

Systemic Diseases
    Primary biliary cirrhosis
    Chronic active hepatitis
    Ulcerative colitis
    Complement deficiency

Connective Tissue Diseases
    Systemic lupus erythematosus
    Rheumatoid arthritis
    Sjögren's syndrome
    Relapsing polychondritis
    Cryoglobulinemia

Malignant Diseases
    Multiple myeloma
    Leukemia
    Lymphoma
    Hodgkin's disease

oglobulins, evaluation of renal function, serum protein electrophoresis, and hepatitis antigen studies. The possibility of finding an answer by blindly performing these tests is very small. Careful follow-up during the course of the disease provides more information and is encouraged.

The histopathologic hallmark of leukocytoclastic vasculitis is leukocytoclasia, which is the fragmentation of polymorphonuclear leukocytes with the scattering of nuclear debris. Other features include fibrin deposition, endothelial cell swelling, blood vessel thrombosis, and extravasated erythrocytes. These are typically identified in biopsies taken within 24 hours of the onset of the skin lesions; biopsies of older lesions can show a predominance of lymphocytes and more severe vessel destruction. Immunofluorescence studies frequently demonstrate immunoglobulins G, M, or A as well as complement (C3) within and around the vessel walls, suggesting a role for immune complex deposition. Histologic variants such as pityriasis lichenoides et varioliformis acuta exist in which the cellular infiltrate is composed of lymphocytes. Even in biopsies taken in the early phases of the disease, dermo-epidermal changes are also present. Another variant is urticarial vasculitis, which shows less severe blood vessel damage, dermal edema, and eosinophils present within the infiltrate. These two variants are forms of cutaneous vasculitis; however, they have distinct clinical presentations and respond to therapeutic modalities not used in the regular treatment of leukocytoclastic vasculitis.

Treatment

The therapy of cutaneous vasculitis must include the removal of the offending antigen if it can be identified, treatment of the underlying disease, and direct treatment of the vasculitic process with anti-inflammatory or immunosuppressive agents. Since the cutaneous vasculitis syndrome is in general a "self-limited" problem, the treatment must be individualized according to severity and the degree of systemic involvement.

When the disease is mild and no systemic involvement exists, the process can sometimes be controlled by bed rest, normal saline compresses to the lesions, and aspirin or other nonsteroidal anti-inflammatory agents such as ibuprofen (Motrin) in doses of 600 to 800 mg 3 times a day. Indomethacin (Indocin), 25 to 50 mg 4 times a day, is effective in the treatment of urticarial vasculitis.

More aggressive therapy may be needed for progressive or persistent skin lesions. In this case, the direct treatment of the inflammatory vascular process can be accomplished with prednisone, which continues to be the mainstay of treatment. It should be started early in doses of 40 to 80 mg per day (1 mg per Kg per day) for two weeks, the dose being halved by the second week. Rarely, the patient will require treatment beyond this period; however, in severe cases, when prednisone needs to be continued, an alternate-day dosing schedule is preferred using the lowest effective dose. At this time, immunosuppressive agents may be useful, including: azathioprine* (Imuran), 50 to 100 mg per day; dapsone,* 50 to 200 mg per day; sulfasalazine,* 500 mg 3 or 4 times a day; and colchicine,* 2 to 3 mg per day. Cytotoxic agents such as cyclophosphamide* in doses of 50 to 100 mg per day have resulted in remissions in those patients with vasculitis associated with rheumatoid arthritis. Although not considered a first-line therapy, plasmapheresis† can improve cutaneous vasculitis by decreasing circulating antibodies, antigens and immune complexes. It is often used in conjunction with anti-inflammatory or immunosuppressive drugs.

---

*This use of these agents is not listed in the manufacturers' directives.

†Still considered experimental for this use.

DISEASES OF THE NAILS

method of
HOWARD P. BADEN, M.D.
Harvard Medical School
Boston, Massachusetts

The nail plate protects the end of the finger but also aids in fine movement of the fingers. Disorders of the nail most commonly result from trauma, infection, or dermatologic disease. Less frequently they may be a manifestation of systemic disease or medications.

Anatomy of the Nail

The nail plate grows out from the matrix, which is the living layer that lies under the proximal nail fold and extends out on some digits and appears as a white half-moon called the lunula. The hardness of the plate results from its compact proteinaceous structure and not from calcium, which is present in trace amounts. The cuticle is the extension of the stratum corneum of the fold, which grows out on the plate and forms a seal between the fold and the plate. The sides of the plate are bounded by the lateral nail fold but no cuticle is present. The plate is firmly attached to the bed, which appears pink due to its rich blood supply. Separation of these two structures occurs at the hyponychium, which appears white in color owing to the presence of air.

Nails grow continuously at about 0.1 mm per day. The most proximal region of the matrix gives rise to the surface of the nail plate and the most distal parts give rise to the deeper portions. The distal end of the matrix also gives rise to the epithelium of the nail bed, which allows the plate to grow over the bed without becoming detached. The dermal papillae run in parallel rows in a longitudinal direction; for this reason, injury to vessels may cause splinter hemorrhages.

ONYCHOLYSIS

Onycholysis is one of the more common nail problems and seems to occur more frequently in women than men. It often involves more than one finger and presents as a white color of the nail. The white color represents separation of the plate from the bed and results from scattering of light by air under the plate. In most patients it is an idiopathic disorder without any other cutaneous changes. However, it may be seen in psoriasis and fungal infections; in the latter, it is most commonly associated with subungual hyperkeratosis. In the idiopathic type, practically no scale is present. Bacteria may grow as saprophytes. *Pseudomonas* is a common one, causing a greenish discoloration of the plate. Similarly, *Candida* species may be isolated; rarely *C. albicans* is found. Specific treatment with ketaconazole topically or systemically does not affect the onycholysis, although the yeast infection may be irradicated.

When spontaneous healing of onycholysis does occur, new nails may become affected. Cutting the nails short does seem to reduce the extent of involvement and reduce the time to healing. In the absence of any known cause or effective treatment, the most practical solution is to use nail polish to hide the cosmetic defect. Patients should be warned not to clean too vigorously under the nail since this may cause a subungual abcess, usually from *Staphylococcus aureus*. If this complication occurs, the nail plate should be removed, a culture obtained, and appropriate antibiotic treatment initiated.

INFECTIONS OF THE NAIL

Paronychia

Acute paronychia commonly follows injury to the nail fold and presents as redness, swelling, and tenderness. Pus is generally present and can be released by elevating the fold with a blade unless it is already draining. A culture should be obtained and the patient started on erythromycin, 250 mg 4 times daily, unless there are systemic signs of infection, when more aggressive treatment should be undertaken. The nail should be soaked in warm water 4 times a day for 15 minutes to encourage drainage of pus, and should be covered with a nonocclusive gauze dressing between treatments and protected from the environment.

Chronic paronychia may follow an acute episode and is particularly common in individuals whose hands are frequently immersed in water. A variety of bacteria may be cultured as well as *C. albicans,* but the condition behaves like an irritant reaction, not an infection.

Treatment of this condition with systemic or topical antibiotics and anti-yeast drugs rarely leads to resolution. The most effective treatment is protecting the hands from excessive wetting and irritants, which is best accomplished with cotton gloves worn inside loose-fitting plastic ones. In resistant cases, partial excision of the nail fold to remove the dead space may be necessary.

Tinea Unguium

Fungal infection of the nails most commonly starts in the toenails and most frequently in the nails of large toes. Subungual hyperkeratosis at the distal or lateral margins of the plate is the earliest change, and fragmentation of the nail plate is a later finding. The infection eventually involves all of the toenails and may spread to the fingernails. Because treatment involves months of systemic drug therapy, it is important to confirm the diagnosis by microscopic examination of scales and culture. To obtain material for mycologic examination, the nail not attached to the bed should be cut off and the scales close to the point of attachment of the plate to the bed collected.

Cure of fingernails is possible but requires high-dose ultramicrosize griseofulvin, 1.0 to 1.5 grams per day. The patient should be followed at 2-month intervals to establish that the dose used is adequate. Treatment can be stopped 1 month after clinical and mycologic cure.

Toenail infections are much more resistant, have a higher recurrence rate, and are ordinarily not treated with griseofulvin. In the occasional young patient with early involvement it may be justified to try this drug.

Warts

Warts commonly affect the fingernails, involving the folds and hyponychium. They can at times be extensive, particularly in the proximal nail fold, and cause pressure on the matrix that leads to a distorted nail plate. In patients with a few and small lesions, fulguration or cryosurgery are the methods of choice. For extensive lesions it is advisable to avoid surgical procedures; the best approach is to paint the lesions with a thoroughly mixed mixture of equal parts of 85 per cent lactic acid and flexible collodion and cover the lesions with waterproof tape for 8 hours. The tape is removed and the treated areas abraded with an emory board while wet. This is repeated nightly until the warts are gone.

Herpes Simplex

Primary and recurrent herpes simplex infection of the ends of the fingers is common in health professionals as a result of exposure to saliva, which contains the virus in 2 to 5 per cent of normal adults. It is important not to confuse these lesions with bacterial infection so as to avoid surgical incision. The indications for use of acyclovir are the same as in treatment of herpes infections in other areas of the body.

Candidiasis

Infection of the nail plate with *C. albicans* occurs as a primary event in the mucocutaneous candidiasis syndrome. *C. albicans* may also be isolated in chronic paronychia and onycholysis, in which it is a secondary invader. Oral ketacon-azole is helpful in the management of primary candidiasis but is not useful for secondary infections in paronychia or onycholysis.

NAIL DISORDERS FROM TRAUMA

Chipping and horizontal and vertical splitting of the nails can result from excessive exposure of the nail to water, and occasionally from nail cosmetics. This problem is aggravated by using the nails as a tool and by incorrect grooming of the nails. The nails should be cut when wet and then smoothed with an emory board when they are dry by filing in one direction and avoiding a back-and-forth movement. The daily application of Brit/tex wax (Liagene Inc., 91 Prescott Street, P.O. Box 524, Worcester, MA 01613–0524), starting at the free edge and sweeping proximally over the cuticle helps fill in any defects, protects the plate, and keeps the cuticle soft. This should be done gently so as not to damage the matrix. Nail wrapping, when done by an experienced manicurist can be very effective for individuals with exceptionally fragile nails.

Trauma to the nail fold by "playing" with it, biting, or excessive manicuring results in defects in the plate that are manifest as variously shaped grooves. Chronic injury may cause permanent injury to the matrix and persistent grooves. The best treatment is avoidance of the injury.

Blunt trauma to the nail can result in a hematoma that may take several days to become apparent if the injury occurs under the nail fold. Unless there is extreme pain, it is best to avoid treatment. There are nail drills designed for making a hole to relieve the pressure, but a hole may be burned in the nail plate using a paper clip heated in an open flame.

Onychogryphosis is a nail dystrophy of the large toes resulting from trauma, usually from poorly fitting shoes. The nail is extremely thick and curved. Clipping and filing the nail is the most conservative treatment, but when the condition becomes too painful the nail should be removed and the matrix permanently destroyed or removed.

Ingrown Nail

Failure to cut the toenail straight across and wearing tight shoes may result in the nail plate growing into the lateral fold. In the early stage this is manifested as pain, redness, and swelling. When the fold is pierced, symptoms and physical findings are magnified and, in addition, granulation tissue becomes apparent. Treatment of the early stage involves packing cotton in the nail groove and under the free edge of the nail. If the changes have progressed beyond the stage when this is possible, then clipping off the offending piece of plate and soaking will give immediate relief. The patient should then be referred to a physician with experience in managing such problems. Skillful podiatrists can also provide excellent care.

CUTANEOUS DISEASE AFFECTING THE NAIL

The most common skin disease affecting the nail is *psoriasis*. It characteristically causes pits or depressions of the nail plate surface. This results from focal involvement of the proximal end of the matrix, causing faulty keratinization. Other changes include a rough surface, onycholysis, subungual hyperkeratosis, and total disintegration of the plate. These changes may be indistinguishable from those caused by a fungal infection of the nails.

Lichen planus also commonly affects the nails. The earliest change is a red to violaceous papule of the fold or bed. When the matrix is involved, roughness of the surface, pits, longitudinal grooves, and splits may appear. With severe involvement there is destruction of the matrix with loss of nail, and one may observe focal attachment of the fold to the plate called *pterygium*.

Pitting and roughness of the surface of the nail plate may be seen in *alopecia areata* and an idiopathic disorder called *twenty-nail dystrophy* in which all of the nails are involved.

Various types of *dermatoses* (e.g., contact dermatitis, atopic dermatitis) that affect the hands may involve the nail folds and extend to the matrix. This results in dystrophy of the nail with horizontal grooves predominating.

Treatment of these nail disorders is difficult, since it is impossible for topical agents applied to the nail folds to reach the involved matrix. Except for some patients with lichen planus, the changes are reversible; with time, new nails will grow out. Corticosteroids (3 mg per ml of triamcimelone acetonide) can be injected under the fold close to the nail; however, this should not be done routinely because of the pain and the risk of infection. It has been advocated in patients with lichen planus whose disease appears to be progressing to scarring, and in this situation it may be indicated. In the dermatoses, topical corticosteroids are helpful for the skin changes, but nail plates will take some time to grow out normally.

KELOIDS

method of
O.G. RODMAN, M.D.
Henry Ford Hospital
Detroit, Michigan

Keloids are benign proliferative cutaneous lesions composed of excessive collagenous tissue. Trauma is the triggering factor in the vast majority of patients with spontaneously arising keloids most commonly noted on the anterior chest. Common areas of keloid formation include the ears, jawline, chest, shoulders, and upper back. There is a higher incidence in black patients. By definition, keloids extend beyond the original trauma site in a crablike configuration, whereas hypertrophic scars are confined within the border of the initial site of trauma.

Prevention

Unnecessary surgery should be avoided in known keloid formers. If surgery is essential, incisions should be parallel to skin tension lines with the final closure under minimal tension. Mid-chest incisions should be minimized and the crossing of joint spaces should be avoided. Pressure garments or devices worn postoperatively further hinder keloid regrowth.

Treatment

There is no single best treatment for keloids. In virtually all patients, combination therapeutic modalities are indicated, including intralesional steroids, surgical excision, pressure dressings, laser therapy, and radiotherapy. My treatment for such patients invariably includes the triad of intralesional steroids, excisional surgery, and pressure devices. Regardless of the therapeutic modality used, the physician should periodically monitor all patients over a period of 18 to 24 months for potential keloid recurrence.

Intralesional Steroids

Intralesional steroid therapy plays a definite role in the improvement of all keloid patients, since it promotes collagen breakdown and overall size shrinkage. Triamcinolone acetonide suspension (Kenalog) is employed in concentrations ranging from 2 to 40 mg per milliliter. A 27-gauge or larger-bore needle should be used to prevent suspension clogging. The use of a Luer-Lok syringe will prevent leakage, thereby significantly enhancing drug delivery.

Most patients will accept a 10- to 15-second freeze with liquid nitrogen prior to steroid injection, because of local anesthetic effects from the cryotherapy. The resultant tissue edema allows for further ease in subsequent steroid injections. All injections should be placed within the substance of the keloid and not sublesionally, to avoid unnecessary cutaneous atrophy. Repeated higher concentrations of triamcinolone acetonide are more likely to produce hypopigmentation that may last 6 to 12 months before resolution.

Earlobe keloids are much more amenable to predictable and successful improvement than are keloids located presternally. Nevertheless, I prefer to treat initially all larger keloids with a steroid injection of 40 mg per ml injection, diluting with 1 to 2 per cent lidocaine to achieve my final desired concentration. After injections for 2 to 4 visits spaced approximately 3 to 4 weeks apart, Kenalog-10 (triamcinolone acetonide) may be used full strength or diluted with lidocaine to a minimum strength of 2 mg per ml. Surgery is virtually never performed on a patient who has not first received a minimum of 3 steroid injections without benefit.

Surgery

The surgical approach to removal of keloids varies depending on the size, location, and configuration of the lesions. In all instances, atraumatic and sterile technique are of paramount importance. It is best to use 6-0 or 5-0 interrupted nylon sutures, carefully avoiding tension and unnecessary trauma to all tissue.

Small, simple posterior pedunculated earlobe keloids may be shaved, followed by postoperative steroid therapy and pressure hemostasis. Keloids with narrow bases may be excised with careful undermining and injected at the base. Larger, dumbbell-shaped keloids may be meticulously cored out, with low-tension interrupted sutures for closure. Sutures generally are removed in 10 to 14 days with subsequent injections of Kenalog-10 two weeks later. Within 2 months, steroid injections may be stopped; however, the patient should return for follow-up at the first sign of recurrence.

Chest or presternal keloids tend to be more painful and much more recalcitrant. However, combining maximum intralesional steroid injections with fine electrocoagulation and postradiation therapy, good-to-excellent results can be obtained. A dose of 250 rads is given postoperatively, followed by four similar treatments every 2 weeks. A youthful patient and the lack of an experienced radiotherapist are relative contraindications to this latter modality because of potential carcinogenesis.

Other Therapeutic Measures

Carbon dioxide laser excision has now been used for treatment of keloids in all anatomic sites. As with other modalities, facial lesions respond best to the carbon dioxide laser. The cutting mode of the laser is controlled to yield minimal thermal damage to uninvolved skin, and the resultant wound is left to heal via secondary intention. Standard wound care and postoperative follow-up with pressure dressings and/or intralesional steroids are recommended.

In the face of failures with the aforementioned treatments, other regimens include methotrexate, colchicine, nitrogen mustard, thiotepa, and beta-aminopropionitrile fumarate. Asiatic acid, topical tretinoin, and zinc therapy have also yielded variable success.

VERRUCA VULGARIS
(Warts)
method of
DAVID P. CLARK, M.D.
University of Missouri Health Science Center
Columbia, Missouri

Despite all efforts, no effective antiviral chemotherapy for verruca has been discovered. All current therapy to eliminate warts is dependent upon tissue destruction and induction of the host's immune system. Some warts are difficult to eradicate; periungual, perirectal, and plantar warts are most resistant to therapy. Immunosuppressed patients are frequently plagued by multiple verrucae and respond poorly to any therapy. Warts are epithelial growths caused by human papilloma viruses (HPV). Over 45 different types of HPV viruses have been isolated from human infections. HPV DNA is incorporated into human DNA. Viral DNA can be recovered in normal-appearing cells up to 15 millimeters from the base of a clinical wart.

Initial Therapy

Simple destructive chemical or cryosurgical methods will eliminate most verrucae and were the first therapeutic measures used to treat warts. Fifty to sixty per cent of common warts will disappear without therapy over a 12 to 18 month period. In evaluating all therapeutic intervention, the risk of scar, pain, infection, and drug side effects must be balanced against the known natural history of warts.

Chemical Destruction

Salicylic acid preparations are an effective first-line therapy. After softening and paring of the wart with a blade or pumice stone, 17 per cent salicylic acid in a collodion base is applied daily. Alternatively, 40 per cent salicylic acid plasters are applied to the treatment area for 48 hours followed by 48 hours of rest and gentle débridement. Daily therapy for 2 to 3 months is needed for elimination of most warts. However, morbidity and cost are low and results are equal to all other methods.

Caustic acids, such as bichloroacetic acid or trichloroacetic acid, may be applied with or without tape occlusion weekly by the physician. An extract from the blister beetle, cantharidin, is used alone or in combination with salicylic acid to cause vesiculation and slough of wart tissue. Although initial application of cantharidin is usually painless, blisters develop over 4 to 8 hours that can be painful or secondarily infected.

Flat Warts. Flat warts are multiple, flat-topped, flesh-colored papules found on the face, arms, and legs. These warts may spread rapidly and are difficult to treat. Retinoic acid (Retin-A)* and 5-fluorouricil* have been used successfully to treat flat warts, but chemical treatments for facial flat warts cause considerable skin irritation. Shaving encourages dissemination and must be stopped.

Condyloma accuminata. These are HPV infections found on mucous membranes and spread primarily through sexual contact. Therapy must start with a complete evaluation of both partners. Podophyllin, an extract of the May apple, is applied as a 20 per cent solution in tincture of benzoin every 5 to 14 days. The surrounding tissue is protected with vaseline and the medication washed off in 2 to 6 hours. Patients vary greatly in response to podophyllin; some patients have little reaction while others have a dramatic inflammatory response. Podophyllin is systemically absorbed after application to mucous membranes. Considerable morbidity and even death have resulted from applications of large amounts of the drug (i.e., greater than 1.4 ml of 25 per cent). Gross visual inspection is insufficient to determine adequacy of therapy. After the wart is not visible on gross inspection, compresses saturated with 3 per cent acetic acid are placed over the treatment site for 10 minutes. Inspection with a hand lens will often demonstrate areas of white scale indicating residual wart tissue.

Cryosurgery

Application of liquid nitrogen ($-320°C$) by a cotton swab or spray device is effective. The area is usually treated until a 1 to 2 ml halo of frost surrounds the wart. A blister develops, causing the slough of wart tissue and adjacent skin. Local pain is usually minimal and rarely requires local anesthesia. Scarring is minimal but cases of hy-

pertrophic scar following cryosurgery have been reported. Due to a high number of nonhealing ulcers, cryosurgery is to be avoided on the lower extremities and over bony prominences. Cryosurgery over the lateral aspects of digits may result in sensory loss. Frequently a wart will require two or three sessions of cryotherapy.

Treatment Modalities for Difficult-to-treat Warts

Chemical Destruction

Dinitrochlorobenzene (DNCB) has been used successfully to treat recalcitrant warts—particularly the difficult-to-treat periungual warts. Although a large experience with physician-applied DNCB has demonstrated few side effects, DNCB is a contact sensitizer and can induce a variety of immune responses. DNCB, in high concentration, has been associated with a positive Ames test for mutagenicity; however, this agent has never been found to be a carcinogen. Currently the drug must be compounded locally because no medical-grade DNCB is marketed in the United States.

Bleomycin, a chemotherapeutic agent, has been injected into verrucae with excellent results. However, the procedure can be associated with considerable pain. Necrosis of digits and induction of Raynaud's phenomenon have been reported after injection of periungual warts with bleomycin.

Use of DNCB and bleomycin for treatment of verrucae is investigational and both drugs have considerably more side effects than any of the initial chemical therapies. Expertise and caution are required.

Surgical Destruction

Surgical methods to treat warts are rapid and often effective but have the potential to scar, require local anesthesia for pain control, and do not have superior cure rates. Cold-steel surgery, electrosurgery, and laser therapy are all used to treat difficult verrucae. Because these nonspecific surgical methods involve considerable destruction of normal tissue and have definite morbidity, they should be reserved for recalcitrant warts.

Carbon Dioxide Laser. The carbon dioxide laser generates high temperatures, 150 degrees Centigrade, with a column of infrared light. The laser beam is focused in a very small area and causes vaporization and destruction of the wart. Due to limited heat transfer to normal tissue and improved accuracy, there is less risk of scarring with laser destruction than with electrosurgical methods. Recent success treating condyloma acuminata with carbon dioxide laser therapy may

---

*This use of these agents is not listed in the manufacturers' directives.

be due to the treatment of an entire "field" rather than isolated lesions. Laser surgery seals nerve endings and lymphatics, which minimizes postoperative discomfort. Laser surgery is not universally available and the technology remains expensive.

Cold-Steel Surgery. Removing wart tissue with a curette or scalpel has been used for many years. However, scalpel excision has been almost wholly abandoned due to unacceptable recurrence rates. The curette is most effectively used following light desiccation with an electrosurgery unit. Cold-steel surgical methods are best used to "debulk" large, exophytic warts prior to chemical or laser therapy.

Electrosurgery. Electrosurgery units destroy tissue with heat produced when current passing through tissue encounters electrical resistance. Electrosurgery involves considerable heat transfer to adjacent normal tissue. If extensive treatment of the wart is necessary, scarring will occur. The amount of scarring is unpredictable due to variable heat transfer. If electrosurgery is performed in the periungual region, permanent nail distortion may occur.

Multiple unsafe or useless therapies are used too often because no one definitive cure for warts is accepted. Patients and families are often less knowledgeable about the long-term consequences of therapy and insist that "something be done." Physicians should persist in conservative treatment and avoid multiple, painful office visits. Fortunately, the large majority of all warts will disappear with simple therapy.

NEVI AND MALIGNANT MELANOMA

method of
RICHARD A. STRICK, M.D.
UCLA Center for Health Sciences
Los Angeles, California

The story of pigmented lesions in the skin is truly a tale of "beauty and the beast," spanning the whole spectrum from the "beauty mark" of nevocellular nevi to the potentially fatal "black mole," malignant melanoma.

The incidence of melanoma has been rising dramatically, having nearly tripled in the last 10 years in the United States. There are now approximately 25,000 cases per year and it is estimated that by the year 2000 the lifetime risk for an American of developing melanoma will be 1 in 90. This is up from 1 in 1500 in 1935, 1 in 800 in 1950, and 1 in 250 in 1980. Although the death rate from melanoma has more than doubled in the United States since 1950, the five-year survival rates have improved from 41 per cent in 1940 to 60 per cent in 1960 and 83 per cent in 1980. Since treatment of melanoma has not improved for comparable lesions, improved survival is based on diagnosis and treatment at earlier stages of disease. Therefore, public education programs have been promoted strongly by the American Academy of Dermatology in order to increase the awareness of melanoma and its importance on the part of both physicians and the lay public.

ACQUIRED NEVI

The most common form of nevus is the acquired variety. The vast majority of individuals have multiple lesions that first occur in early childhood and increase in number until approximately the mid-thirties. Sometime after age 50 they gradually begin to disappear. They may darken or increase in size at puberty and during pregnancy.

There are several clinical types of acquired nevi. The *junction nevus* clinically presents as a flat, macular, hyperpigmented lesion with regular borders. The *intradermal nevus* is a soft, fleshy, papular lesion that may be slightly tan or may be the same color as the surrounding skin. The *compound nevus* is both papular and dark. The hallmark of all of these types is their regularity of both border and surface and relatively uniform color. Most acquired nevi are less than 6 mm in diameter.

The malignant potential of these lesions is particularly low. Approximately 1 in a million will develop into malignant melanoma. However, those who have particularly numerous acquired nevi, especially if the nevi are larger than usual and somewhat irregular (even if not dysplastic), have an increased risk of developing melanoma. This may be due to the increased number of nevomelanocytic cells potentially becoming malignant or it may just be a marker for individuals who are at greater risk for melanoma.

The *halo nevus* is a variant of nevocellular nevus in which the skin surrounding the lesion becomes hypopigmented. This represents a process in which the immune system attacks and eliminates the nevus and melanocytes in the area. In these cases, the halo should be ignored in evaluating the central nevus for its malignant potential, and a thorough search should be made for a primary melanoma located elsewhere on the body, since halo nevi are commonly seen in those who do have a melanoma.

Another variant is the *blue nevus,* in which the melanin pigment is located more deeply in the dermis; due to the differential absorption and scattering of light of different wavelengths, the brown pigment appears blue when viewed through the increased thickness of overlying skin.

The *Spitz tumor,* which has been called by the misnomer "juvenile melanoma," is a red to pink, dome-shaped papule usually occurring on the face of a child. It is a benign nevocellular lesion.

Treatment

Obviously, not all acquired nevi require treatment. Treatment is indicated if the diagnosis of a benign lesion is uncertain or if the lesion is cosmetically objectionable to the patient. In addition, it is generally advisable to remove lesions that the patient says are changing or that are causing undue anxiety to the patient.

If melanoma is considered a possible diagnosis, before a pigmented lesion is removed a full-thickness biopsy should be done. If the lesion is raised and not darkly pigmented, a tangential excision often will minimize the scarring. This may be done with a sterile razor blade, scalpel, or scissors. The base may then be treated with gentle electrocautery, Monsel's solution, aluminum chloride, or direct pressure. Patients treated in this manner need to be forewarned that the lesion may recur, especially if there is a great deal of melanin in the original growth.

Destructive measures, rather than removal of pigmented lesions, should be avoided. It is desirable to have material for histologic examination to ensure that the diagnosis melanoma is ruled out. In addition if there is a recurrence of the lesion and subsequent removal is done, the histology of the lesion is often distorted, resulting in a "pseudomelanoma," which resembles melanoma histologically.

CONGENITAL NEVI

By definition, congenital nevi are present at birth. They tend to be larger than acquired nevi, often greater than 1 cm in diameter. Some may be very large and may be called *giant hairy nevi* or *bathing trunk nevi;* these may involve a large percentage of the body surface. Congenital nevi are classified as small if they can be easily excised, and as medium-sized if they are between "small" and "giant." Although there are exceptions, congenital nevi tend to extend deeper within the skin than do acquired nevi, and they may even involve underlying structures. It is generally accepted that the large lesions carry an increased risk of developing melanomas, which may occur deep within the lesions. Although series vary greatly, the risk of melanoma is generally considered to be at least several per cent. Of those developing into melanoma, they do so before the age of 5 in about 50 per cent of

patients, and they tend to have a particularly poor prognosis.

Treatment

Considerable controversy exists about the treatment of congenital nevi. Although the giant lesions are difficult surgical challenges, many may be removed in stages. The use of tissue expanders may aid in treatment of such lesions. Dermabrasion may be of some cosmetic benefit in these lesions, but since it does not remove the deeper portions, from which melanoma often arises, this therapy is suboptimal and cannot be advocated. The smaller the lesion is, the less the risk of development of melanoma within the lesion, but also the greater the ease of surgical excision. Although the risk of melanoma developing from a small congenital nevus is low, there is some risk. The scar resulting from the removal is often a cosmetic improvement over the original lesion.

DYSPLASTIC NEVI

Dysplastic nevi have been recently characterized as more irregular clinically and histologically than are other nevocellular nevi. The clinical characteristics are an ill-defined, somewhat irregular border, surrounding erythema, truncal location, accentuated skin markings, irregular pigmentation including black foci on a pink background, and diameter greater than 5 mm. Although the diagnosis of dysplastic nevus can be suspected clinically, histologic confirmation of the diagnosis is required.

Less than 5 per cent of adult Caucasians have dysplastic nevi. The main significance of dysplastic nevi is that in those who have multiple dysplastic nevi and who also have family members who have a history of both multiple dysplastic nevi and melanoma, the lifetime risk of development of melanoma approaches 100 per cent. The melanomas may occur in either the dysplastic nevi or on the apparently normal skin, so that in the familial cases these lesions are more a marker for those at increased risk for melanoma than precursors to melanoma.

Treatment

It is neither feasible nor practical to surgically remove all dysplastic nevi. Individual lesions that are growing, or changing in other ways, should probably be excised and examined. It has been advocated by some that extensive photography be done of the lesions when patients have numerous dysplastic nevi and that these be used for comparison on subsequent visits. A practical and economical way to do this is to have the patient obtain multiple Polaroid or other snapshots of the lesions and compare them at home monthly for signs of change; the patient should return for a checkup as soon as any change is noted. This should be done in addition to, but not instead of, regular checkups by a physician at intervals of several months to 1 year.

MALIGNANT MELANOMA

About 20 per cent of melanomas arise from benign nevi. The bulk of the remainder arise without a pre-existing abnormality. In whites the most common locations are the legs in women and the trunk in men; in blacks the palms and soles and mucous membranes are the most common sites of involvement. Approximately 50 per cent of melanoma patients have either dysplastic nevi or other large and unusual nevi. Those who have fair complexion, blue eyes, freckles, and who have increased sun exposure despite a tendency to sunburn easily are the more likely to develop melanoma.

The most reliable early signs of melanoma are the following:

1. Asymmetry of the surface: a raised area at an edge of a pigmented lesion.
2. Border irregularity: indentations and extensions at the border as the battle line between the body's defenses and the tumor is drawn.
3. Colors of red, white, blue, and black found within a pigmented lesion.
4. Diameter greater than 6 mm.

The most reliable prognostic indicator in Stage I (nonmetastatic) melanoma is tumor thickness. This is measured from the granular layer to the base of the tumor. Tumors less than 0.76 mm thick are relatively-low risk lesions with high cure rates and rare metastases; those thicker than 1.5 mm have a much worse prognosis; and those from 0.76 mm to 1.5 mm are in a gray area. Thickness is also useful as a prognostic indicator for length of survival. Metastases may occur in the low-risk group and may be as high as 5 per cent of cases.

Until recently the "BANS" areas (back, arms, neck, scalp) had been thought to be at greater risk for metastases; however, studies have not found this to be the case, and this is not currently felt to be a valid prognostic index.

Controversy still exists as to whether histologic evidence of tumor regression is a good prognostic indicator, but it appears now that it may not be a valuable indication.

Treatment

The optimal biopsy of melanoma is excisional. Any biopsy that does not remove the full thick-ness of the lesion does not allow for accurate determination of the depth of the melanoma and is therefore inadequate. A controversy has existed about whether incisional biopsy of melanoma increases the chance of metastasis. The latest evidence is that when the data are corrected for tumor thickness there is no difference in the rate of metastasis due to the type of biopsy. Rather, those lesions that are larger and deeper, and therefore more advanced and more likely to metastasize, are by their nature more likely to have been biopsied without total removal. This does not cause more metastasis but represents a skewed selection of cases that were already advanced by the time of biopsy. However, total excisional biopsy is the method of choice, since it allows for examination of the entire lesion microscopically.

Although wide excisions of 3 to 5 cm were advocated in the past for melanoma and are still advocated by a minority, the treatment advocated and accepted by most authorities currently is for margins of approximately 1 cm to be taken around melanomas, and for removal to, but not including fascia. Unless the diagnosis is quite certain, this is best done following excisional biopsy rather than at the time of biopsy. Prophylactic node dissection of clinically uninvolved nodes should not be done for low-risk lesions and is probably also unnecessary in higher-risk lesions. If metastasis only to soft tissues has occurred, then aggressive surgical treatment may be helpful; however, if there is visceral involvement, the prognosis is quite poor.

PREMALIGNANT LESIONS

method of
DANIEL M. SIEGEL, M.D.
University of Texas Southwestern
Dallas, Texas

Premalignant lesions of the skin are a diverse group that can be divided into those that can progress to malignant lesions and those that are a marker for the development of malignant lesions either locally or systemically. The incidence of premalignant lesions, especially those associated with sun exposure, is increasing.

Diagnostic Considerations

To diagnose a premalignant lesion of the skin, one must look for it. A thorough examination of the skin can be done methodically in a short period of time. The only instruments needed are a low-power magnifying lens and good lighting. A hair blower is a useful additional tool for looking at the scalp if there is a questionable area in a long haired patient. With the patient standing up, all exposed body areas are examined by the physician. Examination of intertriginous areas including the axillae, inguinal areas, and interdigital areas can be performed at this time. A felt-tipped marking pen is excellent for marking those lesions in need of a biopsy; sequential numbering can eliminate confusion when multiple biopsies are to be performed. The cutaneous examination is completed with a look in the mouth, including under the tongue, for suspicious lesions.

Biopsy Techniques. Biopsy techniques are tailored to specific features and distribution of lesions. When performing a biopsy of a lesion suspected of harboring an invasive malignancy, enough of the dermis must be obtained to allow the diagnosis of invasion if present. If the lesion is small enough, biopsy in toto is recommended, as this will avoid the need for a secondary treatment whether the pathology is benign or premalignant. For pigmented lesions, a full-thickness biopsy is indicated, so that if the lesion is found to be a melanoma, proper therapeutic decisions based on the thickness of the lesion can be undertaken.

Choosing a Pathologist. It is important to work with a pathologist who is knowledgeable about diseases of the skin; a nonspecific report may lead to undertreatment, overtreatment, or inappropriate treatment of a given lesion, which can occasionally lead to litigation.

TREATMENT

Biopsy and treatment can be carried out simultaneously on many lesions. The choice of technique for a given lesion is based on the size, location, and distribution of the lesions and the physician's skill with a given modality. A variety of treatment modalities is available (see Table 1) including (1) cryosurgery with liquid nitrogen, (2) curettage and desiccation, (3) chemical coagulation, (4) laser excision, (5) dermabrasion, and (6) Mohs' micrographic surgery.

Biopsy and Treatment Modalities

Punch biopsies are performed with a trephine under local anesthesia, and a round core of tissue is obtained. This is a very convenient form of biopsy. Disposable punches can be obtained alone or in a small kit that includes disposable scissors and forceps. It is important when doing a punch biopsy to get an adequate specimen including epidermis, dermis, and subcutaneous tissue, if indicated. The specimen should be traumatized as little as possible to avoid architectural disturbance. After the biopsy is obtained, the punch defect may be closed with a suture along relaxed skin tension lines or plugged with a hemostatic agent.

Shave excision is a simple technique that allows rapid treatment of multiple lesions and obtains a flat piece of tissue for pathologic examination. A shave excision going into the dermis at the deepest part of the lesion is necessary to make a diagnosis of invasion if present. To facilitate the pathologist's role in examining the tissue, the shave excision specimen can be placed on a piece of paper for 10 to 15 seconds to dry flat before insertion into formalin, or it can be pressed against the side of the specimen bottle out of the formalin and allowed to dry for 10 to 15 seconds; the bottle is then closed and inverted to allow fixation of the tissue while it remains relatively flat.

Excisional biopsy is a technique that often allows complete removal of the lesions and an easily closed wound with a straight-line scar.

There are no absolute contraindications to biopsy. Relative contraindications include a hemorrhagic diathesis (from therapeutic anticoagulants, nonsteroidal anti-inflammatory agents, or endogenous biochemical disorders such as hemophilia or thrombocytopenia) and granulocytopenia.

Local Anesthesia

Lidocaine 1 per cent with epinephrine is adequate for most biopsies; the use of epinephrine on fingers and toes is contraindicated because of vasoconstriction. If 7 to 10 minutes is allowed to elapse between infiltration of anesthesia and biopsy, the procedure may be almost bloodless. Slow infiltration of anesthesia is desirable, as the patient will experience less discomfort. For most punch or shave procedures, less than one ml of anesthetic is adequate.

Actinic Keratosis

Actinic keratosis, the most commonly diagnosed precancerous lesion, is caused by chronic exposure to sunlight. Actinic keratoses are found on sun-exposed areas, most often the face, dorsum of the hands, and the balding scalp. These lesions range from pinpoint to full facial in size and from rough to markedly hyperkeratotic in texture. Involvement of appendages is not seen. Erythema may or may not be present around a lesion.

Single or Scattered Lesions

Single or scattered lesions may be treated at the time of diagnosis by a variety of methods. If the lesion is very thick and the suspicion of invasion exists, biopsy in toto is indicated. Recognition by the skilled physician is important; often the lesion is treated on a clinical basis without a biopsy being performed. If any suspicion of invasion or uncertainty of diagnosis exists, a biopsy is mandatory.

TABLE 1. **"Low-Technology" Office Biopsy and Therapy Modalities**

Name	Specimen Obtained	Instruments Needed	"Pros"	"Cons"
Punch biopsy	Cylindrical "core"	Trephine punch (>2 mm); wound closure supplies or hemostatic (Gelfoam, lyophilized collagen)	Inexpensive; rapid trephines available in disposable kits	Small specimen, possible sampling error
Shave	Flat specimen	Scalpel or half a double-edged razor; topical hemostatic (Drysol, 25–50 per cent trichloroacetic acid or Monsel's solution)	Removal in toto; inexpensive	Specimen may curl if not flattened prior to fixation (see text); specimen does not allow evaluation of invasion
Excision	Elliptical	Minor surgery tray	Allows evaluation of easily managed tissue by pathologist; allows placement of scar in best cosmetic location	Greater time commitment than above; greater chance of infection, nerve damage, excessive bleeding; longer healing time
Cryosurgery	None	Liquid nitrogen and swab or spray gun	Rapid; inexpensive; well tolerated	Postoperative pigment changes; no specimen
Curettage and Electrodesiccation	Fragmented	Curettes; electrocautery or thermal cautery	Rapid; inexpensive	Specimen architecture distorted; may "rip" extensively sun-damaged skin
Chemical cauterization	None	Chemical cauterant (50 per cent trichloroacetic acid)	Rapid; inexpensive	Difficult to judge depth of damage without extensive experience; no specimen

If the lesion appears to be thin without obvious infiltration on palpation, treatment with liquid nitrogen will result in blistering, mild pain for 8 to 12 hours, and a wound that usually heals in 2 to 3 weeks. Hypopigmentation is a frequent sequela; hypertrophic scarring is uncommon. Liquid nitrogen treatment is inexpensive, rapid, and usually well tolerated by the patient without anesthesia. Treatment can be performed using either a spray bottle or a swab. The patient should be instructed in the care of the wound, including daily cleansing with soap and water and dressings to keep out dirt.

Curettage is a safe and effective method of treatment that allows one to obtain a specimen for pathological examination, although the specimen is fragmented. Electrodesiccation following curettage gives hemostasis and an extra narrow margin of destruction. For premalignant lesions, electrocauterization should be gentle, as there is no need for destruction of deeper structures.

Chemical cautery with phenol or trichloroacetic acid is effective if the physician is properly trained in its use. Trichloroacetic acid is almost fully bound in the epidermis and upper dermis; a concentration of 50 per cent is effective treatment for thin actinic keratoses. Two to three passes of a soaked swab stick is useful on thin lesions. Phenol has much greater penetration than trichloroacetic acid, and treatment of large areas can result in systemic toxicity. Repeated applications cause deeper destruction; the "frosting" that is seen after application of chemical peeling agents has no correlation with the depth of injury.

5-Fluorouracil can be applied as 1 per cent cream on the face or 5 per cent cream on the hands, twice a day for 28 days to obtain clearing of the lesion. Discomfort associated with this treatment often diminishes the patient's compliance (see below).

Focal dermabrasion using ethylchloride or fluoroethyl topical anesthesia can be used for isolated lesions. This treatment has the disadvantage of aerosolizing the specimen and a small amount of associated blood, potentially permitting personnel to inhale this material. Also, no specimen is obtained for pathological examination.

Diffuse Lesions

Diffuse lesions involving the whole face are more difficult to manage. As a greater number of lesions increases the likelihood of development of invasive disease, these patients must be treated more vigorously. A course of 5-fluorouracil, 1 per cent cream, applied to the face twice daily for 28 days can be used if the patient is compliant. Patients must be warned that they will experience mild discomfort for the first week and then severe reddening, crusting, scaling, and burning for the next 3 weeks. Rarely do these symptoms extend beyond the 3- to 4-week healing phase routinely noted after completing therapy. It is important to encourage the patient to follow through with the full course of treatment. Follow-up visits at 10 and 20 days after beginning treatment can help reinforce the importance of a complete course of therapy. The use of one of the brochures issued by the manufacturer of Efudex (Roche) or Fluroplex (Herbert) explaining the severe irritation that will develop is important in enhancing the patient's compliance.

A short, subtherapeutic course of 5-fluorouracil will give temporary, transient results but usually results in full recurrence of all lesions within a short time. At the completion of 28 days of treatment, bland emollients and 1 per cent hydrocortisone cream may be used to speed healing. Infection is an uncommon but possible risk, and scarring in areas that have been infected or traumatized occurs infrequently.

Definitive treatment of widespread lesions may be performed in the office by the physician skilled in full-face dermabrasion or chemical peel. These are surgical procedures that should not be undertaken without adequate training in these procedures. Dermabrasions and chemical peels also serve the effect of rejuvenating aged skin, which may be an added benefit for the patient.

Retin-A Therapy

Retin-A (tretinoin) is becoming a popular "rejuvenation" treatment for aging skin, since it was first shown to aid in the rejuvenation of collagen in animal models a number of years ago. Clinical studies are encouraging, and Retin-A appears to reverse actinic damage to collagen (which may cause a reversal of wrinkling), shrink and eradicate minute actinic keratoses, and abort the development of new lesions. Side effects of Retin-A are minor and include irritation, redness, and increased phototoxicity during use. All patients using Retin-A should be encouraged to use a moisturizing sunscreen in the daytime and avoid excessive sun exposure. The scaling and dryness noted by some patients within 1 to 2 weeks of initiating therapy appears to decrease with continued use of the drug; an occasional patient will experience a severe reaction and will have to have treatment discontinued and then restarted at a lower dosage or lower frequency once symptoms have resolved. Starting patients on Retin-A, 0.05 per cent cream, is a practical approach, as the cream base is less drying than the gel base or liquid. The physician must resist the urging of the patient to begin with a "stronger" preparation, as this will almost certainly result in the side effects noted above.

Leukoplakia/Actinic Cheilitis

These pre–squamous carcinoma lesions arise on the lips from sun exposure and on mucosal surfaces from smoking and snuff dipping. These lesions tend to be more aggressive and have a higher incidence of conversion to invasive squamous carcinomas than actinic keratoses arising on sun-exposed skin. Actinic cheilitis presents as rough or fine scaling, brown, red, or white patches on the lip: the lower lip shows disease more commonly than the upper. Leukoplakia, which can be benign (arising from rubbing, chewing on the lips, chewing on the buccal mucosa, or other nervous habits) or malignant from causes noted, presents as white plaques on mucosal surfaces; erythroleukoplakia, a similar lesion with a reddish hue, has a much higher incidence of malignant degeneration than lesions arising on sun-exposed areas.

Actinic cheilitis, whether focal or diffuse, can be ablated with the CO_2 laser, dermabrasion, or cryosurgery. Disease involving most or all of a lip can be managed with a vermilionectomy and mucosal advancement, a procedure that also supplies the pathologist with a specimen to examine and evaluate for invasive disease.

Lesions of leukoplakia can become quite aggressive, and surgical excision with primary closure with dissolvable sutures is the optimal treatment for these lesions, as it allows the pathologist to evaluate the specimen for invasive disease.

Arsenical Keratoses

These hyperkeratotic papules and plaques are found on the palms and soles of individuals exposed to arsenic compounds therapeutically (Fowler's solution for asthma), in cotton farming (Paris green insecticide for boll weevils) and in industry (metal smelting). Histologically, they are similar to actinic keratoses. These lesions are often numerous in afflicted individuals.

Treatment

Conservative therapy or observation is indicated unless the lesion has undergone recent change or is symptomatic. Treatment is the same as for actinic keratoses, except that 5-fluorouracil is not very effective, possibly because of the thickness of the epidermis of the palms and soles. Patients with arsenical keratoses are at a slightly increased risk for visceral carcinoma, and this should be kept in mind when evaluating these patients.

Giant Condyloma of Buschke and Lowenstein

Genital warts that have persisted for a long time in the normal or immunosuppressed host can undergo malignant degeneration into a verrucous carcinoma.

Infection with certain papilloma viruses appears to be closely correlated with the development of cervical carcinoma in infected women; female sexual partners of males with genital condyloma should be examined closely. Conditions analogous to the Giant condyloma of Buschke and Lowenstein, epithelioma cuniculatum of the hands and feet, and oral florid papillomatosis, are rare disorders that are also locally destructive.

Primary treatment with cryosurgery, 6-hour applications of podophyllin resin in the nonpregnant patient, or conservative local electrofulguration can be used on primary lesions. Nonresponsive disease should be biopsied to rule out malignant degeneration.

Carbon dioxide laser vaporization has become an increasingly popular form of treatment for many types of warts; this modality should only be used by properly trained physicians in a facility with adequate ventilation, as recent studies have shown that potentially infectious viral DNA is found in the smoky plume of vaporized papillomas.

Radiation is absolutely contraindicated in treatment of these lesions, as it enhances their ability to metastasize.

Bowen's Disease

Bowen's disease is a squamous cell carcinoma in situ: the scaly, reddish brown plaques can track along sweat glands and hair follicles and escape destruction by superficial modalities of treatment.

Treatment

Optimal treatment approaches include Mohs' micrographic surgery, full-thickness excision including removal of all epidermal appendages in the area, and full-thickness destruction with cryosurgery using thermocouples to assure freezing of involved tissue. Bowen's disease of the glans penis, also known as erythroplasia of Queyrat, is best managed with Mohs' micrographic surgery, as it is the most tissue-conservative approach, but can also be managed with excisional surgery.

Cutaneous Horns

These hornlike, heaped-up mounds of dead stratum corneum frequently reveal warts, actinic keratoses, squamous carcinomas, or basal cell carcinomas at the base. Appropriate treatment is defined by the lesion found to be the cause of the horn. It is important when biopsying these lesions to obtain epidermis and dermis from beneath the horn; the horn itself frequently will not reveal a pathologic diagnosis. Therapy is that which is most appropriate for the underlying lesion.

Keratoacanthoma

This heaped-up, volcano-like keratotic lesion often contains a central core or plug. These lesions histologically appear to have squamous differentiation and frequently present with a rapid growth phase followed by persistence and later regression. The lesion is considered benign, but a squamous carcinoma can behave very similarly to a keratoacanthoma, and the diagnosis is best determined by a biopsy. If possible, the lesion should be removed totally at biopsy to allow evaluation of the cross-sectional architecture of the lesion and pathologic confirmation of the diagnosis. Some keratoacanthomas can grow to be quite massive and destructive, and occasional lesions have been reported to metastasize. Treatment is indicated to decrease the chance of rapid growth and destruction of nearby tissue and can be undertaken by excision, Mohs' surgery, cryosurgery, or local radiation therapy.

Melanocytic Lesions

Dysplastic Nevi

Nevi with asymmetric configuration, irregular borders ("Coast of Maine" appearance), multiple colors ranging from tan through dark brown to black, and frequently a diameter greater than 1 cm may be dysplastic. Dysplastic nevi are often hereditary but can occur sporadically, especially in individuals with a history of sun exposure resulting in a severe burn. These lesions also appear to arise after Psoralens and UVA light treatment, and in users of tanning salons who give a history of burning in the tanning salon. A controversy exists as to whether these lesions are precursors of melanoma or merely markers for the development of melanoma. In individuals with the hereditary form of the disease, the presence of these lesions increases the likelihood that they will develop a melanoma; in the individual with few lesions and no family history of melanoma, they are often an isolated phenomenon.

Treatment of dysplastic nevi consists of removal of large lesions, lesions that appear to have undergone recent change, lesions that have any associated symptomatology such as pruritus, stinging, or burning, and lesions that are emotionally distressing to the patient. Elliptical excision or deep saucerization shave biopsy to remove the whole lesion and allow pathologic assessment for the presence of melanoma is indicated. Patients with the dysplastic nevus syndrome should be watched closely and all blood relatives of the patient should be examined. Serial photographs of the patient can be used to follow individuals with large numbers of dysplastic nevi.

Congenital Melanocytic Nevi

Congenital pigmented nevi may be precursors of melanoma. The precise frequency of malignant degeneration is unknown but appears to increase dramatically with larger lesions (giant hairy nevus, bathing trunk nevus), and appears to be almost negligible in small lesions. Removal of the small lesions by surgical excision is generally easy to accomplish and can eliminate the small but definite risk of malignant degeneration. The larger lesions, which have a higher incidence of malignant degeneration, are more difficult to remove, but a greater effort should be made to remove them. Treatment of large or giant congenital melanocytic nevi can consist of staged excisions, excision and grafting, or excision after the insertion of tissue expanders that allow additional normal skin to be used for reconstruction, or any combination thereof.

Lentigo Maligna

Lentigo maligna is a malignant melanoma in situ that usually occurs as a dark brown to black hyperpigmented macule on the sun-exposed areas of elderly individuals. Lentigo maligna is an in-situ melanoma that is undergoing a lateral growth phase with no vertical growth. The ideal treatment is removal in toto of the lesion, so that the pathologist may examine the full specimen and rule out the presence of invasive malignant melanoma. If papules or nodules are present within a lesion that cannot be removed in toto, they should be biopsied. Conservative therapy, consisting of shave excision, cryosurgery, or topical 5-fluorouracil, is only indicated in elderly or extremely debilitated patients who cannot tolerate surgical excision.

Paget's Disease

Paget's Disease is an epidermotropic lesion that presents as a scaling, flesh-colored to reddish brown plaque on the nipple and areola or in the anogenital area in extramammary Paget's Disease. This lesion is always associated with an underlying carcinoma when involving the nipple and areola. For disease of the breast, a thorough evaluation of both the ipsilateral and contralateral breast is indicated; ipsilateral mastectomy is also indicated. For extramammary Paget's disease, excision or treatment by Mohs' micrographic surgery is indicated, if a primary underlying malignancy has been ruled out. If an underlying malignancy of the rectum or vagina is found, it should be treated accordingly.

Miscellaneous Conditions

Nevus Sebaceus

Nevus sebaceus is an epidermal nevus that occurs in less than 1 per cent of the population. It appears at birth as an orange-yellow macule or plaque, which can enlarge over time and develop a basal cell epithelioma within it. Treatment is excision of the nevus sebaceus if possible. If malignancy is found, Mohs' surgery is the treatment of choice.

Chronic Ulcers

A chronic ulcer, resulting from venous insufficiency, a burn, or other trauma, may ultimately develop a squamous carcinoma (Marjolin's ulcer). Lesions that remain unhealed for more than one year should be biopsied on a periodic basis to rule out the development of squamous carcinoma.

Large-plaque Parapsoriasis

This chronic, dermatitic inflammatory eruption may progress into frank mycosis fungoides. Treatment can include potent topical corticosteroids, photochemotherapy, and systemic chemotherapy. Extracorporeal photophoresis may eventually play a role in treatment of this disorder.

PREMALIGNANT MARKERS FOR INTERNAL MALIGNANCY

Leser-Trélat Sign. The sudden onset of a large number of seborrheic keratoses with or without inflammation is often a marker for underlying gastrointestinal malignancy. Treatment is that which is indicated for the underlying disease.

Erythema Gyratum Repens. This woody appearing polycyclic and annular scaling eruption is a marker for internal malignancy; treatment is that indicated for the underlying disease.

Skin Tags (Acrochordons). Fleshy pedunculated papules commonly found about the neck and in the axilla that increase in number with age and increasing weight, have recently been noted in association with colonic polyposis. The veracity of this observation is questionable.

PREVENTION

Most premalignant lesions of the skin are sun-induced, and avoidance of exposure to ultraviolet radiation from the sun will prevent many of these. Exposure to sunlight between 10:00 AM and 3:00 PM is most dangerous. It is important to encourage patients to share this knowledge with members of their family, who because of similar skin type may be predisposed to the development of similar lesions.

BACTERIAL DISEASES

method of
MICHAEL T. GOLDFARB, M.D., and
THOMAS F. ANDERSON, M.D.
University of Michigan Medical Center
Ann Arbor, Michigan

IMPETIGO

Impetigo is a common bacterial infection that is found most frequently in children; it is highly contagious. The disease presents as a thick, golden yellow crust on an erythematous base. The majority of the infections (90 per cent) are due to Group A, beta-hemolytic streptococci. Approximately 10 per cent will be coagulase-positive staphylococci, which are often the cause of clinical bullous lesions and are usually penicillin resistant. Culture and sensitivity studies can be reserved for cases that do not respond well to antibiotic therapy.

Treatment

Impetigo should be treated with systemic antibiotics in almost all cases. They offer a much higher cure rate than topical antibiotics (99 per cent vs. 39 per cent, respectively), leading to a much faster healing time, which prevents local spread.

Topical Therapy

Topical therapy still can be a helpful adjuvant for impetigo. The application of warm compresses to the area for 20 minutes 3 times daily is helpful in debriding the crust. Cleansing the area with an antiseptic antimicrobial agent, such as chlorhexidine (Hibiclens), can be useful in decreasing bacterial growth. Finally, bacitracin ointment can be applied topically after the crust has been removed.

Systemic Therapy

Erythromycin, 250 mg orally every 6 hours for a 10-day course, is an excellent first choice. It will cover all streptococci and most community-acquired staphylococci. For children, the proper dosage is 30 to 50 mg per kg per day in divided doses for 10 days. Penicillin VK, 250 mg orally every 6 hours for 10 days, and intramuscular benzathine penicillin (600,000 units in children under 6 years, 1.2 million units for those over 6 years) administered one time only are both effective for streptococcal infections. For bullous impetigo, because of the high possibility of its being a staphylococcal infection, a penicillinase-resistant penicillin such as dicloxacillin (Dynapen), 250 mg orally every 6 hours for 10 days, is effective. Children should receive 12.5 mg per kg per day in divided doses for 10 days. Resistant infections should be cultured and drug sensitivity studies performed to determine the appropriate antibiotics.

FOLLICULITIS

Folliculitis is a superficial bacterial infection usually caused by *Staphylococcus aureus*. Clinically, pustules at the follicular orifices are noted. The pathogenesis is usually plugging of the hair follicles. This may be due to poor personal hygiene, industrial greases, or occlusive cosmetics applied to the skin.

Treatment

Topical Therapy

Cleansing the area twice daily with an antiseptic antimicrobial agent such as chlorhexidine (Hibiclens) is effective in reducing the bacterial growth. Topical antibiotics such as erythromycin 2 per cent solution (T-Stat) or clindamycin 1 per cent solution (Cleocin T) applied twice daily may also be effective.

Systemic Therapy

Erythromycin or tetracycline, 250 mg orally every 6 hours, is effective in patients whose disease does not clear with topical therapy. Occasionally, a more broad-spectrum antibiotic, such as cephalexin (Keflex), 250 mg orally every 6 hours, is useful if all other therapy fails.

FURUNCLES, CARBUNCLES, AND ABSCESSES

A furuncle is a deep form of folliculitis, with inflammation that extends into the subcutaneous tissue. Bacterial isolates are almost always *Staphylococcus aureus*. If several furuncles coalesce, especially on the neck and upper back, it is known as a carbuncle. Suppuration may result in an abscess. Persistent and recurrent disease is known as recurrent furunculosis and is often seen in diabetics.

Treatment

Topical Therapy

Hot compresses applied 3 times daily may lead to resolution or spontaneous drainage of the furuncles and carbuncles. In patients with recurrent disease, bathing twice daily with an antiseptic, antimicrobial soap such as chlorhexidine (Hibiclens) is effective. The application of a topical antibiotic (bacitracin ointment) to the anterior nares is also helpful.

Surgical Therapy

For abscesses that do not undergo spontaneous drainage, surgical incision can rapidly induce resolution. If there are numerous subcutaneous sinus tracts, complete surgical excision may prevent frequent recurrences. Culture and sensitivity studies should be done along with surgical drainage.

Systemic Therapy

Systemic antibiotics should be used to speed resolution and prevent sepsis. Any antibiotic used must be very effective against *Staphylococcus aureus*. Dicloxacillin (Dynapen), 250 mg orally every 6 hours for 10 days, is an excellent first choice because it is a penicillinase-resistant penicillin. Cephalexin (Keflex), 250 mg to 500 mg orally every 6 hours for 10 days, is an effective alternative. For patients who are allergic to penicillin, erythromycin, 250 mg to 500 mg orally every 6 hours for 10 days, is effective against most community-acquired staphylococci. In patients who have evidence of systemic toxicity and sepsis, intravenous antibiotics must be considered. Nafcillin (Nafcil, Unipen), 500 mg intravenously every 4 hours, or cefazolin, 500 mg intravenously every 6 hours, is effective in serious infections. Patients with recurrent furunculosis may require low-dose systemic antibiotics such as erythromycin or tetracycline, 250 mg once to twice daily for up to 3 months, to help prevent further disease.

CELLULITIS

Cellulitis is a bacterial infection of the subcutaneous tissue and skin. It is usually a streptococcal infection, and clinically it appears as edematous, erythematous skin with an advancing border. It is warm and tender to palpation. Systemic signs of fever, lymphadenopathy, and lymphangitis are not uncommon. Trauma to the skin,

diabetes, or use of any immunosuppressant (corticosteroids, chemotherapy) can predispose the patient to cellulitis.

Children under the age of 4 years can develop a more violaceous cellulitis. This is usually secondary to *Haemophilus influenzae* infection.

Treatment

Topical Therapy

The involved area should be elevated if possible to promote drainage. Warm compresses should be applied at least three times daily.

Systemic Therapy

Culture and sensitivity studies may be done by injecting saline solution into the advancing erythematous edge and then aspirating. Gram stains can also be performed on this aspirate. Oral penicillin VK, 250 mg to 500 mg every 6 hours for 10 days, is effective in patients who do not have severe constitutional symptoms. Intravenous penicillin G, 200,000 to 250,000 units every 6 hours, is effective in the septic patient. Patients who are allergic to penicillin should receive erythromycin, 250 mg to 500 mg orally every 6 hours for 10 days. Children with *Haemophilus influenzae* infections commonly have an associated bacteremia, and intravenous therapy is often necessary. Chloramphenicol, 75 to 100 mg per kg per day, or ampicillin, 200 to 400 mg per kg per day administered intravenously in divided doses, is usually adequate.

ERYSIPELAS

Erysipelas is a superficial cellulitis most commonly on the face or legs. It is very erythematous and has sharply defined, indurated margins. The infection comes on rapidly, may be recurrent, and frequently is accompanied by fever. When the infection involves a wide area, death has been reported. The cause is a Group A, beta-hemolytic streptococcal infection. Chronic edema or lymphedema may predispose to this infection.

Treatment

Supportive Therapy

The patient should restrict activity and remain hydrated.

Systemic Therapy

Because streptococcal infection is the underlying cause, penicillin is the treatment of choice. Penicillin VK, 250 mg to 500 mg orally every 6 hours for 10 days, is adequate in patients with a limited area of disease who can maintain adequate hydration orally. Penicillin G, 200,000 to 250,000 units intravenously every 6 hours, is often necessary initially for the patient with severe systemic symptoms. Erythromycin, 250 mg to 500 mg orally every 6 hours for 10 days, is effective for the penicillin-allergic patient. Often patients will have frequent recurrent disease. Erythromycin, 250 mg to 500 mg daily, is often helpful for prophylaxis.

STAPHYLOCOCCAL SCALDED SKIN SYNDROME

The scalded skin syndrome is found almost exclusively in small children, infants, and adults with renal disease. It presents with erythema and flaccid bullae. The patient's skin becomes denuded very early, giving it a scalded appearance. The infecting organism is a Group II *Staphylococcus*, which is highly contagious and leads to epidemics in nurseries. The unique characteristic of the disease is due to bacteria producing exfoliatin, an enzyme that causes separation of the granular layer. The *Staphylococcus* is almost always penicillin resistant. The patients frequently have constitutional symptoms and, because of their young age, require hospitalization.

Treatment

Topical and Supportive Therapy

The patients are usually admitted for bed rest and intravenous hydration. The use of warm compresses may promote débridement of the desquamating skin.

Systemic Therapy

Skin, anterior nares, and nasopharyngeal cultures should be obtained prior to the institution of systemic antibiotic therapy. In patients who have constitutional symptoms, intravenous antibiotic therapy is recommended with a penicillinase-resistant penicillin. Nafcillin (Nafcil, Unipen), 25 mg per kg intravenously every 12 hours, is usually adequate. In very severe infections, nafcillin, 500 mg every 4 hours, may be used. An alternative is oxacillin (Prostaphlin), 10 to 20 mg per kg intravenously every 6 hours to as much as 500 mg every 4 hours. Once the patient is recovering, or in less serious infections, oral antibiotic therapy may be used. Dicloxacillin, 25 mg per kg per day in divided doses, or oxacillin, 25 mg per kg every 6 hours, are both reasonable choices. A minimum of 1 week of therapy is recommended. For the penicillin-allergic patient, erythromycin, 12.5 mg per kg orally every 6 hours, may be used.

ECTHYMA PYODERMA

Ecthyma is a superficial pyoderma that progresses into the dermis, leading to an ulcer with a necrotic eschar. Usually this is due to a persistent primary streptococcal or staphylococcal infection and is called ecthyma pyoderma.

Treatment

Topical Therapy

Warm compresses 3 to 4 times daily are helpful to remove the superficial crust.

Surgical Débridement

Surgical débridement of any necrotic tissue is helpful in allowing the ulcer to heal.

Antibiotic Therapy

Culture and sensitivity studies are recommended initially because these infections are usually longer standing, and it is best to know the underlying organism. If the infecting agent is streptococcal, penicillin VK, 250 to 500 mg orally every 6 hours, is effective. If it is staphylococcal, dicloxacillin, 250 to 500 mg every 6 hours, should be used. For the penicillin-allergic patient, erythromycin, 250 to 500 mg orally every 6 hours, should be used.

ECTHYMA GANGRENOSUM

In some cases ecthyma is due to gram-negative sepsis, usually caused by *Pseudomonas aeruginosa*. This is termed ecthyma gangrenosum and has a grave prognosis in most patients.

Treatment

Supportive Therapy

Because this infection is usually secondary to pseudomonal sepsis, these patients must be hospitalized. Intravenous fluids and hemodynamic monitoring care are essential. Careful evaluation for the underlying cause of the sepsis is necessary. Ultrasound, computed tomography (CT) scans, and gallium scans can be helpful in finding the primary infection.

Surgical Therapy

The involved skin must be débrided to help eradicate the infection.

Systemic Therapy

The ecthyma lesion must be cultured prior to the institution of any antibiotic therapy. However, combination antibiotic therapy against

Pseudomonas must be started immediately before any culture results are available. The combination of tobramycin (Nebcin), 80 mg intravenously every 8 hours, and ticarcillin (Ticar), 3 gm intravenously every 4 hours, is useful.

ERYTHRASMA

Erythrasma is a chronic, localized, superficial infection of the intertriginous area. It is reddish-brown and sharply marginated. The underlying bacterium, *Corynebacterium minutissimum*, produces a porphyrin that fluoresces coral-red under Wood's light (a useful diagnostic test).

Treatment

Topical Therapy

Topical 2 per cent erythromycin (T-Stat) applied twice daily for 14 days is very effective. The topical antifungal agents, clotrimazole 1 per cent cream (Lotrimin) and econazole nitrate 1 per cent cream (Spectazole), are also potent antibacterial agents and are effective when applied twice daily for 7 to 14 days. Keratolytic agents such as a 6 per cent salicylic acid gel (Keralyt Gel) are effective when used twice daily for 7 to 14 days.

Systemic Therapy

Erythromycin, 250 mg orally 4 times daily for 2 weeks, is an effective therapy.

TRICHOMYCOSIS AXILLARIS

Trichomycosis axillaris is characterized by yellow nodules upon the hair shafts of the axillary and pubic areas. The causative organism has been identified as *Corynebacterium tenuis*.

Treatment

Shaving the involved hairs and applying a topical antibiotic, erythromycin 2 per cent solution (T-Stat) or clindamycin 1 per cent solution (Cleocin T), on a twice-daily basis is effective.

ATYPICAL MYCOBACTERIA

Cutaneous atypical mycobacterial infection usually presents as ulcerated granulomas or nodules after inoculation progressing with lymphangiectatic spread. The most common causative organism is *Mycobacterium marinum*, which may be acquired in swimming pools or after cleaning tropical fish tanks. Cultures of the lesions should be performed on Löwenstein-Jensen media at 31°C.

Treatment

Many different therapeutic modalities have been tried, but none are universally accepted. Most lesions will heal spontaneously, but healing may take 2 to 3 years.

Surgical Therapy

If possible, small lesions may be cured by elliptical excision. Electrodessication and cryosurgery have been effective in some cases.

Systemic Therapy

Minocycline (Minocin), 100 mg orally twice daily for 8 weeks or longer, has been effective. Standard antituberculosis antimicrobial therapies are frequently ineffective, and drug sensitivity studies of the isolated organism should be done before these treatments are employed.

HERPES SIMPLEX AND HERPES ZOSTER

method of
PHOEBE RICH, M.D., and
CHERYL BERGER, M.D
The Oregon Health Sciences University

and

CLIFTON R. WHITE, JR., M.D.
The Portland VA Medical Center
Portland, Oregon

HERPES SIMPLEX

Herpes simplex virus (HSV) is one of the most ubiquitous of all viral infections in humans. Some estimates suggest that over 90 per cent of individuals are infected in the United States with HSV by age 15, and approximately 50 million new cases of genital herpes infections occur each year. HSV, a double-stranded DNA virus, consists of two antigenic types of herpesvirus hominis: HSV-1 and HSV-2. Typically, HSV-1 causes most orolabial and nongenital lesions, and HSV-2 causes genital disease. HSV characteristically becomes dormant in sensory nerve ganglia, usually after primary infection by direct mucocutaneous contact with a virus-shedding individual. Recurrent episodes, when the latent virus in the nerve ganglia is reactivated, are usually milder and of shorter duration than primary infections. A variety of stimuli can trigger recurrences including sunlight, stress, illness, and surgery.

TABLE 1. **Management of Herpes Simplex Infections**

Type of Herpes Infection	Symptomatic Care	Specific Treatment
Primary gingivostomatitis	Analgesics; viscous Xylocaine mouthwash	Oral acyclovir, 200 mg 5 times/day for 5–10 days
Recurrent oral-facial	Sunscreens (SPF 15 or opaque) may be useful in preventing recurrences	Oral acyclovir, 200 mg 5 times/day for 5 days
Primary genital herpes	Sitz baths; aluminum acetate (Burow's) soaks; analgesics; xylocaine ointment	1. IV acyclovir, 5 mg/kg q 8 hr for 5 days 2. Oral acyclovir, 200 mg 5 times/day for 5–10 days
Recurrent genital herpes	Analgesics; xylocaine ointment	1. Oral acyclovir, 200 mg 5 times/day for 5 days 2. Chronic suppression, for 6 or more attacks per year—oral acyclovir, 200 mg 3 times/day for up to 6 months
Herpes encephalitis		IV acyclovir, 10 mg/kg q 8 hr for 10 days; or IV vidarabine, 15 mg/kg/day for 10 days
Mucocutaneous herpes in immunocompromised host		1. IV acyclovir, 5 mg/kg q 8 hr for 7 days; or IV vidarabine, 10–15 mg/kg/day for 10 days 2. Oral acyclovir, 200 mg 5 times/day until lesions clear; then 400 mg 2 times/day for up to 6 months (continuous suppression)
Herpetic whitlow	Analgesics	1. Oral acyclovir, 200 mg 5 times/day for 5–10 days 2. Chronic suppression (prophylaxis)—oral acyclovir, 200 mg 3 times/day for up to 6 months
Herpes keratoconjunctivitis	Ophthalmologic consultation recommended	Topical trifluorothymidine 1%; or topical vidarabine 3% for 7–21 days
Neonatal herpes		IV vidarabine, 15–30 mg/kg/day for 10 days; or IV acyclovir, 5–10 mg/kg q 8 hr (or 250 mg/M^2 q 8 hr) for 10 days

Clinical Features

Orofacial Herpes

Primary orofacial herpes simplex is very common, occurring most often in children and adolescents, about 5 to 10 days after exposure. Patients present with fever, pharyngitis, and painful vesicles on the tongue, pharynx, and lips (gingivostomatitis), with mild to severe symptoms including adenopathy, fever, and systemic complaints.

Recurrent herpes labialis (cold sores, fever blisters) afflicts 30 per cent of the United States population, with outbreaks averaging 3 to 4 per year. A prodrome of itching or stinging at the vermilion border often heralds the impending outbreak of grouped vesicles on an erythematous base. The presence of neutralizing antibodies to HSV does not preclude recurrence.

Genital Herpes

Primary genital infections usually occur as the result of sexual exposure to a partner with active HSV lesions. The outbreak begins as small, grouped vesicles that may coalesce to involve a larger surface, often accompanied by constitutional symptoms. Viral shedding continues for 2 weeks, with total duration of disease approximately 3 weeks. Multiple anatomic sites may be affected (labia majora, labia minora, vagina, cervix; glans, prepuce, and shaft), and lesions are usually bilateral. HSV cervicitis occurs in greater than 75 per cent of women with primary genital herpes, whereas 10 to 15 per cent of patients with first-episode genital herpes will have ulcerative pharyngitis. Painful inguinal adenopathy is typical. About one third of patients with primary genital herpes have aseptic meningitis, with headache, stiff neck, and photophobia. Dysuria and urinary retention may be present.

Less severe symptoms and shorter duration of viral shedding characterize recurrent genital HSV infection, with lesions crusting in 5 days and healing in 10 days. A prodrome of tingling, burning, and dysethesia occurs in half of recurrent episodes.

Herpes Proctitis

HSV commonly causes rectal infections in homosexual males, presenting as grouped vesicles and erosions in the perianal region. Anal intercourse is the usual route of transmission. Therapy is the same as for genital herpes simplex infections.

Herpes Encephalitis

Herpes simplex encephalitis is the most common cause of fatal sporadic encephalitis in the world, occurring in 1.5 million people per year. Men and women are equally affected. One third of patients are under age 20, and 40 to 50 per cent are older than age 50. The disease begins in the temporal lobe and leads to hemorrhagic necrosis. Patients may have fever, headache, and altered mentation. Diagnosis must be made by brain biopsy. Mortality is greater than 70 per cent without antiviral therapy.

Herpetic Whitlow

Herpetic whitlow is a major occupational hazard in health care providers. It occurs as primary and recurrent HSV infection on the fingers and hands. The primary infection may last from 2 to 6 weeks and is characterized by painful, grouped vesicles, which may be associated with erythema and edema of the fingers as well as lymphangitis and axillary lymphadenopathy.

Herpetic Keratoconjunctivitis

HSV keratitis, regarded as the leading cause of infectious blindness in the United States, causes recurrent erosions of the conjunctivae and cornea leading to stromal keratitis. Early antiviral therapy can minimize stromal scarring. Ophthalmologic consultation is critical, so that slit-lamp examination, cytology and culture can be accomplished and appropriate therapy initiated.

Erythema Multiforme and Recurrent Herpes Simplex

Erythema multiforme (EM) may occur 7 to 10 days after recurrent herpes simplex infection, usually herpes labialis. EM presents with skin lesions, including macules, papules, bullae, and annular "target" lesions, which are symmetrically distributed on extremities, palms, soles, and sometimes oral mucosa. EM lasts from 1 to 4 weeks, typically occurs in young, healthy males, and probably represents a hypersensitivity reaction to the herpes virus antigen.

Eczema Herpeticum

In patients with widespread denuded cutaneous areas, such as in severe atopic dermatitis, disseminated HSV infection may occur. Apparently, damaged, dermatitic skin allows HSV infection to spread within the denuded area.

Neonatal Herpes Simplex

Primary neonatal HSV infection occurs in about 50 per cent of infants delivered to mothers with active genital herpes lesions. Early detection of HSV infection of skin or mucosa in neonates is essential, as up to 75 per cent of untreated patients develop dissemination with high morbidity and mortality. Infants with neonatal herpes infection may have characteristic facial-oral lesions, or the vesicles may occur at the site of fetal monitoring, such as the buttock or scalp, or elsewhere. Neonatal herpes infection may involve the central nervous system in the absence of skin lesions, presenting a life-threatening diagnostic challenge. When neonatal HSV is treated early with intravenous antiviral drugs, the prognosis is good in 90 per cent of infants.

Herpes Infection in the Immunocompromised Patient

HSV infection in patients who are immunosuppressed can lead to chronic, erosive, nonhealing deep ulcers of the facial and anogenital regions and can progress to herpes esophagitis and herpes pneumonitis. Immunocompromised patients may develop herpes viremia and herpes hepatitis. Systemic antiviral therapy can dramatically reduce morbidity in these patients.

Diagnosis

The standard for diagnosis of HSV is viral culture, with appropriate sample collection and transport. Early vesicles provide higher-yield positive cultures than crusted, almost-healed lesions. Viral identification may take 3 to 7 days and is relatively expensive. The Tzanck smear, a rapid and inexpensive technique for diagnosis of HSV, is obtained by scraping a freshly opened vesicle base and roof, smearing the cells on a slide, and staining it (Giemsa stain). The finding of multinucleated giant or ballooned keratinocytes is pathognomonic for herpes virus, although this does not distinguish HSV from varicella zoster virus. The clinical stage of the lesion affects the sensitivity of the Tzanck test: 70 per cent positivity in vesicles, 50 per cent in pustules, and low return in crusts. The specificity is high if the observer is experienced (i.e., less than 5 per cent false positive rate).

Differentiation of HSV-1 from HSV-2 can be made by a variety of serologic tests, including microneutralization and immunofluorescent (FA) techniques. Restriction endonuclease analysis, a technique that identifies viruses by their DNA composition, may become an important diagnostic tool in the future.

Treatment

Since its release 5 years ago, acyclovir (Zovirax) has dramatically altered the treatment of herpes infections. Acyclovir is an acyclic guanosine derivative that has antiviral properties only when phosphorylated within infected cells. Acyclovir triphosphate interferes with HSV DNA polymerase and inhibits viral DNA replication.

Acyclovir has an excellent safety profile. Because reversible elevations of serum creatinine have been documented, dosages of acyclovir must be decreased in patients with diminished creatinine clearance (<60 cc per minute). Other rare adverse reactions are nausea and vomiting and headaches. Local irritation and phlebitis at intravenous sites can occur. Because there are no adequate studies of acyclovir use in pregnant women and nursing mothers, the drug is best avoided in this group of patients at present.

Acyclovir is available for use topically, orally, and intravenously. Specific doses and therapeutic measures will be discussed for each clinical manifestation.

Orofacial Herpes

For primary herpetic gingivostomatitis, oral acyclovir is the treatment of choice (200 mg 5 times per day for 5 to 10 days). Xylocaine mouthwash may provide symptomatic relief, and analgesics are often necessary.

Similarly, the most effective therapy for recurrent facial oral herpes infection is oral acyclovir, 200 mg 5 times per day for 5 days. Although intermittent oral acyclovir therapy does not alter the frequency of recurrent mucocutaneous herpes, sunscreen protection may be helpful in preventing outbreaks. Topical acyclovir, 5 per cent in polyethylene glycol, does little to alter the clinical course of the infection; however, it may decrease the duration of viral shedding.

Genital Herpes

In extremely severe first-episode (primary or nonprimary) genital infections, characterized by prostration or urinary retention, or requiring hospitalization, intravenous acyclovir, 15 mg per kg per day (in three divided doses) for 5 days, should be administered. In less severe first-episode infections, oral acyclovir capsules, 200 mg 5 times daily for 5 to 10 days, are standard therapy. Oral acyclovir significantly reduces the duration of acute infection (viral shedding) and healing time. However, acyclovir use does not appear to alter the proportion of patients who develop recurrent disease or the frequency of recurrences. Symptomatic treatment with analgesics, sitz baths, and aluminum acetate (Burow's) wet-to-dry soaks may alleviate discomfort.

Therapy for recurrent genital herpes is oral acyclovir, 200 mg 5 times daily for 5 days, and is most effective when initiated early in the course of the outbreak. Often, patients may learn to recognize symptoms that warn of an impending recurrence, enabling them to begin therapy early. In patients who have 6 or more recurrent genital herpes episodes per year, chronic suppressive acyclovir therapy, 200 mg 3 times daily for up to 6 months, is frequently useful, with recurrences prevented in up to 75 per cent of patients. Periodically (every 6 months), a "drug holiday" is suggested to ascertain the continued need for therapy.

Herpes Encephalitis

The treatment of choice for herpes encephalitis is intravenous acyclovir, 30 mg per kg per day in 8 hour intervals for 10 days. In treated patients, the mortality rate remains high (20 per cent at 6 months and 30 per cent at 18 months) for biopsy-proven infections, although it is significantly lower than for untreated patients (>70 per cent mortality). Acyclovir appears to be more effective than vidarabine (Vira-A).

Herpes Infections in the Immunocompromised Patient

Intravenous acyclovir, 5 mg per kg every 8 hours for 7 days, or intravenous vidarabine, 10 to 15 mg per kg per day for 10 days, may be used in immunosuppressed patients. In addition, continuous acyclovir prophylaxis can significantly reduce morbidity. For example, 50 per cent of AIDS patients with frequent recurrent genital herpes infections who received acyclovir, 400 mg orally twice daily, had no recurrences. Similarly, prophylactic oral acyclovir (200 mg every 6 hours for 6 weeks) taken by non-Hodgkin's lymphoma patients during induction chemotherapy reduced the incidence of clinical HSV infection from 60 to 5 per cent.

Herpetic Whitlow

Therapy for herpetic whitlow includes oral acyclovir, 200 mg 5 times daily for 5 to 10 days. Chronic suppressive therapy with acyclovir, 200 mg 3 times daily (see genital herpes section), may be helpful in patients with frequent recurrences.

Herpes Keratoconjunctivitis

Therapy for herpes keratoconjunctivitis includes topical trifluorothymidine, 1 per cent, or topical vidarabine, 3 per cent, for 7 to 21 days. Ophthalmologic consultation is strongly recommended.

Erythema Multiforme and Recurrent Herpes Simplex

While therapy with topical steroids for EM is not effective, the value of systemic steroids has not been documented. Although acyclovir is of no benefit when administered after the herpetic recurrence, suppressive doses of acyclovir, 200 mg 3 to 5 times daily for 6 months, may prevent both herpes and erythema multiforme.

Eczema Herpeticum

Oral acyclovir, 200 mg 5 times daily for 5 days, or intravenous acyclovir, 500 mg 3 times per day for 5 days, is standard therapy for eczema herpeticum.

Neonatal Herpes

When neonatal HSV infection is treated early with intravenous antiviral drugs, prognosis is usually good. Vidarabine, 15 to 30 mg per kg per day, or acyclovir, 250 mg per M^2 every 8 hours or 5 to 10 mg per kg every 8 hours, for 10 days are of equal efficacy in halting the progression of the disease.

HERPES ZOSTER

Varicella-zoster virus (VZV) is another member of the herpesvirus group. Chickenpox (varicella), which is the result of primary infection with the virus, is usually acquired by airborne transmission of varicella respiratory secretions. Ninety per cent of cases of chickenpox occur in children between the ages of 1 and 14 years. Herpes zoster (HZ), or shingles, occurs when latent VZV in sensory ganglia is reactivated, causing the characteristic dermatomal eruption. HZ is seen in all age groups, but there is a direct association between increasing age and increased incidence.

Clinical Features

Ten to twenty per cent of the general population develop reactivation of latent VZV in spinal or cranial sensory ganglia in the form of HZ. Factors triggering reactivation are not well understood but appear to include local trauma, acute illness, and alterations in cell-mediated immune response mechanisms. Patients with lymphoproliferative malignancies who are receiving chemotherapy and/or radiation, and bone marrow recipients commonly develop HZ. However, HZ infection in an otherwise healthy individual does not represent necessarily a sign of increased risk of underlying malignancy. Persons infected with the human immunodeficiency virus (HIV) are also at increased risk for HZ; therefore, otherwise healthy individuals with HZ who are at high risk for the acquired immunodeficiency syndrome (AIDS) should be considered for HIV antibody testing.

Mild to severe radicular pain and hyperesthesia (sometimes mimicking myocardial infarction, cholecystitis, acute appendicitis, or deep vein thrombosis, depending on anatomic location) typically precede the cutaneous HZ exanthem by 1 to 7 days. Skin lesions consist of multiple, grouped vesicles, with surrounding erythema in a unilateral dermatomal distribution. The vesicles usually become pustular in 1 to 2 days, then crust, and may become necrotic and ulcerate. Healing, often with residual scarring, usually occurs within 2 to 3 weeks. The cutaneous lesions are often accompanied by regional lymphadenopathy, malaise, headache, and low-grade fever. Occasionally, two to three contiguous dermatomes are involved, and often there may be a dozen or fewer scattered individual vesicles present at distant skin sites. Neither of these occurrences represents, or is a harbinger of, generalized HZ.

Pain associated with *acute* HZ is the most common complication, seen in both immunocompetent and immunosuppressed hosts. In addition, with increasing patient age, there is a greater incidence (>50 per cent of patients 60 years and older) of the chronic pain syndrome called postherpetic neuralgia, characterized by pain persisting in the involved dermatome for more than 1 month following resolution of cutaneous disease. Fifty per cent of patients have resolution of their neuralgia within 2 months, whereas 70 to 80 per cent experience resolution within 1 year. Attempts to decrease the incidence of postherpetic neuralgia by the use of various modalities during acute HZ have had limited success. Oral corticosteroids taken early in the course of acute infection have shown the most promise.

Other, rarer complications of acute HZ include motor neuropathies, myelitis, encephalitis, ocular manifestations such as keratitis and optic neuritis, visceral involvement, and cutaneous dissemination. Immunosuppressed patients are at higher risk for generalized HZ, which presents 4 to 11 days after a typical HZ outbreak. Cutaneous dissemination and visceral involvement, with pneumonitis, esophagitis, and myocarditis, represent a viremic phase of the illness.

Diagnosis

The diagnosis of HZ can usually be made from the characteristic clinical presentation. Certain laboratory studies can be helpful in those cases with atypical findings, including the Tzanck smear (described in the section on diagnosis of HSV). The presence of rounded, ballooned, and multinucleated keratinocytes confirms infection with a herpes virus (VZV and/or HSV). Viral culture of fluid from a fresh vesicle can specifically identify the varicella-zoster virus (VZV). However, VZV expresses its cytopathic changes more slowly than does HSV (7 to 10 days vs. 1 to 3 days). Acute and convalescent complement fixation titers are occasionally employed, particularly in cases in which few lesions are present clinically. The clinical differential diagnosis of HZ is primarily zosteriform herpes simplex infection, usually distinguishable by viral culture or rapid immunologic detection techniques.

Treatment

Treatment options for HZ, long directed at acute complications and the prevention of postherpetic neuralgia, have been expanded recently by specific antiviral medications. Acyclovir, vidarabine, and leukocyte (alpha) interferon are all clinically effective, but the most experience has been gained with acyclovir. A number of other new antiviral drugs are also being investigated. Indications for the usage of antiviral drugs depend on the immune status of the affected patient, since this is the primary determinant of morbidity and mortality of HZ.

Immunocompetent Host

Cutaneous and visceral dissemination rarely occur in this population. Therapy, therefore, most often consists of local care, such as cleansing and wet-to-dry dressings (Burow's) 2 to 3 times daily to reduce oozing and prevention of secondary bacterial infection. Analgesics appropriate for the degree of pain should be employed. While the use of systemic corticosteroids during acute HZ in patients over age 50 (that is, those at increased risk for postherpetic neuralgia) remains controversial, most evidence suggests that oral corticosteroids taken early in the course of acute HZ can help prevent postherpetic neuralgia. We recommend oral prednisone (in all adult patients with no contraindication) as follows: 60 to 80 mg every morning with breakfast for 7 days, followed by 30 to 40 mg per day for 7 days. Use of corticosteroids in immunocompetent HZ patients does not seem to increase risk of dissemination.

Acyclovir (Zovirax) can effectively influence the course of HZ in normal individuals, but the benefits are not always dramatic. High-dose oral as well as intravenous acyclovir therapy reduces the rate of new lesion formation, decreases viral shedding, improves the rate of healing, and reduces acute pain. Studies to date do *not* demonstrate a reduction in the development of postherpetic neuralgia following either intravenous or oral acyclovir therapy. The dosage of acyclovir is higher for HZ than for HSV infection because of a 10-fold diminished sensitivity of VZV (compared to HSV) to acyclovir, as demonstrated by in vitro drug tests. Oral acyclovir appears to be as effective as intravenous therapy in immunocompetent individuals. The recommended oral dose is 400 to 800* mg every 4 hours, 5 times a day, for 7 to 10 days. Recent evidence suggests that the 800-mg dosage schedule is more effective. Adequate oral hydration (2 to 3 liters daily) is necessary during therapy because acyclovir is metabolized and excreted by the kidneys.

One group of immunocompetent patients who do appear to benefit from oral acyclovir are those with ophthalmic HZ. Treatment with 600 mg every 4 hours, 5 times a day, for 10 days will reduce the likelihood of ocular complications. However, early ophthalmologic evaluation of these patients is essential to reduce sequelae such as scarring and blindness.

Immunocompromised Host

Patients with impaired cellular immune response are at higher risk for serious complications, including dissemination, of HZ. An individual's degree of impaired immune function may be the best indicator of whether oral or intravenous antiviral therapy is necessary. Although controlled studies using oral acyclovir in various immunosuppressed populations have not been done, experience indicates that oral therapy can be effective in patients with less severe immune dysfunction, such as those with AIDS.

In immunosuppressed patients, intravenous acyclovir can decrease the rate of dissemination of virus to skin and visceral organs, decrease viral shedding, speed healing, and decrease acute pain. Intravenous vidarabine is somewhat less effective than acyclovir in effecting acute resolution but does appear to decrease the incidence of chronic pain. Therapy is most effective if instituted within the first several days of onset of infection.

The recommended dose of intravenous acyclovir is 500 mg per square meter, or 10 mg per kg, every 8 hours in 1-hour infusions for 7 days. Dosage should be adjusted for patients with impaired renal function because a reversible obstructive nephropathy can occur during intravenous therapy. Adequate hydration is again essential. The recommended dose of intravenous vidarabine is 10 mg per kg per day for 5 to 7 days.

---

*This dose exceeds the dosage recommended by the manufacturer.

PARASITIC DISEASES

method of
JERRY E. FOOTE, M.D.
Boone Hospital Center
Columbia, Missouri

SCABIES

Sarcoptes scabiei is the etiologic agent of human scabies. The organism completes its life cycle in the human stratum corneum and may persist indefinitely unless the patient, immediate family, and sexual contacts are treated. Actual sensitization to the mite or its fecal material may be required for the development of pruritus or erythema and may take several weeks to emerge. The patient, therefore, may not be aware of the infestation even though burrows are present on the skin. It is for this reason that asymptomatic, close contacts of the patient must be treated. Reinfection of the previously sensitized patient produces pruritus within hours after exposure.

Diagnosis is ideally made by demonstrating the mite in scrapings taken from the burrows containing the organism. Even without the positive scraping, however, a very strong presumptive diagnosis may be made when a patient presents with rather intense pruritus, noted to be worse at night and associated with the presence of burrows, papules, and vesicles in the characteristic locations. The last-mentioned include finger webs, flexor aspects of the wrists, extensor aspects of the elbow, anterior axillary lines, nipples, umbilicus, genitalia and lower buttocks. The lateral edge of the feet may also be involved. In addition, infants may reveal infestation of the scalp as well as the palms and soles. The lesions may vary from a very few to several hundred in neglected cases. Eczematization and excoriations with secondary bacterial infections are common secondary signs.

Scabies incognito is a condition of atypical scabies noted following the topical or systemic use of corticosteroids. The drugs partially suppress many of the secondary signs of the disease such as pruritus, scaling, and erythema.

Treatment

Treatment with scabicides is effective, and toxicity is rare if instructions are rigidly followed and reinfection is prevented. Prescriptions should not be refillable.

Lindane (Kwell, Gamene) lotion is applied to the total skin surface, from the neck to the feet. Particular attention should be given to sites of predilection noted above. The medication is left on for 24 hours (as little as 12 hours may be effective). After this period, wearing apparel and bedclothes should be changed. Reapplication after 5 to 7 days may be advisable to ensure that newly hatched nits are killed. I usually avoid using lindane in infants and pregnant women unless other agents are ineffective.

Crotamiton 10 per cent (Eurax) is applied in the same manner as lindane. Crotamiton has the added benefit of being an antipruritic. This drug should be applied for 2 consecutive nights and again in 7 days.

Precipitated sulfur, 10 per cent, in petrolatum is useful in infants and pregnant women. It should be applied for 3 consecutive nights.

Normal laundering with water at 120°F or cold water with hot iron pressing as well as dry cleaning are effective for treatment of bedclothes and wearing apparel.

Complications

Pruritis and eczematous dermatitis may last days to weeks after successful treatment of the infestation. Treatment should consist of topical steroid creams and oral antihistamines. In severe cases, a short course of oral prednisone is indicated. Secondary bacterial infection such as impetigo, ecthyma and cellulitis are more serious complications and must be treated with appropriate antibiotics.

Nodular Scabies. A small number of infested patients develop dark, erythematous nodules. These lesions may occur on the covered areas of the body, especially the groin, axillae, and genitalia. These lesions are free of mites after 1 month but are very pruritic and do not respond to scabicides. Topical treatment with cortisone cream, cortisone tape, or intralesional steroids may be needed.

PEDICULOSIS

Two species of lice are responsible for pediculosis in humans:

1. *Phthirus pubis,* the pubic louse or "crab" louse.

2. *Pediculus humanus* var. *capitis,* the head louse, and var. *corporis,* the body louse. These organisms require human blood for propagation and will die within a few days without feeding. Nits may remain viable for 30 days. They hatch and become adults within 2 to 3 weeks. The bite of a louse results in a red macule with a central hemorrhagic center. As with scabies, pruritus and inflammation are thought to be due to sensitization to the organism or its excretion.

Pediculosis Capitis

Pruritus of the scalp is the primary symptom. This condition is seen primarily in children. Close inspection will usually reveal nits attached to the hair shafts. These whitish objects are very firmly attached to the hair. Secondary signs such as excoriations, scaling, and bacterial infection may be noted as well as enlarged cervical lymph nodes. Identification of mobile adult lice can be made, but with more difficulty. Erythematous, macular, and sometimes papular lesions may be seen on the smooth skin surrounding the hairy areas; these are caused by the bite of the louse.

Treatment

This condition is highly contagious, and treatment should include all children* who are in close association with those infected.

Treatment is accomplished by applying lindane (Kwell, Gamene) shampoo for 4 to 5 minutes and rinsing thoroughly. Nits may be removed with a fine-toothed comb. The shampoo treatment is repeated in 1 week if viable nits are seen or new nits are noted at the scalp-hair junction. This would indicate new infection.

A pyrethrin compound (A-200 Pyrinate, RID)† is applied to the scalp until wet and left on for 10 minutes, followed by shampooing. A fine-toothed comb may be used to remove the nits.

Pediculosis Corporis

The body louse lives in the seams of clothing, not on the skin. Its favorite feeding sites are the shoulders, trunk, and buttocks. The bite results in a small red macule or papule, in the center of which develops a hemorrhagic point. Excoriation soon results in obliteration of these signs. Secondary bacterial infection is a common result. Nits or lice should be recovered from the clothing for diagnosis.

Treatment

Laundering or dry cleaning of clothing and bedding kills the louse. Also, airtight containment of clothing and bedding in plastic bags for 30 days will kill the organisms. Pruritus may be treated with topical corticosteroids and antihistamines after thorough cleansing of the skin with soap and water. If doubt exists as to the presence of viable organisms on the skin, topical treatment with lindane lotion, as described for scabies, may be used.

---

*Manufacturer's warning: Use with caution in infants and children. Has potential for central nervous system toxicity.

†Safety and efficacy in infants and children have not been established.

Pediculosis Pubis

The "crab" louse attacks not only the pubic area but also the eyebrows, eyelashes, axillae, and occasionally body hair. Pruritus and excoriation result in typical cutaneous signs and possible secondary bacterial infection. Maculae caeruleae, the lingering results of the louse bite, are blue-gray macules 5 to 10 ml in diameter.

Treatment

Lindane shampoo may be applied to the infected area for 4 to 5 minutes as for treatment of pediculosis corporis. Clothing and bedding should be laundered thoroughly or dry cleaned.

Eyelash Infection. Treatment includes yellow oxide of mercury ointment applied 3 times a day for 1 week, petrolatum applied in a thick layer 2 to 3 times a day for 7 to 8 days, and application of 0.025 per cent physostigmine ophthalmic ointment.

CREEPING ERUPTION (CUTANEOUS LARVA MIGRANS)

Penetration and subsequent migration in the skin by the larvae of the dog and cat hookworm (*Ancyclostoma braziliense*) results in creeping eruption. Other helminthic larvae are less common causes in the United States. Erythematous and serpiginous tunnels in the epidermis develop days after the larva penetrates the skin. Pruritus with excoriation results in eczematous changes and secondary bacterial infection. These lesions may spread for weeks to months; however, some lesions clear spontaneously after a few days or weeks. Larvae from the feces of the cat and dog penetrate the exposed skin of people when they are playing on beaches, playgrounds, and so forth. The condition is primarily seen in the warmer, southeastern areas of the United States.

Treatment

Thiabendazole suspension, 10 per cent (Mintezol) is applied 3 or 4 times a day until the activity has ceased. This will usually occur in ten to twelve days. Ethyl chloride or liquid nitrogen—induced sloughing of the areas can be used in cases with a limited number of lesions.

Oral thiabendazole (Mintezol), 10 mg per pound of body weight for patients up to 150 pounds or 1.5 grams for patients over 150 pounds may be given 2 times a day for 2 consecutive days. Familiarity with the toxic side effects of oral thiabendazole should be a prerequisite before prescribing this drug.

FUNGAL DISEASES

method of
MERVYN L. ELGART, M.D.
George Washington University
Washington, D.C.

DERMATOPHYTE INFECTION

Dermatophyte infections are caused by species of *Microsporum, Trichophyton,* and *Epidermophyton.* These organisms have the capacity to grow in keratin, both the soft keratin of the skin as well as the harder keratin of nails and hair. The organisms remain in the keratinized portion of the epidermis and seldom invade the living epidermis. The products of their growth, however, will diffuse down to the epidermis and elicit an immune response in normal individuals. We recognize that immune response as signs of inflammation: a scaling ring of increasing size and itching. Patients who are normally immunocompetent will respond readily to topical and systemic antifungal measures. On the other hand, in immunocompromised individuals, the body's own mechanisms fail to dispose of the organisms and much more aggressive topical or systemic therapy may be necessary.

Fungi proliferate readily in an environment of heat and moisture. Therefore, in many situations, keeping the area dry and cool is very helpful and by itself may be sufficient to diminish or resolve an infection. This is particularly important in the feet and the groin.

In some instances (i.e., tinea corporis, tinea cruris, and tinea pedis), the involved keratin is superficial and can be treated effectively with topical measures. On the other hand, where scalp hair or nails are involved, the infected material is not easily susceptible to topical attack and must be treated with systemic therapy.

Confirmation of a diagnosis of a dermatophyte infection should be made by use of a potassium hydroxide preparation. Epilated hairs or scale scraped from skin or nails may be examined in 10 to 20 per cent potassium hydroxide. Hyphae or, in the case of hair, spores can often be visualized to confirm the diagnosis. Interestingly, this confirmation can be done while the patient waits, and successful therapy can be predicted. Cultures will be useful in situations where the clinical picture is that of a dermatophyte infection, but attempts to demonstrate the organism by potassium hydroxide preparations have failed. The advantage of a culture is that it is easy to do. Media are available for office use and may be kept at room temperature. The problem, of course, is that it may take 7 to 21 days to obtain a positive culture. By that time the clinical situation may very well have changed. I find cultures much more useful in tinea capitis and onychomycosis than in other dermatophyte infections.

Topical Medications

Topical therapy for dermatophyte infections is generally accomplished with the imidazole compounds, including miconazole (Monistat-Derm), clotrimazole (Lotrimin, Mycelex), and, more recently, econazole (Spectazole). Ciclopirox olamine (Loprox) is another antifungal and anti-*Candida* topical medication that is somewhat different from the imidazole structure. These are the most effective topical products currently available and are also effective against *Candida* and the organism that causes tinea versicolor. Their reported efficacy in most situations has been in excess of 80 per cent, and in tinea corporis probably approaches 95 per cent. Older agents, such as tolnaftate (Tinactin) and haloprogin (Halotex) are effective agents but are somewhat less so than the imidazole compounds. Finally, undecylenic acid (Desenex) and combinations of salicylic acid and benzoic acid (Whitfield's ointment, Antitinea) may be used. The latter compounds work, not by inhibiting fungal growth, but by increasing the peeling of the skin. Dermatophytes live in keratin. Consequently, they must grow downward toward the living cell at a rate equal to or greater than the outward growth of keratin. Salicylic acid products attempt to remove the dermatophyte and the keratin at a rate faster than that at which the dermatophyte can grow down into the keratin. They should be used primarily in thick skin such as the palms and soles. All of these compounds are applied about twice a day in small amounts and must be rubbed in well.

Systemic Medications

Griseofulvin (Grifulvin, Fulvicin) is used in doses of approximately 10 mg per kg per day in children and 1 gram per day in adults. The solubility is poor, and grinding the particles down to a smaller size will increase absorption. Micronized griseofulvin (Grisactin, Grifulvin V, Fulvicin U/F) is such a product and is generally given at half the dose as the regular griseofulvin: 5 mg per kg in children and 500 mg per day in adults. The adult dose can be given on a once-a-day schedule. A third form of griseofulvin has the particles suspended in a polyethylene glycol matrix (Gris-PEG, Fulvicin P/G). This is available for adults in a dose of 330 mg, one capsule per day. In my own experience, the micronized griseofulvin seems to be the most consistently effective.

Griseofulvin is related to colchicine and in

laboratory animals has produced changes in spermatogenesis, but this effect has not been observed in humans. The only side effect in humans has been a slight drop (rarely below 4000) in the white blood count, but this is rarely clinically significant. Allergic reactions have been reported, and a few patients have had a photosensitivity reaction. The absorption of griseofulvin from the stomach is related to the presence of fat. The immediate absorption in the presence of a fatty meal produces higher blood levels, but the total 24-hour absorption seems unaffected by diet.

Ketoconazole (Nizoral) interferes with the formation of cellular walls and possibly also with cholesterol production in the liver. A few patients have had liver damage with long use, and instances of cirrhosis have been reported. Ketoconazole has been released for use in mucocutaneous candidiasis at a dose of 200 to 400 mg per day in adults. However, the drug has been reported effective in dermatophyte infections and tinea versicolor as well as some deep mycoses. Because of the toxicity, I do not use ketoconazole in onychomycosis and use it only rarely for other dermatophyte infections. Its success in candidal infections and in tinea versicolor can be dramatic.

Tinea Corporis

Tinea corporis is an infection of the glabrous skin by a dermatophyte. It often represents a situation in which an infection has begun at a point and spread in a centrifugal pattern so that an erythematous scaly ring with clearing in the center is produced. The scale, which is generally farther away from the center than the erythematous ring, contains hyphae, which can usually be demonstrated easily in the early stages of the infection. As the infection progresses in immunocompetent individuals, the erythema and edema become more obvious and often the infection may be stopped by the body's own immune processes. In these later stages, it may be difficult to demonstrate dermatophytes.

Tinea corporis almost always responds to topical imidazole compounds such as miconazole (Monistat-Derm), rubbed in twice a day for 2 to 4 weeks.

In immunocompromised hosts, a normal tinea corporis infection does not stop spontaneously but progresses to large, irregularly shaped, polycyclic infections with persisting scale. Often, there is less inflammation. In these individuals topical therapy with miconazole or clotrimazole (Lotrimin) is helpful, but generally the eruption is fairly widespread and it may be difficult to apply sufficient amounts of medication to cover the entire area of involvement. For that reason, mi-

cronized griseofulvin may be used in combination with topical preparations. Micronized griseofulvin, in a dose of 500 mg daily, plus one of the topical imidazole compounds such as miconazole applied twice daily, is generally effective within 30 days.

Tinea Cruris

Because the scrotum is an area of increased moisture, tinea cruris is primarily a disease of men. Curiously, the infection is almost always limited to the skin of the thighs and does not affect the scrotum itself. Treatment of tinea cruris consists of application of a topical imidazole. In addition, it is helpful to keep the area as dry as possible using compresses that dry the skin, such as Domeboro's solution 1:20 or even plain water for 10 to 15 minutes at a time. Following the compresses a topical antifungal agent can be applied. Clotrimazole (Lotrimin, Mycelex) is sometimes more useful because it is available as a liquid and is therefore less macerating for topical use. Only one antifungal agent, tolnaftate (Tinactin), is available as a powder. In very moist situations a hair dryer turned on low or no heat setting may be useful in drying the area. In immune-compromised individuals treatment with micronized griseofulvin may also be necessary, as with tinea corporis.

Tinea Pedis

Tinea pedis is an infection either between the toes in the webbed spaces or on the soles of the feet. Acute tinea pedis is a severely itching and inflammatory disease. Tinea pedis can easily become secondarily infected, first with gram-positive organisms requiring penicillinase-resistant penicillin (cloxacillin, dicloxacillin) for treatment. Gram-negative bacterial infections are more difficult to eradicate and may require intravenous use of antibiotics for appropriate gram-negative invaders. Secondary irritation by products used by the patient for his own care may play a role in this disease.

The treatment of tinea pedis involves primarily the elimination of moisture and heat. Compresses with water or Domeboro's solution are encouraged, because they help to dry the feet. The use of open shoes or removing the shoes frequently is helpful. The use of Tinactin powder may be helpful in eliminating the moisture: in addition, it is fungistatic. After completion of the soaks, topical treatment with one of the imidazole compounds is generally used. Miconazole nitrate or clotrimazole applied at least twice daily is generally effective. In the immune-compromised individual there is little erythema, but predominantly a chronic dry scaling of the soles of the feet. This is most common in patients with a history of atopy—e.g., asthma, hayfever, urticaria, or topic dermatitis. These individuals seem to have great difficulty in eliminating dermatophyte infections and often will present with bilateral scaly foot in a sandal distribution. This may be accompanied by tinea manuum, a similar scaly process involving generally one hand, but sometimes both, and by onychomycosis, a fungal infection of the nails. Fungal infections in these individuals are quite difficult to eliminate. Griseofulvin may be used and is sometimes helpful, but complete elimination of the infection is almost impossible and frequent repetitions of therapy are often necessary.

Tinea Incognita

"Tinea incognita" is a term for unrecognized fungal infections that are treated inadvertently with topical steroids. As a result of this treatment, inflammation improves but the fungal infection persists. Scrapings after the use of topical steroids are often heavily populated with fungi. The treatment may also cause fungi to invade hair follicles and produce fungal folliculitis (Majocchi's granuloma). For that reason, this infection rarely responds to topical antifungal preparations and generally requires griseofulvin.

Tinea Capitis

In the United States tinea capitis appears in two major clinical forms. With tinea capitis caused by *Microsporum* a discrete area of hair loss is noted. After invasion by the fungus, weakened hairs break off, leaving circumscribed areas of broken hairs. These areas of infection frequently will fluoresce under a Wood's light to produce a bright green color. *Microsporum* infections are becoming much less frequent. The most common cause of tinea capitis in my practice is *Trichophyton tonsurans,* which frequently produces a more diffuse infection resembling seborrheic dermatitis with minimal scaling and inflammation. The only clue is the presence of broken hairs within the infection. No fluorescence is present in *Trichophyton tonsurans* infections, so diagnosis must be made on the basis of hair examination or, more commonly, culture.

Because the invasion of the hair in tinea capitis takes place in the hair follicles below the level of the scalp, topical antifungal agents cannot eradicate the infection. They may, however, be helpful in preventing the spread of the infection because they immobilize and inhibit the growth of spores that are present in the hairs. Therefore, I frequently prescribe topical antifungal agents such as miconazole or clotrimazole in addition to the oral medications. Micronized griseofulvin is the drug of choice for these infections and must be given for at least one month. High doses (1000 mg in adults and proportionately less in children) are needed. Follow-up examinations with culture of the involved area are necessary to ensure that the infection has been stopped.

Tinea capitis may be caused by organisms that produce a swollen, tender, inflammatory area with pus at the surface. Gram staining fails to reveal organisms, and only fungal hyphae are present. This process, called a kerion, is most common with *Microsporum canis* but can be seen with any of the infections. In this instance, griseofulvin is still the treatment of choice. It is worthwhile to add prednisone (30 mg per day in adults and proportionately less in children) to suppress the inflammatory response, which may in some instances lead to permanent scarring of the scalp.

Tinea Barbae

Tinea barbae is frequently caused by organisms that are primarily involved with animal infections. *Trichophyton verrucosum* and the granular forms of *Trichophyton mentagrophytes* are the most frequent offenders. The disease presents as an inflammatory pustular process in the bearded area. The diagnosis is established by examining infected hairs and by culture. Once the diagnosis is established, the treatment is the same as for a kerion in the scalp.

Onychomycosis

Onychomycosis is an infection that first involves the soft underside of the nail, known as the hyponychium. The keratin here is softer than that of the nail itself and is the first to be invaded by dermatophytes. The infection then spreads to the nail plate itself, eventually destroying it. Particular care must be taken in establishing this diagnosis for two reasons. First, not every patient who presents with a destroyed nail plate has onychomycosis. Potassium hydroxide visualization of the organism and culture evidence are necessary to support such a diagnosis, since psoriasis, lichen planus, or trauma may produce a similar clinical picture. Furthermore, infections can be caused by nondermatophyte organisms such as *Scopulariopsis.* Although these infections will clinically resemble onychomycosis, they will not respond to the treatment outlined. Satisfactory treatment, therefore, is dependent on culture of the nail, which should be performed on media both with and without cycloheximide (Actidone), as some organisms that cause onychomycosis may be suppressed by this antibiotic.

For onychomycosis in which dermatophytes have been identified, griseofulvin may be used; I generally use the micronized form. Although the aforementioned dose was 500 mg per day in adults, I will usually prescribe 1000 or even 1500 mg per day, especially in chronic infections that are resistant. I generally treat only fungal infections of the fingernails, because toenail infections are so difficult and respond so poorly. One year of therapy with griseofulvin for toenail infections generally results in a cure rate of less than 25 per cent and a recurrence rate of about 95 per cent by the end of the following year. For these individuals, the continued use of griseofulvin is probably unreasonable. Instead, I prescribe ciclopirox olamine (Loprox cream). There is evidence that there may be some penetration of this compound through the nail plate. Although I have never observed complete resolution of such an infection, there is occasionally some improvement with minimal effort.

When only a single toenail or fingernail is involved, removal of that nail should be considered, as the newly formed nail may grow out more rapidly and produce a faster cure. However, the risks involved are such that I generally do not take this approach. Ketoconazole has been advocated by some for a chronic onychomycosis that has not resolved with griseofulvin therapy. However, because liver damage and toxic hepatitis have been reported, I do not use this drug for this indication.

CANDIDIASIS

Candida albicans causes a superficial infection that principally involves moist areas such as the groin. In these areas it produces the equivalent of an infected contact dermatitis so that biopsy studies of these infections will show vasodilation and a great deal of edema within the epidermis. In addition to the common yeast infections of the skin and nails, *Candida* can also be a more serious problem in immunocompromised individuals. In these, *Candida albicans* and especially *Candida tropicalis* may be involved. Oral or esophageal candidiasis may be the first finding in a patient who develops the systemic form of candidiasis. Some children with a variety of immune defects present with mucocutaneous candidiasis (i.e., progressive scaling and crusting dermatitis around the mouth and genitalia), indicative of infection on both the mucous membrane surfaces and the skin. The dry crusted nature of the eruption is markedly different from the usual candidal infection.

Candida is easy to demonstrate on culture, generally requiring 48 hours or less to grow. Speciation of the *Candida* organisms, however, requires biochemical testing. Potassium hydroxide preparations can be done, but they are somewhat more difficult to see: pseudohyphae, buds that have not completely separated, produce hyphae with pinched-in rather than straight walls.

Candida of the Groin

Candidal infection of the groin in children and adults characteristically produces bright red lesions with satellite lesions at some distance. In males the scrotum is generally involved and may be quite painful. In females a vaginal infection frequently accompanies the cutaneous problem. There may be considerable discomfort and some difficulty in walking.

All of the imidazole compounds mentioned under tinea corporis—e.g., miconazole, clotrimazole, econazole—can be useful when applied several times daily. Additional measures, however, are generally required. Often the patients are quite uncomfortable because of the amount of irritation present. In those individuals, compresses with Domeboro's solution 1:20 or plain tap water may be used for 10 or 15 minutes 2 or 3 times a day. After the compresses are removed the anticandidal preparation can be used. I often mix the anticandidal preparation with 1 per cent hydrocortisone cream for the first few days. This mixing can be done on the skin surface so that a little of the 1 per cent hydrocortisone cream is mixed with a little of the clotrimazole cream on the skin and rubbed into the still-damp compressed area. This helps to relieve the irritation somewhat more quickly and therefore makes the patient more comfortable. A commercial mixture (Lotrisone) consists of clotrimazole and betamethasone dipropionate (Diprosone). This cream is very effective but the steroid is one of the strongest known, and I am afraid to use this product for more than a day or two for fear of excess thinning of the skin and formation of striae. Mycolog is another product that contains an antiyeast product (Mycostatin) and a steroid (triamcinolone), as well as neomycin, bacitracin, and gramicidin. These last three agents are of no use in yeast infections, and only the Mycostatin and triamcinolone have much value. Indeed, the antibacterial agents sometimes cause contact dermatitis. Caution must accompany the use of Mycolog cream, as the mycostatin is suspended in the cream base by ethylenediamine. Ethylenediamine can cause severe contact dermatitis and must be discontinued in the face of a worsening rather than an improving situation. The ointment base does not contain ethylenediamine. A new form, Mycolog II, which contains only the triamcinolone and the Mycostatin, is now available. This is clearly a better product since it does not contain ethylenediamine.

It goes without saying that candidal infections are associated with heat and moisture. Keeping the area cool and perhaps drying with a hair dryer on low setting may be helpful. Dyes such as aqueous gentian violet may be used. Persistent infections may be associated with diabetes. In a woman, candidal infections of the vulva should alert one to the possibility of candidal infections of the vagina, since both must be treated to avoid recurrences.

Candidal Onychomycosis

Candidal onychomycosis is an infection that actually begins as a paronychia, with yeast organisms and bacteria invading the tissue spaces around the nail, the hyponychium, and finally the nail plate. This is in contrast to dermatophytic onychomycosis, in which the fungal infection generally begins at the tip of the nail. Candidal onychomycosis is most common on the fingernails and particularly in individuals whose occupations force them to keep their fingers moist for long periods of time. Topical treatment of candidal onychomycosis with imidazole compounds is generally unrewarding, as these compounds do not penetrate well into the tissue space around the nails. More often the most effective treatment is drying with colorless Castellani's paint, from which the dye (carbol-fuchsin) has been removed. The colorless Castellani's paint is available from the Lannett Company or may be made up from its ingredients (10 per cent resorcinol, 1 per cent boric acid, 4.5 per cent phenol, and 5 per cent acetone in alcohol).

Candidiasis may occur along the lips of people with overlying hanging upper lips or poorly fitted dentures. This is frequently seen in the elderly and can be mistaken for lesions due to vitamin deficiencies. Topical imidazole compounds are extremely helpful, and better-fitting dentures help to eliminate the chronic maceration found in those areas. A novel approach has been the injection of collagen (Zyderm) into those areas in an attempt to eliminate the macerated space.

Mucocutaneous candidiasis is generally treated with ketoconazole for several months. Lesions generally relapse when treatment is discontinued. This is the only FDA-approved use of ketoconazole. Other treatments for mucocutaneous candidiasis depend on the etiology and include iron supplements and appropriate thyroid hormones.

OTHER SUPERFICIAL FUNGAL INFECTIONS

Tinea Versicolor

Tinea versicolor is a superficial mycosis caused by a mold form of a *Pityrosporon* species, *Malassezia furfur*. The disease produces a very fine scale and a slight change in color, with lesions beginning around the hair follicles, spreading peripherally, and becoming confluent. The lesions may appear to change color in the summer as the skin darkens from tanning because the organisms interfere with the tanning response. Treatment of tinea versicolor is generally only temporary since the lesions seem to recur after several months.

All of the topical imidazole compounds are effective against tinea versicolor. This includes miconazole, clotrimazole, econazole, and ciclopirox olamine. In addition, tolnaftate and haloprogin (Halotex) have been effective. All of these products, however, must be applied to the lesions once or twice daily, and this may be mechanically difficult because these infections often are widespread. Nevertheless, if the infections are small, any of these preparations can be used once or twice daily with elimination of fungi within 1 to 2 weeks. The skin color takes weeks to months to return to normal. An easier approach for many patients is to use a 2.5 per cent shampoo of selenium sulfide (Selsun, Excel). The patient gets into the shower and gets wet; following that he or she lathers up with the shampoo on the affected areas, using a back brush to treat hard-to-reach areas on the back. The lather is left on for 5 minutes, and then the skin rinsed off. This can be repeated daily for 2 to 3 weeks, after which time the patient is usually mycologically negative and the scale has disappeared. The skin color will not return to normal for several more weeks. I often have my patients re-treat with Selsun once every month as a way of preventing the recurrence of lesions.

For very extensive cases or for failures from other topical therapies, ketoconazole has been useful. Patients take one tablet (200 mg) a day for 3 days, and the disease generally improves over the next several weeks.

Tinea Nigra Palmaris

Tinea nigra palmaris is a fungal infection of the palm that presents as a brownish macular area. It may be mistaken for a growing nevus but the potassium hydroxide preparation, which shows brown hyphae in the skin, is diagnostic. The disease is caused by *Exophiala wernecki*. The treatment of choice is superficial peeling of the growth of fungal organisms. Preparations of salicylic acid such as Whitfield's ointment or Antitinea usually work well when applied and rubbed in twice daily for 3 to 4 weeks.

Pitted Keratolysis

Pitted keratolysis is a disease of unknown origin that affects very moist sweaty feet. It produces small superficial pits, in which organisms are present. The exact nature of the organisms is unclear since they have not been grown but only seen microscopically. The original reports indicate that they are probably a form of *Corynebacterium*. Other work suggests that they may be a form of fungus *Dermatophilus congolensis*. In any event, simple drying preparations, such as colorless Castellani's paint, are generally helpful. The patient is encouraged to remove his or her shoes several times daily to allow the skin to air out.

Erythrasma

Erythrasma is a bacterial disease caused by *Corynebacterium minutissimum*. It is mentioned here because it is frequently confused with a fungal infection in that it appears in the axilla and groin and may mimic a dermatophyte infection. In the absence of a positive potassium hydroxide preparation, diagnosis is made by using an ultraviolet light. The characteristic coral-red fluorescence is diagnostic of erythrasma.

Because erythrasma is a bacterial disease, it responds to antibiotics. Systemic erythromycin has been recommended as the treatment of choice. Because the lesions are localized I find that the topical erythromycin products available for use in acne (A/T/S solution, Staticin, T-Stat, EryDerm) are effective when used twice daily for 3 weeks.

DISEASES OF THE MOUTH

method of
WILLIAM J. MORAN, D.M.D., M.D.
University of Chicago
Chicago, Illinois

LIP LESIONS

Cleft Lip and Palate

This congenital anomaly may vary from a small notching of the lip or hard palate to exten-

sive deformity of the lip, premaxilla, and palate. It may occur in isolation or in association with other anomalies. The frequency of occurrence is about 1 in 1000 births. A multidisciplinary team approach is necessary in caring for these children. Pediatricians, surgeons experienced in dealing with these defects, dental specialists, otologists, speech therapists, geneticists, and psychologists should work in concert in counseling the family and planning and carrying out treatment.

Cheilitis

Contact cheilitis is manifested by erythema and vesiculation of the lips. It is usually caused by sensitization to lipstick, lip balms, or food and is seen more often in women than in men. Treatment is elimination of the causative agent. Triamcinolone acetonide (Aristocort) ointment is helpful.

Angular cheilitis refers to a condition in which painful fissures develop at the corners of the mouth. This is found most commonly in children and the elderly. It is thought to be related to lip sucking, edentulism, or ill-fitting dentures. Saliva bathes the fissures, producing maceration. Candidiasis may be present. Treatment with an ointment containing nystatin (Mycostatin) is helpful, along with elimination of the causative factors.

In solar cheilitis, keratinization with areas of erosion develops on the lower lip and is due to excessive exposure to the elements, especially the actinic rays of the sun. It occurs more commonly in fair-skinned individuals. Treatment consists of excision with either the CO_2 laser or standard lip shave technique. Patients should avoid sun exposure and use a sun-screen lip balm. Because the lesion may progress to carcinoma, patients must be followed carefully, and any suspicious lesion should be biopsied to rule out carcinoma.

Cheilitis glandularis apostematosa is a condition in which the mucous glands of the lip become inflamed, enlarged, and nodular. The ductal ostia appear as small red papules on the lip, and mucus may seep from these inflamed orifices. Exposure to the elements or other irritants such as tobacco seems to be the cause. Treatment consists of eliminating irritants such as tobacco, careful cleansing of the lips, and use of a sun-screen lip balm. CO_2 laser vaporization of affected areas or lip shaving may be helpful.

Mucous Retention Cyst

Mucous retention cysts usually occur in the lower labial mucosa. They are due to trauma to mucous glands with or without secondary infection, which produces ductal obstruction and results in an expanding collection of mucoid material within the tissues. Treatment is unroofing or excision; incision or aspiration usually results in recurrence.

GINGIVAL AND PERIODONTAL LESIONS

Simple Gingivitis

Inflammation of the gingival tissues surrounding the teeth is known as simple gingivitis. The inflammation is manifested by redness and swelling and is due to irritation from bacterial plaque and calculus, which build up as a result of poor oral hygiene. Treatment should consist of dental referral for complete removal of plaque and calculus, along with patient education regarding oral hygiene.

Acute Necrotizing Ulcerative Gingivitis

Intense erythema and edema of the gingiva with necrosis of the interdental papillae are the hallmarks of acute necrotizing ulcerative gingivitis (ANUG). The patient may have considerable pain, fever, and cervical lymphadenopathy. A mixed fusiform/spirochete etiology has long been proposed; more recently, viral infection and secondary bacterial infection are suspected. Treatment consists of fluids, analgesics, rest, and gentle oral rinses and débridement. Antibiotic therapy may be added.

Desquamative Gingivitis (Gingivosis)

Gingivosis is characterized by vesiculation and desquamation of the gingiva. It occurs most frequently in middle-aged women. The etiology is not known. It may be a manifestation of various disorders such as bullous pemphigoid and pemphigus vulgaris. A biopsy should be obtained for histologic as well as direct immunofluorescent examination. A topical steroid such as fluocinonide (Lidex) gel, 0.05 per cent applied six times a day, may be helpful.

Gingival Enlargement

Generalized gingival enlargement and inflammation that occurs during puberty and pregnancy may arise in response to hormonal changes. A presumed hereditary generalized enlargement known as hereditary gingival fibromatosis may occur at the time of tooth eruption; the gingiva may become quite large and fibrotic. Treatment consists of gingivoplasty and maintenance of excellent hygiene to retard regrowth. A similar type of enlargement that occurs in individuals on phenytoin (Dilantin) therapy may require gingivoplasty if enlargement results in trauma during mastication. Rarely, generalized gingival enlargement is caused by leukemic infiltration. Focal gingival enlargement may be inflammatory or neoplastic in origin; pyogenic granuloma and fibroma are frequently encountered examples. Biopsy, in an excisional manner when possible, is indicated for diagnosis and is often therapeutic.

Eruption Cyst

An eruption cyst is a bluish, translucent, dome-shaped lesion overlying the crown of an erupting tooth. It may be incised to relieve pressure and discomfort. A topical anesthetic ointment may also be of help, especially in young children.

Pericoronitis

In pericoronitis, inflammation surrounds the crown of a partially erupted tooth, due to trapping of plaque and debris beneath a flap of soft tissue overying the crown. Treatment consists of removal of plaque and debris from under the soft-tissue flap and maintenance of good oral hygiene. Antibiotic therapy should be instituted. Occasionally, removal of the overlying soft-tissue flap or tooth extraction is necessary to prevent recurrent infection. Deep space abscess may complicate pericoronitis.

Dental Sinus

A sinus tract may be found in the gingiva. It usually extends from an apical periodontal infection. A panoramic or periapical radiograph may reveal a periapical radiolucency. Dental referral should be made for evaluation and treatment.

TONGUE LESIONS

Median Rhomboid Glossitis

Median rhomboid glossitis is characterized by an irregularly shaped, smooth red patch located on the mid-dorsum of the tongue; it is usually slightly depressed. Histologically one sees stratified squamous epithelium with absence of lingual papillae. This condition may be developmental or perhaps related to chronic low-grade candidiasis. It is usually asymptomatic, but if symptoms are present an antifungal agent may be tried. If symptoms persist, surgical excision is indicated.

Benign Migratory Glossitis

As its name implies, this is a harmless condition characterized by migratory, smooth red patches on the tongue. It is rare and of unknown etiology, although associated occasionally with psoriasis or Reiter's disease. Although this disorder is often asymptomatic, a burning discomfort may occur; this is generally mild and self-limiting. A mild hydrogen peroxide mouth rinse and bland diet may help.

Fissured Tongue

This congenital anomaly may be an isolated finding or associated with Down's, Melkersson-Rosenthal, or Sjögren's syndromes. The tongue is deeply fissured, predisposing to food-trapping, inflammation, and infection. Good oral hygiene, including brushing the tongue with a soft toothbrush and a mild hydrogen peroxide oral rinse after meals and at bedtime, is the only treatment required.

Macroglossia

Enlargement of the tongue may be due to a variety of conditions, including neoplasms, developmental anomalies such as hemangioma and lymphangioma, and metabolic derangements such as amyloidosis. Infection, angioedema, and superior vena cava syndrome may also produce tongue enlargement.

Black Hairy Tongue

In this condition, the filiform papillae of the tongue undergo hyperplasia and elongation and become discolored because of overgrowth of pigment-producing oral flora. The etiology is unknown, although it is associated with prolonged antibiotic therapy; chronic irritation also may play a role. Treatment includes brushing of the tongue with a soft toothbrush and using a mild hydrogen peroxide mouthwash. Use of tobacco and other oral irritants should be avoided. Extremely elongated papillae may be snipped with scissors.

WHITE MUCOSAL LESIONS

Candidiasis (Thrush)

Candida albicans produces infection mainly in immunosuppressed patients. Patients receiving steroid or prolonged antibiotic therapy are also at risk. White, cheesy patches on the mucosa can be wiped off, leaving an eroded and bleeding surface. Treatment includes determining and correction of underlying factors and the use of antifungal agents such as nystatin (Mycostatin) (solution or oral tablets). Ketoconazole (Nizoral) appears to be more effective for cases of *Candida* laryngitis or esophagitis related to radiotherapy.

Nicotinic Stomatitis

The lesions of nicotinic stomatitis occur on the palate and appear to be related to smoking, especially pipe smoking. The palatal mucosa is thickened and gray-white in color, with multiple small red dots that are the inflamed ostia of minor salivary gland ducts. Histologically, hyperkeratosis and inflammation with mild dysplasia are seen. The lesion usually regresses slowly upon cessation of smoking and is not considered premalignant. Atypical lesions should be biopsied.

Oral Burns

Any caustic agent may injure the oral epithelium, leaving a sloughing white membrane; placement of an aspirin in the oral vestibule to relieve toothache is perhaps the most well-known example of this. Healing is usually uneventful and treatment is symptomatic.

Lichen Planus

Lichen planus can affect the mouth or skin, or both. The typical appearance in the mouth is a white reticular network on the buccal mucosa; however, there are many variations, including annular patterns and erosive and bullous lesions. Histologic confirmation is often required. Associated skin lesions most commonly occur on the flexor aspects of the wrists and lower legs bilaterally. Painful lesions may be palliated with topical or intralesional steroids. Fluocinonide (Lidex) gel, 0.05 per cent, may be applied 6 times daily. Triamcinolone acetonide (Aristocort), 5 mg per ml, may be injected 0.1 ml per square cm using a 30-gauge needle. In more severe cases, oral prednisone in daily doses of 40 to 60 mg may be given for 14 days and then tapered over a week. The etiology is unknown.

Leukoedema

This is a variation of normal seen mostly in blacks. The buccal mucosa appears opalescent white. There are no inflammation or symptoms. Histologically, the epithelium is thickened with edema of the spinous layer; dysplasia is absent.

Leukoplakia

Leukoplakia literally means "white patch." The term usually refers to a keratotic plaque that may be premalignant or malignant. If examination suggests an obvious etiology such as infection or trauma from dentition, every effort should be made to resolve these. If the lesion regresses after 2 to 4 weeks, it may be followed up. All other lesions should be examined histologically. Any lesion demonstrating erosion or induration should be considered to be carcinoma until proven otherwise.

Papilloma

Papillomas of the oral cavity, caused by the human papilloma virus, are most frequently seen on the palate, uvula, tongue, and lips. The typical appearance is warty and keratotic. Excisional biopsy is diagnostic and therapeutic.

Squamous Carcinoma

Squamous carcinoma is the most common carcinoma of the upper aerodigestive tract. It may present as a white keratotic lesion or as a red, ulcerated lesion. The most important etiology is heavy tobacco use, including "smokeless" tobacco (snuff); heavy alcohol use seems to have a synergistic effect. A positive family history even in the absence of tobacco use appears to increase risk. While the typical patient is traditionally described as male and in the sixth decade, more women and younger patients are being diagnosed, probably because of changing social habits. Early stage (I and II) carcinomas have a good to fair prognosis. Treatment consists of wide excision or radiotherapy. Advanced stage (III and IV) carcinomas have a poor prognosis (overall 30 per cent 5-year survival) but vary by site. Advanced lesions are usually treated with combination therapy consisting of surgery and radiotherapy, with or without chemotherapy. A multidisciplinary team, including surgical, radiation, and medical oncologists, speech and swallowing therapists, and dental specialists, is required to care for patients with advanced stage lesions.

RED AND PIGMENTED MUCOSAL LESIONS

Denture Stomatitis

Poor oral hygiene in the denture wearer can lead to inflammation beneath the denture, and secondary candidiasis may occur. The mucosa beneath the denture is red and painful. This mucositis occurs most often in the maxilla and corresponds exactly to the area beneath the denture. Treatment consists of thorough daily cleansing of the denture and removal of the denture at night. If secondary candidiasis is present, nystatin (Mycostatin) or ketoconazole (Nizoral) should be prescribed.

Hemangioma

Hemangiomas appear to be hamartomas and may vary greatly in size and resultant deformity. Most congenital lesions regress during childhood; small lesions may be completely excised. Large, deforming lesions that infiltrate structures (e.g., the tongue) can be debulked using CO_2 laser therapy.

Hereditary Hemorrhagic Telangiectasia

This condition has an autosomal dominant pattern of inheritance. Multiple, small telangiectasias may affect the oral cavity, pharynx, and/or nose, producing recurrent bleeding. Cryotherapy, laser therapy, and steroid therapy have been used for treatment.

Amalgam Tattoo

This is an exogenous pigmentation produced when silver amalgam filling material becomes implanted in soft tissue during dental restoration procedures. The tattoo is blue-black in color and asymptomatic. Its nature may be confirmed by a radiograph, revealing radiopaque metallic flecks. If confirmed radiographically further treatment is unnecessary; otherwise, excisional biopsy is indicated. The differential diagnosis includes pigmented nevus and malignant melanoma.

Pigmented Nevus

Benign pigmented nevi of all types may occur in the oral cavity. This includes lentigos and junctional, compound and blue nevi. Except for the blue nevus, they are generally brown in color. They may be raised or flat and are relatively unchanging. These lesions should be excised to exclude the possibility of melanoma. A radiograph may be obtained to exclude amalgam tattoo.

EROSIVE, ULCERATIVE, AND VESICULOBULLOUS LESIONS

Recurrent Aphthous Stomatitis

This condition consists of recurring, painful ulcerations that can occur on any area of the oral mucosa except the gingiva and anterior hard palate. The shallow ulcerations may be single or multiple and can range from less than 2 mm to greater than 10 mm in size. They have a yellowish-gray pseudomembranous base and are surrounded by an erythematous halo. There may be associated fever and lymphadenopathy. The lesions are self-limiting and usually resolve in 7 to 14 days.

The etiology of this condition is unknown. It occurs mainly in adults, more commonly in women than in men.

Only symptomatic treatment is possible. Avoidance of spicy, acidic, and salty foods as well as sharp, hard foods such as crackers promotes comfort. A mixture of diphenhydramine (Benadryl) elixir and Kaopectate in equal parts used as a mouth rinse 6 times a day may be helpful. Tetracycline, 250 mg in 30 ml of water, used as a mouth rinse and then swallowed 4 times a day has been of benefit in some patients.

Behçet's Syndrome

Behçet's syndrome is composed of the triad of recurrent oropharyngeal ulcerations, genital ulcerations, and uveitis. Other manifestations include gastrointestinal lesions, vasculitis, synovitis, and neurologic abnormalities. Patients are generally in their second or third decade, and men are affected more often than women. Treatment consists of symptomatic measures and systemic steroids. Cyclophosphamide (Cytoxan) and other cytotoxic drugs have also been used.

Herpetic Stomatitis

Herpetic stomatitis is due to infection of the oral mucosa with herpes simplex virus, either type 1 or type 2. Primary herpetic stomatitis generally occurs in the pediatric age group, although it may also occur in adults. Vesicular lesions may involve the entire oral mucosa; these then rupture, producing painful ulcerations. Patients usually suffer from fever, lymphadenopathy, malaise, and headache. They may be unable to swallow, with resultant drooling and dehydration. Treatment includes analgesics and antipyretics. Parenteral fluids may be necessary. The course usually lasts from 7 to 14 days.

In secondary herpetic stomatitis, recurring lesions most often involve the lips, hard palate, and attached gingiva. Factors that may precipitate these lesions include upper respiratory infection, trauma, and psychologic stress. Healing usually occurs in 7 to 10 days.

Erythema Multiforme

Erythema multiforme is a disease of the skin and mucous membranes and occurs in two forms.

The minor form lasts 2 to 3 weeks; the major form, known as Stevens-Johnson syndrome, may last up to 6 weeks. The disease occurs in young adults and appears to be more common in men. The etiology is unknown, but precipitating factors include infections, such as herpes simplex and mycoplasma, and drugs, especially sulfonamides. The lesions begin as vesicles or bullae and then slough, leaving large, painful ulcerations with whitish pseudomembranous bases. The lips, buccal mucosa, and tongue are the most frequently involved sites in the oral cavity. In Stevens-Johnson syndrome, there is severe skin, oral, conjunctival, and genital involvement. When oral lesions are the only manifestation, establishing the diagnosis is difficult. Differentiation from bullous pemphigoid and pemphigus vulgaris may require biopsy. Severe lesions may be treated with prednisone, 40 to 60 mg, daily for several weeks.

Herpangina

Herpangina is an infection of the oropharynx caused by Coxsackie virus (groups A and B) and encountered in children. Small vesicles are seen on the soft palate, uvula, and tonsillar pillars symmetrically. They quickly rupture, leaving small painful ulcerations. Fever, lymphadenopathy, headache, and malaise are associated. This disease is distinctive enough to allow clinical diagnosis. Treatment is symptomatic, and healing occurs rapidly.

Pemphigus and Pemphigoid

Pemphigus and pemphigoid appear to be autoimmune diseases and present as oral bullae of varying size that slough, leaving painful ulcerations with a whitish pseudomembranous base. The buccal mucosa, palate, and gingiva are most frequently involved. Patients are usually in the fifth and sixth decades. An important differentiating feature is that pemphigus also affects the skin. However, the oral lesions may precede the skin lesions by years. Conjunctival lesions may occur in pemphigoid. The histologic appearance of the bullae is similar in both disorders; however, in pemphigus, round desquamated epithelial cells (Tzanck cells) may be seen within bullae. Immunofluorescent examination reveals IgG antibodies to intercellular substance in pemphigus, whereas IgG is seen within the basement membrane in pemphigoid.

Systemic steroids are used to treat both diseases. In pemphigus high doses are often necessary and patients may develop steroid complications. Cyclophosphamide (Cytoxan) has been added in severe cases in order to reduce steroid levels. Steroids are not always effective in pemphigoid, and dapsone has been used with some success. Ophthalmologic examination should be done to rule out ocular involvement in pemphigoid.

OTHER LESIONS

Tori

Tori are benign hyperostoses that occur in the midline of the hard palate (torus palatinus) or lingual aspect of the mandible (torus mandibularis). They generally require no treatment.

Fordyce Spots

Fordyce spots are small, discrete, light-yellow papules found in the buccal and labial mucosa of approximately 80 per cent of the general population. They are ectopic sebaceous glands and require no treatment other than patient reassurance.

Orolingual Paresthesia

Orolingual paresthesia most often affects the tongue (glossodynia), but other oral mucosal surfaces may be affected. It is usually encountered in older women. Patients complain of a burning discomfort, yet the mucosa appears normal. Possible causes of this symptom include vitamin deficiency, anemia, referred pain from dental or periodontal disease, and mild candidiasis. It may also be a manifestation of stress. Often no cause can be pinpointed. Treatment includes reassurance, along with counseling regarding good oral hygiene and nutrition. Dental evaluation may be helpful if the patient does not receive regular dental care. Any mucosal changes should be biopsied.

Xerostomia

Xerostomia, or dry mouth, is a bothersome symptom and often causes halitosis. It may have many causes. Virtually all patients who have had radiotherapy to the head and neck have some degree of xerostomia. Systemic illnesses including lymphoproliferative disorders (Mikulicz's disease, Sjögren's syndrome), rheumatoid arthritis, lupus erythematosus, scleroderma, and sarcoid may involve the salivary glands and cause xerostomia. Exogenous substances such as anticholinergics, antihypertensives, antihistamines, and antimotion drugs frequently produce xerostomia. Finally, xerostomia may be related to stress or

may be idiopathic. If a patient has a history of radiotherapy or is on a drug that causes xerostomia, symptomatic relief may be obtained by frequent intake of fluids and use of artificial saliva such as Xerolube. Otherwise, systemic causes should be ruled out. Dental referral should be made, because patients with xerostomia may have an increased incidence of caries and require good oral hygiene and regular dental follow-up.

VENOUS ULCERS AND OTHER CUTANEOUS ULCERATIONS

method of
VINCENT FALANGA, M.D.
University of Miami
Miami, Florida

Ulceration of the lower extremities is a serious clinical problem that has become more common in our ever-increasing elderly population. Table 1 lists many of the causes of chronic leg ulcers by their basic pathophysiologic mechanism.

Clinical Features

When examining the affected extremity, one should note any general abnormality. Dependent rubor, xerosis, and hair loss suggest arterial insufficiency, whereas muscle atrophy and signs of trauma to bony prominences may indicate a neuropathy. The presence of Raynaud's phenomenon suggests systemic sclerosis or other connective tissue diseases. Hyperpigmentation is extremely common in limbs affected by venous disease. The shape of the leg is also important. Thus, while patients with venous disease have an abnormally smaller diameter of the ankle with respect to the calf because of tissue fibrosis, those with lymphedema have a rather characteristic "tubular" appearance of the leg, with little difference in diameters of these two sites.

The location of the ulcer provides important clues to the etiology. Thus, venous ulcers are most common on the medial aspect of the leg, whereas those that are caused by arterial insufficiency tend to occur on the lateral aspect of the leg or over the malleoli. The malleoli are also common sites for neuropathic ulcers, as are the toes and the plantar surfaces. The configuration of the ulcer provides other important clues. Usually, venous ulcers are irregular in appearance, whereas arterial insufficiency or hypersensitivity angiitis leads to well-delineated, "punched out" ulcerations. Pyoderma gangrenosum, in addition to undermined purple edges, may have a cribriform appearance, with strands of re-epithelialization on the ulcer surface. In examining any ulcer, one should note the depth, the presence of exposed tendons or bone, and the extent and quality of granulation tissue. Protuberances or exuberant tissue at the edge or within the ulcer should make one suspect the presence of neopla-

TABLE 1. **Classification of Leg Ulcers**

Vascular	Pressure Necrosis
Venous disease	Diabetes mellitus
Atherosclerosis	Neuropathies
Cholesterol emboli	**Physical Agents**
Hemoglobinopathies	Factitial
Lupus anticoagulant	Heat
Inflammation	Frostbite
Chronic idiopathic	Radiation
hypersensitivity angiitis	**Tumors**
Periarteritis nodosa	Primary skin tumors
Wegener's granulomatosis	Lymphomas
Erythema elevatum	Metastases
diutinum	
Panniculitis	**Infection**
Dysproteinemias	Bacterial
Pyoderma gangrenosum	Fungal
Necrobiosis lipoidica	Mycobacterial
diabeticorum	Tertiary syphilis

sia. Bacterial colonization, evident by sight and odor, may alter the management of the ulcer. The surrounding skin is examined for the presence of erythema, warmth, pitting edema, tenderness, and induration. Contact dermatitis may be noted, in addition to the possibility of cellulitis and the presence of dermatosclerosis. The latter refers to the indurated skin, most commonly observed on the medial aspect of the leg, that is associated with venous disease.

Vascular Ulcers

Venous Ulcers

Regardless of the presence of adequate arterial pulses, Doppler flow studies should be done to exclude significant arterial disease. This has become especially important in our elderly population, where combined venous and arterial disease is present in about 20 per cent of the cases. Compression stockings are not indicated in patients with venous disease if the arterial blood flow is borderline (ankle/brachial blood pressure ratio less than 0.8). A small biopsy of the edge of the ulcer is helpful for a definitive diagnosis of venous ulceration. In typical venous disease, one can demonstrate dermal pericapillary fibrin on direct immunofluorescence examination. This finding, in the absence of other immunoreactants, appears to be specific for venous disease.

Atherosclerosis

Patients who have significant arterial disease should be evaluated as soon as possible for possible vascular reconstruction. Cholesterol emboli may occur in patients with advanced atherosclerosis and may present as a leg ulcer in about 17 per cent of the cases. Patients with cholesterol embolization frequently have fever, myalgias, sudden hypertension, high erythrocyte sedimentation rate, peripheral blood eosinophilia, and

renal disease. Vascular procedures and the use of anticoagulants are risk factors for cholesterol embolization. The most frequent cutaneous lesion in patients with cholesterol emboli is livedo reticularis. A skin biopsy has a high diagnostic yield and shows cholesterol clefts in occluded dermal or subcutaneous arterioles.

Hemoglobinopathies

Diseases affecting the morphology of red blood cells, particularly sickle cell anemia and hereditary spherocytosis, may lead to ulceration of the lower extremities. This is probably due to damage to the venous circulation, since the affected limb usually shows all the clinical signs of venous disease.

Lupus Anticoagulant

It has recently been recognized that a circulating antibody, termed lupus anticoagulant, may be responsible for some cases of vascular thrombosis. This abnormality is not restricted to patients with lupus erythematosus and, paradoxically, the presence of a lupus anticoagulant does not lead to hemorrhage but rather to thrombosis. Its presence is suggested by an abnormal partial thromboplastin time (PTT) and a false-positive serologic test for syphilis. It is thought that the antibody, usually IgG, is directed against phospholipids also present in blood vessels. One should strongly suspect the presence of a lupus anticoagulant when the biopsy specimen of the edge of an ulcer shows thrombosis without any significant degree of inflammation. The lupus anticoagulant may be a cause of recurrent thrombotic episodes and spontaneous abortion.

Ulcers Due to Inflammation

Vasculitis

Vasculitis is an uncommon cause of ulcers of the lower extremities but can lead to indolent and difficult to treat ulcerations. The local treatment of ulcerations due to vasculitis is the same as with ulcers of other etiologies. Specifically, the use of topical antibiotics and occlusive dressings may speed up the healing. In most cases of vasculitis, systemic corticosteroids (e.g., prednisone, 40 to 60 mg per day) are effective in controlling the inflammatory process. Occasionally, systemic corticosteroids alone are not adequate and other immunosuppressive agents have to be added. Biopsy of the edge of the ulcer should extend well beyond the margins of the ulceration so as not to miss the diagnostic changes of vasculitis. It is important to include adequate amounts of fat in the biopsy specimen, since, as in periarteritis nodosa, subcutaneous blood vessels may be the only ones affected.

Pyoderma Gangrenosum

The typical appearance of pyoderma gangrenosum is of a rapidly enlarging ulcer with undermined borders and purple edges. It is associated with rheumatoid arthritis, ulcerative colitis, multiple myeloma, leukemia, Behçet's disease, or IgA monoclonal gammopathy. In many cases it is idiopathic. When the diagnosis of pyoderma gangrenosum is made, fungal or mycobacterial infection must be excluded. The initial lesions of pyoderma gangrenosum may be pustules that quickly ulcerate and enlarge. At the pustular stage, intralesional injections of corticosteroids may be helpful. At times, however, the ulcers may be quite extensive, often involving the subcutaneous tissue and tendons. Systemic corticosteroids are the treatment of choice, and usually doses of 60 to 80 mg of prednisone a day are given. In some cases, this treatment has to be supplemented by the use of immunosuppressive agents. Sulfones have been worthwhile in some cases. One of the most effective treatments is the use of pulse therapy with systemic corticosteroids, in which 1 gram of methylprednisolone is given intravenously daily for 3 to 5 consecutive days. Care must be taken so that electrolyte imbalances do not occur with these large doses of systemic corticosteroids. Pyoderma gangrenosum may respond nicely to the use of hyperbaric oxygen. The combined use of hyperbaric oxygen and systemic corticosteroids may be worthwhile in particularly extensive cases of pyoderma gangrenosum.

Necrobiosis Lipoidica Diabeticorum

This is associated with diabetes mellitus. It has a yellow to orange hue, and is usually confined to the tibial surfaces. When it ulcerates, the use of intralesional corticosteroids in the edges is helpful.

Pressure Necrosis

Most ulcers in patients with diabetes mellitus are due to pressure, although there may also be significant arterial insufficiency. Avoidance of pressure is most important in the management of these ulcers, and this frequently needs repeated emphasis by the physician. Various splints can be devised to shift the pressure away from the ulcers. The same types of ulcers may be seen with other neuropathies.

Ulcers Due to Physical Agents

The agents listed in Table 1 can all lead to extensive leg ulcers. Factitial ulceration is suggested by the presence of geometrically shaped ulcers in atypical places. Many of these patients have severe emotional disturbances, and their treatment is most challenging. It is best to confront patients with the possibility that the ulcer is factitial. The use of an Unna boot to prevent patients from manipulating the ulcer may be helpful diagnostically and therapeutically.

Tumors

In the management of any ulceration, care must be taken to diagnose squamous cell carcinoma or basal cell carcinoma arising from the ulcer bed or from its edge. On occasion, primary skin tumors of the lower extremities ulcerate; this is more commonly seen with squamous cell carcinomas.

Infection

Primary bacterial infections do not usually give rise to chronic leg ulcers. However, fungal and mycobacterial organisms can be a cause of nonhealing ulcers. When these organisms are suspected, biopsy specimens of the edge as well as the bed of the ulcer should be taken, and the specimens sent for histologic studies and appropriate cultures.

General Treatment

Nutritional Aspects

It is uncommon for patients to develop clinically significant vitamin deficiencies. However, ascorbic acid deficiency may develop quickly in elderly individuals, and ascorbic acid (250 mg twice a day) may be helpful. Zinc has been advocated as promoting healing, but one should be cautious with its use because it can interfere with the inflammatory response that is necessary for healing.

Contact Dermatitis

Ulcers of the lower extremities are frequently complicated by the presence of contact dermatitis, either irritant or allergic. This is most common in patients with venous ulcers. Patch testing should ideally be done in all cases of chronic leg ulceration, even in the absence of dermatitis. The results may provide a guide to future therapy with topical agents. Throughout the course of treatment, it is important to minimize the use of topical agents. Patch testing may need to be repeated throughout the course of treatment if the question of contact sensitivity again arises. Severe contact dermatitis is best treated with systemic corticosteroids (prednisone, 40 mg per day) rather than the use of additional topical agents.

Infection

Leg ulcers are commonly contaminated by a variety of organisms, including anaerobic bacteria. When the wound contains considerable amounts of exudate, it becomes difficult to distinguish colonization or superinfection from cellulitis. Fever, new onset of tissue tenderness or warmth, and an elevation of the erythrocyte sedimentation rate are clues to the presence of a cellulitis. Cellulitis should be treated promptly with appropriate systemic antibiotics, but colonization or superinfection of the ulcer bed generally responds to débridement and antimicrobial soaks. Occlusive therapy should not be used in the presence of cellulitis.

Stimulation of Granulation Tissue

Benzoyl Peroxide. In a concentration of no less than 10 per cent lotion, this is used to impregnate a gauze that is left within the ulcer for 12 hours at a time. Normal skin and the edge of the ulcer are protected with petrolatum from the irritant action of benzoyl peroxide.

Tretinoin. There is now considerable rationale for the use of topical tretinoin (Retin-A) in patients on systemic corticosteroids. It tends to counterbalance the stabilizing effect of corticosteroids on lysosomal membranes and, therefore, increases the inflammatory response. Preferably, it should be applied in the lotion form to the bed of the ulcer every night. It is particularly helpful when the granulation tissue is poor in patients on systemic corticosteroids. The use of this agent in patients not on systemic corticosteroids has not been effective.

Unna Boot. This is a form of occlusive therapy and has been used extensively in patients with venous ulcers. The boot should be wrapped around the ulcer in the morning, before the development of significant edema. With the patient supine, the dressing is applied by placing progressively more pressure from the foot to the calf. The Unna boot is changed on a weekly basis. It facilitates ambulatory treatment, since it places no responsibility on the patient for dressing the ulcer. It is also quite helpful in patients who have a factitial component to their ulcerations, since it prevents obvious manipulation of the ulcer. It is probably inadvisable to use an Unna boot in patients with considerable dermatitis because it tends to make the dermatitis worse.

Occlusive Dressings. A variety of synthetic occlusive dressings are now available for the treatment of ulcerations. When applied to chronic

TABLE 2. **Synthetic Occlusive Dressings**

Materials	Trade Name	Adhesiveness
Hydrocolloid	Duoderm	+
	Comfeel Ulcus	+
Polyurethane	Op-Site	+
	Tegaderm	+
	Synthaderm	−
	Bioclusive	+
Polyethylene	Vigilon	−

ulcers, these dressings *relieve pain, cause débridement*, and *stimulate granulation tissue formation*. Since many of these agents are associated with an impressive exudative phase during the first few days of therapy, patients must be warned of this or they will discontinue treatment. A foul-smelling exudate may also develop under these dressings, erroneously suggesting an infection to those not experienced in their use. Thus, considerable teaching is necessary when initiating therapy with occlusive dressings. In choosing a particular occlusive dressing, oxygen permeability is generally not an important variable. Adhesive dressings are generally preferred because they facilitate the ambulatory treatment of patients with chronic ulcerations. However, in elderly individuals with very fragile skin, nonadhesive dressings may be preferred because they cause less trauma to the skin surrounding the ulceration. Occlusive dressings should not be removed until the underlying exudate causes the dressing to be uplifted and to drain at the edges. Untimely removal may cause injury to the re-epithelializing wound. Table 2 lists some of the most common occlusive dressings presently available. One should not use occlusive dressings when cellulitis is present.

Re-epithelialization

The approaches outlined thus far are likely to cause healing of most ulcers. When healing does not occur or is slow in spite of good granulation tissue formation, grafting should be done.

Pinch Grafting. This is an extremely easy way of transplanting tissue to a granulating wound and can be done in the out-patient setting. Grafts are usually taken from the abdomen. The donor site is anesthetized with 2 per cent Xylocaine without epinephrine, and small 2- to 4-mm grafts are taken from the anesthetized area using forceps and a scalpel. Care must be taken to use grafts that are thin and do not include subcutaneous tissue. Larger grafts are less likely to survive. A No. 30 needle may be used to lift up the donor skin, making it easier to cut these small grafts with a scalpel. The grafts are applied dermal side down to the granulating wound and kept in place with gauze that has been impregnated with a topical antibiotic. The leg is dressed with a bulky dressing so as to prevent any dislodgement of the grafts. The dressing is removed after no more than 48 hours. Taking of the grafts is usually evident by their skin-colored appearance, whereas dark grafts are usually necrotic.

Split Thickness Grafts. A keratome is used on a donor site, usually the lateral aspect of the thigh. Again, the donor site is anesthetized with 2 per cent Xylocaine without epinephrine, and the keratome is used to slice a donor graft. The graft is then cut into squares the size of postage stamps, and these are applied dermal side down to the ulceration. Not all of the surface of the ulcer needs to be covered with grafts. Dressing of the grafted ulcer is the same as with pinch grafting.

DECUBITUS ULCERS

method of
LAWRENCE CHARLES PARISH, M.D.,
Jefferson Medical College of Thomas Jefferson University

and

JOSEPH A. WITKOWSKI, M.D.
University of Pennsylvania School of Medicine Philadelphia, Pennsylvania

Decubitus ulcers, known also as pressure ulcers and bed sores, are a poorly understood affliction of the skin, skin structure, and adjacent tissue. The defect in the tissue results from a lack of nutrients or accumulation of toxic products, thus impairing cellular metabolism. How this comes about is not clear. Ostensibly, there has been sufficient pressure to occlude the blood and lymph flow for a long enough period to result in cell necrosis. Metabolic changes, decreased oxygen supply, edema, skin damage, and blood vessel disease are all contributing factors.

Three types of patients may develop decubitus ulcers: (1) the healthy person who is suddenly paralyzed from an accident; (2) the chronic neurologic patient who is otherwise healthy save for the deterioration of the nervous system; and (3) the older patient whose other body systems may be just as debilitated as his skin.

The panorama of the various stages of the decubitus ulcer ranges from minimal redness to destructive ulceration (Figure 1). The process begins with blanchable erythema, in which redness is apparent on the area in question. This may progress to nonblanchable erythema, in which the redness does not disappear on touching. The third stage is that of decubitus dermatitis, in which there may also be scaling and vesicles or bullae. Next, a superficial ulcer may be apparent, with necrosis of the epidermis and dermis. This may worsen into a deep ulcer, with destruction extending into the fat layer and even to the underlying bone.

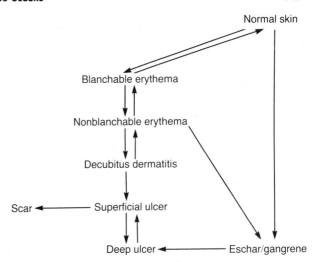

Figure 1. The decubitus ulcer pathway.

Finally, there is the eschar/gangrene stage, in which the tissue is dead but coagulation necrosis holds it intact.

Complications include the development of bacterial infection. This may lead to associated osteomyelitis, septicemia, and even death. Anemia; loss of fluid, electrolytes, and protein; renal disease; amyloidosis; and psychologic effects are other complications.

Prevention

Some ulcers can be prevented by keeping the skin intact and reducing pressure. This can be accomplished by not injuring the skin with abrasive or irritating medicaments such as Merthiolate or Betadine. Pressure may be reduced by utilizing a total support system such as an air-fluidized bed, low airloss bed, or water bed. Although turning the patient would seem helpful, there is no evidence that every patient is the same or that the order for turning every two hours has merit. The duration that pressure can be tolerated may be less than two hours. The patient should be rotated to varying positions as often as is practical. There is no foolproof, safe way to prevent all ulcers.

Treatment

An understanding of the panorama of the decubitus ulcer and of the pathophysiology involved is necessary for selecting rational treatment. All too often the patient is subjected to well meaning regimens that may actually be injurious. Heat lamps aggravate an already inflamed situation. Sugar and egg white may promote bacterial and fungal growth. Some alleged panaceas contain contactants that can create acute dermatitis.

Blanchable Erythema

This represents an early form of dermatitis and can be treated as such. Lidex gel will act as an anti-inflammatory agent; Lassar's paste will mollify the irritated tissue. Both are applied 2 to 3 times a day. An occlusive dressing such as Duoderm, changed Monday, Wednesday, and Friday, will allow epithelial cells to recover and to protect the skin.

Nonblanchable Erythema

The treatment is the same as for blanchable erythema.

Decubitus Dermatitis

The therapy may be the same as for erythema. Sometimes an astringent compress of Burow's solution 1:40 every 8 hours will dry the vesicles or bullae.

Superficial Ulcer

Superficial ulcers need to be cleansed and débrided. If the area is infected, Burow's 1:40 or Betadine may be used in compresses for 20 minutes every 8 hours or as wet-to-dry dressings may be applied every 8 hours. If the area has significant drainage or moisture, dextranomer isomer (Debrisan) or copolymer starch may be used every 8 hours. After the ulcer is clinically clean, a hydrocolloid or polyurethane dressing is used to cover the ulcer. This is changed if the wound fluid leaks or the dressing is displaced; this can occur anytime from 1 to 7 days after cleansing.

Deep Ulcer

The treatment is the same as for superficial ulcers. In deep and undermined ulcers, iodoform gauze packings may be required, but usually destranomer isomer or copolymer starch can be recommended.

Eschar/Gangrene

Although an enzymatic agent would seem ideal for treatment of eschar/gangrene, no effective one is currently marketed that will débride the hard or soggy eschar. Sometimes a wet-to-dry dressing will be helpful; at other times, the use of 5-fluorouracil (Efudex) 5% cream twice daily to the margins of normal skin, sometimes with occlusion, will assist in débridement.

Special Management

Surgery

Surgical débridement of devitalized tissue is recommended when the patient is stable and when surgery can be done. In some institutions, this is done in the operating room and at others, at bedside. More aggressive intervention depends upon the condition of the patient. In a young healthy patient, rotation flaps may expedite healing and a return to a more normal existence. In the older patient whose healing capabilities are diminished, such plastic procedures can constitute cruel and inhuman punishment. In general, each patient has to be considered individually.

Antimicrobial Therapy

Many, if not most, decubitus ulcers are infected with one or more bacteria. Such organisms as *Staphylococcus aureus, Escherichia coli, Proteus mirabilis, Klebsiella pneumoniae,* and *Pseudomonas aeruginosa* may be pathogenic in the ulcer.

Making the diagnosis of an infected decubitus ulcer may require an experienced clinician. The organisms can be cultured by swab, but quantitative analysis is usually not available. Most organisms that are grown are considered to be pathogenic in the ulcer. This can be shown in retrospect, when they have been eliminated by antimicrobial therapy and the ulcer has improved. Similarly, when the ulcer no longer shows any signs of infection and the organism remains, it may then be considered a colonizer.

An infected ulcer may show purulent discharge with odor, necrosis, surrounding induration, and redness. Many decubitus ulcer patients have impaired neurologic activity so that pain and tenderness may not be elicited. Similarly, in such compromised patients, high temperatures, elevated white counts, or increased numbers of polymorphonuclear leukocytes may not be present. These patients may have a normal temperature of 96°F, so that a temperature of 99°F may be a serious fever. Some of this may be confirmed by the use of the Merieux multitest, whereby a lack of any response to the 7 antigens at 48 hours indicates immunologic depression.

In our experience, topical antimicrobial therapy has not been helpful, probably because so much of the tissue is devitalized and the antimicrobial agent lies inertly on the surface of the skin. Systemic use of third-generation cephalosporins such as ceftazidime (Fortaz) or cefataxime (Claforan), 1 gram every 8 hours intravenously, or a new quinolone such as ciprofloxacin (Cipro), 750 mg every 12 hours, is recommended to begin therapy. When cultures and sensitivities are available more specific antimicrobial therapy may then be instituted.

Management of Osteomyelitis

It is not surprising that the underlying tissue and bone can become infected. The diagnosis can be made by a flat plate and possibly a bone scan. A biopsy of the bone may be necessary to yield the offending organism.

Treatment may involve surgical scraping of the

bone and parenteral antibiotics for at least a month. Initiation of therapy is dependent upon the prognosis of the patient. Many times therapy is just not useful and the clinician must judge on an individual basis whether prolonged hospitalization and antimicrobial therapy are worthwhile.

Special Devices

The use of a pressure support system is recommended in ideal situations. Unfortunately, the benefits cannot always be documented. We believe that such beds are useful and use them when it is possible to do so. Whirlpools and other physical modalities may have merit, but we are unaware of any studies confirming their effectiveness.

ATOPIC DERMATITIS

method of
BERNICE R. KRAFCHIK, M.B., Ch.B., F.R.C.P.(C)
University of Toronto
Toronto, Ontario

Since the description of the clinical stages of atopic dermatitis (AD) by Sulzberger and Wise in the 1930s, attempts have been made to understand its cause and pathogenesis. We are no further ahead in delineating these aspects of AD (although strong hereditary patterns are evident), but we have compounded the issues by finding a number of immunologic and cellular defects. In addition, the role of diet in the pathogenesis of the disease is still poorly understood. AD is a disease that has a tendency to improve with time; therefore, treatment is aimed at control of the lesions and comfort of the patient while the disease follows its natural course.

Treatment

General Measures

One of the most important aspects of management is explaining to the parents and patients the course of the disease. Patients are often disappointed because a complete cure is impossible. Therefore, on the first visit, discussion about expectations is essential. Exacerbations are to be expected and their causes, which include fevers, abrupt changes in climate, dryness in the winter months, and sweating from heat in the summer, should be emphasized.

The skin of AD patients is dry. In view of this, a controversy exists regarding the number of baths that patients should take, as water may be both hydrating and dehydrating to the skin. Adding bath oil to the water and patting skin dry and immediately applying an emollient to the normal skin are hydrating. Bathing daily in lukewarm water is preferred. Many brands of bath oil are available that contain cleansing agents, eliminating the need for soap. Mineral oil, although cheap, does not emulsify with the water and is therefore not acceptable. If a soap is used, Lowila or white Dove is recommended. Colloidal oatmeal has been known for years to be soothing to the skin and may be used alone or in addition to bath oil. At times, oatmeal will cause irritation and erythema, in which case its use should be discontinued. Bubble baths should never be used.

Petrolatum and Eucerin are both emollients that are inexpensive, safe (nonsensitizing), and effective; however, they are rather messy and should be reserved for the dry winter months. In summer, with heat and humidity, greasy emollients have the disadvantage of producing a folliculitis; therefore, at this time less oily products such as Keri lotion, Complex 15, or Nivea may be substituted. An emollient or barrier cream applied around the mouth prior to eating can be very helpful in protecting against irritation from food.

Urea is a popular hydrating agent but tends to burn the skin. This effect is minimized by applying the product to moistened skin. Proprietary products are available, and are helpful since formulating 10 per cent urea in Eucerin is difficult.

Both dryness and sweating exacerbate pruritus and are irritating to atopic skin. In extremely hot and/or dry climates, humidifiers and air conditioners are helpful in relieving these problems.

Children should be allowed to follow normal activities. Playing on light-colored or reflective surfaces (like sand) is desirable as it reduces heat and sweating, whereas grass absorbs heat and is irritating. Long pants help protect against this problem. Swimming in chlorinated water is dehydrating. To reduce its effects, affected individuals should shower immediately after leaving the pool and apply emollients both before and after swimming.

Because of the extreme sensitivity of atopic skin, nylon and wool clothing are irritating, and clothing of 100 per cent cotton is preferable. Several layers of cotton may be worn in the winter for warmth. Lining mitts and hats with cotton is most helpful. Clothing should be laundered in mild soap flakes (e.g., Ivory Snow) with no added bleach or fabric softener, because many of these contain perfume that is irritating to the skin. All products containing perfume should be avoided.

Diet and Atopic Dermatitis

Since the first article appeared over fifty years ago, there has been much controversy regarding the importance of diet in the management of AD. This article suggested that prolonged breast-feeding protects the infant against the development of AD. Presently, there is no conclusive proof that this is true, and although nursing should be encouraged, a parent who is unable to breast-feed should not be made to feel guilty.

Later it was also believed that elimination of certain foods in established AD was helpful in controlling the disease. This has been helpful in at best a small percentage of patients. It is never curative. Foods that are commonly implicated include milk, eggs, fish, nuts, citrus fruit, and wheat products. In severe chronic cases, if all else fails, these foods should be eliminated on a trial basis and milk substitutes added to the diet.

Another aspect of diet and AD appears to be the increased propensity for some patients to develop anaphylaxis to certain foods, especially chocolates, eggs, and nuts. It seems prudent to avoid these foods in early life. Because MMR vaccine is cultured on egg cells, egg-sensitive patients should be pretested before MMR vaccination, as anaphylactic reactions have been reported.

It has also been suggested that oil of evening primrose (Efamol) added to the diet of patients with AD may be helpful. However, in a number of double-blind studies this has not been verified.

Specific Measures

The mainstay of treatment of inflamed, eczematous skin is the use of corticosteroid creams and ointments. Lotions contain alcohol and are irritating. The use of hydrocortisone, 1 per cent powder in petrolatum (Cortate 1 per cent ointment) 3 times a day, is often sufficient in mild to moderate cases. In severe cases with chronic lesions on the trunk and extremities, betamethasone-17-valerate (Valisone), applied 3 times a day, can result in resolution. This is more effective when used in an ointment base. Fluorinated topical steroids should not be applied to the face. As the condition improves, either a weaker steroid or an emollient should slowly be substituted, because stopping the treatment suddenly often causes an exacerbation of the initial eruption.

The use of clobetasol 17-propionate (Temovate) or systemic steroids is not advisable because of the side effects from their continued use. The most common side effects of potent topical steroids have been striae formation on the inner thighs and facial eruptions. The scalp in AD is often involved. A mild shampoo with or without tar and the use of a mild corticosteroid cream usually suffice in eliminating the problem. Occasionally, steroid lotions are preferred for the scalp. Tar preparations mainly in the refined form of 5 to 10 per cent liquor carbonis detergens have been available for many years and are useful, particularly in the nummular and lichenified plaques seen in patients with AD.

Antihistamines are often beneficial in treating the associated pruritus; however, none of the available antihistamines eliminate the itching completely. Hydroxyzine is frequently under-prescribed in children at the recommended dose of 2 mg per kg per day. We sometimes double this dose and do not find it causes excessive drowsiness. Terfenadine (Seldane), given in a dose of 30 to 60 mg twice daily, and astemizole (Hismanal), given in a dose of 10 mg once a day, both lack sedating effects. Ketotifen, 1 mg twice a day, has also been found to be effective as an antipruritic agent with potent antihistaminic effects.

Staphylococcus aureus often colonizes the skin of AD patients without overt infection. However, when impetiginization does occur, it should be treated with cloxacillin (Tegopen), 50 to 100 mg per kg per day, or erythromycin, 40 mg per kg per day.

The treatment of Kaposi's varicelliform eruption (infection with herpes simplex virus) with acyclovir* (Zovirax) (100 to 200 mg five times a day for 5 days for children and 200 mg five times a day for 5 days for adults) can minimize the course of the disease.

Ultraviolet light B (UVB) has been used as an adjunct to other treatments with good effect for many years but needs careful monitoring, which makes treatment difficult for children and working adults. Recently ultraviolet light A (UVA) with and without psoralens has been moderately successful, although this is not a suggested treatment in children.

ERYTHEMAS

method of
CHARLES ZUGERMAN, M.D.
Northwestern University
Chicago, Illinois

Erythema, a component of a large number of cutaneous reactions, is caused by an increase in blood within small vessels of the skin that are responsible for skin color. The rate of blood flow does not increase, but dilation of blood vessels occurs, allowing increased flow to the subpapillary plexus of venules and to the

---

*Safety and efficacy of oral acyclovir in children have not been established. Parenteral use is approved.

capillaries of the dermal papillae. The erythemas are a large group of diverse diseases with a multitude of symptoms, etiologies, and epidemiologies all with the common denominator of redness of the skin. Some erythemas defy characterization, whereas others should be placed in more well-defined categories.

ERYTHEMA MULTIFORME

Erythema multiforme is a somewhat common disease that occurs in all age groups but more frequently in young adults. It is rarely a serious illness, but in the extreme form (Stevens-Johnson syndrome), it can be life-threatening.

Clinically, the minor form of erythema multiforme is characterized by typical "iris" or "target" lesions. These consist of concentric rings of variation of color, often with slightly vesicular or necrotic centers. The rash is symmetrical, often distributed on the arms, legs, palms, and soles. In addition to "iris" lesions, macules, papules, vesicles, bullae, and plaques may be present. Erythema multiforme may be a recurrent disease that heals without scarring. Systemic signs and symptoms are often lacking.

At the opposite end of the spectrum is the Stevens-Johnson syndrome, the most severe form of erythema multiforme. This, too, occurs more commonly in young adults and children. In addition to the characteristic lesions described earlier, one often sees large bullae with erosions and crusts, scarring, severe mucous membrane involvement, ocular lesions with blindness, and severe constitutional signs and symptoms.

Erythema multiforme may be induced by a wide range of etiologic agents. These include drugs such as penicillin and sulfonamides; infections, particularly herpes simplex and mycoplasma; connective tissue diseases; ingestants; immunizations; and malignancy in rare cases. Unknown pathogenesis may account for as many as 50 to 80 per cent of cases of erythema multiforme.

Treatment

Mild erythema multiforme may be treated symptomatically. If bullae are present, warm tap water compresses or compresses with normal saline or Burow's stock solution 1:40 dilutions applied for 20 minutes 2 to 3 times daily is helpful. If the lesions are pruritic, an antihistamine such as diphenhydramine hydrochloride (Benadryl), 25 to 50 mg twice daily, or hydroxyzine hydrochloride (Atarax), 10 to 25 mg twice daily, may relieve the symptoms. Terfenadine (Seldane) is helpful for those patients who are oversedated by other antihistamines.

More severe erythema multiforme reactions may involve the mouth and eyes. Oral lesions that are painful should be kept clean with hydrogen peroxide 3 per cent or an oral antiseptic such as Chloraseptic 3 to 5 times per day. Diphenhydramine elixir and viscous lidocaine 2 per cent serve as helpful local anesthetics. Ocular lesions are potentially serious, and under the best circumstances scarring that leads to blindness can occur. Ophthalmology consultation should therefore be obtained early in the course of severe erythema multiforme with ocular involvement.

Patients with severe erythema multiforme with multiple bullous lesions as well as significant mucous membrane involvement may also require parenteral fluids and electrolytes. Potentially superinfected skin should be cultured and appropriate antibiotic therapy initiated. When herpes simplex is thought to be the cause of recurrent erythema multiforme, acyclovir (Zovirax) may be used prophylactically.

Controversy exists as to whether patients with severe erythema multiforme or Stevens-Johnson syndrome should be treated with systemic corticosteroids. Although controlled studies on this point are rare, many dermatologists will give 60 to 100 mg oral prednisone or hydrocortisone intravenously every 8 hours. Nevertheless, in severe Stevens-Johnson syndrome this therapy may be ineffective.

ERYTHEMA NODOSUM

Erythema nodosum is characterized by the sudden onset of erythematous, tender nodules occasionally associated with malaise, arthralgias, and fever. One to four lesions are usually present, although they may be quite numerous. The nodules are frequently located on the anterior lower legs, but they may also occur in other locations including the arms, thighs, face, and scalp.

Although 30 to 50 per cent of cases are idiopathic, one should look carefully for common provoking causes. These include drugs, particularly birth control pills, estrogens, and sulfonamides; inflammatory bowel disease; sarcoidosis; infections, particularly streptococcal, tuberculous, and deep fungal; and, rarely, malignancy.

Treatment

Most young individuals who do not have an ongoing underlying cause of erythema nodosum will have a spontaneous remission in 2 to 6 weeks. In older individuals the disease is more likely to be triggered by serious underlying disorders. A systemic work-up for underlying etiologies is therefore necessary in these cases in order to prevent long-standing erythema nodosum.

Bed rest, elevation of the legs, support hose, and mild sedation are simple but effective therapies for this disease. Aspirin in the largest tolerable dose may also be given. In severe cases, intralesional corticosteroids such as Kenalog, 10 mg per ml diluted 2 to 1 with normal saline, are effective, or intermediate doses of systemic corticosteroids (prednisone, 60 mg per day) may be administered and then tapered over 10 to 14 days.

FIGURATE ERYTHEMAS

The figurate erythemas include a wide variety of eruptions characterized by annular and polycyclic lesions that may be fixed or migratory. These lesions last much longer than those of urticaria and may persist for days, weeks, or months in some cases. There are several diseases classified in this group, the most common of which is *Erythema annulare centrifugum,* which is characterized by slowly enlarging asymptomatic annular and polycyclic rings that spread out gradually and clear centrally. Erythema annulare centrifugum may be associated with various infectious diseases including ascariasis, *Candida albicans* infection, tuberculosis, Epstein-Barr virus infection, and streptococcal disease. Ingestants such as salicylates, blue cheese, and medications have also been associated with this process.

Other more rare figurate erythemas include *Erythema gyratum repens,* which is characterized by scaling erythema with the appearance of wood grain. This form has been associated with internal malignancy. *Erythema chronicum migrans* results from a solitary tic bite and is caused by a rickettsial infection. It has recently been identified as a marker for Lyme disease (see p. 866). *Necrolytic migratory erythema* is a widespread annular or arcuate migrating eruption associated with glucagon-secreting pancreatic tumors. *Erythema marginatum,* which accompanies rheumatic fever, is a widespread, rapidly migrating eruption with a distinctive narrow active border.

Treatment

It is imperative in many of the diseases in this group that a work-up for systemic disease be instituted and a cause be found. Necrotizing migratory erythema and erythema gyratum repens are often associated with malignancy and should be taken very seriously by the examining physician. Also, erythema chronicum migrans may be associated with Lyme disease and spirochetal infection, and it is treatable with penicillin and tetracyclines. Otherwise, diseases in this group are asymptomatic, and if no systemic problems are found, no specific therapy is needed.

BULLOUS DISEASES
method of
LYNNE H. MORRISON, M.D., and
LUIS A. DIAZ, M.D.
The Johns Hopkins Medical Institutions
Baltimore, Maryland

Three major bullous diseases appear to be immunologically mediated: pemphigus vulgaris, bullous pemphigoid, and dermatitis herpetiformis. They may be clinically and histologically distinct, but because of possible overlapping features, skin biopsy specimens and sera should be studied by immunofluorescence to confirm the diagnosis.

PEMPHIGUS VULGARIS

Pemphigus vulgaris (PV) occurs most commonly in middle adulthood, producing flaccid blisters that result in weeping and crusted erosions. Characteristically it involves the oral mucosa, often beginning there. Most patients have circulating anti-epidermal autoantibodies that, in general, correlate with activity of the disease and are helpful in diagnosis.

In the pre-steroid era, PV had a substantial mortality. Presently, the mortality rate in treated patients is about 10 per cent, largely related to steroid and immunosuppressive therapy complications. Although the course of PV is often chronic, treatment can result in long-term remission of the disease.

Treatment

Corticosteroids are the drugs of first choice for treatment of PV, but may need to be combined with an immunosuppressive agent in order to reduce their side effects. Most patients respond to prednisone in doses of 1 to 2 mg per kg daily in divided doses. Initially controlling the disease with higher doses of prednisone (200 to 400 mg per day) has been advocated, but this can increase the risk of life-threatening infection. Response to therapy should be evaluated by assessing healing of existing erosions and reduction of new blister formation. Once the disease is under control, prednisone can be consolidated into a single morning dose and then tapered rather rapidly at first, but more slowly when nearing a dose of 40 mg per day. If the disease remains under control at 40 mg daily, then an attempt to go to alternate-day therapy should be made by gradually tapering the dose given every other day to zero. The 40 mg every other day should then be tapered as tolerated.

If high maintenance doses are required or if the patient is not tolerating prednisone, then addition of an immunosuppressive agent should be considered to aid in the reduction or total elimination of steroid dosage. Immunosuppressive agents that have proved beneficial are cyclophosphamide (Cytoxan*), azathioprine (Imuran*), and methotrexate.* These agents take several weeks to take effect and are not drugs of first choice for treating the acute phase of PV. They are usually not started until the prednisone has been tapered to about 40 mg daily. When the disease is controlled by prednisone and the immunosuppressive agent, attempts should be made to decrease the prednisone by 5 to 10 mg weekly. If the prednisone can be discontinued, the immunosuppressive agent should be tapered over several months as tolerated.

Cytoxan is used in doses of 1 to 2 mg per kg daily. Significant adverse effects include bone marrow suppression, hemorrhagic cystitis and bladder fibrosis, sterility, and increased long-term risk for development of malignancies. These side effects mandate routine monitoring of CBC and routine and microscopic urinalysis. The risk of cystitis can be reduced by encouraging patients to maintain a high fluid intake.

Imuran is also given in doses of 1 to 2 mg per kg daily and can be useful in patients with urinary tract problems or those not responding to Cytoxan. It shares with Cytoxan the side effects of bone marrow suppression and increased risk of developing malignancies and also has been associated with hepatotoxicity. Therefore, chemistry profile as well as a complete blood count (CBC) should be followed routinely.

Less often, methotrexate has been used as adjunctive therapy; 25 to 30 mg are given weekly, either intramuscularly in one dose or orally divided into 3 doses given 12 hours apart. Because of hepatotoxicity, routine chemistry screens are necessary, and liver biopsies, both pretreatment and during therapy, are suggested if long-term treatment is anticipated.

Intramuscular gold sodium thiomalate (Myochrisine*) and gold thioglucose (Solganal*) have both been used successfully as steroid-sparing agents. A test dose of 10 mg is given, followed by a 25-mg dose 1 week later. If the drug is well tolerated, therapy is started, usually with 50 mg weekly. The response is slow, with beneficial effects usually noted after a total dose of 500 mg. When acceptable control is achieved, maintenance therapy may then be instituted. Approximately 40 per cent of patients on gold therapy experience adverse effects. The majority of these are not serious, but life-threatening complications can occur. Side effects include nitroid reactions, mucocutaneous eruptions, nephritis, leukopenia, and thrombocytopenia. A CBC and urinalysis including microscopic examination must be done before each injection.

Plasmapheresis has been of short-term benefit in controlling PV, but its use should be restricted to extraordinary circumstances.

Topical care for the crusted and weeping lesions should include wet Domeboro compresses 3 to 4 times daily, to help remove crusts and decrease discomfort, and silver sulfadiazine cream (Silvadene cream) to reduce the risk of infection. In the acute phase, frequent cultures and appropriate antibiotics are important to minimize infection.

Patients with oral involvement may benefit from a soft diet and viscous lidocaine before meals; topical triamcinolone acetonide in an adherent base (Kenalog in Orabase) may be of some help.

BULLOUS PEMPHIGOID

Bullous pemphigoid (BP) is a blistering disease of the elderly, typically presenting with tense bullae on an erythematous base and often arising in flexural areas. It is a more benign disease than PV, with a relatively low mortality even in untreated patients, and is commonly self-limited. Circulating autoantibodies against epidermal basal cell hemidesmosomes are present in most BP patients. They are useful diagnostically, but their titers are variable and are not helpful in monitoring treatment response.

Treatment

Systemic steroids are the mainstay of therapy for BP. The majority of patients respond to 1 mg per kg per day of prednisone. With this dose, it generally takes more than a week for bullae to heal and new blister formation to stop. The prednisone should be tapered slowly over a period of months. If maintenance doses are unacceptably high or the patient is not responding to or tolerating the prednisone well, addition of an immunosuppressive agent may be necessary. This would be expected in a minority of cases. Azathioprine (Imuran*) in a dose of 1 mg per kg per day appears to be effective and has been the most

---

*This use of this agent is not listed by the manufacturer.

*This use of this agent is not listed by the manufacturer.

widely used immunosuppressive agent for BP. It should be remembered that it takes 4 to 6 weeks for the drug to exert its maximum effect. Alternate agents include cyclophosphamide* and methotrexate.* The significant adverse effects of these medications have been noted previously under Treatment of PV.

Occasionally a patient with mild or localized disease can be managed with topical steroids alone. A mid- to high-potency preparation is usually necessary. Topical therapy for the erosions is the same as in pemphigus vulgaris.

DERMATITIS HERPETIFORMIS

Dermatitis herpetiformis (DH) presents most often in early to mid-adulthood and is characterized by intensely pruritic papulovesicles in an extensor distribution. Many patients with DH have pathologic changes in the small bowel similar to those seen in gluten-sensitive enteropathy, although most lack gastrointestinal symptoms.

Treatment

Dapsone is the drug of choice for treatment of DH. The disease responds promptly, usually within 3 days of starting therapy. Although dapsone controls the disease, it does not cure it or lead to remissions, and discontinuance of therapy will lead to prompt relapse. The usual initial adult dose is 50 to 100 mg orally, given once daily; maintenance doses typically are 100 to 200 mg daily. The most common side effects are hemolysis and methemoglobinemia due to the oxidizing ability of dapsone. It should be anticipated that patients on more than 50 mg of dapsone will experience some degree of hemolysis, causing a fall in hemoglobin level. This is an expected outcome, accompanied by a partially compensatory reticulocytosis, and in itself is not a reason to discontinue the drug. Most patients tolerate the decrease in hemoglobin and methemoglobinemia well, but those with cardiopulmonary disease need to be followed closely. Patients with glucose-6-phosphate dehydrogenase (G-6-PD) deficiency can experience severe hemolysis with dapsone. Therefore, blacks, Asians, and people of Mediterranean descent should have their G-6-PD level checked before starting therapy.

Other less common adverse side effects include toxic hepatitis, cholestatic jaundice, peripheral neuropathy, and rare but potentially fatal agranulocytosis.

Before beginning dapsone therapy, a baseline CBC, chemistry profile, and G-6-PD levels (if

---

*This use of this agent is not listed by the manufacturer.

appropriate) should be obtained. A CBC should be followed weekly for the first month, then monthly for 5 months, and then semiannually thereafter. Liver and renal function should be monitored periodically.

In the majority of patients, a gluten-free diet allows reduction of the dapsone dose, and in some patients it is possible to eliminate medication entirely. The patient needs to be very motivated and follow the diet strictly for 6 to 12 months before benefit can be expected. Assistance of a dietician is very helpful.

Sulfapyridine is an alternate drug that may be used in patients who do not tolerate dapsone, but it is less effective in controlling the disease. The starting dose is 500 mg 2 to 4 times daily; on the average, 1.5 grams is needed for maintenance. Because it can precipitate in the kidneys because of its poor water solubility, patients need to maintain a high fluid intake to minimize this side effect and should have renal function checked regularly.

CONTACT DERMATITIS

method of
JAMES G. MARKS, JR., M.D.
The Milton S. Hershey Medical Center
The Pennsylvania State University
Hershey, Pennsylvania

Contact dermatitis is an inflammatory response of the skin caused by exogenous chemicals. There are two types of contact dermatitis: irritant and allergic. Irritant contact dermatitis, the most frequent type, is produced by a direct toxic effect of the chemical on the skin, whereas allergic contact dermatitis is triggered by an immunologic reaction resulting in a cutaneous inflammatory response. Acids, alkalis, solvents, and detergents are examples of irritants; virtually any chemical has the potential to cause allergic contact dermatitis, the most frequent being poison ivy, nickel, rubber compounds, and preservatives found in topical medicaments and cosmetics. The clinical appearance can range from acute, weeping, crusted vesicles and bullae to chronic, lichenified, scaling plaques. Typically, the rash of contact dermatitis has angular corners and geometric outlines with sharp margins, suggesting an external cause of the dermatitis. Patch tests help in identifying and confirming the responsible allergens in allergic contact dermatitis. There is no standard method to test for irritant contact dermatitis.

Prevention

Prevention of contact dermatitis is the most logical but often the most difficult solution. Avoidance of an irritant or allergen may require a change in occupation or life style. For example, a highly skilled machinist who has irritant contact dermatitis of the hands from cutting oils may not be able to find comparable employment to avoid the cutting oils. On the other hand, if the cutting oil contains an additive to which he or she is allergic, substitution of another cutting oil without the additive can be curative. Sometimes protective clothing, such as gloves and aprons, is helpful in preventing contact dermatitis. Barrier creams, although touted, are of little benefit. Allergens that have high sensitizing potential are best used in closed systems where workers have virtually no contact with the offending chemical. Predictive animal testing for contact irritancy or sensitivity is now a standard procedure used prior to introducing new substances that have significant cutaneous contact. In this way, strong allergens or irritants can be avoided prior to widespread use. For allergic contact dermatitis, immunization is a most promising mode of prevention. Unfortunately, to date, attempts to hyposensitize individuals, particularly to poison ivy or poison oak, have failed.

Treatment

Acute Contact Dermatitis

Acute vesiculobullous contact dermatitis is treated with topical astringents, topical or systemic steroids, and antihistamines. If the area of acute dermatitis is small, wet compresses can be used to reduce oozing, remove crust and necrotic debris, and produce a soothing effect on the skin by reducing inflammation. Compresses can be made of any clean absorbent cloth, such as a washcloth or towel that is very moist but not dripping wet. Plain tap water or the astringent aluminum sulfate, and calcium acetate (Domeboro), 1 or 2 tablets diluted in a pint of water, is used to moisten the compress. When the areas of dermatitis are too extensive for compresses, baths can be used with colloidal oatmeal (Aveeno) or cornstarch. Compresses or baths are used two or three times a day for 20 to 30 minutes for each treatment.

Corticosteroids are the backbone of contact dermatitis treatment. They can be administered topically, intralesionally, or systemically. For extensive or severe acute dermatitis, prednisone, 40 to 60 mg daily, is the treatment of choice. A common mistake is to taper the prednisone too quickly or discontinue it too soon, resulting in a "rebound phenomenon" that allows reappearance of the acute dermatitis. The optimal treatment time is 10 to 14 days, with reduction of the initial dose of prednisone to 20 to 30 mg after 5 to 7 days if

the dermatitis is suppressed. With this short course of prednisone, a slow tapering dosage is not necessary and it can be stopped abruptly. An alternative to prednisone is triamcinolone acetonide (Kenalog), 40 mg intramuscularly, which will have an effect for about 3 weeks. When the acute contact dermatitis is localized, it can be easily treated with a potent topical steroid cream such as fluocinonide (Lidex) or betamethasone dipropionate (Diprosone). Little concern need be given to side effects such as systemic absorption or atrophy of the skin, since the treatment course will be for only 2 to 3 weeks. A cream is used in preference to an ointment because a cream can be rubbed into a weeping area of skin, whereas rubbing in an ointment would result in occlusion and potential maceration.

Itching is a prominent component of contact dermatitis and needs to be reduced to prevent scratching and patient discomfort. Antihistamines such as hydroxyzine (Atarax), 10 or 25 mg, or diphenhydramine (Benadryl), 25 or 50 mg, every 6 hours, should be prescribed.

Chronic Contact Dermatitis

Chronic contact dermatitis is treated more cautiously because therapy may require months. The dry, scaling, thickened skin of chronic dermatitis is better treated with a topical steroid in an ointment than in a cream. The occlusive nature of ointments helps with penetration of the topical steroid as well as retention of moisture and rehydration of dry skin. Patient preference, however, should be taken into account because compliance may be poor if the patient finds ointments greasy and unacceptable. Initially, a potent topical steroid as mentioned previously can be tried, but in the long run, attempts should be made to use weaker topical steroids. Medium-strength steroids, triamcinolone acetonide (Aristocort or Kenalog), or hydrocortisone valerate (Westcort) can be selected, as well as weak topical steroids such as hydrocortisone (Cort-Dome) or desonide (Tridesilone). For resistant plaques that are unresponsive to topical steroids, intralesional injection with triamcinolone acetonide (Kenalog), 10 mg per ml, can be used. Caution must be used, however, since the potential for atrophy is increased with intralesional steroids. For selected resistant cases, systemic steroids, prednisone, 20 to 40 mg daily, or triamcinolone acetonide (Kenalog), 40 mg intramuscularly every 3 to 4 weeks, is useful. It should be remembered that systemic steroids should be used in chronic contact dermatitis only when other forms of treatment fail and should be stopped as soon as possible.

SKIN DISEASES OF PREGNANCY

method of
JO-DAVID FINE, M.D.
University of Alabama at Birmingham
Birmingham, Alabama

Although a number of skin conditions may be aggravated by pregnancy, two disorders, herpes gestationis and pruritic urticarial papules and plaques of pregnancy (PUPPP), are of particular significance to the practitioner, not only because of the extent of maternal morbidity in each, but also because of the increased risk of fetal mortality associated with one of these disorders.

HERPES GESTATIONIS

Herpes gestationis is a rare autoimmune blistering disorder occurring during pregnancy and the postpartum period. The name of this disease is often misleading, since it is unassociated with herpesvirus infection. Herpes gestationis may develop at any time throughout the course of pregnancy, although it most often has its onset during the second and third trimesters and predictably flares just before, during, or very shortly after delivery. Usually the disease diminishes and finally subsides a few weeks to a few months postpartum. Rare patients, however, have been reported to experience significant persistent disease activity for several years after delivery. Some patients also may experience transient flares or recurrences with each menstrual period or following exposure to oral contraceptives, suggesting a definite hormonal influence. In addition, some but not all patients may experience recurrences during subsequent pregnancies, often with earlier onset or greater severity of disease.

Herpes gestationis is characterized clinically by marked generalized pruritus and the development of variably sized tense blisters arising on either normal-appearing or erythematous skin. With time, arcuate or polycyclic lesions with peripheral blistering may be seen. Although lesions usually first develop on the abdomen, widespread involvement may occur later.

Although the precise etiology of herpes gestationis is unknown, it is believed to be hormonally and immunologically mediated. Skin biopsy findings from lesional sites are indistinguishable by light microscopic criteria from those observed in bullous pemphigoid. Examination of perilesional skin by direct immunofluorescence reveals C3 and, less frequently, IgG bound linearly along the skin basement membrane (dermoepidermal junction), a finding that permits ready differentiation from other eruptions of pregnancy. Less frequently, the patient's serum may also contain either circulating autoantibodies or a complement-fixing factor (herpes gestationis factor) directed against normal human skin basement membrane.

Of greatest importance is an associated fetal mortality as high as 30 per cent. There is also an increased rate of premature live births as well as the infrequent occurrence of transient vesiculobullous eruptions in some otherwise healthy infants of affected mothers, the latter presumably due to maternal transmission of the herpes gestationis factor or other autoantibodies to the fetus.

Treatment

Because of the presence of intense pruritus, treatment is necessary in virtually every affected individual. Furthermore, many experts recommend early treatment with oral corticosteroids in hopes of preventing subsequent fetal mortality, although data are lacking as to their efficacy.

Occasional patients respond to simple measures including the topical use of medium- or high-potency fluorinated corticosteroid creams or ointments as well as the administration of oral antihistamines such as diphenhydramine (Benadryl), 25 to 50 mg every 4 to 6 hours. Most patients, however, require treatment with oral prednisone, 20 to 60 mg daily, throughout much of their pregnancy, with intermittent tapering (usually by about 5 mg per week) as tolerated; at the time of delivery, the dose must again be increased. Prednisone is usually given in a single morning dosage, but infrequently it may need to be given in four divided doses. In rare patients unable to tolerate prednisone, oral treatment may be attempted with dapsone (Avlosulfon), starting at 50 to 100 mg daily (this use of this drug is not listed in the manufacturer's directive). If possible, patients are advised not to resume the use of oral contraceptives in the future because of the likelihood of disease exacerbation.

In addition to the use of systemic medications, open erosions and crusts also should be treated with wet compresses of either isotonic saline or 1:40 Burow's solution (Domeboro) 3 to 4 times daily for 15 to 20 minutes, followed by a thin application of an antibiotic ointment such as Polysporin.

PUPPP

PUPPP (pruritic urticarial papules and plaques of pregnancy) is a relatively recently recognized disorder seen during the last few weeks of the third trimester of pregnancy. As the name implies, patients with this disorder develop pruritus and erythematous papules, urticarial plaques, and infrequently small vesicles, initially within the striae distensea of the abdomen but later elsewhere in the abdomen, thighs, buttocks, or arms. The upper chest is rarely involved. In contrast to herpes gestationis, there is no apparent increased fetal morbidity or mortality associated with PUPPP. Similarly, direct immunofluorescence is negative in PUPPP, readily distinguishing it from herpes gestationis. Usually this eruption resolves within the first week or two after delivery and does not recur with subsequent pregnancies.

Treatment

PUPPP in most patients may be controlled with oral antihistamines, medium-potency topical corticosteroids such as fluocinolone acetonide (Synalar cream 0.025 per cent) 3 to 4 times daily, and wet compresses. Infrequently, oral prednisone may also be required for a few weeks, in single or daily divided dosages of 20 to 40 mg, with relatively rapid tapering thereafter. In contrast to herpes gestationis, there appears to be no contraindication to the use of oral contraceptives following delivery and resolution of PUPPP.

PRURITUS ANI AND VULVAE

method of
K. WILLIAM KITZMILLER, M.D.
University of Cincinnati College of Medicine
Cincinnati, Ohio

Pruritus ani is a relatively common affliction, sometimes known as the "Executive Itch." It is characterized by intense, chronic, and protracted itching that is without evident cause. The process is usually limited to the anus and anogenital region. Sometimes it may extend anteriorly over the scrotum, buttocks, and parts of the thighs. In women it is frequently associated with pruritus vulvae.

Early in the course of the disease there is itching (with or without excoriation). However, with repeated trauma, thickening and lichenification appear in the involved areas. Successful management of this condition depends on the etiology of the symptom complex.

Common causes include irritation from dye in cleansing tissue; excessive use of anti-pruritic medications with caine derivatives; and irritation from sanitary napkins, soap, nail polish, and contraceptive devices. Other possible causes include parasitic infestation (e.g., pinworms, pediculosis pubis) and inflammatory dermatoses such as psoriasis, intertrigo, lichen sclerosus et atrophicus, neurodermatitis, and Paget's disease.

Factors that can aggravate the condition include excessive sweating, obesity, occupations that necessitate long periods of sitting (as with executives and truck drivers who use vinyl or leather synthetic seats and seat covers), and synthetic undergarments. Excessive bathing, frequent bowel movements associated with inadequate cleansing, and excessive retention of moisture may also be possible contributory factors. Local factors that may incite pruritus include inadequate cleansing, hemorrhoids, foreign bodies, cryptitis, and fissures. Sensitivity to drugs such as antibiotics and to certain foods (e.g., spicy foods and condiments) should also be considered.

In patients with all forms of pruritus ani, there should be an initial assessment of occupational activities, degree of cleanliness, type and frequency of bowel movements, antibiotic therapy, and oral desensitizations (e.g., poison ivy capsules). General health history, genital cutaneous examination, digital rectal examination, fungal scrapings, urinalysis for glucose, and examination for pinworms should be done.

Examination with Wood's light to rule out fungal infections, biopsy, and patch testing with scotch-tape preparations are all useful diagnostic maneuvers.

Treatment

The majority of cases usually are found to be the result of local irritation that may be caused by compulsive overcleanliness. Common sources of irritation are (1) inadequate cleansing, with fecal matter being retained in the folds of the anal canal; (2) regular and compulsive use of soap on the infected area; and (3) vaginal discharge.

Management of Contributing Habits

It is necessary to instruct the patient in strict personal hygiene. Successful outcome of treatment demands that the affected areas be kept cool; this is best done by wearing cotton underwear. Nylon underwear and pantyhose should be avoided because of the overheating of the vulvar area. Patients who sit at a desk or behind a steering wheel as part of their occupation may benefit from using spring-vented cushions. Attention should be paid to the diet and irritating foods should be avoided. Using soft toilet tissue dampened with water or witch hazel prior to cleansing or applying Tucks afterwards is also helpful. Both soap and frequent rubbing should be avoided.

Medications

Interruption of the itch-scratch cycle is vital. A low-potency topical preparation such as 1 per cent hydrocortisone (Hytone) cream applied frequently and sparingly has been beneficial. On rare occasions, Class-I topical preparations such as diprolene or temovate cream may be needed; however, these should not be used for more than

5 to 7 days. The 1 per cent hydrocortisone cream should be the main topical preparation but Pramosone lotion may also be helpful. Greasy preparations and topical sensitizers such as antihistamines and caine derivatives should be avoided.

Cool compresses are also particularly useful. I instruct patients to dissolve a Domeboro packet in a quart of cool to cold water and use this as a cool compress.

Antipruritics such as hydroxyzine (Atarax), 10 mg once every 4 to 6 hours, or terfenadine (Seldane) during the day in conjunction with the Atarax 4 times a day can also be beneficial. However, systemic therapy used alone is not rewarding.

In my experience, alternate applications of a topical antifungal preparation such as ciclopirox (Loprox) and 1 per cent hydrocortisone cream often provide relief. In certain cases that are more persistent, a diluted solution of triamcinolone acetonide diluted 2 to 4 mg per ml in 1 per cent lidocaine can be injected into the recalcitrant areas. At times this is the only agent that will interrupt the itch-scratch cycle. Tolnaftate (Zeasorb-AF) powder, applied after bathing to reduce moisture, is suggested particularly during the summer months.

URTICARIA

method of
ROBERT B. SKINNER, Jr., M.D., and
DENISE M. BUNTIN, M.D.

University of Tennessee
Memphis, Tennessee

Urticaria is a common cutaneous disorder often referred to as hives or wheals. Lesions consist of raised, well-circumscribed, erythematous pruritic plaques. These are transient and resolve in a few hours. Urticarial lesions range in size from a few millimeters to several inches (giant urticaria). Most urticaria results from an IgE-mediated immune response to a variety of antigens, producing areas of localized cutaneous edema. Urticarial lesions are characterized by edema in the superficial dermis; edema in the deep dermis and subcutaneous tissue produces the condition called angioedema. Evaluation and treatment of urticaria is based on classification into one of the following categories: acute, chronic, physical, or contact urticaria; urticarial vasculitis or angioedema.

Acute Urticaria

Acute urticaria is defined as eruptions lasting less than 6 weeks; it usually responds to oral antihistamines. Work-up consists of a history with particular emphasis on medications and a physical examination. Laboratory tests are not usually necessary unless the urticaria persists for more than 6 weeks. The history should particularly explore drugs, especially aspirin, aspirin-containing products, and penicillin. Aspirin-allergic patients can have cross-sensitivity to nonsteroidal anti-inflammatory agents, azo dyes (tartrazine), and benzoic acid. Over-the-counter medications must be explored, including headache relievers, cold preparations, laxatives, and vitamin supplements.

Foods are a common cause of urticaria. Most commonly associated foods are shellfish, nuts, eggs, chocolate, cheese, peanut butter, tomatoes, and strawberries. Questions should concentrate on food eaten immediately prior to the eruption and foods possibly associated with previous episodes of urticaria.

Treatment

Treatment of acute urticaria usually requires full adult doses of oral antihistamines to control symptoms. Adult doses of oral antihistamines include diphenhydramine (Benadryl), 50 mg; hydroxyzine (Atarax, Vistaril), 50 mg; cyproheptadine (Periactin), 4 mg; chlorpheniramine (Chlortrimeton), 4 mg; trimeprazine (Temaril), 2.5 mg. All should be taken 4 times daily. The main side effect of oral antihistamines is drowsiness. This can sometimes be avoided by using the nonsedating antihistamine terfenadine (Seldane), 60 mg twice daily. Doxepin (Sinequan), 10 mg 3 times daily, can be effective when antihistamines fail.

The goal of treatment in acute urticaria is to control symptoms until the antigen inducing the urticarial eruption is eliminated from the system. Antihistamines should be taken around the clock until symptoms are eliminated. They can then be slowly tapered, with resumption of full dosage if the urticaria recurs. When one antihistamine fails to control symptoms, a second or even a third antihistamine from another pharmacologic class can be added—for example, the combination of diphenhydramine (Benadryl) and hydroxyzine (Atarax, Vistaril).

Topical modalities such as cool compresses or an antipruritic lotion (Sarna) will help to control itching. For severe urticaria or laryngeal edema, subcutaeous or intramuscular administration of 1:1000 epinephrine (0.2 to 0.5 ml) is sometimes required.

Chronic Urticaria

Chronic urticaria is defined as an urticarial eruption lasting longer than 6 weeks. Studies show that laboratory workup for chronic urticaria is not cost effective; however, the studies that seem most productive are complete blood count, multi-channel chemistry profile, erythrocyte sedimentation rate and urinalysis. Thyroid function tests, chest x-ray or sinus films are rarely of benefit. A search for infection should pursue infected teeth, sinuses, gallbladder, and kidney as well as signs and symptoms of viral infections. A food diary may sometimes be helpful; since the urticarial eruption frequently begins within several hours after ingestion of the offending food, the diary may reveal the same food eaten prior to other urticarial attacks. Special diets such as lamb and rice or the food-additive elimination diet may clear the urticaria, and then gradual addition of foods to the diet may reveal the triggering substance.

Treatment

Treatment is with the same agents mentioned above for acute urticaria. General treatment measures include avoidance of aspirin and aspirin-containing products, nonsteroidal antiinflammatory agents, alcohol, exertion, and excessive heat, all of which increase cutaneous vasodilation and exacerbate urticaria.

The Physical Urticarias

The physical urticarias can be diagnosed by history and mechanical tests. *Pressure urticaria* is manifested by development of urticaria several hours after local pressure has been applied to the skin. Common areas are the buttocks after sitting, the feet after walking, and areas subjected to pressure from tight clothes or belts. *Cold urticaria* can be diagnosed by a history of an urticarial eruption of hands and face during rewarming after cold contact. An ice cube placed on the patient's arm for several minutes will produce urticaria after removal of the ice cube and rewarming. *Cholinergic urticaria* is characterized by tiny, highly pruritic, punctate wheals or papules occurring on any part of the skin and lasting from 30 to 90 minutes. Precipitating factors include exercise, increased environment temperature, fever, and emotional stress. Physical urticarias are also reported to occur in association with light, vibration, heat, and water. *Dermographism* is the eruption of a linear wheal when the skin is stroked with a firm object. This differs from *contact urticaria,* which is the production of wheals when the skin is touched by any of a variety of substances. Avoidance of contactants relieves contact urticaria.

Treatment

Treatment of physical urticarias consists of oral antihistamines and avoidance of triggering factors. Dermographism is treated with low-dose antihistamines and avoidance of unnecessary trauma.

Urticarial Vasculitis

Urticarial vasculitis can be suspected when individual urticarial lesions are present in one location for several days instead of several hours and there are associated complaints of fever, abdominal pain, arthralgias, and myalgias. The lesions sometimes hurt rather than itch. A skin biopsy of an urticarial lesion will reveal leukocytoclastic vasculitis. Urticarial vasculitis is frequently associated with medications, hepatitis B, mononucleosis, and systemic lupus erythematosus.

Treatment

Oral antihistamines are ineffective in urticarial vasculitis. Reported treatments include oral prednisone, 40 to 60 mg daily and tapering off in 10 to 14 days; oral colchicine, 0.6 mg twice daily; dapsone, 100 mg daily; and indomethacin (Indocin), 75 to 200 mg daily in divided doses.

Angioedema

Angioedema is a severe form of urticaria involving the deep dermis or subcutaneous tissue and manifested by severe swelling. Usually affected are the more distensible tissues such as the eyelids, lips, ear lobes, external genitalia, oral mucous membranes, tongue, and larynx. The hands and feet can develop severe edema. Urticaria frequently precedes angioedema, and the etiology and treatment of angioedema is the same as for urticaria. In hereditary angioedema, which consists of sudden attacks of gastrointestinal, laryngeal, and pharyngeal edema, there is a functional deficiency of the inhibitor of the activated first component of the complement system. Treatment is with the oral anabolic steroid danazol (Danocrine), 200 mg twice or three times daily.

PIGMENTARY DISORDERS

method of
MARVIN RAPAPORT, M.D.
Beverly Hills, California

HYPERPIGMENTATION

No matter what the cause of hyperpigmentation, whether it be endogenous or exogenous, usually the pigmentation is noted in the sun-exposed areas of the body. The sun exacerbates and perpetuates many pigmentary disorders. Sun exposure induces immediate pigment darkening of the readily available melanocytes in the epidermis and also induces further pigmentation at a later date. This is a protective mechanism and is also the effect desired by the sunbather. Not only do we have the sun to contend with, but artificial sources of ultraviolet B (UVB) (280 to 320 nanometers) and ultraviolet A (UVA) (320 to 400 nanometers) are readily available. Pigmentation problems can also occur with fluorescent and heat lamp light.

The beach, mountains, and sun parlor all provide occasions for exposure to ultraviolet light that causes hyperpigmentation. Prolonged exposure leads to severe photoaging and formation of tumors such as keratoses, basal cell carcinomas, squamous cell carcinomas, and melanomas.

Treatment

Sunscreening agents are available that protect against the UVB rays of the sun and newer ones will be marketed in the near future against UVA radiation. PABA, PABA esters, benzophenone, and salicylates are available as chemical protective agents that absorb ultraviolet light. Physical protection such as titanium dioxide and calamine as well as clothing can also be utilized. In treating any hyperpigmentation disorder, usually adequate sun protection is necessary. An SPF (sun protective factor) of 2 yields minimal protection, and an SPF of 15 or higher yields maximum protection.

Animal studies have demonstrated repeatedly that protection with sunscreens helps avoid tumor formation and slows the aging process. Some animal data also demonstrate that after damage has occurred, protection with sunscreening agents might indeed reverse some of these damaging processes. The damage and hyperpigmentation afforded by sun exposure is heightened with increased humidity, increased altitude, and increased wind velocity. Certain areas of the United States are obviously more at-risk ultraviolet locations. There is also some evidence that acute sunburns acquired during a short vacation may have worrisome sequelae years later, whereas protective pigmentation produced by low-dose exposure probably offers some protection against tumors and aging.

Sunscreening agents such as Sundown, Pre-Sun, Eclipse, and Super Shade, as well as protective cosmetic preparations, offer well-tested, effective protection.

Periorbital Hyperpigmentation

One of the most common complaints is dark circles under the eyes, or periorbital pigmenta-

tion. It has been ascribed to aging, tiredness, diet, nervousness, and cosmetics.

Basically this entity, which causes great concern, has a genetic basis. It is often seen in dark-pigmented individuals, especially of Mediterranean background. It can be seen in individuals as early as puberty.

Treatment

Specific therapy is not helpful, and avoidance of surgical procedures is to be recommended. Change in eating or sleeping habits has not been effective.

Systemic Hyperpigmentation

Listed in Table 1 are drugs and metals and systemic diseases associated with hyperpigmentation.

Treatment

Usually the pigmentation is difficult to treat. However, cessation of exposure to the culprit chemical or metal or treatment of the underlying disease produces therapeutic results. On rare occasions surgical modalities such as dermabrasion or excision aid in making the pigmentation yield.

Melasma (Chloasma)

Melasma is an acquired hyperpigmentation seen on the face, typically in a mottled pattern over the bridge of the nose and on cheeks, upper lip, and forehead. The pigmentation is most discomfiting to patients, who are invariably women. Pregnancy, oral contraceptive use, and heredity (Mediterranean and Central American) are

TABLE 1. **Causes and Clinical Patterns of Systemic Hyperpigmentation**

Culprits	Clinical Pattern
Metals	
Mercury	Generalized
Gold	Randomized
Silver	Photodistribution
Arsenic	Generalized
Drugs	
Antimalarials	Photodistribution
Minocycline	Extremities
Phenothiazines	Photodistribution
Antitumor (bleomycin, busulfan, doxorubicin)	Randomized, nails
Metabolic/endocrine Disorders	
Pellagra	Photodistribution
Addison's disease	Generalized
Acanthosis nigricans	Neck, axilla, groin
Scleroderma	Extremities

among the etiologies of this estrogen/progesterone–induced entity.

Treatment

The best therapy is cessation of the oral contraceptive, if that is indeed the cause, and the judicious and frequent use of sunscreening agents and depigmenting preparations. Dermabrasion, liquid nitrogen, and face peels are to be avoided.

The sunscreening agent should protect against the higher range of exposures and should contain a UVA screen. Better yet are physical screening agents such as zinc oxide and titanium dioxide. It has been shown that when the disorder yields well to therapy, just a bit of sun exposure in one day can cause a recurrence of hyperpigmentation.

Depigmentation creams can provide a fair amount of bleaching. Hydroquinone is often used and is available as a 2 per cent cream (Eldoquin), a 4 per cent cream (Eldoquin Forte), and a 3 per cent solution (Melanex). The liquid application may penetrate better. A compound preparation containing hydroquinone (1 to 3 per cent) mixed with retinoic acid (0.01 per cent to 0.1 per cent) and a mild hydrocortisone (1 to 2 per cent) has been used over the past 10 years with fairly good results. Several studies have demonstrated that steroid preparations as well as retinoic acid have depigmenting qualities; the combination of the three ingredients seems of more benefit than each of the individual ingredients alone.

Monobenzyl ether of hydroquinone (Benoquin) is an effective depigmenting agent but may cause permanent total depigmentation and a confetti-like depigmentation where applied and in distant sites. Its use is not advocated because of poor control.

Mercury compounds have been used in skin-lightening creams in other countries but have been taken off the market in America. Care should always be taken when using imported preparations. Mercury has caused nephropathies in patients many years following application of mercury-containing agents.

Hyperpigmentation Streaks

Pigmentary demarcation lines are commonly seen in individuals of pigmented races. The most frequent lines run along the upper extremities with varying transpectoral extensions. At times streaks are also seen on the extremities. Dorsal skin is more pigmented than ventral skin, possibly providing better protection from the sun.

Pigmented streaks running down the nails are always of great concern to the physician. However, they are invariably normal and benign in pigmented peoples. When a new band appears along one nail in lighter-skinned individuals, there is always the suspicion of a melanoma at the base of the nail. A biopsy of the base and the matrix is appropriate in such cases. Benign nevi are another cause of hyperpigmentation, and flagellate pigmentation from the use of bleomycin has also been seen, especially on the upper extremities.

Treatment

No specific therapy is necessary.

Lentigines

Lentigines ("liver spots"), which typically appear on the backs of the hands and at times on the cheeks—often the left cheek first (sunshine while driving)—are worrisome to the patient because of concern about tumors. However, these are invariably sun-induced and remain benign. Rarely malignant transformation can occur, but variable pigmentation and irregular growth are usually noted in such cases.

Treatment

The cosmetic aspect of these spots can be aided by the judicious use of the hydroquinone creams. Also, very superficial spraying of liquid nitrogen can peel off this pigmented process. Light swabbing of trichloroacetic acid, 20 to 35 per cent, may also be effective. Care should be used to avoid scarring.

Carotenoderma

The ingestion of large amounts of yellow vegetables such as carrots can cause a yellow staining in the skin, or carotinoderma. The ingestion of beta-carotene and canthaxanthin also can give this jaundice-like look to the skin (sclera are normal here). It has been suggested that the carotenoids protect from sun exposure, and they have been used for treatment of erythropoietic protoporphyria.

Some tanning preparations capitalize on the staining ability of certain chemicals to give a yellowish-orange "tan" to the skin when applied externally. These chemicals, usually hydroxyacetones, are shed in the keratin layer.

Treatment

No treatment is necessary, since the stain fades when ingestion of the offending food or agent stops.

HYPOPIGMENTATION

Most areas of blotchy hypopigmentation or leukoderma are caused by prior inflammatory processes in the skin. Usually time and some sun exposure allow the color to return.

Vitiligo

Vitiligo is an idiopathic total loss of pigment of the skin that affects about 1 per cent of the population. On rare occasions it has been associated with autoimmune and endocrine disorders, but history of the vast majority of patients with vitiligo reveals only a familial pattern. Industrial exposure to certain agents such as phenols, quinones, and thiols can cause depigmentation. These chemicals act by killing the melanocytes.

Treatment

The first therapy for vitiligo should be cosmetic. Numerous preparations on the market such as Cover-Mark, Walnut Stain, and Vita Dye serve a useful purpose in hiding this disfiguring depigmentation, especially when it occurs on the face and the hands.

Improvement in vitiligo in response to high-potency topical corticosteroid therapy has been reported. The best results appear to occur in facial lesions of Asian and black patients. Long-term use of steroids should be avoided.

Autografts have been tried in small areas of leukoderma and vitiligo and have shown good success. When the islands of the donor graft are in place, there seems to be a pigment-spreading phenomenon from these melanocyte-intact areas into the vitiliginous areas.

When the problem is more widespread, the use of psoralens should be undertaken. When small areas are involved, topical psoralen therapy may be useful, but great care must be exercised to avoid excessive sun exposure. A 1 per cent solution of 8-methoxypsoralen diluted with 50 per cent ethanol giving a final concentration of 0.1 per cent is usually painted on the vitiliginous areas between 1 and 2 hours before sunlight exposure. Very cautious exposure of 2 to 3 minutes with increasing 30-second intervals to noon sunlight is the best way to start. If an artificial UVA light source is available, then 0.5 to 2.0 joules per square centimeter should be the initiating dose, with slow incremental increases 3 times a week for up to 4 to 6 months. Further exposure to the outdoor sun during the day should be avoided throughout the length of therapy.

Larger areas of vitiligo require the use of systemic psoralen therapy, such as 0.5 mg per kg ingested 2 hours before light therapy (preferably artificial UVA). This combination of psoralens and UVA is called PUVA. It is difficult to control the exposure of natural sunlight, but initial exposures of about 10 minutes can be attempted.

Care must be exercised to protect the eyes with special lenses during therapy and for the rest of the day. Prior to initiating therapy an antinuclear antibody (ANA) test and an eye examination should be performed; those patients who are pregnant, who have photosensitive dermatoses, or who have histories of skin cancers or cataracts should not be treated.

Good repigmentation is usually apparent after 3 months of therapy. If no response is evident after about 20 treatments, then the oral psoralen therapy should be discontinued. Maintenance therapy is usually necessary; care in evaluating vitiliginous areas for cancerous changes should always be part of the treatment.

Total body depigmentation is a final alternative to obtain even coloration. Benoquin is applied for 3 days. If no irritation occurs, then the patient can apply the medication on a twice-daily basis. Depigmentation usually begins after several weeks; rarely, some repigmentation occurs in small areas.

Tinea Versicolor

Tinea versicolor is a superficial fungus infection that commonly occurs on the chest, back, and upper arms in younger individuals. A potassium hydroxide mount will show typical hyphae and spores of *Malassezia furfur*. Often individuals with eczema have similar leukodermic areas on their upper arms, but these have indistinct borders and should be differentiated from this fungus infection.

Treatment

Tinea versicolor responds to Selsun shampoo applied for 30 minutes for 5 consecutive nights. If the area is not extensive, then topical antifungal agents such as clotrimazole (Lotrimin, Mycelex), ciclopirox (Loprox), and econazole (Spectrazole) are very effective. These preparations should be applied twice daily for at least 3 to 4 weeks. Tinver, a sodium thiosulfate preparation, can be applied on a once-a-day basis for about a month. Recently it has been demonstrated that ketoconazole (Nizoral), 200 mg daily for 2 weeks, can also suppress this disease process. Care should also be taken to evaluate liver function if therapy will be prolonged.

Halo Nevus

Commonly, in younger individuals normal benign intradermal nevi will develop a halo of depigmentation. This is thought to represent an autoimmune process in which the body is actively manufacturing antimelanocyte features. Ultimately the nevus is completely gone within a year. Because this phenomenon is sometimes seen in patients with malignant melanoma, the appearance of the halo nevus always is cause for concern.

Treatment

Data and careful follow-up have demonstrated that this process is invariably a benign one in childhood and that excision is not necessary.

OCCUPATIONAL DERMATITIS

method of
HAROLD PLOTNICK, M.D.
Wayne State University School of Medicine
Detroit, Michigan

Occupational dermatoses include a large assortment of cutaneous abnormalities that are primarily caused or aggravated by components in the workplace. Chemical agents by far are the leading cause of occupational skin disease. These agents include an array of primary irritants, allergic sensitizers, photosensitizers, and systemic intoxicants absorbed through the skin.

Despite the introduction of many protective devices, breakthroughs in controls occur. Chemicals that are used and well harnessed in one industry can become unleashed and hazardous in another. The industries with the greatest number of work-related dermatoses are machine tool production, plastic manufacturing, rubber production, food processing, leather tanning and finishing, and metal plating and cleaning.

Most work-related skin diseases affect the exposed areas of the body. The clinical picture of an acute contact eruption is characterized by the appearance of erythema, edema, vesiculation, and weeping. This reaction is the same whether the cause is a primary irritant or an allergic sensitizer.

A primary irritant source produces a direct physical change in the skin. The allergic patient must initially undergo an incubation period to develop antibodies against the specific antigen. Once antibodies are formed, subsequent exposure to the recognized antigen will elicit an eczematous response within 24 hours in the target skin area. Unlike the primary contact dermatitis that is localized to the areas of exposure, the allergic response may appear over other areas of the body besides the locus of contact.

Management

The Physician's Role in Industry

The physician's role in industry is not limited to the diagnosis and treatment of work related skin injuries, but also includes identifying the cause and recommending protective measures to prevent future recurrences. Medical treatment must be prompt and comprehensive to lessen the degree of morbidity and hasten the recovery of the skin to its pre-injury state. When possible, the worker is kept on the job while receiving treatment. If this approach is impractical, the worker should be moved to another area of the workplace or given time off until the skin is clear. A worker who has developed an allergic reaction to a recognized chemical may experience a recurrence of the dermatitis even on minimal re-exposure despite the employment of protective safeguards. In these selected cases, a change in job assignment is mandatory.

Patch Testing

The patch test is not a perfect bioassay but it does possess unique and valuable features since it serves as a miniature model of the disease under investigation. The patch test is recommended for suspected allergens, not for evaluating known or suspected primary irritants. The latter would only contribute to a false positive reaction and confuse the purpose of the test.

The majority of patch testing is performed under a closed system with the exact materials to which the worker is exposed. Dry materials can be utilized as is, but liquids should be diluted with equal parts of a compatible vehicle prior to testing. This cautionary procedure is necessary to avoid a potential primary irritation that could result in a false positive reaction.

The test materials should be covered by a nonallergenic material and fixed in place by an allergy-free adhesive-treated paper tape (3M Micropore, Scanpor) for a period of 48 hours. The patch is then removed and a 45-minute rest period is observed prior to the reading. A positive test is recognized as either erythema and edema (2+), a weak reaction; or as erythema, edema, and vesiculation (3+), a stronger allergic reaction. A negative response indicates the absence of an allergic reaction.

Hand Protection

Hands are the most common site of contact dermatitis. The use of protective gloves or a barrier cream is a necessary part of the working uniform in industries in which corrosive chemicals are encountered. These agents include low pH acids, high pH alkalis, chromates, coolants, cutting oils, some greases, free or uncombined monomers of epoxy and polyester systems, organic solvents, and rust preventatives.

Protection is the key to the avoidance of primary irritants and allergic-sensitizing contact dermatitis in industry. Where hand protection is a must, the choice is the right type of glove for the specific job (e.g., canvas, leather, rubber, or vinyl).

Canvas gloves are suitable for dry work. They do protect the hands from the rough edges on stock and from stains when handling various chemically coated materials. Leather gloves can be used in dry work as well, but their real advantage is in types of work in which there is a need for gripping objects, such as in the buffing and polishing industry.

Wet jobs require the use of rubber or vinyl gloves. Rubber gloves are pliable and supple and are composed of either natural latex or synthetic materials. In some industries in which contact is with organic solvents or uncured plastic monomers, rubber gloves may allow minuscule amounts of chemicals to enter. In these situations, a vinyl glove is preferred because of its alleged nonpermeable nature. The prolonged wearing of rubber or vinyl gloves prevents evaporation of natural sweat, and retention of sweat within the interior of the glove may cause maceration of the epidermal surface. It is advisable that vinyl gloves contain an inner fleece cotton lining to absorb the sweat. Unlined rubber gloves can be worn over absorbent, light-weight cotton gloves. Excessive sweat production within the interior of rubber gloves can sometimes leach out uncombined rubber accelerators and antioxidants that may cause allergic contact dermatitis in susceptible individuals. Workers who develop this problem should wear synthetic rubber (Neoprene) or vinyl gloves.

Protective gloves can be hazardous to workers engaged in machine tool production; the gloves may be grabbed up by the machine and cause injury to the worker. In this type of industry in which manual dexterity is essential, a suitable barrier cream (Kerodex-71) can be used as a protective agent. Kerodex-71 has been used effectively in industries in which coolants and cutting oils are the primary contactants. The barrier cream must be removed every 2 hours and the hands must be washed to free any retained residue and dried. A fresh application of the barrier cream is then applied to all contact areas.

The Problem of Sweaty Hands

Hyperhidrosis (excessive sweat production) with its frequently accompanying pompholyx (dyshidrosis) may precede or become symptomatic from the prolonged use of protective rubber or vinyl gloves. A worker with an active pompholyx may develop a hand dermatitis from materials that normally do not call for gloved protection. The reason for this is that open blisters may provide an easy access to potential irritants and sensitizers to invade the skin and initiate an inflammatory response.

Workers with dyshidrosis or its aggravated form (dyshidrotic eczematous dermatitis) respond favorably to appropriate local care. This includes soaking the hands in Burow's aluminum subacetate (Domeboro) solution, one tablet per quart of water, for 15 minutes twice a day. Following the soaks, a mid-potency glucocorticoid cream (e.g., fluocinolone acetonide (Synalar), desonide (Tridesilon), or betamethasone valerate (Valisone) can be helpful in clearing the dyshidrotic reaction. Workers with active pompholyx who cannot tolerate cotton-lined protective gloves or whose reaction is unresponsive to local medication must be assigned to a dry job.

Physical and Climatologic Influences in Contact Dermatitis

The intact epidermis is provided with a natural lipid-wax protective mantle that can ward off the majority of irritants encountered by the skin. When lipid solvents bathe the skin's surface, the protective layer is washed away. The unprotected keratin layer is free to lose its water content to the atmosphere, a factor that results in a dry stratum corneum and a potential opening for primary irritants to enter the skin.

Climatologic conditions that influence the water content of the skin are recognized as the dew point and humidity. During the colder months of the year, when the ambient water content is low, there is an increase in the loss of water from the skin to the atmosphere. The physical change in the skin is recognized as chapping or dehydration secondary to a low dew point and humidity.

Skin dryness resulting from the coupling of the two examples above can evolve into an eczematous process, a problem often seen in the machine tool industry during the cold winter months. The worker's bare hands are in and out of various lipid solvents (coolants, cutting oils, degreasing agents) many times a day. This sequence of repeated exposure to lipid solvents followed by evaporation of solvent and epidermal water loss to the low water content of the ambient work atmosphere may account for the measurable increase in symptomatic hand eczema during the colder months of the year. The same exposure and work methods usually present little problem during the other seasons of the year.

Treatment

The basic treatment for dehydration-induced eczematoid dermatitis is restoration of water to the thirsty epidermis. This phenomenon can be corrected by avoiding soaps and utilizing a water miscible oil (Alpha Keri) as a hand cleaner and by the after-work use of hygroscopic creams or lotions. These agents restore water to the epidermis and decrease its evaporation to the ambient water deficient atmosphere. The following proprietary medications are suggested: a water-in-oil emollient (Eucerin), and lactic acid derivatives of azelaic acid (LactiCare cream, Lac-Hydrin lotion). These water-holding agents are best applied to a moist skin after work hours and at bedtime.

DERMATOSES INDUCED BY SUNLIGHT

method of
HENRY W. LIM, M.D.
New York University School of Medicine
New York, New York

Electromagnetic radiation, such as that emitted by the sun, can be classified according to wavelength (Table 1). Ultraviolet C (UVC) is absorbed in the atmosphere and does not reach the surface of the earth; it is present only in artificial light sources used primarily as germicidal lamps. By far the most common side effects of sun exposure are from acute and chronic exposure to ultraviolet B (UVB); these side effects range from sunburn to skin cancers (Table 2). Ultraviolet A (UVA) may potentiate the photocarcinogenic effect of UVB and is responsible for the development of photoallergy and phototoxicity. In addition, ultraviolet (UV) light may induce the development of idiopathic dermatoses (e.g., polymorphous light eruption, solar urticaria), and may exacerbate others, such as lupus erythematosus.

SUNBURN

Sunburn results from acute exposure to UVB. It consists of immediate darkening of pigment on exposed sites (during and immediately after UVB exposure), followed by erythema and edema (peaks at 24 hours), and resolves with tanning and desquamation. Blisters and erosions may occur following exposure to high doses of UVB.

Treatment

No treatment is indicated if the patient presents with only mild erythema. Sunburn with

TABLE 1. **Classification of Electromagnetic Radiation from Sun**

Type	Wavelength Range (nm)	Major Biologic Effect
UVC	200–290	Germicidal
UVB	290–320	Sunburn, skin cancers
UVA	320–400	Photoallergy/phototoxicity
Visible	400–800	Illumination
Infrared	800–17,000	Heat

TABLE 2. **Dermatoses Induced by Sunlight**

Dermatosis	Cause
Sunburn	Acute UVB
Photoaging, actinic keratoses, skin cancers	Chronic UV
Photoallergy	Photoallergen + UVA
Phototoxicity	Phototoxic Agent + UVA
Porphyrias	Porphyrins + 400–410 nm radiation
Polymorphous light eruption	Idiopathic, UVB to visible light
Solar urticaria	Idiopathic, UVB to visible light
Lupus erythematosus (exacerbated by sunlight)	Autoantibodies, UVB

moderate erythema, edema, and tenderness should be treated with cool water compresses, for 10 minutes 3 times daily, and topical corticosteroids to reduce the inflammation (hydrocortisone cream 1 per cent twice daily to face and intertriginous areas, triamcinolone acetonide cream 0.1 per cent twice daily to body). Because prostaglandins have been implicated as one of the mediators of UVB-induced erythema, aspirin or one of the nonsteroidal anti-inflammatory agents is the preferred analgesic agent, and therapy should be started as soon as possible to obtain the full therapeutic effect. The blister fluid should be drained without removing the blister roof. Erosions should be treated with hydrogen peroxide, followed by a topical antibiotic such as bacitracin ointment (Baciguent) or polymyxin-bacitracin ointment (Polysporin) twice daily. Systemic steroids should be reserved only for most severe cases; they should be started at 40 to 60 mg of prednisone per day and tapered rapidly over a 5- to 10-day period.

Judicious avoidance of the sun, wearing protective clothings (including hats), and application of sunscreen will prevent the acute as well as the chronic (see below) effects of UV light. Individuals with fair skin who always burn and never tan should use a sunscreen with a sun protective factor (SPF) of 15 or above, while those who are able and have the desire to tan may use a sunscreen of lower SPF. Repeated applications of a sunscreen are necessary following contact with water. It should be emphasized that sunburn occurs not only from direct sunlight but also from UVB light reflected from surfaces such as snow, sand, and water.

PHOTOAGING, ACTINIC KERATOSES, AND SKIN CANCERS

These three conditions are the result of chronic exposure to the sun.

Photoaging

Photoaging is dryness and wrinkling on sun-exposed areas. Results of a short-term (16 weeks) study on the effect of topical tretinoin (Retin-A) 0.1 per cent cream in 30 patients with photoaged skin showed some improvement of fine but not coarse wrinkles. It should be noted that tretinoin cream is a potent topical irritant, and 92 per cent of the patients in the above study developed irritation, some requiring the usage of potent topical steroids. Therefore, until the results of an ongoing, large, multicenter trial are available, photoaging is best managed solely by education on sun-avoidance and the use of sunscreens to prevent further photodamage.

Actinic Keratosis

Actinic keratosis is a rough, skin-colored to erythematous flat spot on sun-exposed areas such as the forehead, nose, and dorsum of hands. It is asymptomatic and is usually multiple. Cryotherapy and electrodesiccation are two very effective therapeutic modalities. In patients with numerous lesions, these modalities may be combined with topical application of 1 or 5 per cent 5-fluorouracil cream or solution (Fluoroplex or Efudex, twice daily for 2 to 3 weeks). Patients should be warned that treated areas will be inflamed and tender, which usually occurs within 1 week of the initiation of therapy, and may take 2 weeks following the completion of therapy to resolve.

Skin Cancers

Squamous cell carcinoma is a rough, skin-colored to erythematous, elevated spot that may bleed occasionally. *Basal cell carcinoma* is an elevated spot with a central crater and a translucent and telangiectatic border; it is asymptomatic aside from occasional bleeding. Both carcinomas are strongly associated with chronic sun exposure. They can be treated by electrodesiccation and curettage, excision, or radiation therapy. There is also evidence that sun exposure is associated with the development of *melanoma,* which usually is a brown-to-black, flat or elevated spot with a variation in surface color and irregular border. Excision with appropriate margin is the treatment of choice, which may be combined with lymph node dissection and chemotherapy.

PHOTOALLERGY AND PHOTOTOXICITY

The clinical manifestations of photoallergy and phototoxicity are erythema, blisters, erosions, hy-perpigmentation, and thickening of the skin in sun-exposed areas. Photoallergy is a type of a delayed hypersensitivity reaction in which the combined presence of photoallergens and UV light is required for the sensitization and elicitation. It occurs only in sensitized individuals. Medications and fragrances are some of the most common photoallergens (Table 3). In contrast, phototoxicity can be elicited in all individuals exposed to adequate doses of phototoxic agents and appropriate radiation. Medications lead the list of the most common exogenous phototoxic agents (see Table 3).

Avoidance of the offending photosensitizers and of sun exposure is essential in the management of photoallergy and phototoxicity. The action spectrum of these two disorders is in the UVA range. Because para-aminobenzoic acid (PABA) is a poor UVA sunscreen, sunscreens containing titanium dioxide, cinnamates, benzophenones, or zinc oxide should be recommended for these patients. Otherwise, treatment is identical to that outlined above for sunburn.

PORPHYRIAS

Porphyrias are examples of phototoxicity induced by endogenous phototoxic agents. Because of enzymatic defects in the heme biosynthetic pathway, patients with porphyrias have elevated levels of porphyrins in their plasma, erythrocytes, urine, and/or feces. The most common type of porphyria is porphyria cutanea tarda, clinically manifested as skin fragility, blisters, and erosion on sun-exposed areas, usually the dorsum of the hands. These patients may also have periorbital mottled hyperpigmentation and hypertrichosis. Treatment modalities include repeated phlebotomies, or low-dose chloroquine (chloroquine base), 125 mg twice weekly. There are several other, less common types of porphyrias. In every instance, diagnosis should be established by careful evaluation of the porphyrin profile in the above-mentioned biologic specimens. Because the action spectrum in porphyrias is in the range of 400 to

TABLE 3. **Common Photosensitizers**

Photoallergens
Phenothiazines
Halogenated salicylanilides
Musk ambrette
Sunscreens
Phototoxic Agents
Furosamide
Thiazides
Tetracyclines
Psoralen
Tar
Hematoporphyrin derivative

410 nm ("Soret band"), only physical blockers (clothing or sunscreens containing zinc oxide) can afford adequate photoprotection for these patients.

POLYMORPHOUS LIGHT ERUPTION

This idiopathic photodermatosis manifests as erythematous macules or urticarial papules that appear within 15 to 30 minutes of sun exposure. Treatment modalities include sun avoidance, sunscreens, hydroxychloroquine (Plaquenil), 200 to 400 mg once or twice daily during spring and summer months, or 8-methoxypsoralen plus UVA (PUVA).

SOLAR URTICARIA

Patients with this condition present with urticaria following sun exposure. The action spectrum can be in the UVB, UVA, or visible range. The cause is unknown. In addition to sun avoidance, other treatment modalities include antihistamines, desensitization by repeated exposure to UV of the appropriate wavelengths, PUVA, and chloroquine, 250 to 500 mg daily, then tapered to 250 mg once weekly.

LUPUS ERYTHEMATOSUS

Sun exposure frequently exacerbates the cutaneous manifestation of lupus erythematosus, consisting of erythema, edema and fine scaling on exposed areas. Frequently, discoid lesions (atrophic patches with hyper- and hypopigmentation, telangiectasia, follicular plugging, and fine scales) also appear on sun-exposed areas. The action spectrum is in the UVB range. Treatment of cutaneous manifestations of lupus erythematosus consists of sunscreens, topical and intralesional steroids, and in severe cases systemic steroids (Prednisone, 20 to 60 mg daily), or antimalarials (hydroxychloroquine, 200 to 400 mg daily).

The Nervous System

BRAIN ABSCESS

method of
SYDNEY M. FINEGOLD, M.D.
VA Wadsworth Medical Center
University of California School of Medicine
Los Angeles, California

Brain abscess begins as a cerebritis, then becomes an abscess, and ultimately becomes encapsulated. The first two stages may often be managed medically.

Etiology

The etiologic agents of intracranial suppuration vary primarily with the site and kind of antecedent infection and also with predisposing host factors. The common isolates are anaerobic bacteria (including anaerobic cocci, *Bacteroides, Fusobacterium, Actinomyces,* and less often, *Clostridium*) and aerobic or microaerophilic gram-positive cocci (*Staphylococcus aureus, Streptococcus pneumoniae, Streptococcus pyogenes,* and viridans group streptococci such as *S. anginosus*). Fastidious bacteria such as *Haemophilus (Actinobacillus) actinomycetemcomitans* and *Haemophilus aphrophilus* may also be found. Although certain organisms such as *S. aureus* are usually found in pure culture, polymicrobial infections are common when other pathogens, such as the anaerobes or Enterobacteriaceae, are involved.

Brain abscesses that arise as a direct extension of infection from the middle ear, mastoids, sinuses, or oropharynx frequently yield anaerobes and microaerophilic streptococci, although other aerobes, such as *S. aureus, H. influenzae,* and Enterobacteriaceae (e.g., *Proteus*), may be encountered. In the compromised host, however, unusual pathogens must be considered. For example, in rhinocerebral zygomycosis, direct extension of fungal infection of the nasopharynx may lead to intracranial abscess. In patients with acquired immune deficiency syndrome (AIDS), *Toxoplasma gondii* must be considered the most likely cause of focal central nervous system infection.

Brain abscesses following hematogenous spread from a preceding lung abscess or other pleuropulmonary infection are commonly caused by anaerobic pathogens and various streptococci. *Nocardia, Aspergillus,* and the zygomycetes may also be found in this setting, especially in the compromised host.

Staphylococcus aureus may cause brain abscess in association with endocarditis, and is the most likely pathogen in brain abscess that follows accidental or surgical trauma to the head. Gram-negative rods are also found in this setting. In patients with congenital heart disease, brain abscesses are most often caused by aerobic or microaerophilic streptococci and anaerobic cocci, less often by *Haemophilus*. Additional, uncommon causes of brain abscess include various Enterobacteriaceae such as *Klebsiella* and *Enterobacter*, which may originate from primary genitourinary or intra-abdominal infections; *Neisseria meningitidis* and *Listeria monocytogenes*, which are usually associated with meningitis; *Mycobacterium* and protozoa, including *Entamoeba histolytica*.

Treatment

Medical Therapy

In the stage of acute suppurative encephalitis or cerebritis prior to the formation of an encapsulated abscess, prolonged antimicrobial therapy may be curative without surgical intervention. When the etiology is known because of a positive culture from a primary source, therapy can be directed specifically. In the case of positive blood cultures, however, bear in mind that not all organisms in the brain abscess may show up in the blood culture. Given the diversity of organisms that may cause brain abscess, particularly in immunocompromised subjects, surgery (burr hole with aspiration) is desirable in order to make a specific bacteriologic diagnosis. It is important that a good anaerobic transport setup be used in sending the specimen to the laboratory. In certain patients with fully formed abscesses, especially those for whom the risk of surgery is prohibitive, treatment with antimicrobial therapy alone may be attempted. Close observation of such patients is obligatory, using serial imaging procedures with monitoring for signs of a decreasing level of consciousness and developing focal neurologic deficits.

Table 1 lists the antimicrobial agents useful in the management of brain abscess, their spectrum of activity, and information concerning dosage and administration. In most situations when the etiology is not known, metronidazole plus penicillin G represents the initial treatment of choice.

Anticoagulation is contraindicated in the presence of brain abscess because of the danger of intracranial hemorrhage. Measures to decrease intracranial pressure may be necessary. Anticon-

TABLE 1. **Antimicrobial Agents Useful in the Treatment of Brain Abscess**

Drug	Susceptible Organisms	Dosage
Penicillin G	Streptococci, many anaerobes	200,000 to 300,000 units/kg/day (given IV every 2 to 4 hr)
Metronidazole (Flagyl)	Anaerobes except *Actinomyces* and *Arachnia*	30 mg/kg/day (given IV every 6 hr)
Chloramphenicol (Chloromycetin)	Gram-negative bacilli, anaerobes	50 to 60 mg/kg/day initially, then 30 mg/kg/day (given IV every 6 hr)
Nafcillin (Nafcil, Unipen)	*Staphylococcus aureus*	100 to 200 mg/kg/day (given IV every 4 hr)
Trimethoprim/sulfamethoxazole (Bactrim, Septra)	*Nocardia*, gram-negative bacilli, methicillin-resistant *S. aureus*	20 mg/kg/day trimethoprim plus 100 mg/kg/day sulfamethoxazole (given IV or orally every 6 hr)
Cefotaxime (Claforan)	Gram-negative bacilli	120 to 175 mg/kg/day (given IV every 4–6 hr)
Vancomycin (Vancocin)	Methicillin-resistant *S. aureus*, streptococci	30 mg/kg/day (given IV every 6 hr)
Rifampin (Rimactane) (use only in combination)	*S. aureus*, anaerobes	15 mg/kg/day (given p.o. every 12 hr)
Amphotericin B (Fungizone)	Fungi	1 mg test dose IV; then gradually build up to 0.5 mg/kg/day by the 5th day

vulsants such as phenytoin (Dilantin), 100 mg intravenously or orally every 8 hours, or phenobarbital, 30 to 60 mg intravenously every 6 to 8 hours, should be used. Blood levels of anticonvulsants should be monitored. Anticonvulsants should be continued until the abscess has definitely resolved. At that point, they may be stopped if the patient has been free of seizures.

Surgical Therapy

Operation is mandatory when neurologic deficits are severe or progressive, particularly when signs of brain stem compression (herniation) are present. This is especially urgent when the abscess is in the posterior fossa. Abscess drainage is by far the most rapid and effective method of reduction of intracranial pressure in the setting of a severe deficit.

When the abscess abuts the ventricular wall, rupture of the abscess into the ventricle is a threat. Drainage is indicated to prevent this possibility, which would lead to disseminated meningeal infection. Operation is also indicated when serial computed tomography (CT) scans or magnetic resonance imaging (MRI) shows progression of an abscess under antibiotic treatment.

Corticosteroids are useful for reduction of edema caused by the operative procedure. Dexamethasone (Decadron), 10 mg intravenously, then 4 mg every 4 to 6 hours, is an effective initial dose. Immunosuppressive effects are minor and temporary with short-term use. Steroids may be tapered rapidly as the patient's neurologic condition improves. They will not usually be required for more than a week following drainage.

Most abscesses can be drained via needle through a burr hole with the patient under local anesthesia. Needle drainage may be repeated as necessary. When the abscess is located in a deep or neurologically sensitive site, CT-guided stereotactic equipment may be used to perform drainage.

If the abscess is large or multiloculated, craniotomy with abscess drainage under direct vision may be needed. A drainage catheter may be left in the cavity and hooked up to a closed-suction system. Significant drainage does not usually continue beyond 48 hours, and the catheter may then be removed.

Craniotomies should be performed, if possible, through an osteoplastic (vascularized) bone flap to minimize the risk of osteomyelitis. Excision of an abscess or of a postabscess scar occasionally may benefit the patient who has seizures that have resisted ordinary treatment.

Antibiotics should be continued for at least 6 to 8 weeks following drainage. CT scans or MRI must be performed to confirm that progressive resolution of the abscess is taking place. Antibiotics may be discontinued even though there is a small residual abnormality on the enhanced CT scan or MRI. Such an abnormality should be re-examined by CT or MRI, about a month after the antibiotics are stopped, to rule out re-emergence of the abscess.

ALZHEIMER'S DISEASE

method of
BALU KALAYAM, M.D., and
CHARLES A. SHAMOIAN, M.D.
*Cornell University Medical College,
New York City, New York*

Alzheimer's disease is the most common form of primary dementia and may have an onset in the presenile (before age 65) or the senile period. The same neuropathology is seen regardless of period of onset, even though the cases with earlier onset have a strong genetic loading and a more rapid course. The illness is invariably a disabling disorder that begins with impairment in activities requiring higher mental functions, such as vocational activities, managing finances, and finding direction in public places. Vegetative functions and tasks of daily living, such as eating, sleeping, bathing, dressing, and continence, are affected as the disease progresses. Life expectancy is considerably shortened, and in advanced stages death may result from infections or seizures.

Treatment

Treatment usually is sought for disturbing and disruptive behavior and emotional states that may manifest as depression, affective outbursts, increased suspicion, fragmented delusions, psychosis, agitation, nocturnal restlessness, wandering, and incontinence; these disturbances occur in association with other symptoms of dementia, including impairment in memory and judgment, poor comprehension, and disorganization of language.

Agitation is a common presenting symptom in patients that may stem from anxiety, psychosis, depression, or delirium. Neuroleptics and sedative drugs are frequently used in the control of agitation. Anxiety may accompany increased awareness of cognitive loss, especially during early stages of the disease. The short-acting benzodiazepines such as lorazepam (Ativan) and oxazepam (Serax) offer the advantage of a renal route of elimination, less accumulation, and fewer complications with drug interactions.

In psychotically disturbed patients, the presence of target symptoms of psychosis, such as agitation, hallucinations, increased suspiciousness and delusions, respond to antipsychotic drugs favorably. However, the core symptoms of dementia such as memory loss are not improved by antipsychotic drugs and may even worsen in some patients, possibly through a blockage of central nervous system (CNS) cholinergic mechanisms. Orthostatic hypotension, pseudoparkinsonism, and sedation may occur as adverse effects of antipsychotic drugs, impairing general functioning of the patient. The individual patient's sensitivity to these side effects is helpful in determining the choice and dose of neuroleptics.

Low-potency phenothiazines such as chlorpromazine and thioridazine are usually associated with sedation, orthostatic hypotension, and less severe parkinsonian symptoms. Comparatively high-potency drugs such as haloperidol infrequently produce sedation and orthostatic hypotension and may lead more frequently to extrapyramidal symptoms. In practice, the physician must weigh the benefit of the low incidence of extrapyramidal symptoms of low-potency neuroleptics against the low sedation but higher incidence of movement disorders of high-potency drugs. The outcome of psychosis in demented patients remains equivocal, and physicians often discontinue neuroleptics after several months of stabilization. If, however, symptoms recur, medications may need to be reinstituted.

Delirium may manifest as a global impairment in functioning, as confusional episodes or agitation, as hallucinations and delusions, or as angry or aggressive outbursts. In patients with Alzheimer's disease, superimposed delirium may manifest as nocturnal confusion or "sundowner's syndrome," which may be triggered by changes in the physical environment or a decrease in sensory input. Although a search for underlying metabolic derangement in delirium and its correction is the first goal in treatment, neuroleptics are often used in relieving behavioral symptoms.

Depression may be the initial manifestation in approximately 20 per cent of patients with Alzheimer's disease (depression of dementia). Cognitive impairment, while seemingly worse during depression, may show some improvement upon recovery from depression. However, the cognitive disturbance may intensify as a result of the anticholinergic side effects of antidepressant drugs. Antidepressant medications are indicated in the presence of major depressions. Differences in the effectiveness of individual tricyclic compounds, however, are not pronounced, and the choice of medication for the elderly may be determined by the side effects of individual drugs. Excess sedation, orthostatic hypotension, cardiac effects, and anticholinergic side effects are of concern in the choice of individual antidepressant drugs in the elderly. With careful follow-up, improvement in depression is usually observed in 3 to 4 weeks of treatment.

The search for a specific treatment to reverse the cognitive loss in dementia still continues. However, current concepts in its pathophysiology, have focused attention on drugs that fit within a cholinergic model—for example, choline, lecithin, physostigmine, tetrahydroaminoacridine, and arecholine. These potentially promising drugs are still experimental.

An important component of care includes the needs of the family, whose members may be devastated by the deterioration of the patient's personality and functioning. Heavy demands may be placed on the time and energy of the caregiver. Depression in these caregivers is not uncommon and monitoring of their health and well-being is crucial. Help may be offered to the caregiver by several disciplines and through various community support groups.

INTRACEREBRAL HEMORRHAGE

method of
J. PHILIP KISTLER, M.D., and
DARYL R. GRESS, M.D.
Massachusetts General Hospital
Boston, Massachusetts

Although there are many causes of intracerebral hemorrhage, four are particularly common: hypertensive and lobar intracerebral hemorrhages, ruptured aneurysm (saccular), and ruptured arteriovenous malformation. Less common are hemorrhage associated with a bleeding disorder and rupture of a mycotic aneurysm.

Rare causes include idiopathic brain purpura, small multifocal hemorrhage associated with hypertensive encephalopathy, and hemorrhage associated with acute hypertension secondary to sympathetic stimulation (e.g., amphetamines, cocaine, antihistamines). These rarely simulate a stroke. Their treatment rests largely on management of the primary disease.

Ruptured saccular aneurysms (usually causing subarachnoid hemorrhage) may rupture into the brain substance, producing intracerebral hemorrhage with mass effect. Two examples are frontal and temporal lobe hematomas from ruptured anterior communicating artery and middle cerebral artery bifurcation aneurysms.

HYPERTENSIVE INTRACEREBRAL HEMORRHAGE

Pathophysiology

Hypertensive hemorrhage typically occurs in four sites: (1) putamen and adjacent internal capsule, often extending into the central white matter (50 per cent of cases), (2) thalamus, (3) pons, and (4) cerebellum. Hypertensive hemorrhage rarely originates in the central white matter. The vessel involved is generally one of the penetrating arteries arising from the middle cerebral artery stem, basilar artery, or circle of Willis—that is, precisely the vessels involved with segmental lipohyalinosis as a consequence of hypertension.

The hemorrhage begins as a small oval mass and then spreads by dissection, growing in volume and displacing and compressing adjacent brain tissue. In these types of hemorrhage, rupture or seepage into the ventricular system almost always occurs; yet rupture from the white matter through the cortical surface gray matter is very rare. Only when the hemorrhage is small (1 to 2 cm) will it be confined to the central gray and white matter and not gain access to the cerebrospinal fluid (CSF) via the ventricular system. Large hemorrhages may compress the ventricular system and displace midline structures to the opposite side, leading to stupor, coma, and death.

Most hypertensive intracerebral hemorrhages develop in a few minutes, but some evolve over 30 to 60 minutes, and others, particularly those associated with anticoagulant therapy, evolve for as long as 24 to 48 hours. In contrast to a ruptured saccular aneurysm, once the bleeding stops, it generally does not start again. However, edema forms in the compressed tissue around the hemorrhage, leading to a greater mass effect and, in some cases, worsening the clinical status. Within 48 hours, macrophages begin to phagocytize the hemorrhage at its outer surface. After 2 months, the hemorrhage mass is generally resolved to a slit-like orange cavity lined with astroglial scar tissue and hemosiderin-laden macrophages.

Clinical Syndromes

The hypertension associated with these strokes is almost always chronic. They are not associated particularly with exertion, but almost invariably the hemorrhages occur when the patients are awake. A hemorrhage may be so rapid that it causes enough mass effect to produce coma in a few moments, but the temporal course is usually slower. The four primary locations of hypertensive hemorrhage produce four respective clinical syndromes: *putaminal, thalamic, pontine,* and *cerebellar.*

As a large *putaminal hemorrhage* begins, the patient often complains that something is wrong in his head. A hemiparesis involving the face, arm, and leg has begun to develop. Speech becomes slurred (dysphasic if the dominant hemisphere is involved). As the hemiplegia worsens, sensation becomes impaired (hemineglect develops if the nondominant hemisphere is involved). The head and eyes deviate laterally away from the hemiplegia, and drowsiness and stupor ensue. With the onset of coma, the ipsilateral pupil dilates and a complete third nerve palsy may develop due to compression by the temporal lobe as it is pushed medially over the tentorium by the expanding mass. Decerebrate posturing occurs and respiration becomes rapid and forced in expiration as compression of the brain stem occurs. Smaller hemorrhages generally produce hemiplegia due to rupture through the internal capsule, but the size and direction of rupture determine the extent of the other neurologic signs. Worsening 12 to 72 hours after the initial hemorrhage is caused by edema formation rather than rerupture.

Thalamic hemorrhages produce a similar picture, except that in addition to hemiplegia, hemisensory deficits are prominent, and the eyes are often displaced downward and medially as coma ensues.

Pontine hemorrhages generally present with coma developing in 1 or 2 minutes. The pupils are miotic but still react to light. Reflex eye movements are lost as coma and quadriplegia develop.

Recognition of the clinical manifestations of *cerebellar hemorrhages* is especially important because of favorable surgical experience with this type. Recurrent vomiting with inability to stand or walk due to truncal ataxia without a hemiparesis is the hallmark neurologic manifestation. Occipital headache, vertigo, and forced deviation of the eyes to the opposite side or the inability to look horizontally to the side of the lesion often occur. Bifacial weakness, stupor, and bilateral Babinski signs warn of impending respiratory cessation due to increased posterior fossa pressure and dictate immediate surgical evacuation.

Laboratory Evaluation

The computed tomography (CT) scan has revolutionized the diagnosis of intracerebral hemorrhage. It reliably detects all hemorrhages in the cerebral or cerebellar hemispheres of 1 cm or more in diameter if they are studied in the first 2 weeks. Because x-ray attenuation values of clotted blood diminish over time, intracerebral hematoma may appear isodense after 2 weeks and may be missed if not associated with surrounding edema or mass effect. In some cases a rim of contrast-enhancing tissue appears after 2 to 4 weeks and may persist for months. Rarely, small pontine hemorrhages may not be identified because of motion and possibly bone artifact. Magnetic resonance imaging (MRI) scans may prove more reliable than CT scanning for detecting either small pontine or medullary hematomas or hematomas in which the clot has become isodense. Early angiography is recommended if the hematoma on CT scan suggests it may have occurred from a ruptured saccular aneurysm at the base of the brain or an arteriovenous malformation (AVM). Subarachnoid blood or a small anterior putaminal or temporal lobe hematoma suggest the former. Any intracerebral hematoma, particularly if it breaks into the subarachnoid space, suggests the latter.

Treatment

The size of the hematoma, in many cases, determines the prognosis. Supratentorial hematomas greater than 5 cm in diameter have a guarded prognosis, and infratentorial pontine hematomas greater than 3 cm in size are almost invariably fatal. The formation of edema for up to a week after the intracerebral hemorrhage often worsens the prognosis. However, in intracerebral hematomas, the tissue surrounding the hematoma is displaced and compressed but not necessarily infarcted. Hence, after the resolution of the hematoma, considerable improvement can result, as the tissue regains its function. Careful management of the patient during the critical phase of the cerebral hematoma can lead to considerable recovery.

Surgical removal of the supratentorial clot in the acute stage is rarely indicated. However, surgical evacuation of a supratentorial clot may prevent temporal lobe herniation in comatose patients who still have reflex eye movements. Surgical evacuation of acute cerebellar hemorrhage is usually the treatment of choice because it is often life saving and offers an excellent prognosis for recovery of function. If patients are alert without focal brain stem signs and if the cerebellar hematoma is small (<2 cm), the physician may elect against acute surgical removal. It must be remembered, however, that deterioration of the clinical state can be rapid. The option for acute surgery must always be available.

Surgical evacuation of pontine hematomas is not an option. Evacuation of putaminal and thalamic hematomas is problematic because the severity of the deficit limits significant recovery. However, if all concerned see a chance for meaningful recovery, surgery should be considered as a life-saving measure. It becomes an option when patients deteriorate 12 to 72 hours after the hemorrhage or present with coma. Then, surgical removal and drainage of the hematoma mass can improve survival. Following surgery, severe hemiparesis usually persists, as do degrees of the other preoperative deficits. On occasion, reasonable recovery occurs, especially when the nondominant hemisphere is involved or when the hematoma has dissected frontally. From the outset, the medical practitioner and the neurosurgeon must plan a therapeutic approach together. The stated wishes of the patient and family, the nature and severity of the initial deficit, and the patient's age and general medical status are most important in the decision making.

Limiting *edema formation* is the most important factor in controlling intracranial pressure. Supratentorial hematomas 3 cm or greater in size and infratentorial hematomas 1 cm or greater in size as seen on the CT scan have the potential to cause lethal elevations in intracranial pressure due to delayed edema formation. Intravenous mannitol is required when there is increasing drowsiness and stupor due to the mass effect of the hematoma and edema. An initial bolus of 20 per cent mannitol is given intravenously 1 gram per kg followed by 100 ml over a few minutes every 4 to 6 hours to raise the serum osmolarity to >310 milliosmols per liter. Intravenous or oral steroids at the outset may be helpful but have not been proved to prevent edema formation or reduce it in this setting. Dexamethasone (Decadron), or its equivalent, 4 mg intravenously or orally every 4 to 6 hours, may be used.

Hypertension at the outset is usually a compensatory mechanism. Cerebral perfusion pressure (mean arterial pressure minus intracranial pressure) is directly related to blood pressure and inversely related to intracranial pressure. Sudden dramatic lowering of the blood pressure may be detrimental. For the most part, hypertensive intracerebral hemorrhages occur over a moment or two or at most a few minutes, and rerupture rarely occurs. By the time the patient arrives in the emergency room, the bleeding has stopped. Therefore, hypertension should be managed conservatively. Systolic blood pressure greater than 190 mm Hg should be treated with diuretics or beta blockers. Intravenous calcium channel blocking agents or vasodilators such as nitroglycerin and nitroprusside may be used. Because of the cerebral vasodilating effect of these agents, they may raise the intracranial pressure if cerebral compliance due to mass effect is on the ascending limb of the pressure volume curve. Therefore, they are best used when the hematoma is small and mass effect is minimal. Parenteral hydralazine (Apresoline) injection may be helpful in reducing the blood pressure safely over a few minutes (25 mg intramuscular every 2 to 4 hours).

Hyponatremia aggravates edema formation and should be avoided. Intravenous solutions should contain no less than half normal saline, and normal saline is often administered to meet the patient's fluid requirements. Patients are best managed in the first few days with fluid restriction so that they have a matched or negative intake versus output.

LOBAR INTRACEREBRAL HEMORRHAGE

As control of hypertension in the general population improves, the relative proportion of hemorrhages outside the basal ganglia and thalamus increases. These "lobar hemorrhages" appear on CT scan as oval or circular clots in the subcortical white matter. The role of chronic hypertension in their genesis is controversial, as many occur without a history of increased blood pressure. A number of other underlying conditions are established in almost half the cases. The most common is arteriovenous malformation. Others are bleeding diathesis, often associated with warfarin administration; hemorrhages into tumor, often a melanoma; aneurysms of the circle of Willis that point upward and bleed into brain substance; and a large number whose causes remain undetermined even after extensive study including arteriography.

Among the latter, the most common is *amyloid angiopathy* which can only be diagnosed at postmortem examination with demonstration that the vessels stain positive with Congo red. Amyloid is deposited in the walls of the cerebral arteries; the angiopathy is unassociated with amyloid deposition elsewhere in the body. The condition seems to account for many lobar hemorrhages among the elderly. Often patients suffer multiple hemorrhages, although months may elapse between occurrences.

Most lobar hemorrhages are small enough to cause a restricted clinical syndrome that simulates an embolus to a vessel supplying one lobe. Larger hemorrhages, associated with stupor or coma, cause larger deficits and affect two or more lobes. Most patients experience focal headaches: occipital hemorrhage afflicts the area around or over the ipsilateral eye; temporal hemorrhage, the area around or anterior to the ipsilateral ear; frontal hemorrhage, the forehead or diffusely in the frontal quadrant; and parietal hemorrhage, the temple region. At the onset, stiff neck or seizures are uncommon, but more than half the patients vomit or are drowsy. The neurologic syndrome appears suddenly, over one to several minutes, not instantaneously as it does in embolus. The clinical syndrome corresponds to the location of the hematoma: the major neurologic deficit of occipital hemorrhage is hemianopia; of left temporal hemorrhage, aphasia and delirium; of parietal hemorrhage, thalamic-like hemisensory loss; of frontal hemorrhage, arm weakness. The region of hemorrhage adds other but less prominent signs to these.

Treatment

Treatment depends upon the underlying condition. Angiography should be performed in most cases, but immediate angiography may not demonstrate a small vascular malformation. If an acute vascular malformation is still suspected, angiography should be performed again after 2 to 4 months, when the vessels adjacent to the clot may have decompressed. In awake or drowsy patients, surgical evacuation offers little benefit over medical management with fluid restriction, corticosteroids, and an osmotic agent if necessary (see Hypertensive Intracerebral Hemorrhage). Stuporous or comatose patients not responding rapidly to medical therapy for raised intracranial pressure should have the clot evacuated immediately. Unlike deep hypertensive intracerebral hemorrhage, lobar hemorrhage often responds to surgical evacuation in this setting, and significant recovery ensues.

ISCHEMIC CEREBROVASCULAR DISEASE

method of
M. J. GAWEL, M.D.
University of Toronto, Sunnybrook Medical Centre
Toronto, Ontario

Although there has been a steady decline in the incidence of stroke over the last 30 to 40 years, it is still the third commonest cause of death in North America. The toll in terms of morbidity is vastly greater and the cost of chronic care makes stroke prevention a vital issue. A stroke is defined as a focal neurologic deficit due to vascular factors lasting more than 24 hours. If the deficit reverses in under 24 hours it is termed a transient ischemic attack (TIA). While this distinction is artificial, it serves to define a population who are at risk for developing a nonreversing stroke and in whom investigation may detect a potentially treatable cause. The definition is clinical. About 25 per cent of patients with a TIA have evidence of a small infarct on the CT scan. In patients in an intermediate category, reversible ischemic neurological deficit (RIND), the deficit clears by 1 week, although some authorities accept 3 weeks. We feel that a TIA and minor stroke (RIND) are risk factors for a further major event and alert the patient's physician to the need for further investigation.

A stroke as defined is due either to infarction of brain tissue or to hemorrhage. Eighty-five per cent of strokes are due to cerebral ischemia. Ischemic stroke can be caused by thrombosis of a major vessel, artery-to-artery embolism, or embolization from the heart; 15 per cent of ischemic strokes are due to occlusion of small penetrating branches of arteries, usually in hypertensive patients. These are called lacunar defects and are small and tend to affect specific areas of the brain, producing recognizable syndromes.

TRANSIENT ISCHEMIC ATTACK (TIA)

Clinical Presentation

A transient focal neurological event *usually* lasts no longer than 4 hours. The symptoms follow the pattern of involvement of the arterial territory involved. For instance, a patient with a left middle cerebral artery TIA would present with dysphasia and weakness and numbness of the right hand. These symptoms clear, and in about 30 per cent of cases the patient is left with a contralateral headache. If the arterial territory is vertebrobasilar, the patient may develop ataxia, slurring of speech, diplopia, or other symptoms suggestive of posterior circulation involvement. A clear description of the symptoms is essential, since there are other events that can produce similar symptoms. Vague symptoms such as dizziness, syncope, and confusion are not specific and should not in themselves lead one to suspect a TIA.

Patients with vertebrobasilar TIAs have a lesser risk of developing stroke later than those with hemispheric TIA. The risk of stroke in a patient with a hemispheric TIA is about 10 per cent a year, being highest in the first 6 months.

Differential Diagnosis

Besides hypoglycemia, the following disorders should be considered in the differential diagnosis of TIA.

Epilepsy. Both sensory and motor phenomena in epilepsy are usually positive (e.g., jerking of a limb, paraesthesia).

Migraines. Migraine causing a focal deficit is much more common in young people. Again, phenomena are positive such as scintillating scotomas. In middle-aged and elderly patients, migrainous deficits may occur in the absence of headache, causing a real diagnostic problem. Here it may be appropriate to treat the condition in the same way as a TIA and investigate risk factors.

Multiple Sclerosis. Either an attack or one of the paroxysmal manifestations can cause transient deficits.

Mass Lesions. These may present initially with transient events either due to irritation of the nerve tissue or because of compression of local vascular structure.

Management

In most instances, the patient is asymptomatic at the time of consultation. If the patient is seen early and has a deficit, it is of course impossible to tell whether he has a TIA or stroke until the deficit either persists or clears up. Once the diagnosis is clear then further investigations are performed.

Clinical Evaluation

Evaluation of the potential sources of emboli is then undertaken. In our hospital we are fortunate to have a sophisticated ultrasonic Doppler laboratory which allows evaluation of both extra- and intracranial vessels. Only if there is significant stenosis do we proceed to angiography, as it is only these patients for whom surgery can be considered. If Doppler studies are unavailable and if the patient is a potential surgical candidate, then cerebral angiography should be performed.

Echocardiography is performed for cardiac evaluation. Valvular lesions, ventricular aneurysms, or atrial clots can all form sites for potential emboli. Old myocardial infarcts or cardiomegaly are also possible risk factors. If there is a history of palpitations associated with the TIA, then a Holter monitor may be valuable.

Angiography carries a small but definite (0.5 to 2.0 per cent) risk of morbidity. Recently, digital subtraction angiography (DSA) has been introduced. This allows a much smaller amount of contrast medium to be used. We perform all (DSA) by the intra-arterial route (IA-DSA). Results with intravenous DSA (IV-DSA) have been disappointing, often not producing views of value to the surgeon. Views of the intracranial portion of the circulation are also necessary to identify tandem lesions.

It is certainly worth obtaining a CT scan if possible; as mentioned, 25 per cent of patients with TIA may have a small infarct and a CT scan may avoid the dangers of anticoagulating a patient who has a small hemorrhage. In practice most patients are given ASA as soon as the diagnosis is confirmed.

It has been shown that a small dose (325 mg) of acetylsalicylic acid (aspirin), is effective in reducing the risk of stroke by 25 per cent in men. Other agents such as ticlopidine are currently being assessed. If the source of embolization is later shown to be cardiac, then anticoagulants are used. When they are used it is wise to keep the prothrombin time between 18 and 20 seconds, as this may reduce the risk of bleeding.

If the local morbidity of carotid endarterectomy is under 3 per cent, then the patient operated on will probably do better than those on medical management (enteric-coated aspirin) after 18 months. The decision for surgery depends on the age of the patient and on geographical location. More sophisticated techniques such as transcranial Doppler studies may allow the identification of higher risk groups. The same applies for asymptomatic patients with carotid bruits. These have a much smaller risk of developing a stroke, but again there may be some patients who are at higher risk.

The management and investigation of vertebrobasilar TIA is essentially the same; however, flow factors may play more of a role than embolic

TABLE 1. **Differential Diagnosis**

Seizure
Subdural
Head injury
Hypoglycemia
Other metabolic factors

Adapted from: Hachinski VC and Norris JW: Misdiagnosis of stroke. Lancet 1:328–331, 1982.

factors. In most patients, subclavian steal, which is readily detected by Doppler studies, is a benign condition.

STROKE

The Hemiplegic Patient

A patients who arrives in emergency with a focal neurologic deficit does not necessarily have a stroke. The commonest misdiagnosis is epilepsy with Todd's paresis. The differential diagnosis is given in Table 1.

"What is the lesion?" is of prime importance. Unfortunately nothing can answer this question better than the CT scan, with the sole exception of isotopic imaging of a subdural hematoma. There are, however, some typical presenting features of stroke depending on arterial territory (Table 2). Neither the clinical history nor the examination will infallibly distinguish between a hemorrhage and an infarct, and exclusion of hemorrhage is vital if anticoagulant therapy is to be considered. Because a CT scan of resolved hemorrhage 2 or more weeks after the event may mimic that of an old infarct, it is not very helpful. Some information may be gained from the isotope scan and electroencephalogram (negative in lacunar and posterior fossa strokes).

Several prognostic factors have been identified. In general, the prognosis is poor for older patients with hemispheric infarcts (as opposed to brain stem) and those with ocular deviation away from the hemiparesis.

Blood pressure on arrival may be high and injudicious treatment of this should be avoided. A precipitous drop in blood pressure may lead to an increase in infarct size. Agents such as hydralazine (Apresoline), or sodium nitroprusside (Nipride) may be used to lower the blood pressure slowly, keeping the diastolic pressure above 100

TABLE 2. **Stroke Syndromes**

Anterior cerebral artery (ACA)—leg weaker than arm
Middle cerebral artery (MCA)—arm weaker than leg
Posterior cerebral artery (PCA)—homonymous hemianopia
Lacunar infarcts
Pure motor stroke
Pure sensory stroke
Clumsy hand and dysarthria

mm Hg. Hyperglycemia predisposes to ischemic cell death and normalization of blood sugar is important in the acute phase.

Protection of the so-called penumbra of viable but metabolically inactive brain tissue is the goal of many studies using a variety of agents, including most recently the calcium channel blockers. Some studies are encouraging but more evidence is necessary before a definite statement can be made.

Optimal conditions must be maintained. The patient must have a good cardiac output and good oxygenation. Subsidary tests include an electrocardiogram, chest x-ray and blood tests for hemoglobin, sedimentation rate, glucose, urea, and electrolytes. Some patients, especially in the context of concomitant chest infection, may develop the syndrome of inappropriate secretion of anti-diuretic hormone.

In the first week death usually is due to cerebral factors such as edema and extension of the infarct. The use of steroids to reduce edema has been shown to be ineffective and even dangerous. After this week, bronchopneumonia and pulmonary embolism become the major causes of death. Some centers advocate low dose subcutaneous heparin to prevent deep vein thrombosis; however, early mobilization and physiotherapy are probably just as effective.

Seizures occur in 7 to 10 per cent of stroke patients in the first week. Patients with cardiogenic emboli are more likely to present with a seizure. Such seizures are managed by loading the patient with 15 mg of phenytoin (Dilantin) per kg of body weight intravenously, no faster than 50 mg per minute. Following this, oral therapy is initiated at an appropriate dose (250 to 350 mg daily). Therapy should be continued for 6 months and then cautiously withdrawn.

Strokes in the Young

Strokes may occur in young people, usually for reasons other than atherothrombotic. Such cases require full investigation for vasculopathologic, cardiac causes such as valvular lesions, mitral valve prolapse, syphilis, and arterial anomalies. In young persons with stroke, migraine headaches, pregnancy, and oral contraceptives are risk factors.

One condition which should be recognized in young individuals is carotid dissection. The patient may complain of pain in the neck or behind the eye. There is a gradual onset of deficit and often Horner's syndrome is seen ipsilateral to the dissection. The angiogram shows a characteristic string sign, a thin, drawn-out line of contrast material. Dissection is usually treated with anticoagulants, initially heparin and then warfarin.

It is probably best to avoid urgent surgery, although this is controversial. The etiology of carotid dissection is unknown but there may be a predisposing anatomic deficit of medial necrosis associated with trauma, at times trivial (e.g., related to tennis, aerobics).

Stroke Prevention

Once the acute phase has passed, the physician should arrange for rehabilitation and prevention of a further stroke. Identification of risk factors is often frustrating. Long term anti-platelet therapy following stroke has been shown to be ineffective. The patient who has survived a stroke has a higher risk of myocardial infarction than of another stroke. Beta blocker and anti-platelet therapy may avert this.

REHABILITATION OF THE PATIENT WITH HEMIPLEGIA

method of
STEVEN R. JARRETT, M.D.
Sunnyview Rehabilitation Hospital
Schenectady, New York

Although hemiplegia may be caused by a variety of conditions, by far the most common cause is cerebrovascular accidents. Approximately 400,000 people in the United States will sustain strokes this year. Stroke is the third leading cause of death in the United States. Approximately 50 per cent of stroke survivors will be left with significant residual neurologic disability. Stroke survivors make up the largest single class of neurologically disabled in the adult population. Its prevalence is more than double the combined prevalence of patients with Parkinson's disease, spinal cord injury, multiple sclerosis and head injuries with neurologic sequelae. Although most stroke patients are over 65 years of age, stroke occurs at all age levels and almost equally between the sexes, with a slightly increased incidence in men.

Acute Management

A number of rehabilitative and preventive measures should be performed early in order to insure an optimal functional outcome.

Deep Vein Thrombosis (DVT)

Deep vein thrombosis is a common and usually silent aspect of stroke. It is estimated that between 30 and 60 per cent of stroke patients will develop lower extremity DVT in their plegic limb. All stroke patients should be given thigh length pressure gradient stockings, which should be worn 24 hours per day. Once the patient is able to ambulate with a cane, the stockings may be discontinued. If there is no contraindication to anticoagulation, then minidose heparin should be given subcutaneously at a dosage of 5000 units every 8 or 12 hours.

Positioning

Proper positioning in bed is necessary to prevent early contracture formation. Initially, the affected extremities are flaccid, but increased tone can occur within the first 24 hours. The affected upper extremity will typically develop abnormal tone which makes it adduct and internally rotate at the shoulder, flex at the elbow with the forearm pronated, and flex at the wrist and fingers. The arm should be positioned with the shoulder abducted and externally rotated, and a rolled washcloth in the hand can prevent complete flexion of the digits. Of utmost importance is the need to prevent shoulder subluxation, a far too common occurrence in stroke patients. Shoulder subluxation occurs in the flaccid arm due to laxity of the rotator cuff muscles and especially the supraspinatus. It is less likely to occur once increased tone has developed in these muscles. Initially the arm should be supported so the humerus does not slip from the glenoid when the patient is being sat up or transferred. When the patient is sitting in a wheelchair, the arm should be supported on a lap board. When the patient is standing, a sling should be used. Positioning of the lower extremity consists of placing sandbags about the leg to prevent external rotation of the hip and the use of a footboard to prevent foot drop. Once tone has returned, the use of the footboard should be discontinued as the plantar stimulation may induce increased flexor spasticity of the foot. Blankets and upper bedsheets should not be tucked in at the foot of the bed.

Inherent in proper positioning is the use of passive range of motion of all affected joints and should be carried out once each nursing shift. In addition frequent turning and repositioning are necessary to prevent decubiti, especially in those patients with sensory loss.

Dysphagia

Swallowing disturbances are frequently encountered in patients with bilateral hemisphere involvement with pseudobulbar palsy or patients with brain stem strokes. Recognition of this problem is mandatory if aspiration is to be prevented. Unfortunately, observation of the patient alone is not always sufficient, as patients with poor gag and cough responses may be aspirating without any overt clues. The state of the art in diagnosing this problem is the use of a modified barium swallow using cineradiographic techniques. Barium is used in different consistencies of liquid and a barium-coated cookie and hamburger are also utilized. The trained speech pathologist can readily evaluate the swallowing mechanism of different consistency liquids and solids, and make proper recommendations about a safe diet and therapeutic compensatory techniques and retraining to prevent aspiration.

Bladder and Bowel Management

Initially, many stroke patients may be incontinent of urine. At times this may be due to the patient's not being able to communicate his or her needs. The vast majority of patients will become continent with time and the use of frequent (every 2 hours) and consistent offers to have the patient void. In men who are initially incontinent but who do not have urinary retention, the use of an external condom collecting device may be used. In men with retention and in females, the use of intermittent catheterization is less likely to cause infection and is therefore preferable to the use of an indwelling catheter.

Patients with bowel incontinence do well with the use of daily stool softeners and daily or alternate day use of a suppository such as bisacodyl (Dulcolax) to provide evacuation.

Postacute Management

Mobility

The greatest initial concern of almost all patients and their families is whether the patient will be able to walk again. The vast majority of stroke patients will return to an ambulatory status. Those that don't usually do not because of severe proprioceptive sensory loss in their limb or significant visual spatial disturbances, hemineglect or other cognitive and perceptual deficits. Rarely, the patient is nonambulatory due to the lack of sufficient motoric return in the lower extremity.

Mobility training is done by the physical therapist and starts at bedside with bed mobility—that is, the ability to roll from side to side and eventually to sit up in bed. This is followed by exercises to improve sitting balance; at the same time training in stand pivot transfers is started. The patient then progresses to standing in the parallel bars, working on weight shifting and standing balance and finally on gait training. The patient finally progresses out of the parallel bars to gait training with assistive devices such as a hemiwalker, quadriped cane, and eventually a straight cane or no assistive devices. The patient then progresses to ambulation on stairs (with and without railings), curbs, ramps and uneven ground.

Motoric return in the lower extremity starts proximally and works its way distally. The fact that as tone returns to the leg, it tends to cause extension of the knee on weight bearing is a definite help. Some patients may initially need bracing of the knee but this can usually be soon discarded. Bracing of the ankle is not uncommon in order for the patient to ambulate with safety. In addition to the timeworn but effective double upright metal braces that have long been used, light weight polypropylene ankle foot orthoses are frequently used. The determining factor in the type of ankle foot orthosis used will depend on the amount of spasticity present, the degree of equinovarus deformity on weight bearing, the amount of edema in the foot, and the condition of the skin of the foot. Patients that require bracing of the knee indefinitely as well as of the ankle are usually not able to be functionally ambulatory.

Patients who are nonambulatory should be fitted with an appropriate wheelchair without a foot rest on their uninvolved side, so that they may propel and steer the chair with their functional arm and leg. Electric wheelchairs are almost never prescribed, since the cognitive and perceptual deficits that have kept the patient from walking will also make it unsafe for him to use a power wheelchair.

Upper Extremity Function and Activities of Daily Living

Approximately 40 per cent of stroke patients will get relatively complete motoric return in their affected upper extremity. This group usually shows some return, both proximally and in the wrist and hand in the first week with almost complete return in the first month. Another 40 per cent will have partial motoric return, with the wrist and hand usually having the least functional return and the extremity being useful only as an assistive limb. Twenty per cent of patients will have no motoric return. Even in the group with full return, many patients will have sensory losses (both peripheral, such as touch and temperature, and cortical, such as two-point discrimination and stereognosis), which makes the extremity useless for functional activities.

Thus it can be seen that the vast majority of patients will have to be taught to perform their activities of daily living (ADLs) one-handed. These include grooming, feeding, toileting, dressing, bathing, and kitchen activities. In most cases adaptive devices will enable the patient to carry out these activities one-handed. Examples are long-handled shoe horns, elastic shoe laces, velcro closures on clothing, front fasteners for bras, and button hooks; elevated toilet seats and railings for tub and shower are devices designed to make transfers easier. A myriad of adaptive devices are commercially available through catalogs, and the occupational therapist can often custom fabricate devices as they are needed. Just as with ambulation, failure to become independent in ADLs is usually more a reflection of cognitive and perceptual disturbances (hemineglect, dressing agnosia, poor short-term memory) than the fact that the patient has only one functional upper extremity.

Communication Disturbances

All stroke patients with communication disorders should be seen by a speech pathologist and should receive a hearing evaluation by an audiologist. Strokes affecting either hemisphere may result in weakness of the oral pharyngeal musculature, resulting in speech which is grammatically correct but often unintelligible (dysarthria). Appropriate exercises provided by the speech pathologist usually will overcome problems of intelligibility.

Aphasia usually results from strokes affecting the dominant hemisphere and therefore is most common in right hemiplegics. Aphasia is a disturbance of language and may be expressive, receptive, or both. In addition, patients with aphasia may have varying degrees of disturbances in reading, writing, and carrying out arithmetic computations. Apraxia (a motoric inability to initiate speech) may also accompany aphasia. The speech pathologist will administer a number of standardized tests to determine the type and severity of the aphasia. The type of specific therapy undertaken will usually depend on the type of aphasia. Some aphasics continue to make improvements with therapy 4 and 5 years post stroke. Global aphasia has the worst prognosis, while anomic aphasia and conduction aphasia usually have the best prognosis for recovery. Broca's and Wernicke's aphasias are generally in the middle prognostically.

The inability to communicate is often the most frustrating component of a stroke to the patient. Families should be involved with the speech therapist early to learn techniques to more easily communicate. These may involve the use of increased voice and facial expression, gestures, pointing to items and slowing speech while simplifying sentences to include only one idea at a time. The family will often be carrying out most of the speech therapy as instructed by the speech pathologist long after the patient is discharged from the hospital. It is important for family, friends, and staff to realize that even though expressive abilities are often severely impaired, receptive abilities may be more functional, so they should never say things in the presence of the patient that they would not say were he not aphasic.

Lesions in the nondominant hemisphere may cause abnormalities in expressive and receptive intonation and inflection called aprosodia. When expressive, the patient's statements will sound flat; the patient may thus appear to be depressed even when this is not the case. Receptive disturbances prevent the patient from understanding statements spoken with different inflections and whose meaning is thus differentiated by how it is said. The speech pathologist plays a key role in the diagnosis and treatment of these disorders.

Behavioral Disturbances

Behavioral disturbances in patients during stroke rehabilitation are fairly common. The rehabilitation staff not only needs to be aware of their presence but why they are present. A person's reaction to a stroke may result in denial, hopelessness, lack of cooperation with the program, unrealistic expectations of recovery, depression, and other behavioral abnormalities. Much of this will be determined by three factors: the patient's premorbid psychological makeup, the response to deficits caused by the stroke, and damage to areas of the brain by the stroke that control behavioral responses.

Premorbid factors include overlearned behaviors (which are more likely to be preserved) and whether the patient believed he had control over life's events or felt he had no control (locus of control theory). Response to deficits of the stroke will depend on how the patient perceives the severity of the deficit. The loss of ability to read may have a significantly different impact on a college professor than it does on a patient who never had a high school education. Last, the patient's coping abilities may be seriously impaired due to damage to the brain areas that affect neurobehavioral coping mechanisms.

In the last few years, post-stroke depression has received a great deal of attention. Approximately 50 per cent of stroke patients will develop a depression. Most of these are reactive and are not long lasting. Other patients may have depression lasting for months or years that may be more endogenous than reactive. Studies have shown that patients who have involvement of the left frontal lobe are at risk for more severe and longer-lasting depression. Many of these patients benefit from antidepressant medication. My first choice is usually trazodone (Desyrel), titrated to therapeutic blood levels, as it has less anticholin-ergic and fewer cardiac side effects than comparable antidepressants. I have not had any instances among my patients of the side effect of priapism.

Neuropsychological Disturbances

It is becoming more common to have all nonaphasic patients undergo neuropsychological testing. Most severe cognitive and perceptual problems will be due to lesions in the nondominant hemisphere (left hemiplegics) and will be readily apparent to the rehabilitation staff. However, more subtle deficits may be present from lesions in either hemisphere; if undetected these may have significant impact on the patient's safety and ability to function properly after discharge. Testing may reveal problems with reaction time that would seriously interfere with driving abilities, although from all outward appearances the patient may appear competent to drive a motor vehicle, based on complete motoric and sensory return. As another example, although a patient may be able to do arithmetic problems presented to him verbally, more complex calculations that have to be done on paper may reveal subtle spatial abnormalities that prevent the patient from correctly doing columnar manipulations; this may have a profound effect on his ability to manage a checkbook or pay bills. Lack of insight into deficits, lack of judgment in solving new or unusual problems, decreased attention span, memory deficits, impulsivity, lack of safety awareness, and reasoning impairments are all areas that should be investigated, as they all may have major impacts on the patient's ability to care for himself safely and return to premorbid vocational or avocational pursuits.

The Family

The stroke patient cannot be treated in isolation. The patient's stroke has also affected the family members. The family needs to be counseled in regard to the residual deficits of the stroke and their implications as to the patient's future role in the family. Family members should be encouraged to take part in the therapy sessions both on the nursing unit with the rehabilitation nurse and in the physical, occupational, and speech therapy departments. Stroke education programs should be provided for family members in group formats. Counseling should be given on an individual basis and should address such problems as depression, role reversal, and sexuality. Arrangements should be made for support services to continue after discharge. These may include ongoing therapy services in the home or as an outpatient in the hospital or a day care or day hospital setting. The family should be apprised of other community support services such as stroke clubs. Financial hardships caused by the stroke should be investigated and attempts made to secure support from available social agencies. The need for home health aides or homemaker services should be assessed and appropriate arrangements made for those services. When applicable, vocational exploration should be undertaken.

Prior to hospital discharge, the entire rehabilitation team should have a meeting with the patient and family and any providers of future services to be sure that all physical, emotional, and social needs have been addressed and provided for. When necessary, arrangements should be available for team members to visit the patient's home to make recommendations for home modifications to improve independence and safety.

Other Considerations

Spasticity

Spasticity is the most common complicating physical factor encountered in stroke rehabilitation. It is often a double-edged sword in that it may help the patient support his weight while standing but may interfere with function of the hand and arm.

Systemic medications used for spasticity include diazepam (Valium), dantrolene (Dantrium), and baclofen (Lioresal). All must be started at low dosage and titrated upward. Unfortunately they all have undesirable side effects ranging from drowsiness to a feeling of weakness of the extremities. Combinations of these drugs will occasionally minimize some of their side effects, but generally they have not proved very useful in treating spasticity in stroke victims. The one instance in which I have found them useful is with the patient who has painful flexion of the toes when ambulating. In this case I have had the best results with Dantrium, building up the dosage usually to approximately 150 mg per day in 3 or 4 divided doses. Liver function studies need to be regularly monitored in these patients because of reported hepatotoxicity, but no fatal reactions have been reported at that dosage level.

More effective for upper extremity spasticity is the use of phenol motor point blocks. These will often reduce spasticity that was masking voluntary muscular function of the antagonist muscles. Results usually last for months, at which time the procedure can be repeated.

Rarely, surgical procedures such as tendon lengthenings and transfers may be useful in producing a more functional extremity.

Shoulder-Hand Syndrome. It is not known why some patients develop shoulder-hand syndrome following stroke and others do not. What is accepted now is that the syndrome is a form of reflex sympathetic dystrophy. It usually starts 1 to 3 months post stroke but can occur up to 6 months post stroke. The shoulder-hand syndrome is characterized by pain in the shoulder, pain and edema of the hand, trophic skin changes, and normal, pain-free elbow motion with limitations in movement of the shoulder and hand. If left untreated, the hand will progress to atrophy of the subcutaneous tissues and severe contractures. Bone scan is extremely helpful in diagnosing this condition early, when there is the best chance for treatment. Treatment should include frequent range-of-motion exercises of the shoulder and hand, elevation of the hand above heart level, and the use of isotonic gloves to prevent edema. A course of oral steroids is usually more effective than stellate ganglion blocks, but the latter can also be employed.

EPILEPSY IN ADOLESCENTS AND ADULTS

method of
THOMAS R. BROWNE, M.D.
Boston University School of Medicine
Boston, Massachusetts

Epilepsy is a common disease with a prevalence estimated at 6 to 34 per 1000 population. Hughlings Jackson put forth the modern definition of a seizure in 1870: ". . . an occasional, excessive, and disorderly discharge of nerve tissue." The points to note are that there is an excessive rate of firing of brain cells, that this firing occurs occasionally (i.e., the firing begins and ends abruptly), and that the usual methods of controlling neuronal discharge break down.

DIAGNOSIS

Determining Type of Epileptic Seizure

The first step in managing a patient who may have epilepsy is establishing definitively whether or not the patient has epilepsy. If a patient who does not have epilepsy is given the diagnosis of epilepsy, he may be unnecessarily subjected to major inconveniences including medication with serious side effects, expensive laboratory tests, loss of driver's license, and even loss of employment.

If a patient *has* epilepsy, it is crucial to determine accurately the type(s) of epileptic seizure the patient has in order that he be given correct therapy. Seizure type diagnosis should be made according to the International Classification of Epileptic Seizures (Table 1). Persons not familiar with this diagnostic system should

TABLE 1. International Classification of Epileptic Seizures

I. Partial (Focal, Local) Seizures
- A. Simple partial seizures (consciousness not impaired)
  1. With motor signs
  2. With sensory symptoms
  3. With autonomic symptoms or signs
  4. With psychic symptoms
- B. Complex partial seizures (temporal lobe or psychomotor seizures) (consciousness usually impaired)
  1. Simple partial onset followed by impairment of consciousness
     - a. With simple partial features (A.1–A.4), followed by impaired consciousness
     - b. With automatisms
  2. With impairment of consciousness at onset
     - a. With impairment of consciousness only
     - b. With automatisms
- C. Partial seizures evolving to secondarily generalized seizures (tonic-clonic, tonic, or clonic)
  1. Simple partial seizures (A) evolving to generalized seizures
  2. Complex partial seizures (B) evolving to generalized seizures
  3. Simple partial seizures evolving to complex partial seizures evolving to generalized seizures

II. Generalized Seizures (Convulsive or Nonconvulsive)
- A. Absence (petit mal) seizures
- B. Myoclonic seizures
- C. Clonic seizures
- D. Tonic seizures
- E. Tonic-clonic (grand mal) seizures
- F. Atonic seizures

consult a textbook on epilepsy. An incorrect seizure diagnosis will often result in the patient's being given medication that will not control his seizure disorder and that may cause serious side effects.

The best way to diagnose the type of seizure is to actually observe a seizure, although the physician usually does not have the opportunity to do so. Often the most important differential diagnostic information is the history obtained from the patient and reliable observers. The physician must elicit the exact details of the aura, ictus, and postictal period of the patient's seizures.

The electroencephalogram (EEG) is a helpful diagnostic tool in the investigation of a seizure disorder. It confirms the presence of abnormal electrical activity, gives information regarding the type of seizure disorder, and discloses the location of the seizure focus. There are instances in which the routine EEG is normal in spite of the fact that the patient has seizures or is suspected of having them. Under these circumstances the study is repeated after the patient is deprived of sleep for an entire night; special (e.g., temporal or nasopharyngeal) leads may also be employed. This procedure is helpful in bringing out the abnormality in many cases. Temporal and nasopharyngeal leads are particularly useful in detecting abnormal discharges from the temporal lobe.

In cases in which the history unequivocally points to a seizure disorder, the patient should be treated despite "normal" waking and sleep-deprived EEGs. The usual EEG study samples only an hour or so of time and is normal in a significant percentage of patients with epilepsy. In cases in which it is not certain if the patient has epilepsy or in which it is not certain which type of seizure a patient has despite a careful history, physical examination, and routine waking and sleep-deprived EEGs, the diagnosis often can be established by prolonged EEG monitoring.

Determining Underlying Causes and Precipitating Factors

Epilepsy is a symptom, not a disease. A seizure can be a symptom of old or recent cerebral trauma, a brain tumor, a brain abscess, encephalitis, meningitis, a metabolic disturbance, drug intoxication, drug withdrawal, and many other disease processes. It is imperative that the underlying cause of a patient's seizures be identified and treated so that a reversible cerebral disease process is not overlooked and in order to facilitate seizure control.

Determining the cause of a patient's seizure disorder involves a combination of history taking, physical examination, and laboratory tests. The history should include questions regarding epilepsy in family history, birth complications, febrile convulsions, middle ear infections and sinus infections (which may erode through bone and cause cerebral focus), head trauma, alcohol or drug abuse, and symptoms of malignancy. The physical examination should look for evidence of past or recent head trauma, infections of the ears and sinuses, congenital abnormalities (e.g., hemiatrophy, stigmata of tuberous sclerosis), focal or diffuse neurologic abnormalities, stigmata of alcohol or drug abuse, and signs of malignancy.

Usually the following laboratory tests should be performed in evaluating the cause of a newly diagnosed seizure disorder: metabolic screen, EEG recording in waking and sleep states, skull radiography (including views of sinuses and/or mastoids if history indicates possible infection), lumbar puncture (for opening pressure, cell counts, protein, glucose, culture, and serology), and magnetic resonance imaging (MRI) or computed tomography (CT).

In addition to determining the underlying cause(s) of a patient's seizure disorder, it is also important to identify and manage factors that precipitate seizures in a given individual, such as anxiety, sleep deprivation, or alcohol withdrawal. Management of such precipitating factors will reduce seizure frequency and reduce the patient's need for medication.

Identifying and Dealing with Psychological and Social Problems

Seizures are a relatively rare phenomenon for most patients. However, the psychosocial consequences of having epilepsy are present all the time. Loss of driver's license, employment, self-esteem, and position in peer groups are all potential problems and may cause more suffering than the seizures themselves. Furthermore, the anxiety associated with these psychosocial consequences of epilepsy may precipitate seizures in some patients. The physician must anticipate that the patient will experience psychosocial problems as a consequence of having epilepsy and must be prepared to assist the patient by carefully explaining the nature of his medical problems and the effect the problems will have on driving and employment, by providing emotional support, by giving the patient an opportunity to "talk through" his problems, and by referring the patient to various resources available to assist individuals with epilepsy (e.g., social workers, epilepsy societies, vocational counselors).

TREATMENT

Begin Monotherapy with the Least Toxic Drug

Once the exact type of seizure(s) a patient has is determined, the physician should initiate monotherapy (single-drug therapy) with the least toxic drug that is likely to produce good long-term seizure control. If a patient has more than one type of seizure, therapy should begin with the least toxic drug for the most bothersome type of seizure. The choice of drug must be made on an individual basis, selecting from available agents the agent that should have the best balance of advantages and disadvantages for a given patient (see below).

The monotherapy approach for initial treatment is based on a growing body of evidence indicating (1) that monotherapy with an appropriately selected drug "pushed" to adequate serum concentration will control seizures in a majority of patients and (2) that polytherapy exposes the patient to several unnecessary risks. Monotherapy of simple partial, complex partial, and tonic-clonic seizures with phenytoin, carbamazepine, phenobarbital, or primidone using the guidelines outlined here will result in satisfactory long-term seizure control in 56 to 88 per cent of patients and complete seizure control in 26 to 80 per cent of patients. Monotherapy of absence seizures with ethosuximide, valproic acid, or clonazepam will result in satisfactory long-term seizure control in 50 to 90 per cent of patients and complete seizure control in 50 per cent of patients. The principal reason for the high rate of success of modern monotherapy trials when compared with older monotherapy trials is the availability of drug-level monitoring that detects low drug serum concentration, which has been the major reason for failure of monotherapy in the past. Factors that appear to be associated with failure of modern monotherapy include persistent noncompliance, drug allergy, large or progressive brain lesions, partial seizures, more than one type of seizure, neuropsychiatric handicaps, and high pretreatment seizure frequency.

The risks of unnecessary polytherapy are many. Chronic toxicity is associated with the use of any antiepileptic drug, and minimizing the number of drugs taken minimizes the risks of toxicity. Unnecessary polytherapy is particularly likely to include barbiturates with their high risk for cognitive and behavioral toxicity. Other risks of unnecessary polytherapy include drug allergy, drug interactions, exacerbation of seizures, and inability to evaluate the effectiveness of individual antiepileptic drugs.

"Push" the First Drug Tried

The first drug tried for a seizure disorder is usually the least toxic drug available, and the physician must be certain he has obtained the maximum possible therapeutic effect from the first drug before adding other drugs. Therapy usually begins with an "average" dose of antiepileptic drug. If the seizures are controlled with this average dose and there are no serious side effects, no changes are necessary. If the seizures are not controlled with this dose and there is no serious drug toxicity, the dosage of the drug should be systematically increased until the seizures are controlled or side effects preclude further dosage increase.

The drug serum concentration should be determined if a patient's seizures are not controlled by an average or high drug dosage. There are many correctable causes of lower than expected drug serum concentration, including inadequate dosing rate, noncompliance, poor absorption, drug interactions, generic drug substitution, pregnancy, and patient error. It would be a serious error to substitute or to add a more toxic drug because the patient has a low serum concentration of the first drug. A drug cannot be said to be ineffective until it is documented that the seizures are not controlled with a high therapeutic serum concentration of the drug unless drug toxicity precludes reaching such concentrations.

The "therapeutic range" of drug serum concentrations represents values applicable to "average" patients. Some patients require higher drug serum concentrations than the therapeutic range for good seizure control. If a patient has a high therapeutic serum concentration of a nontoxic drug, poor seizure control, and no drug side effects, the best approach usually is to increase the dosage of the first drug rather than add a more toxic second drug.

Add Additional Drugs

If the first drug tried is pushed to its maximum tolerated dosage and/or high therapeutic serum concentration and seizures still are not controlled, a second antiepileptic drug should be added. In general, it is best to add the second drug and continue administration of the first drug (at least temporarily) because (1) the first drug will provide protection while the serum concentration of the second drug is being built up, (2) discontinuing the first drug may result in withdrawal activation of the seizure disorder, and (3) there is evidence that two antiepileptic drugs in combination may control seizures in some patients when either drug alone will not.

When a therapeutic serum concentration of the second drug is obtained, the physician should consider tapering the patient off the first drug because of the many hazards of chronic polytherapy. The decision to taper the patient off the first drug must be individualized and take into consideration the antiepileptic effect of the first drug when given alone, the side effects of the first drug, and the psychosocial consequences for the patient of having a seizure if withdrawal of the first drug results in loss of complete seizure control. The many adverse effects of antiepileptic drugs on behavior and cognition argue strongly for attempting to minimize the number of such drugs given to children. In adults, the hazards of polytherapy must be weighed against the risk of loss of job and/or driver's license if withdrawal of the first drug results in a recurrence of seizures. If it is elected to withdraw the first drug, the withdrawal should be done slowly (see below).

A third drug should not be added until it is documented that seizures cannot be controlled with maximum tolerated doses and/or high therapeutic serum concentrations of the first two drugs tried. It is usually better to add a third drug (at least temporarily) than to substitute the third drug for the first and/or second drug, for reasons similar to those cited above for adding rather than substituting the second drug. After a therapeutic serum concentration of the third drug is reached, the physician may elect to withdraw one of the first two drugs using the guidelines outlined above.

Duration of Therapy

Uncontrolled seizures and seizures due to a progressive neurologic illness (e.g., astrocytoma) are indications for continuing antiepileptic drug therapy indefinitely. Antiepileptic drug therapy should usually be maintained for a minimum of 2 to 5 years after diagnosis of epilepsy, even if the patient has no further seizures. When a patient has been free of seizures for 2 to 5 years on antiepileptic drug therapy, the need for continued therapy can be re-evaluated. Risk factors have been identified that help the physician evaluate the likelihood of seizures recurring after medication has been discontinued.

Patients who continue to have an abnormal EEG (spikes, sharp waves, paroxysmal activity, or nonparoxysmal abnormalities) have a 30 to 51 per cent chance of recurrence of seizures if antiepileptic medication is discontinued. Other risk factors include (1) the occurrence of many generalized seizures before control with medication, (2) long duration between onset of therapy and seizure control, (3) presence of a known structural lesion and/or neurologic deficit, (4) mental retardation, (5) onset of seizures before 2 years of age, (6) adult onset of complex partial seizures, and (7) more than one seizure type.

Each decision must be made on an individual basis. A history of seizure frequency and risk factors must be obtained. A routine EEG is mandatory, and a long-term EEG recording is sometimes desirable. The probability of recurrent seizures, the consequences of having another seizure, and the benefits of living without medication must be discussed with the patient. A judgment must be weighted by the needs of the individual.

If it is elected to discontinue antiepileptic therapy, medication should be withdrawn slowly. Elimination of 1 pill per day every 5 elimination half-lives is probably the optimal regimen. More rapid tapering of therapy may precipitate seizures, and more prolonged withdrawal probably does not reduce the risk of seizure recurrence.

Antiepileptic Drug Therapy During Pregnancy

Most antiepileptic drugs appear to possess some teratogenic risk in humans, which may be dose-dependent. Women of child-bearing age should be advised of this risk. If possible, antiepileptic drugs should be discontinued during pregnancy. If not, the lowest effective dose of the least teratogenic drug should be administered. Unfortunately, the relative teratogenicity of antiepileptic drugs in humans has never been established definitively; trimethadione, phenytoin, and valproic acid may possess greater risk than alternative agents. The dosing rate necessary to maintain a given serum concentration increases during pregnancy due to increased volume of distribution, increased biotransformation, and decreased absorption. Phenytoin, phenobarbital, and primidone may lower the maternal folic acid level and increase the risk of third trimester and neonatal hemorrhage. Hydantoins and barbiturates may cause neonatal hemorrhage due to depression of vitamin K–dependent clotting factors.

Antiepileptic Drugs of Choice for Simple Partial, Complex Partial, and Tonic-Clonic Seizures

Simple partial, complex partial, and tonic-clonic seizures are the most common types of seizure disorders in adolescents and adults. Phenytoin (Dilantin), carbamazepine (Tegretol), phenobarbital, and primidone (Mysoline) are the drugs usually employed for treatment (Table 2). Only one study has compared these four drugs in a comprehensive, double-blind efficacy study for partial and tonic-clonic seizures. Treatment success was highest with phenytoin and carbamazepine, intermediate with phenobarbital, and lowest with primidone. Neither this study nor four double-blind comparisons of phenytoin versus carbamazepine for partial and tonic-clonic seizures have demonstrated any statistically significant differences in efficacy of these drugs for these seizure types. Thus, phenytoin and carbamazepine are the two most effective drugs for partial and tonic-clonic seizures and have similar efficacy. The choice between phenytoin and carbamazepine for a given patient depends on weighing the advantages and disadvantages of these two drugs other than efficacy (see below).

Phenytoin (Dilantin)

Advantages. (1) Phenytoin is relatively nonsedating; (2) serious toxicity is rare; (3) parenteral administration is possible; (4) a loading dose may be given by the oral or intravenous route; (5) it need only be taken once a day by a majority of adults; and (6) it is relatively inexpensive.

Disadvantages. (1) Phenytoin may cause some sedation and/or impairment of higher intellectual function; (2) there is a relatively high incidence of annoying side effects with chronic administration, including gingival hyperplasia, hirsutism, acne, and coarsening of facial features.

Pharmacokinetics. (See Table 3.) Approximately 85 per cent of an orally administered dose of

Dilantin, 100-mg extended-release Kapseals, is absorbed slowly over a period of 24 hours. The rate and extent of absorption for generic phenytoin preparations are highly variable. Intramuscular phenytoin is slowly and erratically absorbed. Phenytoin is 69 to 96 per cent protein bound and is biotransformed by the liver. Phenytoin has dose-dependent pharmacokinetics with the following consequences: (1) serum concentration increases (or decreases) faster than dosing rate when dosing rate is increased (or decreased); (2) time to reach steady state after change in dosing rate may vary from 5 to 28 days; (3) serum concentration at one dosing rate does not directly predict serum concentration at another dosing rate.

Usual Adult Dosage. In many adults, 4 to 5 mg per kg of Dilantin, 100-mg Kapseals, may be administered once daily. The daily dosage is usually given at bedtime to minimize side effects associated with peak serum concentration. The following individuals should receive Dilantin Kapseals in at least 2 divided doses daily: (1) persons who have unacceptable toxicity associated with peak serum concentration with once daily administration, (2) children (children have shorter phenytoin elimination half-lives than adults), and (3) persons who do not obtain complete seizure control with once-daily administration (seizures may occur at time of trough serum concentration). Persons receiving a "prompt release" phenytoin preparation (i.e., not an extended-release preparation) should utilize a twice-daily or 3-times daily regimen. Phenytoin is available in 30- and 100-mg capsules and 50-mg tablets. Note that the only extended-release forms of phenytoin are certain 100-mg capsules. A syrup for oral dosage and a parenteral form are also available.

Toxicity

LOCAL. Gastric distress with early treatment (can often be alleviated by taking medication with meals).

DOSE-RELATED. Cerebellar signs (ataxia, limb movement, dysarthria, nystagmus); encephalopathy; changes in mental state ranging from dysphoria and mild confusion to coma; choreiform movements; increased seizure frequency.

IDIOSYNCRATIC. Dermatitis (usually morbilliform and appearing within the first 2 weeks of therapy); agranulocytosis, thrombocytopenia, and aplastic anemia; Stevens-Johnson syndrome; hepatitis; nephritis; lymphoma-like syndrome, thyroiditis; systemic lupus erythematosus; hyperglycemia.

Side Effects. Side effects include hirsutism (in an estimated 5 per cent of patients); gingival hyperplasia (can be minimized with careful den-

TABLE 2. **Antiepileptic Drugs of Choice**

Seizure Type	Drug(s) of First Choice	Alternative Drugs
Simple and complex partial	Phenytoin Carbamazepine	Phenobarbital Primidone
Secondary generalized partial	Phenytoin Carbamazepine Phenobarbital	Primidone
Primary generalized tonic-clonic	Phenytoin Carbamazepine	Phenobarbital[1] Primidone[1] Valproic acid[1,2,3]
Absence	Ethosuximide	Valproic acid[3] Clonazepam

[1]Definitive comparative studies not done; recommended use is based on available non-definitive data.

[2]Not an FDA-approved indication, unless accompanied by absence seizures.

[3]Valproic acid is the drug of choice in patients having both absence and tonic-clonic seizures.

TABLE 3. **Pharmacokinetics of Antiepileptic Drugs***

Drug	Indications†	Starting Dose (mg/day)	Maintenance Dose (mg/day)	Elimination Half-Life (hours)	Time to Steady-State Plasma Concentration (days)	Therapeutic Range of Plasma Concentration (μg/ml)
Phenytoin (Dilantin)	T-C, CP	300	300–500	10–34	7–8	10–20
Carbamazepine (Tegretol)	T-C, CP, SP	200	600–1200	14–27	3–4	4–12
Phenobarbital	T-C, CP, SP	90	90–240	46–136	14–21	10–40
Primidone (Mysoline)	T-C, CP, SP	125	750–1500	6–18	4–7	5–12
Ethosuximide (Zarontin)	A	500	500–1500	20–60	7–10	40–120
Valproic Acid (Depakene, Depakote)	A	1000	1000–4000	6–15	1–2	40–150
Clonazepam (Klonopin)	A, AT, M	1.5	1.5–20	20–40	—	—

*All values are for adults.

†A = absence; AT = atonic; CP = complex partial; M = myoclonic; SP = simple partial; T-C = tonic-clonic.

tal hygiene and avoidance of high serum concentrations); accelerated scar formation; thickening of subcutaneous tissues of face and scalp; Dupuytren's contractures; acne; folic acid, vitamin K, and vitamin D deficiency; low levels of immunoglobulin A; peripheral neuropathy (usually motor and without clinical manifestations).

Drug Interactions. Drug interactions with other antiepileptic drugs are summarized in Table 4. The following other drugs may elevate phenytoin serum concentrations: cimetidine, disulfiram, isoniazid, dicumarol, chloramphenicol, methylphenidate, diazepam, sulfamethizole, phenylbutazone, chlorpromazine, chlordiazepoxide, and propoxyphene. Ethanol, phenylbutazone, and salicylates have been reported to lower phenytoin serum concentration. Phenytoin has been reported to lower the levels of the following drugs: digitoxin, bishydroxycoumarin, metyrapone, DDT, dexamethasone, cortisol, contraceptive steroids, 25-hydroxycholecalciferol, and thyroxine.

Disease States. Phenytoin intoxication is not likely in renal disease, but relatively high concentrations of unbound drug are present and may need to be specifically determined at times. There is some risk of phenytoin intoxication in hepatic dysfunction.

Carbamazepine (Tegretol)

Advantages. (1) Carbamazepine definitely causes less sedation and impairment of intellectual function than phenobarbital or primidone; (2) it probably causes less sedation and impairment of intellectual function than phenytoin; and (3) it does not have the annoying cosmetic side effects of phenytoin.

Disadvantages. (1) Carbamazepine has been reported to cause serious bone marrow depression and other idiosyncratic reactions in a very small percentage of patients; (2) it may cause diplopia, dizziness, drowsiness, ataxia, or nausea, espe-

cially at onset of therapy; (3) parenteral administration is impossible; (4) a loading dose cannot be administered by the oral or intravenous route; (5) it must be given in divided doses; (6) it is more expensive than alternative drugs.

Pharmacokinetics. (See Table 3.) Approximately 75 to 85 per cent of an orally administered dose

TABLE 4. **Effect of Adding a Second Antiepileptic Drug on Serum Concentration of Original Antiepileptic Drug**

Original Drug	Added Drug	Effect of Added Drug on Serum Concentration of Original Drug
Carbamazepine	Clonazepam	No change
	Phenobarbital	Decrease*
	Phenytoin	Decrease*
	Primidone	Decrease*
Clonazepam	Phenobarbital	Decrease
	Phenytoin	Decrease
	Valproic acid	No change
Ethosuximide	Carbamazepine	Decrease
	Phenobarbital	No change
	Phenytoin	No change
	Primidone	No change
	Valproic acid	Increase or no change
Phenobarbital	Carbamazepine	No change
	Clonazepam	Data conflicting
	Phenytoin	Increase
	Valproic acid	Increase*
Phenytoin	Carbamazepine	Increase*
	Clonazepam	Data conflicting
	Ethosuximide	No change
	Phenobarbital	No change
	Primidone	No change
	Valproic acid	Decrease*
Primidone	Carbamazepine	Increased concentration of derived phenobarbital
	Clonazepam	No change
	Ethosuximide	No change
	Phenytoin	Increased concentration of derived phenobarbital
	Valproic acid	Increase
Valproic acid	Carbamazepine	Decrease*
	Clonazepam	No change
	Ethosuximide	No change
	Phenobarbital	Decrease*
	Phenytoin	Decrease*
	Primidone	Decrease*

*Interactions particularly likely to be encountered in clinical practice.

of Tegretol 200-mg tablets is slowly absorbed after oral administration. The bioavailability of generic carbamazepines is usually less than that of Tegretol. Carbamazepine is 70 to 80 per cent protein bound. Carbamazepine is metabolized by the liver into 32 or more metabolites, some of which (especially epoxide) possess antiepileptic activity. Carbamazepine biotransformation exhibits time-dependent pharmacokinetics (self-induction), which is usually complete within 1 to 2 weeks.

Usual Adult Dosage. Initial dosage is 200 mg twice daily, increased at weekly intervals by adding up to 200 mg per day, given in 3 or 4 daily doses until the best response is obtained. Dosage generally should not exceed 1000 mg daily in children 12 to 15 years of age, and 1200 mg daily in patients above 15 years of age. Doses up to 1600 mg daily* have been used in adults in rare instances. Maintenance dosage is adjusted to the minimum effective level, usually 800 to 1200 mg daily. Carbamazepine is available as 200-mg tablets, 100-mg chewable tablets, and 100 mg per 5 ml oral suspension.

Toxicity

LOCAL. Gastric irritability (usually managed by taking the drug after meals).

DOSE-RELATED. Diplopia or blurred vision; dizziness, drowsiness; ataxia; headache; tremor, dystonia, chorea; depression, irritability; psychosis; convulsions; water retention (inappropriate ADH–like syndrome); congestive heart failure; cardiac arrhythmias.

IDIOSYNCRATIC. Anemia, agranulocytosis, leukopenia, thrombocytopenia; hypersensitivity syndrome (dermatitis, eosinophilia, lymphadenopathy, splenomegaly); cholestatic and hepatocellular jaundice. The rate of fatal idiosyncratic reactions with carbamazepine is estimated currently at 1 in 20,000 to 1 in 1 million patients. While a matter of concern, this risk is in a range similar to that of other commonly used drugs such as penicillin.

Drug Interactions. Interactions of carbamazepine with other antiepileptic drugs are tabulated in Table 4. Propoxyphene, erythromycin, chloramphenicol, and cimetidine may elevate serum carbamazepine concentration. Carbamazepine may accelerate the metabolism of warfarin and tetracycline.

Disease States. Carbamazepine may precipitate or enhance congestive heart failure. Its use should be avoided in this setting or where major arrhythmias are a concern. Plasma levels and potential toxicity need to be closely watched if the drug is used in patients with renal or hepatic disease.

Generic Forms of Phenytoin and Carbamazepine

In order for a generic antiepileptic drug to be declared "equivalent" to a brand-name antiepileptic drug by the FDA, the generic drug must pass certain in vitro dissolution tests and must meet two criteria in comparisons in vivo of brand-name drugs versus generic drugs in cross-over studies performed on volunteers. The first in vivo criterion is that mean per cent difference between brand-name and generic drugs should not be more than 20 per cent for values measuring bioavailability (e.g., drug plasma concentration, peak drug plasma concentration, area under the plasma concentration time curve). The second in vivo criterion is that in at least 75 per cent of subjects administered the generic drug, the generic drug has a bioavailability of greater than 75 per cent relative to that of the brand-name drug. Note that these rather loose in vivo criteria would allow a generic antiepileptic drug to be approved as "equivalent" to a brand-name drug by the FDA despite its having a bioavailability considerably different from that of a brand-name drug in a sizeable percentage of individuals. Switching from a brand-name antiepileptic drug to a generic drug of lesser bioavailability may result in a drop in drug serum concentration and a loss of seizure control with resulting loss of driver's license or physical injury. Switching from a brand-name antiepileptic drug to a generic drug with greater bioavailability may result in increased drug serum concentration and drug intoxication.

In the author's opinion, a generic antiepileptic drug should produce a serum concentration that is 90 to 120 per cent of the serum concentration produced by the brand-name antiepileptic drug *in all patients* to ensure there will not be problems with breakthrough seizures or antiepileptic drug intoxication at the time of switching from a brand-name to a generic drug. None of the generic phenytoin or carbamazepine products currently on the market meet this criterion. Thus, none of the currently marketed generic phenytoin or carbamazepine products can be substituted for a brand-name drug without some risk to the patient.

Phenobarbital

Advantages. (1) Serious toxicity is rare; (2) parenteral administration is possible; (3) a loading dose may be given by the oral or intravenous route; (4) phenobarbital is inexpensive; and (5) it need be taken only once a day by a majority of adults.

---

*Exceeds the maximum dose recommended by the manufacturer.

Disadvantages. (1) It is less effective than phenytoin or carbamazepine, and (2) it causes disabling sedation and/or irritability and/or impairment of higher intellectual function in a high percentage of patients.

Pharmacokinetics. (See Table 3.) Phenobarbital is absorbed slowly (over 6 to 18 hours) but completely from the small intestine. The drug is 40 to 60 per cent protein bound. Approximately one third of an administered dose of phenobarbital is excreted unchanged in the urine, and two thirds is excreted as metabolites created by hepatic biotransformation. Phenobarbital exhibits linear (non–dose-dependent) pharmacokinetics.

Usual Adult Dosage. The usual dosage is 3 to 5 mg per kg per day. Because of phenobarbital's long elimination half-life (approximately 4 days), the drug need only be given once daily (usually at bedtime), unless the toxicity associated with attainment of peak serum concentration causes the patient difficulty. In this case, the drug can be given in 2 divided doses. The 4-day elimination half-life means that 14 to 21 days are required for attainment of steady state phenobarbital serum concentration after a change in dosing rate.

Toxicity

DOSE-RELATED. Sedation and slowed mentation; ataxia.

IDIOSYNCRATIC. Dermatitis; agranulocytosis; aplastic anemia; hepatitis.

Side Effects. Side effects include folic acid, vitamin K, and vitamin D deficiency.

Drug Interactions. Interactions of phenobarbital with other antiepileptic drugs are tabulated in Table 4. Folic acid and dicumarol may lower phenobarbital serum concentrations, whereas chloramphenicol may elevate phenobarbital serum concentrations. Phenobarbital may lower serum concentrations of dexamethasone, digitoxin, and chloramphenicol.

Disease States. The risk of phenobarbital intoxication must be monitored carefully in patients with renal or hepatic disease.

Primidone (Mysoline)

Advantage. Serious toxicity is rare.

Disadvantages. (1) It is less effective than phenytoin or carbamazepine; (2) there is a very high incidence of toxicity at time of initiation of therapy (nausea, dizziness, ataxia, somnolence); (3) in a high percentage of patients, it causes disabling sedation and/or irritability and/or impairment of higher intellectual function during chronic administration; (4) parenteral administration is impossible; (5) a loading dose cannot be administered by the oral or intravenous route; (6) it is significantly more expensive than phenobarbital; (7) the patient must pay for monitoring of two blood levels (primidone and phenobarbital) each time blood level is checked; and (8) the drug must be given in divided doses.

Pharmacokinetics. (See Table 3.) Primidone is rapidly absorbed from the gastrointestinal tract. Protein binding is minimal. Biotransformation of primidone leads to the formation of two metabolites, phenobarbital and phenylethylmalonamide (PEMA); each has antiepileptic activity, along with primidone per se. The rate of conversion to phenobarbital is enhanced by concurrent use of inducing drugs such as phenytoin. When primidone is given as a monotherapy drug, the derived phenobarbital concentration may be less than the serum concentration of primidone. Concurrent use of inducing drugs will often provide serum concentrations of primidone that are one third those of the metabolically derived phenobarbital. Concurrent use of primidone and phenobarbital should be avoided to prevent phenobarbital toxicity (this is further enhanced if a third drug with metabolic induction qualities is employed).

Usual Adult Dosage. Special care is needed with the initiation of therapy, particularly in patients who are starting drug treatment for the first time. Previous treatment with phenobarbital (which should be discontinued if primidone is to be used) allows for a smooth introduction of this drug. The patient should take the initial dose at bedtime, and no more than 125 mg (50-mg tablets are available for initiation and it is often best to begin with a dose of this size) should be given. Dosage adjustments are made with the goal of attaining serum concentrations no greater than 15 micrograms per ml (2 hours after ingestion). Primidone is available in 50-mg and 250-mg tablets and a suspension.

Toxicity

DOSE-RELATED. Sedation; ataxia.

IDIOSYNCRATIC. Dermatitis, leukopenia and thrombocytopenia, agranulocytosis and aplastic anemia, lymphadenopathy, hepatitis, lupus erythematosus, personality change.

Side Effects. The patient should be forewarned about side effects such as dizziness, nausea, sedation, and ataxia at the time of initiation of therapy. Rarely, hallucinatory states have also been observed. Thirty per cent of individuals are unable to tolerate this drug and discontinue it during the first 3 months of administration. Prolonged therapy may be associated with folic acid, vitamin D, and vitamin K deficiency.

Drug Interactions. Interactions with other antiepileptic drugs are shown in Table 4. Isoniazid may inhibit primidone metabolism.

Disease States. The risk of primidone toxicity is enhanced in instances of renal disease; its effect on hepatic disease is less clear.

Valproic Acid (Depakene, Depakote)

Valproic acid has never been compared with phenytoin or carbamazepine in a definitive double-blind study of efficacy for initial therapy of partial or tonic-clonic seizures. Valproic acid is an expensive and potentially dangerous drug. Valproic acid is not approved by the FDA for treatment of partial or tonic-clonic seizures unless they are accompanied by absence seizures.

Uncontrolled studies of valproic acid as initial or adjunctive therapy for partial seizures have produced variable results. These studies show that only about 30 per cent of patients with secondary generalized tonic-clonic seizures have good control with valproic acid. Existing medical evidence and medical legal considerations dictate limited usage of valproic acid for partial seizures or secondary generalized tonic-clonic seizures at the present time. However, uncontrolled studies indicate that valproic acid may possess considerable efficacy for primary generalized tonic-clonic seizures. Many experts consider valproic acid the preferred monotherapy drug for patients with the combination of absence and tonic-clonic seizures. Valproic acid also may be effective monotherapy for myoclonic and tonic-clonic seizures of adolescence (syndrome of Janz). (See below for further details.)

Other Drugs for Partial and Tonic-Clonic Seizures

Clorazepate dipotassium, phenacemide, mephenytoin, and ethotoin are less consistently effective and/or more toxic than phenytoin, carbamazepine, phenobarbital, or primidone in the treatment of partial and tonic-clonic seizures. However, an occasional patient whose seizures cannot be controlled with the four first-line drugs may respond to clorazepate dipotassium, phenacemide, mephenytoin, or ethotoin. In particular, ethotoin should be considered for patients who have had a good therapeutic response to phenytoin but were forced to discontinue the drug because of toxicity.

Antiepileptic Drugs of Choice for Absence Seizures

Ethosuximide, valproic acid, and clonazepam are the three drugs used to treat absence seizures (see Table 2). These drugs have been shown to have equal efficacy in treatment of absence seizures in definitive, double-blind studies. The selection among these agents is based upon weighing advantages and disadvantages, aside from efficacy.

Ethosuximide (Zarontin)

Advantages and Disadvantages. Ethosuximide is the drug of first choice for patients with only absence seizures because it is extremely effective and most patients experience little or no side effects during chronic administration. Gastrointestinal upset and drowsiness, the common side effects of ethosuximide, tend to occur early in therapy and then diminish as tolerance develops. The drug seldom causes behavioral or cognitive disturbances. About 1 to 7 per cent of patients taking ethosuximide develop leukopenia, which is reversible if detected early.

Pharmacokinetics. (See Table 3.) This drug is readily and almost completely absorbed in the alimentary tract. There is little or no binding to serum proteins. It is transformed in the liver to either a ketone or an alcohol metabolite, which is then excreted with or without glucuronide conjugation.

Usual Adult Dosage. Initial dosage is 500 mg per day. Dosage thereafter is individualized according to seizure control and serum concentration. Daily dosage may be increased by 250 mg every 4 to 7 days until seizure control is achieved. Optimal dosage is usually 15 to 30 mg per kg per day. Ethosuximide may be administered twice daily unless toxicity associated with peak serum concentration produces unacceptable toxicity, in which case a dosage regimen of 3 or 4 times daily should be employed. Ethosuximide is available as a 250-mg capsule or as a syrup.

Toxicity

LOCAL. Gastric irritation; anorexia; nausea and vomiting.

DOSE-RELATED. Drowsiness; dizziness; headache.

IDIOSYNCRATIC. Pancytopenia, agranulocytosis, and aplastic anemia psychosis; skin rashes; lupus erythematosus; dyskinesia, akathisia, bradykinesia, and parkinsonian changes.

Drug Interactions. Drug interactions of ethosuximide with other antiepileptic drugs are summarized in Table 4. These interactions rarely cause problems in clinical practice.

Disease States. Renal and hepatic disorders do not appear to pose major problems for enhanced toxicity of ethosuximide.

Valproic Acid (Depakene, Depakote)

Advantages and Disadvantages. Valproic acid is extremely effective in controlling absence seizures and also has some activity against tonic-clonic seizures. Valproic acid seldom causes leukopenia. Despite the possible advantages of valproic acid, ethosuximide remains the drug of first choice for patients with only absence seizures because (1) the risk of serious fatal hepatotoxicity as a result of valproic acid administration appears to be greater than the risk of bone marrow depression as a result of ethosuximide administration; (2) the common side effects of valproic acid (gastrointestinal upset, drowsiness, tremor) are more severe and persistent than with ethosuximide; (3) the longer elimination half-life of ethosuximide allows for more constant blood levels with less frequent administration; (4) valproic acid is much more expensive than ethosuximide; (5) valproic acid produces more clinically significant drug interactions with other antiepileptic drugs than does ethosuximide; and (6) the onset of antiabsence effect occurs earlier with ethosuximide than with valproic acid. In patients with both absence and tonic-clonic seizures, valproic acid may be the drug of choice because it has efficacy against tonic-clonic seizures, whereas ethosuximide does not.

Pharmacokinetics. (See Table 3.) Valproic acid is rapidly and completely absorbed after oral administration, with a slight delay in absorption if it is taken after meals. The drug is approximately 90 per cent protein bound. Protein binding varies with drug serum concentration, and the free fraction increases with increasing serum concentration. Primary metabolism is by hepatic hydroxylation and conjugation with glucuronide; valproate also appears in the bowel and undergoes enterohepatic circulation. Beta and omega oxidation may also take place. Excretion as glucuronide in the urine follows, with minor amounts lost in feces and expired air.

Usual Adult Dosage. Therapy is started at 15 mg per kg per day and gradually increased by 5 to 10 mg per kg per day every week until therapeutic success is achieved, a maximum dose of 60 mg per kg per day is reached, or the serum concentration exceeds 150 micrograms per ml. Valproic acid is available (Depakene) in 250-mg and 500-mg tablets and as a syrup; it is also available as enteric-coated divalproex sodium, a stable coordinate compound called Depakote, which is available in 125-mg, 250-mg, and 500-mg tablets. The absorption of this enteric-coated compound is delayed by about 1 hour, with a peak concentration reached in 3 to 4 hours. Depakene must be administered in 3 or more divided doses per day; Depakote can usually be administered twice daily and produces fewer gastrointestinal side effects in many patients.

Toxicity

LOCAL. Anorexia, nausea, and indigestion are common early gastrointestinal symptoms that rarely include vomiting and diarrhea. These symptoms are reduced with the enteric-coated preparation Depakote.

DOSE-RELATED. Elevated serum transaminases (usually transient but could be harbinger of serious hepatic disease); tremor; hyperammonemia.

IDIOSYNCRATIC. Hepatic necrosis; thrombocy-topenia; pancreatitis; stupor and coma; hair loss; "worsened behaviors" and depression. The risk of hepatic fatality is greatest in children younger than 11 years of age and in persons taking valproic acid in combination with other antiepileptic drugs (Table 5).

Side Effects. Weight gain; platelet dysfunction.

Drug Interactions. Interactions with other antiepileptic drugs are summarized in Table 4. Antiepiletic doses of aspirin may displace valproic acid from protein-binding sites and increase valproic acid free fraction by threefold. Also, valproic acid metabolism may be inhibited by aspirin.

Disease States. The use of valproic acid should be avoided in the presence of liver disease. Because of possible effects of valproic acid on hemostasis (thrombocytopenia, platelet dysfunction), persons on valproic acid who are about to undergo surgery should have a thorough hemostatic evaluation.

Clonazepam (Klonopin)

Clonazepam is the third drug of choice for absence seizures, because disabling side effects (drowsiness, ataxia, behavior disturbance) and development of tolerance to the antiepileptic effect of the drug are more common with clonazepam than with ethosuximide or valproic acid.

Pharmacokinetics. (See Table 3.) Clonazepam appears to be well absorbed by the alimentary tract. It is 47 per cent protein bound. Extensive biotransformation takes place, and less than 0.5 per cent is recovered from the urine as clonazepam.

Usual Adult Dosage. The initial dosage is 1.5 mg per day in 3 divided doses. An increase of 0.5 to 1 mg is made at 3- to 4-day intervals until seizure control is attained or a maximum dose of 20 mg per day is reached. A clear correlation between serum clonazepam concentration and seizure control has not been established. Approximately one third of patients receiving clonazepam develop tolerance to the antiepileptic effect of the

TABLE 5. **Rate of Hepatic Fatality by Age Group in Patients Receiving Valproic Acid as Monotherapy or Polytherapy (1978–1984)**

Age Group	Monotherapy		Polytherapy	
	Deaths	*Rate per 10,000*	*Deaths*	*Rate per 10,000*
0–2	1	1.42	15	19.01(1/500)
3–5	1	0.90	3	2.41
6–10	3	1.22	4	1.45
11–20	0	0	5	0.86
21–40	0	0	4	0.60
41–	0	0	1	0.26
Total	5	0.27(1/37,000)	32	1.52(1/6500)

Adapted from Dreifuss FE, Santilli N: Neurology 36 (4, Suppl. 1), 1986.

drug after 1 to 6 months of administration. In some patients the antiepileptic effect of clonazepam can be restored by increasing dosage rate. The drug should be withdrawn very slowly to avoid withdrawal seizures. Tablet sizes include 0.5, 1.0, and 2.0 mg.

Toxicity

DOSE-RELATED. Drowsiness; ataxia; behavioral changes (irritability, depression, psychosis); dysarthria; diplopia.

IDIOSYNCRATIC. Skin rash; hair loss; anemia, leukopenia, and thrombocytopenia.

Drug Interactions.

Interactions of clonazepam with other antiepileptic drugs are summarized in Table 4. Concurrent use of amphetamines and methylphenidate may cause central nervous system depression and respiratory irregularities. Depressant effects may also be enhanced by alcohol, antianxiety and antipsychotic drugs, antidepressants, and other antiepileptic drugs. In some individuals, concurrent use of valproic acid has been associated with the development of absence status.

Disease States.

Renal disease is unlikely to affect the elimination of clonazepam, but the presence of liver disease may require decreased dosage.

Management of Medically "Intractable" Epilepsy

Many cases of "intractable" epilepsy are due to improper seizure diagnosis resulting in use of improper antiepileptic drugs, failure to "push" the drugs used to maximal dosage, or failure to use all available antiepileptic drugs. However, there are some patients who will continue to have seizures despite the proper diagnosis of the type of seizure and despite maximal therapy with conventional antiepileptic drugs. Patients with simple and complex partial seizures should be considered for cortical resection procedures. In patients whose seizures are not controlled with conventional drugs and who are not candidates for cortical resection procedures, there are four therapeutic options: (1) less commonly used antiepileptic drugs, (2) experimental drugs, (3) experimental surgical procedures, and (4) behavioral therapies. Such therapies usually are available only at specialized epilepsy centers.

Management of Tonic-Clonic Status Epilepticus

Status epilepticus is defined as seizures (of any type) occurring so frequently that the patient does not fully recover from one seizure before having another. Tonic-clonic status epilepticus is the most common and dangerous type. The mortality of tonic-clonic status epilepticus is 6 to 20 per cent, and permanent brain damage may result from metabolic exhaustion of neurons.

Maintain Vital Functions

The patient should be positioned to avoid aspiration, suffocation, or falls. A soft plastic oral airway should be taped in place if it is possible to do so without forcing the teeth apart. Forcing an airway between clenched teeth may result in dental injury and aspiration of teeth. Wooden tongue blades may cause injuries from splinters and cuts, and metal spoons may injure teeth. Intubation may be necessary to maintain respirations. A large intravenous catheter should be placed for administration of medication and fluids. Metabolic acidosis is often present and should be corrected promptly with sodium bicarbonate.

Identify and Treat Precipitating Factors

The majority of cases of tonic-clonic status epilepticus do not occur randomly or as a result of a massive new cerebral lesion. Rather, there is a specific precipitating factor that causes a patient with a known seizure disorder to develop status epilepticus at a specific time. The most frequent causes of tonic-clonic status epilepticus are withdrawal from antiepileptic drugs and fever. Other precipitating factors include (1) withdrawal from alcohol or sedative drugs, (2) metabolic disorders (hypocalcemia, hyponatremia, hypoglycemia, hepatic or renal failure), (3) sleep deprivation, (4) acute brain insult (meningitis, encephalitis, cerebrovascular accident, or trauma), (5) diagnostic procedures, and (6) drug intoxication (e.g., cocaine, tricyclic antidepressants, isoniazid).

The precipitating factors in a case of status epilepticus must always be vigorously sought and treated to facilitate seizure control and to be certain any reversible cause of cerebral dysfunction is treated before it results in irreversible cerebral damage.

Antiepileptic Drug Therapy

Loading Dose of a Long-Acting Antiepileptic Drug. To quickly control tonic-clonic status epilepticus and prevent its recurrence, one must immediately obtain a high therapeutic serum concentration of a long-acting antiepileptic drug (phenytoin or phenobarbital in most cases) and then maintain the serum concentration in the therapeutic range. An intravenous loading dose of drug must be given in order to avoid the otherwise long delay in achieving a therapeutic steady-state plasma concentration of the drug if it is given in its usual maintenance dosage.

The usual loading dose of phenytoin is 14 mg

per kg intravenously at a rate no faster than 50 mg per minute, followed in 6 hours by the first maintenance dose of 100 mg. Alternatively, a loading dose of 18 mg per kg at a rate no faster than 50 mg per minute may be administered, followed by a first maintenance dose in 24 hours. The usual loading dose of phenobarbital is 6 to 20 mg per kg intravenously at a rate no faster than 60 mg per minute.

Diazepam (Valium). Intravenous diazepam has a relatively brief duration of action (30 to 120 minutes). It is not a definitive therapy for status epilepticus and can cause life-threatening cardio-respiratory depression. However, intravenous diazepam transiently produces high plasma and brain concentrations of the drug and often brings about immediate (but temporary) control of status epilepticus. Intravenous diazepam is indicated for tonic-clonic status epilepticus (1) if generalized tonic-clonic activity has been occurring without interruption for more than a few minutes or (2) if a tonic-clonic seizure occurs in a postictal patient who is being evaluated and is receiving a loading dose of a long-acting antiepileptic drug.

EPILEPSY IN INFANTS AND CHILDREN

method of
EILEEN P. G. VINING, M.D.
Johns Hopkins Hospital
Baltimore, Maryland

A seizure is a sudden, paroxysmal electrical discharge of neurons in the brain. For us to make the clinical diagnosis of a seizure, this electrical discharge must recruit sufficient surrounding neurons to alter the child's function or behavior. Epilepsy is generally defined as recurring, unprovoked seizures. In recent years, careful attention has been paid to classification of seizures (Table 1) and more recently to classification of the epilepsy syndromes (Table 2). Since etiology, therapy, and prognosis depend upon proper recognition of the disorder, this classification scheme is of great importance.

TREATMENT

Why Seizures Are Treated

Prophylactic medication is prescribed because of fear of the consequences of seizure recurrence, including the fear of neurologic and physical injury. There are no data to support the concept that a few seizures are linked to intellectual deterioration or any other form of neurologic damage, nor is there convincing evidence in hu-

TABLE 1. Seizure Classification

International Classification	"Old Terms"
I. Partial Seizures	Focal or local seizures
A. Simple partial seizures (Consciousness not impaired)	Focal motor seizures
1. With motor symptoms	Jacksonian seizures
2. With somatosensory or special sensory symptoms	Focal sensory seizures
3. With autonomic symptoms	
4. With psychic symptoms	
B. Complex partial seizures (with impairment of consciousness)	Psychomotor seizures
1. Simple partial onset	Temporal lobe seizures
2. With impairment of consciousness at onset	
C. Partial seizures that secondarily generalize	
II. Generalized Seizures (Convulsive or Nonconvulsive)	
A. Absence seizures	Petit mal seizures
1. Absence	
2. Atypical	
B. Myoclonic seizures	Minor motor seizures
C. Clonic seizures	Grand mal seizures
D. Tonic seizures	Grand mal seizures
E. Tonic-clonic seizures	Grand mal seizures
F. Atonic seizures (astatic)	Akinetic, drop attacks

mans of seizures begetting seizures. Although sudden, unexplained death is somewhat more frequent in persons with epilepsy, there are no data to suggest that therapy reduces this occurrence. Obviously there is a risk of physical injury if a seizure should occur in a dangerous or unsupervised setting. The greatest motivation to treat is because of the fear of the psychosocial consequences of recurrence. These risks are best managed by appropriate counseling concerning the nature of seizures, by minimizing the risk of physical or neurologic consequences, and by avoiding overprotection of the child.

TABLE 2. Classification of the Epilepsy Syndromes

1. Localization-related epilepsies
   Benign rolandic
   Benign occipital
2. Generalized epilepsies
   Age-related (benign neonatal convulsion, West's syndrome, childhood absence, benign juvenile myoclonic epilepsy)
3. Undetermined (? focal or generalized)
4. Special syndromes
   Chronic progressive epilepsia partialis continua in children

TABLE 3. **Antiepileptic Drug Therapy for Children**

Drug	Indications	Usual Dose (mg/kg/day)	Usual Dosage Schedule	Half-Life (hr)	Therapeutic Range (μg/ml)	Side Effects
Carbamazepine* (Tetretol)	F, C, G	10–40	bid–qid	12	5–14	Headache, drowsiness, dizziness, diplopia, blood dyscrasia, hepatotoxicity, arrhythmia
Clonazepam (Klonopin)	M, A	0.05–0.03	bid–qid	24–36		Drowsiness, ataxia, secretions, hypotonia, behavioral problems
Ethosuximide (Zarontin)	A (? C, M)	20–40	bid	30	40–100	GI distress, rash, drowsiness, dizziness, SLE, blood dyscrasia
Phenobarbital	F, C, G, S	2–8	qd–bid	48–100	10–25	Drowsiness, rash, ataxia, behavioral and cognitive problems
Phenytoin (Dilantin)	F, C, G, S	4–8	qd–bid	6–30	10–20	Drowsiness, gum hyperplasia, rash, anemia, ataxia, hirsutism, folate deficiency, teratogenicity
Primidone (Mysoline)	F, C, G	12–25	bid–qid	6–12	6–12	Drowsiness, dizziness, rash, anemia, ataxia, diplopia
Valproate (Depakene, Depakote)	F, C, G, M, A	10–60	bid–qid	6–18	50–100	GI distress, hepatitis, alopecia, drowsiness, ataxia, tremors, pancreatitis, thrombocytopenia

Abbreviations: F = focal (partial-simple); G = generalized (tonic-clonic); C = partial-complex; A = absence; M = minor motor (akinetic, atonic, myoclonic); S = status; qd = every day; bid = twice daily; qid = 4 times daily; GI = gastrointestinal; SLE = systemic lupus erythematosus.

*Safety and efficacy for use in children have not been established.

A seizure should be treated when the risk of recurrence and the consequences of that recurrence are clearly greater than the risk of treatment and the consequences of daily prophylactic therapy.

Recent data suggest that an individual with a first seizure, on average, has a 30 per cent chance of having a second seizure. Children with absence seizures, myoclonic seizures, or atonic seizures routinely have had multiple seizures prior to consultation with the physician and will continue to do so unless treated. There is increasing evidence that in children who have had a generalized idiopathic tonic-clonic seizure with a normal electroencephalogram (EEG), the recurrence rate is as low as 15 per cent. However, recurrence rate after a second seizure is closer to 75 per cent.

The Treatment Plan

The decision to treat should be made *after* a discussion of the risk/benefit ratio with the patient and family. This includes the risks of seizure recurrence, the benefit of prophylaxis, and the risks and possible side effects of the medications. The treatment plan must be described to the patient and family to ensure their understanding and knowledgeable participation (see Table 3).

The diagnosis must be certain, since the choice of anticonvulsant is based primarily on the type of seizure (Table 4). This choice also is influenced by possible side effects. In some children, the possible cosmetic side effects of phenytoin (Dilantin) would not be a concern, whereas in others it would be very undesirable. Many medications (carbamazepine* [Tegretol], primidone [Mysoline], valproic acid [Depakene, Depakote]) must be started at suboptimal doses to avoid immediate side effects. The amount of drug is then increased until the desired goal is achieved. That goal is control of seizures without toxicity. Toxicity means evidence of clinical dysfunction and not simply high serum levels. If the drug is not effective, the drug of second choice should be added. When the second drug is in therapeutic range, the first drug should be tapered and discontinued. This will lead to the use of monotherapy. Increasing data indicate that monotherapy has many advantages including equal efficacy, fewer side effects, and easier monitoring. Also it frequently allows less costly treatment of seizures.

Once the medication regimen has been estab-

---

*Safety and efficacy for use in children under 6 years of age have not been established.

TABLE 4. **Treatment**

1. Discuss plan with patient and/or parent.

2. Be sure of diagnosis and classification.

3. Choose the most appropriate drug; consider seizure type and possible side effects.

4. Increase the drug until control of seizures is achieved or there is clinical toxicity (not just high serum levels).

5. If the drug is not effective (i.e., if there is not control of seizures without side effects), add a second drug. When it is in therapeutic range, slowly discontinue first drug. ACHIEVE MONOTHERAPY.

6. MONITOR THOROUGHLY.

7. Provide support, counseling, and education.

8. If seizures are controlled for 2 years, consider tapering off drug.

lished, monitoring of the patient is essential, not only to be certain that the seizures are controlled but, more important, to ascertain that there are no unwanted side effects. This requires going beyond the traditional monitoring of hematologic and hepatic side effects to ensure that physical appearance, motor coordination, learning, and behavior are not being adversely affected. Frequently, the physician will have to rely on more than his or her own observation of the patient, and it may be necessary to carefully question both parents and school regarding any changes they may perceive in the child.

The therapeutic plan must include an awareness that seizures may not be forever. Probably 70 to 75 per cent of children will ultimately have their seizures completely controlled. Once the seizures have been controlled for 2 or more years, it is reasonable to consider discontinuation of medication. Recent studies show that children who have been seizure free for 2 or more years have a 75 per cent chance of remaining seizure free when medication is discontinued. The children who appear to have the greatest likelihood of nonrecurrence are those who have a recent normal EEG.

A therapeutic plan is not complete without dealing with the informational, psychosocial, and emotional needs of the patient and family. This may require considerable counseling that can be augmented by the Epilepsy Foundation of America; the family may request information by calling 800-EFA-1000.

Seizure Types and Epilepsies

Generalized Tonic-Clonic Seizures

The standard anticonvulsants are phenobarbital, phenytoin (Dilantin), carbamazepine* (Tegre-

tol) and valproic acid (Depakene, Depakote). Phenobarbital is inexpensive and well known to pediatricians. Its major disadvantages are hyperactivity, behavioral disorders, cognitive difficulties, and sleep disorders in at least 30 to 40 per cent of children. Data indicate that many patients experience more subtle alterations in learning and behavior. If phenobarbital is used, it is mandatory that the physician pay careful attention to any adverse changes in the child. Phenytoin is also an effective anticonvulsant, but changes in appearance and gingival hyperplasia may occur in up to 90 per cent of children. One must also recall that phenytoin has nonlinear kinetics. As the therapeutic range is approached, small increases in dosage may cause dramatic increases in serum drug levels. Carbamazepine appears to have fewer adverse effects on neuropsychologic function than other drugs. This drug has a fairly short half-life and may need to be given as frequently as 4 times a day in order to smooth the peak and trough levels. Aplastic anemia associated with carbamazepine use is extremely rare and apparently cannot be predicted by routine hematologic monitoring. On the other hand, neutropenia is more frequent but rarely produces clinical problems. Valproic acid is useful in generalized seizures and also appears to have minimal effects on neuropsychological function or behavior. It also has a short half-life. The hepatic side effects of sodium valproate are quite rare but are more frequent in children less than 2 years of age who are receiving polytherapy. Children over 11 years of age and on monotherapy have had no hepatic failures reported.

Partial Seizures

Both simple and complex partial seizures can be effectively treated by phenobarbital, phenytoin (Dilantin), carbamazepine* (Tegretol), and primidone (Mysoline). Primidone is readily converted to phenobarbital. Prior to conversion, primidone and another active metabolite (PEMA) are also active anticonvulsants. Primidone has many of the side effects of phenobarbital and in addition has significant initial toxicity, requiring that it be introduced at very low doses and increased in small increments. Valproic acid (Depakene, Depakote) may be helpful in treating partial complex seizures, especially when there is a significant element of absence. In addition, if the partial seizures secondarily generalize, valproate is a useful medication.

Absence Seizures

Absence seizures are best treated with either succinamides or sodium valproate. Valproate is

---

*Safety and efficacy for use in children under 6 years of age have not been established.

*Safety and efficacy for use in children under 6 years of age have not been established.

probably more effective in atypical absence seizures and would certainly be preferred when a patient has both absence and tonic-clonic seizures. Ethosuximide (Zarontin) is effective in classic absence seizures; side effects include headaches and nausea. Benzodiazepines are frequently used as adjunctive drugs. These drugs include clonazepam (Klonopin), clorazepate (Tranxene) and lorazepam (Ativan).* It is discouraging that the benzodiazepines are effective initially but decrease in efficacy over time. Side effects may be quite intolerable and include sedation, behavior changes, and at times difficulty handling secretions.

Myoclonic and Atonic Seizures

Valproic acid (Depakene, Depakote) is the drug of choice for these seizures. The benzodiazepines also may be effective. The ketogenic diet can play an important role in controlling these seizures. The diet involves fasting the child into ketosis and maintaining this ketosis chronically by using a diet containing a high portion of ketogenic foods (fats). The diet usually consists of a ratio of 4 grams of fat to 1 gram of protein plus carbohydrate, making a 40-calorie unit. Children require 60 to 75 calories per kg per day and at least 1 gram per kg per day of protein. Fluids are restricted to 600 to 1200 ml per day. The diet is deficient in calcium and fat-soluble vitamins and requires supplementation with 1 gram, twice daily, of calcium carbonate and multivitamins with minerals and iron. The child is monitored by examining urinary ketones; the level should be high, especially late in the afternoon.

Febrile Seizures

Febrile seizures occur in 3 to 4 per cent of all children, most commonly between 9 and 20 months of age; 30 to 40 per cent will experience a recurrence. Even with recurrence, there is no increased risk of mental retardation, cerebral palsy, or other significant neurologic sequelae. Only children with two or more risk factors are at a significantly increased risk for epilepsy. These factors include atypical febrile seizure (i.e., lasting longer than 15 minutes, recurring within 24 hours, or focal in nature), a first-degree relative with a history of epilepsy, and abnormal neurodevelopmental status prior to the first febrile seizure. Even with two or more of these risk factors, the risk of afebrile seizures does not exceed 13 per cent.

Therefore, the use of prophylactic therapy should only be considered in the face of these risk factors or multiple recurrences. Daily phenobar-

bital, at a dosage that maintains blood levels of greater than 15 micrograms per ml, will reduce recurrence. However, this therapy frequently produces the previously mentioned behavioral changes. Valproic acid (Depakene, Depakote) is apparently effective, but potentially too toxic to consider for use. For temperatures greater than 38.5°C, rectal diazepam (Valium) (not available in the U.S.), 0.5 mg per kg every 8 hours, is also reported to be effective, producing only mild sedation. The intravenous preparation of diazepam (Valium) can be substituted. *Normally we do not recommend prophylactic therapy for children with febrile seizures.*

Neonatal Seizures

Neonatal seizures are the most reliable predictor of later neurologic deficit. However, the majority of infants with neonatal seizures who survive do well. The most important therapy is the search for the cause and the appropriate treatment. If the neonatal seizures are recurrent or appear to significantly threaten or interfere with the child's well being, therapy with anticonvulsants is utilized.

Phenobarbital is the drug of choice, with a loading dose of 20 mg per kg intravenously as a slow bolus or in divided doses over a short period of time. Phenytoin (Dilantin) can also be used, again with a loading dose of 20 mg per kg. Diazepam (Valium) is a useful agent in its rapidity of action; however, it has a short half-life. It can be used at a dose of 0.2 to 0.5 mg per kg. Concern regarding its diluent does not appear to be warranted any longer. Frequently, we will treat an infant with a loading dose of phenobarbital. If this is effective and ongoing insult to the brain does not appear to be occurring, we will not place the child on maintenance phenobarbital. The long half-life (approximately 100 hours) can be expected to protect the infant over the period of recovery from asphyxia.

Infantile Spasms

These seizures classically consist of sudden flexion of the head, abduction and extension of the arms, and simultaneous flexion of knees. These are the only type of seizures that occur in series or clusters. Frequently the EEG pattern will be that of hypsarrhythmia. Prognosis is generally poor for this group, especially in the two thirds who are considered symptomatic and who are experiencing these seizures owing to a definable underlying pathology.

Treatment should begin promptly since there is some indication that earlier therapy leads to better outcome. ACTH gel, given 20 to 40 units intramuscularly twice daily, is the treatment of

*This use is not listed in the manufacturer's directive.

choice, although variations, including higher doses and alternate-day therapy, have been reported to be successful. Prednisone, 2 mg per kg or 75 mg per M², may be equally effective, but is not used as the first therapy in our center. Duration of treatment varies from 2 weeks to many months. We treat for 4 to 6 weeks and then begin to taper. Side effects of ACTH or prednisone are almost universal and include hypertension and susceptibility to infection. Behavioral disturbances, including severe irritability and transient decrease in psychomotor performance, are not uncommon. Valproic acid (Depakene, Depakote) and benzodiazepines may also be effective.

Lennox-Gastaut Syndrome

The Lennox-Gastaut syndrome consists of an EEG pattern of slow spike-waves and rapid spikes, two or more types of seizures (one of which is usually myoclonic or atonic) and mental retardation. Onset is usually between 1 and 6 years of age and may frequently be seen as part of an evolution from infantile spasms. Valproic acid (Depakene, Depakote) is the treatment of choice but often must be used with additional anticonvulsants. We find the ketogenic diet particularly helpful in this seizure disorder.

Benign Rolandic Epilepsy

This benign form of epilepsy generally begins between 3 and 13 years of age and consists of seizures characterized by facial movements, grimacing, and vocalization, followed by a tonic-clonic component. The EEG frequently shows characteristic repetitive spikes in the midtemporal or parietal area. It is generally much worse in non-REM sleep. Seizures are quite benign and often occur only at night. Often anticonvulsant medication is not necessary. When necessary, carbamazepine (Tegretol) appears to be the drug of choice.

Juvenile Myoclonic Epilepsy of Janz

This disorder begins in late childhood or early adulthood with mild myoclonic seizures, often on awakening. These may then lead to tonic-clonic or absence seizures. This seizure disorder is particularly sensitive to valproic acid (Depakene, Depakote).

Status Epilepticus

While brief tonic-clonic seizures almost certainly do not cause brain damage, there is fear that status epilepticus, or seizures lasting more than 30 minutes, may be a threat to the integrity of the central nervous system, as well as to life itself. In treating status epilepticus, there is a fine line between aggressive therapy to stop the seizures and the production of iatrogenic prob-

lems requiring intubation and ventilation and the potential morbidity associated with these complications. Before medications are given, maintenance of vital functions should be established, including adequate aeration and monitoring of vital signs. An intravenous line should be placed to obtain blood for appropriate studies and to administer glucose (as necessary) as well as anticonvulsant drugs. Diazepam (Valium) is usually the initial drug of choice because of low toxicity and rapid onset of action. It is given as 0.2 to 0.5 mg per kg over a 2-minute period with a maximum single dose of 10 mg. The dose may be repeated in 10 minutes if the seizure persists. This can also be done using rectal diazepam* (Valium). Lorazepam (Ativan),† 0.03 to 0.05 mg per kg, is increasingly being utilized as an alternative because of its longer duration of action. Because diazepam (Valium) is effective for only a short time, the child should also be treated with an intravenous loading dose of phenytoin (Dilantin) or phenobarbital. A loading dose of 15 to 20 mg per kg of phenytoin is infused at a rate not to exceed 50 mg per minute, or phenobarbital can be given in a loading dose of 15 to 20 mg per kg. Simultaneous ECG and blood pressure monitoring is mandatory. Maintenance dosages should be begun within 6 to 8 hours.

Surgical Therapy

Medical therapy is effective in perhaps 75 per cent of children. However, in those individuals whose seizures are intractable and/or who are experiencing life-altering side effects, the search for identifiably abnormal tissue and the potential for surgical remediation should be considered. This frequently requires intensive monitoring to determine the exact focus of the seizure activity. Sometimes a subdural electrode grid is necessary, enabling the clinician to identify the source of the seizure as well as areas that should be spared to preserve important neurologic functions (e.g., movement and speech). In addition, some youngsters have progressive disease of a single hemisphere due to developmental abnormalities, trauma, or Rasmussen's encephalitis. These children should be considered for hemispherectomy.

HEADACHES

method of
JOEL R. SAPER, M.D.
*Michigan Headache and Neurological Institute
Ann Arbor, Michigan*

Headache is a pervasive and widespread illness, estimated to affect more than 70 per cent of American

---

*Rectal diazepam is not available in the United States.
†This use is not listed in the manufacturer's directive.

households. Over 300 medical illnesses can produce headache. The most troubling and chronic of the headache conditions are those referred to as primary headaches, which are characterized by the absence of structural pathology or systemic disease.

PRIMARY HEADACHE DISORDERS

As the perspectives on chronic headache change, the "headache villains" of the past hundred years—the blood vessels and muscles—are coming to be seen more as accomplices. The central hypothesis, which is supported by the current understanding of brain mechanisms, advances the premise that chronic recurring headaches (primary headache disorders) arise in part, if not exclusively, from fundamental disturbances in neuronal, neurotransmitter, receptor, or nerve function. The peripheral muscular or vascular activity is secondary to the central and primary disturbances; as a result, changing attitudes to headache treatment have evolved.

Treatment

The treatment of patients with chronic recurring headache is enhanced by conveying a sincere interest in their distress and by establishing worthwhile and frank communication. Although emotional factors are at times important, psychological and stress-related factors have been overemphasized as the etiological basis for headache. Presumptive and premature emphasis on psychological elements is counterproductive, and may fail to recognize the important physiological changes, usually inherited, that most experts now believe predispose patients to this disorder.

Nonmedical Management

Nonmedical management of headache requires the identification and, if possible, the elimination of provoking influences (see Tables 1 and 2). Often, interventions such as biofeedback and stress management are very important in treatment of patients. Stopping smoking has proved valuable in the treatment of many apparently refractory headache cases; discontinuance of smoking reduces nicotine and carbon monoxide effects, both of which may produce headache. Perhaps the most important of all nonmedical approaches is the elimination of daily or almost daily use of symptomatic medicines such as analgesics or ergotamine tartrate. It is now apparent that too frequent use of ergotamine tartrate or analgesics (more often than 2 days per week) may accentuate headache frequency. Discontinuance of excessively used symptomatic medications may be basic to control and prevention.

Simultaneously present medical conditions, particularly those along the distribution of the trigeminal nerve can aggravate pre-existing primary headache disorders. Therefore, careful evaluation of dental pathology and treatment of disorders such as microabscesses, moderate to severe temporomandibular joint dysfunction, and cracked teeth, as well as treatment of sinus disease or other disturbances about the head and neck, can have a marked beneficial effect on primary headache control.

MIGRAINE HEADACHES

Although traditionally classified into common and classical forms, differences of opinion exist as to whether classical migraine (with a preheadache neurologic aura) and common migraine (without a distinct, identifiable neurologic aura) are different entities. Moreover, it is now apparent that in many individuals, the intermittent migraine during the early course of their head-

TABLE 1. **Migraine-Provoking Influences**

Psychological	Localized or generalized infection
Stress/anxiety	
Anger	Dietary
Let-down	
Exhilaration	Medicines
	Reserpine
Dazzling light	Hydralazine
	MAOIs*
Hormonal	Nonsteroidal anti-inflammatory agents*
Menarche	
Menstruation	Vasodilators*
Menopause	Antiasthmatic agents
Pregnancy (first trimester)	Thiazide derivatives
Delivery	Propranolol*
Birth control pills	Amphetamines, diet pills
Exogenous estrogens	Ephedrine
Sleep	Marked weather changes
Too much	
Too little	Head/neck trauma
Napping	Mild
	Severe
Toxins	
	Smoking

*May also be of benefit.

TABLE 2. **Some Foods That May Trigger Headaches**

Tyramine-containing foods	Onions
Chocolate	Alcohol products
Aged cheeses	Wine/champagne, liquor, beer
Vinegar	
Relishes, dressings, sauces, catsup	Fatty foods
	Nitrite-containing foods
Liver, kidney, other organ meats	Hotdogs, sandwich meats, others
Alcohol	MSG-containing foods
Sour cream	Caffeine
Yogurt	Too much
Yeast extracts	"Rebound" effect
Citrus fruits	Seafood
Milk and milk products	

ache years "transforms" or evolves from the intermittent pattern to a daily or almost daily nonmigraine headache pattern, with superimposed acute exacerbations of typical migraine events. This latter entity, referred to variously as transformed migraine, daily chronic headache, or combined headache, may well represent a progressive disturbance in the pathophysiology of intermittent migraine. Currently, however, migraine is still classified as an intermittent entity, characterized by the absence of headache between acute events.

Treatment

Symptomatic (Rescue) Treatment

Table 3 describes criteria for symptomatic vs. preventive treatment of migraine. The basis for symptomatic treatment is established by frequency. Acute attacks of migraine occurring less than once a week and in the absence of any contraindication to the use of symptomatic therapies warrants this form of treatment. The route of administration for symptomatic therapy may be as critical as the choice of medication. Delay of gastric absorption has been demonstrated in patients during both the preheadache and headache phases and occurs even in the absence of nausea and vomiting. The following interventions are of greatest value.

Ergotamine Alkaloids. Ergotamine alkaloids are estimated to be effective within the first 1 to 2 hours in up to 90 per cent of cases when administered parenterally, in 80 per cent of patients given the rectal form, and up to 50 per cent of patients given the oral form. Recent reports propose that central (brain) effects may be equally or more important than peripheral vasoconstrictive influences. The ergotamine alkaloids ergotamine tartrate and dihydroergotamine (DHE-45) are available in parenteral (intravenous, intramuscular, and subcutaneous), oral, rectal, inhal-

TABLE 3. **Guidelines for Symptomatic Versus Preventive Therapy**

Symptomatic Guidelines
  Frequency less than 1 to 2 headaches/week
  No medical contraindications
  For ergot derivatives: No coronary artery disease, severe
    hypertension, peripheral or cerebrovascular disease
  For analgesics containing aspirin: No peptic ulcer disease,
    anticoagulant use, aspirin-sensitive asthma

Preventive Guidelines
  Frequency greater than 1 to 2 headaches/week
  Medical contraindications for symptomatic therapies
  Failure of symptomatic therapies
  Reliable, predictable regularity of attacks (e.g., at or
    around menstrual period)
  Known substance abuse tendencies

ant, and sublingual forms. The oral and sublingual forms are less effective than those administered by the parenteral or rectal routes. The oral forms (Cafergot, Cafergot P-B, and Wigraine) each contain 1 mg of ergotamine tartrate. They are administered as 2 tablets at the onset of an attack, followed by 1 tablet every half hour until relief is obtained or until 5 mg have been taken. Sublingual tablets (Ergomar, Ergostat, Wigrettes) contain 2.0 mg of ergotamine tartrate and are given as 1 tablet sublingually at the onset of a headache and may be repeated once.

In rectal form, a suppository containing 2 mg of ergotamine tartrate (Cafergot, Cafergot P-B, Wigraine, Wigraine P-B) can be administered initially with a repeat dose in 1 hour, up to a maximum daily dose of 4 mg. I recommend beginning at a dose of one third to one half of a suppository in order to avoid the known adverse effects of ergotamine tartrate when excessive or too rapid absorption occurs. Cafergot P-B (tablets and suppositories) and Wigraine P-B suppositories contain the added ingredients butalbitol and belladonna, considered to enhance efficacy and reduce the gastrointestinal (GI) and other untoward effects of ergotamine tartrate. All preparations of Cafergot and Wigraine also contain caffeine, but sublingual, inhalant, and intravenous preparations do not.

Parenteral treatment with DHE-45 (1 to 2 ml intramuscularly or 0.5 to 1.0 ml intravenously) is effective in most instances and can be combined with parenterally or rectally administered antinauseants. (Treatment regimens using intravenous DHE-45 will be described later.)

Well-known contraindications and untoward reactions are described in easily obtained reference sources. Less widely known, however, is the potential for physical dependence on ergotamine tartrate, reported in patients taking ergotamine as infrequently as 3 times per week, and resulting in "rebound" or "ergotamine headache," a self-sustaining headache/medication cycle in which the next headache represents the withdrawal symptom from the last dose of drug. Therefore, ergotamine tartrate should be used no more than 2 days per week, since greater frequency of usage leads to dependency and increasing headaches.

Isometheptene Mucate. Isometheptene mucate (Midrin) is a sympathomimetic agent combined with acetaminophen and dichloralphenazone (a tranquilizer). It produces less GI distress than ergotamine tartrate and occasionally is more effective.

Midrin is recommended for the symptomatic relief of mild to moderate migraine. Dosage is 2 capsules at the onset of an attack, followed by 1 to 2 capsules 1 hour later, to a maximum of 5 capsules per attack. Usage more than 2 days per week should be avoided.

Nonsteroidal Anti-inflammatory Drugs. Nonsteroidal anti-inflammatory drugs (NSAIDs) have symptomatic as well as preventive properties in migraine therapy. A large number of agents are available, but naproxen sodium (Anaprox) has been most widely evaluated. The dose of naproxen is 275 mg, 1 to 2 tablets, to be taken at the onset of headache. Other agents include meclofenamate sodium (Meclomen), 100 to 200 mg, which can be repeated in 1 to 2 hours.

Other Agents

Although analgesics (narcotic and nonnarcotic) may benefit some patients during an acute migraine attack, overuse risks make these agents unacceptable for routine usage except when proper limits can be established and when other therapies are of little value. Injectable narcotics are more effective than oral medication. Some patients with migraine benefit only from analgesic therapy, given alone or in conjunction with the symptomatic therapies listed above. While physicians must be cautious and alert for the somatic expression of psychological despair and drug-seeking behavior, patients should not be deprived of necessary and available therapy as a result of professional timidity or unfounded prejudice. In selected cases, narcotics may represent the most appropriate and safest treatment.

Other Adjunctive Agents. Antinauseants are administered in conjunction with symptomatic drugs and are most effective by parenteral and suppository routes. The dose of chlorpromazine (Thorazine) is 25 to 50 mg intramuscularly, rectally, or in tablet form. Promethazine (Phenergan) is administered at a dose of 25 mg intramuscularly or rectally or 50 mg orally. Prochlorperazine (Compazine), 25 mg rectally or intramuscularly, should be used with particular caution because of the higher incidence of acute dystonic reactions associated with its use when compared with other agents such as chlorpromazine. Metoclopramide hydrochloride (Reglan), 10 mg orally 3 times a day or in intravenous form (same dose), can have antiemetic effects and may also enhance oral absorption.

Steroids may also be useful for symptomatic treatment of migraine. Patients with prolonged attacks may benefit from prednisone, 40 to 60 mg orally for 3 to 5 days, or dexamethasone, 8 to 16 mg intramuscularly.

Recently, a treatment protocol has been recommended that uses intravenous DHE-45 for refractory migraine. The starting dose is 0.5 to 1.0 mg every 8 hours over a period of 3 to 5 days, after an initial test dose of 0.1 to 0.3 mg. This therapy is best carried out in an inpatient setting and should be reserved for patients in whom standard interventions have been ineffective. Intravenous antinauseant therapy can be given simultaneously for accompanying GI distress.

Similarly, a 4-day protocol of intravenously administered hydrocortisone can be used for severely acute and refractory cases. This regimen consists of 100 mg of hydrocortisone added to 100 cc of an intravenous preparation of dextrose and water, given over 20 to 30 minutes. It is given 4 times a day during the first day; 3 times on the second day; twice on the third day; and once on the fourth day.

Preventive Treatment

The Beta-Adrenergic Blockers. The most important drugs for the prevention of migraine are the beta-adrenergic blocking agents. Their value in chronic daily headache and mixed forms is also recognized. Nadolol* (Corgard) and propranolol (Inderal) are the most widely administered and tested agents, but others may be of similar value. Individual dose determination is required. Nadolol (Corgard) is started at 20 mg per day and increased to tolerance, often to a range 80 to 160 mg per day. Twice-daily dosing may be of added benefit in some patients. The short-acting form of propranolol (Inderal) is used in a range of 20 to 40 mg 3 to 4 times per day, whereas the long-acting form (Inderal LA) is best employed in a twice-daily regimen, beginning at 80 mg once or twice a day and increasing to 160 mg twice daily as tolerated.

Methysergide. Methysergide (Sansert), the oldest of the migraine prophylactic agents, is marred by a history of adverse consequences, but most authorities believe that selective and carefully monitored usage is both appropriate and necessary in difficult-to-manage cases. The drug is given as 2 mg 3 to 4 times a day in equally divided dosages. Treatment should be continued for no more than 6 months. A "drug holiday" of at least one month should separate periods of treatment. A chest x-ray, electrocardiogram, and intravenous pyelography or magnetic resonance imaging of the abdomen is recommended to evaluate for the presence of retroperitoneal, cardiac valvular, and pulmonary changes.

Calcium Antagonists. Of the three available calcium antagonists (verapamil* [Isoptin, Calan], diltiazem* [Cardizem], and nifedipine* [Procardia]), verapamil and diltiazem seem to have the greatest effectiveness for treatment of headache. Calcium antagonists do not appear to be as effec-

---

*This use of these agents is not listed in the manufacturers' directives.

tive as the beta blockers for prophylaxis of migraine but may be very effective in certain instances. They are agents of choice in patients who cannot take beta-adrenergic blockers, such as patients with asthma. Verapamil* is given in a dose range of 40 to 160 mg, 2 to 3 times per day, and diltiazem* is administered in a dose range of 30 to 90 mg, 2 to 3 times per day. Many patients administered nefedipine report increased headache, at least initially, although successful results are occasionally evident.

Nonsteroidal Anti-inflammatory Drugs. The NSAIDs are used for both the symptomatic and preventive treatment of migraine. Naproxen sodium (Anaprox) has been successfully established as an effective preventive agent in dose ranges of 275 mg, 1 to 2 tablets twice daily. Other NSAIDs may also be effective. Appropriate monitoring for untoward reactions, including aggravation of hypertension, is necessary.

Antidepressants. *Tricyclic antidepressants* (TCAs), particularly amitriptyline (Endep, Elavil) and nortriptyline (Aventyl, Pamelor), can be of dramatic benefit in patients with frequently occurring headache. In addition to reducing pain, these agents can ameliorate the frequently present sleep disturbances. Amitriptyline is administered in a dose of 25 to 150 mg per day, often in a single bedtime regimen. Nortriptyline dosages range from 25 to 75 mg at bedtime.

The *Monoamine Oxidase Inhibiting Antidepressants* (MAOIs), particularly phenelzine (Nardil), can dramatically reduce the frequency of migraine and mixed headache forms. The traditional taboo against the simultaneous administration of MAOIs and TCAs has diminished somewhat, and MAOIs and amitriptyline treatment programs are employed for refractory depression and/or headache. Phenelzine, 15 mg 1 to 3 times daily, is usually given before midafternoon.

When simultaneously administering TCAs (amitriptyline, nortriptyline) and MAOIs, both drugs should be started on the same day, gradually increasing dosages to tolerance. Imipramine-related TCAs should not be used in conjunction with MAOIs to avoid hypertensive reactions. Severe orthostatic hypotension can occur in patients taking MAOIs alone or in conjunction with other antidepressants.

Other Preventive Agents. Clonidine hydrochloride* (Catapres), carbamazepine* (Tegretol), and methylphenidate* (Ritalin), are occasionally useful in intractable cases of migraine. Cyproheptadine* (Periactin) may be effective in adults with migraine; it is of considerable importance in the treatment of childhood migraine, and many consider it to be the drug of first choice. Dosages range from 4 to 8 mg, 3 to 4 times a day, in adults and 4 mg, 2 to 3 times a day, in children.

MIXED HEADACHE FORMS (TRANSFORMATIONAL MIGRAINE, DAILY CHRONIC HEADACHE, SO-CALLED TENSION HEADACHE)

Although the term "chronic tension headache" is still used, many experts consider it a variation of migraine or other mixed headache forms. Many authorities doubt that muscular pain is the primary basis for headaches in patients with frequent head and neck pain syndromes. It is possible that *acute* tension headache may be a separate and distinctive entity from that of the chronic form. Distinguishing mild to moderate migraine with muscle components from acute tension headache is not possible clinically and contributes to the disagreement as to whether acute muscular headache actually exists. Many believe that central mechanisms are responsible for the so-called muscular elements seen in the primary headache conditions.

Preventive Treatment

Frequent, recurring headache patterns in which migrainous and nonmigrainous features co-exist are best treated with the pharmacologic and nonpharmacologic programs already described under migraine. Acute tension headache, if such actually exists, can be treated with mild analgesia (e.g., aspirin, acetaminophen) or NSAIDs. Simple muscle relaxants may also be helpful. For acute migrainous elements, symptomatic treatments are appropriate. For the more frequent or daily component, combinations of beta-adrenergic blockers and tricyclic antidepressants are most effective. One such regimen includes nadolol* (Corgard), 60 to 160 mg daily or propranolol (Inderal LA) 80 to 360 mg, and amitriptyline,* 50 to 150 mg at bedtime. The NSAIDs may be added if necessary.

The population of patients suffering frequent mixed element headaches (e.g., daily chronic headache) is a complex and challenging group of headache sufferers. In these patients, even the most appropriate pharmacotherapeutic intervention may be ineffective because of analgesic overuse, psychological distress, and family and other complicating problems. It is the opinion of many authorities that the symptoms in these individuals reflect an endogenous pain syndrome that

---

*This use of these agents is not listed in the manufacturers' directives.

*This use of these agents is not listed in the manufacturers' directives.

manifests as pain and other physiologic and psychological distresses, including periodic depression, sleep disturbance, and substance overuse. Effective treatment often requires multidisciplinary interventions and sometimes hospitalization (see below). Biofeedback, psychotherapy, family involvement, lifestyle regulation, and other nonmedical and medical therapies are often necessary.

CLUSTER HEADACHE

Perhaps the most sinister of the well-recognized headache disorders is cluster headache. Few headaches are a greater challenge to the clinician's knowledge, compassion, and pharmacotherapeutic skills. Cluster headache can be divided into three major forms: episodic, chronic, and variants.

Episodic cluster headache is well known and most commonly characterized by recurring bouts of intensely painful attacks of cephalalgia. The pain is usually centered around an eye or the temple area and accompanied by nasal drainage, lacrimation, and other autonomic disturbances. Each headache lasts between 1 and 2 hours, and cycles of headache occur an average of every 2 to 4 months.

Chronic cluster headache is divided into a primary and secondary form. The term "chronic" is applied when the headache continues day after day, year after year, without remission or an interim period. *Primary chronic cluster headache* occurs without an interim period or remission from the time the first cycle begins; the *secondary chronic cluster headache* is characterized by a pattern of typical, episodic cycles that eventually evolve to a chronic (without an interim period of remission) pattern.

Many variant forms of cluster headache exist, including *chronic paroxysmal hemicrania* (CPH). This disorder, first reported in 1974, is in many ways similar to cluster headache but often affects young women (cluster headache generally strikes adult men). The variant forms of cluster headache, including CPH, may be shorter-lasting than those of a typical cluster headache (less than 1 hour) and generally occur with greater frequency—up to 10 to 12 attacks compared to 2 to 4 cluster attacks per day. These variant forms rarely awaken patients from sleep, which is more typical of cluster headache.

Treatment

The treatment of cluster headache requires persistence, diligence, and innovation. Patients with cluster headache must discontinue all alcoholic products and avoid daytime napping. Dis-

TABLE 4. Ten-Day Protocol for Prednisone Treatment of Cluster Headache

Day	Drug Dose (mg) 8:00 AM	4:00 PM	Bedtime	Total (per day)
1	20	20	20	60
2	20	20	20	60
3	20	20	20	60
4	20	20	20	60
5	20	15	15	50
6	15	15	10	40
7	10	10	10	30
8	5	5	5	15
9	5	0	5	10
10	5	Finished		5

A total of seventy-six 5-mg tablets are needed for this protocol.

continuance of smoking may be extremely important, although this is very difficult to achieve in the cluster headache population.

Symptomatic Treatment

Inhalation of 100 per cent oxygen is an effective means of symptomatically relieving the pain in many patients. Patients are administered 100 per cent oxygen at 7 liters per minute for a period of 15 minutes or more.

Symptomatic medications include rectal ergotamine tartrate or chlorpromazine. Injectible narcotics are discouraged because of the risks of overuse in patients with the daily headache patterns. Risk of overuse of ergotamine is also a concern.

Preventive Treatment

Preventive therapies are most appropriate for cluster headache.

Prednisone. Prednisone is the most reliable and effective drug for the prevention of cluster headache and can dramatically reduce both chronic and episodic varieties within hours of first administration. Several regimens are available, including that listed in Table 4. Although some headache cycles can be terminated with steroids, re-emergence of headaches may occur as dosages decrease to 15 to 20 mg per day.

Lithium Carbonate. Lithium carbonate* (Eskalith, Lithobid, Lithane) is effective in more than 60 per cent of cases. The usual starting dose is 300 mg administered 2 to 4 times daily. Therapeutic response does not necessarily correlate with blood levels, and serum levels exceeding 0.7 mEq per liter are rarely necessary for good results.

Calcium Antagonists. Verapamil* (Isoptin,

*This use of these agents is not listed in the manufacturers' directives.

Calan) can be particularly valuable in dosages ranging from 80 to 160 mg 3 to 4 times per day.

Methysergide. Methysergide can be useful in cluster headache, since many cycles of the episodic form last less than the 6-month limit on continued usage of methysergide. Dosages are the same as those used in migraine treatment.

Nonsteroidal Anti-inflammatory Agents. NSAIDs can be effective for cluster headache but appear to be most useful for the variant forms. Indomethacin (Indocin) at dosages of 25 to 50 mg 3 to 4 times per day is often effective.

Chlorpromazine. Chlorpromazine in dosages ranging from 75 to several hundred mg per day has been reported as useful in cluster headaches, but most authorities have not found this treatment to be acceptable, except rarely. Chlorpromazine can be used as an adjunctive therapy, however.

Other Therapies. Intravenous DHE-45 or hydrocortisone, as described under symptomatic (Rescue) treatment of migraine, can be markedly beneficial to alter cluster headache (reduce the attacks for several days), but its value beyond the actual days of usage cannot be predicted. Nonetheless, the termination, for at least several days, of a severe and disabling pain syndrome can in itself be worthwhile, while allowing other treatments to be started.

Histamine desensitization to alleviate cluster headache is considered by most authorities to be of little value. However, in severely intractable cases, this intervention can be considered.

Surgery and other ablative procedures on the sphenopalatine ganglion, the nervus intermedius, or the branches or ganglion of the trigeminal nerve may be effective and appropriate in some absolutely intractable cases. Surgical treatment is recommended only in the most severe and extreme circumstances.

HEADACHES IN CHILDREN

Children, like adults, suffer headaches. The treatment regimens are generally similar, although greater reliance on nonmedicinal interventions is appropriate. Biofeedback, dietary regulation (e.g., not missing meals and avoidance of headache-provoking foodstuffs) and limiting other provoking factors can be helpful. Cyproheptadine, beta-blocker therapy, tricyclic antidepressants, and NSAIDs are useful for prophylaxis. Symptomatic treatment can be accomplished in a manner similar to that for adults with migraine.

POST-TRAUMATIC CEPHALALGIA

The incidence of headache following closed head injury varies from 33 to 80 per cent and can take one of several forms. Often the headache is a component of the *post-traumatic* or *post-concussion syndrome,* which represents a constellation of symptoms that can follow even mild head or flexion extension neck injury. Among the headache symptoms are generalized throbbing or nonthrobbing cephalgia; unilateral, intermittent, or continuous throbbing (similar to migraine); localized occipital/cervical pain with neuralgic qualities; and unilateral, intense, intermittent cephalagia in the anterior triangle of the neck or in the orbital area, resembling episodic cluster headache. Other mixed forms exist as well.

Treatment

The treatment of these conditions is similar to that of other headache types, emphasizing nonpharmacologic as well as pharmacologic therapies. Transneural stimulation, physical therapy, and nerve-blocking procedures may be additionally helpful. Local tenderness may respond to local anesthetics and/or to neuralgic medication, such as carbamazepine (Tegretol), 100 to 200 mg 3 times daily, or baclofen (Lioresal), 10 to 20 mg 2 or 3 times daily.

Hospital Treatment

Since 1979, when the first inpatient specialty unit for headache was developed in Ann Arbor, patients with severe and refractory headaches have been admitted to the few similar units around the country. The inpatient headache programs provide a comprehensive and intense intervention, and include drug detoxification programs, aggressive pharmacotherapy, milieu treatment, dietary manipulation, identification and reduction of provoking influences, and psychological and family intervention. Admission to such a unit is appropriate for patients with refractory daily or almost daily headache.

EPISODIC VERTIGO

method of
STEPHEN E. THURSTON, M.D.
Geisinger Medical Center
Danville, Pennsylvania

Vertigo is a symptom characterized by abnormal perceptions of motion or of spatial orientation. It results from physiologic or pathologic mismatches between various sensory systems (mainly visual, vestibular, and proprioceptive). These systems subserve stabilization of vision during head movements, spatial orientation, and maintenance of posture and locomo-

TABLE 1. Causes of Acute Vertigo

Physiologic vertigo: motion sickness, height vertigo, head extension vertigo

Benign paroxysmal positional vertigo (cupulolithiasis)

Infection of labyrinth and/or vestibular nerve: viral (including zoster), bacterial, syphilitic, mycotic

Keratoma (cholesteatoma)

Drug toxicity: alcohol, aminoglycosides, anticonvulsants, salicylates, chemotherapeutic agents, heavy metals

Trauma: labyrinthine concussion, temporal bone fracture, perilymph fistula, barotrauma, postsurgical

Ménière's disease

Otosclerosis

Cerebellar, brainstem, or labyrinthine infarction or hemorrhage

Migraine: Bickerstaff's basilar artery migraine, Slater's "benign recurrent vertigo"

Multiple sclerosis

Tumors of middle or inner ear, eighth cranial nerve, brainstem, or cerebellum

Arnold-Chiari malformation and other posterior fossa anomalies

Syringobulbia

Congenital anomalies of the inner ear

Cogan's syndrome

Idiopathic vertigo of childhood

Familial vertigo, ataxia, and nystagmus

Epilepsy

Paget's disease

Diabetes mellitus

Uremia

Hypothyroidism

---

tion. They also connect with autonomic centers in the medulla. Although many different disorders involving any of these systems may produce symptoms, vestibular dysfunction is the most common cause of clinically significant vertigo.

Vestibular vertigo may result from disease of the semicircular canals that sense angular rotation of the head or of the otoliths that sense linear translations of the head and static head position. Involvement of the canals or their central connections produces illusions of turning, spinning, or rotational movement. Disease of the otoliths or their central connections produces illusions of tilt, sway, or linear movement.

Vestibular vertigo is typically associated with nystagmus, postural imbalance, and autonomic symptoms of nausea, vomiting, pallor, diaphoresis, and generalized weakness. Nystagmus may result in blurred vision and oscillopsia, which is the illusory motion of objects due to movement of their images on the retina.

Treatment of vertigo is based on establishing a vestibular cause of symptoms as distinct from the numerous other causes of "dizziness." Therapy may be divided into *general*, with the goal of correcting the vestibular dysfunction, and *specific*, aimed at the underlying cause of dysfunction. Causes of acute vertigo are summarized in Table 1. It should be noted that most causes of acute vertigo may also produce vertigo episodically. Many forms of vertigo can be positionally induced, particularly that due to benign paroxysmal positional vertigo (by definition), labyrinthine concussion, alcohol, multiple sclerosis, Arnold-Chiari malformation and various other structural lesions in the posterior fossa.

General Therapy

General therapy of vertigo is aimed at alleviating acute autonomic symptoms and promoting restoration of normal vestibular function. Although some forms of vertigo may be either very mild or self-limited, requiring only limited intervention, the following approach is applicable to most acute peripheral or central vestibulopathies. In acute episodes, patients are kept at bed rest and allowed to assume their most comfortable head position. Sudden head movements are avoided. Intravenous hydration may be beneficial in patients with protracted vomiting. A clear liquid diet is begun and advanced as tolerated. When indicated, the patient is reassured that symptoms will improve, and every effort is made to decrease anxiety without using anxiolytic drugs.

A wide variety of vestibulosedative and antiemetic drugs are available for the symptomatic treatment of vertigo. Some of the more commonly used agents are listed in Table 2. Although considered helpful empirically, their effectiveness has rarely been evaluated by objective measurement of vestibular function. The variety of agents

TABLE 2. Drugs Commonly Used to Treat Vertigo

Drug	Dose
Anticholinergic	
Scopolamine (Transderm-Scop)	0.6 mg p.o. q 4–6 hr or 0.5 mg transdermally by patch q 3 days
Antihistamine	
Dimenhydrinate (Dramamine)	50 mg p.o. or IM q 4–6 hr or 100 mg rectally q 8 hr
Meclizine (Antivert, Bonine)	25 mg p.o. q 4–6 hr
Promethazine (Phenergan)	25 or 50 mg p.o. or IM or rectally q 4–6 hr
Cyclizine (Marezine)	50 mg p.o. or IM q 4–6 hr or 100 mg rectally q 8 hr
Trimethobenzamide (Tigan)	250 mg p.o. or IM q 6–8 hr
Antidopaminergic	
Prochlorperazine (Compazine)	5 or 10 mg p.o. or IM q 4–6 hr or 25 mg rectally q 12 hr
Droperidol (Inapsine, Innovar)	2.5 or 5 mg IM q 12 hr
Haloperidol (Haldol)	1 or 2 mg p.o. or IM q 8–12 hr
Benzodiazepines	
Diazepam (Valium, Valrelease)	5 or 10 mg p.o., IM, or IV q 4–6 hr
Sympathomimetic amines (adjunctive)	
Ephedrine sulfate	25 mg p.o. q 6 hr with promethazine
Dextro-amphetamine	5 mg p.o. q 6 hr with scopolamine

is indicative of the variability of effectiveness. It is often difficult to predict which patient will be helped by which drug, because our understanding of vestibular neuropharmacology is relatively limited and vestibular disorders encompass pathology in a variety of different anatomic, physiologic and neurochemical systems. Additionally, experimental studies suggest that various central nervous system sedating agents actually inhibit vestibular compensation or produce decompensation. Drug therapy, therefore, should be restricted to the acute phase of the illness and used to relieve only the more severely disabling symptoms. In such settings, parenteral therapy is often necessary.

Prochlorperazine and trimethobenzamide are effective antiemetics with relatively less sedation than promethazine. Promethazine in combination with ephedrine is less sedating and more effective against autonomic symptoms. Scopolamine, which can be administered transdermally with fewer side effects, is a convenient and effective method of preventing motion sickness and is also helpful in acute vertigo due to vestibular tone imbalance. Dextro-amphetamine significantly potentiates the benefit of scopolamine, but has a high abuse potential and is not generally recommended for routine use. The use of papaverine, histamine, betahistamine, nylidrin, and other vasodilators to improve blood flow to the labyrinth and brainstem is of unproven benefit. Vestibulosedative drugs should be used only in acute peripheral and central vestibulopathies and in the prophylaxis of motion sickness. There is no indication for the use of these drugs chronically.

The symptoms of an acute vestibulopathy usually improve significantly within a few days. While drug therapy and immobilization decrease symptoms, they also alter the sensory feedback that the central nervous system requires in order to restore vestibular balance. Experimental studies indicate that immobilization following unilateral peripheral vestibular lesions both prolongs adaptation and limits the ultimate degree of adaptation achieved. It has also been shown that enforced activity increases adaptation. Thus, pharmacotherapy and immobilization are restricted to only the acute phase of illness, and an active program of vestibular rehabilitation is begun as soon as possible. This consists of exercises to elicit the visual and vestibular interactions necessary to promote recovery. In addition to vestibular adaptation, the exercises develop maximal use of other overlapping and compensatory systems. Since these same interactions (mismatches) produce an increase in the offending symptoms, patients will resist therapy. They

must be reassured by explaining the rationale for treatment.

Physical therapy is begun as soon as possible after the severe autonomic symptoms subside. Modifications of the Cawthorne-Cooksey exercises (Table 3) are most commonly used. The patient progresses through the various levels of difficulty as rapidly as possible given the limitations of his or her particular illness. Refractive corrective lenses should be worn during the exercises. Care should be taken with maneuvers done with the eyes closed or when the patient is particularly unstable. The series of exercises is repeated at least three times a day as long as vertigo persists.

In addition to formal exercises, the patient is encouraged to seek out offending head positions and movements, rather than to avoid them, and to actively engage in them as much as possible. Since adaptation tends to be rather stimulus specific, these movements should be practiced over a wide range of frequencies and velocities, particularly those that cause the most symptoms during the patient's daily routines.

TABLE 3. **Modified Cawthorne-Cooksey Exercises**

A. In bed—sitting up if possible
  1. Head stationary
    a. Look up and down
    b. Look from side to side
    c. Repeat a and b, focusing on finger moving up and down, side to side, slowly, then quickly
  2. Head moving—slowly, then quickly while fixating a target; repeat with eyes closed while imagining target
    a. Up and down (pitch)
    b. Rotating head side to side (yaw)
    c. Tilting head side to side (roll)
    d. Repeat a and b, fixating finger on outstretched arm as head and arm move together

B. Sitting
  Repeat 1 and 2
  3. Lean forward and pick up objects from floor
  4. Rotate head, shoulders, and trunk with eyes open, then closed

C. Standing
  5. Practice standing with feet side by side with eyes open, then closed
  6. Change from sitting to standing with eyes open, then closed; repeat 1, 2, and 3
  7. Toss ball from hand to hand above eye level
  8. Pass ball from hand to hand under knees
  9. Change from sitting to standing and turn around in between; repeat 4

D. Walking
  10. Walk across room with eyes open, then closed
  11. Practice making sudden turns while walking
  12. Walk up and down slope with eyes open, then closed
  13. Stand on one foot with eyes open, then closed
  14. Tandem walking with eyes open, then closed
  15. Tandem walking backwards with eyes open, then closed

Persistent vestibular deficits may occur with involvement of central structures important to adaptation, such as the cerebellum and the vestibular commissures in the brainstem. In the case of multiple sensory deficits, spatial orientation may be improved by supplementing proprioceptive and visual function through the use of such devices as canes or refractive correction. Only very rarely is surgical intervention such as vestibular nerve section or labyrinthectomy necessary.

Specific Therapy

Specific therapy of vertigo is aimed at the underlying pathologic process (see Table 1). Benign paroxysmal positional vertigo is the most common cause of positional vertigo. It is believed to be due to detached otoconia from the otoliths adhering to the cupula of the posterior semicircular canal, making it gravity sensitive. It can usually be distinguished from positional vertigo due to central nervous system disease by a careful examination that includes Nylen-Barany positional testing. Brandt and Daroff have demonstrated the effectiveness of head positioning exercises in treating benign paroxysmal positional vertigo. Although adaptation probably plays a role, it is believed that the exercises mechanically disperse the misplaced otoconial debris.

Patients first tilt laterally from the seated position to lying on their affected side and hold that position until the evoked vertigo subsides. They then sit back upright 30 seconds before assuming the opposite head-down position for another 30 seconds. This sequence is repeated until the vertigo subsides, usually after several repetitions. These sessions are carried out every 3 hours while the patient is awake until he or she is free of vertigo for 2 consecutive days. Symptoms usually resolve in 1 to 2 weeks. Very rarely, symptoms will persist and surgical section of the posterior ampullary nerve may be considered. In such a case, vestibular exercises should first be tried for at least 2 to 4 weeks. There is no indication for vestibulosedative drugs in benign paroxysmal positional vertigo.

Some vestibulotoxic agents such as alcohol, salicylates, and anticonvulsants produce predominantly reversible effects that resolve with reducing the dose or discontinuing the drug. Other vestibulotoxic agents such as the aminoglycoside antibiotics (streptomycin, gentamycin, tobramycin, kanamycin, neomycin) produce more permanent effects, and the drug must be promptly discontinued at the first sign of toxicity.

Anticoagulation may be indicated in some unequivocal cases of vertebrobasilar ischemia. Episodic vertigo in isolation, without other evidence of posterior circulation ischemia, is not likely due to vertebrobasilar insufficiency. Cerebellar infarction or hemorrhage requires hospitalization and possible surgical decompression; anticoagulation is contraindicated.

Acute and chronic bacterial, syphilitic, or mycotic infections of the middle or inner ear or meningeal spaces are treated with appropriate antibiotics. Myringotomy and culture may be necessary in bacterial labyrinthitis secondary to acute otitis media. Viral infections of the vestibular nerve, ganglion, or labyrinth are usually treated with the general measures described above. Analgesics and specific antiviral therapy may prove useful in herpes zoster oticus, which is typically associated with ear pain followed in several days by a vesicular eruption in the external auditory canal.

Most perilymph fistulas spontaneously resolve, especially with bed rest and avoidance of Valsalva maneuvers. Surgical repair after definitive diagnosis by exploratory tympanotomy may be necessary if symptoms persist for longer than 3 to 4 weeks. Temporal bone fractures with cerebrospinal fluid otorrhea require close monitoring for the possible development of meningitis. The use of prophylactic antibiotics is now questioned by many.

Meniere's disease is discussed separately. Otosclerosis is suggested by conductive or mixed hearing loss, tinnitus, and vestibular symptoms when examination of the tympanic membrane does not reveal middle ear disease. The recommended treatment has been calcium gluconate, 500 mg orally twice a day (before meals); sodium fluoride, 20 mg orally twice a day (after meals); and vitamin D, 400 units orally daily; however, the necessity for the calcium and vitamin D has been questioned, and the benefit of fluoride therapy must be weighed against the risk of fluorosis.

Tumors involving vestibular pathways often require surgical resection. The use of radiation therapy and/or chemotherapy depends on tumor location and type. Symptoms due to Arnold-Chiari malformation may improve with suboccipital decompression.

Cogan's syndrome (deafness, tinnitus, episodic vertigo, and interstitial keratitis) may respond to steroids and cyclophosphamide.* Certain focal temporal and parietal seizures (vertiginous epilepsy) are rare causes of vertigo that respond to anticonvulsant therapy. Migraine (see article on Headache) may cause vertigo, not necessarily in association with headache. Since there is some anecdotal evidence that vasoconstricting agents

---

*This use is not listed in the manufacturer's directive.

may increase the ischemic complications of migraine, these agents should probably be avoided in treating migraine without headache. Familial recurrent ataxia and nystagmus are controlled with acetazolamide. Idiopathic vertigo of childhood does not need to be treated, given its benign course and the brief duration of symptoms.

In a large number of patients with episodic vertigo, no cause can be found. Although Meniere's disease or some other cause may be identified later, most resolve spontaneously. General therapy and follow-up is appropriate in these cases.

MENIERE'S DISEASE

method of
MICHAEL M. PAPARELLA, M.D.
Minnesota Ear, Head and Neck Clinic and
International Hearing Foundation
Minneapolis, Minnesota

and

SADY S. DA COSTA, M.D.
International Hearing Foundation
Minneapolis, Minnesota

Meniere's disease is a disease of the inner ear characterized by a triad of symptoms that include vestibular symptoms, auditory symptoms, and aural pressure. Usually this triad occurs together, although in many patients vestibular or auditory symptoms can precede the development of other symptoms by many months or years.

The disease is bilateral in at least one out of three patients; males and females are affected fairly equally and the disease is most common in adults, but we have seen many children with the classical picture of Meniere's Disease.

The vestibular symptoms in Meniere's disease include episodic paroxysmal vertigo associated with nausea and/or vomiting, a feeling of imbalance or disequilibrium that can last for a long period of time, and positional vertigo that exacerbates an attack of vertigo or can occur between attacks. Rarely patients also have attacks of such explosive onset that they fall violently to the ground; these have been termed falling spells of Tumarkin.

Classic cochlear symptoms consist of progressive fluctuating sensorineural hearing loss, tinnitus, loudness intolerance, and diplacusis. Lermoyez syndrome is a condition in which a paradoxical improvement of hearing follows the acute attack.

Pressure is a remarkable symptom and it is almost always present in patients with Meniere's disease. Most times it is an aural pressure but the patient may feel it in any part of the head or even the neck.

The course of the disease may be progressive (PMD) or nonprogressive (NPMD). In progressive Meniere's disease the symptoms worsen despite medical treatment and often become incapacitating and intractable. These patients (estimated as one out of four) are candidates for surgery. The remaining three out of four patients, whose disease is nonprogressive (symptoms do not worsen) can be successfully managed with medical treatment.

In addition to the typical presentation of Meniere's disease, two variations of the disorder have been identified: Cochlear Meniere's disease, in which there is hearing loss and pressure without vertigo; and vestibular Meniere's disease, characterized by episodes of vertigo without associated sensorineural hearing loss. Patients with both conditions may develop the full-blown picture of Meniere's disease later in life.

A careful history is the most important guide to a correct diagnosis and, indeed, in 90 per cent of cases a good history makes the diagnosis. An audiogram followed by vestibular studies is helpful. Common audiometric patterns include a peak audiometric configuration, low-frequency losses in early stages, and a flat pattern in advanced Meniere's disease. Auditory brainstem response (ABR) is sometimes used to distinguish a cochlear versus a central lesion. Hypoactivity of the involved labyrinth as recorded by electronystagmography (ENG) is the most common finding of all vestibular tests. Routine mastoid x-rays are used to screen any abnormalities in the mastoid and temporal bone and to assess the position of the lateral sinus.

A computed tomography (CT) scan and magnetic resonance imaging (MRI) should be ordered only when intracranial pathologic conditions have not been completely ruled out. Electrocochleography may be useful in the evaluation of patients with Meniere's disease either pre- or intraoperatively.

The most important pathologic finding in Meniere's disease is endolymphatic hydrops involving both the scala media and the otolitic organs, although hydrops should not be considered synonymous with Meniere's disease. Gross anatomic pathologic findings include decreased mastoid and periaqueductal pneumatization and anterior and medial displacement of the lateral sinus with concomitant reduction of Trautmann's triangle.

From our recent studies it would appear that the etiology of Meniere's disease is a multifactorially (racial, genetic) inherited predisposition to which environmental and individual factors (such as infections, otosclerosis, and trauma) can be added. The pathogenesis subsequently includes the development of endolymphatic malabsorption in the endolymphatic duct and sac; both mechanical and chemical factors appear to provide the best explanation for the pathogenesis and symptoms of Meniere's disease.

TREATMENT

It is of crucial importance in the care of patients with Meniere's disease to establish a good doctor-patient relationship. Psychological support is perhaps the most important medical management. A number of different drugs have been used to treat Meniere's disease, including diuretics, vestibular sedatives, vascular agents, and vestibulotoxic drugs. Since drugs act on an empirical basis, our policy is not to discourage the use of any of them if they minimize symptoms, encourage nonprogressive Meniere's disease, and help prevent progressive Meniere's disease. Medical treatment does not alter the fundamental pathology or pathogenesis of the disease. It does, however, treat the patient and alleviate contributory factors that exacerbate the disease. Our treatment is based on psychological support and a medical trial with a single drug or a combination of drugs, as the status of the patient requires.

The following drugs may be used: Meclizine (Antivert), 12.5 to 25 mg orally 4 times a day; prochlorperazine (Compazine) tablets, 5 to 10 mg orally 3 times a day; transdermal scopolamine patches (Transderm-Scop) 1 every 3 days; diazepam (Valium), 2 to 5 mg orally 2 or 3 times a day.

Acute attacks are managed basically in the same way. If the patient presents with excessive nausea and vomiting, he should be admitted to the hospital, treated with intravenous medicines and fluids, bed rest, and supportive care. The control of underlying etiologic and contributory factors such as stress, allergy, and hormonal disturbances represents an important part of the therapy.

In cases in which the deafness and/or vertigo becomes intractable despite medical therapy, the conservative surgical procedure known as endolymphatic sac enhancement, is considered. The method has been used in approximately 900 patients over a 20-year period. We consider this surgery an extension of conservative treatment because it has minimal risks and appears to reverse the pathogenesis of Meniere's disease. This procedure can be done in patients with either typical or atypical disease; the primary indication is vertigo and deafness. It offers a 90 per cent chance to improve vertigo and a 70 per cent chance to eliminate vertigo. One of three patients has improvement of hearing, whereas hearing is preserved in 90 per cent of patients. The chief risk is deafness, which occurs in 2 per cent of cases.

If a patient experiences a good result for a period of time (years) and then presents with a recurrence of vertigo, an endolymphatic sac revision can be considered. A transmastoid vestibular nerve section can also be considered. Despite inherent risks of intracranial surgery, vestibular nerve section is an effective operation for intractable vertigo. However, in our series of surgical cases, few patients have required vestibular nerve section.

Labyrinthectomy is avoided to enhance the future possible use of a cochlear implant, especially as we have seen complete bilateral deafness occur in certain patients with Meniere's disease.

VIRAL MENINGOENCEPHALITIS

method of
HARLEY A. ROTBART, M.D., and
MYRON J. LEVIN, M.D.
University of Colorado School of Medicine
Denver, Colorado

Many viruses are capable of infecting the central nervous system (CNS) and causing symptomatic disease (Table 1). Several distinct syndromes are recognized, although there is significant overlap in etiologic agents, laboratory findings, and clinical manifestations. *Aseptic meningitis* is the most common CNS viral syndrome, characterized by headache, stiff neck, photophobia and non-specific constitutional signs such as fever, vomiting, and lethargy. *Encephalitis* is the result of parenchymal brain infection and is often associated with a change in level of consciousness and/or affect, frequently with accompanying focal neurologic deficits and seizures. *Myelitis* is a relatively rare syndrome (in the post-polio era) that results from infection of spinal cord neurons, with attendant motor signs and symptoms. Each of these entities is best diagnosed by a combination of clinical findings and cerebrospinal fluid (CSF) analysis. The CSF typically contains leukocytes, usually with a lymphocyte predominance, although polymorphonuclear cells may be in excess early in infection. Glucose levels are usually normal or slightly low, and protein is often modestly elevated (more so in herpes simplex and other necrotizing viral infections).

Most CNS viral disease is acute in onset and of short duration. Chronic (or "slow") infections occur with certain viruses (e.g., Creutzfeldt-Jakob disease, subacute sclerosing panencephalitis) or in certain hosts (e.g., chronic enteroviral infection in hypogammaglobulinemic patients). A postinfectious CNS inflammatory disease has also been described following several viral diseases, including varicella-zoster, measles, and rubella.

Treatment

Approach to therapy is three-pronged: (1) rule out other treatable causes of infection (empiric therapy for nonviral agents may be required while awaiting results of laboratory studies); (2) provide supportive care; and (3) administer specific antiviral therapy when appropriate.

Implicit in the diagnosis of viral CNS infection is the exclusion of other treatable disease. Since that may require hours to days, empiric initiation of antibiotics (for acute bacterial, mycobacterial, or rickettsial infection) or, rarely, antifungal

TABLE 1. **Etiologic Agents of Viral Meningoencephalitis**

	Most Common Clinical Syndrome*		
	Aseptic meningitis	*Encephalitis*	**Comment**
Acute Infection			
Arenaviruses			
Lymphocytic choriomeningitis	X		Rodent handlers at risk
Lassa, Junin, Machupo		X	Hemorrhagic fevers
Bunyavirus			
California encephalitis		X	Arthropod-borne; regional, seasonal
Cytomegalovirus		X	Neonates, immunocompromised patients at risk
Enterovirus	X		Most common cause of aseptic meningitis
coxsackie, echo, polio			
Epstein-Barr virus	X	X	Association still ill-defined
Herpes simplex		X	Type 1 more common
Human immunodeficiency virus		X	Cause of various CNS syndromes
Influenza A	X	X	
Measles		X	
Mumps	X	X	
Orbivirus	X		Colorado tick fever; seasonal
Togaviruses			
Eastern, western, St. Louis encephalitis		X	Regional, seasonal; arthropod-borne
Rubella		X	Part of congenital rubella syndrome
Varicella-zoster		X	Immunocompromised patients at greatest risk; primary infection or reactivation (herpes zoster)
Subacute, Chronic, or Persistent Infections			
Creutzfeldt-Jakob		X	Transmitted by direct inoculation of infected nervous tissue; perhaps by other routes
Enterovirus	X		Hypogammaglobulinemic and agammaglobulinemic patients at risk
Kuru		X	Associated with cananbalism of infected brains
JC and BK viruses		X	Progressive multifocal leukoencephalopathy
Measles		X	Subacute sclerosing panencephalitis
Rabies		X	
Rubella		X	

*The most common syndrome is indicated for each virus, but significant overlap exists, with many agents capable of causing both meningitis and encephalitis. When there is an X in both columns, the syndromes are equally common.

drugs may be indicated. Empiric therapy may also be warranted when parameningeal infections (sinusitis, abscess, epidural and subdural collections) are suspected, as they may be initially indistinguishable from acute viral infection. Noninfectious CNS diseases that may mimic viral infection and require specific therapy include malignancy, collagen-vascular diseases, Reye's syndrome, and lead poisoning. Occasionally antibiotic therapy itself, usually with sulfa compounds, causes an aseptic meningitis-like syndrome.

Supportive therapy, which is directed at the sequelae of severe viral CNS infections, is applicable regardless of the specific pathogen. *Respiratory failure* may result from depression of central pathways, concomitant tracheobronchopulmonary infection, or airway obstruction with or without seizures. An artificial airway, assisted ventilation, and tracheal toilet all may be necessary. *Fluid/electrolyte imbalance* due to dehydration, dilutional hyponatremia, or inappropriate secretion of antidiuretic hormone is common with any CNS infection. Electrolytes and urine/serum osmolality should be monitored and fluid input adjusted regularly. *Brain edema* secondary to the inflammatory response to viral infection should be suspected with the occurrence of new neurologic deficits or changes in pupil size. A computed tomography (CT) or magnetic reso-

TABLE 2. **Specific Therapies for CNS Viral Infections**

	Pathogens	Drug and Dosing	Comment
Established Therapy	Herpes simplex	Acyclovir (Zovirax), 10 mg/kg q 8 hr IV × 10 days	Brain biopsy recommended prior to start of therapy; give acyclovir as 1-hr infusion; adjust dose for renal impairment
	Varicella-zoster	Acyclovir (Zovirax), as above	One hour infusion; adjust dose for renal impairment
	Human immunodeficiency virus	Azidothymidine (Retrovir), 200 mg q 4 hr po; *or* 2.5–5.0 mg/kg q 4 hr IV	Important to exclude other concomitant CNS infection/malignancy; monitor blood counts
	Rabies	Human diploid cell vaccine, 1 ml IM on days 1, 3, 7, 14, 28; *and* human rabies immune globulin, 20 IU per kg (½ given into wound, ½ given IV)	Begin immediately post-exposure; local wound cleansing also recommended
Experimental Therapy	Cytomegalovirus	Ganciclovir, 2.5–7.5 mg/kg q 8 hr IV; *or* 5 mg/kg q 12 hr IV, for duration of symptoms	Available on compassionate use basis from Syntex Corp. Biopsy diagnosis required. Adjust dose for renal impairment or neutropenia
	Epstein-Barr virus	Ganciclovir or Acyclovir, as above	Duration of therapy uncertain
	Influenza A	Amantidine, 200 mg/day po (for >10 years old) × 7–10 days	Adjust dose for renal impairment
	Arenaviruses	Ribavirin, 2 grams IV load, then 1 gram q 6 hr IV × 4 days, followed by 0.5 gram q 6 hr IV × 6 days	Only Lassa fever trials reported; hemolysis may complicate therapy
	Measles Acute encephalitis	Ribavirin, 2.5 mg/kg qid po × 7 days	This dosing reported for acute measles; higher dose may be considered for encephalitis
	Subacute sclerosing panencephalitis	Ribavirin, 10 mg/kg tid po × 3 days followed by 10 mg/kg bid × 6 weeks	
	Enteroviruses Chronic infection	Human immunoglobulin, 200–400 mg/kg q 2–4 weeks IV; duration based on response	Intrathecal therapy may be more effective; gammaglobulin lots may be screened for specific antibody titers to infecting serotype
	Neonatal (high risk)	Human immunoglobulin, 400 mg/kg IV as single dose	High-risk factors include concurrent maternal illness, age at onset <1 week, prematurity

nance imaging (MRI) scan may help in this diagnosis, and an intracranial pressure monitor will confirm and quantitate the elevated pressure and facilitate management. Fluid input should be adjusted to avoid overhydration. Mannitol (0.5 grams per kg of 20 per cent solution given over 20 minutes intravenously) osmotically removes excess CNS fluid, and should be given in repeat doses every 4 to 6 hours as needed. Hyperventilation to constrict CNS blood vessel caliber is generally used after other modalities have failed. The response is usually brisk, but may wane after 24 hours. The use of glucocorticoids is controversial, and in some settings may be harmful.

Seizures may result from direct viral or inflammatory damage of neurons, increased intracranial pressure, or fluid and electrolyte imbalance.

Phenytoin (Dilantin), 15 mg per kg given intravenously as a loading dose at a rate not to exceed 50 mg per minute, while monitoring blood pressure and electrocardiogram (ECG), is the drug of choice, as it does not cloud the sensorium. Maintenance dosing is with 3 to 5 mg per kg daily for adults and 4 to 8 mg per kg for children. Phenobarbital, 5 mg per kg intravenously every 30 minutes, at a rate not to exceed 100 mg per minute, until seizures cease or blood pressure falls (total loading dose not more than 20 mg per kg) is an alternative. Maintenance dosing of phenobarbital is 2 to 3 mg per kg daily for adults and 3 to 5 mg per kg for children. Refractory seizures may require additional antiepileptics or paralysis (to prevent hyperthermia and increased metabolic requirements). We do not recommend prophylaxis against seizures with viral CNS infection.

Bladder atony/hypotony secondary to myelitis or severe encephalitis requires catheterization. Patients with protracted courses may develop malnutrition and require hyperalimentation.

Specific established antiviral therapy is available only for herpes simplex, varicella-zoster, human immunodeficiency virus, and rabies (Table 2). Experimental treatments, however, have shown promise in a number of serious viral CNS diseases (see Table 2), and may be considered on a compassionate basis in certain appropriate settings.

REYE'S SYNDROME

method of
DORIS A. TRAUNER, M.D.
University of California, San Diego School of Medicine
La Jolla, California

Reye's syndrome is an acute metabolic encephalopathy with hepatic dysfunction that occurs almost exclusively in children, although rare cases have been reported in adults of all ages. It is a biphasic illness with characteristic clinical features. In the initial phase, the child has a viral syndrome, most often a flu-like illness, with gastrointestinal or upper respiratory tract symptoms. While influenza B virus is associated with the majority of cases, varicella is the prodromal illness in approximately 10 per cent. The child typically is recovering from this viral ailment when the second phase begins with repeated vomiting, followed by changes in sensorium. These may include lethargy, hyperexcitability, or combativeness; symptoms may progress to obtundation or coma. Hyperventilation is a prominent feature on examination. Seizures may occur at any time during the course of the second phase.

Infants under 1 year of age have a more subtle presentation. Although the prodromal illness is usually present, vomiting may be minimal or absent; respiratory distress is present early, and the initial sign of the second phase may be sudden apnea or seizure activity.

Laboratory abnormalities include evidence of hepatocellular dysfunction with elevated serum transaminase and creatine phosphokinase levels, hyperammonemia and prolonged prothrombin time. Serum bilirubin concentrations are not significantly elevated. Hypoglycemia occurs in about 40 per cent of children. A mixed metabolic acidosis and respiratory alkalosis is typical, with alkalosis predominating. Abnormalities of fatty acid, glucose, and urea cycle metabolism have been demonstrated during the acute illness. All of the metabolic abnormalities are reversible once the acute phase of the illness is over.

Pathologic changes include microvesicular fatty accumulation in the liver, depletion of hepatic glycogen stores, decreased hepatic activity of the succinic acid dehydrogenase enzyme, and mitochondrial swelling and pleomorphism. Massive brain swelling is a potentially fatal complication.

Reye's syndrome affects 0.3 to 3.5 per 100,000 children under the age of 18 years in the United States. The cause of this disorder is unknown. There is evidence of a potential association between salicylate ingestion during the prodromal illness, and subsequent development of Reye's syndrome. No causal relationship has been established.

Treatment

Treatment of the acute illness is limited by a lack of knowledge about causation. Most approaches to therapy are based on intensive supportive care, correction of metabolic abnormalities, treatment of seizures, and reduction of intracranial pressure. In addition, because of experimental evidence of a possible carnitine deficiency state in these patients, we use carnitine as an adjunct to therapy.

A uniform staging system for Reye's syndrome has been proposed by the NIH Consensus Development Conference on the Diagnosis and Treatment of Reye's Syndrome. This consists of five stages:

Stage I: Vomiting; lethargy or sleepiness; responds appropriately to verbal stimuli.

Stage II: Stupor, disorientation, delirium, combativeness; may not respond to verbal stimuli but responds appropriately to painful stimuli.

Stage III: Obtundation or coma; decorticate posturing to painful stimuli; intact brain stem reflexes.

Stage IV: Coma; decerebrate posturing spontaneously or in response to painful stimuli; brain stem reflexes may be impaired, with sluggish pupillary response to light and incomplete oculocephalic (doll's eyes) reflexes.

Stage V: Coma; flaccid quadriparesis; no response to painful stimuli; sluggish or absent oculocephalic and pupillary responses.

General Considerations

Any infant or child with suspected Reye's syndrome should be hospitalized in a pediatric intensive care unit, even if the child is awake and responsive. The clinical condition can deteriorate very quickly, and a child may pass from Stage I to Stage III or IV in a matter of minutes. Continuous cardiac and respiratory monitoring should be instituted immediately. Blood should be drawn for serum glucose, ammonia, bilirubin, transaminase and creatine phosphokinase determinations, and for electrolytes and prothrombin time.

Stages I–II

The child should not be given any oral feedings initially. An intravenous line should be inserted and hypertonic glucose solution (10 to 15 per cent) with appropriate electrolyte concentrations should be administered at low maintenance fluid levels. Serum glucose determinations should be monitored every 8 hours, and the rate of infusion adjusted to maintain serum glucose concentrations between 125 and 175 mg per dl. Treatment should be continued until the child has been clinically stable for 36 to 48 hours and until laboratory confirmation has been obtained that serum ammonia concentrations are stable or decreasing and liver function tests are normalizing. If deterioration in the clinical state occurs, more vigorous therapy as outlined below should be instituted.

Stages III–V

For children in the more advanced stages of Reye's syndrome, the mortality rate is significant, and aggressive therapy is required, including insertion of arterial and central venous lines, elective endotracheal intubation, and mechanical ventilation. Since hyperthermia is a common occurrence, the child should be placed on a cooling blanket to regulate body temperature within the normal range. A nasogastric tube and a Foley catheter should be inserted, and intake and output precisely recorded. Intravenous solutions containing hypertonic (15 per cent) glucose with appropriate electrolyte concentrations should be administered at 75 per cent of maintenance levels. Serum glucose concentrations should be monitored every 4 to 6 hours and kept between 125 and 175 mg per dl. Careful fluid and electrolyte balance should be maintained.

If serum ammonia concentrations exceed 150 micrograms per dl, lactulose and neomycin (25 to 50 mg per kg every 6 hours) can be administered by nasogastric tube, or neomycin by enema. When serum ammonia concentrations exceed 350 micrograms per dl, more aggressive measures such as exchange blood transfusion or peritoneal dialysis may be warranted, since ammonia levels of this magnitude have been correlated with higher mortality rates. Transfusions with fresh frozen plasma are helpful in correcting clotting abnormalities if prothrombin time is markedly prolonged, especially if intraventricular catheter placement is to be considered. We also use L-carnitine, 100 mg per kg every 12 hours intravenously, as an adjunct to therapy.

Seizures can be treated using intravenous phenytoin, with an initial loading dose of 15 mg per kg followed by a daily dose of 5 to 8 mg per kg in 2 divided doses. If the child is to be paralyzed for a prolonged period, it is helpful to use continuous electroencephalogram (EEG) monitoring to identify seizure activity. Alternatively, prophylactic phenytoin may be administered.

Brain swelling and increased intracranial pressure (ICP) may account for significant morbidity and mortality; for this reason, aggressive measures to control ICP appear warranted. An ICP monitoring device should be inserted. We prefer an intraventricular catheter, but many centers use surface recording devices. ICP should be kept within the normal range (under 15 torr). However, perfusion pressure (PP) of the brain is more important than the absolute ICP value. PP is the difference between mean arterial blood pressure (MABP) and ICP. In order to protect the brain from ischemia, PP should be kept above 50 torr. Thus, if MABP is 60, ICP must be 10 or less to ensure adequate PP.

Reduction in ICP may be achieved in several ways. Paralysis with a neuromuscular blocking agent such as pancuronium bromide at a dose of 0.1 to 0.2 mg per kg is useful, not only to reduce ICP but also to prevent the child from fighting the respirator. The child's head should be elevated 30 degrees. Controlled hyperventilation to a P_{CO_2} of 25 to 30 torr will also help to reduce ICP. Administration of an osmotic diuretic such as mannitol, at a dose of 0.25 grams per kg, is also effective. The dose may be repeated or increased to as high as 2 grams per kg per dose every 4 hours as needed to control ICP. Serum osmolality should be monitored and kept below 320 mOsm in order to maintain the effectiveness of mannitol and prevent complications of hyperosmolar states.

The use of high-dose barbiturates to control ICP should be reserved for the most refractory cases, since this mode of therapy is associated with additional complications, including decreased cardiac output and systemic hypotension. The usual method for barbiturate treatment is to administer a loading dose of 3 to 5 mg per kg pentobarbital intravenously, and then 1 to 3 mg per kg per hour to maintain a blood level of 3 to 4 mg per dl and a burst-suppression pattern on EEG. When ICP has remained normal for 24 to 48 hours, the pentobarbital is gradually reduced over 36 to 48 hours.

Outcome

The mortality rate for all cases of Reye's syndrome remains about 30 per cent. There is evidence that the disease is less likely to progress in children who are diagnosed in Stage I and who receive hypertonic glucose therapy. Survivors of Reye's syndrome over the age of 1 year are likely to return to normal levels of function, even in severe cases. Sequelae include mild cognitive dysfunction, seizure disorders, and, rarely, more severe impairment such as psychomotor retardation. Infants less than 1 year of age are more likely to suffer long-term, significant neurologic sequelae such as psychomotor retardation and spastic quadriplegia.

MULTIPLE SCLEROSIS

method of
ANTHONY T. REDER, M.D., and
RAYMOND P. ROOS, M.D.
The University of Chicago
Chicago, Illinois

Multiple sclerosis (MS) is a demyelinating disease of the central nervous system of unknown etiology. Although genetic and environmental factors, including viruses, may play a role in the disease, only therapy that alters immune function appears to reduce the number of attacks and rate of progression. Some forms of treatment have traditionally been used for acute attacks, whereas other modes of therapy, especially those with more pronounced side effects, have been reserved for relatively severe or progressive forms of MS. Although these drugs may slow disease progression, there remains no cure for MS.

Treatment of the Course of the Disease

Adrenocorticotropic hormone (ACTH) reduces the duration of exacerbations in approximately 50 per cent of MS patients, although it does not change the eventual long-term disability. Its beneficial effect is partially due to elevation of serum cortisol, which reduces plaque edema, directly excites neurons, and causes some degree of immunosuppression. In addition, ACTH itself directly inhibits lymphocyte function and may cause redistribution of sodium channels in demyelinated axons, thereby enhancing conduction. ACTH is administered intramuscularly or intravenously for 3 to 10 days. This is followed by an intramuscular taper to prevent a potential rebound in immune function and disease worsening.

A typical protocol for ACTH is 80 units intravenously in 250 ml of 5 per cent dextrose in water over 8 hours each day for 3 days (days 1–3), 40 U intramuscularly (IM) twice a day for 7 days (days 4–10), 35 U IM twice a day for 3 days (days 11–13), 30 U IM twice a day for 3 days (days 14–16), and 20 U IM twice a day for 3 days (days 17–20); tapering off with daily doses IM for 3 days each of 40 U (days 20–22), 30 U (days 23–

25), and 20 U (days 26–28); and concluding with 20 U IM every other day for 6 days (days 30, 32, and 34).

The patient is hospitalized for the initial 3 days and he or an appropriate care-giver is instructed regarding the intramuscular injections. We normally see the patient 2 and 4 weeks after discharge, and obtain a complete blood count and electrolyte and glucose determinations. Improvement may take place within several days or may be delayed for several weeks.

Side effects of ACTH include fluid retention, hypokalemia, hyperglycemia, opportunistic infections, insomnia and manifestations of Cushing's syndrome such as acne, euphoria, and rarely manic or psychotic behavior. The latter usually occurs several weeks after institution of therapy. Some patients may need medications to minimize the side effects. For example, diuretics may be necessary for prominent fluid retention, and sedatives for insomnia. Mild to moderate behavioral problems may be treated with appropriate psychotropic drugs. Severe side effects, such as marked behavioral problems, may necessitate cessation of the drug.

Oral steroids have not been compared with ACTH in a well-controlled trial, and it is possible that they lack the potentially beneficial direct effect of ACTH. Some patients with exacerbations or rapidly progressing MS, however, have a definite reduction in MS symptoms when treated with prednisone. A typical course of oral prednisone is 60 mg daily for 4 days, followed by daily doses for 3 days each of 50 mg, 40 mg, 30 mg, 20 mg, 10 mg, and 5 mg, and tapering off to 5 mg every other day for 4 days.

Side effects are similar to those seen with ACTH. We usually prescribe antacids because of possible dyspepsia or hyperacidity.

When should one treat with ACTH or prednisone and which drug should be used? Our preference is to treat clear-cut, acute attacks, especially when they involve optic neuritis or interfere with normal lifestyle and ambulation. We tend not to treat mild worsening in disease or the frequent fluctuations in neurologic functioning that sometimes occur daily. Although ACTH and steroids are most effective in acute attacks, we occasionally use these drugs for chronic progressive disease, especially when ambulation or employment is in jeopardy. We prefer to use ACTH rather than prednisone for patients with more severe attacks and for those who would benefit from hospitalization for diagnostic testing or social reasons.

If patients continue to have frequent MS attacks, we usually institute chronic azathioprine (Imuran) treatment, since this form of immunosuppression appears to reduce the number of exacerbations in relapsing/remitting MS. Some centers also report slowing of the rate of decline in chronic progressive MS; other studies show little benefit in progressive disease. The dose of azathioprine should be adjusted to allow the MCV to rise to approximately 105 μ^3 while maintaining the white count above 3000 per cubic mm. 100 mg orally per day is usually a satisfactory dose, although some patients may need to take 150 mg or more per day. Liver function and the complete blood count (CBC) should be monitored. Concurrent use of allopurinol should be avoided (azathioprine must be reduced to approximately 25 mg per day if given with allopurinol). Immunosuppression is contraindicated during pregnancy, active infection, and in patients with bone marrow depression. Benefit is long term, and a change in the rate of attacks is often not apparent for 6 to 12 weeks.

In chronic progressive MS, immunosuppressive therapy with cyclophosphamide (Cytoxan) can reduce the rate of progression and sometimes results in clinical improvement. Beneficial effects last for 1 to 2 years. Cyclophosphamide, 100 to 125 mg 4 times per day, is given intravenously in divided doses for 10 to 14 days. Because of the study design in the initial efficacy trials, and because cyclophosphamide alone in some studies is not effective, ACTH is administered concomitantly with cyclophosphamide according to the following protocol: ACTH intravenously (IV), in dosages of 25 U, 20 U, 15 U, 10 U, and 5 U, each for 3 days; then 40 U IM for 3 days and 20 U IM for 3 days; then discontinue. If progression recurs a year or more after this initial treatment, we have had some success with "boosters" of intravenous pulses of cyclophosphamide at 250 mg, four times per day on the second day of a 3 day course of intravenous ACTH, 80 U per day. Monthly pulses of cyclophosphamide, 750 mg per square meter may also reduce relapses or slow progression, but this schedule is still experimental.

Administration of cyclophosphamide should be accompanied by good intravenous hydration to prevent hemorrhagic cystitis. Liver and bone marrow function should be monitored. Cyclophosphamide should be stopped if the white blood count drops below 3500. Nausea, vomiting, and alopecia are common side effects.

Therapies with Less Well-Documented Benefit

High doses of intravenous methylprednisolone are immunosuppressive and have induced a moderate degree of improvement in relapsing or chronic progressive MS in several small trials. Spasticity improved in some patients; weakness was unaffected. This regimen consists of 1 gram of methylprednisolone intravenously for 3 days for 3 months, interspersed with 96 mg of methylprednisolone every other day for 1 month, 72 mg every other day for the second month, 48 mg every other day for the third month, then tapering by 4 mg every 2 weeks (still on an alternate day schedule). This therapy should be considered experimental and may be somewhat dangerous because of the side effects of high-dose steroids.

Intrathecal steroids are not recommended. These can cause serious adhesive arachnoiditis and aseptic meningitis in up to 10 per cent of patients.

The results of a large study of the effects of cyclosporin A completed in January of 1988 will soon be available. Any therapeutic effect must be balanced by the decline in renal function and increase in blood pressure that are common side effects.

Interferon (IFN) α and IFN β may be of some benefit in MS. (Note that IFNγ induces exacerbations, and has effects on immune function that are often opposite those of IFN α and β.) IFN α and β have been shown to reduce the number of exacerbations in relapsing/remitting MS in several small studies; larger trials are in progress at this time. Side effects consist largely of flu-like symptoms.

Copolymer I (COP-I) has been shown to be of minor benefit in mildly affected patients with relapsing/remitting MS. It is only available for experimental use.

Total lymphoid irradiation, 2000 rad over 40 days, slowed deterioration of function in patients with progressive MS. Patients who had a reduction in total lymphocyte count of ≤ 900 per cubic mm did better than those with higher counts.

Plasmapheresis, which potentially could remove antibodies involved in the pathogenesis of MS, has been reported to be moderately effective by several groups, but a number of other centers find no benefit. The results of a large multicenter trial are pending.

Dietary therapy with polyunsaturated fatty acids (PUFA) was initially reported to be beneficial, and in some populations meat-eaters are reported to have a higher incidence of MS than fish-eaters; however, several more recent studies were unable to show benefit from PUFA supplementation. Of course, a well-balanced diet high in unsaturated fats may reduce risks of cardiovascular disease.

Hyperbaric oxygen, snake venom, and calcium chelation are ineffective in the treatment of MS.

Treatment of Symptoms

Disease progression or the frequency of relapse may be slowed by the treatments described above, yet patients often have persisting disability. *Spasticity* and *nocturnal spasms* can be reduced with baclofen (Lioresal). Ten mg orally twice a day can be gradually increased to 40 mg 4 times per day. At higher doses this drug may cause weakness and fatigue, which must be balanced against the reduction in spasticity. If Lioresal is ineffective or not well tolerated, dantrolene (Dantrium) can be administered, beginning with 25 mg orally twice daily and increasing to 100 mg 4 times a day. Weakness and sedation are potential side effects, in addition to prominent alterations in liver function tests. Benzodiazepines such as diazepam (Valium), ranging from 5 mg daily to much higher doses, also reduce muscle spasticity, but are generally less effective than other muscle relaxants.

Physical therapy is helpful in maintaining muscle and joint function after an acute attack. Exercise programs to prevent contractures in chronic MS will also help maintain the peripheral vascular supply and give patients a sense of actively combatting their disease.

Weakness and fatigue are common complaints. The circadian rise in body temperature in the afternoon may amplify these symptoms (Uhthoff's phenomenon). Lowering the body temperature with a cold shower, swimming, or a glass of ice water is sometimes helpful. Amantidine HCl (Symmetrel), 100 mg twice daily, significantly reduces fatigue in one third of patients. This effect is long term, unlike that seen in Parkinson's disease. Livedo reticularis and mental side effects occur infrequently. Note that three fourths of patients show decreased strength or coordination after smoking cigarettes, 4-Aminopyridine, a potassium channel blocker, prolongs action potentials in demyelinated axons and reduces weakness and fatigue in a significant proportion of patients. This drug is awaiting FDA approval.

Tremor often causes severe disability in MS and can sometimes occur when corticospinal symptoms are relatively minor. We have had some success with clonazepam (Klonopin) in patients with cerebellar tremors. This drug is begun at a dosage of 0.5 mg orally at night and very gradually increased to 10 to 20 mg per day in divided doses. Gradual increases help to prevent sedation. Some patients also respond to propranolol (Inderal), 40 to 240 mg per day in divided doses. Isoniazid (INH) may cause slight improvement in postural and action tremors, but patients often prefer to discontinue the drug. Side effects include hepatotoxicity and an occasional increase in spasticity. A large proportion of patients are slow acetylators and should be treated with 12 mg per kg per day; rapid acetylators receive 20 mg per kg per day. Patients should be treated concomitantly with 100 mg per day of pyridoxine (vitamin B_6), and their liver function should be monitored. Rarely L-dopa/carbidopa (Simemet) can be helpful in brain-stem lesions causing a "rubral tremor," but this drug is usually ineffective in more widespread disease.

The bladder is involved in up to 90 per cent of patients with MS. One third have hyporeflexic bladders; two thirds have hyperreflexic bladders, often with sphincter dyssynergia. The abnormal bladder functioning presumably leads to frequent *urinary tract infections*. These infections may in turn exacerbate MS symptoms. Specific antibiotics should be used for short-term management; long-term suppression can be maintained with sulfonamides; nitrofurantoin, 200 to 400 mg per day in divided doses with food; methenamine mandelate, 1 gram 4 times per day; cranberry juice; or vitamin C, 4 grams orally per day.

Vesicular hyporeflexia can be improved with agents that enhance detrusor function, such as bethanechol chloride (Urecholine), 10 to 50 mg every 4 to 6 hours or methacholine Cl (Mecholyl), 200 to 400 mg every 4 to 6 hours. *Sphincter spasticity,* obstructing urinary outflow, can be reduced with phenoxybenzamine HCl (Dibenzyline), 10 mg twice a day, slowly increased to 40 mg 3 times per day, or with diazepam or baclofen.

Bladder hyperreflexia can be reduced with oxybutinin Cl (Ditropan), 5 mg 2 to 4 times per day; propantheline bromide (Pro-Banthine), 30 to 90 mg per day in divided doses with meals; and flavoxate (Urispas), 100 to 200 mg, 3 to 4 times per day. Hyperreflexic bladders are usually more easily treated than hyporeflexic bladders, but if the agents above are ineffective, the following drugs may increase outlet resistance: ephedrine SO_4, 15 to 50 mg 4 times per day; or pseudoephedrine (Sudafed), 30 to 60 mg 4 times per day. Beta adrenergic stimulants such as isoproterenol may also be helpful. If drug therapy fails, self-catheterization has a much lower risk of infection than an indwelling catheter. Bladder residual should be kept below 400 ml. Occasional patients may require permanent catheterization or supravesical urinary diversion. Note that bladder dysfunction will wax and wane along with other MS symptoms, and therapy will need to be reevaluated often.

Sexual counseling can benefit patients with impotence. Penile prostheses may improve sexual functioning.

Depression is a feature in 75 per cent of MS patients. Low doses of amitriptyline (Elavil), 25 to 75 mg at night, often reduce depression and pseudobulbar affect as well as improve sleep and bladder function.

Poorly described *paresthesias* and *dysesthesias*

are common in MS. Neuritic pain, especially that of trigeminal neuralgia, can be treated with carbamazepine (Tegretol), 200 mg initially, gradually increased to 400 mg 3 times per day, or phenytoin (Dilantin), 300 mg per day.

In addition to drug therapy, education and long-term psychological and social support is essential in a disease with frequent changes in neurologic function. Because this is a disease of young adults, advice regarding fitness for employment and child-bearing is important.

MYASTHENIA GRAVIS

method of
CHRISTIAN HERRMANN, JR., M.D.
University of California
Los Angeles, California

Present findings indicate that autoimmune myasthenia gravis is an acquired immune complex disorder of neuromuscular transmission in voluntary striated muscle. Elevated titer of antibody to acetylcholine receptor is detectable in the serum of most patients. There is a break in immunologic tolerance with blocking and degradation of acetylcholine receptors; widening of the synaptic cleft; and partial destruction, simplification, and shortening of the postjunctional membrane. Thymic hyperplasia and/or thymoma may be associated.

Clinically, myasthenia gravis is characterized by variable weakness and easy fatigability. After a short rest of the muscles, there is partial to total recovery of strength. Extraocular, facial, and oropharyngeal muscles are usually affected early, but any of the voluntary striated muscles of the body may be involved. Commonly, its onset in women occurs before the age of 40 years and in men after the age of 40. Either sex may be affected at any time. About 12 per cent of infants born to myasthenic mothers have a transient transmitted form of neonatal myasthenia gravis that remits permanently in days or weeks. Pregnancy is not generally contraindicated in myasthenia gravis.

Treatment

Anticholinesterase Therapy

Anticholinesterase drugs are the usual first line of treatment for myasthenia gravis. Their action is attributed to inhibition of cholinesterase at the neuromuscular junction, allowing acetylcholine to accumulate and facilitate remaining neuromuscular transmission. The three most frequently used are (1) neostigmine bromide (Prostigmin), (2) pyridostigmine bromide (Mestinon), and (3) ambenonium chloride (Mytelase). These partially reduce the defect in neuromuscular transmission and improve strength but are not a cure.

A fourth, very short-acting anticholinesterase agent, edrophonium chloride (Tensilon), is used to aid in the diagnosis of myasthenia gravis and to assess the effectiveness of the dosage of anticholinesterase drugs noted before. It is not useful for ongoing treatment. The diagnostic edrophonium (Tensilon) test is best done when the patient has stopped taking all anticholinesterase drugs for 8 to 12 hours. A detailed test of muscle strength is done throughout the body, with areas of weakness noted, including cranial, oropharyngeal, and respiratory muscles. This is followed by a control injection or protective placebo injection of atropine sulfate, 0.4 mg intravenously. This acts to protect the patient from muscarinic side effects of the edrophonium to be given subsequently, as well as to assess psychological effects of an intravenous injection. A detailed test of muscle strength of the areas previously noted to be weak is done again. This is followed by edrophonium, 2 mg intravenously, with repeated muscle testing in 30 seconds to 2 minutes, as after the atropine injection. Not all areas of weakness may respond equally to the edrophonium. A second injection of edrophonium, 4 to 8 mg intravenously, may be given in 3 to 5 minutes after the first if the first was not definitive and detailed muscle testing of weak areas is done again. In most myasthenics there is a clear-cut, though transient, improvement in strength that may not be uniform in all areas of weakness. This usually lasts 2 to 5 minutes and occasionally longer.

A list of commonly used anticholinesterase drugs and comparable dosage forms and routes of administration is given in Table 1. Anticholinesterase drugs do not occur naturally in man. Excessive anticholinesterase therapy may have adverse effects, increasing weakness and provoking other unpleasant and potentially dangerous side effects. These are listed under the column "Cholinergic Crisis" in Table 2.

Oral anticholinesterase therapy may be started gradually with one half of a 15-mg tablet of neostigmine (7.5 mg) or one half of a 60-mg tablet of pyridostigmine (30 mg) at 4-hour intervals or two to three times daily. Patients with weakness in chewing and swallowing will find it helpful to take the drug 30 to 60 minutes before meals and refrain from talking while eating. Gastrointestinal effects will be fewer if a small amount of milk, bread, crackers, or other bland food is eaten before the anticholinesterase. Foods such as coffee, fruit, tomato juice, or carbonated or alcoholic beverages tend to increase the parasympathetic side effects on the gut, bladder, bronchi, and

TABLE 1. **Anticholinesterase Drugs Used in Diagnosis and Management of Myasthenia Gravis**

Drug	Form	Adult Single Dose and Route	Usual Effective Duration and Range
Tensilon (edrophonium chloride)	10 mg per ml	2–10 mg IV	10 min (2 min to 2 hr)
Prostigmin (neostigmine methylsulfate)	0.25, 0.5, and 1.0 mg per ml	1 mg IM	2 hr (2–4 hr)
Prostigmin (neostigmine bromide)	15 mg tablet	15 mg oral	3 hr (2–5 hr)
Mestinon (pyridostigmine bromide)	10 mg per 2 ml	2 mg IM	2 hr (2–4 hr)
Mestinon (pyridostigmine bromide)	60 mg tablet	60 mg oral	4 hr (3–7 hr)
Mestinon Timespan (pyridostigmine bromide)	180 mg tablet (slow release)	90–180 mg oral	8 hr (6–12 hr)
Mestinon Syrup (pyridostigmine bromide)	60 mg per 5 ml syrup	60 mg per 5 ml (1 tsp oral)	4 hr (3–7 hr)
Mytelase (ambenonium chloride)	10 mg tablet	5–10 mg oral	6 hr (4–8 hr)

mucus glands. They are best avoided or taken at the end of a meal.

The dosage of anticholinesterase drug may be increased gradually at about 2-day intervals and the time shortened to 3 hours only if these changes are followed by objective improvement in symptoms and signs. Increases of one fourth to one half tablet per dose are recommended. Both the physician and patient must realize that anticholinesterase drugs seldom restore muscle strength to more than 80 per cent of normal strength with optimal dosage. Weakness of extraocular, oropharyngeal, respiratory, and other muscles at times selectively or together may show little improvement with anticholinesterase drugs.

Neostigmine and pyridostigmine are quite similar in their action and effectiveness. Some patients note more muscarinic side effects such as abdominal cramps, diarrhea, nausea, salivation, tearing, and sweating with neostigmine than with pyridostigmine. The action of neostigmine is about 30 to 45 minutes shorter than that of pyridostigmine. A few patients find that neostigmine gives more prompt and slightly greater improvement in muscle strength than pyridostigmine.

There are additional helpful forms of pyridostigmine. The syrup contains 60 mg in 5 ml (approximately 1 teaspoonful). This is palatable and easily administered and adjusted for young myasthenic children. Patients with swallowing difficulty may handle this form easier and with greater safety than the tablets. It is also easily given by nasogastric tube. The other useful form of pyridostigmine is Mestinon Timespan tablets. Each contains 180 mg of pyridostigmine. About one third of the dosage is released promptly, and the remainder is released over the next 6 to 12 hours. When a tablet is given at bedtime, it allows the moderate to severe myasthenic to sleep through the night without awakening to take regular anticholinesterase medication. Usually, only patients with moderate to severe myasthenia require medication during sleeping hours and the dosage may be reduced to one half or two thirds of that taken during waking hours. Since the regular forms of pyridostigmine give more

TABLE 2. **Symptoms and Signs of Myasthenic and Cholinergic Crisis**

Myasthenic Crisis	Cholinergic Crisis	
	Muscarinic Symptoms and Signs:	*Nicotinic Symptoms and Signs:*
Ocular ptosis	Sweating	Muscle fasciculations
Dysarthria or anarthria	Salivation	Dysarthric speech
Dysphagia or aphagia	Lacrimation	Dysphagia
Dyspnea or apnea	Abdominal cramping	Trismus
Facial weakness	Nausea	Muscle cramps and spasms
Masticatory weakness	Vomiting	General weakness
Difficulty handling secretions	Diarrhea	
General weakness	Urinary frequency	*CNS Symptoms and Signs:*
	Incontinence of bowel and bladder	
	Miosis	Restlessness
	Blurred vision	Anxiety
	Bradycardia	Vertigo
	Bronchorrhea	Headache
	Substernal pressure	Confusion and stupor
	Dyspnea and wheezing	Coma
	Bronchospasm	Convulsions
	Pulmonary edema	

prompt and dependable release and absorption, Mestinon Timespan is not recommended for daytime use.

When patients are temporarily unable to take anticholinesterase drugs by mouth or are unable to swallow, parenteral forms of neostigmine methylsulfate or pyridostigmine bromide may be substituted. The equivalent of a 15-mg tablet of neostigmine is 1 to 1.5 mg of neostigmine methylsulfate intramuscularly. The equivalent of a 60-mg tablet of pyridostigmine bromide is 2 mg of pyridostigmine bromide intramuscularly. Parenteral anticholinesterase therapy is seldom more effective than oral therapy. It is not practical for long-term care.

Ambenonium chloride (Mytelase) is the third available oral anticholinesterase drug. It is used much less frequently than neostigmine and pyridostigmine. It may be more effective against weakness of the extremities than of the cranial muscles. Duration of action is a bit longer than that of pyridostigmine. Patients not responding well to neostigmine or pyridostigmine may be tried carefully on ambenonium. Muscarinic toxic effects are less prominent, but nicotinic and central nervous system symptoms and signs of toxicity may appear. The nicotinic manifestations include muscle twitching and weakness. The central nervous system manifestations include headache, restlessness, and anxiety. Between 5 and 7.5 mg of ambenonium chloride are equivalent to 15 mg of neostigmine or 60 mg pyridostigmine tablets. One may start with 5 mg of ambenonium every 4 to 6 hours and increase by 2.5 mg per dose if there is objective improvement and no undesirable side effects.

To assess effects of anticholinesterase drugs, it is useful to examine patients just before the next dose of drug and 45 to 75 minutes after it. Helpful areas to test include the following:

1. The patient's inability to sustain upward gaze can reveal fatigue of the lid levators or extraocular muscles.

2. Continuous counting on a single breath gives a rough estimate of respiratory muscle strength and vital capacity.

3. The time the patient is able to keep the arms or legs elevated is an indication of the fatigability of these muscles.

4. The number of times the patient is able to cross and uncross one thigh over the other, squat, and arise or repeatedly compress a partially inflated blood pressure cuff or hand dynamometer are simple tests of strength and fatigability of neuromuscular transmission in these areas.

5. The patient's ability to close the jaw tightly against resistance, to protrude the tongue into each cheek against resistance, to elevate the soft palate, to cough, to swallow, and to speak are useful signs that aid in assessing oropharyngeal strength.

Measurement of the vital capacity is a simple test of respiratory muscle function and reserve. It is weakness in oropharyngeal and/or respiratory muscle strength that constitutes the greatest threat to the myasthenic's life. Treatment should be directed to achieve optimal improvement in these areas.

The edrophonium chloride (Tensilon) test may also be used in an attempt to determine how adequate ongoing anticholinesterase therapy is. One hour after the oral dose of the drug, the patient's strength is tested. The patient is then given 2 mg (0.2 ml) of edrophonium chloride intravenously, and strength is retested in 30 seconds to 2 minutes. If strength is significantly improved, the dosage of oral anticholinesterase may be increased. If strength is unchanged or declines, the oral anticholinesterase dosage is not changed. If muscarinic and nicotinic effects appear after 2 mg of edrophonium chloride, along with increased weakness, the oral anticholinesterase dosage should be lowered.

Although some differences are noted among the effects of neostigmine, pyridostigmine, and ambenonium, overall results are quite similar. Of the three, currently pyridostigmine is the most frequently used oral anticholinesterase drug.

Crisis

Muscle weakness leading to inability to maintain a patent airway free of secretions and/or adequate respiratory exchange constitutes crisis in the myasthenic. It may be caused by increase in the myasthenia gravis itself, too much anticholinesterase drug, or both. Rapid distinction among myasthenic, cholinergic, or mixed or insensitive crisis may be difficult in the acute situation, if not impossible. Promptly providing an adequate airway with tracheal intubation, if necessary, suctioning of excessive tracheobronchial secretions to clear the airway, and positive pressure assisted or controlled respiration may be lifesaving. Bilateral weakness of the abductors of the vocal cords may obstruct the airway, thus limiting exchange. Factors often associated with myasthenic crisis are infections, especially upper respiratory infections, menses, omitting anticholinesterase medication, vigorous physical activity, certain drugs, and emotional upsets.

Drugs having an adverse effect on neuromuscular transmission include most hypnotics, tranquilizers, and antihistaminics, thiazides, quinine, quinidine, procainamide, calcium channel blockers, beta-blockers, ether, d-tubocurarine, pancuronium, succinylcholine, magnesium sulfate, d-penicillamine, adrenocorticotropic hormone (ACTH), adrenocorticosteroids, and aminoglycoside antibiotics. The latter include colistimethate, colistin, dihydrostreptomycin, kanamycin, neomycin, novobiocin, polymyxin B, gentamicin, streptomycin, and tobramycin.

Cholinergic crisis may be caused by too much anticholinesterase medication. It may develop in the course of a spontaneous remission, following thymectomy or an overenthusiastic use of anticholinesterase drugs by the physician or patient. Some patients become unresponsive, insensitive, or resistant to anticholinesterase drugs. This happens particularly when the dosage is gradually increased to high levels over a long period of time. It must be remembered that both the antibody to acetylcholine receptor and anticholinesterase drugs are attacking and acting on the postjunctional membrane of the neuromuscular junction. Each may adversely affect neuromuscular transmission. The symptoms and signs of myasthenic and cholinergic crisis are listed in Table 2.

In the presence of cholinergic crisis or an unresponsive, resistant, or insensitive state, the anticholinesterase drug is stopped for 3 or more days. This is best done in a hospital, since the patient frequently initially becomes still weaker and may require an airway and mechanical ventilation for a time before strength spontaneously improves. This allows junctions that may be damaged and depolarized by excessive prolonged administration of an anticholinesterase drug to recover. Fluid balance and nutrition are maintained parenterally or by nasogastric tube.

If endotracheal intubation is required for more than 3 to 4 days, tracheostomy will be more comfortable for the patient, provide better tracheobronchial toilet, and reduce risk of damage to the larynx. A short, low-pressure cuffed tube is used. At times, patients withdrawn from anticholinesterase drugs and supported improve to the point that they may function for days or weeks without anticholinesterase medication.

Atropine is best used only sporadically or in an emergency to counteract muscarinic side effects of anticholinesterase drugs. Regular use may obscure the signs of cholinergic intoxication. Oral and tracheobronchial secretions are reduced and become thick, tenacious, inspissated, and difficult to aspirate. Bronchial plugging with atelectasis may result. Sedative and tranquilizing drugs are best avoided in the anxious apprehensive myasthenic. These symptoms and signs may be those of failing respiratory function rather than a psychologic reaction to illness. Such drugs may aggravate hypoxia and hypercapnia, setting up a vicious circle of more respiratory depression with

vagal activity already increased by the anticholinesterase drug, leading to arrhythmia and asystole.

The patient in crisis should be turned frequently, given postural drainage, percussion to the chest, and meticulous tracheobronchial toilet. Auscultation of the chest, chest x-rays, and fiberoptic bronchoscopy may help to remove mucus plugs. Smears, cultures, and sensitivities of tracheobronchial secretions, along with appropriate antibiotics, aid in recovery and reduce mortality. Periodic determination of arterial blood gases aid evaluation of adequacy of mechanical ventilation, need for supplemental oxygen, and adjustment of depth and rate of respiration. Automatic periodic sighing, available on some respirators, may help prevent atelectasis and contractures of the chest wall from lack of full range of movement because of weakness. The lung in most myasthenics is normal and compliant once infection and atelectasis are overcome. For this reason, compressed air is best used for long-term operation of the positive pressure respirator.

Thymectomy

Improvement or remission of autoimmune myasthenia gravis following thymectomy has been reported in up to 80 per cent from several centers dealing with large numbers of myasthenic patients. It is most apt to occur in patients without thymoma. However, thymoma, which may occur in 15 per cent of patients with myasthenia gravis, is also an indication for thymectomy, since about 35 per cent of thymomas may become invasive or malignant. Exactly why improvement or remission occurs is not known. Results cannot be predicted in advance in the individual patient. Thymectomy is not helpful in congenital myasthenia. It may be less effective in patients older than 60 years of age in whom the thymus is usually atrophic. It is not recommended for debilitated patients or those showing malignant spread of thymoma. It is not done as an emergency procedure, in the presence of active pulmonary infection, pregnancy, or rapidly worsening myasthenia. Improvement following thymectomy may not occur for weeks or months. Operative risk is small in the hands of a competent thoracic surgeon in a facility where neurologic and medical staff are familiar with the disorder and have intensive care facilities including respiratory support available. The transcervical or suprasternal approach to the thymus has been used at a few centers, but this is not usually satisfactory for removal of thymomas and may not allow removal of all thymic tissue, since the surgeon's operative field is restricted. Most centers continue to use a median sternotomy, which avoids these problems.

Treatment with alternate-day corticosteroid therapy for a few weeks or months before thymectomy is helpful in myasthenic patients with moderate to severe oropharyngeal and/or respiratory muscle weakness. It is not recommended for all patients having thymectomy.

Preoperatively, the patient is allowed to take usual doses of anticholinesterase medication with small sips of water up to the time of surgery. Postoperatively, anticholinesterase medication is resumed in 12 to 24 hours as weakness occurs and dosage requirements are usually less. About one half to three quarters of the preoperative dose is given to start with. Close cooperation with postoperative follow-up by the neurologist is essential. Meperidine (Demerol) rather than morphine is used to relieve pain.

Corticosteroid Therapy

Although some physicians have used alternate-day prednisone as the first choice of treatment even in essentially limited ocular myasthenia gravis, we have generally reserved its use for patients with more generalized weakness not responding favorably to anticholinesterases or thymectomy or both. This regimen may be considered in older patients who are not suitable candidates for thymectomy. However, both the patient and physician should be aware of the long-term commitment, side effects, risks, and complications of chronic use of corticosteroids, since fewer than 10 per cent of patients are able to discontinue them completely in most cases. Strength may greatly improve, but the majority of patients remain dependent upon the corticosteroids for their improvement. Withdrawal is usually followed by recurrent weakness in weeks or months and by the need for even higher doses to reverse the weakness. In some, the improvement may be maintained on a relatively low dose, compared with amounts required to initiate the improvement. Improvement takes place over weeks or months.

Since there may be some paradoxical worsening of the myasthenia gravis when corticosteroids are first begun, they are best started in a hospital setting with staff familiar with this form of treatment in myasthenia gravis and with facilities for mechanical respiratory support and intensive care, should these be needed.

Patients with obesity, hypertension, and/or diabetes mellitus are best not treated with steroids. Patients who are anergic or who have positive skin tests for tuberculosis are best given simultaneously prophylactic isoniazid (INH) and pyridoxine with the corticosteroids.

We recommend that patients taking corticosteroids maintain a diet high in protein, potassium, and calcium; moderate in complex carbohydrates; and low in fat with no added free sugars. Supplemental 10 per cent potassium chloride may be needed to keep the serum potassium in the upper normal levels. We recommend that patients receiving corticosteroids take antacid or nonfat milk 1 to 2 hours after each meal and at bedtime. We prefer to avoid chronic cimetidine or ranitidine therapy.

The blood count, serum potassium, and blood glucose are determined at office visits. Liver function tests are recommended for those on isoniazid; progress chest films are recommended at 6- to 12-month intervals.

We prefer to start alternate-day prednisone at 20 to 25 mg and increase this by 5 mg every second or third dose cycle. When strength begins to improve (which is usually not immediately), the dosage may be maintained at that level. We have seldom needed to exceed 100 mg on alternate days. If the patient already requires mechanical respiratory support, a higher initial starting dose, up to 100 mg, may be used in attempt to reverse severe weakness sooner. This seldom happens before the second or third week. Methylprednisolone, 60 mg intramuscularly, or dexamethasone, 12 mg orally, in divided doses daily, have also been used in such states.

Nonsteroidal Immunosuppressive Therapy

Azathioprine (Imuran),* cyclophosphamide (Cytoxan),* and methotrexate* have been used for long-term treatment in some patients. Those not responding to thymectomy or corticosteroids or those in whom corticosteroids are unacceptable because of side effects or contraindicated may find these drugs helpful. They may also be used to reduce the dosage of corticosteroids required when side effects of these are troublesome. They are useful to provide ongoing immunosuppression in conjunction with plasmapheresis. The major long-term experience with them has been abroad rather than in the United States. Azathioprine, 2 to 3 mg kg daily, is given in single or divided oral doses. Significant response may not be noted for 2 months to 1 year. Maximal improvement may not occur for up to 24 months, but once it is achieved it is quite even, with little fluctuation from day to day. When the patient is stable, dosage may be tapered slowly. Side effects and complications include nausea, vomiting, leukopenia, thrombocytopenia, anemia (often megaloblastic), and hepatotoxicity. Patients receiving this are best followed initially with weekly blood counts and a monthly blood chemistry panel, with particular attention to liver function tests. Low-

---

*This use of this agent is not listed by the manufacturer.

ering or discontinuing the drug usually reverses these. A comparable dose of cyclophosphamide (Cytoxan) is used. Results and side effects are the same except for the added risks of hemorrhagic cystitis and alopecia. Azathioprine and cyclophosphamide are not recommended for women in childbearing years because of possible developmental defects in the fetus. A risk of malignancy, as well as increased susceptibility to infection, is another consideration.

Plasmapheresis Therapy

Exchange of 2 liters of plasma for equal amounts of human albumin and saline every other day three times a week may relieve weakness temporarily. Long-term benefit from this regimen usually requires combining it with corticosteroids, other immunosuppressants, and/or thymectomy. It may be helpful in preparing moderately to severely weak patients for thymectomy or to shorten the time of crisis. Since plasmapheresis requires special facilities and skills and entails other risks, it is best done at centers familiar with both myasthenia gravis and pheresis.

Adjuvant Therapy

Ephedrine sulfate, 25 mg orally two or three times daily, is helpful to some patients. It may make patients wakeful if given late in the day or evening. It should be avoided in men with prostatism, since it inhibits micturition. Potassium chloride, 1 to 2 grams given orally in 10 per cent solution two or three times daily with meals, is helpful to other patients who function better with serum potassium levels at high normal. A few patients appear to benefit from calcium gluconate or lactate, 1 to 2 grams taken orally two to four times daily.

Care for Surgery

Myasthenics may require surgery apart from thymectomy. Preoperative cathartics and enemas are avoided. The patient may take usual anticholinesterase drugs with small sips of water up to the time of surgery. If necessary, this may be converted to a parenteral dose of neostigmine or pyridostigmine. Muscle relaxants and sedatives are best avoided. Spinal, local, or regional anesthesia is preferable. When general anesthesia is necessary, ether is avoided—although it is seldom used for patients at present. Sodium pentothal and inhalation agents, such as nitrous oxide, cyclopropane, or halothane, may be used. In those with significant oropharyngeal and/or respiratory weakness preoperatively, the endotracheal tube may be left in place postoperatively until the patient is well awake and demonstrates stable

respiratory function by adequate measured vital capacity. Meperidine (Demerol) is given to relieve pain. Meticulous care should be given to the respiratory tract to promote full expansion of the lungs using intermittent positive-pressure breathing (IPPB), assisted coughing, and careful tracheobronchial toilet to prevent atelectasis and pulmonary infection. Since patients with myasthenia gravis tend to fatigue with repeated voluntary effort, incentive spirometry is usually counterproductive as compared with IPPB to expand the lungs in someone with pre-existing respiratory muscle weakness. If antibiotics are needed, those listed earlier that are known to interfere with neuromuscular transmission are avoided. Dosage requirements for anticholinesterase are often lower postoperatively. Therapy may be started parenterally as weakness develops. When the patient is able to swallow and is no longer nauseated and bowel sounds are normal, medication may be given by nasogastric tube or orally.

Associated Disorders

The presence of one autoimmune disease increases the likelihood of another in the same patient. As a consequence, one may see such conditions as Graves' disease, Hashimoto's thyroiditis, rheumatoid arthritis, polymyositis, dermatomyositis, scleroderma, vitiligo, pernicious anemia, lupus erythematosus, pemphigus, idiopathic thrombocytopenic purpura, red cell aplasia, autoimmune hemolytic anemia, autoimmune secondary amenorrhea, and multiple sclerosis. The most common are disorders of the thyroid, especially hyperthyroidism. Periodically, tests of thyroid function as well as of creatine phosphokinase are desirable.

Outlook

Better and newer forms of treatment, including improved mechanical respiratory support, antibiotics to combat infection, corticosteroids, other immunosuppressants and current discoveries, and understanding of the immunopathophysiology of neuromuscular transmission, have all helped to reduce mortality and morbidity as well as increase longevity. It is important for patients to learn to pace their physical activities. Patients and their families benefit from learning the nature of myasthenia gravis and general principles of management to reduce unnecessary anxiety, to allow them more control of their care, and to promote a smoother course. Most patients with myasthenia gravis are able to lead gainful, productive, satisfying lives.

TRIGEMINAL NEURALGIA

method of
G. ROBERT NUGENT, M.D.
West Virginia University
Morgantown, West Virginia

Trigeminal neuralgia (tic douloureux) is probably the worst pain afflicting human beings, but fortunately the lightning-like attacks are of brief duration, spontaneous remissions are frequent, and the condition is treatable. As the process progresses, however, one attack follows another, the remissions are shorter, and sometimes the response to medication is less satisfactory.

Trigeminal neuralgia is a stereotyped clinical entity that is easily diagnosed by the history alone. The pain usually affects the older patient, is limited to the distribution of the trigeminal nerve, and is set off by touching a trigger area which is usually in the snout region (side of the nose, nasolabial fold area, upper or lower lip, or chin). The trigger may also be in the gum or, if the first division is involved, in the eyebrow or hairline. It is extremely rare for pain to begin in and remain localized to the first division. The pain is also set off by talking, eating, washing the face, shaving, and especially by brushing the teeth.

There are no abnormal neurologic findings except in those rare cases in which an identical pain may result from a cerebellopontine angle neoplasm or other posterior fossa lesion. Two to 3 per cent of patients with trigeminal neuralgia have multiple sclerosis. An enhanced computed tomography (CT) scan of the head should be performed to rule out other lesions causing the pain if the patient is young, the history is atypical, there are abnormal neurologic findings, or the pain has only been present for a short period of time. Rarely there may be clinical confusion with glossopharyngeal neuralgia, cluster headache, or pain of dental or sinus pathology.

For many years the cause of trigeminal neuralgia was unknown; however, there is evidence now that the pain results from cross compression of the trigeminal nerve, at the point where it enters the pons, by an aberrant blood vessel, usually a branch of the superior cerebellar artery. This artery can often be found compressing, indenting, or otherwise physically injuring the nerve when visualized during surgical approach to the nerve in the posterior fossa.

Medical Treatment

Carbamazepine (Tegetrol) is the treatment of choice and the mainstay of early treatment. This is almost universally successful in stopping the pain, provided side effects do not limit its use. The usual side effects are ataxia, dizziness, drowsiness, nausea, and, in some patients, mental confusion; rarely it may cause a rash. Treatment is started at 200 mg per day and is increased an additional 200 mg in divided dosages until relief of the pain is obtained. Frequently one or two 200-mg tablets per day are adequate to manage the pain. Some patients require 1200 to 1600 mg per day, but side effects may be a limiting factor at this dosage. Rarely carbamazepine may cause aplastic anemia or a fall in the white blood cell or platelet count. Therefore, a complete blood count should be obtained prior to starting therapy and monitored periodically thereafter. Liver function studies should also be monitored and treatment discontinued if there is any alteration in the above studies.

Phenytoin (Dilantin) has been used for many years but is much less effective than carbamazepine. Its use in combination with carbamazepine may prove beneficial; 300 to 400 mg per day is the usual dose.

A better drug than phenytoin is baclofen (Lioresal), which can be used alone or in combination with carbamazepine. The suggested regimen is a starting dose of 10 mg 3 times daily for 3 days, then increasing the dose by 5 mg for 3-day increments to a total of 20 mg 3 times daily. The dosage should not exceed that which provides relief of pain.

In my opinion and experience, acupuncture, treatment for temporomandibular joint dysfunction, and vitamin B_{12} and surgery for gum and bone pathology have no place in the treatment of this disorder.

Nerve Blocks

A traditional therapeutic approach has been to make the trigger area insensitive; to achieve this, various techniques have been in vogue over the years. Second-division pain can be treated by an alcohol or radiofrequency (RF) block of the infraorbital nerve in the cheek; if the gum is a trigger site, the maxillary nerve can be blocked in the pterygomaxillary fissure. Open avulsion of the infraorbital nerve can also be used. For third-division pain, the mandibular nerve may be blocked at the foramen ovale; first-division pain may be treated by open avulsion of the nerves in the supraorbital ridge. These techniques may provide 1 to 2 years of pain relief; however, as the nerve regenerates, the pain recurs.

Surgery

For more permanent pain relief, it is necessary to treat the trigeminal nerve proximal to the gasserian ganglion. Two therapeutic approaches are popular at this time.

The first approach, vascular decompression (popularized by Jannetta), involves a major intracranial procedure to separate from the nerve the blood vessel, usually a branch of the superior cerebellar artery, that is compressing the trigeminal nerve at the root entry zone. An implantable sponge is inserted between the compressed nerve and the artery; this often stops the pain without facial numbness. With this procedure, there is some risk of deafness in the ear on the side of the surgery. Also, the mortality is 1 per cent, the recurrence rate is more than 20 per cent, and in approximately 10 per cent of cases, the offending vessel is not found and the nerve is cut, producing facial numbness.

The second currently popular treatment is RF thermocoagulation of the retrogasserian rootlets, which stops the pain by producing permanent numbness in the trigger area of the face. About 5 per cent of patients experience annoying paresthesias and dysesthesias in the numb area; this is a major problem with any procedure that relieves pain by creation of facial numbness. Most patients, however, are grateful for the numbness, which stops not only the pain but also the necessity for medication. The patient is able to leave the hospital on the day of the RF thermocoagulation procedure. The recurrence rate is about 23 per cent, but this minor procedure can be repeated.

Those patients who are unhappy with the numbness produced by a nerve block should consider the vascular decompression procedure despite the greater risks, greater expense, and extended hospitalization.

GLOSSOPHARYNGEAL NEURALGIA

The pain in glossopharyngeal neuralgia is as severe as that of trigeminal neuralgia but is centered in the area of the tonsil and radiates deeply into the ear. The triggering mechanism is swallowing. It is much less common than trigeminal neuralgia. Carbamazepine (Tegretol) should be used in the same dosage as for trigeminal neuralgia. Temporary relief can be obtained by anesthetizing the posterior oropharynx with 2 per cent lidocaine (Xylocaine) jelly. If topical anesthesia of this area stops the pain, it is also diagnostic. If medication is not helpful, the pain can be eliminated by sectioning the ninth cranial nerve and upper two rootlets of the tenth nerve in the posterior fossa.

OPTIC NEURITIS

method of
BARRETT KATZ, M.D.
University of California, San Diego
La Jolla, California

Optic neuritis is a sporadic, acute, presumedly inflammatory optic neuropathy not consequent to trauma, intoxication, or underlying nutritional deficiency. It is a generic term used to describe a clinical syndrome characterized by acute loss of vision, commonly associated with pain. Optic neuritis implies involvement of the nerve itself as the result of inflammation, demyelination, or infection. When there is swelling of the disc, the term papillitis is used. When the clinical history suggests optic neuritis, but the disc appears perfectly normal, the term retrobulbar neuritis is used. It is important to remember that no clinical or laboratory test can establish the diagnosis of optic neuritis; it is at best a diagnosis of probability, even when made by an experienced observer. Optic neuritis may be an idiopathic disorder, or it may be the initial sign of a more systemic illness, most notably multiple sclerosis.

The majority of patients are between the ages of 20 and 50 at the onset of the disease. Their primary symptom, abrupt visual loss, occurs over hours to days. The degree of visual deficit varies widely and may range from minimally reduced acuity or anomaly of color perception to complete loss of light perception. Commonly, just before the visual loss, patients complain of pain with eye movement. An occasional patient will note positive visual hallucinations such as flashes or sparks of light. The disease ordinarily runs a characteristic course in which visual loss reaches its climax within seven days of its onset. Acuity begins to improve over the next several weeks and may eventually return, albeit incompletely.

Treatment

This is a disease for which efficacy of treatment has not been firmly established, so the physician's task becomes one of prognosis. It is relatively safe to predict that visual function will recover to some degree over the ensuing weeks and months. Many patients have a return of acuity to levels of 20/40 or better, although commonly with residua of subjectively changed vision. While a course of oral corticosteroids may shorten the acute illness and decrease pain, such treatment has not been demonstrated to improve the eventual visual outcome. Treating optic neuritis with corticosteroids may in fact obscure the most important diagnostic indicator of the clinical syndrome—namely, its natural course. Therapy may mask the symptoms of an optic neuropathy that is simulating optic neuritis. Dramatic response to steroids is atypical of optic neuritis and suggests another optic neuropathy. Use of therapeutic steroids therefore demands careful preliminary diagnostic evaluation.

A reasoned approach is to share with the patient the controversy surrounding therapy of optic neuritis—what may be masked, and what the side effects of steroids are. Some cases will argue against such intervention, as when there is glucose intolerance, gastric ulceration, or a history of tuberculosis. Other cases seem appropriate for a short course of oral steroids—for example, when the uninvolved eye is not functional, when the process occurs in each eye at the same time, or when the pain of eye movement is a significant part of the patient's complaint.

My regimen for therapy is 10 days of daily oral prednisone (or equivalent), 60 to 100 mg daily, with rapid taper over the ensuing 10 days. Some centers have tried high doses of intravenous methylprednisolone (Solu-Medrol), 250 mg every 6 hours for 3 to 5 days. Although such therapy is unconventional, it may have merit in selected cases. A collaborative NIH study is underway that hopes to address the controversies surrounding treatment modalities and define what (if any) role corticosteroids serve in the management of optic neuritis.

Relationship of Optic Neuritis to Multiple Sclerosis

Another issue for patient and physician is the relationship between optic neuritis and multiple sclerosis. It is a relationship that is difficult to elucidate. Perhaps 15 per cent of patients with multiple sclerosis had optic neuritis as the heralding event. Almost two thirds of patients with acute idiopathic uncomplicated optic neuritis have multiple white matter brain lesions (presumed focal areas of demyelination) visible on magnetic resonance imaging (MRI), but so do many normal individuals. In one small autopsy series, all patients who died of multiple sclerosis had lesions of the anterior visual pathways; certainly most patients with multiple sclerosis have abnormal pattern visual evoked responses, contrast sensitivity loss, dyschromatopsia, and nerve fiber layer loss.

For the patient who develops optic neuritis in the prime of his life, what is the probability of developing multiple sclerosis in later life? Clinicians have yet to definitively answer this. Many studies suggest that MS develops within two years of the onset of optic neuritis if it is going to develop, and acknowledge that an occasional case will continue to appear after many years. Studies in this country suggest that between 20 and 35 per cent of patients with optic neuritis meet criteria for diagnosis of definite multiple sclerosis within 7 years. Studies overseas show an even higher incidence of multiple sclerosis following optic neuritis. More recent work has suggested that the risk of developing MS following optic neuritis may not necessarily be clustered within those first two years but continues at some constant rate thereafter. Definitive answers are yet to be determined, so clinicians need be cautious and conservative in sharing the partial truths presently available.

ACUTE FACIAL PARALYSIS

method of
STAFFAN EDSTRÖM, M.D.
University of Göteborg,
Gothenburg, Sweden

Facial paralysis may be a symptom of an uncomplicated nerve lesion with spontaneous healing, but it may also signify a dangerous life-threatening condition. A carefully taken history and physical examination are prerequisites for correct management of the patient with facial nerve dysfunction.

Central Lesions

A central nerve lesion is characterized by an injury located above the level of the facial nerve nucleus in the brain stem. This motor nucleus has cerebrocortical connections. These are bilateral for the peripheral facial motor branches directed to the forehead and eye region; however, they are only unilteral for the lower part of the face. This means that an injury affecting motor fibers of the facial nerve at a cortical level in the brain will result in contralateral involvement of the voluntary muscles of the lower part of the face only, since the ipsilateral cortical connection to the upper part of the face remains intact. Most injuries located at a supranuclear level are caused by vascular catastrophes, but neoplastic processes may also occur. The supranuclear lesions are usually accompanied by other neurologic manifestations, such as limb nerve paresis and aphasia.

Peripheral Lesions

A peripheral nerve lesion is characterized by an injury located somewhere between the facial nerve nucleus in the brain stem and the facial muscles. The term "peripheral" facial paralysis may therefore seem somewhat contradictory, since it includes not only the part of the nerve outside the brain but also the part in the brain stem. Peripheral nerve dysfunction is characterized by involvement of all branches, including the upper facial nerve branch. An exception is an injury located distal to the branching region. Such an injury, usually the result of surgical trauma, may cause a single branch dysfunction.

There are basically four different causes of peripheral facial paralysis: trauma, tumors, infections, and unknown etiology (Bell's palsy).

FACIAL PARALYSIS RESULTING FROM TRAUMA

Injuries to the facial nerve may be caused by accidents, assaults, and surgical trauma in the cerebellopontine angle, middle ear, face, and parotid gland. If a nerve dysfunction occurs immediately in association with the injury, it can be assumed that the nerve is cut. On the other hand, the nerve dysfunction may develop gradually, in which case the cause would probably be a hematoma or edema. Surgical nerve exploration in order to reconstruct the nerve transmission is usually more important when a rupture is suspected.

These variations in the development of nerve dysfunction emphasize the importance of thorough clinical assessment of facial nerve function, particularly in patients with multiple injuries. In these cases, facial nerve function may otherwise be overlooked. Therefore, even a normal facial nerve function should be registered in the acute case record.

FACIAL PARALYSIS CAUSED BY TUMORS

If a facial nerve dysfunction gradually develops over several weeks or one or two months, an underlying tumor should be suspected. These tumors may be located in the brain stem and are then extremely uncommon. Sooner or later they give rise to other neurologic manifestations (e.g., abducens paresis or vertigo).

Acoustic neurinoma is the most frequent tumor located in the cerebellopontine angle. This tumor may occasionally be as large as a golf ball and may cause pronounced stretching of the facial nerve. However, it seldom produces a facial nerve dysfunction. Meningioma may also be located in the cerebellopontine angle. Although this tumor is also benign, it more frequently causes a nerve dysfunction.

Tumor invasion of the temporal bone is rare and mostly involves metastases and neurinoma. However, these tumors may occur at any level along the course of the facial nerve. Palpable tumors in the parotid gland in association with a facial dysfunction are almost always malignant and mean a poor prognosis for the patient.

FACIAL PARALYSIS RESULTING FROM INFECTION

Facial paralysis may be caused by acute or chronic otitis media. These infections may also cause pain and hearing loss. Secretion from the ear sometimes occurs. Bone-eroding cholesteatoma may occasionally be the triggering factor.

Not only bacteria but also viruses may cause facial paralysis. The role of herpes zoster virus in this context is well recognized. Vesicles on the eardrum are sometimes present in association with the paralysis as well as periauricular pain, vertigo, and hearing loss (Ramsay Hunt syndrome).

Recently, facial paralysis has been associated with a tick-transmitted *Borrelia* spirochete that causes Lyme's disease. In consecutive studies, it

has been demonstrated that about 20 per cent of patients with facial paralysis demonstrate antibody production against the *Borrelia* antigen.

BELL'S PALSY (PARALYSIS OF UNKNOWN ETIOLOGY)

Bell's palsy was originally described as a facial palsy of unknown etiology. With diagnostic refinements, the percentage of Bell's palsy has ultimately declined, but it is still the most frequent form of facial nerve dysfunction (approximately 75 per cent), the incidence being 1 per 5000 per year. A reactivated herpes simplex virus infection has been proposed as one etiologic factor. There is evidence that Bell's palsy is part of a polyneuropathy, and occasionally an occult stage of multiple sclerosis.

Bell's palsy is characterized by an acute onset within a couple of days. The patients, mostly 30 to 50 years of age, proclaim that the palsy is preceded by an episode of draft. However, there is no significant evidence that draft plays any etiologic role. Sometimes the Bell's palsy patient suffers from a co-existing upper respiratory infection. Pain around the ear is common, and hearing loss and vertigo are infrequent symptoms.

Approximately 75 per cent of patients with Bell's palsy recover completely within a few months without treatment. The remaining patients have a more or less persisting paralysis. It is difficult to assess the outcome in the acute stage of the disease; however, some unfavorable factors exist (Table 1).

Management

A carefully taken history and an appropriate physical examination (Table 2) are prerequisites for correct management of the patient with peripheral facial paralysis. It is important to consult an otolaryngologist immediately in order to plan the further investigation of the patient (Table 3). Investigation programs vary, and some ear, nose, and throat (ENT) departments may admit their patients to the hospital, whereas others have outpatient management.

X-ray examinations are performed in order to reveal trauma, infections, and extensive proc-

TABLE 1. **Unfavorable Prognostic Factors in Bell's Palsy**

Age over 60 years
Slow onset (less than 3 days)
Postauricular pain
Complete paralysis
Diabetes
Herpes zoster
Lack of recovery within 3 weeks of onset

Is the facial nerve dysfunction

1. central or peripheral?

2. an acute disease or has it developed slowly? Have there been previous episodes?

3. associated with trauma?

4. associated with hearing loss or abnormal hearing inspection status?

5. associated with other neurologic manifestations (e.g., abduscens paresis, vertigo, headache, or pain)?

6. associated with a palpable parotid tumor?

7. associated with tick-bites and compatible with a possible *Borrelia* infection?

TABLE 3. **Primary Care Assessment and
Possible Diagnostic Procedures**

I. Primary Care Assessment
  A. Answer the questions in Table 2
  B. Contact your ENT consultant immediately
II. Diagnostic Procedures
  A. Radiologic examination
    1. X-ray of the temporal bone in cases of trauma, middle ear infections and suspicion of tumors
    2. Computed tomography for evaluation of extensive processes in the temporal bone, cerebellopontine angle, and brain stem
  B. Topographic evaluation
    1. Stapedius reflex test
    2. Tear secretory test
    3. Quantification of salivation from the submandibular glands
  C. Neurophysiologic tests
    1. Registration of the degree of nerve degeneration by means of nerve stimulation distal to the level of injury
      a. excitability test (visual registration of muscle contraction)
      b. electroneuronography (objective recording)
    2. Electromyogram (registration of voluntary muscle contraction)
  D. Serologic test
    Borrelia antibody titers (in serum and cerebrospinal fluid)

esses. Topographic tests are of uncertain value because the secretory and taste fibers accompany the facial nerve only along a restricted course in the cerebellopontine angle and the proximal part of the temporal bone; thus, the secretory and taste functions have separate nuclei in the brain stem, which are distinguished from the facial motor nucleus. However, topographic tests may have some value for assessment of the prognosis. This is also true of a variety of neurophysiologic tests.

Serologic examination concerning antibody production against *Borrelia* antigen has attracted much interest during recent years. Some clinics advocate this examination routinely in all patients with facial palsy of unknown etiology. Repeated serology for at least 1 month after the onset of the facial palsy may be needed, since the time taken to develop positive antibody titers differs from one patient to another. It must be emphasized that the specificity of antibody production against *Borrelia* antigen is not yet completely clarified, and a positive antibody titer is not necessarily compatible with a *Borrelia* infection.

Treatment

Traumatic and surgical ruptures of the facial nerve may require surgical recontinuity. Tumors located in the brain stem resulting in facial nerve dysfunction are not surgically accessible. If they are malignant, irradiation may be given. Tumors in the cerebellopontine angle and the facial canal are frequently surgically removed. These tumors are mostly benign. Extracranial tumors, mostly located in the parotid gland, must be evaluated according to histopathology and extension before treatment is started.

Middle-ear infections associated with facial paralysis should be drained. Bacteriologic culture should be performed and antibiotic treatment should then be started. Penicillin-V or cephalosporins are the antibiotics of choice. Mastoidectomy and facial nerve decompression are occasionally needed in cases of persistent facial paralysis.

When there is evidence of *Borrelia* infection, antibiotics, preferably penicillin, should be given. These should be administered intravenously in order to reach sufficient concentrations in the cerebrospinal fluid. Although relief of *Borrelia*-related symptoms has been reported, antibiotic administration does not seem to have any effect on the facial nerve dysfunction. Nevertheless, antibiotics may stop an ongoing infectious process that otherwise might result in Lyme's disease.

The diagnosis of Bell's palsy is established by exclusion. It is important to inform the patient that the prognosis is generally good and to emphasize that there is no evidence of a serious underlying cause. Oral steroid treatment has yet not been proved to have any effect on the paralysis. Treatment is symptomatic. Ear drops (Tears Naturale), 2 drops every hour during the day, and ointment (e.g., Lacri-Lube), at night are recommended. Sometimes a moisture chamber is needed. If a keratitis has developed, an ophthalmologist should be consulted.

If the Bell's palsy persists for 2 months and malignancy has been ruled out, tarsorraphy of the eyelid has to be considered. This can easily be revoked if the muscle function improves. If the Bell's palsy remains complete, other surgical procedures may be considered, such as decompression of the facial canal, nerve grafts, and reconstruction of the facial muscles.

PARKINSONISM

method of
RICHARD F. PEPPARD, M.D., and
DONALD B. CALNE, D.M.
The University of British Columbia
Vancouver, British Columbia

Diagnosis

Parkinsonism is a collection of neurologic features, including tremor, rigidity, akinesia, and loss of postural reflexes. Parkinson's disease, the most important cause of this syndrome, is a chronic progressive disorder of unknown cause. The pathologic hallmarks of Parkinson's disease are degeneration and loss of the pigmented cells of the substantia nigra, with resultant deficiency of the neurotransmitter dopamine in the nigrostriatal pathway.

A number of difficulties may arise in the diagnosis of Parkinson's disease. Essential tremor, particularly if it is of large amplitude and commences or progresses in an elderly person, is sometimes erroneously attributed to Parkinson's disease. Essential tremor is usually an isolated neurologic abnormality, and often there is a family history of this disorder. Characteristically, it appears during a purposeful movement or in maintaining a posture, whereas parkinsonian tremor is present at rest and disappears during action. However, postural or action-related tremor may, on occasion, be seen in association with resting tremor in Parkinson's disease.

In patients in whom tremor is not an early feature, the diagnosis of Parkinson's disease may be delayed. The patient may complain of clumsiness of the hands, slowing down, uncertainty in gait, or falls. Muscular rigidity may produce limb pain suggestive of a rheumatologic disorder. The voice may become soft and indistinct and the handwriting small and cramped.

The physician should be alert to the akinetic features: the difficulty in performing fine hand movements and rapid repetitive movements, loss of arm swing during walking, and poverty of facial expressiveness and gesticulation during speech. An overall impression of stiffness, slowness, and awkwardness of movement is conveyed to the observer.

The stooped posture and shuffling gait of parkinsonism may give an appearance of premature old age in the younger patient. On the other hand, the resemblance of parkinsonian changes to those which occur in aging make the distinction between normal and diseased states more difficult in the elderly.

Other Causes of Parkinsonism

In any patient in whom features of parkinsonism are recognized, inquiry should be made regarding medication. Drug-induced parkinsonism is most commonly due to neuroleptic agents used in the treatment of major psychiatric disorders. These agents are occasionally employed inappropriately for the treatment of chronic nausea, dizziness, and anxiety. After the withdrawal of neuroleptics, parkinsonian side effects may persist as long as a year.

Parkinsonism may also result from the central dopamine depletion induced by tetrabenazine and reserpine. Significant parkinsonian reactions occur rarely with methyldopa and metoclopramide.

The meperidine derivative 1-methyl-4-phenyl-1,2,3,6-tetrahydropyridine (MPTP) is known to produce severe parkinsonism in drug addicts. Other toxic causes include manganese and carbon monoxide poisoning.

In multiple system diseases, parkinsonism may appear alone (striatonigral degeneration) or in conjunction with cerebellar signs (olivopontocerebellar atrophy) or autonomic failure (Shy-Drager syndrome). Progressive supranuclear palsy is characterized by parkinsonism, conjugate gaze paresis, dystonia involving the neck musculature, and dementia.

If there is an abrupt onset or rapid progression of parkinsonism, structural lesions (infarction, neoplasia, arteriovenous malformation) should be considered in the diagnosis.

A parkinsonian disorder may also be seen in Creutzfeldt-Jakob disease and Huntington's chorea. Wilson's disease must be excluded when parkinsonism develops early in life.

The early prominence of dementia may help to distinguish akinetic and rigid features of parkinsonism occurring in association with normal pressure hydrocephalus or Alzheimer's disease.

Informing the Patient with Parkinson's Disease

Explanation of the nature of this disease should be adjusted to the individual's fears and preconceptions. It is important to emphasize the usefulness and variety of currently available therapy and the likelihood of further advances being made over the years.

Prognostic advice is made difficult by the variability of the disease and response to treatment. The rate of progression tends to be maintained in the same individual, but this rate may be difficult to ascertain in the early stages. Some patients are able to maintain an active independent life for many years.

The patient should be made aware of the possible side effects when new drugs are being introduced and when changes are being made in treatment. Communication between patient and physician is more effective if the patient is familiar with such terms as "on" and "off" periods and "descants."

If the patient is intellectually impaired, it is desirable that a family member act as an informant regarding the current status of the patient and be instructed in the administration of medication.

We recommend that, as far as possible, patients stay active and maintain a regular exercise schedule.

Parkinsonism associations may be helpful in alleviating the isolation of the patient and caregivers and in giving the opportunity to share the experience of common problems and the approaches taken to deal with them.

Continuing interest by the physician in the difficulties encountered by patients and their families is as important in Parkinson's disease as in any chronic disabling disorder.

Assessing and Monitoring Parkinson's Disease

On the first and subsequent visits, the patient's occupational and social functioning should be assessed. The physician should be aware of the distress and embarrassment caused by Parkinson's disease. Specific inquiry should be made about problems with commonplace activities of daily life, sleep disturbances, symptoms of depression, and behavioral changes.

Physical examination should include observations of the degree and site of tremor and rigidity. Difficulties with fine and repetitive hand movements, balance, gait, and rising from a chair should be assessed. Supine and standing blood pressure must be taken and current medications recorded.

Fluctuating manifestations, particularly later in the course of the disease, limit the usefulness of observations made on a single occasion.

The reliable patient with relatively stable disease may need to be seen only every 3 or 4 months; obviously, however, more frequent review is necessary following initiation or significant alterations of drug treatment.

Acute deteriorations associated with intercurrent illness and the development of severe central side effects of antiparkinsonian drugs may necessitate admission to hospital. In severely disabled patients with marked fluctuations in disability or prominent dyskinesia, we usually attempt major treatment changes on an in-patient basis.

TREATMENT

Drug Therapy

Anticholinergic Drugs

The reduction of dopaminergic input to the corpus striatum in Parkinson's disease leads to disinhibition of striatal cholinergic interneurons. Anticholinergic drugs oppose this increased cholinergic activity. They may also inhibit the reuptake of dopamine by the presynaptic nerve terminals—which is the major mechanism of inactivation of dopamine.

Pharmacologic treatment of Parkinson's disease may be initiated with anticholinergic agents, especially when tremor or rigidity is the predominant manifestation. These drugs are less effective against the more disabling features of akinesia and loss of postural reflexes. Because of their different mode of action and side effects, they can usefully be combined with other antiparkinsonian agents.

The most common unwanted effects are due to parasympathetic blockade. These include blurred near vision, dry mouth, constipation, urinary retention (especially if there is pre-existing prostatism), and the precipitation of narrow angle glaucoma. Minor peripheral side effects may have to be accepted to allow a useful antiparkinson action. Anticholinergic agents may have a desirable effect on autonomic features of Parkinson's disease, such as drooling, seborrhea, and excessive sweating.

Central side effects, including confusion, delirium, and agitation, will usually resolve within a few days of drug withdrawal but may persist for as long as 2 weeks. Impairment of recent memory due to anticholinergic agents may not be recognized; thus, short-term memory should be assessed before and during therapy, especially in the older patient.

No single agent is universally superior, although some patients exhibit a preference. It is seldom advantageous to give more than one anticholinergic agent at one time. It is best to start with a small dose because tolerance to the peripheral side effects may be observed. The dose is gradually increased until a satisfactory response or unwanted side effects occur.

Some commonly used anticholinergic agents include:

1. Trihexyphenidyl hydrochloride (Artane), 2- and 5-mg tablets and 5-mg (slow release) capsules, initially 4 mg per day; usual maintenance dose range 6 to 15 mg per day.

2. Procyclidine hydrochloride (Kemadrin), 5-mg tablets, initially 5 mg per day; maintenance dose 10 to 30 mg per day.

3. Biperiden hydrochloride (Akineton), 2-mg tablets, initially 6 mg per day; maintenance dose 6 to 30 mg per day.

4. Benztropine mesylate (Cogentin), 0.5-, 1-, and 2-mg tablets, initially 1.5 mg per day; maintenance dose 2 to 6 mg per day.

Antihistamines

The antiparkinsonian action and most of the adverse effects of antihistamines derive from their anticholinergic activity. Because of their sedative properties, they may have a role in treating patients with insomnia and those with severe tremor, which is exacerbated by stress.

Antihistamines used in Parkinson's disease include:

1. Diphenhydramine hydrochloride (Benadryl), 25- and 50-mg capsules and elixer, 12.5 mg per ml; maintenance dose range 50 to 150 mg per day.

2. Orphenadrine hydrochloride (Disipal), 50-mg tablets; maintenance dose range 150 to 250 mg per day. Orphenadrine has little sedative activity and is used in a similar manner to the anticholinergic drugs listed earlier.

Amantadine

The mode of action of amantadine is uncertain. In studies employing higher tissue concentrations than those encountered in routine therapy, it increases the synthesis and release of dopamine and inhibits dopamine reuptake from the synaptic cleft. It also shows anticholinergic activity that may be additive to that of cholinergic drugs so that toxicity may be precipitated.

Amantadine is of limited efficacy but is of some use for akinesia. About 50 per cent of patients derive a worthwhile response; however, loss of benefit often occurs after about 6 months. It may be employed to initiate treatment but more commonly we give it as an adjuvant to anticholinergic or levodopa therapy. Amantadine (Symmetrel) is available as a 100-mg capsule. It is commenced at 100 mg per day and increased to 100 mg twice daily. Further increases are unlikely to be effective.

Amantadine tends to be well tolerated, but because it is largely excreted unchanged in the urine, renal impairment may lead to toxicity. Side effects are mainly related to its anticholinergic activity and include confusion, agitation, hallucinations, and psychosis. Pruritus, headache, nausea, and, rarely, cardiac arrhythmias have been associated with its use. It often produces edema of the dependent limbs and livedo reticularis, a red reticular discoloration of the skin over the legs and feet.

Levodopa and Decarboxylase Inhibitors

In 1961 Barbeau and colleagues and Birkmayer and Hornykiewicz independently developed the principle of dopamine replacement therapy in Parkinson's disease. Recognizing that the deficiency of dopamine in the nigrostriatal system could not be corrected by the administration of dopamine itself because it does not readily cross the blood-brain barrier, they gave its immediate precursor, dopa, which does gain access to the brain where it is converted to dopamine by the enzyme L-aromatic amino acid decarboxylase.

The decarboxylase enzyme located in peripheral tissues is responsible for metabolizing most of any given dose of levodopa. In 1967, Bartholini and others proposed the use of extracerebral decarboxylase inhibitors to reduce the peripheral metabolism of levodopa, which leads to many of the side effects. Preparations of a decarboxylase inhibitor, either carbidopa or benserazide in combination with levodopa, now constitute the standard form of administration and we no longer use levodopa alone.

These combinations allow an 80 per cent reduction in the dosage of levodopa without a fall in plasma level and have significantly reduced the frequency and severity of anorexia, nausea, vomiting, and postural hypotension. They also reduce the risk of cardiac arrhythmias and allow more rapid introduction of therapy.

Levodopa is well absorbed from the upper gastrointestinal tract. Peak plasma levels occur 1 to 3 hours after administration, and the plasma half-life is about 1 to 2 hours. Clinical response commences 15 minutes to 1 hour after an oral dose and lasts 1 to 5 hours.

Levodopa is more effective than anticholinergic agents against all features of parkinsonism, including tremor, rigidity, akinesia, and loss of postural reflexes. Seborrhea and drooling of saliva may also diminish.

About 20 per cent of patients with Parkinson's disease show a dramatic response to treatment with levodopa. Another 60 per cent demonstrate a moderate improvement in functional capacity. However, about 20 per cent of patients either cannot tolerate chronic therapy or respond poorly or not at all. Poor response to levodopa treatment should lead to review of the diagnosis of Parkinson's disease.

Currently available formulations include carbidopa in a 10:1 ratio with levodopa in Sinemet 250/25 (levodopa, 250 mg, with carbidopa, 25 mg) and Sinemet 100/10 (levodopa, 100 mg, and carbidopa, 10 mg) or in a 4:1 ratio in Sinemet 100/25 (levodopa, 100 mg, and carbidopa, 25 mg). Levodopa is combined with benserazide in a 4:1 ratio in Madopar* or Prolopa* capsules, which are available in three sizes: (1) levodopa, 50 mg, with benserazide, 12.5 mg; (2) levodopa, 100 mg, with benserazide, 25 mg; and (3) levodopa, 200 mg, with benserazide, 50 mg. Carbidopa and benserazide are approximately equipotent.

---

*Not available in the United States.

We commence levodopa-carbidopa in low dosage, one-half tablet of Sinemet, 100/25 3 times daily, to minimize gastrointestinal symptoms. Initially, we increase the dose by one half tablet of Sinemet 100/25 every day until the patient is receiving 300 or 400 mg of levodopa per day. When further altering the dose on an outpatient basis, we prefer to allow at least a few weeks for full response to occur before making any change.

Dose increases may be achieved by substituting Sinemet 250 for Sinemet 100/25 or raising the frequency of administration to 5 or 6 times daily or even every 2 hours. Sinemet 100/10 may be added when small adjustments are necessary in patients who do not require an increased amount of carbidopa each day.

We try to maintain most patients on doses of levodopa ranging between 400 and 800 mg per day in combination with carbidopa. If significant parkinsonian disability persists, we will usually introduce bromocriptine at this stage. In patients who cannot tolerate bromocriptine, we increase the total dose of levodopa, if necessary, to 2000 mg per day.

The side effects of levodopa will be discussed later under management problems.

Dopamine Receptor Agonists

Dopamine agonists produce their therapeutic effects by directly acting on dopamine receptors in the striatum. Theoretically, they may remain effective when response to levodopa is limited by the capacity of neurons of the nigrostriatal pathway to synthesize and store dopamine.

Studies with dopamine agonists allow distinction of two major types of dopamine receptors according to whether activation leads to stimulation of adenylate cyclase (D_1 type) or not (D_2 type). The dopaminomimetic ergot derivatives—bromocriptine, lisuride, and lergotrile—are agonists at D_2 receptors and have inhibitory activity at D_1 receptors. Pergolide, a semisynthetic ergot derivative, appears to stimulate both D_1 and D_2 receptors. Bromocriptine is the only dopamine agonist that is currently commercially available.

Bromocriptine is less likely than levodopa to produce dyskinesia and has a more prolonged action (4 to 8 hours). These characteristics give it an advantage in the patient with disabling dyskinesias or fluctuations in response to treatment. However, bromocriptine is more likely to produce psychiatric side effects and probably has more cardiac toxicity than levodopa. It should be avoided in patients with a history of recent myocardial infarction or serious cardiac arrhythmia and in those with mental impairment.

Nausea, headache, dizziness, and postural hypotension can be reduced by very gradual introduction of treatment. Postural hypotension caused by bromocriptine is rarely of such severity as to require drug withdrawal.

Pulmonary infiltrates or pleural effusions may cause respiratory symptoms that usually resolve within a few weeks of cessation of bromocriptine.

Bromocriptine mesylate (Parlodel) is available as 2.5-mg tablets and 5-mg capsules and can be administered 3 or 4 times per day. We commence 1.25 mg (one half tablet) on the first day and increase by 1.25 mg each day until the dose is 2.5 mg three times per day. Further gradual increases are made according to response and adverse effects. Some patients derive benefit from as little as 7.5 mg per day, but we commonly maintain patients in the range of 15 to 30 mg daily. As much as 100 mg per day may be beneficial in patients with severe disease.

Selegiline (Deprenyl)

Selegiline is a selective type B monoamine oxidase inhibitor. Monoamine oxidase type B preferentially metabolizes dopamine, whereas type A has relative specificity for noradrenaline and serotonin. Selegiline reduces the breakdown of dopamine without inducing the hypertensive reaction to levodopa that would occur with monoamine oxidase A inhibitors. It prolongs the duration of action of levodopa and allows a reduction in its dose by 10 to 25 per cent. The dose of selegiline is 5 to 10 mg per day. It is not yet marketed in North America.*

Management Problems

Timing of the Initiation of Pharmacologic Treatment

Following the diagnosis of Parkinson's disease, explanation and observation may be all that are required initially.

It has been suggested that levodopa treatment is characterized by a finite period of usefulness. Levodopa administration theoretically may result in an increased production of deleterious by-products of dopamine metabolism. These concerns have lead to postponement of the initiation of levodopa; however, they remain unproven, and there have been conflicting reports of the influence of treatment on the rate of progression of the disease.

We introduce levodopa when disability interferes significantly with the patient's life, and we attempt to keep the dose as low as is sufficient to produce an acceptable response.

---

*Available under the Orphan Drug Act. For information call 800-336-4797, or in Virginia and Washington D.C. area call 301-565-4167.

Loss of Efficacy

About 50 per cent of mild cases of Parkinson's disease and 80 per cent of severe cases deteriorate after 5 years of treatment. Those with the least initial improvement tend to have the earliest deterioration. However, even in patients who have become severely disabled during the time of their treatment with levodopa, further disability is usually seen on drug withdrawal. There is controversy about why this loss of efficacy occurs, but it is likely that the most important factor is progression of the underlying disease.

Nausea

Anorexia, nausea, and vomiting are infrequent when a decarboxylase inhibitor is used in combination with levodopa. However, gastrointestinal side effects are still a problem in a few patients.

Nausea can be minimized by introducing levodopa gradually and by administering the drug with food. The dose of levodopa may have to be reduced, and smaller, more frequent doses combined with snacks may be given.

Carbidopa or benserazide,* 100 mg per day, is adequate to largely block peripheral decarboxylase in most subjects; however, in those with troublesome nausea, it may be necessary to increase the dose to 200 mg per day. To achieve this without changing the total dose of levodopa, 4:1 levodopa-carbidopa may be substituted for 10:1 preparations. Supplemental carbidopa may be added, but it must be obtained directly from the manufacturer (Merck Sharp and Dohme) because it is not marketed.

Domperidone (Motilium),† a peripheral dopamine receptor (D_2 type) antagonist, may be useful against nausea associated with the use of levodopa or bromocriptine. The usual dose is 10 mg four times per day. Like the dopa decarboxylase inhibitors, it probably penetrates the chemoreceptor zone in the area postrema and reduces centrally mediated nausea.

Postural Hypotension

Levodopa often causes a decrease in supine blood pressure and impairs baroreceptor reflexes. Postural hypotension can usually be controlled by increasing the dose of carbidopa or adding domperidone.

For resistant postural hypotension, consideration should be given to using the mineralocorticoid fludrocortisone, which may be given in doses of 0.1 to 0.3 mg per day. Fluid retention should be monitored during this regimen. A potassium-sparing mild diuretic, such as amiloride or triamterene, is often useful with fludrocortisone.

It may be necessary to use elastic stockings or pants that compress the venous pool of the legs and, preferably, also of the pelvis and lower abdomen.

With chronic hypotension, autoregulatory changes occur that help to maintain cerebral blood flow. Tilting the head end of the bed up at night reduces nocturnal diuresis and enhances these autoregulatory mechanisms.

Severe postural hypotension, particularly if there is other evidence of autonomic failure, suggests a diagnosis of Shy-Drager syndrome.

Psychiatric Disturbances

Levodopa treatment may be associated with confusion, delirium, agitation, paranoia, delusions, hypomania, depression, and pseudodementia. Overt psychotic reaction to levodopa is more common in patients with a history of schizophrenia or paranoid psychosis. The presence of dementia, which develops in about a third of cases of Parkinson's disease, seems to reduce the threshold for the psychiatric side effects of all antiparkinson medication.

A relatively common problem with levodopa therapy is the occurrence of insomnia, vivid dreams, and nocturnal visual hallucinations that are often nonthreatening and that the patient recognizes as unreal. Nocturnal hallucinations and mild, intermittent confusion should lead to consideration of reduction in dosage of levodopa in the evening. However, the benefit of such a decrease must be balanced against the problems of increasing immobility.

More severe psychiatric manifestations necessitate drug withdrawal. In patients on a combination of antiparkinson drugs, consideration should be given to stopping anticholinergic agents, amantadine, and bromocriptine. Levodopa may also have to be reduced or withdrawn temporarily and may be cautiously reintroduced at lower dosage if it still has a significant benefit on motor dysfunction. As with anticholinergic agents, the central side effects of levodopa and bromocriptine usually subside within a few days but may persist for up to 6 weeks.

Depression occurs in about 40 per cent of patients with Parkinson's disease. Diagnosis may be difficult because the psychomotor retardation, restriction of activities, and sleep disturbances that are features of Parkinson's disease overlap with the profile of symptoms by which we recognize depression, so specific inquiry regarding mood alteration should always be made.

Tricyclic antidepressant agents can be used, and their anticholinergic action may be beneficial

---

*Not available in the United States.
†Investigational agent.

against parkinsonian features; however, central toxicity may be precipitated when tricyclics are added to anticholinergic agents or amantadine. They can also exacerbate hypotension. Antidepressants of the nonspecific monoamine oxidase group are contraindicated in patients on levodopa because severe hypertension may ensue.

Fluctuations in Disability

Initially, levodopa produces a smooth antiparkinson effect; eventually, however, dose-related fluctuations in response—"end of dose" deterioration or "wearing-off" phenomena—tend to develop. Further, fluctuations may occur from mobile to immobile states lasting from minutes to several hours that cannot be related to the timing of administration of the drug. These are referred to as the "on-off" phenomena.

There is evidence that the rate of entry of levodopa into the brain is affected by competition with other large amino acids for the same transport system across the blood-brain barrier, so that patients with fluctuating responses are advised to reduce total protein intake. Other measures that are employed in these circumstances are the use of smaller, more frequent doses of levodopa and the addition of bromocriptine, which has a longer duration of action than levodopa. Fluctuations may also be improved by the introduction of selegiline (Deprenyl). Akinesia limiting the ability to roll over in bed during the night may be reduced by an evening dose of bromocriptine.

Slow release formulations of Sinemet and bromocriptine are being developed and will probably have a role in producing a more sustained response to treatment.

"Freezing" and Falls

"Freezing" attacks, sudden brief exacerbations of immobility lasting from a few seconds to a minute or two, are not due to levodopa treatment and should not be confused with the "on-off" phenomenon. Freezing, especially if combined with loss of postural reflexes, is a common cause of falls in Parkinson's disease. Levodopa usually decreases the frequency of freezing episodes; as the disease progresses, however, severe freezing is generally resistant to treatment, and excessive levodopa may actually increase falls by causing postural hypotension.

Dyskinesias

Dyskinesias occur with the use of levodopa and dopamine receptor agonists. They include choreoathetoid movements, dystonia, and less commonly ballism and myoclonus. They often begin around the mouth with grimacing, chewing, or tongue protrusion. Involvement of the limbs and trunk is frequent. Dyskinesias of the respiratory muscles can cause dyspnea and chest discomfort. Blepharospasm and lateral eye deviations may also occur.

It is believed that dyskinesias derive from denervation hypersensitivity that develops in certain of the remaining dopamine receptors consequent upon degeneration of the nigrostriatal pathway. Because of the patchy nature and degree of the pathologic change in Parkinson's disease, dyskinesias and parkinsonian features may be present in different muscle groups at the same time.

Dyskinesias occur in the majority of patients after prolonged treatment with levodopa, but it is not clear whether this increasing prevalence relates to disease progression or to the cumulative dose of levodopa. Once dyskinesias appear, their severity is related to the daily dose of levodopa.

Most commonly, dyskinesias develop in association with peak plasma levels of levodopa. For many patients, the most effective dose of levodopa to control parkinsonian symptoms is at, or just below, that which produces minimal dyskinetic movements. Unfortunately, dyskinesias may come to occupy most of the period during which the patient derives benefit from treatment, and reduction in dosage is accompanied by loss of duration of useful mobility.

For peak-dose dyskinesias and paroxysmal dyskinesias that may occur unrelated to the time of dose, we attempt to reduce the total daily dose of levodopa and to give smaller, more frequent doses. The development of troublesome dyskinesias is an indication to introduce bromocriptine with simultaneous reduction in the dose of levodopa. Diphasic dyskinesias in which involuntary movements are most prominent at the onset and toward the end of the period of therapeutic benefit may also improve with the addition of bromocriptine.

The use of selegiline, again with associated decrease in the dose of levodopa, may be helpful in the management of dyskinesia.

Trends in Management

Over the last several years, there has been extensive effort to develop and evaluate new dopamine agonists, including D_1 receptor agonists.

It is currently the practice of many neurologists to introduce bromocriptine earlier in the course of treatment of Parkinson's disease, before the development of disabling fluctuations and dyskinesias. The combination of levodopa and bromocriptine in lower maintenance doses than would be possible using each agent separately allows effective control of parkinsonism with a low rate of adverse reactions.

POLYNEUROPATHIES

method of
JOHN J. KELLY, M.D.
Boston, Massachusetts

A polyneuropathy can be a difficult diagnostic and therapeutic problem. Sometimes, the cause is clear when the patient, for example, has diabetes or uremia. Frequently, however, no etiology is evident and questions arise as to what constitutes adequate evaluation and management of these patients.

The first step in evaluating these patients is deciding if there is a polyneuropathy, especially if the symptoms are mild and of recent onset. Patients with vascular disease, orthopedic problems, or nerve root disease due to degenerative conditions of the lumbar spine can present special problems since, like polyneuropathy patients, they complain of extremity symptoms with pain and weakness. Words used by patients to describe their symptoms often can be of diagnostic value, since terms such as "tingling," "burning," and "shooting pains" in the extremities suggest peripheral nerve involvement and are not usually due to vascular or orthopedic disease. The findings on examination in polyneuropathy generally reflect involvement of the longest axons, with a gradual spread of the deficit more proximally in a centripetal fashion. Thus, "stocking" sensory loss that gradually fades to normal, distal weakness and muscle atrophy, and distal loss of deep tendon reflexes are characteristic of neuropathy and are generally not seen with other disorders, such as nerve root and spinal cord disease. With chronic and long-standing neuropathies, trophic changes affect the feet and hands.

When the diagnosis is uncertain, nerve conduction studies, needle electromyography (EMG), and nerve biopsy can be very helpful. EMG and nerve conduction studies are useful in the differential diagnosis of polyradiculopathies, plexopathies, and spinal cord disease. Nerve biopsy should be performed in experienced centers since preparation and interpretation are technically difficult.

Treatment of patients can be classed as either symptomatic or specific. Symptomatic therapy including physical therapy and medications to reduce pain and cramping is used for mild neuropathies, those with the uncertain diagnoses, or as an adjunct to specific therapy. Specific therapy is aimed at correcting the primary cause of the polyneuropathy and is usually contingent on discovery of that cause.

One diagnostic approach to polyneuropathies is to look at relative frequency of the types encountered in large series and to concentrate diagnostic energy on those most frequently seen. A compilation of results of several recent large studies is shown in Table 1. Hereditary, inflammatory-demyelinating, and metabolic-toxic neuropathies account for the largest proportion, with undiagnosed neuropathies accounting for approximately 15 to 20 per cent.

HEREDITARY POLYNEUROPATHIES

In several series, this is the commonest recognized cause of polyneuropathy, accounting for about 30 to 40 per cent of cases. Although it would seem relatively easy to recognize these patients, the diagnosis is often difficult. The neuropathies encountered in this category fall into two main types: (1) primarily motor, generally referred to as Charcot-Marie-Tooth disease and its variants, and (2) primarily sensory, generally referred to as the hereditary sensory neuropathies.

Charcot-Marie-Tooth Disease

Patients with Charcot-Marie-Tooth (CMT) disease usually present with progressive weakness of distal legs, with foot drop accompanied by some degree of weakness and atrophy of the hand muscles. The examination discloses distal thinning of legs and arms, with the so-called "inverted champagne bottle" appearance of the legs, and pes cavus and hammer toe deformities of the feet, often with other skeletal abnormalities such as scoliosis. Diagnosis hinges on recognition of the clinical charateristics and extreme chronicity of the disorder. Skeletal deformities frequently suggest that the disease has been present since childhood when the skeleton was developing. CMT disease is often so slowly progressive that patients may be unaware of their deficit or of its onset. Sensory findings are minimal or absent and sensory complaints (tingling, pain) are uncommon, in sharp contrast to patients with acquired neuropathies who can often tell to the week and sometimes to the day when their symptoms began.

Most cases of CMT disease are dominantly inherited, so it would seem that a family history should readily suggest the diagnosis. However, due to the extreme chronicity, slow progression and uncertain age of onset of their disorders, relatives with milder disease are often unrecog-

TABLE 1. **Etiology of Polyneuropathy***

Inherited	30%
Inflammatory—demyelinating (acute and chronic)	20%
Metabolic—toxic (including diabetic)	20%
Associated with monoclonal protein	5%
Polyneuropathy associated with other systemic disorder	5%
Undiagnosed	20%

*Estimates from several studies.

nized. In addition, phenotypic expression is extremely variable, even in the same family, ranging from mild, subclinical disorders to severe, disabling disease. Thus, personal examination and often nerve conduction studies of first-degree blood relatives are usually necessary to establish the inherited nature of the disorder. Nerve conduction and nerve biopsy studies of large kindreds have recognized two main types: a hypertrophic form with enlarged, thickened nerves and very slow nerve conduction velocities, and a neuronal (axonal) form with fairly normal conduction velocities.

Definitive treatment is nonexistent but symptomatic treatment can be effective. Proper shoes, bracing, and physical therapy are important. These patients usually lead fairly normal lives with few restrictions and some have active athletic careers early in life.

Hereditary Sensory Neuropathies

These neuropathies share features in common with CMT disease but are much less common and are essentially purely sensory, with little or no motor involvement. Like CMT disease, and unlike the acquired polyneuropathies, they are very chronic, of obscure onset, and generally not associated with numbness or pain. Skeletal deformities do not occur as frequently as in CMT disease, but trophic changes and foot and hand mutilation are common. Because of altered pain sensation, fractures and ulcers are often unnoticed by the patient or of little concern. In the past, such lesions would become infected and osteomyelitis would develop, resulting in large and weeping ulcers, toe and foot amputation, sepsis, and death in some cases.

Some of these disorders are autosomal dominant, so detection depends on screening relatives as well as recognition of the characteristic pattern. Others are autosomal recessive, so screening of relatives is less productive unless several siblings are available. In patients without a clear family history, reognition of the characteristic pattern alone allows a presumptive diagnosis.

Like CMT disease, only symptomatic therapy is available for these patients. This should consist of meticulous foot care, avoidance of foot trauma, and prompt treatment of any sores or pressure areas on the feet. Patients with these disorders should wear special shoes and should inspect their feet at least twice daily. Special care should be taken to ensure that no objects such as small stones or protruding nails are present in the shoes and that the sock is not bunched up so as to produce a blister or an ulcer. Males with hereditary sensory neuropathy do particularly poorly and proscription of occupations or avocations likely to cause foot traumas is necessary.

INFLAMMATORY DEMYELINATING POLYNEUROPATHIES

Idiopathic inflammatory demyelinating polyneuropathies account for approximately 20 per cent of all neuropathies and are generally thought to be autoimmune disorders in which either sensitized B cells produce antibodies or T cells directly demyelinate peripheral nerves. These polyneuropathies can be acute or chronic. The acute form is generally referred to as Guillain-Barré syndrome (GBS) and the chronic variety as chronic inflammatory demyelinating polyneuropathy (CIDP) or chronic relapsing inflammatory polyneuropathy. Although they share many characteristics, GBS and CIDP are generally thought to be distinct disorders.

Guillain-Barré Syndrome

GBS is relatively common. It is generally triggered by an antecedent event (e.g., viral illness, vaccination, trauma), which somehow perturbs the immune system and leads to a self-limited episode of autoimmunity directed against peripheral nerve myelin. Usually, the neuropathy begins 7 to 21 days after the antecedent event. Patients develop some combination of rapidly progressive gait ataxia, symmetric weakness of distal or proximal muscles and often facial muscles, and minimal sensory loss in hands and feet. The disease can evolve to a maximum deficit in any interval from a few days to 3 to 4 weeks, then stabilizes for a time, and then improves. The vast majority, even those with severe GBS requiring intubation and respiratory therapy, eventually make a satisfactory recovery.

Aside from clinical features, helpful clues to diagnosis include nerve conduction studies, which generally show marked slowing of motor conduction velocities characteristic of diseases affecting the myelin sheath, and cerebrospinal fluid (CSF) examination, which shows an elevated protein-level thought to be due to inflammation of nerve roots.

Treatment is supportive and immunosuppressive. The main danger is respiratory impairment with death. If patients approach respiratory compromise, treatment should include early elective intubation and management in a respiratory intensive care unit by personnel experienced in dealing with these patients. Immunosuppressive therapy at present consists of plasmapheresis. Several recent studies have shown that plasmapheresis is more effective than no pheresis in lessening peak deficit and hastening recovery. Large-volume pheresis 3 times a week for 2 to 3 weeks is the usual regimen. The role of steroids and other immunosuppressive agents is more controversial. There is currently no evidence that drug therapy is effective and some evidence that it may be harmful. As mentioned, most patients make a satisfactory recovery with or without treatment.

CIDP

Chronic inflammatory demyelinating polyneuropathy shares many of the clinical, laboratory, and pathologic similarities of GBS. However, CIDP, as the name implies, is a chronic disease that typically commences without an inciting event; is slowly progressive, often with plateaus and relapses; and remits with or without therapy. These neuropathies are generally thought, like GBS, to represent a chronic autoimmune attack of antibodies and/or cell-mediated immunity against peripheral nerve myelin.

Diagnosis is predominantly clinical since laboratory tests are not definitively diagnostic. However, unlike GBS, the mainstay of treatment is steroids. Patients require high doses of steroids for prolonged periods. Responders have a good prognosis. Nonresponders require stronger immunosuppressive agents and/or plasmapheresis. Occasionally, patients become refractory to immunosuppressive therapy, develop progressive disease, and may die.

DIABETIC NEUROPATHIES

The metabolic neuropathies account for approximately 15 to 20 per cent of all polyneuropathies. The most common cause in this group is diabetes. Neuropathy increases in frequency with longevity of patients with diabetes. The current leading theory is that the neuropathy is due to a vasculopathy of small arterioles and venules provoked by chronic hyperglycemia, with resultant nerve ischemia. Other theories implicate accumulation of sorbitol and deficiency of myoinositol in peripheral nerve. Diabetic neuropathy can present in several ways, including mononeuropathy or mononeuropathy multiplex; proximal diabetic neuropathy (plexopathy, polyradiculopathy, "femoral" neuropathy); small-fiber, painful, distal neuropathy; and large-fiber, areflexic polyneuropathy. Patients often present with a mixture of two or more types, but this distinction is still useful conceptually in deciding whether a neuropathy is due to diabetes.

Treatment of diabetic neuropathy is based on the theory that hyperglycemia is the chief cause.

Therefore, improved diabetic control is generally recommended using frequent insulin injections and frequent blood glucose monitoring. Experimental therapies with aldose reductase inhibitors and myoinositol supplementation, although promising, are of unproved efficacy. Other experimental therapies are designed to increase blood flow and oxygenation to peripheral nerves.

Mononeuropathy or Mononeuropathy Multiplex

This neuropathy generally affects named nerves (oculomotor, facial, median), with the sudden onset of painful nerve dysfunction generally thought to be due to nerve infarction. Prognosis for recovery is generally good.

Proximal Diabetic Neuropathy

The most common presentation is the so-called "femoral" neuropathy, which is a misnomer, since the deficit is never restricted to just the femoral nerve. These patients present with the sudden onset of pain and weakness in the anterior thigh and hip with loss of the knee jerk reflex. However, weakness involves other muscles supplied by the lumbar plexus and/or lumbar nerve roots. Sensory loss is minimal. EMG shows involvement of the plexus and roots. The prognosis is excellent for eventual recovery without treatment. Etiology is also generally thought to be ischemic.

Small-Fiber, Painful, Distal Neuropathy

Patients with this type of neuropathy typically have symptoms out of proportion to findings. Pain is particularly prominent along with autonomic symptoms, but weakness is minimal. The pain is described as burning, aching, or sharp and shooting and is associated with cutaneous hypersensitivity. Autonomic symptoms cause impotence, neurogenic bladder, gastroparesis, nocturnal diarrhea, postural hypotension, and dyshidrosis (decreased or increased sweating). Examination discloses distal sensory loss mainly to pin prick and temperature, with absent ankle jerks. Strength and discriminative sensation are surprisingly well preserved, as are nerve conduction studies due to the relative sparing of large sensory and motor fibers. The neuropathy is generally slowly progressive.

Large-Fiber, Ataxic, Areflexic Polyneuropathy

Patients with the large-fiber typical of metabolic neuropathy present with progressive gait ataxia and distal weakness. Pain and autonomic symptoms are not so prominent as with the small-fiber variant. "Stocking-glove" sensory loss of all modalities occurs. Areflexia is more widespread. Moderate distal weakness, greater in the legs than the arms, also occurs. Nerve conduction studies give evidence of demyelination as well as axonal loss. Nerve biopsy shows thickening of vessel walls and basement membranes of Schwann cells and perineurium. This neuropathy also tends to be slowly progressive.

OTHER TOXIC, DRUG-RELATED AND METABOLIC NEUROPATHIES

Most of these neuropathies are chronic and exposure related. Since most toxins poison the metabolic machinery of the cell body and interfere with production and delivery of essential products to the distal axons (the most vulnerable part), it stands to reason that toxin, drug-related, and metabolic neuropathies are predominantly distal, symmetric, and greater in the legs and that they progress in a distal to proximal fashion. Nerve conduction studies usually show evidence of axonal damage with little evidence of demyelination. Nerve biopsy shows nonspecific changes. Discovery of such a polyneuropathy should prompt a redoubled search for metabolic abnormalities or neurotoxin exposure. A common example of this category is alcoholic polyneuropathy. Although thought to be a complication of chronic alcoholism and chronic malnutrition, with deficiency of multiple essential elements in chronic alcoholics, alcohol itself likely has a toxic effect on peripheral nerves and can cause a mild, distal axonal polyneuropathy mainly affecting the feet.

POLYNEUROPATHIES ASSOCIATED WITH PLASMA CELL DYSCRASIAS

It has been shown in recent years that approximately 5 per cent of all polyneuropathy patients will have an occult plasma cell dyscrasia. About one half of these patients in turn have a polyneuropathy in association with a benign monoclonal gammopathy (or monoclonal gammopathy of undetermined significance, which is now the preferred term for this disorder). Some of these patients have IgM gammopathies and a characteristic primarily sensory, demyelinating polyneuropathy due to an IgM monoclonal protein that is directed at an antigen, myelin-associated glycoprotein, on the surface of the myelin sheath. This neuropathy likely represents a true autoimmune disease and responds to treatment with vigorous immunosuppression designed to lower the concentration of the serum IgM protein level.

About 25 per cent of these patients have primary systemic amyloidosis related to deposition of fragments of the serum monoclonal light chain in peripheral nerve tissue. These patients present with a sensory rather than a motor distal axonal polyneuropathy, with prominent pain and autonomic symptoms. The disease is progressive and fatal owing to cardiac or renal failure within a few years, and no treatment is currently effective.

The remaining 25 per cent of these patients have various neuropathies, the most characteristic of which is that associated with occult osteosclerotic multiple myeloma, which presents as a striking syndrome with polyneuropathy and multiple systemic manifestations suggesting an endocrinopathy or malignancy. Recognition of the osteosclerotic lesions allows treatment of these patients with radiation or chemotherapy, which improves their clinical status.

MONONEURITIS MULTIPLEX

Mononeuritis multiplex refers to a clinical presentation in which multiple named peripheral nerves are involved asymmetrically in the arms and legs. Generally the history is one of progressive, step-wise loss of function of peroneal, median, ulnar, or tibial nerves over days, weeks, or months. The onset of dysfunction in each nerve distribution is generally painful and sudden or subacute. This clinical picture is dramatic and the differential diagnosis relatively limited. The most feared cause of this syndrome is vasculitis, with nerve infarction due to one of the collagen vascular diseases such as periarteritis nodosa, rheumatoid vasculitis, or Wegener's granulomatosis. Nerve conduction studies show axonal neuropathy, and diagnosis is made by recognition of other systemic manifestations of vasculitis and by tissue demonstration of necrotizing arteritis. Biopsy of muscle and sural nerve is also diagnostic.

Patients with diabetes can present with a similar clinical syndrome that is thought to be due to a vasculopathy (see under Diabetic Neuropathies). The prognosis is usually quite good. Patients with CIDP can occasionally present with an asymmetric, mononeuritic form of the disease. EMG generally shows evidence of demyelination rather than axonal degeneration, CSF proteins are elevated, and nerve biopsies show no evidence of vasculitis; these patients usually respond to immunosuppressive therapy. Other rare causes of the mononeuritis multiplex syndrome include Lyme disease, sarcoidosis, AIDS, and leprosy.

UNDIAGNOSED NEUROPATHIES

Despite thorough work-up (see below), the cause of neuropathy in 15 to 25 per cent of patients will not be diagnosed. Most commonly, these patients are elderly, have a mild and distal neuropathy, and are troubled by pain and paresthesias with mild gait imbalance but with little weakness. These neuropathies generally remain mild and progress very slowly over years of follow-up. EMG and nerve biopsy reveal chronic axonal damage without clues to etiology. Prolonged follow-up of these patients will yield a diagnosis in a few (occult cancer, toxin exposure, inherited) but most remain undiagnosed and require symptomatic treatment.

Patient Evaluation

Evaluation of a patient with an undiagnosed polyneuropathy should be a logical step by step process based on the relative likelihood of the various disorders (See Table 1). A suggested approach is shown in Table 2. The first step is to establish that a polyneuropathy is indeed causing the patient's symptoms. Sometimes, history and examination allows for no other diagnosis. On other occasions, orthopedic or vascular disease, radiculopathy, or plexopathy can cause confusion. A careful study of the EMG can facilitate recognition of these disorders. Rarely is nerve biopsy indicated simply to establish the presence of polyneuropathy.

Once the presence of polyneuropathy is estab-

TABLE 2. **Suggested Evaluation of Polyneuropathy Patient**

---

1. Determine whether the patient does have a polyneuropathy and, if so, the type:
   - Clinical history and examination
   - Nerve conduction studies/EMG
   - Family history and drug/toxin history
2. Initial laboratory studies if etiology not evident.
   - CBC, VDRL, BUN, creatinine, calcium, phosphorus, LFT
   - Thyroxin, vitamin B$_{12}$, folate, serum protein electrophoresis
   - Urine porphyrins and heavy metals (Pb, As, Th, Hg)
   - Chest x-ray
3. If diagnosis not apparent, obtain:
   - CSF for cells and protein
   - Lipids, carotene, 72-hour stool fat test
   - Serum immunoelectrophoresis; 24-hr urine protein electrophoresis
   - X-ray skeletal survey (in appropriate clinical setting)
   - Rectal biopsy for amyloid (in appropriate clinical setting)
   - Other tests in selected cases
   - Examination of blood relatives
4. If diagnosis still unclear, consider sural nerve biopsy

Abbreviations: CBC = complete blood count, VDRL = Venereal Disease Research Laboratory test; BUN = blood urea nitrogen; LFT = liver function test; CSF = cerebrospinal fluid.

lished, etiologic investigation should be carried out. Often, the cause is clear. The patient may be diabetic or uremic, or neurotoxins such as vincristine or alcohol may be causative. If the polyneuropathy is otherwise typical of that disorder, no other work-up is necessary. However, if the polyneuropathy is atypical or no obvious cause is present, then further work-up is needed and the necessary laboratory studies are obtained (see Table 2). Following clinical evaluations and laboratory studies, the polyneuropathy is classified depending on features such as degree of symmetry, presence of axonal or demyelinating features, modalities involved, and temporal profile (acute, subacute, or chronic). These various categories have diagnostic significance and are based primarily on clinical and EMG characteristics.

Next, the CSF examination is carried out. High protein levels in the CSF suggest demyelinating disorders or root inflammation. First-degree blood relatives are examined at this point if any suspicion of an inherited disorder exists.

If still no diagnosis is evident, then nerve biopsy should be considered, realizing that there are several caveats regarding this procedure. First of all, the biopsy is often unhelpful, because it is diagnostic in only a minority of disorders in which there are distinct structural changes or infiltration of abnormal material (e.g., vasculitis, amyloidosis). Most often, the changes simply confirm the presence of a polyneuropathy and evidence of axonal degeneration or demyelination, features already known from the clinical and electrical studies. Second, biopsy is unpleasant for some patients. A small minority report disturbing foot or calf dysesthesias that are more bothersome than the neuropathy itself. Third, nerve biopsy preparation is technically difficult and results are often marred by artifacts. Thus, biopsy should be carried out only in centers experienced in nerve biopsy and should be interpreted by an experienced nerve pathologist. Nerve biopsies are undoubtedly overperformed, since they provide information that is useful diagnostically in probably less than 50 per cent of cases.

Treatment

After complete evaluation, if no diagnosis is found, the patient should be followed and treated symptomatically. This includes physical therapy, orthotic devices and pain control. Amitriptyline is useful, as is carbamazepine. Other analgesics are less useful. Prolonged follow-up can sometimes yield a diagnosis.

Patients with moderately severe and disabling

polyneuropathy, however, probably deserve a trial of steroids unless there are major contraindications. These patients should have a careful quantitative examination and then treatment for 2 to 3 months with high-dose steroids. If the patient improves, this suggests that the polyneuropathy is treatable and possibly related to inflammation or immunologic abnormalities. Continued treatment or perhaps use of stronger immunosuppressive therapy such as plasmapheresis or stronger immunosuppressants is then indicated. If steroid therapy is not helpful, the patient should be followed and treated symptomatically and reassessed periodically if the symptoms worsen significantly.

ACUTE HEAD INJURIES IN ADULTS

method of
J. PAUL MUIZELAAR, M.D.
Medical College of Virginia
Virginia Commonwealth University
Richmond, Virginia

Head injuries pose a major health problem in industrialized countries, both in premature death and disability, as well as in sheer numbers. Trauma is the leading cause of death in the male population between 4 and 30 years of age, and many die primarily because of brain injury. It is estimated that 500,000 new cases of head or brain injury with loss of consciousness and post-traumatic amnesia occur each year in the United States, and many more patients seek medical attention for more trivial injuries. There is a wide range in severity of traumatic brain injury, but this is commonly reduced into four categories: trivial, mild, moderate, and severe. Each requires its own clinical and radiologic assessment and its own treatment (Table 1).

TREATMENT

Trivial Injuries

Although the definition of trivial injuries includes radiologic criteria, (i.e., absence of skull

TABLE 1. **Categories of Head Injury Severity**

Trivial:	No loss of consciousness or post-traumatic amnesia; no skull fracture, cerebral contusion, or intracranial hematoma.
Mild:	Loss of consciousness and/or post-traumatic amnesia with a combined duration of less than 30 minutes; no skull fracture, cerebral contusion, or intracranial hematoma.
Moderate:	Loss of consciousness and/or post-traumatic amnesia, for 30 minutes to 24 hours; and/or skull fracture; no intracranial contusion or hematoma.
Severe:	Loss of consciousness and/or post-traumatic amnesia, for more than 24 hours; and/or cerebral contusion, laceration, or intracranial hematoma.

fracture or intracranial contusion or hematoma), it is generally not necessary to obtain skull x-rays or a cerebral computed tomography (CT) scan in these patients. Patients in whom it is justified to obtain skull x-rays are those with extensive hematomas and/or contusions of the forehead or scalp and those with orbital or retromastoid hematomas. These patients should not be left unobserved the first 6 hours after their injury; after that period, they will not have to be awakened for checking. These patients can return to work immediately, and follow-up is scheduled on an as-needed basis only. If a patient later returns complaining of headache, one needs to distinguish between tension headaches and vasomotor headaches. After trivial head injuries, tension headaches are more common, and they can best be treated with diazepam (Valium), 2 mg 3 times a day for 5 days. Vascular headaches, which are often accompanied by complaints of orthostatic dizziness, photophobia, and difficulty in concentrating, are eminently amenable to treatment with a combination of phenobarbital, 40 mg; ergotamine tartrate, 0.6 mg; and belladonna alkaloids 0.2 mg (Bellergal S), two tablets twice daily. Chronic subdural hematomas may occur after trivial head injuries and may remain without neurologic symptoms for a long time. They usually occur only in the elderly, in alcoholics, or in patients using coumadin derivatives; therefore, later CT scans need to be obtained if the patient is in one of these risk groups. If a chronic subdural hematoma has developed, it is best treated by drainage through multiple burr holes made under local anesthesia, with extensive flushing of the hematoma with warm normal saline solution.

Scalp lacerations can be flushed with povidone-iodine (Betadine) solution, cleaned, and closed in one layer with interrupted 3-0 silk sutures. Cutting the ends fairly long will facilitate stitch removal later. The patient can shower his head two days later, and stitches can be removed on the fifth day.

Mild Injuries

For all patients with a mild head injury, a series of skull x-rays should be obtained. If these are normal, no CT scan needs to be obtained, unless the patient is in a high-risk group for intracranial bleeding.

The patient should be observed in the emergency room until 3 to 6 hours post-injury and then can be sent home. Reliable relatives or friends should be instructed to ascertain every 1 to 2 hours that the patient is fully oriented for the first 24 hours, waking the patient up as necessary. If no reliable person is available to carry out this order, or in case of alcohol intoxication, it is often necessary to admit the patient to the hospital overnight.

Further management is similar to that outlined under Trivial Injuries. However, with loss of consciousness, vascular headaches are more common than tension headaches. The patient may have complaints that give the impression of being neurasthenic; however, on neuropsychological testing considerable deficits are sometimes found months after the injury. This may have important legal consequences and the physician should be alert to these sequelae.

Moderate Injuries

If the patient is in this category solely because of a skull fracture, a CT scan should be obtained. The patient with a normal scan is admitted or transferred to a hospital with capacities for neurosurgery, and hourly checks of pupillary status and consciousness are carried out. Moreover, at this time an intravenous line is inserted in order to have immediate access for emergent administration of 500 ml 20 per cent mannitol solution, in case of rapid deterioration. With a strong suspicion of epidural hematoma (skull fracture with ipsilateral unresponsive pupil and lucid interval) any surgeon can do a temporal craniectomy, with chisel and hammer if necessary! Remember, irreparable brain damage may occur in 10 to 15 minutes, whereas even large skull deficits can easily be dealt with later, with most satisfactory cosmetic results.

If a patient in this category has prolonged unconsciousness, a CT scan is obtained, irrespective of whether the patient has regained consciousness or not at the time of being first seen. By definition of the category of "moderate" injuries, this CT scan is normal (except for possible skull fracture); otherwise the patient will be in the "severe" category. Whether the patient needs to be intubated before his CT scan depends to some extent on the level of coma. Any patient not able to follow simple commands such as "stick out your tongue" or "hold up your thumb" is considered to be in coma (unless the cause is aphasia), the depth of which is further assessed with the Glasgow Coma Scale (GCS) (Table 2). In general, intubation and ventilation are necessary, as is insertion of an intra-arterial catheter and a Foley catheter. Ample intravenous fluids are administered; fluid restriction "to prevent cerebral edema" is probably detrimental. Assuming there are no other injuries necessitating blood transfusion or colloid solution administration, the patient is given 2 ml per kg per hour of glucose

TABLE 2. **The Glasgow Coma Scale (GCS)**

Verbal response	
None	1
Incomprehensible sounds	2
Inappropriate words	3
Confused	4
Oriented	5
Eye opening	
None	1
To pain	2
To speech	3
Spontaneously	4
Motor response	
None	1
Abnormal extensor	2
Abnormal flexion	3
Withdraws	4
Localizes	5
Obeys	6

2.5 per cent–half normal saline for the first 24 hours. For sedation one can use 10 mg of morphine intravenously every 3 hours as needed. In case of extreme restlessness or for diagnostic procedures, complete paralysis can easily be obtained by injection of 5 to 10 mg pancuronium bromide (Pavulon). After 24 hours a decision is made as to which category the patient belongs: if the patient follows commands or is localizing briskly, bilaterally, and with eye opening, then ventilatory support is quickly tapered and the patient extubated. During this period, monitoring of intracranial pressure is not necessary; in patients with moderately severe injuries, intracranial pressure (ICP) problems seldom occur, and they develop usually only after 24 hours in patients in prolonged coma but with normal CT scans.

Severe Injuries

The primary goal in the treatment of severe head injuries is the prevention of so-called secondary insults: inadequate cerebral perfusion, high intracranial pressure, cerebral distortion, seizures, or hypoventilation. In all these conditions, the brain—whole or in part—is inadequately supplied with oxygen. Prevention of secondary insults begins at the scene of the accident. By far the most important issue here is to secure the airway and ventilation. In the 1970s in Paris, France, a switch was made to intubation of all comatose head-injured patients at the scene of the accident; the result was an immediate, dramatic reduction of mortality. Therefore, we favor intubation by the rescue squad personnel of patients with GCS of 7 or below (see Table 2). (Incidentally, the rescue squad personnel also should be able to use the GCS.) If intubation is not possible, an oropharyngeal airway should be used, and the patient should be force-ventilated with a face mask. Also, an intravenous line should be inserted, and ample fluid administration is in order. Whether any medication should be given by a rescue squad is controversial. Seizures may be treated by slow intravenous injection of 10 mg of diazepam (Valium). If the patient has an unilaterally wide pupil, 300 ml of mannitol 20 per cent can be administered. Although it is possible that very early administration of corticosteroids is beneficial, we do not favor this until more definite data are available.

Stabilization and Diagnosis

Once in the emergency room, the comatose patient is first intubated (if this had not yet been done). At the same time an intra-arterial catheter is placed for measuring blood pressure and blood gases. At least 50 per cent of all patients with severe head injuries have multiple injuries, and the treatment of those that could result in shock are given priority over the brain injury. At the same time a lateral cervical spine film is obtained; C-7 must be visualized, because in 10 per cent of these patients there is also a fracture or dislocation of the spine. A large-bore multiple-port intravenous access is secured. We prefer a jugular catheter, but a subclavian line is satisfactory. Once ventilation and blood pressure are adequate, the GCS is determined and pupil width and responsiveness to light are assessed. Oculovestibular responses (ice-water test and doll's signs) are tested in cases of more severe injuries if the corneal reflex is absent. A full CT scan is obtained, which obviates the need for obtaining emergency skull x-rays.

In case the patient needs to undergo emergency laparotomy or thoracotomy, it is wise to obtain a two-cut cerebral CT scan. If there is a surgical lesion, this can be dealt with simultaneously with the other operation. If there is no intracranial surgical lesion, an intracranial pressure monitor (ventricular catheter, subarachnoid screw, or intraparenchymal pressure device (Camino) can be employed for intraoperative ICP monitoring.

Surgery

Our indication for surgery is the removal of all hematomas that cause a shift greater than 5-mm of the midline structures. It should be performed as early as possible, not only for epidural hematomas, but also for subdural hematomas. It has been shown that the prognosis is much better in cases in which subdural hematomas are removed within 4 hours post-injury than in cases in which this could not be accomplished within this period. Intracerebral hematomas are also evacuated. The

indication for removal of contusions is less firm. We tend not to remove these unless ICP cannot be controlled under 25 mm Hg with medical measures. Before acute surgery and often even before CT scanning, in cases of suspicion of a surgical lesion, the patient is given 500 ml of mannitol 20 per cent intravenously. During surgery the patient is hyperventilated down to a $PaCO_2$ of 20 to 25 mm Hg. If sudden, severe brain swelling occurs after decompression, the swelling can sometimes be reduced with sodium thiopental (Pentothal) in repeated doses of 100 mg as long as the blood pressure does not fall.

Medical Therapy

The main purpose of the medical treatment of the severely head injured patient is to keep cerebral perfusion pressure (CPP) normal, both by keeping the ICP below 20–25 mmHg and by maintaining mean arterial blood pressure (MABP) above 90 mm Hg. ICP should be monitored in all patients with abnormal admission CT scans and in those patients with normal CT scans whose GCS remains 7 or below after 24 hours. We prefer an intraventricular catheter. The advantages are that it is probably most reliable in regard to ICP recordings and that cerebrospinal fluid (CSF) can be drained as a first measure to treat ICP elevation. The disadvantages are that they are sometimes difficult to place (when the ventricles are compressed), that an intracerebral hematoma can be produced, and that there is a risk of infection (ventriculitis), especially if the catheter is left in place for longer than 3 days. If an intraventricular catheter cannot be inserted, we now prefer to use the Camino monitor, which has its transducer in the tip and thus is very accurate.

Although we do everything we can to keep ICP below 25 mm Hg, we actually start treatment when ICP is consistently greater than 20 mm Hg. The following procedures are used, in sequence, to reduce ICP or to prevent elevations.

Head and Neck Positioning. The head and neck should be kept in a neutral position to prevent flow impediment through the internal jugular veins. In the recent past it was generally thought that raising the head 30 to 45 degrees (reversed Trendelenburg position) would also facilitate venous drainage and thus lower ICP. However, it has been shown that this position can lead to autoregulatory cerebral vasodilation, with ensuing increased cerebral blood volume (CBV) and ICP. Therefore, we keep the patients generally in a neutral flat position; if ICP tends to rise, we try different positions until the best one is found for the particular patient.

Ventilatory Support. For ICP control it is often

necessary to heavily sedate and/or paralyze the patient, mandating artificial ventilation. Moreover, a large proportion of patients hyperventilate spontaneously, while it is preferable to keep their $PaCO_2$ just below normal at 35 mm Hg. Although hyperventilation to 25 mm Hg has been advocated to prevent ICP problems, we have found that this is effective for only 24 hours and after that period may become counterproductive. Thus, normally the patient is ventilated to a $PaCO_2$ of 35 mm Hg, and only in cases in which ICP rises above 25 mm Hg is the $PaCO_2$ brought down to whatever level is necessary; first, by increasing the frequency and second, by increasing the tidal volume of the ventilator.

Of course, good oxygenation is beneficial both for the patient in general and for ICP control. PaO_2 should be kept above 80 mm Hg and saturation above 95 per cent. Initially, 30 per cent O_2 in the inspiratory air mixture is usually sufficient for this goal. Later, however, pulmonary problems often develop, necessitating higher percentages of O_2. To prevent atelectasis, all patients are ventilated with positive end-expiratory pressure (PEEP) of 5 cm H_2O. We have not found this to increase ICP. In patients with poor oxygenation, more PEEP may be needed (up to 25 cm H_2O), and in these cases it is often necessary to find a balance between effects on oxygenation and on ICP.

Sedation. Morphine is used for sedation. Chlorpromazine (Thorazine), 10 mg given as a slow intravenous injection, is often effective for ICP control. The effect on ICP of completely paralyzing the patient with 5 to 10 mg pancuronium bromide (Pavulon) is often dramatic.

Hyperosmolar Agents. Various hyperosmolar agents have been used throughout the years, the prototype being a 20 per cent urea solution. Presently, mannitol 20 per cent and glycerol 10 per cent are used most often. In patients on kidney dialysis, a 30 per cent sorbitol solution can be used, as this is entirely metabolized by the liver and not excreted through the kidneys as are the other hyperosmolar agents. Three different mechanisms are now recognized in explaining their effects. First, because these agents do not cross the blood-brain barrier, an osmotic gradient is created between blood or brain tissue, resulting in withdrawal of water from the brain. Second, these agents decrease blood viscosity, which leads to autoregulatory vasoconstriction while at the same time maintaining cerebral blood flow (in contrast to hyperventilation). In 60 per cent of patients with severe head injuries, autoregulation in the brain is intact. Third, these agents often increase blood pressure slightly, also leading to vasoconstriction, as many pressure waves are set off by vasodilation in response to the gradual decrease of the blood pressure.

Mannitol is used in a dose of 0.25 to 1.0 gram per kg, which translates into doses of 100 to 400 ml for average-size patients. It can be used up to once every 2 hours. However, significant hyperosmolar electrolyte imbalances may develop, threatening cardiovascular and renal functions. Serum osmolality above 325 is not acceptable and limits the use of mannitol. Frequent electrolyte and osmolality determinations are mandatory. Fluid losses should be supplemented, and the patient should not be allowed to be "dried out." When osmolality is too high, 20 mg bolus doses of furosemide (Lasix) can be tried. Its mode of action is not really known and, of course, the same considerations apply about electrolytes and fluid balance as in the use of hyperosmolar agents.

Barbiturates. High-dose intravenous barbiturate therapy is often effective in decreasing high ICP. Most neurosurgeons use pentobarbital. Loading dose is 5 to 10 mg per kg, as 100-mg bolus injections every 5 to 10 minutes until an effect on ICP is obtained or until blood pressure falls. In the latter case, blood pressure may be supported with phenylephrine (Neo-Synephrine), 80 mg in 500 ml of normal saline, the actual infusion rate varying widely. Serum levels around 4 mg per dl (4 mg per cent) are maintained, often requiring 1 to 2 mg per kg of pentobarbital every 1 to 2 hours.

Whether ICP control with barbiturates improves outcome remains unproven. It is a very complicated therapy, requiring Swan-Ganz catheters for monitoring of cardiac output and pulmonary wedge pressure. Fluid volume status must be optimal. In a randomized trial, barbiturate administration to *prevent* ICP problems has been proved ineffective in improving outcome.

Steroids. There is no proof that steroids either improve outcome of severe head injuries or are effective in controlling acute rises in ICP. We never use them.

Nursing. The most common secondary complications in comatose head-injured patients are pulmonary problems (atelectasis, pneumonia, infiltrates) and infection. Pulmonary care should consist of frequent suctioning, chest percussion, and postural drainage. In this respect, we have found the Rotorest kinetic beds to be a helpful adjunct.

We are not in favor of preventive administration of antibiotics. However, frequent temperature measurements and daily white blood cell counts and culturing of urine, sputum, and CSF (in case of a ventricular drain) should be performed in order to begin treatment as early as possible with the appropriate antibiotics in case of infection. It has been shown that early nutritional support by total parenteral nutrition (TPN) rather than by enteral feeding helps to prevent infections as well as improves overall outcome. Therefore, TPN should be instituted by 48 hours post-injury with amino acid/dextrose solutions, multivitamins, trace elements, and lipid emulsions.

Last but not least, close nursing observation of the patient is of paramount importance. The detection of early neurologic changes such as pupillary size or reactions and changes in coma scale parameters and ICP levels may allow treatment intervention in time to avoid the permanent detrimental effect of these events.

ACUTE HEAD INJURIES IN CHILDREN

method of
J. PARKER MICKLE, M.D.
University of Florida
Gainesville, Florida

Head injury is a common occurrence in our pediatric population, and of the five million or so that occur in this country annually, most are minor. However, 10 to 15 per cent of this number are serious and demand an aggressive, multidisciplinary approach for optimal outcome. The most common cause of death in children in this country is trauma. Most children who die of this disease category have associated head injuries, and this often is the primary cause of demise. Head injury in the pediatric patient is age dependent, ranging from the slow deformational forces experienced at birth and early in childhood, to the high-velocity impact with acceleration, deceleration injury experienced in the older child and the young adult.

TREATMENT

General Concepts and Pathophysiology

The first concept in the treatment of pediatric head injury is that the clinical outcome is a result

TABLE 1. **Secondary Insults After Head Injury**

Shock
Anoxia/hypoxia
Diffuse axonal injury
Intracranial hemorrhage
Increased intracranial pressure
Hydrocephalus
Seizures
Infections (CNS, urinary, pulmonary)
Metabolic (inappropriate ADH, nutritional)

of the initial traumatic event and certain secondary events occurring as complications of that primary event. As physicians, we have only a preventive control over the initial event. Certain injuries are not compatible with survival and no amount of intervention can retrieve a patient from the inevitable demise in this situation. However, most head injuries, especially in children, are compatible with survival and if the secondary processes listed in Table 1 are prevented and treated, then a good outcome can be expected in a very high percentage of these children. The concept here is to begin treatment as early as possible after the initiating event, and this necessitates trained personnel at the accident scene with treatment beginning prior to transport to the acute trauma hospital.

The second concept of importance in attending children with head injuries is that neurologic deterioration or improvement is a continuum, and no one single examination can make an accurate prediction of the need for therapeutic intervention or of outcome. This aspect requires frequent and sometimes virtually continuous neurologic assessment. This goal necessitates an accurate and rapid evaluation of the patient's neurologic status at any given time.

The Glasgow Coma Scale (GCS) is the most commonly used quantitative clinical assessment system in defining points along this neurologic continuum to guide the therapeutic decision making of the clinician; it can also provide highly accurate outcome determination. This system, without relying on detailed neurologic examination, gives an excellent idea of the level of neurologic function in the head-injured patient and also gives a good estimate of the prognosis. Using three variables—eye opening, best verbal response and best motor response—this point system can be used in patients of all ages.

It is extremely important, however, no matter which system is used, that frequent neurologic assessment be done in head-injured patients, since rapid changes can occur and a salvageable individual can rapidly deteriorate to a state with high morbidity and high mortality as expected outcome.

The third concept is that children have a better prognosis than the adult head-injured patient with the same degree of apparent injury at the time of initial evaluation. This fact demands an aggressive approach to the treatment in the head-injured child.

The fourth concept important in managing head injury in children involves the fact that the volume of the intracranial contents is fixed (except in very small children) and any mass occurring intracranially must be accommodated by the normal contents of the intracranial cavity; otherwise the intracranial pressure will increase. If the process is general and results in swelling or edema of the brain, then a general rise in intracranial pressure (ICP) will occur. If there is a focal swelling or accumulation of blood, ICP will rise, and various herniation syndromes can occur after the normal compensatory mechanisms have been exhausted. The aggressive multidisciplinary approach to the treatment of head injuries, both at the accident scene and in the emergency ward, is directed toward minimizing these effects as secondary insults on an already injured brain. All of our efforts initially are directed to protecting the injured and vulnerable brain from secondary insults that can change the outlook from excellent to terrible.

A fifth concept is more philosophical and involves prevention. Only recently, with the advent of data collection systems, is society becoming aware of the extent of this problem. We must do everything that we can as physicians and advocates of our patients to identify those activities in society that are highly dangerous and frequently result in serious head injury, such as child abuse.

Minor Versus Serious Head Injury

Most children will sustain a head injury during life. By and large, these are minor events and require no special care. However, especially in children, it is often difficult to decide when an injury should be classified as minor and when it should be classified as serious. Any injury of questionable etiology should be classified as serious, and in the case of the younger child such an occurrence dictates early report and intervention to prevent subsequent serious injury as a result of abuse or neglect. The incidence of child abuse as a cause of head injury is not known, but it appears to be much more frequent than was estimated in the past. Children with minor head injury and no loss of consciousness or significant blood loss, and with a good social situation, can be managed as outpatients. Most children with minor head injuries should have plain skull x-

TABLE 2. Radiologic Assessment of Minor Head Injury

Type	When
None	Minor head injury—good social situation
Skull x-rays	Deformity, point tenderness, scalp hematoma
Long-bone x-rays	Head injury of questionable etiology
CT scan of cranium	Persistent complaints

TABLE 3. Sequence of Events in the Care of the Seriously Head-Injured Child

Event	How
1. Evaluate	General physical examination Examination of central nervous system Radiology (CT scans)
2. Resuscitate	Secure airway, intubate Treat shock Stabilize
3. Triage	Continue resuscitation To operating room To intensive care unit

rays if there is deformity of the skull, significant scalp hematoma, or point tenderness of the skull or if the injury is of questionable etiology (see Table 2).

Minor head injury can have delayed sequelae detrimental to the patient. This necessitates careful evaluation on initial contact as well as adequate follow-up. Often the degree of injury cannot be adequately assessed by the history taken from the family or attending personnel, and only later will the patient continue to complain of headache, memory loss, and difficulty with concentration, all of which signal a more serious injury than initially diagnosed. Minor injuries usually have an excellent outlook, and the family and patient can be assured that most of the minor complaints following these injuries will subside.

Concussive injuries in children—that is, head injuries that cause unconsciousness for a variable period of time—without obvious neurologic deficit on initial evaluation are very important injuries. Clearly these injuries can cause permanent deficit and subsequent injuries are additive. These so-called minor injuries demand thorough radiologic evaluation and careful, regular follow-up. These children should be admitted to the hospital for observation, and family should be educated about possible problems on discharge. If complaints of headache, memory deficit, or inattention persist, computed tomography (CT) scan of the cranium, as well as thorough neuropsychological evaluation, should be made.

This group of patients is by far the most common group that we see as physicians and we are often asked to re-evaluate these individuals be-

TABLE 4. Indications for Emergency/Urgent Surgery of the Head-Injured Child

Condition	Comment
Refractory shock	Usually due to intra-abdominal injury and hemorrhage
Depressed skull fracture	Evaluate with CT scan
Significant intracranial hemorrhage	Rare under 2 years of age

cause of persistent complaints. Only recently has the magnitude of this problem been realized.

Serious head injuries in children range from scalp lacerations with major blood loss, often seen in the young child, to the devastating high-velocity diffuse injury to the brain more common in the older child. Important aspects in the early evaluation and treatment of the comatose child include physical examination, laboratory and x-ray evaluations, resuscitation, pharmacological treatment, monitoring, and triage.

Serious Head Injury

The team approach is essential in caring for the severely head-injured child (Table 3).

At the accident scene or in the emergency room, the child is treated for shock, the airway is secured, and further injury to the head or spine is prevented by adequate immobilization. Careful, frequent assessment of the general neurologic status of the patient is made and recorded. Intravenous access should be central and the fluids administered isotonic. An arterial line is helpful in monitoring the response to resuscitation. The blood pressure must be kept as normal as possible to optimize cerebral perfusion. All patients with serious head injury are assumed to have an unstable cervical spine until proven otherwise. The indications for emergency surgery on the head-injured child are listed in Table 4. This triage is made early and rapidly. The vast majority of patients with serious head injury can be stabilized before being transferred either to the radiology suite for CT scan of the head, chest and abdomen, or to the operating room for exploratory surgery. No patient should be sent to the radiology suite in an unstable condition without adequate monitoring by trained personnel.

Medications that we routinely give to comatose

TABLE 5. Medical Treatment of the Seriously Head-Injured Child

What	How
Dilantin	15 mg per kg loading dose; 5 mg per kg maintenance
Phenobarbital	Same as Dilantin
Valium	1–5 mg IV to stop seizure
Antibiotics	IV; broad-spectrum in contaminated wounds
Mannitol*	1 gram per kg for rapid decompression
Diuretics	1 mg per kg furosemide
Pentobarbital	15 mg per kg loading dose; titrate as needed to control ICP
Dexamethasone	10 mg IV push; 16 mg per day for 3–5 days

*Can push serum osmolarity as high as 310.

TABLE 6. Intensive Care Unit Monitoring of the Seriously Head-Injured Child

1. Monitor vital signs—serial CNS examination (Glasgow Coma Score)
2. Input/Output
3. Central venous pressure (CVP)
4. Arterial blood gases
5. Serum electrolytes
6. Hemogram
7. Intracranial pressure (ICP)
8. Multimodality somatosensory evoked potentials (SSEPs) and brain stem auditory potentials (BAEPs)
9. Serial computed tomography (CT) scans

children are listed in Table 5. Seizures if present, should be treated aggressively; broad-spectrum antibiotics are administered intravenously if grossly contaminated wounds are part of the picture. Mannitol as a dehydrating agent should not be given unless the patient is clearly herniating and needs temporary decompression on the way to the operating room. The loop diuretics and pentobarbitol are medications reserved for the treatment of increasing intracranial pressure of a general nature in the intensive care unit.

The most significant improvement in the care of severely head-injured children has been the development of specialized intensive care units with sophisticated monitoring capability. We utilize routinely the monitoring technologies listed in Table 6. The flow sheet available to the attending staff makes possible a continuous and instantaneous picture of the patient's status. This entire effort is directed toward discovering early and subtle changes in neurologic status, so that early intervention can prevent secondary injury to the brain.

A very important aspect of this monitoring is the accurate measurement of ICP. Various monitors can be used for this procedure and the information obtained is invaluable in making therapeutic decisions concerning the patient's status. We monitor all children with a GCS score of 7 or lower. The ICP must be maintained below 20 torr; this is accomplished utilizing the step-wise decision-making therapeutic regimen outlined in Table 7. Clearly, early detection of increased ICP and its successful treatment is one

TABLE 7. Stepwise Events in the Control of Increased Intracranial Pressure*

1. Hyperventilate to P_{CO_2} of 25 torr
2. Head elevated 30 degrees
3. Sedation/paralysis
4. Keep normothermic
5. Diuresis—loop diuretics vs. Mannitol
6. Cerebrospinal fluid drainage
7. Pentobarbital coma
8. Surgery—decompression

*Greater than 20 mm Hg.

of the most important aspects of the treatment of the seriously head-injured child.

Multimodality somatosensory evoked potentials (SSEPs) and brain stem auditory evoked potentials (BAEPs) are very helpful in detecting early deterioration in a seemingly stable child. Of major importance is the utilization of serial CT scans of the head when a child is experiencing deterioration before a therapeutic plan is decided upon. Delayed intracranial hemorrhage, increased ICP from hydrocephalus, and other causes of increased ICP can be detected and treated by this radiologic technique. ICP monitoring should be continued for as long as the child is in the comatose state and not improving. We usually leave a monitor in for a week before changing it to the opposite side or removing it. We have had no incidences of infection from these transcranially placed monitors in over 100 cases.

BRAIN TUMORS

method of
GRIFFITH R. HARSH IV, M.D., and
PHILIP H. GUTIN, M.D.
University of California
San Francisco, California

Brain tumors are neoplastic lesions that occupy intracranial space. About one half of brain tumors found at autopsy are primary lesions derived from neurons, glia, or their supporting meningo vascular structures, and the remainder are metastatic lesions. Primary brain tumors, which are classified according to the cell type from which they arise, and the most common sites of origin of metastatic tumors are listed in Table 1. The incidence of primary brain tumors in the United States is about 10 per 100,000 persons per year and is increasing; primary brain tumors account for almost 10 per cent of nontraumatic neurologic diseases among the general hospital population and for about 10 per cent of cancer-related deaths. The age-specific incidence of brain tumors has a small peak at 0 to 3 years of age, increases steadily after 30 years of age, and peaks at 70 years of age. Brain tumors are surpassed only by leukemia as a cancer-related cause of death in children, but most brain tumors occur in persons over 50 years of age.

The clinical course is determined by patient age and the histology and location of the tumor; these factors determine the rate of tumor growth, its clinical presentation, and its accessibility and responsiveness to various treatments. The clinical syndrome of brain tumors includes one or more of the following: headache, altered mental status, progressive neurologic deficit, and seizure. The first two usually result from increased intracranial pressure caused by the tumor mass itself and associated cerebral edema or by hemorrhage, blockage of cerebrospinal fluid outflow or absorption,

TABLE 1. **Brain Tumor Frequency**

Primary Brain Tumors	Relative Frequency of Occurrence	
	Adult	*Pediatric*
Glioma	0.60	0.80
Glioblastoma	0.25	0.10
Anaplastic astrocytoma	0.18	0.34
Astrocytoma	0.05	0.10
Oligodendroglioma	0.04	0.01
Ependymoma	0.04	0.05
Medulloblastoma	0.04	0.20
Meningioma	0.18	
Nerve sheath tumors	0.06	
Pituitary adenoma	0.06	
Craniopharyngioma	0.03	0.10
Germinoma	0.01	0.03
Dermoid	0.01	0.02
Others	0.05	0.05

Metastatic Brain Tumors	Relative Frequency of Origin
Lung	0.35
Breast	0.18
Melanoma	0.15
Unknown	0.12
Kidney	0.08
Colon	0.04
Others	0.08

or compromise of venous drainage. The progressive neurologic deficit and seizures result from disruption of focal brain function by local effects of tumor or by mass-induced shifts of brain tissue. Acute neurologic deterioration most often reflects a rapid increase of intracranial pressure secondary to hemorrhage, obstruction of the cerebral ventricles, or seizure and takes the form of lateral or central herniation syndromes. The differential diagnosis of tumor varies with the presentation; although usually idiopathic in children, seizures generally signify a brain tumor in adults. Intracranial abscess, hematoma, and congenital hydrocephalus may produce acute changes that mimic those of brain tumors. Degenerative diseases, the chronic meningoencephalitides, and toxic states may produce chronic changes that resemble those of brain tumors. In most instances, computerized tomography (CT) scans or magnetic resonance imaging (MRI) can be used to differentiate between these conditions and brain tumors.

Treatment

Approaches to the treatment of brain tumors include maintenance medical therapy, surgery, radiation therapy, chemotherapy, and immunotherapy. Preoperative treatment is designed to prevent acute deterioration. Patients with supratentorial tumors are routinely treated prophylactically with anticonvulsants, but this treatment is withheld from patients with posterior fossa tumors unless seizures occur. If the patient has no seizures for 6 to 12 months after complete excision of a tumor, anticonvulsants are discontinued gradually; in the face of recurrent tumor and/or seizures, treatment with anticonvulsants is continued. For seizures that are refractory to treatment, doses of a single drug sufficient to produce a therapeutic level should be given before a second drug is added (Table 2). If there are clinical or radiographic signs of significant mass effect, corticosteroids are given to decrease peritumoral edema. The effects of a standard daily dose are apparent within 24 to 48 hours of beginning therapy. Dose-related symptomatic improvement with minimal side effects has been observed for doses up to 4 times the standard daily dose (see Table 2). If neurologic deterioration continues and, especially if herniation seems imminent, diuretics are employed to decrease the water content of uninvolved brain. The osmotic diuretic mannitol is the drug of choice; its effects may be supplemented with loop diuretics. Intensive diuretic therapy should be accompanied by intracranial pressure monitoring. When it is first administered, the standard dose of mannitol raises serum osmolarity by about 20 milliosmoles per liter and lowers intracranial pressure to approximately half its original value for a maximum of 3 to 4 hours (see Table 2). In the face of imminent herniation, the patient should be intubated and hyperventilated to lower arterial $Paco_2$ to 24 to 26 mm Hg.

Surgery

Surgery is indicated unless severe irreversible neurologic deficit has been sustained. Surgery is performed to obtain material for an histologic diagnosis that can be used to choose adjuvant therapy, to provide a basis for prognosis, and to effect cure by total removal of tumor. If the tumor cannot be resected totally because it is infiltrative or because of its proximity to critical parenchymal or neurovascular structures, as much of the tumor as possible should be removed without causing a significant neurologic deficit. Material for histologic diagnosis can be obtained by stereotaxically directed needle biopsy or by direct excision at open craniotomy. With the exception of predominantly cystic tumors or inaccessible, deep

TABLE 2. **Medical Therapy**

Medication	Adult Dose, Route	Therapeutic Target
Phenytoin (Dilantin)	100 mg IV/PO q 8 hr	10–20 µg/ml
Phenobarbital	30 mg IV/PO qid	20–40 µg/ml
Dexamethasone	4 mg IV/PO q 6 hr	Clinical improvement
Methylprednisolone (Medrol)	20 mg IV/PO q 6 hr	Clinical improvement
Mannitol	0.25 mg/kg IV q 4 hr	310–320 mosm/liter
Furosemide (Lasix)	20 mg IV q 6 hr	310–320 mosm/liter

lesions, open craniotomy or craniectomy is necessary to remove substantial amounts of tumor. Extensive tumor resection may halt or reverse progressive focal neurologic deficit, may prevent acute mass-induced neurologic deterioration, and may enhance the efficacy of adjuvant therapy.

Radiation Therapy

Radiation therapy unequivocally prolongs the survival of patients with most types of malignant primary and secondary tumors in a dose-dependent manner. Usually 50 to 60 Gy from a cobalt-60 source are administered by conventional teletherapy in daily fractions of 180 to 200 cGy over 5 to 6 weeks, beginning 2 to 4 weeks after surgery. These small fractionated doses are chosen to minimize the risk of early, delayed, and late complications of radiation caused by edema, demyelination, and necrosis, respectively. The targeted fields for most types of primary tumors include the tumor bed and a 1- to 3-cm margin. For diffusely infiltrative or secondary malignancies, the whole brain is irradiated; for primary tumors that tend to spread through the cerebrospinal fluid pathways, the entire craniospinal axis is irradiated. Interstitial irradiation (brachytherapy) of tumors with radioisotopes stereotaxically implanted directly into the tumor, heavy particle bombardment by Bragg peak-dependent delivery, radiosurgery using the gamma knife, and dye-concentrated laser phototherapy are being studied in experimental and clinical settings in attempts to deliver higher doses of radiation to tumor with relatively lower risk to normal brain.

Chemotherapy

Agents used for the chemotherapy of brain tumors include prophylactic anticonvulsants and antiedema agents, radiosensitizers, and antineoplastic agents. BCNU (carmustin) is the single most active agent against most primary malignant brain tumors. Chemotherapy rarely cures brain tumors, but progressively longer intervals of palliation are being achieved. Many current chemotherapeutic trials employ combinations of drugs chosen for their different modes of action, cell cycle specificity, and primary toxicities. Experimental techniques of drug delivery designed to improve the efficacy of chemotherapy include intra-arterial injection of drugs, intratumoral implantation of drugs, and osmotic disruption of the blood-brain barrier.

Immunotherapy

Immunotherapeutic approaches using enhancing agents, passive immunity, adoptive immunity, and even intratumoral implantation of lymphocytes treated extracorporeally with various biological response modifiers have theoretical appeal. Immunotherapy is currently limited to experimental studies.

Summary of General Concepts

Aggressive preoperative medical treatment and microsurgical techniques offer the likelihood of cure to most patients with benign brain tumors and the possibility of clinical palliation and increased survival to those with malignant tumors. Rigorous testing of multimodality approaches to treatment including tumor-focused irradiation, combination chemotherapy, immunotherapy, and reoperation is essential to improve the outcome of the latter group of patients. Referral of such patients to centers undertaking these studies is essential to further progress.

Treatment for Specific Tumor Types

Malignant Gliomas. Glioblastomas and the anaplastic forms of astrocytoma, ependymoma, and oligodendroglioma are treated with surgery, irradiation, and chemotherapy. Extensive resection improves survival and radiation therapy is of definite benefit. Currently, the best chemotherapy consisting of hydroxyurea as a radiation sensitizer and BCNU or CCNU (lomustine) combined with procarbazine, vincristine, fluorouracil, or other agents, produces a median postoperative survival of about 1 year in patients with glioblastomas and 2 to 3 years in patients with anaplastic gliomas.

Low-grade Gliomas. When apparently total surgical removal of non-anaplastic gliomas is achieved, the cure rate exceeds 80 per cent. Residual tumor should be irradiated but chemotherapy should be withheld unless there is a malignant recurrence. Patients with recurrent tumors have a median survival from initial presentation of 5 to 10 years.

Medulloblastomas. Medulloblastomas are malignant tumors that occur with greatest frequency in children. Extensive resection of undisseminated tumors lengthens survival. Regardless of the extent of surgical resection, all patients should receive craniospinal irradiation and multiple-agent chemotherapy with agents such as procarbazine, CCNU, and vincristine. Outcome varies with the age of the patient, the stage of the tumor, and the treatment used; overall, the 5-year survival rate exceeds 50 per cent.

Meningiomas. Most meningiomas are benign tumors of adults. They are treated primarily by surgical resection. Apparently total removal is followed by recurrence in fewer than 10 per cent of cases, and subtotal removal is followed by symptomatic regrowth in about 40 per cent of

cases. Radiation therapy is reserved for tumors that cannot be resected completely because of involvement of the tumor with critical neurovascular structures, for those with malignant histology, and for recurrent tumors that could not be resected completely. The rate of cure is about 80 per cent and varies with location and histology.

Nerve Sheath Tumors. Over 90 per cent of intracranial nerve sheath tumors are acoustic schwannomas. They are benign tumors that are often totally resectable by a posterior fossa, transmeatal, translabyrinthine, or middle fossa approach. The probability of preservation of hearing and facial movement is inversely proportional to tumor size and depends critically on the extent that the tumor adheres to the acoustic portion of the eighth and seventh nerves; overall, hearing is preserved in fewer than 25 per cent and facial movement in more than 75 per cent of cases. Radiation therapy is usually reserved for recurrent tumors that cannot be resected completely at a second operation.

Pituitary Adenomas. Pituitary adenomas become clinically apparent from abnormal endocrine activity (Cushing's disease, Nelson's syndrome, hyperprolactinemic amenorrhea, or hypopituitarism) or mass enlargement (chronic visual loss or apoplexy). Although pharmaceutical hormonal manipulation such as the use of bromocriptine (Parlodel) for prolactinomas is palliative in some cases, surgery combined with irradiation of residual tumor offers the best chance of cure. Transsphenoidal microsurgical adenectomy has a lower morbidity and mortality (combined 1 per cent) than craniotomy and achieves a more rapid and complete reduction of tumor mass with less risk to vision and normal hypophyseal function than does irradiation. The cure rate varies with tumor type, size, and invasiveness and with hormone level. In general, 80 to 90 per cent of microadenomas can be cured by transsphenoidal microsurgery alone; about 50 per cent of macroadenomas (greater than 1 cm in diameter) are cured by surgery with or without irradiation.

Craniopharyngiomas. Craniopharyngiomas, although histologically benign, may produce devastating endocrine, visual, and intellectual impairment. Fortunately, more than half of the craniopharyngiomas in children can be completely removed by microsurgery. The remainder of pediatric tumors and most tumors that occur in adults should be subtotally resected; any cystic component should be drained, and the residual mass should be irradiated focally. Cyst recurrence can be treated by repeated percutaneous aspiration or intracavitary instillation of radioisotopes. Clinical stability of at least 10 years can be obtained in 80 to 90 per cent of cases.

Pineal Region Tumors. A great variety of tumors occurs near the posterior third ventricle; these include germinomas, dermoids, epidermoids, teratomas, malignant germ cell tumors, pineocytomas, pineoblastomas, astrocytomas, ependymomas, meningiomas, sarcomas, and metastases. If an unequivocal cytologic diagnosis cannot be made from cells disseminated in the cerebrospinal fluid, a biopsy is required before treatment is initiated. Open surgery by either a supratentorial or an infratentorial supracerebellar approach is preferred to stereotaxic biopsy because benign tumors may be totally resected and malignant lesions may be subtotally resected during the procedure. All malignant tumors are irradiated postoperatively, and some are treated with chemotherapy.

Metastases. Resection of solitary lesions may ameliorate neurologic dysfunction and increase survival. Response to radiation varies with tumor type; compared with radiation therapy for primary lesions, radiation is usually given at lower total doses (20 to 40 Gy) in larger fractions over 2 weeks. Chemotherapy is given for germ cell tumors, small cell lung and breast carcinomas, lymphomas, and malignant melanomas. Patients with extensive systemic disease generally live for fewer than 6 months; those with disease limited to brain metastases have a median survival of 1 to 2 years.

The Locomotor System

RHEUMATOID ARTHRITIS

method of
MARC D. COHEN, M.D.
Mayo Clinic Jacksonville
Jacksonville, Florida

Rheumatoid arthritis (RA) is a chronic, systemic disease of unknown etiology characterized by inflammation, most commonly involving the synovium of peripheral joints. The course of RA is quite variable, and the treatment must be commensurate with the aggressiveness of the disease. No curative treatment is available, but almost all patients benefit from a combined therapeutic program involving medical, rehabilitative, and sometimes surgical expertise. Patient education, the suppression of inflammation in articular and extra-articular sites, the preservation of joint function, and prevention of deformities are important features of any RA treatment plan.

Diagnosis

In its earliest phases RA may be a difficult diagnosis. Fatigue, malaise, and nonspecific musculoskeletal symptoms may be presenting features. Synovitis most often develops gradually, although an acute onset with a more explosive course can be seen. The symmetric involvement of peripheral joints with a chronic disease pattern characterized by exacerbations and remissions is most typical. The American Rheumatism Association has defined criteria for the diagnosis of RA (Table 1). The presence of at least four of these criteria allows the diagnosis of classic RA, if criteria one through four have been present for at least 6 weeks. While these criteria are potentially helpful in establishing a diagnosis, failure to meet all of these, particularly during early phases of the disease, does not exclude the diagnosis.

Management

Once the diagnosis is established, patient and family education is critical. Frank discussions between the physician and the patient are important to provide emotional support, specific points of information, and even sexual and vocational counseling. The patient should be informed of the benefits and risks of drug therapy, the importance of good nutrition and sufficient rest, and the availability of community services. Many pa-tients need continual help in coping with their disease.

Physical and Occupational Therapy

Several physical therapies can be beneficial in the treatment of RA. Systemic and specific articular forms of rest are important and must be individualized. Splinting may be very helpful in resting individual joints and preventing deformities. Sufficient exercise to maintain joint mobility and periarticular muscle strength without causing pain or fatigue must be defined and then encouraged. A combined approach including the services of a physical therapist, occupational therapist, and even a psychosocial professional is often helpful in defining regular active exercises, principles of joint protection, maintenance of muscle strength, and avoidance of activities detrimental to the patient.

Medical Therapy

Medical management must be individualized. Certain medications are helpful in controlling the signs and symptoms of the disease without dramatic effect on underlying disease progression. Other medications are potentially more disease modifying, and in certain patients may be frankly remittive. Nonsteroidal anti-inflammatory drugs including aspirin are helpful in most patients to some degree, although these do not usually induce remission.

Aspirin

Salicylates remain a popular drug for the initial treatment of RA because of their low cost and analgesic and anti-inflammatory properties. Acetylsalicylic acid (aspirin) has anti-inflammatory effects in doses ranging from 3 to 6 grams daily and has analgesic properties at lower doses. For anti-inflammatory effects, blood levels of between 15 and 25 mg per dl are usually required, and constant serum drug levels should be achieved with dosage intervals between 4 and 6 hours. The doses and schedule necessary to achieve therapeutic levels can vary, and determining salicylate levels can be helpful in direct-

TABLE 1. **The 1987 Revised Criteria for the Classification of Rheumatoid Arthritis***

Criterion	Definition
1. Morning stiffness	Morning stiffness in and around the joints, lasting at least 1 hour before maximal improvement
2. Arthritis of 3 or more joint areas	At least 3 joint areas simultaneously have had soft tissue swelling or fluid (not bony overgrowth alone) observed by a physician. The 14 possible areas are right or left PIP, MCP, wrist, elbow, knee, ankle, and MTP joints
3. Arthritis of hand joints	At least 1 area swollen (as defined above) in a wrist, MCP, or PIP joint
4. Symmetric arthritis	Simultaneous involvement of the same joint areas (as defined in 2) on both sides of the body (bilateral involvement of PIPs, MCPs, or MTP is acceptable without absolute symmetry)
5. Rheumatoid nodules	Subcutaneous nodules, over bony prominences, or extensor surfaces, or in juxtaarticular regions, observed by a physician
6. Serum rheumatoid factor	Demonstration of abnormal amounts of serum rheumatoid factor by any method for which the result has been positive in <5% of normal control subjects
7. Radiographic changes	Radiographic changes typical of rheumatoid arthritis on posteroanterior hand and wrist radiographs, which must include erosions or unequivocal bony decalcification localized in or most marked adjacent to the involved joints (osteoarthritis changes alone do not qualify)

*For classification purposes, a patient shall be said to have rheumatoid arthritis if he/she has satisfied at least 4 of these 7 criteria. Criteria 1 through 4 must have been present for at least 6 weeks. Patients with two clinical diagnoses are not excluded. Designation as classic, definite, or probable rheumatoid arthritis is *not* to be made. PIPs = proximal interphalangeal joints; MCPs = metacarpophalangeal joints; MTPs = metatarsophalangeal joints.

From Arnett FC et al. Reprinted from Arthritis and Rheumatism *31*:315, 1988. Used by permission of the American Rheumatism Association.

ing schedules and monitoring compliance. Because of first-order kinetics, a small increase in dose may cause a large increase in the serum salicylate level. Doses must be changed slowly and their effect monitored.

Plain aspirin is inexpensive and should be used with food or an antacid to provide some gastric protection. Buffered tablets that attempt to reduce gastric irritation are also available. Enteric-coated tablets (Ecotrin, Encaprin, ASA Enseals, Easprin) may be better tolerated, but serum salicylate levels should be monitored because of variable absorption. Timed-release or pH-dependent (Zorprin) tablets also delay gastrointestinal absorption but require close monitoring. Sodium salicylate (Pabalate), choline salicylate (Trilisate), and salsalate (Disalcid) are considered to cause less gastrointestinal bleeding and less platelet function inhibition but may be slightly less effective than acetylsalicylic acid.

Gastrointestinal symptoms are common side effects. Dyspepsia, occult bleeding, and peptic ulceration may occur, and routine monitoring of blood counts is appropriate. Tinnitus and deafness can be early indications of salicylate toxicities in adults. Central nervous system (CNS) symptoms such as headache, vertigo, and irritability also tend to occur with high serum levels, particularly in the elderly. High serum levels of salicylates, especially in juveniles, may also cause mild and reversible elevations of serum transaminases and alkaline phosphatase levels. True aspirin allergy is uncommon and usually results in a hypersensitivity reaction. Platelet

adhesiveness and aggregation is inhibited by small amounts of aspirin and is irreversible for the life of the platelets (about 10 days). This effect is potentially important before and after surgical procedures.

Other Nonsteroidal Anti-inflammatory Agents

Other nonsteroidal anti-inflammatory drugs (NSAIDs), of which there are many, are generally felt to be as effective as salicylates in the treatment of RA. Responses to each individual drug tend to be idiosyncratic, so drug selection remains empiric. To evaluate a response, most NSAIDs should be given for 3 to 4 weeks at an adequate dosage. The list of commonly prescribed NSAIDs is summarized in Table 2.

Side effects from NSAIDs include dyspepsia and nausea, although these agents are often touted as having fewer gastrointestinal side effects and less ototoxicity than aspirin. Like aspirin, NSAIDs are prostaglandin inhibitors, and this may be responsible for some of the beneficial effects as well as some of their toxicities. Like aspirin, these medications should be administered with or after food to minimize local gastrointestinal irritation. Patients with pre-existing renal dysfunction, including those who concurrently use diuretics, have hypertension, or are taking other medications that may reduce renal blood flow may be at increased risk for NSAID-induced renal insufficiency. The development of the nephrotic syndrome or acute interstitial nephritis is less common. These agents may cause edema and salt retention; platelet

TABLE 2. **Nonsteroidal Anti-inflammatory Drugs (NSAIDs) for Rheumatoid Arthritis**

Drug	Tablet Size (mg)	Usual Daily Dosage	Dosage Range (mg/day)
Salicylates			
Acetylsalicylic acid (aspirin)	325	3600 mg (three 325-mg tabs q.i.d.)	2400–4800
Aspirin with Maalox (Ascriptin)	325		
Buffered aspirin	325, 500		
Enteric-coated aspirin:			
Ecotrin	325		
ASA Enseals	325, 650		
Encaprin	325, 500		
Easprin	975		
Choline salicylate (Arthrospan liquid)	1 tspn = 650		
Choline trisalicylate (Trilisate)	500, 750		
Magnesium salicylate (Magan)	500		
Salsalate (Disalcid)	500, 750		
Sodium salicylate (Pabalate)	300		
Timed-release Bayer aspirin	650		
Zero-order-release aspirin (Zorprin)	800		
Nonsalicylates			
Diflunisal (Dolobid)	250, 500	500 mg b.i.d.	500–1000
Fenoprofen (Nalfon)	200, 300, 600	600 mg q.i.d.	1200–2400
Ibuprofen (Motrin, Rufen, Advil, Nuprin)	200, 400, 600, 800	600 mg q.i.d.	1600–3200
Indomethacin (Indocin) 75SR:	25, 50	25 mg q.i.d.	100–200
Suppository	50		
Oral suspension	25		
Ketoprofen (Orudis)	50, 75	75 mg t.i.d.	150–300
Meclofenamate (Meclomen)	50, 100	100 mg q.i.d.	200–400
Mefenamid acid (Ponstel)	250	250 mg q.i.d.	1000
Naproxen (Naprosyn)	250, 375, 500	375 mg b.i.d.	500–1000
Phenylbutazone (Butazolidin)	100	100 mg t.i.d.	300–600
Piroxicam (Feldene)	10, 20	20 mg per day	20
Sulindac (Clinoril)	150, 200	200 mg b.i.d.	300–400
Tolmetin (Tolectin)	200, 400	400 mg t.i.d.	600–1800

dysfunction and elevations of liver transaminases can also occur, but these are reversible.

Many NSAIDs have unique properties and toxicities. Indomethacin (Indocin) can cause CNS reactions including headaches and dizziness; phenylbutazone (Butazolidin) has been reported to cause aplastic anemia and generally is not popular for chronic use; meclofenamate sodium (Meclomen) may produce diarrhea; piroxicam (Feldene) has a long plasma half-life; and sulindac (Clinoril) has been reported to cause less nephrotoxicity.

NSAIDs differ in their potency, toxicities, and plasma half-lives. These drugs are generally more expensive than aspirin and are rarely used in combination. There are no clearly definable differences in efficacy. Cost, compliance, and tolerability should be considered for each individual patient. NSAIDs are not recommended during pregnancy or nursing.

Disease-Modifying Drugs

Disease-modifying drugs are available for patients with RA, but they are generally best reserved for patients who have relentless synovitis and definite bony erosions despite therapy with a conservative regimen. These medications are generally slow-acting, requiring weeks to months to achieve maximum benefit. Since these drugs seem to have little local anti-inflammatory or analgesic effects, NSAIDs and aspirin are usually continued during their administration. Regular evaluation of response is imperative, and improvement is demonstrated by reduction of morning stiffness and palpable synovitis and improvement in hematologic evidence of disease activity.

These drugs are all associated with considerable potential toxicity, and careful monitoring of each patient is mandatory. The potential benefits and toxicities are important in determining which to choose initially. Fortunately, lack of response or development of toxicity to one drug does not preclude a beneficial response from another. No clinical or laboratory feature of RA predicts the responsiveness to any of these agents.

Gold. Gold salts are effective in RA and may limit the progression of bony erosions. Approximately two thirds of patients with RA show some therapeutic benefit; however, many patients cannot tolerate gold salts because of the potential toxicities. Parenteral gold salts (Solganal, Myochrysine) require intramuscular injection. Test doses of approximately 10 mg are generally recommended, and if the initial dose is tolerated, 50 mg is usually administered weekly. Any response to this therapy is usually not seen until there is a significant cumulative dose, usually greater than 500 mg and often as much as 1000 mg. If a significant response occurs, the frequency of the 50-mg injections can be reduced slowly. If a relapse occurs, the preceding shorter dosage interval can be retried, although reinitiation of the drug is not always successful. Those patients who respond without adverse effects are often maintained for prolonged periods of time, often indefinitely, on monthly gold injections. If no improvement occurs after a cumulative dosage of more than 1000 mg, the drug is generally discontinued. Oral gold (Ridaura) is also available and may be as effective as parenteral gold. The initial dose is usually 3 mg twice daily. For all gold preparations, serum gold levels do not correlate with drug efficacy.

Gold toxicity occurs often, with some adverse reactions reported in between one third and one half of all those who receive the drug. Discontinuation of the medication because of side effects, however, is much less common. Toxicity occurs most often after 300 mg of the drug has been administered but can be seen at any time during therapy.

Dermatitis is the most common side effect of gold salts. The rash is highly variable but is often associated with pruritus and is reversible with discontinuation of the drug. Dermatitis may be associated with eosinophilia. Stomatitis may also occur and may be painless. These mucocutaneous side effects require withholding gold salts until the lesions clear. Occasionally therapy may then be carefully reinstituted at a lower dose.

Renal toxicity is usually manifested by proteinuria. Nephritis and frank nephrosis are fortunately much less common. If the proteinuria is mild, less than 500 to 1000 mg per 24 hours, gold may be cautiously continued. Proteinuria greater than 1 gram to 1.5 grams per 24 hours mandates cessation of the medication. Even frank nephrosis is usually slowly reversible. Urinalyses must be obtained before each gold injection. Nephropathy is less common in patients treated with oral gold.

Hematologic disorders, including thrombocytopenia, agranulocytosis, and aplastic anemia, are the most potentially serious side effects of gold therapy; fortunately, these are rare. These side effects are not dose related. These potential abnormalities require a complete blood count before each gold injection. Management of severe hematologic toxicity from gold may require the use of corticosteroids and chelating agents, although the efficacy of these therapies has not been clearly established.

Nitritoid reactions of flushing, dizziness, shortness of breath, and even syncope have been reported with the administration of gold salts, particularly gold thiomalate (Myochrysine). Oral gold more commonly causes gastrointestinal side effects, including diarrhea, abdominal pain, and nausea. Gold salts may cause a variety of other adverse reactions, including colitis, pulmonary infiltrates, and cholestatic jaundice. Patients with a severe toxic reaction, such as exfoliative dermatitis, significant cytopenia, or severe nephropathy, should not receive more gold. Patients with less severe toxicity may be able to tolerate lower doses of the drug.

Penicillamine. Penicillamine (Cuprimine, Depen) has been shown to be effective in patients with RA, although perhaps slightly less so than gold. Again, because of potential toxicities, it is reserved for patients who have severe disease or who have not benefited from conservative therapy. Gold toxicity does not preclude use of penicillamine. Penicillamine is a slow-acting, oral drug and is generally begun in a low dosage of 125 to 250 mg daily. Increases in dosage should not be made more frequently than every 2 to 3 months. Toxicity seems to increase with higher doses, and 750 to 1000 mg is considered maximal therapy. Responders generally demonstrate improvement within 6 months of initiation of therapy. Patients who improve without serious toxicities can be maintained on this medication indefinitely.

Side effects from penicillamine are common. Dermatitis is the most common side effect. The rash is highly variable, may be seen soon after the initiation of therapy, often resolves with discontinuation of the drug, and may not recur if the drug is restarted. Rashes seen after months of therapy may be slower to resolve and generally prohibit readministration of the drug. Stomatitis also may occur. Changes in taste perception occur often during the initial weeks of penicillamine therapy but tend to disappear, even with continuation of the drug.

Proteinuria also may occur, and urinalyses should generally be done at monthly intervals. If proteinuria is discovered, then a 24-hour urine protein quantification should be performed. With protein excretion of less than 1 gram per 24 hours, the drug may often be continued. The dosage of penicillamine used should not be increased if there is proteinuria. If proteinuria exceeds 2 grams per 24 hours, the drug should be discontinued. Nephrosis is uncommon and is generally reversible. Renal toxicity may persist up to 1 year after discontinuation of the drug.

Hematologic toxicity is the most serious side effect, and complete blood counts must be obtained monthly. Hematologic toxicities include leukopenia, agranulocytosis, aplastic anemia, and, perhaps most commonly, thrombocytopenia. These reactions are usually reversible when the drug is discontinued.

Other toxicities include the development of other autoimmune syndromes, including myasthenia gravis, polymyositis, systemic lupus erythematosus, and Goodpasture's syndrome. These demand discontinuation of the drug. Uncommon adverse reactions include cholestatic jaundice, yellowing or wrinkling of the skin, and gastrointestinal intolerance. An allergy to penicillin does not preclude the use of penicillamine.

Hydroxychloroquine. Hydroxychloroquine (Plaquenil) is an antimalarial agent that is effective in some patients with RA. The drug is administered orally, generally at a dosage of 200 mg per day, although 200 mg twice daily has been used in patients with extremely aggressive disease. This drug is slow-acting, with months generally required to show improvement. Six months is generally an adequate trial of this medication. Toxicity is perhaps less common than for gold or penicillamine, although hydroxychloroquine can be deposited in the eye. Early retinal lesions may be visualized before symptoms, and every patient taking hydroxychloroquine must have an ophthalmologic examination at 6- to 9-month intervals, including visual field and color vision testing. The drug must be discontinued if there is any visual impairment or change in ophthalmologic testing. Other common side effects include gastrointestinal intolerance and skin rash. The drug should be avoided in patients with porphyria, glucose-6-phosphate dehydrogenase (G6PD) deficiency, or significant renal dysfunction. Complications include neuropathy, hematologic alterations, dizziness, and psychological changes.

Corticosteroids. Corticosteroids are potent antiinflammatory drugs; however, they do not alter the course of RA and have serious potential toxicities. Use of these agents even in small doses must be discussed with the patient, with the potential benefits versus toxicities understood. In RA, corticosteroid therapy should be used only after other treatments have been attempted. Low-dose corticosteroids (less than 7.5 mg of prednisone or equivalent) may be effective in treating sustained, debilitating synovitis involving many joints. Incapacitating systemic symptoms such as fever, weight loss, vasculitis, or serositis may require higher doses, which will produce more toxicity. Toxicities from corticosteroids are clearly dependent both on dosage and duration of therapy. Even low-dose corticosteroids have toxicities, including cutaneous changes, osteoporosis, gastrointestinal side effects, and fluid retention. Moderate doses may be associated with these side effects as well as accelerated cataract formation, insomnia, steroid psychosis, glucose intolerance, centripetal obesity, avascular necrosis of bone, increased risk of infection and aggravation of hypertension, muscle weakness, glaucoma, and hyperlipidemia. If these agents are used to treat synovitis, small dosages must be used, and frequent attempts to lower the dosage should be made. Potentially life-threatening complications such as rheumatoid vasculitis, particularly manifested by end organ ischemia, may justify the use of higher doses of corticosteroids.

Corticosteroids must be tapered very gradually after 6 weeks of chronic use. Patients taking corticosteroids regularly need larger doses parenterally before, during, and after surgery. One acceptable regimen is to administer 100 mg of hydrocortisone sodium succinate or cortisone acetate intramuscularly immediately before anesthesia, an additional dose intravenously during surgery, and again on the first postoperative day. As an oral drug, prednisone is considered the standard corticosteroid. Prednisone, 5 mg, is equivalent to 20 mg of hydrocortisone, 4 mg of methylprednisolone (Medrol), and 0.75 mg of dexamethasone (Decadron).

Intra-articular corticosteroids may be effective in relieving swelling, synovial fluid accumulation, and inflammation in a specific joint. Aseptic technique must be used; currently popular is injection with 0.5 to 2.0 ml of a long-acting crystalline suspension of a corticosteroid such as triamcinolone hexacetonide (Aristospan), betamethasone (Celestone Soluspan), or prednisolone tebutate (Hydeltra TBA Suspension). Relief of symptoms is quite variable, ranging from days to months. Frequent intra-articular injections, particularly more than 3 injections in any joint per year, should be avoided because of possible acceleration of cartilage damage. A post-injection synovitis has been reported, presumably as a result of leukocyte phagocytosis of steroid crystals; this usually subsides within 48 hours. Synovial fluid removed from affected joints should be analyzed, particularly for the possibility of infection. Obviously, joints suspected of infection should not be injected with corticosteroids.

Immunosuppressive Agents. Immunosuppressive drugs have been tried in patients with severe RA whose disease is refractory to more standard drug therapy. Patients must be informed of the many side effects associated with their use and the need for frequent evaluation. In general, these drugs should be reserved for patients who have failed therapy with other potentially remittive agents. Severe extra-articular manifestations such as rheumatoid vasculitis may require more immediate use of a cytotoxic agent. These drugs all have the potential for serious bone marrow suppression, and complete blood counts must be monitored. The lowest dose of these agents necessary to control the disease should be used.

AZATHIOPRINE. Azathioprine (Imuran), in doses approximating 1.5 mg per kg per day, has been used in RA with some effectiveness. Even in responders, it is a slow-acting drug, and often 3 months are required for demonstration of efficacy. Dosage may be increased, but with great care and for short periods of time. Side effects include bone marrow suppression and hepatic toxicity, and complete blood counts, liver function testing, and urinalyses should be performed weekly initially, and later every 2 to 4 weeks. The increased risk of malignancy, particularly of the hematopoietic system, is increased in patients receiving immunosuppressive drugs, including azathioprine. In general, if there is no response after 4 to 5 months on this medication, it should be discontinued. Even if the disease has been controlled for several months, some rheumatologists recommend tapering these agents and attempting to discontinue their use.

METHOTREXATE. Methotrexate* is another immunosuppressive drug found to be efficacious in RA. It is available as an oral or intramuscular medication. Initial dosage ranges from 7.5 to 15 mg per week. This medication works relatively quickly, and if no response has been observed after 12 weeks of therapy, the drug may be discontinued. If the patient does respond, the dosage should be tapered to the smallest effective maintenance dose. Methotrexate is administered on a weekly basis, usually in 2 or 3 divided doses separated by 8 hours. This schedule may reduce toxicity. Methotrexate has many side effects, including bone marrow suppression, hepatotoxicity,

*This use is not listed in the manufacturer's directive.

stomatitis, nausea and other gastrointestinal disorders, and pulmonary complications. Regular monitoring, including complete blood counts and kidney and liver function tests, is mandatory, usually at 2- to 4-week intervals. Increases in liver transaminases may require cessation of the drug, particularly when they are 3 to 4 times normal. Prolonged use of methotrexate has been associated with hepatic fibrosis, and the potential usefulness of liver biopsies in monitoring these patients remains controversial.

CYTOXAN. Cyclophosphamide (Cytoxan) is a cytotoxic agent that is reserved for the most relentless or severe cases of RA. It is an extremely potent medication with many toxicities. The initial dose is generally 1.5 to 2 mg per kg per day orally. In addition to bone marrow suppression, an increased risk of malignancy, and renal and hepatic toxicity, cyclophosphamide has several other severe side effects, including alopecia, sterility, hemorrhagic cystitis, and an increased incidence of bladder carcinoma. Although this medication is effective in controlling severe rheumatoid disease, it must be used with great care and very close monitoring. Lack of response after 12 weeks on this medication warrants discontinuation of the drug. Whether lower-dose cyclophosphamide is effective remains unproven. The efficacy of larger doses at less frequent intervals has also not been established.

Experimental Therapies

Several experimental therapies generally are available only at selected medical centers for those patients who are unresponsive to conventional therapies. These include plasmapheresis, total lymphoid irradiation, and the use of other immunosuppressive agents such as cyclosporine. To date, the efficacy of these modalities remains unproven. Other medications have generated some interest as being of potential benefit in RA. These include sulfasalazine, dapsone, and several other agents initially developed as therapies for alternative diseases. These agents should be used with great care, since clear evidence of their usefulness has not been established. Combinations of different drugs have yet to be completely studied. Controlled studies have not demonstrated any advantage in therapy for RA of diet or vitamin supplements beyond basic and balanced nutritional principles.

Pregnancy and Rheumatoid Arthritis

Pregnancy tends to ameliorate some of the inflammatory symptoms of RA. None of the NSAIDs are particularly recommended for use during pregnancy or lactation, Gold salts, penicillamine, hydroxychloroquine, and immunosuppressive agents must not be used during pregnancy. Even a simple drug such as aspirin, if taken until the time of delivery, may prolong gestation and labor and increase perinatal maternal bleeding.

Surgery

Surgical procedures can be important in the management of patients with RA who have severely affected or damaged joints. Replacement of virtually any affected joint is possible; however, hip and knee replacements are the most successful procedures. Orthopedic surgery of rheumatoid joints requires special expertise. For severe wrist and hand involvement, a combination of tendon repositioning and joint fusion may be necessary. Finger joint prostheses should be reserved for carefully selected patients. Synovectomy, particularly of wrists or knees, may be helpful when involvement is limited to a small number of joints and traditional therapies have been ineffective. This procedure might be best viewed as temporizing. Rupture of extensor tendons, particularly of the fingers, generally requires surgical repair. Carpal tunnel syndrome may require surgical release. C1-2 subluxation rarely requires surgical fixation.

Corrective surgical procedures should have specific goals, usually including pain relief, correction of deformity, and functional improvement; This last goal is the most difficult to achieve.

Diseases Associated with Rheumatoid Arthritis

Several disease associations are important to patients with RA. Sicca syndrome requires topical and local treatment. Felty's syndrome consists of RA, splenomegaly, and granulocytopenia; however, other hematologic abnormalities, recurrent infections, and leg ulcerations are common associations. In patients with RA the development of rheumatoid vasculitis is a bad prognostic sign. There is a significant mortality rate, particularly if tissue necrosis, neuropathy, and severe constitutional features develop. Extremely aggressive therapy is warranted and hospitalization is often required. The pulmonary manifestations of RA often require aggressive therapy also. These too may be life-threatening and require subspecialty expertise.

JUVENILE RHEUMATOID ARTHRITIS

method of
ROBERT W. WARREN, M.D., Ph.D.
Baylor College of Medicine
Houston, Texas

Juvenile rheumatoid arthritis (JRA) is a chronic disease of joints and other tissues that affects approximately 250,000 children in the United States. JRA is subdivided into three major subgroups, based upon the clinical course in the first 6 months of illness. These subgroups are (1) systemic, characterized by spiking fevers, evanescent rash, and other extraarticular disease; (2) pauciarticular, with four or fewer affected joints; and (3) polyarticular, with five or more affected joints. Only a small minority of JRA patients have an illness like adult rheumatoid arthritis (RA); unlike adults with RA, 70 to 90 per cent of children who are treated appropriately recover from JRA without significant disability. The mortality rate in the United States is less than 1 per cent.

JRA must be differentiated from other causes of arthritis. Indeed, more likely etiologies of childhood arthritis include trauma and infectious and postinfectious etiologies. Whereas these processes usually resolve over days to weeks, the arthritis of JRA persists in at least one joint for a minimum of 6 weeks. The formal diagnosis of JRA also requires age at onset under 16 years of age, and exclusion of other inflammatory joint diseases.

General Management

There is no specific cure for JRA. Anti-inflammatory medications improve joint swelling and pain, fever, iritis, and pericarditis, but no medication safely, totally, and instantly quells the inflammation of JRA. Continuing or recurrent inflammation produces secondary phenomena, including joint destruction, soft tissue contractures, and growth abnormalities, with accompanying psychological trauma.

Medical Follow-up

Excellent home and community-based care is critical for the child with JRA, but every child with active JRA should also be evaluated periodically by a health care team that specializes in the care of children with arthritis. The frequency of such visits depends on the diagnosis and the problems of specific patients but should be no less frequent than annually. A systemic JRA flare or acute increased joint symptoms in any JRA patient should command immediate medical attention.

Education and Counseling of Family and Patient

The family's understanding and commitment to the care of the child with JRA is the most critical element in management. Common family concerns are physical deformity and the possible dangers of physical therapy and aspirin. The physician's role in patient and family education should be supplemented by literature on diseases and medication, family support groups (such as those sponsored by the parent-run American Juvenile Arthritis Organization), and professional assistance by rheumatology nurses, social workers, and child psychologists.

Family anxieties and concerns are normal. On the other hand, the JRA-provoked psychosocial dysfunction in the patient and family may far outstrip and outlast active or even residual joint disease. The need for psychosocial intervention must be periodically assessed.

Drug Therapy

Nonsteroidal Anti-inflammatory Drugs (NSAIDs)

These agents are the mainstay of medical therapy for all forms of JRA. Responses to NSAID therapy generally occur in days to weeks. Despite the fact that no one NSAID has proved to be more efficacious than the others, there are differences in chemical structure and unpredictable differences in patient response; thus, changing to another NSAID is reasonable in therapeutic failures. On the other hand, the rare child with aspirin allergy should not be given any other NSAID. Although anecdotally successful, the simultaneous use of two NSAIDs has not been carefully studied in JRA, nor is the practice approved by the FDA, because of the risk of significant additive side effects.

Aspirin. Aspirin is the principal chemotherapeutic agent for all forms of JRA. Used for decades, aspirin is inexpensive and efficacious; no other NSAID is clearly superior. Compliance with aspirin therapy is much easier to measure than with other drugs, although likely more difficult to obtain because of the frequency of administration, and family worries about aspirin's efficacy and about Reye's syndrome. Aspirin is often begun in doses as low as 80 mg per kg per day to decrease the chance of toxicity, but 90 to 100 mg per kg per day (to a maximum dose of 4 grams per day) divided 3 or 4 times daily is usually required for a therapeutic serum salicylate level of 20 to 30 mg per dl. Illnesses affecting gastrointestinal absorption, low serum albumin levels, other medications, and aspirin coating can influence the obtained level. Levels should be obtained 7 to 10 days after the initiation or any change of therapy, including the institution or withdrawal of other drugs, or with the advent of any signs of salicylate toxicity (e.g., tinnitus, hyperpnea). Salicylates should be temporarily discontinued with increased risk for Reye's syndrome (e.g., following exposure to influenza or chickenpox).

A number of prescription salicylate-derivative drugs are now marketed, including choline magnesium trisalicylate (Trilisate), which is approved for use in children. Potential advantages include twice-daily dosing, a liquid form (500 mg per 5 ml), less gastrointestinal intolerance, and the lack of effect on platelet function. Disadvantages include higher cost and the lack of a chewable, small children's tablet. Dose ranges are identical to those for aspirin.

Potential adverse effects of aspirin therapy include gastrointestinal symptoms, such as vomiting, abdominal pain, gastritis, ulcer disease, and constipation. Although children seem less likely to develop these problems than adults, they are not exempt and should take NSAIDs with meals or snacks. Buffered aspirin products offer little additional protection. Antacids and certainly sucralfate (Carafate) are far more efficacious. Parents should report complaints of abdominal pain, vomiting, and hematochezia. A hemoglobin or hematocrit and red cell indices should be performed at least every 4 months to assess occult blood loss. Mild liver function abnormalities are common in children on NSAIDs (transaminases <100 IU); however, rarely children develop significant hepatitis or even liver failure on aspirin, which rapidly resolves with discontinuance of the drug. Liver function studies should be obtained 2 to 4 weeks after beginning or changing therapy, and thereafter, if values are normal, as indicated by careful physical examination. Liver function should be more closely monitored and NSAID therapy changed (e.g., dose decreased) if serum glutamate oxaloacetic transaminase (SGOT) and serum glutamate pyruvic transaminase (SGPT) values consistently exceed 100 IU. Aspirin therapy should be temporarily discontinued when values exceed 300 IU and then restarted at a lower dose after recovery.

Renal effects of aspirin and other NSAIDs include hematuria and decreased creatinine clearance. Urinalysis should be performed every 3 to 4 months, and BUN and serum creatinine every 6 months. Some nephrologists recommend that creatinine clearance be checked yearly. Finally, significant central nervous system effects (e.g., hallucinations) are rare adverse effects of aspirin and other NSAIDs that necessitate discontinuance of the drug.

Other NSAIDs. Only two NSAIDs are currently approved for use in children from 2 to 14 years of age: tolmetin (Tolectin) and naproxen (Naprosyn). Tolmetin is available in 200 mg tablets and 400 mg capsules and should be initiated at 20 mg per kg per day divided into 3 doses, and increased to 30 mg per kg per day (maximum 1.6 grams per day) if well tolerated. Tolmetin bioavailability is decreased by food and milk. Naproxen is available in 250-, 375-, and 500-mg tablets as well as a 125 mg per 5 ml suspension. Naproxen may be given on a twice-daily schedule, with doses of 10 to 15 mg per kg per day (maximum 1 gram per day).

Other NSAIDs can be used in the treatment of older children with JRA, including ibuprofen (Motrin), 35 to 40 mg per kg per day in 3 to 4 divided doses (maximum 2.4 grams per day), sulindac (Clinoril), 150 to 200 mg twice daily, piroxicam (Feldene), 20 mg daily, and indomethacin (Indocin), 1.5 to 3 mg per kg per day, in 2 to 4 divided doses depending on form (maximum 150 mg daily).

Each of these drugs may be useful in specific circumstances. Ibuprofen is relatively less expensive and is available without a prescription. Sulindac may have few renal side effects. Piroxicam's single daily dosing may improve compliance. Finally, indomethacin is likely to be most effective in treating HLA B27–positive pauciarticular JRA; nevertheless, the development of side effects, particularly those affecting the central nervous system, may limit its usefulness.

Slow-Acting Anti-rheumatic Agents

In some patients, NSAIDs alone do not control the polyarticular arthritis of systemic or polyarticular JRA, as judged by the clinical examination and evidence of progressive, erosive joint disease on x-ray. Therapy with slow-acting agents is then indicated, and NSAIDs are continued.

After years of use in JRA, gold remains the supplemental treatment of choice. Gold is available in injectable form as gold sodium thiomalate (Myochrysine) or gold thioglucose (Solganal) and in tablets as auranofin (Ridaura). Although the effectiveness of both forms of gold in JRA has been demonstrated, the use of oral gold in young children is currently not approved by the FDA. Intramuscular injections of gold are begun weekly, with a test dose of 0.25 mg per kg, followed by 0.5 mg per kg, and then 1.0 mg per kg per week thereafter (maximum 50 mg per dose). Since improvement can be slow, treatment is generally continued for 20 weeks. If a positive response is observed, treatment is continued at 1- to 3-week intervals until there is at least 6 months of disease inactivity. Unfortunately, adverse effects limit the use of gold. Significant, relatively common problems include bone marrow suppression, nephrotoxicity, severe rash, and mouth ulcers. Nitritoid reactions are rarely seen in children on thiomalate therapy.

Because the adverse effects are common, a brief history, review of systems, physical examination, and panel of laboratory studies must precede each injection. Laboratory studies should include a complete blood count and urinalysis. The injection should be held at least temporarily and consultation sought if there is significant hematuria, proteinuria, associated rashes and mucosal lesions, an absolute white blood count below 3000 per cu mm or a decrease of 5000, an absolute neutrophil count below 1500 per cu mm or a decrease of 50 per cent, or a platelet count less than 150,000 per cu mm.

Other slow-acting agents used in JRA include penicillamine* (Cuprimine, Depen) and hydroxychloroquine* (Plaquenil); however, neither drug was shown to be more efficacious than NSAIDs in a recent double-blind study done by the Pediatric Rheumatology Collaborative Study Group. Since penicillamine has many of the same side effects as gold, most practitioners are averse to treating a child who could not tolerate gold with the drug.

Hydroxychloroquine is administered in a single oral dose of 200 mg per square meter per day, and is generally well tolerated by children. Eye disease is the most serious potential side effect; thus, children taking hydroxychloroquine should be examined by an ophthalmologist before beginning therapy, and then at least every 6 months.

Corticosteroids

Systemic steroids are rarely used in the treatment of JRA. Intravenous steroids are indicated in the therapy of acutely decreased cardiac function (and other life-threatening complications) in systemic JRA. Methylprednisolone should be given intravenously, 0.25 to 0.5 mg per kg every 6 hours. In addition, systemic oral steroids are occasionally needed to control chronic symptoms in systemic JRA, such as severe anemia and rheumatoid lung disease. They may also be rarely necessary to control extremely active, severe, polyarticular arthritis unresponsive to other medications. In these circumstances, oral prednisone is given daily or preferably every other day, in as low a dose as possible for therapeutic effect. Systemic steroids have no place in the therapy of pauciarticular JRA, except for severe uveitis. Possible benefits of systemic steroids must always be balanced against the well-described major short- and long-term risks, and these should be discussed in detail with the family.

---

*Manufacturer's warnings: Efficacy of penicillamine and safe use of hydroxychloroquine in treatment of JRA have not been established.

Intra-articular steroid injections of triamcinolone hexacetonide (Aristospan) are sometimes used in the therapy of JRA. Although published data is sparse, intra-articular steroid injections have a role in pauciarticular JRA, as well as single and few joint flares of polyarticular disease. The recommended dosage is 5 to 40 mg of triamcinolone (depending upon the age of the child and on the particular joint), which can be mixed with preservative-free lidocaine; this should be injected no more than twice a year per joint. Activity of the joint should be limited for 2 to 3 days thereafter. Although most patients respond well, there are potential problems associated with intra-articular injections. These include minimal or brief overall response, postinjection arthritis flare, and the psychological trauma of intra-articular injection. Risks of bleeding, damage to joint cartilage, and infection should be minimal. Secondary poor bone growth and weakness of surrounding structures near the injected joint have not been confirmed.

Topical steroids are used in the eye for the treatment of uveitis (discussed below).

Experimental Agents

Immunosuppressive agents, such as methotrexate, cyclophosphamide (Cytoxan), azathioprine (Imuran), and chlorambucil (Leukeran), are not approved for the treatment of JRA, although methotrexate and azathioprine are used for severe adult RA. The first controlled trial using one of these agents, methotrexate, in children is currently concluding, but results are not available at this time. Other modalities, including high-dose pulse-dose steroids, sulfasalazine (Azulfidine), plasmapheresis, and immunoglobulin therapy, are also being studied. Use of any of these agents in JRA is strictly experimental.

Physical and Occupational Therapy

Physical and occupational therapy are essential elements in the treatment of JRA. The goals of therapy are to maintain and improve range of motion, strength, and function. Specific guidelines and components for physical therapy of JRA include the following:

1. A home/school/community-based exercise program should be planned and supervised by a licensed physical and/or occupational therapist. Normal activities that accomplish the desired joint motions should be strongly encouraged. Swimming and bicycle and tricycle riding are excellent activities for the child with JRA.

2. Splinting is used for many purposes in JRA, including pain reduction, joint protection, improving contracture and muscle strength, and increasing function. Night splinting is a highly successful and standard technique for reducing peripheral joint contractures, particularly at the wrist and knees. On the other hand, daytime use of immobilizing splints should at most be only a temporizing measure while other therapies are being instituted. Dynamic splints, which hold joint position and yet encourage specific joint motions against resistance to increase strength, are sometimes used in JRA patients. Shoe inserts and other orthotic devices such as metatarsal bars and pads, as well as comfortable, well-supported shoes, reduce pain. Cervical collars may protect the unstable cervical spine that is sometimes a complication of polyarticular and systemic JRA. Serial casting is a technique occasionally used to reduce joint contractures unresponsive to physical therapy and splinting.

3. Localized therapy, and sometimes mild pain relievers such as acetaminophen, can be extremely useful in decreasing joint stiffness and discomfort. Warm baths, local application of moist heat, and frequent changes of position can combat joint stiffness. "Icing" a joint can temporarily decrease discomfort, and is used as an adjunct in serial casting.

Prevention and Treatment of Eye Disease

JRA is a major cause of blindness in children. Chronic, occult iridocyclitis is most common in ANA-positive pauciarticular JRA, and less common in systemic and polyarticular JRA. Risk for eye disease does not correlate with the activity of arthritis. Eye pain and photophobia are uncommon complaints, and ophthalmoscopic examination rarely suggests uveitis until significant eye damage has occurred. Thus, slit-lamp examination must be done as frequently as every 6 weeks in the young, female, ANA-positive, pauciarticular JRA patient; in the patient with systemic or polyarticular JRA, the examination should be performed every 6 months. The consulting ophthalmologist should direct any needed therapy for iritis, which generally includes topical steroids and a mydriatic agent.

Surgery

Orthopedists should see children with severe leg length discrepancy, cervical spine disease, and subluxed and/or extremely restricted joint movement or severe pain. However, surgery is not a cure for JRA; in fact, synovectomy may worsen the disease. On the other hand, surgery can be extraordinarily valuable as a reconstructive modality. Unilateral epiphyseal stapling can improve leg length discrepancy in the growing child with asymmetric, pauciarticular arthritis. Specific operations to be considered in the child with severe deforming polyarticular arthritis include soft tissue releases, metatarsal head resection, pin traction for joint subluxation, and cervical spine stabilization. Selective joint replacement may be considered for the older adolescent and young adult patient.

ANKYLOSING SPONDYLITIS

method of
JOHN H. BLAND, M.D.
University of Vermont College of Medicine
Burlington, Vermont

Ankylosing spondylitis (AS) is an inflammatory arthritis that principally involves the spine and always affects the sacroiliac joints. Derivation of the word is from the Greek *ankylos,* meaning bent or crooked, and *spondylos,* meaning vertebra. Ankylosing spondylitis is the accepted term, but there are many eponyms, the most notable being von Bechterew's or Marie-Strumpell's disease.

The characteristic pathologic pattern is found in the joints of the axial skeleton—namely, the nonsynovial, cartilaginous synchondroses of the intervertebral discs and the diarthroidal, synovial joints (i.e., the zygapophyseal, costovertebral, costotransverse, and neurocentral joints). The sacroiliac joints, having both nonsynovial and diarthrodial articulations, are virtually always involved. Anterior central joints (manubrial sternal, sternoclavicular, and symphysis pubis) are commonly involved. Hips, shoulders, and knees are involved in an estimated 25 per cent of patients. More distal joints may become inflamed during the natural history, but severe involvement of small joints is rare. The anterior uveal tract, the aortic wall, and the upper lobe of lung parenchyma may also be involved.

The major target tissue in the joints is cartilage, particularly fibrocartilage. An obvious osteitis commonly occurs in directly adjacent subchondral bone.

TABLE 1. **Frequency of HLA-B27 in Different Healthy Populations***

Population	Per Cent
Japan	< 1
Black (Africa)	< 1
Black (U.S.)	3–4
London (G.B.)	6
Geneva (Switzerland)	7
Los Angeles (U.S.)	8
Edmonton (Canada)	9
Zagreb (Yugoslavia)	14
Helsinki (Finland)	14
Pima Indians (U.S.)	18
Haida Indians (Canada)	50

*From Calin A: Ankylosing spondylitis. *In* Kelley WN, et al. (eds.): Textbook of Rheumatology, 2nd ed. Philadelphia, W. B. Saunders, 1985, p. 996.

TABLE 2. **Major Differences Between Ankylosing Spondylitis in Men and in Women***

	Males	Females
HLA-B27	> 90%	> 90%
Delay in diagnosis	3 years	10 years
Progress	+ + +	+
Severity	+ + +	+
Peripheral joint disease		
Initial	+	+ +
Subsequent	+	+ + +
Spinal ankylosis†	+ +	+
Cervical spine symptoms	+	+ +
Osteitis pubis	+	+ + +

*From Calin A: Ankylosing spondylitis. *In* Kelley WN, et al. (eds.): Textbook of Rheumatology, 2nd ed. Philadelphia, W. B. Saunders, 1985, p. 1004.

†Skipping thoracic and lumbar spine in females.

The enthesis, the site of entry of tendon, ligament, and capsule into bone and periosteum, is also involved in this disease. The synovitis is only rarely as grossly florid or as clinically significant as in rheumatoid arthritis.

The Human Leukocyte Antigen System (HLA-B27). In 1973 two papers simultaneously published in England and the United States reported a striking association between the histocompatibility antigen HLA-B27 and ankylosing spondylitis. It is now clear that ankylosing spondylitis is a disease spectrum with clinical presentations ranging from the typical and fully expressed picture of spinal inflammation and stiffening to many forme fruste syndromes in which axial involvement may not be prominent. Furthermore, the disease has many clinical, pathologic, and radiographic similarities with other seronegative spondylarthropathies (i.e., Reiter's syndrome and psoriatic arthritis). Patients may display any or all of the features of these seronegative rheumatic syndromes.

With the advent of this genetic marker for susceptibility to ankylosing spondylitis, it became clear that

TABLE 3. **HLA B-27 and Rheumatic Disease in Caucasians**

Group	% Positive
Healthy caucasians	5–14
Ankylosing spondylitis	90–98
Endemic Reiter's syndrome	70–90
Psoriasis	5–10
Psoriatic arthropathy without sacroiliitis	18–22
Psoriatic arthropathy with sacroiliitis	50–60
Seropositive juvenile rheumatoid arthritis	5–10
Juvenile chronic polyarthropathy without sacroiliitis	15–25
Juvenile chronic polyarthropathy with sacroiliitis	40–60
Inflammatory bowel disease	6
Inflammatory bowel disease with peripheral arthropathy	6
Inflammatory bowel disease with sacroiliitis	50–70
Yersinia	10
Yersinia reactive arthropathy	80
Salmonellosis	10
Salmonella reactive arthropathy	80–90

TABLE 4. **Diagnostic Criteria of Ankylosing Spondylitis***

1. Low back pain of over 3 months' duration, unrelieved by rest
2. Pain and stiffness in thoracic cage
3. Limited chest expansion
4. Limited motion in lumbar spine
5. Past or present evidence of iritis
6. Bilateral radiographic sacroiliitis
7. Radiographic evidence of syndesmophytosis

*Diagnosis requires four of the five criteria or No. 6 and one other criterion.

AS is far more common than previously supposed. It was previously thought that AS is primarily a disease of males; the rapid accumulation of knowledge of the natural history of AS and its precise identification has shown that women have AS about as frequently as men, but the disease is less severe in women and thus more difficult to diagnose. The strong familial incidence of AS is now well explained. Table 1 shows the frequency of HLA-B27 in healthy populations; Table 2 lists the principal differences between AS in men and women; and Table 3 shows the frequency of HLA-B27 in healthy individuals and in patients with a broad spectrum of disease.

Clinical and Diagnostic Features (Tables 4 and 5)

Ankylosing spondylitis begins insidiously, usually before the age of 40. The earliest complaints are those of pain and stiffness of the lower back (Table 4). Rarely clinical manifestations are related to iritis, aortic insufficiency, cavitary pulmonary disease of the upper lobes, or peripheral arthritis. The hallmark of AS is sacroiliitis and the consequent low back pain, stiffness, and limitation of motion. The back pain is generally relieved by exercise and made worse by immobilization. Although chronic discomfort occurs, in the insidious onset period, there are usually periods of relief between attacks.

Chest pain is common, frequently being confused with pleuritic symptoms. The pain is exaggerated by inspiration, due to insertional tendonitis of the costosternal and costovertebral insertions (i.e., entheses). The patient may awaken with back pain, which improves when he or she gets out of bed and walks about. Any peripheral joint may become inflamed at any time; peripheral arthropathy is more common in women.

TABLE 5. **Characteristic Features of Back Pain (or Discomfort) in Ankylosing Spondylitis***

1. Age of onset below 40 years
2. Insidious onset
3. Duration greater than 3 months
4. Association with morning stiffness
5. Improvement with exercise

*The presence of all five features confirms the diagnosis of ankylosing spondylitis (AS) in the great majority of patients, differentiating backache and pain of AS from that of other causes, including mechanical.

Achilles tendonitis, as well as other enthesopathies, may occur.

Conjunctivitis and iritis occur in an estimated 25 per cent of patients at some time in the course of the illness. In thirteen per cent of patients there is past or present evidence of iridocyclitis, and over 20 per cent develop this clinical syndrome during a 10-year follow-up period. Physical examination (see Table 6) commonly discloses a decrease in chest expansion (of less than 5 cm). Clinical signs of bilateral sacroiliitis are common. The mobility of the spine is limited, usually in three planes—forward flexion, extension, and lateral flexion. Simple observation of the spine frequently provides the first clue to the diagnosis of AS (i.e., loss of normal lumbar lordosis with a flattening of the lower back). Lower dorsal kyphos is also a reliable diagnostic sign. As the patient bends forward, flexion is seen to occur in the cervical and thoracic spine, with relative rigidity in the lower lumbar area. The Trendelenburg test is commonly positive. Table 7 lists historical and differential characteristics of back pain symptoms of mechanical versus inflammatory etiology.

Treatment

AS is a chronic disease of variable severity, with a relatively good prognosis for long-term function, successful employment, and a normal lifestyle, including athletic activity. Only a few patients progress to severe and total ankylosis. Most patients may continue to participate fully in all work and extra-employment activities. Lifting (i.e., normal use of the back muscles) is encouraged, and special ways of lifting may be taught. Early retirement is to be discouraged, since the evidence is strong that continuing physical activity is tantamount to salvation from this disease.

Since AS is characterized by relatively few chronic complaints, therapy and management should be limited to agents and methods not in themselves worse than the disease. Corticosteroids and immunosuppressive agents are contraindicated. The pain and stiffness of AS can be relieved by appropriate medical management in all stages of the disease. Virtually all studies utilizing drug trials have shown striking differences in pain relief between drug and placebo groups.

Mobility and range of motion can clearly be affected over the short term, and there is evidence that postural and overall exercise programs suppress the tendency toward ankylosis. Also, periods of immobilization as short as 3 months may accelerate the ankylosing ossification process. Thus, therapeutic nihilism is definitely unjustified.

Exercises and Posture

The maintenance of optimum posture and maximum mobility of the cervical, thoracic, and lum-

TABLE 6. **Clinical Examination for Ankylosing Spondylitis**

Test	Maneuver	Interpretation
Occiput-to-wall test	Patient places heels and back against wall and tries to touch wall with back of head without raising the chin above carrying level	Inability to touch head to wall suggests cervical involvement; distance from occiput to wall is measured and compared serially
Fingers to floor	Patient bends forward with knees locked straight; and the distance from middle finger tip to floor is measured, while observing lumbar spine laterally	Inability to touch toes and loss of lumbar lordosis is evidence of early lumbar spine disease
Schober test	Make a mark on the spine at level of L5–S1 (dimples of Venus); make 2 more marks, 5 cm and 10 cm above the first while patient stands erect in best posture; and measure distance between the marks while patient bends forward maximally	An increase of less than 5 cm in the 10 cm distance suggests early lumbar involvement; an increase of less than 3 cm in the 5 cm distance suggests L4–L5 and L5–S1 involvement
Chest expansion	Measure maximum chest expansion at nipple line, while patient clasps hands behind head	Chest expansion less than 5 cm suggests costovertebral and costotransverse joint involvement
Sacroiliac joint compression	Direct compression over sacroiliac joint	Tenderness or pain suggests sacroiliac involvement
Gaenslen's sign	Patient executes maneuver to stress sacroiliac joint	Evokes sacroiliac pain
Thoracic spine motion measurement	Patient bends forward, chin tucked in flexion, and reaches as far as possible toward floor and holds; extend tape measure from spinous process T2 to T10–11; patient returns to upright posture	Failure of tape to fold indicates little or no movement; varying folding indicates a fraction of degree of motion

Modified from Neustadt DH: Postgrad Med 61(1):124–135, 1977.

bar spine is the most important aspect of management of AS. The spinal fusion seen in a few patients definitely seems to be a result of the positions that they have maintained.

Patients should sleep on a firm mattress; sleeping on the back is preferable to a curled-up, fetal position. Special pillows may be useful; for example, a pillow under the lower back may help preserve normal lumbar lordosis and prevent development of forward flexion abnormalities. However, patients with marked cervical spine involvement should avoid using a pillow.

Range-of-motion (ROM) exercises should be regularly performed 3 to 4 times daily. These may be modified according to the constraints of pain but should never be omitted entirely. Serial measurements of height allow early detection of failure to maintain erect posture. Extension and upward stretching exercises are both physically and psychologically advantageous. Breathing exercises, preferably taught by a physiotherapist, should be a part of the daily routine because of their importance in the prevention of lung disease later in the course of AS.

A life-long program of exercise and posture maintenance is mandatory in order to preserve spinal extension, and the strength of extensor muscles in particular. The physical therapy program should include utilization of heat, such as hot showers and baths, whirlpool if available, and infrared therapy; many of these modalities are available in the home. Active participation in sports is encouraged (e.g., jogging, cross-country skiing, cycling, and especially swimming), but activities necessitating a position of flexion for long periods should be avoided.

An experienced physiotherapist should provide initial instruction in the exercise program, and regular repeat visits are recommended for reinforcement. The patient should be instructed about the importance of carrying out the exercises daily at home, emphasizing the fact that, with immobilization, a subtle reduction of spinal extensibility increases by a fraction of a millimeter per day; in time, such minute reductions accumulate significantly.

Frequent follow-up is important in the early stages of AS so that the physician can assess the long-range prognosis and can detect progressive deformity. Objective measurements should be recorded on a regular basis. Loss of spinal extension is reflected in the distance from occiput to wall. In this test the patient places the heel and sacrum against the wall and tries to touch the wall with the back of the head without raising the chin above the normal carrying level, with the cervical spine in a neutral position. Inability to touch the head to the wall indicates cervical involvement and the distance from occiput to wall is measured. This should be done serially.

Maximal chest measurement at the nipple line, done serially, will reveal any reduction in costovertebral and costotransverse joint involvement. In the Schober test, a mark is made on the

TABLE 7. **Differential Historical and Physical Factors in Back Pain of Mechanical versus Inflammatory Origin**

Differential Factor	Mechanical	Inflammatory
Historical		
Past history	+	+ +
Family history	−	+
Onset	Acute	Insidious
Age	15–90	Less than 40
Sleep disturbance	±	+ +
Morning stiffness	+	+ + +
Involvement of other systems	−	+
Effect of exercise	Worse	Better
Effect of rest	Better	Worse
Radiation of pain	Anatomic L4–L5 L5–S1	Diffuse, thoracic, buttock, cervical
Sensory symptoms	+	−
Motor symptoms	+	−
Physical		
Scoliosis	+	−
Decreased range of movement	Asymmetric	Symmetric
Local tenderness	Local	Diffuse
Muscle spasm	Local	Diffuse
Straight leg raising	Decreased	Normal
Sciatic nerve stretch	Positive	Absent
Hip involvement	−	+
Neurologic signs	+	−
Other systems	−	+

midline of the spine at the level of L5, between the dimples of Venus; 5 cm and 10 cm above this, two other marks are made. A mark 5 cm below the initial mark is also useful. The patient then flexes the lumbar spine maximally and the distracted distances between these points are measured. The lower mark represents the lumbosacral joint function; the upper mark, the lumbar spine motion. An increase of less than 5 cm in adults indicates reduced lumbar spine flexion and AS involvement.

Available data permits a reasonable assessment of risk factors for the disease in HLA-B27–positive and HLA-B27–negative family members. It may then become desirable to counsel family members who are at high risk for developing AS. Since the disease carries an excellent prognosis and optimum therapy is available, such family members may profit by counseling.

Other Therapeutic Approaches

All patients with AS must stop smoking cigarettes. A decrease in ventilation, in later years, may result in chronic bronchitis and pulmonary emphysema. Bronchitis should be promptly and vigorously treated.

X-ray therapy was used many years ago, but the potential for the development of leukemia precludes its use. Surgical treatment is rarely indicated. However, surgical consultation is necessary when symptoms include pain radiation in the distribution of the first sacral nerve root or the third, fourth, or fifth lumbar root; pain exaggerated by cough or sneeze; dysesthesia, weakness in the lower limbs; bladder or bowel dysfunction; and neurologic deficits.

Patient Education

The patient should be informed about the natural history of AS and its prognosis. If a patient's disease began at age 20 and he is now in his 40s and has minimal disability, it is reasonable to assure him that his AS is unlikely to show any further progression. In most cases, such a prognosis should be offered cautiously during the first 5 years of follow-up and observation. The dangers of immobilization, perhaps due to some other health problem, and the necessity for maximum activity and adequate rest should be stressed.

Drug Therapy

The role of nonsteroidal anti-inflammatory drugs (NSAIDs) and analgesic agents is the suppression of pain and stiffness, facilitating the exercise program and allowing the patient to continue to be functional. The most potent and popular anti-inflammatory drug remains phenylbutazone (Butazolidine). The maximum daily dose is 400 mg in divided doses. Although symptomatic relief is clearly achieved, there is no evidence that the drug influences the natural history of the disease; therefore, the drug is not taken on a long-term basis. Bone marrow dyscrasia is observed only once in every 125,000 patient-dose-months. The occult development of aplastic anemia occurs mainly in elderly patients. The onset of fever or sore throat after initial treatment with phenylbutazone should alert the patient and the physician to the risk of agranulocytosis and indicates immediate stopping of the drug. The symptoms are far more sensitive indicators than the blood count of this early complication of the drug.

Indomethacin (Indocin), 75 to 175 mg per day orally, is effective in most patients. The 75-mg sustained release preparation is often useful at bedtime. The drug can also be administered as 50- to 150-mg rectal suppositories once or twice daily. Other NSAIDs may have a role in AS and are worth a trial period, the principal goal being to reach a point where drugs are unnecessary.

Aspirin, the mainstay of treatment in rheumatoid arthritis, is not the drug of choice in most patients with AS. The contrast between different anti-inflammatory agents is nowhere more striking than the effect of aspirin on rheumatoid arthritis and AS; patients with the former enjoy striking relief of symptoms, and the reverse occurs in AS patients.

DISORDERS OF THE TEMPOROMANDIBULAR JOINT

method of
WELDEN E. BELL, D.D.S
*University of Texas Southwestern Medical School
Dallas, Texas*

The temporomandibular joint (TMJ) is subject to the ills that afflict other synovial joints plus a few that relate specifically to chewing and other oral functions. Although similar to other synovial joints in most respects, the TMJ has several unique features that should be kept in mind by the treating physician or dentist.

The mandibular joint is the most complex synovial articulation in the body. It is composed of two functionally inseparable TMJs, each of which is a double joint within a single capsule. The upper part is freely movable and capable of extensive sliding movement; the lower part is restricted to hinge movement only. Interposed is an articular disc of dense, avascular fibrous tissue. The temporomandibular disc is a unique structure in that (1) it has true articular facets on its upper and lower surfaces, thus converting an otherwise simple joint into a compound one with four articular surfaces; (2) it is powered independently and therefore moves separately from the osseous parts of the joint during chewing movements; and (3) its chief function is to maintain continuous firm contact of the articulating parts both at rest and during all movements. A damaged articular disc causes loss of stability as well as functional interference and therefore predisposes to degenerative changes in the joint.

The TMJs have a component of function other than that of movement by the muscles—namely the effect of occluding teeth. Each time the teeth are firmly occluded, forces are applied to the joint. Disharmony between the dental occlusion and joint movements sets up conflicting forces that may damage the articular surfaces and thus induce joint dysfunction. Habits such as bruxism and emotional tension accentuate this danger. Also, the occluded dentition establishes a rigid end-point of joint function that is quite different from that of other synovial joints. As a result, a minor dysfunction of the joint may induce a major alteration of occlusal function, and vice versa.

The articular surfaces of the TMJ differ from other joints in that they are composed of dense fibrous tissue rather than hyaline cartilage. Therefore, degenerative joint disease, which ordinarily begins as a cartilaginous change, is somewhat different in TMJs because of the absence of articular cartilage. Since fibrous and cartilaginous tissues have different regenerative capabilities, the articular surfaces of TMJs are more likely to undergo some measure of repair following degenerative change. Disc damage, however, is irreversible.

Within the capsule and lying posterior to the articular disc is a mass of highly vascularized, loose connective tissue that is a major source of synovial fluid to the joint. This tissue is essential for normal joint lubrication and metabolism. Also, its elasticity is needed to permit forward sliding movement of the condyle. Damage to this retrodiscal tissue by trauma, condylar encroachment, or scarring from injudicious surgery may interfere with forward condylar movements as well as with the normal lubrication and metabolism of the articulating parts, thus inviting degenerative changes.

Diagnosis and Classification

Diagnosis and classification of TMJ disorders depend on the proper evaluation of four cardinal symptoms:

1. Chewing pain (that emanates from the joint proper and/or the masticatory muscles).
2. Restricted range of motion.
3. Abnormal sensations, noises, and/or movements.
4. Acute malocclusion (which results from the TMJ disorder).

The clinical diagnosis should identify the complaint as one of the following:

1. A muscle disorder.
2. A disc-interference disorder (noninflammatory degenerative joint disease that impedes disc function).
3. An inflammatory disorder.
4. A chronic mandibular hypomobility.
5. A growth disorder.

Muscle and disc-interference disorders constitute about 90 per cent of all TMJ complaints; inflammatory, hypomobile, and growth disorders make up the other 10 per cent. When a disc-interference disorder becomes inflammatory, it is classified as degenerative arthritis. Rheumatoid arthritis and hyperuricemia occasionally afflict the TMJs initially, and sometimes solely.

Treatment

Palliative Therapy

Palliative therapy may be effective in about 70 per cent of all TMJ complaints. Such treatment may include one or several of the following procedures:

1. Voluntary restriction of chewing within painless limits by smaller bites, softer foods, and slower movements, and by avoiding "testing," strained opening, and clenching the teeth.

2. Nonnarcotic analgesic medications to render the pain tolerable without completely eliminating it, since discomfort is a valuable clue for controlling restricted movements.

3. Short-term use of muscle relaxants such as diazepam (Valium).

4. Relaxation techniques such as meditation or biofeedback.

5. Short-term use of occlusion-disengaging splints.

6. Analgesic blocking to interrupt pain cycling and to permit manipulation of spastic muscles.

7. Nonsteroidal anti-inflammatory drugs (NSAIDs) such as ibuprofen (Motrin, Advil).

8. Judicious application of ultrasound.

9. Exercises that contract antagonist muscles may help resolve acute myospasm; isotonic exercises help extend the range of motion; isometric exercises help resolve disuse atrophy.

Definitive Therapy

A confirmed diagnosis is an essential first step in any definitive therapy. Confirmation of the clinical diagnosis may require one or more of the following:

1. Identification of the pain source by analgesic blocking.

2. Occlusal studies, laboratory tests, consultations.

3. Transcranial radiography, tomography, computed tomography, or fluoroscopy.

4. Arthrotomography.

5. Magnetic resonance imaging (MRI).

6. Arthroscopy.

7. Scintigraphy.

Some disc-interference disorders may require occlusion-correcting or mandibular-repositioning splints. Permanent alteration of the occlusion by selective grinding, orthodontics, occlusal reconstruction, or orthognathic surgery may ultimately be required. Occasionally, operative intervention is justified in the form of arthroscopic surgery, closed condylotomy, laminectomy, disc plication, high condylectomy, or disc excision. Surgery, however, is usually not an option, but rather a necessity. The objective of surgery is not to make a good joint out of a bad one but to make a tolerable situation out of an intolerable one.

Inflammatory disorders of the joint require about the same medical and/or surgical treatment as similar conditions in other synovial joints. Interdisciplinary management is usually needed because special considerations for oral function exist and modify therapy to some extent.

Chronic mandibular hypomobilities and growth disorders of the TMJ are usually surgical conditions.

FIBROSITIS, BURSITIS, AND TENDINITIS

method of
FRANKLIN KOZIN, M.D.
San Diego, California

Fibrositis, bursitis, and tendinitis are the major forms of soft tissue rheumatism. They may occur without an underlying disease process, or they may be secondary to other disorders such as rheumatoid arthritis or crystal-induced synovitis. These are common problems, which often respond to conservative therapies.

FIBROSITIS (FIBROMYALGIA, MYOFASCIAL PAIN SYNDROME)

Fibrositis is a form of nonarticular rheumatism characterized by chronic aching pain, stiffness, and soft tissue tenderness. Studies of patients with fibrositis have failed to find any specific biochemical, serologic, or pathologic abnormalities that might help in diagnosis. Individuals may present at any age (median age 30 to 40 years); women are affected four times more frequently than men.

Patients with fibrositis complain of a deep aching pain, usually in the neck, upper and lower back, and shoulder girdles. They may describe a wide variety of referred sensations both in the painful areas as well as in distant sites, including pressure, tightness, temperature changes (coldness, burning), and paresthesias. Symptoms may be exacerbated by emotional or physical stress, cold drafts, dampness, or immobility. Patients often complain of a diffuse stiffness, which is usually worse in the morning and late afternoon or evening.

Many subjects with fibrositis have a sleep disturbance. While they may fall asleep readily, they awaken several times during the night. As a result patients feel tired or "washed out" on arising and complain of feeling fatigued "all the time."

The physical examination typically discloses a number of tender points. The most common tender points are located in the trapezius muscles, lateral epicondyles, second costochondral junctions, medial fat pads of the knee, and lower cervical and lumbar spinal intervertebral ligaments (midline tenderness). Tender points may be "trigger points" when palpation produces radiating or referred pain. Muscle spasm or tightness is often present and may be diffuse, especially throughout the back.

Patients should be evaluated for other conditions that may produce diffuse myalgias or arthralgias. These include polymyositis, polymyalgia rheumatica, hypothyroidism, or a connective tissue disorder. It is important to evaluate patients for an underlying inflammatory disorder, such as rheumatoid arthritis, or a related painful condition such as cervical spondylosis or radiculitis.

Treatment

Treatment of fibrositis is directed at reducing the pain, muscle spasm, and anxiety produced by the pain syndrome. Patients should be reassured that the pain is not caused by a serious underlying disease; written educational material is often useful for this purpose. Initial treatment should include a simple analgesic agent such as a nonsteroidal anti-inflammatory drug (NSAID) and a physiotherapy program. The latter is helpful in reducing pain and spasm and should consist of hot packs, ice, massage, and ultrasound with or without the use of topical corticosteroids. Occasionally it may be necessary to supplement therapy with local injections, consisting of 1 ml of 1 per cent lidocaine (Xylocaine) combined with 1 ml of 0.25 per cent bupivacaine (Marcaine), into tender/trigger points. A small amount (10 to 20 mg) of corticosteroid suspension (Depo-Medrol or Hydelta TBA) may be added to the local anesthetic injections.

When patients have not improved significantly in 2 to 3 weeks using the aforementioned program, additional drug therapy must be instituted. Muscle relaxants, particularly cyclobenzaprine (Flexeril), 10 mg at bedtime, or the tricyclic antidepressant amitriptyline (Elavil), 10 to 50 mg at bedtime, may be effective. The dose of these medications should be titrated according to symptoms, and they should be used cautiously, especially in elderly patients who may be more susceptible to adverse effects. Biofeedback and transcutaneous nerve stimulation (TENS) may be useful in certain patients.

BURSITIS AND TENDINITIS

Bursitis

It has been estimated that there are over 70 bursa in the human body, many of which are unnamed. Bursae are fluid-filled sacs, lined with synovium, which minimize friction between bony prominences and musculoskeletal tissues. Major bursae are located in the shoulder (subacromial), heel (infra- or retrocalcaneal), knee (anserine, prepatellar, infrapatellar), hip (trochanteric), and other sites.

Pain in a bursa may occur as a result of a systemic rheumatic disease, particularly rheumatoid arthritis, infection, crystal-induced inflammation, trauma, or overuse. Swelling, redness, warmth, and localized tenderness may be present, depending upon the cause and severity of inflammation. Whenever possible, the inflamed bursa should be aspirated and fluid examined for crystals and bacteria.

Subacromial bursitis produces pain in the shoulder and subdeltoid area, especially with elevation of the arm. Olecranon bursitis is almost always associated with an egg-shaped swelling at the tip of the elbow. The olecranon bursa should always be aspirated because of the high frequency of crystal- and bacteria-induced inflammation. Trochanteric bursitis produces pain overlying or posterior to the greater trochanter of the femur; occasionally pain radiates down the lateral thigh and may suggest sciatica. Marked tenderness over the greater trochanter will confirm the diagnosis.

There are several bursae about the knee. Anserine bursitis is often present in patients with osteoarthritis and produces pain beneath the medial joint line. Prepatellar bursitis ("housemaid's knee") or infrapatellar bursitis ("clergyman's knee") will cause pain on or beneath the patella, respectively. The clinician must familiarize him/herself with the locations of these bursae in order to suspect the diagnosis and confirm it by eliciting tenderness in the bursa.

Tendinitis

Tendinitis or tenosynovitis is a common problem, especially with growing participation in exercise and conditioning programs. Trauma, strain, overuse, or calcific deposits may often cause this condition, but it is not rare to see them as complications of a systemic rheumatic disease (rheumatoid arthritis, systemic lupus erythematosus) or infection (*Neisseria gonorrhoeae* or *Staphylococcus aureus*).

Common sites of tendinitis include the rotator cuff tendons about the shoulder, the medial or lateral tendons of the elbow (tennis elbow, epicondylitis), and the tendons of the hand. Flexor tendinitis or tenosynovitis in the hand may produce swelling, palpable nodules, or tendon sheath stenosis; significant loss of function may accompany this problem. Triggering or locking of the finger will often be the presenting complaint of patients, typically after a strenuous day in sports, gardening, or home repairs. Tendinitis of the abductor pollicis longus and extensor pollicis brevis as they pass over the radial styloid produces De Quervain's disease. Patients complain of wrist and thumb pain with pinching or grasping. This disorder is recognized by tenderness and occasional swelling over the radial styloid and by a positive Finkelstein test. The latter is performed by asking the patient to clasp his/her fingers around the abducted thumb (make a fist with the thumb inside). The examiner then deviates the hand toward the ulna, and a "positive" test is present when pain develops in the proximal wrist, distal forearm, or radial styloid.

Treatment

Initial treatment of bursitis and tendinitis consists of rest and ice applications to the affected part. Occasionally an elastic bandage, splint, or brace may be useful. In patients with more intense pain or inflammation, simple analgesics or NSAIDs also should be prescribed. When these measures fail to control symptoms adequately, a physiotherapy program may be helpful and should include ultrasound with or without topical corticosteroids as well as range-of-motion and strengthening exercises.

In patients with persistent pain or functional limitation, local corticosteroid injections may be necessary. Using aseptic technique, the affected bursa or tendon tissue should be infiltrated with 20 to 40 mg of corticosteroid (Hydelta TBA, Depo-Medrol) combined with 1 to 2 ml of 1 per cent lidocaine or 1 to 2 ml of 0.25 per cent bupivacaine or both. Patients should be apprised of the potential risks and complications of such injections and should be instructed to rest the injected area for 5 to 10 days following the injection.

Surgical repair of partially or completely torn tendons and tendons or bursae that fail to respond to less invasive measures should be considered. Rarely, surgical removal of calcium deposits may be useful.

Patients with persisting or recurrent tendinitis or bursitis should be instructed in preventive measures. Every effort should be made to identify and minimize activities that cause the problem. A stretching and strengthening exercise program often is helpful. Icing the affected part before and after sports or other activities also may control symptoms. Use of knee or elbow bands or braces may prevent excess strain of irritated tendons or bursae. In certain patients with chronic symptoms, continual or intermittent NSAID therapy may be necessary. Frequent corticosteroid injections should be avoided whenever possible, as these may lead to tendon rupture.

LYME DISEASE

method of
ROBERT T. SCHOEN, M.D.
Yale University School of Medicine
New Haven, Connecticut

Lyme disease is a complex, multi-system disorder recognized in 1975 in patients living near Lyme, Connecticut. Erythema chronicum migrans (ECM), a characteristic rash seen in 30 to 60 per cent of individuals with Lyme disease, was described in Sweden in 1909. Lyme disease has been reported in 33 states and all continents except Antarctica. In the United States, the number of new cases approximately doubles each year. Lyme disease is a spirochetal infection caused by a newly recognized organism, *Borrelia burgdorferi*, and transmitted primarily by ticks of the *Ixodes ricinus* complex, including *Ixodes dammini*. Lyme disease is now the most commonly reported tick-transmitted illness in the United States.

Diagnosis

As many as 50 per cent of individuals who acquire Lyme disease remain asymptomatic in spite of serologic evidence of recent infection. Like other spirochetal infections, the illness can be divided into three stages or grouped into early and late manifestations. Also like other spirochetal infections, antibiotic therapy is most effective early in the illness and cure becomes less certain in patients with chronic disease. The greatest challenge in the care of patients with Lyme disease is to recognize and treat the illness as early as possible. The diagnosis of Lyme disease depends on (1) a history of potential exposure to ticks in an endemic area, particularly during the spring and summer, (2) recognition of characteristic clinical features, and (3) the use of Lyme disease–specific serologic testing.

The early diagnosis and treatment of Lyme disease is often made difficult by several factors.

1. Not all patients are symptomatic early in the illness. For example, patients may present with arthritis (Stage 3) but even in retrospect have no history to suggest earlier stages of Lyme disease.

2. Currently available serologic testing for Lyme disease by enzyme-linked immunosorbent assay (ELISA) will detect diagnostic antibody titers (IgG and IgM) in most patients with established disease (Stages 2 and 3). Only 40 to 65 per cent of individuals with

Stage 1 disease, however, have disease-specific IgM or IgG antibody titers even when acute and convalescent sera are obtained.

3. ECM, the characteristic rash in Lyme disease, is not always present or may have an uncharacteristic appearance.

4. Diagnosis of Lyme disease is suggested by travel or residence in an endemic area, but the disease is now recognized over an expanding geographic range. Nonetheless, in the United States most cases continue to occur in the northeastern coastal New England and Mid-Atlantic states, in Minnesota and Wisconsin, and in Northern California and surrounding states. It should be remembered that later stages of the illness can begin throughout the year, but Stage 1 disease is most likely during the period from April to July when nymphal ixodid ticks are active and is unlikely to occur during the winter.

5. Increasing information about Lyme disease has led to an expanding clinical spectrum of disease manifestations. For example, uveitis and progressive dementia have recently been attributed to Lyme disease. In most patients, however, the disease has characteristic, well-described disease manifestations.

6. The Centers for Disease Control has reported that 5 of 19 pregnancies in women who acquired Lyme disease during pregnancy were associated with adverse fetal outcomes in spite of antibiotic therapy; this has added uncertainty as to how this disease should be treated during pregnancy.

7. Although *B. burgdorferi* has been cultured from the blood, cerebrospinal fluid, skin, and synovial fluid of patients with Lyme disease and has been visualized in patient specimens, direct identification of the organism requires specialized techniques not routinely used by the clinician.

Stage 1 (Early Disease)

Erythema Chronicum Migrans (ECM). Approximately 30 per cent of individuals remember a tick bite several days to 1 month before they develop Lyme disease. A red macule or papule (ECM) may develop at the site of the bite; when present in its typical form, it is diagnostic of Lyme disease. The rash begins as a red macule or papule and then expands over several days, often to greater than 10 cm in diameter. The advancing ECM rash has a distinct outer border. There may be clearing, bluish discoloration, vesicle formation, or necrosis of the center of the rash. If untreated, the rash usually fades within 1 to 4 weeks, although occasionally it persists for months. During this early period, when Lyme disease is most successfully treated, the organism is thought to disseminate hematogenously; this may explain the presence in some patients of secondary annular skin lesions. These resemble the primary ECM lesion but are usually smaller, lack indurated centers, and wax and wane over short periods independent of the initial ECM lesion. These lesions also occasionally recur during later stages of the illness—for example, with the onset of arthritis.

Constitutional Symptoms. Hematogenous dissemination of *B. burgdorferi* may also explain the constitutional symptoms, which are sometimes, but not always, seen during this stage. Fatigue, malaise, fever, and migratory arthralgias suggest a flu-like illness. Headache and stiff neck may suggest aseptic meningitis. The presence, severity, and duration of these symptoms is highly variable.

Stages 2 and 3 (Late Disease)

Neurologic Manifestations. Weeks to months after the tick bite, about 15 per cent of patients develop neurologic abnormalities. These include meningitis (associated with a lymphocytic pleocytosis), encephalitis, cranial neuropathy (Bell's palsy may be the only manifestation of Lyme disease), peripheral radiculoneuropathies, or myelitis. These manifestations may occur alone or in combination. In untreated patients, neurologic abnormalities usually resolve completely within months, although chronic neurologic disease is increasingly recognized. Patients with late neurologic illness have been reported to have neuropsychiatric symptoms, focal disease of the central nervous system, or a fatigue syndrome. Brain imaging by nuclear magnetic resonance (NMR) scanning has shown demyelinative plaques in some patients.

Cardiac Involvement. About 5 per cent of patients develop cardiac involvement within several weeks after the onset of Lyme disease. In one series, 18 of 20 patients with cardiac disease had fluctuating degrees of atrioventricular block; 8 of these patients developed complete heart block that was more likely to occur when the PR interval was longer than 0.30 second; 13 had acute myopericarditis. These patients did not have valvular heart disease. The duration of Lyme carditis is usually brief (several days to several weeks), but recurrences are possible. Patients usually recover completely, although a cardiac death from Lyme disease has been reported.

Arthritis. Within several days to weeks after disease onset, about 20 per cent of patients develop arthralgias. Typically these are brief episodes of migratory joint, periarticular, and musculoskeletal pain; however, patients may continue to have attacks of arthralgias for up to 6 years without developing objective joint abnormalities. In addition to arthralgias, within days to years following untreated ECM, about 50 per cent of untreated patients develop frank arthritis occurring as single or intermittent attacks of joint swelling lasting from several days up to 1 year. In most patients asymmetric involvement of large joints, particularly the knee, is seen; involvement of more than 5 joints is unusual. About 10 per cent of patients with Lyme disease develop chronic arthritis which can be associated with permanent joint destruction.

Acrodermatitis chronica atrophicans is a late skin manifestation of Lyme disease reported frequently in Europe; however, perhaps because of strain heterogeneity of *B. burgdorferi*, it is an unusual skin manifestation in North America.

Treatment

Stage 1 (Early Disease)

The goals of antibiotic therapy at the onset of Lyme disease are to shorten the duration of ECM and associated symptoms and to prevent the development of later stages of the illness. During Stage 1, the disease can be cured in approximately 90 per cent of patients.

The drug of choice for adults (except pregnant women) and for children with permanent dentition is an oral tetracycline—either tetracycline, 250 to 500 mg 4 times daily, or doxycycline (Vibramycin), 50 to 100 mg twice daily, given for 10 to 21 days. The range of dosages and duration of treatment suggested reflects the variability of severity of symptoms at disease onset. Severe disease at onset correlates with a greater likelihood of late complications such as arthritis than does mild disease at onset. In general, since antibiotic therapy is most effective early in the illness, it is appropriate to treat most patients with more than mild illness at onset for a full 3-week course of antibiotic therapy.

Phenoxymethyl penicillin (penicillin V), 250 to 500 mg 4 times daily, or amoxicillin, 250 to 500 mg 4 times daily, given for 10 to 21 days is also effective therapy for Stage 1 Lyme disease. Phenoxymethyl penicillin is the drug of choice for pregnant and lactating women and for children with deciduous dentition. Since an association between the onset of this infection during pregnancy and fetal malformations has been suggested, and since transplacental infection is postulated to occur very soon after disease onset, it is probably appropriate to treat pregnant women in whom Lyme disease is suspected with a lower threshold than other individuals. There may also be a role for intravenous penicillin in Stage 1 Lyme disease in some pregnant women with relatively severe symptoms, although this is unproven. Children with deciduous teeth should receive phenoxymethyl penicillin, 50 mg per kg per day (not less than 1 gram or more than 2 grams per day).

For adults allergic to tetracyclines or penicillins, erythromycin, 250 to 500 mg 4 times daily for 10 to 21 days, is a slightly less effective alternative. In children allergic to penicillin, erythromycin, 30 mg per kg per day in divided doses for 10 to 21 days, can be used.

Stages 2 and 3 (Late Disease)

Neurologic Manifestations. In patients with mild disease (for example, Bell's palsy alone), tetracycline, 250 to 500 mg 4 times daily for 10 to 31 days, is effective. For individuals with frank meningitis, spinal fluid pleocytosis, and cranial or peripheral neuropathies, intravenous penicillin G, 20 million units daily in divided doses for 10 to 14 days, is usually effective. Cephtriaxone, 2 grams daily for 14 days, is an alternative. In one patient, chloramphenicol at a dose of 1 gram intravenously every 6 hours for 10 days was effective following unsuccessful intravenous penicillin therapy. Patients with Stage 3 neurologic complications of Lyme disease, including neuropsychiatric disease, focal central nervous system disease, and fatigue syndromes, have been treated with variable success with intravenous penicillin G in the regimens suggested for serious Stage 2 neurologic disease.

Cardiac Involvement. Patients with Lyme carditis should probably receive, in addition to antibiotic therapy, aspirin, 6 to 12 325-mg tablets daily, or an equivalent nonsteroidal anti-inflammatory drug (NSAID) in therapeutic dosage. In patients with minor cardiac involvement (first-degree atrioventricular (AV) block, with PR interval less than 0.30 second) and no other significant symptoms, therapy with tetracycline as described for Stage 1 disease is effective. Such patients should restrict their activity, however, and should be monitored closely. Patients with more severe manifestations of Lyme carditis (including first-degree AV block with PR interval greater than 0.30 second) should be hospitalized with cardiac monitoring and treated with intravenous penicillin or cephtriaxone as described for serious neurologic manifestations. Some of these patients will have complete heart block requiring temporary transvenous cardiac pacemaker insertion, usually for less than 1 week. Persistent conduction system abnormalities requiring permanent pacemaker insertion are unusual but have occurred.

Arthritis

Several oral regimens are successful in treating Lyme arthritis in approximately 50 per cent of patients and avoid the morbidity and expense of intravenous antibiotic therapy. In adults these regimens include doxycycline, 100 mg twice daily given for 31 days; and amoxicillin, 500 mg 4 times daily, with probenecid, 500 mg 4 times daily, for 31 days.

Children should receive phenoxymethyl penicillin, 50 mg per kg per day (not less than 1 gram or more than 2 grams per day) in 4 doses for 31 days.

Penicillin G, 20 million units intravenously daily in divided doses for 14 to 21 days, or cephtriaxone, 1 to 2 grams intravenously daily for 14 to 21 days, is effective in approximately 75 per cent of patients with established Lyme arthritis. Children should receive penicillin G, 250,000 units per kg per day intravenously in divided doses every 4 hours for 14 to 21 days.

In some adults who do not respond to antibiotic therapy, especially individuals with chronic knee arthritis, arthroscopic synovectomy has been successful. Other patients require management with NSAID therapy or intra-articular corticosteroid injection. In some patients with arthritis, retreatment with an alternative antibiotic regimen results in an improved outcome. Ultimately, in most patients, Lyme arthritis can be arrested without significant joint destruction.

OSTEOARTHRITIS

method of
GEORGE L. MORTON, M.D.
Portland, Maine

Osteoarthritis is the most common of the rheumatic diseases and is a major cause of limited function in the elderly. Osteoarthritis (degenerative joint disease, hypertrophic arthritis) is a primary or secondary degeneration of the cartilaginous surface of diarthrodial joints. The earliest known changes in the osteoarthritic joint are biochemical, followed by a decrease in tolerance of cartilage to stress resulting in flaking and fissuring of the cartilage. The latter process leads to an asymmetric loss of cartilage within the joint, resulting in irregular joint space narrowing. This is accompanied by radiographic changes of subchondral sclerosis of bone and marginal bony hypertrophy (osteophytosis). Primary osteoarthritis usually occurs in the older population (i.e., greater than 45 years of age), as compared with inflammatory arthritis with its prevalence in the younger population. Secondary osteoarthritis (secondary to mechanical incongruity, metabolic causes, decreased pain perception in the joint, or aseptic necrosis of bone) may occur in any age group.

Treatment

Treatment goals in osteoarthritis are patient education and reassurance, preservation or improvement in the range of motion of the joint, strengthening of muscles about the involved joint, relief of pain and stiffness, and prevention or delay of the progression of the disease process.

Patient Education

Many patients with the diagnosis of osteoarthritis fear a progressive, deforming arthritis with major disability and "crippling." The physician can perform a great service by informing the patient that osteoarthritis, unlike rheumatoid arthritis, does not generally have widespread involvement with progressive destructive changes. Instead, there tends to be involvement of only a few joints, with only a small percentage of patients developing disabling joint deformity. A majority of patients can obtain relief of symptoms and lead productive lives. The booklet "Osteoarthritis," published by the Arthritis Foundation, is a very helpful educational resource material for the patient.

The initial visit is an important time to assess the patient's expectations of treatment and to discuss whether these expectations are realistic. The treatment regimen must be tailored to the extent and severity of the joints involved and to the patient's ability to comply with the regimen. Patients with mild osteoarthritis may need only education, joint protection, and at times use of nonsteroidal anti-inflammatory drugs (NSAIDs), whereas those with severe osteoarthritis require considerable limitation of activities, a more rigorous physical therapy regimen, and more aggressive medical or surgical management.

It is important to dispel the misbelief that continued vigorous use of a joint keeps the joint mobile and functional. This misconception is reinforced by the patient's observation that immobility of an involved joint for a prolonged period of time often causes increased stiffness and discomfort upon using it again. In fact, prolonged and repeated overuse of an involved joint generally leads to an exacerbation of the disease process with increased rate of joint destruction. Specific, concrete recommendations are necessary to prevent overuse of the involved joint. For example, with knee involvement, jogging, deep-knee bending, and bicycling should be avoided and a schedule developed for household activities in order to limit the number of times the patient uses the stairs. With hand involvement, one has to limit repetitive hand activities such as crocheting, knitting, and repetitive grasping activities such as using hammers, saws, or screwdrivers. Both physical and occupational therapists with special training in the treatment of arthritis can provide excellent advice about joint protection.

The current emphasis on nutrition has led to the misconception by some patients that dietary intake may have an effect on arthritis. Patients should be educated that no known dietary changes affect osteoarthritis in a significant manner. Obesity, however, does lead to increased loading on weight-bearing joints, contributing to further damage of cartilaginous surfaces. Weight loss, when indicated, is to be encouraged and is usually best achieved through the use of group counseling services such as Weight Watchers, Diet Workshop, and TOPS. It is important to avoid starvation diets that promote ketosis, as this may lead to increased gastric irritation when used in conjunction with NSAIDs.

Physical Therapy and Occupational Therapy

The objectives of a physical therapy program are to maintain or increase range of motion, improve muscle strength, and provide increased well-being. Range-of-motion exercises should be limited to 10 to 15 repetitions once or twice daily using slow stretching rather than rapid vigorous jerking motion. This is to prevent possible micro-tears with subsequent hemorrhage and increased inflammation. Before exercise, range of motion may be facilitated by the application of hot packs for 15 to 20 minutes to the affected joints. Pro-longed application of hot packs may cause in-creased swelling and flare of symptoms. Cold packs are often helpful immediately following overuse of a joint to prevent a flare of symptoms. If pain continues for more than 20 minutes after the exercise, or if symptoms increase the follow-ing evening or morning, then the program is too vigorous and must be modified. To improve mus-cle strength, isometric rather than isotonic exer-cises should be used. For example, for the knee, straight leg-raising, quadriceps-strengthening exercises should be used rather than isotonic active extension. Besides discussing specific ex-ercises and giving the patient educational mate-rial, the patient should be referred to a physical therapist trained in the principles of arthritis treatment for optimal results in a physical ther-apy regimen.

Some physical and occupational therapists are trained to educate patients about joint protection in daily living and work activities. The occupa-tional therapist can assess and instruct about devices to help protect joints and improve joint function in daily activities. With disease of the hand this might include built-up handles, jar openers, elongating handles of self-care devices, and simple lever faucets. Patients with severe involvement of weight-bearing joints may benefit from assistive devices to decrease joint loading such as the use of a cane, crutches, or a walker. An orthotist or podiatrist may be very helpful in providing inserts or education regarding foot-wear. Elevated seats in chairs and toilets, me-chanical chair elevators, and insertion of grab bars may all be beneficial when lower extremity involvement is severe.

Nonsteroidal Anti-inflammatory Drugs

Nonsteroidal anti-inflammatory drugs (NSAIDs) are the major pharmacologic agents used to treat osteoarthritis. They are effective as an analgesic as well as an anti-inflammatory medication. Since there is a component of intermittent inflam-mation in osteoarthritis, there has been some speculation that NSAIDs may alter the course of the disease favorably if used early and appropri-ately. However, evidence that NSAIDs alter the course of osteoarthritis is still lacking.

Aspirin and the Salicylates. Aspirin is the stan-dard NSAID with efficacy comparable to that of the newer NSAIDs when taken in the appropriate dosage. Aspirin in low dosage (325 to 650 mg three times daily) provides only an analgesic effect. Serum salicylate levels in the range of 20 mg per dl are necessary to obtain an anti-inflam-matory effect; 650 to 1300 mg of aspirin four times a day are required to achieve these thera-peutic levels. The salicylate level in the adult is dependent not upon body weight but upon the rate of metabolism in the liver and excretion through the kidney. Persistent tinnitus and hear-ing loss may indicate the onset of salicylate intoxication, which tends to occur in young or middle-aged patients at salicylate levels exceed-ing 30 mg per dl. Intermittent tinnitus during quiet times is common at low doses and is not an indication to discontinue the drug. In contrast to the young or middle-aged group, the elderly may develop confusion or sedation without tinnitus or hearing loss at serum salicylate levels of above 20 mg per dl.

Aspirin inhibits cytoprotective prostaglandin synthesis in the gastric mucosa, leading to its most common adverse side effect, gastric irrita-tion. Aspirin also inhibits prostaglandin synthe-sis by irreversibly blocking cyclooxygenase in the platelet, causing permanent decreased platelet adhesiveness. Because of this latter effect, aspirin therapy should be discontinued 5 to 10 days before an anticipated surgical procedure. The inhibition of prostaglandin synthesis in the cy-toprotective gastric mucosa and platelets contrib-utes to the increased risk of bleeding in the gastrointestinal tract. This may be lessened by having the patient take the aspirin with meals or use an enteric-coated preparation (Easprin, Ecotrin, Encaprin), zero-order–release aspirin (ZORprin), or the nonacetylated salicylates mag-nesium salicylate (Magan, Mobidin), choline magnesium salicylate (Trilisate), and salsalate (Disalcid). Some of these offer the advantage of twice daily administration.

Elevation of liver enzymes—in particular, as-partate aminotransferase (AST), alanine amino-transferase (ALT), and lactate dehydrogenase (LDH)—may occur with high doses of aspirin and are reversible within a few days of cessation of the drug. The long-term effect of the continued administration of aspirin in the face of low-grade elevation of liver function enzymes is unknown but is thought to be benign. Aspirin allergy is rare and has the unusual property of being dose-related. The classic triad of aspirin allergy is urticaria, asthma, and nasal polyps. However, there is an increased risk of aspirin hypersensi-tivity in individuals who have allergic rhinorrhea and asthma without nasal polyps. Sodium salicylate and salsalate may be used in patients with aspirin allergy.

Other NSAIDs. Since the mid 1970s, several new NSAIDs have been developed with an efficacy comparable to that of aspirin. While they are often better tolerated, they are more expensive than aspirin. These agents are acidic, protein-bound, readily absorbed by the gastrointestinal tract, and rapidly metabolized and excreted by the liver, kidney, or both. Athough one of their known biologic effects is inhibition of prostaglandin, it is not known if this is the major mechanism by which they are effective in the treatment of osteoarthritis.

The newer NSAIDs are divided into several groups based on their chemical structures. The indole derivatives are indomethacin (Indocin, Indocin SR), tolmetin (Tolectin), and sulindac (Clinoril). The propionic acid derivatives include ibuprofen (Motrin, Rufin, Advil, and Nuprin), phenoprofen (Nalfon), naproxen (Naprosyn), and ketoprofen (Orudis). Phenamic acid is the parent compound of meclofenamate (Meclomen). The available oxicam derivative is piroxicam (Feldene). Diflunisal (Dolobid) is a derivative of salicylic acid but is not metabolized to salicylic acid. In a disease in which symptoms are often mild and intermittent, improved patient compliance (and thereby possibly improved efficacy) has been demonstrated with agents administered only once or twice daily. The dosages of the listed agents are indicated in Table 1.

The inhibition of prostaglandin synthesis causes the same types of side effects as aspirin: gastric irritation, erosions, and increased gastrointestinal bleeding. To decrease the risk of gastric irritation, the use of acidic beverages such as coffee, decaffeinated coffee, tea, alcohol, and colas should be avoided. The simultaneous use of aspirin, aspirin-containing compounds, and over-the-counter ibuprofen (Advil, Nuprin) has been shown to decrease serum levels of several of the newer NSAIDs and to increase gastric irritation. Decreased platelet adhesiveness is seen with the newer NSAIDs because of its inhibition of the cyclooxygenase system in the platelet. However, this effect is reversible, in contrast to the permanent inhibition by aspirin. Nephrotoxicity may be manifested by glomerulonephritis, interstitial nephritis, and tubular necrosis, the latter two being the most common. The risk factors for nephrotoxicity are an elderly age, hypertension, diabetes, and decreased renal blood flow such as that seen in congestive heart failure or concomitant use of diuretics. Patients with these risk factors should have blood urea nitrogen (BUN), creatinine, and urine monitored periodically while on NSAIDs. There is cross-reactivity to the newer NSAIDs in aspirin-allergic patients; thus these agents should be used cautiously under supervision in an environment in which anaphylactic regimens can be administered quickly to these patients. Other side effects include skin rash, central nervous system symptoms, headaches and dizziness, hepatitis, and fluid retention. The efficacy of the NSAIDs requires regular

TABLE 1. **Nonsteroidal Anti-inflammatory Drugs (NSAIDs)**

	Tablet Strength (mg)	Usual Daily Dosage (mg)
Salicylates		
Acetylsalicylic acid (aspirin)	325	650–1300 qid
Sodium salicylate (Pabalate)	325	650–1300 qid
Enteric-coated aspirin		
Ecotrin	325 or 500	650–1300 qid
Easprin	975	975 tid to qid
Nonacetylated salicylates		
Magnesium salicylate (Magan)	545	545–1090 tid
Salsalate (Disalcid)	500 or 750	750–1500 bid
Choline magnesium salicylate (Trilisate)	500 or 750	750–1500 bid
Zero-order–release aspirin (ZORprin)	800	800–1600 bid
Indole derivatives		
Indomethacin (Indocin)	25 or 50	25–50 tid to qid
Slow-release (Indocin SR)	75	75 bid
Tolmetin (Tolectin)	200 or 400	200–400 tid to qid
Sulindac (Clinoril)	150 or 200	150–200 bid
Oxicam		
Piroxicam (Feldene)	20	20 once a day
Phenamic Acid		
Meclofenamate (Meclomen)	50 or 100	50–100 tid to qid
Propionic Acid		
Ibuprofen (Motrin, Rufen)	400, 600, or 800	400–800 tid to qid
Ketoprofen (Orudis)	50 or 75	50–75 tid to qid
Naproxen (Naprosyn)	250, 375, or 500	250–500 bid
Fenoprofen (Nalfon)	300 or 600	300–600 tid to qid

rather than intermittent dosages, a fact that often requires reeducation of the patient to maintain optimal benefits. Use of an individual NSAID for 2 to 4 weeks is required before its efficacy can be assessed. The ability of a patient to comply with single or multiple dosing regimens must be taken into consideration in the initial choice of an agent. If the initial drug is ineffective, then other drugs should be tried in sequence, preferably from each of the chemical groups rather than within a group. If a drug is not effective, a review of the patient's compliance with medica tion schedules and joint-protection techniques is necessary.

Analgesics and Muscle Relaxants

Analgesic agents such as acetaminophen, propoxyphene (Darvon, Dolene), and codeine preparations may be helpful as temporary adjuncts to the NSAIDs. Analgesics should not be used primarily instead of NSAIDs. Narcotic analgesics should be restricted to treatment of temporary flares. Muscle relaxants such as cyclobenzaprine (Flexeril), methocarbamol (Robaxin), and diazepam (Valium) may be used to help reduce muscle spasm secondary to osteoarthritis of the cervical and lumbar spine. Muscle relaxants are rarely indicated in the treatment of peripheral joint osteoarthritis.

Intra-articular Corticosteroids

Systemic corticosteroid therapy clearly has no place in the treatment of osteoarthritis. However, intra-articular corticosteroids may be an extremely beneficial adjunct when used in acute flares, particularly if the patient is on a full anti-inflammatory regimen. A careful history and physical examination are important to determine if the acute painful episode is secondary to osteoarthritis or some other musculoskeletal abnormality such as bursitis, tendinitis, or stress fracture. At the knee, anserine bursitis is often confused with a flare of osteoarthritis. Trochanteric bursitis may be confused with a flare of hip joint involvement. With acute shoulder pain, differentiation between acromioclavicular joint involvement, subdeltoid bursitis, supraspinatus tendinitis, and biceps tendinitis must be made. The patient with osteoarthritis of the first carpometacarpal joint may have pain secondary to de Quervain's tendinitis or an unrelated carpal tunnel syndrome. It is extremely important that the patient be instructed to limit weight-bearing

or repetitive motion of the injected joint for one week after injection. The latter has been shown to provide prolonged benefit and prevent rapid exacerbation in the injected joint. A long-acting steroid preparation such as triamcinolone hexacetonide (Aristospan), methylprednisolone acetate (Depo-Medrol), or prednisolone tebutate (Hydeltra-TBA) should be used rather than shorter-acting steroid preparations. A joint should not be injected more than three times a year and preferably not more than once every 3 to 4 months. If there is no benefit after one or two injections, further trials of local injection of steroids should be avoided.

Surgery

Orthopedic surgical intervention in osteoarthritis has provided dramatic relief of symptoms and restoration of function in many patients who have severe end-stage degenerative changes. Total joint arthroplasty of the hip and knee is indicated for those individuals who have failed medical management, have end-stage disease on radiography, continue to have severe incapacitating pain, or have significant instability of the knee. Patients should be cautioned that although they may have significant or complete loss of pain and improved functional status, they should not anticipate return to vigorous physical activities.

The longevity of prosthetic joints has been excellent in the older age group but has had a high failure rate in individuals who may only have involvement of one joint and return to aggressive physical activities. The newer press-fit noncemented prostheses may decrease the failure rate in this latter group of individuals; however, the use of these prostheses has not been long enough to confirm this initial impression. In the younger individual who has only medial-compartment degeneration of the knee, tibial osteotomy may be an excellent procedure providing symptomatic relief for several years before total knee arthroplasty is necessary. Arthroplasty has also been helpful in the first carpometacarpal joint. Arthroplasty of the shoulder and ankle is still in its infancy and is reserved for selected patients.

Arthrodesis may be indicated in failed total joint arthroplasty secondary to repeated loosening or infection, a previously infected joint, or a joint in which heavy weight loading is anticipated. Arthroscopy has provided temporary benefit for patients with loose intra-articular cartilaginous debris.

POLYMYALGIA RHEUMATICA AND GIANT CELL ARTERITIS

method of
JAMES J. CURRAN, M.D., and
DANIEL A. ALBERT, M.D.
University of Chicago
Chicago, Illinois

POLYMYALGIA RHEUMATICA

Polymyalgia rheumatica (PMR) is a disease of the elderly that has a mean age of onset of 70 years and is rare before age 50. Women with the disease outnumber men by 2.5 to 1, and the disease is much more common in whites than in blacks. To date, no specific etiologic agent or immunologic markers have been identified.

Clinically accepted criteria for the diagnosis of PMR include stiffness (morning greater than evening) without weakness in the cervical, pectoral, or pelvic girdles (at least 2 of 3); a Westergren sedimentation rate greater than 50 mm per hour; constitutional symptoms, including weight loss, fever, fatigue, and depression; and a rapid (less than 5 days) response to corticosteroids.

Physical findings may include active synovitis with mild inflammatory joint fluid predominantly in the interphalangeal, metacarpophalangeal, and wrist joints; carpal tunnel syndrome; and more rarely sternoclavicular swelling. Laboratory parameters include hypoalbuminemia; anemia; and elevated erythrocyte sedimentation rate (ESR), C-reactive protein (CRP), alkaline phosphatase, gamma glutamyltransferase (GGT), and globulin levels.

The coexistence of giant cell arteritis (GCA) is 15 to 20 per cent in patients with PMR. Ocular complications are rare in patients with PMR who do not have symptoms of GCA and are being treated for PMR. The differential diagnosis includes late-onset rheumatoid arthritis, polymyositis, systemic lupus erythematosis, thyroid disease, and paraneoplastic syndromes.

Treatment

In mild cases of PMR, a trial of nonsteroidal anti-inflammatory drugs (NSAIDs) may be employed. If this is unsuccessful, or if the patient has marked inflammatory symptoms, prednisone, 5 to 15 mg per day (mean dose 10 mg) given orally in a single morning dose, is recommended. A response should be noted within 4 to 5 days, and usually within 24 hours. The ESR may normalize within 4 weeks. CRP will become normal within 1 week and may be a more sensitive indicator of disease activity and therapeutic response.

The duration of disease is variable, although most patients will require a minimum of 18 to 24 months of therapy and many may be symptomatic for 4 or more years. Relapse commonly occurs during periods of tapering, and the disease may recur within 2 years of discontinuance of treatment. There are no predictors of disease duration or severity. Generally, steroid therapy may be tapered at 1 mg per month when the patient is clinically stable and the ESR is less than 30 mm per hour. Close clinical follow-up with evaluations for the recurrence of symptoms or the evolution to GCA are warranted.

GIANT CELL ARTERITIS

Giant cell arteritis (GCA) is a systemic granulomatous vasculitis affecting the large and medium-sized arteries. As in PMR, there is a female predominance and a mean age of about 70. Up to 40 per cent of patients present with a wasting disorder, with or without fever, that suggests a paraneoplastic process in the absence of clearly demonstrated PMR symptoms. Common clinical manifestations in addition to PMR and wasting are hemicranial headache, scalp tenderness, jaw claudication (pathognomonic for GCA), and synovitis. Less common clinical signs include aortic arch disease, cranial neuropathies, visceral vasculitis, peripheral ischemic disease, and upper respiratory tract complaints (hoarseness, cough, sore throat). Physical findings include transient ophthalmoplegias, scalp and tongue ulcers, hearing loss, visual field loss, thickened and pulseless temporal arteries, and arterial bruits. Laboratory parameters include anemia, elevated liver function tests, ESR, and CRP. Ocular complications occur in 12 per cent of GCA patients. Contralateral temporal artery involvement has been noted in 53 per cent of patients.

High-dose steroid therapy in elderly patients has a potential morbidity; thus a histologic tissue diagnosis is preferable. Occasionally histologic confirmation is difficult to obtain because the disease is focal and segmental; the temporal artery biopsy specimen should be 4 to 6 cm and should be carefully and fully sectioned for histology. If the initial biopsy is negative, the opposite temporal or an occipital artery may be biopsied (up to 40 per cent will be positive).

Treatment

When the diagnosis of GCA is suspected, prednisone should be immediately instituted at 60 mg per day in a single morning dose. The incidence of monocular blindness is 12 to 17 per cent in patients with GCA, and binocular involvement may occur in 18 per cent of these. Visual field loss may progress despite the normalization of the ESR; rarely the ESR is never elevated. Arteritic ischemic optic neuropathy has been successfully treated with high-dose intravenous methylprednisolone, 1000 mg every 12 hours for 5 days, or with oral prednisone, 100 mg per day. One of these drugs should be used when there is established ischemic retinopathy. Therapy should not be delayed to permit a temporal artery biopsy, since tissue obtained 48 to 72 hours after the initiation of therapy is adequate for histologic analysis. Furthermore, therapy for GCA, if strongly suspected on clinical appraisal, should not be withheld from patients with negative biopsies.

Patients with GCA generally respond to prednisone within 2 to 4 days; in 87 per cent the ESR will be normal within 4 weeks. The starting dose of prednisone should be maintained for 4 to 6 weeks; then a slow taper of 10 per cent of the maintenance dose per week is begun until a dose of 10 mg is reached. Prednisone should then be tapered at 1 mg per month. Again, the ESR and CRP are good parameters to follow when assessing for disease recurrence.

Most disease flares occur during steroid tapers. The natural history of active disease is from 18 to 24 months. Some patients may require as long as 5 years of treatment. Complications of steroid therapy in GCA include osteopenia, compression fractures, adrenal suppression and steroid myopathy. In a recent study azathioprine (Imuran), 150 mg per day, was successfully used as a steroid "sparing" agent. Alternate-day steroid therapy has not been found to be effective in GCA.

OSTEOMYELITIS

method of
JENNIFER LI, M.D., and
RALPH COREY, M.D.
Duke University Medical Center
Durham, North Carolina

Osteomyelitis, which is found even in animal and human fossils, was first described in 1831 by Nathan Smith. In this early description he named the disease "Necrosis . . . death of some part of the bony structure" and emphasized its inflammatory nature. Today osteomyelitis is recognized as a disease with a wide spectrum of manifestations related to the site of involvement, the initiating organism, the age and defenses of the host, and the acuteness or chronicity of the illness. Osteomyelitis is caused by a variety of microorgan-

isms, mostly bacterial in nature. Pathogenic organisms gain access to bone, causing infection through either hematogenous spread, inoculation (traumatic or surgical), or direct extension from other sites of infection.

The bacteremia causing acute hematogenous osteomyelitis commonly originates from a urinary, an intravascular, or a dermal focus; however, the source is often not apparent. Patients who have frequent bacteremias are at increased risk, and these include young children, patients on chronic hemodialysis, and intravenous drug abusers. Acute hematogenous osteomyelitis most often involves rapidly growing bone, a highly metabolic tissue with a rich vascular supply. The disease thus has a striking predilection for the long bones of infants and children, particularly the metaphyses of the femur and tibia. Organisms gain access to this area through the nutrient capillary arteries. These arteries make sharp turns in the area of the epiphyseal growth plate to enter a system of large sinusoidal veins connecting the venous network of the medullary cavity. This vascular network is particularly susceptible to infection for several reasons. First, the area lacks phagocytic cells. Second, as the afferent capillaries (8 micrometers in diameter) enter the efferent sinusoidal plexus (15 to 60 micrometers in diameter), blood flow becomes more sluggish, allowing bacterial attachment and growth. Finally, the capillary loops near the vicinity of the epiphyseal plate are nonanastomosing, and any obstruction can lead to avascular necrosis.

In adults, long bones are metabolically more quiescent than in children, and the marrow is largely replaced by fat. These bones are, therefore, rarely a site of acute hematogenous osteomyelitis. On the other hand, the vertebral body adjacent to the intervertebral disk in adults is a richly vascular area and is commonly involved in acute hematogenous osteomyelitis. Organisms reach the spine through nutrient branches of the posterior spinal artery or ascend via retrograde flow from the valveless paravertebral venous plexus of Batson, which drains the body wall and pelvis. Batson's plexus has been implicated as a mechanism by which urinary tract infections cause vertebral osteomyelitis. Infection can spread to other vertebrae by direct extension through the disk space or through communicating venous channels frequently involving two adjacent vertebral bodies and the corresponding intervertebral disk of the thoracolumbar, lumbar, or lumbosacral spine.

Osteomyelitis is also caused by extension from contiguous sites of infection or by inoculation from an exogenous source through trauma or surgery. Contiguous sites of infection include soft tissue (especially burns), teeth and sinuses, infected joints, and prosthetic hardware. Patients with diabetes or atherosclerosis and resulting vascular insufficiency commonly get osteomyelitis of the foot secondary to an infected cutaneous ulcer. Organisms can also invade the bone through open fractures, penetrating wounds, and perioperative contamination of the bone during orthopedic procedures.

Pathology

The pathologic findings are those of acute inflammation with neutrophilic infiltration, edema, and vascular congestion followed by vascular thrombosis, ischemia, and necrosis. After a few days, the devitalized bone forms segments called sequestra. With persistent infections, fibroblastic proliferation and new bone formation occur. Osteogenesis surrounds the inflammation to form the involucrum. Occasionally a fibrous capsule will confine the inflammation to a localized area called a Brodie's abscess.

Clinical Aspects

In children, osteomyelitis classically presents with fever and variable degree of pain, swelling, erythema, warmth of the involved long bone, and decreased range of motion. However, almost one half of patients present with only vague complaints. In 90 per cent of cases the etiologic agent is *Staphylococcus aureus* or *S. epidermidis*, but blood cultures are positive in only 50 per cent. In children with sickle cell anemia, *Salmonella* is isolated in over half of the cases, and this infection is often difficult to distinguish clinically or radiologically from a painful bony vaso-occlusive crisis. Neonatal osteomyelitis represents a distinct clinical entity from childhood osteomyelitis since it is quite subtle and more aggressive and often involves multiple bones. Neonates often have a paucity of systemic signs, and the diagnosis must rest on local findings such as edema or an adjacent joint effusion. However, early diagnosis is essential to prevent permanent sequelae, since the infection rapidly transgresses the epiphyseal growth plate, invading and destroying the joint. The etiologic agent of neonatal osteomyelitis is usually a Group B streptococcus, *Escherichia coli*, or *S. aureus*.

Vertebral osteomyelitis in the adult presents with clinical signs of back pain, stiffness, and fever. There is often tenderness over the affected vertebra, splinting of movement, and paravertebral muscle spasm. The most common causative organisms are *S. aureus*, members of the family Enterobacteriaceae, and *Pseudomonas aeruginosa* (especially in drug addicts). Complications of vertebral osteomyelitis include anterior extension to cause either paraspinal abscess, retropharyngeal abscess, empyema, mediastinitis, or a psoas muscle abscess. A serious complication is posterior extension leading to an epidural abscess, spinal cord compression, or meningitis.

Patients with nonhematogenous osteomyelitis present with few systemic complaints. Local signs usually dominate and include swelling, erythema, and tenderness of the affected area, occasionally accompanied by an overlying cellulitis, ulcer, or draining sinus. Traumatic puncture wounds of the foot may result in an indolent and quiescent but destructive osteomyelitis of the calcaneus or metatarsal; *Pseudomonas aeruginosa* is the most likely etiologic agent. In patients with vascular insufficiency from diabetes mellitus or atherosclerosis, osteomyelitis typically involves the small bones of the feet as a result of long-standing plantar ulcers. Most of these patients have a severe sensory neuropathy, which aids the initiation of ulcer formation while preventing early diagnosis of the infection. There are often two or more infecting organisms including staphylococci, streptococci, Enterobacteriaceae, and anaerobes.

In osteomyelitis resulting from an infected prosthetic device (nails, screws, pins, joints, plates) the infection either may become apparent shortly after surgery (e.g., *S. aureus*) or may have a much later onset (e.g., *S. epidermidis*). Erythema and drainage at the operative site are frequently found, and there is often evidence of loosening of the appliance.

Unusual Clinical Syndromes. The clinical presentation of an *anaerobic osteomyelitis* does not differ markedly from that of an aerobic osteomyelitis. In general, however, anaerobic bone infections result from nonhematogenous spread of organisms usually arising from a contiguous focus of infection. In keeping with this observation, most patients with anaerobic osteomyelitis have few systemic signs. Anaerobic osteomyelitis should be suspected in the following clinical situations: when foul-smelling exudates and subcutaneous gas are present, in chronic indolent diabetic foot ulcers, in infections following a human bite, in osteomyelitis following pelvic infections or decubitus ulcers, in osteomyelitis of the face or skull bones, and in osteomyelitis of the cervical spine.

Tuberculous osteomyelitis generally results from hematogenous spread from a pulmonary focus. As in pyogenic osteomyelitis, the metaphysis of the long bone is the most frequent site in children and the vertebra the most frequent site in adults (Pott's disease). The disease presents either as a primary bone disease with localized swelling and tenderness, as a chronic draining sinus, or as a gibbous deformity of the spine with complications of paraplegia or a paraspinal abscess.

Diagnosis

Laboratory data in osteomyelitis are often nonspecific. Patients with acute hematogenous osteomyelitis frequently have a significant leukocytosis, whereas those with chronic osteomyelitis commonly have only a mild anemia and an elevated sedimentation rate. Although the hematologic values are of no value in predicting the outcome of the disease, they can be useful in following the response to therapy.

The radiologic findings of osteomyelitis are of local destruction (reflected in lytic lesions) and of new bone formation (reflected in periosteal elevation and areas of higher density). In vertebral osteomyelitis there is often narrowing of the intervertebral disk space and loss of anterior vertebral body height. The roentgenographic findings usually lag behind the clinical presentation by at least 10 to 14 days. If bone sclerosis is present, this is evidence that the disease has been present for over a month. Radionuclide scans with technetium pyrophosphate permit earlier visualization of osteomyelitic foci but are less specific, since they cannot distinguish between overlying infection and osteomyelitis. Also, bone scanning does not distinguish osteomyelitis from bone repair after a variety of injuries. Computed tomography (CT) is useful in cases of vertebral osteomyelitis and in defining complications that require surgery.

Cultures to define the pathogenic organism(s) are of primary importance. If blood cultures are negative, bone biopsy or aspiration is mandatory. Cultures of overlying ulcers or draining sinuses are, in general, quite useless.

Treatment

General Principles

1. Prompt therapy to keep bone necrosis to a minimum.
2. Prolonged therapy (4 to 6 weeks) to prevent recurrence.
3. Parenteral therapy is usually the treatment of choice.
4. Necrotic bone and foreign material are often responsible for relapses.

Acute Hematogenous Osteomyelitis

Initial treatment depends on the severity of illness. In acute hematogenous osteomyelitis antibiotic therapy often must be initiated immediately after blood cultures are drawn. The choice of agent then depends on the age and underlying disease of the patient (Table 1). In the nontoxic patient, blood culture results should be awaited before starting antibiotics. In nonbacteremic patients, bone cultures must be obtained to guide therapy.

After culture results have been returned, antibiotic therapy can be adjusted depending on the organism involved (Table 2). Intravenous antibiotics should be used in most cases for 4 to 6 weeks although much of this therapy can be given on an outpatient basis after the infection is well-controlled (i.e., patient is afebrile for 3 to 5 days). Occasionally, oral antibiotics in high doses can be substituted for outpatient parenteral therapy in a reliable, cooperative patient with an uncomplicated infection. Six weeks of oral therapy is the minimum length of treatment, and weekly monitoring of general well being, antibiotic levels, and sedimentation rate is required.

Surgical intervention is empiric and must be individualized. Abscesses, necrotic tissue, and sequestra need prompt excision. Vertebral stabilization is rarely needed.

Chronic Osteomyelitis

Before embarking on therapy, an aggressive diagnostic approach is needed to determine the organism(s) involved. Superficial and sinus tract cultures are of little use, and in the overwhelming majority of cases, invasive biopsy and culture of the infected bone are needed. Only after the pathogenic organism is identified should parenteral antibiotics be started in the same manner as in acute hematogenous osteomyelitis. Much of this therapy can be given on an outpatient basis because of the indolent nature of this infection and the infrequency of complications.

In conjunction with antibiotics, surgical débridement is of utmost importance. Antibiotics alone rarely cure these infections. The guiding principles of surgical therapy include removal of necrotic material and elimination of dead space. Open packing, bone grafting, muscle grafting, and skin grafting are all used to accomplish the latter objective. Occasionally cure is not possible with therapy short of amputation. However, many of these patients do quite well without amputation as long as the infected area is draining and flare-ups of local cellulitis are treated promptly.

The role of hyperbaric oxygen in refractory chronic osteomyelitis has yet to be determined, although it may improve cure rates by stimulating vascular proliferation as well as osteoblastic and osteoclastic activity. This may be important in the refractory osteomyelitis of diabetics in whom amputation is usually the final procedure.

Osteomyelitis involving joint prostheses is a difficult matter. If the organism is quite susceptible to both parenteral and oral antibiotics (e.g., S. aureus) and the prosthesis is stable, a 6-week course of intravenous antibiotics followed by an indefinite course of oral antibiotics is worth a try. When the prosthesis has already loosened, however, removal is necessary. Immediate re-replacement is attempted only when the organism is relatively susceptible, and a 6-week course of parenteral therapy is given at that time. When

TABLE 1. **Factors Affecting Antibiotic Choice in Treatment of Osteomyelitis**

Factors	Usual Organism(s)	Antibiotics
Patient		
Neonate	*Staphylococcus aureus*, Group A or B *Streptococcus*, *E. coli*, *Enterobacter*	Nafcillin and gentamicin
Child	*S. aureus*	Nafcillin
Adult	*S. aureus* and gram-negative bacilli	Nafcillin and gentamicin
Modifying Conditions		
Urinary infection	Gram-negative bacilli	Gentamicin
Intravenous catheter infection	*S. aureus* and *S. epidermidis*	Vancomycin
Sickle cell disease	*Salmonella* and *S. aureus*	Ampicillin and nafcillin
Burns	*S. aureus* and *Pseudomonas aeruginosa*	Vancomycin and tobramycin
Intravenous drug abusers	*S. aureus* and *Pseudomonas aeruginosa*	Vancomycin and tobramycin

TABLE 2. **Antibiotic Therapy for Acute Hematogenous Osteomyelitis**

Organism	Drug	Recommended Daily Dosage		Hours between Doses	Route of Administration
		Children (mg/kg)	*Adults*		
Staphylococcus aureus (methicillin sensitive)	Cefazolin (Kefzol)	40–100	3–6 grams	8	IV
	Clindamicin (Cleocin)	25–40	1.2–2.7 grams	6–8	IV
	Oxacillin (Prostaphlin)	50–100	4–8 grams	4–6	IV
	Nafcillin (Nafcil)	50–100	4–8 grams	4–6	IV
Staphylococcus aureus (methicillin resistant)	Vancomycin (Vancocin)	15–40	1–2 grams	12	IV
Staphylococcus epidermidis	Vancomycin (Vancocin)	15–40	1–2 grams	12	IV
Streptococcus (Groups A, B, C)	Penicillin	50,000–100,000 U	4–12 mU	4–6	IV
Gram-negative bacilli (*E. coli, Klebsiella, Enterobacter, Proteus, Serratia*)	Amikacin (Amikin)	15–20	15 mg/kg	8–12	IV
	Aztreonam (Azactam)	–	3–6 grams	8	IV
	Cefotaxime (Claforan)	50–200	4–8 grams	8	IV
	Ceftriaxone (Rocefin)	100	1–4 grams	12–24	IV
	Gentamicin (Garamycin)	3–7.5	3–5 mg/kg	8	IV
	Imipenem (Primaxin)*	40–100	1–4 grams	6	IV
	Tobramycin (Nebcin)	3–7.5	3–5 mg/kg	8	IV
	Ciprofloxacin (Cipro)†	–	1–1.5 grams PO	12	IV and PO
			200–300 mg IV	12	
Pseudomonas (a)	Amikacin (Amikin)	15–20	15 mg/kg	8–12	IV
	Gentamicin (Garamycin)	3–7.5	3–5 mg/kg	8	IV
	Tobramycin (Nebcin)	3–7.5	3–5 mg/kg	8	IV
Pseudomonas (b)	Aztreonam (Azactam)	–	3–6 grams	8	IV
	Ceftazidime (Fortaz)	30–100	4–6 grams	8	IV
	Imipenem (Primaxin)*	40–100	1–4 grams	6	IV
	Mezlocillin (Mezlin)	200–300	18–24 grams	4–6	IV
	Piperacillin (Pipracil)	200–300	18–24 grams	4–6	IV
	Ciprofloxacin (Cipro)†	–	1–1.5 grams PO	12	IV and PO
			200–300 mg IV	12	
Salmonella	Ampicillin (Principen)	100–300	4–8 grams	4–6	IV
	Chloramphenicol (Chloromycetin)	50–100	1–2 grams	6	IV
	Co-trimoxazole (TMP/SMZ)	10/50	480/2400–640/3200	6–12	IV
Haemophilus influenzae	Ampicillin (Principen)	100–300	4–8 grams	4–6	IV
	Cefotaxime (Claforan)	50–200	4–8 grams	8	IV
	Cefuroxime (Zinacef)	100	2.25–4.5 grams	8	IV
	Chloramphenicol (Chloromycetin)	50–100	1–2 grams	6	IV
	Co-trimoxazole (TMP/SMZ)	10/50	480/2400–640/3200	6–12	IV
Anaerobes	Clindamycin (Cleocin)	10–40	1.2–2.7 grams	6–8	IV
	Metronidazole (Flagyl)	15–35	1–2 grams	6–8	IV
Tuberculosis	Isoniazid (INH)	7–20	300 mg	24	PO
	Rifampin (Rifadin)	10–20	600 mg	24	PO

*Manufacturer states: Safety and efficacy of imipenem have not been established in children younger than 12 years of age.
†Parenteral *and* oral antibiotics; not yet available in the United States.

resistant organisms are encountered, it is prudent to remove the prosthesis and give a 6-week course of therapy. Reinsertion of the prosthesis is accomplished at a later date.

Osteomyelitis involving devices used in the open reduction of fractures is handled in two ways. If the device is intramedullary (e.g., pins, rods), it is left in place as long as healing is being promoted. All other devices (e.g., screws) are left in only if they are stable. If loose, they are removed and replaced with external stabilization.

Tuberculous osteomyelitis usually involves the vertebral column. Treatment with isoniazid and rifampin daily for 9 months is curative. Surgery

is needed only for complications, and immobilization is necessary only if the spine is unstable or neurologic signs are present.

Prophylaxis

Antibiotic prevention of osteomyelitis is possible after a compound fracture by using an antistaphylococcal antibiotic. Also, perioperative antistaphylococcal therapy is effective in preventing infection in cases in which prosthetic material is being inserted. In both of these situations, short-term therapy (1 to 3 days) is optimal, and a first- or second-generation cephalosporin or vancomycin is the antibiotic of choice.

COMMON SPORTS INJURIES

method of
DOUGLAS B. McKEAG, M.D.
Michigan State University
East Lansing, Michigan

Athletes generally are subject to two different injury patterns, according to whether they are sporadic or regular exercisers. The *sporadic* athlete usually participates in a specific, team-oriented activity on a once- or twice-weekly basis and is apt to incur acute injury. The *regular* exerciser, on the other hand, exercises 3 to 6 times a week, participates in individual or paired activities, and is more prone to overuse injury.

TYPES OF ACUTE INJURIES

The various types of injuries seen in high-school athletes are shown, in order of frequency, in Table 1. The most common, discussed below, are sprains and strains, contusions, lacerations, and fractures.

Sprains and Strains (60.5 per cent)

Regardless of anatomic site, the following grading system can be used in the assessment of the common sprain or strain:

First degree/grade 1. Injury to the tissue is usually microscopic with no increase of laxity of either the ligament or musculotendinous unit. Less than 25 per cent of the fibers are involved.

Second degree/grade 2. These injuries result from tears and partial disruption of ligaments and tendons. Between 25 and 75 per cent of the fibers of the particular unit may be involved and result in laxity and loss of function.

Third degree/grade 3. Complete disruption of the ligament or tendon results in immediate pain, disability, and loss of function. Third-degree sprains can actually result in less pain than the second-degree sprain. This results when the lig-

TABLE 1. **Types of High-School Sports Injuries**

	No.	%
Sprains	349	29.5
Strains	366	31.0
Contusions	162	13.7
Lacerations	21	1.8
Fractures	63	5.5
Inflammations	70	5.9
Other	150	12.7
Total	1181	

From Garrick JG, Requa R: Medical care and injury surveillance in the high school setting. Phys Sportsmed 9:115, 1981. Reprinted by permission of The Physician and Sportsmedicine, a McGraw-Hill publication.

ament is torn and there remains no further stretch to initiate pain.

Clinical correlation with an appropriate biomechanical history of the injury remains the cornerstone of diagnosis. Evaluation should be done as soon as possible. If laxity is questioned, a stress x-ray may help to delineate the problem and rule out epiphyseal plate involvement. The majority of young athletes have ligamentous laxity; it is important to always examine and compare the *uninjured* side for what may seem to be an equivocal finding. Frequent sites of sprains include the ankle (anterior talofibular ligament), knee (medial collateral ligament), and finger (interphalangeal ligament). Common sites of strains include the upper leg (biceps femoris, adductor muscles), back (paraspinal muscle), and knee (quadriceps muscles).

Treatment of most sprains and strains involve the following modalities:

R—REST the injured part to allow healing and prevent further injury.

I—Apply ICE to prevent further swelling and extravasation of blood; ice should be applied directly to the skin at frequent intervals, not to exceed 10 to 15 minutes per session). It is more important to have frequent short applications of ice instead of one long application.

C—Create COMPRESSION via an elastic bandage or air splint to prevent movement and further swelling.

E—ELEVATE the injured area when possible to prevent stasis of blood, aid in venous return to the heart, and control swelling.

M—MEDICATE when appropriate. If the athlete is not returning to either practice or a competition, it is beneficial to start anti-inflammatory medication after bleeding has been controlled. Nonsteroidal anti-inflammatory drugs (NSAID) are appropriate but should be used only approximately 48 hours post injury. The effect of most NSAIDs on bleeding makes their use inappropriate immediately post injury.

Contusions and Lacerations

Contusions are inevitable results of athletic activity. Appropriate use of ice and compression is adequate treatment in these injuries. However, *deep* bruising involving muscle and hematoma formation requires special treatment. The area involved needs to be immobilized and the athlete restricted from further play. Complications include further bleeding into the muscle, deep vein thrombosis, and thrombophlebitis. Myositis ossificans can result from repeated injury. This usually occurs in the anterior thigh and lateral upper arm.

Lacerations are common in many contact sports. It is important to prevent blood-borne diseases (e.g., AIDS). Any wound or laceration should be covered before the athlete is allowed to return to participation. In addition, foreign bodies, especially when there are lacerations of the face or eye, need to be suspected when cleaning the wound. Tetanus toxoid may be needed, depending on the state of tetanus prophylaxis.

Fractures (5.5 per cent)

In children, more greenstick and fewer avulsion fractures are seen. Fractures can occur at any site in the body and range from the relatively insignificant fracture of the distal phalanx of the toe, which needs no immobilization or treatment, to life-threatening skull fractures.

Generally speaking, avoid further injury to the neurovascular bundle when evaluating a suspected fracture. Manipulation prior to radiographic examination is normally contraindicated. On rare occasions, when the blood supply appears to be compromised by a fracture, manipulation to relieve vascular pressure by competent personnel may be necessary. For any fracture it is best to immobilize, apply ice and compression, and transport immediately.

Fifteen per cent of childhood fractures of the long bones involve the epiphyseal plate. Such injuries are most common during rapid skeletal growth (adolescent growth spurt). The most frequently involved sites include the epiphyseal plates of the distal radius, distal tibia, and distal femur. The Salter-Harris classification of these fractures is shown in Figure 1. An epiphyseal injury should be suspected in any adolescent who exhibits evidence of a fracture near the end of a long bone. Stress x-rays should be used to differentiate between ligament involvement and Salter I type fractures.

SPECIFIC ACUTE INJURIES

Table 2 lists the anatomic sites, according to frequency, of high-school sports injuries. Following are some general principles that should be kept in mind when evaluating acute injuries to specific parts of the body.

Head and Neck (14.5 per cent)

Intracranial injuries in athletes should be graded. There are many ways to grade such injuries. I prefer Nelson's protocol (see Table 3). Assume that there is involvement of the spine if a head injury occurs. When a head or neck injury is suspected, immobilization for transportation is

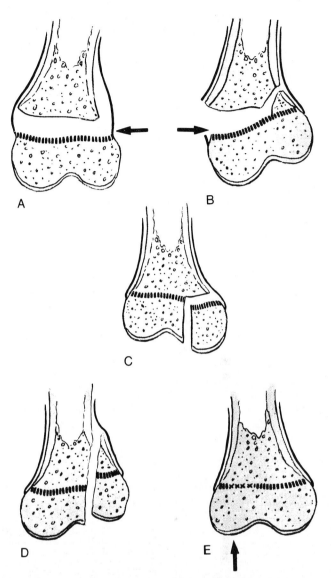

Figure 1. Salter-Harris classification of epiphyseal injury. *A,* Type I, separation of epiphysis. *B,* Type II, fracture-separation of epiphysis. *C,* Type III, fracture of part of epiphysis. *D,* Type IV, fracture of epiphysis and epiphyseal plate. *E,* Type V, crush injury to epiphyseal plate. (From Salter RB, Harris WR: J Bone Joint Surg (Am) *45*:587, 1963.)

absolutely imperative. Injury to the neck in any athlete should always concern the physician, and conservative treatment should be carried out until a diagnosis has been delineated.

The neck and the shoulders are more prone to nerve injuries than any other joint or area of the body. Such injuries can be divided into four groups: (1) brachial plexus traction injuries ("burners"), (2) superclavicular neuropraxias, (3) axillary neuropraxias, and (4) long thoracic neuropraxias. All result from blunt trauma and stretching of the exposed brachial plexus. Pain, tingling, and numbness follow. Severity may

TABLE 2. **Anatomic Sites of High-School Sports Injuries**

	No.	%
Head	60	5.1
Neck/spine	111	9.4
Shoulder	50	4.2
Hand, wrist, and fingers	102	8.6
Other upper extremities	66	5.6
Back/trunk	66	5.6
Thigh	173	14.6
Knee	175	14.8
Ankle	164	13.9
Other lower extremities	214	18.1
Total	1181	

From Garrick JG, Requa R: Medical care and injury surveillance in the high school setting. Phys Sportsmed 9:115, 1981. Reprinted by permission of The Physician and Sportsmedicine, a McGraw-Hill publication.

vary; recovery may be instantaneous or pain and weakness may last for weeks. Injury to the superclavicular nerve can result in loss of function of the supraspinatous (shoulder abductor) and infraspinatous (elevator and external rotator) muscles. Injury to the axillary nerve can cause shoulder dislocation. Injury to the long thoracic nerve may cause "winging" of the scapula. Proper treatment involves rest without return to sports participation. Nearly all such injuries are self-limiting.

Shoulder (4.2 per cent)

Acromioclavicular separation, one of the most frequent shoulder injuries, can be categorized as

shown in Table 4. Treatment consists of ice and early motion following initial rest and use of a simple sling. Surgical repair should not be considered except possibly for a Grade III injury.

Clavicular fracture, another common shoulder injury, is treated with a figure-of-8 strap. Surgery is rarely done and usually only for cosmetic purposes.

Glenohumeral dislocation is most commonly anterior. Posterior dislocation represents less than 10 per cent of all shoulder dislocations. Rapid initial reduction of anterior shoulder dislocations can prevent deltoid muscle atrophy secondary to circumflex artery damage. An aggressive rehabilitation program to strengthen the rotator cuff muscles following such a dislocation can virtually eliminate the problem of recurrent dislocations.

The sternoclavicular joint is commonly injured by forces that drive the shoulder forward. It will usually dislocate anteriorly, but occasionally a posterior subluxation raises the possibility of impingement of the great vessels. Forcible reduction of such a dislocation may be life-saving and can be accomplished with the use of towel clips.

Elbow (5.6 per cent)

Most elbow injuries are relatively minor and involve sprains, strains, and avulsion fractures about the elbow. When treating an elbow injury an x-ray should be taken to rule out a supracondylar fracture, with careful examination of the anterior fat pad.

TABLE 3. **Classification of Concussion**

Grade	Signs and Symptoms	Management
0	Head struck or moved rapidly Not stunned or dazed initially Subsequently complains of headache and difficulty in concentrating	Return to play when sensorium clears Ask about symptoms periodically during remainder of activity Remove from activity if symptoms re-develop
1	Stunned or dazed initially No loss of consciousness (LOC) or amnesia "Bell rung," sensorium quickly clears (less than 1 minute)	Same as for Grade 0
2	Headache, cloudy sensorium (greater than 1 minute) No LOC May have tinnitus or amnesia Irritable, hyperexcitable, confused, dizzy	Remove from practice or game Do not return until symptomatic If symptoms increase or do not clear within 2 days, refer to neurosurgeon
3	LOC (less than 1 minute) Not comatose (arousable with noxious stimuli) Demonstrates Grade 2 symptoms during recovery	Remove from activity Do not return to sports until cleared by neurosurgeon If symptoms increase, urgent consultation is indicated
4	LOC (greater than 1 minute) Not comatose Demonstrates Grade 2 symptoms during recovery	Transport to neurologic trauma center for evaluation and treatment

From Nelson WE, Jane JA, and Gieck JH: Minor head injury in sports: a new system of classification and management. Phys Sportsmed 12(3):103, 1984. Reprinted by permission of The Physician and Sportsmedicine, a McGraw-Hill publication.

TABLE 4. **Classification of Acromioclavicular Separation**

Grade I	The acromioclavicular joint is intact, with point-tender pain or palpation
Grade II	There is laxity of the acromioclavicular joint with traction; however, the joint will return to its normal location
Grade III	The acromioclavicular separation is accompanied by the tearing of all supporting ligaments and displacement of the clavicle from the acromion

Wrist, Hand, and Fingers (8.6 per cent)

Exercise-induced injury of the wrist, hand, and/or fingers can have a profound influence on an athlete's return to sports participation and even a future career. Following are some important points to remember about treatment.

1. Dislocated interphalangeal joints of the fingers can be reduced on site, but always confirm radiographically the presence or absence of associated fracture.

2. Most injuries of both the hand and fingers involve fractures, sprains, and dislocations that are closed and innocuous in nature.

3. Always study the *alignment* and *rotation* of each digit when examining for acute injury. Malalignment and malrotation can cause significant disability.

4. Mallet finger can result if evulsion of the common digital extension tendon is left untreated.

5. Untreated ruptures and evulsions of the superficial and deep digital flexors can cause similar types of deformities.

6. Immobilization of the digits for any length of time is contraindicated unless absolutely necessary.

7. Rupture of the ulnar collateral ligament of the first metacarpal joint (gatekeeper's thumb) is a common injury occurring in down-hill skiers.

8. When treating a "sprained" wrist, always rule out fracture of the carpal navicular bone. It may be necessary to obtain a second x-ray 7 to 10 days post injury, if symptoms persist.

Chest Wall, Back, and Trunk (5.6 per cent)

When dealing with muscle spasm and low back pain in an exercising individual, always rule out

TABLE 5. **Musculoskeletal Overuse Injuries: A Clinical Guide**

	History	Physical Examination	Pathophysiology	Diagnostic Aids	Treatment	Notes
Grade 1	Transient pain—*after* activity (usually hrs.) "Soreness" (Hx < 2 weeks)	Generalized tenderness	+ Lactic acid Muscle breakdown Minor inflammation	None	± Ice	Look at training regimen "New" athlete "Getting in shape"
Grade 2	Longer-standing pain—*late* in activity or immediately *after* activity (Hx 2–3 weeks)	Localized pain, but not discrete point tenderness	Mild musculotendinous (soft tissue) inflammation	None	Ice ↓ Regimen 10–25%	True overuse Wrong environment Wrong equipment
Grade 3	Pain in *early* or *middle* of activity (getting closer to beginning of activity) (Hx 3–4 weeks)	Point tenderness Percussion tenderness Pressure elsewhere produces pain at point Other evidence of inflammation (heat, erythema, swelling, crepitation)	Major musculotendinous inflammation Periostitis Bone microtrauma	X-ray ± Bone scan ⊕ 75%	Ice ↓ Regimen 25–75% Initial 5–7 day rest period with concurrent NSAID course	"Pre-stress" fracture syndrome
Grade 4	Pain *before* or *early* in exercise preventing or affecting performance (Hx >4 weeks)	All Grade 3 signs plus disturbance in function; ↓ ROM; muscle atrophy	Breakdown in soft tissue Stress fracture Compartment syndrome (especially if swelling is major finding)	X-ray Bone scan ⊕ 95%	Ice Rest from exercise NSAID	Immobilization? Usually not

Abbreviations: Hx = history; ROM = range of motion; NSAID = nonsteroidal anti-inflammatory drug.
(From McKeag, DB: The concept of overuse: the primary care aspects of overuse syndromes in sports. Prim Care *11(1)*:43–59, 1984.)

latent scoliosis. During the adolescent growth spurt, young athletes frequently become tight in the lumbodorsal fascia and hamstring muscles. Flexibility needs to be maintained in this group of muscles. Treatment of low back pain is no different in the exercising patient than it is in the non-exercising patient. Frequent use of Williams' exercise is advocated.

Rib fractures usually present little or no problem but may require the use of a "flak jacket" to avoid further injuries. On clinical examination, check for crepitation or immediate shortness of breath to rule out possible pneumothorax or pulmonary tear.

Blunt trauma to the abdomen will occasionally lacerate one of the internal organs. The most common site is the spleen; the most common cause is splenomegaly secondary to infectious mononucleosis.

Knee (14.8 per cent)

Acute knee injury is usually related to (1) medial collateral ligament sprain, (2) anterior cruciate ligament sprain, affecting the anterior-posterior stability of the knee, and (3) meniscal cartilage tear. The swelling pattern after injury and the biomechanics of the injury itself should tell the practitioner how serious the problem is. Treatment of most collateral sprains involves the use of a knee immobilizer with the knee flexed at 10 degrees. Treatment of anterior cruciate tears initially involves appropriate arthroscopy to delineate the extent of the lesion. Treatment of meniscal tears can be conservative (rest, control of swelling) until a partial meniscectomy can be performed at a convenient time.

Lower Leg and Ankle (32.0 per cent)

Many overuse injuries occur in the area of the lower leg. Ankle injuries usually involve the lateral compartment of the ankle and the following ligaments, listed in order of occurrence: (1) anterior talofibular ligament, (2) calcaneofibular ligament, and (3) posterior talofibular ligament. The Achilles tendon can also be involved. Surgical repair of an Achilles tendon rupture is necessary if the rupture involves an area 2 to 6 cm from its calcaneal attachment. Occasionally, the rupture may occur proximally in the musculotendinous unit, in which case the patient is treated with a long leg cast with the ankle in plantar flexion.

CHRONIC INJURY

Chronic injury is usually secondary to overuse, overconditioning, or overtraining. It is a result of a process, not an event, and based upon two major factors: the period of *time* in which the insult has occurred and the amount of *weight* carried by the person (especially in gravity-dependent sports). Overuse injuries are directly related to lack of adequate patient education or overindulgence by the athlete. Regardless of the type of tissue involved or the location, the process and body reaction are similar, varying only in degree. Examples of soft-tissue overuse injuries include tendinitis (tendon), bursitis (bursa), and tenosynovitis (tendon sheath). An example of hard-tissue overuse is stress fracture. A clinical guide to the treatment of overuse injuries is detailed in Table 5.

Obstetrics and Gynecology

ANTEPARTUM CARE

method of
PETER A. T. GRANNUM, M.D., and
JOSHUA A. COPEL, M.D.

Yale University
New Haven, Connecticut

Prenatal care offers the physician an opportunity to involve patients in true preventive medicine. While the overwhelming majority of pregnancies are without complication, only about half of the prenatal complications that develop overall are in pregnancies identified as "high risk" at the onset. The challenge, then, is to identify problems as early as possible. This is a rewarding opportunity for active intervention and the potential for having an impact on the outcome of pregnancy for mother and fetus.

Antepartum care ideally should begin in the first trimester, as soon as the suspicion of pregnancy has been confirmed by blood or urine assay for human chorionic gonadotropin (hCG).

First Visit

History

Age, Gravity, and Parity. Detailed review of all past pregnancies including spontaneous and induced abortions, ectopic pregnancies, preterm and term deliveries; date and method of delivery; sex and weight of children and their current health status, as well as any medical or obstetrical complications.

General Medical History and Review of Systems. Particular attention to allergies, surgery in the past, family history of medical illnesses, genetic diseases (chromosomal, metabolic, structural anomalies) and multiple gestations.

Exposures. Alcohol, tobacco, prescription or over-the-counter medications, environmental or occupational hazards (radiation, anesthetic gases in operating rooms or dental offices, fumes or chemicals in workplaces), vaccinations.

Physical Examination

This should be performed as per usual routine. We shall comment here on specific changes in pregnancy.

General. Height, weight (pre-pregnancy and current), vital signs (pulse, respirations, blood pressure, and fetal heart).

HEENT. Mild thyromegaly without discrete masses or tenderness is normal in pregnancy.

Respiratory. Occasionally bibasilar rales may be present, which should clear with deep inspiration or cough.

Cardiac. A soft systolic ejection murmur may be present owing to the increased flow of pregnancy-induced volume expansion. A third heart sound may also be present without any abnormality.

Abdomen. Starting in the second trimester, palpation of the liver and spleen becomes difficult owing to upward displacement of the viscera by the uterus.

Extremities. A trace of pretibial edema is frequently present. Reflexes often appear brisk (3 +/ 4); the cause of this is not known. Clonus should not be present, although it may appear in the presence of respiratory alkalosis (i.e., an anxious gravida in labor who is hyperventilating).

Pelvic Examination. The external genitalia may appear enlarged owing to hormonal changes of pregnancy. The vaginal walls and cervix often appear blue (Chadwick's sign) because of the increased vascularity of pregnancy. Cervical ectropion often appears pronounced, and the cervix may be quite friable. This may cause bleeding as a consequence of performing a Papanicolaou (Pap) smear or a bimanual examination. Some clear to white discharge is normal, although yeast vaginitis is common and may be treated with a 1-week course of miconazole (Monistat) or clotrimazole (Gyne-Lotrimin, Mycelex).

On bimanual examination pay particular attention to the consistency, angle, effacement, and dilation of the cervix. Early in pregnancy the cervix should be firm, long, closed, and angled posteriorly. Multiparas in the latter half of pregnancy often have a patulous external os, but the internal os should be closed. Cervical length should be maintained, although there may be some slight early effacement in the multipara.

Palpate the bony pelvis, particularly (1) the "obstetric conjugate" (pubic symphysis to sacral promontory), (2) the bispinous diameter (between the ischial spines), (3) the pelvic sidewalls (to determine if convergent, parallel, or divergent), and (4) the pubic arch. These allow characterization of the pelvis into one of four types (gynecoid, android, anthropoid, or platypelloid) and determination of the clinical adequacy of the pelvis.

The adnexae may be palpated until the end of the first trimester. After that the ovaries should be obscured by the bulk of the uterus. Any palpable ovarian masses should be investigated by ultrasonography. If the mass is greater than 5 cm in diameter or is either solid or multiloculated as determined by scan, removal in the second trimester should be considered. A smaller (i.e., less than 5 cm) cystic mass in the first trimester may represent the corpus luteum, which is essential for progesterone synthesis in the first trimester and should be left intact.

Uterine Sizing

Six weeks—The uterus is only slightly enlarged, but the isthmic portion feels soft (Hegar's sign).

Eight to ten weeks—The uterus is the size of a baseball.

Twelve weeks—The uterus is the size of a softball.

Fourteen weeks—The uterus is palpable just above the pubic symphysis abdominally.

Sixteen weeks—The fundus is half-way to the umbilicus.

Eighteen weeks—The fundus is 2 cm below the umbilicus. Fetal heart tones are audible with the unamplified fetoscope.

Twenty weeks—The fundus is at the umbilicus or approximately 20 cm above the pubic symphysis.

For the next 16 weeks the fundus grows at approximately 1 cm per week. At 36 weeks the fundus approaches the level of the xiphoid. After that, the fundal height may appear to decrease as the head engages in the pelvis.

Laboratory Studies

Initial Laboratory Studies. The following studies should be done for all patients: Blood tests include a complete blood count with red blood cell indices, rubella antibody status, and serologic test for syphilis (RPR or VDRL). Also determine the blood type, Rhesus antigen, and antibody screen (the indirect Coombs' test is important, even in those who are Rh positive, as many minor or "irregular" antigens are known to be potential causes of isoimmunization and erythroblastosis fetalis).

Perform a urinalysis (obtain a culture if there are more than 3 to 5 white cells per high-power field or if patient is a carrier of sickle trait).

Finally, obtain a cervical culture for gonorrhea and a cervical smear for cytology (Pap smear).

Supplementary Laboratory Studies. Whether to do the following studies depends on the ethnic group of the patient. A sickle cell screen is important for all black patients, but sickle cell anemia can also occur in Italians and Greeks. Other hemoglobinopathies should be screened for, depending on the patient's origin (e.g., hemoglobin E in Southeast Asians).

Red blood cell mean corpuscular volume can be used to screen for thalassemias in patients of Italian, Greek, and Southeast Asian origin with significant anemia. Hemoglobin electrophoresis can confirm the diagnosis of parental carrier status for these diseases.

Persons of Ashkenazi Jewish ancestry carry a 1 in 14 risk of being carriers of Tay-Sachs disease, a deficiency of the enzyme hexosaminidase A. Carriers can be detected by blood testing, and fetuses at risk can be detected by amniocentesis.

Miscellaneous

Consanguineous marriages are particularly common among couples from Iran, India, and Lebanon. If this is the case, inquire about skeletal or skin disorders.

All patients except those with sickle cell disease should be placed on supplementary iron, either sulfate or gluconate, sufficient to provide at least 60 mg of elemental iron daily (ferrous sulfate, 325 mg). Those with pre-existing anemia (frequently found in any menstruating woman but particularly in women in lower socioeconomic groups) will require higher doses. Women with sickle cell anemia still require supplemental folate to prevent neurologic complications of folate deficiency. All prenatal patients should receive a multivitamin formulation once a day (e.g., Natalins, Stuartnatal 1 + 1).

Follow-up Visits

Follow-up visits should be scheduled every 4 weeks up to 28 weeks, every 2 to 3 weeks until 36 weeks, and weekly thereafter. At each visit weight and blood pressure should be checked and a dipstick urine test for glucose and protein should be obtained. Evaluate fundal height for appropriate growth and listen for fetal heart tones. During the third trimester, the maternal perception of fetal movement is a good screen for fetal well-being, and if movement appears to be diminished, a formal counting system may provide reassurance (i.e., at least 10 movements per half hour while recumbent after a meal). If decreased movement is confirmed, bioelectric or behavioral assessment of the fetus is in order (see Evaluation of Fetal Status, below).

Serum screening for alpha-fetoprotein (AFP) is performed on all patients at our institution who are enrolled for prenatal care. The screening is done between 14 and 17 weeks' gestation (this may not be routinely available in all areas of the United States). Patients with elevated values should undergo ultrasonography to detect twins, wrong dates, fetal demise, or neural tube or ventral wall defects. In some cases the cause will not be evident on routine ultrasonography, and a level II scan along with amniocentesis for AFP and acetylcholinesterase may be indicated.

Low levels of maternal serum AFP have been suggested to be associated with an increased risk of Down's syndrome (trisomy 21) in the fetus. The relative risk for an individual woman is related to her age and the degree of deviation below the median. As laboratory methodology may influence results, each center must develop its own standards. It is important to know the risk assignment of the laboratory running the specimens and to work closely with a genetic counseling service in order to provide appropriate information to the patient.

Recently, the aspiration of a small amount of placental tissue between 8 and 10 weeks' gestation has become available as an additional means of diagnosing certain types of anomalies. Chorionic villus sampling (CVS) is performed under ultrasound guidance, with 10 to 30 mg of placental tissue being aspirated, which can then be used for chromosomal or biochemical analysis. Preliminary studies have shown it to be relatively safe, although the exact risk of fetal loss as a result of the procedure is currently unclear. Even if the risk is higher than that of amniocentesis, CVS will be preferable for some couples because of the prospect of obtaining results early enough in the pregnancy to undergo termination by suction curettage if an abnormality is found.

Amniocentesis for chromosomal studies is routinely offered at our institution to any woman who will deliver after her 34th birthday (at age 35 the incidence of Down's syndrome is 1 per 143 second trimester amniocenteses). Genetic counseling should be given to these women, in addition to any woman who has previously delivered a child with a chromosomal or structural abnormality.

In the third trimester, at approximately 36 weeks, it is useful to recheck the hemoglobin and hematocrit. Depending on the patient population, a repeat of the gonorrhea culture and the serologic syphilis screen may be performed.

Women who are found to be Rhesus group negative should have indirect Coombs' testing (antibody screen) performed every 6 weeks during the late second and third trimesters. Such women are at risk for development of isoimmunization, even in the first pregnancy. If antibodies appear, careful evaluation with ultrasonography and amniotic fluid bilirubin measurement (optical density at 450 nm) are necessary. We now give all women who are Rh negative and who are not isoimmunized a prophylactic dose of 300 micrograms of Rh immune globulin (RhoGAM) at 28 weeks. This is repeated at delivery if the infant is Rh positive. Some centers are recommending an additional prophylactic dose at 34 weeks. Once the prophylaxis has been given, further antibody screening is unnecessary and may be confusing, as the residual antibody may be detectable for 4 to 6 weeks.

Common Patient Concerns

Diet. The recommended diet in pregnancy is designed to provide needed supplemental nutrition without excess. The total weight gained should be about 10 to 12 kg. "Eating for two" will often result in far more. The diet should contain 70 grams of protein per day, preferably in the form of eggs, cheese, meat, poultry, or fish. About 2400 kcal per day should be included in the diet of the pregnant woman who does not show evidence of carbohydrate intolerance. There is no place for routinely recommending salt restriction, as the kidneys increase sodium clearance in pregnancy, although moderation should be recommended for all patients (including the nonpregnant woman).

Drugs. Unnecessary medications should be avoided during pregnancy, and the prenatal record should include all medications taken. Most patients do not consider over-the-counter medications as drugs. Patients should be advised that these, too, are drugs and should be urged to minimize their use. Appropriate use of mild analgesics warrants special attention, as acetylsalicylic acid (aspirin) near term has been associated with neonatal intracranial hemorrhage. Aspirin is found in many products other than the obvious preparations (e.g., Alka-Seltzer, Midol, Coricidin, any APC product). Acetaminophen (Tylenol, Datril) in moderation appears to be safe.

The effects of other drugs in pregnancy are difficult to ascertain because of the reluctance of patients to admit to illegal drug use. In addition, the tendency of many of these patients to use multiple drugs may obscure specific effects. Heroin is known to cause intrauterine growth retardation and to place the neonate at risk of withdrawal. LSD does not appear to cause fetal chromosomal damage. The most frequent questions from patients center on recreational marijuana and cocaine use. General cautions concerning the exposure of the fetus to any unnecessary drugs should be given.

Smoking. Cigarette smoking is clearly associated with an increase in the incidence of low birth weight infants, due both to prematurity and to intrauterine growth retardation. The latter is independent of maternal caloric intake. Children of smokers are smaller in childhood, do less well when tested at mathematics and reading ability, and are more likely to smoke themselves in adulthood. Deleterious effects of smoking on the fetus are seen with as few as five cigarettes per day. The general health consequences of tobacco smoking are so far reaching in terms of chronic lung and heart disease, cancer, and reduced longevity that every pregnant woman should be urged to use her unborn fetus as additional motivation to eliminate smoking.

Caffeine. When used in moderation, caffeine has not been shown to have any adverse effects on pregnancy outcome in terms of teratogenicity, prematurity, or growth. Drinking less than four cups of coffee per day appears to be safe. Patients with concerns should be aware that tea and cola beverages do contain some caffeine, although less than coffee.

Alcohol. Consumption of alcohol in moderation appears to be safe in pregnancy. Moderation in this case is less than two drinks per day (700 ml of beer, 350 ml of wine, or two mixed drinks all contain approximately the same amounts of alcohol). More than this amount is associated with fetal alcohol syndrome. Patients cannot "save up" their drinks because binge drinkers who average less than two drinks per day but who frequently exceed that amount are still at risk for causing fetal alcohol syndrome, a combination of facial abnormalities, intrauterine growth retardation, and central nervous system abnormalities. While the typical appearance of children with this syndrome includes the presence of a hypoplastic philtrum, a short, upturned nose, and a thin upper-lip vermilion border associated with mental retardation, microcephaly, poor coordination, and small stature, there is not a direct relationship between the amount of alcohol consumed and the effect on the child.

Work. Patients who desire to continue to work may be allowed to do so as long as they wish; however, many appreciate "permission" to stop work at about 32 to 36 weeks. Work should not be strenuous, nor should there be any exposure to toxins, teratogens, or ionizing radiation. If the patient is a health care worker, she should take special care to avoid exposure to TORCH infections (*to*xoplasmosis, *r*ubella [unless known to be immune], *c*ytomegalovirus, *h*erpes).

Exercise. Pregnancy is not a contraindication to moderate exercise. Although there appears to be a transient effect of exercise on the fetal heart rate, this seems to be without clinical significance. Core temperature elevation (e.g., prolonged exposure to hot tubs, saunas, or strenuous exercise without adequate rest periods and hydration) should be avoided in the first trimester, since this may be teratogenic.

Sexual Activity. There is no reason to limit sexual intercourse in the normal pregnancy, although those with threatened abortion in the first trimester or with premature labor should avoid coitus. Rupture of the membranes is an absolute contraindication to coitus. Many couples report decreased frequency of coitus as pregnancy progresses, related in large part to a change in the woman's image of herself.

Evaluation of Fetal Status

Ultrasonography

The routine use of ultrasound remains controversial. The American Institute of Ultrasound in Medicine recommends "prudent" use of ultrasonography in pregnancy and avoiding its indiscriminate use. In the patient who is seen in the first trimester and whose uterine size equals the estimated gestational age throughout the pregnancy, little concrete information will be obtained from ultrasonography in most instances. On the other hand, in those who present with vague dates or who develop size-date discrepancies or high-risk problems such as gestational diabetes or hypertension, an early scan can be invaluable. It remains up to the individual practitioner to gauge the risks for each patient. To date, no confirmed biologic effects on patients or operators at intensities typical of diagnostic ultrasound have been defined. No prospective studies of the usefulness of routine ultrasound screening have been able to demonstrate any impact on perinatal outcome, although it has been clearly demonstrated that congenital anomalies and multiple gestations can be detected with a high sensitivity.

Screening, or Level I, ultrasound examinations may be undertaken for any of a variety of indications (Table 1). The examination should include evaluation of a number of areas (Table 2). More detailed examination should be sought if an ab-

TABLE 1. **Indications for Ultrasound Examination**

Accurate gestational age evaluation
Fetal number
Fetal lie
Fetal weight estimation
Fetal viability
Fetal anatomic survey:
    History of previous anomalous infants
    Maternal teratogen exposure
Size-date discrepancy
Fetal activity (behavioral profile)

normality is suspected. This "Level II" scan should be performed by an experienced sonologist using equipment offering a high degree of resolution, preferably at a perinatal center. Thorough evaluation of fetal anatomy should include assessment of the kidneys, bladder, stomach, and spine. Depending on the clinical picture, evaluation of the craniofacial anatomy or the lengths of the proximal and distal long bones, together with the number of digits on each extremity, may be necessary. Patients with risk factors for the presence of fetal congenital heart disease can now be offered fetal echocardiography as a means of detecting structural cardiac lesions.

Antepartum Fetal Heart Rate Testing

A number of tests of fetal well-being based on the normal periodic changes that occur in the fetal heart rate have been developed. Most rely on external monitors that use continuous wave Doppler ultrasound to measure the fetal heart rate. Normal variations in sympathetic and parasympathetic tone cause the heart rate to accelerate, usually at the same time as fetal movements occur. These accelerations can be reliably seen after the 32nd week of gestation and are recorded by means of a strip-chart device.

Healthy fetuses undergo brief periods of activity alternating with quiescence, lasting about 20 to 40 minutes each. Therefore, observation for 30 to 40 minutes may be necessary to obtain a normal "reactive" tracing (non-stress test [NST]).

TABLE 2. **Standard Antepartum Ultrasound Examination (Level I)**

Fetal number
Fetal cardiac activity (after 7 weeks)
Fetal lie
Placental location
Gestational age assessment by multiple parameters:
    Biparietal diameter
    Long bones
    Ocular diameters
Amniotic fluid volume
Fetal anatomic survey:
    Stomach
    Bladder
    Kidneys

This consists of three accelerations of 15 beats per minute over the baseline rate, lasting 15 seconds each, over a 15-minute observation window. A second channel in the fetal monitor records the presence, duration, and relative intensity of uterine contractions. This information should be obtained in all NSTs, as the presence or absence of decelerations in the fetal heart rate with spontaneously occurring uterine contractions may provide important information about the status of the fetus.

If these accelerations are not present (a nonreactive NST), if spontaneous decelerations are seen, or in selected high-risk situations, further evaluation may be indicated. The contraction stress test (CST) requires three contractions over a 10-minute period, whether they occur spontaneously or in response to small doses of intravenous oxytocin (oxytocin challenge test [OCT] or manual breast stimulation (nipple stimulation CST [NSCST]). If no decelerations in the fetal heart rate are seen, the test is normal (negative). The finding of consistent decelerations with contractions (positive) is an ominous sign, often mandating delivery, whereas decelerations with some contractions (suspicious) require close follow-up with further testing within 24 hours.

Behavioral Profile

Each of the fetal heart rate tests mentioned earlier has been found to be highly sensitive to the presence of fetal distress, but with low specificity. In an attempt to improve the specificity of the diagnosis of fetal distress, Platt and Manning proposed the ultrasound observation of multiple parameters of fetal behavior (biophysical profile). This consisted of a traditional NST, as well as evaluation of amniotic fluid volume, presence of fetal limb and trunk motion, fetal breathing movement, and muscle tone. If each was normal, 2 points were assigned, allowing a total possible score of 10. Some improvement in specificity resulted, although the last is time-consuming, as a skilled sonographer must spend up to 30 minutes with each patient in order to perform the test. However, when the biophysical profile is found to be normal in patients with suspicious fetal heart rate testing, it can provide a great deal of reassurance.

High-Risk Pregnancy

Hypertensive Disorders

(see also later article on Hypertensive Disorders of Pregnancy)

The diagnosis of hypertension in pregnancy is defined as a blood pressure of 140/90 torr or greater, or an increase of 30 torr from baseline in the systolic pressure, or 15 torr from baseline in the diastolic pressure, when found by multiple measurements over at least 6 hours.

When the increase in blood pressure is associated with generalized edema and proteinuria after the 20th week of gestation, pre-eclampsia (toxemia of pregnancy, pre-eclamptic toxemia, PET) is considered to be present. The onset of convulsions (without underlying seizure disorder), blindness, or coma in conjunction with the above findings signals the presence of eclampsia. If the woman enters pregnancy with hypertension, or is found to be hypertensive prior to 20 weeks' gestation without edema or proteinuria, the diagnosis is chronic hypertension. Such patients may develop superimposed pre-eclampsia if proteinuria and edema appear later in the gestation.

Toxemia is a condition that affects primarily nulliparous women, particularly teenagers and women over 35 years of age. Multiparous women with multiple pregnancies, chronic hypertension, diabetes mellitus, renal disease, or fetal hydrops are also at increased risk for the disorder. In all of these groups, the precise etiology of the disease remains obscure.

Since both the fetus and the mother are at risk of complications with the onset of toxemia, careful attention should be paid to its identification and management. The onset of seizures increases perinatal morbidity and both perinatal and maternal mortality. If the diagnosis is made at term, delivery should be undertaken, preferably vaginally as long as the fetal heart rate tracing suggests well-tolerated labor induction. During the interval prior to delivery, seizure prophylaxis should be attained. Historically, magnesium sulfate, administered either intravenously or intramuscularly, has been the medication of choice among obstetricians.

Severe pre-eclampsia may also occur, manifested by diastolic blood pressure above 110 torr, thrombocytopenia, oliguria, elevation of the aspartate aminotransferase (AST or SGOT), epigastric pain, and visual disturbances. These patients should be considered to be severely ill, and management should be undertaken only in con-

TABLE 3. **Classification of Diabetes in Pregnancy**

A: Gestational diabetes only
B: Onset after 20 years old and duration less than 10 years
C: Onset between 10 and 20 years old and/or duration 10 to 20 years
D: Onset before 10 years old or duration over 20 years
F: Nephropathy, regardless of duration
R: Proliferative retinopathy, regardless of duration
H: Cardiac involvement, regardless of duration

TABLE 4. **Cut-off Values for Glucose Tolerance Tests (GTT) in Pregnancy**

Test	Plasma (mg/dl)	Whole Blood (mg/dl)
1 hour GTT		
Fasting	95	—
1 hour	130	—
3 hour GTT		
Fasting	95	90
1 hour	180	165
2 hour	160	145
3 hour	135	125

junction with experienced specialists in maternal-fetal medicine. On occasion, because of prematurity, conservative management of some pre-eclamptics may be considered, but such a course is best followed only in tertiary centers at present.

Diabetes Mellitus

Diabetes in pregnancy is traditionally classified according to the system developed by White, given in Table 3. All pregnant women with risk factors for the development of diabetes in pregnancy should undergo glucose tolerance testing at 28 weeks' gestation. These factors include insulin-dependent diabetes in a first-degree relative, previous pregnancy complicated by diabetes, previous unexplained stillbirth or delivery of a macrosomic infant (greater than 4000 grams), or maternal age over 25 years old. We screen with a fasting specimen and another specimen 1 hour after a 50-gram glucose load. If the screen is abnormal, a 3-hour, 100-gram glucose tolerance test is performed (Table 4).

The proper management of gestational diabetes remains open to some question. A properly balanced 2200 to 2400 calorie American Dietetic Association (ADA) diet with careful attention to the glucose levels obtained throughout the day remains the cornerstone of therapy. We use prophylactic insulin (20 U NPH, 10 U regular insulin every morning) as a means of reducing the incidence of macrosomia. Other outcome variables, such as stillbirths and neonatal hypoglycemia, are not affected by this regimen. All Class A diabetics should undergo intensive monitoring of fetal well-being in the third trimester because of the increased incidence of unexplained stillbirths in this group. Careful assessment of fetal growth will also alert the clinician to developing macrosomia.

Higher classes of diabetics require more intensive monitoring of glycemic control, as all of these patients will need insulin throughout the pregnancy. Euglycemia is particularly important in the first trimester, as the incidence of congenital anomalies rises in women with higher homoglobin A_{1c} levels. Those with vascular involvement (Classes D and above) are at risk of intrauterine growth retardation due to poor placental blood supply, as opposed to the macrosomia seen in other diabetic classes. Any diabetic of Class B or above should be managed in conjunction with a perinatologist or an endocrinologist familiar with such patients.

Premature Rupture of the Membranes

Premature rupture of the membranes refers both to rupture prior to 37 weeks' gestation (preterm ruptured membranes) and rupture prior to the onset of labor. The diagnosis is made by a sterile speculum examination of the vagina. Pooling of fluid in the posterior vaginal fornix is highly suggestive of rupture. The diagnosis is further supported by the finding of an alkaline pH by nitrazine paper testing, although blood, semen, and cervical mucus may cause false-positive tests. The most specific test is the microscopic examination of an air-dried specimen of fluid for the presence of a fern pattern of crystallization.

Management of this problem requires balancing the risks to the fetus of intrauterine infection versus those of prematurity. The optimal approach will vary depending on the gestational age of the infant and the experience of the nursery at each hospital with premature infants. We have found amniocentesis to be a useful adjunct, both for chemical assessment of lung maturity and for microbiologic evaluation by Gram stain and culture. Usually, in the absence of signs of infection, expectant management is employed, with bedrest and strict avoidance of manual pelvic examinations. Close cooperation with those providing neonatal care is necessary to ensure that appropriate resources are present should an extremely premature infant be delivered. In general, referral to a regional perinatal center prior to the onset of labor will result in a better outcome than transfer of a mother in labor or of a sick neonate.

Premature Labor

Premature labor is defined as the onset of labor prior to the 37th week of pregnancy. The incidence of premature labor is between 7 and 10 per cent, depending on the patient population observed. Several factors increase the risk for premature labor (Table 5). Patients found to be at risk should be carefully followed in a High Risk Clinic.

Early Recognition. Early detection of premature labor is the best way of reducing the incidence of complications. Education of both patients and medical personnel about the early warning sig-

TABLE 5. **Risk Factors for Premature Labor**

Previous history of premature labor
Socioeconomic factors
Age <20, >35 years
Prepregnancy weight <50 kg
Uterine abnormalities:
Incompetent cervix
Uterine malformations (septa, etc.)
Prior cervical surgery (cone biopsy)
Infections:
Cystitis/pyelonephritis
Chorioamnionitis
Multiple gestations
Fetal anomalies

nals is vital. These include increased vaginal discharge, lower back pain, and uterine irritability. If any of these signs are present in a patient at high risk, she should be evaluated immediately. Frequent antepartum office visits are also useful, so that increased uterine irritability or subtle changes in cervical effacement, dilation, or consistency may be appreciated at the earliest possible opportunity.

Treatment. Once the patient is in premature labor, the success of treatment is related to the frequency and strength of the contractions and the state of the cervix. In patients whose cervix is closed and whose membranes are intact, hydration followed by the use of beta-mimetic agents, such as ritodrine (Yutopar) or terbutaline (Brethine), is recommended (this use of terbutaline is not listed in the manufacturer's directive). Since these drugs have potential harmful maternal effects (and to optimize neonatal care should delivery become unavoidable), transfer to a regional tertiary care center is recommended. Once the cervix has dilated, treatment protocols are not as successful.

An alternative approach, particularly for the mother with diabetes or heart disease that might become aggravated by the use of beta-mimetics, is the use of magnesium sulfate, which may be given intravenously at a rate of 2 grams per hour. Close attention should be paid to the patient's reflexes and breathing rate if this drug is used.

All patients arriving at the hospital in premature labor should have a sterile speculum examination to check for rupture of the membranes. Only if this is negative should a digital examination of the cervix be performed, unless delivery appears imminent. As cystitis or pyelonephritis may cause premature labor, a urinalysis should also be performed.

As for the patient with premature rupture of the membranes, we have found amniocentesis useful in the management of patients with premature labor. Fetal anomalies such as polyhydramnios due to duodenal atresia or multiple gestation may be found at the preliminary ultrasound scan, accounting for the labor. The fluid obtained can be analyzed for the lecithin to sphingomyelin (L/S) ratio or phosphatidylglycerol to assess fetal lung maturity. We also perform a Gram stain and culture of the fluid to rule out the presence of an occult chorioamnionitis.

Incompetent Cervix

Failure of the cervix to remain closed may lead to second trimester pregnancy loss. The patient typically presents with the feeling of pressure in the lower abdomen accompanied by silent dilation of the cervix. Congenital causes of incompetent cervix are uncommon, but may be present in women exposed to diethylstilbestrol (DES) while themselves in utero. Cervical trauma (e.g., following first or second trimester abortions, precipitous delivery, or difficult forceps delivery with cervical lacerations) may lead to cervical incompetence. Cervical surgery (e.g., cone biopsy) may also cause cervical incompetence in some patients.

Once the diagnosis has been made, a cerclage (a suture placed around the cervix at the level of the internal os) may be inserted to help maintain competence. We prefer to perform this procedure electively at 14 weeks' gestation, after the period of major organogenesis and of maximal risk of spontaneous abortion due to chromosomal anomalies has passed. If the diagnosis is made during the gestation, after the cervix has already effaced and dilated, a stitch can still be placed if the membranes have not ruptured and the cervix is dilated less than 4 cm. Such procedures have a much lower success rate and should not be undertaken if contractions are occurring (i.e., if the patient actually has premature labor). In such late cerclages, we also give prophylactic antibiotics, as the risk of infection is higher. The cervix should be checked weekly throughout the second and third trimesters.

The stitch should be removed either electively at 37 to 38 weeks, to allow the spontaneous onset of labor, or if the membranes rupture or premature labor develops and is refractory to therapy, in order to avoid further cervical trauma from the suture ripping through the cervix.

Isoimmunization

Although the availability of rhesus immune globulin (RhoGAM) has reduced the incidence of rhesus (Rh) isoimmunization considerably, there are still some patients who will become sensitized as a result of (1) failure to give RhoGAM to Rh-negative mothers who deliver Rh-positive infants, (2) failure to give prophylactic RhoGAM at 28 weeks' gestation or after amniocentesis, (3) failure to give RhoGAM after first trimester abortions of ectopic pregnancies, (4) administration of an insufficient quantity of RhoGAM to mothers who have had a large feto-maternal hemorrhage at the time of delivery (the standard 300-ml intramuscular dose is sufficient to counteract a feto-maternal hemorrhage of 30 ml of fetal blood or 15 ml of fetal red cells), or (5) sensitization to other red cell antigens, such as Kell or Duffy.

Once the indirect Coombs' test is positive, the fetus is at risk of developing a hemolytic anemia and subsequent hydrops. The IgG antibody produced by the mother's immune system is capable of crossing the placenta and destroying fetal red cells. Indirect bilirubin is produced as a result and can be detected in the amniotic fluid by spectrophotometric methods. An amniocentesis is necessary to obtain the fluid, and the quantity of bilirubin can be measured via the optical density shift at 450 nm (Delta OD 450) and plotted on gestational age-specific curves developed by Liley. These are broken into three zones: Zone I indicates mild or no disease, Zone II indicates moderate disease, and Zone III indicates severe fetal anemia.

Ultrasonography is a particularly useful adjunct, which allows the diagnosis of hydrops and evaluation of its severity. Signs of hydrops include ascites, pleural and pericardial effusions, skin edema, polyhydramnios, and placentomegaly. Hydrops does not usually appear until the end of the second trimester.

Once the Delta OD 450 is in Zone III, treatment of the anemia is mandated until the risks of the treatment are greater than the risks of prematurity at that particular gestational age. In the past, intrauterine transfusions have been given intraperitoneally, with absorption of blood through the subdiaphragmatic lymphatics. More recently, direct intravascular transfusions have been performed via the umbilical cord. Successful performance of such procedures requires specialists highly trained in ultrasound-guided techniques.

ABORTION

method of
WILLIAM D. WALDEN, M.D.
Cornell University Medical College
New York, New York

Classification

Early first trimester—from the first day of the last *normal* menstrual period through the eighth week.

Simple suction evacuation is most appropriate. No fetal parts are recognizable yet; the best correlation with duration of gestation is measurement of tissue volume.

Late first trimester—9 through 12 weeks. Small fetal parts are revealed on close inspection. The appropriate procedure is suction evacuation followed by sharp curettage when necessary to check for retained tissue or uterine anomalies.

Early second trimester—13 through 16 weeks. Termination either involves removal of the fetus by the D & E (dilatation and evacuation) method or expulsion of the intact fetus by initiating labor with prostaglandin vaginal suppositories.

Late second trimester—17 through 24 weeks. Pregnancy may be terminated by the D & E method, the intra-amniotic instillation of abortifacient agents, or the use of prostaglandin vaginal suppositories. Methods involving the expulsion of the intact fetus are preferred when autopsy or genetic studies are needed. It should be emphasized that the D & E procedures should be performed only by the most skilled and experienced operator.

Diagnosis

The new urine or serum pregnancy tests can detect human chorionic gonadotropin (hCG) at the time of a missed menstrual period or anytime thereafter. If a test is positive prior to the missed period, evacuation of the uterus should be delayed to ensure removal of adequate volume of tissue for examination. These judgments must be correlated with a careful pelvic examination to ensure that the patient did not miscalculate her last menstrual period. A quantitative beta subunit serum test should be performed to verify an initial negative test, suspected ectopic pregnancy, or missed abortion. Serum hCG levels double approximately every $2\frac{1}{2}$ days in early intact viable pregnancies; therefore, a repeat test a few days later is necessary to verify a rise or fall in hCG levels.

Pelvic ultrasonography has its limitations in very early pregnancy; however, a fetal sac is usually seen 6 weeks after the last period. At this time the serum hCG levels should be above 5000 mIU per ml. Between 8 and 9 weeks fetal heart activity can be detected.

Office pregnancy tests with a sensitivity of less than 50 mIU per ml on *random* urine samples (not morning urine) are now readily available. Two such tests are the Abbott TESTPACK hCG urine (Abbott Laboratories, North Chicago, Illinois 60064) and the Access ICON pregnancy test (Access Medical Systems, Inc., Branford, Connecticut 06405).

Each patient should receive counseling and detailed information regarding the procedure in a nonjudgmental atmosphere. The patient should be told that the suction method will enhance her fertility and that the rhythm and withdrawal method of contraception will fail and lead to another pregnancy. In my practice information regarding the "morning-after pill" is given to the patient to avoid a similar situation in the future. It is emphasized, however, that this method of pregnancy prevention is *not* a method to be used for routine contraception but only to prevent an inevitable unwanted pregnancy due to contraceptive failure or ac-

cident. The medication must be taken *within 36 hours* after unprotected intercourse. Conjugated estrogen (Premarin) 2.5 mg four times a day for 5 days is most effective. Prior to prescription of the "morning-after pill" the patient must understand the potential for fetal damage and agree to have an abortion if the medication fails. Once the medication is taken, the next menstrual period should occur at approximately the expected time. It is good practice to tell the patient to inform her doctor when she gets her next period or if she misses her period. In that case, an immediate pregnancy test should be performed and if found to be positive, a termination of that pregnancy should be scheduled.

First Trimester Abortion

Most patients with proper psychologic support will do well with local paracervical block anesthesia combined with diazepam (Valium) 5 to 10 mg intravenously. Local is preferred to general anesthesia because there is less bleeding and less risk of major anesthetic complications.

After the preliminary pregnancy testing, counseling, pelvic examination, and blood studies (hematocrit and blood type) have been performed, diazepam (Valium) is injected intravenously slowly. The effect of the medication is immediate in relaxing the patient.

The preferred instrument for exposure is the *small* Graves speculum. The shorter blades on this instrument permit appropriate traction on the uterus, thereby permitting the fundal cavity to be straightened. This in turn provides relatively easy access with dilators and suction cannula and minimizes the possibility of inadvertent perforation. The medium-sized and large specula should only be used on extremely obese patients in whom visualization of the cervix would be impossible with the smaller instrument.

After the speculum is in place, povidone-iodine (Betadine) solution is poured into the vagina and then thoroughly swabbed dry with sterile $4'' \times 4''$ gauze. A sterile drape under the patient is sufficient for placement of the instruments.

The next step involves injecting a 2-ml dose of 1 per cent lidocaine *without* epinephrine submucosally on the anterior lip of the cervix at the site of attachment of the single-toothed tenaculum. The patient will describe a "pulling feeling" as traction is applied but no pain from the bite of the instrument. Vertical application is preferred to the traditional horizontal position because bleeding will be minimal should the tenaculum tear through the cervix. With a retroverted uterus, application on the posterior lip of the cervix not only serves as a reminder of the position of the cavity but also minimizes the risk of perforation by not tenting the anterior lower uterine segment as the dilators are inserted posteriorly. Off-center application (at 11 o'clock on the anterior lip or 7 o'clock on the posterior lip of the cervix for right-handed operators holding the tenaculum in the left hand) permits easier access through the external os with dilators and curettes.

Completion of the cervical block is accomplished with a 10-ml disposable syringe with a 1½-inch, No. 22 needle. Longer needles are absolutely not necessary and can result in intravascular injection with symptoms of mild systemic toxicity with circumoral paresthesias, voices sounding more distant, and a feeling of fearfulness. With an extremely anxious patient, manipulations during the procedure may cause a vasovagal reaction with momentary loss of consciousness. The treatment is simple—stop the procedure temporarily and elevate the patient's legs 45 degrees. She will regain consciousness almost immediately. This reaction is uncommon, and when it occurs the operator should not overreact by giving unnecessary drugs. Once the patient is awake the procedure may be completed.

Injecting the cervix submucosally at the 2, 5, 7, and 10 o'clock positions should produce a distinct wheal that blanches the cervical mucosa from the original pink to white. Occasionally after completion of the block a patient may still feel excessive pain during dilatation. In such cases an extra 5 ml of lidocaine is injected submucosally within the length of the endocervical canal at 3 and 9 o'clock. This usually eliminates the sensation of instrumentation within the cervix.

Pratt dilators are the instruments of choice because of their long, tapered, balanced structure. Hegar dilators should *not* be used in abortion procedures because they are blunt-ended instruments requiring more force during insertion, which can lead to cervical tears and uterine perforation. The Pratt dilator is held with the thumb and third finger, and the little finger is held out and braced against the patient's buttock in order to avoid use of excessive, uncontrolled force. Firm traction on the tenaculum with the operator's opposite hand is essential to perceive the resistance of the internal os. The tenaculum should never be held by a first assistant, since this eliminates all sense of touch for the operator. *Laminaria* are not used in the first trimester.

The use of a metal sound to measure cavity depth is hazardous in a pregnant uterus and can only increase the risk of perforation. The appropriate-sized cannula with centimeter markings etched in the plastic should be gently inserted into the uterine cavity initially without the tubing attached. The cannula used in this way acts as a sound for determining uterine depth which is far safer than a metal sound. A reliable formula for nulliparous patients is:

$$\text{Cavity Depth (cm)} -2 = \text{No. weeks from last menstrual period.}$$

Example: Uterus sounds to 10 cm
minus 2 = 8 weeks.

The choice of the flexible Karmen cannula or the rigid cannula of Berkeley design is based on the operator's preference and experience. Many prefer the flexible cannula for early first trimester abortions and choose the rigid cannula from 9 through 12 weeks. Once the appropriate-sized cannula is in place, the tubing is connected and the aspirator is turned on. Specifically designed machines for abortions provide suction pressure between 500 and 750 mm Hg. The cannula should be rotated 360 degrees within the uterine cavity to cover all surfaces and withdrawn from the cavity to prevent plugging. With the flexible cannula the proximal opening provides the most effective suction and the distal opening acts as a curette. Special attention should be given to ensure that the proximal opening covers all surfaces within the uterus. An occasional complication with the flexible cannula is the breaking off of the suction tip. Tip inspection should be routine, and if it has broken off it can be retrieved with a curette. Once the uterus has contracted a smaller-diameter cannula may be used to complete the procedure. Occasionally one may misjudge the initial size of the cavity and need to step up to a larger size to evacuate the uterus quickly and efficiently. For example, one may start with a No. 6 flexible cannula and find that one needs a No. 7; then, when the contents have been removed, the operator may return to a No. 6 cannula to insure that all the tissue is out and the fundus is well contracted. The decision whether to use a sharp curette is based on the operator's experience. With increasing experience the use of the sharp curette diminishes. When it is used, the operator should avoid overzealous curetting to prevent postabortal amenorrhea and/or Asherman's syndrome.

The usual duration of applied suction is less than 2 minutes and it is during this time that the patient may experience the most severe cramps. The cervical block does not usually relieve the cramping sensations of the contracting uterus. Patients who have cramps during menstruation will also experience cramps with an abortion procedure.

First trimester terminations with local anesthesia do not require continuous intravenous therapy, or routine use of oxytocin (Pitocin) or ergonovine maleate (Ergotrate). Routine prophylactic antibiotics are not used. In patients with cardiac problems such as mitral valve prolapse or a history of endocarditis, prophylaxis with antibiotics is indicated as recommended by the American Heart Association.

Postoperatively the patient is allowed to rest and is given appropriate analgesic medication either by mouth or by injection to relieve cramping. For mild cramps ibuprofen (Motrin) or its equivalent is adequate. Some patients prefer acetaminophen with codeine phosphate (Tylenol with Codeine No. 3). Patients with severe post-abortal cramping need an intramuscular analgesic. My preference is nalbuphine hydrochloride (Nubain), 3 to 4 mg intramuscularly. An ice bag on the lower abdomen also helps to reduce the discomfort of uterine cramps. Within 10 to 15 minutes all cramps have dramatically subsided. Vital signs are checked, and if the patient is Rh-negative and unsensitized, she receives anti-D immune globulin (MiniRhoGam) intramuscularly. The minidose is used for first trimester terminations only. The usual postoperative recovery time is 40 to 60 minutes.

Prior to discharge the patient's chart should be checked to ensure that written consent for the procedure was obtained.

Written postoperative instructions should include:

1. Telephone number to call in case of emergency.

2. Shower only—no baths for at least 5 days.

3. Use ice bag on stomach for 1 hour at a time to control bleeding or to relieve cramping.

4. Avoid sexual activity, douching, tampons, and strenuous exercise like jogging for about 10 days.

5. Next menstrual period should occur in 4 to 6 weeks. If no bleeding occurs by the seventh week, notify your doctor.

6. Use a thermometer to check your temperature if necessary. If there is a fever over 101° F or heavy bleeding or severe cramping, notify your doctor.

7. No alcoholic beverages today because of Valium injection!

During the patient's recovery period the tissue should be examined after it is removed from the suction bottle. All tissue is sent to the laboratory after inspection. Prior to 9 weeks only tissue volume can provide information regarding duration of gestation. Although volume may fluctuate over a wide range, an easy rule of thumb is:

5 to   6 weeks—average volume 7 ml
7 to   8 weeks—average volume 14 ml
9 to 10 weeks—average volume 21 ml

After 9 weeks identification of fetal parts provides information as to length of gestation.

If no tissue is obtained after inspecting the suction bottle, the following six conditions must be considered:

1. False passage created by overzealous dilatation of a stenotic cervix. Avoidance of forceful dilatation reduces the likelihood of this complication. Mechanical devices to dilate the cervix have no place in this procedure.

2. A nonpregnant uterus with a false-positive pregnancy test.

3. Ectopic pregnancy. Scanty decidual tissue with a volume that does not correlate with the history. A quantitative beta subunit serum test is indicated and should be repeated a few days later.

4. Excessive size for dates. In such a case no tissue may be obtained since the suction tip is too small for tissue retrieval. An error in judgment can occur on pelvic examination with a very obese patient, especially when the abdominal hand is below the fundus in a second trimester gestation. Obviously the reported date of last menstruation is completely wrong.

5. Uterine perforation, most commonly occurring in the severely anteverted or retroflexed uterus.

6. Anomalous uterus (incidence 12 per cent). A septate uterus should be considered after the preceding five conditions have been ruled out. A curette is used to evaluate the anomaly. In rare cases, a uterine didelphys—a double vagina, cervix, and uterus—may be missed since the speculum may compress the septum and hide the second vaginal opening. This is another reason for using the *small* Graves speculum. Once this condition is discovered, suctioning of each cavity is necessary using separate sterile instruments for each cavity to prevent possible cross-contamination with different cervical bacterial flora.

Second Trimester Abortion

Ten per cent of all women seeking pregnancy termination in the United States fall in the second trimester group. A special category exists with women who have received unfavorable reports from genetic studies obtained by amniocentesis. For this group the methods involving expulsion of the intact fetus are preferred in order to perform genetic studies on the fetus. Dinoprost tromethamine (Prostin F$_2$ Alpha) is administered intra-amniotically or dinoprostone (Prostin E$_2$) is administered intravaginally to stimulate the myometrium of the gravid uterus to contract in a manner similar to the contractions seen in the term uterus during labor. The first medication can be used only between the 16th and 20th weeks of gestation as calculated from the first day of the last normal menstrual period. The vaginal suppositories may be administered from the 12th through the 20th gestational week. In addition, they may be used to evacuate the uterine contents in the management of missed abortion or intrauterine fetal death up to 28 weeks of gestation. Both medications are potent oxytocic agents and should be administered only in a hospital by trained medical personnel. Intensive care and acute surgical facilities should be available. Contraindications include hypersensitivity to the drug, acute pelvic inflammatory disease, and active cardiac, pulmonary, renal, or hepatic disease. Caution is advised with patients with a history of asthma, hypotension or hypertension, anemia, jaundice, or epilepsy. Vaginal suppositories have a greater tendency to produce a transient pyrexia that may be due to its effect on hypothalamic thermoregulation. The onset is within 15 to 45 minutes of suppository administration. The elevations revert to pre-treatment levels within 2 to 6 hours after discontinuation of therapy.

Prior to initiating therapy, diphenoxylate hydrochloride with atropine (Lomotil), four tablets, is given to reduce the tendency to diarrhea. Also prochlorperazine (Compazine), 10 mg intramuscularly, is given to reduce the tendency to vomit. The suppositories are administered intravaginally every 2 hours. Fifty units of oxytocin (Pitocin) is added to 1000 ml of lactated Ringer's solution 6 hours after the initial insertion. After a latent period of 6 to 8 hours without uterine contractions the patient begins to experience increasing uterine contractions. Demerol may be used in small doses (25 to 50 mg) intramuscularly to ease the discomfort. Labor must be allowed to continue until expulsion of the fetus occurs into a bedpan. The total time from start to finish can vary from 6 to 27 hours. The average is 12 hours. The placenta is not always expelled with the fetus. It is imperative that the physician be informed immediately that expulsion has occurred, and preferably the physician should be present at the time of expulsion. The patient should be examined without delay and removal of the placenta accomplished by fundal pressure with a medium-sized Graves speculum in place in the vagina. Sponge forceps may be necessary to assist in the removal of the placental tissue from the external os. Bleeding is minimal when the placenta is removed as soon as possible after expulsion. No benefit is gained by waiting. The patient is then returned to her bed. The oxytocin (Pitocin)

dosage is reduced to 20 units in 1000 ml of lactated Ringer's solution and kept running at approximately 1 ml per minute until the next morning. The patient is discharged the following day with the same postabortal instructions as listed above. A follow-up visit within 10 days is scheduled. RhoGam if indicated is given prior to discharge.

The D & E procedure is the most common method of midtrimester abortion in the United States, with labor-inducing techniques accounting for most of the remainder. The more advanced the gestation, the greater is the potential for complications such as excessive bleeding and uterine perforation. Only the most experienced physician should perform these procedures.

Since the D & E procedure requires extracting large fetal parts, it is essential that the cervix be adequately dilated by placement of multiple *Laminaria* tents within the cervical canal 12 to 24 hours prior to the procedure. After insertion, the vagina is packed loosely with two 4″ × 4″ Betadine-soaked sponges. With the use of *Laminaria*, prophylactic antibiotics are given orally, usually tetracycline 500 mg four times per day for 7 days. The seaweed in the Japanese Mizutani disposable *Laminaria* is superior to other products. It is thinner, thus permitting easier insertion into a stenotic cervix. It also swells to as much as ten times its original diameter. Precautions when using *Laminaria* are summarized in Table 1.

All second trimester cases should be evaluated as to size by ultrasonography. On the day of surgery, general anesthesia is preferred. Some important points are:

1. A pelvic examination should be performed with the patient under anesthesia.

2. A weighted speculum is preferred to a Graves speculum in those cases that are over 16 weeks.

3. The *Laminaria* are removed with a sponge stick and *counted*.

4. Thorough preparation of the vagina with Betadine is necessary.

5. A sponge forceps is attached to the anterior lip of the cervix; a tenaculum should not be used.

TABLE 1. **Precautions for Use of *Laminaria***

Do Not
— force insertion of *Laminaria*
— insert *Laminaria* into a purulent cervix
— leave in place more than 24 hours
Do
— instruct patient *not* to douche or have intercourse with Laminaria in place
— reassure patient that slight bleeding and cramping is normal
— allow patient to lie recumbent for 10 to 15 minutes following insertion; this may prevent vertigo, weakness, or syncope

6. The cervix should be evaluated as to adequacy of dilatation by the *Laminaria*. Inadequate dilatation is due to placement of the *Laminaria* below the internal os. For early second trimester cases the use of the large Pratt dilators may be sufficient for additional cervical dilatation.

7. The membranes must be ruptured prior to suction. Any instrument may be used to rupture membranes. Once rupture has occurred, suction with a No. 12 or No. 14 Berkeley cannula should be started only to remove the amniotic fluid at this time (to prevent amniotic fluid embolism). Suctioning should be brief at this point, since one wants to *avoid removing the placenta first by suction*. This is to prevent premature contraction of the uterus and trapping of the fetal parts.

8. Once the amniotic fluid has been drained as much as possible by gentle suction, the Bierer forceps or similar instrument should be gently inserted into the uterine cavity to grasp the fetal parts and extract them. Oxytocin and ergonovine maleate should be withheld until the cranium, spine, rib cage, and all four limbs have been identified.

9. The placenta may be removed by use of suction and curettage after all the fetal parts are out. At this point oxytocin may be added to the intravenous solution and ergonovine maleate, 0.2 mg, given intramuscularly. Estimated blood loss may vary from 300 to 1500 ml.

10. The physician should avoid premature removal of the placenta and premature administration of oxytocic medications, which can cause trapping of the fetal parts.

Postoperatively the patient is observed and cared for as with first trimester cases. The recovery from general anesthesia will be prolonged as compared with recovery from local anesthesia.

The saline method utilizing 20 per cent sodium chloride by transabdominal intra-amniotic injection induces fetal death and is preferred in the late second trimester cases beyond 20 weeks. Hypertonic saline generally causes fewer adverse side effects than prostaglandins; however, the induction interval is much longer. In addition, there is a higher risk of serious complications such as tissue necrosis, infection, defibrination, and hypernatremia.

Complications and Their Management

The postabortal syndrome occurs in approximately 1 in 300 cases. The patient begins complaining of severe uterine pain and cramps, usually within an hour or two following an abortion. Examination reveals a tender midline mass extending two to three fingerbreadths above the symphysis that cannot be relieved either by voiding or by catheterization. Rebound tenderness and guarding may lead one to suspect an acute abdomen and to conclude that surgical intervention is necessary. The correct treatment, however, is immediate resuctioning, which results in the removal of 50 to 400 ml of dark blood and clots

TABLE 2. **Clinical Classification and Treatment of Uterine Perforation During Abortion**

Clinical Classification	Treatment
A. *Immediate recognition with cessation of the procedure* (suspected or actual perforation by any instrument including suction cannula *with no suction applied*)	
1. *Completed abortion.* Perforation after contents of uterus completely evacuated	In-hospital observation of clinical status, serial CBCs, for at least 48 hr.
2. *Intact sac.* Gestation undisturbed	As above, then readmit in about 2 weeks for repeat surgical evacuation.
3. *Incomplete abortion.* Perforation occurs during evacuation; uterus partially emptied.	Immediate diagnostic laparoscopy. Laparotomy and repair if needed. Completion of abortion, either transcervically under laparoscopic observation or, if laparotomy, via uterine rent if transcervical approach inappropriate.
B. *Delayed recognition after operative manipulation* (suction or curettage). No abdominal contents identified. Uterine evacuation may have been attempted before possible perforation was recognized.	All require immediate diagnostic laparoscopy with laparotomy if indicated (bowel trauma, uncontrolled bleeding, etc.)
1. *Completed abortion*	
2. *Intact sac*	
3. *Incomplete abortion*	B.2, B.3: Abortion may be completed as in case A.3.
C. *Perforation with identification of abdominal contents* (bowel, omentum, fat, etc.)	All require immediate laparotomy and surgical repair as needed.
1. *Completed abortion*	
2. *Intact sac*	C.2, C.3: Abortion may be completed as in case A.3.
3. *Incomplete abortion*	

Adapted from Walden W, Birnbaum S: Contemp Obstet Gynecol 15:47, 1980.

with no tissue. This procedure brings immediate relief, and ergonovine maleate, 0.2 mg given orally every 4 hours for six doses, should prevent recurrence of the symptoms. A milder form of this syndrome, which may be delayed for as long as 7 days, is frequently associated with a severely retroflexed uterus. Again, resuctioning leads to a dramatic recovery.

Postabortal amenorrhea is more common than the above complication. Cramping occurs at the time of the expected next menses, but there is no sign of blood. The treatment is simple. Probing the cervix either with a No. 5 Karmen cannula or with a plastic disposable uterine sound will open an internal os in which stenosis occurred secondary to trauma of the aspiration. Once the os is open, dark blood will ooze forth, which represents a menstrual period. Cramping subsides almost instantly.

Delayed complications such as retained placental products, postabortal bleeding, fever, and pelvic infection are all managed by re-exploring and emptying the uterine cavity. Ampicillin by mouth as initial therapy usually is effective. However, failure to respond in 24 hours may require hospitalization and parenteral antibiotics.

Uterine perforation, the most serious complication of either first or second trimester procedures, must be evaluated when one of the following occurs:

1. The stenotic cervix, most commonly seen in very early pregnancy. *Correction*: Firm pressure with a No. 5 Karmen cannula with good countertraction will invariably dilate the cervix, and the flexible cannula will find its way through the cervical canal without the risk of creating a false passage.

2. Physical interference of the weighted posterior vaginal speculum in first trimester cases. *Correction*: Remove and replace with a *small* Graves speculum. Since it is mobile it cannot interfere with placement of the dilators.

3. The acutely anteverted uterus or retroflexed uterus. *Correction*: Direct the dilators in the correct direction with good traction on the cervix.

4. Inappropriate use of the metal sound. *Correction*: Substitute the cannula as a sound with appropriate centimeter markings.

5. Overzealous suction with the rigid Berkeley cannula. *Correction*: Make allowances for the shortening of the uterine cavity as it empties.

6. Improper selection of the suction tip, using one far too big for the size of gestation. *Correction*: Re-evaluate using a smaller cannula.

7. Broken tip on the Karmen cannula. *Correction*: Inspect all tips after each withdrawal from the uterine cavity.

8. Unanticipated shortening of the uterine cavity. *Correction*: Avoid forcing the cannula to its original depth on repeated suctioning.

9. Mid-uterine stenosis. *Correction*: Be gentle and use a smaller cannula to pass through the stenotic area to obtain a true sounding of the cavity. Proceed with caution.

10. Improper use of the sharp curette. *Correction*: Do not force into the uterine cavity.

Table 2 summarizes the management of uterine perforation. The classification is concerned with assessing potential maternal injury and pregnancy status. It can be a useful guide to therapy, particularly in centers where many physicians with varied experience and training perform this operation. It can also help in evaluating patients transferred to hospitals from outpatient facilities.

ECTOPIC PREGNANCY

method of
LESLIE A. WALTON, M.D.
University of North Carolina School of Medicine
Chapel Hill, North Carolina

The frequency of extrauterine pregnancy has increased dramatically over the past several years to an incidence of 1.4 per 100 pregnancies. It is still a major cause of morbidity in women of reproductive age and is the fourth leading cause of maternal mortality, particularly in lower socioeconomic groups.

The etiology of extrauterine pregnancy is multifold. Hormonal imbalance, alterations in tubal motility, altered embryo quality, and migration of the embryo are all felt to be causes of ectopic pregnancy. An alteration in pelvic anatomy and/or tubal architecture is seen in 50 per cent of cases. Consequently, the woman at greater risk for ectopic pregnancy has a history of a previous ectopic gestation, tubal surgery, tubal ligation, pelvic inflammatory disease, or use of an intrauterine device. Ninety-five per cent of ectopic gestations occur in the fallopian tube, with 5 per cent occurring in rarer sites, including the abdomen, ovary, and cervix.

Diagnosis

Suspicion is the first important step in diagnosis of ectopic pregnancy. The combined use of the menstrual history and physical examination coupled with beta human chorionic gonadotropin (HCG) titers and pelvic sonography will enable the clinician to arrive at an accurate diagnosis in most cases.

Classically, the patient gives a history of a missed menses followed by abnormal bleeding 1 to 3 weeks later. Early symptoms of pregnancy such as nausea and breast tenderness may be elicited on questioning. Unilateral pelvic pain is present and can take the form of fleeting twinges or sharp, intense, constant pain. An occasional patient with an unruptured ectopic pregnancy may not relate significant pain. Syncope is a late sign and signifies active intra-abdominal hemorrhage and impending profound hypovolemic shock.

Physical findings of a tubal gestation include unilateral adnexal tenderness and perhaps an adnexal mass on pelvic examination. Distention of the cul-de-sac may be present when there is intraperitoneal hemorrhage.

Laboratory studies may reveal a decrease in the hematocrit and hemoglobin. The majority of pregnancy tests utilized today can detect as little as 50 mIU of beta HCG in urine, and virtually yield a positive result in greater than 95 per cent of pregnancies. Furthermore, the normalcy of early pregnancy can be assessed by using serial assays of serum beta HCG titers. A plateau or decrease greater than 85 per cent of basal value indicates a nonviable pregnancy regardless of site. Serial quantitative beta HCG titers in a normal intrauterine pregnancy should exhibit doubling every 3 days or an increase of 65 to 75 per cent of basal values every 48 hours. Titers should be correlated with clinical and sonographic findings. Sonography will confirm the presence or absence of an intrauterine gestational sac. A sac should be present in normal pregnancy when the beta HCG titer exceeds 6500 mIU. Other sonographic findings that are highly suspicious for tubal gestation include an adnexal mass, free fluid in the abdomen, and a "pseudo sac" in the uterus. If blood is obtained at culdocentesis and the patient has classic physical signs and corresponding laboratory studies, there is a high possibility of ectopic pregnancy with intraperitoneal hemorrhage. Failure to obtain blood does not exclude ectopic pregnancy.

Treatment

The availability of beta HCG titers and pelvic ultrasound have enhanced the earlier diagnosis of ectopic pregnancy. Management in selected cases, therefore, is often less radical than in the past. Laparoscopy is a minor procedure of maximal diagnostic accuracy and provides an option for outpatient treatment of the early, unruptured ectopic pregnancy. Tubal gestations can be treated laparoscopically by linear salpingotomy and/or resection or partial salpingectomy by an experienced laparoscopist. After recuperation, microsurgical tubal anastomosis can be performed. Laparoscopic removal obviates the need for laparotomy and a longer recovery period.

Laparotomy is indicated in cases of ruptured tubal gestations and gestations larger than 2 cm. Conservative therapy in the form of linear salpingotomy, with removal or partial resection with delayed anastomosis, separation with a probe from the fimbriated end and removal, or lastly "milking" through the fimbriated end, can be employed to conserve the tube for future fertility. Complications of the above techniques include persistence of viable trophoblastic tissue and hemorrhage.

Before conservative surgery is performed, a number of considerations should be addressed, including extent of tubal damage, status of the contralateral tube and associated pelvic pathology, desire for subsequent pregnancy, availability of in vitro fertilization and embryo transfer, hemodynamic stability of the patient, and prior counseling about the risk of subsequent recurrent ectopic pregnancy.

Radical surgery involving salpingo-oophorectomy is performed when there is involvement of the tube and ovary with inflammation or when the gestation is ruptured. Salpingectomy might also be possible in the latter situation.

When conservative surgery is performed, the recurrence risk with both tubes remaining is 5 to 20 per cent; it is 15 to 40 per cent with a solitary tube. Approximately 40 per cent will have a term live birth following ectopic pregnancy. Many women who have had an ectopic pregnancy do not conceive again.

VAGINAL BLEEDING IN LATE PREGNANCY

method of
DONALD J. DUDLEY, M.D., and
CARL P. WEINER, M.D.
University of Iowa Hospitals and Clinics
Iowa City, Iowa

Vaginal bleeding during pregnancy not associated with term labor is abnormal and is estimated to complicate 2 to 3 per cent of pregnancies. Blood loss may be life-threatening or of minor consequence. Because even scant vaginal bleeding can be the harbinger of maternal or fetal compromise, careful evaluation to determine the etiology is essential.

Abruptio Placentae

Although premature separation of the placenta (abruptio) occurs in only 0.8 per cent of pregnancies, it accounts for 30 per cent of pathologic third trimester bleeding episodes. The separation may be partial, with minor sequelae, or complete, resulting in fetal death and maternal shock. The perinatal mortality rate from a clinically recognizable abruption approaches 30 to 35 per cent.

The precise etiology of abruptio placentae is unknown. There appears to be an underlying vascular defect in the decidua and uterine blood vessels. Contributing factors include chronic hypertension, preeclampsia, trauma, and chronic vasculitis. Consequently, the fetus of a pregnancy complicated by abruptio is often small for gestational age. A shortened umbilical cord, sudden decompression of the uterus, inferior vena caval compression, and folate deficiency have each been unconvincingly implicated. Demographic risk factors include maternal smoking, multiparity, and, independent of parity, advanced maternal age (older than 35 years). A prior history of abruption is also a significant risk factor. The reported recurrence risk ranges between 1 in 6 and 1 in 18. This risk probably reflects an underlying maternal vascular abnormality.

The degree of bleeding at presentation can be misleading, and the extent of maternal hypovolemia is often underestimated. Hemorrhagic shock may occur without evidence of blood loss (concealed abruption). The uterus contains an average of 2500 ml of blood with a concealed abruption. These patients often require massive quantities of crystalloid and blood products to restore their intravascular volume. However, external blood loss is the norm, noted in 80 per cent of women with a placental abruption. Delivery does not necessarily resolve the problem, as the likelihood of postpartum hemorrhage secondary to uterine atony is greatly increased.

A true disseminated intravascular coagulopathy (DIC) occurs in 13 to 28 per cent of women who suffer an abruption. Maternal DIC resolves quickly once the placenta is delivered. Ischemic damage secondary to both fibrin deposition and blood loss affects those organs with extensive microvasculature: the kidneys (acute tubular necrosis or bilateral cortical necrosis), liver, adrenal gland, and pituitary gland (Sheehan's syndrome). A living fetus associated with abnormal clotting studies is uncommon. An abruption exceeding 50 per cent is inconsistent with fetal survival, and fetal hypoxia secondary to placental insufficiency is common in abruptions less than 50 per cent.

Marginal Sinus Separation

Marginal sinus separation of the placenta is a rather ill-defined cause of third trimester bleeding. The exact incidence is difficult to determine. A circumvallate placenta is a common finding. Some authors consider it a "mild" placental abruption, although, clinically, it differs in that the process is usually self-limited. Mild uterine tenderness may occasionally be present. Because the presentation can be identical to that of an early abruption, these patients deserve careful observation for evidence of extension. Marginal sinus separation is a legitimate diagnosis of exclusion if no obvious cause of a self-limited episode of third trimester vaginal bleeding can be elucidated.

Placenta Previa

Placenta previa is defined as placental implantation such that a portion overlies the cervix. Thus, it precedes the presenting fetal part. A complete or total previa covers the entire internal cervical os. A partial previa covers a portion of the internal os. A low-lying or marginal previa lies in the lower uterine segment adjacent to the internal os. Pathologically, the previa differs from placental abruption only in that pressure from accumulating maternal blood is released through the cervical os and a dissecting head of pressure is

prevented. Not surprisingly, abruption frequently complicates previa. Placenta previa is a dynamic diagnosis. Development of the lower uterine segment has the effect of shifting the placenta cephalad. As a consequence, the diagnosis of placenta previa should not be made prior to 20 weeks' gestation, and only a minority of patients with a previa observed sonographically prior to 30 weeks will have one present at term. An exception is the centrally located previa, which is likely to persist.

Placenta previa complicates 0.5 per cent of pregnancies after 28 weeks and accounts for 20 per cent of third trimester bleeding episodes. Predisposing factors include multiparity, a prior uterine scar, and multiple gestation. The etiology is unknown, but may be associated with defective decidual vascularization. The first bleeding episode can occur as early as 20 weeks, and is rarely profuse. As the cervix thins under the normal hormonal milieu of pregnancy, the chance of an intervillous space becoming exposed increases. Bleeding episodes of increasing severity typically occur every 2 weeks. As with abruptio placentae, the blood lost is maternal.

The maternal-fetal consequences of placenta previa are multiple. There are significant risks for premature labor (10 to 30 per cent), intrauterine growth retardation, and abnormal invasion of the placenta into the myometrium (placenta accreta or percreta). Maternal anemia may result from persistent but low-volume vaginal blood loss. Because of the volume of flow and the lack of resistance, life-threatening maternal hypovolemia and shock secondary to hemorrhage can occur with frightening rapidity.

Labor

"Bloody show" results from the tearing of blood vessels as the cervix thins and dilates. Premature labor is likely the most common cause of third trimester bleeding. Unfortunately, it is often overlooked while the possibility of abruption and previa occupy center stage, thus delaying tocolysis.

Trauma and Cervical Lesions

The cervix is highly vascular and friable during pregnancy. Rupture of cervical blood vessels may occur with minor trauma such as that accompanying a Papanicolaou smear, digital examination, or sexual intercourse. The bleeding is rarely profuse. Cervical polyps, condylomata, and infection of the cervix with *Chlamydia trachomatis* increase the risk of minor bleeding with trauma. Cervical carcinoma occasionally presents as bleeding during the pregnancy and should be ruled out in the absence of another source.

Other Causes of Third Trimester Bleeding

Vasa previa is associated with abnormality of umbilical cord development (velamentous insertion) such that fetal vessels precede the presenting part. Although rare, rupture of a vasa previa results in rapid fetal exsanguination unless delivery is prompt. *Uterine rupture* is a rare but potentially catastrophic cause of third trimester bleeding. The external blood loss is usually mild or moderate in degree. Perhaps surprisingly, pain is not a sensitive finding for uterine rupture.

Evaluation and Management

Evaluation

In the Labor and Delivery Unit. Diagnostic evaluation is highly dependent upon clinical presentation. In most instances, a thorough and orderly evaluation of mother and fetus culminates with identification of the cause. A patient with minimal bleeding, no pain, stable vital signs, and without evidence of fetal distress may be approached less urgently than a woman with hemorrhage or fetal distress.

Upon admission to the labor and delivery unit, the patient is rapidly assessed to provide guidelines for the immediate therapeutic steps. Maternal blood pressure and pulse are taken, keeping in mind that significant blood loss may be clinically obscured during pregnancy because of the accompanying hypervolemia. Maternal hypertension can also mask significant blood loss and be revealed only after the patient has been adequately hydrated. External fetal monitoring should be commenced on admission to display the fetal heart rate pattern and aid the identification of uterine contractions. The amount and rapidity of external blood loss should be assessed by weighing the perineal pads. While maternal and fetal vital signs are obtained, a history is taken and physical examination is done. Pertinent details include an estimate of blood loss prior to admission, onset of bleeding, the presence or absence of pain or contractions, a history of bleeding with a prior pregnancy or earlier in this pregnancy, time of last intercourse, the presence or absence of fetal activity, and history of a prior cesarean section. An abdominal examination is performed to assess fundal height, fetal lie and engagement, uterine tenderness, and the presence or absence of contractions. A digital cervical examination should not be done unless either abruption or preterm labor is the obvious cause of bleeding, or placenta previa has been ruled out.

Concomitantly, a 16- to 18-gauge intravenous line is inserted and infusion of lactated Ringer's solution without dextrose is started. Appropriate blood specimens are drawn for laboratory evaluation, including a complete blood count, electrolyte evaluation, liver function tests, uric acid level, and a type and cross-match for packed red blood cells (depending upon blood loss, usually at least 2 units). A bedside clot tube test should always be done. If the blood clots within 7 to 8

minutes, there is at least 50 mg per dl of fibrinogen. If an abruption is suspected, prothrombin time, partial thromboplastin time, and fibrinogen level are often determined, but these values will usually be normal if the fetus is alive. Many delivery units have their own ultrasound equipment. A level I ultrasound examination quickly narrows the differential diagnosis. In the absence of an ultrasound examination, auscultation of the placental souffle may help localize a fundal placenta. Very heavy bleeding (more than 400 to 500 grams in 1 hour) in the absence of pain is likely to be secondary to placenta previa. If the patient is at greater than 32 weeks' gestation and the uterus is not contracting, a double set-up examination should be quickly performed. If labor is present, tocolysis may be considered.

The clinical picture of placenta previa is typically one of painless bleeding associated with an abnormal fetal lie. The uterus is usually soft but can be mildly irritable, and premature contractions may be present. Fetal distress is unlikely unless maternal shock is present. Ultrasonography is highly accurate for diagnosis but clearly depends upon the skill of the sonologist. The sensitivity and specificity of an ultrasound examination for the diagnosis of placenta previa approaches 95 per cent. Conversely, an ultrasound evaluation for suspected abruption has poor sensitivity and specificity. When performing an ultrasound examination for placental location, one must view the cervix both when the bladder is full and when it is empty. A full bladder can cause distortion and rotation of the uterus such that a previa seems apparent, only to have this image disappear after the patient voids. Use of a vaginal or perineal ultrasound transducer eliminates this problem. The posterior placenta previa is the most difficult to identify sonographically. The finding of a fundal placenta on an early scan all but eliminates placenta previa as a cause of third trimester bleeding.

Placental abruption classically, but inconsistently, presents with uterine pain, tenderness, irritability, and, sometimes, tetany. Separation of a posteriorly implanted placenta may be manifested as severe, low back pain. Baseline uterine tonus is usually elevated, and this may be determined either by palpation or by an internal pressure catheter. Abruption is an emergency and its diagnosis demands a decision, if only for close observation. An internal fetal monitor should be placed once the diagnosis is made for all but mild separation in a very preterm pregnancy. The incidence of fetal distress and intrauterine demise is directly related to the length of the delay from diagnosis to delivery. The diagnosis of a mild abruption can be difficult. As long as there is no maternal or fetal distress, conservative management while the final diagnosis is determined is indicated.

After excluding abruption and previa, a gentle speculum examination of the cervix and vagina should be done to observe for polyps or other gross lesions and to perform a Papanicolaou smear and cervical cultures. A speculum examination is probably safe even if a placenta previa is present, but catastrophic bleeding can occur should the cervix be inadvertently manipulated. For this reason, speculum examination prior to ultrasonography is best avoided unless ultrasound equipment is unavailable or premature labor seems likely.

In the Outpatient Setting. Often a patient reports having spotted days or weeks prior to an outpatient visit and not since. A history and physical examination are done as described earlier, although with less urgency. After placenta previa has been excluded, speculum and digital examinations may be done. Often, these episodes of bleeding result from coital trauma or have no other obvious contributing cause.

Management

The management of premature labor is discussed in another article in this section. The ultimate decision to deliver the patient with either a previa or an abruption is based on similar rationale. If there is no evidence of impending maternal or fetal compromise, the blood loss is low (less than 50 to 100 grams per hour), and the etiology is previa or mild abruption, then conservative management of a pregnancy of 32 weeks' gestation or less is advocated. If labor is present, successful tocolysis often results in a slowing or cessation of blood loss. Delivery is indicated regardless of gestational age if there is (1) fetal distress as determined by external or internal fetal monitoring, (2) maternal hypovolemia or shock, or (3) evidence of other maternal compromise (e.g., DIC). The question that should always be considered and ultimately answered is "Is the fetus better off delivered or in utero?"

Gestational age and the type of previa determine the course of action. For a gestation with sure dates at 37 weeks and a central previa, primary cesarean section is indicated. For a previa other than complete or central, an elective double set-up examination should be delayed if possible. The longer gestation continues, the greater the likelihood of successful amniotomy at time of double set-up. If the gestational age is less than 34 weeks and the patient is having contractions, we initiate tocolysis using magnesium sulfate. There is no evidence that tocolysis worsens bleeding, but contractions do. Attempts

at tocolysis are discontinued when the patient reaches 34 weeks' gestation. Ritodrine has not generally been used in this situation because of the theoretic risk of increased hypotension and decreased placental perfusion should bleeding occur. However, recent animal studies fail to identify any added risk of beta-mimetic use after hemorrhage.

The prognoses for both mother and fetus of a pregnancy complicated by previa have improved dramatically with expectant management. Maternal death from excessive bleeding is rare. The fetal mortality rate is 10 per cent and is usually the result of prematurity.

Abruptio Placentae. Prompt delivery for all women with a clinically evident abruption is *not* appropriate, but the number of exceptions are few. Patients with a marginal sinus separation are managed expectantly. Obviously, if there is evidence of severe abruption, tetany, or fetal distress, then cesarean section should be performed if the fetus is viable. If the diagnosis of abruption is clinically firm, then delivery is indicated in almost all instances, and an amniotomy should be performed. It is generally felt that decompression of the uterus allows the fetus to tamponade the separating segment.

For a suspected mild abruption in which the fetal heart rate is without ominous or periodic decelerations, the fetus is appropriately grown, the gestation is greater than 32 weeks, and contractions are occurring, then tocolysis with magnesium sulfate may be initiated. There is no evidence tocolysis extends the abruption, but contractions certainly do. Close observation in the labor and delivery unit is mandated. Should evidence of extension be noted, then tocolysis should be stopped and delivery effected. If tocolysis is successful and there is no evidence of extension or maternal or fetal compromise, the patient should be observed closely on the antepartum unit. Initially, nonstress testing is performed every day.

If the fetus is dead, then vaginal delivery is the treatment of choice. Fetal demise has usually occurred if DIC is present. Vaginal delivery is preferred to avoid the dangers of an abdominal operation in a patient with a coagulopathy.

In women with severe abruption and heavy bleeding, close monitoring of vital signs and urine output is indicated. A central line (a Swan-Ganz line preferably) is helpful. Massive fluid resuscitation, including multiple units of packed red blood cells and fresh frozen plasma, may be required.

Placenta Previa. After the diagnosis of a symptomatic previa, the patient is placed at bed rest in the hospital (acknowledging the likelihood of poor compliance at home). Maternal and fetal vital signs are determined at least three times a day. All vaginal bleeding is weighed. Nonstress fetal heart rate testing is performed semiweekly after 25 weeks' gestation, and periodic fundal height measurements and ultrasound examinations (every 3 to 4 weeks) are made to confirm appropriate fetal growth. A complete blood count is done weekly to detect a developing anemia. A current type and screen is not necessary while the patient is hospitalized unless the blood bank does not have the resources to prepare blood for transfusion within 30 minutes. A screen of the mother for atypical antibodies that might delay the cross-match is important. Continuous intravenous access is not necessary unless the patient is bleeding.

The diagnosis of placenta previa other than one centrally placed should ultimately be confirmed at the time of delivery by a double set-up examination, unless fetal malpresentation precludes vaginal delivery. The patient is prepared fully for cesarean delivery. A gentle speculum examination is performed. If this is normal, a digital vaginal examination is done by feeling first the posterior, then the anterior vaginal fornices for the station of the presenting part and for either a vascular thrill or the spongy resistance of the placenta. At no time should the examining finger be inserted through the cervix if placenta is felt in the fornices. If placenta is not felt, effacement and dilatation of the cervix should be assessed. If placenta is palpated and its location precludes amniotomy, then delivery is effected by cesarean section.

Cervical Lesions. Any venereal disease should be treated appropriately and reported to the health department. Penicillin is used for gonorrhea, and erythromycin for chlamydial infections. Use of tetracycline is contraindicated in pregnancy because of fetal teratogenicity. Condylomata may be safely treated during pregnancy by cryotherapy or laser therapy. Colposcopy with appropriate biopsy studies without endocervical curettage is recommended for any lesion or dysplastic Papanicolaou smear. We generally do not recommend cone biopsy unless invasive cancer is a significant possibility. If early stage invasive cancer is discovered, then a cesarean radical hysterectomy should be performed. Definitive treatment may be delayed until fetal lung maturity is present. The timing of this must be discussed with the patient, as she needs to be fully aware of the risks of delaying therapy.

HYPERTENSIVE DISORDERS OF PREGNANCY

method of
MARSHALL D. LINDHEIMER, M.D., and
ADRIAN I. KATZ, M.D.*
*University of Chicago Medical School
Chicago, Illinois*

In 1974 we were privileged to contribute to the 26th edition of this text edited by the late Dr. Howard F. Conn. At that time data concerning hypertension in pregnancy were scarce, and opinions on management diverse and discordant. Since then advances in perinatal care have materially reduced the number of serious complications associated with high blood pressure during gestation. Still, high blood pressure in pregnancy remains a major cause of maternal and fetal morbidity and mortality, and substantial controversies remain, particularly concerning therapy. We will summarize the status of the hypertensive disorders in gestation as of 1988, focusing on preeclampsia, as well as on our preferred management regimens, especially of acute hypertension near term.

Incidence, Pathophysiology, and Clinical Manifestations

High blood pressure complicates almost 10 per cent of all pregnancies; the incidence approaches 20 per cent if the women are nulliparous and 50 per cent if they carry multiple fetuses. These figures may even be underestimates, as many physicians fail to take into account that the upper limits of normal blood pressure in pregnancy are lower than those for nonpregnant women. Blood pressure starts to decrease soon after conception, diastolic levels reaching 10 mm below prepregnancy values by midtrimester, after which levels increase slowly and approach preconception values near term. Epidemiologic surveys indicate that gestations are at risk when diastolic levels are only 75 mmHg in the second trimester and 85 mmHg in the third trimester, values considered normal in nongravid women. Although pregnant women manifesting these levels do not require immediate intervention, they must be placed in a high risk category and monitored closely throughout gestation.

Classifications of the types of high blood pressure in pregnancy are multiple, and are a source of confusion. We use the classification recommended by The American College of Obstetricians and Gynecologists, which is both sound and concise. Hypertensive gravidas are considered as having elevated blood pressure in one of four categories:

   I. Preeclampsia—eclampsia
   II. Chronic hypertension (of whatever cause)
   III. Chronic hypertension with superimposed preeclampsia
   IV. Late or transient hypertension

*This work is supported by grants from the National Institutes of Health (HD 24498) and the American Heart Association.

Categories I and III represent the greatest danger for the fetus, and are associated with life-threatening maternal syndromes. Women in the second category are primarily those with essential hypertension, who usually do well. However, in rare instances of hypertension secondary to such diseases as pheochromocytoma, scleroderma, and periarteritis, the mother is at considerable risk. The former disease can be managed with alpha- and beta-adrenergic blockade, but pregnancy termination is advisable in women with the collagen diseases mentioned.

Late or transient hypertension (category IV) is a fairly benign disorder, characterized by mild to moderate elevation of the blood pressure in the third trimester, which returns to normal during the first 10 days of the puerperium. Women in this category often have recurrence of hypertension in subsequent gestations, and it appears that they are destined to develop essential hypertension later in life. Because the preeclamptic syndromes and essential hypertension comprise over three fourths of the hypertensive complications during gestation, the remainder of this article focuses on the presentation, pathophysiology, and management of these diseases.

PREECLAMPSIA-ECLAMPSIA

This disease is peculiar to pregnancy, occurs primarily in nulliparas, usually after the 20th gestational week, and most frequently near term. The earlier the onset, the less likely it is that one is dealing with pure preeclampsia, but rather it is probable that there is underlying essential hypertension, or a renal disorder with superimposed preeclampsia. In preeclampsia the high blood pressure is associated with proteinuria, edema, and, at times, coagulation or liver function abnormalities (or both). This disease can progress rapidly to a convulsive phase, eclampsia, which is a dramatic and life-threatening event. The eclamptic convulsion is usually preceded by premonitory symptoms and signs, including headache, epigastric pain, hyperreflexia, and hemoconcentration, but convulsions may appear suddenly in a seemingly stable patient whose blood pressures are only mildly elevated. Therefore, we believe that the practice of categorizing preeclampsia as "mild" or "severe" has limited usefulness (the latter is defined as diastolic and systolic levels of 110 and 160 mmHg or greater, and heavy proteinuria). Because a young gravida with diastolic levels of only 90 to 95 mmHg may rapidly progress to eclampsia, the appearance of de novo third trimester hypertension in a nullipara, even in the absence of other signs, is sufficient reason to suspect preeclampsia and hospitalize the patient.

One should also be aware of a special form of preeclampsia whose clinical appearance may be misleadingly benign. The patient presents with minimal changes in platelet counts and liver function, almost no evidence of hypertension, and little or no proteinuria, so that the physician may be tempted to temporize and observe the patient in the clinic or office. Such patients, however, can rapidly progress to a syndrome characterized by hemolysis and marked signs of both liver dysfunction and coagulation changes. The bilirubin level may rise and transaminase levels increase to values exceeding 1000 U, whereas platelet counts often decrease below 40,000 per microliter and evidence of microangiopathic hemolysis is present on the blood smear. This uncommon form of preeclampsia has been given the acronym HELLP (*H*emolysis, *E*levated *L*iver enzymes, and *L*ow *P*latelet count) and constitutes a medical emergency. Although most patients survive with supportive care, the abnormalities abating 2 to 7 days after evacuation of the uterus, there have been maternal deaths associated with this syndrome, in some instances owing to failure to appreciate the severity of the situation at an early stage.

There is also an entity called *late postpartum eclampsia* (hypertension and convulsions occurring days to weeks after delivery). In some instances, this disorder has been mimicked or elicited by the administration of bromoergocryptine (Parlodel), a drug used to suppress lactation.

Pathophysiology. Hypertension in preeclampsia is characteristically labile when compared with gestational high blood pressure of other causes. This reflects the intense sensitivity of the vasculature to endogenous pressor peptides and catecholamines and represents a reversal of the markedly increased resistance to angiotensin II characteristic of normal pregnancy.

The glomerular filtration rate (GFR) decreases in preeclampsia, partly because of the swelling of intracapillary glomerular cells. Nonetheless, since GFR normally increases in pregnancy, it is often still at, or above, nongravid levels. However, creatinine levels exceeding 1 mg per dl already signal substantial kidney involvement. The increase in protein excretion is usually mild or moderate, but preeclampsia is the major cause of nephrotic-range proteinuria in gestation. In essence, heavy proteinuria and hypertension are most likely due to preeclampsia rather than to another renal disease.

The ability to excrete sodium is also decreased in preeclampsia, but the degree of impairment varies, and very severe disease can occur in the absence of edema. It is important to recognize that even when interstitial edema is present, plasma volume is decreased and hemoconcentration occurs. Furthermore, it appears that the decrement in volume precedes the occurrence of hypertension, and that cardiac output and central venous and pulmonary wedge pressures are low and seem to vary inversely with the severity of the disease. These facts combined with the compromised placental perfusion that also accompanies preeclampsia are the major reasons we discourage the use of diuretics in the treatment of preeclampsia.

Finally, there are disagreements concerning the incidence and importance of clotting abnormalities in preeclampsia and the role of prostaglandins in this pathophysiologic manifestation of the disease. Nevertheless, several encouraging recent reports indicate that antiplatelet or antithromboxane therapy with low-dose aspirin can prevent preeclampsia if started early in pregnancy.

Management

Women in whom preeclampsia is suspected should be hospitalized, an approach that diminishes the frequency of convulsions and other consequences of diagnostic error and enhances fetal survival.

Paradoxically, this approach is cost effective, as in-hospital care delays termination of pregnancy, reducing the high cost incurred by very premature infants in intensive care nurseries. Near-term induction of labor is the treatment of choice, whereas temporization with intensive monitoring of the gravida may be attempted if the pregnancy is at an earlier stage. Under such circumstances several antihypertensive agents that are safe and effective in pregnancy are available. If, however, severe hypertension persists following 24 to 48 hours of treatment, delivery is indicated regardless of the stage of gestation, since the mother is at risk and further delays rarely save the fetus; most infants weighing 1500 grams or more fare better in a premature nursery than in the womb of a woman with preeclampsia. (Survival of infants weighing 1000 to 1500 grams is also quite satisfactory in good neonatal units.) Clotting or liver function abnormalities, decreasing renal function, and signs of impending convulsions (headache, epigastric pain, and hyperreflexia) are indications for termination of the pregnancy, as is, of course, evidence of fetal jeopardy detected by electronic monitoring or ultrasonographic demonstration of severe growth retardation.

Treatment of the Acute Hypertensive Crisis. Authorities disagree on how aggressively they should try to lower the blood pressure when acute hypertension occurs near term. Some are concerned that large, precipitous decrements in

mean arterial pressure jeopardize the fetus because placental perfusion is already compromised in many preeclamptic patients. This view is supported by documented instances in which sudden reductions in blood pressure were accompanied by signs of fetal distress even when diastolic levels remained at or above 80 mmHg. We feel that a moderate approach is the best (Table 1). Antihypertensive medications are withheld as long as maternal diastolic blood pressure is below 105 mmHg. Otherwise, parenteral hydralazine is administered cautiously and is successful in most instances. Diazoxide is also useful in the occasional patient whose condition is resistant to hydralazine therapy and should be administered in small doses (30-mg boluses). Calcium channel blockers are currently undergoing extensive testing following encouraging preliminary observations. Although there have been anecdotal reports of success with sodium nitroprusside, this drug should be avoided as fetal death and cyanide poisoning have been noted in laboratory animals. Parenteral labetalol and clonidine are used at some centers outside the United States.

Use of diuretics to treat acute hypertension in pregnancy is inappropriate because hypovolemia and decreased cardiac output are present in many of these patients, and because of evidence that preeclamptic women treated with diuretics have experienced intrapartum hypotension and puerperal vascular collapse. Likewise, we do not rec-

TABLE 1. **Guidelines for Treating Severe Hypertension Near Term or During Labor**

The degree to which blood pressure should be decreased is disputed. Levels between 90 and 105 mmHg diastolic are recommended (see text).

Drug therapy

Parenteral hydralazine is the drug of choice. Use low doses (start with 5 mg, then give 5 to 10 mg every 20 to 30 minutes) in order to avoid precipitous decreases. Side effects include tachycardia and headache. Neonatal thrombocytopenia has been reported.

Diazoxide is recommended for the occasional patient whose hypertension is refractory to hydralazine. Use 30-mg miniboluses, since maternal vascular collapse and death have been associated with the customary 300-mg dose. Side effects include arrest of labor and neonatal hyperglycemia.

Do not use sodium nitroprusside (fetal cyanide poisoning has been reported in animals), ganglion-blocking agents (meconium ileus has been reported), or loop diuretics (e.g., furosemide). (However, in the final analysis, maternal well-being will dictate the choice of therapy.)

Parenteral magnesium sulfate is the drug of choice for preventing impending eclamptic convulsions. Therapy should continue for 12 (and sometimes 24) hours into the puerperium, since one third of patients with preeclampsia have convulsions after childbirth.

From Lindheimer MD, Katz AI: Current concepts: Hypertension in pregnancy. N Engl J Med 313:675–680, 1985.

TABLE 2. **Antihypertensive Drugs in Pregnancy**

α₁-Receptor agonists	Methyldopa (0.5 to 3 g per day) is the most extensively used drug of this group in the United States; its safety and efficacy have been supported in randomized trials. Neonatal tremors have been reported; other side effects are the same as in the nongravid population. Clonidine appears equally effective, but embryopathy has been described in animals.
β-Receptor antagonists	These agents have undergone considerable testing and appear to be safe and efficacious. Atenolol (50 to 100 mg per day) and metoprolol (50 to 225 mg per day) are used most frequently to date. Small for date infants and fetal and neonatal bradycardia and hypoglycemia have been reported; animal data suggest the possibility of a decreased ability of the fetus to tolerate hypoxic stress.
α- and β-Receptor antagonists	Labetalol appears to be as effective as methyldopa. A possible association with retroplacental hemorrhage is under investigation.
Arteriolar vasodilators	Hydralazine (50 to 200 mg per day) is used frequently as adjunctive therapy with methyldopa and β-receptor antagonists. There has been only fragmentary experience with minoxidil, which is thus not recommended.
Converting-enzyme inhibitors	Captopril, which causes fetal death in several animal species, has been associated with renal failure in the newborn human. Do not use in pregnancy.
Diuretics	Most authorities discourage their use, though some continue these medications if they were prescribed before gestation. We would consider prescribing diuretics when blood-pressure control is poor despite the use of other agents, the fetus is immature, and pregnancy termination is the only alternative.
Miscellaneous	Calcium-channel blockers and serotonin antagonists (e.g., ketanserin) are currently under investigation. Do not use ganglion-blocking agents or nitroprusside.

Modified from Lindheimer MD, Katz AI: Current concepts: Hypertension in pregnancy. N Engl J Med 313:675–680, 1985.

ommend the use of volume expansion in preeclamptic patients, especially with crystalloid solutions. Myocardial performance may be compromised in severe cases, and volume expansion (especially with saline) may further enhance vascular reactivity. More important, the infusion of crystalloid alone decreases oncotic pressure (already markedly decreased in preeclampsia). This can lead to pulmonary and cerebral edema, especially after delivery, when plasma oncotic levels decrease further while central volume and pressure tend to rise. We aim to maintain infusions at rates less than 75 ml per hour, as oliguria and apparently poor renal perfusion usually resolve quickly post partum.

Magnesium sulfate is the therapy of choice in North America for impending convulsions and frank eclampsia. The regimen in use at the University of Chicago Lying-in Hospital consists of a loading dose of 4 to 6 grams of magnesium sulfate in a 10 per cent solution *infused over a 10-minute period* (never as a bolus), after which a sustaining solution (24 grams magnesium sulfate per liter of 5 per cent dextrose in water) is delivered at a rate of 1 gram per hour. Blood levels of magnesium are monitored and are maintained between 5 and 9 mg per dl. The infusion rate may be increased to 2 grams per hour if the patient remains hyperreflexic or if the plasma magnesium level remains below 5 mg per dl. Treatment usually continues for 12 to 24 hours post partum because one third of women convulse after delivery. Deep tendon reflexes are also monitored, and calcium gluconate should be kept at the bedside for the sudden appearance of magnesium toxicity, which can lead to cardiorespiratory arrest.

Special Situations. Monitoring of central venous and pulmonary capillary wedge pressures may be necessary in severe or complicated cases, especially during operative procedures. In our experience, the need for insertion of a Swan-Ganz catheter (a procedure that has a certain morbidity) in preeclampsia is uncommon, and most patients can be managed with good clinical acumen. Patients with marked coagulation changes and severe right upper quadrant pain should be considered for ultrasonographic examination or (postpartum) computed tomographic scanning of the liver, which may reveal unsuspected subcapsular hemorrhages that can rupture and produce an acute emergency.

ESSENTIAL HYPERTENSION UNCOMPLICATED BY PREECLAMPSIA

Most women with essential hypertension alone (85 per cent of hypertensive gravidas) have uncomplicated and successful gestations. The gravida with essential hypertension has a greater propensity to develop superimposed preeclampsia, which in severe cases (fortunately a minority) may lead to placental abruption, acute renal tubular or cortical necrosis, and cerebral vascular accidents. Such complications seem to correlate with age (increased risk after 30 years), the duration of high blood pressure, and prepregnancy evidence of end-organ damage.

Women with essential hypertension often experience reductions in blood pressure during the first two trimesters that may exceed those observed in normotensive gravidas. Failure of this decrement to occur or increases in blood pressure during the early or midtrimester portend a guarded prognosis concerning the patient's ability to complete the gestation successfully.

Management

There is controversy about whether women with chronic hypertension who have only mild blood pressure elevations should be treated during pregnancy. We do not initiate therapy until diastolic levels exceed 90 mmHg in midtrimester and 95 mmHg in the third trimester, and may even wait for levels of 95 and 100 mg, respectively, in selected cases. The use of various antihypertensive drugs in pregnancy is summarized in Table 2. Currently, methyldopa, on occasion combined with hydralazine, is the drug of choice in North America. However, several beta-adrenoceptor agonists, and the combined alpha- and beta-blocking agent labetalol, which are now undergoing protracted testing overseas, are gaining increasing acceptance. These drugs also have the advantage of requiring once or twice daily dosing, thus facilitating patient compliance.

OBSTETRIC ANESTHESIA

method of
BETTYLOU K. MOKRISKI, M.D.
University of Maryland Medical School
Baltimore, Maryland

All drugs have direct and indirect effects on the fetus. After crossing the placenta, drugs or their metabolites may directly affect the fetus. For example, the neonatal respiratory depression caused by narcotics is a direct effect. Drugs cause indirect effects by changing the uteroplacental perfusion. Decreases in uteroplacental perfusion pressure (such as lowering maternal mean arterial pressure) or increases in uteroplacental vascular resistance (such as increases in myometrial tone) decrease uteroplacental blood flow. Decreases in uteroplacental perfusion may cause decelerations or loss of variability in the fetal heart tracing. Some drugs may have both direct and indirect effects. Combined effects complicate the interpretation of studies done to investigate the effects of drugs on neonates.

Factors Governing the Transfer of Drugs

Anesthetic drugs generally cross the placenta by diffusion. Fick's law defines diffusion across the placenta:

$$Q/T = \frac{KA(C_m - C_f)}{D}$$

Fick's law applies to both maternal-to-fetal transfer and fetal-to-maternal transfer. The amount of drug diffused per unit time (Q/T) is directly proportional to the difference between maternal and fetal drug concentrations ($C_m - C_f$), which defines the diffusion gradient. Increases in drug diffusion can occur with increased maternal or decreased fetal "free" drug concentration. Only "free" drug diffuses, not that bound to serum proteins. Maternal and fetal metabolism, protein binding, and excretion of drugs also affect the "free" drug concentration in their respective compartments. K is the drug constant, whose key factors are molecular weight, degree of ionization, and lipid solubility. A is the area for transfer and D is the distance across the membrane. Transfer increases with increasing lipid solubility and decreases with increasing molecular weight.

All local anesthetics and narcotics commonly used in obstetric analgesia/anesthesia have molecular weight less than 500 daltons. The degree of ionization is described by the pKa. The pKa is the pH at which 50 per cent of a drug is nonionized (the only form that can diffuse across a membrane). The pKa of commonly used local anesthetics ranges from 7.7 for lidocaine (Xylocaine) to 9.1 for 2-chloroprocaine (Nesacaine). The pKa for bupivacaine (Marcaine) is 8.1. The closer the pKa is to physiologic pH, the more drug is nonionized and can easily cross the placenta. At physiologic pH 35 per cent of lidocaine is in the nonionized form and 20 per cent of bupivacaine is able to cross the placenta. Q/T is also proportional to the area of the membrane. As the area for diffusion increases or the distance or thickness decreases, more diffusion occurs.

Ion trapping can occur in an acidotic fetus. Local anesthetics may be trapped on the fetal side of the placenta by ionization. Ionized particles do not pass through the placenta. As the molecules available for diffusion are decreased by ionization, the "free" drug concentration in the fetus decreases, allowing more drug accumulation in the fetus.

Indirect Drug Effects

Oxytocin (Pitocin) has indirect effects on the fetus. Increased strength or frequency of uterine contractions may decrease the uteroplacental perfusion below critical levels in a pregnancy with marginally compensated uteroplacental perfusion. Unintentional intravenous administration of large amounts of local anesthetic can also increase uterine tone. Intravenous ketamine (Ketalar) in doses greater than 1.5 mg per kg also increases uterine tone. Uterine artery tone is increased by alpha-adrenergic stimulation. Although the uterine arteries are maximally dilated at term, endogenous catecholamines, as stimulated by maternal pain, may lead to vasoconstriction and decreased uteroplacental perfusion. Hyperventilation associated with pain may also cause a direct uterine artery vasoconstriction thought to be related to decreases in maternal arterial CO_2 tension.

Neonatal Evaluation

Assessment of fetal well-being is necessary to properly evaluate the effects of therapeutic interventions. The common use of electronic cardiotachography has created awareness of the fetal heart rate changes that suggest loss of fetal well-being. Late decelerations and loss of beat-to-beat variability are interpreted as signs of fetal distress. Fetal capillary scalp pH is another method of intrapartum assessment. A scalp pH of less than 7.20 generally indicates fetal metabolic acidosis, while a pH greater than 7.25 signifies fetal well-being. A scalp pH that falls between the two values generally indicates a fetus that requires re-evaluation within 20 minutes. Umbilical cord artery and vein blood gases are used to assess the neonatal intrauterine acid-base status at delivery. Normal umbilical cord gases (Table 1) suggest lack of intrapartum asphyxia. Apgar scoring of the neonate, while commonly performed, does have limitations in the assessment of newborns with anesthetic effects.

Neurobehavioral studies of the neonate have been used to evaluate more precisely the sometimes subtle effects of anesthetics on neonatal behavior. The correlation among various methods of evaluation is high. Neurobehavioral evaluations are also routinely used to evaluate the safety of current obstetric anesthesia practices.

Systemic Narcotics

Narcotics have been used for centuries to relieve the pain of parturition. All narcotics cross the placenta and can be detected in umbilical cord blood. Their ease of administration makes them attractive to those with limited experience in obstetric anesthesia. They can be used safely in situations without an experienced anesthesiologist in attendance. However, their effectiveness is limited. Drugs administered intravenously rather than by the intramuscular route allow more precision in titrating maternal analgesia yet give higher and more rapidly obtained fetal drug levels. Many drugs have been used (Table 2) in the search for an ideal agent.

Morphine, at equipotent maternal doses, has been shown to cause greater neonatal respiratory depression than meperidine (Demerol). For this reason meperidine is frequently used today.

Narcotics lessen the pain of labor. They cannot safely be administered to remove all of the pain of labor. Maternal side effects do occur even at

TABLE 1. **Normal Umbilical Cord Gases**

	Umbilical Artery	Umbilical Vein
pH	7.24	7.32
Po_2	15	30
Pco_2	50	40
Base excess	−7	−5

TABLE 2. **Narcotics Administered During Labor**

Drug	Intravenous Dose (mg)	Intramuscular Dose (mg)
Meperidine (Demerol)	25–50	50–100
Morphine	2–3	5–10
Fentanyl (Sublimaze)	0.025–0.05	0.05–0.1
Butorphanol (Stadol)	1	2

low doses. Nausea and vomiting may be most frequent. Maternal respiratory depression may occur, especially between contractions in the exhausted patient. Maternal respiratory depression has been shown to be associated with maternal hypoxemia. Therefore narcotics can have significant indirect effects on the fetus. Lowered oxygen delivery can lead to a fetal metabolic acidosis. Additionally, direct respiratory depression of the infant may be seen after delivery.

The normal term parturient has a compensated respiratory alkalosis. Increased levels of progesterone cause an increased sensitivity to carbon dioxide. The normal $Paco_2$ in the term parturient is 32 torr. To compensate for this respiratory alkalosis the kidneys excrete bicarbonate to a level of 20 mEq per liter. This allows the pH to return to a near-normal 7.42.

Fetal heart tracing changes are not uncommon after the maternal use of narcotics. Frequently a transient decrease in the beat-to-beat variability is seen.

The fetal/maternal ratio of meperidine approaches 1.0 with time. Meperidine is present in the umbilical cord blood within several minutes of intravenous administration. Fetal blood levels peak sometime between 1 and 3 hours after administration, the period of maximal uptake of meperidine by the fetus. Decreases in respiratory effort are commonly seen in infants born more than 1 hour and less than 3 hours after maternal meperidine administration. Such respiratory depression can be reversed by the neonatal intravenous administration of naloxone (Narcan), 0.01 mg per kg. There is no reason to administer the naloxone to the parturient prior to delivery. The placental transfer of naloxone is unpredictable. In addition, naloxone would reverse any analgesic effect that the parturient has at a time when she may need it most.

The half-life of meperidine is 3 hours in the parturient but 23 hours in the neonate. Normeperidine, a metabolite of meperidine, causes greater respiratory depression than meperidine itself. The neonatal half-life of normeperidine is 62 hours, longer than the half-life of meperidine.

Butorphanol (Stadol) is becoming increasingly popular in obstetric analgesia because of its few maternal side effects. It is comparable to meperidine in regard to analgesia, Apgar scores, and Early Neonatal Neurobehavioral Scale (ENNS) evaluations. A sinusoidal fetal heart rate tracing can be seen after the use of butorphanol.

Intraspinal Narcotics

Narcotics administered in the epidural or intrathecal space provide pain relief through direct stimulation of spinal cord opiate receptors. Their most common use is for the relief of postoperative pain. Injection of 5 mg of preservative-free morphine (Duramorph or Astramorph) in the epidural space provides pain relief for 20 to 36 hours after abdominal delivery. Side effects such as pruritus, nausea, vomiting, and urinary retention are not as worrisome as the rare (1 in 1200) occurrence of late (8 to 16 hours after administration) respiratory depression. The use of a narcotic antagonist such as naloxone in dilute concentrations is effective in reversing all of these side effects while not necessarily affecting the analgesia.

The use of intraspinal narcotics (this term refers to intrathecal and epidural administration) requires appropriate methods of monitoring and response time from the anesthesiologist. Many institutions now commonly employ frequent (every 30 minutes) respiratory rate nursing checks with or without commercially available apnea monitors to detect decreases in respiratory rate. It is believed that the respiratory rate will slow before the patient becomes apneic. Rates of ten or less can thus serve as an indication of a need for naloxone reversal of respiratory depression. Other narcotics, such as fentanyl (Sublimaze), give a shorter duration of pain relief and fewer side effects.

Morphine and fentanyl have also been administered in the subarachnoid space with local anesthetic as part of a spinal anesthetic for abdominal delivery without deleterious effects on the fetus. Intrathecal morphine gives 20 to 30 hours of postoperative pain relief (Table 3).

Intraspinal narcotics have also been administered for labor analgesia. Repeated doses in labor may lead to an increased frequency of side effects (other than respiratory depression). The effectiveness of intraspinal narcotic analgesia may be less than that of continuous lumbar epidural administration of local anesthetics, but the associated maternal hemodynamic changes of sympathetic blockade are prevented. This may be desirable in certain patients with cardiac disease or severe hypertension. The combination of local anesthetic and narcotic is used to improve analgesia, particularly with dilute concentrations of local anesthetic (e.g., bupivacaine 0.0625 per cent and fentanyl 0.0002 per cent). Maternal systemic absorption does occur from administration of intraspinal narcotics, but neonatal effects are minimal. Intraspinal narcotics do not provide analgesia for operative procedures in the second and third stage of labor. An additional anesthetic (local, regional, or general) would be required for episiotomy, forceps delivery, manual removal of the placenta, or abdominal delivery.

Local Anesthetics

Local anesthetics can be used in various ways to obtain pain relief for labor and delivery. Direct neurobehavioral effects from local anesthetics have been reported with lidocaine and recently 2-chloroprocaine but are controversial as evidence is often contradictory. There are no reports of neurobehavioral effects of bupivacaine. Indirect effects of local anesthetics depend on method and site of administration. Fetal heart rate changes associated with local anesthetics are infrequent.

Paracervical block has been used to give pain relief during the first stage of labor. Satisfactory analgesia is obtained in only 50 to 90 per cent of patients, and the rate of fetal complications is relatively high. The large amounts of anesthetic (deposited in close proximity to the umbilical arteries) can cause uterine artery vasoconstriction and fetal bradycardia. Epinephrine must therefore be avoided. Lidocaine 1 per cent or 2-chloroprocaine 1 per cent are the drugs of choice in the United States.

Pudendal nerve block gives perineal anesthesia (spinal nerve roots S2 to S4) with only a 50 per cent effectiveness rate. The high degree of failure makes this an infrequently used procedure, although it can be used to provide anesthesia for a spontaneous delivery or low forceps delivery.

Preparation for Anesthesia

Preparation for maternal anesthesia includes attempts to alter gastric contents, support of uteroplacental perfusion, and proper monitoring of mother and fetus.

Maternal aspiration pneumonitis is a major cause of morbidity and mortality in parturients.

TABLE 3. **Postcesarean Intraspinal Narcotics**

Drug	Site	Dose	Duration (hr)
Morphine	Intrathecal	0.2–0.3 mg	20–36
	Epidural	3–5 mg	20–36
Fentanyl	Intrathecal	6–10 μg	3–4
	Epidural	50 μg	1–4
Butorphanol	Epidural	2–4 mg	2–6

Mechanical factors from the enlarged uterus, as well as hormonal changes that increase gastric volume and acidity and delay emptying, mandate measures that prevent or decrease the risk of aspiration in the parturient. Regional anesthesia maintains maternal protective airway reflexes. It has been shown that increasing the gastric pH lessens the severity of pneumonitis should aspiration occur. A smaller volume also decreases the morbidity of aspiration. It is therefore mandatory for measures to be taken in all pregnant women to minimize the risk of aspiration (Table 4). In addition to nonparticulate antacids, which can be given to all parturients, patients who have scheduled surgery can be given H_2 antagonists to decrease gastric acidity. Ranitidine (Zantac) in an intravenous dose of 2 mg per kg will also decrease gastric volume when given 60 to 90 minutes prior to induction of anesthesia. A two-dose regimen, 6 hours and 1 hour preoperatively, provides the most reliable results. Intravenous metoclopramide (Reglan) can also be given in a parenteral dose of 0.1 mg per kg to increase gastric emptying and thus decrease volume.

Epidural anesthesia causes vasodilation and loss of venous return due to the sympathetic blockade that occurs. Patients who are receiving epidural analgesia should be acutely hydrated with 500 to 1000 ml of a non–dextrose-containing intravenous solution prior to blockade.

Aortocaval compression syndrome occurs in 20 per cent of pregnant women at term. Most of these women compensate for the decrease in venous return that occurs when supine with vasoconstriction, which increases maternal systemic pressure. The administration of an epidural (or spinal) anesthetic with its resultant sympathetic blockade takes away the ability of the parturient to compensate for this decrease in venous return. Acute hydration and avoidance of aortocaval compression through the use of left uterine displacement are mandatory to maintain cardiac output.

Regional Anesthesia for Vaginal Delivery

Continuous Lumbar Epidural Analgesia

Continuous lumbar epidural analgesia is the most effective method of pain relief for labor.

Epidural analgesia decreases circulating maternal catecholamines and thus may improve uteroplacental blood flow. It can be administered at any time after the patient is committed to delivery and can be safely continued until delivery. The same anesthetic can be individualized for spontaneous delivery or operative delivery at any time. Surgical anesthesia can be obtained within minutes.

The epidural space is identified by either the loss of resistance or hanging drop technique. Both of these techniques rely on the negative pressure of the epidural space. After the space is identified, a test dose of local anesthetic is injected to exclude the possibility of intravascular or subarachnoid injection of the complete dose of local anesthetic. The ideal test dose is a controversial issue at the present time. The inclusion of epinephrine is probably not necessary and may actually be dangerous in the laboring woman with borderline uteroplacental perfusion. The pulse rate changes commonly seen with intravascular epinephrine (15 micrograms) are difficult to identify in the woman in labor.

The detection of subarachnoid injection is important to avoid the administration of large volumes of local anesthetics into the subarachnoid space. Volumes that are required to obtain analgesia in the epidural space would give dangerously high levels if administered in the subarachnoid space. Intravenous injection of local anesthetic could lead to systemic toxic levels. The patient should always be asked about circumoral paresthesias, tinnitus, or unusual taste as signs of intravascular injection and systemic toxicity. If these are noted, the needle and/or catheter should be removed and repositioned in another space.

The remote possibility of a toxic systemic reaction or a high level of regional anesthesia requires that resuscitation equipment, including that for intubation and bag and mask ventilation, be immediately available whenever epidural analgesia or anesthesia is administered. A working oxygen supply and effective suction are also necessary.

After the uneventful administration of a test dose, the epidural catheter is placed so that 2 cm

TABLE 4. **Drugs Used in Aspiration Pneumonitis Prophylaxis**

Drug	Dose	Timing before Induction
Sodium citrate (Bicitra), 0.3 M oral	30 ml	Immediate
Ranitidine (Zantac), parenteral or oral	2 mg per kg	60–90 min
		Prior dose at 6 hr increases reliability
Cimetidine (Tagamet), parenteral or oral	4 mg per kg	1 hr
		Prior dose at 6 hr increases reliability
Metoclopramide (Reglan), parenteral	0.1 mg per kg	At least 15 min

remains in the epidural space after the needle is removed. After the catheter is secured, the patient is placed in the supine or semi-Fowler's position with a right hip roll to avoid aortocaval compression.

Incremental doses of 3 to 5 ml of local anesthetic (Table 5) are administered through the catheter until pain relief is obtained. A dermatome level of sensory analgesia to spinal nerve root T10 will usually provide adequate pain relief for the first stage of labor. The pain in the first stage of labor is from the uterus which is innervated from spinal nerve roots T10 to L1. A volume of local anesthetic between 8 and 15 ml is usually given. With additional doses through the catheter (customarily two thirds of the initial dose), sacral anesthesia (the perineum is innervated by spinal nerve roots S2 to S4) necessary for second stage and delivery will be obtained without necessarily giving a dose of local anesthetic just prior to delivery. While certainly given if required, this "delivery" dose exposes the fetus to large doses of local anesthetic just before delivery. Again, while direct neurobehavioral fetal effects are controversial, minimizing the chance of effects by keeping fetal blood levels low seems prudent. Dosing the catheter in a hurried situation with volumes of anesthetic necessary to obtain sacral anesthesia makes the practice of giving a "delivery" dose a situation fraught with danger.

Spinal Anesthesia

Spinal anesthesia is not used for labor but is an excellent method of pain relief for vaginal delivery. The total amount of drug given is small in comparison to that used via the epidural route, which should mean fewer direct neonatal effects.

Spinal anesthesia is most commonly performed with a 26-gauge needle and introducer at the L2–L3 or L3–L4 interspace with the patient in the lateral or sitting position. Acute intravenous hydration has already been discussed. The subarachnoid space is identified with free flow of cerebrospinal fluid (CSF) in at least two quadrants prior to the injection of anesthetic. Hyper-

TABLE 5. **Local Anesthetics Used for Labor and Delivery Analgesia**

	Continuous Infusion	Intermittent Doses
Bupivacaine (Marcaine)	0.0625%	0.25%
	0.125%	0.375%
	0.25%	0.5%
Lidocaine (Xylocaine)	0.5%	1.0%
	1.0%	1.5%
		2.0%
2-Chloroprocaine (Nesacaine)	1.0%	2.0%
		3.0%

baric lidocaine 5 per cent (30 to 40 mg) will give anesthesia to the T10 dermatome for a comfortable delivery and the occasional manual removal of the placenta or exploration of the uterus. The subsequent care and considerations are similar for all patients receiving regional anesthesia.

Sympathetic Blockade

The parturient must be monitored closely in the first 20 minutes for the development of hypotension due to sympathetic blockade. If a decrease in maternal systemic blood pressure of greater than 20 per cent occurs, it should be aggressively treated with intravenous fluids. Vasopressors may be given as required. The vasopressor of choice in the parturient is ephedrine because its primary beta-adrenergic effects do not cause uterine artery vasoconstriction with decreased uteroplacental blood flow. In severe cases of hypotension (usually due to maternal hemorrhage) or certain cardiac diseases a direct-acting alpha-adrenergic agent such as phenylephrine (Neo-Synephrine) may be preferable.

Perinatal Pharmacology

Local anesthetics cross the placenta as previously discussed. The umbilical vein–maternal vein ratio is not affected by the route of administration except for the higher ratio with paracervical block. Similar maternal systemic blood levels are obtained with local perineal anesthesia and continuous lumbar epidural analgesia. If one was to employ both local infiltration and pudendal anesthesia for delivery, maternal blood levels would be expected to be higher than those obtained with epidural analgesia alone. Drug is detectable in the fetal circulation even after the small doses administered with spinal anesthesia.

The amino-ester local anesthetic 2-chloroprocaine is considered safe in the presence of fetal distress because of the absence of ion trapping phenomenon. Accumulation of local anesthetic may occur in the acidotic fetus. Such accumulation is less likely to occur with 2-chloroprocaine because of its short half-life (43 seconds) in the neonatal plasma.

Effects on the Progress of Labor

Numerous studies have shown that the first stage of labor is not prolonged, and may even be shortened, by the use of continuous lumbar epidural analgesia. The second stage may be prolonged by less than 30 minutes. The incidence of forceps delivery, particularly "outlet" forceps, may be slightly increased owing to the ease and maternal comfort of such a delivery with functioning epidural analgesia.

Contraindications

Contraindications to spinal or epidural anesthesia include patient refusal or lack of cooperation, the presence of coagulopathy, hypovolemia, septicemia, and infection over the lumbar area. Increased intracranial pressure may be a relative contraindication to epidural anesthesia. Increased intracranial pressure is an absolute contraindication to spinal anesthesia.

Complications

Complications related to regional anesthesia include the postdural puncture headache (PDPH). The incidence of headache after a spinal anesthetic with a 26-gauge needle is less than 5 per cent for all anesthetics and even less in experienced hands. The incidence of headache is much higher after an unintentional dural puncture with a 17-gauge epidural needle. The incidence of headache is not changed by the practice of requiring the supine position after anesthesia, so this is not a requirement in our hospital. All patients who have had a dural puncture should be encouraged to drink fluids. Those complaining of postural headache are treated initially with high-dose anti-inflammatory drugs such as ibuprofen (Motrin) up to 800 mg four times per day. If this regimen is not effective after 24 hours, an epidural blood patch is performed by injecting 12 to 15 ml of a patient's own blood (obtained in a sterile fashion) into the epidural space at the same interspace as the previous dural puncture. Epidural blood patch is effective up to 99 per cent of the time. Prophylactic blood patches are not done as their effectiveness at preventing headache is limited.

The incidence of PDPH after accidental puncture with a 17-gauge epidural needle appears to be less if an epidural catheter is placed in another interspace and used for analgesia. The amount of drug needs to be carefully titrated to the degree of blockade, as some of the drug may diffuse across the rent in the dura. The drug may function at least partially as a spinal anesthetic. Care must be taken in choice and dosage of drug.

Backache is a common complaint in postpartum patients. It generally resolves in several days with symptomatic therapy. Postpartum paresthesias may occur owing to root, plexus, or peripheral nerve damage. Most are not due to regional anesthesia, but careful investigation should be made to delineate the lesion and to arrange proper follow-up care. Again, most of these resolve in days to weeks. Extremely rare but potentially devastating, epidural hematoma must be considered in anybody with motor and/or sensory deficit that does not recover with regressing anesthesia.

Anesthesia for Abdominal Delivery

Regional Anesthesia

Abdominal delivery requires a higher dermatome level of anesthesia with a more profound block than does vaginal delivery. Complete sympathetic blockade leads to a higher incidence of hypotension than in regional anesthesia for vaginal delivery. Parturients should be hydrated acutely with larger amounts of intravenous crystalloid (1000 to 1500 ml). Other considerations are nearly identical to those already discussed.

Epidural anesthesia can be obtained with the use of lidocaine 2 per cent with epinephrine 1:200,000, bupivacaine 0.5 per cent, or 2-chloroprocaine 3 per cent. All doses are 18 to 25 ml based on the patient's height.

Spinal anesthesia can be induced with lidocaine 5 per cent (60 to 80 mg), bupivacaine 0.75 per cent (8 to 12 mg), tetracaine (Pontocaine, 7 to 11 mg) or a mixture of procaine (Novocain) 10 per cent in water (60 to 100 mg) and tetracaine 1 per cent in water (6 to 10 mg). All drugs are used in hyperbaric solutions. The procaine-tetracaine mixture is also hyperbaric. Narcotics can be used for postoperative pain relief as already discussed. Sedation after delivery, while not often necessary, may be accomplished with small doses of diazepam (Valium) or fentanyl. Midazolam (Versed) is not often used with regional anesthesia, as it frequently gives retrograde amnesia for delivery. Intravenous droperidol (Inapsine), 0.625 mg, or metoclopramide, 10 mg, is often given to prevent the nausea and vomiting that may occur with peritoneal traction.

General Anesthesia

With the current techniques of general anesthesia, neonatal outcome after abdominal delivery is as good as with regional anesthesia. Regional anesthesia may still be preferred because of the maternal participation in the delivery and the decreased risk of maternal complications such as aspiration. The use of previously discussed drugs to minimize the risk of maternal aspiration is mandatory.

Induction of general anesthesia after preoxygenation with 100 per cent oxygen is safely accomplished with intravenous thiopental (Pentothal) 4 mg per kg pregnant body weight (PBW). Doses of 8 mg per kg have been shown to increase the number of infants with low Apgar scores. The lower dose reliably induces anesthesia in the parturient because of the lower concentration of anesthetics necessary to anesthetize her brain. Changes in progesterone and beta-endorphin levels are theorized to cause this decreased anesthetic requirement.

Ketamine (Ketalar) increases uterine tone in doses greater than 1.5 mg per kg. An intravenous dose of 1 mg per kg in a hypovolemic patient will induce general anesthesia with minimal hemodynamic effect.

Intubation is facilitated by intravenous succinylcholine (Anectine), 1 mg per kg. Induction is carried out in a "rapid sequence" fashion with cricoid pressure to minimize the risk of maternal aspiration. General anesthesia should not be induced without endotracheal intubation. Muscle relaxation can be maintained with an intravenous succinylcholine infusion (0.1 per cent) titrated with the use of a neuromuscular blockade monitor. Nondepolarizing neuromuscular blocking agents can be used for maintenance of paralysis if preferred. All neuromuscular blocking agents have been shown to cross the placenta. The high degree of ionization limits their transplacental passage to clinically insignificant amounts.

Increasing maternal inspired oxygen concentration increases maternal PaO_2, but does not increase fetal umbilical vein PaO_2 beyond 60 torr. Generally, the use of 50 per cent oxygen provides maximal fetal benefit. Increased concentrations can be used if maternal indications exist.

Nitrous oxide is commonly added to deepen maternal anesthesia. It rapidly crosses the placenta and is taken up by the fetus. After 3 minutes, the umbilical vein–maternal artery ratio is 0.8. The umbilical artery–umbilical vein ratio tends to plateau after 15 to 19 minutes, which indicates rapid uptake by the fetus. If there is prolonged induction to delivery time the nitrous oxide effect may add to neonatal depression. Oxygen and positive-pressure ventilation will enable the neonate to excrete the nitrous oxide rapidly through the lungs. Oxygen must be given to prevent diffusion hypoxia as nitrous oxide fills the alveoli.

The addition of a volatile agent during the period between induction and delivery does not affect Apgar scores, maternal and fetal blood gases, lactate levels, or the ENNS. The incidence of maternal recall decreases to 0 per cent from 17 per cent with the addition of 0.5 MAC (minimal alveolar concentration) of isoflurane, halothane, or enflurane.

After delivery of the neonate, left uterine displacement can be discontinued as the anesthetic is deepened with intravenous morphine (10 to 20 mg) or other narcotic. The nitrous oxide can be increased to 70 per cent if no maternal contraindication exists and the volatile agent can be discontinued. Intravenous oxytocin (Pitocin) is infused. A 1- to 2-mg dose of midazolam may be given to enhance amnesia.

Complications

Complications of general anesthesia generally involve airway problems. The difficult intubation is associated with risk of maternal aspiration. Inability to ventilate leads to hypoxia, which is disastrous for mother and infant. A well-rehearsed "failed intubation" protocol should be mandatory for all delivery suites.

POSTPARTUM CARE

method of
DOTTIE L. WATSON, M.D.
Wayne State University
Detroit, Michigan

The puerperium is that period of time in which both anatomic and physiologic processes return to the nonpregnant state. This period lasts approximately 6 to 8 weeks.

The methods of patient care during this time have evolved from a conservative approach to one that is more conducive to today's society. In recent years postpartum management has also changed to accommodate patients who are discharged early from the hospital (less than 48 hours). A visiting nurse program specifically geared to postpartum care and recognition of complications is important to the success of early hospital discharge.

The puerperium is divided into immediate and late periods for purposes of identifying specific complications.

Delivery Room

After delivery of the baby and expulsion of the placenta, the uterus contracts to the level of the umbilicus. Intravenous oxytocin, 20 units, is placed in 1000 ml of dextrose Ringer's lactate (D5RL) and titrated to decrease uterine blood loss. Uterine massage is performed simultaneously. In most cases this is adequate therapy to prevent excessive blood loss. Careful inspection of the cervix, vagina, and perineum for lacerations should also be performed.

If excessive bleeding (greater than 500 ml for a vaginal delivery) is observed, the following should be considered: lacerations (cervix, vagina, perineum), retained placental fragments, uterine atony, uterine rupture, and disseminated intravascular coagulation (Table 1).

Any patient with the diagnosis of postpartum hemorrhage should at least have (1) insertion of a large intracatheter (No. 18) needle with instillation of appropriate fluids (normal saline or Ringer's lactate), and (2) blood typed and crossmatched (depending on the patient's risk factors,

TABLE 1. **Postpartum Hemorrhage**

Source	Diagnosis	Treatment
Lacerations (cervix, vagina, perineum)	Tear visualized, active bleeding	Suture (absorbable)
Retained placenta	Grossly incomplete placenta, fragments palpated, succenturiate lobe, manual removal	Gauze-covered, gloved, manual exploration; may require curettage
Uterine atony	Soft to palpation	Bimanual massage; 20–40 units of oxytocin in 1000 ml D5RL (titrate) IV. Additional therapy: 1. 0.2 mg methylergonovine IM 2. 0.25 mg of 15-methyl PG-F$_{2\alpha}$ IM or PG-E$_2$ suppository per rectum For persistent bleeding (if above fails): Bilateral hypogastric artery ligation, ovarian artery ligation and/or hysterectomy

Uterine rupture	Traumatic: forceps, version and extraction, excessive fundal pressure
	
	 Spontaneous: grand multiparity, cephalo-pelvic disproportion, oxytocin stimulation, prior uterine surgery
	
	 Physical: maternal tachycardia, hypotension, uterine atony
		1. Uterine exploration
		 2. Exploratory laparotomy
		 3. Repair or hysterectomy, depends on:
		    a. Extent of the tear
		    b. Amount of blood lost
		    c. Status of patient
		    d. Desire for future childbearing

as listed in Table 1, this should be performed on admission). Blood should be replaced as needed.

Recovery Room

After delivery, the patient is transferred to the recovery room for close observation. Vital signs are taken every 15 minutes for 1 hour, every 30 minutes for the second hour, and then hourly until the patient is transferred to the postpartum floor. The patient is observed for uterine atony, excessive vaginal bleeding, episiotomy hematoma, bladder distention, or any abnormality of vital signs. This is also an important time for maternal-infant bonding.

Postpartum Floor

After 2 to 4 hours in the recovery room, the patient is transferred with a specific set of orders to the postpartum floor. The orders, as described below, may be used for an uncomplicated vaginal delivery.

Hospital Orders

Vital Signs. The following vital signs should be monitored every 4 hours.

TEMPERATURE. Puerperal fever is defined as a temperature higher than 100.4° F (38° C) on two separate occasions 24 hours apart (exclusive of the first 24 hours postpartum). Maternal infection should be suspected.

PULSE. Tachycardia that is persistent should

be investigated. This may be a sign of acute hemorrhage, cardiac disease, thyroid disease, infection, or thromboembolic disease.

RESPIRATION. Persistent tachypnea should also be investigated. This may be a sign of pneumonia, pulmonary embolus, or another serious medical condition.

BLOOD PRESSURE. Hypotension may be secondary to blood loss. Hemoglobin and hematocrit should be measured and blood replaced as needed. Hypertension may be secondary to pre-eclampsia or chronic hypertension. The treatment for these conditions is discussed under the appropriate topic.

Activity. Patients may ambulate immediately unless conduction anesthesia was used. In this case bed rest is recommended for up to 24 hours. Early ambulation has been shown to reduce maternal morbidity by decreasing the incidence of thrombophlebitis, and stimulating earlier bowel and bladder functions. The patient may require assistance initially but should soon be able to ambulate on her own. A postpartum exercise routine may be initiated. Overexertion should be prohibited, and periods of rest should be encouraged.

Diet. Patients should be allowed to eat regular meals unless their medical condition dictates otherwise. Fluids should be encouraged, especially for breast-feeding mothers.

Medication. For pain relief, acetaminophen 600 mg with codeine 60 mg is given every 4 hours orally as needed. For insomnia, secobarbital (Seconal) 100 mg orally at night is given as needed. The intravenous line may be discontinued, if the patient's condition is stable.

Bowels. Constipation is commonly encountered post partum, and the following may be used to alleviate this condition starting on postpartum day 2: (1) milk of magnesia, 30 ml orally as needed, or (2) Fleet's Enema or Dulcolax suppository per rectum as needed. If the patient has had a repaired fourth-degree laceration, nothing should be given per rectum. The patient should be placed on a soft diet and given stool softeners such as docusate sodium (Colace), 100 mg orally twice a day.

Perineum Care. This area should be cleansed several times a day and a sterile perineal pad applied. If an episiotomy was performed, the area may be swollen and tender for several days. Treatment may include sitz baths three times a day, anesthetic spray, or Tucks as needed. The area should be observed daily for signs of infection.

Breast Care

BREAST FEEDING. Although lactogenesis begins approximately 2 to 5 days after delivery, the infant should be allowed to suckle on each breast for 10 minutes starting in the immediate postpartum period. Prolonged suckling or direct suckling on the nipple may cause cracking and bleeding. Aids in breast care at the bedside include lanolin cream, breast pump (hand or electric), and nipple shields.

NON-BREAST FEEDING. The best method to prevent lactation is use of the orally administered agent bromocriptine (Parlodel), 2.5 mg twice a day for 2 weeks. If the patient refuses or is not a candidate for this medication, she may use a tight binder or bra, analgesics, or ice packs if engorgement is evident.

Urinary Tract. The most common complications post partum are related to the urinary tract. Urinary retention may be secondary to swelling of the episiotomy site, vulva, or vagina. Conduction anesthesia may also contribute to urinary retention. If the patient has a full bladder or is unable to void 8 hours after delivery, straight catheterization is initially performed. If a second catheterization is required, a Foley catheter is placed until her condition has improved. This usually takes less than 24 hours. A urine culture is obtained on removing the catheter.

Laboratory Tests. Each patient should be tested for blood type, Rh factor, and antibody screen. Rh-negative patients should be evaluated for possible RhoGAM injection. Each patient should also have blood drawn to measure hemoglobin or hematocrit on postpartum day 2 or prior to discharge.

Hospital Course

The patient's hospital course should consist of daily rounds to assess her general status, vital signs, and physical examination of her breasts, abdomen, fundus, perineum, lochia, and legs.

Maternal fever (as previously defined) should be promptly investigated. The patient should have a physical examination and an appropriate history should be taken, which should include the following: breasts, lungs, costovertebral angles, heart, abdomen, fundus, perineum, lochia, pelvis, and legs. Laboratory tests such as a complete blood count with differential, blood cultures, and urine cultures are often ordered. The evaluation should rule out the following: breast engorgement, atelectasis, pneumonia, urinary tract infection, endometritis, infected episiotomy, and thrombophlebitis.

Discharge to 6 Weeks Post Partum

Today patients are discharged earlier from the hospital than in the past. They may leave as early as 24 to 48 hours post partum, which gives the physician less time to observe for the previously described possible complications. If patients are discharged early, a good ambulatory back-up program is advised, such as a visiting nurse program, to monitor the patient for possible complications.

At the time of discharge, instructions are given to each patient. For example, the patient is taught how to take her temperature. She should be advised to notify her physician of possible late postpartum complications, including fever, heavy vaginal bleeding, mastitis, uterine tenderness, and amenorrhea. The patient is advised to rest but to continue a postpartum exercise routine and progressively increase her physical activity at home. Contraception should be discussed and appropriate counseling given. For example, the patient may start oral contraceptives the Sunday after discharge from the hospital. She should abstain from sexual intercourse for at least 2 weeks. She may shower or bathe but should avoid douching. Patients may continue prenatal vitamins and iron supplements if needed. An appointment in 4 to 6 weeks should be scheduled for a postpartum examination, which should include assessment of the patient's general well-being, weight, vital signs, and breasts, and a pelvic examination and Papanicolaou (Pap) smear. Contraception should be discussed and the need for an annual pelvic examination emphasized.

NEONATAL RESUSCITATION

method of
THOMAS F. MYERS, M.D., and
CRAIG L. ANDERSON, M.D.
Loyola University Perinatal Center
Maywood, Illinois

Pathophysiology of Perinatal Asphyxia

Asphyxia is the cessation of oxygen and carbon dioxide exchange with the concomitant arrest of cellular aerobic metabolism. It is manifested by hypoxemia, hypercarbia, and a combined respiratory and metabolic acidosis. Asphyxia results in a marked increase in activity of the sympathetic nervous system and release of catecholamines by the adrenal medulla. The unique features of perinatal asphyxia relate fetal-neonatal anatomy and physiology.

The fetus is totally dependent upon the maternal-uteroplacental-umbilical circulatory axis for respiratory function, nutrition, and excretion of toxic wastes. An interruption of this circulation immediately jeopardizes the fetus. Fetal circulation is designed to maintain placental perfusion and to preserve the flow of oxygenated blood to the cerebral hemispheres and the myocardium. The musculoskeletal and cutaneous circuits are expendable, whereas the gastrointestinal, renal, and pulmonary circulations are negotiable. The ductus venosus, foramen ovale, and ductus arteriosus, coupled with pulmonary vasoconstriction, direct oxygenated umbilical venous blood to the cerebral and coronary circulations. Under the stress of fetal asphyxia, blood flow is severely curtailed in the expendable and negotiable circulations by a combination of the fetal "diving reflex," baroreceptor responses, and a surge of norepinephrine. Vagal reflexes contribute to the fetal-neonatal predisposition to bradycardia and apnea.

The cardiorespiratory transition from fetus to newborn is the metamorphosis from placental to pulmonary gas exchange. A rapid increase in oxygenation at birth induces pulmonary vasodilation, a reduction in pulmonary arterial pressure, and functional closure of the foramen ovale and ductus arteriosus with resultant massive increases in pulmonary blood flow. In the presence of fetal-neonatal hypoxemia and acidosis, pulmonary vasoconstriction persists or recurs and right to left shunting occurs through the foramen ovale and ductus arteriosus, a condition called persistent fetal circulation. The resultant pulmonary ischemia increases hypoxemia, setting up a vicious circle. The transition from a fetal fluid-filled to a neonatal gas-filled lung is dependent upon the establishment of functional residual capacity, which improves lung compliance. This is normally accomplished in the first several minutes of breathing. The newborn's initial breaths require tremendous negative intrathoracic pressures (minus 20 to minus 35 cm H_2O). Achievement of pulmonary function is dependent upon adequate alveolarization for gas exchange and pulmonary surfactant, which reduces the collapsing force of intra-alveolar surface tension.

TABLE 1. **Perinatal Asphyxia: Risk Factors**

Maternal Factors
Primipara, age > 35 years
Maternal diabetes mellitus
Chronic maternal disease
Preeclampsia
Maternal hypertension
Maternal circulatory collapse
Maternal sedatives or analgesics

Intrapartum Factors
Fetal distress
Abnormal prepartum monitoring
Abnormal presenting part
Instrumented delivery
Dystocia
Abnormal uterus
Oligohydramnios
Polyhydramnios
Chorioamnionitis
Placenta previa
Abruptio placentae
Abnormal placenta
Umbilical cord prolapse

Fetal Factors
Prematurity
Immature fetal lungs
Intrauterine growth retardation
Multiple gestation
Hydrops fetalis (immune and nonimmune)
Fetal ascites
Fetal pleural effusion
Fetal arrhythmia
Fetal anomalies (other)

The fetal-neonatal cardiovascular and respiratory systems are both "rate dependent." The immature myocardium appears to be relatively incapable of increasing cardiac output via stroke volume, while alveolar ventilation in the volume-compliance compromised neonatal lung is dependent on respiratory rate. Cerebral blood flow in the stressed neonate appears to be dependent upon systemic arterial pressure. This apparent defect in autoregulation renders the neonate susceptible to cerebral ischemia when hypotensive and to intracranial hemorrhage when hypertensive.

Perinatal asphyxia interrupts the fetal-neonatal cardiorespiratory transition. Fetal-neonatal circulatory reflexes may induce renal, gastrointestinal, and he-

TABLE 2. **Perinatal Asphyxia: Fetal Distress**

Prepartum Monitoring
Abnormal stress test
Nonreactive nonstress test
Abnormal biophysical profile
Lack of fetal movement (>12 hours)

Intrapartum Fetal Monitoring
Fetal bradycardia (<120 bpm)
Fetal tachycardia (>160 bpm)
Fetal scalp pH < 7.20
Fetal scalp Po_2 < 25 mmHg
Late deceleration
Severe variable deceleration
Decreased heart rate variability
Meconium passage
Sinusoidal heart rate pattern

TABLE 3. **Neonatal Resuscitation Team**

Title	Role
Delivering physician	Identifies high-risk mother Recognizes fetal distress Alerts other personnel Delivers infant Manages mother
Infant resuscitator #1	Manages infant's airway
Infant resuscitator #2	Dries and warms infant Positions infant Assigns Apgar scores External cardiac massage Intravenous medications
Infant care support person	Keeps time Prepares medications Prepares surgical trays Keeps records Coordinates lab specimens Coordinates transfer Has no maternal reponsibilities Assists with medications

patic ischemia in moderately prolonged asphyxia. Prolonged asphyxia can easily overwhelm protective reflexes, resulting in cerebral and myocardial ischemia.

Resuscitation Technique

Delivery suite preparation, staff education, and anticipation and recognition of the high-risk pregnancy are key elements in successful neonatal resuscitation. The delivery suite must be equipped for resuscitation during every delivery. Resuscitation equipment must be located in an accessible central location in each delivery area. Supplies must be replenished and the function of critical items checked before and after each delivery. The staff should be well versed in the resuscitation set-up protocol. Infant cardiopulmonary resuscitation training, including, if possible, animal model practice, should occur every 6 months.

The physician managing the pregnant woman is charged with early prenatal risk assessment and the recognition of fetal distress (Tables 1 and 2). When recognized early, the high-risk pregnancy can be carefully monitored, and appropriate consultation with a regional perinatal center can be obtained. Recent advances in prenatal monitoring techniques, such as the fetal biophysical profile, have permitted early recognition of

fetal distress and timely delivery. Fetal ultrasound diagnosis of congenital anomalies has facilitated appropriate referral to specialized facilities. Intrapartum fetal monitoring and intervention can prevent prolonged fetal asphyxia.

Division of labor is essential to orderly neonatal resuscitation. Ideally, the neonatal resuscitation team consists of four members (Table 3). The delivering physician will anticipate the high-risk delivery, recognize the signs of fetal distress, alert the other members of the team, and choose the optimal mode of delivery. One team member must have primary responsibility for securing the airway and initiating assisted ventilation. A second team member will dry and position the infant as well as suction the pharynx. This team member will also assign the Apgar scores, perform external cardiac massage, and order medications. It is particularly important that a circulating nurse (infant care support person) be assigned to resuscitation with no duties related to maternal care. Gloves should always be worn by team members and protective goggles employed when a history of maternal intravenous drug abuse or AIDS exposure is documented.

All infants should be dried and placed under a radiant warmer at birth. Evaporative heat loss from the infant's large skin surface area relative to body mass is the most common cause of neonatal hypothermia. Cold stress is extremely harmful in the asphyxiated infant owing to the increase in oxygen consumption that accompanies all but deep (operating room) hypothermia. A warming mattress is particularly useful during prolonged resuscitation and for low-birth-weight infants. Warming the delivery room to 80° F and heating and humidifying respiratory gases are useful adjuncts for preventing hypothermia. The infant is placed on the warming platform in a 30-degree Trendelenburg's position with the neck slightly extended. The nasal and oral pharynx are briefly suctioned and the 1-minute Apgar score is assigned prior to initiating assisted ventilation. Excessive hyperextension of the neck or neck flexion will occlude the newborn's airway, and prolonged suctioning will cause bradycardia.

The cornerstone of the resuscitative effort is restoration of ventilation; alleviation of hypoxemia and hypercarbia will reverse the patho-

TABLE 4. **Apgar Scores**

Sign	0	1	2
Heart rate	Absent	Below 100/min	Above 100/min
Respiratory effort	Absent	Weak/irregular cry	Strong cry
Muscle tone	Flaccid	Slightly flexed extremities	Well-flexed extremities
Reflex activity	No response	Grimace	Cry, cough, sneeze
Color	Blue, pale	Body pink, extremities blue	Completely pink

TABLE 5. Neonatal Resuscitation Time Line
(Minutes After Birth)

Apgar Score					
0	1	2	3	5	10
All Infants					
Dry, radiant heat, briefly suction	7–9: Observe				
No Meconium					
Proceed as per Apgar score	3–6: Mask ventilation	5–9: Improving, no bradycardia, wean ventilation	7–10: Observe	7–10: Good prognosis	
Meconium					
Pharyngeal suction, direct laryngoscopy, tracheal suction, then proceed as per Apgar score	0–2: Intubate, assisted ventilation	0–4: Not improving, bradycardia and cyanosis, intubate, reposition tube, treat pneumothorax	0–6: Give bicarbonate, if bradycardia give epinephrine, if shock give volume	0–6: Apnea, poor prognosis	
	Initiate external cardiac massage if bradycardia > 30 sec	Continue external cardiac massage if bradycardia	Continue external cardiac massage if bradycardia		

physiologic processes of asphyxia. Given adequate ventilation, medications will rarely be required; without ventilation, pharmacologic agents are futile. The initial procedures employed in resuscitation depend upon the presence or absence of meconium-stained amniotic fluid and upon the initial (1 minute or less) Apgar assessment (Table 4).

The meconium-stained infant must undergo pharyngeal suction immediately upon delivery of the head. Direct laryngoscopy with tracheal suction is performed following birth. An 8 Fr or 10 Fr DeLee catheter, a conventional suction catheter, or an appropriate-sized endotracheal tube with ET-to-wall suction adapter may be used for this purpose. The frequency of maternal AIDS infection precludes use of mouth suction devices. These procedures have significantly reduced the incidence and severity of meconium aspiration pneumonia. Further resuscitative efforts proceed according to the 1-minute Apgar assessment (Table 5).

Infants with 1-minute Apgar scores of 0 to 2 require immediate assisted ventilation, preferably by endotracheal intubation. The extremely immature infant and the infant with a suspected anomaly affecting ventilation should also be considered for immediate intubation (Table 6). A 1-minute trial of mask ventilation is probably not detrimental. A No. 0 straight laryngoscope blade with the tip placed in the vallecula will produce adequate tracheal visualization in most infants; a No. 1 blade may be needed in large infants (over 3.5 kg). An appropriate diameter endotracheal tube with retracted guide is advanced to the mid-trachea (Table 7). The most common intubation errors include insertion of the laryngoscope blade beyond the vallecula, with occlusion of the trachea by the blade tip, and advancing the endotracheal tube beyond the carina into the right mainstem bronchus. The former error results in bradycardia and esophageal intubation, and the latter error causes persistent bradycardia and asymmetrical lung expansion. Pre-cut endotracheal tubes will obviate the latter complication.

A flow-inflating (anesthesia) bag with adapter, blended air-oxygen gas source, and airway pressure gauge with pop-off valve is most suitable for neonatal assisted ventilation. A self-inflating bag (Ambu) is kept in readiness for use in cases of gas source failures. Ventilation is begun with 100 per cent oxygen, a flow rate of 5 to 8 liters per minute, inflating pressures of 20 cm H_2O, and a rate of 40 to 60 breaths per minute. Although

TABLE 6. Indications for and Timing of Endotracheal Intubation

Indication	Time (Minutes After Birth)
Meconium-stained amniotic fluid	0–1
Apgar score 0–2	0–1
Extreme immaturity, gestational age less than 28 weeks or birth weight less than 900 grams	0–2
Suspected anatomic/surgical anomaly (e.g., diaphragmatic hernia)	0–1
Obvious upper or lower airway obstruction	0–1
Poor response (heart rate less than 100 bpm) after hand (mask) ventilation	2–3
Peristent apnea-hypopnea	5–10
Persistent respiratory distress (prior to transport to nursery)	10

TABLE 7. **Endotracheal Tube Size and Insertion Distance**

Birth Weight (Grams)	Size (ID, mm)	Orotracheal Insertion Distance (cm)*	Gestational Age (weeks)
Below 1000 grams	2.5	5.5–6.5	24–28
1001–2000 grams	3.0	6.5–8.0	29–33
Above 2000 grams	3.5	8.0–10.0	34 weeks and above

*A simple rule for orotracheal insertion distance is crown-heel length times 0.2 minus one centimeter ([Lt $\times$ 0.2] $-$ 1 cm).

assessment of breath sounds is commonly employed, resolution of bradycardia within 30 seconds, visible chest wall movement, and improved skin color are the most reliable signs of successful intubation and adequate ventilation. Inflating pressures may be increased in increments of 5 cm H_2O every three to five breaths until adequate ventilation is achieved; pressures as high as 35 cm H_2O may be necessary initially. Careful observation for overinflation (barrel chest) and monitoring of inflating pressure will prevent pneumothorax. Delivered oxygen concentration and inflating pressures are reduced as the infant's ventilation and skin color improve. We have found that noninvasive oxygen saturation moni-

TABLE 8. **Differential Diagnosis and Management of Infant who Responds Poorly to Initial Resuscitation**

Diagnosis	Management
Ineffective Ventilation	General: cardiac massage, medications
Mechanical Causes	
Mask not tightly sealed to face*	Reseal or intubate
Head-neck position not optimal*	Reposition or intubate
Inadequate inflating pressure	Increase pressure
Esophageal intubation	Reintubate
Intubation right mainstem bronchus*	Reposition tube
Anatomic-Surgical Causes	Chest roentgenogram
Pneumothorax*	Transillumination
Tracheoesophageal fistula	Evacuate
Diaphragmatic hernia	Intubate
Abdominal distention	Intubate
Ascites	
Pleural effusion	Evacuate stomach
Tracheal atresia/obstruction	Paracentesis
Pulmonary hypoplasia	Thoracentesis
Cystic adenomatoid malformation	Tracheostomy
Severe fetal acidosis	Lethal
	Intubate
	Bicarbonate, epinephrine
Cyanosis Without Bradycardia	
Shock	Plasma expansion
Sepsis	Work-up/antibiotics
Persistent fetal circulation	Hyperventilation
Cyanotic congenital heart disease	Work-up
Arrhythmia	ECG, treatment
Apnea Without Cyanosis or Bradycardia	
Narcosis	Naloxone
Central hypoventilation syndrome	Ventilation
Severe central nervous system disorder	Ventilation
Spinal cord injury	Ventilation
Muscle disorder	Ventilation

*Primary causes.

toring (pulse oximetry) is useful in assessing the progress of resuscitation. In the normal term newborn, arterial oxygen saturation gradually increases from 70 per cent to 90 per cent over the first 7 minutes of life.

External cardiac massage should be initiated if bradycardia (heart rate less than 100 beats per minute) persists for more than 30 seconds after assisted ventilation is initiated. This procedure is performed by encircling the chest with both hands so that the interlocking fingers are behind the infant's back and the thumbs meet on top of the mid-sternum, which is depressed 1.0 to 1.9 cm in a regular rhythm at a rate of 100 to 120 times per minute. The operator must be careful to fully release the sternum during the "diastolic" phase of each compression (without losing contact) in order to allow complete cardiac filling. Assisted breaths are inserted during the "diastolic" phase of every third sternal compression. The operator allows his thumbs to "ride up" with each breath. The procedure is continued until the 2- to 3-minute Apgar assessment.

The infant with a 1-minute Apgar score of 3 to 6 will have had fetal distress for 10 minutes or less. Spontaneous respirations can be expected within 1 minute. Brief nasopharyngeal and oropharyngeal suctioning will clear the airway. An appropriate-sized mask is then placed over the mouth and nose, and several inflations with the above-mentioned flow-inflating (anesthesia) bag are delivered. Adequate spontaneous respirations will frequently ensue, and the infant may be quickly weaned to a continuous positive airway pressure of 4 to 6 cm H_2O. The delivered oxygen concentration should be reduced as the infant's color improves. The infant who deteriorates or who remains apneic should be managed as indicated for Apgar scores of 0 to 2.

Infants who have 1-minute Apgar scores of 7 to 10 should be carefully observed. A deterioration in status warrants etiologic investigation and management as outlined earlier for infants with lower Apgar scores. Among the most frequent causes for such deteriorations are maternal anesthetics or analgesics and bacterial sepsis.

The 2- to 3-minute Apgar score serves to assess the adequacy of initial resuscitative efforts and

TABLE 9. **Neonatal Resuscitation Medications**

Medication	Dose	Time After Birth (Minutes)	Administration	Indication
Sodium bicarbonate (0.5 mEq/ml = 4.2%)	2–3 mEq/kg	5–10	Term infant: administer slowly IV Preterm infant: dilute 1:1, slowly IV	Metabolic acidosis with adequate ventilation, bradycardia at 5 minutes, or apnea at 8–10 minutes
Epinephrine (1:10,000 = 0.1 mg/ml)	0.1–0.5 ml/kg	3–5	IV, intracardiac, endotracheal	Persistent bradycardia at 3–5 minutes
Naloxone (0.02 mg/ml)	0.01–0.02 mg/kg	5–10	IV, IM, repeat doses: 5–10 minutes, prn	Antagonizes narcotic depression
Plasma expander (5% albumin, Plasmanate 0.9% saline, blood)	5–20 ml/kg	5–10	IV slowly in 5 ml/kg increments	Shock, pulselessness, especially with antecedent maternal hemorrhage

the response of the neonate. Bradycardia resolves within 30 seconds with adequate ventilation. Cyanosis is replaced by a pink appearance within 2 minutes. Spontaneous respirations return within 30 seconds to 1 minute in the infant with an Apgar score of 3 to 6 and within 2 to 4 minutes for each minute of asphyxia in the severely asphyxiated infant whose Apgar score is 0 to 2.

TABLE 10. **Perinatal Asphyxia: Postnatal Problems**

Respiratory
  Respiratory distress*
  Apnea*
  Pneumothorax*
  Pulmonary hemorrhage

Metabolic
  Hypothermia
  Hypoglycemia*
  Hypocalcemia
  Inappropriate antidiuretic hormone
  Hyperkalemia

Cardiovascular
  Shock*
  Persistent fetal circulation*
  Cardiac ischemia
  Congestive heart failure

Neurologic
  Hypoxic-ischemic encephalopathy*
  Stupor, coma
  Cerebral edema*
  Seizures*
  Intracranial hemorrhage

Renal
  Acute renal failure*
  Acute renal tubular necrosis*
  Acute cortical necrosis

Hematologic
  Hemolysis
  Disseminated intravascular coagulation

Gastrointestinal
  Peptic ulcer
  Necrotizing enterocolitis
  Hepatic necrosis, failure
  Cholestasis

*Most common complications of asphyxia.

Muscle tone and reflex activity return after spontaneous respirations. Persistence of bradycardia and cyanosis at 2 to 3 minutes indicates inadequate ventilation due to either ineffective resuscitative technique or an underlying congenital abnormality (Table 8).

The most common technical problems include esophageal or right mainstem bronchus intubation, an inadequate seal between the mask and face, hyperextension of the neck, and iatrogenic pneumothorax. These problems must be quickly diagnosed and corrected. If there is doubt concerning tracheal intubation, direct laryngoscopy or reintubation should be performed. A 1- to 2-cm retraction of the endotracheal tube will correct right mainstem bronchus intubation and allow rapid recovery of the infant. Pneumothorax may be diagnosed by transillumination. Thoracentesis with a 50-ml syringe and a 20-gauge intravenous catheter at the anterior axillary line of the fourth or fifth intercostal space will correct the problem. Ineffective mask ventilation must be quickly corrected or replaced by endotracheal intubation and assisted ventilation. Less common conditions that can cause an infant to respond poorly to initial resuscitation are listed in Table 8. External cardiac massage must be continued simultaneously with these corrective measures; pauses for assessments and procedures should be minimized. Correction of technical problems should produce rapid improvements in heart rate and color.

The infant who continues to manifest bradycardia and cyanosis can be assumed to have a profound metabolic acidosis and will require pharmacologic resuscitation. The most expedient route for the initial administration of epinephrine is via the endotracheal tube (Table 9). Umbilical vein catheterization is necessary for administration of sodium bicarbonate. We suggest that an initial endotracheal dose of epinephrine be given at 4 to 5 minutes after birth to those infants who continue to manifest bradycardia (Table 9). Since the drug will be more effective after correction of metabolic acidosis, we would suggest a second dose of epinephrine following umbilical vein catheterization and sodium bicarbonate administration (Table 9). Briefly, an umbilical tie ligature is placed around the base of the umbilical cord, and the cord is transected at a point 1 cm above the abdomen. A saline-filled umbilical catheter (5 Fr) is introduced into the transected umbilical vein and advanced just 3 to 5 cm to a point where blood can be easily aspirated. The appropriately diluted doses of sodium bicarbonate and epinephrine can then be administered. Dilution of sodium bicarbonate is important in the preterm infant because of the risk of hyperosmolar-induced intraventricular hemorrhage.

The administration of intracardiac medications is fraught with potential complications and should be reserved for "last ditch" resuscitative efforts or for infants in whom congenital anomalies preclude umbilical vessel catheterization. Volume resuscitation should be considered in the infant with weak pulses or documented hypotension, especially when there is an antecedent history of maternal bleeding. Plasma expansion should be used sparingly in the preterm infant owing to the risk of intraventricular hemorrhage, which may be associated with surges in blood pressure. Naloxone is indicated when a possible history of maternal analgesic administration is known.

Postnatal Management

The distressed newborn should be moved from the delivery suite to the nursery as soon as adequate ventilation, heart rate, pulses, and color have been assured. If the infant was temporarily intubated during resuscitation, a 2- to 5-minute period of post-extubation observation in the delivery room should be allowed prior to transfer to the nursery. In the intubated infant the endotracheal tube must be carefully secured prior to transfer. The transport Isolette will have been prewarmed and should have its own oxygen source, air source, respiratory gas blender, flow-inflated (anesthesia) and self-inflated (Ambu) hand ventilator bags, an airway pressure gauge, oxygen analyzer, appropriate-sized ventilation masks, spare endotracheal tubes, a laryngoscope and blades, a mouth suction device, stethoscope, and emergency medications (see Table 9). Other helpful transport items include a warming mattress, cardiorespiratory monitor, transcutaneous oxygen monitor, noninvasive oxygen saturation monitor, an intravenous infusion pump, and an infant transport respirator. Similar equipment should be in readiness in the admission nursery.

Both physician and nurse should accompany the infant to the nursery.

Upon arrival in the nursery, the airway should once again be secured, ventilation maintained by a hand or mechanical ventilator, cardiorespiratory monitoring instituted or maintained, and vital signs, including blood pressure, taken. An intravenous infusion, generally 10 per cent dextrose at 2 to 4 ml per kg per hour, may be initiated and a nasogastric tube may be passed. Immediate laboratory studies include arterial blood gases, fasting blood sugar (and Chemstrip or Dextrostix), hematocrit, and a chest-abdominal roentgenogram. Transcutaneous oxygen–carbon dioxide or noninvasive oxygen saturation monitoring may be helpful. A thorough etiologic investigation should be undertaken in cases of unexplained asphyxia. An evaluation for and treatment of bacterial sepsis—meningitis should be included, especially in those cases complicated by prolonged rupture of membranes (greater than 24 hours), maternal chorioamnionitis, respiratory distress, shock, neutropenia, or thrombocytopenia.

The clinician caring for the resuscitated newborn must be vigilant; the list of possible postnatal problems in the resuscitated newborn is prodigious (Table 10). The frequent occurrence of acute renal tubular necrosis and acute renal failure mandates that the initial intravenous fluid administration be limited to the replacement of insensible water losses (35 ml per kg per day for the term infant, 50 to 100 ml per kg per day for the preterm infant). Potassium should be withheld, and only one dose should be given of any drug whose primary route of clearance is renal excretion (e.g., gentamicin). Hypoglycemia induced by stress and anaerobic metabolism is a frequent complication. Dextrose must be administered in constant infusions of 4 to 12 mg per kg per minute. Hypertonic dextrose may be required in cases of fluid restriction. Enteral feedings should be avoided for 24 to 48 hours in the severely asphyxiated infant because of the risk of necrotizing enterocolitis. Cerebral edema and seizures are frequent components of hypoxic-ischemic encephalopathy at 12 to 24 hours after birth. Prompt recognition of seizures and treatment with appropriate intravenous phenobarbital are required (loading dose, 20 mg per kg daily; maintenance dose, 5 mg per kg divided every 12 hours). Appropriate consultation with a regional perinatal center should be sought.

Outcome

Accurate prediction of the long-term neurologic outcome of perinatal asphyxia has been hindered by imprecise diagnostic criteria. Nevertheless, a few general conclusions can be drawn. The asphyxiated newborn has a tenfold increase in mortality risk. The majority of infants with low Apgar scores will be totally normal. Although a frequently used resuscitation assessment tool, Apgar scores correlate poorly with outcome. The absence of spontaneous respiration for more than 5 to 10 minutes after birth is a more powerful correlate of mental retardation and cerebral palsy. Later signs include an abnormal neurologic examination at discharge, poor feeding, and inadequate temperature regulation at an appropriate gestational age. The occurrence of neonatal seizures, especially status epilepticus, doubles the risk of neurologic sequelae. Two electroencephalographic findings, the burst-suppression pattern and any persistently abnormal pattern when seen with neonatal seizures, portend a poor outcome. Direct evidence of cerebral injury may be demonstrated by ultrasonography or computed tomography. While intraventricular hemorrhage in the preterm infant and intracortical hemorrhage in the term infant may be demonstrated early, periventricular leukomalacia and parasagittal cortical atrophy will not be apparent until 3 to 4 weeks postnatally.

CARE OF THE HIGH-RISK NEONATE

method of
LAWRENCE J. FENTON, M.D.
University of South Dakota
Sioux Falls, South Dakota

The care of a high-risk neonate actually begins prior to birth. Therefore, it is important to recognize when such an infant may be born so that steps can be taken to prevent or minimize serious complications. Table 1 summarizes the reasons to anticipate ill health in the neonate and the typical problems associated with each risk category. The scoring system developed by Creasy and colleagues is also helpful in determining the risk of premature labor (Table 2). Most problems arise from either the failure to recognize potential problems or lack of aggressiveness in diagnostic evaluation and treatment.

One can sometimes begin to assume that a baby is well until a crisis is reached, even though signs and symptoms may have been pointing toward a problem for several hours. It is helpful, especially during the first 6 hours after a birth, to maintain an attitude that all newborn babies are in a recovery phase and must *prove* themselves to be well. Of course, infants can become ill after the first 6 hours of life, but in most cases clues to the diagnosis of ill health appear in the first 6 hours, or at least during the first 48 hours.

History and Physical Examination

Many of the risk factors listed in Table 1 can be recognized by taking a careful, thorough history. Others can be found in the physical examination performed soon after birth. If there are any questions about the normality of findings on the physical examination, these should be pursued immediately by consultation, appropriate diagnostic tests, or a concrete plan for re-examination in a short time. Close attention should be paid to instability of temperature, poor sucking, or any major change in behavior.

General Appearance. Any unusual aspects of the baby's activity or facial appearance should be noted. The baby's gestational age and physical maturity should be assessed and plotted on a graph to determine percentile rankings (Figures 1 and 2).

Head. The head should be examined for anomalies, including palpation of the hard palate to determine whether there is a submucosal cleft. The ears, eyes, nose, and throat should also be examined.

Respiration. Sounds should be equal bilaterally at the base of the lungs and at the axillae. Abnormalities such as grunting or retraction or a respiratory rate above 60 may also indicate a problem. If there is any reason for doubt about the health of the lungs, transillumination, a chest x-ray, and a complete blood count should be performed to determine whether there is spontaneous pneumothorax, pneumonia, or a congenital pulmonary or cardiac anomaly.

Cardiovascular System. Peripheral perfusion can be tested by pressing on the chest, abdomen, or thigh and timing the return of blood to the skin. If the return of blood takes more than 3 seconds, peripheral perfusion should be considered diminished. Possible causes of this include hypovolemia, infection, hypoplastic left heart syndrome, hypoglycemia, and hypothermia. A chest x-ray, complete blood count, and blood glucose measurement are helpful in pursuing the cause of diminished peripheral perfusion.

The baby should also be examined for signs of congenital heart disease. Bilateral inequality of pulses and blood pressure in the arms or legs may suggest coarctation. Other signs of congenital heart disease include an unusual second heart sound (single, widely split, or loud) and central cyanosis as evidenced by blue coloration of the trunk, face, or lips.

Abdomen. The examiner should palpate the abdomen carefully for the presence of masses and to locate the liver, spleen, and kidneys. If the liver is more than 2 cm below the right costal margin, infection, heart failure, or hemolytic disease may be present. If more than the tip of the spleen is palpable, bacterial or viral infection or hemolysis should be suspected. A complete blood count and a platelet count should be obtained. The examiner should be able to feel both kidneys clearly. If this is not possible despite repeated palpation, renal ultrasonography is indicated.

Genitalia. Careful inspection for genital abnormalities should be performed routinely.

Extremities. In addition to checking the pulses and blood pressure as mentioned earlier, the examiner should look carefully for anomalies of the extremities. A thorough examination of the hips should include both the Barlow and Ortolani maneuvers.

TABLE 1. **Major Categories of Risk of Ill Health in the Neonate**

Risk Category	Reasons to Anticipate High-Risk Birth	Typical Problems
Prematurity (less than 38 weeks' gestation)	Premature labor Premature rupture of membranes Vaginal bleeding after 12 weeks' gestation History of previous premature delivery or abortion Multiple gestation Maternal infection, e.g., of urinary tract Maternal smoking Low income Uterine anomaly Placenta previa Abdominal surgery History of cesarean section Maternal diabetes	Hyaline membrane disease Apnea and bradycardia Hypoglycemia Hypocalcemia Intraventricular hemorrhage Feeding problems Necrotizing enterocolitis Other fluid and electrolyte disorders Infection Anemia
Postmaturity (more than 42 weeks' gestation) and intrauterine growth retardation	Poor uterine growth Maternal hypertension or other vascular disease Maternal illness during pregnancy possibly compatible with the TORCH group of infections Maternal smoking Oligohydramnios	Birth asphyxia and brain damage Hypoglycemia Polycythemia Clotting disorders, e.g., thrombocytopenia Necrotizing enterocolitis
Birth asphyxia	Postmaturity Intrauterine growth retardation Meconium-stained amniotic fluid Fetal distress, e.g., persistent fetal heart rate greater than 160, loss of beat-to-beat variability, persistent abnormal pattern, fetal acidosis	Brain damage Seizures Meconium aspiration Apnea and bradycardia Necrotizing enterocolitis Feeding disorders Persistence of fetal circulation Hypoglycemia Clotting disorders Renal failure (acute tubular necrosis) Poor cardiac output hypotension

Infants of diabetic mothers	Maternal diabetes, either pre-existing or appearing during pregnancy	Hypoglycemia
		Polycythemia
		Hypocalcemia
		Feeding problems
		Congenital anomalies
		Respiratory problems
		  Hyaline membrane disease
		  Transient tachypnea

Congenital anomalies	Intrauterine growth retardation Oligohydramnios Polyhydramnios Elevated or depressed alpha-protein Breech presentation	Surgical Life-threatening Major handicaps Need for genetic counseling Parental guilt With elevated alpha-protein: neural tube defect, omphalocele, gastroschisis, congenital nephrosis, upper gastrointestinal obstruction, Turner's syndrome With depressed alpha-fetoprotein: chromosomal anomalies, especially trisomy 21
Infection	Maternal infection, e.g., of urinary tract Chorioamnionitis Birth asphyxia Premature labor Premature rupture of membranes Prematurity Membranes rupture longer than 24 hours	Respiratory failure Hypotension Hypoglycemia Anemia Hyperbilirubinemia Persistent fetal circulation Clotting disorders

TABLE 2. **Scoring System for Risk of Preterm Delivery**

Points*	Socioeconomic Status	Past History	Daily Habits	Current Pregnancy
1	Two children at home Low socioeconomic status	One abortion less than 1 year since last birth	Work outside home	Unusual fatigue
2	Younger than 20 years Older than 40 years Single parent	Two abortions	Greater than 10 cigarettes per day	Less than 13-lb gain by 32 weeks Albuminuria Hypertension Bacteriuria
3	Very low socioeconomic status Shorter than 150 cm Lighter than 45 kg	Three abortions	Heavy work Long, tiring trip	Breech at 32 weeks Weight loss of 2 kg Head engaged Febrile illness
4	Younger than 18	Pyelonephritis		Metrorrhagia after 12 weeks' gestation Effacement Dilatation Uterine irritability
5		Uterine anomaly Second-trimester abortion Diethylstilbestrol (DES) exposure		Placenta previa Hydramnios
10		Premature delivery Repeated second-trimes- ter abortion		Twins Abdominal surgery

*Score is computed by addition of the number of points given any time. 0–5 = low risk; 6–9 = medium risk; greater than or equal to 10 = high risk.
Adapted from Creasy R, Gummer B, Liggins G: Obstet Gynecol 55:692, 1980.

Nervous System. Neurologic problems may be indicated by asymmetry of facial movements during crying, or asymmetry of movement or tone of the arms or legs. The overall vigor of the infant's tone, suck, and cry should also be assessed.

PREMATURE BIRTH

Fluid and Electrolyte Treatment

Intravenous administration of fluids and electrolytes should be started if the baby weighs less than 2500 grams, is less than 36 weeks of gestational age, is unable to suck or swallow, needed resuscitation by intubation or by prolonged bag-and-mask ventilation in the delivery room, or has an Apgar score less than 4 at 1 minute or less than 6 at 5 minutes. If an intravenous line is needed, use of a peripheral vein is preferable if it is possible. A 23- or 25-gauge scalp vein needle may be very useful. In an emergency, an umbilical vein catheter can be used, positioned just above the diaphragm as located on an x-ray or placed in just far enough to allow blood return. No hypertonic solutions should be infused through the umbilical vein catheter unless the tip is known to be above the diaphragm in the inferior vena cava.

In general, 80 ml per kg per 24 hours is a safe amount of fluid to administer when beginning intravenous therapy for premature babies. For babies weighing more than 1200 grams, 10 per cent dextrose in water (D10W) should be used.

For infants weighing 1200 grams or less, 5 per cent dextrose in water (D5W) is preferable. Rates of administration can be adjusted on the basis of electrolyte levels, weight changes, urinary output, and specific gravity of urine; however, specific gravity is an unreliable indicator for several weeks or longer in premature babies because of their inability to concentrate urine. If weight increases or fails to decrease, the baby may be overloaded with fluid (unless there was a major loss of volume at delivery). If weight decreases by more than 2 per cent per day, the baby probably needs more fluids.

Usually no electrolytes are needed for the first 6 to 12 hours after birth unless there is reason to suspect electrolyte abnormalities in the mother, as could occur if the mother received a large volume of hypotonic fluid prior to delivery. Serum sodium and potassium levels should be measured at 12 hours of age. Maintenance sodium chloride (3 mEq per kg per day) should be added if the sodium level is below 135 mEq per liter; the desired range for serum sodium is 135 to 145 mEq per liter. Maintenance potassium chloride (2 mEq per kg per day) should be added if the potassium level is less than 4.5 mEq per liter and urine output is established.

Hypocalcemia is common in premature babies. A serum calcium level of less than 7 mg per dl in a premature baby is usually considered a deficiency. The serum calcium level usually reaches its lowest point at about 48 hours of age.

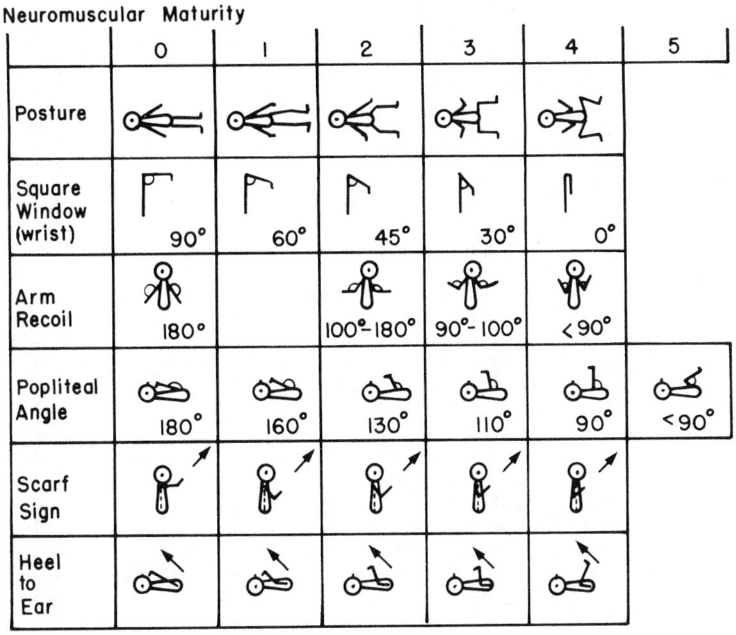

Neuromuscular Maturity

	0	1	2	3	4	5
Posture						
Square Window (wrist)	90°	60°	45°	30°	0°	
Arm Recoil	180°		100°-180°	90°-100°	< 90°	
Popliteal Angle	180°	160°	130°	110°	90°	< 90°
Scarf Sign						
Heel to Ear						

PHYSICAL MATURITY

Skin	gelatinous red, transparent	smooth pink, visible veins	superficial peeling &/or rash few veins	cracking pale area rare veins	parchment deep cracking no vessels	leathery cracked wrinkled
Lanugo	none	abundant	thinning	bald areas	mostly bald	
Plantar Creases	no crease	faint red marks	anterior transverse crease only	creases ant. 2/3	creases cover entire sole	
Breast	barely percept.	flat areola no bud	stippled areola 1–2 mm bud	raised areola 3–4 mm bud	full areola 5–10 mm bud	
Ear	pinna flat, stays folded	sl. curved pinna; soft with slow recoil	well-curv. pinna; soft but ready recoil	formed & firm with instant recoil	thick cartilage ear stiff	
Genitals ♂	scrotum empty no rugae		testes descending, few rugae	testes down good rugae	testes pendulous deep rugae	
Genitals ♀	prominent clitoris & labia minora		majora & minora equally prominent	majora large minora small	clitoris & minora completely covered	

MATURITY RATING

Score	Wks
5	26
10	28
15	30
20	32
25	34
30	36
35	38
40	40
45	42
50	44

Figure 1. Assessment of gestational age. (Modified from Ballard JL, Novak KK, and Driver M: J Pediatr 95:769, 1979.)

I usually begin treatment of hypocalcemia by adding maintenance calcium gluconate to the intravenous fluids at a dose of 1 mEq of elemental calcium per kg per day or 200 mg of calcium gluconate per kg per day. (This is equivalent to 2 ml of 10 per cent calcium gluconate per kilogram per day.) An alternative to adding the calcium gluconate to the intravenous fluid is to give it as four divided boluses; this should be done very slowly with the infant on a cardiac monitor to allow quick recognition of bradycardia. We prefer this latter method because we

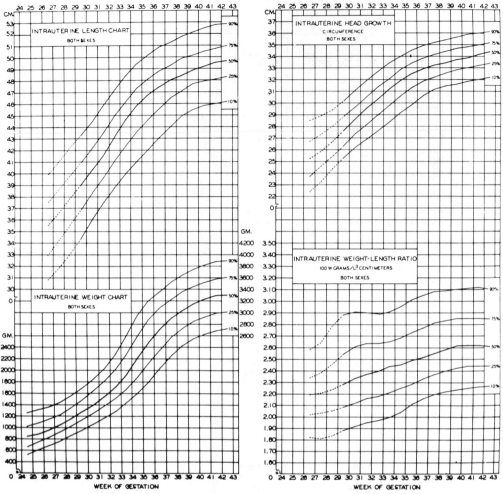

Figure 2. Intrauterine growth curves for length, head circumference, and weight for singleton births in Colorado. (From Lubchenco L, Hansman C, and Boyd, E. Reproduced by permission of Pediatrics 37:403, 1966.)

occasionally substitute sodium bicarbonate for sodium chloride in the intravenous line when there is significant metabolic acidosis; the sodium bicarbonate and calcium cannot be kept in the same solution, so the calcium in these cases must be administered separately. Another approach is to "drip" the calcium and push bicarbonate "very slowly" if needed. The major risk of rapid pushing of sodium bicarbonate is intraventricular hemorrhage.

The pharmacist should be asked to make up these solutions on a per kilogram basis, rather than giving the electrolytes as a specified measurement per 100 ml. The amount of sodium, potassium, or other electrolyte a baby may need can be quite independent of the baby's need for fluids. Therefore, whenever the rate of infusion of fluid is changed, the electrolyte concentration of the fluid should be adjusted to maintain the desired level of electrolyte administration based on the baby's weight.

A constant weight, typically the birth weight, should be used as the reference weight for determining how much fluid to administer. Otherwise, the normal loss of weight during the first days of life may offset to some extent any increase in fluid administration ordered on a per kilogram basis, or cause an unwanted reduction in total fluid administration in an infant who started out receiving an adequate amount of fluid when infusion was originally based on birth weight.

Fluid intake and output should be carefully monitored and totaled at least every 8 hours. Measurement of urine specific gravity and testing with a urine test-tape should be done frequently, in some cases with every void.

If the baby can tolerate it, weight should be measured once or twice a day. The baby should be kept warm during the weighing process. Emerson lights over the scale are helpful, and adequate staff should be assigned to the procedure to assure that it is done quickly. Respiratory stability should never be compromised for the sake of monitoring weight.

Basic Laboratory Assessment

Blood glucose levels can be monitored by using Chemstrips or Dextrostix every half hour for 2 hours, then hourly for 2 hours, then 2 hours later, and then at 4-hour intervals until the patient is stable. If the blood sugar reading is 40 mg per dl or lower, a blood sample should be taken for laboratory analysis to confirm the finding. If the laboratory finding is also below 40 mg per dl, an intravenous line should be started.

A complete blood count should be taken. Findings should be compared with normal values as listed in Table 3.

Arterial blood gases should be assessed if birth asphyxia occurs or if resuscitation is needed in the delivery room. If arterial blood gas measurements cannot be obtained, a warmed capillary heel puncture in conjunction with transcutaneous monitoring of PaO_2 or monitoring of oxygen saturation may be helpful.

A chest radiograph should be obtained if there is respiratory distress or an abnormal blood gas value found on laboratory study. A chest radiograph should also be taken prior to transportation of the infant, especially if air transportation is anticipated.

Routine Care

The infant should be placed on a cardiorespiratory monitor if he or she is of less than 36 weeks' gestational age, has any respiratory distress or cyanosis, or needs intravenous therapy, or if there is a historical factor indicating that the baby is at risk for infection. We monitor *all* babies in the newborn intensive care unit from admission to discharge. The monitoring unit should be set to give an alarm if an episode of apnea continues for 15 seconds or if the heart rate rises above 180 or falls below 100. (The lower limit of the heart rate can be adjusted to 80 when the baby is fully stabilized or becomes a "grower"; the upper limit may need to be adjusted to over 200 if the baby is active or crying frequently.)

If the infant is less than 35 weeks' gestational age or has an unstable temperature, a neutral thermal environment should be provided (Table 4). An open warmer or an Isolette can be used. If the baby weighs less than 1500 grams and is placed in an open warmer, use of a plastic shield to enclose the baby and addition of warmed humidity (not enough to cause condensation or to form fog) will greatly reduce insensible water loss and preserve the skin. This is especially useful for very small babies. If the baby is in an Isolette that is being opened frequently, Emerson lights may be used to add heat. A double-walled Isolette can also be used to preserve heat, and in some cases a warming mattress is essential.

Vital signs and blood pressure should be monitored every 15 minutes for 2 hours, then every 30 minutes for 2 hours, then 2 hours later, and at 4-hour intervals thereafter. However, if a baby is very unstable, these orders should be modified to keep disturbances to a minimum.

Respiratory Distress

Assessment of respiratory distress should begin with a chest x-ray to rule out pneumothorax and congenital anomalies. If the distress is sustained or is initially fairly significant, blood should be drawn for culture and antibiotic therapy should be started (see Table 6). Monitoring should include arterial blood gas measurements taken every 1 to 4 hours or, if this is not practical, monitoring by warmed heel puncture and transcutaneous PaO_2 measurement or monitoring of oxygen saturation. The PaO_2 should be maintained in the range of 60 to 80 torr. A PCO_2 measurement greater than 50 torr may indicate impending respiratory failure.

If pH is below 7.25 and PCO_2 is above 50 torr, the patient should be intubated and placed on a ventilator or ventilated with a bag. If endotracheal intubation is not feasible, an orogastric tube should be placed and bag-and-mask ventilation should be instituted. A tertiary referral center should be consulted in these cases.

Any sudden adverse change in a premature infant's respiratory status should indicate the need for a repeat physical examination as well as a chest x-ray or transillumination of the chest or both. The endotracheal tube should be checked to ensure that it has not become dislodged or plugged; direct visualization of the tube's position may be needed. If there is doubt, the tube should be pulled and bag-and-mask ventilation begun.

Pneumothorax

If transillumination of the chest unquestionably shows pneumothorax, measures to relieve this condition should be instituted without delay for chest x-rays. This is especially true if the baby is doing poorly. If the baby is unstable, an 18-gauge scalp vein needle can be inserted at the second intercostal space in the midclavicular line. The needle should be connected to a three-way stopcock and a 12- to 35-ml syringe and inserted to a depth of approximately 5 to 10 mm, depending

TABLE 3. **Hematologic Values in the Newborn**

NORMAL HEMATOLOGIC VALUES*

Value	Gestational Age (wks) 28	34	Full-term Cord Blood	Day 1	Day 3	Day 7	Day 14
Hb (gm/dl)	14.5	15.0	16.8	18.4	17.9	17.0	16.8
Hematocrit (%)	45	47	53	58	55	54	52
Red cells (mm³)	4.0	4.4	5.25	5.8	5.6	5.2	5.1
MCV (μ^3)	120	118	107	108	99	98	96
MCH (pg)	40	38	34	35	33	32.5	31.5
MCHC (%)	31	32	31.7	32.5	33	33	33
Reticulocytes (%)	5–10	5–10	3–7	3–7	1–3	0–1	0–1
Platelets (1000s/mm³)			290	192	213	248	252

WHITE CELL AND DIFFERENTIAL COUNTS IN PREMATURE INFANTS*

Birth Weight	Less than 150 gm			1500–2500 gm		
Age in weeks	1	2	4	1	2	4
Total count ($\times 10^3$/mm³)						
Mean	16.8	15.4	12.1	13.0	10.0	8.4
Range	6.1–32.8	10.4–21.3	8.7–17.2	6.7–14.7	7.0–14.1	5.8–12.4
Per cent of total						
Polymorphs						
Segmented	54	45	40	55	43	41
Unsegmented	7	6	5	8	8	6
Eosinophils	2	3	3	2	3	3
Basophils	1	1	1	1	1	1
Monocytes	6	10	10	5	9	11
Lymphocytes	30	35	41	9	36	38

LEUKOCYTE VALUES AND NEUTROPHIL COUNTS IN TERM AND PREMATURE INFANTS†

Age (hrs)	Total White Cell Count	Neutrophils	Bands/Metas	Lymphocytes	Monocytes	Eosinophils
Term Infants						
0	10.0–26.0	5.0–13.0	0.4–1.8	3.5–8.5	0.7–1.5	0.2–2.0
12	13.5–31.0	9.0–18.0	0.4–2.0	3.0–7.0	1.0–2.0	0.2–2.0
72	5.0–14.5	2.0–7.0	0.2–0.4	2.0–5.0	0.5–1.0	0.2–1.0
144	6.0–14.5	2.0–6.0	0.2–0.5	3.0–6.0	0.7–1.2	0.2–0.8
Premature Infants						
0	5.9–19.0	2.0–9.0	0.2–2.4	2.5–6.0	0.3–1.0	0.1–0.7
12	5.0–21.0	3.0–11.0	0.2–2.4	1.5–5.0	0.3–1.3	0.1–1.1
72	5.0–14.0	3.0–7.0	0.2–0.6	1.5–4.0	0.3–1.2	0.2–1.1
144	5.5–17.5	2.0–7.0	0.2–0.5	2.5–7.5	0.5–1.5	0.3–1.2

MCV, mean corpuscular volume; MCH, mean corpuscular hemoglobin; MCHC, mean corpuscular hemoglobin concentration.
*From Klaus MH, Fanaroff AA: Care of the High-Risk Neonate. 3rd ed. Philadelphia, W. B. Saunders Co., 1986.
†Oski F, Naima J: Hematologic Problems in the Newborn. Philadelphia, W. B. Saunders Co., 1972.

on the thickness of the chest wall. Air should be aspirated, and preparation should be done for placement of a chest tube. If a chest tube cannot be inserted, needle aspiration can be used to maintain control until more definitive treatment can be instituted.

The chest tube can be inserted either in the second intercostal space in the midclavicular line or at the fourth or fifth interspace in the anterior axillary line. The axillary approach avoids anterior scarring, which is more noticeable than axillary scarring. The insertion of a chest tube requires sterile technique, including use of a gown and gloves. A ¼-inch incision should be made over the rib, with care taken to avoid blood vessels that run along the inferior edge. A small,

curved hemostat ("mosquito") is used to spread the skin, and pressure by the index finger on top of the curve of the hemostat will "pop" the hemostat through the pleura. The hemostat is then spread gently to allow a No. 10 French (for a small baby) or a No. 12 French (for a baby weighing more than 2000 grams) chest tube to be inserted without use of a stylet. If the axillary approach is used, the tip of the tube should be aimed anteriorly. The tube should be inserted no more than 3 cm, but should be placed far enough in so that it "steams up" with each expiration. A purse-string suture should be tied, with use of 4-0 nonabsorbable suture material.

When the chest tube is sutured in place it should be attached to a suction apparatus with a

TABLE 4. **Neutral Thermal Environmental Temperatures**

Age and Weight	Range of Temperature (°C)	Age and Weight	Range of Temperature
0–6 hours		72–96 hours	
Under 1200 gm	34.0–35.4	Under 12 gm	34.0–35.0
1200–1500 gm	34.0–35.4	1200–1500 gm	34.0–35.0
1200–1500 gm	33.0–34.4	1200–1500 gm	33.0–34.0
1501–2500 gm	32.8–33.8	1501–2500 gm	31.1–33.2
Over 2500 (and > 36 weeks)	32.8–33.8	Over 2500 (and > 36 weeks)	29.8–32.8
6–12 hours		4–12 days	
Under 1200 gm	34.0–35.4	Under 1200 gm	33.0–34.0
1200–1500 gm	33.5–34.4	1501–2500 gm	31.0–33.2
1501–2500 gm	32.2–33.8	Over 2500 (and > 36 weeks)	
Over 2500 (and > 36 weeks)	31.4–33.8	4–5 days	29.5–32.6
12–24 hours		5–6 days	29.4–32.3
Under 1200 gm	34.0–35.4	6–8 days	29.0–32.2
1200–1500 gm	33.3–34.3	8–10 days	29.0–31.8
1501–2500 gm	31.8–33.8	10–12 days	29.0–31.4
Over 2500 (and > 36 weeks)	31.0–33.7	12–14 days	
24–36 hours		Under 1500 gm	32.6–34.0
Under 1200 gm	34.0–35.0	1501–2500 gm	31.0–33.2
1200–1500 gm	33.1–34.2	Over 2500 (and > 36 weeks)	29.0–30.8
1501–2500 gm	31.6–33.6	2–3 weeks	
Over 2500 (and > 36 weeks)	30.7–33.5	Under 1500 gm	32.2–34.0
36–48 hours		1501–2500 gm	30.5–33.0
Under 1200 gm	34.0–35.0	3–4 weeks	
1200–1500 gm	33.0–34.1	Under 1500 gm	31.6–33.6
1501–2500 gm	31.4–33.5	1501–2500 gm	30.0–32.7
Over 2500 (and > 36 weeks)	30.5–33.3	4–5 weeks	
48–72 hours		Under 1500 gm	31.2–33.0
Under 1200 gm	34.0–35.0	1501–2500 gm	29.5–32.2
1200–1500 gm	33.0–34.0	5–6 weeks	
1501–2500 gm	31.2–33.4	Under 1500 gm	30.6–32.3
Over 2500 (and > 36 weeks)	30.1–33.2	1501–2500 gm	29.0–31.8

Adapted from Scopes J, Ahmed I: Arch Dis Child 41:417, 1966. For his table, Scopes had the walls of the incubator 1° to 2° warmer than the ambient air temperatures.

Generally, the smaller infants in each weight group will require a temperature in the higher portion of the temperature range. Within each time range, the younger the infant, the higher the temperature required.

negative pressure of approximately 10 cm of water. (A Heimlich valve can also work very well for a short time. Excessive drainage can cause rubber to stick together.) Once the tube is in place, its position should be checked radiographically. A lateral view is helpful. Cross-table supine films can often be taken with minimal disturbance to the baby.

Hypoglycemia

Chemstrips can be used to monitor for hypoglycemia. They should be checked at least once every 4 hours until feeding is well established and the baby is stable. If readings on Chemstrips indicate blood sugar less than 40 or greater than 150 mg per dl, a blood sample should be drawn for laboratory analysis of blood sugar.

If blood sugar is confirmed as being less than 40 mg per dl and the baby is stable, an increase in the amount of sugar in the intravenous line can be considered. I usually do not exceed D10W in a peripheral vein because the hypertonicity

will decrease the time that the intravenous line will remain usable. However, D12.5W can be used on a temporary basis. Unless there is a contraindication, the rate of fluid infusion can be increased by 20 ml per kg per day to increase sugar intake.

If the blood sugar level is below 30 mg per dl or if there are symptoms (seizures, lethargy, excessive tremors) with blood sugar below 40 mg per dl, a bolus of D10W at 2 to 4 ml per kg (or 0.2 to 0.4 grams of glucose per kg) can be given intravenously over a 15-minute period. Chemstrips should be rechecked every 30 to 60 minutes until the patient is stable. No bolus with a sugar concentration greater than D10W should ever be given.

Feeding

Overly aggressive feeding of small babies, babies with respiratory distress, or babies recovering from birth asphyxia may cause aspiration or necrotizing enterocolitis. A lethargic or tachypneic baby may frequently aspirate liquid feedings, and this may greatly complicate any other problems the baby has had. Adequate time for recovery and stabilization should be allowed before feeding is attempted. The first feeding should always be plain sterile water.

The first feeding should be delayed in a number of situations. If the infant is less than 36 weeks' gestational age, or less than 2500 grams birth weight, the first feeding should be given 24 hours after birth if no problems have developed. If the infant has had respiratory distress, the first feeding should be delayed until the distress is nearly gone—that is, when the respiratory rate is less than 60 and the infant appears comfortable. For infants affected by birth asphyxia, hypotension, acidosis, hypothermia, or severe anemia, the first feeding should not be given until the child is at least 7 days old in order to avoid necrotizing enterocolitis. If the infant has been unstable for any reason, the first feeding should be delayed until the infant has been stable for at least 24 hours; delay of as much as 7 days may be advisable if the instability involved prolonged hypoxia, hypotension, acidosis, or hypothermia.

If the infant is younger than 35 weeks' gestational age, has impaired ability to suck or swallow, or appears to lack vigor, a conservative approach to feeding is advisable. The first feeding, as for all babies, should be sips of sterile water. If aspiration should occur, water will do no damage to the airway. D5W is as harmful to the airway as formula. If there are no problems with the first feeding, the next feeding is with quarter-strength to half-strength sterile formula; smaller or sicker babies should receive the more diluted formula. Babies weighing less than 1500 grams should receive a specially designed formula for the premature that contains 24 kcal per ounce. The first feeding of formula should be approximately 2 to 3 ml per kg. Subsequent feedings can be given every 2 hours for the infant weighing less than 1500 grams or every 3 hours for the infant weighing more than 1500 grams.

The feedings should be adjusted gradually so that full-volume, full-strength feedings are being given at the end of the seventh day of feeding. Table 5 shows a typical 7-day regimen designed for a 2-kg infant who needs gavage feeding and was quite sick for the first 3 to 4 days of life. In this example, the infant's eventual need is 120 kcal per kg per day, which would require 180 ml per kg per day using a formula providing 20 kcal per ounce. The eventual amount of the daily feedings should therefore be 360 ml (180 ml per kg, times 2 kg), divided into eight feedings of 45 ml per feeding. This example assumes that there is no requirement to limit water intake; in some situations, such as bronchopulmonary dysplasia, water intake may need to be limited.

If feeding is not tolerated, as may be indicated by abdominal distention, diarrhea, or vomiting, feeding should be stopped and the baby should be reassessed. If the baby seems well, feeding can be resumed in 24 hours at reduced strength and/or reduced volume. This schedule is cautious and conservative, and rarely is followed by necrotizing enterocolitis.

Oxygen

Oxygen should be used liberally but monitored closely, especially if the baby is less than 35 weeks' gestational age. If the baby is unstable, continual transcutaneous monitoring of PaO_2 or monitoring of oxygen saturation is indicated. If oxygen needs remain greater than 40 per cent for a sustained period, an arterial line is generally indicated. If the baby is unstable, arterial gases should be checked every 1 to 4 hours. Also, when the transcutaneous monitor is changed, arterial gases should be measured so that the values provided by the monitor can be compared for appropriateness and accuracy.

Apnea

Apnea and bradycardia are very common problems that affect most premature babies at some time. Several possible causes of apnea should be considered. A complete blood count, blood culture, and possibly a lumbar puncture should be performed to rule out infection. We have found sepsis due to coagulase-negative staphylocci an important cause of apnea that may be associated with normal results of the blood count. Blood sugar and electrolytes should be measured. A chest x-ray may reveal any of a variety of causes of respiratory disturbances. A careful physical examination should focus on new findings that might change pulmonary dynamics, such as a patent ductus arteriosus, excessive weight gain, or increased fluid in the lungs. An electroencephalogram should be considered to rule out seizures. Computed tomography or ultrasonography of the head may reveal an intracranial malformation or hemorrhage. Conduction abnormalities may be discovered by electrocardiography. A 12-hour pneumogram may be helpful in quantitating and documenting events. Gastroesophageal reflux should be considered as a cause; an esophageal pH study and a barium esophagogram may be required to rule out anomalies.

In practice, the main early work-up should focus on new physical changes, infections, glucose and electrolyte levels, and seizures, because im-

TABLE 5. **Sample Regimen for Increasing Feeding for a Premature Infant**

Day	Strength	Initial Volume	Volume by End of Day
Day 1	¼	5 ml—advance 1 ml per feeding	12 ml
Day 2	¼	12 ml	20 ml
Day 3	½	20 ml (hold volume for 2 feedings after strength change)	26 ml
Day 4	½	26 ml	34 ml
Day 5	¾	34 ml (hold volume after 2 feedings again)	40 ml
Day 6	¾	40 ml	45 ml
Day 7	Full strength	45 ml	45 ml

See text for details of sample case this regimen applies to.

mediate treatment of these problems is necessary, available, and curative.

In most cases apnea in premature infants has no discernible cause. Mild cases of idiopathic apnea are handled merely by stimulation. Low-dose oxygen (22 to 23 per cent) may be helpful, but careful monitoring is required. If apnea is associated with feeding, helpful techniques may include reducing the volume of feeding, adding oxygen, or positioning the baby on the abdomen with the head up. When these methods fail or when spells are significant with associated brady-cardia, cyanosis, or pallor, aminophylline is our drug of choice. A loading dose of 5 mg per kg, orally or intravenously, can be followed with 5 to 6 mg per kg per day in four divided doses to achieve a therapeutic level. In our experience, this level usually ranges from 7 to 14 micrograms per ml. Occasionally lower levels are effective, and in some infants higher levels may be needed. After the baby has been stable for several weeks, weaning may be attempted. Some infants will require aminophylline for 2 to 4 months after discharge from the hospital. Levels must be closely followed. Peak levels must be kept below 20 micrograms per ml. Toxic symptoms may appear at levels greater than 10 micrograms per ml.

Home Monitors

Although there is no certain relationship between apnea and sudden infant death syndrome, we tend to use home monitoring if apnea has been a significant problem in the nursery or if a baby requires theophylline after discharge to control apnea. We insist that all babies be free of apnea for at least 1 week prior to discharge. Home monitoring is then frequently carried through for a 6-month period and discontinued if there have been no apneic spells for at least 2 months and the infant has tolerated an infection without having any apneic spells.

POSTMATURITY AND INTRAUTERINE GROWTH RETARDATION

If the fetus is older than 42 weeks' gestation or if there is evidence of intrauterine growth retardation, delivery room personnel and equipment should be prepared for major resuscitation.

Monitoring of blood sugar is mandatory. Chemstrips should be checked every 1 to 2 hours for the first 6 hours, then intermittently until feeding is established. It is especially important to check the sugar level prior to feeding, when blood glucose may be at its lowest value.

A complete blood count should be obtained. Thrombocytopenia may be found in association with intrauterine infection or with toxemia of pregnancy. Polycythemia is frequently seen, and its management is controversial. The presence of polycythemia should be verified by at least two measurements and by use of a central venous or central arterial puncture. If the central hematocrit (Hct) is 65 to 70 and the baby is perfectly well, no treatment is indicated. Higher Hct values may indicate the need for aggressive management. If the central Hct is 70 to 75 and the baby is symptomatic, for example showing neurologic abnormalities, respiratory distress, or signs compatible with congestive heart failure, such as hepatomegaly, tachypnea, cardiomegaly, or pulmonary edema on x-ray, partial exchange transfusion may be indicated. If the central Hct is greater than 75, a partial exchange transfusion may be indicated even if the baby shows no symptoms. If the baby is symptomatic or if the

Hct is above 75, the case should be discussed with a specialist from a tertiary care center.

A postmature baby who is well can be fed ad libitum as for a normal term infant. If there is extreme growth retardation, cautious feeding as for a premature baby is advisable, because of the risk that chronic hypoxia may have affected the gut.

BIRTH ASPHYXIA

Clinically birth asphyxia can be defined as having occurred when there is an Apgar score of less than 3 at 1 minute after birth or an Apgar score of less than 5 at 5 minutes. Severe birth asphyxia, which places the baby at high risk for cerebral palsy, can be recognized when the Apgar score is less than 5 at 10 minutes, when cord blood gases indicate metabolic acidosis, when the baby is hypotonic for more than 30 minutes (hypotonicity for more than 2 hours is an ominous sign), or when seizures develop.

Following birth asphyxia the baby must not be fed. An intravenous line should be started, with fluids restricted to 60 ml per kg per day. Blood sugar levels should be kept fairly high, in the range of 75 to 100 mg per dl. Oxygen levels should be monitored closely. The baby must be kept *well oxygenated*; it is essential to avoid a second episode of hypoxia. If the baby is having apnea or a seizure and begins to become hypoxic, mechanical ventilation may be necessary to maintain good oxygenation until the spell is brought under control. Severely asphyxiated babies should be cared for in a tertiary care center because the chance of deterioration is so great. If further hypoxic events can be avoided and metabolic normality can be maintained, there is a reasonable possibility of a favorable outcome.

Seizures

If the baby is having seizures, a tertiary care center should be contacted. I use phenobarbital to control seizures, with a loading dose of 10 to 20 mg per kg intravenously, followed by a maintenance dose of 3 to 5 mg per kg per day given in two divided doses. The loading dose may be increased to as much as 30 mg per kg, but if a dose this large is given, the physician must be prepared to institute ventilation. The blood level of phenobarbital should be measured in 24 hours. Therapeutic levels are usually achieved between 20 and 30 micrograms per dl, but sometimes higher levels are used in the first several days. Blood levels of sugar, calcium, and sodium must be checked.

Counseling of Parents

In counseling parents of babies with birth asphyxia, I am as honest as I can be. If I have great concern over the prognosis, I say so. However, until the effects of the cerebral edema are gone and the seizures are controlled, the baby cannot be adequately assessed. Prognostic discussions are more valid after about 7 days. Parents should be encouraged to be with their baby and should be given as much emotional support as possible. The health care team should be prepared for the parents' feelings of anger, guilt, and frustration. Parents need to know that no matter what the outcome, the health care team will help them with every step and every difficult decision and will be available to talk with them as frequently as possible. Criticism of the delivering physician, either by direct statements or as implied by attitude, should be avoided.

CONGENITAL ANOMALIES

If surgical anomalies such as omphalocele, gastroschisis, or meningomyelocele are present, the baby must be transported immediately to an appropriate surgical center. The exposed tissues of a meningomyelocele should be covered with moist gauze soaked in sterile saline and then covered with plastic (Saran Wrap, Op-site) and a large, bulky dressing. Exposed bowel can be managed with a commercially available plastic bowel bag. As is done for any major intestinal problem, the stomach should be decompressed with a gastric tube.

Babies with syndromes and malformations that are diagnostic puzzles should also be transferred to a tertiary care center so that a diagnosis can be obtained as soon as possible. A great deal of parental anxiety is frequently relieved when a "name" can be put on something, a definite prognosis given, and genetic counseling obtained. If an infant with multiple anomalies dies, a careful autopsy should be performed that includes blood or tissue sampling for chromosomal analysis as well as x-rays of the chest and skeleton.

INFECTION

The key to successful management of an infection is to begin an appropriate work-up and treatment long before the signs and symptoms have reached a critical point. This requires a prompt and aggressive response to early signs and symptoms or major risk factors.

Signs and Symptoms Requiring Prompt Attention

Diagnostic procedures should be instituted promptly if the baby has respiratory distress of any kind. Disturbances in breathing should not be assumed to be due to transient tachypnea. Grunting should be considered abnormal. A normal appearance on a chest x-ray does not rule out pneumonia, since pneumonia in the newborn is often diffuse and may be difficult to distinguish from hyaline membrane disease or transient tachypnea of the newborn. Cyanosis or an oxygen requirement after 20 minutes of age should *always* be considered abnormal.

Unstable body temperature with axillary temperatures above 37.4° C (99.4° F) or below 36.7° C (98° F) require prompt diagnosis and adequate treatment. Gastrointestinal signs and symptoms necessitating work-up without delay include poor feeding, vomiting, distention, diarrhea, and bloody stools. Also, lethargy, unexplained metabolic acidosis, unexplained hypoglycemia, pallor, or hypotension demands prompt attention.

A number of findings on blood tests may indicate sepsis. A white blood count of less than 5000 per microliter, an absolute neutrophil count of less than 1200 polymorphonuclear leukocytes per microliter, or a ratio of bands to total polymorphonuclear leukocytes (including bands) greater than 0.4 should be considered as evidence of sepsis until proved otherwise.

Risk Factors

Some risk factors require prompt treatment even if the baby is perfectly asymptomatic. Birth trauma, perinatal asphyxia, maternal infection, chorioamnionitis, and prematurity are the major risk factors. Prolonged rupture of membranes becomes of major importance only when the above factors coexist.

The approach to infants with other risk factors depends to some extent on the maturity of the baby. Observation alone is sufficient initially for a term infant with prolonged rupture of membranes, fetal distress, or difficult or traumatic delivery as the sole risk factor. Any one of these accompanying risk factors in a preterm infant is sufficient reason for investigating by obtaining a blood culture, complete blood count, and platelet count. These studies should also be performed in a term infant with prolonged rupture of membranes plus either fetal distress or traumatic delivery, with maternal infection, or with minimal or questionable amnionitis, and in the baby who has required invasive resuscitation.

Work-Up for Sepsis

The suspicion of sepsis is a medical emergency. There may be less than 1 hour between the development of minimal symptoms and respiratory failure with shock. A complete work-up for sepsis should be done for any term infant with any risk factor accompanied by abnormal laboratory data indicating sepsis, with frank (purulent) chorioamnionitis, or with any risk factor in combination with a history of maternal infection. A complete work-up for sepsis is also indicated for any preterm infant with abnormal laboratory data and any risk factor, with two or more risk factors, with early or questionable chorioamnionitis, or with a history including maternal infection or invasive resuscitation.

A blood culture study using a sample of 2 ml of blood and a complete blood count should always be included in the work-up when sepsis is suspected. If the baby is symptomatic, a spinal tap should also be done; however, the spinal tap may have to be delayed if the baby is unstable. In most cases of meningitis, culture will not become negative for 1 to 3 days, and abnormalities of cells, protein, and sugar usually persist for a much longer time. A suprapubic urine collection for culture is indicated if the baby is more than 7 days of age. If the baby is ill but appropriate specimens cannot be obtained, it is advisable to begin treatment; it is better to have a good outcome with an uncertain diagnosis than a poor outcome with a known diagnosis.

Treatment

Initial therapy, especially if the baby is less than 7 days of age, should include both ampicillin and gentamicin (Table 6). Ampicillin covers Group B streptococci, which are the most common cause of infection in the newborn, *Listeria*, some gram-negative organisms, and some anaerobes. Gentamicin covers most gram-negative organisms. *Bacteroides* and *Staphylococcus* infections are not covered by this regimen. Staphylococci rarely cause infection in the first week of life. If an anaerobic infection with *Bacteroides* is suspected, cefoxitin can be added to the ampicillin-gentamicin regimen. An older baby has an increased risk for nosocomial infections, which are commonly caused by coagulase-negative staphylococci. Vancomycin and cefotaxime can be used empirically in this situation.

If sepsis is proven or clinically likely, therapy should be continued for 7 to 10 days. If pneumonia is present, with or without positive cultures, treatment for 10 to 14 days is indicated. Meningitis should be treated for a minimum of 14 days if the infecting organism is a Group B streptococcus. Meningitis involving *Escherichia coli* or other gram-negative organisms should be treated for at least 21 days.

If cultures are negative, antibiotic treatment

TABLE 6. **Commonly Used Drugs for Infections in Neonates**

Drug	Usual Dose	Comment
Ampicillin	Less than 7 days of age: 50 mg per kg every 12 hours intravenous push Greater than or equal to 7 days of age: 70 mg per kg per dose every 8 hours intravenous push	For babies less than 7 days of age, increase to 100 mg per kg per dose every 12 hours if Group B streptococcal infection or meningitis is suspected
Gentamicin	2.5 mg per kg per dose every 12 hours given intravenously over 20 minutes	Measure levels to keep peak less than 8.00 micrograms per ml and trough between 1.5 and 2.5 micrograms per ml. Frequency of dose decreased for premature babies or those with decreased creatinine clearance (as with birth asphyxia)
Cefotaxime	50 mg per kg per dose every 8 hours intravenous push	May be substituted for gentamicin, especially if gentamicin levels cannot be measured. May be used empirically with vancomycin in baby with suspected nosocomial infection
Vancomycin	10 mg per kg per dose every 8 to 12 hours (less frequent if premature). Give intravenously over 45 minutes to 1 hour	Must monitor drug levels. Keep peak at 20 to 30 micrograms per ml. Keep trough at 5 to 10 micrograms per ml. Watch for flushing, hypothermia, and tachycardia. Indicated for proven or suspected resistant staphylococcal infections
Cefoxitin	40 mg per kg per dose intravenously every 6 to every 8 hours	Indicated for empiric treatment of anaerobic infection

can be discontinued if (1) the initial reason for treatment was a risk factor only, the baby was asymptomatic, and laboratory values were normal, or (2) the baby was symptomatic but review of clinical circumstances indicates that the symptoms were probably due to another cause and laboratory values did not support the diagnosis of infection. Antibiotic treatment should be continued for a full 7-day course despite negative cultures if (1) initial signs and symptoms were clinically convincing, (2) the baby was asymptomatic but laboratory values were highly abnormal, or (3) the baby was asymptomatic but at high risk and the mother received intrapartum antibiotics.

INFANT OF A DIABETIC MOTHER

If the mother is diabetic, the infant's blood sugar level should be monitored by use of Chemstrips, which should be checked every 10 minutes for the first 2 hours, then hourly for the next 2 hours, and at 2-hour intervals thereafter. If the level is questionable or is below 40 mg per dl, blood should be obtained for measurement of blood sugar. If blood sugar is less than 40 mg per dl, there are no contraindications to feeding, and the initial feeding with sips of sterile water has been handled without difficulty, 3 to 4 ml of D5W per kg can be offered to the baby. If the sugar level remains above 30 mg per dl and the baby is asymptomatic, D5W or formula can be fed as tolerated.

If the baby will not take feedings or if there are contraindications to feeding, such as prematurity or respiratory distress, an intravenous line should be started with D10W infused at 80 ml per kg per day. Intravenous boluses of sugar should be avoided, as they may exacerbate the problem that was the initial contraindication to feeding. However, if the baby is showing symptoms such as lethargy, seizures, or apnea or seems jittery and the sugar level is remaining below 40 mg per dl and not responding to the intravenous infusion, 4 ml of D10W per kg can be given by intravenous push over 5 to 10 minutes and the intravenous infusion rate can be increased to 100 ml per kg per day. If there is still no response to this therapy, a central line will be needed to increase the blood sugar concentration. The central line can be established with either an umbilical venous catheter with the tip above the diaphragm, or an umbilical artery catheter with the tip between the levels of the sixth and tenth thoracic vertebrae.

TRANSFER TO A TERTIARY CARE CENTER

A baby should be transported to a tertiary care center whenever the baby's current problems exceed the capabilities of either the physician or the hospital to manage them. Similarly, the baby should be transferred if there is a high likelihood that such problems will develop. The goal of transportation is to avoid a crisis rather than being forced to treat one with inadequate resources.

The following items should be considered in

the decision of whether to transport the baby to a tertiary care center, even if the physician in charge of the case has the medical skills to care for the baby:

1. Can an intravenous line be maintained 24 hours per day by in-hospital personnel?

2. Is in-house resuscitation available with staff skilled in intubation?

3. If the baby is at high risk for an air leak (for example, due to hyaline membrane disease, meconium aspiration, or any form of mechanical ventilation), is there an in-house team capable of treating acute pneumothorax?

4. Are facilities for x-rays, blood gas testing, and most basic laboratory tests available in the hospital 24 hours per day?

If the answer to any of the above questions is no, transportation to a tertiary care center may be advisable.

NORMAL INFANT FEEDING

method of
JAMES L. SUTPHEN, M.D., Ph.D., and
ANA ABAD SINDEN, M.S., R.D.
The University of Virginia
Charlottesville, Virginia

Breast Feeding

Human breast milk is the ideal nourishment for the healthy full-term infant. Human milk offers nutritional, immunologic, psychosocial, and economic advantages over commercial formulas. From a nutritional standpoint, human milk is the ideal species-specific nourishment for the human infant. The protein is of high biologic value and provides a low renal solute load. The presence of the saturated fatty acids in the 2 position of the triglycerides and the action of lipase enhance fat digestibility. Lactose, the predominant form of carbohydrate in human milk, enhances calcium and mineral absorption. Milk from a well-nourished healthy woman provides adequate levels of almost all micronutrients; moreover, the nutrients in human milk have a high bioavailability.

Although breast feeding is a natural act, it is not totally instinctive. Women who wish to breastfeed should be encouraged to do so and should receive procedural instruction during the prenatal and early postnatal period. Successful breast feeding depends on supportive obstetric, pediatric, and nursing care. Parental attitudes, including those of the father, should be discussed during the prenatal period. A breast examination should be conducted to identify problems with the nipple, areola, or breast itself. Several manipulation techniques such as nipple rolling, as well as the wearing of a breast shield, can help flat or inverted nipples become more protractile. Sometimes an infant with a strong healthy suck can help bring out inverted nipples. Breast care should also be addressed with emphasis on the avoidance of the use of strong soaps or ointments on the nipples. Sufficient lubrication for the areola and nipples is provided by the glands of Montgomery during pregnancy and lactation.

The mother should have the opportunity to nurse her infant as soon as possible after the delivery. Feedings initially should be offered every 2 to 4 hours and adjusted according to infant demand. For a proper grasp and seal, the nipple should be drawn up against the roof of the infant's mouth with the tongue stroking the bottom of the nipple. The infant's lips should almost completely surround the areola while the jaw applies pressure, forcing the milk out through the pores in the nipple during the act of suckling. The infant should be allowed to suck for at least 4 to 5 minutes, at which time the mother can break the seal by inserting a clean finger in the corner of her infant's mouth. The infant should then be offered the second breast. A normal healthy infant should demonstrate appropriate rooting, grasping, and suckling behaviors. Gradually the feeding period will increase, taking up to 10 minutes or more on each side by the third postpartum day. Bottle feeding should not be offered to an infant during the first 2 weeks until lactation is well established. Since bottle feeding requires a different tongue and jaw motion, introducing it too early could lead to nipple confusion. Moreover, an infant who bottle feeds may take less from the breast, especially when an entire feeding is substituted with a bottle feeding. This will lead to decreased milk production.

Successful lactation is also dependent on the establishment of the letdown reflex. To establish letdown a mother should be encouraged to relax and establish a comfortable nursing environment. If letdown does not proceed, the woman should be encouraged to massage her breast in a circular pattern with her fingertips in order to help promote the emptying of her breasts through an external means. Awareness of letdown can be felt in a variety of ways, such as through tingling sensations during nursing, uterine contractions, or thirst.

Monitoring the breast fed infant involves checking feeding frequency, number of wet diapers, and weight gain. During the first few weeks of life the breast fed infant will nurse at least 6 times a day, but more frequently 8 to 12 times a day, and will produce 6 to 8 wet diapers per day. The infant should regain birth weight by 3 weeks of age. As the infant becomes older and requires more milk, there will be an increased emptying and sucking stimulation which will promote increased milk production. For the older infant who has been introduced to solid foods, the nursing interval may lengthen with a simultaneous shortening of the nursing period, resulting in less milk production.

The quantity and quality of human milk is affected by maternal diet and nutritional status. The lactating mother needs approximately 500 to 600 extra kilocalories and 20 extra grams of protein per day. Precise needs depend upon maternal age, metabolism, and activity as well as duration of lactation and number of infants being breast fed. A balanced, varied diet consisting of four servings of milk or milk products, two servings of meat or high-protein meat substitutes, four servings of fruits and vegetables, including a source of vitamins A and C, and four servings of breads and cereals should promote adequate nutritional support. As traces of anything consumed can show up in breast milk, foods suspected of causing infant colic or congestion should be gradually eliminated from the diet, one at a time, to identify if the food is indeed causing the symptoms.

Women who anticipate returning to work should be encouraged to continue breast feeding. Those women who work part-time may be able to breast feed totally, while full-time working mothers may be able to provide their infant's nutritional needs by various combinations of breast milk, stored breast milk, or supplemental formula feedings. Women who wish to feed their infants breast milk while they are working need to express their milk with a breast pump. Breast pumps have a funnel-shaped flange which comes in contact with the nipple and removes the milk by suction. Breast milk not intended for immediate use should be properly stored for maintenance of its safety and nutritional quality. Breast milk can be safely frozen in new plastic bags or disposable liners from baby bottles and then thawed under cold running water. To ease the transition, the infant should be offered a bottle a few times a week before the mother returns to work.

Common deterrents to successful breastfeeding include lack of maternal confidence, incorrect nursing techniques, improper positioning of the infant's lips onto the areola, or maternal stress caused by fatigue, inadequate nutrition, or postpartum depression. Breast problems such as engorgement, sore nipples, and infections also prevent successful lactation. Appropriate emptying of the engorged breast via manual expression and nursing often can help alleviate maternal discomfort. Painful or cracked nipples may be caused by improper positioning of the infant on the breast or consistently nursing in the same position. Dry heat is quite effective in healing sore nipples, and varying nursing positions can vary nipple stress points. Mastitis, or a localized breast infection, produces systemic flu-like symptoms. Nursing on the unaffected side to promote letdown, followed by manual expression or nursing on the affected side is often effective. A 10-day course of an appropriate antibiotic may be prescribed to minimize recurrence.

Certain drugs are contraindicated for the mother's use while nursing, such as radioactive agents, antimetabolites, atropine, metronidazole, and tetracycline, while others are viewed as potentially harmful if used inappropriately. Prolonged breast feeding beyond the sixth month to the exclusion of other important nutrient sources has been associated with malnutrition and iron deficiency. The introduction of solid foods, including iron-fortified cereals, between the fourth and sixth month and gradual reduction in breast milk intake through the first year will provide the appropriate nutrient blend to meet an infant's nutritional needs.

Formula Feeding

The decision to breast feed is a personal one and should be reached with freedom from guilt or pressure. Information on formula feeding as an acceptable substitute should be provided by the physician or health care professional in the event that the decision not to breast feed is made. In the developed world the advantages of breast feeding relative to formula feeding are less pronounced, assuming a clean water supply is available. The usual reason for instituting formula feedings is parental preference. Occasionally, parents will prefer to substitute formula feeding completely when mothers return to work.

When bottle feeding is initiated, parents may find that infants have marked preferences for different commercially available nipples. Before abandoning one type of nipple, the parents should be certain that the hole in the nipple is adequately patent. There is little reason to recommend one style of bottle over another, although advantages are claimed by manufacturers. When the infant is fed, there should be few distractions and the parents should be discouraged from making rapid or jerking motions during feeding. Children should be fed in a semi-inclined position. Supine feeding and bottle propping should be discouraged, as they could promote aspiration of the formula. When bottle feeding is initiated, it is reasonable to involve the father in the feeding. There is no reason to isolate feeding as a strictly maternal duty. The mother's work schedule is often as demanding as the father's. We suggest that mothers and fathers share responsibility for nighttime feedings as well.

All formulas are available as liquid or powdered concentrate, or ready-to-feed varieties. Formula should be prepared with a clean water supply. Parents may prefer to use boiled water for this purpose. If the water supply is a public treated water supply in the United States, there is little advantage provided by boiling. However, other water sources probably should be boiled. After each feeding, equipment should be washed in hot soapy water with a bottle and nipple brush, followed by rinsing in hot water. If an automatic dishwasher is used, the heated drying cycle should be used.

Prior to feeding, the formula should be warmed. It is convenient to do this in a pan of warm water, but faster to use a microwave oven. Different microwave ovens heat at dramatically different rates. Parents who microwave should be cautioned that the temperature of the formula may exceed that of the glass or plastic bottle. It is therefore advisable to test the actual temperature of the formula prior to feeding the baby.

During feedings the infant should be periodically burped. It is best to do this by supporting the child in a sitting position with one hand holding both the chest and the lower chin. The back is gently tapped and rubbed, and occasionally the infant may be moved up and down or gently side to side to facilitate the passage of air from the stomach. This process will require considerable practice but is absolutely essential. Finally, it is best to warn parents that normal infants will often spit even if burping is done adequately. Therefore, several washable blankets and towels should be within reach in the area where infant feeding is performed.

Cow's Milk Formula

In the United States there are three common cow's milk formulas—SMA, Enfamil, and Similac. For the full-term normal infant, there is little advantage of one over the other. In fact, infants generally accept these formulas interchangeably. Therefore, parents are best advised to look for the lowest price in their local market.

Soy Formula

Soy formulas provide protein from soy. The carbohydrate component is derived from corn syrup solids and/or sucrose in various combinations. These formulas are intended to be used when there is proven cow's milk protein sensitivity or lactose intolerance. The absorption of calcium in soy formula is adequate but less than with cow's milk formula. Full-term infants fed soy milk grow at rates equal to those fed cow's milk formulas. It is best for parents to try once or twice to reintroduce cow's milk formula to be certain that there is indeed an allergy or intolerance to cow's milk. If there is a true allergy to cow's milk, it is not uncommon for allergies to develop to soy milk as well. If this is the case, a protein hydrolysate formula should be used.

Protein Hydrolysate Formula

Protein hydrolysate formulas generally are somewhat less palatable than soy or cow's milk formulas. Two varieties are currently on the market—Nutramigen and Pregestimil. Both are milk protein hydrolysates. A third soy protein hydrolysate will be introduced in the near future. The major difference between currently available formulas is that Pregestimil contains a portion of its fat as medium-chain triglycerides. Either formula may be used when there is proven allergy to both cow's milk and soy protein. However, both are expensive and their use should be limited. For infants who have had recurrent episodes of gastroenteritis, and are not tolerating soy or cow's milk formulas, a switch to Pregestimil for several weeks may be useful until adequate weight gain is once more achieved. However, the expense of these formulas dictates that other, less expensive formulas be periodically tried. If they must be used on a prolonged basis, the physician should begin a preliminary investigation into the etiology of the persistent intolerance (e.g., sweat test). Generally, even infants who have severe cow's or soy milk sensitivity will ultimately be able to accept cow's milk. It may take several months or even years for tolerance to develop. Often by one year of age the other protein sources can be safely introduced.

Evaporated Milk Formula

Evaporated milk formula was at one time popular in the United States. These formulas are now discouraged for many reasons. The renal solute load is unacceptably high. The vitamin content is not standardized and is often inadequate. The amount of phosphorus is excessive. The can that is used to package some evaporated milks has a lead seam—a possible source of contamination.

Formula Volume

Infants are generally started on 1 to 2 ounces of formula per feeding. The frequency initially should be every 2 to 4 hours. Gradually the frequency should be decreased to every 4 hours and the volume slowly increased to 6 to 8 ounces per feeding. When the infant is consuming 800 to 1000 ml of formula per day, it is reasonable to introduce solid foods. Generally this occurs somewhere between 4 and 6 months of age. If the infant attains this goal earlier and is not obese or the child of obese parents, it is acceptable to introduce solids earlier. This is sometimes necessary for infants who are adjusting or rechanneling their linear growth curve from a low percentile to a higher percentile. This rechanneling is common in the first year of life, and if the growth velocity is extremely rapid, it is not uncommon for formula feedings to become inadequate before the usual time of 4 to 6 months. The same can be said of breast feeding in this situation. If the infant or the parents are obese, early feeding of solids should be discouraged.

Solid Foods

Solid foods can be made by grinding regular foods in a babyfood grinder, or they may be purchased in prepared form. If parents elect to prepare their own solid foods, they should be warned that the feedings should be well pureed because a coarse texture may be unacceptable to an infant. Generally, infants do not switch to home-prepared solids if they have first been introduced to ready-made solids. Solid foods are difficult to feed before 4 months of age, as the extrusion reflux of the tongue makes it difficult for the infant to consume them. Parents should be cautioned that the infant will inevitably spit out a small amount in the course of learning how to swallow from a spoon. This does not mean that the infant does not tolerate that particular food.

Solid feedings are progressed along a common (but unproven) schedule. Cereal is started first, followed by yellow vegetables and fruits, then green vegetables, and finally meats. No mixed foods are provided until the components of the mixture have been previously introduced. No more than one new food should be introduced every 3 to 7 days so that food intolerances may be detected. We generally discourage the feeding of strained egg yolks and strained desserts at any age. The concentrated cholesterol in the former and sugar in the latter are unnecessary and potentially harmful.

Cow's Milk

Whole cow's milk feedings should not be introduced before 9 to 12 months of age. There is evidence that allergy to cow's milk protein may be more common if it is introduced too early.

Late introduction of whole cow's milk decreases the tendency toward iron deficiency anemia seen with early introduction. When parents introduce cow's milk they should be cautioned against defatted milk. This is especially true for skim milk, which has been shown to cause nutritional deficiencies when given to infants who were less than 6 months of age and consuming little solid food. Two per cent fat cow's milk has not been tested on an extensive basis as a substitute for whole cow's milk, but it is probably adequate for infants over 2 years of age who are consuming an adequate amount of solid foods. Between 1 and 2 years of age whole cow's milk is preferable. Beyond 2 years of age, the American Heart Association encourages the use of lower-fat-concentration milks to limit dietary fat to 30 per cent of total calories in an effort to prevent atherosclerotic heart disease. This recommendation is still not formally accepted by the American Academy of Pediatrics. Pediatricians should monitor the growth of children fed fat-restricted diets. The use of 2 per cent milk is undesirable if limited solid foods are being consumed or if the child is underweight.

Vitamin and Mineral Supplements

Infants should receive supplemental iron by the age of 6 months. This can be given most easily in the form of iron-fortified cereals. Alternatively, iron-fortified formula is available. Fluoride drops should be given to infants who live in an area where the water supply does not contain fluoride. Infants who are formula fed require no additional vitamin supplements. Infants who are breast fed probably require no vitamin supplements as well, assuming that the mother's diet is adequate. There is a relatively low concentration of vitamin D in human milk. However, rickets is very uncommon in full-term infants who are breast fed, especially if solids are introduced at the usual time and there is adequate exposure to sunlight and adequate maternal vitamin D intake. If this is not the case, 400 IU of vitamin D should be provided daily to the infant.

DISEASES OF THE BREAST

method of
SHARON GRUNDFEST-
BRONIATOWSKI, M.D., and
ROBERT E. HERMANN, M.D.
Cleveland Clinic Foundation
Cleveland, Ohio

In the newborn, the breast is usually mildly enlarged as a result of the stimulation from the mother's hormones. Occasionally this even causes nipple discharge. The engorgement subsides in a few days, and the breast glands stay in a quiescent state until puberty. At this time, the breast glands differentiate and proliferate under the influence of estrogen, progesterone, and other hormones. Occasionally the mother of an adolescent girl will become concerned that the developing breast bud represents a tumor. The practitioner must not fall into the trap of removing this area, since it contains all the developing cells of the new breast. With the onset of menstruation, the breast will be periodically engorged and tender during the luteal phase of the cycle. These changes are physiologic and should not be a cause for concern.

The normal breast is a mixture of glandular tissue, supporting stroma, and fat. In younger women, the proportion of glandular tissue and stroma to fat is increased, as compared with the breasts of older women, in whom fatty replacement is predominant. Therefore, in premenopausal women one should expect the breast to feel rather granular. After menopause (in the absence of exogenous estrogens) the breast becomes softer and more homogeneous.

CONGENITAL DISORDERS

Rarely, the breast may be completely absent (amastia), or the gland may be present with an absent nipple (athelia). More commonly, the nipple is present, but the breast is hypotrophic (hypoplasia). Breast hypoplasia may be associated with absence or hypoplasia of the pectoral muscles, deformities of the rib cage, and deformities of the ipsilateral upper extremity (synbrachydactyly). These deformities may all be corrected by reconstructive surgery.

Supernumerary breasts or nipples may appear anywhere along the embryologic milk line. Generally these do not require excision unless they are large or tender.

ACQUIRED DISORDERS

Breast development may sometimes be seen at an early age, along with other signs of early sexual maturation (precocious puberty). Such cases should be referred to an endocrinologist for evaluation to exclude hormone-secreting tumors. Premature development may also occur in the absence of any other signs of puberty, such as axillary and pubic hair, clitoral and labial pigmentation, and pigmentation of the areolae. In such cases, only observation and reassurance are required.

Asymmetry in growth may also occur because of chest wall deformities (e.g., pectus excavatum) or to an abnormal growth spurt in one breast (probably as a result of end-organ hypersensitivity). When gigantomastia occurs during puberty it generally requires reduction mammoplasty for correction. Most authorities recommend that this be delayed until the growth spurt has ended. Gigantomastia may also occur during pregnancy or lactation. There have been some case reports of regression after danazol treatment.

In males the breast usually remains undeveloped; however, benign gynecomastia may be encountered at puberty, in senescence, or after administration of certain drugs (e.g., digitalis, cimetidine, isoniazid, and spironolactone). It has also been associated with liver disease, testicular tumors, androgen or estrogen excess, thiamine deficiency, and Klinefelter's syndrome. Removal of the enlarged tissue (subcutaneous mastectomy) is indicated for pain or for cosmetic reasons. It may also be performed as a diagnostic measure in older men to exclude carcinoma. For men undergoing estrogen therapy for prostatic carcinoma, prophylactic breast irradiation is useful to prevent subsequent breast engorgement.

Breast pain (mastodynia) may occur as a result of hormonal stimulation of the breast, in which case it is usually cyclical. Most women do not require medical treatment, and wish only to be reassured that no damaging pathologic process is involved. In more severe cases, medical therapy may be tried. A wide range of treatments have been advocated, including dietary manipulation (e.g., abstention from caffeine), cold compresses, thiamine, vitamin E, diuretics, iodine, thyroid hormone, and danazol. Caffeine in large doses can cause breast pain in susceptible women, and abstention is sometimes beneficial. Vitamin E has not been shown effective in double-blind trials. Danazol (Danocrine) is helpful (in doses of 100 mg twice a day), but it is expensive and causes virilizing side effects at high doses. Further, its effects on fetal development are not known. The other treatments have not been the subjects of rigorous testing. Noncyclical mastodynia is often associated with stress or depression, but may be caused by neuritis, arthritis, or post-traumatic inflammation. When inflammation or arthritis is suspected, an anti-inflammatory medication may be tried. Costochondritis is frequently mistaken for breast pain.

Inflammatory Disorders (Mastitis)

During lactation an area of edema and erythema may develop in the breast as a result of incomplete emptying of milk. This usually responds to emptying the breast by massage or with a breast pump.

The most common inflammatory condition is a breast abscess. Abscesses frequently occur as a result of trauma to the nipple during lactation and are usually caused by Staphylococcus aureus.

Typically the breast is red, swollen, and tender. The patient may be febrile and has an elevated white blood cell count. Fluctuance is slow to develop owing to the many septations in the breast. An initial trial of antibiotics directed against penicillin-resistant staphylococci and warm compresses should be tried. If the woman is breast feeding, she should stop using the abscessed breast and empty it with a breast pump. If these measures do not resolve the problem, incision and drainage will be necessary. Skin abscesses and infected sebaceous cysts are also common.

Squamous metaplasia of the lactiferous ducts (Zuska's disease) may cause an inflammation in the subareolar tissues with secondary infection. Anaerobes are found in 20 to 30 per cent. Initially this presents as a tender, erythematous swelling adjacent to the edge of the areola and may be accompanied by a nipple discharge. The infection will sometimes resolve with warm compresses and oral antibiotics. If incision and drainage is performed a *chronic mamillary duct areolar fistula* will frequently be the result. Treatment consists of wide excision of the diseased lactiferous ducts from beneath the nipple. Many authors have remarked on the high recurrence rates if diseased tissue is left behind.

A variety of other infections have been reported to involve the breast, including tuberculosis, blastomycosis, cryptococcosis, and actinomycosis. Tubercular infection is rare in the United States. It presents as a mass accompanied by multiple draining sinuses and adenopathy. There is almost always a primary lung infection. Antibiotic therapy is indicated, with surgery being reserved for residual masses.

Another common inflammatory process is *duct ectasia* or *plasma cell mastitis*. Its etiology is unknown, and it may occur at any age. Typically it presents as a multicolored, sticky discharge that can be expressed from several ducts in both breasts. It may also be noted incidentally at operation as a grayish green material within the ducts. Occasionally it produces itching. No therapy is needed for this condition, although if the patient finds it bothersome, or if the physician has some doubt as to the nature of the nipple discharge, an excision of the subareolar ducts will relieve symptoms and establish the diagnosis.

A rare cause of breast pain is *superficial thrombophlebitis (Mondor's disease)* of the thoracoepigastric vein. The condition is self-limited and requires no treatment.

Traumatic Disorders

An injury to the breast may result in *fat necrosis*. Clinically this presents as a firm, irregular mass. There may be overlying erythema. The lesion may be indistinguishable from carcinoma on mammography. The history of trauma may not always be obtained and, even if it is clear that there has been an injury, biopsy is necessary to exclude the presence of cancer. Generally a core needle biopsy or fine needle aspiration cytology will be sufficient. However, if excision is not performed, it is imperative that the patient be maintained under observation to be sure that the mass is resolving (which it generally does within a month).

Neoplastic Disorders

Benign Lesions

In teenagers and women in their early twenties the most common breast tumor is a *fibroadenoma*. This lesion may also arise later in life. These tumors are easily recognized; they are firm, rounded, and usually mobile. They are solid on aspiration. Breast cancers are rare in women below the age of 25, and small fibroadenomas in this age group may be safely observed for a period. Usually they are slow growing, and with time some lesions actually involute. They are not generally considered to be premalignant. Fibroadenomas may occasionally grow rapidly under the influence of estrogen during adolescence or pregnancy, or with the use of exogenous hormones. Occasionally, these tumors may achieve a large size accompanied by an exuberant overlying vasculature. Simple excision is sufficient, and mastectomy is never indicated.

As women enter their late twenties and thirties the increased nodularity and thickening that was primarily seen during the luteal phase *(physiologic nodularity)* may develop into a persistent two-dimensional thickening *(mastoplasia)*. These areas may be distinguished from carcinoma by their tendency to vary in size with the menstrual cycle and the presence of tenderness. In general, carcinomas present as a three-dimensional thickening and are nontender, but this is not invariably the case. Histologically, mastoplasia may include areas of glandular hypertrophy or hyperplasia *(adenosis, or epithelial hyperplasia)* or of stromal hypertrophy. These diagnoses are often lumped together under the rubric "fibrocystic disease"; however, it is better to attach a more precise diagnosis whenever possible. Adenosis and epithelial hyperplasia do not carry an increased risk of future malignancy unless atypia is present.

As women enter the decade before menopause, cysts become more frequent. These are usually easily diagnosed by aspiration, although mammography and ultrasound may be helpful. Cysts are not associated with an increased risk of malignancy unless there is a strong family history of breast cancer (e.g., in a mother or a sister) and are treated by evacuating the fluid with a syringe. If there is a persistent mass after aspiration or if the cyst recurs, biopsy should be performed to exclude the presence of carcinoma. Although some have advocated abstention from methylxanthines, there has been no double-blind study that unequivocally shows a reduction in cyst formation after such dietary manipulation.

Benign papillary lesions such as an *intraductal papilloma* may present as palpable masses, but more commonly cause a nipple discharge. They can occur at any age. Unlike the discharge associated with duct ectasia, only one breast and one duct are usually involved, and the discharge is usually spontaneous. The discharge may be clear, serous, or bloody. Because there is no way to distinguish such a discharge from that seen in association with carcinoma, biopsy is mandatory if the nipple fluid cytology does not yield malignant cells. Simple excision is sufficient. Rarely an *adenoma of the nipple* may be seen. This tumor also presents with a bloody nipple discharge. On inspection of the nipple, a raised area with multiple fissures is seen. The diagnosis is easily made by biopsy, and excision is curative.

A rare tumor usually found in middle-aged women is the *phyllodes tumor*, also called *cystosarcoma phyllodes*. These lesions usually present as bulky, multilobulated tumors. They have a strong tendency to invade locally, but only 10 per cent are malignant. Microscopically they bear a resemblance to the fibroadenoma; however, the stroma is more cellular. The malignant potential depends on the number of mitotic figures and the cytologic characteristics of the stromal cells. Wide excision is the treatment of choice. Since this tumor almost never metastasizes to lymph nodes, axillary dissection is unnecessary.

Noninvasive Carcinomas

There is great debate over the management of in situ lesions. *Intraductal carcinoma* (also called *in situ ductal carcinoma, comedocarcinoma,* and *cribriform carcinoma*) may present as a palpable lump or a cluster of microcalcifications. Occasionally, the tumor will attain a very large size (3 cm or more) and axillary involvement will be found despite the diagnosis of "noninvasive" cancer. At other times, no mass will be palpable, but mammography will demonstrate widespread calcifications. Small (less than 2 cm) intraductal lesions not associated with a nipple discharge and not located beneath the nipple areolar complex have been treated by wide excision and radiotherapy with acceptable short-term results.

No data are available as to the long-term results of conservative therapy, and mastectomy remains an option. Larger lesions should be treated by mastectomy and axillary sampling (if not a total axillary clearance).

Lobular carcinoma in situ, also called lobular neoplasia, is not considered a malignancy by some authors. Nevertheless, it is associated with an increased risk of carcinoma in both breasts (25 to 30 per cent at 20 years). There is a 30 per cent incidence of multicentricity in this condition. It is interesting to note that the carcinoma that may eventually develop is more likely to be ductal than lobular in origin. Treatment options include careful follow-up with a physical examination of the breast three times a year and a yearly mammography, or bilateral "prophylactic" mastectomy removing all the glandular tissue and the nipple areolar complex. Which choice is taken depends on the age of the patient, the family history, the ease of examination of the breasts, and the preference of the patient.

Invasive Carcinoma

Carcinoma of the breast is the leading cause of cancer mortality among American women. Carcinomas may arise in either the ductal or lobular portions of the breast glands. The most common malignancy (90 per cent) is the *infiltrating ductal cancer.* Well-differentiated forms of this tumor are sometimes called tubular carcinomas. About 10 per cent of tumors are *infiltrating lobular carcinomas.* Other invasive carcinomas include medullary, mucinous, metaplastic, and adenoid cystic carcinomas.

Cancer should be suspected when the patient presents with a three-dimensional, irregular, hard mass; skin retraction or nipple inversion of recent onset; a unilateral nipple discharge coming from one duct; nipple ulceration; or a mammogram showing a spiculated density or a cluster of microcalcifications.

Screening Techniques. Physical examination and mammography remain the principal means of detecting carcinomas of the breast. Breast self-examination is to be encouraged, but unfortunately it has not been shown to improve cancer detection rates.

Palpation of the breast will rarely detect tumors less than 1 cm in size. A number of studies have shown a decrease in mortality when women are regularly screened by mammography (Swedish National Board of Health, the New York Health Insurance Plan trial, the Nijmegen Project, and the Breast Cancer Detection Demonstration Project). The American Cancer Society recommends the following guidelines: (1) women should have a baseline mammogram between the ages of 35 and 40, (2) biannual screening between the ages of 40 and 49, and (3) annual mammography thereafter for life. Women with a history of breast cancer in a first-degree relative should have annual mammography beginning at 40 years of age. Only about 0.5 per cent of asymptomatic women screened will actually have a cancer.

Mammography alone will miss approximately 20 to 30 per cent of palpable tumors. However, mammography when combined with physical examination will detect 95 per cent or more of cancers. Biopsy of a suspicious breast lump should always be performed regardless of the mammographic findings. Mammography helps the surgeon to ascertain the presence of multicentric disease, improves the estimation of tumor size, and may detect unsuspected tumors in the contralateral breast.

Other techniques such as thermography, ultrasound, and diaphanography have not been shown to be sufficiently accurate to be used for cancer screening at this time.

Biopsy Techniques. Histologic samples of vast majority of breast masses may be obtained in the office using either a fine needle aspiration for cytology or a core needle biopsy (e.g., Tru-Cut or drill biopsy). Where the diagnosis is equivocal, an open excisional biopsy should be performed. Care should be taken when planning the biopsy incision so as not to interfere with subsequent surgical therapy. Nonpalpable lesions found by mammography are localized first by Kopan's hook-wire technique, and the surgeon follows the wire to the mass.

In past years it was popular to combine biopsy and subsequent mastectomy during one period of general anesthesia because of fears that the tumor would spread if definitive therapy was not immediately carried out. However, it appears that a delay of even 3 weeks does not carry any increased risk. Further, the use of the two-step biopsy procedure allows the surgeon to fully discuss all the options with the patient. A one-anesthesia procedure is still useful when the planned therapy is a partial mastectomy for a small lesion or when a clinically suspicious lesion cannot be diagnosed by needle biopsy and the patient has agreed to undergo mastectomy if the frozen section is positive for carcinoma.

Prognosis of Breast Cancer. The prognosis for an invasive carcinoma of the breast is determined by the size of the tumor, its histologic grade, and the number of axillary nodes involved. Unlike some tumors, breast cancer may appear to be dormant for many years, only to reappear as a systemic or local recurrence. TNM staging is given in Table 1. Five-year survival rates are as

TABLE 1. **Clinical TNM Staging for Breast Cancer (UICC—AJC)**

Stage I	T_1—Tumor size 2 cm or less
	N_0—No suspicious lymph nodes
	M_0—No distant metastases
Stage II	T_2—Tumor size 2–5 cm and/or
	N_1—One or more palpable, suspicious nodes
	M_0—No distant metastases
Stage III	T_3—Tumor larger than 5 cm or
	N_2—Ipsilateral nodes fixed to one another or other structures or
	N_3—Ipsilateral supraclavicular or infraclavicular suspicious nodes, or arm edema
	M_0—No distant metastases
Stage IV	T_4—Tumor of any size with fixation to chest wall, edema or ulceration of breast skin, satellite skin nodules, or inflammatory carcinoma, or
	M_1—Any distant metastasis

follows: Stage I, 80 to 95 per cent; Stage II, 70 to 75 per cent; Stage III, 38 to 42 per cent; and Stage IV, 25 per cent.

Treatment of Operable Breast Cancer. The treatment of invasive carcinoma is a matter of great controversy at present. Treatment options include radical mastectomy; modified radical mastectomy (with or without immediate reconstruction); segmental mastectomy and axillary dissection (with or without radiotherapy); and local excision, axillary dissection, and radiotherapy. The vast majority of clinical trials have shown that survival for Stages I and II breast cancer is the same regardless of the local treatment, whether it be radical mastectomy, modified radical mastectomy, segmental mastectomy, or excision and radiotherapy. Dissection of the internal mammary nodes does not appear to confer any benefit. Axillary dissection is usually performed for staging information and to control possible local recurrence in the axilla, but it has not been shown to improve survival. Local recurrence may be higher after local excision and axillary dissection than after local excision, axillary dissection, and radiotherapy (NSABP trial B-06). This, too, is controversial since the local excision in this trial may not have been extensive enough to have eradicated nearby foci of intraductal cancer found in the vicinity of a primary tumor.

Radical mastectomy is rarely performed for Stage I and II lesions in the United States now. Modified radical mastectomy (removal of the breast and axillary nodes with conservation of one or both pectoralis muscles) is usually the treatment of choice for tumors that are centrally located or are larger than 2.5 cm. It is accomplished with little morbidity, with a minimal hospital stay, and at relatively little expense. It also alleviates the concern about multicentric tumors. Breast reconstruction often provides a satisfactory cosmetic result, although the older woman may not wish to be subjected to the added operative time and expense. There are many satisfactory external breast prostheses available. Breast reconstruction can often be accomplished at the time of mastectomy using either a silicone implant or an expandable prosthesis. Where skin coverage is a problem, a latissimus dorsi or a rectus muscle myocutaneous flap may be used. Some surgeons prefer to delay reconstruction for several months after mastectomy, but there is no evidence that reconstruction adversely affects local recurrence or survival.

Partial mastectomy with breast conservation is preferred for small (less than 2 cm), peripheral lesions. The addition of radiotherapy to surgery is generally thought to reduce the risk of local recurrence; however, it adds 6 weeks of treatment time and almost doubles the cost of treatment. If a salvage mastectomy is needed after radiotherapy, the skin may be more prone to wound healing problems, making breast reconstruction more difficult. Finally, there is some concern about late morbidity and even mortality as a result of radiation damage to the heart, lungs, and other structures in the radiation field. Ultimately the choice of treatment depends on the size of the tumor, its histology, the stage of the disease, the size of the breast, the location of the tumor in the breast, and the preferences of the patient after a detailed discussion of the options.

Adjuvant Therapy. Adjuvant therapy is given in an effort to improve either local or systemic control of disease. In 1985 the National Institute of Health convened a Consensus Conference which recommended that adjuvant chemotherapy be reserved for premenopausal women with positive nodes. There is still debate as to whether chemotherapy in this group results in an improvement in survival, but there is a prolongation in disease-free survival.

Premenopausal women with positive nodes are usually given adjuvant cytotoxic chemotherapy utilizing three or more drugs (e.g., cyclophosphamide, 5-fluorouracil, and methotrexate [CMF]; cyclophosphamide, 5-fluorouracil, methotrexate, vincristine, and prednisone [CMFVP]; or 5-fluorouracil, doxorubicin (Adriamycin), and cyclophosphamide [FAC]) for a period of 6 to 12 months. Patients with estrogen-receptor-positive tumors may undergo hormonal manipulation in addition. Adjuvant castration alone has not been shown to improve survival over that produced by chemotherapy.

Postmenopausal women with Stage II receptor-positive tumors are treated with tamoxifen (Nolvadex) 10 mg twice a day for at least 2 years.

Several trials have demonstrated an improvement in the disease-free interval, and one trial appears to show a small survival advantage in postmenopausal women treated with this estrogen blocker. Toxicity is minimal. No benefit for adjuvant chemotherapy in postmenopausal women with estrogen-receptor-negative tumors has been established.

Adjuvant radiotherapy is used to reduce local recurrence in women with poorly differentiated tumors, multiple lymph node involvement, angioinvasion, or neural invasion.

Post-Treatment Follow-up. Patients with Stage I or II breast cancer should probably be seen by a physician every 3 months for the first year, every 6 months for the next 4 years, and yearly thereafter. Mammograms and chest x-rays are obtained once a year, and liver function tests and a complete blood count are usually drawn twice a year. There is little justification for yearly bone and liver scans unless the patient is in an experimental protocol. These tests are usually reserved for patients with symptoms or an abnormal alkaline phosphatase level, or patients who presented with more advanced disease.

Advanced Breast Cancer. The treatment of advanced breast cancer is dependent on the menopausal status of the patient, the presence or absence of nodal involvement, the presence of systemic disease, and the degree of local involvement.

Patients with bulky chest wall disease but without overt systemic disease are usually treated by modified radical mastectomy followed by chemotherapy and radiation. Alternatively, radiotherapy may be given first to reduce the size of the tumor before resection.

Many different chemotherapy regimens have been advocated. Slightly higher response rates are found for those containing doxorubicin, but no clear survival advantage has been demonstrated for any combination therapy or single agent.

Inflammatory breast cancer is a relatively rare form of breast cancer (1.5 to 4 per cent of all breast carcinomas) characterized by diffuse swelling, erythema, tenderness, warmth, and peau d'orange. Pathologically there is invasion of the dermal lymphatics. Multimodal therapy is recommended. There is a very high rate of local recurrence when surgery alone is used, and 75 per cent of patients develop systemic disease when radiotherapy is used alone. Therefore, the initial treatment is usually a combination of chemotherapy (e.g., FAC) for two or three cycles, followed by mastectomy if the tumor has significantly decreased in size, and postoperative radiotherapy. If no initial response to chemotherapy is seen, radiotherapy is added. Surgery may then be performed at a later time if residual disease is present and appears resectable.

Local Recurrence. Patients presenting with a local recurrence are at significant risk for subsequent systemic disease and should have a complete metastatic evaluation (chest x-ray, bone scan, liver scan, and laboratory studies). Excision and radiotherapy or radiotherapy alone will initially control most local and regional recurrences, but there is a high rate of relapse. The addition of chemotherapy should be considered for patients with widespread or large deposits.

Systemic Recurrence. Radiotherapy provides useful palliation for patients with metastases to bone, brain, spinal cord, orbit, or the brachial plexus. Malignant pleural effusions are treated by chest tube drainage with instillation of tetracycline for pleurodesis. Where possible, biopsy for hormone receptor data should be accomplished in patients with systemic disease. If the tumor is hormone receptor–positive, oophorectomy or treatment with tamoxifen, medroxyprogesterone, or aminoglutethimide may be helpful. A significant number of patients will be palliated by combination chemotherapy, although it has not been shown that such treatment improves survival.

ENDOMETRIOSIS

method of
JOHN A. ROCK, M.D., and
SANFORD M. MARKHAM, M.D.*
*The Johns Hopkins Hospital,
Baltimore, Maryland*

Incidence and Etiology

Endometriosis is a unique gynecologic entity in which endometrium-like tissue and cells are found outside the uterus. This ectopic location is most common in and around the ovary, fallopian tube, and the peritoneum of the posterior and anterior cul de sac, but is also reported in most locations of the body. Endometriosis currently represents one of the most common gynecologic pathologies, with a current rate of 5 to 50 per cent. Some feel that this rate is increasing. The etiologies of endometriosis include the transport theory (tubal regurgitation or lymphatic and hematogenous spread) and the coelomic metaplasia theory. Endometriosis causes symptoms because it disrupts normal tissue and causes development of fibrosis

*The opinions and assertions contained herein are the private views of the authors and are not to be construed as official views of the Department of the Air Force or the Department of Defense.

and adhesions. The diagnosis should be suspected if there is a history of dysmenorrhea, dyspareunia, and premenstrual low backache with or without infertility. Physical findings include adnexal masses with decreased mobility of the adnexa, thickening and nodularity of the cul de sac, and the presence of a retroflexed uterus. The diagnosis can only be substantiated by laparoscopy or laparotomy.

Treatment

It is important to correctly assess not only the presence of but also the extent of the disease. Use of a staging system such as the revised classification of endometriosis of the American Fertility Society (1985) is recommended and is most helpful in defining the extent of disease. The treatment modalities utilized are shown in Table 1.

Individual treatment for endometriosis should be based on the extent of the disease, the patient's desire for childbearing, age, and other coexisting medical and surgical factors. When early endometriosis (minimal to mild) is present in a woman desiring to become pregnant, expectant therapy is most beneficial, provided an infertility evaluation is within normal limits. If, however, pregnancy has not occurred within a reasonable period of time, or the patient becomes more symptomatic, then a medical treatment plan is recommended utilizing one of the medical approaches (Table 2). In young women who have early endometriosis with minimal or no symp-

TABLE 1. **Treatment Modalities for Endometriosis**

Expectant therapy:	Complete medical evaluation without therapy
Medical therapy:	Pseudopregnancy regimens using acyclic combined oral estrogen-progesterone, such as birth control pills (Lo/Ovral, Ovral), or continuous progestin (Provera, Depo-Provera, Aygestin, Norlutate, Megace)
Surgical therapy:	Conservative surgery

Laparoscopy with electrocoagulation or laser vaporization of endometriosis and lysis of adhesions

Laparotomy with excision, vaporization, or electrocoagulation of endometriosis; lysis of adhesions; suspension of uterus; and, possibly, uterosacral plication or presacral neurectomy

Semiconservative surgery
Total abdominal hysterectomy with ovarian conservation, usually unilateral oophorectomy

Definitive surgery
Total abdominal hysterectomy with bilateral salpingo-oophorectomy, excision of endometriosis, and lysis of adhesions

Combined therapy:	Utilization of conservative surgery with medical adjunct either before or after surgery

TABLE 2. Medical Therapy of Endometriosis

1. Acyclic combined oral estrogen/progesterone, using a low estrogen dose with an androgenic progesterone such as ethinyl estradiol and norgestrel (Lo/Ovral, Ovral). Begin with 0.03/0.3 mg pill, and increase to 0.05/0.5 mg should breakthrough bleeding occur.

2. Continuous progestins using medroxyprogesterone acetate (Provera, Depo-Provera), norethindrone acetate (Aygestin, Norlutate), or megestrol acetate (Megace). Provera should be given in the range of 40 to 60 mg per day orally, or Depo-Provera, 150 mg, should be given parenterally every 1 to 3 months. Aygestin, 15 mg per day; Norlutate, 30 mg per day; Megace, 40 to 60 mg per day. In the case of Provera, Aygestin, Norlutate, and Megace, the total dose should be achieved in increments, with lower doses being given over several weeks.

3. Methyltestosterone (Metandren). Given as 5 to 10 mg linguets (buccal) daily.

4. Ethinyltestosterone (danazol). Given orally at a dose of 400 to 800 mg per day.

5. 19-Nortestosterone derivatives (Gestrinone). Given orally at a dose of from 2.5 to 5.0 mg two or three times a week.

6. Gonadotropin-releasing hormone agonists. Given as a daily subcutaneous injection of 0.05 mg or a variable dose regimen intranasally of 800 micrograms each.

toms, and in whom childbearing is not yet a consideration, the use of a standard low-dose birth control pill is felt to retard progression of the disease.

Mild to moderate endometriosis is best treated with a medical approach or with conservative surgery including excision, coagulation, or vaporization of all visible endometriosis and lysis of adhesions. Of the medical modalities listed in Table 2, only three are currently available as prescription medications. These are birth control pills with a low estrogen dose and a potent androgenic progestin (Lo/Ovral and Ovral), progestins (Provera, Depo-Provera, or Megace), and synthetic ethinyl-testosterone (danazol). Methyltestosterone (Metandren) and testosterone propionate have been used successfully as hormonal regimens. However, these drugs are not yet approved by the FDA for routine therapy. Significant success has been recorded in Europe with the 19-nortestosterone derivative (Gestrinone) but it is not yet available in the United States. Gonadotropin-releasing hormone agonists hold great promise for improved therapy in the near future, but they are also not available for general use in the United States. Of the medications currently available, estrogen-progesterone medications that have a low estrogen dose and an androgenic progesterone (Lo/Ovral or Ovral) create a pseudopregnancy state and are effective when given on a continuous basis for 6 to 9 months. The side effects, however, have prevented this regimen from being as widely used

as others. The use of a continuous progestin, such as Provera, in doses of 40 to 60 mg per day orally for 6 months, or Megace, 40 to 60 mg daily orally, has been useful in mild to moderate disease as an alternative to danazol therapy.

The most commonly used medical therapy is synthetic ethinyltestosterone (danazol) given orally, 400 to 800 mg per day for 6 months. The most effective dose is in the range of 600 to 800 mg per day. In either of the cases listed earlier, medical therapy is interrupted after 6 months in order for the patient to attempt to become pregnant or for the benefits of management to be assessed. Consider, however, that endometriosis is cured only by ablation of ovarian function and that all other forms of management are usually only temporary. Hormonal therapy may cause regression or may arrest the progression of endometriosis for a variable period of time.

Moderate to severe endometriosis is best treated surgically with or without a medical adjunct. Endometriosis in the presence of an endometrioma of 1 cm or more seldom responds to medical therapy alone. The treatment of choice in patients who have severe or extensive endometriosis and who no longer desire pregnancy is definitive surgery, including total abdominal hysterectomy with bilateral salpingo-oophorectomy and with excision of, coagulation of, or vaporization of all endometriotic foci and lysis of adhesions. In patients with moderate disease who have one uninvolved ovary, a unilateral oophorectomy may be performed, provided all visible endometriosis can be surgically extricated or adequately coagulated. Patients who have undergone bilateral oophorectomy should receive estrogen replacement postoperatively; however, a waiting period of approximately 3 to 6 months may be beneficial in severe disease if there has been a question as to the completeness of eradication of endometriotic implants.

DYSFUNCTIONAL UTERINE BLEEDING

method of
RANDLE S. CORFMAN, Ph.D., M.D., and
ALAN H. DECHERNEY, M.D.
Yale University School of Medicine
New Haven, Connecticut

Dysfunctional uterine bleeding (DUB) is defined as uterine bleeding that results from a cause other than uterine pathology. Inherent in this diagnosis, then, is the obligation to exclude pathologies that could account for the bleeding in question.

A thorough medical history and physical examination, bearing in mind the differential diagnosis of vaginal bleeding, are mandatory for correct and expedient assessment of the patient. The history helps in differentiating between the various causes of vaginal bleeding, including those that might not be primary to the reproductive system. Physical examination includes a thorough examination of the lower reproductive tract, with care taken to ascertain whether the bleeding is uterine in origin. This includes careful examination of the external genitalia, a gentle speculum examination, and palpation of the pelvic organs.

Upon completion of the history and physical examination, serious attention can be directed toward the differential diagnosis of DUB (Table 1). The age of the patient dictates the direction of both the subsequent diagnostic evaluation and the treatment. Although DUB occurs most frequently during puberty and the perimenopausal years, a high index of suspicion for pregnancy-related complications and malignancies, respectively, must be maintained.

Information is then sought from various tests that might shed light upon the etiology of the bleeding. The need to establish that the patient is not pregnant cannot be overstated. Laboratory testing, then, includes a sensitive pregnancy test, complete blood count, coagulation profile, and, if indicated by the history and physical examination, thyroid function testing.

Evaluation of the uterine cavity can be accomplished by either biopsy or endoscopy, and should be performed if the patient is at risk for uterine neoplasia. Biopsy is performed either in the office, using a Novak curette, or in the hospital setting, using cervical dilatation and uterine curettage (D & C). Hysteroscopy, while allowing evaluation of the uterine cavity, is more difficult in patients with acute bleeding, owing to poor visibility. It can be utilized either in the office or in the hospital setting.

Having gathered this information one can, by exclusion, arrive at the diagnosis of DUB. Table 1 presents the diagnoses that must be considered in differentiating DUB from organic pathologies. Many of these diagnoses are rare, but proper and expedient care of the patient dictates an awareness of the various possibilities, even before beginning the initial evaluation of the patient.

The pathophysiology of DUB is attributed to anovulation in 90 per cent of cases. Classically, this disorder occurs at the extremes of the reproductive years. Bleeding is from estrogen withdrawal or estrogen breakthrough, resulting either from an immature hypothalamic-pituitary-ovarian axis or from ovarian failure. These imbalances result in unopposed estrogenic stimulation of the endometrium, with continual proliferation. Without progesterone, which is derived from the corpus luteum and acts to stabilize the endometrium and to limit endometrial growth, the endometrium becomes thick and disorganized and spontaneous superficial hemorrhage occurs. The resulting endometrium is fragile, a function of both unopposed estrogen stimulation and deficient progesterone production.

Treatment

The immediate objective of therapy is to halt the bleeding episode and to re-establish cyclic

TABLE 1. **Differential Diagnosis of Dysfunctional Uterine Bleeding**

Dysfunctional uterine bleeding
Pregnancy complications
  Abortion, threatened vs. incomplete
  Ectopic pregnancy
  Trophoblastic disease
  Second or third trimester bleeding
  Puerperal complications
Benign and malignant lesions of the genital tract
  Vagina
    Carcinomas, sarcomas
    Adenosis
  Cervix
    Polyps
    Carcinomas
  Uterus
    Polyps
    Leiomyomas
    Carcinomas, sarcomas
    Intrauterine device
Systemic disorders
  Coagulopathies
  Thyroid dysfunction
  Diabetes mellitus
  Liver disease
  Renal disease
  Nutritional deficiencies
Trauma, foreign bodies

hormonal events in order to prevent recurrence. The treatment of DUB is medical in nature (Figure 1), and surgery should be reserved for those patients who do not respond to a medical therapeutic regimen that has been based upon a sound understanding of the pathophysiology of the disorder.

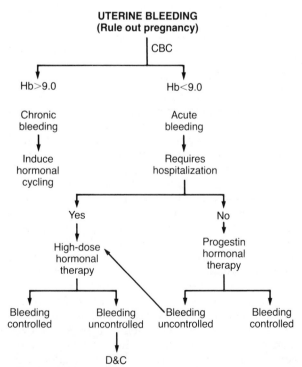

Figure 1. Management of dysfunctional uterine bleeding.

It is important to acknowledge that the therapeutic regimen chosen must be tailored to the patient, taking into account her age, her desire for pregnancy, and the odds of underlying pathology. At all stages of therapy it is necessary to re-evaluate the patient in order to avoid overlooking a previously undetected pathology. This is particularly true in the perimenopausal patient.

The mode by which cyclical hormonal stimulation of the endometrium is achieved is dictated by the patient's desire for pregnancy. In the patient who desires contraception, combined progestin-estrogen therapy in the form of low-dose birth control pills containing less than 50 micrograms of synthetic estrogen is recommended. This is continued until pregnancy is desired, and therapy is altered to a form of ovulation induction.

In the patient who desires pregnancy, therapy is directed toward correcting the basic underlying problem, anovulation. The use of ovulation induction agents, including clomiphene citrate and human menopausal gonadotropins, requires careful monitoring of the patient and should be managed only by a physician who is knowledgeable of the benefits and side effects of these drugs.

The patient who is not at risk for, and who does not desire, pregnancy can be treated with an orally active progestin, after pregnancy has been ruled out. Medroxyprogesterone acetate, taken 10 mg orally every day for 10 days monthly, can be prescribed in order to establish a monthly menstrual flow, thereby counteracting the effects of unopposed estrogen stimulation. It is the physician's obligation to rule out underlying pathology if unscheduled bleeding occurs on this, or any other, regimen.

Although not classically considered as DUB, estrogen breakthrough bleeding on low-dose birth control pills often occurs, owing to the minimal estrogen effect of the pills. Use of an estrogen-dominant pill, or supplementation with 0.02 mg ethinyl estradiol, often eliminates this problem.

Management of acute, excessive DUB is directed toward restoring structural stability, with accompanying vasoconstrictive rhythmicity, to the endometrium. In the hemodynamically stable patient, in whom neoplasia and pregnancy have been ruled out, treatment consists of oral estrogen-progesterone combination pills administered as one tablet four times per day, for 5 to 7 days. Bleeding usually ceases within 12 to 24 hours, and is followed in 5 to 7 days by another menstrual flow. If the bleeding is not controlled, or if the patient's hemoglobin level is less than 9.0 grams per dl, the patient is hospitalized and given intravenous conjugated estrogens in 25-mg doses every 6 hours until bleeding ceases. The estrogen therapy is then followed by progestin support as outlined above. If these measures fail to control the bleeding the patient is taken to dilatation and curettage, in order to definitively establish whether an organic cause is present.

AMENORRHEA

method of
SANDRA ANN CARSON, M.D
University of Tennessee, Memphis
Memphis, Tennessee

and

ANTONIO SCOMMEGNA, M.D.
University of Chicago
Chicago, Illinois

Primary amenorrhea is the absence of menarche by age 16 or absence of both menarche and development of breast buds by age 14 in females. Secondary amenorrhea is also defined as the absence of menstrual periods for 6 months or three usual cycle lengths in a woman who has previously been menstruating regularly. The menstrual cycle results from the coordinated integration of a functioning hypothalamus, pituitary, ovary, and uterus and is influenced by higher cortical centers. Disorders at any of these levels may result in amenorrhea, and treatment focuses on eliminating the cause.

Physiologic Causes

Amenorrhea occurs normally during pregnancy and lactation, and after the menopause. Treatment of physiologic amenorrhea is, of course, not warranted except to prevent consequences of estrogen deprivation after the menopause.

Anatomic Causes

The most common anatomic cause of amenorrhea is the *imperforate hymen*. Located at the introitus, this thin transparent membrane will prevent passage of menstrual effluvium. The membrane will bulge with a Valsalva maneuver, and the blood-filled vagina can be felt below the uterus during rectal examination. The imperforate hymen must be differentiated from the *transverse vaginal septum,* which forms when the point of fusion between the urogenital sinus and müllerian tubes fails to cannulate. The transverse septum is thicker and higher in the vagina than the imperforate hymen. Both of these disorders may be corrected by surgical incision of the membrane or septum.

Vaginal atresia occurs when the urogenital sinus fails to develop into the lower portion of the vagina. These patients do exhibit müllerian differentiation and have a uterus. Therefore, once the vagina is surgically created, they are fertile, unlike those patients who lack a vagina owing to müllerian aplasia. *Müllerian aplasia* occurs when the müllerian tubes fail to differentiate into the fallopian tubes, uterus, and upper vagina. Although hormonal function in patients with müllerian aplasia is normal, even those who have a rudimentary uterus (Rokitansky-Küster-Hauser syndrome) do not have menstrual periods.

Uterine Factors

Intrauterine synechiae (Asherman's syndrome) usually result after an abortal or postpartum dilatation and curettage (D & C). They can also result from a D & C performed for anovulatory bleeding. The diagnosis is suggested by failure to bleed after estrogen and progesterone (E_2 + P) replacement and is confirmed by either hysterosalpingography or hysteroscopy. Lysis of the adhesions may be performed under direct division through the hysteroscope. After lysis, estrogen therapy and placement of an intrauterine device or intrauterine Foley catheter may retard further adhesion formation. Infectious disorders such as tuberculosis or schistosomiasis have also been reported to cause intrauterine synechiae. In such cases treatment should be augmented with appropriate antibiotics.

Ovarian Factors

Polycystic Ovarian Disease. Anovulation resulting in amenorrhea may arise from polycystic ovarian disease (PCOD), a disorder that includes a spectrum of abnormalities from hyperthecosis to large sclerocystic ovaries. The disorder is characterized by multiple ovarian follicules in various stages of development leading to an altered hormonal milieu in which the normal hormonal fluctuations are replaced by constant steady-state levels. Ovarian androgens are usually elevated, as is the luteinizing hormone/follicular stimulating hormone (LH/FSH) ratio. Insulin resistance is also commonly noted. Besides amenorrhea, which presents in about half of these patients, infertility, hirsutism, obesity, and irregular bleeding may also be present.

Treatment of patients with PCOD revolves around their desire for pregnancy. In patients not desiring or at risk for pregnancy, cyclic progestin withdrawal is mandatory to prevent unopposed estrogenic stimulation of endometrial growth and resultant hyperplasia. Those patients desiring contraception are best treated with a combined oral contraceptive. The estrogen-progesterone action will control endometrial growth and sloughing as well as provide the needed contraception. Hirsutism is also ameliorated by the estrogen-progestin treatment. Patients who desire a pregnancy and are not ovulating require ovulation induction with first clomiphene citrate and then a trial of human menopausal gonadotropin, either combined LH/FSH (Pergonal) or pure FSH (Metrodin). Recently, pulsatile gonadotropin releasing hormone (GnRH) therapy has been used for induction of ovulation in these patients, but results have been disappointing.

Gonadal Failure. Gonadal failure from a variety of reasons will lead to amenorrhea. The absence of viable ovarian follicles will result in loss of estradiol production and, thus, amenorrhea. Patients with gonadal dysgenesis have a reduced number of primordial follicles, which, by the time of puberty, have usually become atretic. This disorder is associated with a variety of chromosomal complements. Most patients with gonadal dysgenesis have a 45,X karyotype and extragenital somatic anomalies constituting Turner's syndrome. Some patients with gonadal dysgenesis who have a history of menstruation may have follicles deep in the ovarian medulla that can be stimulated to ovulate. Weekly blood samples drawn and saved over 4 weeks can be assayed for LH, FSH, and estradiol. A drop in gonadotropins with a simultaneous rise in estradiol may signal follicular activity. These patients may be followed with ultrasound during cyclic estrogen/progesterone replacement for detection of follicular growth.

IDIOPATHIC PREMATURE MENOPAUSE. Premature menopause is ovarian failure prior to the age of 40. In idiopathic cases patients have elevated gonadotropin levels and low levels of estrogens as a result of absence of ovarian follicles. These patients may actually represent an end point of 46,XX gonadal dysgenesis and are difficult to distinguish from patients with gonadotropin-resistant ovaries (Savage syndrome). Patients require hormonal replacement therapy (Table 1) to prevent the consequences of estrogen deficiency syndrome.

Gonadotropin-Resistant Ovaries. Patients with gonadotropin-resistant ovaries (Savage syn-

TABLE 1. **Regimens of Estrogen-Progesterone Replacement Therapy**

17-beta-estradiol skin patch (continuous) + 14 days medroxyprogesterone acetate, 10 mg q.d.
Micronized 17-beta-estradiol 2 mg q.d. continuously + 14 days medroxyprogesterone acetate, 10 mg q.d.
Conjugated estrogens 0.625 mg q.d on days 1 to 25 of each month + medroxyprogesterone acetate 10 mg q.d. on days 16 to 25 of each month

drome) have ovarian follicles that do not respond to gonadotropin and thus do not produce estradiol. These patients may have secondary sexual characteristics or may require exogenous estrogen to enter puberty. In addition, they have a 46,XX karyotype, elevated gonadotropins, and amenorrhea. The follicles that are present are deep within the ovarian medulla, unreachable by laparoscopic biopsy and insensitive to gonadotropins. The etiology of ovarian resistance to gonadotropin remains obscure. Theories range from an FSH receptor defect to autoimmune antibodies directed against the FSH receptor or the gonadotropin itself. No evidence as to its cause exists; it may be just a point in the spectrum of idiopathic premature ovarian failure as described above. Pregnancies have been reported during the administration of estrogen/progestin replacement therapy.

Male Pseudohermaphroditism

Male pseudohermaphrodites have a 46,XY karyotype but are phenotypically female. This disorder has a variety of causes, all involving disorders of either testosterone metabolism or its receptor.

Testicular Feminization. Patients with testicular feminization are male pseudohermaphrodites who lack testosterone receptors. Although these patients have normal testes producing normal amounts of testosterone, they cannot respond to any of the androgens that they make. Not only do they have female external genitalia, but they also feminize at puberty. Even in women pubic and axillary hair is a result of androgen production, and therefore these patients have no or scanty pubic or axillary hair. In addition, because their normal testes produce müllerian inhibitory factor, these patients do not have a uterus or fallopian tubes. Their intra-abdominal testes are at risk for hilar cell adenomas, seminomas, and Sertoli-Leydig cell tumors. Thus, they require gonadectomy after puberty. Estrogen/ progesterone replacement therapy is necessary after gonadectomy.

Adrenal Enzyme Deficiencies. 17-Alpha-hydroxylase deficiency, 17,20-desmolase deficiency, and 17-alpha-ketosteroid reductase deficiency may all lead to male pseudohermaphroditism. When these enzymes, which are important in testosterone synthesis, are absent, the hormone cannot be produced and thus is not available to masculinize a fetus. Patients with 17-alpha-hydroxylase deficiency, in addition, may have hypertension from the buildup of adrenal mineralocorticoids. Treatment with corticosteroids will suppress adrenal mineralocorticoid overproduction as well as replace cortisol deficiency.

Pituitary Factors

Hyperprolactinemia is found in 13 to 30 per cent of patients who have secondary amenorrhea. Prolactin influences ovarian steroid production directly, influences pituitary gonadotropin release, and also interferes with ovarian steroid modulation of hypothalamic pituitary function. Normally under tonic inhibition by dopamine from the hypothalamus, prolactin is also controlled by histamine inhibition and serotonin and thyrotropin-releasing hormone (TRH) stimulation. Factors that physically obstruct the inhibition from the hypothalamus, such as craniopharyngioma, sarcoidosis, and surgical ablation, will increase prolactin levels. Similarly, prolactin levels will also be increased by direct stimulation, such as in primary hypothyroidism, in which TRH is elevated. Drugs such as phenothiazines, exogenous sex steroids, and many antihypertensives and antidepressants can cause hyperprolactinemia. Prolactin-secreting pituitary adenomas must be ruled out in patients with hyperprolactinemia. Computed tomography and magnetic resonance imaging are important tools to detect the presence of pituitary adenoma. Bromocriptine is the mainstay of treatment of patients with hyperprolactinemia. This ergot alkaloid directly suppresses prolactin secretion by the lactotroph and will also shrink tumors. Those patients whose hyperprolactinemia results from hypothyroidism need only be treated with thyroid replacement.

Patients with pituitary necrosis after a previous postpartum hemorrhage, cerebral radiation, or surgical ablation will have no gonadotropin to stimulate ovarian steroid production. In addition, no other tropic hormones for the adrenal and thyroid will be made. Besides replacing needed ovarian steroids, both thyroid and adrenal hormones must be replaced. Human menopausal gonadotropins may be administered in patients desiring pregnancy.

Hypothalamic Factors

Hypothalamic amenorrhea is the second most frequent cause of amenorrhea in reproductive age women. It is associated with stress, vigorous athletic participation, or severe weight loss. Its etiology is unknown but involves the inability of the hypothalamic-pituitary axis to respond to ovarian steroid feedback. Endocrine regulation of gonadotropin-releasing hormone (GnRH) involves dopamine, serotonin, and opioids. The exact role of these neural peptides is unknown; however, alteration of their secretion, synthesis, or action by psychotropic and antihypertensive agents will result in hypothalamic amenorrhea. The diagnosis is one of exclusion, and treatment centers on removing the cause of stress.

Anorexia nervosa is one example of severe psychologic stress that results in a loss of gonadotropin pulsatility. Affected patients are usually in the middle to upper social economic classes and younger than 25 years. They exhibit a prepubertal LH and FSH response to GnRH, which can be reversed by pulsatile administration of GnRH. This suggests that the disorder lies in the hypothalamus or higher cortical centers. Anorexia nervosa combines psychologic stress with severe weight loss. However, weight loss alone to less than 70 per cent of ideal body weight can also result in amenorrhea. Women seem to require a fat content equal to about 22 per cent of body weight to maintain menstrual function. Patients who begin to gain weight will resume menstruating at about 90 per cent of ideal body weight. However, patients with anorexia nervosa may not begin having menses even if their weight increases.

Hypogonadotropic Hypogonadism

Patients who have hypogonadotropic hypogonadism actually have an altered GnRH synthesis or metabolism. This results in a lack of pituitary secretion of LH and FSH. Thus the gonads are not stimulated to produce sex steroids. This disorder is autosomal recessive. If hypogonadotropic hypogonadism is associated with decreased ability or inability to smell, it is termed Kallmann syndrome. This syndrome is inherited in either an autosomal dominant or X-linked recessive fashion. It is the most common type of hypogonadotropic hypogonadism and may also be associated with other midline somatic abnormalities such as cleft palate. Estrogen/progesterone replacement therapy is necessary for the initiation of puberty and menses. Human menopausal gonadotropins are required if pregnancy is desired.

Traumatic or exudative processes disrupting the hypothalamic-pituitary axis can result in amenorrhea. Tumors such as craniopharyngioma, granulomas from tuberculosis, or sarcoid tumors are examples. These diseases usually present with symptoms other than amenorrhea alone.

Thyroid Causes

Both hyper- and hypothyroidism may result in amenorrhea. Hyperthyroidism is associated with an increase in sex hormone–binding globulin (SHBG) and therefore a reduced metabolic clearance rate of testosterone. Such an effect leads to increased levels of androstenedione and estrone, and anovulation results. On the other hand, hypothyroidism decreases SHBG, and more testosterone and estradiol are free to interfere with ovulation. In addition, TSH is elevated in hypothyroidism and may increase levels of prolactin, which itself can interfere with ovulation. Treatment of the amenorrhea necessitates elimination of the thyroid problem.

Adrenal Causes

Amenorrhea may also result from adrenal steroid enzyme deficiency. In the congenital forms, the resulting adrenal hyperandrogenism causes hirsutism, virilization, and, if not treated, primary amenorrhea. In the adult type of adrenal hyperplasia, caused by an attenuated enzyme deficiency, secondary amenorrhea gonadotropin profiles and steroid hormone levels similar to those seen in PCO are encountered. Patients with this form of enzyme deficiency usually have hirsutism. Serum dehydroepiandrosterone sulfate (DHEA-S) and testosterone (T) concentrations will help differentiate adrenal from ovarian causes of excess androgens. Furthermore, an adrenocorticotropic hormone (ACTH) stimulation test will identify the level of the enzyme block, and the disorder is treated with corticosteroid replacement. Androgen-secreting tumors of either the adrenal or ovary must be excluded in patients after abrupt onset of hirsutism, virilization, and amenorrhea. A testosterone level greater than 200 ng per dl is highly suggestive of an ovarian tumor, which can be excluded only by means of exploratory laparotomy. A DHEA-S concentration greater than 700 ng per ml may signal an adrenal tumor. A CAT scan of the adrenals is a very sensitive test for diagnosing an adrenal tumor.

Management

The clinical evaluation of the patient with amenorrhea begins with a careful history and physical examination. Historical inquiry to elicit symptoms of pregnancy, chronic disease, and severe psychologic stress should be made. Physical examination should pay particular attention to breast development, pelvic examination, hirsutism, virilization, and extragenital congenital anomalies. Laboratory work-up should include routine blood chemistry, complete blood count, pregnancy test, prolactin, and TSH. A karyotype should be included in most patients who have never menstruated and in those who have ovarian failure but are younger than 35 years of age. LH and FSH levels will help distinguish between hypothalamic pituitary disorders and ovarian failure. The schematic diagram in Figure 1, which is described below, is a logical approach to interpreting these laboratory tests.

We begin by determining if the patient has a uterus. In the patient who has experienced previous menstrual periods, the presence of the uterus is obvious. However, in the young adolescent or pediatric patient, pelvic examination with the patient under anesthesia, ultrasonic evaluation, or even laparoscopy may be required to ascertain the answer to this very important ques-

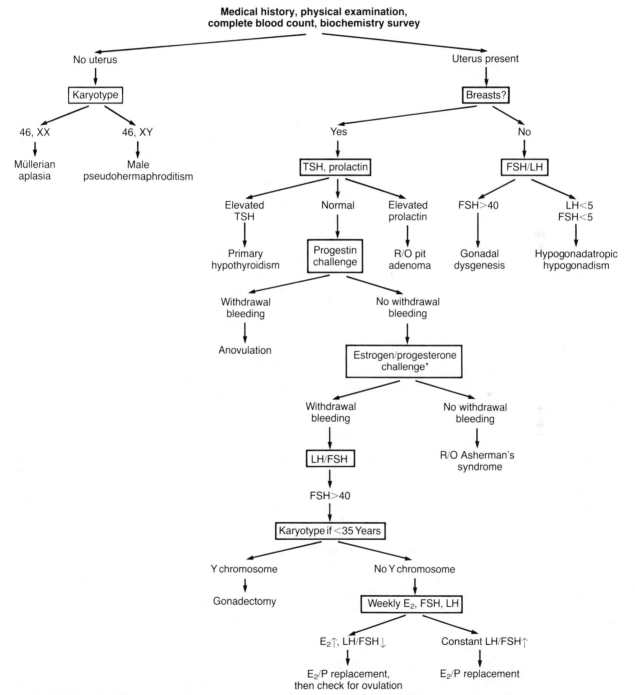

Figure 1. Work-up of patients with amenorrhea. *Estrogen/progesterone challenge may be omitted in patients with primary amenorrhea. TSH = thyroid-stimulating hormone; FSH = follicle-stimulating hormone; LH = luteinizing hormone; E_2 = 17 beta-estradiol; R/O = rule out.

TABLE 2. Regimens for Progestin Challenge or Cyclic Progestin Withdrawal

Progesterone in oil 100 mg IM
Medroxyprogesterone acetate 10 mg PO q.d. for 10 days
Norethindrone acetate 5 mg PO q.d for 10 days

tion. If a patient does not have a uterus, then she either has müllerian aplasia or is a male pseudohermaphrodite with müllerian inhibitory factor preventing uterine development. The easiest way to differentiate between these disorders is by karyotype. A patient without a uterus who has a 46,XX karyotype has müllerian aplasia. A patient with a 46,XY karyotype without a uterus is a male pseudohermaphrodite, and the differential diagnosis of male pseudohermaphroditism must be approached.

The patient with a uterus who presents with amenorrhea must then be evaluated for estrogen status. Breast development is a convenient, available biologic assay for endogenous estrogen. This presumes, of course, that the patient has never been given exogenous estrogen. Breast development does not require much estrogen, and if the patient does have breasts this reflects the presence, at some point in her life, of endogenous estrogen. A quick pelvic examination will then rule out any anatomic abnormality causing amenorrhea.

The next question becomes, "Does the patient still have enough endogenous estrogen to continue cycling?" A progestin challenge with either intramuscular progesterone in oil, medroxyprogesterone acetate, or oral norethindrone acetate will induce menses in a patient who has sufficient estrogen to permit endometrial stimulation and growth. Bleeding after a progestogen challenge makes the diagnosis of anovulation. Gonadotropin levels will confirm a diagnosis of polycystic ovaries if the LH/FSH ratio is greater than 3 and will also suggest hypothalamic amenorrhea if the gonadotropin levels are low to normal. Failure of bleeding after a progestogen challenge in a patient who has previously experienced menstrual periods suggests either uterine unresponsiveness or estrogen levels too low to provoke endometrial proliferation. The patient should then be given a course of estrogen followed by another progestin challenge. After both hormones are provided, if the patient does not bleed, she most likely has intrauterine synechiae, a diagnosis that can be confirmed by either hysterosalpingography or hysteroscopy. The patient who bleeds after estrogen and progesterone therapy and also the patient with primary amenorrhea who fails to bleed after progesterone alone is estrogen-deficient. Gonadotropin levels will distinguish the patient with an ovarian disorder from a patient with hypothalamic-pituitary disorder. Patients with elevated gonadotropin levels have ovarian failure, which results in lack of estrogen and no feedback to inhibit gonadotropin secretion. Such patients who are younger than 35 years of age require a karyotype test to rule out the presence of a Y chromosone. If the gonadotropins are low, the patient has a hypothalamic-pituitary disorder and the ovaries are not being stimulated to make estrogen. These patients should have a pituitary MRI or CT scan to rule out tumor.

Treatment of amenorrhea depends on both its cause and the desires of the patient. Patients desiring a pregnancy must be treated differently than patients not interested in fertility. Nonetheless, all patients must be protected from the hazards of unopposed estrogen (Table 2) or estrogen deficiency. It cannot be stressed too greatly that pregnancy must be the first condition ruled out before any medical therapy or invasive diagnostic measures are undertaken.

DYSMENORRHEA

method of
RONALD L. YOUNG, M.D.
Baylor College of Medicine
Houston, Texas

Dysmenorrhea, or painful menstruation, is a condition that may affect women at any time during their reproductive lives. At least 50 per cent of women responding to inquiries about their periods describe some degree of pain or discomfort associated with menstruation. This number reaches 75 per cent in the case of adolescents and teenagers. Ten to 15 per cent of these women suffer some degree of incapacitation, impairing their ability to function at work, in school, or in society. Again, teenagers tend to be at the upper ranges of these numbers.

While menstrual pain is the principal element, the condition actually encompasses a broader range of symptoms, including nausea, vomiting, diarrhea, headache, dizziness, and blurred vision. Symptoms may precede the menses by a few hours or coincide with the onset of flow. They may last for only a few hours or throughout the entire menstruation. Pain is usually colicky, intense, and, as with any pain of pelvic origin, it may radiate to the legs or lower back.

From a functional standpoint, dysmenorrhea is caused by or associated with increased prostaglandin in the menstrual fluids. Prostaglandins F_2 alpha and E_2 have been cited in the etiology of dysmenorrhea. These compounds gain access to the general circulation in the process of degeneration of endometrial tissue. This, in turn, leads to the additional symptoms mentioned. Dysmenorrhea, on the other hand, may also be associated with a variety of organic lesions of the pelvic organs or the genital outflow tract. These lesions may be congenital, such as imperforate hymen, vaginal septum, total or partial absence of vagina, or noncommunicating uterine horn. Acquired lesions that are most frequently encountered are endometriosis, leiomyomas, adenomyosis, or chronic pelvic inflammatory disease. Elevated prostaglandin levels may also be found in patients in whom organic lesions are present. Together they may bring about painful increases in uterine contractility.

Primary dysmenorrhea is associated with the onset of ovulatory cycles and therefore mainly affects younger, nonparous women. Organic lesions are far less frequently encountered. If present, they are likely to be of the congenital type. The pain is generally maximal early in the period and is associated with the more severe generalized symptoms. *Secondary dysmenorrhea* is seen in older women and is associated to a far greater degree with acquired organic lesions. The pain is usually consistent throughout the duration of menstrual flow, and associated symptoms may be absent, or far less frequent and intense.

History and physical examination are generally the only steps necessary in the evaluation of the dysmenorrheic patient. Laboratory tests are seldom of value, except in cases in which questions concerning differential diagnosis exist. Particular attention must be paid to separating the problem of premenstrual syndrome from the broader dysmenorrhea picture, since some of the symptoms may be shared.

A functional cause is to be assumed in primary dysmenorrhea if no obvious congenital anomaly is found on physical examination. When conservative therapy fails in these cases, further investigation, including laparoscopy, may be indicated. This may lead to a previously unsuspected finding of uterine anomaly or even endometriosis. In cases of secondary dysmenorrhea, if organic lesions are suspected, more aggressive early investigation, including radiologic or endoscopic procedures, is indicated. However, even secondary dysmenorrhea may be functional in nature.

Treatment

Surgical Management

If adenomyosis is present to a significant degree and is associated with severe dysmenorrhea, then conservative therapy is often fruitless. Hysterectomy may be the only option if there is no desire for further reproduction. In the surgical management of endometriosis, adjunctive presacral neurectomy is advocated in various centers but remains controversial. As more cases of surgical endometriosis are being handled by laparoscopy and laser, the issue of presacral neurectomy is being shunted aside.

Medical Management

Medical therapy such as danazol (Danocrine), gonadotropin-releasing hormone (GnRH) agonists, or pseudopregnancy is also available. If the patient is wearing an IUD and it appears to be causing or exacerbating dysmenorrhea, then its removal is advisable.

In the adolescent who is experiencing emotional as well as physical problems and is incapacitated by her painful periods, dysmenorrhea requires special attention. Around 15 per cent of teenagers suffer significant school absences as a result of this condition. The initial negative experience is known to have potential lasting sequelae in the lives of these women. Although the analgesic effects of the compounds listed later may be of benefit here, it is often advisable to use low-dose oral contraceptives for 4 to 6 months. This regimen shifts the patient back to an anovulatory status, thereby neutralizing many of the physical and emotional impacts of dysmenorrhea. Without the fear of the impending menses, more attention can be directed toward counseling and educating the patient.

Modern medical management involves the use of newer nonsteroidal anti-inflammatory agents that act as prostaglandin synthetase inhibitors. These have generally replaced salicylates, indomethacin, phenylbutazone, and narcotic analgesics as first line agents. Nonsteroidal anti-inflammatory agents are begun with the onset of symptoms and may be continued for the duration of the pain. Naproxen (250 mg) and naproxen sodium (275 mg) are recommended every 6 to 8 hours. An initial loading dose of two tablets enhances the overall effect. Five tablets daily is the maximum dose for each drug. Mefenamic acid, 250 mg every 6 hours, can also be used after a loading dose of 500 mg. Treatment extending beyond 1 week is not advised. Ibuprofen, 300 or 400 mg every 4 to 6 hours, is usually effective. A 600 mg dose exists and may be necessary. Nonsteroidal agents are effective in 80 to 90 per cent of the cases. If they are ineffective and organic pathology has been ruled out, then narcotic analgesics or oral contraceptives may be employed. Investigation continues with other drugs such as calcium channel blockers and beta-mimetic agents.

MENOPAUSE

method of
DANIEL R. MISHELL, JR., M.D.
University of Southern California School of Medicine
Los Angeles, California

The mean age of menopause is about 51 years, with a normal distribution curve and 95 per cent confidence limits between ages 45 and 55. The average life expectancy for a woman in the U.S. is about 78 years, and about one third of a woman's life will be spent postmenopausally. This time of life should be considered an estrogen deficiency state, and improvement in both the quality as well as the quantity of life can be obtained with the use of estrogen replacement during the postmenopausal years.

Genitourinary Effects

Atrophy in the genitourinary tract can produce symptoms of atrophic vaginitis with itching, burning, dyspareunia, and possibly vaginal bleeding. Local estrogen therapy rapidly relieves these symptoms, but because vaginal administration of estrogen results in irregular systemic absorption, estrogen is best administered systemically for long-term prevention of vaginal atrophy as well as osteoporosis. Estrogen deficiency may also cause uterine prolapse as the supporting ligaments lose their tonicity. In addition, cystocele and rectocele may develop as a result of estrogen deficiency. These changes can be prevented or alleviated by administering estrogen. The trigone of the bladder and the urethra are embryologically derived from estrogen-dependent tissue, and postmenopausal estrogen deficiency can cause atrophy of these structures producing symptoms of urinary urgency, incontinence, dysuria, and urinary frequency. Because of atrophy of the vaginal elastic tissue, urinary stress incontinence can also occur. If these symptoms develop postmenopausally, they are best initially treated with estrogen replacement.

Central Nervous System Changes

The pathognomonic symptom of the menopause is the hot flush or flash, which is caused by a decrease in circulating estrogen levels. The best treatment for the hot flush is estrogen, which has been shown to alleviate symptoms better than placebo. It is best to administer the estrogen at bedtime to alleviate the hot flushes that can interfere with sleep. The usual dosage is 0.625 mg of conjugated estrogen, although higher doses may be necessary, especially when the ovaries are removed in a premenopausal individual. For women with contraindications to estrogen therapy, specifically, cancer of the breast or endometrium, other medications that are effective in treating hot flushes include oral medroxyprogesterone acetate (Provera) in a dosage of 20 mg per day. Hot flushes can also be relieved by a single injection of Depo-Provera 150 mg given once every 3 months. In addition, clonidine in a dosage of 150 μg per day can also reduce the incidence of hot flushes.

Symptoms such as anxiety, depression, irritability, and fatigue increase after the menopause and it has been shown that estrogen replacement significantly relieves these symptoms even in women who do not have hot flushes that interfere with their sleep.

Skin Changes

Recent studies have shown that postmenopausal estrogen users have a significantly thicker skin and a greater amount of collagen in the dermis than do postmenopausal women who do not use estrogen. Thus systemic estrogen use can retard wrinkling and thinning of the skin which occurs postmenopausally.

Osteoporosis

Postmenopausal osteoporosis affects about 25 per cent of women but is uncommon in blacks and in obese and tall women. In thin white and Oriental women, about 1 to 1.5 per cent of bone mass is lost each year after the menopause. Bone loss is more rapid in trabecular bone, which is found mainly in the thoracic spine, than in cortical bone, which is present in the axial skeleton. Beginning about age 60, fractures occur in the vertebral spine as well as the distal portion of the radius, which is also composed of trabecular bone. Fractures in the neck of the femur, made up mainly of cortical bone, usually start about age 70 to 75 and increase at a logarithmic rate thereafter. Estrogen replacement therapy will reduce the bone loss associated with postmenopausal osteoporosis and thus reduce the fracture rate in women, prolonging women's productive life span as well as providing a tremendous saving in health care costs. Supplemental calcium therapy and weight-bearing exercise are ancillary measures that by themselves without estrogen will not prevent postmenopausal bone loss. To determine if a patient is at risk for osteoporosis, a careful history and physical examination should be performed. The following factors are known to increase the risk of osteoporosis: (1) white or Oriental race; (2) reduced weight for height, (3) early spontaneous menopause or early surgical menopause, (4) family history of osteoporosis, (5) diet low in calcium, high in caffeine, or high in alcohol, (6) cigarette smoking, and (7) sedentary lifestyle. Routine screening by densitometry or CT scanning is not cost effective and is not recommended.

Osteoporosis is associated with an increased rate of bone resorption, and the administration of estrogen will return the resorption rate to normal. Numerous prospective and retrospective

TABLE 1. **Age-Adjusted All-Cause Mortality Rates (per 1000 per year)**
by Hysterectomy Status and Estrogen Use*

Hysterectomy Status	Estrogen Use		Total
	Nonuser	*User*	**Total**
Intact uterus and ovaries	9.0	4.9	8.2
	(6.5–12.0)	(1.8–10.7)	(6.1–10.8)
Hysterectomy	8.2	2.8	5.7
	(3.3–16.8)	(0.3–10.0)	(2.6–10.8)
Oophorectomy	11.8	1.4	7.2
	(5.9–21.2)	(0.0–7.6)	(3.7–12.6)
Total	9.3	3.4	
	(7.2–11.9)	(1.5–6.4)	

From Bush TL, Cowan LD, Barrett-Connor E, et al: JAMA 249:903, 1983. Copyright 1983, American Medical Association.
*Ninety-five percent confidence limits on rate.

epidemiologic studies have shown that estrogen therapy reduces the amount of postmenopausal bone loss as well as the incidence of fractures. Once estrogen therapy is stopped, bone loss resumes at the same rate as it does immediately postmenopausally. Therefore, estrogen replacement therapy should be maintained as long as a woman is ambulatory. The minimum dosage of estrogen needed to prevent osteoporosis is 0.625 mg of conjugated equine estrogen. Bone density studies with other estrogen formulations have not been published. It is recommended that in addition to estrogen, 1.5 grams of calcium should be ingested daily, and weight-bearing exercise should be encouraged. Supplemental use of vitamin D is of no benefit.

Cardiovascular Effects

Because estrogen replacement regimens have a minimal effect on liver globulins, postmenopausal estrogen users do not have an increase in mean blood pressure compared with women not ingesting estrogen. It is safe to provide estrogen replacement for postmenopausal women with or without hypertension. Because natural estrogens do not produce a hypercoagulable state, there is no evidence that postmenopausal women with or without a past history of thrombophlebitis have an increased incidence of thrombophlebitis with estrogen replacement therapy. Use of estrogen replacement has been shown in numerous retrospective as well as prospective epidemiologic studies to reduce the risk of myocardial infarction by about 50 per cent. Oral estrogen increases levels of the protective high-density lipoprotein cholesterol. Although it has not been determined that this is the mechanism by which estrogen prevents myocardial infarction, the demonstrated reduction of this entity, the major cause of mortality in women, is a major beneficial effect of estrogen. Age-adjusted data indicate that mortality from all causes is significantly lower in estrogen users than nonusers regardless of whether their uteri are intact or have been removed (Table 1).

Neoplastic Effects

Only a few of many epidemiologic studies investigating the relation of estrogen use and breast cancer have shown an increased risk of breast cancer in some subsets of postmenopausal estrogen users, while the majority of studies show no effect of estrogen on this cancer. Since estrogen can stimulate the growth of a nonpalpable breast cancer, it is advisable that all women have mammograms performed before initiation of estrogen therapy. If no tumor is found, current evidence indicates that oral estrogen use will not increase the risk of developing breast cancer. Epidemiologic data indicate that there is a significant increased risk of developing endometrial cancer in postmenopausal women who are ingesting estrogen without progestins. This risk increases with increased duration of use of estrogen as well as with increased dosage. The endometrial cancer that develops in estrogen users is usually well differentiated and is usually cured by performing a simple hysterectomy. The risk of developing this endometrial carcinoma in women receiving estrogen replacement can be markedly reduced by also administering progestins. The duration of progestin therapy is more important than the dosage, and it is now recommended that the progestin be administered for at least 12 days per month. The addition of progestin to the estrogen therapy acts synergistically to cause a slight increase in bone density. However, progestins reverse some of the beneficial effects of estrogen on serum lipids and thus should not be given to women without a uterus. There are no well-controlled epidemiologic studies yielding evidence that the use of progestins with estrogen alters the risk of breast cancer.

Treatment Regimens

The treatment regimen most commonly used in the United States is the sequential regimen of 0.625 mg of estrogen orally for the first 25 days each month. Beginning on day 12 to 15 of estrogen treatment, 5 to 10 mg of medroxyprogesterone acetate (MPA) is added daily for 10 to 13 days. With this regimen more than half the women have regular withdrawal bleeding, an annoying problem for the postmenopausal woman. It is not necessary to have withdrawal bleeding to slough the endometrium to reduce the risk of cancer. A continuous regimen in which the estrogen is given daily together with a small dose of oral progestin such as 2.5 to 5 mg of MPA reduces the chance of developing uterine bleeding as well as avoiding a week off treatment, in which symptoms may appear. Data from several recent studies indicate that most women do not bleed on this regimen and the endometrium usually remains atrophic. A routine pretreatment endometrial biopsy is unnecessary, as it is not cost effective, and routine annual endometrial biopsies are not necessary unless breakthrough bleeding occurs.

Estrogen replacement therapy is indicated for nearly all postmenopausal women because of its numerous beneficial effects. Contraindications to estrogen replacement are uncommon. These include a history of breast cancer, recent history of endometrial cancer, active liver disease, or the presence of thrombophlebitis. A past history of thrombophlebitis is not an absolute contraindication for estrogen replacement.

VULVOVAGINITIS

method of
SEBASTIAN FARO, M.D., Ph.D.
Baylor College of Medicine
Houston, Texas

The most frequent gynecologic complaint addressed by the physician rendering ambulatory care to the female patient is vulvovaginitis, which may be due to an allergic reaction, infection, or lack of hormones. The three most common causes of vaginitis are bacteria, *Candida albicans*, and *Trichomonas vaginalis*. Although a variety of bacteria may cause vaginitis, the two most common types of bacterial vaginitis are *Gardnerella vaginalis* and anaerobic vaginitis (bacterial vaginosis). The latter is a polymicrobial infection due to an overgrowth of anaerobic bacteria but may also involve *G. vaginalis*. In addition to *T. vaginalis*, other parasites may cause vulvovaginitis.

Vulvovaginitis due to a lack of estrogen is referred to as atrophic vaginitis, whereas inflammation due to the application of an external irritant is referred to as contact vulvovaginitis. The differentiation of microbial and nonmicrobial vulvovaginitis can be established by performing colposcopically directed biopsy of the vulva and a macroscopic as well as a microscopic examination of the vaginal discharge. The vaginal discharge reflects the status of the lower genital tract environment. In an asymptomatic or healthy or normal vagina, the discharge has a pH of 3.2 to 4.5, is white to slate-gray, and does not have an odor. Microscopic examination reveals squamous epithelial cells that are estrogenized and not covered with bacteria, thus obliterating the nucleus and cell membranes. There is not an abundance of white blood cells. The bacteria seen in the surrounding milieu are usually not clumped together and consist mainly of bacilli.

The examination of a patient complaining of vaginal burning, discomfort, dyspareunia, or abnormal vaginal discharge should begin with a detailed history. It is often helpful to show the patient a photograph or diagram of the vulva, vestibule, introitus, and vagina, then asking her to indicate on the diagram where her symptoms are located. Frequently, the patient states she has vaginal itching when in reality the inflammation is localized to the introitus. Questions should be asked as to whether or not she douches; if so, how often, and with which agent? Does the douching agent contain perfume? Is the patient utilizing a new soap or a new laundry detergent? Questions should be asked regarding her sexual habits. Is she using a new form of birth control? For example, has she begun to use a spermicidal cream or jelly or a coital lubricant? Does she allow cunnilingus, which may result in excessive moisture on the vulva and clitoris, thus resulting in maceration of the tissue and inflammation?

Patients with contact vaginitis will present with complaints of itching or burning that involves the vulva but usually does not involve the vagina. The vagina will be involved only if the inflammatory agent is introduced into the vagina. The tissues appear erythematous and excoriated. Inspection of the vulva with the aid of a colposcope does not reveal any discrete lesions. The vagina frequently has a normal pH, unless the patient has been douching repeatedly with either an acidic or an alkaline solution. Elimination of the suspected agent will often result in resolution of the patient's symptoms. In some instances, the patient may require the use of a topical steroid ointment or cream. The patient should be advised to apply the cream lightly and rub it into the affected area thoroughly. It should not be applied for longer than 10 days, since prolonged administration of a topical steroid may result in thinning of the tissues. This process will result in continuing symptoms.

ATROPHIC VAGINITIS

Postmenopausal patients not on estrogen replacement therapy often develop atrophic vaginitis. The hallmark of this condition is regression of the genital structures; the labia become less prominent, the vaginal mucosa becomes smooth owing to the loss of the rugae, and the epithelium thins. The pink color gives way to a pale pink to white coloration. The pH often is above 4.5 and may be as high as 7.5. There is a change in the bacterial flora, with the lactobacilli no longer being dominant. The patient often complains of burning, dyspareunia, and vaginal spotting. In addition, the patient may complain of urinary incontinence and burning when she urinates. The latter complaint is due to the passage of urine over the atrophic tissue.

Pelvic examination reveals the vulva to be smooth with loss of definition of the external genitalia, especially loss of the labia minora. The vagina is as described above. The vaginal discharge is scant and appears gray. The pH is between 5.0 and 7.5. Microscopic examination of the discharge reveals few epithelial cells; those present tend to be elliptical to round and are referred to as parabasal cells. The bacteria tend to be few in number, and there may be numerous white blood cells present. If a specimen of the vaginal discharge is cultured for aerobes and anaerobes, there will be a noticeable decrease in or absence of lactobacilli as well as an increase in anaerobic colonization. It is important to remember that the same presentation will be found in patients who have had a total hysterectomy with bilateral salpingo-oophorectomy.

It is extremely important in those patients with vaginal bleeding or spotting that the origin of the bleeding be determined. The etiology of the bleeding should be established before estrogen therapy is instituted. If the patient has a uterus, an endometrial biopsy should be performed. Other possible sites of origin are the lower urinary tract and rectum, which should be investigated.

Treatment for this condition is not systemic or topical antibiotics, but hormonal replacement. This can be accomplished by applying topical estrogen cream or oral estrogen or a combination of both. If topical estrogen cream is utilized after the acute phase has been corrected, the patient may require a maintenance program of once weekly or as-needed use of the estrogen cream.

MICROBIAL VAGINITIS

The physician attempting to treat the patient with complaints of vaginal itching or burning or discomfort must be familiar with the normal status of the healthy or asymptomatic vagina. The symptomatic vagina has a pH of greater than 4.5 and usually above 5. The discharge is usually a cream color, green, yellow, or dirty gray. The odor is usually offensive, and described as fishlike or foul (fetid). The discharge is frequently frothy; that is, it appears to contain air bubbles. The amount of discharge may vary from scant to copious, depending on the phase of the menstrual cycle, the concentration of estrogen and progesterone influencing the vagina, and the number of growing microbes present.

The lower genital tract has an endogenous microflora made up primarily of aerobic and anaerobic bacteria. The predominant bacterium of an asymptomatic vagina is *Lactobacillus*. This bacterium may play a pivotal role in maintaining the equilibrium of the healthy vagina by maintaining a pH of 3.8 to 4.2 by the production of lactic acid. This pH is not favorable to the growth of other more pathogenic bacteria, such as the facultative and obligate anaerobes. In addition, it is theorized that the ability of lactobacilli to produce hydrogen peroxide may also play a role in suppressing the growth of anaerobic bacteria. Thus, when a patient is found to have vaginitis, the pH is often above 5 and there is a marked reduction in the number of lactobacilli.

Prior to examining the patient, the physician should ask questions focusing on factors that may influence the normal vaginal environment. The patient should attempt to describe the characteristics of the initial episode and how the episodes have changed over time. Has there been a use of antibiotics? Have they been used for maintenance or therapeutic indications? Does the patient douche? If so, how often and with what agent? Questions regarding sexual habits should be asked. How many sexual partners does she have? Does she know if her partner has sexual contact with others? Does she practice cunnilingus, fellatio, or rectal intercourse? The patient should be asked to localize her symptoms; that is, are they located at the opening of the vagina or in the vagina proper? Finally, she should be asked to characterize her discharge with regard to color, consistency, and odor.

HUMAN PAPILLOMA VIRUS VESTIBULITIS

The examination should begin with the external genitalia. Attention should be paid to the medial aspect of the labia minora and majora, especially the area of the vestibule and introitus. Patients often complain of itching or burning and dyspareunia in this area. Examination of this area often reveals a horseshoe-shaped area of erythema, which is often painful or tender to palpation. Examination under magnification often reveals the presence of glistening papules. Application of 5 per cent acetic acid will turn this epithelium white, which is characteristic of human papilloma virus (HPV) infection. It is best to refer this patient for further evaluation to a gynecologist specializing in infections of the genital tract. Colposcopically directed biopsies will be required to establish a diagnosis. Treatment is usually initiated with laser ablation of this area followed by intravaginal application of 5-fluorouracil cream. The patient should undergo colposcopic examinations of the vulva, vagina, and cervix every 3 to 4 months for the next 2 years to determine if there is a recurrence. The patient's partner will require a similar examination to determine if there are HPV lesions present on his penis.

YEAST VAGINITIS

Typically, yeast favors a pH of 4.5 or lower, but not always. There are usually white blood cells present, and the number of free-floating bacteria is usually reduced. The discharge is white and tends to be pasty but may be liquid. Classically, the discharge is cottage cheese–like and clings to vaginal epithelium. The microscopic picture may be that of elliptical yeast cells, budding cells, cells with germ tubes present, or long strands of pseudohyphae. These different forms of the yeast can easily be seen when the vaginal discharge is mixed with potassium hydroxide (KOH). It is not necessary to culture routinely for yeast except in those instances when the patient's symptoms suggest a yeast infection but no fungal forms are seen microscopically.

Atypically, the patient may have a pH above 4.5 and there may be an increase in the number of bacteria seen in a wet preparation of the vaginal discharge. The physician should rely on a wet preparation mixed with KOH to rule out the presence of yeast.

Initial treatment should be with an intravaginal cream, ointment, or suppository such as clotrimazole (Lotrimin, Gyne-Lotrimin, Mycelex G), miconazole (Monistat), candicidin (Vanobid), or nystatin. These are all beneficial in treating yeast vulvovaginitis. There are different dosing regimens ranging from a single dose to 3-day and 7-day regimens. A patient with an initial infection may do well with a short treatment schedule if the precipitating factors can be established. Patients with recurrent infection will require longer treatment regimens and the possible use of maintenance therapy. Some patients will benefit from gentian violet applied as a vaginal paint or tampon. In addition, consideration should be given to examination and treatment of the patient's sexual partner. Ketaconazole (Nizoral) has been used in single doses of 400 mg with good results. However, hepatic and renal toxicity have been reported, and use of ketaconazole for vaginal yeast infection has not been encouraged.

BACTERIAL VAGINITIS

The examination of the patient with bacterial vaginitis begins with localizing the symptoms to the vagina. The characteristics of the discharge are noted, including pH, color, consistency, odor, and microscopic appearance. The macroscopic characteristics are not pathognomonic of a specific bacterial vaginitis. However, a pH above 5 and no specific odor may be indicative of a bacterial vaginitis that developed in a patient who has been treated repeatedly with antibiotics.

One or two drops of vaginal discharge should be mixed with 1 to 2 ml of normal saline and examined microscopically. The presence of clue cells, the absence of white blood cells, and the presence of floating clumps of bacteria are suggestive of G. vaginalis vaginitis, whereas the presence of clue cells, numerous white blood cells, and individual free-floating bacteria is indicative of bacterial vaginosis. A drop or two of the vaginal discharge should be mixed with concentrated KOH and if either G. vaginalis or bacterial vaginosis is present, a fishlike odor will be given off.

Another bacterium that has generated interest is Mobiluncus, a anaerobic gram-negative curved rod. However, its role as a cause of vaginitis is not firmly established. The strength of this organism's role in vaginitis is based on identification by either a wet preparation or a Gram stain of a vaginal specimen. This is a very tenuous identification at best, since it is difficult to identify the genus of a bacterium on a Gram stain from a mixed preparation, especially of a vaginal specimen.

Patients who fail to respond to treatment with an agent that is effective against anaerobic bacteria should be referred for further evaluation. The most accepted treatment at present is metronidazole, 250 mg given orally three times daily for 7 days. If the wet preparation is indicative of G. vaginalis and not bacterial vaginosis, then I will treat the patient with a first-generation cephalosporin (e.g., cephradine [Velosef] or cephalexin [Keflex]) in a dose of 250 mg, four times daily for 7 days. All patients should return for follow-up examination to determine if the pH has returned to 3.8 to 4.2 and if the microscopic picture reflects the normal vaginal state. Patients should also be advised to use condoms when having sexual intercourse until the follow-up examination establishes that the environment of the vagina has been restored to the healthy state. Following unprotected intercourse, if the patient's infection returns, then consideration should be given to treating her partner. If she has more than one partner, then a program of education concerning the transmission of these bacteria is needed.

Patients with persistent recurrent bacterial vaginitis should be referred to a physician experienced in treating vaginitis, who can evaluate the patient with appropriate bacterial culturing capabilities. It has been our experience that many of these patients, because they have had several repeated courses of antibiotics, may have an unusual microflora. The bacteria present may have unusual antibiotic sensitivity patterns. In these instances, I have found amoxicillin plus clavulanic acid (Augmentin) in a dose of 250 mg given orally three times daily for 7 days to be helpful.

PARASITIC VULVOVAGINITIS

The most common parasitic genital infection is *Trichomonas vaginalis*. Other common, but less frequent parasitic infections are *Phthirus pubis*, *Sarcoptes scabiei*, and *Enterobius vermicularis*.

Phthirus pubis, commonly referred to as "the crabs," is one of three species of lice that infect humans; the others are *Pediculus humanus humanus*, the body louse; and *Pediculus humanus capitis*, the head louse. Lice are transmitted by person-to-person contact. Although the pubic louse is most commonly transmitted via sexual contact, cases have been documented in which transmission has occurred from toilet seats, bed linen, and infected loose hairs. The incidence of infection is highest among those individuals with gonorrhea and syphilis. The patient presents with itching, evidence of excoriation, erythema, irritation, and inflammation. Patients who have a large number of bites may even develop a mild elevation in body temperature, malaise, and irritability.

The diagnosis is established by taking a detailed history and carefully examining the patient. The adult crab louse and nits (eggs) can be seen by the naked eye. A simple magnifying glass will facilitate examining the pubic area. The pubic lice may appear as scabs; however, when the scab is removed and examined microscopically, the crab louse becomes easy to identify. If no adults are present, the eggs or nits can be identified.

Treatment must be effective against both the adult lice and the nits. The partner of the infected patient must also be examined, as well as other household members. Several agents are available, including preparations with pyrethrins and piperonyl butoxide (Rid [liquid and shampoo]; Triple X [liquid and shampoo]; A-200 Pyrinate [shampoo]; and Barc), copper oleate (Cuprex), lindane (Kwell [lotion, shampoo, and cream]), crotamiton (Eurax), 20 per cent benzyl benzoate, and 10 per cent sulfur ointment. The pediculicide should remain in contact with the infected area for at least 1 hour to be ovicidal. Kwell is probably the most commonly used pediculicide. The proper use of this agent requires the patient to shower before applying the Kwell (1 per cent gamma benzene hexachloride), which then remains on the body surface for 8 hours. This process should be followed for three applications of Kwell, and each 8-hour application is followed by a shower. The patient should wash thoroughly with soap and water to remove the Kwell. After the final shower, no further treatment should be necessary.

Kwell is absorbed, especially if the skin has been severely excoriated, and may result in neurotoxicity. This agent should not be used on children and pregnant women.

The patient's clothing and fomites should also be treated for adult lice and nits. Clothes should be washed in hot water (125° F), and nonwashable items should be dry cleaned; either process will kill adult lice, nymphs, or nits. Inanimate or nonwashable items that cannot be processed by dry cleaning can be treated with disinfectants containing pyrethrin and piperonyl butoxide.

Sarcoptes scabiei is the causative agent of scabies, which is transmitted via close personal contact. The organism is transmitted by sexual and nonsexual contact. The hands and feet are initially infected. The female breast may have lesions resembling Paget's disease. Infection may occur in skin folds such as the umbilicus, the groin, and where the buttocks meet the thigh. The characteristic lesion is a burrow. Most sites are erythematous and excoriated, as is most frequently seen in the web between the fingers.

The infection can be diagnosed by taking skin scrapings and examining them microscopically for the presence of the mite. Other diagnostic modalities include needle extraction of a mite from a burrow; epidermal shave biopsy of a burrow or papule; covering the burrow with ink and wiping with alcohol (if a mite is present, it will be stained by the ink); scraping the burrow and mixing the scrapings with mineral oil and examining microscopically; punch biopsy; and placing topical tetracycline to the infected area and wiping, then examining under ultraviolet light for fluorescence.

Treatment of scabies is best accomplished with topical agents such as 1 per cent gamma benzene hexachloride (Lindane cream or lotion, Kwell, or Scabene), crotamiton (Eurax), or sulfur.

TRICHOMONAS VAGINALIS

Trichomonas vaginalis is a protozoan with five flagella, four located anteriorly and one located in an undulating membrane. The organism has the ability to adhere to epithelial cells. The hallmark of *T. vaginalis* infection is vaginal discharge, which may vary in color from a dirty gray to a yellow-green color. The discharge appears frothy owing to the presence of gas bubbles. The pH of the discharge is usually greater than 5. The patient may complain of dyspareunia, dysuria, pruritus, and a foul vaginal odor. The patient may note an exacerbation of her symptoms shortly following her menses.

Pelvic examination may reveal the vulva to be erythematous, slightly edematous, and excoriated. Petechiae may be present on the cervix and vaginal walls. A urine specimen may also reveal the presence of trichomonads. One or two drops of the vaginal discharge mixed with 1 to 2 ml of normal saline and examined microscopically typically will show numerous bacteria, white blood cells, and mobile trichomonads. However, if no protozoans are seen, it would be beneficial to inoculate a medium designed for the growth of *T. vaginalis* (e.g., Diamond's medium), since this is a more sensitive method for detecting *T. vaginalis* than microscopic examination of vaginal discharge.

Treatment should be instituted with metronidazole, 250 mg given orally three times daily for 7 days. I prefer this regimen over intravaginal suppositories, since the organism commonly infects extravaginal sites such as the bladder, urethra, or periurethral glands. I have found that the single 2-gram dose is not well tolerated by the patient because of gastric upset. The male partner should be treated to achieve a cure in the female patient. Condoms should be utilized during the treatment period. The patient should be re-examined to determine if the organism has been eradicated and the vaginal environment restored to a healthy state.

Patients who present to the physician with vulvovaginitis of microbial etiology should be considered to have a sexually transmitted disease. Consideration should be given to obtaining a culture specimen to test for the presence of *Neisseria gonorrhoeae* and *Chlamydia trachomatis*. In addition, serologic study for syphilis should be performed. These recommendations should be followed especially for the patient who is between the ages of 15 and 30, unmarried, and sexually active.

TOXIC SHOCK SYNDROME

method of
JOHN L. WHITING, M.D., and
ANTHONY W. CHOW, M.D.
University of British Columbia
Vancouver, British Columbia

Toxic shock syndrome (TSS) is an acute multisystemic illness characterized by sudden onset of high fever; diarrhea; hypotension; hyperemia of the conjunctival, oropharyngeal, and urogenital mucous membranes; and a diffuse scarlatiniform rash followed by desquamation from the hands and feet. Other organ systems, including the hepatic, renal, muscular, hematologic, gastrointestinal, cardiopulmonary, and central nervous systems, may also be involved, Since a definitive diagnostic test for TSS currently does not exist, recognition of the syndrome is primarily based on clinical findings (Table 1) and epidemiologic considerations (Table 2). Although TSS was primarily described in menstruating women and was associated with tampon use and vaginal *Staphylococcus aureus* infection, nonmenstrual cases are increasingly recognized. Nonmenstrual TSS has been associated with use of contraceptive diaphragms or sponges and with any of the myriad infections caused by *S. aureus*. Many such infections are acquired in the hospital, particularly infections associated with postoperative wounds, parturition, and nasal packing. The overall mortality of TSS remains high (3 to 7 per cent). Recurrence of disease is frequent in menstrual TSS, but is quite rare in nonmenstrual cases.

Etiology and Pathogenesis

The precise etiology and pathogenesis of TSS remain unclear. Since bacteremia rarely occurs despite multisystemic involvement, it is widely believed that staphylococcal exotoxin(s) are implicated. Among these staphylococcal products, the toxic shock syndrome toxin-1 (TSST-1), a 24 kilodalton protein that can be demonstrated in over 95 per cent of vaginal *S. aureus* strains associated with menstrual TSS, is a leading candidate as a causative agent of TSS. However, since up to 30 per cent of *S. aureus* strains associated with nonmenstrual TSS may be negative for TSST-1 production, other staphylococcal exotoxins may be responsible in these latter cases. The exact mechanisms for cellular injury by these exotoxins remain unknown, but the most important pathophysiologic effect is extensive capillary leakage of intravascular fluid resulting in rapidly progressive hypovolemia and end organ dysfunction. Whether staphylococcal exotoxins act directly on target organ sites or indirectly by triggering major biologic mediator systems such as interleukins, cachectin, prostaglandins, kallikrein, complement, and coagulation cascades remains to be determined. Answers to these important questions could provide new therapeutic options.

Diagnostic Approach

TSS should be considered in the differential diagnosis in any patient who is febrile, is in shock, and

TABLE 1. **Clinical Manifestations of Toxic Shock Syndrome**

Almost Always Present (>80%)	Commonly Present (20–80%)	Rarely Present (<20%)
Temperature ≥38.9°C	Headache	Arthritis
Rash and desquamation	Confusion or agitation	Lymphadenopathy
Hypotension	Meningismus	Hepatosplenomegaly
Nausea or vomiting	Pharyngitis	Pulmonary infiltrates
	Vaginitis	Pericarditis
	Conjunctivitis	Photophobia
	Strawberry tongue	Seizure
	Nonpitting edema	
	Myalgia	
	Arthralgia	
	Diarrhea	

has a rash. This applies not only to previously healthy, menstruating women, but also to anyone with a suspected *S. aureus* infection. A diligent effort should be made to uncover any occult focus, particularly since infected wounds associated with nonmenstrual TSS often show only minimal signs of local inflammation. Presence of a characteristic sunburn-like rash is particularly helpful in the differential diagnosis; however, the rash may be evanescent or atypical. Laboratory findings, although striking, are nonspecific, and are useful only for monitoring target organ dysfunction and the severity of complications (Table 3). Blood should be drawn for baseline investigations, and cultures from blood, urine, wounds, or other body sites should be obtained. Although the distinction between TSS and other illness can be quite difficult at times, a careful history and physical examination in combination with a strong index of suspicion and appropriate laboratory tests of exclusion will usually provide the correct diagnosis.

Treatment

The major goals of treatment in TSS are (1) resuscitative measures for hypovolemia and shock, (2) eradication of toxin-producing *S. aureus*, (3) removal or neutralization of preformed toxin(s), and (4) treatment of complications.

Resuscitation

Supportive and resuscitative measures should be commenced as soon as the patient has been examined. In patients who have mild hypotension and are otherwise stable, the insertion of a wide-bore intravenous catheter may be all that is necessary. Those with profound hypotension, however, will require rapid infusions of intravenous fluids. As hypotension is largely due to increased capillary wall permeability and leakage of fluids into extravascular compartments, colloid should be included in the intravenous fluid regimen. Oxygen is administered and a urinary catheter is inserted for monitoring of urine output. Many patients will quickly respond and can then be managed under close observation in a general ward.

If the hypotension persists and the patient is oliguric after 1 or 2 hours of aggressive intravenous fluid management, the patient is best moved to an intensive care facility where hemodynamic parameters can be closely monitored and more effectively controlled. Monitoring devices such as a central venous pressure line, a Swan-Ganz catheter, or an intra-arterial catheter should be inserted if responses remain inadequate after reasonable fluid challenge, or if significant renal impairment or pulmonary edema is present. If the patient remains unresponsive to fluid management, a pressor agent such as dopamine hydrochloride should be considered. It is worth noting that cardiac indices in most patients with TSS usually indicate a state of high cardiac output. If a diminished cardiac output is observed, a toxin-mediated cardiomyopathy causing

TABLE 2. **Risk Factors for Toxic Shock Syndrome***†

High	Moderate	Low
Absence of antibody to TSS toxin-1	Regular absorbency tampons used	Contraceptive diaphragm
Infection with TSST-1 positive *S. aureus*	regularly during menstruation	Intrauterine contraceptive
Menstruating female less than 35 years of age	Alternating use of tampons and pads	device
	Contraceptive sponge	Surgical wound infections
Super absorbency tampon used continuously during menstruation		Early postpartum state
Nasal surgery with packing		

*Oral contraceptives may be protective.
†Modified with permission from Smith CB, Jacobson JA: Toxic shock syndrome. Disease-a-Month, Year Book Medical Publishers, Chicago, 1986.

depressed myocardial contractility should be suspected. In this instance, alternative management, including decreased fluid volume and reduction of cardiac afterload, should be instituted. Dobutamine (Dobutrex) rather than dopamine is preferable when myocardial damage is evident.

High-dose corticosteroids (e.g., methylprednisolone, 10 to 20 mg per kg every 6 to 8 hours), although commonly used, have not been prospectively evaluated in acute TSS. A retrospective study of a limited number of patients did suggest that corticosteroids are of some benefit when administered within the first 2 to 3 days of illness. Such therapy should be considered for the critically ill patient, but is probably unnecessary for most patients. Similarly, there has been only limited experience with the use of naloxone (Narcan) (0.4 mg intravenously followed by an infusion at a rate of 0.05 mg per kg per hour), and such investigational treatment should be reserved for patients with refractory shock.

Antimicrobial Therapy

Although antimicrobial therapy has not been shown to affect the course of the acute illness in menstrual TSS, it definitely reduces the frequency of recurrent episodes. Antimicrobial therapy is clearly important in the management of nonmenstrual TSS. There is no unique susceptibility profile of TSS-associated *S. aureus* compared with strains not associated with TSS. The choice of specific antistaphylococcal agents is therefore based on other considerations, such as tissue penetrance, bactericidal activity, and known history of hypersensitivity reactions. Beta-lactamase stable penicillins and cephalosporins such as nafcillin, cloxacillin, and cefazolin (100 mg per kg per day given every 6 hours), and other agents such as clindamycin (Cleocin) (25 mg per kg per day every 8 hours), or vancomycin (Vancocin) (30 mg per kg per day every 6 hours) are all appropriate choices.

Interestingly, clindamycin, at subinhibitory concentrations for bacterial growth, can "switch off" in vitro production of TSST-1 by toxin-positive strains of *S. aureus,* presumably by its action at the ribosomal level where protein synthesis

takes place. However, the therapeutic implication of this observation is unknown. Antistaphylococcal therapy should be administered intravenously and at maximal doses. In addition, if gram-negative sepsis cannot be ruled out clinically, empiric coverage with an aminoglycoside may be prudent until blood culture results are available. Therapy should be continued until the patient is afebrile and clinically stable. The benefit of additional oral antimicrobial therapy after this time is unproved, but many physicians prefer to complete a 10- to 14-day course of total treatment. Obviously, antibiotics alone may be ineffective in the presence of a loculated infection. Such areas should be adequately drained or débrided as indicated.

Toxin Removal and Neutralization

Apart from antimicrobial therapy to eliminate a continuing reservoir of toxin-producing bacteria, measures to minimize systemic absorption of preformed toxin from infected wounds or vagina may be worthwhile. Surgical wounds, if present, should receive special attention, since most cases of postoperative TSS occur in the absence of obvious local signs of infection. Thus, any surgical wound, even if grossly uninfected, should be closely examined and probably surgically explored. Any foreign body, such as an infected prosthesis, intravenous catheter, tampon, diaphragm, or contraceptive sponge, should be removed and cultured. Some clinicians have advocated liberal irrigations of wounds or douching the vagina with saline or povidone-iodine. This is of unproved benefit but unlikely to be harmful.

Since seroprevalence studies in humans and animal protection studies in experimental TSS suggest that antibody to TSST-1 is protective, attempts to rapidly neutralize systemically absorbed TSST-1 by hyperimmune serum appear promising. Human immune globulin has been shown to have high antibody titer to TSST-1, and the protective and therapeutic efficacy of such immune serum has been demonstrated in a rabbit model of TSS. Whether immune globulin will be effective in patients with established disease remains to be ascertained.

Treatment of Complications

While the relative contribution of hypotension versus direct toxin effect to multiple organ dysfunction in TSS is uncertain, it is clear that close attention to the potential for such late complications will be particularly important (see Table 3). Severe electrolyte and acid-base disturbances such as hyponatremia, hypocalcemia, hypomagnesemia, and acidosis should be corrected. Seizure and arrhythmias should be controlled. Pa-

TABLE 3. **Complications of Toxic Shock Syndrome**

Common (>20%)	Rare (<20%)
Acute renal failure	Disseminated intravascular
Adult respiratory distress	coagulation
syndrome	Ataxia
Hypocalcemia	Toxic encephalopathy
Hypomagnesemia	Memory impairment
Menorrhagia	Cardiomyopathy
Alopecia	Protracted malaise
Nail loss	

tients with acute renal failure may require hemodialysis, whereas those with adult respiratory distress syndrome will need aggressive ventilatory support. Although such complications are rare, patients with late and debilitating sequelae such as persistent neuromyasthenia, severe depression, lack of concentration, and memory loss will require continued support and psychologic counseling.

Prevention

Recurrence of TSS is primarily limited to women with menstrual TSS who had received inadequate antimicrobial therapy. With antibiotic treatment and appropriate precautions, fewer than 5 per cent of patients will have a second episode of TSS. Subsequent episodes may be mild or severe, and generally occur under circumstances similar to the initial illness. Recurrence is rare in nonmenstrual TSS. Serologic studies have indicated that women who developed TSS during menses may take many months to acquire an antibody titer to TSST-1, whereas patients with nonmenstrual TSS generally develop a significant antibody response soon after their illness.

Until more is understood about the nature of the disease and its relationship to menstruation and tampon use, patient education remains the mainstay of prevention. Women need to be aware of the symptoms of TSS, and should be instructed to remove tampons and seek medical attention at the first sign of such symptoms. Women who have not developed TSS but wish to reduce future risk should diminish tampon use to a minimum, and wear sanitary pads as an alternative. For those in whom total abstinence from tampon use is impractical, frequent changes and choice of the lowest absorbency compatible with their needs should be recommended.

The value of routine vaginal cultures and screening for serum antibody titers to TSST-1 in the general population is unclear at present. Certainly among women who have had a recent episode of menstrual TSS, surveillance culture of the vagina, nares, oropharynx, and perineum for recurrence of toxin-positive *S. aureus* could be obtained at regular intervals. Colonization by such strains should be eliminated by oral antibiotics until serum antibody titer to TSST-1 has clearly developed. The ability to detect TSST-1 production by *S. aureus* and serum antibody levels to TSST-1 is now readily available at a number of medical centers.

Since TSS is likely to be a continuing problem and probably occurs more frequently than is currently recognized, there is clearly the need for effective screening methods to identify the susceptible population and for effective vaccines or toxoids for the individuals at risk.

CHLAMYDIA TRACHOMATIS

method of
LEWIS H. HAMNER, III, M.D., and
JOHN H. GROSSMAN, III, M.D., PH.D.
George Washington University
Washington, DC

Genitourinary infections caused by the bacterial pathogen *Chlamydia trachomatis* are now recognized to be the most common sexually transmitted disease in the United States. It is estimated that 3 to 4 million or more cases occur annually, making chlamydial infections more common in the United States than the estimated number of new cases of gonorrhea, syphilis, and herpes simplex infection combined. The incidence of cervical colonization in the general population is 3 to 5 per cent. However, among certain high-risk patient populations, cervical carriage rates may approach 15 to 20 per cent.

Chlamydia trachomatis is the leading cause of pneumonia in infants less than 6 months of age and has replaced gonococcal infection as the leading cause of neonatal conjunctivitis. Neonatal chlamydial pneumonia is thought to affect 3 to 10 per 1000 live births. However, in populations with a high prevalence of cervical infection this may be as high as 50 to 60 per 1000 live births. In the United States, estimates suggest that in low-prevalence populations (3 to 5 per cent), 26,000 cases of pneumonia and 29,000 cases of conjunctivitis due to *Chlamydia* will occur each year. The number of infections attributed to *Chlamydia* in populations with a higher prevalence of disease will be even greater. The risk to the infant of an infected mother is 60 to 70 per cent for acquiring the disease, with 10 to 20 per cent risk of pneumonia and 25 to 55 per cent risk for conjunctivitis.

Microbiology

The genus *Chlamydia* contains two species, *C. psittaci* found in avian species and some lower mammals, and *C. trachomatis*. *C. trachomatis* is a bacterium; DNA and RNA are present, as is a cell wall. These bacteria lack the enzymes necessary for oxidative phosphorylation, however, and so they are obligate intracellular parasites for at least a portion of their life cycle. During the extracellular portion of their life cycle, infectious particles (called "elementary bodies") are extremely small, approximately 0.3 microns in diameter. These elementary bodies attach to columnar epithelium and gain entry to the cell through phagocytosis. During the intracellular portion of their life cycle, chlamydiae utilize the adenosine triphosphate (ATP) and amino acids of the cell to replicate via binary fission and produce new infectious particles that are released with cell lysis.

Fifteen serotypes of *C. trachomatis* have been identified. Serotypes A, B, Ba, and C are associated with blinding trachoma in adults, and serotypes L1, L2, and L3 are the causative agents in lymphogranuloma venereum (LGV). Serotypes D to K are most commonly found in genitourinary infections. The remainder of this article will deal specifically with these infectious organisms.

Epidemiology

Chlamydial infections are most prevalent in young, promiscuous, indigent patient populations. As would be expected from this profile of risk factors, they are more likely to occur among unmarried, inner-city women, especially those who are concomitantly infected with or who have a prior history of other sexually transmitted diseases. Women with positive endocervical cultures for gonorrhea, for example, have a 25 to 50 per cent incidence of simultaneous chlamydial infections.

Clinical Presentation

Many adult women with genital chlamydial infection are either asymptomatic or minimally symptomatic. Diagnostic testing in the former group may be prompted by discovery of another sexually transmitted disease. Mucopurulent cervicitis has been associated with a 50 per cent incidence of chlamydial infection. The diagnosis of mucopurulent cervicitis is established by visualization of yellowish mucopurulent endocervical secretions on a white swab and the presence of ten or more polymorphonuclear leukocytes per field in a Gram-stained smear of secretions at $1000\times$ magnification. Women with symptoms of urethral irritation and pyuria whose urine specimens show no evidence of infection by Gram stain or conventional bacteriologic culture are at high risk for chlamydial infection as well.

Chlamydial infection has been found to cause 5 to 10 per cent of cases of acute salpingitis in the United States. When compared with women who have gonococcal or mixed aerobic/anaerobic salpingitis, women with chlamydial salpingitis are often less clinically ill, with minimal or even no leukocytosis. Subsequent scarring of the fallopian tubes can lead to infertility and an increased risk for ectopic pregnancy.

The majority of cases of acute epididymitis in men under the age of 35 are caused by *Chlamydia*. Infertility has been described as a long-term complication, as a result of scarring and occlusion of the vas deferens.

Chlamydial infection is the leading cause of conjunctivitis and afebrile interstitial pneumonitis among infants less than 6 months of age. Recent experience suggests that prior or concomitant chlamydial infection may be associated with a significantly higher prevalence of neonatal otitis media and gastroenteritis in the same childhood population.

Follow-up examination of children 7 to 8 years after hospitalization for chlamydial pneumonia during infancy has shown long-term pulmonary changes. Obstructive pulmonary function studies and a significantly greater rate of physician-diagnosed asthma have been reported in these children.

Laboratory Diagnosis

The isolation of *Chlamydia trachomatis* using tissue culture from presumptively infected individuals remains the "gold standard" for definitive laboratory diagnosis. In addition to being somewhat expensive and cumbersome, the tissue culture methodologies that assure reliable recovery are relatively stringent and, consequently, few health care facilities are optimally equipped to perform cultural isolation on a large scale.

Diagnostic methods other than isolation in tissue culture are less sensitive and slightly less specific but are appropriate and may be preferable as cost-effective alternatives in certain patient populations. There are two major rapid direct antigen kits commercially available. One utilizes an ELISA (immunoperoxidase) and the other an immunofluorescent indicator system. The sensitivity of either method in testing endocervical specimens ranges from 70 to 90 per cent and the specificity ranges from 94 to 98 per cent. A recent study comparing the immunofluorescent method with tissue culture in a patient population with a 13 per cent prevalence of infection noted a predictive value of a positive (PVP) rapid test of only 65 per cent. Lower-prevalence populations would have even lower PVPs. Of more importance may be the potential 20 to 30 per cent incidence of false negative results of rapid direct tests of specimens from the cervices of asymptomatic individuals subjected to screening. Nevertheless, the cost and labor of tissue culture isolation makes it an impractical albeit scientifically desirable alternative. The rapid direct methods seem most useful for large-scale screening in high-risk, high-prevalence populations.

Papanicolaou smears are not acceptable substitutes for either screening or diagnosis, since their sensitivity ranges from 40 to 60 per cent among culture-positive individuals. Serologic testing is of little clinical value, since neither seropositives nor seronegatives reliably correlate with infection or absence of infection.

Perinatal Implications

The extent to which chlamydial infection adversely affects pregnancy and causes perinatal complications remains controversial. Several retrospective studies have demonstrated a significantly higher incidence of stillbirth, premature delivery, and neonatal death

TABLE 1. **Treatment of *Chlamydia trachomatis* Infection**

Tetracycline 500 mg orally four times a day for 7 days
or
Doxycycline 100 mg orally twice a day for 7 days
Pregnancy or patients unable to tolerate tetracycline derivatives
Erythromycin base 500 four times a day for 7 days
or
Erythromycin ethylsuccinate 400–800 mg four times a day for 7 days

among pregnant women with chlamydial infection compared with uninfected, matched controls. However, the most recent prospective information shows no statistical difference between cases and controls for premature rupture of the membranes, preterm delivery, amnionitis, intrapartum fever, delivery of infants that are small for gestational age, postpartum endometritis, and neonatal sepsis. In a subset of women with recent or invasive chlamydial infection, indicated by the presence of IgM antibody against *C. trachomatis*, preterm delivery and premature rupture of the membranes occurred in 19 per cent of patients, which was statistically higher than in controls. Further prospective studies are needed to determine whether there is an association between perinatal chlamydial infection and preterm labor or amniorrhexis.

At present, it seems reasonable to screen certain "high-risk" obstetric populations for chlamydial infection. Adolescents, women with "sterile" pyuria or mucopurulent cervicitis, women with other venereal diseases, and contacts of individuals with chlamydial infections should be included in such testing, either for diagnosis or for follow-up after treatment. Some studies have suggested that obstetric populations with a prevalence of infection greater than 12 per cent are groups in which such screening is likely to be cost effective.

Treatment

The treatment of choice for genitourinary chlamydial infections is tetracycline, 500 mg orally, four times daily for 7 days or doxycycline (Vibramycin), 100 mg orally, twice daily for 7 days (Table 1). Since treatment with tetracycline derivatives during pregnancy should be avoided, erythromycin is the obstetric treatment of choice. Erythromycin base, 500 mg, or erythromycin ethylsuccinate, 400 to 800 mg, four times daily for 1 week is the preferred treatment for pregnant women. A recent study has been associated with a cure rate in excess of 90 per cent when the ethylsuccinate regimen was employed in 400-mg dosages. Erythromycin in the ethylsuccinate form seems to be well tolerated, with better patient compliance and less nausea than erythromycin base. Since the neonatal infection rate among offspring of untreated infected women approaches 50 per cent, all women in whom chlamydial infection is diagnosed during gestation should receive treatment, follow-up with culture testing, and appropriate testing for other associated sexually transmitted disease.

In the patient hospitalized for parenteral treatment of pelvic inflammatory disease, therapy should include coverage for *Chlamydia*. Penicillin derivatives, cephalosporins, and aminoglycosides are generally not effective against *Chlamydia*. Although some of the broad-spectrum antibiotics such as ticarcillin, mezlocillin, and clindamycin have antichlamydial activity, resolution of clinical symptoms does not correlate with eradication of the chlamydial organism. Recent experience with fluorinated quinolones (e.g., ofloxacin) suggests that these agents may be an effective treatment alternative, although the safety of such agents in pregnancy has not yet been established. Current STD treatment guidelines suggest the use of cefoxitin (Mefoxin), 2 grams intravenously 4 times daily, plus doxycycline (Vibramycin), 100 mg intravenously twice daily for at least 4 days and at least 48 hours after the patient improves. Doxycycline 100 mg by mouth twice a day is then used to complete 10 to 14 days of total therapy.

PELVIC INFLAMMATORY DISEASE

method of
MICHEL E. RIVLIN, M.D.
University of Mississippi Medical Center
Jackson, Mississippi

Pelvic inflammatory disease (PID) is a broad term which includes a variety of upper genital tract infections, unrelated to pregnancy or surgery, such as salpingitis, salpingo-oophoritis, endometritis, peritonitis, and tubo-ovarian inflammatory masses. Usually the patient has had a lower genital tract infection, generally via sexual transmission, which ascends through intermediate stages of cervicitis and endometritis to the fallopian tubes. Recurrence of PID is common but must be differentiated from periodic lower abdominal pain without reinfection, which occurs in nearly 20 per cent of women after an initial episode. Primary infection is due to virulent organisms, such as *Neisseria gonorrhoeae* or *Chlamydia trachomatis* and probably *Mycoplasma hominis* and *Ureaplasma urealyticum*, introduced by sexual contact. Once the cervical barrier has been overcome, secondary colonization by virulent organisms that usually colonize the vagina occurs within a few days. These organisms create a polymicrobial infection including facultative gram-negative bacilli such as *Escherichia coli* and anaerobic bacteria such as *Bacteroides* species and, rarely, *Actinomyces israelii*. Once damaged, the genital tract often does not recover completely, and many women thereafter have recurrent infections with their own endogenous vaginal or rectal organisms. True chronic disease, for instance with tuberculosis, is very rare in the United States.

The important risk factors frequently overlap. These include young age, early coital debut and promiscuity, single status, low socioeconomic class, and nonwhite race. The intrauterine device (IUD) increases the relative risk two to nine times, whereas oral contraceptives and barrier methods appear to exert some protective effect. Bacterial vaginosis (nonspecific vaginitis) may predispose to PID, but this is still hypothetical.

Clinical Picture

Symptoms include abdominal pain and dyspareunia, fever, vaginal discharge and irregular bleeding, urinary and rectal symptoms, nausea, and vomiting. Signs include pyrexia, vaginal discharge, cervical excitation tenderness, and tenderness and adnexal masses evident on bimanual examination. Investigations include endocervical Gram stain for gonorrhea, complete blood count, urinalysis, serum pregnancy test, erythrocyte sedimentation rate test, serology, and culture for aerobes, anaerobes, *Chlamydia*, and *N. gonorrhoeae* from the cervix, urethra, and rectum. In selected cases, culdocentesis, ultrasound, or laparoscopy should be performed. All these investigations would be extremely expensive if done routinely, and clinical judgment must therefore be used. Differential diagnoses include acute appendicitis, endometriosis, ectopic pregnancy, mesenteric adenitis, and complications of ovarian cysts. *Chlamydial* infection is probably a more common cause of PID than gonorrhea, and while the older division of PID into gonococcal and nongonococcal variants is no longer emphasized, it is true that gonococcal infections tend to cause a more florid clinical picture, usually within a week of menstruation. By contrast, chlamydial infections are more insidious and as a result the sequelae of infection are greater in nongonococcal PID, probably because of delay in recognition and therapy. Anaerobic infections are clinically the most severe and are relatively more resistant to therapy. They usually occur in patients using an IUD or with a previous history of PID.

Diagnosis and Sequelae

The clinical diagnostic accuracy using classic criteria is low, with the diagnosis being incorrect in 17 to 63 per cent of cases. This is because all the hallmark signs and symptoms are very variable. Standardized criteria have been proposed to improve diagnostic accuracy, but have probably not entered general use as yet. Laparoscopy is thought to be the definitive technique for diagnosis, but routine use of the procedure is impractical in most circumstances. It should probably be reserved for situations in which more information is necessary, for example, if appendicitis or ectopic pregnancy is suspected or for pelvic pain of unknown origin.

The sequelae of PID include involuntary infertility from tubal occlusion, which is related to the number and severity of the infections. Twelve per cent, 35 per cent, and 75 per cent of women were found to be infertile after one, two, or three episodes of PID, respectively. Chronic abdominal pain, possibly related to adhesions, occurs in 20 per cent and recurrent infection in approximately 25 per cent of women who have had PID. Tubal damage from previous PID is the most common cause of ectopic pregnancy, increasing the risk six to ten fold. This risk is also increased with recurrent infections.

Treatment

Medical Management

Infertility is probably less frequent when PID therapy is started early. Uncomplicated cases

TABLE 1. Centers for Disease Control Recommendations for Outpatient Treatment of Pelvic Inflammatory Disease

Non—penicillin-allergic patients
  After 1 gram probenecid orally:
    Amoxicillin, 3 grams PO
    Ampicillin, 3.5 grams PO
    Aqueous procaine penicillin G, 4.8 mU IM
    Cefoxitin, 2 grams IM
  Ceftriaxone or equivalently effective cephalosporins
Penicillin-allergic patients
  Spectinomycin, 2 grams IM
  Tetracycline loading dose plus maintenance dose as indicated below
All patients also receive a 7-day course of:
  Tetracycline, 0.5 gram qid
  Doxycycline, 0.1 gram bid
  Erythromycin base, 0.5 gram qid
  Erythromycin stearate, 0.5 gram qid
  Erythromycin ethylsuccinate, 0.8 gram qid

(Grade I, limited to tubes and ovaries) are usually treated as outpatients although there is a move toward more liberal hospitalization criteria. Patients with cases complicated by inflammatory adnexal masses and/or pelvic peritonitis (Grade II) and patients with suspected ruptured abscess (Grade III) must be hospitalized. Other suggested criteria for inpatient management include temperature greater than 38° C; uncertain diagnosis; pregnancy; inability to follow or tolerate outpatient regimen or lack of response to outpatient management; inability to arrange follow-up within 48 to 72 hours; and disease in a prepubertal or adolescent patient.

As no single antibiotic is active against all possible pathogens, combination regimens directed against *N. gonorrhoeae*, including PPNG (penicillinase-producing *Neisseria gonorrhoeae*), and *C. trachomatis* are recommended by the Centers for Disease Control (CDC) (Table 1). Cefoxitin (Mefoxin), or an equally effective cephalosporin plus either doxycyline (Vibramycin) or tetracycline provides this activity. If nongonococcal polymicrobial infection is suspected, the patient can be treated with metronidazole (Flagyl), 500 mg orally four times daily and trimethoprim

TABLE 2. Centers for Disease Control Recommendations for Inpatient Treatment of Pelvic Inflammatory Disease

Regimen A
  Cefoxitin, 2.0 grams IV q 6 hr
  Doxycycline, 0.1 gram IV q 12 hr
  Doxycycline, 0.1 gram PO q 12 hr for 6 to 10 days
Regimen B
  Clindamycin, 0.6 gram IV q 6 hr
  Gentamicin
    2 mg/kg IV, loading dose
    1.5 mg/kg IV q 8 hr
  Clindamycin, 0.45 gram po q 6 hr for 6 to 10 days

plus sulfamethoxazole (Bactrim DS or Septra DS) twice daily. Bed rest, sexual abstinence, analgesics, referral of sexual partners, removal of IUD if present, and contraceptive counseling are further important aspects of management. If specific pathogens are cultured, the cultures should be repeated 7 days after therapy is completed.

The CDC recommends two regimens for inpatient PID therapy (Table 2). Intravenous therapy is recommended for at least 4 days and at least 48 hours after the patient improves. In practice, patients who require hospitalization but who do not have an adnexal mass are often treated with single-agent regimens with results equal to those of the CDC recommendations and with lower costs and side effects. Thereafter, outpatient therapy with an agent active against *Chlamydia* (doxycycline, erythromycin) is commonly prescribed. Many of the newer broad-spectrum cephalosporins have proven efficacious against PID; these include ceftizoxime, 1 gram every 8 hours. The expanded-spectrum penicillins (mezlocillin [Mezlin], piperacillin [Pipracil]) are effective in doses of 3 to 4 grams every 6 hours, but probably should be reserved for therapy of *Pseudomonas* infections. Good results are also reported with other agents, such as ticarcillin-clavulanic acid and imipenem (Primaxin).

Adnexal abscesses are generally treated with combination regimens including an aminoglycoside or aztreonam (Azactam), and an agent with specific antianaerobic activity (clindamycin, chloramphenicol, metronidazole). Patients with true abscess formation as distinct from inflammatory complexes require surgery for clinical cure in a significant number of cases.

Surgical Management

Indications for surgery include ruptured tubo-ovarian abscess, failure to respond to appropriate antibiotic therapy within 48 to 96 hours, a persistent pelvic mass, or persistent pelvic pain. Surgical cure may be expected with removal of the uterus and adnexa; however, this is a procedure usually reserved for older, parous women. Advances in tubal microsurgery and in vitro fertilization provide some hope of childbearing even in patients with badly damaged tubes, so that conservative surgery, such as unilateral adnexectomy, is recommended for younger patients who have not completed their families.

LEIOMYOMAS OF THE UTERUS

method of
DONALD C. CHAMBERS, M.D.
Howard University College of Medicine
Washington, D.C.

Leiomyomas of the uterus are solid benign tumors that are also known as fibroids, myomas, and fibro-myomas. They are the most common masses of uterine origin and are found in 30 per cent of white women and 50 per cent of black women over age 50. Grossly, they appear as ovoid masses of varying sizes formed from smooth muscle and connective tissue, in a whorl-like pattern surrounded by a pseudocapsule of compressed myometrium. Their presence in the uterus creates an enlarged, nodular, irregularly shaped mass in the pelvis. Leiomyomas may be found outside the uterus in the fallopian tubes, vagina, peritoneal cavity, and broad ligament. Their growth appears to be related to estrogen production, as they are rarely seen before puberty and regress after the menopause. Additionally, their size can increase dramatically in pregnancy and retrogress after delivery.

Diagnosis

Leiomyomas can be easily diagnosed on pelvic examination. The symptom complex generated by these pelvic masses is related to the size, number, and location of the masses. Submucous tumors are located in the endometrial cavity, causing hypermenorrhea and intermenstrual bleeding. This bleeding may be heavy and painful, and it may result in a significant degree of anemia. Intramural fibroids lead to a large nodular uterus with resultant pelvic pressure on bladder and large intestines. Subserosal leiomyomas also cause uterine enlargement, but may be solitary and pedunculated. Pelvic and intra-abdominal pain and pressure are the usual symptoms. Additionally, these can cause acute abdominal pain from degeneration and torsion. Solitary, pedunculated tumors must be distinguished from solid or cystic ovarian masses that could be malignant.

The clinical impression of leiomyomas of the uterus can be substantiated by the use of sonography and an intravenous pyelogram. Asymptomatic fibroids can cause significant distortion of the genitourinary system, leading to hydroureter and obstruction. Fibroids may undergo degenerative changes during pregnancy, leading to pain or obstruction of the descent of the fetus in labor. Intramural fibroids in pregnancy can lead to premature labor or abnormal fetal presentations such as transverse lie.

Degeneration of leiomyomas occurs when they outgrow their blood supply. If the process is acute, the pain will be severe and the patient will require hydration and sedation. Other degenerative changes include hyalinization, calcification, and sarcomatous proliferation. Although malignant degeneration is rare, it should be suspected when there is rapid change in the size of a previously small tumor or increasing size of a myomatous uterus in a postmenopausal patient.

Fibroids can also cause reproductive problems such as infertility from tubal obstruction and an increased incidence of spontaneous abortion and premature labor.

Treatment

The management of uterine leiomyomas can be conservative or surgical, depending on the symptoms, size, age, and reproductive plans of the patient. The small, asymptomatic mass (less than 5 cm) in the young patient can be observed and followed with biannual pelvic examinations. Baseline sonograms and intravenous pyelograms should be obtained on all patients with pelvic masses. Patients who desire continued reproductive capacity and are asymptomatic may also be observed regardless of uterine size. These patients should be counseled as to the risks of pregnancy.

Tumors with a conglomerate size of 12 weeks or more should be treated surgically because of the insidious changes to the surrounding organs and the relative inability to evaluate the ovaries on pelvic examination. Patients who have significant bleeding should have surgery after appropriate endometrial sampling to rule out other endometrial pathology. This pathologic bleeding is more often seen with submucous tumors even though the uterus may not be increased in size.

Hysterectomy is the procedure of choice, especially in patients over 40 years of age or in those whose reproductive careers have ended. In patients in whom infertility or poor pregnancy outcome has been attributed to myomas, myomectomy is the recommended procedure. Care should be taken to remove as many tumors as possible with minimal blood loss. Fifty per cent of patients undergoing myomectomy will need repeat surgery within 5 years for recurrence or for growth of new tumors.

The use of oral contraceptives and estrogens in the presence of uterine fibroids is to be approached with caution, and careful follow-up to assess tumor size is needed. Preliminary reports of the use of luteinizing hormone–releasing hormone (LH-RH) agonists as a nonsurgical method of decreasing the size of myomas have been encouraging. These medications decrease the level of circulating estrogens. The use of intra-abdominal laser has recently been advocated as a technique for myomectomy with a resultant decrease in the intraoperative and postoperative blood loss.

CANCER OF THE ENDOMETRIUM

method of
JAMES S. HOFFMAN, M.D.
*University of Connecticut Health Center
Farmington, Connecticut*

Cancer of the endometrium is the most frequent invasive malignancy of the gynecologic tract. The incidence in North America has steadily increased in the past 20 years. This appears to be a result of the aging of the population as well as the use of exogenous estrogen. Ninety-five per cent of cases occur after 40 years of age, and 80 per cent occur beyond the menopause. Women remain at significant risk through to advanced years, with a cumulative lifetime risk of 2 to 3 per cent. Certain factors identify women who are at greatly increased risk. These include obesity, low parity, history of irregular bleeding, hypertension, diabetes, hypothyroidism, and the use of unopposed estrogen. All of these factors are associated with high serum levels of estrogen. History of use of birth control pills protects against carcinoma of the endometrium. This is presumably due to the inclusion of progestational hormone.

Diagnosis

Vaginal bleeding is the cardinal symptom that raises the suspicion of endometrial cancer. Depending on the patient's age and circumstance, it may be described as intermenstrual, irregular, or postmenopausal. If the vagina appears normal on examination, it is acceptable to offer teenage girls a trial of birth control pills as therapy for irregular bleeding. All other patients require biopsy for diagnosis of unexplained bleeding once pregnancy and infection have been excluded. Diagnosis can usually be made by office biopsy, but examination under anesthesia and dilatation and curettage may also be employed. Only occasionally do these methods fail to explain the cause of the bleeding. If the symptoms persist and the cause remains undetermined, hysteroscopy or hysterectomy may be necessary.

Considerable study has been given to the pathologic prediction of cancer and precursor endometrial lesions from the biopsy specimen. High levels of serum estrogen may lead to endometrial hyperplasia. The lowest grade of hyperplasia is cystic hyperplasia. There is little architectural change in the glands and no cytologic atypia. This rarely progresses to cancer. Adenomatous hyperplasia is characterized by branched, complex, crowded glands. This is seen with varying degrees of nuclear atypia and loss of cellular polarity within glands. Patients with significant atypia are at increased risk of developing cancer. They need to be treated with hormonal therapy and repeat biopsy or with hysterectomy. The former is to be preferred if further childbearing is desired.

Cytologic features may help to distinguish invasive cancer from hyperplastic lesions. Overall, this is not as accurate as recognition of stromal invasion on the biopsy specimen. Stromal invasion is recognized by a fibroblastic reaction to the abnormal glands, a cribriform pattern of replacement of the stroma, or complex branching of the glandular material. There is only scanty experience with hormonal treatment of invasive cancer, and this should only be undertaken if fertility is desired and the malignancy is very well differentiated. Cancer should be suspected even in patients found to have atypical adenomatous hyperplasia, as cancer is found in up to 20 per cent of hysterectomy specimens from patients with atypical hyperplasia.

Evaluation

After histologic diagnosis of endometrial cancer, the patient requires evaluation to determine the stage of disease and to search for a synchronous second primary tumor. We routinely perform a thorough physical examination, sounding of the uterus and endocervical curettage, chest radiography, and mammography. Barium enema and sigmoidoscopy may be useful among older patients, but the most common sites for second primary tumors are the breasts and ovaries. All patients are assigned a stage according to the International Federation of Gynecology and Obstetrics (FIGO) (Table 1).

There are several histologic types of endometrial cancer. The most common are adenocarcinoma and adenocarcinoma with squamous change. The prognosis of these varies greatly with the differentiation of the glandular elements. Two less common forms of endometrial cancer are the clear-cell type and the papillary serous type. These lesions have a worsened prognosis even when well differentiated.

Treatment

The most effective and most generally employed treatment of endometrial cancer is total hysterectomy and bilateral salpingo-oophorectomy. Additional treatment has been given to patients with Stage I disease who are judged to be at increased risk of recurrence. Other factors that influence prognosis include grade, stage, depth of myometrial invasion, and presence of extrauterine disease.

Stage I

We have not found a role for preoperative radiation of Stage I cases. Careful abdominal exploration, aortic nodal dissection, and omental biopsy have been helpful additions to the hysterectomy and bilateral salpingo-oophorectomy for grade 2 and 3 cases. If the need for adjuvant

TABLE 1. **FIGO Classification of Endometrial Carcinoma**

Stage I	The carcinoma is confined to the corpus
Stage 1a	The length of the uterine cavity is 8 cm or less
Stage 1b	The length of the uterine cavity is more than 8 cm

Stage I cases should be subgrouped with regard to the histologic type of adenocarcinoma as follows:

Grade 1	Highly differentiated adenomatous carcinomas
Grade 2	Differentiated adenomatous carcinomas with partly solid areas
Grade 3	Predominantly solid or entirely undifferentiated carcinomas
Stage II	The carcinoma involves the corpus and cervix
Stage III	The carcinoma extends outside the corpus but not outside the true pelvis (it may involve the vaginal wall or the parametrium but not the bladder or the rectum)
Stage IV	The carcinoma involves the bladder or rectum or extends outside the pelvis

pelvic radiation has been determined by severe anaplasia or extensive invasion, then pelvic node dissection is not necessary. Otherwise, pelvic node dissection should be done as a screening tool for extrauterine spread. Five-year survival has been noted in 20 to 40 per cent of treated patients with nodal metastasis. Thus careful surgical exploration is important in improving cure rates without having to give external radiation to an inordinate number of patients. In addition to those patients with biopsy-proven extrauterine disease, we use adjuvant radiation therapy in patients with invasion to greater than 50 per cent of the myometrial depth. Recently, the CA-125 serum antigen has been found to be a marker for extrauterine disease.

Stage II

Endometrial cancers with extension to the cervix have also been noted to present increased risk of recurrence if treated with hysterectomy alone. It is sometimes difficult to identify cases with cervical extension, as cells from the endometrial cancer may break away from their site of origin and be presented as "floaters" in the endocervical curettage. Only cases with cervical stromal involvement can be considered as Stage II. (Magnetic resonance imaging has been reported to assist in distinguishing true cervical involvement.) If the patient's health and habitus permits, a radical hysterectomy may be utilized as therapy. We have also utilized preoperative cesium treatment with the Fletcher-Suit apparatus, followed by total hysterectomy and bilateral salpingo-oophorectomy with aortic node dissection, followed by external beam radiation.

Stages III and IV

In most Stage III cases, the only extrauterine site of involvement is the ovary. Patients with this type of disease have a favorable outlook and have been managed with adjuvant hormonal therapy, radiation therapy, or chemotherapy after primary surgery. Careful consideration should be given to the possibility of a coincident second primary tumor rather than metastasis of the endometrial cancer. Occasional cases are found with direct extension of endometrial cancer to other pelvic tissues. Radiation is the mainstay of therapy in these cases and is usually begun as external beam therapy to the whole pelvis for about 5000 rads. We have had occasion to employ radioisotopic therapy, hysterectomy, hormonal therapy, and chemotherapy as additional treatments in this setting. None of these treatments have been shown to be curative, but all may provide palliation. Metastasis may occur through a variety of mechanisms, including transceolomic spread to peritoneal surfaces, nodal involvement, and hematogenous spread principally to lung and liver. Progestational hormone therapy is effective in inducing a remission in fewer than 10 per cent of cases of metastatic endometrial cancer. This is probably explained by the predominance of poorly differentiated cases among metastatic cases. Hormone receptors are known to be infrequent in poorly differentiated cases. We have had some success with cisplatin (Platinol), doxorubicin (Adriamycin), and cyclophosphamide (Cytoxan) as therapy for metastatic and advanced recurrent cases. We have not noted any cures, and responses have generally been short-lived.

CANCER OF THE UTERINE CERVIX

method of
R. GERALD PRETORIUS, M.D.
San Diego, California

The mean age of women with invasive cancer of the cervix is 53 years, with a range of 20 to 75 years. Women at high risk for the development of cervical cancer are those with early age of first coitus, multiple sexual partners, or a history of herpes type II or condyloma virus infection, and women who smoke. Most women with cervical cancer present with abnormal vaginal bleeding, that is, postmenopausal bleeding, irregular menstrual periods, or postcoital bleeding. Vaginal discharge, abnormal Papanicolaou (Pap) smear, and asymptomatic cervical lesions are less common presentations. Most women with invasive cervical cancer have cervical lesions and diagnosis is obtained by biopsy. The diagnosis of cervical cancer can be excluded by the absence of a cervical lesion, a normal Pap smear, and a negative endocervical curettage. *A negative Pap smear does not exclude the diagnosis of cervical cancer, as 10 to 35 per cent of women with cancer of the cervix have negative Pap smears.* Some cervical cancers are located within the cervical canal and are not visible on speculum examination. Such endocervical cancers may be diagnosed by endocervical curettage. Women with abnormal Pap smears but without cervical lesions should receive colposcopic evaluation.

Many cervical cancers are preceded by precancerous lesions, which include cervical intraepithelial neoplasia (CIN), dysplasia, and carcinoma in situ (CIS). CIN I is equivalent to mild dysplasia, CIN II to moderate dysplasia, and CIN III to severe dysplasia and CIS. CIN, dysplasia, and CIS are precancerous. They are more common and occur in women who are 10 to 20 years younger than women with invasive cervical cancer. Women at high risk for CIN, dysplasia, and CIS are the same as those at risk for invasive cervical cancer. Three to 71 per cent of women with CIN, dysplasia, or CIS will develop invasive cancer of the cervix if untreated. Eradication of CIN, dysplasia, and CIS prevents the development of cervical cancer. Unlike women with invasive cervical cancer, most women with precancerous cervical lesions are asymptomatic. The majority of precancerous lesions come to the attention of physicians through routine screening with Pap smears. The need for annual screening with Pap smears has been questioned both by the American Cancer Society and the American College of Obstetricians and Gynecologists. Women with three consecutive negative Pap smears should have a routine Pap smear every 2 years. Women who have undergone hysterectomy with removal of the cervix should have Pap smears every 3 to 5 years. Women with a history of CIN, invasive cervical cancer, or cervical condyloma should have Pap smears performed every 3 to 6 months for 2 years and then annually.

The International Federation of Gynecology and Obstetrics (FIGO) has defined the stage of cervical cancer (Table 1). Staging of cervical cancer is clinical, that is, the stage is assigned prior to operative intervention. Evaluation of patients

TABLE 1. **FIGO Stage of Cervical Cancer**

Stage	0	Carcinoma in situ, intraepithelial carcinoma
Stage	I	Carcinoma confined to the cervix
	Ia1	Minimal microscopically evident stromal invasion
	Ia2	Stromal invasion less than 5 mm deep and less than 7 mm wide
	Ib	Limited to the cervix but not meeting requirements for Ia
Stage	II	The carcinoma extends beyond the cervix but has not extended onto the pelvic wall, or the cancer involves the vagina, but not the lower third
	IIa	No obvious parametrial involvement
	IIb	Obvious parametrial involvement
Stage	III	The carcinoma has extended onto the pelvic wall; on rectal examination there is no cancer-free space between the tumor and the pelvic wall, or the tumor involves the lower third of the vagina
	IIIa	No extension to the pelvic wall
	IIIb	Extension onto the pelvic wall and/or hydronephrosis or nonfunctioning kidney
Stage	IV	The carcinoma has extended beyond the true pelvis or has clinically involved the mucosa of the bladder or rectum
	IVa	Spread of growth to adjacent organs
	IVb	Spread to distant organs

with invasive cervical cancer includes history, physical examination, chest radiography, intravenous pyelography, and serum studies for creatinine, calcium, and hemoglobin. In patients with advanced disease, computed tomography, cystoscopy, sigmoidoscopy, or retroperitoneal lymphadenectomy may be indicated.

Stage 0 is composed of precancerous lesions, none of which invade or metastasize, and all of which are amenable to local ablation by excision (conization of the cervix), freezing (cryotherapy), burning (hot cautery), or vaporization (laser). Conization of the cervix with clear margins has the greatest chance of success (97 per cent), but has complications of increased infertility, cervical stenosis, and bleeding. Cautery, cryotherapy, and laser vaporization are less likely to eradicate precancerous lesions (around 90 per cent), but all are less morbid than is conization of the cervix. The danger in treating precancerous lesions of the cervix is that the diagnosis may have been missed with the result that invasive cancer is being treated with local ablation. Excluding invasive cancer in a woman with an abnormal Pap smear requires evaluation with colposcopically directed biopsies and a negative endocervical curettage. As none of the current treatments is completely effective, appropriate follow-up after treatment of precancerous lesions is important. Follow-up is individualized, but minimum requirements would be Pap smears at 3, 6, 12, 18, and 24 months. The presence of cervical stenosis may invalidate the results of Pap smears and indicate the need for endocervical curettage.

Stage Ia, or microinvasive cancer of the cervix, is invasive cancer in which the risk of spread of disease beyond the cervix is small enough to be ignored. Appropriate therapy for microinvasive cancer is conization of the cervix including clear margins, or hysterectomy. Though the concept of microinvasive cancer is clear, the definition is not. The risk of metastatic disease depends on tumor size, and may be dependent upon histologic variants such as vascular space invasion and the presence of small undifferentiated tumor cells. The definition for Stage Ia cancer adopted by FIGO uses two tumor dimensions; it is not easily applied, and it is not universally accepted. The definition for microinvasion adopted by the Society of Gynecologic Oncologists is invasive squamous cancer to a depth less than 3 mm without vascular space invasion. The diagnosis of microinvasive cancer requires a cone biopsy in which there is no invasive cancer at the margin. Review of histologic slides by specialists is strongly recommended prior to instituting therapy for microinvasive cancer of the cervix.

Stage Ib cervical cancers are limited to the cervix, but do not meet the requirements for microinvasion. Stage IIa cancers involve the cervix and the upper two thirds of the vagina, but do not involve the parametrium. Stage Ib and IIa cervical cancers may be treated by radical hysterectomy, partial vaginectomy, and lymphadenectomy with or without oophorectomy; by radiation therapy including both external pelvic and internal brachytherapy; or by a combination of radiation and surgery. There is controversy concerning which treatment should be used for Stage Ib and IIa cancers. Women less than 65 years of age with lesions less than 4 cm in diameter are often treated with radical surgery. Other indications for surgical extirpation are the presence of a pelvic or adnexal mass, a pelvic kidney, or a history of pelvic abscess. Women over 65 years of age or with lesions greater than 4 cm in diameter and those with significant medical illnesses are usually treated with radiation therapy. Combinations of hysterectomy and radiation are used when cancer expands the lower uterine segment, or when positive nodes are found at the time of radical surgery. Serious complications follow radical hysterectomy in 2 to 5 per cent of cases, approximately the same percentage as following radiation therapy. Survival following radiation and surgery are also equivalent; for Stage 1 the 5-year survival is 80 per cent.

In Stage IIb through IVa the cancer has involved the tissues adjacent to the cervix, but metastatic disease has not been documented. In this situation, radiation therapy is employed. External radiation to a pelvic field that encompasses all of the local disease plus the pelvic lymph nodes is administered first. This is followed by application of a hollow implant that surrounds the cervix and is afterloaded with cesium. The dose, fractionation, and timing of the implant vary with each patient. Serious complications of radiation therapy include vesicovaginal and rectovaginal fistulas, small or large bowel obstruction, and radiation cystitis and proctitis. The complication rate is dependent upon the dose and technique of radiation therapy, with higher rates when large field size and higher doses are used. Survival following radiation therapy is dependent upon the stage and the size of the tumor. Patients with small Stage IIb cancers have a 5-year survival of 75 per cent, while those with large Stage IIIb cancers have a 5-year survival of only 20 per cent.

Stage IVb cervical cancer involves metastatic disease, usually to the lungs. Metastatic cervical cancer responds to a number of chemotherapeutic agents, including cisplatin (Platinol), methotrexate, and bleomycin (Blenoxane). Response rates are between 20 and 50 per cent; long-term survival is unusual.

Cervical cancer recurrent after surgery is treated with radiation if the recurrence is within the pelvis, and with chemotherapy if the recurrence is distant. Recurrence after radiation therapy is treated with pelvic exenteration if disease is confined to the central pelvis. Recurrence following radiation therapy that is not amenable to exenteration may be reirradiated if sufficient time has lapsed since the original treatment. In patients in whom radiation therapy fails, response to chemotherapy is rare.

NEOPLASMS OF THE VULVA

method of
LARRY J. COPELAND, M.D.
The Ohio State University College of Medicine
Columbus, Ohio

Vulvar tumors are rare. Squamous carcinoma, the most common, comprises less than 5 per cent of neoplasms arising in the female genital tract. Although invasive squamous carcinoma is a disease most commonly seen in women older than 50 years of age, preinvasive lesions are detected in younger women, those under age 50.

For many years standard therapy for both preinvasive and invasive vulvar lesions consisted of various forms of aggressive surgery. Surgical complications such as wound breakdown, lymphedema of the lower extremities, and patient dissatisfaction with the cosmetic results have encouraged a more conservative trend in planning treatment for patients with vulvar neoplasia.

PREINVASIVE LESIONS

Vulvar Dystrophy

Various terminologies for dystrophic lesions of the vulva have contributed to confusion in our understanding of the types of vulvar dystrophy and their clinical significance. The current classification (Table 1) simplifies the terminology. Although approximately one third of patients with invasive squamous carcinoma of the vulva have an associated focus of dystrophy, the percentage of patients with a vulvar dystrophy who

TABLE 1. **Classification of Vulvar Dystrophy**

Hypertrophic dystrophy
without atypia
with atypia
Atrophic dystrophy (lichen sclerosus)
Mixed dystrophy
without atypia
with atypia

develop an invasive lesion is small, less than 5 per cent.

Since dystrophic lesions of the vulva develop after menopause, the lack of estrogen may play a role. Complaints of pruritus and chronic irritation are common. Undergarments and tight-fitting clothes contribute to the vulvar irritation, often leading to an itch-scratch-itch cycle. This chronic abrasive trauma may encourage malignant transformation.

In patients with extensive vulvar dystrophy, particularly of the hypertrophic type, identifying a focus of invasion can be clinically difficult. Areas of ulceration or friable tissue should be regarded as suspect and biopsies should be performed. A nuclear stain (1 per cent toluidine blue with a 1 per cent acetic acid wash) may help identify abnormal areas. A colposcopic evaluation of the vulva with 3 per cent acetic acid may also identify abnormal areas of white epithelium, but if the skin is inflamed or atrophic, or if there are areas of denuded epithelium, the acetic acid may cause unacceptable discomfort. However, since most dystrophic vulvar lesions are best managed by topical medication, the generous use of biopsy studies to rule out invasion is recommended.

Treatment

Hypertrophic dystrophy is treated with topical corticosteroids and estrogen therapy (topical or systemic). Although most patients will respond promptly and satisfactorily, symptoms persist in a few. In such situations an occult carcinoma must be considered, and repeat tissue sampling may be prudent. Performing a wide excision of the dystrophic area (sometimes requiring a complete vulvectomy) or ablating the superficial epidermis with laser vaporization may be appropriate in the rare symptomatic patient with hypertrophic dystrophy unresponsive to more conservative forms of therapy. Should biopsy studies reveal cellular atypia in addition to hypertrophic dystrophy, laser or surgical treatment is the method of choice.

Atrophic dystrophy is treated differently. If the lesion contains a significant inflammatory or pruritic element, treatment is best begun with a 2-week course of topical corticosteroids. Although this does not remedy the problem of a thin epithelium, it provides the patient with immediate relief of symptoms. Many topical steroid preparations are commercially available; however, I often use a combination of 0.25 per cent menthol, 0.25 per cent camphor, 0.25 per cent phenol, and 0.05 per cent betamethasone in an ointment base applied sparingly twice daily. This preparation causes some stinging on application, especially if any of the epithelium is denuded or split; however, this combination seems to relieve the inflammatory symptoms and breaks the pruritic cycle very effectively. When the inflammation has decreased, the patient should be treated with a topical testosterone preparation, 2 per cent testosterone propionate, twice daily. This treatment enhances restoration of the normal epithelial thickness. Side effects related to the topical testosterone therapy are rare. Topical estrogen therapy, however, does not usually reverse the atrophic dystrophy.

Vulvar Intraepithelial Squamous Neoplasia

Possibly related to the recent increase in human papilloma virus infections, squamous neoplasia of the vulva is becoming more common among younger women. Although it used to occur predominantly in older women, vulvar intraepithelial squamous neoplasia (VIN) is now common in patients in their 20s. Patients may be asymptomatic, but generally they complain of pruritus or vulvar irritation. Preinvasive lesions may be flat, white, pigmented, or reddened, or the epithelium may appear normal. The toluidine stain or a colposcopic assessment with acetic acid may help the physician to identify occult lesions. Small lesions (those with a diameter of less than 2 cm) can be excised using local anesthesia. Larger lesions should be evaluated by taking punch biopsy specimens of the most suspect areas. Condylomatous lesions, both condylomata acuminata and flat condyloma, may conceal neoplastic areas, and for this reason they should be generously sampled.

Vulvar intraepithelial squamous neoplasia can range from mild to severe dysplasia to carcinoma in situ (CIS). Lesions can be isolated or multifocal. The term Bowen's disease is often applied to multifocal CIS lesions, especially those in younger women. Adding further confusion to the terminology, a similar term, Bowenoid papulosis, has recently been applied to lesions that appear to be associated with the human papilloma virus.

Since intraepithelial squamous lesions of the genital tract frequently involve multiple areas, it is important to assess carefully the vaginal and cervical epithelium of all patients with vulvar lesions. Similarly, patients with CIS of the cervix frequently develop vulvar lesions, either concurrently or a number of years later.

Treatment

Multiple treatments are available for preinvasive squamous lesions of the vulva. Small focal areas are most simply treated by wide local excision. However, excising large or multifocal lesions can cause significant cosmetic and functional problems, although split-thickness skin grafting offers an acceptable method of reconstruction.

Laser vaporization is a popular treatment for patients with large or multifocal lesions. This treatment method produces excellent cosmetic results, and it is particularly advantageous for lesions of the clitoris or periclitoral skin, areas where surgical excision may alter clitoral sensation and compromise sexual enjoyment. However, when lesions are extensive, laser vaporization does have drawbacks, the most significant of which is discomfort during the healing phase. The depth of epithelial destruction is critical: if too superficial, treatment is ineffective, but if too deep, recovery is prolonged and discomfort is excessive. Because the healing interval after laser therapy is painful, most physicians tend to destroy relatively superficial tissue, using a braising technique, and to simply re-treat the focal, persistent abnormal areas. Regardless of the efficacy of the initial treatment, it is the nature of the disease for de novo lesions to develop subsequently.

Since laser vaporization, in contrast to excision (either by scalpel or laser), does not provide tissue for confirmation of diagnosis, it is important that the physician be confident the disease process is preinvasive. For this reason, it is prudent to obtain multiple biopsy specimens prior to vaporization. Likewise if a focal area demonstrates persistent disease after two laser treatments, the area should be excised for diagnostic purposes as well as for the therapeutic benefit.

Topical chemotherapy has also been advocated as a treatment of multifocal or large lesions. Five per cent 5-fluorouracil (Efudex) is applied twice daily until it causes an inflammatory response (described to the patient as a sunburn effect), usually in about 7 days. Over the next 4 to 6 days the skin reaction worsens and then culminates with an exfoliative end stage. The patient may be less than impressed with the symptoms associated with this inflammatory response, especially when she is told that two or three treatment courses may be necessary and that areas of persistent disease may require additional surgical treatment. However, warning the patient of the expected reaction before beginning treatment enhances the probability that she will complete the therapy.

Whatever treatment is chosen, it is important to emphasize the necessity of a reliable follow-up to detect persistent disease foci and to identify new lesions.

Paget's Disease

Extramammary Paget's disease of the vulva occurs most frequently in the sixth and seventh decades of life. During its early phase the patient is often asymptomatic; by the time symptoms—most frequently pruritus—are evident the lesion extends over much of the vulva. The typical appearance is that of a velvety red epithelium with interspersed white patches.

Treatment

As opposed to the multifocal nature of squamous lesions, Paget's disease is a continuum of one lesion. Although it is primarily intraepithelial, approximately 20 per cent of patients have an adenocarcinoma of the underlying apocrine glands. Therefore a "skinny" vulvectomy or laser vaporization is not advised because it will not remove an unrecognized apocrine gland carcinoma. The treatment of choice is a "simple" vulvectomy, one in which the superficial subcutaneous tissue (1 to 1.5 cm) is excised in addition to the skin. Since this lesion is notorious for extending onto the clinically normal skin, the surgical specimen should be clearly oriented for the pathologist, who should evaluate all the surgical margins.

When an underlying apocrine gland adenocarcinoma is identified, a bilateral inguinal lymphadenectomy is usually recommended. However, when nodal metastasis has occurred, the likelihood of curative therapy is very low. Therefore the lymphadenectomy is of prognostic, not of therapeutic, value.

Paget's disease of the vulva carries associated risks for a concurrent or subsequent adenocarcinoma of the colon and breast neoplasia. Therefore in addition to initial colon (air-contrast barium enema) and breast (mammogram) evaluations, a close surveillance program is recommended.

INVASIVE SQUAMOUS CELL CARCINOMA

Risk factors for squamous carcinoma of the vulva include age (over 60), squamous carcinoma (in situ or invasive) of other areas of the genital tract, vulvar dystrophy, and a history of chronic vulvar irritation. Symptoms include pruritus, pain, burning on urination, and a bloody discharge. Physical examination often reveals a nodule or raised ulceration; however, since benign

TABLE 2. Incidence of Regional Node Metastases by Depth of Tumor Invasion

Depth of Invasion (mm)	Per Cent of Positive Inguinal Nodes
<1	1–5
1–3	10–15
3–5	15–30
5–10	30–45
>10	≥40

TABLE 3. Incidence of Regional Node Metastases by Tumor Diameter

Tumor Diameter (cm)	Per Cent of Positive Inguinal Nodes
≤1	0–15
1–2	5–20
2–3	25–35
3–5	35–50
>5	≥50

conditions can simulate carcinoma, histologic confirmation is necessary.

This tumor may be relatively slow growing and spreads both by direct infiltration of adjacent tissue and through the lymphatics. The lymphatic spread is usually orderly—first to superficial inguinal lymph nodes, then to deep inguinal nodes (femoral lymph nodes), to pelvic nodes (external and common iliac nodes), and then to paraaortic, mediastinal, and supraclavicular nodes. The incidence of regional node metastasis varies with depth of invasion (Table 2), diameter of the lesion (Table 3), and FIGO (International Federation of Gynecology and Obstetrics) stage (Table 4).

Staging. Vulvar tumors are staged using both the tumor, node, metastasis (TNM) classification (Table 5) proposed by the International Union Against Cancer and the less cumbersome FIGO classification, which can be summarized in terms of the TNM system (Table 6). After examination of a biopsy specimen has confirmed the presence of invasion, a physical examination and chest radiogram provide staging information. For Stage I or II lesions, neither a pretreatment lymphangiogram nor an intravenous pyelogram is likely to alter the treatment plan.

Treatment

Therapy is influenced by the depth of invasion, the location of the lesion with respect to laterality, and the extent (stage) of the disease.

Stages I and II Lesions

Microinvasion and "Good-Prognostic" Lesions. Authors have used various criteria to describe microinvasive vulvar carcinoma. The risk of lymph

TABLE 4. Incidence of Regional Node Metastases by FIGO* Stage

FIGO Stage	Per Cent of Positive Inguinal Nodes
I	5–10
II	20–30
III	55–70
IV	40–100

*International Federation of Gynecology and Obstetrics.

TABLE 5. **TNM* Classification for Vulvar Carcinoma**

T Primary tumor
  TIS   Carcinoma in situ
  T1   Confined to vulva, diameter ≤2 cm
  T2   Confined to vulva, diameter >2 cm
  T3   Adjacent spread to urethra, vagina, perineum, or
        anus (any size)
  T4   Infiltration of upper urethral mucosa, bladder
        mucosa, or rectal mucosa, or fixed to bone

N Regional lymph nodes
  N0   Nodes not palpable
  N1   Nodes palpable but not clinically suspicious
  N2   Clinically suspicious nodes
  N3   Fixed or ulcerated nodes

M Distant metastases
  M0   No clinical metastases (disregarding inguinal
        lymph nodes)
  M1a   Palpable deep pelvic lymph nodes
  M1b   Other distant metastases

*TNM = tumor, node, metastasis.

node metastasis is significant if invasion is deeper than 1 mm; for lesions invading 1 to 5 mm, the incidence of nodal spread is estimated to be between 10 and 30 per cent. Although a wide local excision could be considered treatment for a tumor invading no more than 1 mm, the associated risk of lymph node metastasis is between 0 and 5 per cent. If the tumor invades more than 1 mm, the ipsilateral inguinal nodes are at significant risk and must be addressed in the treatment plan.

Recently, a trend toward conservative surgical management has resulted in the use of wide local excision and ipsilateral superficial inguinal lymphadenectomy (tissue superior to the cribriform fascia) for "favorable" lesions, those well lateralized, invading to a depth of less than 5 mm, and with a diameter less than 1 cm. If the ipsilateral superficial lymph nodes contain metastases, identified on either frozen sections or permanent sections, then the deep ipsilateral inguinal lymph nodes and the contralateral inguinal lymph nodes must be either surgically evaluated, treated with adjuvant radiation, or both. Midline lesions of the clitoris or perineum should be treated with a bilateral superficial lymphadenectomy, since there is a risk of occult bilateral spread.

High-Risk Lesions. Stage I and II lesions that invade more deeply than 5 mm are being treated by various methods. The time-honored therapy has been radical vulvectomy and bilateral inguinal lymphadenectomy, a surgical procedure with considerable morbidity. Wound healing of the vulva and groins can be prolonged, sexual function is severely affected, and lymphedema of the lower extremities can be problematic. For these reasons, there has been a trend toward combining radiotherapy with less radical sur-

gery. Unilateral lesions are treated with a wide local excision, ipsilateral inguinal lymphadenectomy (bilateral if the ipsilateral nodes are positive on frozen section or the lesion extends close to the midline), and postoperative radiation to the vulva and inguinal areas. The radiation field is extended to include the pelvic lymph nodes when lymphatic spread is evident. Although the long-term results from this combination therapy are not available, the short-term results are favorable. Disease control appears similar to that of radical sugery, and the morbidity is less severe. The radiation therapy, consisting of 45 to 50 Gy over 5 weeks, produces significant desquamation and skin excoriation, but once this acute reaction subsides, the cosmetic results and patient satisfaction are better than with radical surgery. Adjuvant local radiation in the form of a perineal boost or iridium needle implantation is indicated if there is uncertainty about the margins of the primary lesion.

Currently, pelvic lymphadenectomy probably has no role in the management of invasive vulvar tumors. If the inguinal nodes are free of metastases, spread to the pelvic nodes is rare. If the inguinal nodes have certain metastases, adjuvant radiotherapy offers an equal or better survival rate than that of patients who have undergone a pelvic lymphadenectomy.

Stage III and IV Lesions

Tumors that are classified as Stage III on the basis of the presence of clinically suspicious (N2) nodes are usually treated similarly to high-risk Stage I and II lesions—with either a radical vulvectomy and bilateral inguinal lymphadenec-

TABLE 6. **FIGO* Classification and Corresponding TNM Classification**

FIGO	TNM		
Stage 0	TIS		
Stage I	T1	N0	M0
	T1	N1	M0
Stage II	T2	N0	M0
	T2	N1	M0
Stage III	T3	N0	M0
	T3	N1	M0
	T3	N2	M0
	T1	N2	M0
	T2	N2	M0
Stage IV	T1	N3	M0
	T2	N3	M0
	T3	N3	M0
	T4	N0	M0
	T4	N1	M0
	T4	N2	M0
	T4	N3	M0
	All M1 lesions		

*International Federation of Gynecology and Obstetrics.

TABLE 7. **Survival Rate by FIGO* Stage for Patients with Invasive Squamous Cell Vulvar Carcinoma**

FIGO Stage	Per Cent Surviving 5 Years
I	70–90
II	50–80
III	30–50
IV	10–15

*International Federation of Gynecology and Obstetrics.

tomy or combination therapy (wide local excision, ipsilateral or bilateral inguinal lymphadenectomy, and adjuvant radiation). Tumors that are classified as Stage III or IV on the basis of extension beyond the boundaries of the vulva, involving the urethra, vagina, anus, or adjacent bony structures, have traditionally been treated with radical surgery such as the various forms of pelvic exenteration. However, the preferred therapy today is a combination of preoperative radiation to the vulva, inguinal areas, and pelvic nodes followed by excisional surgery and, in some circumstances, a regional lymphadenectomy.

Survival and Recurrences

Survival rate by stage is outlined in Table 7. When regional lymph nodes contain metastases, the survival rates are half those of patients without regional nodal disease.

Local recurrence of a squamous carcinoma in the vulva is potentially curable with excision and, if the patient has not had previous radiotherapy, adjuvant irradiation. Although recurrences involving regional lymph nodes are more difficult to treat, they also have been successfully managed with surgery and irradiation. When recurrent tumor cannot be excised, irradiation alone may provide local control.

Chemotherapy. Chemotherapy for either metastatic or recurrent squamous cell carcinoma of the vulva has had limited success. Although chemotherapy regimens containing cisplatin (Platinol) have induced responses, the responses are usually short.

TABLE 8. **Clark's Classification of Cutaneous Melanoma**

Clark's Level	Description of Depth of Invasion
I	Intraepithelial
II	Into papillary dermis
III	Filling dermal papillae
IV	Into reticular dermis
V	Into subcutaneous fat

UNCOMMON VULVAR NEOPLASMS

Malignant Melanoma

Malignant melanomas constitute 3 to 6 per cent of vulvar neoplasms. They are usually pigmented and raised, and may ulcerate. When amelanotic, they may be confused with poorly differentiated squamous carcinoma. The prognosis is related to the histologic type of the lesion, lesion size, and depth of invasion. Nodular melanomas carry a worse prognosis than the superficial spreading or lentigo variants. The Clark classification describes the depth of a melanoma as related to the microanatomy of the skin (Table 8). However, since the vulvar mucosa has no papillary dermis, the Clark classification has been replaced by direct measurement. When the lesion invades beyond a depth of 0.75 mm (similar to Clark's level III), the risk of lymphatic spread increases.

For lesions invading to a depth of 0.75 mm or less, the usual treatment is wide local excision. When invasion is deeper than 0.75 mm, a regional lymphadenectomy (ipsilateral inguinal lymphadenectomy for lateralized lesions and bilateral inguinal lymphadenectomy for lesions near the midline) is performed, although probably only a small number of patients derive a therapeutic benefit if metastases are present in the regional lymph nodes. Adjuvant therapy, in the form of either biologic modifiers or radiotherapy, has not been shown to be of therapeutic value; however, further clinical trials are in progress.

Bartholin's Gland Carcinoma

Various neoplasms, including squamous cell carcinoma, transitional carcinoma, adenocarcinoma, and adenoid cystic carcinoma, develop from Bartholin's gland and duct. These tumors frequently are misdiagnosed as Bartholin's gland abscesses, resulting in inappropriate therapy or delays in treatment.

The current therapy of choice is a wide local excision, often necessitating a hemivulvectomy, ipsilateral inguinal lymphadenectomy, and postoperative radiation. Because the gland is located deep in the labium majus, an extensive dissection into the ischiorectal fossa and partial resection of the rectum or vagina may be necessary to obtain clear surgical margins. With current therapy, the expected 5-year survival rate is approximately 80 per cent.

Basal Cell Carcinoma

This tumor exhibits local growth only and is best treated by wide local excision. The lesion should be carefully evaluated pathologically, since the presence of a squamous element changes the diagnosis to a basosquamous cell carcinoma. For this lesion, prognosis and therapy are the same as for a squamous cell carcinoma of the vulva.

Verrucous Carcinoma

This tumor is a variant of squamous cell carcinoma but lacks malignant histologic features and appears similar to condyloma acuminatum. Since verrucous carcinoma invades locally and does not metastasize, the recommended treatment is wide local excision with careful attention to obtaining tumor-free margins. This tumor is considered relatively resistant to radiation.

Vulvar Sarcomas

Sarcomatous lesions rarely occur in the vulva. There are multiple histologic types. The fibroid sarcoma (desmoid tumor) and leiomyosarcoma usually do not metastasize early; however, following wide local excision they are prone to recur locally. Epithelioid sarcomas tend to recur locally and are also prone to metastasize to the lungs. Alveolar rhabdomyosarcoma occurs in adolescents and may be confused with a benign Bartholin's gland problem. These tumors are characterized by early occult spread; therefore, the best hope for cure is an early diagnosis.

THROMBOPHLEBITIS IN OBSTETRICS AND GYNECOLOGY

method of
JAMES O. MENZOIAN, M.D.
Boston University
Boston, Massachusetts

The management of deep vein thrombosis (DVT) in pregnancy represents an especially difficult task because of the difficulty in making the diagnosis and the potential hazards of the various methods of therapy to both the mother and the fetus.

Incidence

The exact incidence of DVT in pregnancy is difficult to assess, and there is considerable variability in the literature relative to its frequency. This probably relates to the various modalities by which the diagnosis is made. Earlier reports probably overestimated the incidence of this disease because many of these evaluations were based solely on clinical impression. A swollen leg in a pregnant woman was assumed to be DVT. More recent studies have pointed out that making the diagnosis of DVT on clinical impression alone is extremely unreliable and is probably erroneous at least 50 per cent of the time. In addition, some of the more recent modalities for diagnosing this disease, although far more accurate than clinical impression, still suffer from lack of specificity and sensitivity to some degree.

The true incidence is probably low and may be in the range of 1 to 18 cases per 5000 deliveries. Although DVT is not very common, it represents a significant cause or contributing factor to maternal death.

Pathophysiology

In 1856, Virchow described a triad of hypercoagulability, endothelial injury, and stasis that he thought were significant in the development of DVT. All of these factors may exist during pregnancy. Stasis may be related to physical compression by the uterus on the iliac and pelvic veins. Thrombin-mediated fibrin generation has been shown to be increased in pregnancy, resulting in the possibility of hypercoagulability. These changes are especially evident in the third trimester. Endothelial damage can occur at the time of delivery. It is believed that thrombosis is initiated by an injury to the endothelium of the vessel, which could be either a mechanical injury at the macroscopic level or a biochemical abnormality at the ultrastructural level. This injury will result in platelet adhesion, the release of various platelet substances, and further clot propagation.

Diagnosis

Diagnostic modalities include noninvasive and invasive methods. There has been increasing enthusiasm for noninvasive methods because of advances in the technology in this area.

Clinical Evaluation. The classic clinical findings of DVT usually are warmth, tenderness, and a swollen, heavy extremity, often with a palpable cord representing a thrombosed vein. In addition, Homans's sign, in which calf pain is elicited by dorsiflexion of the foot, is often mentioned as a frequent finding. However, diagnosis of DVT based on clinical examination alone is extremely inaccurate, as revealed by a number of studies, and probably is helpful only 50 per cent of the time.

Doppler Ultrasonography. This is performed by placing a Doppler probe over the extremity at various levels and listening to alterations in venous flow related to respiratory excursion. DVT is characterized by absence of venous flow signals, loss of respiratory fluctuation in this signal, and a diminished signal in response to distal compression or a proximal Valsalva maneuver. This test is reasonably accurate but is extremely dependent upon the skill of the examiner.

Plethysmography. Both impedance plethysmography (IPG) and phleborrheography (PRG) can be used. IPG is based on the principle that temporary venous occlusion in an extremity by a cuff results in a marked increase in venous volume followed by rapid venous outflow when the obstruction is released. Blood is a good conductor of electricity, and thus measurement of electrical resistance or impedance to the passage of a weak current through the extremity provides a sensitive measurement reflective of changes in blood volume. A positive test would show obstruction to venous emptying by the clot once the cuff is released.

PRG is based on the principle of changes in venous volumes related to respiratory variations. Recording cuffs are placed around the thorax, thigh, upper calf, mid-calf, and ankle. A positive test is obtained if compression of an extremity distal to the recording cuff causes a rise in the baseline or if there is an absence or diminution of respiratory waves.

Both plethysmographic techniques are portable and accurate. However, these techniques cannot distinguish between active thrombosis, old thrombosis, and mechanical obstruction of veins unrelated to venous thrombosis. Compression of the vena cava or iliac veins by the gravid uterus could yield a false-positive result. Thus, plethysmography has some limited value during pregnancy. In addition, plethysmographic evaluations have been shown to be inaccurate in diagnosing calf DVT. Although some feel that calf DVT does not represent a clinical entity requiring treatment, our own studies have revealed that some patients with calf DVT can develop either clot propagation or a pulmonary embolism.

Invasive Techniques

Radioactive Fibrinogen. This test involves the injection of ^{125}I fibrinogen followed by scanning of the extremity. The test depends upon incorporation of the labeled fibrinogen into actively forming thrombus, which is then detected by measuring the increased radioactivity in the extremity. The test is extremely sensitive and many investigators wonder about its clinical significance, as it may overdiagnose DVT. In addition, unbound ^{125}I crosses the placenta and has been found in the fetal circulation and also in breast milk. For this reason, ^{125}I fibrinogen scanning is contraindicated during pregnancy and lactation.

Contrast Venography. This test involves the injection of radiopaque contrast material into the venous system. A positive venogram is one in which filling defects are seen in the veins of the deep venous system. In my opinion, this is the most accurate technique available for diagnosing DVT. With appropriate protection of the fetus, the entire lower extremity, including the external and common iliac veins, may be evaluated. This test can differentiate external compression from true intrinsic thrombosis.

The best approach to the diagnosis of DVT would be the use of noninvasive testing, if possible. A combination of the plethysmographic techniques and venous Doppler ultrasonography is most often used. If the plethysmographic or Doppler studies are negative, one can be reasonably certain that significant DVT does not exist. If a patient has a swollen, tender calf and normal noninvasive test results, we recommend contrast venography. If a patient has a positive noninvasive test, we also recommend contrast venography since the results of the noninvasive techniques may be abnormal owing to external compression of the venous system by the gravid uterus.

Treatment

Once the diagnosis of DVT is established, local and systemic therapeutic measures should be instituted. We suggest bed rest and elevation of the involved extremity to help reduce the swelling. In addition, local measures such as warm packs or Ace wraps may reduce symptoms. The optimal period of bed rest is unclear but should probably be approximately 3 to 5 days while anticoagulant therapy is being administered and the local thrombus becomes more adherent to the venous wall.

Anticoagulant Therapy

Anticoagulant therapy results in inhibiting the synthesis or enhancing the inactivation of clotting factors. Anticoagulants themselves do not cause lysis of established thrombi. Intrinsic fibrinolytic activity will lyse the clot with time.

Full-dose intravenous heparin therapy for established DVT should be initiated. A loading dose in a range of 5000 to 10,000 units of heparin followed by 1000 units per hour is recommended. Adjustment of the hourly dose should be based upon the monitoring of the activated partial thromboplastin time (APTT). This should be in the range of 1.5 to 2.5 times control to maintain heparin at a therapeutic level. I recommend heparin therapy by the intravenous route until delivery, if possible. Nonpregnant patients could be started on oral coumarin derivatives at approximately 5 days following heparin therapy. However, I *do not recommend* the use of these coumarin derivatives in pregnancy, because they pass through the placenta to the fetus and may cause fetal death. In addition, coumarin derivatives during the first trimester carry a teratogenic risk as well as a risk for neurologic defects in the second and third trimesters. However, heparin does not cross the placental barrier. Intravenous heparin and prolonged hospitalization can pose considerable expense and inconvenience to the patient, and the subcutaneous route of heparin administration in an outpatient setting has been shown to be effective. A loading dose of 5000 to 15,000 units every 8 to 12 hours has been shown to be effective. Again, the APTT should be checked at the mid-interval between subcutaneous heparin injections.

Potential complications related to heparin therapy by either route of administration include hemorrhage from the gastrointestinal tract, urinary system, retroperitoneum, and central nervous system. In addition, heparin-induced thrombocytopenia may occur in 30 per cent of treated patients. Platelet counts should be obtained before and during the course of heparin administration. Mild drops in platelet counts are well tolerated. However, if the platelet count falls significantly, heparin therapy must be discontinued. Another less frequent complication of heparin therapy is osteoporosis, which apparently reflects heparin inhibition of dehydroxylation of vitamin D in the kidney. A frequent clinical presentation of this is back pain.

Heparin therapy should be discontinued prior to delivery. The half-life of heparin is approximately 90 minutes. The APTT should be checked prior to delivery or proposed cesarean section and, if not normal, may be treated with protamine sulfate. One milligram of protamine will neutralize 100 units of heparin. Once the patient has been delivered, postpartum heparin is indicated. The exact duration of postpartum anticoagulant therapy is unclear. It is generally recommended that patients be treated for 6 to 12 weeks. Subcutaneous heparin seems to be best tolerated in the postpartum period. In addition, graded full length venous compression in the form of thigh-high support hose or waist-high hose is recommended.

At all subsequent pregnancies, the patient should be treated with heparin prophylaxis at a dose of 5000 units subcutaneously every 12 hours.

Fibrinolytic Therapy

While anticoagulant therapy is aimed at preventing extension of an already established thrombus and protecting against recurrence of DVT, the goal of fibrinolytic therapy is dissolution of the thrombus. The two currently available agents are streptokinase and urokinase. Fibrinolysis is activated by these agents by converting plasminogen to plasmin. Plasmin is the proteolytic enzyme that depolymerizes fibrin in intravascular clot. Streptokinase is derived from streptococcal bacterial cell cultures and urokinase is extracted from human urine or fetal kidney cell cultures. Allergic side effects of streptokinase are due to its bacterial source. Urokinase is nonantigenic.

The use of thrombolytic agents in pregnancy is *contraindicated*. Although streptokinase and urokinase have not been found to pass the placental barrier, the fibrinopeptides that are formed as a result of the breakdown of fibrinogen and fibrin have been shown to pass the placenta. These fibrinopeptides may cause bleeding. In addition, children born of mothers treated with streptokinase prior to delivery were found to have elevated levels of antistreptococcal antibodies. For these reasons, pregnancy is considered a contraindication to thrombolytic therapy, and until more data are available these agents should be withheld.

Aspirin Therapy

There is no evidence that aspirin therapy is effective for venous clotting during pregnancy. In addition, although aspirin therapy was found to reduce the incidence of thromboembolic disease in men undergoing hip replacement, no beneficial effect was found in women. There is no role for aspirin in DVT of pregnancy.

Prophylactic Therapy

Prophylactic anticoagulant therapy is indicated in pregnant patients who have had a history of DVT during previous pregnancies or in those patients who have had DVT in the recent past. The recommended therapy is heparin, 5000 units subcutaneously every 12 hours. There is evidence that the heparin dose needs to be increased as the pregnancy continues. It is recommended that the dose be increased to 7500 units every 12 hours at about 13 weeks' gestation and then 10,000 units every 12 hours after 30 weeks' gestation. The APTT is usually not prolonged with this form of therapy.

Complications of low-dose heparin are the same as those for full heparin therapy. There is no evidence that heparin treatment will result in an overall increase in preterm delivery, placental abruption (abruptio placentae), or increased blood loss at delivery.

There is no role for aspirin therapy for prophylaxis against DVT during pregnancy.

Venous Thrombectomy

Patients with extensive iliofemoral DVT may develop phlegmasia alba dolens (this has often been called milk leg). At this stage, arterial flow is normal and the clinical picture is one of an acutely edematous leg. This may progress to phlegmasia cerulea dolens, at which point arterial flow is impeded by the tightness of the swollen leg from extensive venous thrombosis. This condition may progress to venous gangrene of the extremity. The usual treatment is elevation and anticoagulant therapy. In rare instances, this medical management may not be sufficient and venous thrombectomy is indicated. Following venous thrombectomy, anticoagulant therapy should be continued.

Complications of DVT

Postphlebitic Syndrome. Patients who develop deep vein thrombosis have been shown to have a higher incidence of leg swelling, pigment changes in the medial aspect of the lower leg, and ulceration. This is related to the damage of the venous valves that results in pooling of the blood in the lower extremity and can often be confused with active deep vein thrombosis. A venogram may reveal that there is no active clot present but might show absence of some veins that have become totally obliterated or could show pooling of contrast material in veins that emptied poorly.

The treatment for this condition is long-term venous compression in the form of properly fitting graded elastic stockings. If this therapy is unsuccessful and if venous ulcers recur, ligation of incompetent perforating veins in the lower extremity should be considered.

Recurrent DVT. It has frequently been shown that the incidence of recurrent DVT in patients who have had DVT in the past is higher than the incidence of new cases of DVT in patients with no past history of the disorder. For this reason, patients with a history of DVT should be treated with heparin prophylaxis during pregnancy.

Pulmonary Emboli. Propagation and embolization of thrombus from the extremities to the lung results in a pulmonary embolism (PE). The exact incidence of this is unclear but it can occur even in the presence of adequate anticoagulant therapy for DVT. The usual clinical presentation is shortness of breath, hypoxemia, chest pain, tachypnea, and tachycardia. Just as in the diagnosis of DVT, these clinical findings do not firmly establish the diagnosis, and a 50 per cent error is also made by relying only on the signs and symptoms.

DIAGNOSIS. Chest x-ray film, electrocardiogram, and arterial blood gas determination may be helpful but are not in themselves diagnostic. Lung scanning techniques are helpful but, again, have unacceptable sensitivity and specificity. If a lung scan is normal, no further evaluation need be done because many studies have shown that these patients, when studied by angiography, do not have PE. Pulmonary arteriography is the most accurate method of diagnosing PE. We have found an unacceptable sensitivity and specificity in the diagnosis of PE when relying on ventilation/perfusion scanning techniques alone. In view of the low incidence of complications associated with pulmonary angiography, we recommend its use in patients suspected of having PE, particularly when weighed against the risks of anticoagulant therapy on the one hand and the risks of not treating pulmonary emboli on the other. Lung scanning techniques may be useful in alerting the angiographer to suspicious areas and possibly in reducing the duration of angiography and the contrast load administered.

TREATMENT. The treatment for PE is the same as that for DVT. A loading dose of heparin followed by continuous infusion of intravenous heparin should be initiated. The APTT should be maintained between 1.5 and 2.5 times normal. The heparin therapy should be continued for the duration of the pregnancy by either the intravenous or the subcutaneous route as previously outlined and then continued for 6 to 12 weeks post partum. As with DVT, patients who develop a PE during one pregnancy should be treated with heparin prophylaxis during subsequent pregnancies.

INFERIOR VENA CAVAL INTERRUPTION. In those patients in whom there is a contraindication to or a complication of anticoagulant therapy, vena caval interruption should be considered. Previous direct approaches to the inferior vena cava involved a transabdominal laparotomy or retroperitoneal approach to the inferior vena cava with the application of a clip. Recently, transvenous filters have been shown to provide a safe and much simpler alternative method of caval interruption. If caval interruption is indicated, we would recommend the placement of a Kimray-Greenfield filter.

CONTRACEPTION

method of
MARIAN BLOCK, M.D.
University of Pittsburgh School of Medicine
Pittsburgh, Pennsylvania

The risk of any contraceptive method must be understood in the context of the risk of pregnancy and childbirth; in general, with the exception of oral contraceptive use by women over age 40 or with certain risk factors, the morbidity and mortality of childbearing far outweigh that of any contraceptive method. In addition to those methods reviewed below, sterilization and fertility awareness are reasonable choices for certain patients.

Effectiveness rates vary widely among studies, particularly for barrier methods; published data should, therefore, be interpreted with caution, and reliable patients who have used a method successfully for years should not be switched to some theoretically more effective method. The riskiest time for unwanted pregnancy is when a method is initiated or changed. It is frequently helpful to combine methods for added effectiveness; a common example is the simultaneous use of foam and condoms. All patients should be instructed in a backup method of contraception, such as a barrier method, for use when the patient experiences a problem with her usual method, such as forgotten pills or expulsion of an IUD. All patients should be counseled on the utility of condoms in preventing sexually transmitted diseases, regardless of the method they ultimately choose.

Barrier Methods

Vaginal Spermicides and Condoms. These non-prescription methods include condoms, vaginal spermicides (foam, jellies, suppositories, and creams containing nonoxynol 9 or octoxyinal 9 as the spermicide), the newer sponge, or some combination of these methods (e.g., the frequently recommended use of foam and condoms). The only contraindication to the use of these methods is allergic sensitivity of either partner to the active ingredient or to the vehicle of the spermicide, in which case another spermicide can be tried. Patients should be educated as to their correct use. Repeated episodes of intercourse require repeated applications of the spermicide.

The sponge is more costly and has a higher incidence of irritation associated with its use. It is best for those couples who engage in multiple episodes of intercourse within a 24-hour period, as it is effective for that period of time even if intercourse is repeated because it contains a very much larger dose of spermicide and also acts as a mechanical barrier. The sponge is more effective for nulliparous than for parous users; it is contraindicated in women who have a history of toxic shock syndrome.

Diaphragm. Although the diaphragm has highly variable effectiveness rates in different studies depending on age, parity, and user reliability, it is an excellent method of contraception for the woman who is motivated and who can achieve a good fit. Users should be counseled that its effectiveness is related to the proper placement of adequate amounts of spermicide; used alone as a barrier, its effectiveness is poor.

To fit the diaphragm, the patient is placed in the usual position as for a pelvic examination; a mirror held by the patient greatly aids teaching, as the patient must be familiar and comfortable with her anatomy in order to use the method successfully. A series of sample diaphragms (sterilized after each patient) of each marketed size is then inserted by the clinician until a comfortable fit is achieved. Fit is determined by the ability of the diaphragm to cover the cervix and at the same time fit snugly but comfortably (that is, the patient has no sense of bladder pressure anteriorly or pain posteriorly) between the pubic bone and the posterior fornix. The patient then practices insertion and removal in the office. Most women find the arcing spring type effective and comfortable; the flat spring rim is better suited to the nulliparous woman with very firm vaginal muscle tone or with a shallow notch behind the pubic bone, and the coil spring rim for those who want a more gentle spring feel or who wish to use an introducer. A starter kit with instructions and samples of cream and gel allows the patient to experiment with different preparations. Gels are more lubricating, a plus for some patients, but too slippery for others who will experience difficulty with insertion.

Some women will require a larger size as their muscles relax with familiarity of use. Therefore, the patient is instructed to practice insertion daily regardless of intercourse for 1 month (during which time she continues to use additional contraception), then return with the diaphragm in place for a recheck of the fit. Some women cannot achieve a comfortable safe fit, particularly those with extensive vaginal relaxation following childbirth or those with a narrow arch behind the pubic ramus. The method is contraindicated in the woman who has a history of toxic shock syndrome, repeated urinary tract infections, uterine prolapse or extreme retroversion, a history of vaginal delivery within the past 3 months, and allergy to the latex or spermicide. It is not a good method for the woman who is sexually active for the first time unless an additional method is used until the patient is comfortable with using the diaphragm.

The Intrauterine Device

Currently the only intrauterine devices (IUD) marketed in the United States are the Progestasert (containing progesterone), which must be changed annually, and the copper-containing T380A (marketed as ParaGard), effective for 4 years but causing more bleeding and pain. The copper-containing Cu-7 and Tatum-T, no longer marketed, are not effective after 3 years. Because of the risk of pelvic inflammatory disease, the IUD is not a good choice for the woman who desires future fertility or who has a history of or is at risk for pelvic inflammatory disease because of multiple sexual partners. It is also contraindicated in the woman at risk for subacute bacterial endocarditis, in pregnancy or suspicion of pregnancy, and in active pelvic infection. It must be removed in those patients who experience recurrent infections (endometritis, salpingitis), menorrhagia or abnormal bleeding patterns, pelvic pain, perforation, partial expulsion, or uterine or cervical malignancy or who become pregnant with the IUD in place. If pregnancy occurs it is more likely to be ectopic. The asymptomatic woman with a Lippes Loop or Saf-T-Coil (which are no longer marketed) can keep her IUD with annual surveillance until menopause. Annual surveillance includes a gynecologic history and examination, with a check of IUD position by noting length of string, and a Pap smear with a check for *Actinomyces* infection. Any woman with a Dalkon Shield (which may be identified by history or by its thick knotted black string protruding from the os) should have it removed promptly.

Oral Contraceptives

The newer low-dose (containing a progestin and 30 or 35 micrograms of estrogen) combination oral contraceptive pills offer an excellent profile of safety and efficacy, particularly for young, nonsmoking women. These pills all contain ethinyl estradiol as the estrogen and varying amounts of four progestins—norethindrone, norethindrone acetate, ethynodiol diacetate, and norgestrel. The cardiovascular risk of these compounds is dose-related to both the estrogen (with its adverse effect on blood coagulation) and to the progestin (with its adverse effect on blood lipids and possibly blood pressure). Higher rates of thromboembolic disease, myocardial infarction, and stroke have been demonstrated in users, particularly in older women who smoke. On the other hand, certain noncontraceptive health benefits accrue to users, including decrease in menstrual flow and premenstrual symptoms, decrease in functional ovarian cysts and benign breast disease, decrease in incidence and severity of pelvic inflammatory disease, and decrease in incidence of endometrial and ovarian carcinoma. No change in the incidence of breast carcinoma is associated with use of these contraceptive compounds.

The physician's assessment should identify those women for whom the risk of taking the pill outweighs its benefit in preventing pregnancy. Such an assessment includes past and current medical history, family history, a physical examination with particular attention to the breast and pelvic structures, and appropriate laboratory studies to rule out contraindications. A woman's age, general health, and smoking status are the most critical factors. Absolute contraindications include thromboembolic disease, previous cerebrovascular accident, coronary artery disease, hyperlipidemia, impaired liver function and/or history of obstructive jaundice in pregnancy, pregnancy, known or suspected breast cancer or other estrogen-dependent neoplasia, hepatic adenoma, and undiagnosed abnormal vaginal bleeding.

Strong relative contraindications function as additive risk factors and a challenge to the patient's physiologic reserve. These include delivery of term pregnancy within 14 days, severe vascular or migraine headaches, hypertension with resting diastolic pressure greater than 95, diabetes mellitus or history of gestational diabetes, gallbladder disease, age greater than 40, major injury to lower limb, long leg cast (risk of phlebitis), lactation, hemoglobin SS or SC disease, uterine myoma (which may grow with use of contraceptive hormones), and age greater than 35 in a smoker.

Less strong relative contraindications are those for which the clinician will want to inform the patient about the available evidence; one may start an oral contraceptive regimen but monitor carefully for adverse effects. These contraindications include strong family history of early cerebrovascular or coronary artery disease; cardiac or renal disease, especially congestive heart failure or renal failure; unreliable patient; obesity associated with a strong family history of diabetes mellitus; clinically significant depression (which contraceptive use may make better or worse or neither); prior pregnancy on oral contraceptives (use of a higher-dose pill should be considered); recurrent vomiting or diarrhea that may interfere with absorption of the pill; resting diastolic blood pressure 90 to 95 mmHg; age greater than 35 years; chloasma; varicose veins; recent hepatitis (including infectious mononucleosis) with normal liver function tests; duration of pill use greater than 5 years in a smoker over age 30 years; elective surgery in the next 4 weeks; and use of medications such as phenytoin or rifampin that accelerate the metabolism of oral contraceptives.

The initial choice of a pill for a particular patient is arbitrary; one approach is to select a pill with an excellent profile of safety and efficacy containing 35 micrograms of ethinyl estradiol and the lowest dose of progestin as 0.4 mg of norethindrone (Ovcon-35). No benefit of the triphasic and biphasic pills has yet been demonstrated, a 20-microgram estrogen pill has a higher failure rate, and the "minipill" containing only a progestin has an unacceptably high rate of pregnancy and breakthrough bleeding. All women should read the package insert and/or have it explained to them. Some women experience breast tenderness, nausea, and unexpected bleeding in the first months, but these effects usually disappear with continued use. For those patients who continue to have breakthrough bleeding or who fail to have withdrawal periods, it is reasonable to try different pills by varying the amount and/or the type of progestin in the pill. If this does not work one may increase the dose of estrogen to 50 micrograms, counseling the patient that there is a greater (although still small) risk of cardiovascular side effects at this dose. For refractory cases of breakthrough bleeding, some clinicians recommend a natural estrogen (such as Premarin) in a dose of 1.25 to 2.5 mg per day for 7 days when the bleeding starts;

often one cycle of therapy corrects the problem and allows the patient to continue the same low-dose pill.

Surveillance consists of seeing the patient 2 to 3 months after the initial prescription to review any problems or side effects and to check the blood pressure, and then every 6 months to monitor blood pressure and symptoms, and yearly for history and physical examination with particular attention to blood pressure, abdomen, breasts, pelvis, Pap smear, and urinalysis to detect glycosuria. The pill should be stopped in any woman who develops hypertension. Patients should be evaluated for serious complications due to the pill if they develop severe vascular-type headaches; pain in the legs, chest, or abdomen; or visual symptoms. To permit accurate dating of pregnancy, the pill should be stopped in anticipation of pregnancy to permit at least one spontaneous cycle to occur.

Psychiatric Disorders

ALCOHOL-RELATED PROBLEMS

method of
LOU GOLDMAN, M.B., B.S.
Sydney, Australia

The term alcoholism as a disease entity has in recent years been replaced by the term alcohol-related disorders. This term prevents the degrading use of alcoholic or alcoholism to describe an unfortunate sufferer of this disorder.

Alcohol-Related Problems

Such problems may be physical, affecting any one of the body's systems. In addition, they may be psychologic or social.

Alcohol-related problems affecting the patient in a physical sense may involve the gastrointestinal tract with gastritis, reflux esophagitis, or pancreatitis. The effect may be on the central nervous system with Wernicke-Korsakoff's syndrome; on the peripheral nerves, producing peripheral neuropathy; or on the cardiovascular system, with production of cardiomyopathy or hypertension. Endocrine and metabolic disorders may occur, leading to impotence, gout, and lactic acidosis.

Trauma is a common related problem, particularly with fractures and head injuries. The fetus may be affected in pregnancy, with the development of fetal alcohol syndrome, and second trimester abortion is commonly associated with an alcohol-related problem.

Common alcohol-related psychologic problems are anxiety and depression and confusion and paranoia. Social problems related to alcohol use may occur in family systems, with divorce and separation and marital deterioration or occur in the workplace, with dismissal or failure to gain promotion.

Legal problems commonly associated with alcohol use are drunk driving offenses and in some cases assault, homicide, and child abuse.

The Alcohol Dependent Syndrome

The major elements of the alcohol dependent syndrome are the following:
1. A narrowing of the pattern of drinking.
2. The importance of drinking over all other activities preferred by the patient.
3. An awareness of a loss of control to drinking.
4. An increased tolerance to alcohol. This often presents with increased speed of drinking or an ability to drink large amounts of alcohol without intoxication.
5. Repeated symptoms of withdrawal (e.g., tremor and nausea).
6. Relief of withdrawal symptoms by the use of alcohol.
7. The recurrence of drinking problems after abstinence.

The Diagnostic Dilemma

Epidemiologic studies in many countries indicate a high incidence of alcohol-related disorders in communities throughout the world. In Australia, recent studies indicate that 9.5 per cent of men and 5.8 per cent of women can be identified as in medium to very high risk groups related to alcohol consumption and as dependent upon the frequency and amount consumed.

Despite the size of these risk groups, morbidity studies both in hospital and community practice reveal that a much lower number of cases are recognized by physicians in their practice. Probable causes of the discrepancy between expected community studies and the diagnosed and reported cases may relate to the following:
1. The difficulty in recognition of alcohol-related disorders.
2. Physician ignorance of diagnostic indicators.
3. The attitude of physicians to this disorder and in some cases the presence of personal or family problems with alcohol and drug abuse.

Diagnosis of Alcohol-Related Problems

The first step in diagnosis is the development of a high index of suspicion. The disorder has been likened to syphilis in previous decades because of its protean and varied modes of presentation.

The major part of the diagnostic process is the use of a systematic drinking history-taking technique. This technique is required to be both quantitative and qualitative. The physician needs to establish both the drinking pattern and the average daily consumption of alcohol and to translate this with a knowledge of the ethanol content of common alcoholic drinks. This will lead to an accurate measure of the daily consumption of alcohol.

Further information can be revealed by recognizing symptoms that indicate alcohol-related disorders and the alcohol dependent syndrome. In particular the physician needs to recognize the following hallmarks of dangerous drinking behavior.

Alcohol Intake. Regular drinking of more than 60

grams of alcohol per day for males and 40 grams per day for females. Episodes of intoxication occurring more frequently than twice a month should be suspect.

A dangerous drinking behavior would include the gulping of first drinks of alcohol and the difficulty to stop drinking once started. One would find that most leisure activities are involved in drinking and that most of the friends of the patient are heavy drinkers.

In most cases those with dangerous drinking behavior will eat lightly or skip meals, and their previous attempts to cut down on their drinking will have had limited success. Physical examination may reveal scarring and bruising due to injury and some coating of the tongue. Conjunctival injection and facial telangiectasia may be obvious. In many cases the demeanor of the patient is of an anxious and agitated state. Tachycardia and hypertension are common, and a soft and often tender hepatomegaly may be found on abdominal examination.

The routine use of simple screening investigations is helpful in diagnosis, especially the mean corpuscular volume, blood alcohol levels, and serum glutamic-pyruvic transaminase (SGPT) and other liver function tests.

Role of the Family in Alcohol-Related Problems

It is axiomatic that families play a large part in the etiology of alcohol-related problems. In addition, a patient with such a disorder will affect most of that family group directly or indirectly. In many instances the presentation is made by the spouse, the sibling, or a child in an "indirect" fashion. The challenge to the physician is to motivate the "patient" to accept treatment. Within the family, some indicators that may lead to the suspicion of problem drinking include the following:

1. Inability to take appropriate responsibility within the family.
2. A lack of self-discipline.
3. Overdependence on others.
4. Preoccupation with oneself.
5. A sense of inadequacy.
6. Limited outside interests.
7. Superficial relationships with others in the family group.

Treatment

Early Intervention

Once a problem drinker has been recognized, what can the physician do to help? Recent reports of a multicentric study by the World Health Organization in 11 countries indicate that early intervention is effective.

The methods used are a brief counseling session with some patient education and education material being given to the patient following the consultation. This information describes the effects and consequences of dangerous levels of consumption of alcohol.

Abstinence and Controlled Drinking

For the past few decades a controversy has raged related to the feasible goal for the management of problem drinkers. Abstinence as the only goal has previously been regarded as the most acceptable. This is certainly the goal of those who follow the concepts and ideas of Alcoholics Anonymous.

In the past decade and a half the concept of controlled drinking as an acceptable goal has gained favor, particularly among those with a behavioral orientation. Controlled drinking attempts to limit consumption to no more than three drinks per day with at least two alcohol-free days per week.

The use of either goal appears most likely to be related to the presence or absence of the alcohol dependent syndrome. Long-term studies of patients with alcohol dependence have confirmed that only a small number of those who are dependent can resume social or controlled drinking.

Most physicians now involved in the therapy of problem drinkers will, however, advise an initial period of abstinence for the first 3 months or so. Following this period, provided there has been no relapse or sign of the alcohol dependent syndrome, controlled drinking may be commenced.

Continuing Care of the Problem Drinker

There seems no doubt that the most important part of the management of the problem drinker is to follow up and have frequent contact with the patient. This will assist in the continuance of a safe drinking behavior.

In the early stages there may be need for weekly visits, but gradually the visits may be reduced and they should be continued over a period of 12 to 18 months.

The nature of this disorder is that relapse may occur. This should not be regarded as a failure by the patient and/or the physician. Continued support and counseling should be reintroduced if relapse should occur.

NARCOTIC POISONING

method of
ELIZABETH T. KHURI, M.D.
Cornell Medical Center
New York, New York

Few conditions in medicine are as dramatic and respond so swiftly to appropriate treatment as narcotic poisoning. These cases are therefore often gratifying to manage. Since narcotic overdose is a common emergency and a leading cause of death, especially in young urban males, it is essential that all physicians be at ease with the principles of evaluation, specific basic treatment, and possible complications of the condition. Rapid diagnosis and intervention are frequently lifesaving.

It is important to recognize that heroin abuse and addiction are now seen in a broad spectrum of patients, including those who are affluent, female, suburban, and rural. The stereotype of the male inner city "junkie" no longer holds true. The physician must maintain a high index of suspicion in a wide variety of clinical settings.

Agents

Acute narcotic reactions may be caused by various opioid preparations, both those directly derivative of opium and those synthetically produced, such as methadone and propoxyphene (Table 1). Death is primarily due to central respiratory depression and arrest. This is common to pharmacologic overdose of all narcotic preparations. Cardiac arrhythmias secondary to hy-

poxia and aspiration of gastric contents have been frequently implicated as fatal factors. However, socalled overdose is seldom pure in a pharmacologic sense. It is often an allergic or hypersensitive response to injected adulterants or contaminants of street drugs or the concomitant presence of other mood-altering drugs. The synergistic reaction with other drugs, especially alcohol, barbiturates, sedative-hypnotics, and antidepressants, is of enormous importance, both because it is so common and because it confuses the clinical presentation, deepening the respiratory depression, which is then unresponsive to simple treatment. The concomitant use of alcohol or cocaine is so frequently a cofactor in narcotic poisoning that these substances should always be kept in mind.

Clinical Presentation

The clinical triad of coma, pinpoint pupils, and depressed respiration strongly suggests opioid poisoning. Accidental narcotic overdoses are most often seen in a setting of illicit narcotic use, usually of intravenous heroin, but severe reactions can occur after intranasal use ("snorting" or "sniffing") or oral ingestion.

TABLE 1. **Representative Narcotic Preparations**

Generic Name	Trade Names	Street Names	Toxic Dose (mg)*	Plasma Half-Life (hr)	Comments
Morphine		Dreamer, Miss Emma	10	2.5–3.0	Oral, subcutaneous, intramuscular, intravenous routes.
Heroin (diacetylmorphine)		Smack, H, Scag, Dope, Junk, DooJee, Horse (caballo, manteca, tecaté), Speedball (with cocaine)	3	2.5–3.0	Snorted, smoked; subcutaneous, intravenous, intramuscular routes. Appears in urine as morphine.
Hydromorphone	Dilaudid	Little D	1.5	3	Oral, rectal, subcutaneous, intramuscular, intravenous routes.
Meperidine	Demerol	Pethidine, Big D	75	3	May cause seizures and mydriasis.
Opium	Pantopon	Big O, Black stuff	PO or RR only		May be smoked as powder. Overdose usually oral.
Codeine	Codeine	Cough medicine	120	2.5–3.0	Oral, subcutaneous, intramuscular routes.
Oxycodone	Percodan, Percocet	Perks	15	3	Oral route only; abuse common.
Hydrocodone	Hycodan	Hyke	5–10 (oral only)	2–4	Common cough syrup.
Propoxyphene	Darvon	Dummies		10–12	Oral only. Seizures in overdose.
Methadone	Dolophine	Meth, Fizzies	10	24–48	Common mixed overdose. Extended treatment necessary.
L-α-Acetylmethadol	LAAM	LAAM	10	48–72	Ultra–long-acting methadone congener. Extended treatment necessary.
Diphenoxylate	Lomotil		300 (oral only)		Overdose seen in children. Concomitant atropine poisoning.
Fentanyl	Sublimaze	Sub, China white	0.1	0.5	Common anesthetic.

*Dose based on equivalent to 10 mg of morphine subcutaneously.

Unintentional poisoning can occur in nontolerant rec- reational, novice, sporadic, or chronic users, often com- plicated by simultaneous use of alcohol, cocaine, or sedative-hypnotics. Variability of the purity of illicit street heroin or the injection of a previously well- tolerated dose after a period of abstinence can lead to unintentional overdose. Poisoning may also be the result of a suicide attempt. Because a good history is frequently unavailable at the time of crisis, it is im- portant to examine the patient for signs of chronic abuse: the skin for old tracks, scars, cellulitis, or fresh needle marks; and the nasal mucosa for edema, inflam- mation, ulcers, or perforation. The respiratory rate is low and the patient may be comatose. The hypoxia may produce cardiac arrhythmias and, due to impair- ment of capillary permeability, pulmonary edema. Al- lergic reaction to adulterants of heroin may also cause the pulmonary edema as well as electrocardiographic repolarization changes (ST segment and T wave alter- ations), predisposing the patient to ventricular ar- rhythmias. Pupillary constriction is usually present, but in severe hypoxia or the presence of other factors, dilation may occur. Seizures may also cloud the picture, especially in poisoning due to meperidine (Demerol) or propoxyphene (Darvon).

Narcotic poisoning occurs in children who have taken adult doses of methadone or other opiates. Be- cause of high cross-tolerance to all opiates, patients on methadone rarely have simple narcotic poisoning but rather succumb to the combined effects of polydrug overdose, especially alcohol or sedative-hypnotics. In a hospital setting, poisoning may result from failure to verify an alleged methadone maintenance dose or in- accurate assessment of the relative potencies, phar- macokinetics, and interactions of various agents. El- derly patients and those with chronic liver disease are particularly susceptible to overdose with narcotic drugs.

Treatment

The primary treatment of narcotic poisoning may be divided into administering supportive care and specific intervention.

The principles of treatment of narcotic overdose are the same for all narcotic agonists. However, when either methadone or levo-alpha-acetyl- methadol (LAAM) is suspected, management must consider their much longer plasma half- lives (see Table 1), and specific treatment must continue for days rather than hours.

Supportive Care. Unfortunately, the majority of deaths from narcotic poisoning occur before med- ical care is available or after unsuccessful home remedies have been attempted.

As soon as rapid examination has suggested the diagnosis of acute narcotic reaction, treat- ment should start immediately. There is seldom time for laboratory confirmation of suspicion. The patient should be rapidly transported to a medical facility, with maintenance of an open airway,

oral passages cleared, and administration of ar- tificial respiration if necessary. In the presence of acute pulmonary edema, endotracheal intuba- tion or even tracheotomy may be required for adequate ventilation. Oxygenation by an Ambu bag or respirator may be neeeded. An intravenous line should be established and a bolus of 50 ml of 50 per cent glucose should be administered. Acidosis (pH less than 7.2) should be treated with 50 ml of sodium bicarbonate and repeated if necessary.

In the case of an oral narcotic overdose in an awake patient, emesis may be induced by admin- istering 15 ml of ipecac followed by 200 to 300 ml of water, then 50 mg of activated charcoal in 500 ml of water. Emesis should be induced even if ingestion occurred hours earlier, since opiates slow gastrointestinal motility and absorption may be delayed. If the patient is obtunded or comatose after oral ingestion of narcotic, he or she should be intubated with a cuffed endotra- cheal tube (to prevent aspiration) and gastric lavage performed with tap water or isotonic sa- line solution (100 to 500 ml).

Specific Intervention. The specific short-acting narcotic antagonist naloxone (Narcan) should be intravenously administered as soon as possible to the patient in a 0.4-mg bolus. Intramuscular or subcutaneous routes may be used if rapid intra- venous access is not possible. Electrolytes, blood gas levels, electrocardiographic monitoring, and blood acid urine for toxicology should be obtained. If narcotic poisoning is present, the response to naloxone is dramatic, within 15 to 30 seconds, marked by lightening of coma, pupillary dilation, and marked increase in respiratory rate. Nalox- one may be repeated every 2 to 3 minutes up to a maximum dosage of 1.2 mg. If no response is observed, the central nervous system depression must have other causes that must be sought.

Naloxone hydrochloride is a pure short-acting narcotic antagonist with no narcotic agonist ef- fects such as respiratory depression. It is much to be preferred over the older, formerly used mixed agonist-antagonist drugs nalorphine (Nal- line) and levallorphan (Lorfan), which may deepen depression. In fact, naloxone may be used safely in mixed drug overdoses and other clinical situations without compromising ventilation. It may indeed even produce central nervous system arousal in patients suffering pure alcohol over- dose alone. It is crucial to remember that the duration of action of naloxone is only 2 to 3 hours and *all* narcotic agonists have a plasma half-life longer than naloxone (Table 2). Therefore, the patient must be closely monitored. Naloxone should continue to be administered (0.2 to 0.4 mg) every 3 hours as a bolus or continuously

TABLE 2. **Representative Narcotic Antagonists**

Generic Names	Trade Names	Street Name	Dose (mg)*	Plasma Half-Life (hr)
Mixed Agonist Antagonists				
Pentazocine	Talwin	Ts and Blues (with Pyribenzamine)	20 (agonist equivalent)	2
Nalorphine	Nalline		—No longer drug of choice for overdose—	
Buprenorphine†	Buprenex			
Butorphanol	Stadol			
Antagonists				
Naloxone	Narcan		0.4–1.2 mg intravenously or intramuscularly (needed to reverse narcotic overdose)	1–2
Naltrexone‡	Trexan		100 mg on Monday and Wednesday; 150 mg on Friday	13

*Dose based on equivalent to 10 mg of morphine subcutaneously.
†Safety and efficacy for use of this drug in children have not been established.

infused at a rate of 1.2 to 1.6 mg per hour as long as necessary to maintain proper respiration and consciousness. This may be as long as 24 to 48 hours with methadone or 2 to 3 days with LAAM. There have been no episodes of overdose or significant adverse effects reported with administration of naloxone. In the absence of narcotics, this antagonist produces no notable physiologic effects.

Since the initial response to naloxone is quite dramatic, it is important not to be deceived that the patient is out of danger. Indeed, patients often relapse after initial treatment and, if ignored or discharged, may die. Therefore, all patients should be observed for at least 24 hours or longer, depending on the drugs involved.

Naloxone can precipitate a painful acute narcotic withdrawal syndrome ("instant cold turkey") in a methadone-maintained patient. The comatose person may suddenly become agitated, begin retching, and be miserable and unmanageable. If this occurs, the state can be reversed by judicious "renarcotization" with morphine, 2 mg every 3 to 5 minutes until symptoms are tolerable. Naloxone should therefore not be used to arouse an obtunded person with normal ventilation. Rather, it should be made instantly available for use while the patient is being monitored with an intravenous line in place and other causes for the sedation sought. Naloxone reversal of narcotic overdose in nondependent patients may result in hypoglycemia. Hypoglycemic restlessness and agitation may be controlled by giving 50 ml of 50 per cent glucose intravenously.

The patient maintained on 80 to 100 mg of methadone is highly tolerant to narcotics and rarely loses consciousness because of opiate poisoning. If such patients present with respiratory depression or coma, they are usually suffering from alcohol or sedative-hypnotic mixed over-doses. Naloxone may induce partial arousal or muscle twitching in such patients. Other causes of the clinical picture must be avidly sought and supportive treatment maintained.

If the patient is unresponsive to specific treatment, other conditions must be considered. Various infections, pneumonia, meningitis, subacute bacterial endocarditis, and septicemia may confuse the clinical picture with alteration of vital signs. Head trauma may be present with irregular breathing, elevated blood pressure, and unequal pupils. Metabolic abnormalities, such as hypoglycemia, diabetic coma, adrenal insufficiency, hepatic coma, and uremia, must also be included in the differential diagnosis of unresponsiveness.

Seizures have been reported in overdoses due to meperidine and propoxyphene or situations marked by hypoxia. Usually, relief occurs with naloxone therapy and oxygenation. Antiseizure drugs, such as a rapidly acting benzodiazepine, may be used if necessary.

Aftercare. Narcotic poisoning usually implies some associated or underlying addictive disorder or psychiatric illness that requires appropriate treatment after the acute emergency has been managed. The patient should also be evaluated for suicidal risk, and hospitalization should be continued if the overdose was intentional. If the narcotic abuse has been sporadic, counseling or psychotherapy is indicated. Opiate addiction is a chronic disease that requires judicious referral to methadone maintenance treatment, therapeutic detoxification, self-help groups, or drug-free therapeutic communities. In addition to narcotic abstinence syndrome, other concomitant drug dependencies, such as alcohol, sedative-hypnotics, and cocaine, must be recognized and appropriately treated.

Narcotic Poisoning in Children. Children may

accidentally ingest a take-home dose of methadone in its fruit-flavored vehicle, although the introduction of child-proof caps has helped to prevent this tragedy. Occasionally, the antidiarrheal agents Lomotil (diphenoxylate hydrochloride with atropine sulfate) and Imodium (loperamide) have caused poisoning. Also implicated are codeine in antitussive syrups or other palatable forms. Propoxyphene (Darvon), pentazocine (Talwin), and meperidine (Dermerol) are "household narcotics" that pose a risk of overdose. Ingestion by children is a real emergency, since respiratory depression, coma, and cardiovascular collapse may occur extremely rapidly (within 1 hour). If the patient is conscious, emesis should be induced by giving ipecac and water, 5 ml for infants and 15 ml if over 1 year of age. Activated charcoal in water should then be administered. If the patient is comatose, intubation with an inflatable cuffed endotracheal tube and gastric lavage should be performed. Prompt treatment with intravenous naloxone, 0.01 mg per kg, is imperative. This dose should be repeated every 5 minutes up to three times until adequate respiration is restored. Naloxone should be administered every 3 hours and the child monitored closely in a hospital setting for at least 72 hours. During this time it is important to arrange counseling for family members to devise strategies to prevent recurrence of such accidents and to assess the need for further family intervention.

ANXIETY DISORDERS

method of
WILLIAM E. FANN, M.D.
*Baylor College of Medicine and Veterans
   Administration Medical Center
Houston, Texas*

All humans experience anxiety, and not all anxiety is pathologic, even when it is severe. Nevertheless, some individuals suffer from anxiety persistently, severely, and in a manner that effectively disables them. Severe, chronic anxiety is probably induced or learned, but there may be a primary neurophysiologic (perhaps familial or genetic) component to the condition. It is often mixed with moderate depression and as such is the most frequent psychiatric diagnostic category with which the primary physician is confronted.

Anxiety is an unpleasant affect manifesting in its free-floating form as fear, apprehension, or even terror, with physical concomitants of tremor, sweating, tachycardia, dry mouth, urgency to micturate, diarrhea, paresthesias, inability to concentrate, insomnia, and easy fatigue. The revised third edition of the American Psychiatric Association's Diagnostic and Statistical Manual (DSM-III-R) can be consulted for extensive categorizations and manifestations.

Anxiety, like syphilis, is one of medicine's great imitators and can manifest itself in the guise of many physical diseases. Thus, the anxious patient may present with weakness, easy fatigue, or multiple aches and pains. Symptoms may be referable to one or more organ systems.

Approach to the Patient

A complete evaluation of the patient's physical complaints is necessary to establish the diagnosis of generalized anxiety disorder. Diminishing the severity of the patient's experience of discomfort as "nerves" or "all in your mind" will neither resolve the problem nor strengthen the therapeutic alliance necessary for its resolution. If the patient has (or believes that he has) a significant physical illness, his anxiety may be a response to the disease and may be associated with fears of pain, disability, or death. He may suffer from one of the many physical diseases in which anxiety is a prominent symptom, or he may have an anxiety disorder that looks like a physical disease. It is usually helpful to explain to the patient that anxiety exists in everyone, that for reasons we do not always understand it may become severe enough to affect functioning, that it may have an underlying neurophysiologic cause, and that it can be treated.

Generalized anxiety disorder is typically experienced at a persistent relatively low but nevertheless uncomfortable level, as opposed to the periodic intense highly uncomfortable attack, with physiologic components of tachycardia, diaphoresis, and flushing that are characteristic of panic disorder. Although reassurance that the unpleasant feelings of anxiety will not result in death can be helpful, medication is indicated as a therapeutic adjunct when anxiety is chronic and appears to exceed the limits of normal response to environmental threats. Panic disorder, with associated phobia, was once believed to represent an extreme manifestation of generalized anxiety. It is now better understood as a complex neurophysiologic disease that does not respond to the treatment regimens usually prescribed for relief of other anxiety disorders.

Treatment

There are several types of medications that are effective in relieving symptoms of generalized anxiety disorder and associated anxiety conditions such as posttraumatic stress disorder. These are benzodiazepines, tricyclic antidepressants, buspirone, and beta-adrenergic blockers. Each of these medications has limitations as well as advantages and should be used only after careful evaluation of the patient's mental and physical status.

The benzodiazepines are highly effective and safe but can produce euphoria and are therefore susceptible to abuse. They have the potential for physiologic dependency when used at high doses for protracted periods. When dependency does develop, drug withdrawal symptoms can include seizures, insomnia, irritability, and increased anxiety. Patients with a history of drug abuse should not be given benzodiazepines if other therapeutic modes are available. For the patient with generalized anxiety disorder, a longer-acting benzodiazepine such as diazepam (Valium) may be preferable, providing symptomatic relief for up to 6 hours. Compounds with shorter half-lives, such as alprazolam (Xanax), may quickly quell a period of acute anxiety but may lose effectiveness between scheduled doses. It is often useful to advise the patient to take one 5-mg diazepam tablet when anxiety symptoms are first felt and a second if symptoms remain intolerable after 30 minutes. Ten mg of diazepam is ordinarily sufficient to control the symptoms of even intense anxiety; if this dosage is ineffective, the patient may be suffering from a physical disease such as hyperthyroidism, which manifests with anxious symptoms that do not respond to anxiolytics. Subsequent dosages should be administered in response to symptoms rather than on a fixed schedule. This dosing schedule puts the patient in control of his condition and avoids a constant condition of medication intoxication. On return office visits the patient should bring the bottle for a pill count as an index of the frequency and severity of the anxiety.

Tricyclic antidepressants are the medication of choice for patients who may be at risk for dependency on benzodiazepines. Imipramine (Tofranil-PM), doxepin (Sinequan), or amitriptyline (Elavil) should be administered on a regular basis (usually 25 mg three times daily), rather than on an as needed basis. Tricyclics are potent sedatives that can interfere with daytime functioning until the patient becomes accustomed to their effects. Doses at supper and bedtime will minimize interference with regular activities and will help the anxious patient to sleep. A steady-state blood level will usually be achieved in about 2 weeks, with anxiolytic effect evenly distributed around the clock. In some cases tricyclic antidepressants can paradoxically worsen the symptoms of anxiety, and the physician should be alert to this possibility.

Buspirone (BuSpar) is a new compound differing in most respects from other antianxiety agents now on the market. Its principal advantages are that it does not appear to produce euphoria or dependency; its chief disadvantage is that it may require 1 week to 10 days to achieve therapeutic effect. It is neither cross-tolerant nor cross-sensitive to sedative medication and therefore cannot be used to treat the effects of withdrawal from alcohol, sedatives, or benzodiazepines. The usual prescribing pattern is 5 mg four times daily.

Beta-adrenergic blocking agents have some antianxiety efficacy, primarily in patients with a strong cardiovascular component to their symptomatology. It is helpful in reducing tachycardia and tremor, especially in situations such as public speaking, where there may be a powerful anticipatory anxiety element. Propranolol (Inderal), 20 mg, can be given three to four times daily beginning 2 to 3 days before the anticipated triggering event. Beta blockers can cause hypotension, bradycardia, and impairment of short-term memory and are specifically contraindicated in asthmatics.

BULIMIA NERVOSA

method of
HARRISON G. POPE, Jr., M.D., and
JAMES I. HUDSON, M.D.
Harvard Medical School
Boston, Massachusetts

Bulimia nervosa is a syndrome of compulsive eating binges, usually followed by self-induced vomiting or laxative abuse. The disorder afflicts primarily women between the ages of 13 and 40 years; it appears to be increasingly common in the United States. Studies have estimated that 2 to 5 per cent of young American women suffer from the syndrome; prevalence estimates vary depending on how "broadly" or "narrowly" the disorder is defined.

Clinical Features

In its Diagnostic and Statistical Manual of Mental Disorders, third edition revised (DSM-III-R), the American Psychiatric Association has proposed operational diagnostic criteria for bulimia nervosa. These are shown in Table 1.

In the patient who has developed full-blown bulimia nervosa, the syndrome is characteristic and often severe. Preoccupation with food and body weight, planning and carrying out binge eating episodes, and associated feelings of depression and guilt (particularly in the wake of binges), may dominate the patient's life. These patients may be eager to be rid of their symptoms and anxious to see a physician and to obtain treatment.

More often, however, bulimic patients may be surreptitious, keeping their symptoms secret from their closest friends, their spouses, and their physicians. Such cases may be difficult to identify, since such patients may appear physically and psychologically healthy. In the authors' experience, several clues on physical examination may help to recognize such cases: (1) some patients may develop parotitis (possibly as a result of reflux of vomitus down the parotid ducts),

TABLE 1. **DSM-III-R Criteria for Bulimia Nervosa**

1. Recurrent episodes of binge eating (rapid consumption of a large amount of food in a discrete period of time).
2. A feeling of lack of control over eating behavior during the eating binges.
3. The person regularly engages in either self-induced vomiting, use of laxatives or diuretics, strict dieting or fasting, or vigorous exercise in order to prevent weight gain.
4. A minimum average of two binge eating episodes a week for at least 3 months.
5. Persistent overconcern with body shape and weight.

leading to a chipmunklike appearance; (2) tooth enamel may be severely eroded by exposure to the acid in vomitus (a feature sometimes first noticed by the patient's dentist); and (3) patients may display abrasions on the dorsal aspects of the fingers due to the insertion of the hand into the mouth to induce vomiting (Russell's sign). Laboratory tests may offer further clues: (1) on electrolyte determinations, reduced potassium, reduced chloride, and increased CO_2 may all reflect the effects of self-induced vomiting, with loss of stomach acid. (2) Disturbances of acid-base balance caused by vomiting may also be reflected in an unusually high urinary pH. A urinary pH of 8.0 or higher is unusual in normal young women but may occur in 20 to 40 per cent of patients with bulimia nervosa.

In the presence of any of the above signs, a history of bulimia nervosa should be carefully sought. Even in the absence of such signs, a question about bulimic symptoms should probably be routinely included when taking the medical history of a female patient between the ages of 13 and 40 years.

Associated Disorders

Bulimia nervosa may be associated with a number of other psychiatric disorders. *Anorexia nervosa,* in which the patient deliberately diets to a weight well below appropriate body weight, may coexist with bulimia nervosa. Indeed, 10 to 40 per cent of bulimic patients experience anorexia nervosa at some time during their lives. Patients with both disorders may present with profound cachexia complicated by severe electrolyte and electrocardiogram (ECG) abnormalities, sometimes necessitating hospital admission in order to manage the patient's medical condition.

Depressive illness and occasionally *bipolar disorder* (manic-depressive illness) occur frequently in individuals with bulimia nervosa, suggesting that the eating disorders may share etiologic features in common with depressive illness. Fortunately, the medications used to treat depression and bipolar disorder are frequently effective for bulimia nervosa as well (see the following treatment recommendations). In bulimic patients with severe depressive symptoms, suicide attempts are not uncommon, and hospitalization may be necessary until sufficient control of the depressive symptoms is achieved.

Anxiety disorders, including *panic disorder* (the syndrome of spontaneously occurring panic attacks), *agoraphobia,* and *obsessive-compulsive disorder* are also much more frequent in bulimic patients than in the general population. Fortunately, these disorders may also respond to antidepressant medications used to treat the bulimic symptoms.

Drug and alcohol abuse are also more common in bulimic patients than in the general population. These syndromes may improve with effective treatment of the eating disorder but more often require additional therapeutic intervention.

Kleptomania (impulsive shoplifting or stealing) may occur in as many as a third of bulimic women.

Medical disorders associated with bulimia nervosa include the fluid, electrolyte, and acid-base abnormalities caused by vomiting, laxative abuse, and diuretic abuse. The more common of these abnormalities have been enumerated already; it is rare that these are of sufficient magnitude to be life-threatening or to require inpatient medical treatment. However, it should be noted that occasional bulimic patients may use ipecac on a regular basis to induce vomiting and may develop cardiac and skeletal muscle myopathy as a result of chronic emetine poisoning. Very rarely, such cases have resulted in death.

Treatment

Because of the surreptitious nature of bulimic behavior, treatment depends heavily on successfully identifying the bulimia and securing the patient's consent to treatment. Identification of cases may come from direct historical information furnished by the patient (or sometimes by her family), recognition of the various physical and laboratory signs enumerated previously, or recognition of one of the various psychiatric syndromes, also listed above, that may accompany bulimia.

Once the patient feels comfortable in describing her (or occasionally his) symptoms to the physician, treatment can proceed promptly. The great majority of patients can be treated on an outpatient basis. In general, only patients with (1) concomitant anorexia nervosa and severe cachexia, (2) severe electrolyte or ECG abnormalities, or (3) severe depression and suicidal ideation require inpatient treatment.

Whether the patient is an inpatient or an outpatient, antidepressant medication is the initial treatment of choice under most circumstances. However, many bulimic patients are initially reluctant to take antidepressant medications, and some education and reassurance by the physician is often required. In particular, patients often need to be reassured (1) that antidepressants are not "tranquilizers" or stimulants that will cause them to feel "drugged" in some way; (2) that these drugs are not addictive; (3) that side effects are mild, especially with the newer antidepressants; (4) that these drugs rarely cause bulimic patients to gain weight; and (5) that taking these drugs is not incompatible with psychotherapy. Indeed, a good antidepressant response may improve the patient's progress in subsequent psychotherapy. When these issues are reviewed with the patient, compliance with medication is often improved.

In most cases, we suggest starting with the antidepressant fluoxetine (Prozac), raising the dose to 60 mg per day by the end of the first week. Although some patients will respond to doses of less than 60 mg per day, bulimic patients are generally young and capable of metabolizing antidepressants rapidly; hence, it may be wise to use a full 60 mg except in cases in which patients show difficulty tolerating this dose. Fluoxetine may be given all at once, morning or evening, since the drug has a half-life of several days. Side effects are usually modest with fluoxetine (gastrointestinal upset, sedation, or stimulation being most common), but in a small percentage of patients allergic rash may develop, necessitating discontinuation of the drug and substitution of another medication.

Although controlled data with fluoxetine in bulimia are not available at the time of this writing, the authors' experience suggests that at least 50 per cent of patients will experience a remission or at least a major improvement (greater than 75 per cent reduction in frequency of eating binges) after 21 to 28 days of treatment. For those who show no improvement or inadequate improvement, lithium carbonate, starting at 300 mg three times a day, may be added to fluoxetine and the lithium dose raised to achieve a blood level (measured 12 hours after the previous dose of lithium has been administered) of about 1.0 mEq per liter. For patients who still show no improvement after about 2 weeks of lithium plus fluoxetine treatment, another antidepressant is usually required.

In such cases, fluoxetine and lithium may be stopped abruptly without adverse effects, since both drugs in effect "taper themselves" as they are slowly removed from the central nervous system. A tricyclic antidepressant with a low incidence of side effects, such as desipramine (Norpramin) or nortriptyline (Aventyl), may then be begun immediately and raised to full doses within a week. Since bulimic patients are generally young and metabolize tricyclics rapidly, larger-than-average doses of these drugs may be required: at least 3.5 mg per kg of body weight for desipramine and about 1.5 mg per kg for nortriptyline. Because of wide differences in individual metabolism of these drugs, it is important to measure plasma levels after 5 to 7 days at full doses. Desipramine dose should then be adjusted to achieve plasma levels of at least 200 ng per ml; nortriptyline levels should be adjusted to be between 50 and 140 ng per ml. If plasma levels are not determined, a fair number of patients will not receive an adequate trial of tricyclics.

Other tricyclic antidepressants, such as imipramine (Tofranil-PM), amitriptyline (Elavil), and doxepin, and the related drug maprotiline, also appear effective in bulimia. However, these drugs generally have more side effects than desipramine and nortriptyline, and plasma levels, although commercially available, are more difficult to interpret, since (with the exception of imipramine) there is less agreement in the literature as to what constitutes the optimum therapeutic range for these drugs.

In patients who fail both fluoxetine and a tricyclic trial, a monoamine oxidase inhibitor such as tranylcypromine (Parnate) may succeed where previous drugs have failed. Although manufacturers of monoamine oxidase inhibitors generally recommend a 14-day washout period between the discontinuation of tricyclics and the initiation of the monoamine oxidase inhibitors, many authorities feel that this is not necessary and will administer the latter drugs within only a few days or even immediately upon discontinuing tricyclics. However, monoamine oxidase inhibitors should not be given until 5 weeks after discontinuation of fluoxetine. Of course, patients must be counseled to avoid foods such as aged cheeses, Chianti wine, beer, sour cream, broad bean pods, and chicken livers, since these may cause hypertensive reactions with monoamine oxidase inhibitors. Although bulimic patients rarely binge on such foods, the physician should satisfy himself that the patient can adhere to a tyramine-free diet before prescribing these agents.

As in the case of fluoxetine and tricyclics, young bulimic patients frequently require and tolerate surprisingly large doses of monoamine oxidase inhibitors, such as 40 to 80 mg per day* of tranylcypromine (Parnate) or 75 to 105 mg per day* of phenelzine (Nardil). Typically, these drugs are started at modest doses (say, 10 mg twice daily of tranylcypromine or 15 mg twice daily of phenelzine), with the dose raised every couple of days until the patient notices some lightheadedness. At this point the dose can usually be raised no further, or disabling postural hypotension ensues.

Severe insomnia may occur with tranylcypromine and, to a lesser extent, with phenelzine. This can often be treated with trazodone, usually 100 to 400 mg at bedtime. Trazodone is a potent sedative, rarely causes a "hangover" in the morning, and has clear antidepressant effects of its own. Thus, it may act synergistically with mono-

---

*Exceeds the maximum dosage recommended by the manufacturer.

amine oxidase inhibitors in the treatment of bulimia.

A substantial majority of bulimic patients will respond to one of the above three sequential antidepressant strategies with either a remission or marked reduction of bulimic symptoms. Another small group of bulimic patients, as mentioned earlier, display symptoms of concomitant bipolar disorder and may respond to lithium, carbamazepine, or valproate. Finally, occasional patients refractory to standard medication may respond to anorexigenic drugs, such as fenfluramine (Pondimin).

However, even among patients who respond well to pharmacologic treatment, there are some who will require, or who at least wish to obtain, some form of psychotherapy. Psychotherapeutic treatments for bulimia nervosa are generally not in the domain of the general physician. However, several principles should be noted. First, groups for women with eating disorders, often organized by local self-help organizations, are available in many areas. These are often inexpensive and offer powerful support and reassurance, particularly to women who have not had a chance to share their experiences with fellow sufferers. Patients wishing to participate in such support groups should be encouraged to contact self-help organizations for individuals with eating disorders in their area.

On a more formal level, psychodynamic psychotherapy, various forms of group psychotherapy, and cognitive behavioral therapy all enjoy wide use in the treatment of bulimia nervosa. The last of these techniques has been shown effective in controlled studies and may produce beneficial effects in relatively short periods of time (a few weeks to a few months). In referring a bulimic patient to a behavioral therapist, it is helpful to ensure that the individual is experienced with treating bulimic patients.

On the other hand, several recent studies suggest that formal behavioral techniques may not be demonstrably superior to nondirective individual or group psychotherapy, whether outcome is measured in terms of the frequency of eating binges per se or in terms of associated symptoms of the eating disorder. If these findings are correct, then it may be that specialized psychotherapeutic intervention does not offer any particular advantage over ordinary individual or group support for most patients and should be reserved primarily for those patients who have failed both pharmacologic treatment and standard psychotherapy.

DELIRIUM

method of
ALAN STOUDEMIRE, M.D.
Emory University School of Medicine
Atlanta, Georgia

Delirium is the behavioral manifestation of cerebral dysfunction. It is almost always the result of an "acute" process, which distinguishes it from chronic degenerative brain diseases such as Alzheimer's disease. In addition, delirium is generally reversible and is usually caused by acute toxic or metabolic processes that have disrupted normal cerebral metabolic functioning and electrophysiologic activity. In addition to toxic and metabolic causes, abnormal electrophysiologic activity such as seizures may cause delirium, as can the acute sequelae of physical injury and mass effects (e.g., head trauma and brain tumors).

An essential clinical feature of delirium is an acute change in mental status resulting in a clouding or diminution in the patient's level of consciousness that fluctuates with time. Even though "clouding" of consciousness is the most frequently cited symptom of delirium, patients may also at times appear to be hyperalert, anxious, and agitated. Since consciousness levels in delirium typically fluctuate in a sine wave fashion over a 24-hour period, patients may at times essentially return to baseline and have lucid intervals during which mental status even appears normal.

Delirium is always accompanied by abnormalities in the patient's cognitive functioning as exhibited by problems in orientation (to place, time, or circumstance), attention, concentration, and memory. The *behavioral* abnormalities associated with delirium, however, may be the earliest and most obvious sign of cerebral dysfunction that will come to the medical staff's attention. The behavioral manifestations of delirium include hostility, belligerence, irritability, paranoia, insomnia, illusions, hallucinations (auditory, tactile, or visual), agitation, and combativeness. More times than not these disturbances are initially attributed to an "acute psychotic break" or "functional" psychiatric causes before more detailed assessment reveals gross underlying cognitive abnormalities. Delirious patients may also be quietly withdrawn and apathetic and have their cognitive disruption go completely unrecognized.

EVALUATION

The bedside evaluation of delirium involves not only careful notation of the patient's current behavioral cognitive state but also a review of the course of the patient's mental status over the past 24 to 72 hours or greater. A chart review with special attention to nursing notes is essential in this regard. A brief mental status examination should be performed and can be completed in 5 minutes. Standard questions to ask include having patients state (1) the date, place, and reason for being in the hospital or office; (2) the current full date; (3) their name, place, and date of birth; (4) their parents, siblings, and children's names; (5) their address and telephone and social security numbers; and (6) the names of the past six presidents in order. In addition, they should be asked (1) to perform serial subtractions by 7s or 3s from 100 or, alternatively, simple money-change exercises; (2) to remember three objects after a 5-minute delay; (3) to draw the face of a clock on a sheet of paper; and (4) to repeat a set of digits (usually six) both forward and in reverse. In my experience any substantial problem with any of the above exercises, coupled with behavioral abnormalities and fluctuations in the level of consciousness, indicates the presence of delirium.

There exists a vast differential diagnosis for the etiology of delirium. Disturbances in almost *any* organ system may cause physiologic abnormalities leading to delirium (neurologic, cardiovascular, renal, hepatic, pulmonary, endocrine, gastrointestinal). As will be discussed later, medications are perhaps the most common cause of delirium (particularly in the elderly) and should receive primary attention in the diagnostic evaluation.

The diagnostic evaluation of delirium begins with careful observation and mental status examination to confirm the diagnosis. A physical and neurologic examination is essential as well as a review of the patient's vital signs. A drug review of both medical and psychotropic agents is the next *essential* step, with particular note of any drugs the patient may have taken prior to admission and that may have been stopped—from which a withdrawal syndrome may have developed (alcohol, barbiturates, benzodiazepines, opiates). A urine drug screen may be indicated based on the patient's history, physical examination, and clinical history to detect occult drug abuse.

Medication Side Effects

The most common causes of delirium in the elderly are the side effects of medication. The most common offenders are narcotics and sedative hypnotics such as benzodiazepines. Alcohol intoxication and alcohol withdrawal (delirium tremens) are common drug-related causes of deliria. Iatrogenic causes of delirium may be related to the use of digoxin, quinidine, theophylline, narcotics, anticonvulsants, and histamine-blocking agents such as cimetidine and ranitidine. Delirium may also be induced by the anticholinergic effects of tricyclic antidepressants or other drugs with anticholinergic effects. If drug levels are available, these may be obtained, but even a therapeutic serum level does not necessarily mean the agent in question is not responsible, since delirium may be observed with some drugs (such as digoxin) even at "therapeutic" levels.

Differential Diagnosis

After medication/drugs have been considered as possible causes, the next step is a systematic organ system approach to the differential diagnosis. In this approach one assesses the diagnostic possibilities in a sequential systemic manner: neurologic (stroke, infection, tumor, seizures, posttraumatic effects), cardiovascular (congestive heart failure), pulmonary (hypoxia, pneumo-nia), endocrine (hypoglycemia, hyperthyroidism, hypothyroidism, adrenal dysfunction, hypo- or hypercalcemia), gastrointestinal (intestinal obstruction, hepatic failure), and renal (uremia, fluid and electrolyte abnormalities, especially hyponatremia). Systemic or focal infections should also be considered, especially if mental status changes occur during febrile episodes. Abrupt environmental changes and stresses, such as placement in the intensive care unit, may cause disorientation in the elderly.

Although the differential diagnosis for delirium is extensive, the laboratory assessment is relatively straightforward. The standard laboratory assessment includes a complete blood count, SMA-18 (or an equivalent metabolic screen), erythrocyte sedimentation rate, arterial blood gases, appropriate drug levels or drug screens, and urinalysis as well as a search for local or systemic infections. A chest radiograph and electrocardiogram should be routinely performed if the clinical evaluation dictates, and if a primary central nervous system disorder is suspected, an EEG, CT scan, and lumbar puncture may be indicated. Other tests may be ordered depending on the clinical history and the patient's presentation, such as an evaluation for cerebritis in patients with systemic lupus erythematosus.

Treatment

The treatment of delirium primarily involves a vigorous search for the underlying etiology of the patient's cerebral dysfunction in order that it may be corrected or stabilized. In the interim, behavioral control is best achieved by the use of (at least initially) carefully titrated low doses of antipsychotic agents. Haloperidol (Haldol) is the most frequently used medication in this regard, usually at doses of 2 mg orally, intramuscularly, or intravenously every hour or two until the patient is sedated. The 24-hour requirement to achieve the desired level of sedation is then determined and the medication can then be given on a regularly timed basis. The dose is tapered as rapidly as possible as the underlying cause for the patient's cerebral dysfunction is identified and treated. Patients should be monitored carefully for the development of extrapyramidal symptoms (dystonia, muscle rigidity, drooling, masklike faces, tremor, dysphagia, and dysarthria) and have either the dose of phenothiazine reduced or anticholinergic agents instituted (trihexyphenidyl [Artane] 2 mg every 4 hours orally or intramuscularly every 6 hours). Alternatively, benztropine mesylate (Cogentin), 2 mg every 6 hours, may be used. These drugs are tapered concurrently with the phenothiazine but may need to be continued longer than the phenothiazine itself to bring about full resolution of the extrapyramidal symptoms. It is essential to keep the use of phenothiazines to a minimum both in terms of dosage and duration of therapy. Patients undergoing alcohol or drug withdrawal should be treated with the appropriate detoxification protocols, which usually obviate the need for adjunctive phenothiazines.

Delirium usually resolves with correction and stabilization of the underlying disorder. Simple environmental strategies may be as helpful as the psychopharmacologic techniques noted above and include (1) placing the patient near the nurses' station, (2) providing a room with a (secured) window to allow the patient to follow light/dark patterns, (3) making available sitters—preferably family members—especially at night, (4) utilizing easily visible clocks and calendars to help patients mark the passage of time, (5) displaying family objects or family photographs from home to be kept at the bedside, and (6) using nightlights.

AFFECTIVE DISORDERS

method of
DAVID L. DUNNER, M.D.
University of Washington
Seattle, Washington

Affective disorders is a term denoting disorders of mood with particular reference to depression. Although the prevalence of the depressive disorders is unknown, several estimates suggest that depression is perhaps the most frequent psychiatric condition and that 15 to 20 per cent of the population will experience a significant depression at some time. Most depressions are extremely responsive to treatment. However, inaccurate clinical diagnosis results in many depressed patients being inadequately treated. In this article, I will review classifications of depression that are useful in delineating specific treatments for depressed patients, with emphasis on the recently revised nomenclature of the revised third edition of the American Psychiatric Association's Diagnostic and Statistical Manual (DSM-III-R).

Depression is a word that has both psychiatric and commonplace meanings. Thus, people will use the word depression to mean that they are upset about a particular life event. Depressed mood in the absence of specific symptoms of depression is essentially not of sufficient significance to be clinically treatable. Depression as a psychiatric disorder consists of depressed mood plus depressive symptoms. Other terms for depressed mood include feeling sad, blue, hopeless, low, down in the dumps, and irritable. Typical depressive symptoms include change in appetite and weight, with either poor appetite and weight loss or increased appetite and weight gain; change in sleeping habits, with either insomnia or hypersomnia; change in motor activity, with either agitation or motor retardation; loss of interest in usual activities and in sexual rela-

tions; loss of energy; feelings of worthlessness, self-reproach, or guilt; decreased ability to think or concentrate; and recurrent thoughts of death or suicide or suicide attempts. In this article, I will use depressed mood plus symptoms to define psychiatric depression in contrast to depression without symptoms.

Subclassification

It is generally recognized that there is affective response to the death of a close friend or relative. This depression, which is termed "uncomplicated bereavement," is associated with depressed mood and depressive symptoms. Bereavement tends to be prompt in onset and relatively short lived. Feelings of worthlessness and psychomotor retardation are uncommon with this disorder. In general, bereavement is not treated by psychiatrists but is usually treated by internists or family physicians. Bereavement is often not treated except with supportive care. Brief courses of small doses of antianxiety agents may be of benefit. It is unusual for psychiatrists to treat bereaved persons. However, when the syndrome fails to respond to brief therapy or the symptoms persist for several months, one should consider a major depression as a diagnostic possibility.

Depression occurring shortly after a traumatic life event is termed "adjustment disorder with depressed mood." Such depressions are usually time limited and often respond to supportive measures. By definition in DSM-III-R, adjustment disorder with depressed mood lasts less than 6 months. If the mood disorder persists, rediagnosis to major depression should be considered.

Depression (or elated mood) occurring with evidence of a specific organic factor that is judged to be etiologically related to the mood disturbance is termed "organic mood syndrome." Such etiologic factors may include stroke, endocrine disturbance, medication or drug use or abuse, or cancer. Treatment of the etiologic factor is the main therapeutic approach.

The primary mood disorders can be divided into those with mania or hypomania (bipolar disorder) and those with depression only (unipolar disorder or depressive disorders).

Mania is defined as a change in mood state (euphoria or irritability) and presents with symptoms such as increase in activity, increase in talkativeness, flight of ideas or racing thoughts, grandiosity, decreased need for sleep, distractability, and impulsive behavior. The severe form of this disorder, which is often accompanied by delusions of grandeur or frank psychosis, usually results in the patient being hospitalized specifically for the manic condition. Such patients have been termed bipolar I. In DSM-III-R these patients would be termed as having a bipolar disorder. Patients who have manic symptoms but not to the degree resulting in hospitalization (i.e., hypomanic symptoms) are termed bipolar II. Bipolar II patients typically have recurrent depressions and hypomania. Their hypomanic symptoms are rarely incapacitating and may be productive or beneficial to their life status. In DSM-III-R, bipolar II patients are classified as "bipolar disorder, not otherwise specified." Patients with less severe forms of bipolar and unipolar depression, cyclothymic personality and depressive personality, respectively, were defined as those who had mood disorder but not of sufficient severity to require treatment. The DSM-III-R terms "cyclothymic" and "dysthymic" would probably correspond well to the older terms cyclothymic and depressive personality, respectively.

One other point of diagnostic clarification regards the presence of Schneiderian first rank symptoms in affective disorders. These symptoms, such as bizarre delusions, somatic delusions, auditory hallucinations such as a voice commenting on the patient's behavior or two or more voices conversing with one another, and delusions such as audible thoughts and thought broadcasting, represent psychotic symptoms, which in the past have been used synonymously with schizophrenia. However, in the past few years schizophrenia has been narrowly defined to include patients who have the above psychotic symptoms associated with a chronic course and absence of affective symptoms. Research studies clearly demonstrate a high prevalence of Schneiderian first rank symptoms during manic epidoses.

The term "schizoaffective disorder" is defined in DSM-III-R in such a way that psychotic symptoms occur in the absence of symptoms of mood disorder in patients who also have prolonged periods of mood disorder. Such patients clearly are complicated to treat and require symptomatic treatment for both mood and psychotic symptoms.

In contrast to the rather clearly defined bipolar and unipolar disorders, there are other disorders in which the illness is presumably affective, although the data to support this assumption may be scant. An example is "masked depression," in which a patient will present clinically with somatic complaints rather than depressive symptoms. Masked depressions may be more frequently seen among older patients. The recognition of this problem is important, since it is felt that masked depression represents a significant portion of patients with depression and that most frequently such patients do not have their psychiatric problems adequately recognized or treated. Another less well-defined illness is depression occurring in a patient whose psychiatric disorder becomes complicated by a second psychiatric illness, for example, alcoholism or polydrug abuse. An underlying depression is often suspected in such patients, particularly if they have positive family histories of depression and if there are atypical features to the course of their secondary illness.

Bipolar-Unipolar Differentiation

Recent data support the separation of bipolar from unipolar primary affective disorders. In general, bipolar I illness is a well-characterized clinical condition in comparison to other primary affective disorder subtypes. Patients with bipolar I illness tend to have extreme psychomotor retardation and often have hypersomnia when depressed, whereas patients with unipolar depression may either be agitated or have psychomotor retardation. Futhermore, the age of onset of illness tends to be earlier in life in bipolar disorders than in unipolar disorders, with the former occurring at a mean age of approximately 30 years and the latter

occurring at a mean age of 40 years. Of some interest is the fact that bipolar disorders may have a more frequent postpartum onset than unipolar disorders. There is considerable evidence relating genetic and biologic factors to the etiology of bipolar depression, although these factors have not been elucidated to the point at which a clear biologic-genetic etiology has been determined. Recent studies have pointed toward a possible genetic defect on chromosome 11 or the X chromosome in certain selected families with bipolar illness. Bipolar depression tends to be familial, and approximately 25 per cent of the first degree relatives of a patient with bipolar disorder will experience either bipolar or unipolar depression. In contrast, unipolar depression probably represents a very heterogeneous group of patients, with various causes for their disorders. For example, the genetic and biologic factors associated with bipolar disorder are not nearly as well delineated among families of patients with unipolar disorders, and the relationship of unipolar disorders to other psychiatric illnesses such as alcoholism is often striking.

Clinical Course

The course of affective disorders can be recurrent attacks or single episodes. The bipolar disorders tend to be marked by recurrent episodes, sometimes on a regular cyclic basis in such a way that the timing of subsequent attacks is quite predictable. Unipolar disorders tend not to be recurrent, and the frequency of attacks tends to be much reduced in unipolar depression as compared with bipolar depression. Rapid cycling (four or more episodes per year) occurs in about 10 per cent of bipolar disorders, and such patients present particular treatment problems. Mania usually begins early in bipolar illness, with about 80 per cent of patients having experienced a manic attack at the onset of their disorder. About one third of patients have a significant premanic depression, and almost 100 per cent of patients have a significant postmanic depressive episode. Indeed, the concept of "unipolar mania" (defined as patients who have only recurrent manic episodes) was studied and found not to be useful in that most patients who have recurrent manic episodes also have some depressive features. Between episodes of illness, patients with bipolar and unipolar illness tend to be free of affective symptoms.

Treatment

Treatment considerations should relate to diagnosis, current mood state, and the clinical history. For example, one could be treating a patient with bipolar disorder who is manic or who is depressed or who is euthymic but prone to recurrent cycles. Similarly, one could be treating a patient with unipolar disorder who is depressed or who is prone to recurrent attacks.

Finally, it should be noted that the suicide risk in depressive illness is considerable. About 15 to 20 per cent of patients with depression die from suicide, and approximately 30 to 50 per cent of primary affective disorder patients have a history of suicide attempts. Suicide generally occurs during the depressed phase of illness. Although it has been stated that suicide is unusual early in the course of depression and more common later in the course of depression, we suggest that the clinician should be carefully aware of suicidal behavior during any phase of the depressive illness. Suicide during mania and during the interim euthymic phases between depressions is unusual. Suicidal behavior tends to occur more frequently among men, among older patients, and among patients who are single, widowed, or divorced. It should be noted that there has been a considerable increase in the reported suicides among adolescents in the past few years.

Most patients who have committed suicide have indicated their intent to commit suicide to other people, and such communication of suicidal intent should be taken quite seriously in the depressed patient. In terms of assessing suicidal risk in an individual patient, it is important to have an underlying assumption that all patients with depression are suicidal but that their tendency to commit suicide at any given point in time may be contingent upon a number of factors. For example, very few patients with depression will have active suicidal plans. A higher percentage of patients will have thoughts of death or suicide, and a majority of patients with depression will wish they would not wake up in the morning or will wish they were dead. The recognition of this hierarchy of suicidal behavior is important in order to establish rapport with the patient and to apply appropriate treatment. It should be stressed that hospitalization should be advocated for any patient in whom the suicidal risk is felt to be high at that period of time. Depression is a highly treatable disorder, and the suicide of a patient during the course of a severe depression might have been prevented with appropriate treatment.

In the following section I will discuss modes of treatment for various types of depression. In general, these modes include electroconvulsive therapy, pharmacotherapy, and various forms of psychotherapy. The decision about which mode or combination of modes to use is often based upon the severity of the depressive symptoms as well as diagnostic considerations. It should be emphasized that the best guide to treatment is the past response to treatment.

Modes of Treatment

Electroconvulsive Therapy. Electroconvulsive therapy (ECT) was widely used in the 1940s, but the beneficial effects of other forms of treatment as well as some attempts to regulate its use legally have resulted in decreased use of ECT. However, it should be noted that ECT is the most effective of all the forms of antidepressant treatment.

ECT is usually administered to hospitalized patients, although patients who have family members to take care of them can receive this treatment on an outpatient basis. A course of therapy usually consists of a series of 8 to 12 treatments, with a frequency of approximately one every other day. Before the treatment is administered, the physician should have good knowledge of the patient's medical condition, including cardiovascular and pulmonary status. The only absolute contraindication to ECT is a space-occupying brain lesion. During ECT, there is a temporary increase of intracranial pressure, which could result in brain stem herniation if a space-occupying lesion is present.

The patient is prepared for ECT by maintaining an empty stomach for at least 8 hours prior to ECT. Approximately half an hour before ECT a small dose of atropine is administered in order to reduce bronchial secretions. Prior to ECT, the patient should void, and dentures should be removed. Furthermore, hairpins should be removed, and any constricting garments around the chest should be removed or loosened. Immediately before administering ECT, the patient should receive an anesthetic intravenously, usually a short-acting barbiturate. The patient is then given succinylcholine in a dose sufficient to cause relaxation of all muscles but not so excessive as to reduce spontaneous respiration for too prolonged a period after ECT. The usual dose of succinylcholine is about 20 to 40 mg intravenously. It is important to maintain the airway and respirate the patient during the succinylcholine-induced paralysis. With bilateral ECT the electrodes are placed on both temples; with unilateral ECT both electrodes are placed over the nondominant hemisphere. In either case a short period of electrical current is applied to the electrodes, usually at the point of maximal muscle depolarization from the succinylcholine. This current application induces a grand mal convulsion characterized by a tonic phase, followed by a brief clonic phase. It is important to respirate the patient with oxygen until the effects of succinylcholine wear off and the patient begins to breathe spontaneously. At this point the patient will be drowsy and somewhat confused. The patient's airway should be protected, and the patient should be observed for approximately half an hour after ECT or until such time as confusion has cleared sufficiently for the patient to resume usual functioning. There is a considerable amount of confusion that occurs just after each treatment; as the number of treatments increases, the patient may become confused for longer periods of time between treatments. Usually, a course of eight treatments suffices to treat a severe depression, at which time a few days are necessary to enable the confusion to clear up sufficiently so that the patient can return home. Although much has been made recently of permanent brain damage resulting from ECT, ECT remains the safest and most effective treatment for severe depression. ECT is useful in the treatment of acute depression. There is no reliable evidence that chronic ECT prevents occurrence of future attacks of depression.

ECT has also been used successfully to treat acute manic episodes. Lithium carbonate therapy should be discontinued about 1 week prior to ECT in order to reduce the risk of neurotoxicity.

Antidepressant Medication. Antidepressant medication can be divided into three types: the tricyclic antidepressants, newer antidepressants, and monoamine oxidase inhibitors. The tricyclic antidepressants (Table 1) have become the most widely used treatment of depression and are efficacious in approximately 80 per cent of depressed patients. Recently, measurement of these compounds in the blood has become available, and for most compounds there seems to be some relationship with either a threshold or range of blood levels and therapeutic response. Thus, if a patient is not responding to a tricyclic antidepressant and is felt to have an adequate dose, it may be useful to obtain a plasma tricyclic level approximately 12 hours after the last dose of tricyclic medication to determine whether the blood level is in the adequate range.

The tricyclic antidepressants can be generally divided into two types: sedating (such as amitriptyline [Elavil], nortriptyline [Pamelor], trimipramine [Surmontil], and doxepin [Adapin]) and alerting (such as imipramine [Tofranil], desipramine [Norpramin], and protriptyline [Vivactil]).

TABLE 1. Tricyclic Antidepressant Medication

Generic Name	Trade Names	Dose Range*
Amitriptyline	Amitid, Amitril, Elavil, Endep	150–300 mg/day
Imipramine	Imavate, Janimine, Presamine, SK-Pramine, Tofranil	150–300 mg/day
Nortriptyline	Aventyl, Pamelor	50–150 mg/day
Trimipramine	Surmontil	75–300 mg/day
Desipramine	Norpramin, Pertofrane	150–200 mg/day
Protriptyline	Vivactil	10–60 mg/day
Doxepin	Adapin, Sinequan	150–300 mg/day

*Some doses may be higher than those listed in the manufacturer's official directive.

TABLE 2. Newer Antidepressant Medication

Generic Name	Trade Names	Dose Range*
Amoxapine	Asendin	150–300 mg/day
Maprotiline	Ludiomil	150–225 mg/day
Trazodone	Desyrel	300–600 mg/day
Fluoxetine	Prozac	20–60 mg/day
Bupropion	Wellbutrin	Up to 450 mg/day

*Some doses may be higher than those listed in the manufacturer's official directive.

"Newer" antidepressants (Table 2) include amoxapine (Asendin), maprotiline (Ludiomil), trazodone (Desyrel), fluoxetine (Prozac), and bupropion (Wellbutrin). All of these agents have advantages and disadvantages as compared with the standard tricyclic compounds. Amoxapine is sedating, but this compound has a major metabolite that has dopamine-blocking effects. Concern for the development of tardive dyskinesia might limit its use to patients who are refractory to other agents. Maprotiline is similar to imipramine; however, an increased risk for seizures has been associated with this compound. Trazodone is among the most frequently prescribed antidepressants. It seems safer than the tricyclic antidepressants, in that the effects of overdose are less severe with trazodone. A small percentage of males will develop priapism with trazodone, and we have therefore not recommended this drug for initial treatment of male patients. Fluoxetine has been recently released, and this compound lacks the anticholinergic side effects and weight gain associated with the tricyclic compounds. The suggested dose of fluoxetine is 20 mg in the morning, and the drug is activating. Side effects include nausea and tremulousness. Bupropion has at this time not been rereleased by the Food and Drug Administration for prescription use. The compound is activating and seems not to cause cycling among bipolar depressives. Cardiovascular and anticholinergic side effects are lacking, but seizures are reported with bupropion if administered at too high a dose, if the dose is increased too rapidly, or if certain patients (e.g., bulimics) are treated with bupropion.

Monoamine oxidase inhibitors (MAOI) (Table 3) were introduced to psychiatry before the tricyclic antidepressants and in the early years of their use were noted to be quite effective. A potentially serious side effect of these drugs re-

TABLE 3. Monoamine Oxidase Inhibitors

Generic Name	Trade Names	Dose Range
Isocarboxazid	Marplan	10–30 mg/day
Phenelzine	Nardil	15–75 mg/day
Tranylcypromine	Parnate	10–60 mg/day

sults from inhibition of MAO in liver. Tyramine, which is present in many food substances, is ordinarily metabolized by liver MAO. If tyramine-containing foods are ingested while the patient is treated with an MAOI, tyramine enters the blood stream, and sudden increases in blood pressure may occur. Because of these potentially serious side effects (headache, strokes) MAOIs were little used for many years. They have been reintroduced recently and are gaining considerable popularity for the treatment of refractory depressions, "atypical" depressions, anxious patients, and postmanic depressive episodes in bipolar patients.

There are two general types of MAOIs. Tranylcypromine (Parnate) has a structure very similar to that of amphetamine and is stimulating, whereas phenelzine (Nardil) is somewhat less stimulating. MAOI drugs have the usual side effects of tricyclic antidepressants, and orthostatic hypotension is the most frequent serious side effect. Hypertensive crisis can be avoided completely if patients follow a low tyramine diet and avoid medication that affects biogenic amines. The appropriate dose of the medication can be determined by the dose required to inhibit MAO in platelets. In general, a dose of 45 mg per day of phenelzine inhibits this enzyme in about 50 per cent of patients, and thus a somewhat higher dose is required of this medication.

Approaches to Treatment

General Principles. As a general principle of psychopharmacology, it is inadvisable to use fixed dose regimens. Thus, patients who are outpatients should be encouraged to alter the dose frequently, within certain guidelines, depending on symptoms or side effects, and for hospitalized patients the physician should carefully assess the dose on a daily basis, balancing therapeutic effect with side effects.

In treating unipolar depression one should be cognizant of two general types of depression: those patients with agitation and insomnia and those patients with psychomotor retardation and hypersomnia. For the former patients, who also may experience anxiety as a prominent feature of the depression, a sedating antidepressant often given at bedtime seems to be most effective. For the latter patients, a more alerting antidepressant, often given toward morning hours in divided doses, seems to be the most logical choice of medication. The target dose for hospitalized patients should be approximately 3.5 mg per kg (imipramine or amitriptyline). It should be noted that protriptyline is given in approximately one fifth the dose of the other tricyclic antidepressants.

In considering the starting dose, one should take into account previous responses to antidepressants, the general medical state of the patient, and the patient's age. Patients who are older should be started on lower doses of antidepressants than younger patients, and older patients have a lower target dose. The initial dose should be increased progressively toward the target dose with an attempt to achieve the target dose within the first 2 weeks of treatment. During the first week of treatment, there is usually no apparent improvement in depression. Toward the end of this period the patient, when questioned carefully, may experience very brief periods of feeling well, followed by a feeling of sinking back into the depressive condition. The patient should be encouraged to see this as a beneficial sign that the antidepressant will be working, and the dose should be increased appropriately. For outpatients the general starting dose of amitriptyline or imipramine is approximately 25 to 100 mg per day, and the dose should be increased by the patient every 3 to 4 days as tolerated.

It is advisable, considering the suicidal potential of such patients, to have the patient seen or phone in during the first week of treatment so that the dose can be adjusted upward or downward, depending on therapeutic response or side effects. In general, outpatient depressives have less severe depression than hospitalized patients and often require less antidepressant total dosage, although many depressed outpatients will require doses in the range of 3.5 mg per kg.

At times, inpatients or outpatients will not respond to antidepressants at the target dose, and the dose will have to be increased, perhaps even above the therapeutic levels recommended in the *Physician's Desk Reference*. For example, it is not uncommon to have patients respond to 350 mg of amitriptyline, whereas they had not responded to a daily dose of 300 mg. Special attention should be paid to the patient's cardiovascular status when doses are increased, and in general outpatients should be told that they should reduce the dose and increase their salt and food intake if they feel dizzy. The typical side effects of tricyclic antidepressants are dry mouth, constipation, blurring of vision, and orthostatic hypotension (experienced as dizziness when one changes position). Later in the course of treatment patients may experience a craving for sweets and weight gain.

Patients tend to respond within 2 to 4 weeks of instituting treatment, although on close questioning they may not feel 100 per cent back to normal. At this point the patient should be maintained on the antidepressant for 2 to 6 months. Frequently, toward the end of this interval the dose can be gradually reduced with approximately 10 per cent reduction in dose every week or every other week. Having the patient reduce the dose and then waiting a week or two to see if symptoms recur is a satisfactory way of determining whether the patient still requires that dose of medication. The patient should be advised not to stop the dose suddenly, as a brief confusional episode may ensue.

The acute depressions of bipolar patients are often somewhat refractory to treatment with tricyclic antidepressants. In general, such patients have retarded depression, and imipramine-like drugs seem to be more indicated than amitriptyline-type drugs. The patient often will improve somewhat but not completely, and the depression in general will take several months to improve in spite of using maximal doses. For this reason, it may be preferable to treat the acute postmanic depressive phase of a bipolar patient with a monoamine oxidase inhibitor rather than with a tricyclic antidepressant. The premanic depressive phase of bipolar patients often spontaneously ends in manic or hypomanic episodes. Thus, the patient should be alerted to the possibility of a manic occurrence during the course of tricyclic treatment, and it may be advisable to treat the patient simultaneously with lithium carbonate. In general, tricyclic antidepressants seem to accentuate mania and are contraindicated during manic or hypomanic episodes. Lithium carbonate has an antidepressant effect, but treatment of the acute depressed phase of bipolar or unipolar depression with lithium carbonate alone is not recommended, although some favor lithium for bipolar depressions because of the tendency for tricyclic antidepressants to cause rapid cycling.

It has been claimed that low doses of antipsychotic agents may be useful in treating some depressive episodes. Furthermore, it has been suggested that patients with psychotic depression often are nonresponders to antidepressant therapy and that antipsychotic drugs should be added to the tricyclic antidepressant. In general, antipsychotic drugs are not the treatment of choice for depression. The addition of an antipsychotic drug to antidepressant therapy in psychotic depressives is of clinical benefit at times. However, ECT should also be considered in these patient.

Prophylaxis of Depression. Recently, tricyclic antidepressants such as amitriptyline and imipramine have been administered on a long-term basis to patients with recurrent unipolar depression to effect a reduction in the frequency of future attacks of this disorder. Such reduction in frequency and/or severity of future episodes with long-term treatment is termed prophylaxis or maintenance therapy, and several studies support the efficacy of chronic tricyclic antidepressants in unipolar recurrent depression. However, it should be noted that some of these studies report a high incidence of manic or hypomanic failures while supposedly unipolar patients are being treated with tricyclic antidepressants. The bipolar II category includes patients who have brief hypomanic episodes before or after their depression, and such patients probably were included as unipolar in those studies mentioned above, resulting in the reported hypomanic failures with chronic tricyclic treatment. Lithium carbonate has also been shown to have a prophylactic effect for recurrent unipolar and bipolar depression, and lithium carbonate is preferred over tricyclic antidepressants for such treatment.

The appropriate dose of tricyclic antidepressants in prophylactic treatment has not been established, although most physicians seem to prefer a maintenance dose of approximately 100 to 150 mg daily of amitriptyline or imipramine. Other antidepressants have not been systematically studied for their long-term prophylactic effect. Lithium carbonate maintenance will be discussed later in this article. Maintenance efficacy for recurrent depression may not become clinically apparent until the patient has been in treatment for about 2 years.

Patients with the rapid cycling form of bipolar illness will experience recurrent depressions and hypomanic episodes. Their depressions are seen as illness, whereas the hypomanic episodes are not viewed by the patient as being clinically significant. However, treating such patients with tricyclic antidepressants alone or in combination with lithium carbonate seems to result in a perpetuation of the cyclic process, whereas treating rapid cyclers with lithium carbonate alone or perhaps with a small dose of antipsychotic agent (such as thioridazine) may be of benefit.

Special Uses in Depression. The use of tricyclic antidepressants in the secondary depressions and in bereavement has not been systematically studied. In my experience if such patients require an antidepressant based on the presence of depressive symptoms, they usually respond at relatively low doses of the antidepressant, such as 50 mg daily of amitriptyline. One should be cautious in treating depression associated with alcoholism, since the antidepressants are sedating, as is alcohol, and the sedative effects of alcohol may be potentiated. Also, particular attention should be paid to treating depression in the elderly, as such patients are particularly prone to the hypotensive and cardiovascular effects of tricyclic antidepressants. The beginning dose for elderly patients is low, on the order of 10 to 25 mg of amitriptyline daily, and very slow increments of the dose are advised, along with careful assessment of blood pressure and cardiovascular status. New antidepressants lacking the cardiovascular side effects of the tricyclic compounds may be of particular benefit in the treatment of the elderly depressed patient.

An important drug-drug interaction of the tricyclic antidepressants occurs with guanethidine, an antihypertensive agent. The antihypertensive effects of guanethidine can be blocked with the administration of tricyclic antidepressants. Thus, if patients are hypertensive and prone to depression, it is advised that they be treated with an antihypertensive agent other than guanethidine. In addition, antidepressants are not advocated during the first trimester of pregnancy.

Acute Mania. Acute manic disturbances may present particular problems because the patient may not be willing to be hospitalized for treatment. Treating manic patients on an outpatient basis is difficult because of the lack of control regarding medication that can be exercised in such circumstances. Thus, the optimal plan is to hospitalize the patient for treatment of an acute manic disorder. ECT is effective in the treatment of acute manic disturbances. Lithium should be discontinued about 1 week before administering ECT because neurotoxicity has been noted with combined treatment. The usual method of treating acute mania is with lithium carbonate, antipsychotics, or a combination of lithium carbonate and antipsychotics. In general, treatment of acute mania consists of beginning either a benzodiazepine or an antipsychotic drug and instituting lithium carbonate as soon as the patient is willing to take medication orally. The severity of the acute manic disorder and cooperation of the patient are the critical factors in the choice of the antipsychotic drug. For example, patients who are uncooperative in taking oral medication will require intramuscular medication, such as haloperidol or chlorpromazine. Chlorpromazine (Thorazine) can be given in 25 to 50 mg doses intramuscularly every 1 to 3 hours, with careful attention being paid to blood pressure, since orthostatic hypotension often accompanies this route of administration. Haloperidol (Haldol) has been used more recently as an acute antimanic drug and is often given as 5 to 10 mg intramuscularly every 1 to 2 hours. Haloperidol has a great propensity for causing parkinsonian symptoms, which should be treated with antiparkinsonian drugs. Haloperidol has very little effect on blood pressure, and although it is not as sedating as chlorpromazine, manic patients can be successfully sedated with haloperidol. For patients who are more cooperative or whose manic episodes are less severe, thioridazine is an excellent drug in that it has very few blood pressure effects or parkinsonian side effects. The thioridazine dose should not exceed 800 mg per day. Starting doses on the order of 200 to 400 mg per day can be used in combination with lithium carbonate to treat the acute manic episode. Two serious side effects can occur with antipsychotic medication—tardive dyskinesia and neuroleptic malignant syndrome. Therefore, sedating benzodiazepines may be useful to reduce the doses of antipsychotic drugs.

Lithium carbonate is perhaps more effective in treating acute manic episodes than are the antipsychotic agents. However, lithium carbonate cannot be given in an intramuscular form, and thus the patient must be cooperative to be treated with lithium carbonate. Prior to treatment with lithium carbonate it is advisable to have a medical work-up, which would include physical examination, electrocardiogram, thyroid studies, white blood count, urinalysis, blood urea nitrogen, and creatinine. There have been several regimens described for determining the dose of lithium carbonate. These involve giving a "test dose" of 600 to 900 mg of lithium carbonate and determining a blood lithium level at a fixed time thereafter. This blood level is used to select a "therapeutic" dose. In our experience these projected doses often result in a high daily dose being administered to the patient with resulting lithium toxicity. We prefer to start lithium carbonate at 300 to 600 mg the first day and increase the dose daily until therapeutic blood concentrations of lithium result. This method requires frequent blood levels but is safe for the patient and produces fewer acute side effects, such as nausea and vomiting. The therapeutic blood lithium concentration for acute mania is about 1.0 to 1.5 mEq per liter. Blood levels should be taken frequently on hospitalized patients who are undergoing increasing doses of lithium treatment, particularly older patients or patients with borderline renal function. Patients should be examined daily for the presence of lithium side effects, such as nausea, vomiting, diarrhea, or tremor. Signs of neurotoxicity for lithium should also be observed; these would include confusion, gross tremor, ataxia, slurring of speech, and sedation. These neurotoxic symptoms may occur in some patients at doses within the therapeutic range, particularly if the patient is receiving high doses of antipsychotic drugs concomitantly. It is vital that the patient have an adequate fluid and salt intake during lithium treatment because lithium urinary excretion is dependent on sodium metabolism. In many but not all cases, manic symptoms will improve at about 10 to 14 days, at which time the dose of the antipsychotic drug can be tapered. The dose of lithium may also have to be reduced somewhat, as while manic, the patient may be drinking copious amounts of fluid, and this phenomenon will decrease as the mania abates. The physician should be cautioned about premature discharge of the manic patient from the hospital, as insight and judgment seem to be the last manic symptoms to improve in contrast to sleep and activity. Patients who are discharged from the hospital prematurely may stop their medication and have a relapse of manic symptoms. As a general guide, the manic episode has not been completed until the patient enters into a postmanic depressive phase.

Patients who are refractory to lithium treatment may respond to treatment with anticonvulsants such as carbamazepine or benzodiazepines. These compounds, although effective in the treatment of acute mania, have been less studied than lithium or antipsychotic medication.

Lithium Carbonate Maintenance. Prophylaxis of manic episodes is the most striking reason why lithium carbonate became the accepted drug of the 1970s. It was found that the administration of this simple salt on a long-term basis reduced the frequency and intensity of subsequent manic episodes in patients who are prone to bipolar cyclic manic-depressive illness. The maintenance dose is that dose sufficient to produce a blood level of 0.7 to 1.0 mEq per liter. During proper administration of chronic lithium treatment, there are minimal side effects, mainly occasional diarrhea or occasional tremor. A slight polyuria is frequently found, but this is usually not of clinical significance.

There are several medical concerns about long-term administration of lithium. An antithyroid effect is often noted early in the course of administration and can be corrected by giving thyroid supplements if clinical manifestations of hypothyroidism persist. Cardiac effects, especially in older patients, have been noted during lithium treatment. Sinus node dysfunction may be accentuated during lithium therapy. A third effect has been related to severe polyuria and the possibility of renal disease in patients undergoing chronic lithium treatment or who have experienced lithium toxicity. For this reason, patients should have monitoring of medical status, including thyroid tests, blood urea nitrogen, creatinine, and electrocardiogram at least yearly while undergoing lithium treatment. If symptoms develop referable to a primary medical illness, appropriate consultations should be obtained. It should not be too lightly stressed that patients must be carefully monitored during long-term lithium treatment and that it is important to obtain blood lithium levels at least several times a year. Blood

for lithium concentrations should be obtained 8 to 12 hours after a lithium dose. It is best to keep the interval between the patient's taking the medication and the blood level being determined constant from visit to visit. During steady-state lithium treatment, the blood level generally does not vary more than 0.1 mEq per liter, and variations greater than this are probably due to irregularities in the patient's taking the medication. The most likely time for a relapse during lithium treatment is in the initial 6 months of treatment, based on actuarial life table statistics. Patients have a risk of developing an affective episode when starting lithium treatment of about 5 per cent per month through the initial 6 months of treatment, and subsequent to that the risk is about 1 per cent per month. Maintenance lithium treatment for outpatients (who are generally euthymic) is usually initiated with low doses, i.e., one capsule per day. The dose is increased on a weekly basis until the therapeutic blood level is achieved. Patients are generally seen every 1 to 2 weeks initially, and when they are stable, the interval visits can be lengthened to once per month.

While it is clear that lithium has an effect on reducing manic and hypomanic episodes very dramatically in the first year of treatment, its effect against depression in both bipolar and unipolar recurrent depression takes longer to achieve. Recent data suggest that it takes approximately 1½ to 2 years of treatment before the prophylactic effect of lithium against recurrent depression can be statistically demonstrated. However, the data also suggest that there may be subclinical beneficial effects on mild mood states during this initial period. Thus, in starting patients on lithium one should carefully explain that it is likely that they will have recurrent depressions at least for 1 to 2 years in spite of treatment and that these depressions initially may seem as severe as their prior depressions before they began taking lithium. Second, patients should notice a decrease in the frequency and severity of manic and hypomanic attacks, although manic episodes may not be completely obliterated during lithium treatment. Those patients who have had a recurrence of severe manic episodes at least once every 7 years or at least two recurrent depressive episodes in 5 years are candidates for lithium prophylactic treatment. It should also be noted that the prophylactic efficacy of lithium carbonate in unipolar recurrent depression is controversial, although its use has been supported by several research studies. Patients frequently feel well for long intervals during lithium treatment, and some may wish to stop their medication. This should not be advised, since on stopping medication patients tend to return to their previous rate of episodes, and the failure rate on stopping lithium treatment seems to be the same as if the patient never was on lithium treatment.

Although there are few drug-drug interactions with lithium, diuretics should be avoided. Lithium excretion requires sodium, and concomitant diuretic administration often results in lithium retention and can provoke episodes of lithium toxicity. Thus, patients should be cautioned not to change their sodium intake or their sodium metabolism in any way while taking lithium carbonate. Lithium toxicity, in contrast to lithium side effects, tends to be a fairly acute onset illness. Usually, the symptoms occur over a week or so, and these symptoms are characterized by polyuria, confusion, agitation, and tremor and may eventually progress to coma and death. As the patients continue to take lithium they become progressively dehydrated because of polyuria resulting from lithium toxicity. The treatment of lithium toxicity is to stop lithium and to rehydrate the patient, particularly with water, sodium, and potassium.

Rapid-cycling patients who continue to cycle in spite of lithium maintenance therapy may benefit from long-term treatment with carbamazepine or valproic acid. Laboratory tests for blood counts and liver function should be obtained regularly if these compounds are prescribed. Neurotoxicity from the combination of lithium carbonate and carbamazepine has been reported.

Barbiturates and Stimulants. Barbiturates should be avoided as sleeping medications for patients with depression. Barbiturates are totally unneeded for treatment of depressed patients with insomnia because such patients can be treated with a sedating antidepressant such as amitriptyline. In addition, barbiturates tend to activate liver enzymes that metabolize tricyclic antidepressants. Thus, the effect of a barbiturate in combination with a tricyclic antidepressant would be to lower the dose of the antidepressant. Stimulants such as methylphenidate or amphetamine are of only temporary benefit in depression and should be avoided.

Psychotherapy. Although psychotherapy is generally felt to be of importance in the treatment of depression, there has been a considerable change in the emphasis on psychotherapy for depressed patients over the past several years. In the late 1960s in some centers, analytically oriented psychotherapy was considered the treatment of choice for both bipolar and unipolar affective disorders. The efficacy of psychopharmacologic agents resulted in the need for greater specificity and efficacy in the psychotherapies employed for affective disorders.

Educational and supportive psychotherapies are helpful for the depressed patient. It is very important to have the patient understand his illness as thoroughly as possible and to understand the need for and the role of medication and therapy. The patient should be taught to recognize early symptoms and to adjust medication according to agreed-upon guidelines. Decisions that could alter life situations, such as job changes, marital changes, moves, and the like, should be avoided if at all possible until the depression is over. It is important to have the patient try to get out of the house as much as possible, even if only for an hour a day. Physical exercise, such as jogging, may be of benefit to some patients. However, patients should be cautioned that physical exercise is usually of only brief benefit in depression. More specific psychotherapies, such as cognitive-behavioral psychotherapy and interpersonal psychotherapy, have been used successfully with some depressives.

Psychotherapy of a manic patient during such episodes is extremely difficult, as the patient attempts to maintain control of the therapy situation. Family and/or marital therapy may be indicated in some manic patients after remission of the manic episode. A flexible approach to psychotherapy is probably best. Some patients may benefit from certain types of therapy but not other types, and some patients may need little psychotherapy.

SCHIZOPHRENIC DISORDERS

method of
ROBERT CANCRO, M.D.
New York University
New York, New York

The origin of the schizophrenic disorders is unknown. For at least some of the patients, there is evidence of a genetically loaded vulnerability that, if exposed to the appropriate environmental stresses, will cause a decompensation into a schizophrenic psychosis. The vulnerability is an outcome of gene-environment interaction and may or may not be the product of an abnormal gene.

TREATMENT

Psychosocial Treatments

Psychosocial *interventions* in schizophrenia remain important in several ways. The patient and the family need emotional support during the psychotic and postpsychotic states. Patients and families also require encouragement concerning such issues as medication and hospitalization. These kinds of interventions are often best done by the family physician, who is perceived in a more positive and trusting fashion by both the patient and the family. The psychosocial *treatment* of schizophrenia, whether on an individual, group, or family basis, is highly specialized and requires expert administration.

While behavior modification techniques can be helpful, particularly in chronic schizophrenia, they require specialized resources not usually available to the office-based clinician. They are not usually useful in the hands of a general practitioner.

Somatic Treatments

Electroconvulsive Therapy (ECT)

Electroconvulsive therapy has been of limited utility in the treatment of schizophrenia since the advent of the antipsychotic drugs. There are occasional patients who are resistant to or not suitable for medication therapy and who, therefore, are candidates for ECT. The usual course of treatment consists of 20 ECTs administered three times a week. Care must be used in giving repeated courses of treatment. Electroencephalographic monitoring of the treatment is useful. Patients who are resistant to drug therapy are often more responsive to continuing treatment with psychopharmacologic agents after a course of ECT.

Insulin Treatment

Insulin treatment has been dropped almost completely from our therapeutic armamentarium. When administered, it should be done in a specialized hospital facility.

Psychosurgery

The indications for psychosurgical intervention in schizophrenia are indeed rare. For all practical purposes it can be ignored as a treatment method and reserved for the exceptional patient in whom all else has failed and in whom there is an urgent need for symptom control.

Renal Dialysis

The early positive reports on the use of renal dialysis have not withstood carefully controlled clinical studies.

Pharmacotherapy

Under the topic of pharmacotherapy, the principles involved in the use of antipsychotic agents will be included. Megavitamins have not proved to be helpful in the treatment of schizophrenia and will not be discussed. The antipsychotic drugs are not to be considered as anxiolytics. They are substances that have major and diffuse effects on the central nervous system and must be used judiciously and cautiously. There is a bewildering array of antipsychotic agents available, and it is pointless for the physician to attempt to develop expertise in the use of all of them. It is much wiser that several drugs be learned well. At the very least, one should be familiar with a drug from each of the major groups: aliphatic, piperidine, and piperazine phenothiazines; thioxanthenes; butyrophenones; dihydroindolones; and dibenzoxazepines. Widely used agents in these groups are listed in Table 1.

Before instituting therapy with any of these drugs, baseline blood pressure measurements with the patient in both the standing and reclining positions should be recorded. Initial laboratory work-up should include a complete blood count, liver profile, and electrocardiogram in older patients. These tests should be repeated at 6-month intervals.

A comprehensive drug history must be obtained from each patient, including sensitivity, drugs taken in the past, and side effects. Target symptoms and goals should be identified so that dosage can be titrated against clinical response. After maximal control of the target symptoms has been obtained, the patient should be maintained at the lowest effective dose possible for at least 1 year.

Only one antipsychotic agent should be used at a time. It is better pharmacologic practice to use an adequate dose of one drug than inadequate doses of two or more. Homeopathic doses should be avoided, because they expose the patient to the risks of antipsychotic drug treatment without the potential benefits. There is no evidence that any one antipsychotic drug is inherently superior to any other. The consensus is that they all are essentially equivalent clinically if enough medication is given. Drug choice in the absence of a good prior response to a particular agent should be based on side effect profile and cost. Nevertheless, individual responses are sufficiently common that the physician should be familiar with several such compounds. The routine addition of antidepressive or antianxiety drugs to antipsychotic medication is to be sharply discouraged.

Patients who show severe schizophrenic symptomatology should have rapid drug treatment. In the case of hospitalized patients, their control dosage should be reached in 3 to 7 days. There is nothing to be gained by building up the medication levels very slowly. Obviously, if the patient has a history of idiosyncratic drug effects, ar-

TABLE 1. **Antipsychotic Drugs in Common Use**

Generic Name	Trade Name	Type	Daily Dosage Range	Potency Equivalent	Comments
Chlorpromazine	Thorazine	Aliphatic	100–1200 mg	1	High sedation, low EPS
Thioridazine	Mellaril	Piperidine	100–600 mg	1	High Sedation, lowest EPS, a strong anticholinergic agent, inhibits ejaculation, Ca^{++} channel blocker
Perphenazine	Trilafon	Piperazine	8–64 mg	10	Low sedation, high EPS including dystonia
Trifluoperazine	Stelazine	Piperazine	5–30 mg	20	Low sedation, high EPS including dystonia
Fluphenazine	Prolixin	Piperazine	5–20 mg	50	Low sedation, high EPS including dystonia, low hypotensive effect
Thiothixene	Navane	Thioxanthene	6–30 mg	20	High EPS including dystonia, low hypotensive effect
Haloperidol	Haldol	Butyrophenone	4–15 mg	50	High EPS including dystonia, low hypotensive effect
Loxapine	Loxitane	Dibenzoxazepine	50–100 mg	10	High EPS including dystonia, low hypotensive effect
Molindone	Moban	Dihydroindolone	20–250 mg	5	High EPS, lowest weight gain

rhythmia, or hypotension, more care is necessary, and a level of caution must be exercised that is more stringent than that practiced in routine situations. Occasionally megadoses that are in the equivalent range of 2 to 3 grams of chlorpromazine may prove necessary. Such occasions are infrequent and are best handled in concert with a consultant. The refractory patients who may respond to megadoses are usually under age 40 and have spent less than 10 years in the hospital.

Antipsychotic drugs are best administered on a once or twice a day basis after the initial symptoms are controlled. Patients who have a paradoxical reaction and become restless or have difficulty sleeping should be given approximately two thirds of the daily dose in the morning. Most patients who are placed on a twice a day schedule should get at least two thirds of the dose at night and the remainder in the morning. If the patient can tolerate the full dose at bedtime, he or she obtains the benefits with the least feelings of discomfort, particularly drowsiness, dry mouth, and blurred vision. There is no value in the use of sustained-release forms.

It is wise to use medication in parenteral form during early phases of hospitalization when patient cooperation is often low. At least 20 per cent of hospitalized mental patients do not actually take their oral medication. Urine or blood tests can be very helpful in identifying which patients are taking their drugs. It should be remembered that parenteral medication is from two to four times more powerful than the oral form, and the dosage level must be corrected accordingly. Slower acting fluphenazine (both the enanthate and the decanoate forms) is not useful for rapid control of psychotic symptoms because

it takes 2 to 4 days to act. Its use is primarily in the management of patients who cannot be relied upon to take oral medication. There are also situations in which the patient's life circumstances are such that it is more realistic to have him return for an injection than to try to take medication on a daily basis. Antipsychotic agents in liquid form can also be useful in the hospital as a transition from parenteral medication to the tablet form.

Ideally, an inpatient with acute symptoms should have a 6- to 8-week trial on a particular drug before a shift to a different medication can be justified on the grounds of clinical failure. Unfortunately, in an era of reimbursement by diagnosis related groups (DRGs), this may not be possible. Patients with chronic conditions, particularly those whose hospitalization is long-term, may require a 4- to 6-month trial before a particular drug is abandoned. Should the need to change drugs appear, the estimated potency equivalence can be used as an approximate guideline (see Table 1). It is best to decrease one medication over time while adding increasing doses of the second. It is certainly more feasible to change medications abruptly or very rapidly in a hospital setting than it is in an outpatient setting. Drug holidays are no longer in vogue. It is best to maintain the patient at the lowest dose consistent with the best clinical response.

Contraindications. Severe cardiovascular disease is a significant contraindication to antipsychotic medication. Extreme caution is warranted in the face of serious liver damage. The use of these agents in early pregnancy involves a calculated risk.

Side Effects. *Drowsiness* is a common side effect, particularly with the aliphatic and piperidine side chain compounds. Tolerance is rapidly achieved by the patient, and usually at the end of 1 week drowsiness is markedly diminished.

Depression frequently appears as the psychotic symptoms improve with medication. These symptoms are not a consequence of medication and, usually, antidepressant drugs are not necessary. Rather, they reflect an awareness on the part of the patient of the seriousness of the illness. A feeling of despair is a common complication in psychosis, and the use of antidepressant medications should be discouraged because tricyclic antidepressants may worsen the schizophrenic symptomatology. In those situations in which the combined use of antidepressants and antipsychotics is warranted, psychiatric consultation is in order.

Some *skin* side effects may occur. Urticaria, contact dermatitis, and photosensitivity may all appear.

Metabolic side effects may also appear. Weight gain is a frequent side effect of these drugs. Molindone is the drug of choice in patients in whom weight gain is a problem. Weight gain can be a particular problem in young, female patients who stop taking medication out of concern for the changes in their appearance. Rigid dietary management is to be encouraged, and the use of appetite suppressants is strongly discouraged. Other metabolic changes include gynecomastia, galactorrhea, and amenorrhea.

Ocular changes may occur. Pigmentation of the lens and cornea is frequently seen in chlorpromazine therapy, particularly when it is at a high dosage (greater than 2500 mg per day for more than 2 years).

Electrocardiographic changes occur in 2 to 3 per cent of patients and are usually seen as Q and T wave alterations. Dysrhythmias also occur. Syncope is not uncommon and is related to the hypotensive effects of these drugs. Syncope is more of a problem in patients over the age of 40. Thiothixene has the least hypotensive action. Many patients adapt to this side effect fairly rapidly, whereas others must have their dosage reduced.

Jaundice is a possible side effect of all these drugs. They must be discontinued if jaundice develops.

Hematologic changes may occur. Leukocytosis, leukopenia, and eosinophilia are all common. Agranulocytosis occurs only rarely, usually between 4 and 10 weeks after the onset of treatment. Medication must be stopped in the presence of agranulocytosis, but this disorder should not be diagnosed simply because of a reduced white blood cell count. In the presence of a white count below 4000 per microliter or a superimposed infection on a lowered white cell count, agranulocytosis should be assumed. Antibiotics and cortisone must be administered rapidly in the case of an infection.

Extrapyramidal signs (EPS) are a frequent concomitant of antipsychotic drug treatment. They are particularly common in elderly patients, women, and individuals with central nervous system disease. The treatment of choice is with anticholinergic drugs such as benztropine mesylate (Cogentin), 0.5 to 8 mg* per day by mouth. Benztropine mesylate can also be used intramuscularly in a dose of 1 to 2 mg. If there is doubt as to the presence of EPS, then an intramuscular dose can be given; if the symptoms clear within 30 minutes, the probability of their being extrapyramidal in origin is very high. Diphenhydramine (Benadryl) in the dosage of 25 to 50 mg intramuscularly is also useful as a diagnostic test.

Akathisia is a very common manifestation of extrapyramidal involvement and should not be confused with agitation. It most frequently involves the lower limbs and takes the form of regular and rhythmical motor movements, e.g., tapping or rocking. The use of anticholinergic drugs or the reduction in the dosage level of antipsychotic drugs is indicated in the presence of akathisia.

Dystonic reactions are also common and are usually manifested by torticollis and oculogyric crises. The treatment of a dystonic reaction is to reduce the dosage of antipsychotic medication or to add anticholinergic drugs. Anticholinergic drugs should not be given routinely as a prophylactic measure; they should only be used when extrapyramidal side effects appear. They should be given in divided doses because their action is short. After about 3 months, the anticholinergic drug should be reduced and discontinued over approximately 1 week. About 90 per cent of patients who have shown EPS will not continue to do so after this course of medication. The other 10 per cent will show a return of symptoms within 2 to 4 weeks and will require further anticholinergic treatment.

A tricyclic antidepressant has strong anticholinergic effects and can be used as a substitute for antiparkinsonian medication with the constraints indicated earlier. Anticholinergic agents must be used very cautiously or not at all in patients with glaucoma or prostate hypertrophy. Urinary retention is also common with the use of anticholinergic drugs. The tricyclic antidepressants and thioridazine are powerful anticholin-

---

*Exceeds the maximum dose recommended by the manufacturer.

ergic agents, and their combined use is quite risky.

Persistent tardive dyskinesia is a disorder primarily of buccolingual movements. It is particularly common in elderly patients, and there is no established treatment. It is sometimes associated with rapid discontinuance of antipsychotic medication, particularly after prolonged use.

Increased susceptibility to convulsive disorders has been reported with these drugs. All these agents potentiate the effects of central nervous system depressants such as alcohol, anesthetics, barbiturates, and narcotics. They tend to slow the breakdown of tricyclic antidepressants in the body.

Rehabilitation

Virtually all schizophrenic patients require both social and vocational rehabilitation in order to return to effective membership in society. These forms of rehabilitation require specialized facilities.

PANIC DISORDER AND AGORAPHOBIA

method of
MICHAEL R. LIEBOWITZ, M.D.
New York State Psychiatric Institute and
  Columbia University
New York, New York

Imagine yourself walking alone down a dark street at night, and someone comes up behind you in a menacing way. Your heart starts to race and pound, and you find it harder to breathe, your palms get sweaty, and you have a strong urge to flee as quickly as possible. These are panicky feelings but not a panic attack, because the response is appropriate to the situation. Now imagine yourself walking down a broad sunny street chatting with a friend about pleasant subjects, and you begin to feel the same physical and emotional sensations. This is a panic attack.

The importance of panic attacks is that they are a source of great distress to the affected individuals, who usually think they are having a heart attack or going insane. Panic attacks are common; single attacks may occur in 6 per cent of adults, recurrent attacks in 4 per cent, and panic disorder in 2 per cent. Untreated, they lead to agoraphobia, depression, and alcoholism.

History

Panic attacks were first recognized in treatment studies of imipramine in the 1970s. At the same time, British investigators noted the association of phobic anxiety (panic attacks) and depersonalization. Also

around this time phobias were divided into agoraphobia (see following), social phobia (excessive embarassment or anxiety with public speaking or meeting people), and simple phobias (heights, insects). In the 1980 psychiatric classification (DSM-III), the older and broader concept of anxiety neurosis was subdivided into panic disorder and generalized anxiety disorder.

Diagnosis

Panic disorder is characterized in the current DSM-III-R by one or more panic attacks (discrete periods of intense fear or discomfort). At least four attacks must occur within a 4-week period, or one or more attacks must be followed by a month or more of persistent fear of having another attack (anticipatory anxiety). At least four of the following symptoms have to occur rather suddenly during at least one of the attacks: dyspnea; feeling unsteady, dizzy, or faint; palpitations or tachycardia; trembling or shaking; sweating; choking; nausea or abdominal distress; depersonalization or derealization; numbness or tingling; hot flushes or chills; chest pain or discomfort; fear of dying; or fear of going crazy or doing something uncontrolled. The anxiety attacks occur unexpectedly (not immediately before or on exposure to a situation that almost always causes anxiety) to distinguish them from simple phobias. To distinguish the panic attacks from social phobia, the anxiety episodes in panic disorder cannot be triggered by being the focus of others' attention. These distinctions are supported by pathophysiologic and treatment differences. To meet criterion for panic disorder, the anxiety attacks cannot be initiated and maintained by some ongoing organic disturbance such as hyperthyroidism or caffeine or amphetamine abuse. Mitral valve prolapse is frequently associated and does not preclude the diagnosis.

Course

Patients with recurrent panic attacks often become fearful of traveling any distance alone, hence developing agoraphobia. They also fear being places where it is hard to leave or to leave unobtrusively should a panic attack develop, and so begin to avoid theaters (especially nonaisle seats), restaurants, crowded stores, planes, tunnels, bridges, and highway driving. Any activity that resulted in a panic attack, such as driving a car, also becomes feared because of a possible recurrence. Dependency on others often becomes extreme and is especially troubling for people who were once quite independent. Depression and generalized anxiety are frequent complications, as are alcohol and sedative abuse.

Treatment

The essence of treatment is to block the panic attacks. A number of medication regimens have proved highly effective.

Tricyclic antidepressants have had the longest use. Imipramine (Tofranil) is quite effective but must be started at a low dosage because initially it can make panic disorder patients very jittery and nervous.

Start with 25 mg at night for the first 3 days,

then increase the dosage by 25 mg every fourth day. An alternative is to begin with 10 mg and increase by 10 mg every 2 days until 50 mg is reached, then proceed by 25-mg increments. The endpoint is when panic attacks cease, which is usually readily apparent once the therapeutic dose for that patient is achieved. For patients with infrequent panic attacks but substantial phobic avoidance, the dosage can be increased to 150 mg per day, after which the patient should go out alone to test the degree of antipanic blockade. Medically stable patients can be raised to 300 mg per day if needed unless adverse side effects occur. Nonresponders to this dose should have blood levels checked for rapid metabolism, in which case the dose can be raised further. At high doses electrocardiogram and blood pressure monitoring for heart block and postural changes are advisable.

Perhaps 80 per cent of patients with panic attacks will respond to imipramine with full panic blockade. Anticipatory anxiety and travel restrictions may persist even with panic blockade, requiring additional time or exposure-based behavior therapy. Antipanic medication should be maintained for 6 to 12 months after panic is blocked, at which time a cautious tapering can be attempted. Relapse rates are uncertain; we tell patients that a third will remit permanently, a third will relapse at some future point, and the remaining third will relapse on tapering and require further treatment.

Other tricyclics have not been extensively studied, but desipramine (Norpramin, Pertofrane) also seems effective and has fewer anticholinergic side effects.

The older benzodiazepines such as chlordiazepoxide (Librium) and diazepam (Valium) do not routinely block panic attacks in well-tolerated doses. However, alprazolam (Xanax) and clonazepam (Klonopin) seem effective and act more quickly than the tricyclics. Alprazolam can be started at 0.25 mg three or four times per day and increased gradually to 3 to 6 mg* per day as needed for full antipanic blockade. Side effects other than drowsiness are uncommon, but sudden discontinuation of the upper dose range can cause grand mal seizures. Even gradual discontinuation is sometimes poorly tolerated. Clonazepam is longer acting and thus somewhat easier to withdraw but seems to lower mood at times. The dose range is similar to that for alprazolam. These drugs are often used in lower doses adjunctively with the tricyclics.

Monoamine oxidase inhibitors (MAOIs) also effectively block panic attacks but should be reserved for cases that are refractory to other treatments. Phenelzine (Nardil) is indicated if there are symptoms indicating associated atypical depression such as overeating, oversleeping, environmentally responsive dysphoria, or lethargy. Beta blockers are not dramatically helpful, and neuroleptics are not indicated. Fluoxetine (Prozac) seems to block panic attacks but must be initiated very slowly, beginning at 5 mg per day, to avoid increasing anxiety.

Behavioral therapy for panic attacks is now being studied. Procedures aim at reducing acute and chronic hyperventilation through slow abdominal breathing, cognitive retraining to prevent overreaction to disturbing physical sensations, and desensitization to physical arousal through a variety of exposure procedures. Insight-oriented psychotherapy does not seem to relieve panic attacks in many patients.

---

*Exceeds the maximum dose recommended by the manufacturer.

Physical and Chemical Injuries

BURNS

method of
DAVID M. HEIMBACH, M.D.
University of Washington
Seattle, Washington

Each year in the United States approximately 2 million individuals are burned seriously enough to see a physician; about 70,000 of these require hospitalization, and about 7000 die. It has been estimated that more than 90 per cent of burns are completely preventable and are caused by carelessness or ignorance. While prevention of burns is the obvious long-term solution to burn care, advances in the care of burned patients during the past 20 years have been among the most dramatic in all of medicine. The development of specialized treatment centers staffed by highly trained individuals from many disciplines has improved the medical, physical, and psychosocial outlook of the burned patient and has served as a model for care in other complex diseases. As with other forms of trauma, burns frequently affect children and young adults. The hospital expenses and the social costs related to time away from work or school are staggering. Although most burns are limited in extent, a significant burn of the hand or foot may keep manual workers away from work for a year or more, and in some cases may permanently prevent them from returning to their former activity. The eventual outcome for the burned patient is related to the severity of the injury, individual physical characteristics of the patient, the motivation of the patient, and, very importantly, to the quality of the treatment of the acute burn. Because of space limitations, this article will deal only with the initial assessment, initial treatment, and the proper triage of the severely burned patient, and the principles of care for burns on an outpatient basis.

The primary rule for the emergency physician is "Forget About The Burn." As with any form of trauma the "ABCs"—Airway, Breathing, Circulation—must be followed. Although a burn is usually readily apparent and is a dramatic injury, a careful search for other life-threatening injuries must take priority. Only after an overall assessment of the patient's general condition is made should attention be directed to the specific problem of the burns.

TREATMENT

Smoke Inhalation

In the burned patient, the airway and breathing may be compromised by smoke inhalation. Any patient with flame burns that occurred in a closed space who has carbonaceous sputum and a carboxyhemoglobin level in the fire (see following discussion) of greater than 9 per cent is at risk and should be closely watched for progressive airway obstruction or compromise of oxygenation. Anyone suspected of having smoke poisoning should have a set of arterial blood gases drawn. One of the earliest indicators is an improper ratio (P/F ratio) of the arterial PaO_2 to the inspired oxygen concentration (FiO_2). A ratio of 400 to 500 is normal, whereas patients with impending pulmonary problems have a ratio of less than 300 (e.g., a PaO_2 of less than 120 with an FiO_2 of 0.40). A ratio of less than 250 is an indication for vigorous pulmonary therapy. All surgeons agree that in the presence of increasing laryngeal edema, nasotracheal or orotracheal intubation is indicated. A tracheostomy is never an emergency procedure.

Mild cases of smoke poisoning are treated with highly humidified air, vigorous pulmonary toilet, and bronchodilators as needed. Blood gases are drawn at least every 4 hours, and the P/F ratio is calculated. Increasing symptoms, difficulty in handling secretions, and a falling P/F ratio are all indications for intubation and respiratory assistance with a volume ventilator. The decision for hospital admission and the need for specialized care rests on the severity of symptoms from the smoke and the presence and magnitude of associated burns. Any patient who is symptomatic following smoke inhalation and has more than trivial burns should be admitted. If the burns cover more than 15 per cent of the total body surface area (TBSA) (see following discussion), the patient should probably be referred to a special care unit.

Carbon Monoxide Poisoning

Carbon monoxide (CO) poisoning is the most common cause of death in fires and may be a source of long-term morbidity in survivors. Carbon monoxide has an affinity for hemoglobin 200 times that of oxygen, and reversibly displaces oxygen on the hemoglobin molecule. Carboxyhemoglobin levels are reported as the percentage of hemoglobin bound to CO and are easily measured in the emergency room. Levels less than 10 per cent do not cause symptoms and may be found in heavy smokers or in people living in polluted cities. At levels of 20 per cent, healthy persons complain of headache, nausea, vomiting, and loss of manual dexterity. At 30 per cent, they become confused and lethargic and may show depressed S-T segments on the electrocardiogram. In a fire, this level may lead to death as the victim loses both the interest in and the ability to flee the smoke. At levels between 40 per cent and 60 per cent the patient lapses into coma, and levels much above 60 per cent are usually fatal. In very smoky fires, levels of 40 to 50 per cent may be reached after only 2 to 3 minutes of exposure.

Carbon monoxide is reversibly bound to the heme pigments and enzymes and, despite its intense affinity, readily dissociates according to the laws of mass action. The half-life of carboxyhemoglobin in room air is between 4 and 5 hours. In an individual breathing 100 per cent oxygen, the half-life is reduced to 45 to 60 minutes. Thus, a patient seen in the emergency room after 1 hour on 100 per cent oxygen who has a carboxyhemoglobin level of 10 per cent can be assumed to have had levels of greater than 20 per cent in the fire. There is clear agreement that all patients burned in an enclosed space or having any suggestion of neurologic symptoms should be administered 100 per cent oxygen while awaiting measurement of carboxyhemoglobin levels. This should be instituted in the field by the paramedics, using a tight-fitting mask or, when necessary, endotracheal intubation if the personnel are adequately trained in tube insertion. Anecdotal reports of spectacular successes with hyperbaric oxygen treatment have never been subjected to a scientific study.

Burn Severity

Prognosis and all treatment plans, including initial resuscitation, are directly tied to the size of the burn. A general idea of burn size is provided by the "Rule of Nines." Each upper extremity accounts for 9 per cent of the total body surface area (TBSA); each lower extremity accounts for 18 per cent; the anterior and posterior trunk each accounts for 18 per cent; the head and neck account for 9 per cent; and the perineum accounts for 1 per cent. While the Rule of Nines provides a reasonably accurate estimate of burn size, a number of more precise charts have been developed and are available in nearly every emergency room. For smaller burns an accurate assessment can be made of burn size by using the hand of the patient. The palmar surface, including the fingers, amounts to 1 per cent of the TBSA.

Burns are classified by increasing depth as First Degree, Superficial Dermal, Deep Dermal, Full Thickness and Fourth Degree.

First Degree Burns

First degree burns involve only the epidermis. First degree burns do not blister. They become erythematous because of dermal vasodilation, and they are quite painful, both spontaneously and when touched. Over 2 to 3 days both the erythema and the pain subside. By about day 4 the injured epithelium desquamates in the phenomenon of "peeling," which is known to everyone following a sunburn.

Superficial Dermal Burns

Superficial dermal burns include the upper layers of dermis and characteristically form blisters with fluid collection at the interface of the epidermis and dermis. Blistering may not occur for some hours following injury, and burns originally appearing to be first degree may, in fact, be diagnosed as superficial dermal burns after 12 to 24 hours. Once blisters are removed the wound is pink and wet and is quite painful as currents of air pass over it. The wound is hypersensitive, and the burns blanch with pressure. If infection is prevented, superficial dermal burns will heal spontaneously in less than 3 weeks and will do so with no functional impairment. They rarely cause hypertrophic scarring, but in pigmented individuals the healed burn may never completely match the color of the surrounding normal skin.

Deep Dermal Burns

Deep dermal burns also blister, but the wound surface is usually a mottled pink and white color immediately following the injury. The patient complains of discomfort rather than pain. When pressure is applied to the burn, capillary refill occurs slowly or may be absent. The wound is often less sensitive to pin prick than the surrounding normal skin. By the second day the wound may be white and is usually fairly dry. If infection is prevented, such burns will heal in 3 to 9 weeks, but invariably do so with considerable scar formation. Unless active physical therapy is continued throughout the healing process, joint function may be impaired and hypertrophic scarring, particularly in pigmented individuals and children, is common.

Full Thickness Burns

Full thickness burns involve all layers of the dermis and can heal only by wound contracture, by epithelialization from the wound margin, or by skin grafting. Full thickness burns are classically described as being leathery, firm, depressed when compared with adjoining normal skin, and insensitive to light touch or pinprick. Unfortunately, the difference in depth between a deep dermal burn and a full thickness burn may be less than a millimeter. Full thickness burns can masquerade with many of the clinical findings of a deep dermal burn. Like deep dermal burns they may be mottled in appearance. They rarely blanch on pressure, and they may have a dry, white appearance. In some cases the burn may be translucent with clotted vessels visible in the depths. Some full thickness burns, particularly immersion scalds, may have a red appearance, and can be confused by the uninitiated with a superficial dermal burn. They can be distinguished, however, because these red, full thickness burns do not blanch with pressure. Full thickness burns develop a classic burn *eschar*. An eschar represents the structurally intact but dead and denatured dermis that, over days and weeks, will separate from the underlying viable tissue.

Fourth Degree Burns

Fourth degree burns involve not only all layers of the skin but also subcutaneous fat and deeper structures. These burns almost always have a charred appearance, and frequently only the etiology of the burn gives a clue to the amount of underlying tissue destruction. Electrical burns, contact burns, and burns sustained by patients who are unconscious at the time of burning may all be fourth degree.

While these descriptions appear to separate burns nicely into categories, many burns have a mixture of characteristics, giving the observer a very imprecise diagnostic ability. Considerable research is currently underway to devise instruments that will more precisely diagnose the depth of injury. Much of current burn treatment depends upon knowledge of the depth of the burns.

Electrical Burns

Electrical burns are in reality thermal burns from very high intensity heat. Electricity as it meets the resistance of body tissues is converted to heat in direct proportion to the amperage of the current and the electrical resistance of the body parts through which it passes. The smaller the size of the body part through which the electricity passes, the more intense the heat and the less the heat is dissipated. Therefore, fingers, hands, forearms, feet, and lower legs are frequently totally destroyed by high voltage current (>1000 volts), whereas larger volume areas, like the trunk, usually dissipate the current enough to prevent extensive damage to the viscera, unless the entrance or exit wound is on the abdomen or chest. Although cutaneous manifestations may appear limited, the skin injury is only the tip of an iceberg, as massive underlying tissue destruction may take place.

Electrical burns cause a particular set of other injuries and complications that must be considered during initial evaluation. Injuries related to a fall are common. The intense associated muscle contractions may cause fractures of the lumbar vertebrae, humerus, or femur, and may dislocate shoulders or hips. Electrical cardiac damage may present in a similar manner to a myocardial contusion or infarction. Alternatively, the conduction system may be deranged; in some cases, actual rupture of the heart wall or rupture of papillary muscle, leading to sudden valvular incompetence and refractory cardiac failure, can occur. Household current at 110 volts generally either does no damage or induces ventricular fibrillation. If the patient has no cardiac abnormalities that are detected in the emergency room following shocks of 110 to 220 volts, the likelihood that they will appear later is small; if the initial electrocardiogram is normal, the patient can usually go home. However, we believe that patients with higher voltage exposure should be admitted and their cardiac state monitored for 24 to 48 hours.

Chemical Burns

Chemical burns, usually caused by strong acids or alkalies, are most often the result of industrial accidents, drain cleaners, assaults, and the improper use of harsh solvents. In contrast to a thermal burn, chemical burns cause progressive damage until the chemicals are inactivated by reaction with the tissue or dilution by flushing with water. Although individual circumstances vary, acid burns may be more self-limiting than alkali burns. Acid tends to "tan" the skin, creating an impermeable barrier that limits further penetration of the acid. Alkalies, on the other hand, combine with cutaneous lipids to create soap and thereby continue "dissolving" the skin until they are neutralized. A full thickness chemical burn may appear deceptively superficial, clinically causing a mild brownish discoloration of the skin. The skin may appear to remain intact during the first few days postburn, and only then begin to slough spontaneously. Unless the observer can be absolutely sure, chemical burns should be considered deep dermal or full thickness until proved otherwise. Initial treatment consists of copious rinsing with tap water for as long as 30 minutes—this should be encouraged at the site of the accident before transport to the emergency room. Patients with chemical burns of the eye should have a copious saline lavage until the pH of the eye returns to normal.

Burn Resuscitation

All patients with dermal or full thickness burns greater than 15 per cent TBSA should be considered candidates for intravenous fluid replacement to prevent the decreased plasma volume that is a universal accompaniment of the capillary permeability resulting from the burn. Because of its simplicity, its ease in administration, and its need for little blood chemistry monitoring, the formula developed by Baxter, known as the "Baxter" or "Parkland" formula, has been adopted by most hospitals. The Baxter formula recommends the administration of crystalloid as Ringer's lactate solution (or equivalent) during the first 24 hours while the capillaries are still permeable to albumin, and colloid-containing solutions should be given during the second 24 hours after the capillary leak has presumably sealed. The formula calls for the administration of 4 ml of Ringer's lactate solution per kg of body weight for each 1 per cent of body surface burned during the first 24 hours post-injury. One half of this fluid should be given in the first 8 hours and the second half during the next 16 hours. Fluid therapy during the second 24 hours consists of the administration of free water in a quantity sufficient to maintain a normal serum sodium concentration, and plasma (or other colloid) in order to maintain normal vital signs and urine output.

The Baxter formula is merely a guideline, and adjustments in fluid rate are made based on the clinical response of the patient. The adequacy of resuscitation can be judged by frequent measurements of vital signs, hourly urine output, and observation of general mental and physical response. Despite the myriad of new monitoring devices, urine output remains one of the most sensitive and reliable assessments of fluid resuscitation. A urine output of 30 to 50 ml per hour in adults and 1.5 ml per kg per hour in children assures that renal perfusion is adequate. The patient should be alert and cooperative; confusion and combativeness are signs of inadequate resuscitation or warn of other causes of hypoxia.

Other Considerations

Paralytic ileus is a common accompaniment of burns greater than 20 per cent TBSA. In all such patients a nasogastric tube should be placed and gastric contents evacuated. Burns are tetanus-prone wounds. The need for tetanus prophylaxis is determined by the patient's current immunization status. The treating physican should follow the recommendation of the American College of Surgeons. All medications administered during the "shock phase" of burn care should be given intravenously. Subcutaneous and intramuscular injections are undependably absorbed and should be avoided. Pain control is best managed with small intravenous doses of morphine, usually in the range of 2 to 5 mg, given every 5 to 10 minutes until pain control is adequate without affecting blood pressure.

All patients undergoing intravenous resuscitation should have a Foley catheter placed for hourly monitoring of urine output. Arterial lines may be useful in patients who will need frequent blood gas determinations or repeated blood sampling; however, necessary laboratory work during the resuscitation phase is relatively minimal. Blood for baseline chemistry studies should be drawn. Only if major operative procedures, such as fasciotomy or multiple escharotomies, are contemplated should it be necessary to type and cross match blood. Blood gas determinations are mandatory in any patient with a suspected inhalation injury, and arterial pH measurement is useful as an assessment of the overall treatment of shock. If the Baxter formula is used for resuscitation, frequent electrolyte determinations are not necessary since they will remain in the normal range.

The blood glucose level is commonly elevated because of the glycogenolytic effect of elevated catecholamines, the gluconeogenic effect of elevated glucococorticoids, elevated glucagon, and relative insulin resistance. This well-described form of "stress diabetes" can become a problem in normal patients if glucose-containing solutions are given during resuscitation, and it frequently becomes a serious problem in patients with preexisting diabetes. All diabetic patients require careful monitoring of blood and urine glucose levels, and most will need supplemental insulin during resuscitation.

Psychosocial care should begin immediately. The patient and family must be comforted, and a realistic outlook regarding the prognosis of the burns should be given, at least to the patient's family. In house fires, loved ones, pets, and many or all possessions may have been destroyed. If the family is not available, some member of the team, usually the social worker, should find out the extent of the damage in hopes of being able to comfort the patient. If the patient is a child and if the circumstances of the burn are suspicious, physicians are required by law to report any suspected case of child abuse or neglect to local authorities.

Burn Severity—Transfer Protocols

Severity of injury is proportionate to the size of the total burn, the depth of the burn, the age of the patient, and associated medical problems or injuries. Burns have been classified by the American Burn Association and the American College of Surgeons Committee on Trauma into categories of minor, moderate, and severe. Moderate burns are defined as partial thickness burns of 15 to 25 per cent TBSA in adults (10 to 20 per cent in children); full thickness burns of less than 10 per cent TBSA; and burns that *do not* involve the face, hands, feet, or perineum. Because of the significant cosmetic and functional risk, all but very superficial burns of the face, hands, feet, and perineum should be treated by a physician with a special interest in burn care in a facility that is accustomed to dealing with such problems. Major burns and most full thickness burns in infants, the elderly, or in patients with associated disease or injuries should also be cared for in a specialized facility. Patients with moderate burns can be cared for in a community hospital by a knowledgeable physician as long as the *other* members of the health care team have the resources and knowledge to ensure a good result. Newer techniques of early wound closure have made burn care more complex, and an increasing number of patients with small but significant burns are being referred to specialized care facilities to take advantage of these concepts.

The criteria for admission of patients with minor and moderate burns to the hospital vary according to physician preference, the patient's social circumstances, and the ability to provide close follow-up care. In rare circumstances, patients with superficial burns as large as 15 per cent TBSA can be successfully managed as outpatients. In other circumstances, patients with burns as small as 1 per cent TBSA may require admission because of the patient's inability or unwillingness to care for the wound. In general, the physician should have a low threshold for admission of elderly patients and infants. Any patient (child or adult) in whom abuse is suspected *must* be admitted.

Once an airway is established and resuscitation under way, burned patients are eminently suitable for transport. Resuscitation can continue en route, and, for the most part, the patient will remain stable for several days. This was well proved during the Viet Nam war; military burn victims were first transported from Viet Nam to Japan, and then from Japan to the military Burn Center in San Antonio, Texas. The transport was generally accomplished during the first 2 weeks post-burn, and very few complications occurred in over 1000 patients transferred.

Hospitals without specialized burn care facilities should decide where they will refer patients, and work out transfer agreements and treatment protocols with the chosen Burn Center well in advance of need. If this is done, definitive care can begin at the initial hospital and continue without interruption during transport and at the Burn Center. In general, transfer should be from physician to physician, and contact should be established between them as soon as the patient arrives in the emergency room of the initial hospital. The mode of transport, and the arrangements for procuring it, should be well known to all involved.

Treatment of Burns in Outpatients

Using the guidelines described earlier, the severely burned patient should be stabilized and well on his or her way to get optimal care. However, the vast majority of patients who sustain burns do not require hospitalization at all. In many cases, the burn, if merely kept clean, heals spontaneously in less than 3 weeks with acceptable cosmetic results and no functional impairment. Unfortunately, good results in treating superficial minor burns may entice the unwary physician to treat more complex burns by the same methods. For the patient, the consequences of such a mistake can be unnecessary hospitalization, joint dysfunction, hypertrophic scarring that may be difficult to correct, and loss of considerable time from work or school.

First Degree Burns

Although first degree burns are very painful, victims rarely seek medical attention unless the area burned is extensive. These patients do not require hospitalization, but control of the pain is extremely important. Aspirin or codeine may be adequate for small injuries, but for large burns, liberal use of a more potent narcotic for 2 to 3 days is indicated. For topical medication we recommend one of the many proprietary compounds containing extracts of the aloe vera plant in concentrations of at least 60 per cent. Aloe vera has some antimicrobial properties and is an effective temporary analgesic. Anecdotal evidence suggests that it may decrease subsequent pruritus and peeling.

Burns from ultraviolet rays (sunlight, sunlamp) may initially appear to be only epidermal, but the injury may in fact be a superficial dermal burn with blistering apparent only after 12 to 24 hours. Therefore, the patient with such a burn should be cautioned about blisters and should be asked to return if they form, since wound management then becomes more important because of the potential for infection and subsequent scarring.

Superficial Dermal Burns

Treatment of superficial dermal burns presents little problem. If the wound is kept clean, the patient is kept comfortable, and the joints are kept active, these wounds heal in less than 3 weeks with minimal scarring and no joint impairment.

Initially, the wound should be cleansed and gently débrided, with loose skin removed. Small blisters may be left intact. Larger blisters are difficult to protect, and blister fluid is a reasonable culture medium for bacteria that live in the skin appendages. Therefore, blisters should usually be totally removed with forceps and scissors. In some instances, the blister fluid can be aspirated with a large-bore needle, allowing the blistered epidermis to remain on the wound as a biologic dressing. This dead epidermis, however, is fragile, tends to contract, and rarely stays in place except over small areas. After débridement, these wounds are ideally managed with a biologic dressing such as porcine xenograft (pig skin). Pig skin is available frozen or treated with gluteraldehyde, permitting a long shelf life. Once applied the burn pain is markedly diminished, and if the xenograft "sticks," no further treatment is necessary except for a periodic wound check. When the burn reepithelializes, the xenograft desiccates and peels away from the new epidermis. Other synthetic dressings, such as those made from plastic film (Op-Site or Epigard), or those with composite materials (Biobrane), have achieved some popularity, but the author has little experience with them.

The most common treatment is wound coverage with silver sulfadiazine and a light dressing. Some very small burns do not require topical agents. For small facial burns, antibiotic ointment may be a better choice than silver sulfadiazine cream, because it is less drying. Our home-treatment regimen is to have the patient cleanse the wound daily with tap water and reapply the topical agent and a light dressing. During dressing changes, and as often as possible, all involved joints should be put through a full range of motion. The dressing may be unnecessary while the patient is at home, but we recommend that the patient dress the wound before leaving the house. This method is highly successful, but it is inconvenient and the dressing changes may be fairly painful, requiring good patient cooperation.

If a biologic or synthetic dressing is chosen, we generally give the patient an oral anti-staphylococcal antibiotic for 5 to 7 days, since these dressings have no antibacterial action of their own. Pain is managed as with first degree burns, and the patient usually should return every 2 to 3 days until the wound heals or the patient has demonstrated the ability to manage the wound without supervision.

Deep Dermal and Full Thickness Burns

Treatment of these burns is a matter of much graver concern than treating superficial burns. Full thickness burns heal only by contraction and epithelialization from the periphery. Epithelium does not begin to migrate until the eschar is removed; the growth rate then is only about 1 mm per day. Thus, healing of even a small full thickness burn may involve many weeks of discomfort and disability. Deep dermal burns may take 4 to 8 weeks to heal and then leave an unacceptable scar. If a joint is involved, some loss of joint function is the rule rather than the exception. Thus, we have adopted a policy of early excision and grafting for such wounds.

Initial outpatient treatment can be followed by elective surgery as soon as it can be scheduled. Small wounds can be treated through day surgery; larger wounds over dynamically important areas can be closed with only a day or two of hospitalization. The excision and grafting procedures should be done by a surgeon experienced in burn wound excision. We believe that the advantages of this aggressive approach—a pain-free patient with normal joint function, a better cosmetic result, and a rapid return to work or school—more than compensate for the brief hospitalization and the very small risk associated with minor operation.

Should the excision and grafting plan not be acceptable to the patient or the treating physician, the standard method of daily cleansing and application of silver sulfadiazine cream is used. Most full thickness burns eventually need grafting at about 3 to 4 weeks. Deep dermal burns should be seen by the physician frequently during the healing process; active physical therapy is crucial to ensuring a successful outcome.

DISTURBANCES DUE TO COLD

method of
C. MEL WILCOX, M.D., and
THOMAS W. SHEEHY, M.D.
University of Alabama at Birmingham
Birmingham, Alabama

The major entities associated with cold injury are frostbite, nontropical immersion foot, and hypothermia. Each of these entities may exist alone or in combination. Immersion foot results from cold stasis and ischemia. The tissue is not frozen. Frostbite results when the tissue is frozen. Hypothermia is a systemic manifestation of multifactorial etiology defined as a core body temperature below 35° C (95° F).

Local cold injuries are classified into two major types: (1) *frostbite*, the acute freezing injury and (2) *immersion foot*, the nonfreezing injury.

FROSTBITE

Frostbite has been classified into three types: mild (frostnip), superficial, and deep. The last two classifications are largely descriptive of the late results of frostbite and are of little help to the clinician who first sees the patient.

The major pathophysiologic events causing frostbite and triggered by freezing temperatures are vasospasm and extracellular ice-crystal formation. Tissue damage follows in their wake. Freezing temperatures lead to local and reflex arterial and venous constriction, increased venous pressure, decreased capillary perfusion, erythrocyte sludging, thrombus formation, and finally tissue ischemia. The latter is fostered by extracellular ice-crystal formation, which increases the extracellular osmotic gradient leading to intracellular dehydration, enzyme destruction, and death unless the condition is relieved.

Factors relative to the extent and severity of frostbite include (1) the degree of cold exposure, (2) the duration of cold exposure, (3) wind speed, (4) immobilization, (5) race, and (6) lack of acclimatization and proper clothing. Peripheral vascular disease and drugs (e.g., alcohol and tobacco) have been cited as additional factors.

The Degree of Cold Exposure. At −25° C (−13° F), the skin temperature drops to subfreezing levels within 1 minute. The majority of frostbite cases occur at temperature ranging from −4° F to 10° F and after 6 to 12 hours exposure.

The Duration of Cold Exposure. Prolonged exposure to subfreezing levels enhances the chance for frostbite.

Wind Speed. As it increases at a constant ambient temperature, the amount of body heat lost by convection increases. At an ambient temperature of 10° F, a wind speed of 20 miles per hour results in an equivalent temperature on exposed flesh of −25° F. Wind chill is helpful in predicting the risk of injury to exposed flesh.

Immobilization. In the Korean conflict, 67 per cent of 1000 patients with cold injury were immobilized by enemy fire, riding in open vehicles, or sleeping in foxholes.

Race. Blacks are several times more susceptible to cold injury than whites, as are individuals born in subtropical or tropical climates.

Lack of Acclimatization and Proper Clothing. Thorough weather education, acclimatization, and proper clothing are essential for individuals who must spend considerable time outdoors in frigid weather. Factors that increase susceptibility to the cold such as age must also be given consideration.

Chilblains

Chilblains is a very mild form of cold injury that is classically seen in young women, who present with red, tender, pruritic areas of involvement that blanche with pressure. Swelling is common.

Treatment

Therapy consists of local measures such as heat and massage and application of lubricants to prevent breaks in the skin. Prevention is important and is best accomplished by keeping the hands and legs warm and dry at all times.

Frostnip

Frostnip (mild frostbite) affects areas such as the nose, ears, fingers and toes and other exposed body parts. Initially, it leads to a feeling of severe cold with progression to numbness and pain. A distinct "ping" has been described at the time of extracellular water crystallization. The skin is red but not distorted.

Treatment

Usually, warming the affected tissue, relief from the cold, and removal of wet clothing are ample treatment.

Superficial and Deep Frostbite

Superficial frostbite affects the skin and upper subcutaneous tissue. The skin becomes waxy white in appearance and is cold to the touch. *Deep* frostbite involves the skin, subcutaneous tissue, and muscle. Progression from superficial to deep can be assumed when the patient's sensation of cold discomfort is replaced by a feeling of warmth in the affected part. The flesh becomes hard and cold to the touch, bluish gray in color, and painless. The fingers and limbs lose their dexterity and with continued cold exposure become paralyzed. Finally, when freezing occurs, the cold-induced anesthesia obliterates all awareness of these changes.

Treatment

Patients with frostbite should be managed in a facility that is capable of offering definitive care. Thawing is to be avoided in the field unless evacuation is imminent. It should be discouraged if refreezing is a possibillity, because freeze-thaw-freeze injuries lead to extensive tissue loss.

Rapid rewarming is the pivotal point of definitive therapy. The frozen part should be immersed in a circulatory water bath or simply placed in a plain tub or basin at water temperatures ranging from 38° to 42° C (101° to 109° F). Thawing within this temperature range leads to less tissue loss than thawing at 37° C or lower. If a thermometer is not available, warm water comfortable to the normal hand may be used.

The clinical effects of the pathologic changes occasioned by freezing become obvious during the rewarming period. Signs of thawing appear after 15 to 30 minutes at the above temperatures, with complete thawing occurring within 30 to 60 minutes. With thawing there is a gradual return of sensation to the frozen tissue. Unfortunately, this is not a reliable end point.

With deep frostbite, throbbing pain of marked severity develops and a narcotic may be necessary. As the tissue warms, it assumes an erythematous reddish color indicating vasodilatation and reestablishment of the circulatory flow. Swelling or edema develops as a result of the increased capillary fragility and/or vascular thrombosis. Within a period of 30 to 60 minutes, a demarcation line develops separating revascularized from avascular tissue. Warming is stopped when this line fails to progress.

Clear blisters may form shortly thereafter or may not appear until 12 to 36 hours later. Blisters should be left intact and not débrided unless they have ruptured spontaneously. Early débridement is to be discouraged because it increases tissue loss and enhances the chance for infection. Usually, the intact blisters dry into hard black eschars within 1 to 2 weeks. The appearance of multiple, large hemorrhagic blisters on thawing indicates severe and deep tissue injury.

Unfortunately, the final depth of the serious frostbite injury cannot be assessed with any certainty until after the appearance of gangrenous demarcation. Recently, scintigraphy with technetium-99m pertechnate has been found helpful in differentiating viable from nonviable tissue.

Daily hydrotherapy is useful for cleansing the tissue and for general débridement of superficial sloughing tissue. It also aids the circulation and encourages limb motion. Following whirlpool therapy, the tissue should be gently blotted dry to avoid abrading fragile tissue and to decrease the chances for tissue infection. Lamb's wool, cotton pledgets, or sterile gauze is used to separate injured digits. Sterile dressings are applied to those areas in need of protection from injury. Hands should be bandaged with fluffy gauze, and arms should be placed in a functional position and elevated to decrease edema. Bed rest is essential to avoid further tissue injury if the feet or lower extremities are affected. Cradles are used to keep the sheets and covers from touching affected parts.

Therapy for severe frostbite is painful, expensive, and lengthy. Mummification, or gangrenous demarcation, requires 60 to 90 days. Occasionally, spontaneous amputation occurs, obviating the need for surgical removal. Débridement must always be conservative to avoid premature removal of potentially viable tissue. When amputation is necessary, reconstructive surgery may be necessary, along with continued rehabilitation and physiotherapy. For planning purposes, these facts should be brought to the attention of both the patient and the family early in the treatment course.

Analgesics may be necessary for pain and mobilization of joints. Frostbite injuries are susceptible to infection, and antibiotics are used for specific and, when possible, cultured infections. Prophylactic and topical antibiotic usage has not been efficacious. Aseptic techniques in management are essential. Normally acceptable indications govern the use of tetanus toxoid.

Clinical trials with the anticoagulant heparin and low molecular weight dextran have not been efficacious. These agents have usually been given to patients after thawing and during the period of potential thrombosis. In contrast, when they were given to experimental animals prior to rewarming, these agents were considered helpful by some but not all investigators. Data are not available on the use of thrombolytic agents in frostbite. However, aspirin, 324 mg twice daily, plus dipyridamole, 50 mg twice daily, has been given to patients prior to thawing because of their known platelet-inhibitory effects.

IMMERSION FOOT

Immersion foot (trench foot or lifeboat leg) occurs with prolonged exposure of the feet to wet but not freezing cold. Water conducts heat 25 times faster than air; hence, the colder the water, the more rapid the onset. Unlike frostbite, the vascular tissue is not irreparably damaged. The primary cause of injury is severe and prolonged vasoconstriction. Therefore, the muscles and nerves are affected earlier than is the skin.

Cold-induced vasoconstriction leads to tissue ischemia manifested locally by cold, numb feet that become pale and pulseless as the condition evolves. The situation is made worse by dependency, stasis, constriction by footwear, and dehydration. The resulting vascular injury causes the feet to become red, swollen, and painful. Sensory and motor deficits may develop that later may cause muscle atrophy or vasomotor instability. The injured tissue is prone to infection, and cellulitis and wet gangrene are common.

Treatment

Rewarming is essential, but at much lower temperatures than used for treatment of frostbite.

Room temperature is adequate. This is a critical point because overheating the tissue during the ischemic phase may enhance thrombus formation and lead to extensive injury, even to gangrene. The feet should be kept elevated to reduce edema and to prevent further vascular injury. Blebs should be left intact and not débrided unless they have ruptured spontaneously. Physiotherapy is encouraged for more severe cases in order to restore muscle and vascular tone.

Antibiotics are given early when there is extensive tissue sloughing because of the propensity for infection in this condition. Anticoagulants are used only if there is evidence of thrombophlebitis or subsequent thrombosis. Surgical intervention is conservative and is used primarily for superficial débridement or relief of strictures.

HYPOTHERMIA

Hypothermia can be defined as a central or core body temperature (CBT) of 35° C (95° F) or less. Classification has been based on either the etiology or the severity of the hypothermia. Three forms of hypothermia have been distinguished etiologically: (1) *immersion hypothermia* results when cold stress exceeds maximum body heat production (e.g., in inadequately clothed snow skiers); (2) *exhaustion hypothermia* results from depletion of the body's readily available energy sources (e.g., in long-distance runners); and (3) *subclinical hypothermia* results from impairment of the central thermal regulatory center and occurs frequently in the elderly.

Exposure is a common denominator for all types of hypothermia, although the duration may be quite brief. Based on the depression of CBT, hypothermia can also be classified as mild (CBT of 90° to 95° F, or 32° to 35° C), moderate (CBT of 86° to 89° F, or 30° to 32° C), and severe (CBT below 86° F, or 30° C).

Pathophysiology

The general physiologic responses to cold are governed by peripheral afferent thermorecepters, which send stimuli via the spinal thalamic tracts to the temperature-regulatory center in the anterior hypothalamus. This center coordinates and controls CBT. From here, impulses are sent to the sympathetic nervous system, the extrapyramidal tract, and the anterior pituitary gland. Stimulation of the autonomic nervous system increases the heart rate, vasoconstricts the dermal blood vessels, and vasodilates muscle blood vessels. Extrapyramidal tract stimulation induces shivering, leading to vasodilation of muscular arteries. Thyroxine and corticosteroid release are increased indirectly, due to stimulation of the anterior pituitary gland. Through these complex mechanisms, body heat loss is decreased and heat production increased.

Etiology

The predisposing conditions for hypothermia are numerous. When prolonged exposure is excluded, especially in the elderly, patients should be evaluated carefully for evidence of an acute process such as an infection or central nervous system lesion. A careful drug history should also be elicited.

Clinical Manifestations

All patients in whom the diagnosis of hypothermia is suspected should have the temperature recorded with a high rectal thermometer to ensure an accurate reading. With mild hypothermia, the skin is pale and cold to the touch. Shivering may be present unless this response is lost because of age. As the CBT falls further, the "slowing phase" of hypothermia ensues, manifested by decreases in respiratory rate, heart rate, cardiac output, and blood pressure. Altered mentation occurs when the CBT declines to 86° F (30° C), and neurologic deficits such as hyperreflexia and decreased pupillary light reflexes may be observed. When the CBT approaches 80.6° F (27° C) a rigor mortis–like appearance develops even though the patient is still alive.

Treatment

General Supportive Care

Given the high mortality rate, especially in the elderly, moderate to severe hypothermia should be considered a medical emergency and treatment must not be delayed. All wet clothing should be removed, and the patient should be placed in a warm room and wrapped in blankets or other insulating material. The pulse may not be palpable or blood pressure may not be obtainable owing to bradycardia, especially with a CBT less than 86° F (30° C). The rectal temperature should be taken and monitored continuously. A thorough physical examination should be undertaken to look for evidence of a precipitating cause.

A Foley catheter should be placed to monitor urine output. Intravenous access should be in a peripheral location; however, a central venous line may become necessary in the elderly when vigorous fluid resuscitation is needed. The central line catheter should not enter the heart, as myocardial stimulation may precipitate ventricular fibrillation.

Initial laboratory studies should include serum electrolytes, glucose, creatinine, complete blood count including platelets, urinalysis, and an arterial blood gas measurement. A chest radiograph should be obtained, as aspiration pneumonia is not uncommon.

A dextrose-containing crystalloid solution, preferably normal saline, should be administered initially at 150 ml per hour, since volume depletion is a constant finding. Naloxone and thiamine should be given; steroids are not indicated unless adrenocortical failure is suspected. Broad-spectrum antibiotics are controversial, but again can be given if indicated by clinical suspicions.

Oxygen should be given after the blood gas measurement is obtained. Since the respiratory rate may be low but sufficient to support the lowered metabolic requirements, endotracheal intubation should not be done unless apnea or severe hypoxia is present. If intubation is needed, the patient should be ventilated and oxygenation improved prior to the procedure; this will reduce the possibility of ventricular irritability from the stimulation of endotracheal intubation. Acid-base balance is also critical and should be monitored frequently until the patient is stabilized.

Cardiovascular Considerations

Careful attention to the cardiovascular system is paramount. The initial electrocardiogram will dictate appropriate interventions and should be monitored continuously in an intensive care unit. Prolonged Q-T interval, bradycardia, and Osborn or J waves (positive deflection in the left ventricular leads at the junction of the QRS and ST segments) may be seen and are correlated with the degree of hypothermia; these abnormalities will become attenuated as the CBT is normalized.

Atrial fibrillation may occur with a CBT of 28° to 32° C (82° to 89.6° F); spontaneous ventricular fibrillation is common at a CBT less than 28° C (82° F) and can be induced by cardiac stimulation or irritation. If asystole or ventricular fibrillation is the initial cardiac rhythm, cardiopulmonary resuscitation (CPR) should be instituted in the usual fashion. Although the hypothermic heart is relatively unresponsive to electrical countershock, atropine, lidocaine, and electrical pacing, each of these resources should be instituted accordingly when required. However, if no effect is realized, CPR should be continued until the CBT is 30° to 32° C (86° to 89.6° F); defibrillation may become effective at this point. The patient should not be pronounced dead until the CBT has been increased to 30° to 32° C (86° to 89.6° F).

Rewarming Techniques

The most important therapy involved in both the initial and continued management of the hypothermic patient is rewarming. A variety of methods have been utilized with different degrees of practicality, efficacy, and safety. In any case, the technique employed should depend on the severity of the hypothermia. *Passive external rewarming* is the traditional method and consists of placing the patient in a warm room and covering him or her with blankets. Warmed intravenous fluids may also be used. Fluids can be warmed in a water bath, in a microwave oven, or with a warming sleeve. In this fashion, the patient warms at his or her own pace using the heat generated by the body. This method provides gradual rewarming (0.5° C or 0.9° F per hour) and should be the primary technique for warming those with mild hypothermia. Although moderate to severe hypothermia may warrant more aggressive maneuvers, many patients with severe hypothermia have been successfully managed with passive external rewarming alone.

Active rewarming techniques can be divided into external and core rewarming. *Active external rewarming* consists of using hot water bottles, electric blankets, or even immersion in hot water (40° to 45° C or 104° to 113° F). Although effective, this method is not without risk. Cutaneous vasodilation may result from active external rewarming, leading to hypotension, myocardial ischemia, and shunting of cool blood to the myocardium, resulting in arrhythmias. Thus, this technique should be used cautiously in the elderly and those with an already compromised circulation; however, its use in younger patients may be of less risk.

Active core rewarming is the most aggressive form of rewarming and should be reserved for those with moderate to severe hypothermia. Proponents of active core rewarming claim that this approach provides preferential warming of the myocardium, leading to an increase in cardiac output, a decrease in cardiac irritability, and a rapid return of CBT to normal. It must be remembered, however, that these invasive procedures may cause cardiac irritability and ventricular fibrillation. Techniques are numerous and include inhalation of heated oxygen, peritoneal dialysis or hemodialysis, partial cardiac bypass, and irrigation of the stomach, colon, and mediastinum. Heated humidified oxygen can raise CBT by 1° F per hour; this is useful and of low risk and thus should be done. Peritoneal dialysis is equal in efficacy to partial cardiac bypass; however, peritoneal dialysis is probably the procedure of choice, given its availability in most institutions. Although the active core rewarming techniques have been used successfully in the elderly, these methods (other than heated humidified oxygen) should be considered only in those with severe hypothermia and cardiac instability.

Follow-up

Once hemodynamic stabilty and rewarming have been achieved, attention must be directed to associated frostbite, trauma, and premorbid disease. Volume status and acid-base and electrolyte balance should be monitored. Continued vigilance for infection, especially pneumonia, must be maintained, as this complication is common after recovery. In the elderly, a tendency to recurrent hypothermia is common.

DISTURBANCES DUE TO HEAT

method of
T. MICHAEL HARRINGTON, M.D.
The University of Alabama
Birmingham, Alabama

Heat-related fatalities occur more commonly than deaths due to any other natural phenomenon in the United States. From 1962 to 1986, 1000 to 2000 excess deaths per year in this country were attributable to heat. In comparison, during the same 25-year period the annual rate of deaths due to flooding was 151; 94 deaths per year resulted from lightning, 87 from tornados, and 31 from hurricanes. The 1980 heat wave in the southwestern United States claimed over 1265 lives. In July 1987, in Greece, 878 people died during a 6-day heat wave when daily temperatures approached 115° F.

Physiology

An understanding of heat physiology is essential for the adequate treatment of the heat-related disorders. Homeostatic mechanisms limit the human temperature range to 96.5° to 99° F. This narrow range is essential for proper bodily functions and enzymatic processes. There is a constant interchange between heat production and heat loss maintained through complex hormonal, caradiovascular, renal, and neural influences. The largest producers of heat in the human body are the muscles. Muscles produce heat through exercise or shivering. However, the body remains only 25 per cent efficient in fuel consumption, with 75 per cent of metabolic energy converted into heat. Without *any* ability to lose heat the human body would increase core temperature by 1° C (1.8° F) every 5 minutes.

Heat loss is largely accomplished by four separate mechanisms: radiation, convection, conduction, and evaporation. Radiation is the photon emission of electromagnetic energy from the skin and accounts for approximately 50 per cent of heat loss. Convection is heat transfer to an air current, and conduction is heat loss by direct contact. These mechanisms account for about 15 per cent of the body's heat loss. Evaporation (conversion of a liquid to a vapor) is responsible for around 25 per cent of heat loss. Several other factors account for the remaining 10 per cent, such as loss in stool and urine. When ambient temperature exceeds skin temperature (92° F), radiation, convection, and conduction are largely nonoperative. In addition, when relative humidity exceeds 60 per cent, heat loss by evaporation is reduced, and there is very little heat loss when the relative humidity exceeds 75 per cent.

It becomes clear then that in a hot, humid environment, the body's heat loss mechanisms are largely impaired. Any cardiovascular, renal, neural, or endocrine abnormality that hinders the body's capacity to dissipate heat compounds the situation.

HEAT CRAMPS

Heat cramps, also known as miner's, stoker's, logger's, or fireman's cramps, are incapacitating but *not* life-threatening. They generally occur in an acclimatized individual during or after heavy labor. The diagnosis is suspected when the large muscle groups of the abdomen or legs sustain severe cramps occurring during or after exercise. The patient's temperature and vital signs are normal, the skin is moist, and there are no central nervous system (CNS) symptoms (Table 1). Pathophysiologically, there is sodium loss in excess of water loss.

The treatment of choice is oral hydration with salt water. This can be easily made with a teaspoon of salt added to 500 to 1000 ml of water. This is a simple, safe, and effective treatment. Alternatively, normal saline via an intravenous route can be used, but generally is not necessary. It is important to have the patient liberally salt his or her food for the next 2 to 3 days and recognize that residual soreness may be present for 24 to 48 hours.

Current recommendations do not include use of salt tablets. Adverse effects of salt tablets include gastric pooling of oral fluid, vomiting, and potassium depletion. At times salt tablets remain undigested and pass through the gastrointestinal tract with little or no therapeutic benefit.

HEAT EXHAUSTION

Heat exhaustion is also known as heat prostration and heat collapse. This is the most common heat disorder. The diagnosis is suspected when the patient develops nausea, vomiting, dizziness, or a headache. The patient may also be confused or disoriented. Occasionally muscle cramps may intervene. Vital signs can vary from normal to elevated pulse and a normal or low blood pressure. Body temperature may be elevated, but is less than 104° F.

Pathophysiologically, both salt and water are depleted in the patient. At times salt depletion is in excess of water depletion, and at other times the reverse is true. There are some clinical differences between heat exhaustion with salt depletion (hypotonic) and heat exhaustion with water depletion (hypertonic), yet these distinctions have minimal significance for treatment.

Treatment includes moving the patient to the shade, removing any constricting garments, and keeping him or her recumbent. Oral hydration with salt and water is adequate if the patient is conscious and the airway is maintained. If this is not achievable, then intravenous hydration with either hypotonic or isotonic solution can be used. The patient should be hospitalized if he or she is elderly, has another chronic disease, or has a severe case of heat exhaustion. If there is *any*

TABLE 1. **Signs, Symptoms, and Treatment of Heat Disorders**

	Vital Signs	Central Nervous System Symptoms	Skin Signs	Treatment
Heat cramps	Temperature: usually normal Blood pressure: normal Pulse: usually normal	None	Sweaty	Oral salt replacement, outpatient
Heat exhaustion	Temperature: less than 104° F Blood pressure: normal to low Pulse: elevated	Headache Nausea Dizziness Confusion	Sweaty or cool and clammy	Oral or IV salt and water replacement, outpatient or inpatient
Heat stroke	Temperature: greater than 104° F (often 106°–108° F) Blood pressure: low, normal, or high Pulse: elevated	Seizure Delirium Coma	Hot and dry (classic) Sweaty (exertional)	Rapid cooling ICU admission

concern whatsoever about heat stroke, that would constitute a clear-cut need for hospitalization.

HEAT STROKE

Heat stroke is also known as heat pyrexia, sun stroke, or siriasis. Heat stroke is a true medical emergency. It is generally accepted that therapy must be instituted within 30 minutes to make an impact on the disease. Mortality ranges from 10 to 80 per cent depending on other factors, most notably the patient's age, general health, and other chronic diseases.

The diagnosis is entertained when a patient has significant CNS dysfunction coupled with extreme hyperthermia. The CNS disturbance may present as seizures, delirium, or coma. The skin can be hot and dry (classic heat stroke) or moist (exertional heat stroke). Blood pressure can be normal, elevated, or decreased, and the pulse is generally normal or elevated. Temperature is greater than 104° F, and the 106° to 108° range is not unusual. (The highest recorded temperature in a surviving patient was 115.7°.)

There are important differences in presentation between classic and exertional heat stroke that are worthy of discussion. Classic heat stroke is typically found in an older patient after a 3- to 5-day prodrome of headache, nausea, lassitude, and confusion. It is often found during a heat wave in the summer months. The differential diagnosis would include other CNS disorders, stroke, sepsis, and other causes of shock, but the key feature is the extremely elevated core temperature.

Exertional heat stroke is more commonly found in the young, active patient and with no prodrome. It is more typically found in the military recruit or the athlete. Pathophysiologically there is total hypothalamic and/or sweat gland failure. There is a complete inability to lose body heat.

Primary Treatment

The fundamental treatment for acute heat stroke is rapid cooling. The patient should be removed to a cool, shady area and his or her clothing should be removed. Ice packs, ice bags, or iced sheets or towels can be placed on the patient if available. Fans will promote evaporation and aid cooling. The airway should be secured, oxygen supplied, and intravenous access established. A Foley catheter and nasogastric tube may be used; however, they can be inserted later in the hospital. En route to the hospital, the patient should be splashed or cooled with cold water and either the windows of the vehicle left open or the air conditioning turned on to provide the coldest environment for transportation.

The optimal and recommended method of cooling is total immersion in an ice bath with active muscle massage. This is the most reliable, time-honored, and effective method. The patient is placed in a tub of ice and water and a minimum of four people actively and vigorously massage the skeletal muscles and extremities. Muscle massage is critical to prevent vasoconstriction and paradoxical temperature rise. It will also promote effective heat exchange.

In many larger hospitals, the physical therapy department has a whirlpool tank that is quite adequate. Ice can be delivered from the cafeteria. In the smaller community hospital, an emergency facility should have the availability of a large tub (a small rubber boat or children's wading pool works nicely) and a planned means of securing ice for the tub. Body cooling units are being developed that deliver a cool mist and a fan for rapid cooling by evaporation, yet these should be considered investigational and are not universally available. Ice bath massage remains the only specific treatment for heat stroke.

The core temperature should be monitored with a rectal probe and the patient removed from the tub when the temperature reaches 101° F. This will prevent overcooling of the patient with subsequent hypothermia. If shivering due to the ice bath presents a major problem (and thus increases heat production) small doses of chlorpromazine, 25 to 50 mg intravenously, can be used.

Hospital Care

Once the temperature is reduced, attention is directed toward the complications of heat stroke. Organ systems that may sustain damage include the CNS, cardiac, respiratory, renal, hepatic, pancreatic, and skeletal muscle systems. Several laboratory tests should be ordered on admission to assess for organ damage (Table 2).

Central nervous system problems include seizures and cerebral edema. Seizures can be controlled in the acute setting with small doses (5 to 10 mg) of intravenous diazepam (Valium). Cerebral edema can be managed with mannitol (12.5 to 25 grams intravenously) and careful fluid management.

Cardiac manifestations include hypotension and myocardial damage. While not all patients with heat stroke are hypotensive and volume-depleted, many are. The volume-depleted patients usually respond well to volume replacement guided by monitoring of urine output and central venous pressure (CVP). If fluid resuscitation is not completely successful, an intravenous drip of dopamine or isoproterenol drips may be used.

Respiratory complications include pulmonary edema. This can result from myocardial damage or fluid overload from overhydration. Monitoring is done with physical examination and central venous pressure (CVP) readings. Management

TABLE 2. **Initial Laboratory Assessment for Heat Stroke**

Complete blood count (CBC) with platelet count
Blood urea nitrogen (BUN), creatinine
Creatine phosphokinase (CPK), serum glutamic-oxaloacetic transaminase (SGOT), serum glutamic-pyruvic transaminase (SGPT), bilirubin
Electrolytes, glucose
Prothrombin time (PT), partial thromboplastin time (PTT)
Amylase, arterial blood gases, serum lactate
Chest x-ray, electrocardiograph
Urinalysis

includes careful fluid resuscitation, diuretics, and digitalis as for classic pulmonary edema.

Renal complications include acute tubular necrosis and myoglobinuria. Extensive rhabdomyolysis can occur secondary to heat stroke. The resulting colored urine is related to the myoglobin pigment from the muscle destruction. Myoglobin is thought to be nephrotoxic, at least in part resulting from a direct toxic affect on the renal tubule. Therefore, adequate renal blood flow should be maintained. Furosemide (Lasix) and mannitol are used to minimize renal damage. Early dialysis might be carried out in some situations.

Hepatic, pancreatic, and skeletal muscle damage is monitored with liver function tests and measurements of amylase levels and total creatine phosphokinase (CPK). Damage to these systems is managed supportively. Disseminated intravascular coagulopathy (DIC) may appear within the first 48 to 72 hours. Prothrombin time (PT), partial thromboplastin time (PTT), and platelet counts are used to monitor for DIC. Treatment is supportive.

Steroids or antibiotics are not indicated for the general care of the heat stroke patient. Their use would be predicated upon a specific indication only.

PREVENTION

It is apparent from this discussion that an "at risk" population can be defined and preventive measures should be employed prior to the onset of one of the heat disorders. Athletes, laborers, and military personnel are at risk when working in a hot environment. Obese and nonacclimatized people are at risk. The elderly patient is at risk owing to reduced cardiovascular ability to respond to a heat challenge. A large group of medications impair an individual's ability to respond to heat. Anticholinergics, phenothiazines, tricyclics, and antihistamines can all promote hypohidrosis. Dehydration is aggravated by diuretics. Alcohol and drug withdrawal promote increased muscular activity (and thus increased heat). Vasoconstrictors decrease cutaneous blood flow, and myocardial reserve is reduced by beta blockers. Finally, hot, humid, and windless days add to everyone's risk.

Anyone working or exercising in a warm environment should have adequate acclimatization. This is generally achieved after 10 to 14 days of gradually acclimatizing to the heat. There are definite renal and hormonal adaptations made to the heat. Salt and water conservation mechanisms are enhanced, and the sweating apparatus is modified so that there is more extracellular fluid volume for sweating. Sweating can increase up to two and one-half times. Under aldosterone influence salt and water are conserved at the kidney and sweat gland level. After acclimatization it is still necessary to maintain hydration. The best solution for this is cool or cold water. Cold water is more rapidly absorbed from the gastrointestinal tract, and solutions with high concentrations of electrolytes and sugar are generally not needed (one exception to this might be the endurance athlete, such as the marathon runner or bicycle racer). In addition, hypotonic solutions empty more rapidly from the stomach than isotonic or hypertonic solutions. Other common-sense approaches would be to wear light-colored and loose-fitting clothing, to avoid the midday heat, and to pay attention to the temperature-humidity index provided by the National Weather Service. Temperature-humidity indexes, wet-bulb thermometers, and wet-bulb globe thermometer (WBGT) indexes all provide useful information for predicting and avoiding heat disorders.

SPIDER BITES AND SCORPION STINGS

method of
PHILIP C. ANDERSON, M.D.
University of Missouri—Columbia
Columbia, Missouri

The principal mischief in the diagnosis and treatment of spider bites results from erroneously considering all necrotic infarcts of the skin to be spider bites. Real spider bites are single, seasonal, and seldom dangerous. Far more likely to cause trouble are infections, focal vasculitis, artifacts, emboli, and the much more common stings or bites of the Hymenoptera (bees, wasps, hornets) and of ticks, fleas, mites, and some other arthropods. Perhaps a dozen species of spiders can inflict a tender, sometimes necrotic lesion in skin, but of North American spiders, only the bite of *Loxosceles*, the infamous Missouri brown recluse spider, causes major necrosis of skin and severe systemic disease.

Reports by patients that a spider bit them are more often erroneous than true, and the physician must be skeptical, considering the season, local environment, and the proved density of *Loxosceles* spiders in that neighborhood.

Recovery of the actual biting spider adds precision to what is usually only a presumptive diagnosis. Lacking such recovery, a careful search of the locale should recover additional recluse spiders. Consultants employed to find and identify spiders should be bona fide experts, not enthusiastic amateurs. If an arachnid is recovered, it should be preserved carefully on cotton in 90 per cent ethanol for expert verification. (Recovered spiders suspected of causing loxoscelism can be sent to us* for expert identification by our staff entomologist, by arrangement, for physicians only, and at no cost. Several agencies can assist.)

SPIDER BITES

Brown Recluse Spider

Between the Eastern mountains and the arid plains of Kansas and Nebraska, in the South Central plains, bites of *Loxosceles reclusa* are common enough to study. Within 2 to 6 hours a bite may cause extensive, painful, rapid necrosis of the skin (cutaneous loxoscelism), but systemic loxoscelism is a rare complication. This systemic disease is a sudden hemolysis with intravascular coagulation, sudden renal failure, confusion, coma, and perhaps even death, although no reports of deaths have been proved and published.

The diagnosis of systemic loxoscelism is best made early by finding hemoglobin in the urine or by laboratory documentation of the early signs of a consumptive coagulopathy.

Treatment

Overtreatment, often surgical, seems to be the main source of disability following cutaneous loxoscelism. Treatment should be conservative and should include prompt rest, cooling and padding the injury, elevation and splinting, and excellent hydration of the patient. Ordinarily, antibiotics are not needed, but tetanus immunization should be ensured. Hasty, wide excisions are ill-advised, of unproven value, and unnecessary.

Follow-up is important. If hemolysis develops, the routine procedure practiced in your hospital for consumptive coagulopathy should be employed. Such treatment usually includes hydration; prednisone, 100 mg daily (adult); coagulation monitoring; and sometimes heparin. Caution about transfusion is important. If the patient is seen long after hemolysis and renal function is lost, peritoneal dialysis may be necessary, and during coagulopathies it is preferable to hemodialysis. The venom is rapidly inactivated in tissue, so the overall strategy is to reverse or limit the secondary effects of the initial venomous injury while nature cures the patient. If loxoscelism is uncommon in your community, seek expert advice.

Even when the necrotic site of the spider bite is large and ugly, débridement and grafting are not necessary, as demonstrated in our very large experience. Natural healing is excellent. Early

*Department of Dermatology, University of Missouri—Columbia, Columbia, MO 65212.

skin grafts often fail entirely because envenomation causes poor wound healing. The worst cosmetic results I have seen have been from hastily excised and grafted presumed bites.

Prevention

Prevention of bites is a matter of interest. For several reasons, pesticides cannot be used safely to rid a building of spiders. Spiders will re-enter buildings readily. *Loxosceles* prefers to avoid humans and therefore shaking out shoes, towels, and bathrobes is of some benefit. Immunity to spider venom is known in animals and humans. How extensive the protection is in humans has not been studied, but it appears to suffice. Among Missourians who know the spider and the bites well, severe second bites are rare.

Black Widow Spider

An understanding of the severe envenomation by a different arachnid, the Sydney funnel web spider (*Atrax robustus*), is needed to understand the very mild variant which is lactrodectism (the bite of the black widow spider) in North America. Compared to ataxotoxin, the venom of the black widow spider is only a moderately potent neurotoxin that does not induce necrosis in skin or systemic hemolysis. Healthy adults almost never react severely to it. Children may experience painful muscle spasm, parasthesias, hypertension, abdominal discomfort, heart irregularities, salivation, agitation, confusion, or even coma within 10 to 90 minutes after a bite; more often, the reaction is milder and brief.

The physician should not be gullible about a report of a bite by a black widow spider but should consider other neurologic or psychiatric disorders as well as infectious and metabolic ills until the details of the report are better known. Most reports of lactrodectism are not well proved.

Treatment

Most real envenomations respond quickly to sustained intravenous infusions of calcium gluconate, beginning with 50 ml of a 10 per cent solution given slowly, with intermittent doses of a benzodiazepine. Intramuscular calcium gluconate is not advisable, especially in infants and children. Recurrences of symptoms and signs after 48 hours ought not occur. The need for tetanus toxoid ought not be neglected. Antivenin is available for the rare severe envenomation but may be of little help once the illness has progressed and unnecessarily risky if given routinely for mild bites. Children, the very elderly, and persons with hypertensive disease or other medical conditions of risk need special attention, including hospitalization and possibly antivenin.

SCORPION STINGS

The natural habitat of the dangerous species of scorpion in the United States is Arizona and New Mexico, but they can appear unexpectedly in neighboring states, and even in the Northern urban centers, because people keep strange pets.

Scorpions are arthropods, like spiders, and have a similar neurotoxic venom. The exquisitely poisonous scorpions of legend are found in India and Africa and, it is hoped, are never pets. Almost all stings of scorpions in the United States prove to be harmless. In the United States, bad scorpion stings are very rare. Within hours after a true sting the area of skin is red and painful.

Treatment

A pressure dressing is worth more and is much safer than ice packs or tourniquets. Avoid morphine, epinephrine, and antihistamines. Calcium gluconate and diazepam are not helpful. For the rare severe sting, correct therapy includes atropine, phenobarbital, and even antivenin. Expert advice is valuable because this disease is rare today.

SNAKEBITE

method of
SHERMAN A. MINTON, M.D.
Indiana University School of Medicine
Indianapolis, Indiana

Poisonous snakes exist in most tropical and temperate lands. Nearly all belong to two families, the Elapidae, which include the cobras, mambas, coral snakes, kraits, and numerous Australian snakes, and the Viperidae. One subfamily of the latter, the pit vipers, includes the rattlesnakes, neotropical lanceheads, Asian habus, and several others; the other, the Old World vipers, includes the puff adder, Russell's viper, and the saw-scaled vipers. Of minor importance are the Hydrophidae or sea snakes and an unknown number of species in the family Colubridae, which includes more than half the world's snakes. Snakebite as a medical problem is greatest among agricultural peoples in Third World nations. In the United States and Europe, it is of minor importance and often is associated with deliberate contacts with venomous snakes. Pit vipers, the copperhead, cottonmouth, and 15 species of rattlesnakes, cause most of the snakebites seen in the United States.

Snake venoms contain numerous biologically active substances, some of which are enzymes and others nonenzymatic polypeptides. Among them are proteases (endopeptidases), found mostly in viperid venoms and accounting for much of their hemorrhagic and necrotizing activity; arginine ester hydrolases, which contribute to hypotensive and anticoagulant activity;

phospholipase A, which is associated with myolytic activity; and hyaluronidase, which facilitates spread of venom in tissues. Polypeptide toxins of elapid and sea snake venoms have pre- and postsynaptic blocking activity at the neuromuscular junction. Other toxins originally described as hemolysins and cardiotoxins actually are toxins with wide activity against cell membranes. It must be emphasized, however, that effects of snake envenomation result from many venom components acting in concert. The classification of venoms as neurotoxic, hemorrhagic, or myotoxic is usually an oversimplification. Also, venoms of many snake species show individual, ontogenic, and geographic variation in their properties.

First Aid

Numerous measures have been advocated in both medical and popular literature. Those with some claim to effectiveness attempt either to remove venom mechanically or to localize its effects. Local application of cold by ice or chemical refrigerants is ineffective in reducing venom activity and may add cold injury to that done by venom. Ligatures and constricting bands on extremities used alone or in conjunction with chilling or incision and suction do inhibit absorption of some venoms and venom components, but their potential for increasing local damage, particularly under field conditions, is great. Excision of the area around a snakebite has not proved effective and carries unacceptable risk. High-voltage, low-amperage electric current applied to the area of a bite has not been adequately evaluated and cannot be recommended at present. However, some type of first aid is desirable for the individual bitten by a venomous snake in a situation where definitive medical help will be delayed an hour or more. The pressure-immobilization technique involves application of a wide elastic bandage (Ace or Coban) bound as tightly as for a sprained ankle to cover as much as possible of the bitten limb. The limb is then immobilized with a splint. Bandage and splint are left in place until a medical facility has been reached, the patient's condition has been evaluated, and definitive treatment, including establishment of an intravenous line, has been initiated. This procedure effectively localizes venom and does no damage if the bite is not accompanied by envenomation. However, local damage produced by venoms of pit vipers and other species may be increased. The "Sawyer Extractor" is a small, hand-held vacuum device capable of producing a negative pressure of one atmosphere. It is packaged for field use. It is applied to the fang punctures without incision or use of a ligature. When it is used within 5 to 15 minutes, appreciable amounts of venom can be removed.

Evaluation in the Emergency Room

This involves (1) differentiation of snakebite from wounds made by thorns and other inanimate objects, (2) differentiation of snakebite from arthropod stings and other injuries by animals, (3) differentiation of snakebite with envenomation from snakebite without envenomation, and (4) differentiation of mild envenomation from envenomation likely to result in death or serious injury.

With injuries by inanimate objects, pain and swelling are usually proportionate to mechanical damage and are not progressive. Arthropod bites and stings rarely bleed, and puncture wounds are difficult to detect. One or more tooth punctures, often with profuse and persistent bleeding, are nearly always seen with snakebites. Number and pattern of puncture wounds is of little value in differentiating venomous from nonvenomous snakebites or in determining the size of the snake inflicting the bite. Local pain, swelling, and discoloration often begin within 10 minutes following a snakebite with envenomation and tend to progress. However, pain may be difficult to evaluate if the patient is badly frightened or under the influence of alcohol or drugs. Swelling in serious envenomation may occasionally be difficult to detect during the first hour. Measurement of circumference at corresponding points on the bitten and unbitten limb should be made. With bites by coral snakes, sea snakes, and a few other species, tooth punctures are very small and there are no local signs of envenomation. Tenderness of regional lymph nodes can often be detected within an hour after a snakebite and is a reliable indicator of envenomation. Nausea, vomiting, sweating, thirst, muscle fasciculations, tingling of the face, and metallic taste are common symptoms of systemic envenomation by North American pit vipers. Evidence of cranial nerve palsy, particularly ptosis and dysphagia, are early signs of envenomation by snakes with neurotoxic venoms. With cobra envenomation, these may appear within 30 minutes; however, a delay of several hours may be seen with coral snake bites. With bites by sea snakes and a few Australian elapids, muscle pain remote from the bite and dark urine due to myoglobinuria are the first definite signs of envenomation.

Although it is impossible to anticipate all eventualities, four general situations are usually seen:

1. The injury can definitely be ascribed to an arthropod, other animal, or inanimate object. Treatment appropriate for the situation is administered.

2. The snake is identified as nonvenomous or circumstances strongly suggest such; for example, if the bite was inflicted outdoors in a locality where venomous snakes do not occur naturally,

and the patient is without symptoms of envenomation. In these cases treatment appropriate for the mechanical damage should be given. The patient can be sent home with orders to return immediately if unexpected symptoms develop.

3. The snake is identified as venomous and tooth punctures are present. There is slight to moderate pain plus swelling and discoloration not extending more than 10 to 15 cm from site of bite. No systemic symptoms are present, and vital signs are normal. The patient should be observed for 12 to 24 hours, preferably in the hospital. Routine laboratory values, including coagulation parameters, should be obtained. Symptomatic treatment is indicated without use of antivenom. The patient can be discharged if asymptomatic at the end of the observation period. If symptoms worsen and progress during the observation period, more definitive therapy must be initiated.

4. The snake is identified as venomous and tooth punctures are present. There is slight to intense pain; swelling and discoloration spread 10 to 15 cm beyond the site of the bite within 2 hours; and regional lymph nodes are tender. Systemic symptoms and signs of envenomation are present. The patient should be admitted to the hospital, preferably to an intensive care unit. Two No. 18 French intravenous lines should be established in uninjured extremities with crystalloid solution or 5 per cent dextrose in water. Appropriate antivenom must be obtained. A particularly difficult situation occurs when snakebite is suspected but the snake was not seen or not identified. In the absence of a rapid and specific ELISA for venom, careful observation of the patient for signs and symptoms of snake envenomation for at least 12 hours is the best management. Treatment corresponds to that for the apparent degree of envenomation. Detailed knowledge of the local snake fauna is often helpful. In the United States nearly all envenomations by free-living snakes are due to pit vipers.

Laboratory

Routine procedures include urinalysis, hemoglobin count, hematocrit, leukocyte count, blood typing and crossmatching, serum electrolyte measurements, and a coagulation profile including platelet count, prothrombin, partial thromboplastin time, and fibrinogen and fibrin split product levels. In systemic envenomation, coagulation parameters may change markedly, and determinations should be repeated every 6 to 8 hours for the first 24 to 48 hours after admission. An electrocardiogram should be obtained in patients age 45 or older. Serum levels of creatine phosphokinase and lactic dehydrogenase are markedly elevated in snakebite patients with myonecrosis, and this may sometimes be helpful in differential diagnosis. ELISA tests for detection of snake venoms are generally available in Australia and are under development in some other nations. Venom is most readily detected in aspirate from tissue around a suspected fang puncture, serum, and concentrated urine. Such tests can help in differentiating snakebites from other envenomations and in determining the type of snake responsible.

Antivenoms

Antivenoms prepared from serum of hyperimmunized horses are produced by about 50 laboratories worldwide. Antivenoms may be monovalent against venom of one snake species (but often effective against closely related species) or polyvalent against several species, usually of a particular geographic area. Antivenin Crotalidae Polyvalent (Wyeth Laboratories) is generally available in the United States and is effective against venoms of all North American pit vipers. Eastern coral snake antivenin produced by the same manufacturer is available in states where this coral snake occurs. Zoos are the best source of antivenoms for bites by nonnative snakes. Consultation should be obtained regarding type of antivenom and dose.

Antivenoms in adequate dosage usually neutralize life-threatening systemic effects of snake venoms; they are less effective against local effects. There are no firm indications for initiating antivenom therapy. With pit viper bites the indications for antivenom include hypotension or markedly unstable blood pressure; abnormal coagulation parameters combined with bleeding gums, hemoptysis, hematuria, or melena; widespread fasciculations; diarrhea; or angioneurotic edema. Ptosis, oculomotor palsy, and dysphagia are early signs of neurotoxic envenomation. However, with some bites such as those of coral snakes or kraits, antivenom should be started before signs of envenomation appear. In the United States, a preliminary skin test for horse serum sensitivity should be done, although a negative test does not ensure that anaphylactoid reactions will not occur, nor does a positive test indicate they will be inevitable. Antivenom diluted 1 to 10 with crystalloid or glucose solution is given intravenously over a 15- to 30-minute period. Five vials (50 ml) is the initial dose for North American pit viper antivenom; repeat doses of 40 to 50 ml may be given every 30 to 60 minutes if needed. Dilution should be reduced for children to avoid fluid overload. Bolus injection of antivenom is not recommended. The total response of the patient rather than a single parameter should determine the quantity of antivenom given. Doses to 400 to 500 ml may be necessary. Antivenom is most effective if begun within 4 hours after a bite; however, some venom effects, including coagulopathy, may be reversed after more than 24 hours. Epinephrine 1:1000 in a syringe should be available when antivenom infusion is begun, and 0.3 to 0.5 ml should be administered subcutaneously for acute anaphylaxis. A positive skin test for horse serum is a relative contraindication to antivenom. If gravity of envenomation makes administration of antivenom mandatory, the patient should be given a subcutaneous dose of 0.3 ml epinephrine and 50 to 100 mg diphenhydramine hydrochloride (Benadryl) intravenously before administration of antivenom. Some 70 to 80 per cent of patients receiving antivenom develop serum sickness, which responds to conventional management.

Surgical Procedures

Marked swelling is common with pit viper bites. Usually this is comparatively benign and subsides in 48 to 72 hours without sequelae. However, with deep injection of venom, a compartment syndrome is possible. If intracompartment pressure measured with a wick catheter reaches 30 mmHg, surgical consultation should be obtained and fasciotomy considered. When intense swelling affects the hand, a digit dermatotomy from the web distally should be performed. Incisions are packed open for 24 hours, and secondary closure is not done.

Supportive Treatment

Intravenous fluids are usually necessary in the early stages of envenomation, and intake should be adequate to maintain a urinary output of at least 50 ml per hour in adults. In viper envenomation with severe blood loss into tissues and externally as indicated by low red cell count and hemoglobin count, whole blood transfusion is indicated. Profound thrombocytopenia may require infusion of 4 to 6 units of platelets, and hypofibrinogenemia may require 2 to 4 units of fresh frozen plasma or up to 12 units of cryoprecipitate. Adequate antivenom usually corrects coagulopathy, however.

Impending respiratory paralysis from venom neurotoxins may be difficult to reverse with antivenom. Artificial respiratory support and tracheostomy may be required for several days. Edrophonium hydrochloride (Tensilon) counteracts the neuromuscular blocking action of cobra venom more rapidly than antivenom, although its action is temporary. The intravenous dose is 0.25 mg per kg with 0.6 mg of atropine sulfate. It may be followed by neostigmine methyl sulfate, 25 micrograms per kg per hour. Antivenom may be used concomitantly. Effectiveness of this regimen against other snake venoms with neurotoxic activity (coral snake, krait, mamba, etc.) has not been established.

Renal failure in snakebite may be secondary to hypovolemia, disseminated intravascular coagulation, myolysis, or unknown factors. Dialysis and correction of electrolyte imbalance follow conventional lines. Permanent renal damage is rare.

Pain in snakebite may be severe enough to require analgesics such as meperidine hydrochloride (Demerol), 50 mg intravenously or intramuscularly repeated at 3- to 4-hour intervals. In many cases less potent analgesics suffice. Salicylates should be avoided because of anticoagulant effect. Oral diazepam (Valium), 5 to 10 mg repeated at 3- to 4-hour intervals if necessary, may be given for anxiety.

Prophylactic antibiotic therapy is not recommended unless circumstances, such as necrosis around the bite or deep incisions made with a probably contaminated instrument, make infection highly likely. Ampicillin and cephalosporins are suitable. Culture and sensitivity should determine the choice of an antibiotic for infections developing after a snakebite. These are uncommon and usually are caused by gram-negative organisms. Appropriate tetanus prophylaxis is mandatory even with minimal envenomation.

ACUTE POISONINGS

method of
HOWARD C. MOFENSON, M.D.
THOMAS R. CARACCIO, Pharm.D., and
JOSEPH GREENSHER, M.D.
Long Island Regional Poison Control Center
East Meadow, New York

BASIC MANAGEMENT OF POISONINGS

The severity of the manifestations of acute poisoning exposures varies greatly with the age and intent of the victims. Accidental poisoning exposures make up 80 to 85 per cent of all poisoning episodes and are most frequent in children under 5 years of age. Many of these episodes are actually ingestions of relatively nontoxic substances that require minimal medical care. Intentional poisonings constitute 10 to 15 per

The assistance of Lauren Leader and Helene Jacobs in the preparation of this manuscript is gratefully acknowledged.

cent of poisonings, and often these patients require the highest standards of medical and nursing care and the occasional use of sophisticated equipment for recovery. Suicide deaths are a significant number, and the use of toxic substances is often involved. The majority of the drug-related suicide attempts involve a central nervous system depressant, and "coma management" is vital to the treatment.

Sixty per cent of patients who take a drug overdose do so with their own prescribed medication and 15 per cent with drugs prescribed for relatives. The top poisoning categories for all ages are over the counter analgesics, sedative-hypnotics, benzodiazepines, cleaning agents and petroleum products, alcohol and abuse substances, pesticides, tricyclic antidepressants, plants, carbon monoxide, and opioids.

Assessment and Maintenance of Vital Functions

Upper airway obstruction is the most common cause of death in intoxicated patients outside the hospital. Any patient who is comatose and has absent protective airway reflexes is able to tolerate an endotracheal tube (cuffed for those over ages 7 to 9 years) and should have it inserted as soon as possible.

Ventilation is required if the respiratory rate and depth are inadequate.

The circulatory status is best assessed by the blood pressure and heart rate and rhythm. The circulatory clinical status and tissue perfusion may be inferred from the skin temperature, the return of color after pressure blanching (capillary filling), and the urine output. Intra-arterial blood pressure measurements are essential for adequate monitoring.

If the circulation fails to improve after adequate ventilation and oxygenation, then a 15- to 20-cm elevation of the foot of the bed may aid by increasing the venous return to the heart. A fluid challenge also may improve the circulatory status if hypovolemia is the cause. If these measures fail, plasma expanders and similar products may be required. As a last resort vasopressors may be needed. If these measures fail to produce a response, a central venous pressure (CVP) or a pulmonary artery wedge pressure (PAWP) line should be inserted to monitor for heart failure and fluid overload.

The level of consciousness of all intoxicated patients should be assessed and the time of assessment recorded. The Glasgow Coma Score used in head trauma is not useful in intoxications, as alcohol, depressant drugs, and hypotension may give falsely lowered scores. The Reed Coma Scale is preferred (Table 1).

Prevention of Absorption and Reduction of Local Damage

Ocular exposure should be immediately treated with water or saline irrigation for 20 minutes with eyelids fully retracted. Do not use neutralizing chemicals. All caustic and corrosive injuries should be evaluated by an ophthalmologist.

Dermal exposure is treated immediately with rinsing, not a forceful flushing in a shower, which might result in deeper penetration of the toxic substance. The skin should be rinsed with copious amounts of water for at least 30 minutes. Hair shampoo, cleansing of fingernails and navel, and irrigation of the eyes are necessary in an extensive exposure. The clothes may have to be discarded. Leather goods are often irreversibly contaminated and must be abandoned. Caustics (alkali) often require hours of irrigation until the "soapy" feeling of the burn is gone. Dermal absorption may occur with pesticides, hydrocarbons, and cyanide.

Injected exposures to drugs and toxins or those introduced by envenomation may require a proximal tourniquet and early incision and suction. (See Antidotes 4 through 6 in Table 4.)

Inhalation exposures to toxic substances are treated by immediately removing the victim from the contaminated environment.

Gastrointestinal exposure is the most common route of poisoning, and an estimate of what, when, and how much of the toxic substance was ingested must be made. If there is a possibility of potential intoxication, gastrointestinal decontamination is performed rather than waiting for symptoms to develop.

Gastrointestinal Decontamination

To decrease gastrointestinal absorption, emesis should be induced or gastric aspiration and lavage performed. Neither of these methods is completely effective; each removes only 30 to 50 per cent of the ingested substance. They are recommended up to 3 to 4 hours postingestion; however, to elect *not* to remove a potential toxin after 4 hours requires reliance on an often unreliable history of the substance and the time of ingestion. Therefore, it is safer to evacuate the stomach up to 12 hours after an ingestion in most significant intoxications.

Emesis

Relative contraindications to the induction of emesis are (1) in petroleum distillate ingestion of high-viscosity agents; (2) with agents that are likely to rapidly produce coma (short-acting barbiturates) or convulsions (propoxyphene, camphor, isoniazid, strychnine) in less than 30 minutes and therefore may predispose to aspiration during emesis; and (3) prior significant vomiting.

Absolute contraindications to the induction of emesis are (1) in caustic (alkali) or corrosive

TABLE 1. **Level of Consciousness (Reed Coma Scale)**

Stage	Conscious Level	Pain Response	Reflexes	Respiration	Circulation
0	Asleep	Normal	Normal	Normal	Normal
1	Coma	Decreased	Normal	Normal	Normal
2	Coma	None	Normal	Normal	Normal
3	Coma	None	None	Normal	Normal
4	Coma	None	None	Abnormal	Abnormal

Patients in *Stages 3 and 4* require intubation and placement in an intensive care unit.
Patients in *Stage 4* need intervention to sustain life.

(acid) ingestions; (2) in convulsions because of the danger of aspiration and possible induction of laryngospasm; (3) in coma because of the possibility of aspiration with the loss of protective airway reflexes; (4) in absence of a cough reflex; absence of the gag reflex is not a reliable indication of lack of airway protection, since a number of healthy people lack gag reflexes; (5) in hematemesis, in which vomiting may produce additional damage; (6) in an infant under 6 months of age, because of immature protective airway reflexes; and (7) with foreign bodies—emesis is ineffective and risks obstruction or aspiration.

Inducing Emesis. *Syrup of ipecac* is the preferred method; but never fluid extract of ipecac, which is too potent, or salt water, which has produced fatal hypernatremia. Emesis is not recommended to be induced at home in children under 1 year of age but can be performed in a medical facility under supervision when indicated. The dose of syrup of ipecac in the 6- to 9-month-old infant is 5 ml; in the 9- to 12-month-old, 10 ml; and in the 1- to 12-year-old, 15 ml. In children over 12 years and in adults, the dose is 30 ml. The dose may be repeated *once* if the child does not vomit in 15 to 20 minutes. The vomitus should be inspected for remnants of pills or toxic substances and the appearance and odor noted.

Apomorphine is a parenteral emetic that must be freshly prepared. Its use is fraught with complications, although it produces more rapid onset of emesis than syrup of ipecac. We do not recommend its use in the cooperative patient. Naloxone should be available to reverse CNS depression.

Gastric aspiration and lavage may be preferable to the induction of emesis in cooperative adolescents or adults because a large tube can be introduced through the oral cavity. *Contraindications* to gastric aspiration and lavage in intoxicated patients are (1) caustic (alkali) and corrosive (acid) ingestions, because of the risk of esophageal perforation, (2) uncontrolled convulsions, because of the danger of aspiration and injury during the procedure, (3) petroleum distillate products, (4) coma or absent protective airway reflexes, which require the insertion of an endotracheal tube to protect against aspiration, (5) significant cardiac dysrhythmias, which should be controlled first, and (6) hematemesis, which may be a relative contraindication.

The best results with gastric aspiration and lavage are obtained with the largest possible orogastric tube that can be reasonably passed (nasogastric tubes are not large enough for this purpose). In adults, use a large bore orogastric Lavacuator hose or a No. 36 Fr Ewald tube; in children, use a No. 22–28 Fr orogastric-type tube.

The amount of fluid used will vary with the patient's age and size, but in general 300 ml per lavage is used in an adult and 100 ml in a child.

Continuous gastric suction has been used for substances that have an enterohepatic recirculation or are actively secreted into the gastrointestinal tract, such as tricyclic antidepressants (Tofranil) and local anesthetics such as mepivacaine (Carbocaine) (Table 2).

Activated charcoal is produced by combustion of organic material in the absence of air until the carbon particle is formed. There are few *relative contraindications* to the use of activated charcoal: (1) it should not be administered prior to, concomitantly with, or shortly after syrup of ipecac since it may adsorb the ipecac and interfere with its emetic properties; (2) it should not be given prior to, concomitantly with, or shortly after oral antidotes unless proved not to interfere significantly with their absorption; and (3) it does not effectively adsorb caustics and corrosives and may produce vomiting or cling to the esophageal or gastric mucosa and falsely appear as a burn on

TABLE 2. **Substances with Enterohepatic Recirculation**

Chloral hydrate
Colchicine
Digitalis preparations (digoxin, digitoxin)
Glutethimide
Halogenated hydrocarbons (DDT derivatives)
Isoniazid
Methaqualone
Phenothiazines
Phenytoin
Salicylates
Tricyclic antidepressants

endoscopy. Activated charcoal has no *absolute contraindications,* but it does not effectively absorb alcohols, boric acid, caustics, corrosives, cyanide, metals, and drugs insoluble in aqueous acid solution (Table 3). Activated charcoal is a stool marker, indicating that the toxin has passed through the gastrointestinal tract and that no further significant absorption from the original ingestion will occur.

The dose of activated charcoal is 1 gram per kg per dose orally with a minimum of 15 grams. The usual adolescent and adult dose is 60 to 100 grams. It is administered as a slurry mixed with water or by orogastric tube. It is too thick to get down by nasogastric tube. It should not be mixed with milk, marmalade, or starch because these interfere with charcoal's adsorptive action. Charcoal should be mixed with sorbitol, which acts as a cathartic, enhances palatability, and does not interfere with charcoal's adsorptive capacity.

Activated charcoal may be administered orally every 4 hours as long as bowel sounds are present, and may be especially beneficial in intoxications that have an enterohepatic recirculation (see Table 2). Repeated dosing with oral activated charcoal has been shown to increase the clearance of many drugs without enterohepatic recirculation (see individual poisonings).

Catharsis is used to hasten the elimination of any remaining toxin in the gastrointestinal tract. Cathartics are *relatively contraindicated* (1) when ileus is indicated by absence of bowel sounds, (2) in intestinal obstruction or evidence of intestinal perforation, and (3) in cases with a pre-existing electrolyte disturbance. Magnesium sulfate (Epsom salts) is contraindicated in renal failure; sodium sulfate (Glauber's salts), in heart failure or diseases requiring sodium restriction. Magnesium sulfate or sodium sulfate is administered in doses of 250 mg per kg per dose as 20 per cent solutions. The adolescent and adult doses are 30 grams. Sorbitol, 2.8 ml per kg to a maximum of 214 ml of a 70 per cent solution, can be used in adults. The cathartic should be given with the initial dose of activated charcoal. *Note:* Super Char with sorbitol (Gulf Biosystems, Inc.) has

TABLE 3. **Toxic Substances Not Effectively Adsorbed by Activated Charcoal**

Alcohols
Aliphatic hydrocarbons
Boric acid
Caustic alkali
Corrosive acids
Cyanide
Glycols
Metals—iron, lead, lithium, mercury
Mineral acids
Saline cathartics—sodium, magnesium

been shown to be a more efficacious charcoal preparation because it has three times the surface area as compared with standard activated charcoal preparations.

Dilutional treatment is indicated for the immediate management of caustic and corrosive poisonings but is otherwise not useful. *Contraindications* to dilution are (1) inability of the patient to swallow, resulting in aspiration of the diluting fluid, and (2) signs of upper airway obstruction, esophageal perforation, and shock. The administration of large quantities of diluting fluid—above 30 ml in children and 250 ml in adults—may produce vomiting, re-exposing the vital tissues to the effects of local damage and possible aspiration.

Neutralization has not been proved to be scientifically effective.

The Use of Antidotes

Antidotes are available for only a relatively small number of poisons. An available antidote should be administered only after the vital functions are established. Table 4 summarizes the commonly used antidotes and their indications and methods of administration. Most informational, so-called first aid measures and antidotes on commercial product labels are notorious for their inaccuracy; it is preferable to contact the regional poison control center rather than follow recommendations on these labels.

Enhancement of Elimination

The medical methods for elimination of the absorbed toxic substances are diuresis, dialysis, hemoperfusion, exchange transfusion, plasmapheresis, enzyme induction, and inhibition. The methods to increase urinary excretion of toxic chemicals and drugs are being studied extensively, but the other modalities have not been well evaluated.

In general, these methods are needed in only a minority of instances and should be reserved for life-threatening circumstances or when a definite benefit is anticipated.

Diuresis. Diuresis increases the renal clearance of compounds that are partially reabsorbed in the renal tubules. *Forced-fluid diuresis* is based on the principle that it will shorten exposure for reabsorption at the *distal* renal tubules. The risks of diuresis are fluid overload, with cerebral and pulmonary edema, and disturbances in acid-base and electrolyte balance. Failure to produce a diuresis may imply prerenal or renal failure. If renal failure is present, dialysis should be considered.

TABLE 4. **Antidotes***

Medications	Indications	Comments
1. *N*-Acetylcysteine (NAC, Mucomyst), Bristol. Glutathione precursor that prevents accumulation and helps detoxify acetaminophen metabolites. **Dose:** *Adult,* 140 mg/kg PO of 5% solution as loading dose, then 70 mg/kg PO every 4 hr for 17 doses as maintenance dose. *Child,* same as adult. **Packaged:** 10 and 20% solution in 4, 10, and 30 ml vials.	Acetaminophen toxicity. Most effective within first 8 hr (to make more palatable, administer through a straw inserted into closed container of citrus juice) **AR:** Stomatitis, nausea, vomiting. See Acetaminophen in text. The full course of therapy is required in any patient whose level falls in the toxic range.	IV preparation experimental. The dose of NAC should be repeated if the patient vomits within 1 hr after administration. Methods to stop vomiting of the NAC are: (a) placement of a tube in the duodenum, (b) slow administration over 1 hr, (c) one half hour before NAC dose use metoclopramide (Reglan) 1 mg/kg intravenously over 1–2 min (max dose 10 mg) every 6 hours or droperidol (Inapsine) 1.25 mg IV; for extrapyramidal reactions use diphenhydramine (see 18, Diphenhydramine).
2. **Ammonium chloride**, USP, usually given via nasogastric tube. **Dose:** *Adult,* 2 grams every 6 hr in 60 ml dose to maximum of 12 grams/day or 1.5 grams as 1–2% IV q 6 hr up to 6 grams/day. *Child,* 75 mg/kg (2.75 mEq/kg) 4 times/day to maximum of 2–6 grams IV or PO. **Packaged:** 325, 500, and 1000 mg tablets: 2.14% in 500 ml, 21.4% in 30 ml, 26.75% in 20 ml	Acidification of urine may enhance the elimination of phencyclidine and other weak bases (amphetamines and strychnine), but the danger of rhabdomyolysis and precipitation of myoglobin in the renal tubules in an acid milieu indicates this therapy is too dangerous to recommend routinely.	Goal in acid diuresis is to keep urine pH 4.5–5.5 and output 3–6 ml/kg/hr. Monitor blood pH, keep at 7.2–7.3. A diuretic may be used to enhance acid diuresis. Contraindications: weak acid drugs, rhabdomyolysis and myoglobinuria, liver dysfunction, renal dysfunction, closed head injury.
3. **Amyl nitrite.**	See 14, Cyanide kit	
4. **Antivenin Black Widow Spider** (*Latrodectus mactans*) **Dose:** 1–2 vials infused over 1 hr. **Packaged:** 6000 units/vial with 2.5 ml sterile watering and 1 ml horse serum 1:10 dilution.	Black widow spider; all *Latrodectus* species with severe symptoms. Most healthy adults will survive with supportive care. Used in elderly or infants or if underlying medical condition causing hemodynamic instability. **AR:** Same as antivenin polyvalent because derived from horse serum.	Preliminary sensitivity test. Supportive care alone is standard management.
5. **Antivenin Polyvalent** for Crotalidae (pit vipers), Wyeth. IV only. **Dose:** depends on degree of envenomation—minimal: 5–8 vials, moderate: 8–12 vials, severe: 13–30 vials. Dilute in 500–2000 ml of crystalloid solution and start IV at a slow rate, increasing after the first 10 min, if no reaction occurs. **Packaged:** 1 vial (10 ml) lyophilized serum, 1 vial (10 ml) bacteriostatic water for injection, 1 vial (1 ml) normal horse serum.	Venoms of crotalids (pit vipers) of North and South America. **AR:** (Shock anaphylaxis) Reaction occurs within 30 min. Serum sickness usually occurs 5–44 days after administration. It may occur less than 5 days, especially in those who have received horse serum products in the past. Symptoms include fever, edema, arthralgia, nausea, and vomiting, as well as pain and muscle weakness.	Consider consulting with Regional Poison Control Center and herpetologist. Administer IV. Preliminary sensitivity test. Never inject in fingers, toes, or bite site.
6. **Antivenin**, North American coral snake. Wyeth. IV only. **Dose:** 3–5 vials (30–50 ml) by slow IV injection. First 1–2 ml should be injected over 3–5 min. **Packaged:** 1 vial antivenin, 10 ml. 1 vial bacteriostatic water 10 ml for injection.	*Micrurus fulvius* (Eastern coral snake); *Micrurus tenere* (Texas coral snake) **AR:** Anaphylaxis (sensitivity reaction). Usually 30 min after administration. Signs/Symptoms: Flushing, itching, edema of face, cough, dyspnea, cyanosis. Neurologic manifestations: Usually involve the shoulders and arms. Pain and muscle weakness are frequently present, and permanent atrophy may develop.	Same as for Antivenin Polyvalent: for Crotalidae. Will not neutralize the venom of *Micrurus euryxanthus* (Arizona or Sonoran coral snake).

*This is for information purposes and is not intended to substitute for independent judgment. It is always advisable to review the package insert for the most up-to-date information. Contact Regional Poison Control Center for additional details on use.
AR = adverse reactions to antidotes. MP = monitor parameters.

TABLE 4. **Antidotes*** *Continued*

Medications	Indications	Comments
7. **Atropine** (various manufacturers). Antagonizes cholinergic stimuli at muscarinic receptors. **Dose:** *Adult*, initial dose 2–4 mg IV. Dose every 2–5 min as necessary until cessation of secretions. Severe poisoning may require doses up to 2000 mg. *Child*, initial dose of 0.05 mg/kg to a max of 2 mg every 2–5 min as necessary until cessation of secretions. **Packaged:** 0.3 mg/ml in 30 ml; 0.4 mg/ml in 0.5, 1, 20, and 30 ml vials; 1 mg/ml in 1 and 10 ml vials.	Therapy in carbamate and organophosphate insecticide poisonings. Rarely needed in cholinergic mushroom intoxication (*Amanita muscaria, Clitocybe, Inocybe* spp.). Lack of signs of atropinization confirms diagnosis of cholinesterase inhibition. **AR:** Flushing and dryness of skin, blurred vision, rapid and irregular pulse, fever, and loss of neuromuscular coordination.	If cyanosis, establish respiration first because atropine in cyanotic patients may cause ventricular fibrillation. If severe signs of atropinization, may correct with physostigmine in doses equal to one-half dose of atropine. If symptomatic, administer until the end point of drying secretions and clearing of lungs. Hallucinations, flushing of the skin, dilated pupils, tachycardia, and elevation of body temperature are not end points and do not preclude atropine administration. Atropinization should be maintained for 12 to 24 hours, then taper dose and observe for relapse. Atropine has successfully been administered by IV infusion, although this method has not received FDA approval. **Dose:** Place 8 mg of atropine in 100 ml D5W or saline. Conc. = 0.08 mg/ml Dose range = 0.02–0.08 mg/kg/hr or 0.5 ml/kg/hr. Severe poisoning may require supplemental doses of intravenous atropine intermittently in doses of 2–4 mg until drying of secretion occurs.
8. **BAL**	See 17, Dimercaprol	
9. **Bicarbonate**	See 35, Sodium bicarbonate	
10. **Botulism antitoxin**, Connaught Med. Research Labs. **Dose:** *Adult*, 1 vial IV stat then 1 vial IM repeat in 2–4 hr if symptoms appear in 12–24 hr. *Child*, Check with state health department.	Prevention or treatment of botulism.	Contact local or state health department for full management guidelines.
11. **Calcium disodium edetate** (EDTA), Versenate, Riker. **Dose:** *Adult*, Max 4 grams. *Child*, 1 gram. Moderate toxicity, IM or IV, 50 mg/kg day for 3–5 days. Severe toxicity, IV or IM, 75 mg/kg day for 4–5 days, divided into 3–6 doses daily. Dilute 1 gram in 250–500 ml saline or D5W, infuse over 4 hr twice daily for 5–7 days. Max 1 gm. For lead levels over 69 µg/dl or if symptoms of lead poisoning or encephalopathy: Add BAL alone initially, 4 mg/kg, then combination BAL and EDTA at different sites. EDTA dose: 12.5 mg/kg IM. (See Lead in text for latest recommendations.) Modify dose in renal failure. **Packaged:** 200 mg/ml. 5 ml amps.	For chelation of cadmium, chromium cobalt, copper, lead, magnesium, nickel, selenium, tellurium, tungsten, uranium, vanadium, and zinc poisoning. **AR:** 1. Thrombophlebitis. 2. Nausea, vomiting. 3. Hypotension. 4. Transient bone marrow suppression. 5. Nephrotoxicity, reversible tubular necrosis (particularly in acid urine). 6. Fever 4–8 hr after infusion. 7. Increased prothrombin time.	Hydrate first and establish renal flow. Avoid plain sodium EDTA since hypocalcemia may result. Procaine 0.25–1 ml of 0.5% for each ml of IM EDTA to reduce pain. Do not use EDTA orally. Limit use to 7 days (otherwise loss of other ions and cardiac dysrhythmias may occur). **MP:** Calcium levels, urinalysis, renal profile, erythrocyte protoporphyrin, blood lead, and liver profile. Contraindicated in iron intoxication, hepatic impairment, and renal failure.

*This is for information purposes and is not intended to substitute for independent judgment. It is always advisable to review the package insert for the most up-to-date information. Contact Regional Poison Control Center for additional details on use.

AR = adverse reactions to antidotes. MP = monitor parameters.

Table continued on following page

TABLE 4. **Antidotes*** *Continued*

Medications	Indications	Comments
12. (A) **Calcium gluconate** (various manufacturers). **Dose:** *Adult:* 10 grams in 250 ml of water PO or by NG tube. 30 grams max daily dose. **Packaged:** 500, 650 mg, 1 gram tabs.	To precipitate fluorides, magnesium, salts, and oxalates after oral ingestion.	
(B) **Calcium gluconate** 10%. **Dose:** IV 0.2–0.5 ml/kg of elemental calcium up to maximum 10 ml (1 gram) over 5–10 min with continuous ECG monitoring. Titrate to adequate response. **Packaged:** 10% in 10 ml vial.	Calcium channel blocker poisoning, e.g., nifedipine *(Procardia)*, verapamil *(Calan)*, diltiazem *(Cardizem)*. It improves the blood pressure but does not affect the dysrhythmias. Hypocalcemia as result of poisonings. Black widow spider envenomation.	Repeat dose as needed. Monitor calcium levels. Contraindicated with digitalis poisoning.
(C) **Calcium chloride.** **Dose:** IV 0.2 ml/kg up to maximum 10 ml (1 gram) with continuous IV monitoring. Titrate to adequate response.	Hydrofluoric acid (HF) (if irrigation with cool water fails to control the pain). **AR:** IV bradycardia, asystole, necrosis with extravasation.	Infiltration with calcium gluconate should be considered if HF exposure results in immediate tissue damage and erythema and pain persists following adequate irrigation.
(D) **Infiltration of calcium gluconate.** **Dose:** Infiltrate each square cm of the affected dermis and subcutaneous tissue with about 0.5 ml of 10% calcium gluconate using a 30-gauge needle. Repeat as needed to control pain. **Packaged:** 10% in 10 ml vial.		
(E) **Calcium Gel** 3.5 gm USP, calcium gluconate powder added to 5 oz of KY jelly.	Dermal exposures of hydrofluoric acid less than 20%.	Gel must have direct access to burn area. If pain persists, a calcium gluconate injection may be needed.
13. **Chlorpromazine** (various manufacturers). Phenothiazine derivative. **Dose:** *Adult,* 1 mg/kg dose IV/IM or 0.5 mg/kg dose if taken with barbiturate or if exhausted. **Packaged:** 25 mg/ml in 1, 2, and 10 ml vials.	Only in *pure* amphetamine OD, with life-threatening manifestations. (Diazepam [Valium] is preferred.) Toxicity: CNS depression, coma, hypotension, extrapyramidal syndrome, agitation, fever, convulsions, dry mouth, cardiac arrhythmias, ECG changes.	Do not use if any signs of atropinization or "street drug" amphetamines are present. Watch for hypotension. In general it is safer to use diazepam (Valium) or haloperidol (Haldol).
14. **Cyanide antidote kit**, Lilly. Nitrite-induced methemoglobinemia attracts cyanide off cytochrome oxidase and thiosulfate forms nontoxic thiocyanate. **Doses:** *Adult,* amyl nitrite. Inhale for 30 sec of every min. Use a new ampule every 3 min. Reapply until sodium nitrite can be given. Then inject IV 300 mg (10 ml of 3% solution) of Na nitrite at a rate of 2.5 to 5 ml/min. Then inject 12.5 grams (50 ml of 25% sol.) of Na thiosulfate. *Child,* use the following chart for children's dosage. **Packaged:** 2–10 ml ampules Na nitrite injection: 2–50 ml ampules Na thiosulfate injection; 0.3 ml amyl nitrite inhalant.	Cyanide poisoning. **AR:** Hypotension, methemoglobinemia.	*Note:* If a child is given the adult dose of Na nitrite, a fatal methemoglobinemia may result. *Do not use methylene blue* for methemoglobinemia in cyanide therapy. Observe for hypotension and have epinephrine available. Cyanide kits should have amyl nitrite changed annually. Administer oxygen 100% between inhalations of amyl nitrite. Monitor hemoglobin, arterial blood gases, methemoglobin concentration (nitrite given to obtain a methemoglobin of 25%). Some add cyanide ampule to resuscitation bag.

*This is for information purposes and is not intended to substitute for independent judgment. It is always advisable to review the package insert for the most up-to-date information. Contact Regional Poison Control Center for additional details on use. AR = adverse reactions to antidotes. MP = monitor parameters.

TABLE 4. **Antidotes*** Continued

Medications	Indications	Comments
Hemoglobin	*Initial Child Dose of Sodium Nitrite 3% (do not exceed 10 ml)*	*Initial Child Dose of Sodium Thiosulfate (do not exceed 12.5 grams)*
8 grams	0.22 ml/kg (6.6 mg/kg)	1.10 ml/kg
10 grams	0.27 ml/kg (8.7 mg/kg)	1.35 ml/kg
12 grams	0.33 ml/kg (10 mg/kg)	1.65 ml/kg
14 grams	0.39 ml/kg (11.6 mg/kg)	1.95 ml/kg

If signs of poisoning reappear, repeat above procedure at one-half the above doses.

15. **Deferoxamine mesylate** (DFOM, Desferal), Ciba. Has a remarkable affinity for ferric iron and chelates it.
 Therapeutic Dose: *Adult*, 90 ml/kg IM or IV every 8 hr to a max of 1 gram per injection, may repeat to maximum of 6 grams in 24 hr. *Child*, same as adult. IM or IV. IV administration should be given by slow infusion at rate not exceeding 15 mg/kg/hr.
 Packaged: 500 mg/amp (powder).

DFOM is useful in the treatment of symptomatic iron poisoning or cases where the serum iron is greater than 500 µg/dl.
A positive result of a DFOM challenge test is not a definite indication that therapy is necessary in the asymptomatic patient. Oral DFOM is not recommended.
Iron intoxication.
Therapeutic: see dose in left column.
Diagnostic trial. Give deferoxamine, 50 mg/kg IM (up to 1 gram). If serum iron exceeds TIBC, unbound iron is excreted in urine, producing a "vin rose" color of chelated iron complex in the urine (pink orange). However, may be negative with high serum iron exceeding TIBC.
AR: Flushing of the skin, generalized erythema, urticaria, hypotension, and shock may occur. Blindness has occurred rarely in patients receiving long-term, high-dose DFOM therapy.
Contraindicated in patients with renal disease or anuria.

Therapy is usually continued until urine color and/or iron levels are normal. Therapy is rarely required over 24 hr.
Establish a good renal flow.
To be effective DFOM should be administered in first 12–16 hr.
In mild to moderate iron intoxication, IM or IV route. In severe intoxication or shock, IV route only.
Monitor serum iron levels, urine output, and urine color.

16. **Diazepam** (Valium), Roche.
 Dose: *Adult*, 5–10 mg IV (max 20 mg) at a rate of 5 mg/min until seizure is controlled. May be repeated 2 or 3 times. *Child*, 0.1–0.3 mg/kg up to 10 mg IV slowly over 2 min.
 Packaged: 5 mg/ml, 2 ml, 10 ml vials.

Any intoxication that provokes seizures when specific therapy is *not* available, e.g., amphetamines, PCP, barbiturate and alcohol withdrawal.
Chloroquine poisoning.
AR: Confusion, somnolence, coma, hypotension.

Intramuscular absorption is erratic. Establish airway and administer 100% oxygen and glucose.

17. **Dimercaprol** (BAL), Hynson, Westcott, and Dunning.
 Dose: Recommendations vary, contact Regional Poison Control Center. Prevents inhibition of sulfhydryl enzymes. Given deep IM only. For *severe lead poisoning:* see 11, EDTA. For *mild arsenic or gold:* 2.5 mg/kg every 6 hr for 2 days, then every 12 hr on the third day, and once daily thereafter for 10 days. For *severe arsenic or gold:* 3–5 mg/kg every 6 hr for 3 days, then every 12 hr thereafter for 10 days. For *mercury:* 5 mg/kg initially, followed by 2.5 mg/kg 1 or 2 times daily for 10 days.

For chelation of antimony, arsenic, bismuth, chromates, copper, gold, lead, and mercury nickel.
AR: 30% of patients have reactions: fever (30% of children), hypertension, tachycardia, may cause hemolysis in G6PD deficiency patients. Doses greater than recommended may cause various adverse effects: nausea, vomiting, headache, chest pain, tachycardia, and hypertension.

Contraindicated in instances of hepatic insufficiency, with the exception of postarsenic jaundice.
Should be discontinued or used only with extreme caution if acute renal insufficiency is present.
Monitor blood pressure and heart rate (both may increase), urinalysis, qualitative urine excretion of heavy metal.
Contraindicated in iron, silver, uranium, selenium, and cadmium poisoning.

---

*This is for information purposes and is not intended to substitute for independent judgment. It is always advisable to review the package insert for the most up-to-date information. Contact Regional Poison Control Center for additional details on use.
AR = adverse reactions to antidotes. MP = monitor parameters.

Table continued on following page

TABLE 4. **Antidotes*** *Continued*

Medications	Indications	Comments

Packaged: 100 mg/ml 10% in oil in 3 ml amp.

18. **Diphenhydramine** (Benadryl), Parke-Davis. Antiparkinsonian action.
   Dose: *Adult,* 10–50 mg IV over 2 min. *Child,* 1–2 mg/kg IV up to 50 mg over 2 min. Maximum 24 hr 400 mg.
   Packaged: 10 mg/ml in 10 and 30 ml vials. 50 mg/ml in 1, 5, 10, and 30 ml vials. Caps, tab 25.50 mg. Elixir, syrup 12.5 mg/5 ml.

Used to treat extrapyramidal symptoms and dystonia induced by phenothiazines and related drugs.
AR: Fatal dose, 20–40 mg/kg
Dry mouth, drowsiness.

Continue with oral diphenhydramine 5 mg/kg/day to 25 mg 3 times a day for 72 hr to avoid recurrence.

19. **EDTA**

See 11, Calcium disodium edetate

20. **Ethanol** (ETOH). Competitively inhibits alcohol dehydrogenase.
   Dose: *Loading:* Administer 7.6–10.0 ml/kg of 10% ETOH in D5W over 30 min IV or 0.8–1.0 ml/kg 95% ETOH PO in 6 oz of orange juice over 30 min. While administering loading dose start maintenance.
   Maintenance Dose: Volume of 10% ETOH needed IV or 95% oral solution (not in dialysis). (See table of maintenance dose below.) If patient is on dialysis, add 91 ml/hr in addition to regular maintenance dose. See comments to prepare 10% solution if not commercially available.
   Packaged: 10% ethanol in D5W 1000 ml; 95% ethanol. May be given as 50% solution orally.

Methanol, ethylene glycol.
Ethanol infusion therapy may be started in cases of suspected methanol and ethylene glycol poisoning presenting with increased anion gap and osmolal gap, or if the urine shows the crystalluria of ethylene glycol poisoning or the hyperemia of the optic disc of methanol intoxication.
AR: CNS depression, hypoglycemia.

Monitor blood ethanol 1 hr after starting infusion and every 4–6 hr. Maintain a blood ethanol concentration of 100–200 mg/dl. Monitor blood glucose, electrolytes, blood gases, urinalysis, and renal profile at least daily. Continue infusion until safe concentration of ethylene glycol or methanol is reached. Ethanol-induced hypoglycemia may occur. Dialysis, preferably hemodialysis, should be considered in severe intoxication not controlled by ethanol alone.
To prepare 10% ethanol for infusion for infusion therapy: Remove 100 ml from 1 liter of D5W and replace with 100 ml of tax-free bulk absolute alcohol after passing through 0.22 micron filter. 50 ml vials of pyrogen-free absolute ethanol for injection are available from Pharm-Serve, 218–20 96th Avenue, Queen's Village, NY 11429. Telephone 718–475–1601.

Maintenance Dose: Patient Category	ml/kg/hr using 10% IV	ml/kg/hr using 50% oral
Nondrinker	0.83	0.17
Occasional drinker	1.40	0.28
Alcoholic	1.96	0.39

21. **Fab** (antibody fragment) (Digibind).
   Dose: The average dose used during clinical testing was 10 vials. Dosage details are specified by the manufacturer. It should be administered by the IV route over 30 min. Calculate on basis of body burden either by known amount ingested or by serum digoxin concentration.
   Calculation of dose of Fab:
   1. Known amount ingested multiplied by bioavailability (0.8) = body burden. Body burden divided by 0.6 = number of vials.

Digoxin, digitoxin, oleander tea with life-threatening intoxications, refractory dysrhythmias, hyperkalemia. 40 mg binds 0.6 mg digoxin.

Contact Regional Poison Control Center.
Preliminary sensitivity test.
Administer through a 0.22 micron filter. It causes a rise in measured bound digoxin but a fall in free digoxin.

*This is for information purposes and is not intended to substitute for independent judgment. It is always advisable to review the package insert for the most up-to-date information. Contact Regional Poison Control Center for additional details on use.
AR = adverse reactions to antidotes. MP = monitor parameters.

TABLE 4. **Antidotes*** *Continued*

Medications	Indications	Comments
2. Known serum digoxin (obtained 6 hr postingestion) multiplied by volume distribution (5.6 liters/kg) and weight in kg divided by 1000 = body burden. Body burden divided by 0.6 = number of vials.		
22. **Glucagon**. Works by stimulating production of cyclic adenyl monophosphate. **Dose:** 50–150 µg/kg over 1 min IV followed by a continuous infusion of 1–5 mg/hr in dextrose and then taper over 5–12 hr. **Packaged:** 1 mg (1 unit) vial with 1 ml diluent with glycerin and phenol; also in 10 ml size.	Propranolol and other beta blocker intoxication. **AR:** Generally well tolerated—most frequent are nausea, vomiting.	Do not dissolve the lyophilized glucagon in the solvent packaged with it when administering IV infusion because of possible phenol toxicity. Effects of single dose observed in 5–10 min and last for 15–30 min. A constant infusion may be necessary to sustain desired effects.
23. **Labetalol hydrochloride** (Normodyne) Schering; (Trandate) Glaxo. Nonselective beta and mild alpha blocker. **Dose:** IV 20 mg over 2 min. Additional injections of 40 or 80 mg can be given at 10 min intervals until desired supine blood pressure achieved. Max dose 300 mg. Alternative: Slow IV infusion: 200 mg (40 ml) is added to 160 or 250 ml of D5W and given at 2 mg/min. Titrate infusion according to response. **Packaged:** Solution 5 mg/ml in 20 ml.	Hypertensive crises secondary to cocaine. **AD:** GI disturbances, orthostatic hypotension, bronchospasm, congestive heart failure, A-V conduction disturbances, and peripheral vascular reactions.	Concomitant diuretic enhances therapeutic response. Patient should be kept in a supine position during infusion. **MP:** Monitor blood pressure during and after administration.
24. **Methylene blue**, Harvey and others. Physiologically transformed to reduced form, leukomethylene blue, which is then oxidized to methylene blue in the presence of methemoglobin. The methemoglobin is converted to hemoglobin. **Dose:** *Adult,* 0.1–0.2 ml/kg of 2% solution (1–2 mg/kg over 5 min IV). *Child,* Same as adult. **Packaged:** 1% 10 ml ampules. May repeat in 1 hr if necessary.	Methemoglobinemia **AR:** GI (nausea, vomiting), headache, hypertension, dizziness, mental confusion, restlessness, dyspnea when IV dose exceeds 7 mg/kg. Treatment is unnecessary unless methemoglobin is over 30% or respiratory distress.	Saliva, urine, and other body fluids may turn blue. *Contraindications:* Renal insufficiency, cyanide poisonings when sodium nitrite is used to induce methemoglobinemia in G6PD deficiency patients. Monitor hemolysis, methemoglobin level, and arterial blood gases. Avoid extravasation because of local necrosis.
25. **Naloxone** (Narcan). Pure opioid antagonist. **Dose:** *Adult,* 0.4–2.0 mg IV and repeat at 3-min intervals until respiratory function is stable. Before excluding opioid intoxication on the basis of a lack of naloxone response a minimum of 2 mg in a child or 10 mg in an adult should be administered. *Child,* Initial dose is 0.01 mg/kg IV. If no response, a subsequent dose of 0.1 mg/kg may be administered.	Narcotic, opiate, CNS depression. This drug is relatively free of adverse reactions. Rare report of pulmonary edema. Should be administered with caution in pregnancy. It is used only to reverse depression and hypoxia.	Naloxone infusion therapy should be used if a large initial dose was required, repeated boluses are necessary, or a long-acting opiate is involved. In infusion therapy the initial response dose is administered every hour and may need to be boostered in a half hour after starting. The infusion may be tapered after 12 hr of therapy. Naloxone infusion: calculate daily fluid requirements, add initial response dose of naloxone multiplied by 24 to the solution. Divide fluid by 24 to determine ml/hr of naloxone infusion.

*This is for information purposes and is not intended to substitute for independent judgment. It is always advisable to review the package insert for the most up-to-date information. Contact Regional Poison Control Center for additional details on use.
AR = adverse reactions to antidotes. MP = monitor parameters.

Table continued on following page

TABLE 4. **Antidotes*** *Continued*

Medications	Indications	Comments
Packaged: 0.02 mg/ml. 0.4 mg/ml ampule, and 10 ml multidose vial.		Dose not cause CNS depression. Routes: IV or endotracheal are preferred routes. Pentazocine (Talwin), dextromethorphan, propoxyphene (Darvon), and codeine may require larger doses.
26. **Nicotinamide** (various manufacturers). **Dose:** *Adult*, 500 mg IM or IV slowly, then 200–400 mg q 4 hr. If symptoms develop, the frequency of injections should be increased to every 2 hr (max 3 grams/day). *Child*, one half suggested adult dose. **Packaged:** 100 mg/ml: 2, 5, 10, 30 ml vials; 25 and 50 mg tablets.	Vacor poisoning: phenylurea pesticide intoxication. *Note:* Vacor 2% is now available only to professional exterminators. 0.5% Vacor is available to the general public and can be toxic to children if swallowed. **AR:** Large doses: flushing, pruritus, sensation of burning, nausea, vomiting, anaphylactic shock.	Nicotinamide is most effective when given within 1 hr of ingestion. Do not use niacin or nicotinic acid in place of nicotinamide. Monitor liver profile.
27. **Oxygen** 100%. **Dose:** *Adult*, 100% oxygen by inhalation or 100% oxygen in hyperbaric chamber at 2–3 atm. *Child*, same as adult.	Carbon monoxide, cyanide, methemoglobinemia. Any inhalation intoxication.	Half-life of carboxyhemoglobin is 240 min in room air 21% oxygen; if a patient is hyperventilated with 100% oxygen, half-life of carboxyhemoglobin is 90 min; in chamber at 2 atm, half-life is 25–30 min.
28. **Pancuronium bromide** (Pavulon). Nondepolarizing (competitive) blocking agent. **Dose:** *Adults and children*, initially, 0.1 mg/kg IV; for intubation, 0.1 mg/kg IV, repeated as required (generally every 40 to 60 minutes). **Packaged:** Sol 1 mg/ml in 10 ml; 2 mg/ml in 2 and 5 ml containers.	Neuromuscular blocking agent. Used for intubation and seizure control act in 2 min, last 40–60 min. **AR:** Main hazard is inadequate postoperative ventilation. Tachycardia and slight increase in arterial pressure may occur owing to vagolytic action.	The required dose varies greatly and a peripheral nerve stimulator aids in determining appropriate amount. Should monitor EEG, since motor effect may be abolished without decreasing electrical discharge from brain.
29. **D-Penicillamine** (Cuprimine) Merck; (Depen) Wallace. Effective chelator and promotes excretion in urine. **Dose:** 250 mg 4 times daily PO for up to 5 days for long-term (20–40 days) therapy: 30–40 mg/kg/day in children. Max 1 gram/day. For chronic therapy 25 mg/kg/day in 4 doses. **Packaged:** 125 and 250 mg capsules.	Heavy metals, arsenic, cadium, chromates, cobalt, copper, lead, mercury, nickel, and zinc. **AR:** Leukopenia (2%); thrombocytopenia (4%); GI: nausea, vomiting, anaphylactic shock, diarrhea (17%); fever, rash, lupus syndrome, renal and hepatic injury.	This is not considered standard therapy for lead poisoning after chelation therapy. May produce ampicillin-like rash, allergic reactions, neutropenia, and nephropathy. Contraindication: hypersensitivity to penicillin. **MP:** Routine urinalysis, white differential blood count, hemoglobin determination, direct platelet count, renal and hepatic profiles. Collect 24 hr urine, quantify for heavy metal.
30. **Physostigmine salicylate** (Antilirium), Forest. Cholinesterase inhibitor. A diagnostic trial is not recommended. **Dose:** *Adult*, 1–2 mg IV over 2 min: may repeat every 5 min to max dose of 6 mg. *Child*, IV, 0.5 mg over 2 min to a max dose of 2 mg. Once effect accomplished give lowest effective dose every 30–60 minutes if symptoms recur. **Packaged:** 1 mg/ml 2 ml/amp.	Used if conventional therapy fails for coma, convulsions, severe cardiac dysrhythmias, severe hypertension, hallucinations secondary to anticholinergics, antihistamines, and anticholinergic plants. **AR:** Death may result from respiratory paralysis, hypertension/hypotension, bradycardia/tachycardia/asystole, hypersalivation, respiratory difficulties/convulsions (cholinergic crisis).	Do not consider for the following: antidepressants, amoxapine, maprotiline, nomifensine, bupropion, trazodone, imipramine. IV administration should be at a slow controlled rate, not more than 1 mg/min. Rapid administration can cause adverse reactions. Can be reversed by atropine. Lasts only 30 min. Contraindicated in asthma, cardiovascular disease, intestinal obstruction.

*This is for information purposes and is not intended to substitute for independent judgment. It is always advisable to review the package insert for the most up-to-date information. Contact Regional Poison Control Center for additional details on use.

AR = adverse reactions to antidotes. MP = monitor parameters.

TABLE 4. **Antidotes*** *Continued*

Medications	Indications	Comments
31. **Pralidoxime chloride** (2-PAM, Protopam), Ayerst. Cholinesterase reactivator by removing phosphate. **Dose:** *Adult*, 1 gram IV at 0.5 gram/min or infused in 150 ml saline over 30 min. Repeat every 8–12 hr when needed; if severe, 0.5 gram/hr infusion. *Child*, 25–50 mg/kg IV over 30 min, no faster than 10 mg/kg/min. **Packaged:** 1 gram/20 ml vials.	Organosphosphate insecticide poisoning. Not usually needed in carbamate insecticide poisoning. Most effective if started in first 24 hr before bonding of phosphate. **AR:** Rapid IV injection has produced tachycardia, muscle rigidity, transient neuromuscular blockade. IM: conjunctival hyperemia, subconjunctival hemorrhage, especially if concentrations exceed 5%. Oral: nausea, vomiting, diarrhea, malaise.	Should be used only after initial treatment with atropine. Draw blood for RBC cholinesterase level prior to giving 2-PAM. The use of 2-PAM may require a reduction in the dose of atropine. **MP:** Monitor renal profile and reduce dose accordingly.
32. **Propranolol** (Inderal). Nonselective beta blocker. **Dose:** *Adult*, 0.1–0.15 mg/kg IV, administered in increments of 0.5–0.75 mg every 1–2 min with continuous ECG and blood pressure monitoring up to 10 mg. *Child*, 0.01–0.015 mg/kg dose slow IV with repeat dose every 6–8 hr as needed. **Packaged:** 1 mg/ml; tab: 10, 20, 40, 60, 80, 90 mg; cap: 20, 80, 160 mg.	Cocaine intoxication. Has not been scientifically proved to be safe and effective. Anecdotal reports only. Labetalol is theoretically preferred agent for cocaine intoxication. **AR:** Bradycardia, hypotension, pallor; neurologic effects include hallucinations, coma, and seizures.	Not a specific antidote; used for catecholamine storm and dysrhythmias. Increased mortality has been reported in animals that received propranolol for cocaine poisoning, and hypertension has occurred in humans following its use in cocaine intoxication.
33. **Protamine sulfate.** **Dose:** 1 mg neutralizes 90–115 units of heparin. Maximum dose = 50 mg IV over 5 min at 10 mg/ml. **Packaged:** 5 ml = 50 mg; 25 ml = 250 mg.	Heparin overdose. **AR:** Rapid administration causes anaphylactoid reactions.	**MP:** Monitor thromboplastin times. Doses of up to 200 mg have been tolerated over 2 hr in an adult.
34. **Pyridoxine (Vitamin B₆).** Gamma-aminobutyric acid agonist. **Dose:** *Unknown amount ingested:* 5 gm over 5 min IV. *Known amount:* Add 1 gram of pyridoxine for each gram of INH ingested IV over 5 min. **Packaged:** 50 and 100 mg/ml; 10, 30 ml.	Isoniazid (INH), hydrazine. **AR:** Unlikely owing to the fact that vitamin B₂ is water soluble. However, nausea, vomiting, somnolence, and paresthesia have been reported from chronic high doses.	Pyridoxine is given as 5–10% solution IV mixed with water. It may be repeated every 5–20 min until seizures cease. Some administer pyridoxine over 30–60 min. **MP:** Correct acidosis, monitor liver profile, acid-base parameters.
35. **Sodium bicarbonate.** **Dose:** IV 1–3 mEq/kg as needed to keep pH 7.5 (generally 2 mEq/kg every 6 hours). When alkalinization is desired to correct acidosis to a pH of 7.3, use 2 mEq/kg to raise pH 0.1 unit. **Packaged:** 50 ml, 44.6 mEq, 50 mEq ampule.	To promote urinary alkalinization for salicylates, phenobarbital (weak acids with low volume of distribution excreted in urine unchanged). To correct severe acidosis. To promote protein-binding and supply sodium ions into Purkinje cells in cyclic antidepressant intoxication. **AR:** Large doses in patients with renal insufficiency may cause metabolic alkalosis. In patients with ketoacidosis, rapid alkalinization with sodium bicarbonate may result in clouding of consciousness, cerebral dysfunction, seizures, hypoxia, and lactic acidosis.	Alkaline diuresis. The assessment of the need for bicarbonate should be based on both the blood and urine pH. Maintain the blood pH at 7.5. Keep the urinary output at 3–6 ml/kg/hr. May use a diuretic to enhance diuresis. Potassium is necessary to produce alkaline diuresis. Monitor electrolytes, calcium, pH of both urine and blood, arterial blood gases.
36. **Sodium nitrite.**	See 14, Cyanide kit	
37. **Sodium thiosulfate.**	See 14, Cyanide kit	

*This is for information purposes and is not intended to substitute for independent judgment. It is always advisable to review the package insert for the most up-to-date information. Contact Regional Poison Control Center for additional details on use.

AR = adverse reactions to antidotes. MP = monitor parameters.

Table continued on following page

Table 4. **Antidotes*** *Continued*

Medications	Indications	Comments
38. **Vitamin K** (AquaMEPHYTON) Merck. Promotes hepatic biosynthesis of prothrombin and other coagulation factors. Competitive antagonist of warfarin. It may be administered orally in the absence of vomiting. **Dose:** *Adult,* 2.5–10 mg IV, depending on potential for hemorrhage. Severe bleeding, 5–25 mg slow IV push. Rate 1 mg/min. Repeat every 4–8 hr depending on prothrombin time. *Child,* 1–5 mg IV may be given orally when vomiting ceases. **Packaged:** 2 mg/ml in 0.5 ml ampules. 2.5 or 5 ml vials.	Warfarin (coumarin), salicylate intoxication.	Fatalities from anaphylactic reaction have been reported following IV route. It takes 24 hr for vitamin K to be effective. The need for further vitamin K is determined by the prothrombin time test. If severe bleeding, fresh blood or plasma transfusion may be needed.

*This is for information purposes and is not intended to substitute for independent judgment. It is always advisable to review the package insert for the most up-to-date information. Contact Regional Poison Control Center for additional details on use. AR = adverse reactions to antidotes. MP = monitor parameters.

Osmotic diuresis is meant to increase the osmotic gradient and prevent reabsorption from the *proximal* loop and *distal* tubules. Mannitol is used to initiate this type of diuresis, and then fluids are added in sufficient amounts to produce a diuresis similar to forced-fluid diuresis.

Acid and alkaline diuresis is based on the principle that to inhibit reabsorption of certain toxic agents the urinary pH can be adjusted so the substance is maintained in its ionized form, which interferes with its passage back into the blood. Electrolyte and acid-base monitoring is necessary. Hypokalemia and hypocalcemia are frequent complications. *Acid diuresis* is accomplished by using ammonium chloride (Antidote 2, Table 4). Ascorbic acid may be used as an adjunct. It enhances the elimination of weak bases such as amphetamines and fenfluramine (Pondimin). Ammonium chloride is contraindicated if rhabdomyolysis is present. *Alkaline diuresis* with sodium bicarbonate can be utilized in the therapy of weak acids, such as salicylates, and long-acting barbiturates, such as phenobarbital (Antidote 35, Table 4).

Dialysis. Dialysis is the extrarenal means of removing certain toxins from the body or can substitute for the kidney when renal failure occurs. Dialysis is never the first measure instituted; however, it may be life-saving later in the course of the severe intoxication. It is needed only in a small minority of intoxications (Table 5). *Peritoneal dialysis* is only one twentieth as effective as hemodialysis. It is easier to use and less hazardous to the patient but also less reliable in removing the toxin. *Hemodialysis* is the most effective means of dialysis but requires experience with sophisticated equipment. *The patient-related criteria for dialysis* are anticipated prolonged coma and the likelihood of complications, renal impairment, and deterioration despite careful medical management.

Hemoperfusion. Hemoperfusion is the extracorporeal exposure of the patient's blood to an adsorbing surface (charcoal or resin). This procedure has extended extracorporeal removal to a large range of substances that were either poorly dialyzable or nondialyzable. *Hemoperfusion may be used for agents that have* high protein-binding, low aqueous solubility, and poor distribution in the plasma water. In these cases hemodialysis is relatively ineffective. Hemoperfusion has proved useful in glutethimide (Doriden) intoxication, barbiturate overdose even with short-acting barbiturates, theophylline, cyclic antidepressants, and chlorophenothane (DDT). The commonly used types are activated charcoal and resin cartridges. In general, supportive care is all that is required. Analysis of studies with hemodialysis and hemoperfusion does not indicate that they reduce morbidity or mortality substantially except in certain cases (Table 6).

Supportive Care, Observation, and Therapy of Complications

The comatose patient is on the threshold of death and must be stabilized initially by establishing an airway. Intubation should be attempted in any comatose patient. This is the best means to check for the presence of the protective airway reflexes.

An intravenous line should be inserted in all

TABLE 5. **Indications and Contraindications for Dialysis**

Immediate Consideration of Dialysis
    Ethylene glycol with refractory acidosis
    Methanol with refractory acidosis and levels
        consistently over 50 mg/dl
    Lithium levels consistently elevated over 4 mEq/liter
    Amanita phalloides

Indications on Basis of Patient's Condition (Coma
    greater than Stage 3 of Reed Coma Scale)

Alcohol*	Iodides
Ammonia	Isoniazid*
Amphetamines	Meprobamate
Anilines	Paraldehyde
Antibiotics	Potassium*
Barbiturates* (long-acting)	Quinidine
Boric acid	Quinine
Bromides*	Salicylates*
Calcium	Strychnine
Chloral hydrate*	Thiocyanates
Fluorides	(Certain other drugs also dialyzable)

*Most useful

Indicated for General Supportive Therapy
    Uncontrollable metabolic acidosis or alkalosis
    Uncontrollable electrolyte disturbance, particularly
        sodium or potassium
    Overhydration
    Renal failure
    Hyperosmolality not responding to conservative therapy
    Marked hypothermia
    Nonresponsive Stage 3 or greater coma
        (Reed Coma Scale)

Contraindicated on Pharmacologic Basis
  Except for Supportive Care
    Antidepressants (tricyclic and MAO inhibitors)
    Antihistamines
    Barbiturates (short-acting)
    Belladonna alkaloids
    Benzodiazepines (Valium, Librium)
    Digitalis and derivatives
    Hallucinogens
    Meprobamate (Equanil, Miltown)
    Methyprylon (Noludar)
    Opioids (heroin, Lomotil)
    Phenothiazines (Thorazine, Compazine)
    Phenytoin (Dilantin)

TABLE 6. **Plasma Concentrations above Which Removal by Extracorporeal Means May Be Indicated**

Drug	Plasma Concentration (mg/dl)	Method of Choice
Phenobarbital	10	HP>HD
Other barbiturates	5	HP
Glutethimide	4	HP
Methaqualone	4	HP
Salicylates	80	HD>HP
Ethchlorvynol	15	HP
Meprobamate	10	HP
Trichloroethanol	5	HP
Paraquat	0.1	HP>HD
Theophylline	6 (chronic), 10 (acute)	HP
Methanol	50	HD
Ethylene glycol	unknown	HD
Lithium	4 mEq/liter	HD
Ethanol	500	HD

Modified from Haddad L, Winchester JF (eds): Clinical Management of Poisoning and Drug Overdose. Philadelphia, WB Saunders Company, 1983, p 162.

comatose patients and blood collected for appropriate tests, including toxicologic analysis (10 ml of clotted blood, initial gastric aspirate, 100 ml of urine). The initial management of the comatose patient should include the administration of 100 per cent oxygen, 100 mg of thiamine intravenously, 50 per cent glucose as an intravenous bolus, and 2 to 10 mg of naloxone (Narcan) intravenously. Other causes associated with coma and mimicking intoxications should be eliminated by examination and laboratory tests (trauma, infection, cerebrovascular accident, hypoxia, and endocrine-metabolic causes).

Pulmonary edema complicating poisoning may be cardiac or noncardiac in origin. Fluid overload during forced diuresis may cause the cardiac variety, particularly if the drugs have an antidiuretic effect (opioids, barbiturates, and salicylates). Some toxic agents produce increased pulmonary capillary permeability, and other agents may cause a massive sympathetic discharge resulting in neurogenic pulmonary edema (opioids and salicylates). Management consists of minimizing the fluid administration, diuretics, and oxygen. If renal failure is present, dialysis may be necessary. The noncardiac type of pulmonary edema occurs with inhaled toxins such as ammonia, chlorine, and oxides of nitrogen or with drugs such as salicylates, opioids, paraquat, and intravenous ethchlorvynol (Placidyl). This type does not respond to cardiac measures, and oxygen with intensive respiratory management using mechanical ventilation with positive end-expiratory pressure (PEEP) is necessary.

Hypotension and circulatory shock may be caused by heart failure due to myocardial depression, hypovolemia (fluid loss or venous pooling), decrease in peripheral vasculature resistance (adrenergic blockage), or loss of vasomotor tone caused by central nervous system depression.

Renal failure may be due to tubular necrosis as a result of hypotension, hypoxia, or a direct effect of the poison on the tubular cells (salicylate, paraquat, acetaminophen, carbon tetrachloride). Hemoglobinuria or myoglobinuria may precipitate in the renal tubules and produce renal failure.

Cerebral edema in intoxications is produced by hypoxia, hypercapnia, hypotension, hypoglycemia, and drug-impaired capillary integrity. Computed tomography may aid in diagnosis. Therapy consists of correction of the arterial blood gas and metabolic abnormalities and the hypotension. Reduction of the increased intracranial pressure may be accomplished by 20 per cent mannitol, 0.5 gram per kg, run in over a 30-minute period, and hyperventilation to reduce the $PaCO_2$ to 25 mm Hg. The head should be elevated, and intracranial pressure monitoring should be considered. Fluid administration should be minimized.

Seizures are caused by many substances, such as amphetamines, camphor, chlorinated hydrocarbon insecticides, cocaine, isoniazid, lithium, phencyclidine, phenothiazines, propoxyphene, strychnine, tricyclic antidepressants, and drug withdrawal from ethanol and sedative-hypnotics. Isolated brief convulsions require no therapy, but recurring or protracted seizures require intravenous diazepam (Valium) and phenytoin.

Cardiac dysrhythmias occur with poisoning. A wide QT interval occurs with phenothiazines and a wide QRS interval occurs with tricyclic antidepressants, quinine, or quinidine overdose. Digitalis, cocaine, cyanide, propranolol, theophylline, and amphetamines are among the more frequent toxic causes of dysrhythmias. Correction of metabolic disturbances and adequate oxygenation will correct some of the dysrhythmias; others may require antidysrhythmic drugs or a cardiac pacemaker or cardioversion.

Metabolic acidosis with an increased anion gap is seen with many agents in overdose. Assessment of the arterial blood gases, electrolytes, and osmolality may be a clue to the etiologic agent. Intravenous sodium bicarbonate may be needed when the pH is below 7.1.

Hematemesis can be produced by caustics and corrosives, iron, lithium, mercury, phosphorus, arsenic, mushrooms, plant poisons, fluoride, and organophosphates. Therapy consists of fluid and blood replacement and iced saline lavage if there is no esophageal damage.

Toxicokinetics for the Practicing Physician

Toxicokinetics is clinical pharmacokinetics from the viewpoint of the toxicologist. Pharmacokinetics is a mathematical description of what the body does to a drug. Knowledge of the toxicokinetics of a specific toxic agent will allow the physician to plan a rational approach to the definitive management of the intoxicated patient after the vital functions have been stabilized.

The LD_{50} (the lethal dose for 50 per cent of experimental animals) and the *MLD* (the minimum lethal dose) are seldom relevant in human intoxications but indicate potential toxicity of the substance. *Protein-binding* of toxic agents influences the volume distribution, elimination, and action of the drug. Diuresis and dialysis are usually reserved for drugs with less than 50 per cent protein-binding. The *therapeutic blood range* is the concentration of any drug at which the majority of the treated population can be expected to receive therapeutic benefit. The *toxic blood range* is the concentration at which this majority would be expected to have toxic manifestations. The range is not an absolute value. *Blood concentrations* are a quantitative aid in determining whether more specific measures need to be instituted in correlation with the clinical manifestations. The *apparent volume distribution (Vd)* is the percentage of body mass in which the drug is distributed. It is determined by dividing the amount absorbed by the blood concentration. When a substance has a large volume distribution, as in most lipid-soluble chemicals (above 1 liter per kg), and is concentrated in the body fat, it will not be available for diuresis, dialysis, or exchange transfusion. *Elimination routes* of detoxification will allow the physician to make therapeutic decisions, such as using ethanol to interfere with the metabolism of methanol and ethylene glycol into more toxic metabolites. *Urine identification* is qualitative and allows only the identification of an agent.

Never manage a poisoned patient solely by laboratory tests, and always treat according to the manifestations of poisoning, not the laboratory test results. The laboratory toxicology analyst should be given whatever historical information is available so the agent can be sought and identified as rapidly as possible. Toxicologic analysis is like a miniresearch project, unlike most other laboratory tests. *Specimens* for toxicologic analysis require the patient's name, date, time of ingestion, time specimen was drawn, therapeutic drugs administered, patient's manifestations, and other relevant data. The toxicologic specimens that should be obtained for analysis are (1) vomitus or initial gastric aspiration, (2) blood, 10 ml (ask the analyst about the type of container and anticoagulant), and (3) urine, 100 ml.

COMMON POISONS AND THERAPY

Abbreviations Used in Following List of Common Poisons

t½	= half-life (time required for blood level to drop by 50 per cent of the original value)
Vd	= volume of distribution (liter per kg)
TLV	= threshold limit value in air
TWA	= time-weighted average
PPM	= parts per million in air and water

Conversion Factors

1 gram	= 1000 milligrams (mg)
1 milligram (mg)	= 1000 micrograms (μg)

1 microgram (μg)   = 1000 nanograms (ng)
Blood levels:
1 microgram per ml = 100 micrograms per dl
                   = 1 milligram per liter
                   = 1000 nanograms per ml
100 mg per dl   = 0.1 gram per dl
                   = 1000 mg (1 gram) per liter
                   = 1.0 mg per ml

Acetaminophen, APAP (Tylenol). *Toxic dose:* Child, 3 or more grams; adult, 7.5 or more grams. Liver toxicity, 140 mg per kg. *Toxicokinetics:* Absorption time, 0.5 to 1 hour. Vd, 0.9 liter per kg. Route of elimination by liver. Draw peak blood level after 4 hours in overdose. *Manifestations:* First 24 hours: malaise, nausea, vomiting, and drowsiness, followed by a latent period of 24 hours to 5 days; then hepatic symptoms, disturbances in clotting mechanism, and renal damage. *Management:* (1) Activated charcoal has been contraindicated when *N*-acetylcysteine is contemplated; use gastric lavage. However, recently activated charcoal may be given in the first few hours or alternated 2 hours after the *N*-acetylcysteine. (2) *N*-Acetylcysteine for toxic overdose (Antidote 1, Table 4). Start and give a full course if a toxic dose has been ingested or if blood concentrations are above the toxic line on the nomogram shown in Figure 1. (3) In this instance, a saline sulfate cathartic is preferred to sorbitol. *Laboratory aids:* APAP level, optimally at 4 to 6 hours. Plot levels on nomogram in Figure 1 as a guide for treatment. Monitor liver and renal profiles daily.

Acids. See Caustics and Corrosives.

Alcohols

1. *Ethanol* (grain alcohol). *Manifestations:* Blood ethanol levels over 30 mg per dl produce euphoria; over 50, incoordination and intoxication; over 100, ataxia; over 300, stupor; and over 500, coma. Levels of 500 to 700 mg per dl may be fatal. Chronic alcoholic patients tolerate higher levels, and the correlation may not be valid. *Management:* (1) Gastrointestinal decontamination up to 1 hour postingestion. Activated charcoal and cathartics are not indicated. (2) 0.25 gram per kg of dextrose, 25 to 50 per cent, intravenously if the blood glucose level is less than 60 mg per dl. (3) Thiamine, 100 mg intravenously, if chronic alcoholism is suspected, to prevent Wernicke-Korsakoff syndrome. (4) Hemodialysis is indicated in severe cases when conventional therapy is ineffective (rarely needed). (5) Treat seizures with diazepam (Valium) followed by phenytoin (Dilantin) if unresponsive. (6) Treat withdrawal with hydration and chlordiazepoxide (Librium) or diazepam. Large doses of sedatives may be required for delirium tremens. *Laboratory aids:* Arterial blood gases, electrolytes, blood ethanol levels, glucose, determine anion and osmolar gap, and check for ketosis. Chest radiograph to determine whether aspiration pneumonia is present. Liver function tests and bilirubin levels.

2. *Isopropanol* (rubbing alcohol). Normal propyl alcohol is related to isopropanol but is more toxic. *Manifestations:* Ethanol-like intoxication with acetone odor to breath, acetonuria, acetonemia without systemic acidosis, gastritis. *Management:* (1) Gastrointestinal decontamination. Activated charcoal and cathartics not indicated. (2) Hemodialysis in life-threatening overdose (rarely needed). *Laboratory aids:* Isopropyl alcohol levels, acetone, glucose, and arterial blood gases.

3. **Methanol** (wood alcohol). *Toxic dose:* One teaspoonful is potentially lethal for a 2-year-old and can cause blindness in an adult. The toxic blood level of methanol is above 20 mg per dl, the potentially fatal level over 50 mg per dl. *Manifestations:* Hyperemia of optic disc, violent abdominal colic, blindness, and shock. *Management:* (1) Gastrointestinal decontamination. Activated charcoal and cathartics are not indicated. (2) Treat acidosis vigorously with sodium bicarbonate intravenously. (3) Initiate ethanol therapy (Antidote 20, Table 4). (4) Folinic acid and folic acid have been used successfully in animal investigations. (5) Consider hemodialysis if the blood methanol level is greater than 50 mg per dl or if significant metabolic acidosis or visual or mental symptoms are present. *Note:* The ethanol dose has to be increased during dialysis therapy. (6) Ophthalmology consultation. *Laboratory aids:* Methanol and ethanol levels, electrolytes, glucose, and arterial blood gases.

Alkali. See Caustics and Corrosives.

Amitriptyline (Elavil). See Tricyclic Antidepressants.

Amphetamines (diet pills, various trade names). *Toxicity:* Child, 5 mg per kg; adult, 12 mg per kg has been reported as lethal. *Toxicokinetics:* Peak time of action is 2 to 4 hours. t½, 8 to 10 hours in acid urine (pH less than 6.0) and 16 to 31 hours in alkaline urine (pH, 7.5). *Route of elimination:* Liver, 60 per cent; kidney, 30 to 40 per cent at alkaline urine pH; at acid urine pH, 50 to 70 per cent. *Manifestations:* Dysrhythmias, hyperpyrexia, convulsions, hypertension, paranoia, violence. *Management:* (1) Gastrointestinal decontamination up to 4 hours. (2) Control extreme agitation or convulsions with diazepam. Chlorpromazine (Thorazine) may be dangerous if ingestion is not pure amphetamine. (3) Treat hypertensive crisis with diazoxide. (4) Acidification diuresis is not recommended. (5) Treat hyperpyrexia symptomatically. (6) If unusual neurologic symptoms, consider cerebrovascular accident. (7) Observe for suicidal depression that may follow intoxication. (8) In life-threatening agitation use haloperidol (Haldol). *Laboratory aids:* Monitor for rhabdomyolysis (creatine phosphokinase), myoglobinuria, hyperkalemia, and disseminated intravascular coagulation. Toxic blood level, 10 μg per dl.

Aniline. See Nitrites and Nitrates.

Anticholinergic Agents. Examples are antihistamines—hydroxyline (Atarax), diphenhydramine (Benadryl); antipsychotics (neuroleptics)—phenothiazines (Thorazine); antidepressant drugs (tricyclic antidepressants)—imipramine (Tofranil); antiparkinson drugs—trihexyphenidyl (Artane), benztropine (Cogentin); over-the-counter sleep, cold, and hayfever medicine (methapyrilene); ophthalmic products (atropine); plants—jimsonweed *(Datura stramonium),* deadly nightshade *(Atropa belladonna),* henbane *(Hyoscyamus niger);* and antispasmodic agents for the bowel (atropine). *Toxicokinetics:* See Table 7. *Manifestations:* Anticholinergic signs—hyperpyrexia, dilated pupils, flushing of skin, dry mucosa, tachycardia, delirium, hallucinations, coma, and convulsions. *Management:*

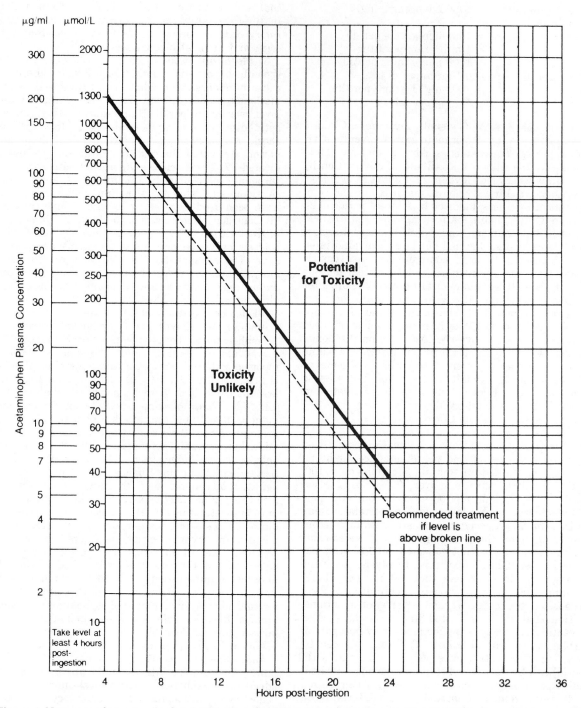

Figure 1. Nomogram for acetaminophen intoxication. Start *N*-acetylcysteine therapy if levels and time coordinates are above the lower line on the nomogram. Continue and complete therapy even if subsequent values fall below the toxic zone. The nomogram is useful only in acute, single ingestions. Serum levels drawn before 4 hours may not represent peak levels. (From Rumack BH, Matthew H: Acetaminophen poisoning and toxicity. Reproduced by permission of Pediatrics 55:871, 1975.)

(1) Gastrointestinal decontamination up to 12 hours postingestion. (2) Control seizures with diazepam. (3) Control ventricular dysrhythmias with lidocaine. (4) Physostigmine (Antidote 30, Table 4) for life-threatening anticholinergic effects refractory to conventional treatments. (5) Treat urinary retention. (6) Treat cardiac dysrhythmias only if patient tissue fusion is not adequate or if the patient is hypotensive.

Anticonvulsants. See Table 8. *Toxic dose:* Specific anticonvulsant blood levels and the clinical manifestations will indicate toxicity. In general, the ingestion of five times the therapeutic dose is expected to have

TABLE 7. **Toxicokinetics of Anticholinergic Agents**

Drug	Potential Fatal Dose	Peak Effect	Vd	t½	Excretion Route
Atropine	Child: 10–20 mg; adult: 100 mg	1–2 hours, may be prolonged in overdose	2.3 liters/kg	2–3 hr	Renal (30–50%) hepatic (50–70%)
Diphenhydramine	20–40 mg/kg; 2 oz has been fatal in 2-year-old	3–4 hours, may be prolonged in over-dose	3–4 liters/kg	5–8 hr	Renal (some hepatic)

the potential for toxicity. *Management:* (1) Gastrointestinal decontamination up to 12 hours postingestion. (2) Monitor specific anticonvulsant blood levels. (3) The effectiveness of hemoperfusion and dialysis has not been established.

Antidepressants. See Tricyclic Antidepressants.

Antifreeze. See Alcohols (Methanol) and Ethylene Glycol.

Antihistamines. See Anticholinergic Agents.

Arsenic and Arsine Gas. Toxic dose: In humans, the inorganic arsenic trioxide toxic dose is 5 to 50 mg; the potential fatal dose is 120 mg. Organic arsenic is less toxic. The maximum allowable concentration for prolonged exposure is 0.05 ppm. See Table 9. Humans are more sensitive than rodents to arsenic. Acute poisoning results from accidental ingestion of arsenic-containing pesticides. (Ant traps sold in some states contain arsenic.) *Toxicokinetics:* Rapidly absorbed by inhalation and ingestion. Crosses placenta and can cause fetal damage. Distributes into spleen, liver, kidneys. *Excretion:* In urine, 90 per cent. Following acute ingestion, it takes 10 days to clear a single dose; chronic ingestion takes up to 70 days. *Arsine gas:* Forms when active hydrogen comes in contact with arsenic. This may occur when zinc, antimony, lead, or iron is contaminated with arsenic and comes in contact with acid.

This causes arsine inhalation intoxication characterized by a latent period of 2 to 48 hours and a triad of abdominal pain, jaundice (due to hemolysis), and hematuria. *Manifestations:* Gastroenteritis, neurologic and cardiac abnormalities, subsequent renal involvement. A garlic odor to the breath may be a clue. Smaller doses and prolonged low level exposure produce subacute (stomatitis) and chronic (peripheral neuropathy) symptoms.

Management: (1) Gastrointestinal decontamination. Follow with abdominal radiographs, as arsenic is radiopaque. (2) Intravenous fluids to correct dehydration and electrolyte deficiencies. (3) Treat shock with oxygen, blood, and fluids as needed. (4) In severe cases, administer BAL (dimercaprol) (Antidote 17, Table 4). (5) In chronic poisoning, D-penicillamine (Antidote 29, Table 4) may be used to chelate arsenic. Therapy should be continued until the urine arsenic is less than 50 μg per liter. (6) Hemodialysis is effective in acute poisoning and can be used concurrently with chelation therapy in severe cases, especially if renal failure develops. (7) Arsine intoxication is treated by exchange transfusion and hemodialysis if renal failure occurs. BAL is ineffective. *Laboratory aids:* Blood arsenic and 24-hour urine arsenic levels. Excessive exposure is indicated by a level of 50 μg per liter of arsenic in

TABLE 8. **Anticonvulsants**

Drug	Peak Time of Action/Hrs (steady state)	Vd (liters/kg)	t½ (hr)	Route of Elimination (per cent)	Protein-Binding (per cent)	Blood Level (μg/ml)	Comment*
Carbamazepine (Tegretol)	6–12 (2–4 days)	0.8–1.4	30–60	Liver (98)	70	Therapeutic, 5–12	Related to tricyclic antidepressants, can cause dysrhythmias
Ethosuximide (Zarontin)	24–48 (5–8 days)	0.6–0.8	24–56	Liver (80–90) Renal (10–20)	0	Therapeutic, 40–100	
Phenytoin (Dilantin)	Oral, 6–12 IV, 1 (5–10 days)	0.6–1.0	20–30; varies in toxic doses: zero order kinetics	Liver (95)	87–93	Therapeutic, 10–20; toxic, 20–30; nystagmus only, 30–40; ataxia, 40 +; coma, convulsions	Dysrhythmias with parenteral use only
Primidone (Mysoline)	3–4? (4–7 days)	0.6	Parent, 3–12; metabolites, 30–36	Liver	70–80	Therapeutic, 8–12 primidone and 10–25 phenobarbital (PB); toxic, over 50 primidone and over 40 PB (see Barbiturates)	Metabolized to active metabolites phenylethylmalonamide and PB; overdose gives white crystals in urine†
Valproic acid (Depakene)	? (1–4 days)	0.3–0.5	8–15	Liver (80–100)	20	Therapeutic, 60–100	Produces nausea and vomiting, changes in liver function
Clonazepam (Clonopin)	? (4–12 days)		20–60	Liver (98)	90	Therapeutic, 20–70 ng/ml	

*Manifestations: The major manifestations of these agents are depression of consciousness and respiratory depression. Other significant manifestations are mentioned in this column.

†Primidone produces whorls of shimmering white crystals in the urine from precipitation of intact primidone in massive overdose.

TABLE 9. **Comparative Acute Toxicities of Some Common Arsenicals**

Arsenical	Oral LD$_{50}$ in Rats *(mg/kg)*	Estimated Mortality in Human Poisoning *(%)*
Arsenic trioxide	385	12
Sodium arsenite	42	65
Calcium arsenite	ca. 275	?
Lead arsenite	1500 +	5
Ortho Crabgrass Killer*	3719	None known

*Product containing 8 per cent each of only mildly toxic octyl NH$_4$ and dodecyl NH$_4$ methanearsonate.

From Done AK: . . . And old lace. Emergency Med 5:246, 1973.

urine, but persons whose diets are rich in seafood may excrete 200 µg per day. View values over 100 µg per day with suspicion. Monitor electrocardiogram (ECG) and renal function. Normal blood arsenic level is less than 7 µg per dl (false values occur in inexperienced laboratories).

Aspirin. See Salicylates.

Atropine. See Anticholinergic Agents.

Barbiturates. See Table 10. *Management:* (1) Gastrointestinal decontamination up to 8 to 12 hours. Activated charcoal and a cathartic in repeated doses have been shown to reduce the serum half-life and increase the nonrenal clearance over 50 per cent. Give every 4 hours while the patient is comatose. (2) Supportive and symptomatic care are all that are necessary in the majority of cases. (3) Forced alkaline diuresis (if the patient is not in shock) for phenobarbital intoxication. Sodium bicarbonate, 44 to 88 mEq/liter, and potassium chloride, 20 mEq/liter, should be given at a rate to produce a urine flow of 3 to 6 ml per kg per hour and a urine pH of 7 to 8. Additional sodium bicarbonate (1 to 2 mEq/kg) and potassium chloride (20 to 40 mEq/liter) may be needed to achieve an optimal urine pH. Assure adequate hydration and renal function prior to alkalinization. Not useful for other barbiturates (Antidote 35, Table 4). (4) In severe cases that do not respond to conservative measures, consider hemodialysis and hemoperfusion. (5) Treat any bullae as a local second degree skin burn. (6) Give intensive care monitoring to comatose patient. *Treatment of withdrawal: In an emergency,* use pentothal or diazepam intravenously. If the patient is stable, a pentobarbital tolerance test may be given; 200 mg of pentobarbital is given orally and the patient examined after 1 hour for signs of intoxication (nystagmus, slurred speech, and ataxia). If none are present, the dose is repeated every 3 hours until these signs develop. This is the stabilizing dose; the patient is maintained on this dose for 72 hours and then changed to phenobarbital, 30 mg substituted for each 100 mg of pentobarbital. The phenobarbital is tapered, decreasing by 10 per cent or 30 mg every 3 to 5 days. *Laboratory aids:* Emergency plasma barbiturate concentrations rarely alter management.

Benzene. See Hydrocarbons.

Benzodiazepines (BZP). See Table 11. *Toxicity:* Low toxic potential. More than 500 mg has been ingested without respiratory depression. Benzodiazepines have an additive effect with sedatives such as alcohol and barbiturates. Most patients intoxicated with BZP alone recover within 24 hours. Many of these agents have

TABLE 10. **Barbiturates: Examples and Elimination***

	Long-Acting		Intermediate	Short-Acting	
Generic name	Barbital	Phenobarbital	Amobarbital	Pentobarbital	Secobarbital
Trade name	Veronal	Luminal	Amytal	Nembutal	Seconal
Slang name	—	Purple hearts	Blue heaven	Yellow jackets	Red devils
pK$_a$	7.74	7.24	7.25	7.96	7.9
Detoxification	Renal	Renal 30% Hepatic 70%	Hepatic 98%	Hepatic 90–100%	Hepatic 90–100%
Onset: IV	22 min	12 min	—	0.1 min	0.1 min
PO	Over 6 hr	3–6 hr (peak 12–18 hr)	Less than 3 hr (peak 3–4 hr)	10–15 min (peak 2–4 hr)	10–15 min (peak 2–4 hr)
Protein-binding (%)	5	29	—	35	44
Hypnotic dose (mg)	300–500	100–200	50–200	50–100	50–100
Fatal dose (grams)	10	8	5	3	3
Toxic dose (mg/kg)	8	8	3–5	3–5	3–5
Therapeutic level (µg/ml)	5–8	15–35	5–8	1–4	3–5
Toxic level (µg/ml)	Over 30	Over 40	10–30	Over 10	Over 10
Lethal level† (µg/ml)	Over 100	Over 100	Over 50	Over 35	Over 35
Duration of action	Over 6	Over 6	Less than 3	Less than 3	Less than 3
Half-life (hr)	58–96	24–96	16–24	36–50	25–50
Rate of metabolism (hr)	—	0.7	2.5	—	—
Volume distribution, liter/kg	—	0.75	0.5–1.1	0.65–1.5	0.65–1.5

Manifestations
    Low dose: Euphoria, ataxia, incoordination, nystagmus on lateral gaze
    High dose: Flaccid coma, hypotension, respiratory depression, pulmonary edema (particularly with the short-acting barbiturates), subcutaneous bullae (6%), dermatographia

*Classification into long-acting, intermediate, and short-acting has no relationship to the duration of coma.
†These levels are not absolute, and tolerance occurs.

TABLE 11. **Benzodiazepines (BZP)**

Drug	Oral Dosage Range	Peak Oral Plasma Levels (hr)	Half-Life (hr)	Major Active Metabolites (half-life in hr)	Elimination Rate
ANXIOLYTICS					
Diazepam (Valium)	6–40 mg/day	1–2	20–50	Desmethyldiazepam (30–60)	Slow
Chlordiazepoxide (Librium, Libritabs, various others)	15–100 mg/day	2–4	5–30	Desmethylchlordiazepoxide, demoxepam, desmethyldiazepam	Slow
Clorazepate (Tranxene)	15–60 mg/day	—	30–60	Desmethyldiazepam	Slow
Prazepam (Centrax)	20–60 mg/day	6	78	3-Hydroxyprazepam, desmethyldiazepam	Slow
Halazepam (Paxipam)	60–160 mg/day	1–3	7	N-3-Hydroxyhalazepam, desmethyldiazepam	Slow
Oxazepam (Serax)	30–120 mg/day	1–2	5–10	None	Rapid to intermediate
Lorazepam (Ativan)	2–6 mg/day	2	10–20	None	Intermediate
Alprazolam (Xanax)	0.75–4 mg/day	0.7–1.6	12–19	α-Hydroxyalprazolam	Intermediate
HYPNOTICS					
Flurazepam (Dalmane)	15–60 mg	—	50–100	Desalkylflurazepam (50–100)	Slow
Flunitrazepam (Rohypnol—investigational, Roche)	1–2 mg	< 1	—	7-Aminoflunitrazepam (23) N-Desmethylflunitrazepam (31)	—
Temazepam (Restoril)	15–30 mg	2–3	9–12	None	Intermediate
Triazolam (Halcion)	0.125–0.5 mg	0.5–1.5	2.3	α-Hydroxytriazolam	Rapid

active metabolites with a long plasma t½, so performance in skilled tasks such as driving may be impaired. Withdrawal may be delayed. *Manifestations:* Central nervous system depression. Deep coma leading to respiratory depression suggests presence of other drugs. *Management:* (1) Gastrointestinal decontamination. (2) Supportive and symptomatic care. (3) Withdrawal, if it occurs, is treated with a long-acting benzodiazepine on a tapering schedule. *Laboratory aids:* Document benzodiazepines in urine. Quantitative blood levels are not useful.

Bleach. Household bleaches are 4 to 6 per cent sodium hypochlorite. Commercial types are 10 to 20 per cent. *Manifestations:* Difficulty in swallowing; pain in mouth, throat, chest, or abdomen. General household strength bleach does not produce burns; commercial strength bleach may. Inhalation of gases produced by mixing chlorine bleach with acids (toilet bowl cleaner and rust removers—chlorine gas) or with household ammonia (chloramine gas) is irritating to mucous membranes, eyes, and upper respiratory tract. *Management:* (1) Ingestion—Do not induce emesis. Dilute with water or milk. Avoid acids. (2) Esophagoscopy only if unusually large amounts have been ingested, the patient is symptomatic, or the product was stronger than the average household bleach. (3) Inhalation—Remove from contaminated area. Observe for pulmonary edema.

Botulism. See article on Foodborne Illnesses in Section 2.

Brake Fluid. See Ethylene Glycol.

Calcium Channel Blockers. Used in treatment of effort angina and supraventricular tachycardia. See Table 12. *Manifestations:* Hypotension, bradycardia within 1 to 5 hours, central nervous system depression, and gastric distress. *Management:* (1) Gastrointestinal decontamination. (2) Treat hypotension and bradycardia with calcium gluconate or chloride. See Antidote 12B, Table 4. Dopamine may be used if necessary. (3) Heart block—may respond to IV calcium, atropine sulfate, 0.5 to 1 mg, or isoproterenol. (4) Ventricular pacing may be required in the severely intoxicated patient. (5) Patients receiving digitalis run the risk of toxicity and should be carefully monitored. *Laboratory aids:* Specific drug levels, blood sugar and calcium, electrocardiogram.

Camphor (External analgesic rubs, Vicks Vaporub

TABLE 12. **Calcium Channel Blockers**

	Nifedipine	Verapamil	Diltiazem
Trade name	Procardia	Calan, Isoptin	Cardiazem
Onset of action	Oral: < 20 min sublingual: < 3 min IV: < 1 min	Oral: < 1 hr — IV: < 2 min	Oral: < 15 min — —
Peak effect	Oral: 1–2 hr	5 hr	30 min
Half-life (hr)	2.5–5	2–7	2–6
Route of elimination	Liver/kidney	Liver/kidney	Liver/kidney
Toxic level (ng/ml)	> 100	> 300	> 200

4.8 per cent, Campho-Phenique 11 per cent). Many camphorated oil products were removed from the marketplace in September, 1982. Five milliliters of camphorated oil (20 per cent camphor) equals 1 gram of camphor. *Toxicity:* Adult, 5 grams; child, 1 gram has been fatal. *Toxicokinetics:* Onset of manifestations, 5 to 90 minutes. Readily and rapidly absorbed through the skin, mucous membranes, and gastrointestinal tract and crosses the placenta. Route of elimination: Rapidly metabolized in liver to the glucuronide form, which is excreted in urine. Pulmonary excretion causes a distinctive odor on the breath. *Manifestations:* Nausea, vomiting, and burning epigastric pain. Seizures may occur suddenly and without warning within 5 minutes of ingestion. Apnea and vision disturbances may occur. *Management:* (1) Induction of emesis is contraindicated because of early seizures. (2) Remove residual drug by gastric lavage. (3) Administer activated charcoal and a saline cathartic. Avoid giving oils or alcohol. (4) Treat seizures with IV diazepam. (5) Treat apnea with respiratory support.

Carbon Monoxide (CO). This is an odorless gas produced from incomplete combustion; it is found also as an in vivo metabolic breakdown product of methylene chloride (paint removers). Observe for the symptoms described in Table 13. Contrary to popular belief, the skin rarely shows a cherry-red color in the live patient. *Toxicokinetics:* CO is rapidly absorbed through the lungs. The rate of absorption is directly related to alveolar ventilation. Elimination occurs through the lungs. The t½ in room air equals 5 to 6 hours; in 100 per cent oxygen, 90 minutes; in hyperbaric oxygen, 20 minutes. The nomogram pictured in Figure 2 can be used to decide quickly whether serious CO intoxication is likely to have occurred and to select patients at high risk or who need early management in the intensive care unit or hyperbaric oxygen.

Management: (1) Remove the patient from contaminated area and expose to fresh air. Establish vital functions. (2) Give 100 per cent oxygen to all patients until the carboxyhemoglobin level falls to 5 to 10 per cent. Assisted ventilation may be necessary. (3) Monitor arterial blood gases and carboxyhemoglobin levels. Determine carboxyhemoglobin level at time of exposure by using nomogram. *Note:* A near normal carboxyhemoglobin level does not rule out significant CO poisoning. (4) Only if pH is below 7.1 after correction of hypoxia and adequate ventilation, give sodium bicarbonate to correct acidosis. (5) Consider hyperbaric oxygen for patients with carboxyhemoglobin over 25 per cent, or over 15 per cent if patient is pregnant, is a child, has cardiac or liver disease, or has a disturbance in mentation. (6) Treat seizures with intravenous diazepam. (7) Monitor electrocardiogram, chest radiograph and serum creatinine phosphokinase (CPK) and lactate dehydrogenase (LDH) levels. (8) Treat cerebral edema with elevation of the patient's head, minimizing intravenous fluid, hyperventilation, and, if needed, mannitol and intracranial pressure monitor. (9) Re-evaluate after recovery for neuropsychiatric sequelae. *Laboratory aids:* Arterial blood gases show metabolic acidosis and normal oxygen tension but reduced oxygen saturation.

Carbon Tetrachloride. See Hydrocarbons.

Caustics and Corrosives. Common acid substances are hydrochloric acid, sulfuric acid (battery acid), carbolic acid (phenol), nitric acid, oxalic acid, hydrofluoric acid, and aqua regia (mixture of hydrochloric and nitric acids). These are used as cleaning agents. Common alkali substances are sodium or potassium hydroxide (lye), sodium hypochlorite (Clorox) (bleach), sodium carbonate (nonphosphate detergents), potassium permanganate, ammonia, electric dishwashing agents, cement, and flat disk batteries. *Toxicity:* Acids produce mucosal coagulation necrosis. They usually do not penetrate deeply (exception: hydrofluoric acid). The gastric mucosa is the primary site of injury. Alkalis produce liquefaction necrosis and saponification and penetrate deeply. Oropharyngeal and esophageal damage by solids is more frequent than by liquids. Liquids are more likely to produce gastric damage. *Toxic dose:* Adult potential fatal dose of concentrated acid/alkali is 5 ml. The absence of oral burns does not exclude the possibility of esophageal burns (10 to 15 per cent).

TABLE 13. **Carbon Monoxide (CO)**

CO in Atmosphere	Duration of Exposure	Saturation of Blood (per cent)	Symptoms
Up to 0.01	Indefinite	1–10	None
0.01–0.02	Indefinite	10–20	Tightness across forehead, slight headache, dilation of cutaneous vessels
0.02–0.03	5–6 hr	20–30	Headache, throbbing temples
0.04–0.06	4–5 hr	30–40	Severe headache, weakness and dizziness, nausea and vomiting, collapse, leukocytosis
0.07–0.10	3–4 hr	40–50	Above, plus increased tendency to collapse and syncope, increased pulse and respiratory rate
0.11–0.15	1.5–3 hr	50–60	Increased pulse and respiratory rate, syncope, Cheyne-Stokes respiration, coma with intermittent convulsions
0.16–0.30	1–1.5 hr	60–70	Coma with intermittent convulsions, depressed heart action and respirations, death possible
0.50–1.00	1–2 min	70–80	Weak pulse, depressed respirations, respiratory failure and death

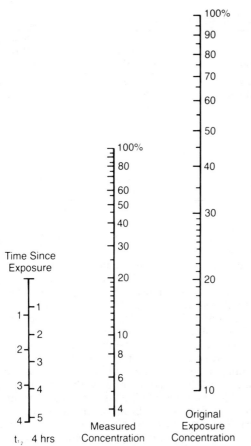

100%
90
80
70
60
50
40
30
20
10

100%
80
60
50
40
30
20
10
8
6
4

Time Since
Exposure

1 — 1
2 — 2
  — 3
3 — 4
4 — 5

t_{1_2} 4 hrs

Measured
Concentration

Original
Exposure
Concentration

Figure 2. Nomogram for calculating carboxyhemoglobin concentration at time of exposure. The time since exposure is given on two scales to allow for the effects of previous oxygen administration on the half-life of carboxyhemoglobin (left-hand scale assumes a half-life of 3 hours). *Note:* The nomogram assumes a half-life of carboxyhemoglobin of 4 hours in a subject breathing room air. Most patients will not have received supplementary oxygen before admission, and at best this will have been administered via a face mask, giving a maximum fractional inspired oxygen concentration of 50 to 60 per cent with little effect on carboxyhemoglobin elimination. The scale on the left side of the time column makes allowances for prior oxygen supplements by assuming a short half-life of 3 hours. The nomogram may help decide quickly whether serious carbon monoxide intoxication is likely to have occurred and may help select patients at high risk for early management in the intensive care unit. The nomogram may be an oversimplification because patients usually are not resuscitated with constant concentrations of oxygen, and many patients may hyperventilate, thus changing elimination characteristics. (Redrawn from Clark et al: Blood carboxyhemoglobin and cyanide levels in fire. Lancet *1*:1332, 1981.)

Management: (1) Dilute with milk or water immediately up to 30 ml in children or 250 ml in adults. Neutralization with acidic or alkalinic agents is contraindicated. Dilute only if patient can swallow. (2) Gastrointestinal decontamination is contraindicated. However, in acid ingestions some authorities advocate nasogastric intubation and aspiration in the early postingestion phase. Patient should receive only intravenous fluids following dilution until surgical consultation is obtained. Dermal and ocular decontamination

should be carried out. (3) Esophagoscopy may be indicated postingestion to assess severity of burn. (4) Steroids are controversial. Some recommend administration of steroids if burns are found or esophagoscopy is not performed. (5) Antibiotics are not useful prophylactically. (6) Barium swallow may be necessary at 10 days to 3 weeks to assess severity of damage. (7) Esophageal dilation may need to be performed at 2- to 4-week intervals if evidence of stricture is found. (8) Intraposition of the colon may be necessary if dilation fails to provide an adequate-sized esophagus. (9) Inhalation management requires immediate removal from the environment, and clinical, x-ray, and arterial blood gas evaluation when appropriate. Oxygen and respiratory support may be required.

Chloral Hydrate. See Sedative Hypnotics.

Chlordane. See Organochlorine Insecticides.

Chlordiazepoxide (Librium). See Benzodiazepines.

Chlorine Gas. Chlorine gas is a yellow-greenish gas with an irritating odor used in bleach, in manufacture of plastics, and for water purification. Exposure usually results from transportation mishaps, industrial accidents, chemistry experiments, the mixing of household cleaners with bleach containing hypochlorite, and accidental release around swimming pools. Its density is greater than that of air, and an odor is detected at concentrations of less than 0.5 PPM. Chlorine acts as an oxidizing agent and also acts with tissue water to form hypochlorite and hydrochloric acid and generate free oxygen radicals. *Toxic dose and management:* The threshold limit value is less than 1 PPM; 4 PPM is tolerated for 0.5 hour; 15 PPM immediately irritates mucous membranes of eyes, ears, nose, and throat; 30 ppm produces choking and chest pain; 60 ppm produces pulmonary edema; 400 PPM for 30 minutes is lethal; and 1000 PPM is fatal in a few minutes.

Management: (1) Remove the patient from contaminated environment and stabilize vital functions. Decontamination procedures for dermal and ocular contamination as indicated. Protect rescue personnel with breathing apparatus. Classification—If symptomless or with a cough that clears up in less than 1 hour, rest for 12 hours and report if symptoms occur; no vigorous exercise for 24 hours. If symptoms persist beyond period of exposure, admit to hospital and treat with bronchodilators (use theophylline, not epinephrine) and humidified oxygen. Noncardiac pulmonary edema is treated with positive end-expiratory pressure; corticosteroids are controversial; furosemide (Lasix) may be used. For conjunctival irritation, copious water irrigation and fluorescein stain for corneal damage. For dermal burns, copious water irrigation and conventional treatment of burns. *Laboratory aids:* Chest radiograph (may not reflect damage for 24 hours), arterial blood gases, cardiac monitor for dysrhythmias.

Chlorpromazine (Thorazine). See Phenothiazines.

Clinitest Tablets. See Caustics and Corrosives.

Cocaine (Benzoylmethylecgonine). Toxic dose: The potential fatal dose is 1200 mg, but death has occurred with 20 mg parenterally. *Toxicokinetics:* See Table 14. *Manifestations:* Hypertension, convulsions, hyperthermia, and cardiac dysrhythmias. *Management:* (1) Supportive care. Cardiac and thermal monitoring. Phenytoin may be effective for ventricular dysrhyth-

TABLE 14. **Pharmaco-Toxicokinetics of Cocaine**

Type	Route	Onset	Peak	Duration t½ (min)	Possible Fatal Dose (Adult)
Hydrochloride	Insufflation	1–5 min	20–60 min	60–75	750–800 mg
	Ingested	Delayed	30–90 min	60–75	1.4 grams
	IV	2–3 min	30–60 min	60–75	20–800 mg
Free base	Smoked	<2 min	seconds	<20	750–800 mg
Coca paste	Smoked			Not known	
Crack	Smoked	(Fastest) 4–6 sec	seconds	<20 5–7	Not known

mias, whereas lidocaine may be ineffective and enhance toxicity. Control anxiety and convulsions with diazepam. Labetalol intravenously (Antidote 23, Table 4) has been used to control life-threatening hypertension and tachycardia. A nonthreatening environment to reduce all sensory stimuli and protect patient from injury is required.

Codeine. See Opioids.

Corrosives. See Caustics and Corrosives.

Cyanide. See Table 15. Hydrocyanic acid and sodium and potassium salts act rapidly and are extremely poisonous. The acid is extremely volatile, producing cyanide, which has a distinctive odor of bitter almonds and can produce death within minutes after inhalation. Cyanide interferes with the cytochrome oxidase system. *Classes of cyanides and derivatives*: (1) Hydrogen cyanide and simple salts in large doses act to produce death in 15 minutes. (2) Halogenated cyanides such as cyanogen chloride produce irritant and vesicant gases that may cause pulmonary edema. (3) Nitriles such as acrylonitrile and acetonitrile. Cyanides are used as fumigants (hydrogen cyanide), in synthetic rubber (acrylonitrile), in fertilizers (cyanamide), in metal refining (salts), and in the home in some silver and furniture polishes. Cyanide in the seeds of fruit stones is harmful only if the capsule is broken. *Manifestations*: Seizures, stupor, cardiac dysrhythmias, pulmonary edema, lactic acidemia, decreased arterial venous oxygen difference. Bright red venous blood.

Management: Attendants should not administer mouth to mouth resuscitation. (1) Immediately, 100 per cent oxygen. If inhaled, remove patient from contaminated atmosphere. (2) Cyanide antidote kit (Antidote 14, Table 4). Use antidote only if certain of diagnosis and significant toxicity (impairment of consciousness). (3) Gastrointestinal decontamination by gastric lavage. *No* syrup of ipecac. Activated charcoal not very effective (1 gram binds only 35 mg of cyanide). (4) Treat seizures with intravenous diazepam. (5) Correct acidosis. (6) Other antidotes: In Europe, dicobalt edetate, 600 mg, is used intravenously, followed by 300 mg if the response is not satisfactory. Hydroxycobalamin (vitamin B_{12}) is a useful antidote but must be given immediately after exposure in very large doses. Dose: 1800 mg of vitamin B_{12} per dl of KCN is usually required (forms cyanocobalamin).

DDT and Derivatives. See Organochlorine Insecticides.

Desipramine (Norpramin, Pertofrane). See Tricyclic Antidepressants.

Diazepam (Valium). See Benzodiazepines.

Digitalis Preparations. See Table 16. *Manifestations*: Abdominal pain, nausea, vomiting, diarrhea, dysrhythmias, heart block, central nervous system depression, colored-halo vision. *Management*: (1) Gastrointestinal decontamination. Repeated doses of activated charcoal may interrupt enterohepatic recirculation. (2) Treat ventricular premature contractions, including bigeminy, trigeminy, quadrigeminy, ventricular tachycardia, and atrial tachycardia, with phenytoin. Lidocaine also may be administered for ventricular dysrhythmias. (3) Treat bradycardia and second and third degree AV block with atropine. External pacing may be needed. (4) Treat hyperkalemia (above 6 mEq/liter with intravenous glucose 5 to 10 per cent, intravenous sodium bicarbonate, intravenous insulin (insulin is not used in children), and Kayexalate retention enema (25 per cent in sorbitol 25 per cent) in severe cases. If hyperkalemia is present (ominous sign), insertion of a pacemaker should be seriously considered. Hemodialysis is treatment of choice for severe or refractory hyperkalemia. (5) Direct current countershock may cause life-threatening dysrhythmias. (6) Specific Fab antibody fragments (Digibind) (Antidote 21, Table 4) have been used for life-threatening cardiac dysrhythmias, hyperkalemia, and cases refractory to conventional measures. *Laboratory aids*: Monitor electrocardiogram and potassium and digitalis levels. Draw digoxin levels 6 to 8 hours postingestion.

Diphenhydramine (Benadryl). See Anticholinergic Agents.

Doxepin (Sinequan, Adapin). See Tricyclic Antidepressants.

Ethchlorvynol (Placidyl). See Sedative Hypnotics.

Ethyl Alcohol. See Alcohols.

Ethylene Glycol (solvent, antifreeze). *Toxic dose*: Death has occurred after a 60 ml ingestion; fatal dose = 1.4 ml per kg of 100 per cent solution. The threshold limit value (TLV) is 50 PPM. *Toxicokinetics*: Time of onset, 30 minutes to 12 hours for central nervous system and metabolic abnormalities to occur (Phase I). Twelve to 36 hours postingestion, cardiopulmonary depression (Phase II). In Phase III (2 to 3 days postingestion), renal failure occurs. The t½ is 3 hours (during ethanol therapy this is prolonged to 17 hours). *Management*: (1) Gastrointestinal decontamination up

TABLE 15. **Forms of Cyanide and Their Toxicity**

Common Forms	Toxicity
Hydrocyanic acid	PFD* = 50 mg (0.5 mg/kg)
Potassium/sodium cyanide	PFD = 150–300 mg (2 mg/kg)
Calcium and ferric or ferrocyanides	Low order of toxicity; PFD = 50 grams
Sodium nitroprusside	5 mg/kg causes acute toxicity; PFD = 3–4 grams (195–260 mg)
Bitter almonds	
Oil	2 oz kills immediately
Almonds	50–60 bitter almonds; each contain 0.001 gram of hydrogen cyanide
Pulp	240 grams
Peach seed	100 grams of moist seeds = 88 mg of cyanide
Apricot	
Wild	100 grams of moist seed = 217 mg of cyanide
Cultivated	100 grams = 8.7 mg of cyanide
Laetrile (amygdalin); cyanogenic glycoside in kernels of apricots	
Laetrile strengths:	HCN in mg/gram
tablets: 250 mg	2.7
tablets: 500 mg	29–51.5
parenteral 10 ml, 3 gram vial	23.2–27.9
Amygdaline, parenteral, 10 ml, 3 gram vial	8.3–51.3
Hydrogen cyanide inhalation; acrylonitrile, cyanamide, cyanogen chloride, cyanides, nitroprussides (produced in fire involving polyurethane foams)	Maximum allowable concentration, 10 PPM TLV* = 5 mg/m³ in air for cyanide salts 0.2–0.3 mg/liter is immediately fatal 0.13 mg/liter (130 PPM) is fatal in 1 hour
Hydrogen cyanide liquid	Rapidly absorbed through skin

*PFD, Potential fatal dose; TLV, Threshold limit values.

TABLE 16. **Digitalis Preparations**

	Digoxin	Digitoxin
Trade name	Lanoxin	Crystodigin
Onset time po	1.5–6 hr	3–6 hr
Peak	4–6	6–12
Half-life	31–40 hr	4–6 days
Protein-bound (%)	25	90
Vd	7–8 liters/kg	0.6 liter/kg
Route of elimination	Renal, 75%	Liver, 80%
Toxic blood levels	2.4 ng/ml	> 30 ng/ml
Enterohepatic route	Small	Large

to 2 to 4 hours postingestion. Activated charcoal and cathartics are not indicated. (2) Treat seizures with intravenous diazepam. Exclude hypocalcemia. (3) Correct acidosis with intravenous sodium bicarbonate. (4) Initiate ethanol therapy to block metabolism (Antidote 20, Table 4). (5) Early hemodialysis is indicated if the ingestion was large; if the blood ethylene glycol level is greater than 50 mg per dl; if severe acid-base or electrolyte abnormalities occur despite conventional therapy; or if renal failure occurs. (6) Thiamine and pyridoxine have been recommended but not extensively studied. *Laboratory aids*: Complete blood count, electrolytes, urinalysis (look for oxalate crystals), and arterial blood gases. Obtain ethylene glycol and ethanol levels, plasma osmolarity (use freezing point depression method). Calcium, creatinine, and BUN studies. An ethylene glycol level of 100 mg per dl is usually toxic (levels are very difficult to obtain).

Flurazepam (Dalmane). See Benzodiazepines.

Glutethimide (Doriden). See Sedative Hypnotics.

Hallucinogens

1. *LSD* (lysergic acid diethylamide). *Toxic dose*: ≥ 35 µg. Street doses are typically 50 to 300 µg. *Toxicokinetics*: Peak effect, 1 to 2 hours. Duration, 12 to 24 hours. t½, 3 hours. Route of elimination, bile.

2. *Morning-Glory Seeds* (*Rivea corymbosa* or *Ipomoea*). These have one-tenth the potency of LSD.

3. *Mescaline/Peyote* (trimethoxyphenylethylamine or *Lophophora williamsii*). *Toxic dose*: ≥ 5 mg per kg. Each button of mescaline contains 45 mg (4 to 12 produce symptoms). *Toxicokinetics*: Peak effect, 4 to 6 hours. Duration, 14 hours.

4. *Psilocybin*. Similar in effect to LSD but short-acting. Peak effect, 90 minutes. Duration, 5 to 6 hours.

5. *Nutmeg (Myristica)*. *Toxic dose*: 5 to 15 grams (1 to 3 nutmegs). Peak effect, 3 to 6 hours. Duration, up to 60 hours.

6. *Marijuana* (*Cannabis sativa*) (δ-9-tetrahydrocannabinol, THC). One joint equals 500 mg of marijuana; when smoked, 50 per cent is destroyed. *Toxicokinetics*: Time of onset, 2 to 3 minutes (smoked). Duration, 2 to 3 hours. t½, 28 to 47 hours (shorter for chronic user). *Note*: 1 per cent of the metabolite can be detected in urine up to 2 weeks after use. *Manifestations*: Visual illusions, sensory perceptual distortions, depersonalization, and derealization. *Management*: "Talk-down" technique.

7. *Inhalants*. Nitrites (amyl and isobutyl nitrite)—act immediately; aromatic hydrocarbon in airplane model glues, plastic cements (benzene, toluene, xylene)—see hydrocarbons; *nitrous oxide* and *halogenated hydrocarbons*.

8. *Tryptamine Derivatives* (DMT, dimethyltryptamine; DET, diethyltryptamine; DPT, dipropyltryptamine). Rapid onset of action, but duration is only 1 to 2 hours.

9. *STP* or *DOM* (2,5-dimethoxy-4-methyl-amphetamine). Acts like LSD but lasts 72 hours or longer.

10. *MDA* (3-methoxy-4,5-ethylenedioxy amphetamine). Related to amphetamine, produces a mild LSD-like reaction lasting 6 to 10 hours (love pill).

See also Alcohols, Amphetamines, Anticholinergic Agents, Barbiturates, Cocaine, Opioids, Phencyclidine, Phenothiazines, and Tricyclic Antidepressants.

TABLE 17. **Common Examples of Aliphatic Halogenated Hydrocarbons**

	Estimated Fatal Dose (Ingested)	TLV-TWA (PPM)	Synonyms
Trichloroethane 1, 1, 1	5.7 grams/kg	350	Methyl chloroform, Triethane, chlorethane, Glamorene Spot Remover, Scotchgard
Trichloroethane 1, 1, 2	580 mg/kg	10	Vinyl trichloride
Trichloroethylene	Controversial, 3–5 ml/kg	50	—
Tetrachloroethanene	Not known	5	Acetylene tetrachloride
Dichloromethane	25 ml	100	Methylene chloride
Tetrachloroethylene	5 ml	50	Tetrachloroethene Perchloroethylene
Dichloroethane	0.5 ml/kg	200	—
Carbon tetrachloride	3–5 ml	5	—

Haloperidol (Haldol). See Phenothiazines.

Heroin. See Opioids.

Hydrocarbons

1. *Petroleum Distillates.* Gasoline (petroleum spirit), 2 to 5 per cent benzene; kerosene (coal oil, kerosene, jet aviation fuel No. 1, charcoal lighter fluid); petroleum naphtha (cigarette lighter fluid, ligroin, racing fuel); petroleum ether (benzine); turpentine (pine oil, oil of turpentine); and mineral spirits (Stoddard solvent, white spirits, varasol, mineral turpentine, petroleum spirit). *Manifestations*: Materials aspirated during the process of ingestion may produce pneumonitis. Hypoxia associated with aspiration is the cause of central nervous system depression, not absorption. It is *unlikely* that a child accidentally or an adult during siphoning would ingest a sufficient quantity to warrant the induction of emesis.

2. *Aromatic Hydrocarbons. Benzene*, a solvent used in manufacturing dyes, phenol, and nitrobenzene, has a threshold limit value (TLV) of 10 PPM by inhalation according to the Occupational Safety and Health Administration (OSHA). The National Institute for Occupational Safety and Health (NIOSH) value is 1 PPM. The adult ingested toxic dose is 15 ml. Chronic exposure may cause leukemia. Two hundred PPM is fatal in 5 minutes. *Toluene*, used in manufacturing TNT, has an OSHA TLV of 200 PPM by inhalation; the NIOSH figure is 100. The adult ingested toxic dose is 50 ml. *Styrene* has an OSHA TLV of 100 PPM by inhalation. *Xylene,* used in the manufacture of perfumes, has an OSHA TLV of 100 PPM by inhalation. The adult ingested toxic dose is 50 ml. *Manifestations*: Asphyxiation, central nervous system depression, defatting dermatitis, and aspiration pneumonitis. A bite into a tube of household plastic cement by a young child does not warrant the induction of emesis. Ingestion of hydrocarbon with a benzene fraction over 5 per cent may warrant induction of emesis.

3. *Aliphatic Halogenated Hydrocarbons.* See Table 17 for common examples. *Manifestations*: Myocardial sensitization and irritability, hepatorenal toxicity, and central nervous system depression. Dichloromethane may be converted into carbon monoxide in the body. Trichloroethylene concentrates in the fetus (pregnant women should not be exposed) and causes a disulfiram (Antabuse) reaction ("degreaser's flush")

when associated with ingestion of ethanol. The decision to induce emesis must be based on the toxicity of the agent.

4. *Dangerous Additives.* Dangerous additives to the hydrocarbons, such as heavy metals, nitrobenzene, aniline dyes, insecticides and demothing agents, may warrant the induction of emesis.

5. *Heavy Hydrocarbons.* These have high viscosity, low volatility, and minimal absorption, so emesis is unwarranted. Examples are asphalt (tar), machine oil, motor oil (lubricating oil, engine oil), diesel oil (engine fuel, home heating oil), petrolatum liquid (mineral oil, suntan oils), petrolatum jelly (Vaseline), paraffin wax, transmission oil, cutting oil, and greases and glues.

6. *Products Treated as Petroleum Distillates.* Essential oils (e.g., turpentine, pine oil) are treated as petroleum distillates. Mineral seal oil (signal oil), found in some furniture polishes, is a heavy, viscous oil that *never* warrants emesis; it can produce severe pneumonia if aspirated. It has minimal absorption. *Management*: Dermal decontamination. Removal from the environment in inhalation.

First Aid Treatment. See Table 18. *The use of activated charcoal, oils, and cathartics is not advised in petroleum distillate ingestions. General management*: (1) In the asymptomatic patient: observe several hours for development of respiratory distress. (2) In the symptomatic patient: supportive respiratory care for respiratory distress. Bronchospasm may be treated with intravenous aminophylline. Avoid epinephrine. Monitor ECG; arterial blood gases; liver, pulmonary, and renal function; serum electrolytes; serial radiographs. Observe for intravascular hemolysis and disseminated intravascular coagulation. If cyanosis is present that does not respond to oxygen or the arterial Pa_{O_2} is normal, suspect methemoglobinemia that may require therapy with methylene blue. Steroids have not been shown to be beneficial. Antimicrobial agents are not useful in prophylaxis. (Fever or leukocytosis may be produced by the chemical pneumonitis itself.) It is not necessary to treat pneumatoceles. Most infiltrations resolve spontaneously in 1 week except for lipoid pneumonia, which may last up to 6 weeks.

Imipramine (Tofranil). See Tricyclic Antidepressants.

Iron. The iron content of some preparations appears in Table 19. *Toxic dose*: Range, 20 to 60 mg per kg or

TABLE 18. **First Aid Treatment for Hydrocarbon Ingestion**

Symptoms	Contents	Amount	First Aid
None	Petroleum distillate only	Less than 2 ml/kg	None
None	Heavy hydrocarbon Mineral seal oil	More than 2 ml/kg	None* None
	Petroleum distillate	Minimum, 30 ml	Consider emesis induction†
None	Petroleum distillate with dangerous additive	Depends on toxicity of additive	Consider emesis induction†
	Aromatic and halogenated hydrocarbons	Depends on toxicity of hydrocarbon	Consider emesis induction†
Loss of protective airway reflex; convulsions	Petroleum distillate with dangerous additive	Depends on toxicity of additive	Consider endotracheal intubation prior to gastric aspiration and lavage
Breathing difficulty	Aromatic and halogenated hydrocarbons	Depends on toxicity of individual hydrocarbon	Consider endotracheal intubation prior to gastric aspiration and lavage

*Emesis may be necessary if machine oil contains triorthocresyl phosphate (TOCP), which causes weakness, sensory impairment, and "partially reversible damage to the spinal cord."

†Emesis induction is rarely indicated if the patient has already vomited. Emesis usually should be induced with proper positioning.

greater of elemental iron. Dose to induce emesis, ≥ 20 mg per kg. The potential fatal dose is 180 mg per kg (600 mg of elemental iron). *Toxicokinetics*: Absorption occurs chiefly in the small intestine. For excretion there is no normal route except blood loss or gastrointestinal desquamation. *Manifestations*: Phase I—Mucosal injury possibly with hematemesis (1 to 6 hours postingestion). Phase II—patient appears improved (6 to 48 hours). Phase III—cardiovascular collapse and severe metabolic acidosis. Phase IV—sequelae of intestinal stricture and obstruction or anemia (weeks to months). Patients asymptomatic for 6 hours rarely develop serious intoxication manifestations.

Management: (1) Gastrointestinal decontamination. Emesis should be induced in ingestions of elemental iron of over 20 mg per kg. Emesis should be followed by gastric lavage if large amounts have been ingested (over 60 mg per kg). The solution to be used for lavage is 1 to 1.5 per cent sodium bicarbonate to form ferrous carbonate salts, which are poorly absorbed. One hundred milliliters of this solution should be left in the stomach (prepared by dilution of a sodium bicarbonate ampule with saline). The use of deferoxamine (Desferal) in the gastrointestinal tract is controversial. The use of diluted Fleet's enema solution risks severe hypertonic phosphate poisoning. (2) Postlavage abdominal radiograph—if significant amounts of residual

TABLE 19. **Iron Content of Some Preparations**

Salt	Elemental Iron Content (%)	Average Tablet Strength (mg)	Iron Content Per Tablet (mg)
Ferrous sulfate	20	300	60
Ferrous sulfate (dried)	29.7	200	65
Ferrous gluconate	11.6	320	36
Ferrous fumarate	33	200	67

radiopaque material are present, consider removal by endoscopy or surgery since coalesced tablets have produced hemorrhagic infarction and perforation peritonitis. (3) Protect the mucosal surfaces with demulcents if damage is evident. (4) Diagnostic chelation test—deferoxamine not reliable. (5) Indications for chelation therapy with deferoxamine are serum iron greater than total iron binding capacity, or positive diagnostic chelation test; serum iron over 500 mg per dl; and systemic signs of intoxication independent of serum iron level. Chelation should be performed within 12 to 18 hours to be effective.

Laboratory aids: Serum iron levels correlate with the clinical course. Iron levels drawn at 2 to 6 hours that are below 350 mg per dl predict an asymptomatic course; levels of 350 to 500 are associated with mild gastrointestinal symptoms (rarely serious); and levels greater than 500 suggest the possibility of serious Phase III manifestations. White blood cell counts greater than 15,000 per μl, blood glucose levels over 150 mg per dl, radiopaque material present on abdominal radiograph, vomiting, and diarrhea predict iron levels greater than 300 mg per dl. Monitor complete blood counts, blood glucose, serum iron, stools, and vomitus for occult blood; electrolytes; acid-base balance; urinalysis and urinary output; liver function tests; BUN; and creatinine. Obtain type and match of blood in severe cases. Abdominal radiographs. Follow-up is necessary for sequelae in significant intoxications—gastrointestinal series for intestinal strictures and anemia secondary to blood loss. Patients who develop fever or toxic symptoms following iron overdose should have blood and stool cultures checked for *Yersinia enterocolitica*.

Isoniazid (INH, Nydrazid). This is an antituberculosis drug frequently used in suicides by American Indians and Eskimos. *Mechanism of toxicity:* It produces pyridoxine deficiency (doubles excretion of pyridoxine). *Toxic dose:* 1.5 grams, 35 to 40 mg per kg, produces convulsions; severe toxicity is seen at 6 to 10 grams; 200 mg per kg is an obligatory convulsant. *Toxicoki-*

netics: Absorption is rapid, with a peak in 1 to 2 hours (clinical symptoms may start in 30 minutes). Volume distribution is 0.6 liter per kg. It passes the placenta and into breast milk at 50 per cent of the maternal serum level. Not protein-bound. Elimination is by the liver, which produces a hepatotoxic metabolite, acetylisoniazid. The t½—slow acetylators (2 to 4 hours) may develop peripheral neuropathy (50 per cent of blacks and whites). Fast acetylators (0.7 to 2 hours) may develop hepatitis (90 per cent of Orientals and a majority of patients with diabetes). Excreted unchanged, 10 to 40 per cent. *Major toxic manifestations:* Visual disturbances, convulsions (90 per cent or more with one or more seizures), coma, resistant severe acidosis (due to lactate secondary to hypoxia, convulsions, and metabolic blocks).

Management: (1) Control seizures with large doses of pyridoxine, 1 gram for each gram of isoniazid ingested (Antidote 34, Table 4). If the dose ingested is unknown, give at least 5 grams of pyridoxine intravenously. (2) Correct acidosis with fluids and sodium bicarbonate (pyridoxine may spontaneously correct the acidosis). (3) Diazepam may be used as a supplement to control the seizures. (4) After patient is stabilized or if asymptomatic, gastrointestinal decontamination procedures may be carried out, keeping in mind the rapid onset of convulsions. Asymptomatic patients should be observed for 4 hours. (5) Hemodialysis is rarely needed but may be used as an adjunct for uncontrollable acidosis and seizures. Hemoperfusion has not been adequately evaluated. Diuresis is ineffective. *Laboratory aids:* Isoniazid toxic levels are above 8 μg per ml. Monitor the blood glucose (often hyperglycemia), electrolytes (often hyperkalemia), bicarbonate, and arterial blood gases. Monitor the temperature closely (often hyperpyrexia).

Isopropyl Alcohol. See Alcohols.

Kerosene. See Hydrocarbons.

Lead. *Acute* lead poisoning is rare. *Acute toxic dose:* 0.5 gram. *Management:* (1) Gastrointestinal decontamination. (2) Supportive care, including measures to deal with the hepatic and renal failure and intravascular hemolysis. (3) Ethylenediaminetetraacetic acid (EDTA) in all severe cases if lead levels confirm absorption. **Chronic** lead poisoning occurs most often in children 1 to 6 years of age who are exposed in their environment and in adults in certain occupations or from illicit whiskey. *Chronic toxic dose:* Determined by blood lead level and clinical findings. Over 25 μg per dl indicates excess body burden. A chronic dose of 0.6 mg a day will increase the body burden, 2.5 mg a day will result in toxicity in 4 years, and 3.5 mg a day will cause toxicity in a few months. *Toxicokinetics:* Absorption—10 to 15 per cent of the ingested dose is absorbed in adults; in children up to 40 per cent is absorbed with iron deficiency anemia. Inhalation absorption is rapid and complete. Vd—95 per cent present in bone. In blood, 95 per cent is in red blood cells. t½, 35 days; in bone, 10 years. The major elimination route for inorganic lead is renal. Organic lead is metabolized in the liver to inorganic lead; 9 per cent is excreted in the urine per day. *Manifestations of acute symptoms of chronic lead poisoning* (ABCDE): Anorexia, apathy, anemia; behavior disturbances; clumsiness; develop-

mental deterioration; and emesis. Manifestations of encephalopathy are "PAINT:" *P,* persistent forceful vomiting; *A,* ataxia; *I,* intermittent stupor and lucidity; *N,* neurologic coma and convulsions; *T,* tired and lethargic. In adults one may see peripheral neuropathies and "lead gum lines."

Management: (1) Gastrointestinal decontamination with enemas if radiopaque foreign bodies are noted. Do not delay therapy until clear. (2) Remove from exposure. For children, see Table 20. *Laboratory aids:* (1) Provocation mobilization test—50 mg per kg of EDTA intramuscularly for 1 dose and collect the urine for 6 to 8 hours. A ratio of micrograms excreted in the urine to milligrams of Ca-EDTA administered greater than 0.6 represents an increased lead body burden, and chelation should be administered. (2) Evaluate complete blood count, levels of serum iron, or ferritin; repeat blood lead levels and erythrocyte protoporphyrin. (3) Flat plate of the abdomen and long bone radiographs (knees usually). (4) Renal function tests. (5) Monitor electrolytes, serum calcium, phosphorus, blood glucose.

Lindane. See Organochlorine Insecticides.

Lithium (Eskalith, Lithane). Most cases of intoxication have occurred as therapeutic overdoses. The toxic dose is determined by serum levels, although intoxication has occurred with levels in the therapeutic range.

Toxicokinetics: Absorption is rapid, with complete peaking in 1 to 4 hours. Vd is 0.5 to 0.9 liter per kg. It is not protein bound. The t½ therapeutically is 18 to 24 hours. Eighty-nine to 98 per cent is excreted by the kidney unchanged, one third to two thirds in 6 to 12 hours. Excretion is decreased in the presence of hyponatremia and dehydration. The cerebrospinal fluid concentration is one half the plasma concentration. The breast milk level is 50 per cent of the maternal serum level—toxic to the nursling. *Manifestations:* The first sign of toxicity may be diarrhea. Fine tremor of hands, lethargy, weakness, polyuria and polydipsia, goiter and hypothyroidism, and fasciculations are side effects. Severe toxicity is manifest by ataxia, impaired mental state, coma, and seizures (limbs held in hyperextension with eyes open in "coma vigil"). Cardiovascular manifestations are dysrhythmias, hypotension, flat T waves, and increased QT interval.

Management: (1) Gastrointestinal decontamination may not be useful after 2 hours because of rapid absorption. In slow-release preparations, decontamination may be useful up to 24 hours postingestion. Activated charcoal is not indicated. (2) Hospitalize if intoxication is suspected because seizures may occur unexpectedly. (3) Restore normothermia and fluid and electrolyte balance, particularly sodium. If diabetes insipidus is present, an infusion of sodium may cause hypernatremia. Current evidence supports saline infusion as enhancing excretion of lithium. (4) Forced diuresis has no role, unless the glomerular filtration rate is low. Consider only when the lithium level is not above 2.5 mEq per liter and fails to fall below 1 mEq per liter within 30 hours. (5) Hemodialysis is the treatment of choice for severe intoxication. Lithium is the most dialyzable toxin known. Long runs of 12 hours or longer should be used until the lithium level

TABLE 20. **Choice of Chelation Therapy Based on Symptoms and Blood Lead Concentration**

Clinical Presentation	Treatment	Comments
Symptomatic children		
Acute encephalopathy	BAL, 450 mg/M²/day CaNa₂-EDTA, 1500 mg/M²/day (EDTA not used alone if blood Pb >72 μg/dl or symptoms present)	Start with BAL, 75 mg/M² IM every 4 hours After 4 hours start continuous infusion of CaNa₂-EDTA, 1500 mg/M²/day Therapy with BAL and CaNa₂-EDTA should be continued for 5 days Interrupt therapy for 2 days Treat for 5 additional days, including BAL if blood Pb remains high Other cycles may be needed depending on blood Pb rebound.
Other symptoms	BAL, 300 mg/M²/day CaNa₂-EDTA, 1000 mg/M²/day Monitor BUN, creatinine, AST, ALT, urine	Start with BAL, 90 mg/M² IM every 4 hours After 4 hours start CaNa₂-EDTA, 1000 mg/M²/day, preferably by continuous infusion, or in divided doses IV (through a heparin lock) Therapy with CaNa₂-EDTA should be continued for 5 days BAL may be discontinued after 3 days if blood Pb <50 μg/dl Interrupt therapy for 2 days Treat for 5 additional days, including BAL if blood Pb remains high (>50 μg/dl) Other cycles may be needed depending on blood Pb rebound
Asymptomatic children		
Before treatment, measure venous blood lead		
Blood Pb >70 μg/dl	BAL, 300 mg/M²/day CaNa₂-EDTA, 1000 mg/M²/day	Start with BAL, 50 mg/M² IM every 4 hours After 4 hours start CaNa₂-EDTA, 1000 mg/M²/day, preferably by continuous infusion, or in divided doses IV (through a heparin lock) Treatment with CaNa₂-EDTA should be continued for 5 days BAL may be discontinued after 3 days if blood Pb <50 μg/dl Other cycles may be needed depending on blood Pb rebound
Blood Pb 56 to 69 μg/dl	CaNa₂-EDTA, 1000 mg/M²/day	CaNa₂-EDTA for 5 days, preferably by continuous infusion, or in divided doses (through a heparin lock) Alternatively, if lead exposure is controlled, CaNa₂-EDTA may be given as a single daily outpatient dose IM or IV Other cycles may be needed depending on blood Pb rebound
Blood Pb 25 to 55 μg/dl		
Perform CaNa₂-EDTA provocation test to assess lead excretion ratio		
If ratio >0.70	CaNa₂-EDTA, 1000 mg/M²/day	Treat for 5 days IV or IM, as above
If ratio 0.60 to 0.69		
Age <3 years	CaNa₂-EDTA, 1000 mg/M²/day	Treat for 3 days IV or IM, as above
Age >3 years	No treatment	Repeat blood Pb and CaNa₂-EDTA provocation test periodically
If ratio <0.60	No treatment	Repeat blood Pb and CaNa₂-EDTA provocation test periodically

From Piomelli S., et al.: Management of childhood lead poisoning. J. Pediatr. *105*:523–532, 1984.

is less than 1 mEq per liter because of extensive re-equilibration rebound. Follow levels every 4 hours after dialysis. Dialysis may have to be repeated. Expect a time lag in neurologic recovery. If hemodialysis is not available or delayed, peritoneal dialysis can be used but is less effective. (6) Monitor ECG. Refractory dysrhythmias may be treated with magnesium sulfate and sodium bicarbonate. (7) Aminophylline may increase lithium excretion and decrease lithium reabsorption but has not been extensively studied. (8) Avoid thiazides and spironolactone diuretics, which increase lithium levels.

Laboratory aids: Lithium level determinations should be performed every 4 hours. Although they do not always correlate with the manifestations at low levels, they are predictive in severe intoxications. Levels of 0.6 to 1.2 mEq per liter are usually therapeutic. Levels over 4.0 mEq per liter are severely toxic. Other tests to be monitored are complete blood count (lithium causes leukocytosis), renal function, thyroid, ECG, and electrolytes. Factors that predispose to lithium toxicity are febrile illness, sodium depletion, concomitant drugs (thiazide and spironolactone diuretics), impaired renal function, advanced age, and fluid loss in vomiting and diarrheal illness.

Lomotil (Diphenoxylate and Atropine). See Opioids and Anticholinergic Agents.

LSD (Lysergic Acid Diethylamide). See Hallucinogens.

Marijuana. See Hallucinogens.

Meperidine (Demerol). See Opioids.

Meprobamate (Equanil, Miltown). See Sedative Hypnotics.

Mercury. *Management:* (1) Inhalation of elemental mercury—remove from exposure. (2) Ingestion of mercuric salt—gastrointestinal decontamination. A protein solution such as egg white or 5 per cent salt-poor albumin can be given to reduce salt to mercurous ion (less toxic). Give activated charcoal and cathartic. (3) Chelating agents (do not use Ca-EDTA because of nephrotoxicity): Dimercaprol (BAL) enhances mercury excretion through the bile as well as the urine and would be the choice if there were renal impairment from the mercury (Antidote 17, Table 4). Penicillamine (Antidote 29, Table 4) or N-acetyl DL-penicillamine (investigational use). Use of BAL in methyl mercury intoxication increases the brain mercury and appears to be contraindicated; penicillamine and its analogue should be used (decreases mercury in brain). A new chelator, 2,3-dimercaptosuccinic acid, holds promise of less toxicity and more specific therapy and is now available under the Orphan Drug Program.* (4) Monitor fluid and electrolyte levels, renal function, hemoglobin levels. Obtain blood and urine mercury levels (consult the laboratory for proper collection technique and containers). (5) Hemodialysis early in the symptomatic patient is useful. (6) New but not established approaches are Polythiol resin to bind the methyl mercury excreted in the bile; heat and sauna treatment to increase mercury excretion through perspiration; and a regional dialyzer system using L-cysteine. (7) Surgical excision of *local injection sites*.

Laboratory aids: (1) Blood levels are below 2 to 4 µg per dl and urine levels below 10 to 20 µg per liter in 90 per cent of adult population. Levels above 4 µg per dl in blood and 20 µg per liter in urine probably should be considered abnormal. Blood levels are not always reliable. Exposed industrial workers' urine levels are 150 to 200 µg. (2) In asymptomatic patients with urine levels under 300 µg per liter, a chelating challenge with BAL or penicillamine may bring a significant increase that may aid in establishing the diagnosis. (3) Approximately 150 µg per liter of mercury in urine is equivalent to 3.5 µg per dl in blood. (4) Methyl mercury is excreted mainly through the feces, so urine mercury would not be a reliable measurement. (5) Mercury is also excreted in the sweat and saliva. The parotid fluid level is approximately two thirds that of the blood. Since the hair is porous, it may absorb mercury from the atmosphere; however, hair concentrations of 400 to 500 µg are likely to be associated with neurologic symptoms.

Methadone. See Opioids.

Methanol. See Alcohols.

Methaqualone. See Sedative Hypnotics.

Methyprylon (Noludar). See Sedative Hypnotics.

Narcotic Analgesics. See Opioids.

Neuroleptics. See Phenothiazines.

Nitrites (NO$_2$) and Nitrates (NO$_3$). These are readily available in both inorganic and organic forms. Organic nitrates used for angina pectoris are listed in Table 21. Inorganic nitrates have more toxicologic importance in natural foods and contaminated well water. *Potential fatal doses:* Nitrite, 1 gram; nitrate, 10 grams; nitrobenzene, 2 ml; nitroglycerin, 0.2 gram; and aniline dye (pure), 5 to 30 grams. *Toxicokinetics:* Onset of action of nitroglycerin sublingually is 1 to 3 minutes,

*Inquiries can be made to the National Information Center for Orphan Drugs and Rare Diseases, 800-336-4797.

TABLE 21. Organic Nitrates for Angina Pectoris

Drug and Route	Trade Name	Onset (min)	Duration (hr)
Nitroglycerin			
Oral	Many	Varies	4–6
Sublingual	Many	1–3	¼–½
2% ointment	Nitrobid Nitrol	Varies	3–6
Isosorbide dinitrate	Isordil		
Sublingual		1–3	1.3–3
Oral		2–5	4–6
Chewable		2–5	2–3
Timed release		varies	—
Pentaerythritol tetranitrate, oral	Peritrate	2–5	3–5
Erythrityl tetranitrate, oral	Cardilate	2–5	4–6

with a peak action of 3 to 15 minutes and a duration of 20 to 30 minutes. Other routes have a slower onset (2 to 5 minutes) and longer duration of action (1.5 to 6 hours). Nitrites are potent oxidizing agents converting ferrous to ferric iron, which cannot carry oxygen. Normally, humans have 0.7 per cent of methemoglobin, which is converted by methemoglobin reductase into oxygen-carrying hemoglobin. Liver detoxification by dinitration is the route of elimination. *Toxic manifestations* depend on the level of methemoglobinemia. At 10 per cent, "chocolate cyanosis" occurs; at 10 to 20 per cent, headache, dizziness, and tachypnea occur; and at 50 per cent mental alterations are present and coma and convulsions may occur. Headache, flush, and sweating are due to the vasodilatory effect; hypotension, tachycardia, and syncope may also occur. Severe hypoxia may produce pulmonary edema and encephalopathy. Levels above 50 per cent produce metabolic acidosis and ECG changes; cardiovascular collapse occurs at levels of 70 per cent.

Management: (1) Dermal decontamination, if indicated. Aniline dyes may be removed with 5 per cent acetic acid (vinegar). (2) Gastrointestinal decontamination if ingested. (3) Hypotension can be treated by the Trendelenburg position and fluid challenge. Vasoconstrictors (dopamine or norepinephrine) are rarely needed. (4) Methylene blue (Antidote 24, Table 4) is indicated for methemoglobin levels above 40 per cent, dyspnea, metabolic acidosis (lactic acidosis), or an altered mental state. (5) Oxygen, 100 per cent, or a hyperbaric chamber should be used in symptomatic patients if methylene blue fails or is not effective, e.g., chlorate intoxication or G6PD deficiency. *Laboratory aids:* Methemoglobin levels, arterial blood gases. Blood has a chocolate-brown appearance and fails to turn red on exposure to oxygen.

Nortriptyline (Aventyl, Pamelor). See Tricyclic Antidepressants.

Opioids (Narcotic Opiates). See Table 22. The major metabolic pathway differs for each opioid but they are 90 per cent metabolized in the liver. Patients should be observed for central nervous system and respiratory

TABLE 22. **Opioids (Narcotic Opiates)**

Drugs Generic	Trade	Equivalent IM Dose* (mg)	Oral* (mg)	Peak Action (hr)	Half-Life (hr)	Duration (hr)	Potential Toxic Dose (mg)
Alphaprodine	Nisentil	45	—	0.5	—	1–2	—
Butorphanol	Stadol	2	12	—	3	3–4	—
Camphorated tincture of opium	Paregoric		25 ml	—	—	4–5	—
Codeine	Various	120	200	—	3	3–6	800
Diacetylmorphine	Heroin	3.0	60	—	0.5	3–4	100
Dihydrocodeine	Hycodan	5–10	—	—	—	—	100
Diphenoxylate	Lomotil	40–60	—	Delayed by atropine	—	—	—
Fentanyl	Sublimaze	0.2	—	0.5	—	1–2	—
Hydromorphine	Dilaudid	1.5	6.5	0.5–0.75	2–3	4–5	100
Meperidine	Demerol	75–100	300	0.5–1	3	4–6	1000
Methadone	Dolophine	10.0	20	4	—	4–6	120
Morphine	Various	10.0	60	0.75–1	2–3	4–6	200
Nalbuphine	Nubain	10.0	60	—	5	3–6	—
Oxycodone	Percodan	15	30	—	—	3–4	—
Oxymorphone	Numorphan	1.0	6.5	1	2–3	4–5	—
Pentazocine	Talwin	60	180	0.75	2	4–7	—
Propoxyphene	Darvon	240	—	2–4	12–36	2–4	500

"Ts and blues" are a combination of pentazocine (Talwin) and tripelennamine (Pyribenzamine) used intravenously. Pentazocine now has naloxone added to it to counter this abuse. Innovar is fentanyl plus droperidol, used as an IV anesthetic.

*Dose equivalent to 10 mg of morphine.

depression and hypotension. Pulmonary edema is a potentially lethal complication of mainlining (intravenous use). *Manifestations:* All opiate agonists produce miotic pupils (except meperidine and Lomotil early), respiratory and central nervous system depression, physical dependence, and withdrawal. *Management:* (1) Supportive care, particularly an endotracheal tube and assisted ventilation. (2) Gastrointestinal decontamination up to 12 hours postingestion, as opiates delay gastric emptying time, but this is of no benefit if overdose is by injection. Convulsions occur rapidly with propoxyphene (Darvon) and codeine overdose, and this may be an indication not to use an emetic for gastrointestinal decontamination in this drug overdose. (3) Naloxone (Narcan) (Antidote 25, Table 4) may be given in bolus intravenous doses and by continuous drip. Naloxone must be titrated against the clinical response and precipitation of withdrawal in narcotic addicts. It should be repeated as often as necessary, since many opioids in overdose can last 24 hours to 48 hours, whereas the action of naloxone lasts only 2 to 3 hours. *Larger doses are needed for codeine, pentazocine, and propoxyphene.* (4) Pulmonary edema does not respond to naloxone and needs respiratory supportive care. Fluids should be given cautiously in opioid overdose, because these agents stimulate antidiuretic hormone effect and pulmonary edema is frequent. (5) *If the patient is comatose, give 50 per cent glucose* (3 to 4 per cent of comatose narcotic overdose patients have hypoglycemia). (6) *If the patient is agitated,* consider hypoxia rather than withdrawal and treat as such. (7) *Observe for withdrawal* (nausea, vomiting, cramps, diarrhea, dilated pupils, rhinorrhea, piloerection). If these occur, stop naloxone.

OPIOID ADDICT WITHDRAWAL SCORE. Symptoms of withdrawal are diarrhea, dilated pupils, gooseflesh, hyperactive bowel sounds, hypertension, insomnia, lacrimation, muscle cramps, restlessness, tachycardia,

and yawning. Each sign or symptom is given 0, 1, or 2 points, depending on the severity. A score of 1 to 5 is mild; 6 to 10, moderate; and 11 to 15, severe. Seizures are very unusual with withdrawal. They indicate severity regardless of the rest of the score. *Management:* Mild withdrawal is treated with diazepam orally, 10 mg every 6 hours; moderate withdrawal, with intramuscular diazepam; and severe withdrawal, with diazepam and diphenoxylate (Lomotil) for the diarrhea. Methadone orally may be used, 20 to 40 mg every 12 hours, decreased by 5 mg every 12 hours. When 10 mg is reached, add Lomotil. Clonidine (Catapres), 6 µg per kg every 6 hours, can be used with informed consent. (This is an unlisted use of clonidine; the manufacturer states that relief from withdrawal symptoms has been reported with 0.8 mg/day.)

PROPOXYPHENE (Darvon). *Manifestations:* Onset may be as early as 30 minutes after ingestion. Convulsions occur early. Patients may develop diabetes insipidus, pulmonary edema, and hypoglycemia. *Elimination:* Metabolism is 90 per cent by demethylation in the liver. Peak plasma level of 1 to 2 hours after oral dose. Half-life is 1 to 5 hours. As little as 10 mg per kg has caused symptoms, and 35 mg per kg has caused cardiopulmonary arrest. Therapeutic blood level is less than 200 µg per ml. *Treatment* (in addition to the general management): (1) Emesis can be dangerous because of the rapid onset of seizures. (2) Indications for naloxone are respiratory depression, seizure activity, coma, and miotic pupils. Signs of naloxone effect are dilation of pupils, increased rate and depth of respirations, reversal of hypotension, and improvement of obtunded or comatose state. (3) Naloxone and intravenous glucose should be tried first to control seizures. If these fail, diazepam may be tried.

Organochlorine Insecticides (DDT Derivatives). See Table 23 for a listing of these agents. The *toxic dose* varies greatly. Chlorophenothane (DDT), 200 to 250

TABLE 23. **Organochlorine Pesticides (DDT Derivatives)**

Chemical Name	Trade Name	Toxicity Rating	Elimination Time	Comment
Endrin	Hexadrin	Highest	hrs–days	Banned
Lindane	1% in Kwell; Benesan; Isotox; Gamene	Moderate to high	hrs–days	Scabicide; general garden insecticide
Endosulfan	Thiodan	Moderate	hrs–days	
Benzene hexachloride	BHC, HCH	Moderate	wks–mos	Banned, produces porphyria (cutanea tarda)
Dieldrin	Dieldrite	High	wks–mos	
Aldrin	Aldrite	High	wks–mos	
Chlordane (10% is heptachlor)	Chlordan	High	wks–mos	Restricted; termiticide
Toxophene	Toxakil Strobane-T	High	hrs–days	
Heptachlor	—	Moderate	wks–mos	Malignancy in rats
Chlorophenothane	DDT	Moderate	mos–yrs	Banned in 1972
Mirex	—	Moderate	mos–yrs	Banned; red anticide
Chlordecone	Kepone	Moderate	mos–yrs	Tidewater, Virginia, contamination
Methoxychlor	Marlate	Low	hrs–days	
Perthane	—	Low	hrs–days	
Dicofol	Kelthane	Low	hrs–days	
Chlorobenzilate	Acaraben	Low	hrs–days	Banned

mg per kg, is fatal; 16 mg per kg causes seizures. Methoxychlor, 500 to 600 mg per kg, is fatal. Chlordane, 200 mg per kg, is fatal (chlordane house air guidelines are below 5 μg per M³; the occupational threshold limit value [TLV] is 500 μg per M³). These insecticides interfere with axon transmission of nerve impulses. Metabolism varies; they resist degradation in human tissue and the environment. They accumulate in adipose tissue; the elimination route is via the liver. *Manifestations:* Central nervous system stimulation, convulsions, late respiratory depression, increased myocardial irritability. Endrin produces liver toxicity with guarded prognosis. Chronic exposure causes liver and kidney damage. *Management:* (1) Dermal decontamination, discard contaminated leather goods. Protect personnel. Gastrointestinal decontamination, no oils. Emesis can be dangerous owing to rapid seizures. Many are dissolved in petroleum distillates, presenting an aspiration hazard. (2) No adrenergic stimulants (epinephrine) should be used because of myocardial irritability. (3) Cholestyramine, 4 grams every 8 hours, has been reported to increase the fecal excretion. (4) Anticonvulsants, if needed.

Organophosphate Insecticides (OPI). These may cause (a) irreversible inhibition of cholinesterase, either direct (TEPP) or delayed (parathion or malathion), or (b) reversible inhibition of cholinesterase (carbamates). Examples of OPI are listed in Table 24. Absorption is by all routes. The onset of acute toxicity is usually before 12 hours and always before 24 hours. *Toxic manifestations:* Early, cholinergic crisis—cramps, diarrhea, excess secretion, bronchospasms, bradycardia. Later, sympathetic and nicotine effects occur—twitching, fasciculations, weakness, tachycardia and hypertension, and convulsions. Central nervous system effects are anxiety, confusion, emotional lability, and coma. Delayed respiratory paralysis and neurologic disorders have been described.

Management: (1) Basic life support and decontamination with careful protection of personnel. (2) Atropine (Antidote 7, Table 4), if symptomatic, every 10 to 30 minutes until drying of secretions and clear lungs occur. Maintain for 12 to 24 hours, then taper the dose and observe for relapse. (3) Intravenous pralidoxime (2-PAM) may be required after atropinization (Antidote 31, Table 4). It should be given in the first 24 hours. It is used in the presence of weakness, respiratory depression, or muscle twitching. Its use may require reduction in the dose of atropine. (4) Careful dermal and gastrointestinal decontamination when stable. (5) Suction secretions until atropinization drying is achieved. Intubation and assisted ventilation may be needed. (6) *Do not* use morphine, aminophylline, phenothiazine, or reserpine-like drugs or succinylcholine. *Laboratory aids:* Draw blood for red blood cell cholinesterase determination before giving pralidoxime. Levels are usually more than 50 per cent depressed for severe symptoms. Monitor chest radiograph, blood glucose, arterial blood gases, ECG, blood coagulation status, liver function, and the urine for the metabolite alkyl phosphate p-nitrophenol. *Note:* If the diagnosis is probable, do not delay therapy until it is confirmed by laboratory tests. Atropine is both a diagnostic and a therapeutic agent. A test dose of 2 mg in adults and 0.05 mg per kg in children may be administered parenterally. In the presence of severe cholinesterase inhibition, the patient fails to develop signs of atropinization.

It is not medically advisable to administer atropine or pralidoxime prophylactically to workers exposed to organophosphate pesticides.

CARBAMATES (esters of carbonic acid). Carbamates cause reversible carbamylation of acetylcholinesterase. Pralidoxime is usually not indicated in the management but atropine may be required. The major differences from OPI are (1) toxicity is less and of shorter

TABLE 24. **Examples of Organophosphate Insecticides (OPI)**

Common Name	Synonym	EFD*
Agricultural Products (highly toxic; LD_{50} is 1–50 mg/kg)		
Tetraethyl pyrophosphate	TEPP, Tetron	0.05
Phorate	Thimet	
Disulfoton†	Di-Syston	0.2
Demeton†	Systox	
Terbufos	Counter	
Chlortriphos	Calathion	
Mevinphos	Phosdrin	0.15
Parathion	Thiophos	0.10
Methamidophos	Monitor	Delayed neuropathy
Monocrotophos	Azodrin	
Octamethyl-diphosphoramide	OMPA, Schradan	
Azinphosmethyl	Guthion	0.2
Ethyl–nitrophenyl thiobenzene PO_4	EPN	
Animal Insecticides (moderately toxic; LD_{50} is 50–500 mg/kg)		
DEF	DeGreen	
Dichlorvos	DDVP, Vapona	
Coumaphos	Co-ral	
Trichlorfon	Dylox	
Ronnel	Korlan	10.0
Dimethoate	Cygon, De-Fend	
Fenthion	Baytex	Long-acting
Leptophos	Phosvel	
Chlorfenvinophos (tick dip)	Supona, Dermaton	
Household and Garden Pest Control (low toxicity; LD_{50} is 500–1300 mg/kg)		
Malathion	Cythion	60.0
Diazinon‡	Spectracide, Dimpylate	25.0
Chlorpyrifos‡	Lorsban, Dursban	
Temephos	Abate	

*EFD, Estimated fatal dose (grams/70 kg).
†Most OPI degrade in the environment in a few days to nontoxic radicals. These are taken up by the plants and fruits.
‡Some classify these as moderately toxic.

duration; (2) they rarely produce overt central nervous system effects because of poor penetration; and (3) cholinesterase returns to normal rapidly so that blood values are not useful in confirming diagnosis. Some common examples of carbamates are Ziram, Temik (alkicarb) (taken up by plants and fruit), Matacil (aminocarb, carazol), Vydate (oxamyl), Isolan, furadan (Carbofuran), Lannate (methomyl, Nudrin), Zectran (mexacarbate), and Mesural (methiocarb). These agents are all highly toxic. Moderately toxic are Baygon (propoxur) and Sevin (carbaryl). Some of these agents may be formulated in wood alcohol and have the added toxicity of methyl alcohol.

Paradichlorobenzene. See Hydrocarbons.

Paraquat and Diquat. Paraquat is a quaternary ammonia herbicide rapidly inactivated in the soil by clay particles. Nonindustrial preparations of 0.2 per cent are unlikely to cause serious intoxications. *Toxic dose:* Commercial preparations such as Gramoxone 20 per cent are very toxic; one mouthful has produced death. Systemic absorption in the course of occupational use is apparently minimal. Paraquat on marijuana leaves is pyrolyzed to nontoxic dipyridyl. *Toxicokinetics:* "Hit and run" toxin. Less than 20 per cent is absorbed. The peak is 1 hour postingestion. The route of elimination is the kidney. Most of the dose is eliminated in the first 40 hours; it is detected in urine for 15 days. Volume distribution is over 500 liters per kg. *Manifestations:* Local corrosive effect on skin and mucous membranes. Acute renal failure in 48 hours (often reversible). Pulmonary effects in 72 hours are progressive, and oxygen aggravates the pulmonary fibrosis. Diquat does not produce effects on the lungs but produces convulsions and gastrointestinal distention. Long-term exposure may cause cataracts. Chlormequat's target organ is the kidney.

Management: (1) Gastrointestinal decontamination despite corrosive effects should be done cautiously with a nasogastric tube; administer local adsorbent. Repeated doses of activated charcoal are recommended. Dermal and ocular decontamination as needed. (2) Hemodialysis and hemoperfusion may be carried out in tandem. Hemoperfusion with charcoal alone is the present choice; however, the results are still poor. Continue hemoperfusion until blood paraquat levels cannot be detected. (3) Diuresis may be of value but consider the risk of fluid overload. (4) Niacin and vitamin E have not been effective. (5) Avoid oxygen unless absolutely necessary (PaO_2 below 60 mm Hg) because this aggravates fibrosis. Some use hypoxic air, FiO_2 10 to 20 per cent. (6) Corticosteroids may help prevent adrenocortical necrosis. *Laboratory aids:* Blood levels above 2 µg per ml at 4 hours or above 0.10 at 16 hours are usually fatal. Blood level testing and advice may be obtained from ICI American, (800) 327-8633. Monitor renal, liver, and pulmonary functions and chest radiographs. Urine test for paraquat exposure: alkalinization and sodium dithionite give an intense blue-green color in exposure.

Parathion. See Organophosphate Insecticides.

Pentazocine (Talwin). See Opioids.

Perphenazine. See Phenothiazines.

Petroleum Products. See Hydrocarbons.

Phencyclidine (Angel Dust, PCP, Peace Pill, Hog). This is the "drug of deceit" because it is substituted for many other drugs, such as THC and mescaline. There are now at least 38 analogues. Smoking may give cyanide poisoning. Improper mixing has caused explosions. *Toxic dose:* Two to 5 mg smoked or "snorted" produces drunken behavior, agitation, and excitement. Five to 10 mg produces stupor, coma, and myoclonus convulsions. Ten to 25 mg smoked, snorted, or taken orally results in prolonged coma and respiratory failure. It is usually fatal over 25 mg (250 ng per ml blood concentration). *Toxicokinetics:* Weak base. Rapidly absorbed when smoked, snorted, or ingested and secreted into stomach gastric juice. Absorbed in alkaline intestine, but ion-trapping takes place in acid gastric media. Half-life is 30 to 60 minutes. Lipophilic drug with extensive Vd. The onset of action if smoked is 2 to 5 minutes (peak in 15 to 30 minutes); orally, 30 to 60 minutes. The duration at low doses is 4 to 6 hours and normality returns in 24 hours. At large overdoses coma may last 6 to 10 days (waxes and wanes). An adverse reaction in overdose occurs in 1 to 2 hours. *Route of elimination:* By liver metabolism (50 per cent). Urinary excretion of conjugates and free PCP. *Manifestations:* Sympathomimetic, cholinergic, cerebellar. Observe for violent behavior, paranoid schizophrenia, self-destructive behavior. Clues to diagnosis are bursts of horizontal, vertical, and rotary nystagmus, coma with eyes open.

Management (avoid overtreatment of mild intoxications): (1) gastrointestinal decontamination up to 4 hours postingestion, but this may not be effective because PCP is rapidly absorbed. Insert nasogastric tube into stomach for administration of activated charcoal every 6 hours, because PCP is secreted into the stomach even if it is smoked or snorted. (2) Protect patient and others from harm. "Talk down" is usually ineffective. Low sensory environment. Diazepam (Valium) may be used orally or intramuscularly in the uncooperative patient. (3) For behavioral disorders and toxic psychosis—haloperidol (Haldol), 2 to 5 mg, or diazepam or both. (4) Seizures and muscle spasm—control with diazepam, 2.5 mg, up to 10 mg (Antidote 16, Table 4). (5) Dystonia reaction—diphenhydramine (Benadryl) intravenously (Antidote 18, Table 4). (6) Hyperthermia—external cooling. (7) Hypertensive crisis (dopaminergic)—diazoxide, 3 to 5 mg per kg intravenously up to 300 mg bolus, or nitroprusside. (8) Acid diuresis ion-trapping (controversial). Ammonium chloride use is not routinely recommended. If rhabdomyolysis occurs, myoglobin may precipitate in the renal tubules. (Antidote 2, Table 4): (9) No phenothiazines in the acute phase of intoxication because they lower the convulsive threshold. May be needed later for psychosis.

Laboratory aids: (1) CPK level will be clue to the amount of rhabdomyolysis occurring and the chance of myoglobinuria developing. Values up to 20,000 units have been reported. (2) Test urine for myoglobin and pigmented casts. Test urine with ortho-toluidine; a positive test without red blood cells on microscopic examination suggests myoglobinuria. (3) Monitor urine and blood pH and urinary output if acidifying patient. (4) Measure phencyclidine level. (5) Evaluate BUN, ammonia, electrolytes, blood glucose (20 per cent have hypoglycemia) levels. (6) Test for PCP in gastric juice; levels are 40 to 50 times higher than in blood. *Complications:* Rhabdomyolysis, myoglobinuria, and renal failure. Dopaminogenic—hypertensive crisis, cerebrovascular accident (CVA), encephalopathy, and malignant hyperthermia. Schizophrenic paranoid psychosis (induced in chronic users or precipitated in acute users). Loss of memory for months. Teratogenic cases have been reported. Children have been intoxicated from inhalation in a room where adults were smoking PCP. PCP-induced depression and suicide.

Phenobarbital. See Barbiturates.

Phenothiazines and Other Major Neuroleptics. Phenothiazines are represented by aliphatic compounds: chlorpromazine (Thorazine), promethazine (Phenergan), promazine (Sparine), triflupromazine (Vesprin), methoxypromazine (Tentone); piperazine compounds (dimethylamine series); acetophenazine (Tindal), fluphenazine (Prolixin), prochlorperazine (Compazine),

perphenazine (Trilifon), trifluoperazine (Stelazine); and piperidine compounds: mepazine (Pacatal), mesoridazine (Serentil), thioridazine (Mellaril), pipamazine (Mornidine). Nonphenothiazines are the thioxanthines: clorprothixene (Taractan), thiothixene (Navane); butyrophenones: haloperidol (Haldol), droperidol (Inapsine); dibenzoxazepines: loxapine (Loxitane, Daxolin); and dihydroindolones: molindone (Moban, Lidone). These have pharmacologic properties similar to those of the phenothiazines. *Manifestations:* Clues to phenothiazine overdose are miosis, tremor, hypotension, hypothermia, respiratory depression, radiopaque pills on radiograph of abdomen, and increased QT waves in the ECG. Anticholinergic actions are also present. Major problems are respiratory depression, myocardial toxicity (quinidine-like), neurogenic hypotension (antidopaminogenic), and idiosyncratic reaction, which may occur at therapeutic levels. Idiosyncratic reaction consists of opisthotonos, torticollis, orolingual dyskinesis, and oculogyric crisis (painful upward gaze) and can be mistaken for a psychotic episode. Extrapyramidal crisis is frequent in children and women. Death is usually due to cardiac effects. Phenothiazines are metabolized by the liver into many metabolites. Some remain in the body longer than 6 months.

Management: (1) Gastrointestinal decontamination. Emesis induction may be useful if symptoms have not occurred. If symptoms are already present, many of these agents have antiemetic action, so lavage may be required. Always provide gastric lavage to comatose patients after the airway is protected regardless of the time of ingestion because of inhibition of gastric motility. (2) Extrapyramidal signs (idiosyncratic reaction) can be treated with diphenhydramine (Benadryl) (Antidote 18, Table 4), or benztropine (Cogentin), 1 to 2 mg intravenously slowly. Symptoms recur, and these drugs should be continued orally for 2 to 3 days. *This is not the treatment of overdose,* only of the idiosyncratic reaction. (3) Monitor ECG for dysrhythmias and treat with antidysrhythmic agents. (4) Hypotension is treated with the Trendelenburg position or fluid challenge or both. Vasopressors are used only if these fail. Dopamine (Intropin) should not be used to treat the hypotension because these drugs are antidopaminogenic. If a pressor agent is needed, use norepinephrine (Levarterenol, Levophed). (5) Physostigmine may be used for life-threatening anticholinergic symptoms. (6) A radiograph of the abdomen is useful to detect undissolved tablets, which may be radiopaque. (7) Treat hypo- or hyperthermia with external physical measures (not drugs).

Laboratory aids: A ferric chloride test of urine can confirm exposure to phenothiazines if there is a sufficient blood level. Blood levels are *not* useful in management.

Phenylpropanolamine (PPA). See Amphetamines.

Primidone. See Anticonvulsants.

Propoxyphene. See Opioids.

Propranolol and Beta Blockers. Some of these agents available in the United States at this time are listed in Table 25. *Toxic dose:* Varies considerably. *Toxicokinetics:* Peak action is 1 to 2 hours orally and lasts 24 to 48 hours. In drugs with long half-lives, e.g., nadolol, it may take many days to recover from overdose toxicity (Table 25). *Manifestations*: Observe for bradycardia and hypotension. Fat-soluble drugs have more CNS effects. Partial agonists may produce tachycardia and hypertension (oxprenolol, pindolol).

Management: (1) Gastrointestinal decontamination up to 2 hours postingestion. (2) Treat hypoglycemia (frequent in children) and hyperkalemia. (3) Control convulsions. (4) Cardiovascular manifestations: Bradycardia—if hemodynamically stable and asymptomatic, no therapy. If unstable (hypotension or atriovenous block), use atropine, isoproterenol, glucagon, and pacemaker. Ventricular tachycardia or premature beats—use lidocaine, phenytoin, or overdrive pacing. Myocardial depression and hypotension—correct dysrhythmias, institute Trendelenburg positioning, and fluids. Monitor with pulmonary arterial wedge pressure (PAWP) catheter. If low cardiac output with low PAWP, give more fluids. If low cardiac output with normal PAWP, use glucagon (Antidote 22, Table 4). Avoid quinidine, procainamide, and disopyramide (Norpace). Glucagon is probably the drug of choice since it works through adenyl cyclase mechanism not affected by the beta blockers. It is given as a bolus and may be continued as an infusion (Antidote 22, Table 4). If bronchospasm, give aminophylline. Hemodialysis or hemoperfusion for low volume distribution drugs that are low protein binding and watersoluble (nadolol and atenolol), particularly with evidence of renal failure. If hypoglycemia, give intravenous glucose. *Laboratory aids*: Moni-

tor blood glucose, potassium, ECG, PAWP. Fatal blood level of propranolol is 0.8 to 1.2 mg per dl (8 to 12 µg per ml).

Quinidine and Quinine (Antidysrhythmic and Antimalarial Agents). *Toxic dose* in child is 1 gram; in adult it is 2 to 8 grams. There is 95 to 100 per cent absorption, peak action in 2 to 4 hours. Half-life is 3 to 4 hours (quinidine gluconate, 8 to 12 hours). Large Vd. Metabolized predominantly by the liver. *Manifestations*: Cinchonism (headache, nausea, vomiting, tinnitus, deafness, diplopia, dilated pupils). Myocardial depression, dysrhythmias, ECG changes—prolongation of PR, QRS, and QT intervals. Skin rashes and flushing. Hemolysis in G6PD deficiency. Dementia reported. *Management*: (1) Gastrointestinal decontamination. (2) Monitor ECG and liver function. (3) May need antidysrhythmic drugs and pacemaker and alkalinization.

Salicylates. *Toxic dose:* See Table 26. Methyl salicylate (oil of wintergreen): 1 ml equals 1.4 grams of salicylate. One teaspoonful equals 21 adult aspirins. *Toxicokinetics*: Plasma concentration is significant in 30 minutes and peaks in 1 to 2 hours. Half-life is 3 to 6 hours (therapeutic) to 12 to 36 hours (toxic). Urine pH influences urine salicylate elimination. *Manifestations of acute ingestion* (see Table 26): The metabolic disturbance in adults and older children is usually respiratory alkalosis; in children under 5 years of age the initial respiratory alkalosis will usually change to metabolic or mixed metabolic acidosis and respiratory

TABLE 25. **Propranolol and Beta Blockers**

Drug	Solubility and Absorption (%)	Membrane Stabilizer	Relative Potency (Propranolol = 1)	Plasma Half-life	Elimination	Protein-Bound	Vd (liter/kg)
Atenolol (Tenormin) Dose: 50–100 mg MDD = 100 mg	Water (46–62)	no	1.0	6–9	95% renal	3–10	0.7
Metoprolol (Lopressor) Dose: 50–400 mg MDD = 450 mg	Fat (over 95)	no	1.0	3–4	Hepatic	10	5.6
Nadolol (Corgard) Dose: 40–320 mg MDD = 320 mg	Water (15–25)	+/−	1.0	17–23	70% renal	25	2.1
Pindolol* (Visken) Dose: 20–60 mg MDD = 60 mg	Fat (over 90)	no	6.0	3–4	Hepatic (40% renal)	57	2.0
Propranolol† (Inderal) Dose: 40–160 mg MDD = 480 mg	Fat (100)	+ +	1.0	2–3	Hepatic (less than 1% renal)	90–95	3.6
Timolol‡ (Blocadren) Dose: 20 mg MDD = 60 mg Ophthalmologic (Timoptic, 0.25–0.5%) Dose: 1 drop twice daily	Fat (over 90)	no	6.0	3	Hepatic (20% renal)	<10	1.5

*Partial agonists.
†Substantial first pass.
‡Mitochondrial calcium protection during ischemia.
MDD, maximum daily dose.

TABLE 26. **Quantities of Aspirin Ingested: Deposition and Manifestations***

Category	Amount Ingested (mg/kg)	Toxicity Expected	Gastrointestinal Decontamination	Manifestations Anticipated
Nontoxic	<150	No	No	None
Usually nontoxic	>150	No	Yes (home)	None
Mild intoxication	150–200	Yes	Yes (ECF)	Vomiting, tinnitus, mild hyperventilation
Moderate intoxication	200–300	Yes	Yes (ECF)	Hyperpnea lethargy or excitability
Severe intoxication	300–500	Yes	Yes (ECF)	Coma, convulsions, severe hyperpnea
Very severe intoxication	>500	Yes	Yes (ECF)	Potentially fatal

*See toxic dose indications for gastrointestinal decontamination.
ECF, emergency care facility.

alkalosis with acidosis predominating within a few hours.

Management: (1) Gastrointestinal decontamination is useful up to 12 hours postingestion, as some factors delay absorption (food, enteric-coated tablets, other drugs); pylorospasm may delay emptying; and concretions may form. Activated charcoal should be administered every 4 hours until stools are black. Concretions may be removed by lavage, endoscopy, or gastrostomy. (2) Intravenous fluid should be given as recommended in Table 27. Alkalinization enhances salicylate excretion. Potassium is essential to produce adequate alkalinization. Monitor *both* the urine and blood pH. Do not use the urine pH alone to assess the need for alkalinization (Antidote 35, Table 4). (3) Fluid retention can be treated with mannitol (20 per cent), 0.5 gram per kg over 30 minutes, or furosemide, 1 mg per kg intravenously. (4) Hyperpyrexia should be treated with external cooling. (5) Abnormal bleeding or hypoprothrombinemia will need vitamin K, 10 mg intramuscularly, and, if bleeding continues, fresh blood or platelet transfusion (Antidote 38, Table 4). (6) Dialysis (hemodialysis) or hemoperfusion is indicated if there is persistent acidosis (pH<7.1) and lack of response to fluid or alkali in 6 hours; if serum salicylate levels are initially greater than 160 mg per dl or greater than 130 mg per dl at 6 hours postingestion

(do *not* use the salicylate level as the sole criterion for dialysis); or if there are coma and uncontrollable seizures, congestive heart failure, acute renal failure, or progressive deterioration despite good management. (7) Chronic toxicity is usually a more severe intoxication because of the cumulative pharmocokinetics of salicylates. Management needs are outlined in Table 28.

Laboratory aids: The metabolic acidosis of salicylism has a moderately elevated anion gap. Hyper- or hypoglycemia may exist. Serum salicylate levels used in conjunction with the Done nomogram (Figure 3) are useful predictors of expected severity following *acute single ingestions.* The Done nomogram is *not* useful in chronic intoxications, methyl salicylate, phenyl salicylate, or homomethyl salicylate ingestions. The salicylate level for use in the Done nomogram should be obtained 6 hours postingestion. Before 6 hours, levels in the toxic range should be treated, and patients with levels below the toxic range should be retested if a potentially toxic dose is ingested. Monitor urine output, urine pH, electrolytes, arterial blood gases, blood glucose, prothrombin time, renal function, serum salicylate level, and urine salicylate with the ferric chloride test. Arterial blood pH should be kept at 7.5. *Prognosis:* Persistent vigorous treatment of salicylate ingestion is

TABLE 27. **Recommendations for Fluid Management for Moderate or Severe Salicylism**

Purpose	Rate (ml/kg/hr)	Duration (hr)	Na	K	Cl	HCO$_3$	Glucose (%)
					(mEq/L)		
Volume expansion	20	0.5–1.0	100	0	77	23	5–10
Administered as 0.45 per cent saline with 23 mEq/L sodium NaHCO$_3$							
Hydration Ongoing losses Alkalinization	4–8	Until therapeutic BCS 30 mg/dl	56	40	56	1–2 mEq/kg child; 50–100 mEq adult	5–10
Administered as .33 per cent saline and NaHCO$_3$ to obtain urine pH 7.5–8.0, blood pH 7.5							
						mEq/day	
Maintenance	2–6	—	56	30	40	20	

For severe acidosis pH <7.15 may require 1–2 mEq/kg every 1–2 hours. Usual fluid loss is 200–300 ml/kg, but carefully monitor for fluid overload. Potassium may be needed in excess of 40 mEq/L when alkalinizing.

TABLE 28. **Management of Chronic Salicylate Intoxication**

Classification	Urine pH	Blood pH	Hydration	NaHCO₃ (mEq/L)	Potassium (mEq/L)
Mild	Alkaline	Alkaline	Yes	Yes	20
Moderate	Acid*	Alkaline	Yes	pH 7.5†	40
Severe	Acid	Acid	Yes	pH 7.5	40‡ 80§

*Paradoxical acid urine and alkaline blood indicate potassium depletion.
†Bicarbonate administered to keep blood pH 7.5 and urine pH 7.5–8.0.
‡Normal serum potassium and ECG.
§Low serum potassium and/or abnormal ECG indicating potassium deficiency.

essential, as recovery has occurred despite decerebrate rigidity.

Sedative Hypnotics, Nonbarbiturate. See Table 29. *Management* is primarily supportive (especially intubation and ventilator therapy with continuous positive airway pressure (CPAP) for adult respiratory distress syndrome) and with the use of hemoperfusion or hemodialysis in patients who are severely intoxicated and fail to respond to good supportive care and whose intoxication is life-threatening. (1) *Chloral hydrate* management includes cautious gastrointestinal decontamination. Avoid the use of epinephrine and catecholamines that may produce dysrhythmias. Propranolol, 0.1 mg per kg in 1 mg increments, appears to be more effective than lidocaine for ventricular dysrhyth-

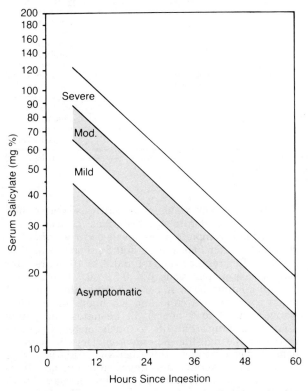

Figure 3. The Done nomogram for salicylate intoxication. For limitations of use, see *Laboratory aids.* (Redrawn from Done A: Salicylate intoxication: Significance of measurements of salicylate in blood in cases of acute ingestion. Pediatrics 26:800, 1960. © American Academy of Pediatrics, 1960.)

mias. (2) *Ethchlorvynol* management includes gastrointestinal decontamination up to 12 hours postingestion. Resin hemoperfusion (Amberlite XAD-4) is the best method of extracorporeal removal when other measures fail in a life-threatening situation (ingestion of over 10 grams or 100 mg per kg, with serum levels of over 100 μg per ml in the first 12 hours or 70 μg per ml after 12 hours in patients with prolonged life-threatening coma). External rewarming if temperature is below 32° C. (3) *Glutethimide* management includes gastrointestinal decontamination up to 24 hours postingestion. Concretions may form. Resin hemoperfusion appears to be the best method of extracorporeal removal in life-threatening protracted coma when the patient has ingested over 10 grams and has a serum level of over 30 μg per ml. Treat hyperthermia with external cooling. (4) *Meprobamate* management includes gastrointestinal decontamination up to 12 hours postingestion, with charcoal hemoperfusion in prolonged coma with life-threatening complications. Concretions may form in the stomach and may require breaking up or surgical removal. (5) *Methaqualone* management includes gastrointestinal decontamination. Forced diuresis, dialysis, and hemoperfusion are not indicated. Fatalities are rare. (6) *Methyprylon* management includes gastrointestinal decontamination and may require treatment of the hypotension with vasopressors of the alpha adrenergic variety—levarterenol (Levophed). The hypotension usually does not respond to position or fluids alone. This is a dialyzable drug, but dialysis usually is not necessary. Fatalities are rare.

Strychnine. Primarily available as a rodenticide and component of cathartics and "tonics." Adulterant of "street drugs," particularly marijuana and cocaine. *Toxic dose*: 5 to 10 mg; fatal in doses of 15 to 30 mg. *Toxicokinetics*: Rapid absorption. Manifestations may occur within 15 to 30 minutes. Low protein-binding. Hepatic metabolism, which appears to be saturable. Twenty per cent is excreted in urine. Has been found in the urine up to 48 hours after a 700 mg dose. *Manifestations*: Interferes with postsynaptic neurotransmitter inhibition by glycine. Hyperacusis is often the first sign. Mild cases—face stiffness (trismus and risus sardonicus). Moderate cases—extensor muscle thrusts. Severe cases—tetanic convulsions with opisthotonos. Death occurs within 1 to 3 hours after ingestion. The prognosis for survival improves if the patient survives beyond 5 hours. The complications of intoxication are lactic acidosis, hyperthermia, rhabdo-

TABLE 29. **Nonbarbiturate Sedative Hypnotic Drugs**

	Absorption and Toxic Dose	Peak Hours	Vd (L/kg)	Protein-Bound (%)	Elimination Route	Serum Half-life (hr)	Toxic Level (μg/ml)	Manifestations and Comment*
Chloral hydrate (Noctec)	Rapid TD, 2 grams FD, 4–10 grams	1–2	0.6	40	Hepatic 90% to active metabolite trichloroethanol (TCE)	4–8	100 (80 TCE—very toxic)	Pearlike odor; dysrhythmias (especially ventricular), hepatotoxic, irritant to mucosa of GI tract; ARDS; radiopaque capsules
Ethchlorvynol (Placidyl)	Rapid TD, 2.5 grams	2–4	3–4	35–50	Hepatic 90%	(1–6) 21–105 in toxic dose	20–80	Prolonged coma up to 200 hr, apnea, hypothermia, pulmonary edema, pink gastric aspirate, pungent odor
Glutethimide (Doriden) (highest mortality of all sedative hypnotics, 14%)	Slow, erratic TD, 5 grams FD, 10 grams	6	Large, 10–20	50	Hepatic 98% to toxic metabolite 4-hydroxyglutarimide (4HG)	10	20–80	Prolonged, cyclic coma up to 120 hr, anticholinergic signs, convulsions, recurrent apnea, hyperthermia
Meprobamate (Equanil, Miltown)	Rapid TD, 10 grams	4–8	1.0	20	Hepatic 90%	6–16	30–100, 200	Coma, convulsions, pulmonary edema, apnea, concretions in stomach
Methaqualone (Quaaludes, "love drugs")	Rapid TD, 800 mg FD, 125 mg/kg	1–3	2–6	80	Hepatic 90%	10–40	8–10	Hypertonia, hyperreflexia, convulsions, apnea, acts "drunk," bleeding tendencies
Methyprylon (Noludar)	Rapid TD, 3 grams	2–4	1–2		Hepatic 97%	3–6; over 8 in toxic dose	30	Hyperactive coma lasts 30 hr, miosis, persistent hypotension, pulmonary edema. Mortality rare

*Comment includes other features besides the typical manifestations of all these agents—coma, respiratory depression, psychologic and physiologic withdrawal, hypotension, hypothermia (except glutethimide hyperthermia).

TD, toxic dose; FD, fatal dose; ARDS, adult respiratory distress syndrome.

myolysis and renal damage from precipitation of myoglobin in the renal tubules, and death from hypoxia. *Management*: (1) Emesis appears contraindicated because of rapid absorption and the early onset of seizures. Gastric aspiration and lavage may be used after the seizures are controlled. Activated charcoal should be given and repeated. (2) Control convulsions with diazepam or phenobarbital. (3) Supportive care for respiratory depression. (4) Acid diuresis and dialysis do not appear to be justified on the basis of available studies. (5) Paralysis with assisted ventilation is useful.

Tear Gas (Lacrimators). CS (chlorobenzylidine), "riot control;" CN powder (chloroacetophenone, 1 per cent); Mace (chloroacetophenone). *Management:* Dermal and ocular decontamination. Protect attendants from contamination. Ophthalmologic evaluation. Oxygen therapy may be needed for dyspnea and respiratory distress.

Theophylline. *Toxic dose*: Acute, single dose greater than 10 mg per kg yields mild toxicity. Greater than 20 mg per kg, moderate manifestations. *Toxicokinetics*: Absorption is complete. Peak levels occur within 60 to 90 minutes after ingestion of liquid preparations; 1 to 3 hours after regular tablets; and 3 to 10 hours after slow-release preparations. Vd, 0.3 to 0.7 liter per kg. Protein-binding, 15 to 40 per cent. Half-life varies: 3.5 hours average in a child and 4.5 hours in an adult (range from 3 to 9 hours). In neonates and young infants the drug's half-life is much longer. Overdose increases the half-life. *Elimination*: Hepatic metabolism, 90 per cent (demethylation and oxidation); 8 to 10 per cent is excreted unchanged in the urine. *Manifestations*: Acute toxicity generally correlates with blood levels; chronic toxicity does not. Ten to 20 μg per ml is the therapeutic range, but some mild gastrointestinal toxicity may occur. Twenty to 40 μg per ml is moderate toxicity, with gastrointestinal and CNS stimulation. Over 50 μg per ml—seizures and dysrhythmias may occur, but they may also occur at lower levels and without gastrointestinal symptoms. Children tolerate higher serum levels. Chronic intoxication is more serious and difficult to treat. Many factors increase theophylline concentration.

Management: (1) Gastrointestinal decontamination in acute overdose, up to 4 hours with regular preparations and up to 8 to 12 hours with slow-release preparations. Test aspirate or vomitus for blood. Give activated charcoal every 4 hours. Do not induce emesis if hematemesis exists. (2) Monitor ECG, obtain theophylline levels every 4 hours until in the therapeutic range of 10 to 20 μg per ml. (3) Control seizures with diazepam. If coma, convulsions, or vomiting exists, intubate immediately. (4) Hypotension is treated with fluid challenge and if this fails, vasopressors. (5) Hematemesis is managed with iced saline lavage and blood replacement if needed. (6) Charcoal hemoperfusion is the management of choice in life-threatening convulsions, dysrhythmias, hematemesis, or intractable vomiting refractory to conventional measures. Differences in slow release preparations from regular preparations: little or no gastrointestinal symptoms with high levels; peak concentration times may be 10 to 24 hours postingestion; and onset of seizures may occur 10 to 12 hours postingestion. *Laboratory aids*: Monitor theophylline levels, check for occult blood in vomitus and stools, monitor vital signs and hemoglobin and hematocrit (for hemorrhage). Monitor cardiac, renal, and hepatic function, electrolytes, blood glucose, arterial blood gases, and acid-base balance.

Toluene. See Hydrocarbons.

Tranquilizers. See Sedative Hypnotics.

Trichloroethylene. See Hydrocarbons.

Tricyclic Antidepressants (TCAD). These agents are generally rapidly absorbed from the gastrointestinal tract, but absorption may be prolonged in overdose owing to anticholinergic action. Their bioavailability has considerable variation among patients, and they are highly bound to plasma and tissue proteins. Protein-binding decreases with decreasing pH. The Vd is large, usually 10 to 20 liters per kg. The TCAD are metabolized primarily in the liver. *N*-Demethylation of the tertiary amines yields the active secondary amine metabolites; hydroxylation gives rise to inactive metabolites. Forty per cent is excreted in the feces and only 3 per cent in the urine unchanged. The t½ varies from 9 to 198 hours. In an overdose, the half-life may be much longer. Tricyclic tertiary amines (metabolized to active metabolites) are amitriptyline (Elavil), imipramine (Tofranil), and doxepin (Sinequan). Tricyclic secondary amines (metabolized to nonactive metabolites) are desipramine (Norpramin, Pertofrane), protriptyline (Vivactil), and nortriptyline (Aventyl). Tricyclic dibenzoxazepine (metabolized to a major metabolite) is amoxapine (Asendin).

Manifestations: The onset of action varies from less than 1 hour to 12 hours after ingestion. The phases of intoxication are (1) consciousness with dry mouth, mydriasis, ataxia, increased deep tendon reflexes, and changes in the ST segment; (2) Stages I and II coma with hypertension, tachycardia above 160, mydriasis, and supraventricular tachycardia; and (3) Stages III and IV coma with hypotension, heart rate under 120,

respiratory depression, tonic-clonic seizures, and ventricular dysrhythmias. The central nervous system effects occur early, and seizures are common. *Cardiovascular toxicity* is frequent in the serious poisonings and results from anticholinergic effects, sympathomimetic activity (by blocking reuptake of catecholamines), quinidine activity, catecholamine depletion, and alpha adrenergic blockage. Cardiotoxic effects include cardiac dysrhythmias, hypertension, hypotension, and pulmonary edema.

Toxic dose: The TCAD have a narrow margin of safety. In a child, a 375-mg dose and in adults, as little as 500 to 750 mg has been fatal. The following dosages may serve as a guide to the degree of toxicity: Less than 10 mg per kg produces light coma, mydriasis, and tachycardia and has a good prognosis. At 20 mg per kg, Stage III manifestations are produced. At 30 mg per kg, fatalities may result. At 50 mg per kg, the mortality rate is increased. Over 70 mg per kg is rarely survived. Therapeutic blood levels are in the range of 50 to 170 ng per ml. If the QRS interval is less than 0.10 sec for 6 hours, the prognosis is good. If it is greater than 0.10 sec, seizures may occur, and if it is over 0.16 sec, serious dysrhythmia may occur.

NEWER ANTIDEPRESSANTS. Amoxapine (Asendin) allegedly has less cardiotoxicity. Patients with amoxapine overdose may develop the syndrome of seizures, rhabdomyolysis, and acute renal tubular necrosis. Recent reports indicate more fatalities with amoxapine than with TCAD. Maprotiline (Ludiomil) is a tetracyclic compound with cardiac toxicity similar to the existing tricyclic antidepressant drugs. Trazodone hydrochloric acid (Desyrel) is an antidepressant chemically unrelated to the other antidepressants. It produces less serious toxicity, although orthostatic hypotension, vertigo, and priapism have been reported. Bupropion (Wellbutrin) is a phenylaminoketone antidepressant that produces dose-related seizures. Nomifensine (Merital) was withdrawn in 1986 because of reports of hemolytic anemia associated with it.

Management: (1) Maintenance of vital functions. ICU care until there are no abnormalities in the ECG for 24 to 48 hours. (2) Gastrointestinal decontamination (omit emesis) if the patient is alert. Intact pills have been recovered by lavage up to 18 hours after ingestion. Suspected cases should have ECG monitoring. (3) Activated charcoal cathartic every 4 to 6 hours and continuous nasogastric suction for the first 48 hours may interrupt enterohepatic recycling of tricyclic antidepressants. (4) Control seizures with intravenous diazepam. Intravenous phenytoin (Dilantin) may be added for seizures not responding to diazepam alone. For refractory seizures, physostigmine may be used (Antidote 30, Table 4). (5) Life-threatening delirium and hallucinations can be treated with physostigmine. Physostigmine was the drug of choice, but recently its use has been advocated only when conventional therapy has failed. (6) All cardiovascular complications of TCAD should *first* be treated by alkalinization of blood with sodium bicarbonate to a pH of 7.5 to 7.55 (Antidote 35, Table 4). Serum potassium levels should be followed, as a sudden increase in blood pH can aggravate or precipitate hypokalemia. Specific cardiovascular complications should be treated as follows: *Hypo-*

tension—norepinephrine (Levophed), a predominantly alpha-adrenergic drug, is preferred over dopamine. (Hypertension that occurs early rarely requires treatment.) *Serious conduction defects* are best managed with phenytoin, and patients may need a temporary transvenous pacemaker. *Sinus tachycardia* usually does not require treatment. If the tachycardia persists despite alkalinization and the patient is unstable, physostigmine may be used. *Supraventricular tachycardia* that does not respond to alkalinization alone may be treated with phenytoin, physostigmine, or synchronized cardioversion. *Ventricular tachycar-*

dia—after alkalinization and phenytoin, intravenous lidocaine (for one dose only) may be required for persistent ventricular tachycardia. Synchronized cardioversion may be needed if lidocaine fails. *Ventricular fibrillation* should be treated with DC countershock. *Laboratory aids*: Arterial blood gases with blood pH, ECG, serum electrolytes, BUN and creatinine, serum phenytoin level, urine output, and, in severe cases, central venous pressure and/or pulmonary wedge pressure should be monitored.

Turpentine. See Hydrocarbons.

Xylene. See Hydrocarbons.

Appendices and Index

LABORATORY VALUES OF CLINICAL IMPORTANCE

method of
REX B. CONN, M.D.
Thomas Jefferson University
Philadelphia, Pennsylvania

INTRODUCTION

The quantitative procedures carried out in a clinical laboratory represent measurements of substances normally present within rather narrow ranges of concentration. In order to use such data, we must know the values to be expected in a normal individual and what is considered a significant deviation from normal. Actually, there can be no sharp dividing line between abnormal and normal values, since there is a gradual transition during any pathologic process from what is clearly normal to what is clearly a pathologic condition.

In medicine, it is a logical impossibility to define normality, and the term "reference values" has replaced the earlier term "normal values." Reference values are derived from statistical studies on subjects believed to have no condition that might affect the measurements under consideration. The traditional and most widely used statistical approach is to carry out the measurement on a large group of subjects and to set the reference limits at the mean value plus or minus two standard deviations. Since values obtained for many measurements are not Gaussian in distribution, additional steps are frequently used in calculation of the reference ranges. The important consideration is that the reference ranges derived by these statistical methods contain only 95 per cent of the reference population. Thus, a value slightly outside the reference range might be due either to chance distribution or to an underlying pathologic process.

A single reference range for all individuals may be inadequate for some clinical measurements. Values obtained on presumably normal persons may vary because of age, sex, body build, race, environment, and state of gastrointestinal absorption. A universal caveat in the use of reference values is that for many procedures the reference range will vary with the method used. This is particularly true for enzyme measurements and measurements based upon immunochemical principles.

THE INTERNATIONAL SYSTEM OF UNITS FOR LABORATORY MEASUREMENTS (LE SYSTÈME INTERNATIONAL D'UNITÉS)

An extensive modification of the metric system has been adopted by clinical laboratories in many countries. This adaptation is the International System of Units (Le Système International d'Unités), usually abbreviated S.I. units. Whereas the metric system utilizes the centimeter, the gram, and the second as basic units, the International System uses the meter, the kilogram, and the second as well as four other basic units.

The International System is a coherent approach to all types of measurement that utilizes seven dimensionally independent basic quantities: mass, length, time, thermodynamic temperature, electric current, luminous intensity, and amount of substance. Each of these quantities is expressed in a clearly defined *base unit* (Table 1).

Two or more base units may be combined to provide *derived units* (Table 2) for expressing other measurements such as mass concentration (kilograms per cubic meter) and velocity (meters per second). Standardized prefixes (Table 3) for base and derived units are used to express fractions or multiples of the base units so that any measurement can be expressed in a value between 0.001 and 1000.

TABLE 1. **Base Units**

Property	Base Unit	Symbol
Length	metre	m
Mass	kilogram	kg
Amount of substance	mole	mol
Time	second	s
Thermodynamic temperature	kelvin	K
Electric current	ampere	A
Luminous intensity	candela	cd

TABLE 2. **Derived Units**

Derived Property	Derived Unit	Symbol
Area	square metre	m²
Volume	cubic metre	m³
	litre	l
Mass concentration	kilogram/cubic metre	kg/m³
	gram/litre	g/l
Substance concentration	mole/cubic metre	mol/m³
	mole/litre	mol/l
Temperature	degree Celsius	C = K − 273.15

TABLE 3. **Standard Prefixes**

Prefix	Multiplication Factor	Symbol
atto	10^{-18}	a
femto	10^{-15}	f
pico	10^{-12}	p
nano	10^{-9}	n
micro	10^{-6}	μ
milli	10^{-3}	m
centi	10^{-2}	c
deci	10^{-1}	d
deca	10^{1}	da
hecto	10^{2}	h
kilo	10^{3}	k
mega	10^{6}	M
giga	10^{9}	G
tera	10^{12}	T

Medical Applications

The most profound change in laboratory reports will result from expressing concentration as amount per volume (moles per liter) rather than mass per volume (milligrams per 100 milliliters). The advantages of the former expression can be seen in the following:

Conventional Units

1.0 gram of hemoglobin
 Combines with 1.37 ml of oxygen
 Contains 3.4 mg of iron
 Forms 34.9 mg of bilirubin

S.I. Units

1.0 mmol of hemoglobin
 Combines with 4.0 mmol of oxygen
 Contains 4.0 mmol of iron
 Forms 4.0 mmol of bilirubin

Chemical relationships between lactic acid and pyruvic acid and the glucose from which both are derived, as well as the relationship between bilirubin and the binding capacity of albumin, are other examples of chemical relationships that will be clarified by using the new system.

There are a number of laboratory and other medical measurements for which the S.I. units appear to offer little advantage, and some that are disadvantageous because the change would require replacement or revision of instruments such as the sphygmomanometer. The cubic meter is the derived unit for volume; however, it is inappropriately large for medical measurements, and the liter has been retained. Thermodynamic temperature expressed in kelvins is not more informative for medical measurements. Since the Celsius degree is the same as the kelvin degree, the Celsius scale is used. Celsius rather than centigrade is the preferred term.

Selection of units for expressing enzyme activity presents certain difficulties. Literally dozens of different units have been used in expressing enzyme activity, and interlaboratory comparison of enzyme results is impossible unless the assay system is precisely defined. In 1964, the International Union of Biochemistry attempted to remedy the situation by proposing the International Unit for enzymes. This unit was defined as the amount of enzyme that will catalyze the conversion of 1 micromole of substrate per minute under standard conditions. Difficulties remain, however, as enzyme activity is affected by temperature, pH, the type and amount of substrate, the presence of inhibitors, and other factors. Enzyme activity can be expressed in S.I. units, and the katal has been proposed to express activities of all catalysts, including enzymes. The katal is that amount of enzyme that catalyzes a reaction rate of 1 mole per second. Thus, adoption of the katal as the unit of enzyme activity would provide no more information than is obtained when results are expressed in International Units.

Hydrogen ion concentration in blood is customarily expressed as pH, but in S.I. units it would be expressed in nanomoles per liter. It appears unlikely that the very useful pH scale will be discarded.

Pressure measures, such as blood pressure and partial pressures of blood gases, would be expressed in S.I. units using the pascal, a unit that can be derived from the base units for mass, length, and time. This change probably will not be adopted in the early phases of the conversion to S.I. units. Similarly, a proposed change in expressing osmolality in terms of the depression of freezing point is inappropriate, because osmolality may be calculated from vapor pressure as well as freezing point measurement.

Conventions

A number of conventions have been adopted to standardize usage of S.I. units:

1. No periods are used after the symbol for a

unit (kg not kg.), and it remains unchanged when used in the plural (70 kg not 70 kgs).

2. A half space rather than a comma is used to divide large numbers into groups of three (e.g., 5 400 000 not 5,400,000).

3. Compound prefixes should be avoided (nanometer not millimicrometer).

4. Multiples and submultiples are used in steps of 10^3 or 10^{-3}.

5. The degree sign for the temperature scales is omitted (38 C not 38°C).

6. The preferred spelling is metre not meter, litre not liter.

7. Report of a measurement should include information on the system, the component, the kind of quantity, the numerical value, and the unit. For example: *System,* serum. *Component,* glucose. *Kind of quantity,* substance concentration. *Value,* 5.10. *Unit,* mmol/l.

8. The name of the component should be unambiguous; for example, "serum bilirubin" might refer to unconjugated bilirubin or to total bilirubin. For acids and bases, the maximally ionized form is used in naming the component; for example, lactate or urate rather than lactic acid or uric acid.

Tables of Reference Values

Tables accompanying this article indicate "normal values" for most of the commonly performed laboratory tests. The title of the tables has been changed from the "normal values" of previous years to "reference values" to conform to current usage. The reference value is given in conventional units, and the value in S.I. units is calculated from these figures. Notes (page 1077) provide additional information.

Reference Values in Hematology

	Conventional Units		S.I. Units		Notes
Acid hemolysis test (Ham)	No hemolysis		No hemolysis		
Alkaline phosphatase, leukocyte	Total score 14–100		Total score 14–100		
Carboxyhemoglobin	Up to 5% of total		0.05 of total		a
Cell counts					
Erythrocytes					
Males	4.6–6.2 million/cu mm		$4.6\text{–}6.2 \times 10^{12}/l$		
Females	4.2–5.4 million/cu mm		$4.2\text{–}5.4 \times 10^{12}/l$		
Children (varies with age)	4.5–5.1 million/cu mm		$4.5\text{–}5.1 \times 10^{12}/l$		
Leukocytes					
Total	4500–11,000/cu mm		$4.5\text{–}11.0 \times 10^9/l$		
Differential	*Percentage*	*Absolute*			
Myelocytes	0	0/cu mm	0/1		b
Band neutrophils	3–5	150–400/cu mm	$150\text{–}400 \times 10^6/l$		
Segmented neutrophils	54–62	3000–5800/cu mm	$3000\text{–}5800 \times 10^6/l$		
Lymphocytes	25–33	1500–3000/cu mm	$1500\text{–}3000 \times 10^6/l$		
Monocytes	3–7	300–500/cu mm	$300\text{–}500 \times 10^6/l$		
Eosinophils	1–3	50–250/cu mm	$50\text{–}250 \times 10^6/l$		
Basophils	0–0.75	15–50/cu mm	$15\text{–}50 \times 10^6/l$		
Platelets	150,000–350,000/cu mm		$150\text{–}350 \times 10^9/l$		
Reticulocytes	25,000–75,000/cu mm		$25\text{–}75 \times 10^9/l$		b
	0.5–1.5% of erythrocytes				
Bone marrow, differential cell count					
	Range	*Average*	*Range*	*Average*	
Myeloblasts	0.3–5.0%	2.0%	0.003–0.05	0.02	a
Promyelocytes	1.0–8.0%	5.0%	0.01–0.08	0.05	
Myelocytes: Neutrophilic	5.0–19.0%	12.0%	0.05–0.19	0.12	
Eosinophilic	0.5–3.0%	1.5%	0.005–0.03	0.015	
Basophilic	0.0–0.5%	0.3%	0.00–0.005	0.003	
Metamyelocytes	13.0–32.0%	22.0%	0.13–0.32	0.22	
Polymorphonuclear neutrophils	7.0–30.0%	20.0%	0.07–0.30	0.20	
Polymorphonuclear eosinophils	0.5–4.0%	2.0%	0.005–0.04	0.02	
Polymorphonuclear basophils	0.0–0.7%	0.2%	0.00–0.007	0.002	
Lymphocytes	3.0–17.0%	10.0%	0.03–0.17	0.10	
Plasma cells	0.0–2.0%	0.4%	0.00–0.02	0.004	
Monocytes	0.5–5.0%	2.0%	0.005–0.05	0.02	
Reticulum cells	0.1–2.0%	0.2%	0.001–0.02	0.002	
Megakaryocytes	0.3–3.0%	0.4%	0.003–0.03	0.004	
Pronormoblasts	1.0–8.0%	4.0%	0.01–0.08	0.04	
Normoblasts	7.0–32.0%	18.0%	0.07–0.32	0.18	

Table continued on following page

Reference Values in Hematology *Continued*

	Conventional Units	S.I. Units	Notes
Coagulation tests			
Antithrombin III (synthetic substrate)	80–120% of normal	0.8–1.2 of normal	
Bleeding time (Duke)	1–5 min	1–5 min	
Bleeding time (Ivy)	Less than 5 min	Less than 5 min	
Bleeding time (template)	2.5–9.5 min	2.5–9.5 min	
Clot retraction, qualitative	Begins in 30–60 min Complete in 24 hrs	Begins in 30–60 min Complete in 24 h	
Coagulation time (Lee-White)	5–15 min (glass tubes) 19–60 min (siliconized tubes)	5–15 min (glass tubes) 19–60 min (siliconized tubes)	
Euglobulin lysis time	2–6 hrs at 37°	2–6 h at 37 C	
Factor VIII and other coagulation factors	50–150% of normal	0.50–1.5 of normal	a
Fibrin split products (Thrombo-Wellco test)	Less than 10 mcg/ml	Less than 10 mg/l	
Fibrinogen	200–400 mg/dl	5.9–11.7 μmol/l	c
Fibrinolysins	0	0	
Partial thromboplastin time, activated (APTT)	20–35 sec	20–35 sec	
Prothrombin consumption	Over 80% consumed in 1 hr	Over 0.80 consumed in 1 h	a
Prothrombin content	100% (calculated from prothrombin time)	1.0 (calculated from prothrombin time)	a
Prothrombin time (one stage)	12.0–14.0 sec	12.0–14.0 sec	
Tourniquet test	Ten or fewer petechiae in a 2.5 cm circle after 5 min	Ten or fewer petechiae in a 2.5 cm circle after 5 min	
Cold hemolysin test (Donath-Landsteiner)	No hemolysis	No hemolysis	
Coombs' test			
Direct	Negative	Negative	
Indirect	Negative	Negative	
Corpuscular values of erythrocytes (values are for adults; in children, values vary with age)			
MCH (mean corpuscular hemoglobin)	27–31 picogm	0.42–0.48 fmol	d
MCV (mean corpuscular volume)	80–96 cu micra	80–96 fl	
MCHC (mean corpuscular hemoglobin concentration)	32–36%	0.32–0.36	a
Haptoglobin (as hemoglobin binding capacity)	100–200 mg/dl	16–31 μmol/l	d
Hematocrit			
Males	40–54 ml/dl	0.40–0.54	a
Females	37–47 ml/dl	0.37–0.47	
Newborn	49–54 ml/dl	0.49–0.54	
Children (varies with age)	35–49 ml/dl	0.35–0.49	
Hemoglobin			
Males	14.0–18.0 grams/dl	2.17–2.79 mmol/l	d
Females	12.0–16.0 grams/dl	1.86–2.48 mmol/l	
Newborn	16.5–19.5 grams/dl	2.56–3.02 mmol/l	
Children (varies with age)	11.2–16.5 grams/dl	1.74–2.56 mmol/l	
Hemoglobin, fetal	Less than 1% of total	Less than 0.01 of total	a
Hemoglobin A$_{1c}$	3–5% of total	0.03–0.05 of total	a
Hemoglobin A$_2$	1.5–3.0% of total	0.015–0.03 of total	a
Hemoglobin, plasma	0–5.0 mg/dl	0–0.8 μmol/l	d
Methemoglobin	0–130 mg/dl	4.7–20 μmol/l	e
Osmotic fragility of erythrocytes	Begins in 0.45–0.39% NaCl Complete in 0.33–0.30% NaCl	Begins in 77–67 mmol/NaCl Complete in 56–51 mmol/l NaCl	
Sedimentation rate			
Wintrobe: Males	0–5 mm in 1 hr	0–5 mm/h	
Females	0–15 mm in 1 hr	0–15 mm/h	
Westergren: Male	0–15 mm in 1 hr	0–15 mm/h	
Females	0–20 mm in 1 hr	0–20 mm/h	
(May be slightly higher in children and during pregnancy)			

Reference Values for Blood, Plasma, and Serum
(For some procedures the reference values may vary depending upon the method used)

	Conventional Units	S.I. Units	Notes
Acetoacetate plus acetone, serum			
Qualitative	Negative	Negative	
Quantitative	0.3–2.0 mg/dl	3–20 mg/l	
Adrenocorticotropin (ACTH), plasma			
6 AM	10–80 picogm/ml	10–80 ng/l	
6 PM	Less than 50 picogm/ml	Less than 50 ng/l	
Alanine aminotransferase, *see* Transaminase			
Aldolase, serum	0–11 milliunits/ml (30°)	0–11 units/l (30 C)	f
Aldosterone			
Adult, supine	3–10 nanogm/dl	0.08–0.3 nmol/l	
standing			
male	6–22 nanogm/dl	0.17–0.61 nmol/l	
female	5–30 nanogm/dl	0.14–0.8 nmol/l	
Alpha amino nitrogen, serum	3.0–5.5 mg/dl	2.1–3.9 mmol/l	
Ammonia (nitrogen), plasma	15–49 mcg/dl	11–35 μmol/l	
Amylase, serum	25–125 milliunits/ml	25–125 units/l	
Anion gap	8–16 mEq/liter	8–16 mmol/l	
Ascorbic acid, blood	0.4–1.5 mg/dl	23–85 μmol/l	
Aspartate aminotransferase, *see* Transaminase			
Base excess, blood	0 ± 2 mEq/liter	0 ± 2 mmol/l	
Bicarbonate, serum	23–29 mEq/liter	23–29 mmol/l	
Bile acids, serum	0.3–3.0 mg/dl	3.0–30.0 mg/l	
Bilirubin, serum			
Direct	0.1–0.4 mg/dl	1.7–6.8 μmol/l	
Indirect	0.2–0.7 mg/dl (Total minus direct)	3.4–12 μmol/l (Total minus direct)	
Total	0.3–1.1 mg/dl	5.1–19 μmol/l	a
Calcium, serum	4.5–5.5 mEq/liter	2.25–2.75 mmol/l	
	9.0–11.0 mg/dl		
	(Slightly higher in children)	(Slightly higher in children)	
	(Varies with protein concentration)	(Varies with protein concentration)	
Calcium, ionized, serum	2.1–2.6 mEq/liter	1.05–1.30 mmol/l	
	4.25–5.25 mg/dl		
Carbon dioxide content, serum			
Adults	24–30 mEq/liter	24–30 mmol/l	
Infants	20–28 mEq/liter	20–28 mmol/l	
Carbon dioxide tension (PCO_2), blood	35–45 mm Hg	35–45 mm Hg	g
Carotene, serum	40–200 mcg/dl	0.74–3.72 μmol/l	
Ceruloplasmin, serum	23–44 mg/dl	230–440 mg/l	h
Chloride, serum	96–106 mEq/liter	96–106 mmol/l	
Cholesterol, serum			
Total	150–250 mg/dl	3.9–6.5 mmol/l	
Esters	68–76% of total cholesterol	0.68–0.76 of total cholesterol	a
Cholinesterase			
Serum	0.5–1.3 pH units	0.5–1.3 pH units	f
Erythrocytes	0.5–1.0 pH unit	0.5–1.0 pH unit	f
Copper, serum			
Males	70–140 mcg/dl	11–22 μmol/l	
Females	85–155 mcg/dl	13–24 μmol/l	
Cortisol, plasma			
8 AM	6–23 mcg/dl	170–635 nmol/l	
4 PM	3–15 mcg/dl	82–413 nmol/l	
10 PM	Less than 50% of 8 AM value	Less than 0.5 of 8 AM value	
Creatine, serum	0.2–0.8 mg/dl	15–61 μmol/l	
Creatine kinase, serum (CK, CPK)			
Males	12–80 milliunits/ml (30°)	12–80 units/l (30 C)	f
	55–170 milliunits/ml (37°)	55–170 units/l (37 C)	f
Females	10–55 milliunits/ml (30°)	10–55 units/l (30 C)	f
	30–135 milliunits/ml (37°)	30–135 units/l (37 C)	f
Creatine kinase isoenzymes, serum			
CK-MM	Present	Present	
CK-MB	Absent	Absent	
CK-BB	Absent	Absent	
Creatinine, serum	0.6–1.2 mg/dl	53–106 μmol/l	
Cryoglobulins, serum	0	0	
Fatty acids, total, serum	190–420 mg/dl	7–15 mmol/l	i
nonesterified, serum	8–25 mg/dl	0.30–0.90 mmol/l	
Ferritin, serum	20–200 nanogm/ml	20–200 μg/l	

Table continued on following page

Reference Values for Blood, Plasma, and Serum *Continued*
(For some procedures the reference values may vary depending upon the method used)

	Conventional Units	S.I. Units	Notes
Fibrinogen, plasma	200–400 mg/100 ml	5.9–11.7 µmol/l	c
Folate, serum	1.8–9.0 nanogm/ml	4.1–20.4 nmol/l	
Erythrocytes	150–450 nanogm/ml	340–1020 nmol/l	
Follicle-stimulating hormone (FSH), plasma			
Males	4–25 milliunits/ml (I.U.)	4–25 IU/l	
Females	4–30 milliunits/ml (I.U.)	4–30 IU/l	
Postmenopausal	40–250 milliunits/ml (I.U.)	40–250 IU/l	
Gamma glutamyltransferase			
Males	6–32 milliunits/ml (30°)	6–32 units/l (30 C)	f
Females	4–18 milliunits/ml (30°)	4–18 units/l (30 C)	f
Gastrin, serum	0–200 picogm/ml	0–200 ng/l	
Glucose (fasting)			
Blood	60–100 mg/dl	3.33–5.55 mmol/l	
Plasma or serum	70–115 mg/dl	3.89–6.38 mmol/l	
Growth hormone, serum	0–10 nanogm/ml	0–10 µg/l	
Haptoglobin, serum	100–200 mg/dl	16–31 µmol/l	d
	(As hemoglobin binding capacity)	(As hemoglobin binding capacity)	
Hydroxybutyric dehydrogenase, serum (HBD)	0–180 milliunits/ml (30°)	0–180 units/l (30 C)	f
17-Hydroxycorticosteroids, plasma	8–18 mcg/dl	0.22–0.50 µmol/l	j
Immunoglobulins, serum			
IgG	550–1900 mg/dl	5.5–19.0 g/l	
IgA	60–333 mg/dl	0.60–3.3 g/l	
IgM	45–145 mg/dl	0.45–1.5 g/l	
IgD	0.5–3.0 mg/dl	5–30 mg/l	
IgE	<500 nanogm/ml	<500 µg/l	
	(Varies with age in children)	(Varies with age in children)	
Insulin, plasma (fasting)	5–25 microunits/ml	36–179 pmol/l	
Iodine, protein bound, serum	3.5–8.0 mcg/dl	0.28–0.63 µmol/l	k
Iron, serum	75–175 mcg/dl	13–31 µmol/l	
Iron binding capacity, serum			
Total	250–410 mcg/dl	45–73 µmol/l	
Saturation	20–55%	0.20–0.55	a
Lactate, blood, venous	4.5–19.8 mg/dl	0.5–2.2 mmol/l	
arterial	4.5–14.4 mg/dl	0.5–1.6 mmol/l	
Lactate dehydrogenase, serum (LD, LDH)	45–90 milliunits/ml (I.U.) (30°)	45–90 units/l (30 C)	f
	100–190 milliunits/ml (37°)	100–190 milliunits/ml (37 C)	
LDH₁	22–37% of total	0.22–0.37 of total	
LDH₂	30–46% of total	0.30–0.46 of total	a
LDH₃	14–29% of total	0.14–0.29 of total	
LDH₄	5–11% of total	0.05–0.11 of total	
LDH₅	2–11% of total	0.02–0.11 of total	
Leucine aminopeptidase, serum	14–40 milliunits/ml (30°)	14–40 units/l (30 C)	f
Lipase, serum	0–1.5 units (Cherry-Crandall)	0–1.5 units (Cherry-Crandall)	f
Lipids, total, serum	450–850 mg/dl	4.5–8.5 g/l	m
Lipoprotein cholesterol, serum			
LDL cholesterol	60–180 mg/dl	600–1800 mg/l	
HDL cholesterol	30–80 mg/dl	300–800 mg/l	
Luteinizing hormone (LH), serum			
Males	6–18 milliunits/ml (I.U.)	6–18 IU/l	
Females, premenopausal	5–22 milliunits/ml (I.U.)	5–22 IU/l	
midcycle	3 times baseline	3 times baseline	
postmenopausal	Greater than 30 milliunits/ml (I.U.)	Greater than 30 IU/l	
Magnesium, serum	1.5–2.5 mEq/liter	0.75–1.25 mmol/l	
	1.8–3.0 mg/dl		
5'-Nucleotidase, serum	3.5–12.7 milliunits/ml (37°)	3.5–12.5 units/l (37 C)	f
Nitrogen, nonprotein, serum	15–35 mg/dl	10.7–25.0 mmol/l	
Osmolality, serum	285–295 mOsm/kg serum water	285–295 mmol/kg serum water	n
Oxygen, blood			
Capacity	16–24 vol % (varies with hemoglobin)	7.14–10.7 mmol/l (varies with hemoglobin)	o
Content Arterial	15–23 vol %	6.69–10.3 mmol/l	o
Venous	10–16 vol %	4.46–7.14 mmol/l	o
Saturation Arterial	94–100% of capacity	0.94–1.00 of capacity	a
Venous	60–85% of capacity	0.60–0.85 of capacity	a
Tension, P_{O_2} Arterial	75–100 mm Hg	75–100 mm Hg	g
P_{50}, blood	26–27 mm Hg	26–27 mm Hg	g

Reference Values for Blood, Plasma, and Serum *Continued*
(For some procedures the reference values may vary depending upon the method used)

	Conventional Units	S.I. Units	Notes
pH, arterial, blood	7.35–7.45	7.35–7.45	p
Phenylalanine, serum	Less than 3 mg/dl	Less than 0.18 mmol/l	
Phosphatase, acid serum	0.11–0.60 milliunit/ml (37°) (Roy, Brower, Hayden)	0.11–0.60 units/l	f
Phosphatase, alkaline, serum (ALP)	20–90 milliunits/ml (30°) (Values are higher in children)	20–90 units/l (30 C) (Values are higher in children)	f
Phosphate, inorganic, serum			
Adults	3.0–4.5 mg/dl	1.0–1.5 mmol/l	
Children	4.0–7.0 mg/dl	1.3–2.3 mmol/l	
Phospholipids, serum	6–12 mg/dl (As lipid phosphorus)	1.9–3.9 mmol/l (As lipid phosphorus)	
Potassium, serum	3.5–5.0 mEq/liter	3.5–5.0 mmol/l	
Prolactin, serum			
Males	1–20 nanogm/ml	1–20 μg/l	
Females	1–25 nanogm/ml	1–25 μg/l	
Protein, serum			
Total	6.0–8.0 grams/dl	60–80 g/l	m
Albumin	3.5–5.5 grams/dl	35–55 g/l	q
	52–68% of total	0.52–0.68 of total	a
Globulin			
Alpha$_1$	0.2–0.4 gram/dl	2–4 g/l	m
	2–5% of total	0.02–0.05 of total	a
Alpha$_2$	0.5–0.9 gram/dl	5–9 g/l	m
	7–14% of total	0.07–0.14 of total	a
Beta	0.6–1.1 grams/dl	6–11 g/l	m
	9–15% of total	0.09–0.15 of total	a
Gamma	0.7–1.7 grams/dl	7–17 g/l	m
	11–21% of total	0.11–0.21 of total	a
Protoporphyrin, erythrocyte	27–61 mcg/dl packed RBC	0.48–1.09 μmol/l packed RBC	
Pyruvate, blood	0.3–0.9 mg/dl	0.03–0.10 mmol/l	
Sodium, serum	136–145 mEq/liter	136–145 mmol/l	
Sulfates, inorganic, serum	0.8–1.2 mg/dl	83–125 μmol/l	
Testosterone, plasma			
Males	275–875 nanogm/dl	9.5–30 nmol/l	
Females	23–75 nanogm/dl	0.8–2.6 nmol/l	
Pregnant	38–190 nanogm/dl	1.3–6.6 nmol/l	
Thyroid-stimulating hormone (TSH), serum	0–7 microunits/ml	0–7 milliunits/l	
Thyroxine, free, serum	1.0–2.1 nanogm/dl	13–27 pmol/l	
Thyroxine (T$_4$), serum	4.4–9.9 mcg/dl	57–128 nmol/l	
Thyroxine binding globulin (TBG), serum (as thyroxine)	10–26 mcg/dl	129–335 nmol/l	
Thyroxine iodine, serum	2.9–6.4 mcg/dl	229–504 nmol/l	k
Triiodothyronine (T$_3$), serum	150–250 nanogm/dl	2.3–3.9 nmol/l	
Triiodothyronine (T$_3$) uptake, resin (T$_3$RU)	25–38% uptake	0.25–0.38 uptake	a
Transaminase, serum			
SGOT (aspartate aminotransferase, AST)	8–20 milliunits/ml (30°) 7–40 milliunits/ml (37°)	8–20 units/l (30 C) 7–40 units/l (37 C)	
SGPT (alanine aminotransferase, ALT)	8–20 milliunits/ml (30°) 5–35 milliunits/ml (37°)	8–20 units/l (30 C) 5–35 units/l (37 C)	f f
Triglycerides, serum	40–150 mg/dl	0.4–1.5 g/l 0.45–1.71 mmol/l	r
Urate, serum			
Males	2.5–8.0 mg/dl	0.15–0.48 mmol/l	
Females	1.5–7.0 mg/dl	0.09–0.42 mmol/l	
Urea			
Blood	21–43 mg/dl	3.5–7.3 mmol/l	
Plasma or serum	24–49 mg/dl	4.0–8.3 mmol/l	
Urea nitrogen			
Blood	10–20 mg/dl	7.1–14.3 mmol/l	k
Plasma or serum	11–23 mg/dl	7.9–16.4 mmol/l	
Viscosity, serum	1.4–1.8 times water	1.4–1.8 times water	
Vitamin A, serum	20–80 mcg/dl	0.70–2.8 μmol/l	
Vitamin B$_{12}$, serum	180–900 picogm/ml	133–664 pmol/l	

Reference Values for Urine
(For some procedures the reference values may vary depending upon the method used)

	Conventional Units	S.I. Units	Notes
Acetone and acetoacetate, qualitative	Negative	Negative	
Albumin			
Qualitative	Negative	Negative	
Quantitative	10–100 mg/24 hrs	10–100 mg/24 h	q
		0.15–1.5 μmol/24 h	
Aldosterone	3–20 mcg/24 hrs	8.3–55 nmol/24 h	
Alpha amino nitrogen	50–200 mg/24 hrs	3.6–14.3 mmol/24 h	
Ammonia nitrogen	20–70 mEq/24 hrs	20–70 mmol/24 h	
Amylase	1–17 units/hr	1–17 units/h	f
Amylase/creatinine clearance ratio	1–4%	0.01–0.04	
Bilirubin, qualitative	Negative	Negative	
Calcium			
Low Ca diet	Less than 150 mg/24 hrs	Less than 3.8 mmol/24 h	
Usual diet	Less than 250 mg/24 hrs	Less than 6.3 mmol/24 h	
Catecholamines			
Epinephrine	Less than 10 mcg/24 hrs	Less than 55 nmol/24 h	
Norepinephrine	Less than 100 mcg/24 hrs	Less than 590 nmol/24 h	
Total free catecholamines	4–126 mcg/24 hrs	24–745 nmol/24 h	s
Total metanephrines	0.1–1.6 mg/24 hrs	0.5–8.1 μmol/24 h	t
Chloride	110–250 mEq/24 hrs	110–250 mmol/24 h	
	(Varies with intake)	(Varies with intake)	
Chorionic gonadotropin	0	0	
Copper	0–50 mcg/24 hrs	0–0.80 μmol/24 h	
Cortisol, free	10–100 mcg/24 hrs	27.6–276 mmol/24 h	
Creatine			
Males	0–40 mg/24 hrs	0–0.30 mmol/24 h	
Females	0–100 mg/24 hrs	0–0.76 mmol/24 h	
	(Higher in children and during pregnancy)	(Higher in children and during pregnancy)	
Creatinine	15–25 mg/kg body weight/24 hrs	0.13–0.22 mmol·kg⁻¹body weight/24 h	
Creatinine clearance			
Males	110–150 ml/min	110–150 ml/min	
Females	105–132 ml/min	105–132 ml/min	
	(1.73 sq meter surface area)	(1.73 m² surface area)	
Cystine or cysteine, qualitative	Negative	Negative	
Dehydroepiandrosterone	Less than 15% of total 17-ketosteroids	Less than 0.15 of total 17-ketosteroids	a
Males	0.2–2.0 mg/24 hrs	0.7–6.9 μm/24 h	
Females	0.2–1.8 mg/24 hrs	0.7–6.2 μm/24 h	
Delta aminolevulinic acid	1.3–7.0 mg/24 hrs	10–53 μmol/24 h	
Estrogens			
Males			
Estrone	3–8 μg/24 hrs	11–30 nmol/24 h	
Estradiol	0–6 μg/24 hrs	0–22 nmol/24 h	
Estriol	1–11 μg/24 hrs	3–38 nmol/24 h	
Total	4–25 μg/24 hrs	14–90 nmol/24 h	u
Females			
Estrone	4–31 μg/24 hrs	15–115 nmol/24 h	
Estradiol	0–14 μg/24 hrs	0–51 nmol/24 h	
Estriol	0–72 μg/24 hrs	0–250 nmol/24 h	
Total	5–100 μg/24 hrs	18–360 nmol/24 h	u
	(Markedly increased during pregnancy)	(Markedly increased during pregnancy)	
Glucose (as reducing substance)	Less than 250 mg/24 hrs	Less than 250 mg/24 h	
Hemoglobin and myoglobin, qualitative	Negative	Negative	

Reference Values for Urine *Continued*
(For some procedures the reference values may vary depending upon the method used)

	Conventional Units	S.I. Units	Notes
Homogentisic acid, qualitative	Negative	Negative	
17-Hydroxycorticosteroids			
Males	3–9 mg/24 hrs	8.3–25 μmol/24 h	j
Females	2–8 mg/24 hrs	5.5–22 μmol/24 h	
5-Hydroxyindoleacetic acid			
Qualitative	Negative	Negative	
Quantitative	Less than 9 mg/24 hrs	Less than 47 μmol/24 h	
17-Ketosteroids			
Males	6–18 mg/24 hrs	21–62 μmol/24 h	l
Females	4–13 mg/24 hrs	14–45 μmol/24 h	
	(Varies with age)	(Varies with age)	
Magnesium	6.0–8.5 mEq/24 hrs	3.0–4.3 mmol/24 h	
Metanephrines (see Catechol-amines)			
Osmolality	38–1400 mOsm/kg water	38–1400 mmol/kg water	n
pH	4.6–8.0, average 6.0	4.6–8.0, average 6.0	p
	(Depends on diet)	(Depends on diet)	
Phenolsulfonphthalein excretion (PSP)	25% or more in 15 min	0.25 or more in 15 min	a
	40% or more in 30 min	0.40 or more in 30 min	
	55% or more in 2 hrs	0.55 or more in 2 h	
	(After injection of 1 ml PSP intravenously)	(After injection of 1 ml PSP intravenously)	
Phenylpyruvic acid, qualitative	Negative	Negative	
Phosphorus	0.9–1.3 gram/24 hrs	29–42 mmol/24 h	
Porphobilinogen			
Qualitative	Negative	Negative	
Quantitative	0–0.2 mg/dl	0–0.9 μmol/l	
	Less than 2.0 mg/24 hrs	Less than 9 μmol/24 h	
Porphyrins			
Coproporphyrin	50–250 mcg/24 hrs	77–380 nmol/24 h	
Uroporphyrin	10–30 mcg/24 hrs	12–36 nmol/24 h	
Potassium	25–100 mEq/24 hrs	25–100 mmol/24 h	
	(Varies with intake)	(Varies with intake)	
Pregnanediol			
Males	0.4–1.4 mg/24 hrs	1.2–4.4 μmol/24 h	
Females			
Proliferative phase	0.5–1.5 mg/24 hrs	1.6–4.7 μmol/24 h	
Luteal phase	2.0–7.0 mg/24 hrs	6.2–22 μmol/24 h	
Postmenopausal phase	0.2–1.0 mg/24 hrs	0.6–3.1 μmol/24 h	
Pregnanetriol	Less than 2.5 mg/24 hrs in adults	Less than 7.4 μmol/24 h in adults	
Protein			
Qualitative	Negative	Negative	
Quantitative	10–150 mg/24 hrs	10–150 mg/24 h	m
Sodium	130–260 mEq/24 hrs	130–260 mmol/24 h	
	(Varies with intake)	(Varies with intake)	
Specific gravity	1.003–1.030	1.003–1.030	
Titratable acidity	20–40 mEq/24 hrs	20–40 mmol/24 h	
Urate	200–500 mg/24 hrs	1.2–3.0 mmol/24 h	
	(With normal diet)	(With normal diet)	
Urobilinogen	Up to 1.0 Ehrlich unit/2 hrs	Up to 1.0 Ehrlich unit/2 h	
	(1–3 PM)	(1–3 PM)	
	0–4.0 mg/24 hrs	0–6.8 μmol/24 h	
Vanillylmandelic acid (VMA) (4-hydroxy-3-methoxymandelic acid)	1–8 mg/24 hrs	5–40 μmol/24 h	

Reference Values for Therapeutic Drug Monitoring

Drug	Therapeutic Range	Toxic Levels	Proprietary Names
Antibiotics			
Amikacin, serum	15–25 mcg/ml	Peak: >35 mcg/ml Trough: >5–8 mcg/ml	Amikin
Chloramphenicol, serum	10–20 mcg/ml	>25 mcg/ml	Chloromycetin
Gentamicin, serum	5–10 mcg/ml	Peak: >12 mcg/ml Trough: >2 mcg/ml	Garamycin
Tobramycin, serum	5–10 mcg/ml	Peak: >12 mcg/ml Trough: >2 mcg/ml	Nebcin
Anticonvulsants			
Carbamazepine, serum	5–12 mcg/ml	>12 mcg/ml	Tegretol
Ethosuximide, serum	40–100 mcg/ml	>100 mcg/ml	Zarontin
Phenobarbital, serum	10–30 mcg/ml	Vary widely because of developed tolerance	
Phenytoin, serum (diphenylhydantoin)	10–20 mcg/ml	>20 mcg/ml	Dilantin
Primidone, serum	5–12 mcg/ml	>15 mcg/ml	Mysoline
Valproic acid, serum	50–100 mcg/ml	>100 mcg/ml	Depakene
Analgesics			
Acetaminophen, serum	10–20 mcg/ml	>250 mcg/ml	Tylenol Datril
Salicylate, serum	100–250 mcg/ml	>300 mcg/ml	
Bronchodilator			
Theophylline (aminophylline)	10–20 mcg/ml	>20 mcg/ml	
Cardiovascular drugs			
Digitoxin, serum	15–25 nanogm/ml (Specimen obtained 12–24 hrs after last dose)	>25 nanogm/ml	Crystodigin
Digoxin, serum	0.8–2 nanogm/ml (Specimen obtained 12–24 hrs after last dose)	>2.4 nanogm/ml	Lanoxin
Disopyramide, serum	2–5 mcg/ml	>5 mcg/ml	Norpace
Lidocaine, serum	1.5–5 mcg/ml	>5 nanogm/ml	Anestacon Xylocaine
Procainamide, serum	4–10 mcg/ml *10–30 mcg/ml (*Procainamide + N-Acetyl Procainamide)	>16 mcg/ml *>30 mcg/ml	Pronestyl
Propranolol, serum	50–100 nanogm/ml	Variable	Inderal
Quinidine, serum	2–5 mcg/ml	>10 mcg/ml	Cardioquin Quinaglute Quinidex Quinora
Psychopharmacologic drugs			
Amitriptyline, serum	*120–150 nanogm/ml (*Amitriptyline + Nortriptyline)	*>500 nanogm/ml	Amitril Elavil Endep Etrafon Limbitrol Triavil
Desipramine, serum	*150–300 nanogm/ml (*Desipramine + Imipramine)	*>500 nanogm/ml	Norpramin Pertofrane
Imipramine, serum	*150–300 nanogm/ml (*Imipramine + Desipramine)	*>500 nanogm/ml	Antipress Imavate Janimine Presamine Tofranil
Lithium, serum	0.8–1.2 mEq/liter (Specimen obtained 12 hrs after last dose)	>2.0 mEq/liter	Lithobid Lithotabs
Nortriptyline, serum	50–150 nanogm/ml	>500 nanogm/ml	Aventyl Pamelor

Reference Values in Toxicology

	Conventional Units	S.I. Units	Notes
Arsenic, blood	3.5–7.2 mcg/dl	0.47–0.96 μmol/l	
Arsenic, urine	Less than 100 mcg/24 hrs	Less than 1.3 μmol/24 h	
Bromides, serum	0	0	
	Toxic levels: Above 17 mmol/l	Toxic levels: Above 17 mmol/l	
Carbon monoxide, blood	Up to 5% saturation	Up to 0.5 saturation	
	Symptoms occur with 20% saturation	Symptoms occur with 0.20 saturation	a
Ethanol, blood	Less than 0.005%	Less than 1 mmol/l	
Marked intoxication	0.3–0.4%	65–87 mmol/l	
Alcoholic stupor	0.4–0.5% mcg/dl	87–109 mmol/l	
Coma	Above 0.5%	Above 109 mmol/l	
Lead, blood	0–40 mcg/dl	0–2 μmol/l	
Lead, urine	Less than 100 mcg/24 hrs	Less than 0.48 μmol/24 h	
Mercury, urine	Less than 100 mcg/24 hrs	Less than 50 nmol/24 h	

Reference Values for Cerebrospinal Fluid

	Conventional Units	S.I. Units	Notes
Cells	Fewer than 5/cu mm; all mononuclear	Fewer than 5/μl; all mononuclear	
Chloride	120–130 mEq/liter	120–130 mmol/l	
	(20 mEq/liter higher than serum)	(20 mmol/l higher than serum)	
Electrophoresis	Predominantly albumin	Predominantly albumin	
Glucose	50–75 mg/dl	2.8–4.2 mmol/l	
	(20 mg/dl less than serum)	(1.1 mmol/less than serum)	
IgG			
Children under 14	Less than 8% of total protein	Less than 0.08 of total protein	a,m
Adults	Less than 14% of total protein	Less than 0.14 of total protein	
Pressure	70–180 mm water	70–180 mm water	g
Protein, total	15–45 mg/dl	0.150–0.450 g/l	m
	(Higher, up to 70 mg/dl, in elderly adults and children)	(Higher, up to 0.70 g/l, in elderly adults and children)	

Reference Values for Gastric Analysis

	Conventional Units	S.I. Units	Notes
Basal gastric secretion (1 hour)			
Concentration	(Mean ± 1 S.D.)	(Mean ± 1 S.D.)	
Males	25.8 ± 1.8 mEq/liter	25.8 ± 1.8 mmol/l	
Females	20.3 ± 3.0 mEq/liter	20.3 ± 3.0 mmol/l	
Output	(Mean ± 1 S.D.)	(Mean ± 1 S.D.)	
Males	2.57 ± 0.16 mEq/hr	2.57 ± 0.16 mmol/h	
Females	1.61 ± 0.18 mEq/hr	1.61 ± 0.18 mmol/h	
After histamine stimulation			
Normal	Mean output 11.8 mEq/hr	Mean output 11.8 mmol/h	
Duodenal ulcer	Mean output 15.2 mEq/hr	Mean output 15.2 mmol/h	
After maximal histamine stimulation			
Normal	Mean output 22.6 mEq/hr	Mean output 22.6 mmol/h	
Duodenal ulcer	Mean output 44.6 mEq/hr	Mean output 44.6 mmol/h	
Diagnex Blue (Squibb):			
Anacidity	0–0.3 mg in 2 hrs	0–0.03 mg in 2 h	
Doubtful	0.3–0.6 mg in 2 hrs	0.3–0.6 mg in 2 h	
Normal	Greater than 0.6 mg in 2 hrs	Greater than 0.6 mg in 2 h	
Volume, fasting stomach content	50–100 ml	50–100 ml	
Emptying time	3–6 hrs	3–6 h	
Color	Opalescent or colorless	Opalescent or colorless	
Specific gravity	1.006–1.009	1.006–1.009	
pH (adults)	0.9–1.5	0.9–1.5	p

Gastrointestinal Absorption Tests

	Conventional Units	S.I. Units
D-Xylose absorption test	After an 8 hour fast, 10 ml/kg body weight of a 0.05 solution of D-xylose is given by mouth. Nothing further by mouth is given until the test has been completed. All urine voided during the following 5 hours is pooled, and blood samples are taken at 0, 60, and 120 minutes. Normally 0.26 (range 0.16–0.33) of ingested xylose is excreted within 5 hours, and the serum xylose reaches a level between 25 and 40 mg/100 dl after 1 hour and is maintained at this level for another 60 minutes.	No change
Vitamin A absorption	A fasting blood specimen is obtained and 200,000 units of vitamin A in oil is given by mouth. Serum vitamin A level should rise to twice fasting level in 3 to 5 hours.	No change

Reference Values for Feces

	Conventional Units	S.I. Units	Notes
Bulk	100–200 grams/24 hrs	100–200 g/24 h	
Dry matter	23–32 grams/24 hrs	23–32 g/24 h	
Fat, total	Less than 6.0 grams/24 hrs	Less than 6.0 g/24 h	
Nitrogen, total	Less than 2.0 grams/24 hrs	Less than 2.0 g/24 h	
Urobilinogen	40–280 mg/24 hrs	40–280 mg/24 h	
Water	Approximately 65%	Approximately 0.65	a

Reference Values for Immunologic Procedures

	Conventional Units
Lymphocyte subsets	
T cells	60–85%
B cells	1–20%
T-helper cells	35–60%
T-suppressor cells	15–30%
T-H/S ratio	1.5–2.5
Complement	
C3	85–175 mg/dl
C4	15–45 mg/dl
CH_{50}	25–55 H_{50} units/ml
Tumor markers	
Carcinoembryonic antigen (CEA)	
(Roche)	Less than 5 nanogm/ml
(Abbott)	Less than 4.1 nanogm/ml
Alpha-fetoprotein (AFP)	Less than 10–30 nanogm/ml (depends on method)

Reference Values for Semen Analysis

	Conventional Units	S.I. Units	Notes
Volume	2–5 ml; usually 3–4 ml	2–5 ml; usually 3–4 ml	
Liquefaction	Complete in 15 min	Complete in 15 min	
pH	7.2–8.0; average 7.8	7.2–8.0; average 7.8	p
Leukocytes	Occasional or absent	Occasional or absent	
Count	60–150 million/ml	60–150 million/ml	
	Below 60 million/ml is abnormal	Below 60 million/ml is abnormal	
Motility	80% or more motile	0.80 or more motile	a
Morphology	80–90% normal forms	0.80–0.90 normal forms	a

Oral Glucose Tolerance Test

The oral glucose tolerance test (OGTT) may be unnecessary if the fasting plasma glucose concentration is elevated (venous plasma ≥140 mg/dl or 7.8 mmol/l) on two occasions. The OGTT should be carried out only on patients who are ambulatory and otherwise healthy and who are known not to be taking agents that elevate the plasma glucose (see reference 10). The test should be conducted in the morning after at least 3 days of unrestricted diet (≥150 grams of carbohydrate) and physical activity. The subject should have fasted for at least 10 hours but no more than 16 hours. Water is permitted during the test period; however, the subject should remain seated and should not smoke throughout the test.

The dose of glucose administered should be 75 grams (1.75 grams per kg of ideal body weight, up to a maximum of 75 grams for children). Commercial preparations containing a suitable carbohydrate load are acceptable. If criteria for gestational diabetes are used, a dose of 100 grams of glucose is required.

A fasting blood sample should be collected, after which the glucose dose is taken within 5 minutes. Blood samples should be collected at 30 minute intervals for 2 hours (for gestational diabetes, fasting 1, 2, and 3 hours). The following diagnostic criteria have been recommended by the National Diabetes Data Group:

Normal OGTT in Nonpregnant Adults	Fasting venous plasma glucose <115 mg/dl (6.4 mmol/l); ½ h, 1 h, and 1½ h OGTT venous plasma glucose <200 mg/dl (11.1 mmol/l); 2 h OGTT venous plasma glucose <140 mg/dl (7.8 mmol/l)
Diabetes Mellitus in Nonpregnant Adults	Both the 2 hour sample *and* some other sample taken between administration of the 75 gram glucose dose and 2 hours later must show a venous plasma glucose ≥200 mg/dl (11.1 mmol/l)
Impaired Glucose Tolerance in Nonpregnant Adults	Three criteria must be met: Fasting venous plasma glucose <140 mg/dl (7.8 mmol/l); ½ h, 1 h, or 1½ h OGTT value ≥200 mg/dl (11.1 mmol/l); 2 h OGTT venous plasma glucose between 140 and 200 mg/dl (7.8 and 11.1 mmol/l)
Gestational Diabetes	Two or more of the following values after a 100 gram oral glucose challenge must be met or exceeded: (values are for venous plasma glucose)

Fasting	105 mg/dl	5.8 mmol/l
1h	190 mg/dl	10.6 mmol/l
2h	165 mg/dl	9.2 mmol/l
3h	145 mg/dl	8.1 mmol/l

NOTES

a. Percentage is expressed as a decimal fraction.

b. Percentage may be expressed as a decimal fraction; however, when the result expressed is itself a variable fraction of another variable, the absolute value is more meaningful. There is no reason, other than custom, for expressing reticulocyte counts and differential leukocyte counts in percentages or decimal fractions rather than in absolute numbers.

c. Molecular weight of fibrinogen = 341,000 daltons.

d. Molecular weight of hemoglobin = 64,500 daltons. Because of disagreement as to whether the monomer or tetramer of hemoglobin should be used in the conversion, it has been recommended that the conventional grams per deciliter be retained. The tetramer is used in the table; values given should be multiplied by 4 to obtain concentration of the monomer.

e. Molecular weight of methemoglobin = 64,500 daltons. See note d above.

f. Enzyme units have not been changed in these tables because the proposed enzyme unit, the katal, has not been universally adopted (1 International Unit = 16.7 nkat).

g. It has been proposed that pressure be expressed in the pascal (1 mm Hg = 0.133 kPa); however, this convention has not been universally accepted.

h. Molecular weight of ceruloplasmin = 151,000 daltons.

i. "Fatty acids" includes a mixture of different aliphatic acids of varying molecular weight. A mean molecular weight of 284 daltons has been assumed in calculating the conversion factor.

j. Based upon molecular weight of cortisol 362.47 daltons.

k. The practice of expressing concentration of an organic molecule in terms of one of its constituent elements originated when measurements included a heterogeneous class of compounds (nonprotein nitrogenous compounds, iodine-containing compounds bound to serum proteins). It was carried over to expressing measurements of specific substances (urea, thyroxine), but the practice should be discarded. For iodine and nitrogen 1 mole is taken as the monoatomic form, although they occur as diatomic molecules.

l. Based upon molecular weight of dehydroepiandrosterone 288.41 daltons.

m. Weight per volume is retained as the unit because of the heterogeneous nature of the material measured.

n. The proposal that osmolality be reported as freezing point depression using the millikelvin as the unit has not been received with universal enthusiasm. The milliosmole is not an S.I. unit, and the unit used here is the millimole.

o. Volumes per cent might be converted to a decimal fraction; however, this would not permit direct correlation with hemoglobin content, which is possible when oxygen content and capacity are expressed in molar quantities. One millimole of hemoglobin combines with 4 millimoles of oxygen.

p. Hydrogen ion concentration in S.I. units would be expressed in nanomoles per liter; however, this change has not received general approval. Conversion can be calculated as antilog ($-$pH).

q. Albumin is expressed in grams per liter to be consistent with units used for other proteins. Concentration of albumin may be expressed in mmol/l also, an expression that permits assessment of binding capacity of albumin for substances such as bilirubin. Molecular weight of albumin is 65,000 daltons.

r. Most techniques for quantitating triglycerides measure the glycerol moiety, and the total mass is calculated using an average molecular weight. The factor given assumes a mean molecular weight of 875 daltons for triglycerides.

s. Calculated as norepinephrine, molecular weight 169.18 daltons.

t. Calculated as metanephrine, molecular weight 197.23 daltons.

u. Conversion factor calculated from molecular weights of estrone, estradiol, and estriol in proportions of 2:1:2 daltons.

REFERENCES

1. AMA Drug Evaluations, 6th ed. Chicago, American Medical Association, 1986.
2. AMA Council on Scientific Affairs: J.A.M.A. *253*:2552, 1985.
3. Goodman, A. G., Gilman, L. S., Rall, T. W., and Murad, F.: Goodman and Gilman's The Pharmacological Basis of Therapeutics, 7th ed. New York, Macmillan, 1985.
4. Henry, J. B.: Clinical Diagnosis and Management by Laboratory Methods, 17th ed. Philadelphia, W. B. Saunders Company, 1984.
5. Henry, R. J., Cannon, D. C., and Winkleman, J. W.: Clinical Chemistry—Principles and Techniques, 2nd ed. New York, Harper & Row, 1974.
6. International Committee for Standardization in Hematology, International Federation of Clinical Chemistry and World Association of Pathology Societies: Clin. Chem. *19*:135, 1973.
7. Lundberg, G. D., Iverson, C., and Radulescu, G.: J.A.M.A. *255*:2247, 1986.
8. Miale, J. B.: Laboratory Medicine—Hematology, 6th ed. St. Louis, C. V. Mosby, 1982.
9. National Diabetes Data Group: Diabetes *28*:1039, 1979.
10. Page, C. H., and Vigourex, P.: The International System of Units (S.I.). U.S. Department of Commerce, National Bureau of Standards, Special Publication 330, 1974.
11. Physicians' Desk Reference, 42nd ed. Oradell, N.J., Medical Economics Company, 1988.
12. Scully, R. E., McNeely, B. U., and Mark, E. J.: N. Engl. J. Med. *314*:39, 1986.
13. Tietz, N. W.: Clinical Guide to Laboratory Tests. Philadelphia, W. B. Saunders Company, 1983.
14. Tietz, N. W.: Textbook of Clinical Chemistry. Philadelphia, W. B. Saunders Company, 1986.
15. Williams, W. J., Beutler, E., Erslev, A. J., and Lichtman, M. A.: Hematology, 3rd ed. New York, McGraw-Hill Book Company, 1983.

Some of the values have been established by the Clinical Pathology Laboratories, Emory University Hospital, Atlanta, Georgia, or by the Clinical Laboratories, Thomas Jefferson University Hospital, Philadelphia, Pennsylvania, and have not been published elsewhere.

NOMOGRAM FOR THE DETERMINATION OF BODY SURFACE AREA OF CHILDREN AND ADULTS*

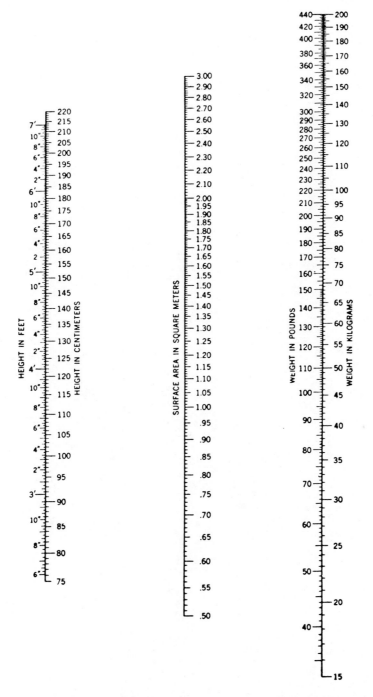

*From Boothby, W. M., and Sandiford, R. B.: Boston Med. Surg. J. *185*:337, 1921.

Index